Surgery for GASTROINTESTINAL CANCER

Surgery for GASTROINTESTINAL CANCER

EDITED BY

Harold J. Wanebo, MD, PhD

Professor of Surgery
Director
Division of Surgical Oncology
Brown University
Providence, RI

with 131 contributors

Lippincott - Raven
PUBLISHERS
Philadelphia • New York

Acquisitions Editor: Lisa McAllister
Developmental Editor: Emilie M. Linkins
Project Editor: Bridget H. Meyer
Production Manager: Caren Erlichman
Production Coordinator: David Yurkovich
Design Coordinator: Melissa G. Olson
Indexer: Julia Figures
Compositor: Maryland Composition Company, Inc.
Printer: Courier Book Company/Westford

Library of Congress Cataloging-in-Publication Data

Surgery for gastrointestinal cancer : a multidisciplinary approach / edited by Harold J. Wanebo ; with 131 contributors.
p. cm.
Includes bibliographical references and index.
ISBN 0-397-51518-9 (alk. paper)
1. Gastrointestinal system—Cancer—Surgery. 2. Gastrointestinal system—Cancer. I. Wanebo, Harold J., 1935– .
[DNLM: 1. Gastrointestinal Neoplasms—surgery. 2. Combined Modality Therapy. WI 149 S961 1996]
RD668.S87 1996
616.99′433059—dc20
DNLM/DLC
for Library of Congress 96-14257
CIP

Care has been taken to confirm the accuracy of the information presented and to describe generally accepted practices. However, the authors, editors, and publisher are not responsible for errors or omissions or for any consequences from application of the information in this book and make no warranty, express or implied, with respect to the contents of the publication.

The authors, editors, and publisher have exerted every effort to ensure that drug selection and dosage set forth in this text are in accordance with current recommendations and practice at the time of publication. However, in view of ongoing research, changes in government regulations, and the constant flow of information relating to drug therapy and drug reactions, the reader is urged to check the package insert for each drug for any change in indications and dosage and for added warnings and precautions. This is particularly important when the recommended agent is a new or infrequently employed drug.

Some drugs and medical devices presented in this publication have Food and Drug Administration (FDA) clearance for limited use in restricted research settings. It is the responsibility of the health care provider to ascertain the FDA status of each drug or device planned for use in their clinical practice.

9 8 7 6 5 4 3 2 1

Contributors

James D. Ahlgren, MD
Professor of Medicine and Pharmacology
The George Washington University Medical Center
2150 Pennsylvania Avenue, NW
Washington, DC 20037-2396

Takayuki Akasu, MD
Staff Surgeon of Surgery
Department of Surgery
National Cancer Center Hospital
1-1, Tsukiji
5-Chome, Chuo-Ku
Tokyo 104, Japan

Hiroshi Akiyama, MD, PhD, FACS(Hon), FRCS(Eng) (Hon)
Head, Division of Gastrointestinal Surgery
Department of Surgery
Toranomon Hospital
2-2-2 Toranomon, Minato-ku
Tokyo 105, Japan

Nasser Altorki, MD
The New York Hospital
Cornell University Medical College
525 East 68th Street
New York, NY 10021

Shigeki Arii, MD
First Department of Surgery
Faculty of Medicine
Kyoto University
54-Shogoin Kawara-cho
Sakyo-ku
Kyoko 606, Japan

Dan A. Avradopoulos, MD
Surgical Oncology Fellow
Department of Surgical Oncology
Brown University School of Medicine
Roger Williams Medical Center
825 Chalkstone Avenue
Providence, RI 02908

Robert W. Bailey, MD, FACS
Chief of General Surgery
Greater Baltimore Medical Center
6569 North Charles Street, Suite 708
Towson, MD 21204

David J. Bertsch, MD
Surgical Oncology Fellow
Division of Surgical Oncology
Department of Surgery
Ohio State University and
The Arthur G. James Cancer Hospital and Research Institute
410 West 10th Avenue, Doan N-911
Columbus, OH 43210-1236

Leslie H. Blumgart, MD, FRCS, FACS
Chief, Hepatobiliary Service
Memorial Sloan-Kettering Cancer Center
1275 York Avenue
New York, NY 10021-6098

John S. Bolton, MD
Ochsner Medical Institutions
1514 Jefferson Highway
New Orleans, LA 70121

James H. Bond, MD
Chief, Gastrointestinal Section
Minneapolis VA Medial Center
One Veterans Drive
Minneapolis, MN 55417

K. Böttcher, MD
Chirurgische Klinik und Poliklinik
Klinikum rechts der Isar der Technician Universität München
Ismaningerstr. 22
0-81675 München, Germany

John L. Cameron, MD
Alfred Blalock Professor and Chairman
Department of Surgery
Johns Hopkins University School of Medicine
720 Rutland Avenue, Ross 759
Baltimore, MD 21205

Brian I. Carr, MD, FRCP, PhD
Professor
Department of Surgery/Liver Transplant
University of Pittsburgh
Biomedical Science Tower, E1552
200 Lothrop Street
Pittsburgh, PA 15213-3442

Carlos Fernández-del Castillo, MD
Massachusetts General Hospital
Harvard Medical School
Wang Ambulatory Care Center, Suite 336
Boston, MA 02114

Helena R. Chang, MD
Associate Professor of Surgery and Pathobiology
Department of Surgery
Brown University/Roger Williams Hospital
825 Chalkstone Avenue
Providence, RI 02908

Chusilp Charnsangavej, MD
Department of Diagnostic Radiology
The University of Texas
M.D. Anderson Cancer Center
1515 Holcombe Boulevard
Houston, TX 77030

Gar-Yang Chau, MD, MPH
Instructor of Surgery
National Yang-Ming Medical University
Veterans General Hospital—Taipei
Taipei, Taiwan, R.O.C. 217

Nathan I. Cherny, MBBS, FRACP
Pain and Palliative Medicine Physician
Department of Internal Medicine
Shaare Zedek Medical Center
Jerusalem, ISRAEL

Maureen Chung, MD, FRCS(C)
Surgical Oncology Fellow
Rogers Williams Medical Center
Department of Surgery
825 Chalkstone Avenue
Providence, RI 02908

James M. Church, BSc, MB ChB, MMed Sci, FRACS, FACS
Staff Colorectal Surgeon
Director
David G. Jagelman Inherited Colorectal Cancer Registries
Department of Colorectal Surgery
Cleveland Clinic Foundation
Cleveland Clinic Hospital
9500 Euclid Avenue
Cleveland, OH 44195-5044

Jeffrey W. Clark, MD
Assistant Professor of Medicine
Harvard Medical School
Hematology-Oncology
Massachusetts General Hospital
100 Blossom Street
Boston, MA 02114

Harold O. Douglass, Jr., MD, FACS
Surgical Oncology
Roswell Park Cancer Institute
Elm and Carlton Streets
Buffalo, NY 14263

E. Henry Ellis, Jr., MD, PhD
Clinical Professor of Surgery, Emeritus
Department of Cardiothoracic Surgery
Deaconess Hospital, Harvard Medical School
110 Francis Street, Suite 2C
Boston, MA 02215

Steven Eustace, MD
Boston University Medical Center
88 East Newton Street
Boston, MA 02215

David R. Farley, MD
Assistant Professor of Surgery
Mayo Medical School
Senior Associate Consultant
Department of Surgery
Mayo Clinic
200 First Street, SW
Rochester, MN 55905

John L. Flowers, MD
Assistant Professor of Surgery
Department of Surgery
University of Maryland School of Medicine
22 South Greene Street
Baltimore, MD 21201

Kathleen M. Foley, MD
Chief, Pain Service
Department of Neurology
Memorial Sloan-Kettering Cancer Center
1275 York Avenue
New York, NY 10021-6094

Michael A. Friedman, MD
Office of Operations
Food and Drug Administration
5600 Fishers Lane
Rockville, MD 20857

David Fromm, MD
Professor of Surgery
Chairman, Department of Surgery
Wayne State University
University Health Center
Detroit, MI 48201

George M. Fuhrman, MD
Ochsner Medical Institutions
1514 Jefferson Highway
New Orleans, LA 70121

Cedric F. Garland, DrPH, FACE
Associate Professor
Department of Family and Preventive Medicine
University of California, San Diego
9500 Gilman Drive 0631C
La Jolla, CA 92093-0631

Frank C. Garland, PhD
Assistant Adjunct Professor
Department of Family and Preventive Medicine
University of California, San Diego
9500 Gilman Drive 0631C
La Jolla, CA 92093-0631

Ralph George, MD
Assistant Professor of Surgery
Memorial University of Newfoundland
St. Johns, Newfoundland, Canada A1C 5B8

Leonard Girardi, MD
The New York Hospital Cornell University Medical College
525 East 68th Street
New York, NY 10021

Philip H. Gordon, MD, FRCSC, FACS
Director, Colon and Rectal Cancer
The Sir Mortimer B. Davis Jewish General Hospital
3755 Chemin De La Cote-Sainte-Catherine
Departments of Surgery and Oncology
McGill University
Montreal, Quebec H3T 1E2, Canada

Edward D. Gorham, MPH
Department of Family and Preventative Medicine
University of California, San Diego
9500 Gilman Drive 0631C
La Jolla, CA 92093-0631

James S. Goydos, MD
Section of Surgical Oncology
Cancer Institute of New Jersey
303 George Street, Suite 501
New Brunswick, NJ 08901

Frederick L. Greene, MD
Professor of Surgery
Department of Surgery
University of South Carolina School of Medicine
Two Medical Park Road, Suite 402
Columbia, SC 29203

Bruce D. Greenwald, MD
Assistant Professor
University of Maryland School of Medicine
Division of Gastroenterology
University of Maryland Hospital, Room N3W62
22 South Greene Street
Baltimore, MD 21201-1595

J. Michael Hamilton
NCI-Navy Medical Oncology Branch, DCS
National Cancer Institute
National Naval Medical Center, Bldg 8
Room 5101
Bethesda, MD 20889-5105

Marquis Hart, MD
Assistant Professor
Department of Surgery
University of Southern California, San Diego
UCSD Medical Center
200 West Arbor Drive
San Diego, CA 92103-8401

John P. Hoffman, MD
Department of Surgery
Fox Chase Cancer Center
7701 Burholme Avenue
Philadelphia, PA 19111-2497

Ryan F. Holbrook, MD
Surgical Oncologist
Former Fellow in Surgical Oncology at Roswell Park Cancer Institute
910 West 5th Avenue, Suite 680
Spokane, WA 99204

J. Milburn Jessup, MD
Associate Professor
Department of Surgery
Deaconess Hospital/Harvard Medical School
110 Francis Street
Boston, MA 02215-6915

Robert A. Kane, MD
New England Deaconess Hospital
110 Francis Street
Boston, MA 02215

Hitoshi Katai, MD
Department of Surgical Oncology
National Cancer Center Hospital
5-1-1, Tsukiji, Chou-ku
Tokyo, Japan

David Paul Kelsen, MD
Professor of Medicine
Cornell University Medical College
Chief, Gastrointestinal Oncology Service
Department of Medicine
Memorial Sloan-Kettering Cancer Center
1275 York Avenue
New York, NY 10021-6094

M. Margaret Kemeny, MD, FACS
Chief, Division of Surgical Oncology
North Shore University Hospital
300 Community Drive
Manhasset, NY 11030

B. J. Kennedy, MD
Regents' Professor of Medicine, Emeritus
Masonic Professor of Oncology, Emeritus
University of Minnesota Medical School
University of Minnesota Hospital and Clinic
Division of Oncology—Box 286
420 Delaware Street, SE
Minneapolis, MN 55455

Jila Khorsand, MD
Department of Pathology
Brown University and Roger Williams Medical Center
Providence, RI, 02908

Taira Kinoshita, MD
Department of Surgical Oncology
National Cancer Center Hospital
5-1-1, Tsukiji, Chou-ku
Tokyo, Japan

R. James Koness, MD
Department of Surgical Oncology
Brown University/Roger Williams Medical Center
825 Chalkstone Avenue
Providence, RI 02908

Jonathan B. Kruskal, MD, PhD
Assistant Professor of Radiology
Radiological Sciences
Harvard Medical School/Deaconess Hospital
One Deaconess Road
Boston, MA 02215

Alessandro Laviano, MD
Department of Clinical Medicine
Laboratory of Clinical Nutrition
viale dell-Universita, 37
00185 Rome, ITALY

Alan T. Lefor, MD
Associate Professor of Surgery and Oncology
Department of Surgery and the University of Maryland Cancer Center
University of Maryland
22 South Greene Street
Baltimore, MD 21201-1595

Edward H. Livingston, MD, FACS
Associate Professor of Surgery/Assistant Dean
Department of Surgery
UCLA Medical School and UCLA Medical Center
10833 Le Conte Avenue
Los Angeles, CA 90095-6904

Michael T. Lotze, MD
Professor of Surgery
Molecular Genetics and Biochemistry
Department of Surgery
University of Pittsburgh
Biomedical Science Tower
200 Lothrop Street—WI540
Pittsburgh, PA 15261

Kirk A. Ludwig, MD
Assistant Professor of Surgery
Department of Surgery
Duke University Medical Center
Box 3479
Durham, NC 27710

Wing-Yiu Lui, MD
Associate Professor of Surgery
Department of Surgery
Veterans General Hospital—Taipei
Shie-pai Road
Taipei, Taiwan, Republic of China

Russell E. Luke, III
Surgical Oncology
State University of New York at Buffalo
Roswell Park Cancer Institute
Elm and Carlton Street
Buffalo, NY 14263

Henry T. Lynch, MD
Professor and Chairman
Professor of Medicine
Department of Preventive Medicine
Creighton University School of Medicine
2500 California Plaza
Omaha, NE 68178

Jane Lynch, BSN
Instructor
Department of Preventive Medicine
Creighton University School of Medicine
2500 California Plaza
Omaha, NE 68178

Thomas H. Magnuson, MD
Assistant Professor of Surgery
Department of Surgery
Johns Hopkins Bayview Medical Center
4940 Eastern Avenue
Baltimore, MD 21224

David M. Mahvi, MD, FACS
Assistant Professor of Surgery
Department of Surgery
University of Wisconsin School of Medicine
H4/724, CSC
600 Highland Avenue
Madison, WI 53792

Gerald J. Marks, MD
Edgar Deissler Professor of Surgery
Department of Surgery
Director of Gastrointestinal Surgical Endoscopy
Director of Comprehensive Rectal Cancer Center
Medical College of Pennsylvania and Hahnemann University
Broad and Vine Streets MS 413
Philadelphia, PA 19102-1192

John H. Marks, MD
Instructor—Department of Surgery
Medical College of Pennsylvania and Hahnemann University
Broad and Vine MS 413
Philadelphia, PA 19102-1192

Edward W. Martin, Jr., MD
Associate Professor
Division of Surgical Oncology
Department of Surgery
Ohio State University and
The Arthur G. James Cancer Hospital and Research Institute
410 West 10th Avenue
Doan N-911
Columbus, OH 43210-1236

Ronald F. Martin, MD
Assistant Clinical Professor of Surgery
University of Vermont
Staff Surgeon
Divisions of General Surgery
Maine Medical Center and Mercy Hospital
72 West Street
Portland, ME 04102

Keiichi Maruyama, MD
Professor of Surgery
Head, Department of Surgical Oncology
National Cancer Center Hospital
5-1-1, Tsukiji, Chou-ku
Tokyo 104, Japan

Michael M. Meguid, MD, PhD, FACS
Professor of Surgery
State University of New York
Health Science Center
750 East Adams Street
Syracuse, NY 13210

Steven J. Meltzer, MD
Associate Professor of Medicine and Molecular Biology
Department of Medicine
University of Maryland and Baltimore VA Hospital
22 Greene Street
Baltimore, MD 21201-1598

Neal J. Meropol, MD
Assistant Professor of Medicine
State University of New York at Buffalo
Division of Medicine
Roswell Park Cancer Institute
Elm and Carlton Street
Buffalo, NY 14263

Jeffrey W. Milsom, MD
Staff Surgeon
Head, Section of Colorectal Research
The Cleveland Clinic Foundation
Department of Colorectal Surgery, Desk A111
9500 Euclid Avenue
Cleveland, OH 44195-5044

Bruce D. Minsky, MD
Associate Professor of Radiation Oncology
Cornell University Medical College
Department of Radiation Oncology
Memorial Sloan-Kettering Cancer Center
1275 York Avenue
New York, NY 10021

Mohammed Mohiuddin, MD
Professor and Chair
Department of Radiation Oncology
University of Kentucky
800 Rose Street
Lexington, KY 40536

A. R. Moossa, MD
Professor and Chairman
Department of Surgery
University of California, San Diego
UCSD Medical Center
200 West Arbor Drive
San Diego, CA 92103-8400

Yoshihiro Moriya, MD
Head of Surgery
Department of Surgery
National Cancer Center Hospital
1-1, Tsukiji 5-Chome, Chuo-Ku
Tokyo 104, Japan

Gordon F. Murray, MD
Professor and Chairman
Department of Surgery
West Virginia University School of Medicine
Robert C. Byrd Health Sciences Center
P.O. Box 9238
Morgantown, WV 26506-9238

Isha A. Mustafa, MD
Fellow
Division of Surgical Oncology
Brown University
Providence, RI

Takukazu Nagakawa, MD
The Second Department of Surgery
School of Medicine, Kanazawa University
Takaramachi 13-1
Kanazawa, 920 Japan

Hector R. Nava, MD, FACS
Research Assistant Professor of Surgery
Department of Surgery
State University of New York at Buffalo
Roswell Park Cancer Institute
Elm and Carlton Streets
Buffalo, NY 14263

Amy Noffsinger, MD
Department of Pathology & Laboratory Medicine
University of Cincinnati College of Medicine
231 Bethesda Avenue
Cincinnati, OH 45267-0529

Bernard Nordlinger, MD
Centre de Chirurgie Digestive
Hospital Saint-Antoine
184 Rue du Faubourg Saint Antoine
75571 Paris, France Cedex 12

Nicholas J. Petrelli, MD
Professor of Surgery
State University of New York at Buffalo
Chief, Department of Surgical Oncology
Roswell Park Cancer Institute
Elm and Carlton Streets
Buffalo, NY 14263

Theodore L. Phillips, MD
Professor and Chairman
Department of Radiation Oncology
University of California, San Francisco, L-08
San Francisco, CA 94143-0226

Rudolf Pichlmayr, MD
c/o Burckhardt Ringe, MD
Medizinische Hochschule Hannover
Klinik für Abdominal- und Transplantationschirurgie
Konstanty-Gutschow-Strasse #8
30625 Hannover, Germany

Peter W. T. Pisters
Assistant Professor of Surgical Oncology
M. D. Anderson Cancer Center
1515 Holcombe Boulevard
Houston, TX 77030

Henry A. Pitt, MD
Professor and Vice Chairman
Department of Surgery
Johns Hopkins Hospital, Blalock 679
600 North Wolfe Street
Baltimore, MD 21287-4679

Tyvin A. Rich, MD
Department of Radiation Oncology
University of Virginia
Circle Drive, P.O. Box 383
Charlottesville, VA 22908

Burckhardt Ringe, MD
Medizinische Hochschule Hannover
Klinik für Abdominal- und Transplantationschirurgie
Konstanty-Gutschow-Strasse #8
30625 Hannover, Germany

Miguel A. Rodriguez-Bigas, MD
Assistant Professor of Surgery
State University of New York at Buffalo
Associate Chief, Colorectal Surgery
Roswell Park Cancer Institute
Elm and Carlton Streets
Buffalo, NY 14263

Jerry C. Rosenberg, MD
Professor of Surgery
Department of Surgery
Chief of Surgery
Hutzel Hospital
4707 St. Antoine
Detroit, MI 48201

Ricardo L. Rossi, MD
Professor of Surgery
Hospital Clinico
Pontifica Universidad Catolica de Chile
Escuela Medicina, Marcoleta 347
Casilla 114D, Santiago, Chile

Theodore John Saclarides, MD
Associate Professor of Surgery
Head, Section of Colorectal Surgery
Department of General Surgery
Rush-Presbyterian-St. Luke's Medical Center
1653 West Congress Parkway
Chicago, IL 60612

Takeshi Sano, MD
Department of Surgical Oncology
National Cancer Center Hospital
5-1-1, Tsukiji, Chou-ku
Tokyo, Japan

Michael G. Sarr, MD
Professor of Surgery
Mayo Medical School
Chair, Division of Gastroenterologic & General Surgery
Mayo Clinic
200 First Street, SW
Rochester, MN 55905

Mitsuru Sasako, MD
Department of Surgical Oncology
National Cancer Center Hospital
5-1-1, Tsukiji, Chou-ku
Tokyo, Japan

J. R. Siewert, MD, FACS
Professor of Surgery
Head, Department of Surgery
Chirurgische Klinik und Poliklinik
Klinikum rechts der Isar der Technischen Universität München
Ismanigerstr. 22
D-81675 München, Germany

William F. Sindelar, MD, PhD
Senior Investigator
Surgery Branch
National Cancer Institute
National Institutes of Health
Bethesda, MD 20892

Steven R. Smalley, MD
Clinical Professor of Radiation Oncology
Radiation Oncology Department
University of Kansas Medical School
20375 W 151 Street, Suite 180
Olathe, KS 66160-7321

Judy L. Smith, MD, FACS
Surgical Oncology
State University of New York at Buffalo
Roswell Park Center Institute
Elm and Carlton Streets
Buffalo, NY 14263

Thomas Smyrk, MD
Clarkson Hospital
Department of Pathology
Omaha, NE 68178

Michio Sowa, MD, PhD, FACS
Professor
First Department of Surgery
Osaka City University Medical School
1-5-7, Asahimachi, Abenoku
Osaka 545, Japan

H. J. Stein, MD
Chirurgische Klinik and Poliklinik
Klinikum rechts der Isar der Technischen Universität München
Ismaningerstr. 22
0-81675 München, Germany

Grant N. Stemmermann, MD
Department of Pathology & Laboratory Medicine
University of Cincinnati College of Medicine
231 Bethesda Avenue
Cincinnati, OH 45267-0529

F. Kristian Storm, MD, FACS
Professor of Surgery and Human Oncology
Associate Director, Comprehensive Cancer Center
University of Wisconsin School of Medicine
CSC H4/724
600 Highland Avenue
Madison, WI 53792

Paul H. Sugarbaker, MD
Director
Surgical Oncology
The Washington Cancer Institute
Washington Hospital Center
110 Irving Street, NW
Washington, DC 20010-2975

Zhao-You Tang, MD
Professor of Surgery
Liver Cancer Institute
Zhong Shan Hospital
136 Yi Xue Yuan Road
Shanghai 200032, China

Emmanuel Tarla, MD
Centre de Chirurgie Digestive
Hospital Saint-Antoine
184 Rue du Faubourg
75571 Paris, France, Cedex 12

Joel E. Tepper, MD
Professor and Chairman
Department of Radiation Oncology
University of North Carolina
School of Medicine
Campus Box 7512
Chapel Hill, NC 27599-7512

Norman W. Thompson, MD
Henry King Ransom Professor of Surgery
Department of Surgery
University of Michigan
University Hospital
Room 2920 Taubman
1500 Medical Center Drive
Ann Arbor, MI 48109

Takayoshi Tobe, MD, FACS (Hon)
Doctor of Medical Science
Professor Emeritus
General Director
Hamamatsu Rosai Hospital
25 Shogencho
Hamamatsu 430, Japan

Ronald K. Tomkins, MD, MSc
Professor of Surgery
Surgery/General Surgery
UCLA School of Medicine
10833 Le Conte Avenue
Los Angeles, CA 90095-6904

Masahiko Tsurumaru, MD, PhD, FACS
Department of Surgery
Toranomon Hospital
2-2-2 Toranomon, Minato-ku
Tokyo 105, Japan

Peter Turk, MD
Teaching Faculty
Department of Surgery
Carolina's Medical Center
Randolph Surgical Associates
2300 Randolph Road
Charlotte, NC 28207

Günther Tusch, PhD
c/o Burckhardt Ringe, MD
Medizinische Hochschule Hannover
Klinik für Abdominal- und Transplantationschirurgie
Konstanty-Gutschow-Strasse, #8
30625 Hannover, Germany

Harushi Udagawa, MD, FACS
Department of Surgery
Toranomon Hospital
2-2-2 Toranomon, Minato-ku
Tokyo 105, Japan

Jacques Van Dam, MD, PhD, FACP, FACG
Assistant Professor of Medicine
Harvard Medical School
Director, Endoscopic Gastrointestinal Oncology
Associate Director, Gastrointestinal Endoscopy
Brigham and Women's Hospital
75 Francis Street
Boston, MA 02115

Alexander Vasilakis, MD
Assistant Professor
West Virginia University School of Medicine
Robert C. Byrd Health Sciences Center
P.O. Box 9238
Morgantown, WV 26506-9238

Alan P. Venook, MD
Department of Medicine
Division of Hematology/Oncology
University of California, San Francisco
400 Parnassus Avenue
Suite 502, Mail Stop 0342
San Francisco, CA 94143

Michael P. Vezeridis, MD, FACS
Professor of Surgery
Department of Surgery
Brown University/Roger Williams Medical Center
825 Chalkstone Avenue
Providence, RI 02908

Sidney Wallace, MD
Department of Diagnostic Radiology
The University of Texas
M. D. Anderson Cancer Center
1515 Holcombe Boulevard
Houston, TX 77030

Harold J. Wanebo, MD
Professor of Surgery
Director of Surgical Oncology
Brown University Department of Medicine
Chief of Surgery—Roger Williams Medical Center
825 Chalkstone Avenue
Providence, RI 02908

Robert S. Warren, MD
Chief of Surgical Oncology
Associate Professor of Surgery
Department of Surgery
University of California, San Francisco
533 Parnassus Avenue
Room U-373, Box 0790
San Francisco, CA 94143-0790

Andrew L. Warshaw, MD
Harold and Ellen Danser Professor of Surgery
Harvard Medical School
Chief of General Surgery
Massachusetts General Hospital
Wang Ambulatory Care Center, Suite 336
Boston, MA 02114

Arved Weimann, MD
c/o Burckhardt Ringe, MD
Medizinische Hochschule Hannover
Klinik für Abdominal- und transplantationschirurgie
Konstanty-Gutschow-strasse #8
30625 Hannover, Germany

Russell E. White, MD, MPH
Staff Surgeon
Department of Surgery
Tenwek Hospital, P.O. Box 39
Bomet, Kenya

Stephen Williamson, MD
Associate Professor of Medicine
Clinical Oncology Department
University of Kansas Medical Center
3901 Rainbow Boulevard
Kansas City, KS 66160-7353

Chew-Wun Wu, MD
Professor of Surgery
Section of General Surgery
Department of Surgery
National Yang-Ming University School of Medicine
Veterans General Hospital—Taipei
Shih-Pei Road
Taipei, Taiwan, Republic of China

Ye-Quin Yu, MD
Liver Cancer Institute
Shanghai Medical University
136 Yi Xue Yuan Road
Shanghai 200032, China

Xin-Da Zhou, MD
Professor of Surgery
Liver Cancer Institute
Zhong Shan Hospital
Shanghai Medical University
136 Yi Xue Yuan Road
Shanghai 200032, China

Foreword

The challenges presented to the surgeon by gastrointestinal cancers are multiple and complex. In virtually all instances surgical removal of the cancer represents the only hope of long-term survival. Although radiotherapy and chemotherapy may play a significant role, it is usually in the adjuvant setting. Occasionally with lymphomas involving the stomach or pancreas, radiotherapy and chemotherapy may assume a primary role, with long-term survival and even cure possible. In most instances, however, surgical extirpation is necessary. The surgical procedures required for extirpating many gastrointestinal cancers are among the most challenging that face surgeons today. Esophagectomy, pancreaticoduodenectomy, major liver resections, and resection of proximal cholangiocarcinomas are difficult operative procedures that in the past have carried substantial mortality and significant morbidity. Over the past decade great strides have been made, the operative procedures are now safe, and in some instances we are on the verge of multidisciplinary approaches that will allow many patients to survive for long periods of time after being treated for gastrointestinal cancer.

The current multi-authored text edited by Dr. Harold J. Wanebo brings together world experts on managing gastrointestinal cancers. The first part of the book is an overview of the current state of our understanding of gastrointestinal cancers. Outstanding discussions on epidemiology and screening, as well as the genetics of gastrointestinal cancer, are included. Superb discussions of the molecular events that precede the development of gastrointestinal cancers, as well as the biology of the primaries and their metastases, are included. In the later sections of the book, the multidisciplinary approaches to the management of esophageal, gastric, pancreatic, liver, biliary and gall bladder, and colo-rectal cancers are discussed. The chapters are well written, readable, and complete without being encyclopedic. Superb bibliographies are included for those who require even more extensive review. The editor has made an attempt to include not only authors from the United States but also from the rest of the world to give the text an international flavor.

The approach is distinctly multidisciplinary. In essentially all of these diseases, gastroenterologists, medical oncologists, and radiotherapists are involved in the management of these patients, as well as surgeons. The successful management of most of these tumors requires a team approach. Institutions with the lowest operative mortality and morbidity and best long-term result are generally those who have developed over a period of years a team that includes not only gastroenterologists, surgeons, medical oncologists, and radiotherapists, but also radiology interventionists, critical care intensivists, experienced nursing, strong departments of nutrition, rehabilitation, and social work, all of which may be required to manage patients with complex gastrointestinal cancers. In the current climate of cost effectiveness in the United States, such a complex team might appear to be an extravagance not affordable. Most studies to date, however, have demonstrated that such a team approach results in lower hospital mortality and morbidity, shorter hospitalization, and better long-term results, all at a reduced cost, when compared to a less structured approach.

This text is beautifully edited and should present not only to the surgeon but also all other physicians an easily readable, readily understood reference that outlines clearly the current multidisciplinary approaches required for gastrointestinal cancer.

John L. Cameron, MD

Preface

The purpose of this book is to present the current surgical management of gastrointestinal cancer from a multidisciplinary perspective. Strong collaboration with medical and radiation oncologists is emphasized, as well as the vigorous interaction with the interventional gastroenterologist and radiologist. The clinical approaches described are well-grounded in the authoritative introductory sections on current epidemiology, molecular and tumor biology, and diagnostic and monitoring approaches. Although the major thrust is to provide an updated reference for the surgeon, it should also prove useful to the gastroenterologist, medical oncologist, and radiation therapist. We have recruited the acknowledged experts in the field to address the major problem areas of surgical treatment for gastrointestinal cancer. Each was encouraged to emphasize his or her own viewpoint and experience on a particular topic and to synthesize this with the findings in the current literature. We feel that an opinion based on the expertise of an authoritative figure in the field imparts a seasoned and informed judgment on the topic discussed. Differences of opinion will be reflected in the discussion of the same topic by the radiation therapist or medical oncologist or to provide counterbalance to the surgical opinion. The continued flow of data from the numerous cooperative study groups is especially noted in the views of the medical and radiation oncologists. The continued expansion of the oncologic database related to clinical trials is an ongoing process that always frustrates the definitiveness of any textbook. The current work, however, will allow the practicing clinician to develop a reasonable plan on an individual problem based on current expertise and knowledge. This can be readily supplemented by the ready access to the current literature as provided by computer access in most medical libraries and the various ''online'' services.

Acknowledgments

I am indebted to all of the authors and co-authors who have contributed to this book. They are like virtuosos in a symphony orchestra, who essentially are gathered together by a well-meaning conductor (in this case, myself), but who perform in the superior manner they are accustomed to (with or without the man at the podium).

I am also indebted to the residents, fellows, and colleagues of our oncology division who continue to question what we do as senior faculty and who enlighten us with the current scientific literature. My thanks to my patients who continue to instruct me by their successes and failures, and who constantly remind me of my limitations.

I am also thankful for the continued emotional support of my wife, Claire, and the editorial assistance of Katherine B. Terrell, who devoted countless hours to this project.

Introduction

One of the most exciting rewards for an editor is having the privilege of interacting with a large number of experts who have national and international reputations and to entice their interest in collaborating in a publication of this type. Gastrointestinal cancer has worldwide implications and yet, from the perspective of a westerner, we often have limited knowledge of certain types of GI malignancies which are very common in other parts of the world, especially in Asia. I have been gratified by the contributions of numerous authors from around the world which greatly enhances the international status of this effort. Indeed, we have much to learn from our colleagues abroad. We are all aware of the contributions in the current literature, but frequently we may not be aware of their viewpoints on these topics as these are frequently censored out by the objective nature of individual reports in the scientific literature. I have asked them to strongly emphasize their viewpoints in the light of their own experience and that of others so that this distillate is available to the reader of this text.

ESOPHAGEAL CANCER

Esophageal cancer affects only 12,000 patients in the United States annually, but has a very high death rate (>80%); yet it is the third most frequent GI cancer in the world, responsible for over 310,000 new cases.[2] Experience varies drastically worldwide with a greater than a hundredfold difference in incidences between high and low areas.[2] This disease often remains occult until late in its course at which time its discovery presents a formidable challenge for the clinician and the patient. Screening with esophageal cytology has been explored in high risk areas of China with some success. Unfortunately, the disease is commonly advanced when seen by the surgeon. Perhaps the most exciting aspect in this country has been the promising results with preoperative chemotherapy and radiation, which are still under evaluation. The assessment, staging, and surgical management of esophageal cancer are explored by experts with a long history of interest in this disease. Dr. Ellis reviews his long experience with the transthoracic resection and the alternative transhiatal approach is given by Dr. John Bolton. The enbloc radical resection is presented by the Cornell group (Altorki and Girardi). The Japanese experience of radical resection with aggressive cervical, mediastinal, and upper abdominal lymphadenectomy is presented by Dr. Akiyama. Primary radiation is presented by Drs. Minsky and Phillips, which perhaps brings back into focus the long-standing confrontation between surgery and radiation for thoracic esophageal cancer. The value of combined therapy is discussed by Dr. Kelsen, reflecting both an institutional and national experience with chemotherapy and radiation. Does this therapy-induced tumor reductive approach, which facilitates surgical resection, contribute to long-term control? The area continues to be controversial, however, and it is being addressed by clinical trial. Complications of esophageal cancer, including the dreaded broncho-esophageal fistula and other complications, are discussed by Drs. Murray and Vasilakis. The management of Barrett's esophagus, a precursor of adenocarcinoma, is reviewed by Dr. Jerry Rosenberg. The potential for endoscopic laser therapy, its indications and limitations, are represented by Dr. Hector Nava, reflecting on his extensive endoscopic experience at Roswell Park Cancer Center.

GASTRIC CANCER

Although gastric cancer has declined in incidence worldwide, it still the most common GI cancer globally. In 1980 there were over 669,000 cases estimated, of which 550,000 deaths occurred.[2] It occurs in high incidence in Japan, the Far East, and Chile, is of intermediate incidence in Russia and Europe, and relatively low incidence in the US. The outcome is highly dependent on stage. In Japan screening programs employing upper gastrointestinal double contrast barium studies complemented by endoscopy and biopsy have permitted diagnosis at an early stage with an increasing probability of long-term survival after surgical resection. The Japanese have also emphasized and popularized the use of lymph node dissection to surgically improve outcome. Retrospective data suggests that there has been some improvement in outcome stage by stage. Centers in Europe and in the East (Taiwan and Japan) have used lymph node dissection in an effort to improve outcome. We have asked both Western and Eastern authors to explore the various aspects of gastric cancer including the staging by BJ Kennedy, problems associated with proximal gastric lesions addressed by JR Siewert, and the value of lymph node dissection from both the Japanese and Chinese perspective (Drs. Keiichi Maruyama, of the National Cancer Center Hospital in Tokyo, and Chew-Wun Wu, of Veterans General Hospital in Taipei, Taiwan) respectively. The problems associated with management of early gastric cancer uncommonly seen in Western countries, but diagnosed frequently in Japan, has been addressed by Dr. Michio Sowa. The clinical trial results of adjuvant therapy for stomach cancer are addressed by Drs. Harold Douglass and Judy Smith of Roswell Park. Dr. Douglass, who was involved with the clinical trials by the Gastrointestinal Study Group (GITSG), and his associate have pointed out the findings and the limitations of the adjuvant therapy of American and European trials. Unfortunately, no clear cut message has resulted and further studies are needed. The frequency of an advanced gastric cancer and the need for surgical palliation have been addressed by Dr. Michael Vezeridis, including the role of palliative gastrectomy. The value of radiation for both palliation and its use as an adjuvant with some reflection on some of the current studies are pointed out by Dr. Steven Smalley. The potential use of intraoperative radiation is also addressed.

GASTRIC LYMPHOMA

The issues related to the histologic classification, its natural history, the role of *H pylori* and the difficulties in assessing the MALT versus other lymphomas of the stomach, and the numerous questions and controversies that result are pointed out. Indeed, is this disease treatable with antibiotics, which is suggested in some studies? The role of surgery, chemotherapy, and radiation in the current management of this confusing entity is reviewed in detail by Drs. Mustafa, Khorsand, Clark and Wanebo.

CANCER OF THE PANCREAS

Cancer of the pancreas is the second most common GI cancer in the United States. Over 26,000 cases are projected for 1996 with a very high death rate in all patients unless surgical resection can be done. Unfortunately, only small numbers are amenable to resection and there are yet no screening programs of value. It is the fifth most common malignancy in the world (137,000 cases in 1980). Drs. Michael Sarr and David Farley have addressed the operative management of "apparent" malignancy in the head of the pancreas and have reviewed the questions of diagnosis, bypass, and resection. Many problems face both the gastroenterologist and surgeon in making the diagnosis of cancer of the pancreatic head. The limitations and questionable risk of CT directed needle aspiration biopsy and the problems related to obtaining a definitive tissue diagnosis intraoperatively are discussed. Decision making in patients in the absence of obtaining a definitive diagnosis (should resection be done in absence of a tissue diagnosis) are some of the issues addressed. The treatment of cancers of the ampulla and periampullary area, terminal bile duct, and duodenum area are addressed by Drs. Ronald Tompkins and Edward Livingston. Here there is more ground for optimism both diagnostically and therapeutically. There is the potential for obtaining long-term control in perhaps a third of these patients. Laparoscopic staging is another important issue, especially in the current era of pancreatic surgery, and is discussed by Drs. Fernandez-del Castillo and Andrew Warshaw, representing the long experience with this technique at the Massachusetts General Hospital. Laparoscopy does provide the opportunity to assess operability and perhaps to bypass and provide nutritional access for those patients who may get preoperative therapy as is discussed later. The use of pylorus preserving pancreaticoduodenectomy is addressed by Drs. Ricardo Rossi and Ronald Martin. Dr. Martin's group, more than any other, has studied the role of pylorus preserving surgery in pancreatic cancer and has demonstrated that with good patient selection the hazard of histologic invasion of the pylorus can be minimized and a more conservative resection, which preserves the gastric function, can be permitted. Certainly, in more limited cancers of ampulla, periampullary area, and bile duct, this is an optimum technique and in the hands of these authors it appears to be of value in most of their patients seen with pancreatic head cancers. At the opposite extreme total pancreatectomy is a logical though controversial solution for a potentially multicentric disease. It is ably addressed by Dr. A. R. Moossa and his associate, Dr. Marquis Hart. Regional pancreatectomy, a surgically encompassing but formidable procedure pioneered by Dr. Joseph Fortner over two decades ago, is discussed by another pioneer, Dr. Takukazu Nagakawa, who has updated his experience, which began in the early seventies. Dr. William Sindelar of the Surgery branch at the NCI pioneered the addition of intraoperative radiation to regional resection in an effort to extend control, and has updated his experience with the combined approach. Lastly, the value of preoperative therapy for pancreatic cancer has been addressed by Dr. John Hoffman from Fox Chase Cancer Center. Dr. Hoffman and his colleagues have pioneered the use of preoperative chemotherapy and radiation therapy in an effort to achieve long-term control. They have demonstrated that this technique can be adapted with relatively low morbidity and low mortality in their hands. This study was adopted by ECOG, which demonstrated the feasibility of the protocol in a cooperative group setting. The ECOG study has been presented in abstract form in the American Society of Clinical Oncology Proceedings and we are awaiting the final manuscript publication. Similar studies have also been done at the M. D. Anderson Cancer Center in Houston, Texas. The use of this type of approach to assess the effect of chemoradiation is exciting. It permits coupling of the Phase II aspect of drug assessment of untreated pancreatic cancer with the potential of down staging and increasing resectability. Radiation provides excellent palliation for unresectable pancreatic cancer and is discussed by Dr. Mohammed Mohiuddin who has made a major contribution in the way radiation is used in the management of these difficult patients. Chemotherapy of upper GI cancer, including the esophagus, stomach, and pancreas, is addressed by Dr. James Ahlgren, who has recently edited a superb tome entitled, *Gastrointestinal Oncology*.[4] Dr. Ahlgren and his colleagues have had a long association with the former GI Tumor Study Group and with the Mid-Atlantic Oncology Program which heavily focused on the therapy of gastrointestinal cancer. He brings to bear his extensive experience as well as reflecting the results presented in the literature. The treatment of endocrine tumors of the gastrointestinal tract, including the pancreas and carcinoid tumors, is presented by Dr. Norman Thompson, whose group has had extensive experience in neuroendocrine surgery.

LIVER, BILE DUCT, AND GALL BLADDER

Hepatocellular cancer (HCC), although uncommon in the United States (<3 persons per 100,000), is one of the most common malignancies worldwide, with the estimated incidence in 1980 of 251,000 cases making it the fourth most common gastrointestinal cancer. Approximately 85% of the cases are fatal. Extreme high-risk areas occur in Africa and Asia, ranging up to a standardized incidence of 100 per 100,000 in Mozambique and Taiwan. In Japan it is the third most frequent cause of cancer deaths among males and fifth among females.[2] Viral infection with hepatitis B (HBV) is considered the major cause of hepatocellular carcinoma. Hepatitis C is equally carcinogenic and is a prevalent cause in Japan. Although less common in the West, it is not inconsequential and major large series representing both the Western and the Eastern experience have been presented. The Western experience is addressed by Dr. Bernard Nordlinger and Emmanuel Tarla of Centre de Sainte-Antoine Hospital in Paris and the Eastern (Japanese) experience has been ably discussed by Dr. Takayoshi Tobe and his associate, Dr. Shigeki Arii. The resection of small HHC cancer is discussed by Dr. Zhao-You Tang and his colleagues from Shanghai, who relate their unique surgical experience with treatment of small HCC. The selection of transplantation versus resection has been addressed by one of the premiere surgeons in this area, Dr. Burckhardt Ringe, who has an enormous experience in transplant with his mentor and colleague, Dr. Pichlmayer, during his tenure at Hanover. The problems and the limitations of the operative approach in the cirrhotic patient are discussed by Drs. Wing-Yiu Lui and Gar-Yang Chau of Veterans General Hospital in Taipei, which has a enormous institutional experience with hepatocellular carcinoma. The value of resection from metastases, specifically colorectal cancer, are reviewed by Dr. Margaret Kemeny. The concept of regional chemotherapy for hepatic neoplasms is overviewed by Drs. Alan Paul Venook and Robert Warren of the University of California who are highly experienced in this area and reflect the need to have alternative approaches for these high risk patients, most of whom are not resectable. The use of other techniques including hyperthermia and cryosurgery are reviewed by Dr. Kristian Storm and his associate, Dr. David Mahvi. Dr. Storm pioneered the use of hyperthermia for liver tumors almost two decades ago. He has had extensive experience with the alternative methods for treatment of liver tumors and provides perspective of the use of these methods, especially as alternatives to resection.

Bile duct cancer is a much lesser common entity, often included in the listing of 19,100 hepatobiliary cancers reported nationally. Probably only a third of these are bile duct cancers. The selection of therapy for this disease ranging from resection to biliary intubation and the survival results are reviewed by the Hopkins group (Drs. Magnuson, Pitt and Cameron), who have had a long-term experience with this entity. Resectional approaches to proximal bile duct cancer can be formidable procedures and are addressed by one of the experienced pioneers in this type of surgery, Dr. Leslie Blumgart and colleague Dr. Peter Pisters of the Memorial Sloan-Kettering Cancer Center. The question of patient selection, the limitations of resection, the perioperative mortality and morbidity, and long-term sequelae are pointed out by a true expert in this field. Lastly, considering the limitations of resection for these tumors, radiation either as a supplement or alternative to surgery is commonly needed. Radiation therapy of the bile duct by interstitial intraoperative or external beam techniques are discussed by Dr. Joel Tepper, an experienced therapist with this entity. The radiologic access to bile duct tumors facilitates the use of interstitial radiation (brachytherapy) by inserting radiation sources into hepatobiliary stents. This should be considered in those patients who may not be treatable by resectional techniques. Additional issues meriting discussion in the liver and biliary system include the management of gall bladder cancer, which is also a relatively uncommon malignancy, but which is currently being frequently diagnosed with the advent of laparoscopic cholecystectomy. Considering the high incidence of gall stones in most Western centers and the strong relationship to gall bladder cancer, the need to have a positive approach to these patients is emphasized by Dr. Harold J. Wanebo. The issue of resection of the hepatic bed, node dissection, and adjuvant therapies are reviewed. The inadvertent discovery of gallbladder cancer during laparoscopic cholecystectomy is a new challenge facing the surgeon and is also addressed in this chapter. The role of combination chemotherapy for hepatobiliary cancer is addressed by Dr. Brian Carr, who has extensive experience in this area. He has pioneered the use of preoperative chemotherapy for hepatocellular cancer and has attempted to define the role of chemotherapy prior to either resection or transplant. Lastly, the use of interventional radiologic techniques to diagnose and treat hepatobiliary malignancy are addressed by Drs. Sidney Wallace and Chusilp Charnsangavej of the M. D. Anderson Cancer Center. This group has had extensive experience with interventional radiologic techniques in the diagnosis and treatment of hepatobiliary cancers and reflect on this in addressing the technical considerations, ongoing clinical trials, and future directions with this technique.

COLORECTAL CANCER

Colorectal cancer is the second most common GI malignancy worldwide with over 572,000 cases estimated in 1980, resulting in 330,000 deaths.[2] It is the most common GI malignancy in the United States with an estimated 134,000 patients being diagnosed in 1996. Colorectal cancer has been the most extensively studied of the GI malignancies from the prospective of its genetic, molecular, biologic, environmental, and dietary factors. The genetic factors have been identified in specific families as well as in the rare inherited forms, such as familial polyposis. The role of dietary factors, however, is a dominant concern in the sporadic cases. In recent years the role of diet is emphasized by the changing incidence of this disease in certain populations related to intake of defined dietary sustenance in the patient. For example, in Japan, the incidence has more than doubled in the last three decades with strong implication of diet, especially in the consumption of meat and animal fat. The low intake of dietary fiber has also been implicated as contributing to the high incidence in Western society as initially suggested by Dr. Dennis P. Burkitt.[2] The application of molecular biologic techniques by Vogelstein and his associates at Johns Hopkins has shown that a specific tumor suppressor gene p53 is inactivated in many colorectal cancers. A second tumor suppressor gene deleted in colorectal cancer (DCC) appears also to participate in this process. Mutations in the ras protooncogene are also implicated and, in conjunction with deleted or deactivated p53 and DCC and perhaps other tumor suppressor genes, result in a transition of normal mucosal epithelium to polyps and eventually cancer. The accumulative carcinogenic steps are strongly suggested by the works of Vogelstein and his colleagues, and others provide the important information not only for the understanding of the disease, but by perhaps suggesting ways to diagnose at an earlier stage, as well as provide ways for chemoprevention. Because of the silence of this disease until the advanced stage, the need for screening has been addressed by many groups, with the same level of emphasis as screening for gastric cancer in Japan, although this has not been achieved. For example, the screening programs have relied heavily on testing for occult blood and subsequent diagnostic steps by fluoroscopy, colonoscopy, or both. The potential for recognizing early genetic changes or for detecting the presence of oncogene products in the stool may increase the sensitivity of testing. The important goal of identifying cancer at an early non-metastatic stage has the greatest chance for achieving long-term control with simplified surgical techniques.

The role of endoscopy and associated techniques are discussed by Dr. Frederick Greene from the University of South Carolina, who presents some basic technical considerations regarding patient selection in the testing of precursor lesions for incidence of colorectal cancer. The discussion of laparoscopic surgery in the management of large bowel cancer is addressed by an individual who is strongly identified with the Society of Gastrointestinal Endoscopic Surgery (SAGES). This group probably has done more than any other to advance the cause of laparoscopic surgery in the United States. The polyposis syndromes which have now become a more formidable issue for surgeons and gastroenterologist alike are reviewed by Dr. James Church, the Director of the Heritable Rectal Registry at the Cleveland Clinic. The emphasis on prophylaxis, optimal surgical approach, patient selection, and technique in managing these patients are reviewed. The selection of patients for colorectal resection with coloanal or ileoanal anastomotic procedures and the efforts to preserve bowel function in these commonly young patients are addressed by a surgical expert in this area. This may even be more important in the future with earlier diagnosis pending the success of some of the new molecular biologic techniques in screening and the potential for earlier detection of patients at risk to develop invasive cancer.

Surgical resection for colon cancer is reviewed by Dr. Philip Gordon, the Director of Colon and Rectal Cancer at the Mortimer B. Davis Jewish Hospital in Montreal. The discussion of no-touch wide field resection, management of tumors, and extension to other structures are all reviewed. Rectal cancer is discussed by Dr. Jeffrey Milsom with special emphasis on the management of low and mid-rectal cancers. Questions regarding the use of the stapler, other sphincter saving techniques, and technical considerations in low rectal resections including APR are addressed. The valve of pelvic node dissection which has been long popularized in Japan by Dr. Yoshihiro Moriya and his predecessor, Dr. HoJo, are reviewed by Dr. Moriya. This is a controversial area, but one that merits an open discussion by an expert who focuses on both the limitations and the potential for obtaining better local and regional control. Dr. Moriya has also emphasized the use of the nerve sparing technique to preserve urogenital function, which is an area of major concern considering the current emphasis by other pelvic surgeons, that is nerve sparing radical prostatectomy. The use of preoperative radiation for the high risk patient with low lying rectal cancer is addressed by Dr. Gerald Marks, an individual with perhaps the greatest experience in this area. Drs. Gerald and John Marks and Dr. Mohiuddin have popularized the technique of preoperative radiation and resection with coloanal anastomosis for low lying rectal cancer and have achieved an enviable record regarding local and regional control and survival in these patients. Whether this technique can be broadly applied remains to be determined, but the awareness of surgeons of this approach and their having an open mind in adapting these techniques may be of value when applied to the highly selected patients. At the other end of the spectrum is the patient with the small mobile cancer which can be treated by a lesser technique. This is reviewed by Dr. J. Milburn Jessup of the New England Deaconess Hospital in Boston. Dr. Jessup has had a long interest in local excision of rectal cancer which no longer is considered controversial. The application of this technique to properly selected patients merits emphasis. A clinical trial is underway in the cooperative study groups to examine this issue and to sort out the usefulness of local excision per se or local excision plus radiation. The willingness to adapt this technique in the properly selected patients, preserving anorectal function with achievement of good long-term tumor control, is being increasingly adapted by general surgeons and colorectal surgeons. There are technical issues for local resection and we have asked Dr. Theodore Saclarides, Head of Colon and Rectal Surgery at Rush Hospital in Chicago, to address these issues. The adjuvant therapy for colorectal cancer is reviewed by Drs. J. Michael Hamilton and Michael A. Friedman, who provide an overview of the clinical trial results, as well as the status of ongoing clinical trials. The use of pre- and postoperative radiation for rectal cancer, both in the adjuvant setting and in the circumstance of advanced disease, is addressed by Dr. Ty Rich, formerly of M.D. Anderson. The coupling of radiation with chemotherapy merits discussion in view of the insights gained from the labeling studies to assess the therapeutic effects of sensitizing chemotherapy. There are questions regarding dose and timing of fractionation to effect local and regional control. Some studies suggest that modifying the fractionation may reduce the regrowth fraction and perhaps this, combined with chemotherapy, may improve tumor control. These areas all merit attention. Anal canal cancer, a rather uncomon entity representing only 1% of all neoplasms of the anorectum, is still a clinical issue. There are issues regarding etiology, epidemiology, natural history, and of course, the role of multimodality therapy. It is a disease that is amenable to preoperative therapy with the potential for inducing tumor regression and down staging allowing for more conservative anorectal resection (addressed by Drs. James Koness and Harold J. Wanebo). The role of monitoring colorectal cancer patients with carcinoembryonic antigen is addressed by one of the premiere authorities in this area, Dr. Edward Martin. Dr. Martin and a former colleague, the late Dr. John P. Minton, were pioneers in monitoring with carcinoembryonic antigen and advancing the concept of CEA directed second-look surgery. This group has expanded their techniques coupled with radioimmune guided surgery in selecting the sites within the abdomen and pelvis which harbor occult metastases. The value of this approach in not only detecting recurrence, but perhaps in improving the staging of these patients, merits clinical attention. Ongoing trials will hopefully define the role of radioimmune guided surgery in staging patients, but it also appears that this technique may allow one to salvage patients with second look surgery who otherwise might not be salvaged because not all disease is resected. The management of pelvic recurrence and other alternatives is addressed by Drs. Peter Turk and Harold J. Wanebo. Pelvic recurrence is an ominous event after apparent curative resection of rectal cancer and is a formidable problem facing the patient and his physician. The technique of interim management with radiation therapy and pain control is highly important. The potential for resecting these patients merits discussion. There are limitations to this technique and certainly pitfalls, but there are opportunities for curative resection in highly selected patients. Perhaps one third of highly selected patients may survive five years. The importance of adequately staging these patients is essential. In the patient not amenable to resection the potential for other considerations such as pelvic perfusion is also discussed. Perineal and pelvic pain are major consequences of rectal cancer. These and other issues of pain management for advanced disease are cogently discussed by Dr. Nathan Cherny of the pain service at Memorial Sloan-Kettering Cancer Center. Probably in no other group of cancer patients is there such a need for pain control. Certainly other diseases have associated pain, such as cancer of the pancreas, but because of the short life span of these patients it is less of a formidable problem. In patients with recurrence following rectal cancer, survival is commonly measured in terms of several months, if not longer, and the need for pain control is very important. The listing of new techniques and improved understandings of the pharmacology and the use of other drug delivery systems, for example epidural blockade to improve the outcome of these patients, is addressed. Intraperitoneal chemotherapy, a new application of a technique long in use in ovarian cancer, is addressed by a pioneer in this area, Dr. Paul Sugarbaker. Patient selection and the limitation, morbidity, and potential for future directions are addressed. The value of chemotherapy for advanced GI cancer is addressed by Drs. Nicholas J. Petrelli and Miguel Rodriguez-Bigas. The development of new drugs, new delivery systems, and consideration of new concepts of therapy merit careful consideration. There is probably nowhere that the advances are more rapidly made than in examining the results of Phase I and Phase II trial results in these groups of patients. The differential responses in patients with upper versus lower GI malignancies and malignancies involving certain organ systems cannot be ignored. The potential for modulating drugs with leucovorin and other active modulators, which had been pioneered by Dr. Petrelli and his associates at Roswell Park, merits attention.

Lastly, a chapter is devoted to biologic therapy, a scientific area which is literally exploding. The use of tumor vaccines, immune potentiation with cytokines, and gene therapy are reviewed by Dr. Michael T. Lotze and Dr.

James S. Goydos. Dr. Lotze pioneered many of the advances in cytokine therapy with his mentor Dr. Rosenberg at the NCI Surgery branch for over a decade and contributed greatly to the development of knowledge in this area. He has provided an update of ongoing studies, as well as indicating future directions for therapy, making this a fitting concluding chapter.

REFERENCES

1. Parker SL, Tong T, Bolden S, Wingo PA (eds). Cancer Statistics 1996. CA Vol 1996;46:5.
2. Schein P. Gastrointestinal cancer: a global perspective. In: Ahlgren J, McDonald J (eds). Gastrointestinal Oncology, 1992:3.
3. DeVita VT Jr, Hellman S, Rosenberg SA (eds). Cancer: Principles and Practice of Oncology, 4th ed. Philadelphia: JB Lippincott, 1993.
4. Ahlgren JD, Macdonald JS (eds). Gastrointestinal Oncology. Philadelphia: JB Lippincott, 1992.
5. Additional Reference Sources:
   National Cancer Institute (NCI)—Phone 1-800-422-6237.
   Physician's Data Query—Phone 1-800-624-7890
   World Wide Web—http://cancernet.nci.nih.gov
6. Suggested journals for access to current literature: All are listed in the Index Medicus available in all medical school libraries (italics indicate how Index Medicus list the journal)
   New England Journal of Medicine—*N Eng J Med*
   Journal of Clinical Oncology—*J Clin Oncol*
   Journal of the National Cancer Institute—*JNCI*
   Journal of the American Medical Association—*JAMA*
   Cancer—*Cancer*
   Cancer Research—*Cancer Res*
   Clinical Cancer Research—*Clin Cancer Res*
   Annals of Surgery—*Ann Surg*
   American Journal of Surgery—*Am J Surg*
   Journal of Surgical Oncology—*J Surg Oncol*
   Archives of Surgery—*Arch Surg*
   Journal of Clinical Oncology—*J Clin Oncol*
   International Journal of Cancer—*Int J Cancer*
   World Journal of Surgery—*World J Surg*
   Lancet—*Lancet* (London)
   British Journal of Surgery—*Br J Surg*

Contents

I. Introduction and Overview

II. Esophageal Cancer

III. Gastric Cancer

IV. Pancreatic Cancer

V. Liver, Bile Duct, and Gallbladder

VI. Lower Gastrointestinal Cancer

Surgery for
GASTROINTESTINAL CANCER

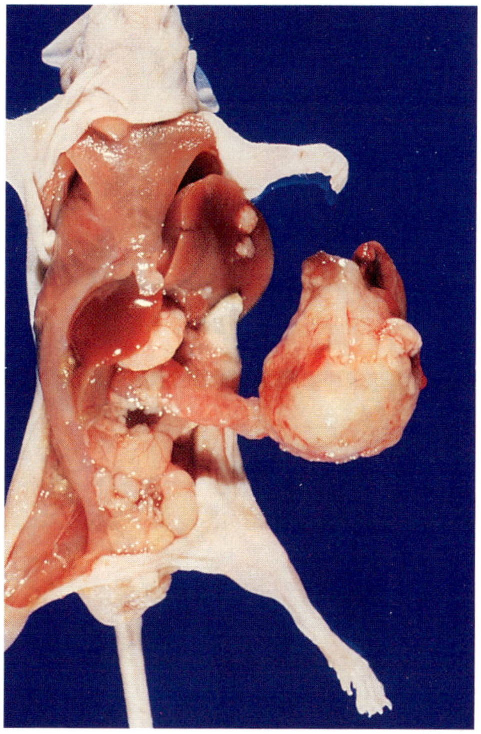

COLOR FIGURE 4-4. Autopsy findings in a mouse transplanted with L3.3 large growth at the site of the transplantation and metastatic nodules in the liver. (From Vezerides MP, Doremus CM, Tibbetts LM, et al. Invasion and metastasis following orthotopic transplantation of human pancreatic cancer in the nude mouse. J Surg Oncol 1989;40:261.)

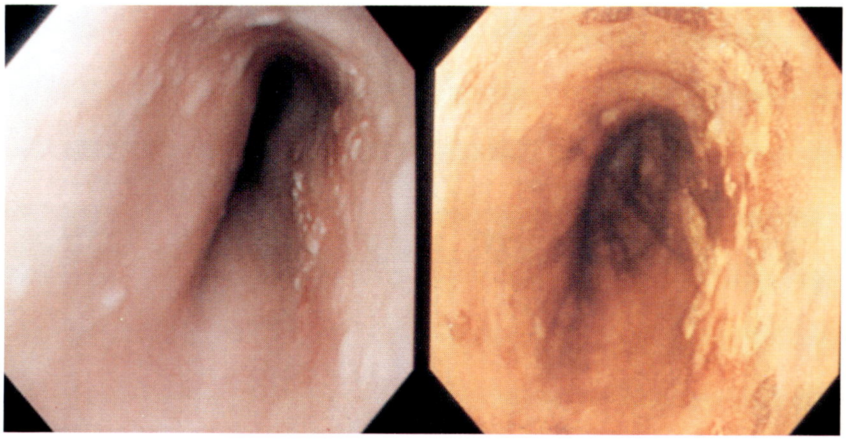

A B

COLOR FIGURE 18-1. (**A**) Endoscopic finding of slightly depressed type (0-11c) of intraepithelial cancer of the esophagus. (**B**) Margin of cancer is well demarcated by iodine vital staining.

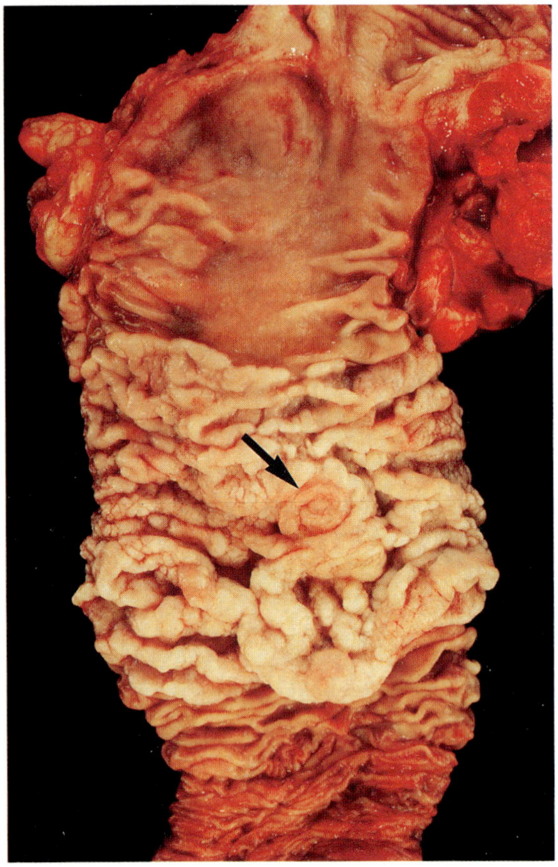

COLOR FIGURE 33-8. Gross specimen removed by standard Whipple procedure from a patient with a villous adenoma of papilla of Vater (*arrow*). The mucosal field defect extends proximally and distally from the papilla and the margins would not be adequate if the pylorus preservation technique had been used (Pylorus is at top of figure).

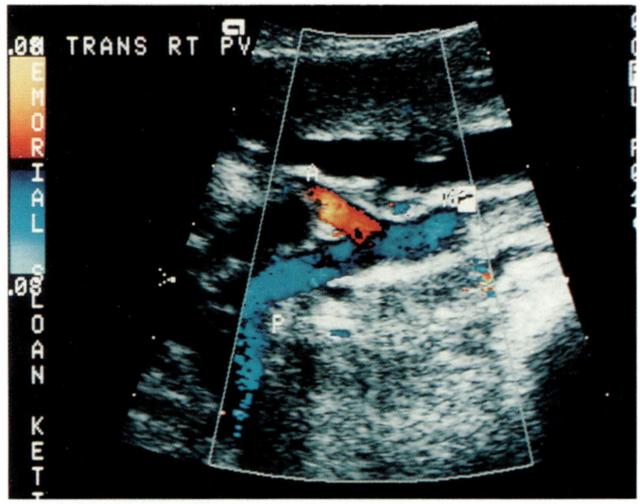

COLOR FIGURE 52.2. Transverse sonographic view through the hepatic hilus demonstrating dilated bile ducts anteriorly with right anterior and posterior sectoral branches of the right portal vein. The significant anatomic detail that can be imaged using this technique is apparent.

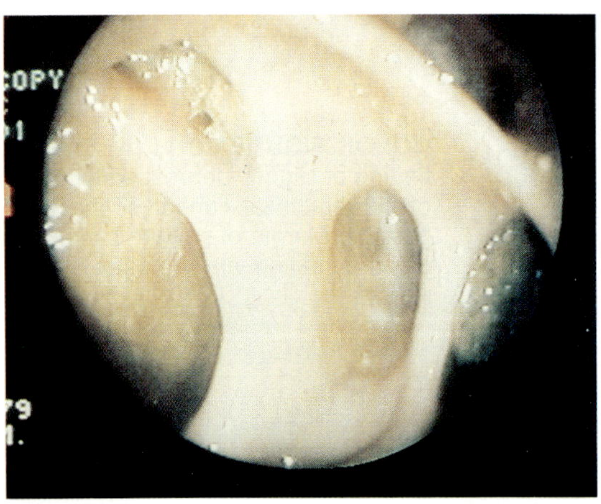

COLOR FIGURE 57-1. Intraluminal view showing extensive diverticulosis.

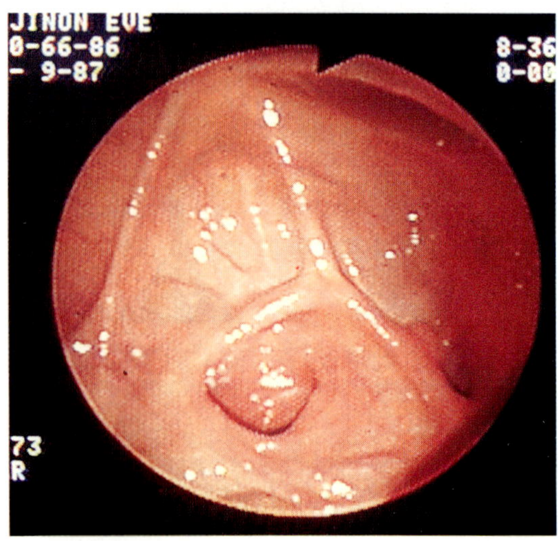

COLOR FIGURE 57-4. Appearance of cecum, showing "vaulted-church" appearance.

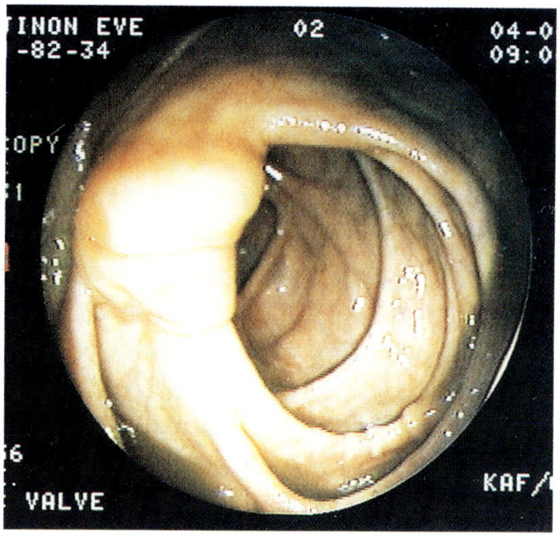

COLOR FIGURE 57-5. Prominent ileocecal valve may mimic polypoid lesion.

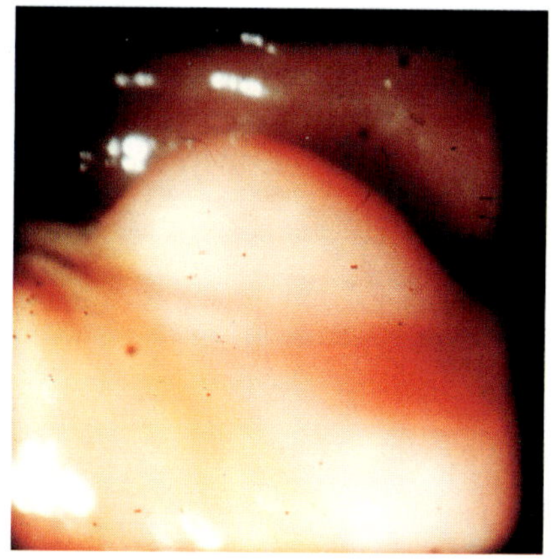

COLOR FIGURE 57-6. Diminutive, hyperplastic polyp of colon.

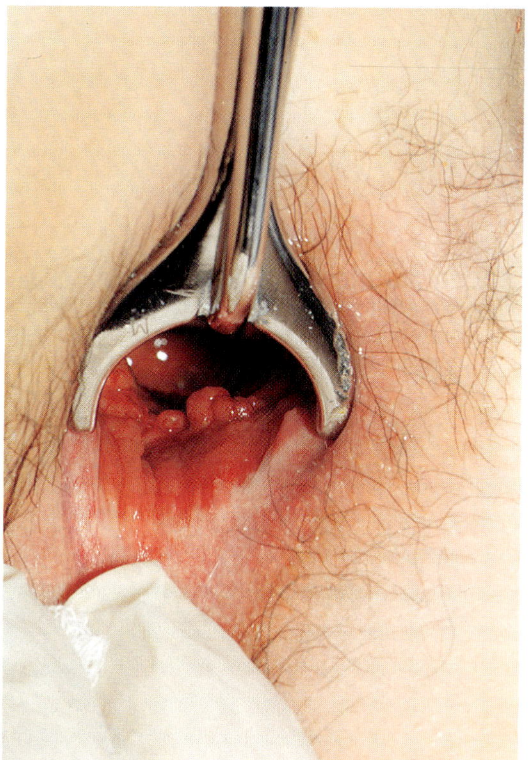

COLOR FIGURE 58-4. A villous adenoma growing in the small strip of residual rectum after stapled IPAA.

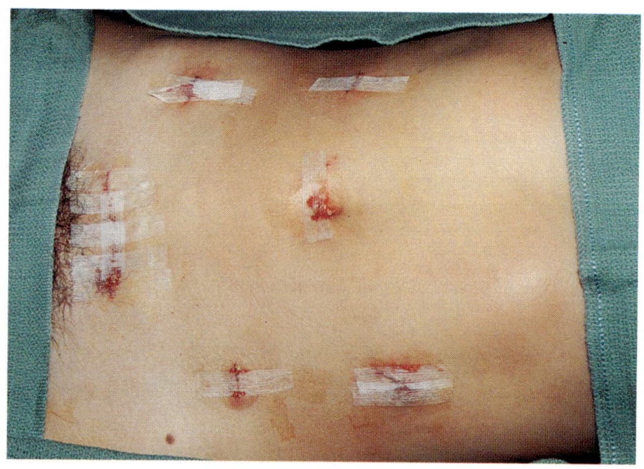

COLOR FIGURE 58-6. The incisions made for laparoscopic colectomy and IRA in a 13-year-old girl with mild, asymptomatic FAP.

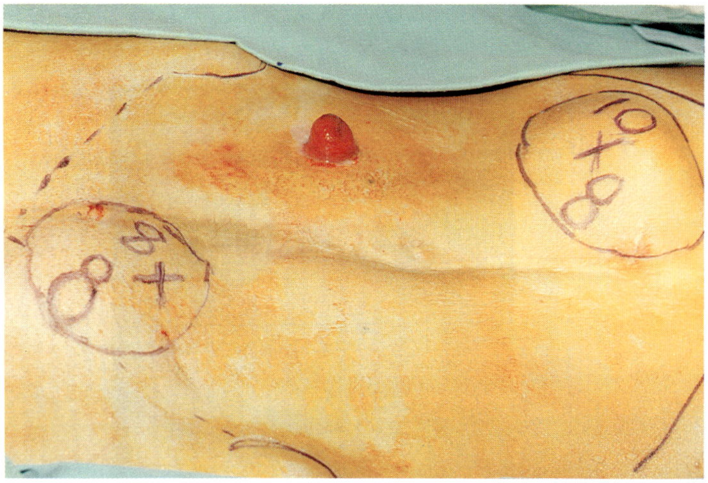

A

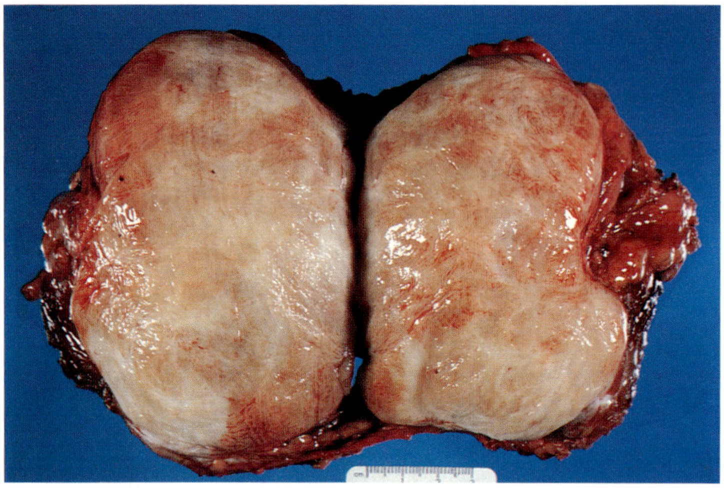

B

COLOR FIGURE 58-8. (**A**) Abdominal wall desmoid tumors ready for excision. After 4 years there has been no recurrence. (**B**) Excised abdominal wall desmoid; this patient's desmoid is different from that shown in (**A**).

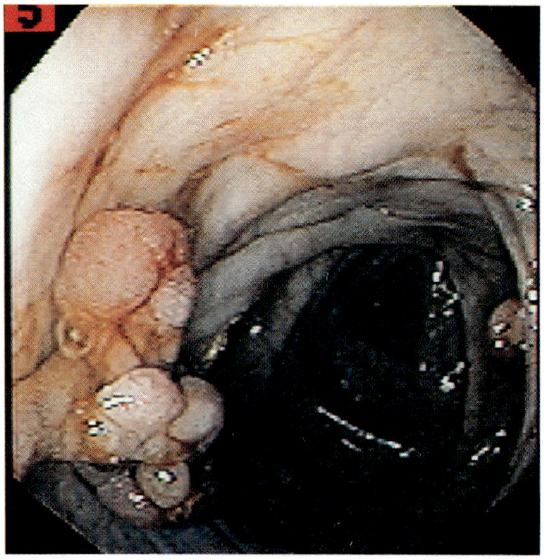

COLOR FIGURE 58-9. Juvenile polyposis. Note the light red, multi-lobular appearance of the polyps. This patient presented with a colon cancer and was initially diagnosed as having familial adenomatous polyposis.

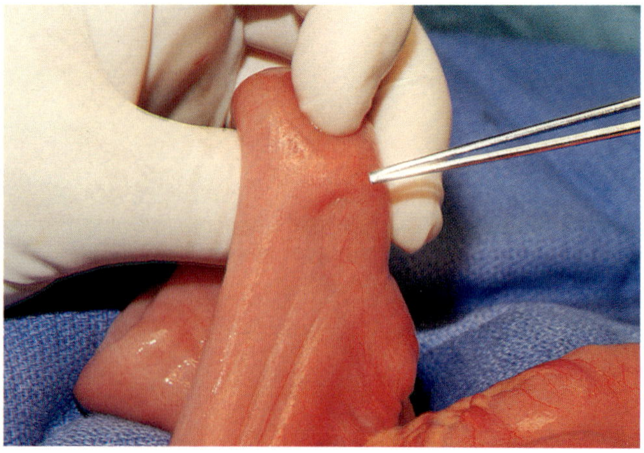

COLOR FIGURE 58-10. The mid-small bowel in a patient with Peutz-Jeghers syndrome. Note the serosal dimpling caused by traction on a polyp stalk.

PART I

Introduction and Overview

Surgery for Gastrointestinal Cancer: A Multidisciplinary Approach, edited by Harold J. Wanebo.
Lippincott-Raven Publishers, Philadelphia, © 1997.

CHAPTER 1

Etiology, Epidemiology, and Potential Prevention of Gastrointestinal Cancer

Cedric F. Garland, Frank C. Garland, and E. D. Gorham

Approximately 223,000 Americans are diagnosed with cancers of the digestive system each year (Table 1-1), 1 accounting for 124,330 deaths in the United States in 1994. The most common digestive system malignancy in the United States, colorectal cancer, accounts for 138,200 new cases per year, ranking it the third most common major malignancy after cancer of the lung (169,900 cases) and breast (183,400 cases). This chapter reviews the epidemiology of the major digestive system cancers—esophagus, stomach, pancreas, liver, colon, and rectum—and suggests possible avenues for prevention.

CANCER OF THE ESOPHAGUS

Like most other digestive tract cancers, esophageal cancer shows marked international variation in incidence and mortality rates. However, even in developed countries where risk is generally low, esophageal cancer often exhibits a distinct regional pattern, with steep gradients and marked variation among neighboring areas within short distances. This microvariation suggests an etiologic role of environmental risk factors that vary over relatively short distances.[2]

International Comparisons

Esophageal cancer is the 6th most common cause of cancer mortality worldwide[3] and the 13th most common cause of cancer mortality in the United States.[1] It ranks as the second most common cause of cancer death after stomach cancer in China,[4] and in some provinces accounts for nearly half of all deaths from cancer.[5] In the Chinese provinces of Linxian and Henan, the longstanding endemicity of this dreaded disease has led to worship of a "God of the Throat."[4] Incidence of esophageal cancer in these regions of China, and in certain former Soviet republics (Kazakhstan and Turkmenistan), Northern Afghanistan, and the Caspian region of Iran, has been so high that these regions are referred to collectively as the "Asian esophageal cancer belt."[6–8]

According to incidence data for 1992 from the International Agency for Research on Cancer, the annual age-standardized incidence rate per 100,000 for esophageal cancer in men in the Gombad region of Iran was 166; in Linxian, China, it was 161; and in Guryev, a region in the former Soviet republic of Kazakhstan, it was 132.[9] The rate in Kazakhstan is in marked contrast to rates as low as 4 per 100,000 in other former Soviet republics such as Latvia, Lithuania, and Estonia.[7]

Increasing incidence rates that are now nearly half as high as those in the Asian esophageal cancer belt have been reported in some populations in southern Africa, including annual rates in Bulawayo men of Zimbabwe (formerly Rhodesia) of 64 per 100,000 and in men of Natal, South Africa of 41 per 100,000. High rates also are present in men in Miyagi, Japan (14 per 100,000) and Hong Kong (18 per 100,000).[9]

In general, countries in Western Europe and the Americas have low incidence rates of esophageal cancer. Low annual incidence rates in Europe, ranging from 2 to 3 per 100,000 population, have been reported for Norway, Sweden, and Denmark. The lowest incidence rate in Europe was 1 per 100,000 in Romania. The highest annual incidence rate, 30 per 100,000, was in Calvados, France.

Mortality rates vary greatly within the Americas. The highest age-standardized annual mortality rates occur in Uruguay (12 per 100,000), Puerto Rico (11 per 100,000), and Argentina (9 per 100,000), and the lowest in Mexico (2 per 100,000), the Dominican Republic (1 per 100,000) and Peru (1 per 100,000).[10]

Steep local regional gradients have been reported in Iran, the

Cedric F. Garland, Associate Professor, Department of Family and Preventive Medicine, University of California, San Diego Cancer Center, 9500 Gilman Drive 0631C, La Jolla, CA 92093-0631.

Frank C. Garland, Assistant Adjunct Professor, Department of Family and Preventive Medicine, University of California, San Diego Cancer Center, 9500 Gilman Drive 0631C, La Jolla, CA 92093-0631.

Edward D. Gorham, Department of Family and Preventive Medicine, University of California, San Diego Cancer Center, 9500 Gilman Drive 0631C, La Jolla, CA 92093-0631.

TABLE 1-1. *Number of new cases per year, annual incidence rate, and overall relative 5-year survival rates of digestive system cancers, United States, 1995**

Site	Estimated no. of new cases per year	Annual incidence rate per 100,000 population		Overall 5-year relative survival rate (%), whites, 1983–1990†
		Men	Women	
Colon	100,000	17	11	61
Rectum	38,200			58
Pancreas	24,000	8	6	3
Stomach	22,800	5	2	18
Liver and biliary tract	18,500	2	1	7
Esophagus	12,100	5	2	11
Small intestine	4600	1	1	—
Other and unspecified digestive system cancers	2800	1	1	—
Total	223,123	39	24	

* Survival rates are based on Surveillance, Epidemiology, and End Results data from Connecticut, New Mexico, Utah, Iowa, Hawaii, Atlanta, Detroit, Seattle, and San Francisco–Oakland. Survival rates were lower in blacks.

† Overall relative survival rates include distant–metastatic, regional, and localized malignancies. Relative survival rates were higher for localized malignancies than overall.

Data for numbers of new cases from Wingo PA, Tong T, Bolden S. Cancer statistics, 1995. CA Cancer J Clin 1995;45: 8; data for survival rates from Miller BA, Ries LAG, Hankey BF, et al. SEER cancer statistics review: 1973–1991. NIH Publication 94-2789. Bethesda, MD: National Cancer Institute, 1994; Whelan SL, Parkin DM, Masuyer E. Patterns of cancer incidence in five continents. IARC Publication No. 102. Lyon France: International Agency for Research on Cancer, 1990.

Linxian and Hunan provinces, Bretagne and Calveros, France, and in Japan and South Africa.[2] Notable differences in risk were present within Bretagne even among neighboring communes.[2] The small South African nation of Transkei (whose dimensions are only 100 × 150 miles) has regional incidence rates that varies by greater than fourfold.[11] A similar fourfold magnitude of variation in incidence rates exists in men, and nearly an eightfold difference in women among the 13 regions of Kazakhstan, with striking differences between adjacent regions.[12]

Demographic Factors

Sex

Esophageal cancer is more frequent in men than women throughout most of the world. The age-standardized mortality rate for esophageal cancer in the United States was 4 per 100,000 men and 1 per 100,000 women during 1985 to 1988.[10] Despite a 10-fold variation in age-standardized mortality rates for esophageal cancer among 16 countries in the Americas for both men and women, rates in men were approximately four times those in women.

One of the highest male-to-female ratios for esophageal cancer was reported in the Bulawayo tribe of Zimbabwe. Bulawayo men were reported to have an annual age-adjusted incidence rate of 64 per 100,000 population, whereas Bulawayo women had an annual incidence of only 2 per 100,000. In contrast, Bantu men of the South African Cape had an annual incidence rate of 38 per 100,000, compared to 14 in Bantu women.[6] Overall, the sex ratio for esophageal cancer tends to be high in areas with high incidence rates. In striking contrast to this general rule, annual incidence of esophageal cancer among women in Kazakhstan was 174 per 100,000, whereas in men it was 133 per 100,000.[13]

Race

Incidence rates of esophageal cancer in blacks have increased since the mid-1960s in the United States, but have remained stable in whites.[1] In 1992, the incidence rate of esophageal cancer in black men in Connecticut was nearly five times that of white men. In Los Angeles, the incidence rate in black men was three times the rate in white men. The annual incidence rate in Chinese Americans living in Los Angeles was 3 per 100,000, whereas the incidence rate in Chinese living in Shanghai was 21 per 100,000.[7]

Age

The incidence of esophageal cancer worldwide is logarithmically associated with age, and the disease is rare at ages younger than 40 years.[9]

Nutritional Deficiencies

The marked gradients within countries for esophageal cancer, as well as variation within countries according to social class, point to the possibility of nutritional factors playing an important role in esophageal cancer. A review of the role of nutritional factors has identified particular foods and micronutrients associated with decreased risk.[14] Ten of 11 case–control studies found a significant protective effect of intake of fresh fruits and vegetables on risk of esophageal cancer.[15]

A review of studies in which smoking and alcohol intake also were examined indicated that the effect of fresh fruits and vegetables was independent of the effect of smoking and alcohol use.[16] An early epidemiologic study detected a halving of risk of esophageal cancer in women associated with frequent intake of citrus fruits.[17] This was followed by 12 epidemiologic studies that found beneficial effects of intake of citrus fruits[18] and vitamin C on risk of esophageal cancer, with odds ratios in the range of two to three for subjects in the lowest tertiles of intake.[19]

Although reports concerning possible effects of vitamin A have been mixed, a case–control study in Italy reported an inverse association between intake of carotene (but not retinol) and risk.[20] Riboflavin deficiency has been suspected as a risk factor for esophageal cancer on ecologic grounds,[21,22] and this association was supported by a study of black men that found that those in the lowest tertile of riboflavin intake had 1.7 times the baseline risk of esophageal cancer.[23]

Nutritional Risk Factors

Alcohol

Alcohol intake is an acknowledged factor for esophageal cancer, particularly in industrialized countries. Typical of results supporting such an association is a study from Italy reporting that drinkers of more than 6 alcoholic drinks per day were 10 times more likely than nondrinkers to contract the disease.[20] Consistent results have been reported from France, where intake of more than 40 g/d of ethanol (heavy drinking) was associated with significantly increased risk.[24] Although alcohol plays an important role in the etiology of esophageal cancer in the United States and Europe, it may be of considerably less importance in areas such as the Asian esophageal cancer belt.

Other Factors

Silica fragments have been found in bread in Iran[25] and in millet in Linxian, China,[26] two of the highest-risk areas of the world for esophageal cancer. These appear to be a result of harvesting and milling practices that introduce silica into the food. Thermal injuries from hot beverages have also been suggested as a factor in the etiology of esophageal cancer in areas where tea and other beverages are consumed while very hot.

Tobacco

Men who smoke more than 30 cigarettes per day are 3 times as likely to contract esophageal cancer as those who do not smoke, a finding that remains significant after adjustment for intake of alcohol.[27]

Prevention

Esophageal cancer is a highly preventable disease. Its incidence could be greatly reduced by avoidance of heavy intake of alcohol and cigarette smoking, and inclusion in the diet of fresh citrus fruit, vegetables rich in carotenoids, and adequate sources of riboflavin, such as milk and enriched flour. Fortification of alcoholic beverages with vitamin C and riboflavin would be a first step toward prevention on a population-wide basis, combined with programs to limit the advertising for and widespread availability of alcohol, and provision of adequate nutritional support to adults who drink alcohol heavily, including the homeless. Extension of public health laws against cigarette smoking in places frequented by heavy consumers of alcohol, such as bars, would help to lower the combined risks of cigarette use and alcohol drinking. Efforts by national and international agencies to test milled grains for silica particles and elimination of practices associated with these and other particle contaminants in food also would be desirable.

CANCER OF THE STOMACH

International Comparisons

Cancer of the stomach is the most common cancer in men in many countries in Latin American and Asia, and ranks second in incidence after breast cancer in women in these countries.[28] The highest annual incidence rates worldwide in men are in Nagasaki (82 per 100,000) and Miyagi, Japan (80 per 100,000). High rates are also present in Costa Rica (59 per 100,000), Shanghai (58 per 100,000), São Paulo, Brazil (54 per 100,000), Cali, Colombia (50 per 100,000), and Varese, Italy (39 per 100,000). The lowest annual incidence rates for men are in Kuwaitis (4 per 100,000) and in whites in Los Angeles (9 per 100,000). Incidence rates in women range from a high of 36 per 100,000 in Nagasaki and Miyagi, Japan, to 4 in Los Angeles whites, 3 in Iowa, and 2 in Kuwait.

Demographic Factors

Sex

The sex ratio of stomach cancer is nearly identical in high-incidence areas such as Nagasaki and Miyagi Japan, where it affects 2.3 men per woman affected, and in low-incidence areas such as the United States and Kuwait, where it is 2.2 to 1 and 2.3 to 1, respectively.[28]

Race

The incidence of gastric cancer in the United States in blacks and other nonwhites is approximately double that in whites, whereas that in Hispanics in California is approximately 1.5 times that in non-Hispanic whites.[29,30]

Age

Incidence rates of stomach cancer increase logarithmically with age in most countries, including the United States, with patients younger than 35 years of age being rare.[28] Possible exceptions are in residents of Geneva, Switzerland, and Maori residents of New Zealand, for whom annual incidence rates above 1 per 100,000 have been reported beginning at age 15 years. The rate of increase in risk at age 75 years and older is less steep than at ages 35 to 74 years in most countries, including the United States.

Time Trends

Stomach cancer was the leading cause of cancer death in the United States in the early part of the 20th century, accounting in 1913 for 4 of 10 cancer deaths.[31] The annual death rate from cancer of the stomach was 31 per 100,000 population, triple that of colorectal cancer and twice that of breast cancer. Age-adjusted mortality rates in men and women declined steeply throughout the century, dropping to an overall rate of 5 per 100,000 by the beginning of the 1990s.[32] A similar decline occurred in Australia and several other countries.[33]

Migrant Studies

Immigrants from Japan (where the risk is highest) to Hawaii and other areas of the United States that have low overall incidence rates had risks of stomach cancer that were only slightly lower than those in Japan, even if they were young when they migrated.[34,35] Children of these immigrants, however, had incidence rates that were closer to those of native-born residents of the United States. Similar results were present in immigrants to Australia from high-risk areas in Europe,[33] and in immigrants from Puerto Rico to New York, where incidence rates are approximately half those in Puerto Rico.[36] These studies suggest the possibility of a factor present or absent in childhood that may establish lifelong risk.

Pathologic Types

Although there are numerous pathologic classifications pertinent to cancer of the stomach, the Lauren classification of stomach cancer as either intestinal or diffuse has emerged as having the greatest epidemiologic significance.[37] Historically, the predominant type of stomach cancer throughout the world has been the intestinal type (epidemic form), so named because the gastric epithelium takes on the appearance of the intestinal epithelium, with distinct, polarized glandularity. This type of gastric cancer usually begins in the gastric antrum, and is two to three times more common in men than women.[38] The historically less common diffuse form consists of an infiltration of malignant single cells or clusters of cells without the distinct glandular lumina present in the intestinal type. The diffuse type of gastric cancer usually arises in the cardia or fundus of the stomach, and incidence rates are similar in men and women. Occasional cases of gastric cancer in the young tend to be of the diffuse type, and the diffuse type is suspected of having a genetic component based on an unfavorable association with blood group A.[38] It is almost exclusively the intestinal type that has declined in incidence during the 20th century, leaving the two types of stomach cancer according to the Lauren classification with approximately equal incidence rates.

Helicobacter pylori

Evidence has emerged that *H pylori*, a common microorganism that colonizes the stomach in populations in many areas of the world, is involved in gastritis and peptic ulcer,[39] and may be implicated in stomach cancer.[40,41] *H pylori* organisms attach to the gastric mucosa and thrive beginning in childhood.[42] *H pylori* infection is relatively uncommon in affluent areas and in young whites in the United States, but is more common in developing areas of the world, where infection may be nearly universal, in lower social classes, where most people may have serologic evidence of prior or current infection, and in blacks.[42] The infection is contracted by the fecal–oral route. Swallowing of the organism by volunteers results in an acute gastritis with vomiting and epigastric discomfort, shifting to chronic gastritis with a relative hypochlorhydria after about 2 weeks.[42] *H pylori* can colonize the stomach for months to years, but can be eliminated with antimicrobial agents. Reinfection occurs at a rate of about 1% per year.[43] The source appears to be the spouse in about half the cases, and other sources in the rest.[44]

The evidence for a role of *H pylori* infection in gastric cancer suggests that infection in childhood may be more important than in adulthood. Incidence of gastric cancer is high in countries where *H pylori* infection is endemic and affects essentially the whole population, including children, such as Colombia, Peru, and Mexico.[38] Infection rates are also particularly high in areas of Colombia and Louisiana where gastric cancer rates are high.[38] Also, three nested case–control studies of serum banked from 6 to 14 years indicated odds ratios from 2.8 to 6.0 for seropositivity to *H pylori*.[40,45,46] The serologic evidence for a role of *H pylori* in gastric cancer has previously been summarized.[47]

Evidence against a role of adult *H pylori* infection in stomach cancer has included a study that examined tissue from gastric malignancies and found the organism present only in about 10% of patients.[48] Also arguing against the role of *H pylori* in both duodenal ulcer and gastric cancer is the existence of populations with high incidence rates of gastric cancer but apparently low prevalence rates of duodenal ulcer.[49]

Nutritional Deficiencies

B Vitamins

Gastric cancer has long been linked epidemiologically with nutritional deficiencies and diseases that result from them. In 1926, Minot and Murphy discovered that pernicious anemia could be treated with liver, leading to some of the earliest discoveries of concerning the roles of the B vitamins.[50] Identification of the causal role of vitamin B_{12} deficiency in pernicious anemia was one of the scientific triumphs of the early 20th century. It was important with respect to gastric cancer because it provided a simple means to eradicate the anemia and thereby minimize the the elevated risk of gastric cancer that was associated with it.[50] The sex ratio for pernicious anemia was two cases in men for every case in a woman, which is identical to the sex ratio in gastric cancer.

Vitamin C

A number of studies have identified a favorable association between diets high in fresh fruits and vegetables and lower risk of gastric cancer.[38] Consistent with these, a study of serum levels of vitamin C in gastric cancer cases and noncases found an association between low levels of serum ascorbate and risk of gastric cancer.[51]

Calcium

Studies have suggested that low intake of calcium may be associated with increased risk of gastric cancer.

Fatty Acids

The intake of fats from plant sources, such as corn, soybean, and cottonseed oil, has accelerated rapidly throughout the 20th century. The shift from exclusively animal fats and olive oil to industrial oils extracted by large-scale industrial processes was accelerated by the need of the U.S. population for fats and oils diverted to soldiers overseas during World War I. The dramatic historical increase in use of vegetable oils was paralleled by declining death rates from gastric cancer in the United States. Such changes did not occur in most other countries until later, and major reductions in incidence rates from gastric cancer still have not occurred in developing countries or in Japan, where use of industrial oils is far lower than in the United States and the industrialized areas of Western Europe. Dietary fatty acids such as linoleic acid serve as substrates for the synthesis of prostaglandins, including the E series prostaglandins that appear to protect the gastric mucosa from damage, and may inhibit bacterial colonization of the gastric mucosa.

Nutritional Risk Factors

Long-term intake of salted and pickled foods[52] and those rich in nitrosamines and their precursors[53] is associated with increased risk of gastric cancer.[45] Correa has proposed that salt causes gastric irritation and induces superficial and atrophic gastritis, which is followed by a rise in gastric pH and bacterial overgrowth; the overgrowth is believed to contain organisms that convert nitrites from the diet to mutagenic *N*-nitrosamines, ultimately causing malignancy.[54,55]

Prevention

Epidemiologic studies have suggested several elements of a strategy to prevent gastric cancer. Briefly, these involve changes to the diet to eliminate high intake of salted and pickled foods, an increase in intake of fresh fruits and vegetables to at least five servings per day, with high intake of citrus fruits and other foods containing vitamin C, and an increased (but not excessive) intake of linoleic acid. Because serologic evidence of infection with *H pylori* appears to be associated with risk of gastric cancer, it is important that food hygiene standards be maintained at a level that reduces to a minimum the prevalence of infections transmitted by the fecal–oral route. This can be accomplished by universal enforcement of the sanitation measures that help to minimize the prevalence of gastroenteritis and diarrheal disease in Western countries. In areas where B vitamin deficiencies may be present, particularly in developing countries, such deficiencies should be addressed by dietary programs or use of supplements.

CANCER OF THE PANCREAS

International Comparisons

The incidence of pancreatic cancer varies by about 10-fold around the world. Places with low incidence are Nigeria, Bombay, South Africa, and Colombia. Japan has intermediate rates. The highest annual rates occur in New Zealand Maoris (>20 per 100,000, age-standardized to the world population), who also have a very high male-to-female ratio (nearly 4 : 1).[56] Curiously, the group with the second highest incidence rate, native Hawaiians, has a sex ratio barely greater than 1 : 1. Jews, particularly Ashkenazi Jews, in Israel have high incidence rates.[6]

An estimated 24,000 new cases of cancer of the pancreas occur in the United States each year, and 97% are fatal.[1] Mortality rates for pancreatic cancer were exceeded only by those for lung, colorectal, and prostate cancer in men, and lung, breast, and colorectal cancer in women.

The pattern of mortality from pancreatic cancer is essentially uniform throughout the the United States. There is no north-to-south or east-to-west gradient, as is present for colon cancer[57] and breast cancer.[58] Mortality rates by county show a positive correlation with degree of urbanization,[59] and a higher urban incidence in New York State.[60] Urban–rural ratios greater than one have been reported in Denmark,[61] Norway,[6] and Finland.[62] A study by Pickle and Gottlieb[63] reported a geographic cluster of cases in Louisiana.

Demographic Factors

Sex

The male-to-female incidence ratio for all Surveillance, Epidemiology, and End Results (SEER) study areas in the United States was 1.6 for whites and 1.4 for blacks from 1973 to 1977. From 1978 to 1981, the sex ratio was 1.5 for both races.[64] Sex ratios above 1.0 occur at all ages for both whites and blacks in the SEER population,[64] although the ratio declines at older ages.[65] However, among Hispanics in El Paso, Texas, the sex ratio is below 1.0.[56]

Incidence rates for smoking-related cancers and cancers related to occupational exposures have traditionally been higher among men (although this is changing because increasing numbers of women have taken up smoking and are involved in hazardous occupations). Historical differences in occupation and smoking behavior may partially account for the higher incidence of pancreatic cancer observed in men.[66]

Race

Blacks had 1.6 times the incidence, and 1.3 times the age-adjusted mortality rates of whites in the U.S. SEER population from 1973 to 1981.[64] Blacks also had higher mortality rates than Native Americans and Chinese, and slightly lower rates than Japanese in two studies, one using national data[56] and one using data from Alameda County, California.[67]

Age

As with most neoplasms, incidence and mortality from pancreatic cancer increase with age.[64] This is true for whites and blacks of both sexes, although mortality rates for blacks drop slightly after age 70 years, particularly in black men. More than 80% of all pancreatic cancer occurs at ages 60 to 79 years. The tumor is rare before age 40 years, but can occur at earlier ages in association with hereditary chronic calcifying pancreatitis. Rare case reports describe this association in very young people.[66]

Religion

Pancreatic cancer has been studied in several religious groups.[68–76] Mormons and Seventh-Day Adventists differ from the general U.S. population in diet, chiefly in their abstinence from or reduced consumption of alcohol, cigarettes, coffee, and tea. Most Seventh-Day Adventists also refrain from eating meat. Mormons[56,69] and Seventh-Day Adventists[74,75] have 27% and 35% lower mortality from pancreatic cancer, respectively, than would be expected based on U.S. general population age-specific mortality rates. Mortality rates in men in both religious groups were particularly reduced compared to the general U.S. male population, probably reflecting sex differences in smoking and alcohol use. Incidence rates in Mormons were 35.8% lower than expected compared to non-Mormons. Unlike mortality, however, the reduction in incidence was greatest in Mormon women.[71] Jewish men have higher age-adjusted mortality rates than the general population.[70,76]

Time Trends

In Connecticut, where incidence data have been available since the 1930s, average annual age-adjusted incidence rates in men increased 62%, from 8 per 100,000 population in 1935 to 1939 to a high of 12 in 1975 to 1977, but dropped slightly thereafter. In women, incidence rates increased 41%, from 6 per 100,000 population in 1935 to 1939 to 9 in 1975 to 1977, but also dropped slightly thereafter.[64,65] The increase in age-adjusted incidence rates has been more evident in men than women, and in blacks than whites.[64,77] Incidence rates in the United States reached a plateau during the early 1990s.[77]

Migrant Studies

Migrant studies of pancreatic cancer are few and have dealt mostly with Japanese populations. The results have been less clear than for stomach or breast cancer. Recent immigrants from Japan had higher mortality rates than U.S. whites, native Japanese, or Japanese born in the United States.[78,79] Pancreatic cancer mortality rates in Japanese residents of Hawaii and the United States were found to be higher than in whites and nonwhites, but not significantly so.[80] Japanese residents of Hawaii had lower mortality rates than native Hawaiians.[81]

Alcohol, Pancreatitis, and Pancreatic Cancer

Pancreatic cancer has been reported more frequently than expected in patients with a history of pancreatitis,[82] and pancreatitis is often associated with alcoholism.[83,84] The relationship between alcohol intake and pancreatic cancer may be a consequence of the increased risk of pancreatitis in alcoholics. However, even the association between pancreatic cancer and chronic pancreatitis is not entirely clear, and there are discrepant studies of this association.[85]

A longitudinal study of 245 patients with chronic pancreatitis followed for 20 years[86] found 7 cases of pancreatic cancer, significantly more than expected (less than 1 was expected), but when the analysis was stratified by alcohol consumption, there were no differences in risk of pancreatic cancer between the two groups, implying that the high pancreatic cancer risk conferred by pancreatitis was independent of alcohol use. A second prospective study of patients with chronic calcific pancreatitis also suggested that risk of pancreatic cancer is increased by pancreatitis, regardless of the etiology of the pancreatitis.[87]

A retrospective study by Gold and colleagues,[88] which excluded pancreatic cancer cases with pancreatitis diagnosed within 2 years of the cancer, did not find an association between pancreatic cancer and chronic pancreatitis. There are even greater discrepancies in studies of alcohol use and pancreatic cancer. Four case–control studies in the United States found no increased risk,[88–91] but two positive case–control studies were reported from France and Japan.[92,93] All but one of the U.S. studies[88] used hospital control subjects.

Alcohol and Nutritional Risk Factors

Alcohol

There have been a number of case–control studies of the association between alcohol intake and risk of pancreatic cancer. Lin and Kessler[89] reported no significant association between pancreatic cancer and alcohol use in a multihospital-based study using one cancer-free hospital control subject matched to each case by age, race, sex, marital status, and hospital. MacMahon and associates[90] found a slightly decreased risk from alcohol use based on cases and control subjects hospitalized for diseases unrelated to tobacco and alcohol identified from hospitals in Boston and Rhode Island. Controls were matched to cases based on date of hospitalization, and attending physician.

Wynder and associates[91] studied a large number of histologically confirmed cases from U.S. hospitals and unmatched control subjects with or without cancer, excluding only smoking and alcohol-related hospitalizations. They detected a relative risk for alcohol use of 1.6 for men and 1.1 for women, but neither association was significant. Gold and colleagues[88] used hospital and population control subjects. The relative risk from alcohol use was 1.1, using hospital control subjects, and was not statistically significant. Population control subjects were selected by random digit dialing, and matched by sex, age, race, and telephone prefix; the relative risk compared to these control subjects was only 0.6, also not significantly different from 1.0. Ishii and coworkers in Japan[81] reported on histologically confirmed cases of pancreatic cancer in men older than 40 years of age from 100 Japanese hospitals, and compared their responses to a questionnaire with results of a national survey of more than 100,000 adults. Estimated relative risks attributable to alcohol use were low (1.1 to 1.5) but statistically significant; however, no adjustment for smoking was made. Durbec and colleagues[92] interviewed cases from three hospitals in Marseille and control subjects selected by a door-to-door method. Cases were matched to control subjects by age and sex. The estimated relative risk for ethanol intake greater than 40 g/d was 2.7 (95% confidence interval, 1.7 to 4.3).

There also have been a number of prospective studies of the association between intake of alcohol and risk of pancreatic cancer. Dean and associates[94] followed 3600 male blue-collar workers from a large Dublin brewery, who drank an average of 58 g/d of alcohol, and compared their mortality rates with age-specific mortality rates from the Dublin cancer registry and Republic of Ireland cancer registry. There were 17 cases of pancreatic cancer in the brewery workers, compared to an expected number of 14 based on Dublin county rates and 11 based on Ireland's national rate.

Jensen[95] studied male brewery workers in the Danish Brewery Workers Union. Workers in Danish breweries received free beer, consuming an equivalent of 78 g/d of ethanol. The relative risk of pancreatic cancer mortality was 1.1, which was not statistically significant. Other prospective studies have found relative risks in the range of 0.9 to 1.3.[83,96]

Coffee

Hsieh and colleagues[97] reported an association between intake of coffee and risk of pancreatic cancer. The report, an extension of an earlier study by MacMahon and coworkers,[90] suggested that the effect of coffee was present but weak, because it was absent unless at least four cups per day were consumed.

The influence of coffee on risk of pancreatic cancer continues to be a concern. Studies other than those of MacMahon and coworkers[90] and Hsieh and colleagues[97] have reached mixed conclusions, but the study by Gold and colleagues reported a statistically significant association between intake of coffee and risk of pancreatic cancer in women, and indicated a dose–response relationship.[88] A case–control study in California found a positive association between both regular and decaffeinated coffee use and pancreatic cancer that was almost completely limited to cigarette smokers. Smokers who drank more than three cups of regular coffee per day had 4.3 times the risk for development of pancreatic cancer of smokers who drank fewer cups, a statistically significant difference. An estimated relative risk of 5.5 was found for smokers drinking more than one cup per day of decaffeinated coffee, but this association was of borderline statistical significance.[98]

CANCER OF THE LIVER

International Comparisons

Liver cancer has an estimated annual incidence of 500,000 to 1 million cases worldwide. It is also among the most variable malignancies in terms of worldwide incidence.[28] Populations with particularly high incidence of liver cancer include South African natives (65 per 100,000)[99] and Chinese living in Shanghai (34 per 100,000), Hong Kong (323 per 100,000), and Singapore (32 per 100,000).[28] Low-risk regions include England, Scotland, and Wales, the United States, Australia, and Canada, where annual incidence rates range from 1 to 3 per 100,000.[28] Intermediate incidence rates have been reported in Japan (11 per 100,000), New Zealand Maoris (11 per 100,000), Spain (8 per 100,000), native Hawaiians (7 per 100,000), Italy (7 per 100,000), France (7 per 100,000), India (5 per 100,000), and Sweden (5 per 100,000).[28]

Demographic Factors

Sex

Liver cancer occurs approximately twice as frequently in men as women. In Shanghai, the male-to-female ratio is 3 : 1, and it is slightly higher in Hong Kong and Singapore. The male-to-female ratio usually is higher in areas with high incidence rates. The sex differences in incidence of liver cancer probably reflect underlying sex differences in exposures; however, the frequency of chemically induced liver tumors in rats can be increased by administration of testosterone.[100]

Age

Age at onset of liver cancer varies importantly by region, suggesting that distinct etiologic factors are present in different regions and that these act at different ages. In African men in Mozambique, for example, incidence of liver cancer increases rapidly beginning at an early age. In the 10- to 15-year-old age group, incidence rates of over 50 per 100,000 have been reported. These rates steadily increase until ages 35 to 45 years, when incidence rates approach 200 per 100,000 men, then gradually decline to about 85 per 100,000 men at age 60 years and older. A similar pattern of age-specific incidence is present for African women in Mozambique, although their age-specific incidence rates are in general three to five times lower than those of men.[99]

In Japan, age-specific incidence rates increase more gradually, although more rapidly than in the United States or Europe.[101] Incidence rates in the first three decades of life are low in Japan. However, by the end of the fourth decade, the age-specific incidence rate approaches 20 per 100,000 in men. It doubles in the next 5 years and continues to rise steadily to over 100 per 100,000 men at age 85 years and older. In the United States, liver cancer is rare before age 50 years, but incidence rates slowly increase until reaching a plateau at about 20 per 100,000 in men 70 years of age and older.[101]

Time Trends

Since the 1970s, incidence of liver cancer has remained stable in most of the United States and Europe, but incidence rates have increased in Japan, with rates having doubled in Osaka during one decade.[102]

Migrant Studies

There are major differences in incidence rates between Japanese and Japanese American immigrants and their offspring. The annual incidence rate of liver cancer in Japanese men living in Miyagi, Japan is 11 per 100,000, whereas that of Japanese men living in Los Angeles is 2.5 per 100,000.[28] Chinese living in Shanghai, Hong Kong, and Singapore have annual incidence rates ranging from 32 to 34 per 100,000, but Chinese Americans in Los Angeles have approximately half that level of incidence (16 per 100,000).[28]

Risk Factors by Region

United States and Europe: Alcohol and Hormones

In developed countries, where incidence rates generally increase at ages greater than 70 years, alcoholic cirrhosis of the liver is the best known precursor lesion for liver cancer.[103] Alcohol consumption, although associated with liver cancer, does not seem to increase risk more than cirrhosis alone.[104] High doses of anabolic steroids or long-term use of oral contraceptives have also been associated with increased risk of liver cancer.[105–107]

Japan: Hepatitis C Virus and Tobacco

In Japan, increased incidence of liver cirrhosis due to chronic hepatitis C virus infection may be associated with an increased risk of liver cancer at younger ages.[108] Tobacco smoking may increase risk of liver cancer in adults with cirrhosis in association with hepatitis C or excessive alcohol use, which may also contribute to increased incidence rates of liver cancer in Japan.[102]

Africa and China: Hepatitis B Virus and Aflatoxins

In the high-risk regions of Africa and China, nearly all liver cancer is associated with liver cirrhosis due to chronic hepatitis B virus infection.[109] High dietary intake of aflatoxin B_1 is also associated with liver cirrhosis and may increase susceptibility to liver cancer, particularly in carriers of hepatitis B virus.[110] This etiology is consistent with the younger peak in age-specific incidence for liver cancer in these regions compared to more developed countries.[111]

Prevention

A good control measure in developing countries would be to take measures to limit spread of endemic hepatitis B infection. Much of the transmission of hepatitis B virus in developing countries occurs through vertical transmission from the infected carrier-mother to the infant,[112] but some transmission occurs horizontally through blood contact, skin piercing, and sexual transmission. These forms of transmission might be amenable to control. Increased use of hepatitis B vaccines in high-risk areas should also be considered.

CANCER OF THE COLON AND RECTUM

International Comparisons

Colorectal cancer is the second leading cause of death from cancer, after lung cancer, in the United States, Canada, the United Kingdom, Ireland, New Zealand, and almost all Western countries with population centers at latitudes north of 37° N, or south of that latitude in the southern hemisphere.[1] It is surprisingly uncommon at low latitudes, virtually vanishing within 10° of the equator,[7,9] and also historically has been relatively uncommon in Asia.

Although overall rates are low, colorectal cancer in China has a distinctive pattern of lower occurrence in rural areas. Incidence rates are higher along river courses, where it may be associated with intestinal parasitism.[113] In Japan, colon cancer was relatively rare until the mid-1960s, but the incidence rate approximately doubled between the 1960s and the mid-1970s,[7,9] bringing it to the low end of the range characteristic of Western countries.

There are approximately 138,200 new cases and 55,300 deaths from colorectal cancer annually in the United States.[1] Death rates from colorectal cancer have risen steadily in men and declined steadily in women since 1930. Age-adjusted death rates of colon cancer in women in the United States declined 23% during 1930 to 1986, whereas they increased 39% in men.[1] The death rate per 100,000 men climbed from 18 in 1930 to 25 in 1986; in women it declined from 22 in 1930 to 17 in 1986.[1] The opposing trends in male and female death rates are intriguing, and have occurred only in certain countries, including the United States and Canada. The pattern is unlikely to be the result of any change in genetic factors.

The divergent trends suggest that the decline is caused by a practice adopted almost exclusively by women since 1930. One possibility, the increased use of calcium supplements by women, is discussed elsewhere in this review. The pattern cannot be explained by any overall change in dietary calcium consumption.[114] The decreased mortality rates in women also cannot be readily attributed to later ages for childbirth, because early age at first birth is associated with reduced incidence of colon cancer and age at first birth has been increasing in recent years.[115] The possibility that increased use of exogenous female hormones might have produced this effect through a favorable influence on calcium metabolism should be considered.

Incidence Rates

The highest incidence rate of colon cancer in 137 population-based cancer registries worldwide reporting to the World Health Organization was in Connecticut.[28] The rate in Connecticut white men was 34 per 100,000, and in white women it was 27 per 100,000. Annual incidence rates of 25 per 100,000 or higher in white men were also reported in Los Angeles (non-Hispanic whites), and in Geneva, Switzerland; and rates of 20 per 100,000 or higher were reported in white women in Canada and New South Wales, Australia. Incidence rates of 25 or higher in men also were reported in Japanese Americans in Hawaii, blacks in Connecticut, and Los Angeles Chinese Americans, Japanese Americans, and blacks. The lowest incidence rates were in Kuwait, where the rate was 0.2 per 100,000 population. Incidence rates in both sexes were 5 or less per 100,000 population in residents of Bombay, India; Romania; the Philippines; and Costa Rica. The incidence rates in men and women in Japan[9] (Miyagi prefecture) were 9.8 and 9.4 per 100,000 population, respectively, slightly less than one third those in Connecticut.

Mortality Rates

Age-adjusted mortality rates in the United States are characterized by marked geographic variation. Northeastern U.S. counties in general have three to five times higher mortality rates than southwestern counties.[57]

Demographic Factors

Sex

One of the more intriguing aspects of colorectal cancer is its sex distribution. In the United States, the age-adjusted death rate in men is 17 per 100,000, whereas in women it is 11 per 100,000.[116,117] Death rates in men and women were similar in 1960, but the rates declined steadily in women since then, although they remained stable in men. A possible reason for the decline in death rates in women has emerged. Use of replacement estrogens has become more popular since 1960, and has been associated with lower risk of colon cancer.[118]

Race

Colorectal cancer incidence and death rates are similar in whites and blacks in the United States, but were historically lower in blacks than whites when the black population was mainly limited to the southern tier of states. The most marked racial difference in the United States now is the difference between the high rates in non-Hispanic whites compared to low rates in Hispanics and Native Americans.[119]

Age

Incidence rates of colorectal cancer increase logarithmically with age until approximately age 70 years, then continue to increase thereafter but in an arithmetic rather than logarithmic fashion.[28] Colorectal cancer is extremely rare before age 40 years throughout the world.

Time Trends

Time trends in colorectal cancer in the United States have been distinctly different in men and women, as noted earlier, with a steady decrease since 1960 in women in contrast to slightly rising rates in men.[119] The dichotomy between trends in the two sexes suggests the possibility that the drop in incidence in women may result from estrogen replacement and calcium supplementation, as discussed in a subsequent section.

Migrant Studies

There are major differences in mortality rates of colorectal cancer by race and ethnicity. At ages 65 to 69 years, for example, the age-specific mortality rate in California Hispanics was 38 per 100,000 population, compared to 74 per 100,000 in non-Hispanic whites.[30] The lower rate in Hispanics in part is associated with their status as migrants from Mexico and Central America. The death rate from colorectal cancer in migrants from Mexico is markedly lower than in Hispanics born north of the Mexican Border.[30]

Role of Nutritional and Environmental Deficiencies

Calcium and Vitamin D

Calcium and vitamin D have become important subjects of interest in studies of the etiology and pathogenesis of colorectal cancer.[120,121] The idea that vitamin D and its metabolites might play a beneficial role arose from observation of the unusual geographic distribution of colon cancer mortality rates in the United States,[122] and the interest in calcium arose from its strong physiologic association with vitamin D and its metabolites. This area of interest has now expanded to include examination of the possible role of vitamin D receptors in the pathogenesis of colorectal cancer.[123]

Death rates from cancers of the colon and rectum were observed to be markedly lower in areas of the United States that receive high levels of sunlight, particularly ultraviolet B (295 to 320 nm), a geographic characteristic that persisted after adjustment for age and stratification by race.[122]

The close physiologic relationship between vitamin D and calcium metabolism suggested that the low death rates from colorectal cancer in the sunnier areas of the United States might might be the result of a possibly beneficial influence of higher levels vitamin D or its metabolites on absorption of calcium by the colon.[120]

Age-adjusted death rates from colon cancer in white men in the extreme northeastern counties of the United States, for example, were nearly three times those in the sunniest counties of the United States in the south and southwest.[120] The effect was present both in urban and rural areas.

Epidemiologic studies that helped to establish a role of calcium and vitamin D in prevention of colorectal cancer are summarized in Table 1-2. A 19-year prospective study of men in Chicago observed that those who had a dietary intake of 150 + IU/d of vitamin D had half the incidence of colorectal cancer ($P < 0.05$) associated with consumers of less vitamin D,

TABLE 1-2. *Summary of observational epidemiologic studies of the relationship between calcium and colon cancer*

Author, year, location	Summary
Garland and Garland, 1980, United States[122]	Geographic epidemiology study of colon cancer, in both sexes, all ages, in the United States, 1995–61. This study proposed that a favorable influence of vitamin D metabolites on metabolism of calcium may reduce the death rate from colon cancer. The study was based on a detailed geographic analysis of vital statistics data.
Garland et al, 1985, Chicago[124]	Prospective study of colorectal cancer in white men aged 40–55 y at baseline. This 19-y study of a cohort of 1954 men enrolled in 1957–59 was based on 28-d dietary histories obtained using plastic food models. The histories were administered by dietitians on two occasions 1 y apart. Follow-up rate was 99.9%. By the 20th anniversary of the initial examination, there were 29 cases of colon cancer (ICD-9 code 153) and 20 of rectal cancer (ICD-9 code 154). Quartiles of calcium intake, in mg/d, were 316–749, 750–949, 950–1189, and 1190–2808. Incidence of colon cancer decreased with increasing intake of calcium. Odds ratios for calcium intakes from the lowest to highest quartiles were 1.0, 0.6, 0.6, and 0.3 (P trend < 0.05). Quartiles of vitamin D intake were 6–94, 95–149, 150–229, and 230–652 IU/d. Odds ratios for vitamin D intakes from lowest to highest quartiles were 1.0, 1.3, 0.5, and 0.5 (P trend < 0.05). Similar results were obtained from a combined calcium–vitamin D index calculated as 5.0 plus the sum of standard (z) scores for calcium and vitamin D intakes. This index ranged from 1.8 to 13.0 units, with a mean of 5.0 units. Odds ratios from the lowest to the highest quartile of the index were 1.0, 0.6, 0.6, and 0.4. This is the only study to date of the association between dietary vitamin D and colorectal cancer. It reported that the incidence of colorectal cancer was reduced by half in those who consumed 150+ IU/d (3.8+ μg/d) compared to those who consumed less.
Slattery et al, 1988, Utah[181]	Case–control study, both sexes, whites, ages 40–79 y. This population-based study used a 99-category food frequency interview. Intake was requested for the period 2 y previous to the date of onset (cases) or interview (control subjects). There were 231 cases of colon cancer and 391 control subjects. The control subjects were obtained by random digit dialing. No results were reported for vitamin D. *Men.* Quartiles of calcium intake, in mg/d, were 0–641, 642–975, 976–1401, and 1402+. There was a linear inverse dose–response relationship beginning with the third quartile, with increased calcium intake above that level associated with decreased risk of colon cancer. Crude odds ratios, from highest to lowest quartile of calcium intake, were 1.0, 1.1, 0.8, and 0.5. Odds ratios were similar after adjustment for age, religion (Mormon/non-Mormon), crude fiber, and calories (ie, 1.0, 1.3, 0.8, and 0.4). The effect of calcium was reported as statistically significant for the highest quartile compared to the lowest ($P < 0.05$, one-tailed). *Women.* Quartiles of calcium intake, in mg/d, were 0–592, 593–826, 827–1141, and >1141. Crude odds ratios, from lowest to highest quartile, were 1.0, 0.6, 0.8, and 0.8. Odds ratios after adjustment for age, religion, crude fiber, and calories were 1.0, 0.5, 0.5, and 0.5. These odds ratios were reported as not being statistically significant. However, a statistically significant effect was present when calcium was examined as mg/1000 kcal. Quartiles of this variable were 0–408, 409–525, 516–667, and >667. Crude odds ratios, from lowest to highest quartile, were 1.0, 0.9, 0.6, and 0.5. Odds ratios after adjustment for age, religion, crude fiber, and calories were 1.0, 0.9, 0.6, and 0.4. The effect of calcium was statistically significant in either of the two highest quartiles compared to the lowest ($P < 0.05$, one-tailed).
Kune et al, 1987, Melbourne, Australia[136]	Case–control study of colon cancer, both sexes, ages 40–79 y. This study used a dietary interview conducted by a dietitian concerning the previous 20 y. It included approximately 300 foods. The authors reported results for calcium, milk, and dairy products, but not vitamin D. Community controls were obtained by random digit dialing. *Men.* There were 388 male cases, including 202 of colon and 186 of rectal cancer, and 398 control subjects. Overall median calcium intake was 851 mg/d. Quintiles of calcium intake were 0–597, 598–771, 772–928, 929–1150, and 1151+ mg/d. Odds ratios, from lowest to highest quintile of calcium intake, were 1.00, 0.61, 0.51, 0.62, and 1.06. *Women.* There were 327 female cases, including 190 of colon and 137 of rectal cancer, and 329 control subects. Overall median calcium intake was 758 mg/d. Quintiles of calcium intake were 0–529, 530–686, 687–829, 830–1043, and 1044+ mg/d. Odds ratios, from lowest to highest quintile of calcium intake, were 1.00, 1.04, 0.73, 0.78, and 0.56.
Heiburn et al, 1986, Hawaii[182]	Nested case–control study, Japanese American men, ages 46–68 years. The results of this study have been superseded by a site-specific prospective study of this cohort by Stemmermann and colleagues[183] based on 277 cases (see following).

TABLE 1-2. *Continued.*

Author, year, location	Summary
Stemmermann et al, 1990, Hawaii[183]	Prospective study of colon, rectosigmoid, and rectal cancer (ICD-8 codes 153.0–153.9, 154.0–154.9) in 7,472 Japanese American men, ages 40–55 y at baseline 1957–59. The study was based on 24-h dietary recall interviews administered by dieticians using food models and utensils to estimate portion sizes. Ascertainment of cases was based on a cancer registry and other linked records. By December 31, 1987, approximately the 22nd anniversary of accession to the study, there were 189 cases of colon cancer (ICD-8 codes, 153.0–153.04), 39 of rectosigmoid cancer (ICD-8 codes, 154.0–154.1), and 49 of rectal cancer (ICD-8 codes 154.1–154.9). Mean calcium intake in this cohort was only about half that in other studies reported here (ie, 503 mg/d). The standard deviation of total calcium intake was 303 mg. In the sigmoid, where most of the cancers were located, (113/189, or 60% of cancers), incidence decreased significantly with increasing intake of calcium. Relative risks for calcium intakes from the lowest to highest tertiles were 1.0, 0.8, and 0.6 (P trend <0.02). No statistically significant effect of calcium intake was observed for other sites.
Garland et al, 1989, Maryland[125]	Serum was collected in Washington County, MD, from 25,620 volunteers aged 18 y and older in August–November, 1974, and frozen at −73°C. Serum was analyzed from 34 individuals (17 men, 17 women; median age 55–64 y) who contracted colon cancer (ICD-8 codes 153.0–153.8) between 1975 and 1983, and 67 control subjects matched by race, sex, age, and month blood was taken. Quintiles of serum 25-hydroxyvitamin D, in ng/mL, were 4–19, 20–26, 27–32, 33–41, and 42–91, respectively. Estimated relative tasks, by quintile from lowest to highest 25-hydroxyvitamin D were 1.0, 0.5, 0.2, 0.2, and 0.7. The relationship was statistically significant ($P < 0.05$, one-tailed).

ICD, International Classification of Diseases.

whereas an intake of approximately 1200 + mg/d of calcium was associated with one quarter the incidence rate of colorectal cancer ($P < 0.05$) associated with an intake of less than approximately 625 mg/d.[124]

A nested case–control analysis of sera collected in 1974 to 1975 from a cohort of 25,620 healthy community volunteers in Washington County, Maryland observed that moderately elevated levels of 25-hydroxyvitamin D, in the range 27 to 41 ng/mL (which is well within the usual adult range of approximately 10 to 59 ng/mL), were associated with reduction by 75% to 80% ($P < 0.05$) in the incidence of colorectal cancer over an 8-year period of observation. Low levels of 25-hydroxyvitamin D result primarily from inadequate exposure to sunlight.[125]

Dietary calcium was also associated with reduced incidence of colon cancer in several epidemiologic studies. These results are supported by clinical and laboratory studies, particularly those of Lipkin and Newmark[126,127] and Wargovich and Lointier.[128]

Reviews of the epidemiology of calcium, vitamin D, and colorectal cancer indicate a pattern of increasing support for the inverse association between calcium intake and risk of colorectal cancer[120,121,129–132] and the potential anticarcinogenic role of vitamin D.[120–122,124,125]

The geographic distribution of colorectal cancer and its association with relative deficiencies of ultraviolet light, vitamin D status, and calcium intake has a historical parallel in nutritional rickets.[133] A notable site of high incidence of rickets was the heavily industrialized midlands of England surrounding the city of Manchester.[134,135] A comparison of death rates from colorectal cancer in Manchester, which is located at 53.5°N, and San Diego, California, which is located at 32.7°N, revealed that death rates in women in Manchester were twice those in women in San Diego, and death rates from rectal cancer in women in Manchester were eight times higher in Manchester than in San Diego (11.2 per 100,000 population in Manchester women compared to 1.4 per 100,000 in San Diego).[134,135] The differences in rates in men were slightly less pronounced, but still approximately fourfold for rectal cancer.

Other Studies of Calcium, Vitamin D, and Colorectal Cancer

A positive finding concerning calcium intake and colorectal cancer was reported in women but not men in Melbourne, Australia by Kune and associates, who observed a statistically significant decrease in risk of colorectal cancer with increasing calcium consumption in women ($P < 0.01$).[136]

Consumption of calcium was in general low in this population. About 50% of men and 75% of women consumed less than 800 mg/d of calcium.[136] These levels of calcium consumption may not provide a sufficient range to detect the full impact of calcium intake. Vitamin D status was not assessed in this study, but vitamin D intake in New Zealand is low (Sylvester K, personal communication, 1990).

Some results of this study suggest that vitamin D or another micronutrient in fish may have some beneficial role in risk. Fish consumption was found to be significantly and independently associated with reduced risk of colorectal cancer (men, $P < 0.001$; women, $P < 0.05$). Fatty marine fish are good sources of vitamin D, but data on types of fish consumed were not reported.

One of the clearest findings of this study was the independent protective effect of vitamin supplementation (estimated relative risk, 0.32; 95% confidence interval, 0.21 to 0.50). No description of the vitamin D or calcium content of any supplements was provided. Vitamin D supplementation in multiple vitamins could have been an important source of vitamin D in vitamin takers, because dietary intake of vitamin D is low in New Zealand, and cool winters discourage exposure of the skin to sunlight. In Australia and New Zealand, milk is not fortified with vitamin D, unlike in the continental United States, where 400 IU (10 μg) is routinely added per liter.

A mildly supportive case–control study was reported from Marseille,[137] and a negative case–control study was reported from Canada.[138] Case–control studies are not well suited in general to studies of diet and cancer because they often contain recall and other biases that can hide real associations.[139] When a cohort study demonstrates a statistically significant association, particularly if a dose–response relationship is present, case–control studies usually cannot provide adequate evidence to indicate that the association found in the prospective study was absent.[139] Such a conclusion could be reached only after additional cohort studies or experiments.

Risk and Benefit

Issues of risk and benefit will need to be addressed when recommending increased levels of dietary consumption of calcium and vitamin D. Vitamin D administered orally maintains normal calcium levels in the blood of rats even in the face of calcium starvation,[140] a result that emphasizes the ability of vitamin D to mobilize calcium stores. A possible adverse effect of increasing vitamin D intake in the absence of adequate calcium intake would be depletion of these calcium stores and decreases in skeletal mass.

Historically, rickets in infants and children was associated with deficiencies of sunlight and dietary calcium.[133,141,142] Nutritional rickets all but disappeared from the United States after vitamin D supplementation of milk,[143,144] and elsewhere in the industrialized world after adoption of cod liver oil supplementation in children (cod liver oil provides 425 IU, or 11 μg of vitamin D_3 per teaspoonful).[145]

Since the fortification of milk and infant formulas in the United States, the vitamin D intake of children has been sufficient to control rickets, but most adults continue to be deficient in dietary intake of vitamin D by all existing standards. Even now, rickets can develop in children who do not drink fortified milk or take cod liver oil[144] if they are kept from ultraviolet light by indoor habits or excessive clothing, even in sunny climates.[142–145] Particularly low intakes of calcium may paradoxically increase the rate of excretion of some vitamin D metabolites, which may also play an as yet undetermined role in the pathogenesis of rickets.[146] The levels of 25-hydroxyvitamin D in serum needed to prevent rickets (3 to 5 ng/mL)[142] are far lower than those associated in one report with reduced incidence of colon cancer (27 to 41 ng/mL).[122]

Sunlight, Vitamin D, and Colorectal Cancer

The amount of sunlight reaching the ground varies markedly in the United States from a mean daily solar radiation level of approximately 300 g-cal/cm^2 in the northernmost states to 500 g-cal/cm^2 in the southwest and 450 g-cal/cm^2 in the south.[120] Age-adjusted mortality rates of colon cancer have been reported by the National Cancer Institute for all 506 state economic areas,[147] and the highest rates occurred in the high latitudes of the industrial northeast, whereas the lowest were in the south and southwest.

Elsewhere in the world,[9] countries with the highest age-adjusted death rates from colon cancer tend to be located at high latitudes. The lowest rates tend to occur in countries nearer the equator (although there are some exceptions, notably Japan).

Filtration of ultraviolet light by stratospheric ozone and air pollution selectively reduces transmission of ultraviolet B light through the atmosphere.[148] This may be important because ultraviolet B light in the range of 290 to 310 nm is needed to create vitamin D in the skin.[149] Gorham and colleagues proposed in 1989 that the notably high death rates from colon cancer in northeastern North America may be associated with diminished levels of transmission of ultraviolet B light due to precursors of acid rain known as acid haze.[148] Acid haze is composed primarily of sulfur dioxide.[148] Similar north–south and acid haze-related gradients are associated with colon cancer incidence and mortality rates in Italy[150] and the former Soviet Union.[151]

Nutritional Risk Factors

Fats

Fat intake has long been a suspected risk factor for colorectal cancer, but the geographic distribution of fat intake cannot explain the geographic distribution of colorectal cancer in the United States, where dietary fat intake as measured by regional consumption patterns varies in the opposite direction to the geographic distribution of colon cancer.[120] The role of total dietary fat in colon carcinogenesis within the ordinary dietary range found in the United States is problematic.[152,153] Six case–control studies cited in one review reported a positive association between total and saturated fat and risk of colon cancer, but five similar studies found no association.[153] The studies that reported no association included a 19-year prospective study that found that intake of energy as total fat was 42% in colon cancer cases and 43% in control subjects.[124] Mean dietary intake of total fats in this cohort was 145 g/d.[124] Four studies, all case–control, found no association between total dietary fat and risk of colon cancer.[136,154–156]

Although many people have decreased their intake of saturated fat in an effort to reduce risk of heart disease, estimates of consumption of total fats have in general increased throughout this century. Consumption in the United States of dietary fat was 127 g/person/d in 1909, 145 g/d in 1950, 158 g/d in 1974, and 170 g/d in the 1980s.[114]

Fiber, Fruits, and Vegetables

It has long been surmised that cereal fiber protects against colon cancer.[157] Although some epidemiologic studies have reported a beneficial effect of cereal fiber on risk of colon cancer,[158] others are negative.[159,160] Regional differences in crude cereal fiber intake within the United States cannot explain variations in colorectal cancer mortality rates.[161]

Countries with low intake of cereal fiber tend to have higher incidence and death rates from colon cancer,[159] but most are located at relatively high latitudes where serum levels of vitamin D metabolites may be low[162,163] and absorption of calcium may be poorer, especially in the elderly. Deficiency of 25-hydroxyvitamin D[164] can result in reduced serum levels of 1,25-dihydroxyvitamin D, an especially active metabolite of vitamin D.[165] Alternatively, deficiency of 25-hydroxyvitamin D might itself be the critical factor.

Japan has had low intake of crude cereal fiber and simultaneously low incidence[166] of and mortality rates[167] from colon cancer. Polished rice is the staple carbohydrate in Japan, and the bran fiber has been removed from this food. Furthermore, intestinal transit times[168] and stool mass[169] are similar in people eating a traditional Japanese diet to those of people on a presumably high-risk British diet.[7,167] Intake of fruits and vegetables is surprisingly uniform throughout the United States[170] and cannot explain the north–south gradient in rates of colorectal cancer.

Alcohol

A role of alcohol in colorectal cancer has long been suspected, but has been difficult to demonstrate in prospective studies. For example, a major U.S. prospective study found no effect of alcohol intake, with an average intake of 17 mL/d of ethanol in the cases and 15 mL/d in the noncases.[124]

Genetic Factors

A detailed investigation of patients with colorectal cancer revealed that 1% to 2% were from hereditary nonpolyposis coli kindreds.[171] Because at most 5% of cases arise in patients with familial polyposis or inflammatory bowel disease, most (at least 93%) cases of colorectal cancer are sporadic. Consistent with this was a study of the incidence of colorectal cancer in a cohort of health professionals that provided data indicating that the attributable risk associated with a family history of colorectal cancer was only 6%.[172] These studies are also consistent with migrant studies showing that immigrants from low-risk to high-risk areas acquire the risk present in the high-risk areas.[173,174]

Cigarette Smoking

Cigarette smoking does not appear to play a major role in risk of colorectal cancer. In a major prospective study, average intake of cigarettes was 7 per day in cases and 10 per day in noncases. Cigarette smoking was also inversely related to risk of colorectal cancer in the Framingham cohort.[175]

Aspirin

Several studies have suggested that intake of aspirin is associated with reduced risk of colorectal cancer,[176,177] consistent with a hypothesis described by by Rosenberg and associates.[178] However, one clinical trial reported a small but significant increase in the risk for colon cancer associated with use of aspirin.[179]

Role of Estrogen

The lower risk of colorectal cancer in women taking replacement estrogens was described previously. Because estrogen increases calcium flux across the intestine,[180] its effect appears to be consistent with parallel effects of calcium and vitamin D.

Prevention

The epidemiologic evidence suggests that there are several approaches available that may help to prevent the occurrence of colorectal cancer. Major relevant studies are summarized in Table 1-2. Two large studies, one cohort[124] and one case-control,[181] have suggested that a linear dose–response relationship may exist between intake of calcium and risk of colon cancer. Similar reductions in risk have been reported for dietary vitamin D in Chicago men[124] and serum 25-hydroxyvitamin D in Washington County, Maryland men and women.[125] No epidemiologic studies of colon cancer incidence or mortality are available on the effect of intakes above 1200 mg/d of calcium.

Because no epidemiologic data are available on calcium intakes above 1200 mg/d, attempts to model the dose–response relationship above this level may be premature. However, modeling was attempted as a hypothesis-generating exercise and heuristic tool to assist in planning further studies. Such modeling, although theoretical, may help to define the questions that remain to be answered and the studies needed to answer them.

Given this caveat, it is possible that the dose–response relationship between intake of calcium and risk of colorectal cancer is linear. Other theoretical models may be equally plausible, including those that assume the existence of various thresholds or plateaus beyond which further intake of calcium offers no marginal benefit or even has an adverse effect on risk of colonic cancer.

Results regarding calcium reported by Garland and coworkers[124] fit a linear approximation reasonably well in the range of 700 to 1200 mg/d of calcium, with a Pearson product moment correlation of −0.94 (Fig. 1-1). If the association between in-

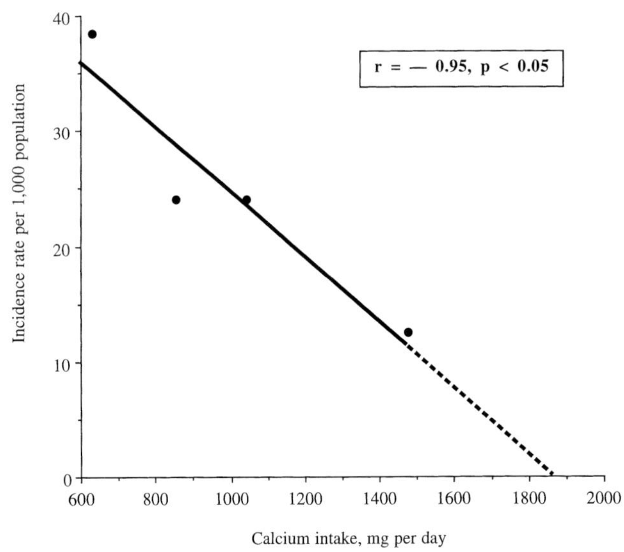

FIG. 1-1. Incidence rate of colorectal cancer according to calcium intake, men aged 40 to 55 years at baseline, Chicago, 1957 to 1977. (Garland F. Shekelle RB, Barrett-Connor E, et al. Dietary calcium and vitamin D and risk of colorectal cancer: 19-year prospective study. Lancet 1985;1:307.)

take of calcium and risk of colon cancer is linear, which is only one of several possibilities, then extrapolation from these results suggests the possibility that incidence might approach a very low level at a calcium intake of 1800 mg/d (see Fig. 1-1). Even if the drop in incidence of colon cancer is not linear, however, the data from this study suggest that a 75% reduction in incidence could be achieved with intake of 1200 + mg/d of calcium.[121]

The study by Slattery and colleagues in Utah[181] used a different methodologic approach than that used in the Chicago study,[124] but results from it also can be used to estimate the intake of calcium at which incidence of colon cancer might be markedly reduced. The Utah study was a case–control study, so incidence rates could not be computed. Instead, a simple linear extrapolation was performed of the Utah data to the level of calcium intake at which the expected relative risk would become 0.05. This point represents a theoretical reduction of risk to 5% of that of the current lowest quartile of lowest calcium intake. Such a linear extrapolation is shown for men in Figure 1-2. This result is essentially the same as that derived from the prospective study of Chicago men.[121] Vitamin D was not assessed in the Utah study.

For women in the Utah study, intake of calcium in milligrams per 1000 kilocalories was also linearly related to estimated relative risk (Fig. 1-3). A simple linear extrapolation suggests the possibility that a major reduction of risk might be achievable at a dietary level of 900 mg/1000 kcal. This amounts to approximately 1500 mg/d of calcium in women who consume the mean energy intake, 1670 kcal/d.

The study by Heilbrun and colleagues,[182] which failed to detect a favorable association between calcium intake and incidence of colorectal cancer in Japanese American men in Hawaii, has been superseded by another study of Japanese American men, from the same research group, showing that higher calcium intake is now associated with a statistically significant decreased incidence of cancer of the sigmoid, which is the site of most colonic cancers.[183]

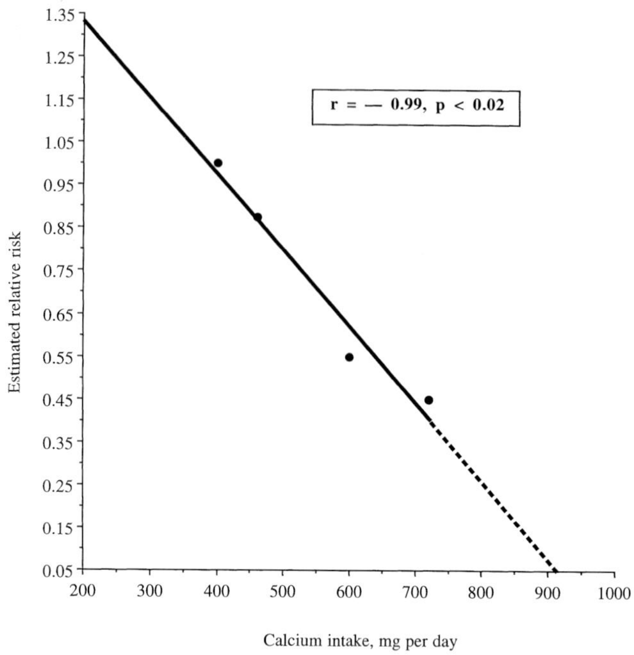

FIG. 1-3. Estimated relative risk of colon cancer according to calcium intake per 1000 kcal, women aged 40 to 79 years, Utah, 1979 to 1982. (Slattery ML, Sorenson AW, Ford MH. Dietary calcium intake as a mitigating factor in colon cancer. Am J Epidemiol 1988;128:504.)

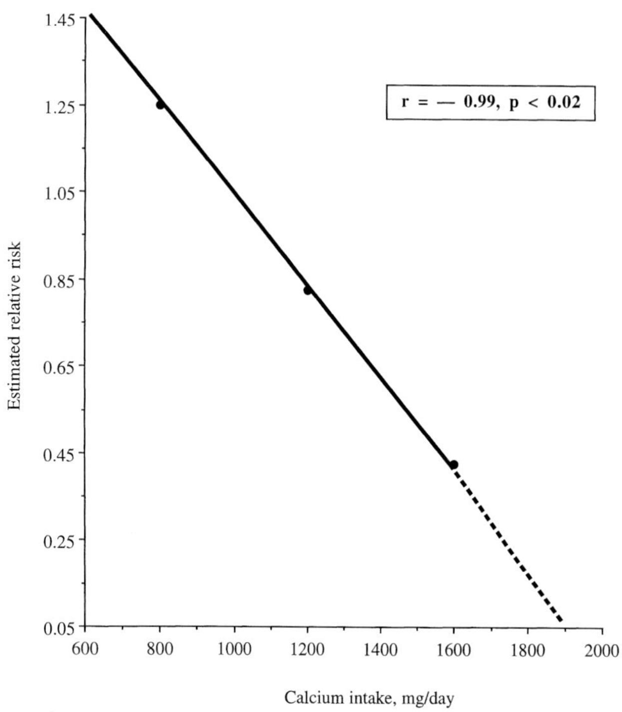

FIG. 1-2. Estimated relative risk of colon cancer according to calcium intake, men aged 40 to 79 years, Utah, 1979 to 1982. (Slattery ML, Sorenson AW, Ford MH. Dietary calcium intake as a mitigating factor in colon cancer. AM J Epidemiol 1988;128:504.)

A positive finding concerning calcium intake and colorectal cancer was reported in women but not men in Melbourne, Australia by Kune and associates, who observed a statistically significant decrease in risk of colorectal cancer with increasing calcium consumption in women ($P < 0.01$).[136]

Consumption of calcium was in general low in this population. About 50% of men and 75% of women consumed less than 800 mg/d of calcium.[136] These levels of calcium consumption may not provide a sufficient range to detect the full benefit of calcium intake. Vitamin D status was not assessed in this study, but vitamin D intake in New Zealand is low (Sylvester K, personal communication, 1990).

Dietary calcium deficiency continues to be widespread in adults in the United States. The National Health and Nutrition Examination Survey II reported that women aged 45 to 54 years consumed a median of 474 mg/d of calcium, and men of the same age a median of 733 mg/d.[184,185] These amounts are below the current recommended dietary allowance of 800 mg/d of calcium.[186] They are also well below the daily calcium intakes recommended by the National Institutes of Health Consensus Conference on Osteoporosis, 1500 mg/d for women past the menopause and not taking replacement estrogens, and 1200 mg/d for those taking estrogens.[187] In the elderly, current levels of intake of calcium are seriously deficient both for prevention of hip fractures[188] and mitigation of hypertension.[189,190]

Supplementation has historically played only a small role in calcium and vitamin D intake. During 1971 to 1975, 77.2% of the U.S. population took no vitamin or mineral supplement, and less than 2% of the population in any 10-year age group took a calcium or vitamin D supplement daily.[191] Corresponding data on frequency of use of specific supplements were collected for 1976 to 1980, but have not been reported.[191] These data suggest that calcium supplementation alone may not have been sufficient to produce the decrease in colon cancer death rates in women, although this possibility cannot be excluded.

Nutritional vitamin D deficiency is also widespread in adults in the United States. Middle-aged women consume a median of only 86 IU/d (2.2 μg/d) of vitamin D,[185] and middle aged men, 125 IU/d (3.1 μg/d).[192]

Sunlight exposure and dietary sources of vitamin D are both effective means of increasing circulating blood levels of vitamin D metabolites, but the relative importance of each varies by geographic location and the amount of dietary vitamin D consumed. Casual exposure to sunlight is the primary source of vitamin D in the United States.[193–195]

Women in Massachusetts consume a median of only 408 mg/d of calcium and 112 IU/d (2.8 μg/d) vitamin D[164]; other studies in industrial countries have shown similarly low vitamin D intakes. Vitamin D intakes have been assessed as deficient in older adults in the United States,[196,197] Canada,[198] Holland,[199] and Northern Ireland.[200] Intake of vitamin D in New Zealand adults is only 60 to 100 IU/d (1.5 to 2.5 μg/d; Sylvester K, personal communication, 1990). Neither New Zealand nor Australia fortifies milk with vitamin D, which is the reason for the unusually low dietary intake in these countries (Radford G, personal communication).

A relatively higher median intake of vitamin D, 186 IU/d (4.6 μg/d), was reported in Finnish elderly (mean age, 76 years),[201,202] although even this is below the U.S. recommended daily allowance.[186] Except for the relatively high dietary intake of vitamin D in Finland, intakes in the United States, Canada, and Europe are markedly below the 200 IU of vitamin D per day (5 μg/d) recommended daily allowance[186] and greatly below the 800 IU/d (20 μg/d) recommended for the elderly.[203,204] Low intakes of dietary vitamin D such as those present in most of Europe and North America are associated with prominent seasonal variations in serum vitamin D,[205] 25-hydroxyvitamin D,[205] and 1,25-dihydroxyvitamin D.[206,207] Seasonal variations in 25-hydroxyvitamin D and 1,25-dihydroxyvitamin D are also present in Finland, despite its relatively high oral intake of vitamin D.[202] It remains uncertain whether seasonal variations in 1,25-dihydroxyvitamin D are present in the United States. One survey of children and adults (ages 18 months to 35 years) reported a low of 29 pg/mL of 1,25-dihydroxyvitamin D in the serum near the beginning of winter, 40 to 43 pg/mL in the spring, and a high of 49 pg/mL by the end of summer.[208] These findings were, however, interpreted as consistent with lack of a seasonal effect because the result was not statistically significant.[208]

Vitamin D Precautions

The main caution about vitamin D use concerns the fact that with higher plasma levels of 25-hydroxyvitamin D and dietary levels of calcium, there might be greater calcium flux through the intestine and higher concentrations of calcium in the urine. Adverse effects might include increases in the incidence of renal stones in those predisposed by various metabolic defects to lithogenic urine (ie, urine that contains high levels of oxalates or other anions that precipitate calcium). If this occurs, it would most likely happen in a setting of dehydration, and would be more likely in men than women. This possibility must be weighed against the potential benefits of reducing death rates from colon cancer, which accounts for vastly greater mortality than renal stones or their complications. This concern may not be overwhelming, because Netelenbos and associates[209] have shown that subjects who formed renal stones had no higher serum concentrations of vitamin D metabolites than did control subjects.

Precautions can be taken to shift the benefit–risk ratio in a more favorable direction. As a starting point, the recommendation could be made that no one with a personal or family history of oxalate renal stones or stones of mixed or unknown composition should modify calcium or vitamin D intake without investigation and correction of any hyperoxaluria that may be present. If the hyperoxaluria is dietary in origin, it may often be controlled with a low-oxalate diet (less than 50 mg/d of oxalates). This would require limitation of intake of high-oxalate foods such as spinach, rhubarb, beets, and Swiss chard,[210] resulting in a total intake of 50 mg/d or less of oxalate. Fluid intake of 2 L/d would be needed to ensure adequate renal hydration.

The usual precautions regarding vitamin D toxicity at high supplemental intakes, especially in children, may be warranted, and supplementation with vitamin D must be well controlled. Vitamin D from foods (naturally occurring or supplemented) is the safest source of dietary vitamin D. For example, Japanese adults routinely consume foods that contain 800 to 1000 IU (20 to 25 μg) of vitamin D per day, albeit in a population with lower daily intake of calcium (380 to 400 mg/d).[138] Establishing safe and effective ranges of human intake of calcium and vitamin D will be a task requiring the expertise and work of many investigators and worldwide scope.

Intake of calcium in the United States is too little, and too late for the prevention of several diseases.[211] For example, adults aged 50 to 79 years at baseline in Rancho Bernando, California who consumed less than 283 mg of calcium per 1000 kcal had 3.7 times the incidence of hip fractures as those who consumed 440 + mg/1000 kcal ($P < 0.05$).[212] No other risk factor was consistently associated with risk of hip fracture.[212]

Recommended levels for human consumption of calcium and vitamin D are well below those for animals. For example, standard laboratory animal diets for mammals require a minimum of 1.5 mg/kcal of calcium and 0.4 IU/kcal (0.01 μg/kcal) of vitamin D.[213] This would correspond to 3750 mg/d of calcium and 1000 IU/d (25 μg/d) of vitamin D in a person who consumed 2500 kcal/d. These amounts are well above known human intakes of calcium at the present time, but similar to the present human dietary intake of vitamin D in many low-risk populations.[214]

Recommendations

From a viewpoint limited to efficacy, calcium intakes of 1800 mg/d in men and 1500 mg/d (or 900 mg/1000 kcal) in women would appear to be suitable targets for reducing the incidence of colon cancer. These intakes are consistent with calcium intakes of humans throughout evolution.[209] The epidemiologic data suggest that amounts of vitamin D from ultraviolet light or diet sufficient to raise the serum 25-hydroxyvitamin D level to the 27- to 41-ng/mL range would reduce the incidence of colon cancer markedly,[122] because dietary vitamin D intakes above 150 IU/d (3.8 μg) are associated with a drop by half in the incidence rate.[121] Therefore, it would seem wise to recommend that all adults consume the current recommended daily allowance of vitamin D of 200 IU (5 μg). Exceptions might include people with a personal or family history of kidney stones or with conditions that predispose to stone formation.

Large-scale trials are needed to examine the efficacy of calcium in doses above 1200 mg/d, vitamin D in doses above 400 IU/d, and combinations of these micronutrients in the prevention of colon cancer. Possible adverse long-term effects of calcium and vitamin D intake at these levels should be investigated, along with the anticipated benefits, to provide the full risk–benefit data needed for making nutritional policies.

These trials should not be used to delay the public health interventions urgently needed to ensure that every child and adult receives adequate calcium and vitamin D in countries where high incidence and death rates of colon cancer are endemic, such as the United States, Canada, the United Kingdom, New Zealand, Denmark, the Netherlands, Norway, Sweden, northern Italy, and other developed nations.

A reasonable definition at this point would be 1200 mg/d of calcium and 200 to 400 IU/d of vitamin D. Because these are two to four times the current intake, the goal of calcium and vitamin D adequacy can be achieved only through supplementation of foods. Newmark has suggested fortification of flour with calcium, a practice with historical precedent in the United States (Newmark HL, personal communication, 1993). Most people eat bread, so this may be an ideal means of raising calcium intake. Other possibilities include fortification of popular beverages with calcium. Adequate vitamin D status is probably best achieved in late spring, summer, and early fall with moderate (10 to 15 min/d) exposure to sunlight during the period from 11:00 AM to 2:00 PM. Sunscreens, such as paraaminobenzoic acid and its esters, inhibit synthesis of previtamin D in the skin and should be avoided. Overexposure to ultraviolet light (>10 to 15 minutes) should be carefully avoided by use of clothing, or, on exposed areas, physical sunscreens such as zinc or titanium oxides, if well tolerated.

When trials are conducted, data collected should include measures of dietary intake of oxalate, and dietary and supplemental intake of ascorbate, phosphate, and citrate, because these may influence risk of kidney stones. Daily oral intake of fluids should be ascertained, with appropriate proxy measures of hydration. Measures should also be obtained of urinary oxalates and other anions that are common in renal stones in the geographic areas and populations studied, as well as appropriate indices of urinary concentration and pH.

REFERENCES

1. Wingo P, Tong T, Bolden S. Cancer statistics, 1995. CA Cancer J Clin 1995;45:8.
2. Munoz N, Day N. Oesophagus. In: Schottenfeld D, Fraumeni JJ, eds. Cancer epidemiology and prevention. 2nd ed. New York: Oxford University Press, 1992:596.
3. Parkin D, Laara E, Muir C. Estimates of the world-wide frequency of sixteen major cancers in 1980. Int J Cancer 1988;41:184.
4. Yeng C. Research on esophageal cancer in China: a review. Cancer Res 1980;40:2633.
5. Cheng K. The etiology of esophageal cancer in Chinese. Semin Oncol 1994;12:411.
6. Waterhouse J, Muir C, Correa P, et al. Cancer incidence in five continents. vol 3. IARC Scientific Publication No. 15. Lyon, France: International Agency for Research on Cancer, 1976.
7. Muir C, Waterhouse J, Mack T, et al. Cancer incidence in five continents. vol 5. IARC Scientific Publication No. 88. Lyon, France: International Agency for Research on Cancer, 1987.
8. Munoz N. Epidemiological aspects of oesophageal cancer. Endoscopy 1993;25(Suppl):609.
9. Parkin D, Muir C, Whelan S, et al. Cancer incidence in five continents. vol 6. IARC Scientific Publications No. 120. Lyon, France: International Agency for Research on Cancer, 1992.
10. Boffetta P, La Vecchia C, Levi F, et al. Mortality patterns and trends for lung cancer and other tobacco-related cancers in the Americas, 1955–1989.
11. Van Rensburg S, Benade A, Rose E, Du Plessis J. Nutritional status of African populations predisposed to esophageal cancer. Nutr Cancer 1983;4:206.
12. Serenko A, Tserkovnogo G. Malignant tumours: statistical data from the USSR. Int J Epidemiol 1993;22:377.
13. Nugmanov S, Kolycheva N. Age, sex, and ethnic characteristics of patients with esophageal carcinoma in Kazakhastan. In: Epidemiology of malignant tumors. Alma Ata, Kazakhstan: 1970:272.
14. Franceschi S. Role of nutrition in the aetiology of oesophageal cancer in developed countries. Endoscopy 1993;25(Suppl):613.
15. Steinmetz K, Potter J. Vegetables, fruit, and cancer: I. epidemiology. Cancer Causes Control 1991;2:325.
16. Greenwald P, Kelloff G, Kalagher S, McDonald S. Research studies on chemoprevention of esophageal cancer at the United States National Cancer Institute. Endoscopy 1993;25:617.
17. Wynder E, Bross I. A study of etiological factors in cancer of the esophagus. Cancer 1967;14:389.
18. Tuyns A, Riboli E, Doornbos G, Pequignot G. Protective effect of citrus fruit on esophageal cancer. Nutr Cancer 1983;4:195.
19. Block G. Vitamin C and cancer prevention: the epidemiologic evidence. Am J Clin Nutr 1991;53:270s.
20. DeCarli A, Liati P, Negri E. Vitamin A and other dietary factors in the etiology of esophageal cancer. Nutr Cancer 1987;10:27.
21. Yeng C. Research on esophageal cancer in China: a review. Cancer Res 1980;40:2633.
22. Zaridze D, Blettner M, Trapeznikov N, et al. Survey of a population with high incidence of oral and esophageal cancer. Int J Cancer 1985; 36:153.
23. Ziegler R, Morris L, Blot W, et al. Esophageal cancer among black men in Washington DC: II. role of nutrition. J Natl Cancer Inst 1981; 67:1199.
24. Tuyns A, Riboli E, Doornbos G, Pequignot G. Diet and esophageal cancer in Calvados, France. Nutr Cancer 1987;9:81.
25. Ghadirian P. Food habits of the people of the Caspian littoral of Iran in relation to esophageal cancer. Nutr Cancer 1987;9:147.
26. Guo W, Li J, Blot W, et al. Correlations of dietary intake and blood nutrient levels with esophageal cancer mortality in China. Nutr Cancer 1990;13:121.
27. Brown L, Blot W, Schuman S. Environmental factors and high risk of esophageal cancer in men in coastal South Carolina. J Natl Cancer Inst 1988;80:1620.
28. Whelan S, Parkin D, Masuyer E. Patterns of cancer incidence in five continents. IARC Scientific Publication No. 102. Lyon, France: International Agency for Research on Cancer, 1990.
29. Young J. Surveillance, epidemiology, and end results: incidence and mortality data, 1973–77. National Cancer Institute Monograph No. 57. Bethesda, MD: National Cancer Institute, 1981.
30. Coye M, Young J, Bal D, Lyman D. Cancer mortality in California, 1985–1989. Sacramento, CA: California State Department of Health Services, 1991.
31. Hoffman F. The mortality from cancer throughout the world. Newark, NJ: Prudential Press, 1915:111.
32. U.S. National Center for Health Statistics. Vital statistics of the United States, 1991. Washington, DC: Government Printing Office, 1994.

33. Rohan T, McMichael A. Alimentary tract cancer mortality in Australia, 1908–1978. Med J Aust 1981;1:232.
34. Haenszel W, Kurihara M, Mitsuo S, et al. Stomach cancer among Japanese in Hawaii. J Natl Cancer Inst 1972;49:96.
35. Kmet J. The role of migrant population in studies of selected cancer sites. J Chronic Dis 1970;23:305.
36. Rosenwaike I. Cancer mortality among Puerto Rican-born residents in New York City. Am J Epidemiol 1984;119:177.
37. Lauren P. The two histological main types of gastric cancer: diffuse and so-called intestinal type of carcinoma. Acta Pathol Microbiol Scand 1965;64:31.
38. Parsonnet J. *Helicobacter pylori* and gastric cancer. Gastroenterol Clin North Am 1993;22:89.
39. Marshall B, Warren J. Unidentified curved bacilli in the stomach of patients with gastritis and peptic ulceration. Lancet 1984;1:1311.
40. Parsonnet J, Friedman G, Daniel M, et al. *Helicobacter pylori* and the risk of gastric carcinoma. N Engl J Med 1991a;325:1127.
41. Parsonnet J, Vandersteen D, Goates J, et al. *Helicobacter pylori* infection in intestinal- and diffuse-type gastric adenocarcinomas. J Natl Cancer Inst 1991;83:640.
42. Marshall B. *Helicobacter pylori*: a primer for 1994. Gastroenterologist 1993;1:241.
43. Borody T, Andrews P, Mancuso N, et al. *Helicobacter pylori* infection 4 years post-eradication. Lancet 1992;339:1295.
44. Costas M, Owen R, Bickley J, Morgan D. Molecular techniques for studying the epidemiology of infection by *Helicobacter pylori*. Scand J Gastroenterol 1991;181(Suppl):20.
45. Forman D, Newell D, Fullerton F, et al. Association between infection with *Helicobacter pylori* and risk of gastric cancer: evidence from a prospective investigation. Br Med J 1991;302:1302.
46. Nomura A, Stemmermann G, Chyou P, et al. *Helicobacter pylori* infection and gastric carcinoma in a population of Japanese-Americans in Hawaii. N Engl J Med 1991;325:1132.
47. Munoz N. Is *Helicobacter pylori* a cause of gastric cancer? An appraisal of the seroepidemiological evidence. Cancer Epidemiol Biomarkers Prev 1994;3:445.
48. Robey-Cafferty S, Ro J, Cleary K. The prevalence of *Campylobacter pylori* in gastric biopsies from cancer patients. Mod Pathol 1989;2: 473.
49. Burstein M, Monge E, Leon-Barua R, et al. Low peptic ulcer and high gastric cancer prevalence in a developing country with a high prevalence of infection by *Helicobacter pylori*. J Clin Gastroenterol 1991;13:154.
50. Thompson G, vanHeerden J, Sarr M. Adenocarcinoma of the stomach: are we making progress? Lancet 1993;342:713.
51. Nomura A, Stemmermann G, Heilbrun L, et al. Serum vitamin levels and risk of cancer of specific sites in men of Japanese ancestry in Hawaii. Cancer Res 1985;45:2369.
52. Chen V, Abu-Elyazeed R, Zavala D, et al. Risk factors for gastric precancerous lesions in a high risk Colombian population: I. salt. Nutr Cancer 1990;13:59.
53. Chen V, Abu-Elyazeed R, Zavala D, al. Risk factors for gastric precancerous lesions in a high risk Colombian population: II. nitrate and nitrite. Nutr Cancer 1990;13:67.
54. Correa P. The gastric precancerous process. Cancer Surv 1983;2:437.
55. Correa P. Is gastric carcinoma an infectious disease? N Engl J Med 1991;325:1171.
56. Fraumeni JF, Jr. Cancers of the pancreas and biliary tract: epidemiological considerations. Cancer Res 1975;35;3437.
57. Garland CF, Garland FC. Do sunlight and vitamin D reduce the likelihood of colon cancer? Int J Epidemiol 1980;9:227.
58. Garland FC, Garland CF, Gorham ED, Young JF. Geographic variation in breast cancer mortality in the United States: a hypothesis involving exposure to solar radiation. Prev Med 1990;19:614.
59. Blot WJ, Fraumeni JF Jr, Stone BJ. Geographic correlates of pancreas cancer in the United States. Cancer 1978;42:373.
60. Burnett WS, Greenwald P, Nasca PC, et al. Population density as an indicator of urban-rural differences in cancer incidence, upstate New York, 1968–72. Am J Epidemiol 1980;112:362.
61. Clemmesen J. Statistical studies in the etiology of malignant neoplasms: IV. lung/bladder ratio for Denmark 1943–67. Acta Pathol Microbiol Scand 1974;(Suppl 247):1.
62. Klintrup HE. Carcinoma of the pancreas: a statistical, clinical, and pathological study. Acta Chir Scand 1966;(Suppl 362):1.
63. Pickle LW, Gottlieb MS. Pancreatic cancer mortality in Louisiana. Am J Public Health 1980;70:256.
64. Horm JW, Asire AJ, Young JL, Pollack ES, eds. Cancer incidence and mortality in the United States: Surveillance, epidemiology, and end results (SEER), 1973–81. NIH Publication No. 85–1837. U.S. Department of Health and Human Services, Public Health Service. Bethesda, MD: National Cancer Institute, 1985.
65. Levine DL, Connelly RR, Devesa SS. Demographic characteristics of cancer of the pancreas: mortality, incidence, and survival. Cancer 1981;47:1456.
66. Gordis L. Epidemiology of pancreas cancer. In: Lilienfeld AM, ed. Reviews of cancer epidemiology. vol 1. New York: Elsevier, 1980: 84.
67. Arellano MG, Linden G, Dunn JE Jr., Cancer patterns in Alameda County, California. Br J Cancer 1972;26:473.
68. Enstrom JE. Cancer and total mortality among active Mormons. Cancer 1978;42:1943.
69. Enstrom JE. Cancer mortality among Mormons in California during 1968–75. J Natl Cancer Inst 1980;65:1073.
70. Greenwald P, Korns RF, Nasca PL, et al. Cancer in United States Jews. Cancer Res 1975;35:3507.
71. Lyon JL, Gardner JW, West DW. Cancer incidence in Mormons and non-Mormons in Utah during 1967–75. J Natl Cancer Inst 1980;65: 1055.
72. Lyon JL, Klauber MR, Gardner JW, Smart CR. Cancer incidence in Mormons and non-Mormons in Utah, 1966–1970. N Engl J Med 1976;294;129.
73. Lyon JL, Klauber MR, Gardner JW, Smart CR. Low cancer incidence and mortality in Utah. Cancer 1978;39:2608.
74. Phillips RL. Mortality among Seventh-Day Adventists for selected cancer sites. J Natl Cancer Inst 1980;65:1097.
75. Phillips RL. Role of life-style and dietary habits in risk of cancer among Seventh-Day Adventists. Cancer Res 1975;35:3513.
76. Wynder EL, Hall NEL, Polansky M. Epidemiology of coffee and pancreatic cancer. Cancer Res 1983;43:3900.
77. Murr MM, Sarr MG, Oishi AJ, van Heerden JA. Pancreatic cancer. CA Cancer J Clin 1994;44:304.
78. Haenzel W, Kurihara M. Studies of Japanese migrants: I. mortality from cancer and other diseases among Japanese in the United States. J Natl Cancer Inst 1968;40:43.
79. Hirayama T. Prospective studies on cancer epidemiology based on census population in Japan. In: Nieburgs HE, ed. Prevention and detection of cancer. vol 1. New York; Marcel Dekker, 1978:1139.
80. Maruchi N, Brian D, Ludwig J, et al. Cancer of the pancreas in Olmsted County, Minnesota, 1935–1974. Mayo Clin Proc 1979;54: 245.
81. Ishii K, Takeuchi T, Hirayama T. Chronic calcifying pancreatitis and pancreatic carcinoma in Japan. Digestion 1973;9:429.
82. Gambill EE. Pancreatitis associated with pancreatic carcinoma: a study of 26 cases. Mayo Clin Proc 1971;46:174.
83. Robinette CD, Hrubec Z, Fraumeni JF Jr. Chronic alcoholism and subsequent mortality in World War II veterans. Am J Epidemiol 1979; 109:687.
84. Yen S, Hsieh C-C, MacMahon B. Consumption of alcohol and tobacco and other risk factors for pancreatitis. Am J Epidemiol 1982;116:407.
85. Velema JP, Walker AM, Gold EB. Alcohol and pancreatic cancer: insufficient evidence for a causal relationship. Epidemiol Rev 1986; 8:28.
86. Ammann RW, Akovbiantz A, Largiader F. Course and outcome of chronic pancreatitis: longitudinal study of a mixed medical-surgical series of 245 patients. Gastroenterology 1984;86:820.
87. Lowenfels AB, Patel VP, Pitchumoni CS. Chronic calcific pancreatitis and pancreatic cancer [abstract]. Dig Dis Sci 1985;30:982.
88. Gold EB, Gordis L, Diener MD, et al. Diet and other risk factors for cancer of the pancreas. Cancer 1985;55:460.
89. Lin RS, Kessler II. A multifactorial model for pancreatic cancer in man: Epidemiological evidence. JAMA 1981;245:147.
90. MacMahon B, Yen Y, Trichopoulos D, et al. Coffee and cancer of the pancreas. N Engl J Med 1981;304:630.
91. Wynder EL, Mabuchi K, Maruchi N, Fortner JG. A case control study of cancer of the pancreas. Cancer 1973;31:641.
92. Durbec JP, Chevillotte G, Bidort JM, et al. Diet, alcohol, tobacco and risk of cancer of the pancreas: a case control study. Br J Cancer 1983; 47:463.

93. Ishii K, Nakamura K, Ozaki H, et al. Epidemiological problems of pancreas cancer. Jpn J Clin Med 1968;26:1839.
94. Dean G, MacLennan R, McLoughlin H, et al. Causes of death among blue-collar workers at a Dublin brewery, 1954–73. Br J Cancer 1979; 40:581.
95. Jensen OM. Cancer morbidity and causes of death among Danish brewery workers. Int J Cancer 1979;23:454.
96. Schmidt W, Popham RE. The role of drinking and smoking in mortality from cancer and other causes in male alcoholics. Cancer 1981;47: 1031.
97. Hsieh C-C, MacMahon B, Yen S, et al. Coffee and pancreatic cancer [letter]. N Engl J Med 1986;315:587.
98. Gorham ED, Garland CF, Garland FC, Benenson AS, Cottrell L. Coffee and pancreatic cancer in a rural California county. West J Med 1988;148:48.
99. Waterhouse J, Muir C, Correa P, et al, eds. Cancer incidence in five continents. vol 3. IARC Scientific Publication No. 15. Lyon, France: International Agency for Research on Cancer, 1976.
100. Falk H., Thomas LB, Popper H, et al. Hepatic angiosarcoma associated with androgenic-anabolic steroids. Lancet 1979;2:1120.
101. Fugimoto I, Hanai A. Cancer statistics in Japan and in Osaka: incidence, therapy, and survival. Gann Monogr Cancer Res 1979;22:201.
102. Tsukuma H, Hiyama T, Tanaka S, et al. Risk factors for hepatocellular carcinoma among patients with chronic liver disease. N Engl J Med 1993;328:1797.
103. Martini GA. The role of alcohol in the etiology of cancer of the liver. In: Nieburgs HE, ed. Prevention and detection of cancer. Part 2: Detection, vol 2: Cancer detection at specific sites. New York: Marcel Dekker, 1980:2163.
104. Adami H-O, Hsing AW, McLaughlin JK, et al. Alcoholism and liver cirrhosis in the etiology of primary liver cancer. Int J Cancer 1992; 51:898.
105. Edmonson HA, Henderson B, Benton B. Liver cell adenomas associated with use of oral contraceptives. N Engl J Med 1976;294:470.
106. Klatskin G. Hepatic tumors: possible relationship to use of oral contraceptives. Gastroenterology 1977;73:386.
107. Blum HE, Liang TJ, Wands JR. Hepatitis B virus carriers and hepatocellular carcinoma. In: Bianchi L, Gerok W, Maier K-P, Deinhardt F, eds. Infectious diseases of the liver. Dordrecht, The Netherlands: Kluwer Academic, 1990:261.
108. Munoz N, Bosch X. Epidemiology of hepatocellular carcinoma. In: Okuda K, Ishak KG, eds. Neoplasms of of the liver. Tokyo: Springer-Verlag, 1987:3.
109. Wands JR, Blum HE. Primary hepatocellular carcinoma. N Engl J Med 1991;325:729.
110. Hollstein M, Sidransky D, Vogelstein B, Harris CC. p53 mutations in human cancers. Science 1991;253:49.
111. Maupas P, Chiron JP, Barin F, et al. Efficacy of hepatitis B vaccine in prevention of early HBsAg carrier state in children: controlled trial in an endemic area (Senegal). Lancet 1981;1:289.
112. Norkrans G. Epidemiology of hepatitis B virus (HBV) infections with particular regard to current routes of transmission and development of cirrhosis malignancy. Scand J Infect Dis 1990;(Suppl 69):43.
113. Li J, Liu B, Li G, et al. Atlas of cancer mortality in the People's Republic of China. Shanghai: China Map Press, 1979.
114. Gortner WA. Nutrition in the United States, 1900 to 1974. Cancer Res 1975;35:3246.
115. Tutton PJM, Barkla DH. Steroid hormones as regulators of the proliferative activity of normal and neoplastic intestinal epithelial cells [review]. Anticancer Res 1988;8:451.
116. Jacobs EJ, White E, Weiss NS. Exogenous hormones, reproductive history, and colon cancer (Seattle, Washington, U.S.A.). Cancer Causes Control 1994;5:359.
117. Newcomb PA, Storer BE. Postmenopausal hormone use and risk of large bowel cancer. J Natl Cancer Inst 1995;87:1067.
118. Calle EE, Miracle-McMahill HL, Thun MJ, Health CW Jr. Estrogen replacement therapy and risk of fatal colon cancer in a prospective cohort of postmenopausal women. J Natl Cancer Inst 1995;87:517.
119. Chow WH, Devesa SS, Blot WJ. Colon cancer incidence: recent trends in the United States. Cancer Causes Control 1991;2:419.
120. Garland CF, Garland FC, Gorham ED. Can colon cancer incidence and death rates be reduced with calcium and vitamin D? Am J Clin Nutr 1991;54(Suppl 2):193S.
121. Garland CF, Garland FC, Gorham ED. Colon cancer parallels rickets. In: Lipkin M, Newmark HL, Kelloff G, eds. Calcium, vitamin D, and prevention of colon cancer. Bethesda, MD: National Cancer Institute, and Boca Raton, FL: CRC Press, 1991:81.
122. Garland CF, Garland FC. Do sunlight and vitamin D reduce the risk of colon cancer? Int J Epidemiol 1980;9:227.
123. Lointier P, Meggouh F, Pezet D, et al. Specific receptors for 1,25A dihydroxyvitamin D3 (1,25-DR) and human colorectal carcinogenesis. Anticancer Res 1989;9:1921.
124. Garland C, Shekelle RB, Barrett-Connor E, et al. Dietary calcium and vitamin D and risk of colorectal cancer: a 19-year prospective study in men. Lancet 1985;1;307.
125. Garland C, Comstock GW, Garland FC, Helsing KJ, Shaw EK, Gorham ED. Serum 25-hydroxyvitamin D and colon cancer: eight-year prospective study. Lancet 1989;2:1176.
126. Lipkin M, Newmark HL. Effect of added dietary calcium on colonic epithelial cell proliferation in subjects at high risk for familial colonic cancer. N Engl J Med 1985;313:1381.
127. Newmark HL, Wargovich MJ, Bruce WR. Colon cancer and dietary fat, phosphate, and calcium: a hypothesis. J Natl Cancer Inst 1984; 72:1323.
128. Wargovich MJ, Lointier PH. Calcium and vitamin D modulate mouse colon epithelial proliferation and growth characteristics of a human colon tumor cell line. Can J Physiol Pharmacol 1987;65:472.
129. Spitz MR, Paolucci MJ, Newell GR. Occurrence of colorectal cancer: focus on Texas. Cancer Bull 1988;40:187.
130. Wargovich MJ. Calcium and colon cancer. J Am Coll Nutr 1988;7: 295.
131. Sorenson AW, Slattery ML, Ford MH. Calcium and colon cancer: a review. Nutr Cancer 1988;11:135.
132. Vogel VG, McPherson RS. Dietary epidemiology of colon cancer. Hematol Oncol Clin North Am 1989;3:35.
133. Palm TA. The geographical distribution and aetiology of rickets. Practitioner 1890;45:271.
134. California Department of Health Services. Cancer incidence and mortality, California, 1988. Sacramento, CA: California Tumor Registry, 1987.
135. Registrar General of England and Wales. Mortality data, 1985.
136. Kune S, Kune GA, Watson LF. Case-control study of dietary etiological factors: the Melbourne colorectal cancer study. Nutr Cancer 1987; 9:21.
137. Macquart-Moulin G, Riboli E, Cornie J, et al. Case-control study on colorectal cancer and diet in Marseille. Int J Cancer 1986;38:183.
138. Jain M, Cook GM, Davis FG, et al. A case-control study of diet and colo-rectal cancer. Int J Cancer 1980;26:57.
139. Lilienfeld DE, Garland CF, Lilienfeld AM. Gastric cancer [letter]. J Natl Cancer Inst 1976;57:9.
140. Kramer B, Howland J. Factors which determine the concentration of calcium and inorganic phosphorus in the blood serum of rats. Johns Hopkins Hosp Bull 1992;33:313.
141. DeLuca HF. The transformation of a vitamin into a hormone: the vitamin D story. Harvey Lect 1981;75:333.
142. Hayward I, Stein MT, Gibson MI. Nutritional rickets in San Diego. Am J Dis Child 1987;141:1060.
143. Edidin DV, Levitsky LL, Schey W, Dumbovic N, Campos A. Resurgence of nutritional rickets associated with breast-feeding and special dietary practices. Pediatrics 1980;65:232.
144. Eliot MM, Nelson EM, Barnes DJ, Browne FA, Jenss RM. A study of the comparative value of cod liver oil, viosterol, and vitamin D milks in the prevention of rickets. J Pediatr 1936;9:355.
145. Lawson DEM, Cole TJ, Salem SI, et al. Aetiology of rickets in Egyptian children. Hum Nutr Clin Nutr 1987;41:199.
146. Clements MR, Johnson L, Fraser DR. A new mechanism for induced vitamin D deficiency: 1,25-dihydroxyvitamin D enhanced hepatic inactivation of vitamin D. Nature 1987;325:62.
147. Pickle LW, Mason TJ, Howard N, et al. Atlas of U.S. cancer mortality among whites: 1950–1980. NIH Publication No. 87–2900. Washington, DC: U.S. Government Printing Office, 1987.
148. Gorham ED, Garland CF, Garland FC. Acid haze air pollution and breast and colon cancer in 20 Canadian cities. Can J Public Health 1989;80:96.
149. Holick MF. The photobiology of vitamin D and its consequences for humans. Ann NY Acad Sci 1985;453:1.
150. Garland FC, Garland CF, Gorham ED, et al. Sunlight, sulfur dioxide,

and breast and colonic cancer in Italy. Abstracts of the San Diego Epidemiology Research Exchange, April, 1989.
151. Gorham ED, Garland CF, Garland FC. Sunlight and breast cancer incidence in the U.S.S.R. Int J Epidemiol 1990;19:820.
152. Kolonel L, Le Marchand L. The epidemiology of colon cancer and dietary fat. In: Dietary fat and cancer. New York: Alan R. Liss, 1986: 69.
153. Willett W. The search for the causes of breast and colon cancer. Nature 1989;338:389.
154. Macquart-Moulin G, Riboli E, Cornee J, et al. Case-control study on colorectal cancer and diet in Marseille. Int J Cancer 1986;38:183.
155. Berta JL, Coste T, Rautureau J, et al. Diet and rectocolonic cancers. Results of a case-control study. Gastroenterol Clin Biol 1985;9:348.
156. Tuyns AJ, Haelterman M, Kaaks R. Colorectal cancer and the intake of nutrients: oligosaccharides are a risk factor, fats are not: a case-control study in Belgium. Nutr Cancer 1987;10:181.
157. Burkitt DP. Epidemiology of cancer of the colon and rectum. Cancer 1971;28:3.
158. Modan B, Barell V, Lubin F, et al. Low-fiber intake as an etiologic factor in cancer of the colon. J Natl Cancer Inst 1975;55:15.
159. McKeown-Eyssen GE. Fiber intake in different populations and colon cancer risk. Prev Med 1987;16:532.
160. Potter, McMichael AJ. Diet and cancer of the colon and rectum: a case-control study. J Natl Cancer Inst 1986;76:557.
161. Patterson B, Block G. Food choices and the cancer guidelines. Am J Public Health 1988;78:282.
162. Webb AR, Kline L, Holick MF. Influence of season and latitude on the cutaneous synthesis of vitamin D_3: exposure to winter sunlight in Boston and Edmonton will not promote vitamin D_3 synthesis in human skin. J Clin Endocrinol Metab 1988;67:373.
163. Punnonen R, Gillespy M, Hahl M, et al. Serum 25-hydroxyvitamin D, vitamin A, and vitamin E concentrations in healthy Finnish and Floridian women. Int J Vitam Nutr Res 1988;58:37.
164. Krall EA, Sahyoun RD, Tannenbaum S, Dallal G, Dawson-Hughes B. Effect of vitamin D intake on seasonal variations in parathyroid hormone secretion in postmenopausal women. N Engl J Med 1989; 321:1777.
165. Bouillon RA, Auwerx JH, Lissens WD, et al. Vitamin D status in the elderly: seasonal substrate deficiency causes 1,25-dihydroxycholecalciferol deficiency. Am J Clin Nutr 1987;45:755.
166. Segi M. Graphic presentation of cancer incidence by site and area and population, compiled from the data published in Cancer Incidence in Five Continents, Volume III. Nagoya, Japan: Segi Institute of Cancer Epidemiology, 1977:13.
167. Muir C, Waterhouse J, Mack T, et al. Cancer incidence in five continents. vol 5. IARC Scientific Publication No. 88. Lyon, France: International Agency for Research in Cancer, 1987.
168. Glober GA, Klein KL, Moore JO, Abba BC. Bowel transit-times in two populations experiencing similar colon-cancer risks. Lancet 1974; 2:80.
169. Glober GA, Kamiyama S, Nomura A, et al. Bowel transit-time and stool weight in populations with different colon-cancer risks. Lancet 1977;2:110.
170. United States Department of Agriculture. Dietary levels of households in the northeast, north central, south, and west. Washington, DC: U.S. Government Printing Office, 1970.
171. Kee F, Collins BJ. How prevalent is cancer family syndrome? Gut 1991;32:5409.
172. Willett W, et al. Familial aggregation of colorectal cancer. N Engl J Med 1995.
173. Haenszel W, et al. Migrant studies of colorectal cancer.
174. Ziegler R, Fraumeni J, et al. Migrant studies of colorectal cancer.
175. Williams RR, Sorlie PD, Feinleib M, McNamara PM, Kannel WB, Dawber TR. Cancer incidence by levels of cholesterol. JAMA 1981; 245:247.
176. Thun MJ, Namboodiri MM, Heath CW, Jr. Aspirin use and reduced risk of fatla colon cancer. N Engl J Med 1991;325:1593.
177. Paganini-Hill A, Chao A, Ross RK, Henderson BE. Aspirin use and chronic diseases: a cohort study of the elderly. Br Med J 1989;299: 1247.
178. Rosenberg L, Palmer JR, Zauber AG, et al. A hypothesis: nonsteroidal anti-inflammatory drugs reduce the incidence of large bowel cancer. J Natl Cancer Inst 1991;83:355.
179. Gann PH, Manson JE, Glyn RJ, et al. Low-dose aspirin and incidence of colorectal cancers in a randomized trial. J Natl Cancer Inst 1993; 85:1220.
180. Arjmandi BH, Hollis BW, Kalv DN. In vivo effect of 17-beta estradiol on intestinal calcium absorption in rats. Bone and Mineral 1994;26: 181.
181. Slattery ML, Sorenson AW, Ford MH. Dietary calcium intake as a mitigating factor in colon cancer. Am J Epidemiol 1988;128:504.
182. Heilbrun LK, Hankin JH, Nomura A, et al. Colon cancer and dietary fat, phosphorus, and calcium in Hawaii Japanese American men. Am J Clin Nutr 1986;43:306.
183. Stemmermann GN, Nomura A, Chyou PH. The influence of dairy and nondairy calcium or subsite large-bowel cancer risk. Dis Colon Rectum 1990;33:190.
184. National Center for Health Statistics. Dietary intake source data [from the Health and Nutrition Examination Survey II]: 1976–1980. Vital and health statistics series 11, no. 231. DHHS Publication No. 83-1681. Washington, DC: 1983.
185. Murphy SP, Calloway D. II. Nutrient intakes of women in NHANES II, emphasizing trace minerals, fiber, and phytate. J Am Diet Assoc 1986;86:1366.
186. National Academy of Sciences—National Research Council, Food and Nutrition Board, Subcommittee on the Tenth Edition of the RDAS. Recommended dietary allowances. 10th ed. Washington, DC: National Academy Press, 1989.
187. National Institutes of Health, Osteoporosis Consensus Panel. Consensus conference on osteoporosis. JAMA 1984;252:799.
191. Block G, Cox C, Madans J, et al. Vitamin supplementation use, by demographic characteristics. Am J Epidemiol 1988;127:297.
192. Subar AF, Bowering J. The contribution of enrichment and fortification to the nutrient intake of women. J Am Diet Assoc 1988;88:1237.
193. Webb AR, Holick MF. The role of sunlight in cutaneous production of vitamin D_3. Annu Rev Nutr 1988;8:375.
194. Holick MF. In Norman T, et al, eds. Vitamin D, chemical and clinical update. New York: Walter de Gruyter, 1988:925.
195. Lawson DEM, Paul AA, Black AE, Cole TJ, Mandal AR, Davie M. Relative contribution of diet and sunlight to vitamin D status of the elderly. Br Med J 1979;2:303.
196. Omdahl JL, Garry PJ, Hunsaker LA, Hunt WC, Goodwin JS. Nutritional status in a healthy elderly population: vitamin D. Am J Clin Nutr 1982;36:1225.
197. Lukert BP, Carey M, McCarty B, et al. Influence of nutritional factors on calcium-regulating hormones and bone loss. Calcif Tissue Int 1987; 40:119.
198. Delvin EE, Imbach A, Copti M. Vitamin D nutritional status and related biochemical indices in an autonomous elderly population. Am J Clin Nutr 1988;48:373.
199. Lips P, van Ginkel FC, Jongen MJ, Rubertus F, van der Vigh WJ, Netelenbos JC. Determinants of vitamin D status in patients with hip fracture and in elderly control subjects. Am J Clin Nutr 1987;46:1005.
200. Vir SC, Love AH. Nutritional status of institutionalized and noninstitutionalized aged in Belfast, Northern Ireland. Am J Clin Nutr 1979; 32:1934.
201. Lambert-Allardt C. Vitamin D intake, sunlight exposure and 25-hydroxyvitamin D levels in the elderly during one year. Ann Nutr Metab 1984;28:144.
202. Lambert-Allardt C, von Knorring J, Slatis P, Holmström T. Vitamin D status and concentrations of serum vitamin D metabolites and osteocalcin in elderly patients with femoral neck fracture: a follow-up study. Eur J Clin Nutr 1989;43:355.
203. Parfitt AM, Gallagher JC, Heaney RP, Johnson CC, Neer R, Whedon GD. Vitamin D and bone health in the elderly. Am J Clin Nutr 1982; 36(Suppl):1014.
204. McKenna MJ, Freaney R, Meade A, Muldowney FP. Prevention of hypovitaminosis D in the elderly. Calcif Tissue Int 1985;37:112.
205. Holmberg I, Larsson A. Seasonal variation of vitamin D3 and 25-hydroxyvitamin D_3 in human serum. Clin Chim Acta 1980;100:173.
206. Bouillon RA, Auwerx JH, Lissens WD, Pelemans WK. Vitamin D status in the elderly: seasonal substrate deficiency causes 1,25-dihydroxycholecalciferol deficiency. Am J Clin Nutr 1987;45:755.
207. Juttmann JR, Visser TJ, Buurman C, et al. Seasonal fluctuations in serum concentrations of vitamin D metabolites in normal subjects. Br Med J 1981;282:1349.
208. Chesney RW, Rosen JF, Hamstra AJ, et al. Absence of seasonal variation in serum concentrations of 1,25-dihydroxyvitamin D despite a rise in 25-hydroxyvitamin D in summer. J Clin Endocrinol Metab 1981;53:139.
209. Netelenbos JC, Jongen MJM, van der Vijgh, et al. Vitamin D

status in urinary calcium stone formation. Arch Intern Med 1985; 145:681.
210. Ney DM, et al. The low oxalate diet book for the prevention of oxalate kidney stones. San Diego, CA: University of California at San Diego Medical Center, 1981.
211. Barrett-Connor EL. The RDA for calcium: too little, too late. Calcif Tissue Int 1989.
212. Holbrook TL, Barrett-Connor E, Wingard DL. Dietary calcium and risk of hip fracture: 14-year prospective study. Lancet 1988;2:1046.
213. National Research Council. Nutrient requirements of laboratory animals. No. 10. 3rd ed. Washington, DC: National Academy of Sciences, 1978.
214. Marcus R, Plimpton J. Guide to Japanese food. Tokyo: Shufunotomo, 1984:75.

Surgery for Gastrointestinal Cancer: A Multidisciplinary Approach, edited by Harold J. Wanebo.
Lippincott-Raven Publishers, Philadelphia, © 1997.

CHAPTER 2

Screening, Detection, and Early Diagnosis of Gastrointestinal Cancer

John H. Bond

Attempts to reduce the great mortality from gastrointestinal (GI) malignancies are hindered by the fact that, as a group, these cancers tend to be at an advanced stage when they cause symptoms.[1] In most GI malignancies, however, diagnosis at an earlier, asymptomatic stage greatly improves survival. This chapter discusses strategies of screening, surveillance, and early diagnosis of GI malignancies that are designed either to prevent cancer altogether or reduce cancer morbidity and mortality. This approach is based on the careful assessment of risk factors, accurate and prompt evaluation of early symptoms, cost-effective screening, and appropriate posttreatment surveillance.

SYMPTOMS OF GASTROINTESTINAL MALIGNANCY

Table 2-1 lists the most common presenting symptoms of upper and lower tract malignancy. Early symptoms of upper GI tumors include dysphagia, nausea and vomiting, early satiety, abdominal discomfort, and GI bleeding. Early signs and symptoms of colorectal cancer (CRC) include rectal bleeding, a change in bowel movement pattern, and cramping abdominal pain. The presence of these signs or symptoms in cancer-age patients, especially if unexplained by other obvious causes, should prompt an immediate evaluation for possible GI neoplasia. Signs and symptoms of advanced cancer include weight loss, abdominal pain, bowel obstruction, perforation, and a palpable abdominal mass. Surgical cure is rarely possible when diagnosis is delayed until the onset of these advanced manifestations of GI malignancy.

Abdominal pain, colicky or steady, is the most common symptom of small bowel malignancy. About one third of patients have symptoms of partial or complete small bowel obstruction due to constricting growth of the tumor, blockage of the lumen by the tumor itself, or, rarely, as the result of intussusception. Initially, obstructive symptoms are often intermittent. Weight loss and bleeding occur in about half of patients with small bowel malignancy, and a palpable abdominal mass or perforation occurs in about 40% and 10%, respectively. Periampullary tumors usually present with painless obstructive jaundice.[2] Malignant carcinoids most often present with local obstructive symptoms due to the growth of the tumor or to the desmoplastic reaction that occurs in the mesentery as the tumor begins to spread. Rarely, these patients present with symptoms of the carcinoid syndrome as the result of compounds released by tumor metastases into the circulation.[3]

DIAGNOSIS OF GASTROINTESTINAL MALIGNANCY

Upper GI tract malignancies are diagnosed either by barium radiographic studies or endoscopy. Double-contrast barium upper GI series, when properly carried out, can detect the presence of most cancers of the esophagus and stomach. However, because of its greater accuracy, especially for small or superficial lesions, as well as its capability for obtaining tissue samples for histologic or cytologic study, esophagogastroduodenoscopy has become the primary diagnostic method for detecting or ruling out early upper tract malignancy or premalignant conditions.[4] Although initially more costly than radiographic studies, esophagogastroduodenoscopy is highly accurate and definitive, and the procedure is safe and well tolerated by most patients.

Colonoscopy is the procedure of choice for detecting early colorectal neoplasia. It is more accurate than double-contrast barium enema (DCBE), especially in the diagnosis of superficial lesions or smaller polypoid tumors. The entire large bowel can be examined at one sitting with a single preparation in over 95% of patients.[5] Performed by well trained and experienced gastroenterologists or GI surgeons, the procedure is safe and usually well tolerated. A carefully controlled, single-blinded study comparing the accuracy of colonoscopy and DCBE performed at the same time period in the same patients demonstrated an accuracy for detecting polyps of 94% and 67%, re-

Professor of Medicine, University of Minnesota, Chief, Gastrointestinal Section (111D), Minneapolis VA Medical Center, One Veterans Drive, Minneapolis, MN, 55417.

TABLE 2-1. *Signs and symptoms of gastrointestinal malignancy*

	Early	Late
Upper tract	Dysphagia	Weight loss
	Nausea and vomiting	Obstruction
	Abdominal discomfort	Mass
	Satiety	Abdominal pain
	GI bleeding	
Small bowel	Cramping pain	Weight loss
	GI bleeding	Mass
		Perforation
		Abdominal pain
Lower tract	GI bleeding	Weight loss
	Change in bowel habits	Obstruction
		Mass
	Cramping pain	Perforation
		Abdominal pain

GI, gastrointestional.

spectively.[6] In an investigation of colonoscopy accuracy, tandem colonoscopies performed by two different examiners in 96 patients indicated a miss rate of 14.7% for polyps of 8 mm diameter or less, but no larger lesions went undetected by the first colonoscopy.[7] An additional advantage of colonoscopy over DCBE is the ability immediately to take biopsy samples of suspect lesions and resect most detected polyps.

Complications of bleeding or perforation, although rare, occur more frequently during colonoscopy (0.1% to 0.4%) than with DCBE (0.02%).[8,9] The cost of colonoscopy is appreciably greater than the cost of the alternative evaluation with DCBE plus proctosigmoidoscopy (needed to assess accurately the rectosigmoid colon). Although these cost and risk differences may appear to favor DCBE over colonoscopy, the need to do a subsequent colonoscopy in the 30% to 40% of patients suspected of colorectal neoplasia who will be found to have an abnormality detected by DCBE, makes the two alternative diagnostic strategies, on the average, equally expensive and risky.

Barium radiographic studies are used to diagnose most malignancies of the small bowel.[10] Enteroclysis is 20% to 30% more accurate than conventional small bowel follow-through, even when abdominal compression is used, and should be requested if a suspected tumor is not detected by small bowel follow-through. Barium enema with reflux into the terminal ileum may detect ileal lesions, especially during the evaluation of distal small bowel obstruction. Arteriography may be indicated when the cause of gastrointestinal bleeding is not revealed by barium studies and endoscopy. Noninvasive scanning studies, computed tomography and ultrasonography, may help delineate the nature of a palpable abdominal mass. Standard upper GI endoscopy, or upper endoscopy using a side-viewing endoscope, diagnoses lesions of the first and second parts of the duodenum, including the periampullary area. Colonoscopy allows examination of about 10 cm of the terminal ileum in about 85% of cases. "Push-enteroscopy," a procedure in which a colonoscope or one of the newly available long upper GI endoscopes is passed though the mouth into the small bowel, is capable of detecting tumors located up to 30 to 40 cm beyond the ligament of Treitz.[11] Finally, a few reports indicate successful diagnosis of more distal lesions with very long "Sonde endoscopes," which are passively advanced through the small bowel over several

TABLE 2-2. *Premalignant disorders of the upper gastrointestinal tract*

Disorder	Malignancy
Achalasia	Esophagus (squamous)
Lye stricture	Esophagus (squamous)
Tylosis	Esophagus (squamous)
Barrett's esophagus	Esophagus (adenocarcinoma)
Gastric polyps	Stomach (adenocarcinoma)
Postgastrectomy	Stomach (adenocarcinoma)
Familial adenomatous polyposis	Duodenum (adenocarcinoma [ampullary])

hours and then are withdrawn while the lumen is visualized. This procedure is used mainly for patients with unexplained intestinal bleeding, is expensive and not widely available, cannot be used in the presence of bowel obstruction, and requires further outcome analysis.

UPPER GASTROINTESTINAL TRACT MALIGNANCIES

Upper GI tract malignancies are often associated with diseases or disorders that are considered premalignant conditions. Considerable indirect information suggests that surveillance of selected people with these conditions may lead to early diagnosis of cancer and improved survival, although results of randomized, controlled trials are lacking. Likewise, there has been very little evidence that mortality from upper GI tract malignancy has been favorably affected by current efforts. Table 2-2 lists possible premalignant upper GI tract disorders.

Achalasia

Squamous cell carcinoma of the esophagus occurs in a small percentage of patients with longstanding achalasia.[12,13] Inadequate or delayed initial treatment of achalasia is reported in many of these patients with esophageal malignancies; however, the cancers may not be entirely prevented by successful dilatation or surgical therapy. On the average, cancers develop 15 to 20 years after diagnosis.[14] Chronic stasis and inflammation are believed to cause dysplasia and subsequent malignant degeneration. These cancers are usually advanced by the time they cause symptoms of dysphagia, probably because they grow in a chronically dilated esophagus and therefore obstruct late. Although data are lacking to prove the efficacy of surveillance in patients with achalasia, some experts recommend periodic endoscopy with biopsies every 2 to 3 years in selected patients.[15] This surveillance may be considered for the rare patient who has longstanding disease without effective treatment, or for the patient who is successfully treated late in the course of disease.

Lye Stricture

People with lye strictures of the esophagus have a high frequency of development of squamous cell carcinoma of the esophagus many years after caustic ingestion. The risk of cancer is estimated to be at least 1000 times greater than that of the average population.[16,17] Cancers developing 15 to 50 years after the initial lye ingestion (mean, 40 years) tend to occur in the mid-esophagus, and produce symptoms early, probably because the esophageal lumen is already compromised by longstanding fibrosis. Postsurgical resection prognosis is therefore relatively good for these esophageal cancers, with a reported 5-year survival of about 33%.[18] Esophagoscopy is recommended for these patients every 2 to 3 years, beginning 15 to 20 years after the lye ingestion. Any new symptoms of dysphagia occurring in these patients should also be promptly evaluated with endoscopy.

Tylosis

Tylosis is a rare autosomal dominant genetic disorder causing hyperkeratoses of the palms and soles, and a high predisposition for squamous cell carcinoma of the esophagus.[19] Similar to the patient with lye stricture, endoscopic surveillance is recommended every 2 to 3 years beginning at age 30 years for affected members of tylosis families.

Barrett's Esophagus

Barrett's esophagus is the replacement of normal esophageal squamous epithelium with a specialized columnar epithelium in response to longstanding, severe gastroesophageal reflux.[20] The disease is usually defined as the displacement of the normal squamocolumnar junction at least 3 cm above the lower esophageal sphincter. The incidence of the condition is increasing and is reported in 5% to 10% of patients with reflux symptoms, 11% to 36% in patients with documented esophagitis, and over 40% of patients with peptic esophageal strictures.[21] Adenocarcinoma of the esophagus or the gastroesophageal junction has been reported in 8% to 15% of patients with Barrett's esophagus. Endoscopic surveillance studies suggest a cancer incidence of one in 52 to 175 patient years.[22] Surgical and medical treatment of reflux does not appear to reduce the risk of cancer.

There is a high correlation between the presence of high-grade dysplasia and carcinoma in patients with Barrett's esophagus. This has led to the widespread practice of performing periodic surveillance endoscopy every 1 to 2 years in patients with histologically documented Barrett's esophagus.[23] Because foci of dysplasia may be small and scattered throughout the abnormal metaplastic epithelium, multiple biopsies are usually recommended at each surveillance endoscopy. Although the efficacy and cost effectiveness of surveillance have not been documented in prospective trials, current guidelines recommend surveillance endoscopy with multiple biopsies for patients who are good surgical risks every 2 years.[24] Surgical esophagectomy is recommended for those found to have confirmed high-grade dysplasia or early cancer. Preliminary reports of ablative photodynamic therapy for patients at high risk for surgical intervention are promising.

Gastric Polyps

Most gastric polyps (70% to 90%) are hyperplastic and, like their counterpart in the colon, have little, if any, malignant potential.[25] Gastric adenomas, on the other hand, have a malignant potential similar to that of adenomas of the large bowel. Over 10% of gastric adenomas develop foci of carcinoma within 3 to 5 years. The American Society for Gastrointestinal Endoscopy has recommended endoscopic surveillance for gastric cancer only in patients who have had gastric adenomas resected.[26] When feasible, all gastric adenomas detected by endoscopy should be excised, especially if they are greater than 1 cm in diameter when the malignant risk becomes appreciable. Repeat surveillance endoscopy should then be done every 2 to 3 years to check for recurrences or the development of dysplasia in the gastric mucosa.

Postgastrectomy

Gastric cancer is reported in increased incidence in the gastric remnant after partial gastric resection for peptic ulcer disease.[27] Cumulative data from available series suggests a twofold to fourfold risk of gastric cancer beginning 15 years after the original surgery. Periodic endoscopic surveillance with biopsies has detected early cancer or dysplasia in 4% to 6% of these patients.[28] Some recommend periodic surveillance endoscopy with biopsies every 1 to 3 years beginning 15 to 20 years after gastric resection.[29] Outcome studies are needed to determine if this approach is cost effective and prevents death from gastric cancer.

Familial Adenomatous Polyposis

In patients with familial adenomatous polyposis (FAP), gastroduodenal polyps develop in 40% to 100% of reported cases.[30] Gastric polyps are usually fundic gland or hyperplastic polyps with little or no malignant potential. Duodenal polyps are usually adenomas that occur primarily in the periampullary region. These lesions carry a high risk for dysplasia and subsequent carcinoma.[31] Periodic endoscopic surveillance with multiple biopsies of any periampullary or duodenal lesion is indicated in patients with FAP. The detection of high-grade dysplasia is an indication for endoscopic ablative therapy or possibly more extensive surgical resection.[32] Further studies are needed to determine the frequency of surveillance endoscopy and the best treatment for adenomas and dysplasia.

MALIGNANCIES OF THE SMALL BOWEL

Malignant tumors of the small intestine comprise only 1% to 1.5% of all GI malignancies (annual age-adjusted incidence, 1/100,000 population).[33] In order of decreasing frequency, the four primary malignant tumors of the small bowel in the United States are adenocarcinoma, carcinoid, lymphoma, and leiomyosarcoma. Table 2-3 gives the relative frequency and location of each of these small bowel tumors.[34,35]

A number of primary conditions increase the risk of small bowel malignancies (Table 2-4). As discussed earlier, adenocarcinomas of the upper small bowel, especially the duodenum and periampullary region, occur in about 5% of patients with FAP.[36] These adenocarcinomas appear to arise from benign adenomas, which occur in about 40% of FAP patients. Adeno-

TABLE 2-3. *Relative frequency and location of small bowel malignancies*

	Relative frequency (%)	Location (%)		
		Duodenum	Jejunum	Ileum
Adenocarcinoma	42	40	38	22
Carcinoid	29	18	4	78
Lymphona	18	6	38	58
Leiomyosarcoma	11	3	53	44

carcinoma also is more common in patients with mucosal disease due to celiac sprue and Crohn's disease.[37,38] Longstanding inflammation, penetration of the mucosa by harmful antigens, and bacterial overgrowth in stagnant bowel may lead to dysplastic changes and cancer in patients with these conditions. Primary small bowel lymphomas are more common in patients with celiac sprue (T-cell lymphomas), and in those with diffuse nodular lymphoid hyperplasia and acquired immunodeficiency syndrome (AIDS).[39] Adenocarcinomas occasionally develop in patients with longstanding ileostomies, urinary ileoanastomoses, and neurofibromatosis.

With the exception of patients with FAP, no screening or surveillance strategies have been effective in patients with these predisposing small intestinal disorders. Rather, careful attention to symptoms of possibly complicating malignancy should prompt early evaluation, which may improve survival from these rare small bowel malignancies.

MALIGNANCIES OF THE LARGE BOWEL

Colorectal adenocarcinomas comprise nearly 99% of all large bowel malignancies. The disease is common (over 160,000 new cases in the United States annually) and lethal (over 65,000 annual deaths), yet readily curable when detected at an early stage (overall 5-year survival about 50%).[40] Complete surgical resection of all malignant tissue offers the only reasonable chance for cure, and postsurgical survival is roughly proportional to the anatomic extent of the tumor at the time of resection (Table 2-5). When detected before the development of symptoms, most CRCs are localized to the bowel wall (Dukes' A and B cancers), and the 5-year survival averages about 80%. By the time most CRCs cause symptoms, however, they have spread to regional lymph nodes or beyond, and the chance of cure is less than 40%.[41] Because no major curative advances in surgical, radiotherapeutic, or medical therapy are anticipated in the near future, the best hope for improving survival once cancers develop is to detect them at an earlier stage, preferably before they produce symptoms.

The Polyp–Cancer Sequence

Nearly all CRCs appear to arise in a previously benign neoplastic polyp (adenoma).[42] In a discontinuous sequence, colorectal neoplasia proceeds from normal mucosa, cellular proliferation, oncogene activation, and chromosomal deletion, to adenoma formation, growth, increasing dysplasia, and then adenocarcinoma. Pathologic correlations indicate that malignancy does not occur in hyperplastic polyps, rarely occurs in tubular adenomas, and is more common in tubulovillous and villous adenomas.[43] The larger an adenoma is, the more likely it is to contain invasive cancer.

Early detection and removal of colonic polyps should prevent the development of CRC in the first place (secondary prevention). Gilbertsen and Nelms reported that removal of rectal polyps during screening proctosigmoidoscopy decreased the subsequent incidence of rectal carcinoma by 85% in 21,000 subjects and totally eliminated mortality from rectal cancer.[44] More recently, Winawer and colleagues reported results from the National Polyp Study, a prospective multicenter trial of postpolypectomy surveillance, that showed that removal of polyps and postpolypectomy surveillance in over 1400 patients with adenomas reduced the subsequent incidence of CRC by up to 90%.[45]

Risk Factors for Colorectal Cancer

The major recognized risk factors for CRC include age over 50 years, a family history of colorectal neoplasia, a personal history of colorectal neoplasia, and longstanding inflammatory bowel disease. Most people are at "average risk" for colorectal neoplasia simply because they are older than 50 years of age, the time in life when the incidence begins to increase appreciably (Table 2-6). After age 50 years, the incidence approximately doubles with each decade of life.[40] A small fraction of the population are at lower-than-average risk because they have known cancer-free families or follow restricted life patterns (eg, Seventh-Day Adventists).

TABLE 2-4. *Conditions that increase the risk of small intestinal malignancy*

Condition	Tumor	Usual location
Familial adenomatous polyposis	Adenocarcinoma	Duodenum
Crohn's disease	Adenocarcinoma	Ileum
Celiac sprue	Adenocarcinoma, non-Hodgkin's lymphoma	Jejunum
Urinary-ileo anatomosis	Adenocarcinoma	Ileum
Ileostomy	Adenocarcinoma	Ileocutaneous junction
Nodular lymphoid hyperplasia, immunodeficiency syndromes	Non-Hodgkin's lymphoma	Ileum

TABLE 2-5. *Prognosis after surgical resection related to Dukes' stage*[14]

Duke's stage	5-Year survival (%)
Stage A (invasion of muscle)	80–90
Stage B (invasion of serosa)	70–80
Stage C (involvement of regional lymph nodes)	30–50

TABLE 2-7. *Hereditary risk for colorectal cancer*

1. Polyposis syndromes
   - Familial adenomatous polyposis
   - Gardner's syndrome
2. Hereditary nonpolyposis colorectal cancer
   - Site-specific colorectal cancer (Lynch syndrome I)
   - Cancer family syndrome (Lynch syndrome II)
3. Familial genetic risk for "sporadic" colorectal cancer

Inherited genetic factors have also been strongly implicated in the pathogenesis of CRC.[46–48] Table 2-7 lists the three types of genetic/familial patterns currently recognized. The most intriguing and potentially important discovery in this area is the likelihood that even the ''sporadic cancers,'' which previously were believed to be environmentally induced, may have an underlying genetic predisposing cause. Epidemiologic studies show a threefold increased risk of CRC for people with one first-degree relative with the disease, and pedigree studies of polyp incidence patterns by Burt and colleagues suggest that 50% to 100% of sporadic cancers may be ultimately caused by a genetic predisposition to the disease.[49] Whether a cancer develops in a given person may depend on the combination of the inherited genetic trait plus superimposed environmental factors. Hereditary CRC syndromes are discussed in detail in Chapter 5.

Besides age and a family history of CRC cancer, the two main risk factors for the disease are a personal past history of CRC or adenomas, and chronic ulcerative colitis. Two studies from the Mayo Clinic provide estimates of the risk of cancer after polypectomy. Spencer and coworkers in 1984 reported the results of 10,000 person-years of follow-up of 751 patients who had undergone fulguration of small colorectal polyps.[50] They found no increased incidence of subsequent cancer in this group. In contrast, the same investigators reported in 1986 that patients with larger polyps (>1 cm) had a risk for development of metachronous cancer that was 2.7 times greater than expected, and those with multiple polyps had a relative risk 5 times greater than expected.[51]

Another study of the risk of CRC after excision of rectosigmoid adenomas was reported from St. Mark's Hospital, London.[52] A group of 1618 patients who had rectosigmoid adenomas resected during proctoscopy with no further surveillance were followed a mean of 14 years (22,462 person-years). The incidence of subsequent rectal cancer was similar to that of the general population. However, 80% of the rectal cancers occurred in people who had incompletely resected index adenomas. Patients with index adenomas that were tubulovillous, villous, or large (≥1 cm) had a 3.6-fold increased subsequent incidence of colon cancer, and those with multiple index adenomas of this type had a 6.6-fold increased incidence of metachronous cancer. Those with only small tubular adenomas (≥1 cm), whether single or multiple, had a subsequent incidence of cancer similar to that of the general population.

TABLE 2-6. *Age-specific incidence rates (per 100,000 population) for cancers of the colon and rectum*

Age (y)	Men	Women
30–34	2.5	2.4
40–44	12.3	11.9
50–54	57.2	46.3
60–64	169.9	105.7
70–74	320.5	226.9
80–84	463.5	365.5

In another Mayo Clinic study, Stryker and associates performed a retrospective evaluation of 226 patients with large polyps (≥1 cm) detected by barium enema before the availability of colonoscopy.[53] Follow-up of these untreated patients showed that 37% of the polyps enlarged, 21 invasive carcinomas developed at a polyp site, and 11 carcinomas developed at another site. The cumulative risk of cancer at 5, 10, and 20 years was 2.5%, 8%, and 24%, respectively. This study supports the need to excise all colorectal polyps 1 cm or greater in size, and the need for periodic surveillance to identify metachronous neoplasms as a site in the colon remote from the index polyp.

A prospective study by Grossman and colleagues showed that patients with a single index tubular adenoma 10 mm or less in size who had no first-degree relatives with CRC, had only a 3% prevalence of clinically significant metachronous neoplasms on follow-up colonoscopy.[54] Subgroups with more advanced adenomas (≥10 mm, tubulovillous or villous, severely dysplastic, or invasive carcinoma) had a prevalence of subsequent adenomas of 8% to 18%. The incidence of synchronous cancers and adenomas in a patient with one known cancer is 2% to 7% and 25% 50%, respectively. Metachronous cancers and adenomas develop in 3% to 10% and 20% to 40%, respectively.[55] Pathologic reviews and an analysis by the National Polyp Study indicate that it takes an average of 10 years for a gross cancer to develop from a ''clean'' colon.[42,56] Surveillance for patients undergoing a curative resection for CRC is discussed in detail in Chapter 6.

Carcinoma of the colon and rectum occurs much more frequently in patients with chronic ulcerative colitis than in the general population.[57] Clinically, risk of cancer is strongly related to both the duration and extent of disease. Patients with pancolitis appear to have minimal risk until after 8 to 10 years of disease activity. Thereafter, the excess risk increases rapidly to over 20 times that of the general population by 20 years of disease, and to over 30 times by 30 years. Patients with left-sided colitis are also at increased risk; however, cancers tend to develop about 10 years later than in patients with universal colitis. People with ulcerative colitis limited to the rectum and sigmoid colon appear to have no appreciably increased risk. In ulcerative colitis, the distribution of cancer is uniform throughout the colon, and at times is multifocal.[58]

Histologic dysplasia often precedes or occurs with the malignant transformation in the mucosa, and colonoscopic surveillance with multiple mucosal biopsies therefore has the potential to identify those people at greatest risk. Surveillance usually is recommended every 2 years in most patients. Detection of significant dysplasia is considered an indication for colectomy. Efficacy and cost effectiveness of colonoscopic surveillance in ulcerative colitis has not yet been demonstrated in prospective clinical trials. The risk of cancer and the limitations of surveillance, especially after 20 years of colitis, must be presented for careful consideration by each patient in whom surveillance is planned.

Carcinoma of the colon also occurs more frequently in patients with longstanding Crohn's colitis. However, the risk appears to be less than that seen in ulcerative colitis, and because it may not be as consistently associated with mucosal dysplasia, surveillance usually is not recommended.[59]

Postpolypectomy Surveillance

Because of the increased subsequent risk of CRC, most patients undergoing colonoscopic polypectomy are advised to have periodic colonoscopic surveillance to detect metachronous polyps. A report from the National Polyp Study indicates that an initial follow-up colonoscopy 3 years after polypectomy will protect the patient from advanced neoplasia.[60] The American College of Gastroenterology has developed a comprehensive guideline for polyp management and follow-up that is based on available scientific data, including those of the National Polyp Study.[61] As outlined in this guideline, subsequent postpolypectomy surveillance should be tailored to the individual needs and situation of each patient. After an initial negative follow-up examination, subsequent colonoscopy usually is not needed for 5 years. People with only a single small tubular adenoma have such a small subsequent risk of cancer that no follow-up surveillance may be indicated. Last, it is important to discontinue surveillance according to advanced age and comorbidity when further follow-up is unlikely to benefit the patient.

Screening for Colorectal Cancer

Colorectal cancer is highly suitable for a screening approach. The disease is common and lethal, and therefore warrants the expenditure of public health resources. As discussed earlier, it has an unusually long preclinical phase during which it is readily detectable and treatable. Accurate, safe, and well tolerated diagnostic tests are available for the disease, and without question, early detection improves survival.

Only two methods—flexible sigmoidoscopy and fecal occult blood tests (FOBT)—are available for screening for CRC that are potentially capable of satisfying the criteria established by the World Health Organization for a screening test.[62] According to this standard, a test may be promoted for general public health screening if it satisfies the following criteria:

1. It improves mortality and function; this should not be confused with apparent prolongation of survival due to earlier diagnosis
2. It is simple and inexpensive so as to be widely available to the target population
3. Adequate compliance is achievable
4. Long-term benefits outweigh long-term detriments
5. There is proof of benefit to the screened community
6. The cost–benefit and cost–effectiveness ratios are known, and the harmful effects of the disease must be a measurable burden and must compare favorably to the known cost, sensitivity, specificity, and acceptance of the screening test

Flexible sigmoidoscopy performed by experienced, well trained examiners is safe, well tolerated, accurate, reasonably inexpensive, and capable of detecting 50% to 70% of all colorectal neoplasia.[63] All that is known about the procedure suggests that its widespread use in the average-risk population should reduce mortality from CRC. However, efficacy for CRC screening remains unproven because there has never been a definitive, randomized, controlled trial performed. Long-term descriptive studies using rigid proctoscopy suggested that screening examinations of the rectum can greatly reduce the incidence and mortality of rectal cancer.[44] Two more recent case-controlled studies suggested that screening with flexible sigmoidoscopy every 10 years or less might reduce mortality from cancer of the distal colon and rectum by 60% to 70%.[64,65] A large, National Cancer Institute-funded multicenter trial using flexible sigmoidoscopy is underway.

Five long-term controlled trials are evaluating the efficacy of FOBT screening for CRC.[66–70] All have published preliminary data that indicate that the method is feasible, high compliance can be achieved, cancers are detected at an earlier stage, and survival from cancer appears to be increased.[71,72] Because of the confounding effects of length and lead-time bias, neither stage nor survival are considered valid indicators of screening efficacy for this disease. The method will have proven efficacy only if it is shown to reduce mortality from CRC. All of the five prospective trials use the Hemoccult (SmithKline Diagnostics, San Jose, California) guaiac slide test.

The Minnesota fecal occult blood screening trial, begun in 1975, reported the first definitive mortality results in May, 1993.[73] Using largely a rehydrated Hemoccult screening method that has a higher sensitivity for detecting blood than the standard Hemoccult slide, a 33% reduction in mortality was demonstrated in participants screened annually compared to control subjects. This highly statistically and clinically significant result was accompanied by improved survival in those with CRC, and by a marked reduction in the number of incurable stage D cancers.

The results of the Minnesota trial have been corroborated by the New York study, which reported a marginally significant 43% reduction in CRC mortality when FOBTs were added to sigmoidoscopy screening compared to sigmoidoscopy alone.[74] In addition, a U.S. case–control study reported a mortality reduction of 31% as the result of FOBT screening.[75]

In conclusion, definitive scientific data are now available supporting the efficacy of screening for CRC. Widespread use of these methods in the average-risk population has the ability to detect early curable cancers, and to detect and remove premalignant polyps. These data strongly support the current recommendations of the American Cancer Society, the National Cancer Institute, and the World Health Organization Collaborating Center for Colorectal Cancer. These recommendations are as follows:

1. People concerned about cancer should undergo a general health evaluation with a careful search for possible symp-

toms of early cancer and an assessment of special risk factors.
2. Asymptomatic, average-risk patients should undergo flexible sigmoidoscopy and FOBT at age 50 years.
3. Primary colonoscopy is recommended for symptoms or for a positive screening test.
4. Average-risk, asymptomatic patients with negative screening tests should have annual FOBTs and flexible sigmoidoscopy every 5 years.
5. As with every medical strategy, this approach should be modified appropriately depending on age, comorbidity, and the individual desires or anxieties of patients.

Cost Effectiveness of Screening

Preliminary analyses by the Congressional Office of Technology and by the National Cancer Institute assessed the cost effectiveness of FOBT screening for CRC.[76,77] These analyses indicate that this approach would cost between $25,000 and $35,000 per year of life saved. This figure is similar to that for screening mammography for breast cancer, as well as other services currently deemed cost effective. Thus, although screening for CRC is costly, when balanced against the higher cost of missing a curable cancer, it appears to be cost effective.

REFERENCES

1. Luk GD. Cancer surveillance strategies. In: Sleisenger M, Fordtran J, eds. Gastrointestinal disease. 5th ed. Philadelphia: WB Saunders, 1993: 115.
2. Galandiuk S, Hermann RE, Jagelman DG, et al. Villous tumors of the duodenum. Ann Surg 1988;207:234.
3. Creutzfeld W, Stockmann F. Carcinoids and carcinoid syndrome. Am J Med 1987;82:4.
4. Tytgat GN. Benign and malignant tumors of the esophagus. In: Sivak M, ed. Gastroenterologic endoscopy. Philadelphia: WB Saunders, 1987:373.
5. Knutson CO, Max MH. Diagnostic and therapeutic colonoscopy: a critical review of 663 examinations. Arch Surg 1979;114:430.
6. Hogan WJ, Stewart ET, Geenen JE, et al. A prospective comparison of the accuracy of colonoscopy vs air-barium contrast exam for detection of colonic polypoid lesions. Gastrointest Endosc 1977;23:230.
7. Hixson LJ, Fennerty MB, Sampliner RE, et al. Prospective blinded trial of the colonoscopic miss-rate of large colorectal polyps. Gastrointest Endosc 1991;32:125.
8. Rankin GB. Indications, contraindications, and complications of colonoscopy. In: Sivak MV, ed. Gastroenterologic endoscopy. Philadelphia: WB Saunders, 1987:874.
9. Dodd GD. The radiologic diagnosis of carcinoma of the colon in gastrointestinal cancer. In: Stroehlein JR, Romsodahl MM, eds. Gastrointestinal cancer. New York: Raven Press, 1981:311.
10. Nolan DJ. Barium examination of the small intestine. Gut 1981;22: 682.
11. Lewis BS, Waye JD. Small bowel enteroscopy in 1988: pros and cons. Am J Gastroenterol 1988;83:799.
12. Chuong JJH, DuBovik S, McCallum RW. Achalasia as a risk factor for esophageal carcinoma: a reappraisal. Dig Dis Sci 1984;29:1105.
13. Aggestrup S, Holm JC, Sorensen HR. Does achalasia predispose to cancer of the esophagus? Chest 1992;102:1013.
14. Carter R, Brewer LA. Achalasia and esophageal carcinoma: studies in early diagnosis for improved surgical management. Am J Surg 1975; 130:114.
15. Eckardt VF, Junginger T, Gabbert HE, Bettendorf U. Superficial esophageal carcinoma in achalasia, detected by endoscopic surveillance. Z Gastroenterol 1992;30:411.
16. Leape LL, Ashcraft KW, Scarpelli DG, et al. Hazard to health: liquid lye. N Engl J Med 1971;248:232.
17. Applegvist P, Salmo M. Lye corrosion carcinoma of the esophagus. Cancer 1980;45:2655.
18. Hopkins RA, Postlethwait RW. Caustic burns and carcinoma of the esophagus. Ann Surg 1982;194:146.
19. Marger RS, Marger D. Carcinoma of the esophagus and tylosis: a lethal genetic combination. Cancer 1993;72:17.
20. Reid BJ. Barrett's esophagus and esophageal adenocarcinoma. Gastroenterol Clin North Am 1992;20:817.
21. Cameron AJ, Zinsmeister AR, Ballard DJ, Carney AJ. Prevalence of columnar lined (Barrett's) esophagus: comparison of populations-based clinical and autopsy findings. Gastroenterology 1990;99:912.
22. Spechler SJ. Endoscopic surveillance for patients with Barrett's esophagus: does the risk justify the practice. Ann Intern Med 1987;106:902.
23. Robertson CS, Mayberry JF, Nicholson DA, James PD, Atkinson M. Value of endoscopic surveillance in the detection of neoplastic change in Barrett's oesophagus. Br J Surg 1988;75:760.
24. Levine DS, Haggitt RC, Blount PL, Rabinovitch PS, Rusch VW, Reid BJ. An endoscopic biopsy protocol can differentiate high-grade dysplasia from early adenocarcinoma in Barrett's esophagus. Gastroenterology 1993;105:40.
25. Cristallini E, Ascani S, Bolis G. Association between histologic type of polyp and carcinoma in the stomach. Gastrointest Endosc 1992;28: 481.
26. The role of endoscopy in the surveillance of premalignant conditions of the upper gastrointestinal tract. Guideline of the American Society for Gastrointestinal Endoscopy. Gastrointest Endosc 1988;34:18S.
27. Stalnikowicz R, Benbassat J. Risk of gastric cancer after gastric surgery for benign disorders. Arch Intern Med 1990;150:2022.
28. Greene FL. Gastroscopic screening of the post-gastrectomy stomach. Am Surg 1989;55:12.
29. Stael von Holstein C, Eriksson S, Huldt B, Hammar E. Endoscopic screening during 17 years for gastric stump carcinoma: a prospective clinical trial. Scand J Gastroenterol 1991;26:1020.
30. Sarre RG, Frost AG, Jagelman DG, Petras RE, Sivak MV, McGannon E. Gastric and duodenal polyps in familial adenomatous polyposis: a prospective study of the nature and prevalence of upper gastrointestinal polyps. Gut 1987;28:306.
31. Johan G, Offerhaus A, Giardiello M, et al. The risk of upper gastrointestinal cancer in familial adenomatous polyposis. Gastroenterology 1992; 102:1980.
32. van Stolk R, Sivak MV Jr, Petrini JL, Petras R, Ferguson DR, Jagelman D. Endoscopic management of upper gastrointestinal polyps and periampullary lesions in familial adenomatous polyposis and Gardner's syndrome. Endoscopy 1987;19(Suppl 1):19.
33. Darling RC, Welch CE. Tumors of the small intestine. N Engl J Med 1959;260:297.
34. Zollinger RM, Sternfeld CW, Schreiber H. Primary neoplasms of the small intestine. Am J Surg 1986;151:654.
35. Wilson JM, Melvin DB, Gray GF, Thorbjarnarson B. Primary malignancies of the small bowel: a report of 96 cases and review of the literature. Ann Surg 1974;180:175.
36. Kurtz RC, Sternberg SS, Miller HH, DeCosse JJ. Upper gastrointestinal neoplasia in familial polyposis. Dig Dis Sci 1987;32:459.
37. Swinson CM, Slavin G, Coles EC, Booth CC. Coeliac disease and malignancy. Lancet 1983;1:111.
38. Petras RE, Mir-Madjilessi SH, Farmer RG. Crohn's disease and intestinal carcinoma. Gastroenterology 1987;93:1307.
39. Cooper BT, Holmes GKT, Ferguson R, Cookie WT. Celiac disease and malignancy. Medicine (Baltimore) 1980;59:249.
40. Silverberg E, Lubera J. Cancer statistics, 1988. CA Cancer J Clin 1988; 38:5.
41. Falterman KW, Hill CB, Markey DC, et al. Cancer of the colon, rectum, and anus: a review of 2313 cases. Cancer 1974;34:951.
42. Morson BC. Evolution of cancer of the colon and rectum. Cancer 1974; 34:845.
43. Fenoglio CM, Pascal RR. Colorectal adenomas and cancer: pathologic relationships. Cancer 1982;50:2601.
44. Gilbertsen VA, Nelms JM. The prevention of invasive cancer of the rectum. Cancer 1978;41:1137.
45. Winawer SJ, Zauber AG, Ho MN, et al. Prevention of colorectal cancer by colonoscopic polypectomy. N Engl J Med 1993;329:1977.
46. Bodmer WF, Bailey CJ, Bodmer J, et al. Localization of the gene for

familial adenomatous polyposis on chromosome 5. Nature 1987;328: 614.
47. Lynch HT, Watson P, Kriegler M, et al. Differential diagnosis of hereditary nonpolyposis colorectal cancer (Lynch syndrome I and Lynch syndrome II). Dis Colon Rectum 1988;31:372.
48. Anderson DE. Risk in families of patients with colon cancer. In: Winawer S, Schottenfeld D, Sherlock P, eds. Colorectal cancer: prevention, epidemiology, and screening. New York: Raven Press, 1990:109.
49. Burt RW, Bishop DT, Cannon LA, et al. Dominant inheritance of adenomatous colonic polyps and colorectal cancer. N Engl J Med 1985; 312:1540.
50. Spencer RJ, Melton LJ III, Ready RL, et al. Treatment of small colorectal polyps: a population-based study of risk of subsequent carcinoma. Mayo Clin Proc 1984;59:305.
51. Lotfi AM, Spencer RJ, Illstrup DM, et al. Colorectal polyps and the risk of subsequent carcinoma. Mayo Clin Proc 1986;61:337.
52. Atkin WS, Morson BC, Cuzick J. Long-term risk of colorectal cancer after excision of rectosigmoid adenomas. N Engl J Med 1992;326:658.
53. Stryker SJ, Wolff BG, Culp CE, et al. Natural history of untreated colonic polyps. Gastroenterology 1987;93:1009.
54. Grossman S, Milos ML, Tekawa IS, et al. Colonoscopic screening for persons with suspected risk factors for colon cancer: II. past history of colorectal neoplasms. Gastroenterology 1989;96:299.
55. Lockhart-Mummery HE, Heald RJ. Metachronous cancer of the large intestine. Dis Colon Rectum 1972;15:261.
56. Winawer SJ, Zauber A, Diaz B. Temporal sequence of evolving colorectal cancer from the normal colon. Gastrointest Endosc 1987;33:167.
57. Yardley JH, Ransohoff DF, Riddell RH, et al. Cancer in inflammatory bowel diseases: how serious is the problem and what should be done about it? Gastroenterology 1983;85:197.
58. Lennard-Jones J. Cancer risk in ulcerative colitis: surveillance or surgery. Br J Surg 1985;72:584.
59. Sachal DB. Cancer in inflammatory bowel disease. In: Goebell H, Peskar BM, Malchow H, eds. Inflammatory bowel disease: basic research and clinical implications. New York: MTP Press, 1988:289.
60. Winawer SJ, Zauber AG, O'Brien MJ, et al. Randomized comparison of surveillance intervals after colonoscopic removal of newly diagnosed adenomatous polyps. N Engl J Med 1993;328:901.
61. Bond JH. Polyp guideline: Diagnosis, treatment, and surveillance for patients with nonfamilial colorectal polyps. Ann Intern Med 1993;119: 836.
62. Snauck R. World Health Organization for screening. In: Winawer S, Schottenfeld D, Sherlock D, eds. Colorectal cancer: prevention, epidemiology, and screening. New York: Raven Press, 1980:175.
63. Winnan G, Berci G, Panish J, et al. Superiority of the flexible to the rigid sigmoidoscope in routine proctosigmoidoscopy. N Engl J Med 1980;302:1011.
64. Selby JV, Friedman GD, Quesenberry CP Jr, et al. A case-control study of screening sigmoidoscopy and mortality from colorectal cancer. N Engl J Med 1992;326:653.
65. Newcomb PA, Norfleet RG, Storer BE, et al. Screening sigmoidoscopy and colorectal cancer mortality. J Natl Cancer Inst 1992;84:1572.
66. Flehinger BJ, Herbert E, Winawer SJ, et al. Screening for colorectal cancer with fecal occult blood test and sigmoidoscopy: preliminary report of the colon project of Memorial Sloan-Kettering Cancer Center and PMI-Strang Clinic. In: Chamberlain J, Miller AB, eds. Screening for gastrointestinal cancer. Toronto: Huber, 1988:9.
67. Kronborg O, Fenger C, Sowdergaard O, Pedersen KM, Olsen J. Initial mass screening for colorectal cancer with fecal occult blood test. Scand J Gastroenterol 1987;22:677.
68. Gilbertsen VA, McHugh R, Schuman L, et al. The early detection of colorectal cancers: a preliminary report of the results of the occult blood study. Cancer 1980;45:2899.
69. Hardcastle JD, Thomas WM, Chamberlain J, et al. Randomized controlled trial of fecal occult blood screening for colorectal cancer: the results of the first 107,349 subjects. Lancet 1989;1:1160.
70. Kewenier J, Bjork S, Haglind E, et al. Screening and rescreening for colorectal cancer: a controlled trial of fecal occult blood testing in 27,700 subjects. Cancer 1988;62:645.
71. Winawer SJ, St. John J, Bond JH, et al. Screening of average-risk individuals for colorectal cancer. Bull WHO 1990;68:505.
72. Winawer SJ, Schottenfeld D, Flehinger BJ. Colorectal cancer screening. J Natl Cancer Inst 1991;83:243.
73. Mandel JS, Bond JH, Church TR, et al. Reducing mortality from colorectal cancer by screening for fecal occult blood. N Engl J Med 1993; 328:1365.
74. Winawer SJ, Flehinger BJ, Schottenfeld D, Miller DG. Screening for colorectal cancer with fecal occult blood testing and sigmoidoscopy. J Natl Cancer Inst 1993;85:1311.
75. Selby JV, Friedman GD, Quesenberry CP Jr, et al. Effect of fecal occult blood testing on mortality from colorectal cancer: a case-control study. Ann Intern Med 1993;118:1.
76. Wagner JL, Herman RC, Wadhwa S. Cost effectiveness of colorectal cancer screening in the elderly. Ann Intern Med 1991;115:807.
77. Brown ML. Screening for colorectal cancer [letter]. N Engl J Med 1993;329:1352.

Surgery for Gastrointestinal Cancer: A Multidisciplinary Approach, edited by Harold J. Wanebo.
Lippincott-Raven Publishers, Philadelphia, © 1997.

CHAPTER 3

Molecular Biology of Gastrointestinal Cancer: Current Relevance

Bruce D. Greenwald and Stephen J. Meltzer

THE MOLECULAR GENETIC BASIS OF CARCINOGENESIS

In contrast to normal tissue, which is composed of cells from many different progenitors (polyclonal), tumor tissue arises from the clonal expansion of a single cell. This cell is believed to expand because it has undergone a genetic alteration yielding a growth advantage over other cells. Over time, additional genetic alterations accumulate in offspring of this clone, giving rise to cells with an even greater growth advantage. Eventually, this process of genomic instability culminates in the formation of a malignant tumor. Further alterations may lead to tumor cell invasion and metastasis.

The stepwise events by which a cell becomes transformed from normal to malignant are the subject of intensive scientific study. One of the first abnormalities studied is a change in the amount of DNA within malignant cells. Normal human cells are diploid, carrying two copies of each chromosome, one from each parent. Abnormal cells may be aneuploid, containing a greater or lesser amount of DNA than their normal counterparts. Aneuploidy represents a gross difference in chromosome number; it does not directly reflect more subtle alterations in individual genes. Individual gene alterations, or mutations, have been studied carefully since the 1970s. At least three or four classes of genes are known to be involved in the malignant process: protooncogenes, tumor suppressor genes (TSGs), DNA repair genes, and the newest class of cancer-related genes, those that control entry into the cell cycle. Alterations in the structure, function, or expressed quantity of these genes promote carcinogenesis. These mutational events are discussed later.

Bruce D. Greenwald, Assistant Professor, University of Maryland School of Medicine, Division of Gastroenterology, University of Maryland Hospital, Room N3W62, 22 South Greene Street, Baltimore, MD 21201-1595.

Stephen J. Meltzer, Associate Professor, University of Maryland School of Medicine, Division of Gastroenterology, University of Maryland Hospital, Room N3W62, 22 South Greene Street, Baltimore, MD 21201-1595.

The paradigm for research in this field has been neoplasms of the colorectum, for several reasons: the high prevalence of colorectal carcinoma and colonic polyposis allows a large number of samples to be collected and creates pressure for improved clinical management; adenomatous polyps are easily obtainable through colonoscopy and are routinely removed during surveillance for carcinoma; these adenomatous polyps are believed to be the precursors of carcinoma; and two forms of colorectal cancer—familial adenomatous polyposis (FAP) and hereditary nonpolyposis colorectal cancer (HNPCC)—are hereditary, allowing for the search for specific genes that predispose to or cause these forms of cancer.

Abnormal DNA Content (Aneuploidy)

Much of the groundwork for evaluation of neoplastic progression in the human gastrointestinal (GI) tract was first laid with work on DNA content. DNA content, or ploidy, can be determined using flow cytometry of disaggregated nuclei. This is a valuable tool in detecting clonality of tissues or cells. For example, neoplastic progression in Barrett's esophagus is associated with a process of genomic instability and clonal evolution similar to that postulated by Nowell.[1] Early in this process, genetic instability develops. For example, Reid and colleagues showed that the evolution from normal esophagus to premalignant Barrett's metaplasia is frequently associated with abnormal DNA content, or aneuploidy, of the metaplastic epithelial cells.[2,3] In these seminal mapping studies, biopsy samples were taken in meticulous fashion from the entire area of Barrett's-lined epithelium in each patient. Large, irregularly shaped clonal areas were delineated by precise, exhaustive ploidy analysis of biopsy specimens. It was evident from these studies that clonal expansion of single progenitor cells (all with the same abnormal DNA content, or aneuploidy) had occurred, and that repopulation of large areas of mucosa could take place from these single parent cells. All of this clonal growth, highly characteristic of fully developed malignancies, was happening in nonmalignant, metaplastic Barrett's mucosa. This work was corroborated by other groups.[4] In patients who have been prospectively evaluated by DNA content flow cytometry, the evolution from diploid to single aneuploid cell populations and then to multiple aneuploid cell populations is a common occurrence. In some patients, this clonal evolution has been documented by cytogenetic analysis of mucosal biopsy specimens.[5]

Similar work has been performed in other premalignant GI conditions, such as ulcerative colitis. The earliest reports of flow cytometric DNA analysis in ulcerative colitis were published from Stockholm in 1984[6] and in a later survey by the same group.[7] The prevalence of aneuploidy in this series of 51 patients correlated with disease duration and the presence of histologic dysplasia or carcinoma. Similar findings were reported by other investigators.[8,9] In one of these studies,[8] a higher prevalence of DNA aneuploidy was found in dysplastic than in nondysplastic tissues, but this difference did not achieve statistical significance. A prospective study was published in 1987.[10] In this study, 53 patients with longstanding universal ulcerative colitis were followed for a mean of 3.5 years. Dysplasia developed in four of five patients with aneuploidy; aneuploidy preceded dysplasia by 1 year in one patient and antedated a Dukes' stage A carcinoma by 1 year in another patient.

Unfortunately, the precise predictive value of aneuploidy has not been consistently substantiated.[11,12] More recent publications on aneuploidy in ulcerative colitis have included elegant mapping studies, some of which combine ploidy studies with molecular analyses.[13–17] These systematic investigations have often demonstrated large, expansive areas of colonic mucosa containing cells with precisely identical aneuploid DNA contents. This evidence strongly suggests that these large areas of epithelium arose from a single abnormal progenitor cell, in agreement with the clonal theory of cancer proffered earlier.

In summary, measurement of DNA content is a well established technique that has been shown to correlate often, if imperfectly, with the clinical behavior of premalignant GI conditions. In this respect, it shows promise as a potential clinical tool to be used in conjunction with conventional histologic analysis.

Protooncogenes

Protooncogenes were the first major group of genes to be intensively studied in GI cancers and premalignant lesions. This term now encompasses a diverse group of over 200 genes encoding proteins that control cell growth and differentiation, including such classic genes as *MYC*, *SRC*, *ERBB2*, *MYB*, *FOS*, *JUN*, *ABL1*, *PDGFB*, and many others. Proteins encoded by these genes span the cell from its exterior to the nucleus, including growth factors and their receptors, G-protein–like transducers, tyrosine kinases, intracellular messengers, transcription factors, DNA-binding proteins, and DNA replication-related substances. The prefix ''proto'' connotes normality: that is, normal versions of all members of this group are present as growth controls in every normal body cell. They become oncogenic only when activated by various mutational events; when this happens, they are known as oncogenes. Oncogenes function as ''dominant'' cancer genes. That is, one activated version of this type of gene can exert a cancer-promoting effect, even in the presence of one normal version of the same gene in the same cell. Activation of protooncogenes into oncogenes may occur by a number of molecular genetic mechanisms, including point mutation, chromosomal translocation or rearrangement, viral insertion, DNA amplification, or simply overexpression.

Perhaps the most important of the protooncogenes from the GI standpoint is the *RAS* family. This includes three principal members, *KRAS*, *HRAS*, and *NRAS* (named for their discoverers or tissues of discovery). Some of the first molecular abnormalities described in GI cancer were very frequent point mutations in codons 12, 13, and 61 of *KRAS*, *HRAS*, or *NRAS* in colon cancers and adenomas.[18,19] The two research groups discovering these alterations noted that *RAS* mutations were more common in more advanced tumors, but could also occur early in small adenomas. These findings were corroborated in a larger follow-up study.[20] Subsequently, the role of *RAS* family gene mutations was expanded to include a large variety of tumor types.[21] *RAS* family protooncogene mutations were evaluated in the premalignant conditions ulcerative colitis and Barrett's esophagus and were found to be rare.[22] However, in the GI tract, in addition to being so common in colorectal cancer, they are extremely frequent in pancreatic carcinomas. In two studies, *KRAS* mutations were present in 72% to 95% of carcinomas of the exocrine pancreas.[23,24] One study used tissue obtained by fine-needle aspiration of pancreatic masses, potentially making this a useful diagnostic tool in the diagnosis of pancreatic adenocarcinoma.[24]

Tumor Suppressor Genes

Tumor suppressor genes (TSCs), like protooncogenes, function in normal cells to regulate cell growth. Their presence was first hypothesized after the discovery of regions of chromosomal deletion in many tumors (see section on Allelic Deletion). This finding led to a famous hypothesis proposed by Alfred Knudson.[25] In this ''two-hit'' model, both copies of a TSG must be inactivated for its tumor-suppressive effect to be abolished. For example, one copy of the TSG may be lost by allelic deletion, whereas the second copy is mutated, resulting in a dysfunctional or nonfunctional protein. Much research has focused on identifying areas of frequent allelic deletion at given chromosomal regions in specific tumor types. As these target areas are identified, researchers then direct their efforts toward identifying and characterizing TSGs in these regions and identifying mutations that occur in these genes. Simultaneously, investigations into the function of the proteins encoded by the TSGs have often been performed.

In certain tumors occurring at an early age, such as hereditary retinoblastoma, one allele of the TSG is missing or nonfunctional at birth, leaving only one intact copy of the gene, which undergoes mutation somatically after birth. In other tumor types, inactivation of one copy (for example, by allelic deletion) occurs later in life, often accompanied by mutation of the remaining copy of the TSG in question. Many additional TSG examples conforming to the Knudson hypothesis and important in GI tract tumors have subsequently been identified.

Allelic Deletion

Loss of one of the two alleles of a gene or chromosomal locus is known as allelic deletion. Frequent allelic deletion at a specific locus occurring in a given tumor type suggests the presence of a TSG at that locus that is important in the tumor under study.

The allelic deletion studies of Vogelstein and colleagues in colorectal cancer were perhaps the first in a series of steps toward appreciating the fundamental importance of TSGs.[20] These investigators analyzed the frequency and timing of allelic deletion in colorectal carcinoma and adenomas. Chromosomes 5, 17, and 18 were investigated. Allelic loss was seen in 36% of carcinomas at chromosome 5, in 75% at chromosome 17, and in 73% at chromosome 18. The rate of allelic loss on chromosome 5q for adenomatous polyps was similar to the rate in carcinomas, whereas the rates of loss on chromosomes 17 and 18 were lower in polyps compared to carcinomas. This early evidence suggested that genetic alterations in these tumors were progressive, with some (such as losses on chromosome 5) occurring early in tumor development, and others (such as losses on chromosome 17) occurring only after polyps had become advanced. This group systematically studied allelic loss by examining each arm of all chromosomes in search of deletions, termed allelotypes.[26] A large number of deletions on many chromosomes was found; the median "fractional allelic loss" (FAL) score was 20%; that is, an average of 20% of the chromosomal arms evaluated showed allelic deletions in any given tumor.

Studies of allelic loss have since been performed on many types of GI tumors and premalignant lesions, including squamous cell carcinoma and adenocarcinoma of the esophagus, Barrett's esophagus, gastric carcinoma, hepatocellular carcinoma, and pancreatic carcinoma. The prevalence of allelic loss differs somewhat among histologic tumor types, but it occurs to some extent in all GI malignancies.

Specific Tumor Suppressor Genes

P53

The most commonly mutated gene in all human cancers is *P53*.[27,28] This gene is located on the short arm of chromosome 17 (17p) and encodes a 53-kd nuclear phosphoprotein. The gene is composed of 11 exons and contains 5 domains that are highly conserved across species. The P53 protein was first discovered in 1979, when it was identified bound to the large transforming antigen of the SV40 virus.[29,30] Detailed discussion of the normal and abnormal function of *P53* is beyond the scope of this chapter, but several excellent reviews of this topic have been published.[27,28,31–34]

The P53 protein is normally undetectable in cells because of its short half-life, approximately 6 to 20 minutes.[28] The exact function of the normal protein is still under investigation. However, it is known to be involved in regulating cell growth and initiating programmed cell death, or apoptosis. It does this by regulating the transcription of many other genes, both through up- and down-regulation of specific gene transcription and by controlling DNA repair.[31] The P53 protein arrests cell growth in the G1 phase, when DNA repairs are undertaken before DNA synthesis and mitosis,[35] and insertion of wild-type *P53* into a colon cancer cell line has been shown to cause reversion to a nonmalignant state in vitro.[36] The mutant gene often loses these critical functions.

In the most common type of *P53* mutation, known as missense mutation, one amino acid is substituted for another, producing an abnormal but full-length protein. This mutated protein frequently has a prolonged half-life, up to 6 hours,[28] allowing it to be detected by immunohistochemical methods. Thus, P53 protein that is detectable in nuclei by antibody staining is usually mutated. The site of amino acid substitutions varies, but at least four "hot spots," or sites of frequent mutation, are recognized across many different tumor types.[33,36] The exact cause of these mutations is unknown, but proposed etiologic agents include chemical carcinogens,[33,36] human papillomavirus,[37] *Helicobacter pylori*,[38] and aflatoxin B1, a food contaminant produced by *Aspergillus* species.[39] In tumor development, a common scenario consists of loss of the normal or wild-type *P53* gene by allelic deletion (see previous discussion), whereas the mutant gene remains and may exert a "negative dominant" abnormal effect on cell growth.

Gastrointestinal tract tumors in which mutations in *P53* have been reported include both squamous cell carcinoma[40–45] and Barrett's-associated adenocarcinoma[45–49] of the esophagus, gastric carcinoma,[50–53] sporadic,[54,55] hereditary,[56,57] and ulcerative colitis-associated[58–60] colorectal carcinoma, hepatocellular carcinoma,[61–67] and pancreatic cancer.[68–71] Hepatocellular carcinomas from the region of South Africa and Qidong, China, but not other countries, are characterized by a high-frequency "signature" mutation at codon 249 of *P53*.[62,64,66] However, *P53* mutations this specific are rare in human cancers.

APC

Familial adenomatous polyposis is an autosomal dominant disorder characterized by the development of hundreds to thousands of adenomatous colonic polyps and colon carcinoma at an early age. Cytogenetic analysis of a patient with FAP[72] and subsequent linkage analysis[73,74] localized the gene for this disease to the long arm of chromosome 5 (5q). In 1991, the gene responsible for FAP was identified by two groups.[75–78] The *APC* (adenomatous polyposis coli) gene codes for 2843 amino acids. It comprises 16 exons, 15 of which code for amino acids, and one that is noncoding.

Patients with FAP inherit a germline mutation in *APC*. The types of mutations that occur include base pair deletions and insertions, as well as point mutations (alterations of a single base). Greater than 90% of these mutations cause a shift in the reading frame of the DNA, yielding a premature stop codon. This event results in the production of a truncated protein product. Over two thirds of the *APC* mutations reported thus far have occurred in the 5′ half of exon 15.[79] This clustering of mutations could have significant implications in the development of screening tests for FAP.

Screening for *APC* mutations is made difficult by the large size of the gene and its protein product, and the widespread distribution of mutations in the gene in different families. Powell and associates have developed a novel method of screening. By analyzing proteins synthesized in vitro from the *APC* gene DNA and applying an allele-specific expression assay, 87% of 62 patients with FAP were correctly identified.[80] This is discussed in more detail later.

APC has been found to be deleted or mutated in a variety of tumors. Frequent allelic deletions in this region have been noted in esophageal cancer,[81] ulcerative colitis-associated colorectal cancer,[82] and hepatocellular carcinoma.[83,84] Mutations have been found to occur early and frequently in sporadic colorectal cancer,[85,86] but also in gastric carcinoma[87,88] and pancreatic cancer.[89] In colon cancer, *APC* mutation has been seen in adenomatous polyps as small as 0.5 cm in size and remained constant from polyp to carcinoma, suggesting that *APC* mutation is an early event in tumorigenesis.[90] Nevertheless, *APC* mutation was rare in esophageal carcinoma.[91]

The precise function of the APC protein is not yet completely elucidated. Immunohistochemical analysis of the APC protein in normal colonic mucosa shows it to be present in the basolateral portion of the cytoplasm in colonocytes. Staining is increased in the upper portion of crypts, suggesting a relationship between APC protein and cell maturation.[92] Studies have shown that the APC gene product interacts with catenin, a member of the cell adhesion-related gene family known as cadherins.[93,94] In fact, down-regulation[95] and mutation[96] of E-cadherin have been noted in gastric cancer, a neoplasm characterized by prominent involvement of *APC*. Therefore, it is also possible that *APC* plays a role in inhibiting the invasion and metastasis of tumor cells.

DCC

The deleted in colon cancer (*DCC*) gene was identified within a frequently deleted region on chromosome 18q in colorectal carcinomas.[97] Various abnormalities affecting *DCC* have subsequently been described in GI and other tumors, including reduced messenger RNA expression,[98–104] alternative splicing,[105,106] mutation,[107] and allelic loss.[100,104,108,109] Blockage of *DCC* expression by antisense RNA malignantly transforms fibroblasts.[110,111] This gene, like *APC*, may also play a role in cell-to-cell communication; it is expressed on the cell surface[112] and bears some resemblance to neural cell adhesion molecules.[97,113]

MTS1

A putative new TSG has been described by Kamb and colleagues.[114,115] This gene plays an important role in regulating the cell cycle, which controls cell division. Its existence was suspected when a high prevalence of loss of heterozygosity involving chromosome 9p was observed in a wide variety of tumors. Tumor types characterized by a very high frequency of allelic loss at this locus include glioma,[116–119] leukemia,[119,120] bladder cancer,[121–126] lung cancer,[119,127–130] mesothelioma,[131] head and neck carcinoma,[132] and melanoma.[119,133,134] Moreover, linkage studies of familial melanoma assigned this syndrome to chromosome 9p13–p22.[135]

One gene located on chromosome 9p21 is named *MTS1* (multiple tumor suppressor 1). It contains three exons and encodes the 16-kd protein p16, which is known to play a crucial role in regulating the cell cycle that governs cell division. The cell cycle is tightly controlled by a large family of enzymes known as the cyclins, which are in turn regulated by the cyclin-dependent kinases (CDK).[136] CDK4, one of several such enzymes, is activated by binding to a member of the large cyclin family, cyclin D. Protein P16 binds to and inhibits CDK4, preventing it from interacting with cyclin D and allowing the cell cycle to proceed. Thus, cell growth is regulated by a fine balance between activation of the CDKs by cyclins and inhibition by proteins such as P16.[137]

The *MTS1* gene itself is altered in a wide variety of cancer cell lines. Kamb and colleagues studied 12 tumor types for deletions or mutations directly affecting *MTS1*.[115] Only one GI tumor type, colon carcinoma, was studied. No microdeletions were seen in colon cancer lines; however, point mutations were not specifically examined. A simultaneous report described frequent deletion or rearrangement of this gene in melanomas, gliomas, lung cancers, and leukemias; no point mutations were described in primary tumors.[138] Subsequent to these reports, the *MTS1* gene has been studied extensively. In the GI tract, its importance has been established in esophageal squamous cell carcinoma[139,140] and pancreatic carcinoma.[141] In general, however, in other tumor types, *MTS1* mutation is very rare.[142,143] This finding implies that another gene on chromosome 9p functions as a tumor suppressor in these cell types. In fact, a second CDK4 inhibitor has just been found in close proximity to *MTS1/P16*: this gene is known as *P15*.[144] Other members of the cyclin kinase inhibitor family will probably be isolated; thus, this part of the GI TSG story is becoming increasingly complex.

Microsatellite Instability

Found throughout the human genome are repeating simple sequences of nucleotides known as microsatellites. The repeating unit is usually less than four or five nucleotides in length.[145] In humans, tandem repeats of only two nucleotides are widely distributed throughout the genome.[146,147] The number of tandem repeats at each site is polymorphic, or variable between individuals, and thus may serve as a unique genetic marker for an individual. Genetic instability, in the form of missing or extra copies of tandem repeats, has been described in many different tumor types, including sporadic and HNPCC,[148–150] gastric carcinoma,[151–153] and pancreatic carcinoma.[153] The widespread genomic phenomenon of microsatellite instability appears to be caused by mutation in any one of a number of DNA repair genes.

DNA Repair Genes

Four human DNA repair genes involved in hereditary colon cancer have been cloned. They are located on chromosomes 2p, 2q, 3p, and 7p.[154–160] These DNA mismatch repair genes are responsible for locating and repairing nucleotide sequences that have been improperly replicated during DNA synthesis. Mutations in these genes are responsible for the microsatellite instability observed in tumors of patients with HNPCC. The resultant mutations impair the normal DNA repair function, leading to widespread DNA repair errors. In HNPCC, a germline mutation is present in one of these four genes. Somatic (ie, acquired; nongermline) mutations have also been identified in some sporadic colorectal cancers.[156,159] It is likely that other human DNA repair genes will be found to be mutated in hereditary cancer syndromes; each one of the four genes isolated thus far accounts for only a portion of the total HNPCC cases.

Stepwise Progression of Carcinogenesis

No single gene loss or mutation is sufficient to allow a cell or group of cells to escape the normal controls on growth and proliferate in a malignant fashion. Instead, genetic alterations occur in a stepwise fashion, until enough changes have occurred to allow the uncontrolled growth of a particular clone of cells. That no oncogene or TSG has been shown to be altered in 100% of tumors studied suggests that different pathways involving different genes allow tumorigenesis to occur.

The stepwise progression of tumor development has best been studied in colorectal tumors, for reasons mentioned earlier. An early study by Vogelstein and colleagues[20] examined alterations in the *RAS* gene and allelic deletions in three chromosomes, 5, 17, and 18, in 92 colorectal carcinomas and 80 colonic adenomas. They showed that *RAS* gene mutations were present in approximately half of all carcinomas and large adenomas (>1 cm) but in only 9% of adenomas smaller than 1 cm. Chromosome 5 deletions were not significantly different between adenomas and carcinomas in cases of sporadic colorectal carcinoma. Chromosome 18 deletions were present in adenomas, but were more common in carcinomas. The prevalence of chromosome 17 deletions was statistically more frequent in carcinomas than in adenomas. These data suggest that tumorigenesis occurs in a stepwise fashion, with *RAS* oncogene mutations occurring early, followed by stepwise losses of chromosome 5, 18, then 17. This order is not invariate and not all genes necessarily are altered. Carcinomas of the left colon are twice as likely to show allelic loss as right colon tumors.[161] The order of these genetic alterations differs with different tumor types. In comparison to sporadic colorectal carcinoma, *P53* mutations occur early in ulcerative colitis-associated tumorigenesis.[162–164] In esophageal adenocarcinoma, inactivation of *P53* and *LOH* involving chromosome 17p are early events, whereas inactivation of *APC* is a rarer and later event.[165] In comparison, in gastric cancer, allelic deletions involving both *P53* and *MCC/APC* occur late in the development of carcinoma, with allelic losses seen only rarely in adjacent gastric dysplastic mucosa.[52] In theory, early events should have potential as early detection markers, whereas late events should have some bearing on tumor progression and offer potential as prognostic markers. This theory is being actively investigated in many laboratories.

CLINICAL APPLICATIONS

Diagnosis

Genetic Screening for Familial Adenomatous Polyposis

Familial adenomatous polyposis syndrome is a condition characterized by the presence of hundreds of adenomatous colorectal polyps that inevitably progresses to colorectal cancer. The syndrome is inherited in an autosomal dominant fashion, and the responsible gene, *APC*, is located on chromosome 5q21 (discussed earlier).

Screening for *APC* mutations is made difficult by the large size of the gene and its protein product and the widespread distribution of mutations in the gene in different families. However, researchers have taken advantage of the finding that most *APC* mutations produce a truncated protein to produce a useful method of screening. By analyzing proteins synthesized in vitro from *APC* gene DNA, Powell and associates correctly identified 51 of 62 patients with known FAP (82%) by identifying truncated APC protein. A second assay uses differences in expression levels of natural polymorphisms (substitutions) of a single base in one allele of the *APC* genome in FAP. By applying this allele-specific expression assay, three additional FAP patients were identified, increasing the yield of the combined tests to 87%.[166]

This test is commercially available through Roche Biomedical Laboratories. It should be used only in patients with suspected FAP, because the significance of a positive test in the general population is unknown.

Screening of Stool for RAS *Mutations in Colorectal Carcinoma Detection*

In theory, the DNA from cells shed by colonic neoplasia should be detectable in stool. This would provide a noninvasive means of screening patients for colorectal malignancy. Inherent difficulties in screening for DNA in stool include the heterogeneous composition of stool, the risk of degradation of DNA, and the unknown concentration of abnormal DNA present. Nonetheless, this method has been applied to a small sample of patients with colorectal carcinomas and adenomas. Because *KRAS* mutations are present in approximately half of colorectal carcinomas and large adenomas, and because most mutations occur in codons 12 or 13,[20] they were chosen as the targets for study. Sidransky and coworkers[167] examined previously collected stool for *KRAS* mutations in nine patients found later to have adenocarcinoma or an adenoma greater than 1 cm in diameter. Using a Southern blot assay, eight of nine stool samples were positive for the same *KRAS* mutation found in the tumor. The one negative tumor was a 1 cm rectal carcinoma.

This assay is not yet ready for widespread application. Seven of the nine tumors studied were in the colon or rectum, so the consistent success of this assay in right colon malignancies is unproven. In addition, the sample size of this pilot study was small. Success as a screening tool would require that stool be examined for all likely *KRAS* mutations, because the exact mutation present would not be known prospectively. Even this would identify only half of all malignancies, because this is the proportion of carcinomas known to carry a *RAS* mutation. However, this technique holds promise as a potential screening tool for colorectal carcinomas and large adenomas. Intraluminal recurrence of tumor could also be screened, because it is likely that the recurrence would contain the same *KRAS* mutation as the primary tumor. However, this has not been tested.

RAS *Mutations in the Early Detection and Diagnosis of Pancreatic Cancer*

Because *RAS* mutations were originally reported to occur in 75% to 90% of pancreatic ductal adenocarcinomas,[68,69] but not in benign conditions of the pancreas, they are a good potential tool for distinguishing between pancreatic neoplasms and benign pancreatic enlargement or nonpancreatic neoplasms.[168] *KRAS* point mutations may serve as clonal markers; in one study, most pancreatic carcinomas contained one single mutation.[169] In addition to being highly specific for clonal pancreatic adenocarcinomas, *KRAS* mutations have shown promise as an early detection marker. They were seen in most preinvasive pancreatic cancers[170] and fine-needle pancreatic aspirates from cancers.[24] *RAS* mutations have been easily detectable in paraffin-embedded biopsy sample as well as surgical resection specimens.[171]

Microsatellite Instability as a Potential Global Tool to Screen Bodily Fluids

As discussed earlier, microsatellite instability is present in many different types of cancer. Mao and colleagues examined microsatellite alterations in head and neck, bladder, and lung cancer patients.[172] Twenty-six percent of tumors demonstrated microsatellite instability. The authors hypothesized that tumor cells present in sputum, urine, or surgical margins could be detected by searching for the same microsatellite alterations. This in fact proved to be the case. Identical microsatellite alterations were found in the urine of one patient and sputum of two patients considered negative for malignancy by cytologic examination. In addition, examination of histologically negative surgical margins in two patients with lung cancer revealed the presence of cells containing microsatellite alterations identical to those of the primary tumor.[172]

Although preliminary, this technique is promising for the early detection of tumors before they become obvious microscopically. Rather than searching for specific gene mutations that may be unique for a tumor, this technique detects microsatellite alterations that may be common in a large number of tumors. This may make it a better screening tool.

Prognosis

Attempts have been made to use alterations in the genes discussed earlier to improve prognosis for different GI malignancies. This would be especially helpful, for example, in Dukes' stage B and C colorectal carcinomas, where adjuvant chemotherapy has been shown to improve survival in some cases. Specific markers have also been searched for that may predispose to metastasis of the primary tumor. Efforts in this area have centered on several approaches—allelic loss, detection of mutations in specific genes, and immunohistochemical staining for detection of abnormal protein.

Aneuploidy

Measurement of the total nuclear DNA content has been studied extensively.[173] In colorectal cancer, early studies showed that aneuploid tumors were associated with a poor prognosis and shortened survival.[174–177] However, more recent studies have yielded conflicting results.[178–180] To date, evaluation of DNA ploidy has not become a widespread tool in clinical use because of the conflicting data in this area as well as the expense and technical expertise required in the proper preparation and interpretation of this type of data.

Allelic Loss

Allelic loss has been shown to carry prognostic information in different tumor types. Vogelstein and colleagues[26] characterized the allelic losses on all chromosomal arms and called this an allelotype. In the colorectal tumors of the 56 patients evaluated, they found that a median of 20% of evaluable chromosomal arms were lost (the FAL). The patients were then divided into two groups: those with less than the median FAL (group I) and those with greater than the median FAL (group II). The groups were well matched by demographic and histologic features, Dukes' stage of the tumor, and frequency of *RAS* mutation. However, group II patients were more likely to have recurrent disease, including distant metastases, and die from their disease than group I patients. In a separate report, multivariate analysis of a subgroup of these patients showed that allelic loss of chromosomes 17p and 18q, as well as fractional allelic loss, were statistically significant predictors of survival and development of metastatic disease.[181] A study by a different group examined *KRAS* mutation, DNA content, and allelic loss on chromosomes 17p, q8q, 5q, and 1p as potential prognostic factors in 109 patients with colorectal cancer. In multivariate analysis, only allelic loss of 17p was associated with shorter survival.[182] Unfortunately, applicability of this approach is limited because it relies on fresh frozen tissue as a source of DNA and on many different genetic probes for the detection of losses.

The same group published a simplified method of detecting allelic deletion on 18q in paraffin-embedded tissues and has examined the role of 18q loss in prognostication for stage II and III (Dukes' stages B and C) sporadic colorectal carcinomas.[183] Loss of 18q was seen in 67% of tumors, and was more common in tumors distal to the splenic flexure. Five-year survival in patients with stage II tumors with loss of 18q was significantly worse than in stage II tumors without 18q loss (54% vs. 93%). In the former group, survival was no different than in stage III tumor patients. Thus, it will be important to investigate whether the former group benefits from adjuvant chemotherapy, as has been shown for stage III tumors.[184]

Immunohistochemical Staining

As mentioned earlier, the half-life of normal P53 protein is only minutes, so the normal protein is not detectable in tissue. Some types of *P53* mutation, however, result in an abnormal protein product that persists for hours in tissue. This protein is detectable by tissue staining. Expression of P53 protein in malignancies has been extensively studied in the hopes of finding a correlation between *P53* expression and the clinical behavior of a specific tumor.[185–191] Variable correlations between *P53* protein expression and survival and tumor recurrence have been shown. In colorectal cancer, an early study showed no correlation with *P53* expression and survival.[178] Other studies have shown positive results[177–182]; however, only certain studies have shown correlation when controlled for pathologic stage.[179,183,184] Two studies[183,184] have shown that survival correlated only with cytoplasmic P53 staining rather than nuclear staining. Three studies have examined the prognostic significance of P53 staining in gastric carcinoma. Two studies demonstrated decreased survival in P53-positive patients,[181,192] whereas one showed increased risk of lymph node metastasis in these patients.[193]

The conflicting results are likely caused by several reasons. First, not all *P53* mutations produce a protein identifiable by immunohistochemical staining. Up to 20% of *P53* mutations do not produce a detectable protein.[194] Second, antibodies against different epitopes on the p53 protein have been used. These include monoclonal antibodies (PAb 240, PAb 421 PAb 1801) and a polyclonal antibody (CM1). The sensitivity and specificity of these markers is not well defined, although one study using only 19 colorectal cancers showed wide variation between different antibodies.[195] Third, all of the studies investigating this issue are retrospective, the number of tissues studied in each was relatively small, and multivariate analysis was infrequently performed to assess the relationship of P53 staining to other variables. Therefore, at present, immunostaining for P53 protein expression remains experimental.

Mutations

Only one study has specifically examined survival in patients with a specific TSG mutation rather than allelic loss or abnormal staining.[196] This may be important, because in some cases allelic loss of chromosome 17p may not include the *P53* locus, and in others the mutated *P53* gene may not produce a protein that is overexpressed, and hence detectable by staining in malignant cells.

In this study, mutant *P53* genes were identified and sequenced. Mutations were found in 44 of the 85 tumors studied (52%). Of these 44, 32 tumors could be assessed for allelic loss, which was found in 28 (88%). Allelic loss of 17p and *P53* mutation were both more common in left-sided tumors, and both were predictive of shorter survival. However, when controlled for tumor stage, *P53* mutation remained a significant predictor of poor survival, whereas in this study, 17p loss did not remain significant.

Thus, identification of a mutation in *P53* may serve as a predictor for survival in patients with colorectal cancer. Unfortunately, detection of specific mutations is time consuming and is not ready for wide application as a screening tool.

Novel Approaches

Circulating P53 Antibodies

Serum antibodies against the P53 protein have been detected in some patients with carcinoma. A host response against mutated P53 protein is believed to develop because of the prolonged half-life of the abnormal protein in the malignant cells. These antibodies have been detected in patients with GI cancers,[197] as well as cancer of the liver,[198] breast,[199–201] and lung,[202,203] in approximately 20% of cases studied. In one case, P53 antibody was detected in a patient without diagnosed malignancy who died 6 months later of lung carcinoma.[203] There are inadequate data to determine whether circulating P53 antibodies are useful either for the early diagnosis of malignancy or as a prognostic tool.

Treatment

Treatment of GI neoplasms using the knowledge described in this chapter remains speculative. The most obvious approaches would include ''turning off'' oncogenes abnormally activated and repairing or replacing mutated or lost TSGs, DNA repair genes, and cell cycle control genes—essentially ''turning them on'' again. This latter approach has been realized experimentally, with suppression of in vitro colon cancer cell growth achieved by transfection of a wild-type *P53* gene.[36] However, gene therapy of this type is still in its infancy. As an alternative approach, analogs to these gene products could be developed, which could be administered to patients known to have tumors with defective genes. These approaches await improvements in gene therapy and systems of delivery targeted specifically to tumor cells.

REFERENCES

1. Nowell PC. The clonal evolution of tumor cell populations. Science 1976;194:23.
2. Rabinovitch PS, Reid BJ, Haggitt RC, Norwood TH, Rubin CE. Progression to cancer in Barrett's esophagus is associated with genomic instability. Lab Invest 1988;60:65.
3. Reid BJ, Blount PL, Rubin CE, Levine DS, Haggitt RC, Rabinovitch PS. Flow-cytometric and histological progression to malignancy in Barrett's esophagus: prospective endoscopic surveillance of a cohort. Gastroenterology 1992;102:1212.
4. McKinley MJ, Budman DR, Grueneberg D, Bronzo RL, Weissman GS, Kahn E. DNA content in Barrett's esophagus and esophageal malignancy. Am J Gastroenterol 1987;82:1012.
5. Raskind WH, Norwood TH, Levine DS, Haggitt RC, Rabinovitch PS, Reid BJ. Persistent clonal areas and clonal expansion in Barrett's esophagus. Cancer Res 1992;52:2946.
6. Hammarberg C, Rubio C, Slezak P, Tribukait B, Ohman U. Flow-cytometric DNA analysis as a means for early detection of malignancy in patients with chronic ulcerative colitis. Gut 1984;25:905.
7. Hammarberg C, Slezak P, Tribukait B. Early detection of malignancy in ulcerative colitis: a flow-cytometric DNA study. Cancer 1984;53:291.
8. Fozard JBJ, Quirke P, Dixon MF, Giles GR, Bird CC. DNA aneuploidy in ulcerative colitis. Gut 1986;27:1414.
9. Melville DM, Jass JR, Shepherd NA, et al. Dysplasia and deoxyribonucleic acid aneuploidy in the assessment of precancerous changes in chronic ulcerative colitis: observer variation and correlations. Gastroenterology 1988;95:668.
10. Lofberg R, Tribukait B, Ost A, Brostrom O, Reichard H. Flow cytometric DNA analysis in longstanding ulcerative colitis: a method of prediction of dysplasia and carcinoma development? Gut 1987;28:1100.
11. Rutegard J, Ahsgren L, Stenling R, Roos G. DNA content in ulcerative colitis: flow cytometric analysis in a patient series from a defined area. Dis Colon Rectum 1988;31:710.
12. Cuvelier CA, Morson BC, Roels HJ. The DNA content in cancer and dysplasia in chronic ulcerative colitis. Histopathology 1987;11:927.
13. Levine DS, Rabinovitch PS, Haggitt RC, et al. Distribution of aneuploid cell populations in ulcerative colitis with dysplasia or cancer. Gastroenterology 1991;101:1198.
14. Meling GI, Clausen OPF, Bergan A, Schjolberg A, Rognum TO. Flow cytometric DNA ploidy pattern in dysplastic mucosa, and in primary and metastatic carcinomas in patients with longstanding ulcerative colitis. Br J Cancer 1991;64:339.
15. Rubin CE, Haggitt RC, Burmer GC, et al. DNA aneuploidy in colonic biopsies predicts future development of dysplasia in ulcerative colitis. Gastroenterology 1992;103:1611.
16. Offerhaus GJ, De Feyter EP, Cornelisse CJ, et al. The relationship of DNA aneuploidy to molecular genetic alterations in colorectal carcinoma. Gastroenterology 1992;102:1612.
17. Brentnall TA, Crispin DA, Rabinovitch PS, et al. Mutations in the

p53 gene: an early marker of neoplastic progression in ulcerative colitis. Gastroenterology 1994;107:369.
18. Bos JL, Fearon ER, Hamilton SR, Verlaan-de Vries M, van Boom J, van der Eb AJ, Vogelstein B. Prevalence of ras gene mutations in human colorectal cancers. Nature 1987;327:293.
19. Forrester K, Almoguera C, Han K, Grizzle WE, Perucho M. Detection of high incidence of K-*ras* oncogenes during human colon tumorigenesis. Nature 1987;327:298.
20. Vogelstein B, Fearon ER, Hamilton SR, et al. Genetic alterations during colorectal-tumor development. N Engl J Med 1988;319:525.
21. Bos JL. *ras* oncogenes in human cancer: a review. Cancer Res 1989; 49:4682.
22. Meltzer SJ, Mane SM, Wood PK, et al. Activation of c-Ki-*ras* in human gastrointestinal dysplasias determined by direct sequencing of polymerase chain reaction products. Cancer Res 1990;50:3627.
23. Almoguera C, Shibata D, Forrester K, Martin J, Arnheim N, Perucho M. Most human carcinomas of the exocrine pancreas contain mutant c-K-ras gene. Cell 1988;53:549.
24. Shibata D, Almoguera C, Forrester K, et al. Detection of c-K-ras mutations in fine needle aspirates from human pancreatic adenocarcinomas. Cancer Res 1990;50:1279.
25. Knudson AG. Hereditary cancer, oncogenes, and anti-oncogenes. Cancer Res 1985;45:1437.
26. Vogelstein B, Fearon ER, Kern SE, et al. Allelotype of colorectal carcinomas. Science 1989;244:207.
27. Vogelstein B, Kinzler KW. p53 function and dysfunction. Cell 1992; 70:523.
28. Levine AJ, Momand J, Finlay CA. The p53 tumour suppressor gene. Nature 1991;351:453.
29. Lane DP, Crawford LV. T antigen is bound to a host protein in SV40-transformed cells. Nature 1979;278:261.
30. Linzer DI, Levine AJ. Characterization of a 54K dalton cellular SV40 tumor antigen present in SV40-transformed cells and uninfected embryonal carcinoma cells. Cell 1979;17:43.
31. Harris CC, Hollstein M. Clinical implications of the p53 tumor-suppressor gene. N Engl J Med 1993;329:1318.
32. Chang F, Syrjänen S, Kurvinen K, Syrjänen K. The p53 tumor suppressor gene as a common cellular target in human carcinogenesis. Am J Gastroenterol 1993;88:174.
33. Hollstein M, Sidransky D, Vogelstein B, Harris CC. p53 mutations in human cancers. Science 1991;253:49.
34. Frebourg T, Friend SH. The importance of p53 gene alterations in human cancer: is there more than circumstantial evidence? J Natl Cancer Inst 1993;85:1554.
35. Lin D, Shields MT, Ullrich SJ, Apella E, Mercer WE. Growth arrest induced by wild-type p53 protein blocks cells prior to or near the restriction point in the late G1 phase. Proc Natl Acad Sci U S A 1992; 89:9210.
36. Baker SJ, Markowitz S, Fearon ER, Willson JK, Vogelstein B. Suppression of human colorectal carcinoma cell growth by wild-type p53. Science 1990;249:912.
37. Chang F, Syrjänen S, Shen Q, Wang L, Wang D, Syrjänen K. Human papillomavirus (HPV) involvement in esophageal precancer lesions and squamous cell carcinomas as evidenced by microscopy and different DNA techniques. Scand J Gastroenterol 1992;27:553.
38. Parsonnet J, Friedman GD, Vandersteen DP, et al. *Helicobacter pylori* infection and the risk of gastric carcinoma. N Engl J Med 1991;325: 1127.
39. Hsu IC, Metcalf RA, Sun T, Welsh JA, Wang NJ, Harris CC. Mutational hotspot in the p53 gene in human hepatocellular carcinomas. Nature 1991;350:427.
40. Hollstein MC, Metcalf RA, Welsh JA, Montesano R, Harris C. Frequent mutation of the p53 gene in human esophageal cancer. Proc Natl Acad Sci U S A 1990;87:9958.
41. Hollstein MC, Peri L, Mandard AM, et al. Genetic analysis of human esophageal tumors from two high incidence geographic areas: frequent *p53* base substitutions and absence of *ras* mutations. Cancer Res 1991;51:4102.
42. Bennett WP, Hollstein MC, He A, et al. Archival analysis of p53 genetic and protein alterations in Chinese esophageal cancer. Oncogene 1991;6:1779.
43. Wagata T, Shibagaki I, Imamura M, et al. Loss of 17p, mutation of the *p53* gene, and overexpression of p53 protein in esophageal squamous cell carcinomas. Cancer Res 1993;53:846.
44. Audrézet MP, Robaszkiewicz M, Mercier B, et al. *TP53* gene mutation profile in esophageal squamous cell carcinomas. Cancer Res 1993; 53:5745.
45. Huang Y, Meltzer SJ, Yin J, et al. Altered messenger RNA and unique mutational profiles of *p53* and Rb in human esophageal carcinomas. Cancer Res 1993;53:1889.
46. Casson AG, Mukhopadhyay T, Cleary KR, Ro JY, Levin B, Roth JA. *p53* gene mutations in Barrett's epithelium and esophageal cancer. Cancer Res 1991;51:4495.
47. Huang Y, Yin J, Meltzer SJ. A unique *p53* intragenic deletion flanked by short direct repeats results in loss of mRNA expression in a human esophageal carcinoma. Carcinogenesis 1994;15:1653.
48. Greenwald BD, Huang Y, Baum R, Meltzer SJ. Barrett's carcinoma in a 25-year-old man with point mutation of the p53 tumor suppressor gene. Int J Oncol 1992;1:271.
49. Blount PL, Ramel S, Raskind WH, et al. 17p allelic deletions and p53 protein overexpression in Barrett's adenocarcinoma. Cancer Res 1991;51:5482.
50. Yamada Y, Yoshida T, Hayashi K, et al. p53 gene mutations in gastric cancer metastases and in gastric cancer cell lines derived from metastases. Cancer Res 1991;51:5800.
51. Renault B, van den Broek M, Fodde R, et al. Base transitions are the most frequent genetic changes at P53 in gastric cancer. Cancer Res 1993;53:2614.
52. Rhyu M-G, Park W-S, Jung Y-J, Choi S-W, Meltzer SJ. Allelic deletions of *MCC/APC* and *p53* are frequent late events in human gastric carcinogenesis. Gastroenterology 1994;106:1584.
53. Mironov NM, Aguelon MA-M, Potapova GI, et al. Alterations of $(CA)_n$ DNA repeats and tumor suppressor genes in human gastric cancer. Cancer Res 1994;54:41.
54. Baker SJ, Fearon ER, Nigro JM, et al. Chromosome 17 deletions and p53 gene mutations in colorectal carcinomas. Cancer Res 1989;244: 217.
55. Baker SJ, Preisinger AC, Jessup JM, et al. p53 gene mutations occur in combination with 17p allelic deletions as late events in colorectal tumorigenesis. Cancer Res 1990;50:7717.
56. Shirasawa S, Urabe K, Yanagawa Y, Toshitani K, Iwama T, Sasazuki T. *p53* gene mutations in colorectal tumors from patients with familial polyposis coli. Cancer Res 1991;51:2874.
57. Kikuchi-Yanoshita R, Knoishi M, Ito S, et al. Genetic changes of both *p53* alleles associated with the conversion from colorectal adenoma to early carcinoma in familial adenomatous polyposis and non-familial adenomatous polyposis patients. Cancer Res 1991;52:3965.
58. Yin J, Harpaz N, Tong Y, et al. p53 point mutations in dysplastic and cancerous ulcerative colitis lesions. Gastroenterology 1993;104:1633.
59. Taylor HW, Boyle M, Smith SC, Bustin S, Williams NS. Expression of p53 in colorectal cancer and dysplasia complicating ulcerative colitis. Br J Surg 1993;80:442.
60. Harpaz N, Peck AL, Yin J, et al. p53 protein expression in ulcerative colitis-associated colorectal dysplasia and carcinoma. Hum Pathol 1994;25:1069.
61. Hsu IC, Metcalf RA, Sun T, Welsh JA, Wang NJ, Harris CC. Mutational hotspot in the p53 gene in human hepatocellular carcinomas. Nature 1991;350:427.
62. Bressac B, Kew M, Wands J, Ozturk M. Selective G to T mutations of p53 gene in hepatocellular carcinoma from southern Africa. Nature 1991;350:429.
63. Debuire B, Paterlini P, Pontisso P, Basso G, May E. Analysis of the p53 gene in European hepatocellular carcinomas and hepatoblastomas. Oncogene 1993;8:2303.
64. Coursaget P, Depril N, Chabaud M, et al. High prevalence of mutations at codon 249 of the p53 gene in hepatocellular carcinomas from Senegal. Br J Cancer 1993;67:1395.
65. Ng OLN, Chung LP, Tsang SWY, et al. p53 gene mutation spectrum in hepatocellular carcinomas in Hong Kong Chinese. Oncogene 1994; 9:985.
66. Scorsone KA, Zhou Y-Z, Butel JS, Slagle BL. *p53* mutations cluster at codon 249 in hepatitis B virus-positive hepatocellular carcinomas from China. Cancer Res 1992;52:1635.
67. Hosono S, Chou M-J, Lee C-S, Shih C. Infrequent mutation of p53 gene in hepatitis B virus positive primary hepatocellular carcinomas. Oncogene 1993;8:491.
68. Almoguera C, Shibata D, Forrester K, Martin J, Arnheim N, Perucho

M. Most human carcinomas of the exocrine pancreas contain mutant c-K-ras genes. Cell 1988;53:549.
69. Smit VTH, Boot AJM, Smits AMM, Fleuren GJ, Cornelisse CJ, Bos JL. K-ras codon 12 mutations occur very frequently in pancreatic adenocarcinomas. Nucleic Acids Res 1988;16:7773.
70. Mariyama M, Kishi K, Nakamura K, Obata H, Nishimura S. Frequency and types of point mutation at the 12th codon of the c-Ki-ras gene found in pancreatic cancers from Japanese patients. Jpn J Cancer Res 1989;80:622.
71. Nagata Y, Abe M, Motoshima K, Nakayama E, Shiku H. Frequent glycine-to-aspartic acid mutations at codon 12 of c-Ki-ras gene in human pancreatic cancer. Jpn J Cancer Res 1990;81:135.
72. Herrera L, Kakati S, Gibas, Pietrzak E, Sandberg AA. Brief clinical report: Gardner syndrome in a man with an interstitial deletion of 5q. Am J Med Genet 1986;25:473.
73. Bodmer WF, Bailey C, Bodmer J, et al. Localization of the gene for familial adenomatous polyposis on chromosome 5. Nature 1987;328: 614.
74. Leppert M, Dobbs M, Scambler P, et al. The gene for familial polyposis coli maps to the long arm of chromosome 5. Science 1987;238: 1411.
75. Groden J, Thliveris A, Samowitz W, et al. Identification and characterization of the familial adenomatous polyposis coli gene. Cell 1991; 66:589.
76. Joslyn G, Carlson M, Thliveris A, et al. Identification of deletion mutations and three new genes at the familial polyposis locus. Cell 1991;66:601.
77. Kinzler KW, Nilbert MC, Su L-K, et al. Identification of FAP locus genes from chromosome 5q21. Science 1991;253:661.
78. Nishisho I, Nakamura Y, Miyoshi Y, et al. Mutations of chromosome 5q21 genes in FAP and colorectal cancer patients. Science 1991;253: 665.
79. Miyoshi Y, Ando H, Nagase H, et al. Germ-line mutations of the APC gene in 53 familial adenomatous polyposis patients. Proc Natl Acad Sci U S A 1992;89:4452.
80. Powell SM, Petersen GM, Krush AJ, et al. Molecular diagnosis of familial adenomatous polyposis. N Engl J Med 1993;329:1982.
81. Boynton RF, Blount PL, Yin J, et al. Loss of heterozygosity involving the *APC* and *MCC* genetic loci occurs in the majority of human esophageal cancers. Proc Natl Acad Sci U S A 1992;89:3385.
82. Greenwald BD, Harpaz N, Yin J, et al. Loss of heterozygosity affecting the p53, Rb, and mcc/apc tumor suppressor gene loci in dysplastic and cancerous ulcerative. Cancer Res 1992;52:741.
83. Ding SF, Habib NA, Dooley J, Wood C, Bowles L, Delhanty JD. Loss of constitutional heterozygosity on chromosome 5q in hepatocellular carcinoma without cirrhosis. Br J Cancer 1991;64:1083.
84. Fujimori M, Tokino T, Hino O, et al. Allelotype study of primary hepatocellular carcinoma. Cancer Res 1991;51:89.
85. Kinzler KW, Nilbert MC, Vogelstein B, et al. Identification of a gene located at chromosome 5q21 that is mutated in colorectal cancers. Science 1991;251:1366.
86. Nishisho I, Nakamura Y, Miyoshi Y, et al. Mutations of chromosome 5q21 genes in FAP and colorectal cancer patients. Science 1991;253: 665.
87. Horii A, Nakatsuru S, Miyoshi Y, et al. The APC gene, responsible for familial adenomatous polyposis, is mutated in human gastric cancer. Cancer Res 1992;52:3231.
88. Nakatsuru S, Yanagisawa A, Ichii S, et al. Somatic mutation of the APC gene in gastric cancer: frequent mutations in very well differentiated adenocarcinoma and signet-ring cell carcinoma. Hum Molec Genet 1992;1:559.
89. Horii A, Nakatsuru S, Miyoshi Y, et al. Frequent somatic mutations of the APC gene in human pancreatic cancer. Cancer Res 1992;52: 6696.
90. Powell SM, Zilz N, Beazer-Barclay Y, et al. APC mutations occur early during colorectal tumorigenesis. Nature 1992;359:235.
91. Powell SM, Papadopoulos N, Kinzler KW, Smolinski KN, Meltzer SJ. APC gene mutations in the mutation cluster region are rare in esophageal cancers. Gastroenterology 1994;107:1759.
92. Smith KJ, Johnson KA, Bryan TM, Hill DE, et al. The *APC* gene product in normal and tumor cells. Proc Natl Acad Sci U S A 1993; 90:2846.
93. Rubinfeld B, Souza B, Albert I, et al. Association of the APC gene product with beta-catenin. Science 1993;262:1731.
94. Su L-K, Vogelstein B, Kinzler KW. Association of the APC tumor suppressor protein with catenins. Science 1993;262:1734.
95. Mayer B, Johnson JP, Leitl J, et al. E-cadherin expression in primary and metastatic gastric cancer: down-regulation correlates with cellular dedifferentiation and glandular disintegration. Cancer Res 1993;53: 1690.
96. Oda T, Kanai Y, Oyama T, et al. E-cadherin gene mutations in human gastric carcinoma cell lines. Proc Natl Acad Sci U S A 1994;91:1858.
97. Fearon ER, Cho KR, Nigro JM, et al. Identification of a chromosome 18q gene that is altered in colorectal carcinoma. Science 1990;247: 49.
98. Kikuchi-Yanoshita R, Konishi M, Fukunari H, Tanaka K, Miyaki M. Loss of expression of the *DCC* gene during progression of colorectal carcinomas in familial adenomatous polyposis and non-familial adenomatous polyposis patients. Cancer Res 1992;52:3801.
99. Höhne MW, Halatsch M-E, Kahl GF, Weinel RJ. Frequent loss of expression of the potential tumor suppressor gene DCC in ductal pancreatic adenocarcinoma. Cancer Res 1992;52:2616.
100. Gao X, Honn KV, Grignon D, Sakr W, Chen YQ. Frequent loss of expression and loss of heterozygosity of the putative tumor suppressor gene *DCC* in prostatic carcinomas. Cancer Res 1993;53:2723.
101. Scheck AC, Coons SW. Expression of the tumor suppressor gene *DCC* in human gliomas. Cancer Res 1993;53:5605.
102. Porfiri E, Secker-Walker LM, Hoffbrand AV, Hancock JF. *DCC* tumor suppressor gene is inactivated in hematologic malignancies showing monosomy 18. Blood 1993;81:2696.
103. Miyake K, Inokuchi K, Dan K, Nomura T. Expression of the *DCC* gene in myelodyplastic syndromes and overt leukemia. Leuk Res 1993;17:785.
104. Thompson AM, Morris RG, Wallace M, Wyllie AH, Steel CM, Carter DC. Allele loss from 5q21 (*APC/MCC*) and 18q21 (*DCC*) and *DCC* mRNA expression in breast cancer. Br J Cancer 1993;68:64.
105. Nigro JM, Cho KR, Fearon ER, et al. Scrambled exons. Cell 1991; 64:607.
106. Reale MA, Hu G, Zafar AI, Getzenberg RH, Levine SM, Fearon ER. Expression and alternative splicing of the deleted in colorectal cancer (*DCC*) gene in normal and malignant tissues. Cancer Res 1994;54: 4493.
107. Cho KR, Oliner JD, Simons JW, et al. The *DCC* gene: structural analysis and mutations in colorectal carcinomas. Genomics 1994;19: 525.
108. Huang Y, Boynton RF, Blount PL, et al. Loss of heterozygosity involves multiple tumor suppressor genes in human esophageal cancers. Cancer Res 1992;52:6525.
109. Uchino S, Tsuda H, Noguchi M, et al. Frequent loss of heterozygosity at the *DCC* locus in gastric cancer. Cancer Res 1992;52:3099.
110. Narayanan R, Schaapveld RQJ, Cho KR, et al. Antisense RNA from DCC transforms fibroblasts. Oncogene 1992;7:553.
111. Lawlor KG, Telang NT, Osborne MP, et al. Antisense RNA to the putative tumor suppressor gene "deleted in colorectal cancer" transforms fibroblasts. Ann NY Acad Sci 1992;660:283.
112. Hedrick L, Cho KR, Boyd J, Risinger J, Vogelstein B. *DCC*: a tumor suppressor gene expressed on the cell surface. Cold Spring Harb Symp Quant Biol 1992;57:345.
113. Cunningham BA, Hemperly JJ, Murray BA, Prediger EA, Brackenbury R, Edelman GM. Neural cell adhesion molecule: structure, immunoglobulin-like domains, cell surface modulation, and alternative RNA splicing. Science 1987;236:799.
114. Serrano M, Hannon GJ, Beach D. A new regulatory motif in cell-cycle control causing specific inhibition of cyclin D/CDK4. Nature 1993;366:704.
115. Kamb A, Gruis NA, Weaver-Feldhaus J, et al. A cell cycle regulator potentially involved in genesis of many tumor types. Science 1994; 264:436.
116. Olopade OI, Jenkins RB, Ransom DT, et al. Molecular analysis of deletions of the short arm of chromosome 9 in human gliomas. Cancer Res 1992;52:2523.
117. James CD, Collins VP, Allalunis-Turner MJ, Days RS. Localization of chromosome 9p homozygous deletions in glioma cell lines with markers constituting a continuous linkage map. Cancer Res 1993;53: 3674.
118. Ichimura K, Schmidt EE, Yamaguchi N, James CD, Collins VP. A common region of homozygous deletion in malignant human gliomas

lies between the IFNα/ω gene cluster and the D9S171 locus. Cancer Res 1994;54:3127.
119. Coleman A, Fountain JW, Nobori T, et al. Distinct deletions of chromosome 9p associated with melanoma versus glioma, lung cancer, and leukemia. Cancer Res 1994;54:334.
120. Diaz MO, Ziemin S, Le Beau MM, et al. Homozygous deletion of the α- and β-1 interferon genes in human leukemia and derived cell lines. Proc Natl Acad Sci U S A 1988;85:5259.
121. Tsai YC, Nichols PW, Hiti AL, Williams Z, Skinner D, Jones PA. Allelic losses of chromosomes 9, 11, and 17 in human bladder cancer. Cancer Res 1990;50:44.
122. Ruppert JM, Tokino K, Sidransky D. Evidence for two bladder cancer suppressor loci on human chromosome 9. Cancer Res 1993;53:5093.
123. Cairns P, Shaw ME, Knowles MA. Preliminary mapping of the deleted region of chromosome 9 in bladder cancer. Cancer Res 1993;53:1230.
124. Devlin J, Keen AJ, Knowles MA. Homozygous deletion mapping at 9p21 in bladder carcinoma defines a critical region within 2cM of IFNA. Oncogene 1994;9:2757.
125. Cairns P, Tokino K, Eby Y, Sidransky D. Homozygous deletions of 9p21 in primary human bladder tumors detected by comparative multiplex polymerase chain reaction. Cancer Res 1994;54:1422.
126. Orlow I, Lianes P, Lacombe L, Dalbagni G, Reuter VE, Cordon-Cardo C. Chromosome 9 allelic losses and microsatellite alterations in human bladder tumors. Cancer Res 1994;54:2848.
127. Olopade OI, Buchhagen DL, Malik K, et al. Homozygous loss of interferon genes defines the critical region on 9p that is deleted in lung cancers. Cancer Res 1993;53:2410.
128. Mead LJ, Gillespie MT, Irving LB, Campbell LJ. Homozygous and hemizygous deletions of 9p centromeric to the interferon genes in lung cancer. Cancer Res 1994;54:2307.
129. Merlo A, Gabrielson E, Mabry M, Vollmer R, Baylin SB, Sidransky D. Homozygous deletion on chromosome 9p and loss of heterozygosity on 9q, 6p, and 6q in primary human small cell lung cancer. Cancer Res 1994;54:2322.
130. Merlo A, Gabrielson E, Askin F, Sidransky D. Frequent loss of chromosome 9 in human primary non-small lung cancer. Cancer Res 1994; 54:640.
131. Cheng JQ, Jhanwar SC, Lu YY, Testa JR. Homozygous deletions within 9p21-p22 identify a small critical region of chromosomal loss in human malignant mesotheliomas. Cancer Res 1993;53:4761.
132. van der Riet P, Nawroz H, Hruban RH, et al. Frequent loss of chromosome 9p21-22 early in head and neck cancer progression. Cancer Res 1994;54:1156.
133. Fountain JW, Karayiorgou M, Ernstoff MS, et al. Homozygous deletions within human chromosome band 9p21 in melanoma. Proc Natl Acad Sci U S A 1992;89:10557.
134. Holland EA, Beaton SC, Edwards BG, Kefford RF, Mann GJ. Loss of heterozygosity and homozygous deletions on 9p21-22 in melanoma. Oncogene 1994;9:1361.
135. Cannon-Albright LA, Goldgar DE, Meyer LJ, et al. Assignment of a locus for familial melanoma, MLM, to chromosome 9p13-p22. Science 1992;258:1148.
136. Xiong Y, Zhang H, Beach D. D type cyclins associate with multiple protein kinases and the DNA replication and repair factor PCNA. Cell 1992;71:505.
137. Marx J. Research news: new tumor suppressor may rival p53. Science 1994;264:344.
138. Nobori T, Miura K, Wu DJ, Lois A, Takabayashi K, Carson DA. Deletions of the cyclin-dependent kinase-4 inhibitor gene in multiple human cancers. Nature 1994;368:753.
139. Mori T, Miura K, Aoki T, Nishihira T, Mori S, Nakamura Y. Frequent somatic mutation of the MTS1/CDK4I (multiple tumor suppressor/cyclin-dependent kinase 4 inhibitor) gene in esophageal squamous cell carcinoma. Cancer Res 1994;54:3396.
140. Zhou X, Tarmin L, Yin J, et al. The *MTS1* gene is frequently mutated in primary human esophageal tumors. Oncogene 1994;9:3737.
141. Caldas C, Hahn SA, da Costa LT, et al. Frequent somatic mutations and homozygous deletions of the p16 (MTS1) gene in pancreatic adenocarcinoma. Nat Genet 1994;8:27.
142. Cairns P, Mao L, Merlo A, et al. Rates of p16 (MTS1) mutations in primary tumors with 9p loss. Science 1994;265:415.
143. Spruck CH III Gonzalez-Zulueta M, Shibata A, et al. p16 gene in uncultured tumours. Nature 1994;370:183.
144. Hannon GJ, Beach D. $p15^{INK4B}$ is a potential effector of TGF-β-induced cell cycle arrest. Nature 1994;371:257.
145. Cleaver JE. It was a very good year for DNA repair. Cell 1994;76: 1.
146. Jeffreys AJ, Wilson V, Neumann R, Keyte J. Amplification of human minisatellites by the polymerase chain reaction: towards DNA fingerprinting of single cells. Nucleic Acids Res 1988;16:10953.
147. Weber JL, May PE. Abundant class of human DNA polymorphisms which can be typed using the polymerase chain reaction. Am J Hum Genet 1988;44:388.
148. Aaltonen LA, Peltomäki P, Leach FS, et al. Clues to the pathogenesis of familial colorectal cancer. Science 1993;260:812.
149. Thibodeau SN, Bren G, Schaid D. Microsatellite instability in cancer of the proximal colon. Science 1993;260:816.
150. Ionov Y, Peinado MA, Malkhosyan S, et al. Ubiquitous somatic mutations in simple repeated sequences reveal a new mechanism for colonic carcinogenesis. Nature 1993;363:558.
151. Rhyu M-G, Park W-S, Meltzer SJ. Microsatellite instability occurs frequently in human gastric carcinoma. Oncogene 1994;9:29.
152. Mironov NM, Aguelon A-M, Potapova GI, et al. Alterations of $(CA)_n$ DNA repeats and tumor suppressor genes in human gastric cancer. Cancer Res 1994;54:41.
153. Han H-J, Yanagisawa A, Kato Y, Park J-G, Nakamura Y. Genetic instability in pancreatic cancer and poorly differentiated type of gastric cancer. Cancer Res 1993;53:5087.
154. Peltomäki P, Aaltonen LA, Sistonen P, et al. Genetic mapping of a locus predisposing to human colorectal cancer. Science 1993;260: 810.
155. Fishel R, Lescoe MK, Rao MRS. The human mutator gene homolog MSH2 and its association with hereditary nonpolyposis colon cancer. Cell 1993;75:1027.
156. Leach FS, Nicolaides NC, Papadopoulos N, et al. Mutations of a *mutS* homolog in hereditary nonpolyposis colorectal cancer. Cell 1993;75: 1215.
157. Parsons R, Li G-M, Longley MJ, et al. Hypermutatability and mismatch repair deficiency in RER + tumor cells. Cell 1993;75:1226.
158. Papadopoulos N, Nicolaides NC, Wei Y-F, et al. Mutation of a *mutL* homolog in hereditary colon cancer. Science 1994;263:1625.
159. Bronner CE, Baker SM, Morrison PT, et al. Mutation in the DNA mismatch repair gene homologue *hMLH 1* is associated with hereditary non-polyposis colon cancer. Nature 1994;368:258.
160. Nicolaides NC, Papadopoulos N, Liu B, et al. Mutations of two *PMS* homologues in hereditary nonpolyposis colon cancer. Nature 1994; 371:75.
161. Delattre O, Olschwang S, Law DJ, et al. Multiple genetic alterations in distal and proximal colorectal cancer. Lancet 1989;2:353.
162. Burmer GC, Rabinovitch PS, Haggitt RC, et al. Neoplastic progression in ulcerative colitis: histology, DNA content, and loss of a p53 allele. Gastroenterology 1992;103:1602.
163. Greenwald BD, Harpaz N, Yin J, et al. Loss of heterozygosity affecting the p53, Rb, and mcc/apc tumor suppressor gene loci in dysplastic and cancerous ulcerative colitis. Cancer Res 1992;52:741.
164. Yin J, Harpaz N, Tong Y, et al. p53 point mutations in dysplastic and cancerous ulcerative colitis lesions. Gastroenterology 1993;104:1633.
165. Blount PL, Meltzer SJ, Yin J, et al. Clonal ordering of 17p and 5q allelic losses in Barrett's dysplasia and adenocarcinoma. Proc Natl Acad Sci U S A 1993;90:3221.
166. Powell SM, Petersen GM, Krush AJ, et al. Molecular diagnosis of familial adenomatous polyposis. N Engl J Med 1993;329:1982.
167. Sidransky D, Tokino T, Hamilton SR, et al. Identification of *ras* oncogene mutations in the stool of patients with curable colorectal tumors. Science 1992;256:102.
168. Motojima K, Tsunoda T, Kanematsu T, Nagata Y, Urano T, Shiku H. Distinguishing pancreatic carcinoma from other periampullary carcinomas by analysis of mutations in the Kirsten-*ras* oncogene. Ann Surg 1991;214:657.
169. Motojima K, Urano T, Nagata Y, Shiku H, Tsurifune T, Kanematsu T. Detection of point mutations in the Kirsten-*ras* oncogene provides evidence for the multicentricity of pancreatic carcinoma. Ann Surg 1993;217:138.
170. Lemoine NR, Jain S, Hughes CM, et al. Ki-*ras* oncogene activation in preinvasive pancreatic cancer. Gastroenterology 1992;102:230.
171. Hruban RH, van Mansfeld ADM, Offerhaus GJA, et al. K-*ras* oncogene activation in adenocarcinoma of the human pancreas: a study of

82 carcinomas using a combination of mutant-enriched polymerase chain reaction analysis and allele-specific oligonucleotide hybridization. Am J Pathol 1993;143:545.
172. Mao L, Lee DJ, Tockman MS, Erozan YS, Askin F, Sidransky D. Microsatellite alterations as clonal markers for the detection of human cancer. Proc Natl Acad Sci U S A 1994;91:9871.
173. Seckinger D, Sugarbaker E, Frankfurt O. DNA content in human cancer: application in pathology and clinical medicine. Arch Pathol Lab Med 1989;113:619.
174. Wolley RC, Schreiber K, Koss LG, et al. DNA distribution in human colon carcinomas and its relationship to clinical behavior. J Natl Cancer Inst 1982;69:15.
175. Armitage NC, Robins RA, Evans DR, et al. The influence of tumour cell DNA abnormalities on survival in colorectal cancer. Br J Surg 1985;72:828.
176. Kokal W, Sheibani K, Terz J, Harada JR. Tumor DNA content in the prognosis of colorectal carcinoma. JAMA 1986;255:3123.
177. Quirke P, Dixon MF, Clayden AD, et al. Prognostic significance of DNA aneuploidy and cell proliferation in rectal adenocarcinomas. J Pathol 1987;151:285.
178. Bauer KD, Lincoln ST, Vera-Roman JM, et al. Prognostic implications of proliferative activity and DNA aneuploidy in colonic adenocarcinomas. Lab Invest 1987;57:329.
179. Offerhaus GJA, De Feyter EP, Cornelisse CJ, et al. The relationship of DNA aneuploidy to molecular genetic alterations in colorectal carcinoma. Gastroenterology 1992;102:1612.
180. Bosari S, Lee AKC, Wiley BD, et al. Flow cytometric and image analyses of colorectal adenocarcinomas: a comparative study with clinical correlations. Am J Clin Pathol 1993;99:187.
181. Kern SE, Fearon ER, Tersmette KWF, et al. Allelic loss in colorectal carcinoma. JAMA 1989;261:3099.
182. Laurent-Puig P, Olschwang S, Delattre O, et al. Survival and acquired genetic alterations in colorectal cancer. Gastroenterology 1992;102:1136.
183. Jen J, Kim H, Piantadosi S, et al. Allelic loss of chromosome 18q and prognosis in colorectal cancer. N Engl J Med 1994;331:213.
184. Moertel CG, Fleming TR, MacDonald JS, et al. Levamisole and fluorouracil for adjuvant therapy of resected colon carcinoma. N Engl J Med 1990;332:352.
185. Scott N, Sagar P, Stewart J, Blair GE, Dixon MF, Quirke P. p53 in colorectal cancer: clinicopathological correlation and prognostic significance. Br J Cancer 1991;63:317.
186. Yamaguchi A, Nakagawara G, Kurosaka Y, Nishimura G, Yonemura Y, Miyazaki I. p53 immunoreaction in endoscopic biopsy specimens of colorectal cancer, and its prognostic significance. Br J Cancer 1993;68:399.
187. Remvikos Y, Tominaga O, Hammel P, et al. Increased p53 protein content of colorectal tumours correlates with poor survival. Br J Cancer 1992;66:758.
188. Starzynska T, Bromley M, Ghosh A, Stern PL. Prognostic significance of p53 overexpression in gastric and colorectal carcinoma. Br J Cancer 1992;66:558.
189. Yamaguchi A, Kurosaka Y, Fushida S, et al. Expression of p53 protein in colorectal cancer and its relationship to short-term prognosis. Cancer 1992;70:2778.
190. Sun X-F, Carstensen JM, Zhang H, et al. Prognostic significance of cytoplasmic p53 oncoprotein in colorectal adenocarcinoma. Lancet 1992;340:1369.
191. Bosari S, Viale G, Bossi P, et al. Cytoplasmic accumulation of p53 protein: an independent prognostic indicator in colorectal adenocarcinomas. J Natl Cancer Inst 1994;86:681.
192. Joypaul BV, Hopwood D, Newman EL, et al. The prognostic significance of the accumulation of p53 tumour-suppressor gene protein in gastric adenocarcinoma. Br J Cancer 1993;69:943.
193. Kakeji Y, Korenaga D, Tsujitani S, et al. Gastric cancer with p53 overexpression has high potential for metastasising to lymph nodes. Br J Cancer 1993;67:589.
194. Jego N, Thomas G, Hamelin R. Short direct repeats flanking deletions, and duplication insertions in p53 gene in human cancers. Oncogene 1993;8:209.
195. Baas IO, Mulder J-WR, Offerhaus JA, Vogelstein B, Hamilton SR. An evaluation of six antibodies for immunohistochemistry of mutant p53 gene product in archival colorectal neoplasms. J Pathol 1994;172:5.
196. Hamelin R, Laurent-Puig P, Olschwang S, et al. Association of p53 mutations with short survival in colorectal cancer. Gastroenterology 1994;106:42.
197. Muller M, Volkmann M, Zentgraf H, Galle PR. Clinical implications of the P53 tumor-suppressor gene (letter; comment). N Engl J Med 1994;330:865.
198. Volkmann M, Muller M, Hofmann WJ, et al. The humoral immune response to p53 in patients with hepatocellular carcinoma is specific for malignancy and independent of the alpha-fetoprotein status. Hepatology 1993;18:559.
199. Crawford LV, Pim DC, Bulbrook RD. Detection of antibodies against the cellular protein p53 in sera from patients with breast cancer. Int J Cancer 1982;30:403.
200. Mudenda B, Green JA, Green B, et al. The relationship between serum p53 autoantibodies and characteristics of human breast cancer. Br J Cancer 1994;69:1115.
201. Davidoff AM, Iglehart JD, Marks JR. Immune response to p53 is dependent upon p53/HSP70 complexes in breast cancers. Proc Natl Acad Sci U S A 1992;89:3439.
202. Winter SF, Minna JD, Johnson BE, Takahashi T, Gazdar AF, Carbone DP. Development of antibodies against p53 in lung cancer patients appears to be dependent on the type of p53 mutation. Cancer Res 1992;52:4168.
203. Schlichtholz B, Tredaniel J, Lubin R, Zalcman G, Hirsch A, Soussi T. Analyses of p53 antibodies in sera of patients with lung carcinoma define immunodominant regions in the p53 protein. Br J Cancer 1994;69:809.

Surgery for Gastrointestinal Cancer: A Multidisciplinary Approach, edited by Harold J. Wanebo.
Lippincott-Raven Publishers, Philadelphia, © 1997.

CHAPTER 4

Biology of Metastasis

Michael P. Vezeridis and Dan A. Avradopoulos

Metastasis is a complex and fascinating biologic phenomenon that represents the most prominent feature and the main cause of mortality and morbidity associated with malignant tumors. Although uninhibited growth of the primary tumor can result in invasion of vital structures and unresectability, most human primary tumors can be controlled locally by available treatment modalities, and metastasis is responsible for the eventual demise of the host in most cancer deaths.[1,2] The treatment of metastasis is a challenging problem for clinicians involved in the care of patients with cancer.

Reasons for treatment failure include the dispersed anatomic location of the metastatic deposits, their variation in age and size, the inability to detect micrometastases, and the heterogeneity of human tumors.[1–5] Unfortunately, many human tumors give rise to metastatic dissemination by the time diagnosis of the primary lesion is made.[6–8] The lack of effective imaging techniques for the detection of micrometastases creates the false impression that the disease has been eradicated by the removal of the primary tumor. The inability to detect micrometastases is a severe limitation of potential antimetastatic strategies. Despite the significant implications of metastasis in cancer treatment, research in this area has been disproportionately limited. In the last two decades, however, a considerable amount of knowledge regarding the pathogenesis of the metastatic process has been generated for both murine and human solid tumors. In this chapter, the biology of metastasis is reviewed briefly and its implications on cancer management are discussed, with particular emphasis on gastrointestinal neoplasms.

PATHOGENESIS OF METASTASIS

Gastrointestinal cancers, much like other human malignant tumors, can spread by direct invasion and growth into adjacent organs and by migration into the peritoneal cavity. The two most common routes of dissemination are lymphatic and hematogenous metastases. Metastasis is a multistep process that includes the following steps: growth of the primary tumor, invasion into adjacent tissues, invasion of lymphatic or blood vessels, lymphatic or hematogenous dispersal of cancer cells, entrapment of cells in lymph nodes or in the microvasculature of distant organs, extravasation (invasion) of the cells from the microvasculature into organ tissues, and growth of the metastatic deposits (Fig. 4-1). To succeed in producing a metastatic tumor, a cancer cell must complete all the sequential steps of the metastatic process and survive through adverse conditions. Few tumor cells survive this perilous journey and develop into metastatic tumors, fully deserving of Fidler's characterization as "decathlon champions."[9]

Despite its devastating effects on the host, metastasis is an inefficient process.[10,11] Although large numbers of tumor cells may enter the circulation, most are eliminated. Fidler observed that less than 1% of radiolabeled tumor cells were viable 24 hours after placement into the bloodstream and less than 0.1% survived to produce metastases.[12] From a clinical viewpoint, the multistep nature of metastasis may be seen as an advantage, at least theoretically, because it offers the opportunity for intervention at each step.

INVASION

Tumor cell invasion and penetration through lymphatics and blood vessels is a fundamental step in the metastatic process and has been the focus of considerable scientific investigation during the last two decades. The mechanical theory of invasion predominated before 1970.[13] According to this theory, invasion is a passive process caused by mechanical pressure that is the result of rapid growth of the primary tumor.[14] This mechanical pressure is responsible for atrophy, destruction of tissues surrounding the tumor, and penetration into blood vessel walls. Tumor cells then become detached, because of reduced cohesiveness, and disseminate through the circulation.[13,15]

The mechanical theory of invasion cannot explain the fact that although some benign neoplasms can expand rapidly and compress surrounding tissues, they do not invade or metastasize. Furthermore, some extremely invasive tumors grow somewhat slowly.[8,16] The fact that tumor cells can infiltrate organ explants when added to the surface of these explants raises further doubts about the role of mechanical pressure in the process of invasion.[1,17–19] Considering the contradictions sur-

M. P. Vezeridis: Professor of Surgery, Division of Surgical Oncology, Brown University School of Medicine, Roger Williams Medical Center, 825 Chalkstone Avenue, Providence, RI 02908
D. A. Avradopoulos: Fellow, Department of Surgical Oncology, Brown University School of Medicine, Roger Williams Medical Center, 825 Chalkstone Avenue, Providence, RI 02908

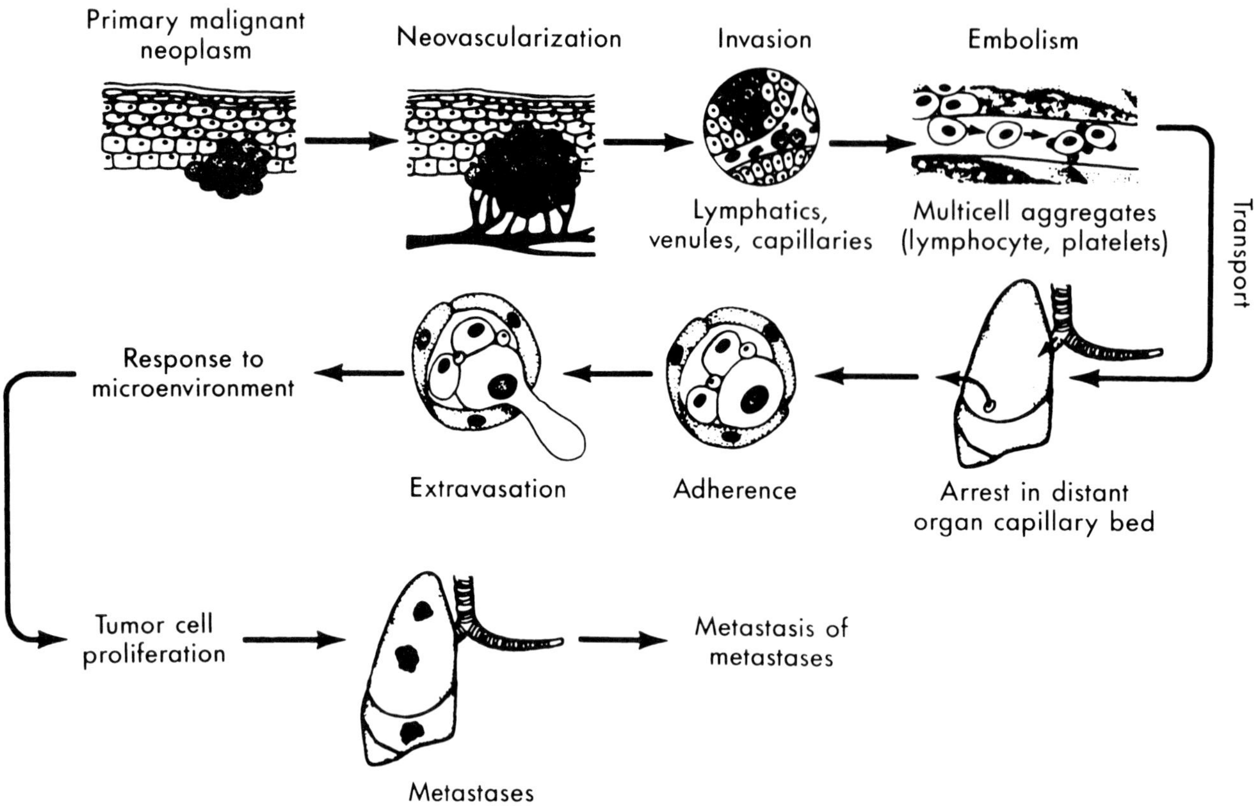

FIG. 4-1. The sequential steps of the metastatic process. (From Fidler IJ. Critical factors in the biology of human cancer metastasis: twenty-eighth GHA Clowes Memorial Award Lecture. Cancer Res 1990; 50:6131.)

rounding the mechanical theory, it is not surprising that the focus of investigation in the last two decades has shifted toward active mechanisms of invasion.

The role of cell motility in invasion has not been firmly established.[1,20–22] Although an association exists between in vitro cell motility and tumorigenic potential, no correlation has been found between in vitro motility and the malignant capacity in vivo of variant murine tumor lines with different invasive behavior.[23–26] Work by Raz showed a correlation between the expression of gp78, a cell-surface glycoprotein, and higher tumor grade, recurrence, and metastasis in human bladder cancer specimens.[27] The expression of this protein was stimulated by autocrine motility factor, suggesting that gp78 may play a role in increasing tumor cell motility. This increase in gp78 also was associated with a decrease in the expression of E-cadherin adhesion molecules. In a separate experiment, polyomavirus-transformed murine endothelioma cell lines were found to secrete a soluble protein, endothelioma-derived motility factor, that stimulates chemotaxis, haptotaxis, and chemoinvasion. This factor is believed to play a role in stimulating and directing endothelial cell migration, and may play a role in the motility of endothelial cells and metastasis.[28] Ladsin, a large cell-adhesive protein that may support metastasis by stimulating tumor cells and surrounding endothelial cells, has been isolated from gastric adenocarcinoma cell lines.[29] Finally, Yabkowitz and colleagues showed a relation between the metastatic potential of tumor cells and response to thrombospondin, a glycoprotein common to the extracellular matrix.[30] Considerable work is needed to clarify further the mechanisms and the role of cell motility in inducing invasion.

The biochemical mechanisms involved in the process of invasion are better defined. Liotta and colleagues proposed a three-step theory describing the sequence of biochemical events during invasion of the extracellular matrix by tumor cells.[13,31,32] The three steps (Fig. 4-2) are tumor cell attachment to the matrix, local degradation of the matrix, and locomotion of tumor cells into the proteolytically modified region of the matrix.[13] During the first step, tumor cells attach to the extracellular matrix through glycoprotein attachment factors and specific receptors to matrix components such as laminin, the integrins, and the fibronectins.[13] Laminin is a basement membrane component synthesized by different cell types.[33–36] Laminin receptors have been found in a variety of normal and neoplastic cells,[37–41] and appear to influence hematogenous metastases.[13,42,43] Significant inhibition of pulmonary metastases was observed after the hematogenous introduction of tumor cells treated with the receptor-binding fragment of laminin.[42] Tumor cells with the capability to attach through laminin showed a tenfold higher production of metastases after intravenous injection.[43] Jaskiewicz and associates showed a relation between the downregulation of laminin production and poorly differentiated tumors in patients with hepatocellular carcinoma.[44] Using a human melanoma model, one study found a positive correlation between the expression of laminin receptors and disease progression.[45]

The fibronectins are large extracellular glycoproteins involved in many biologic functions related to cell adhesion and

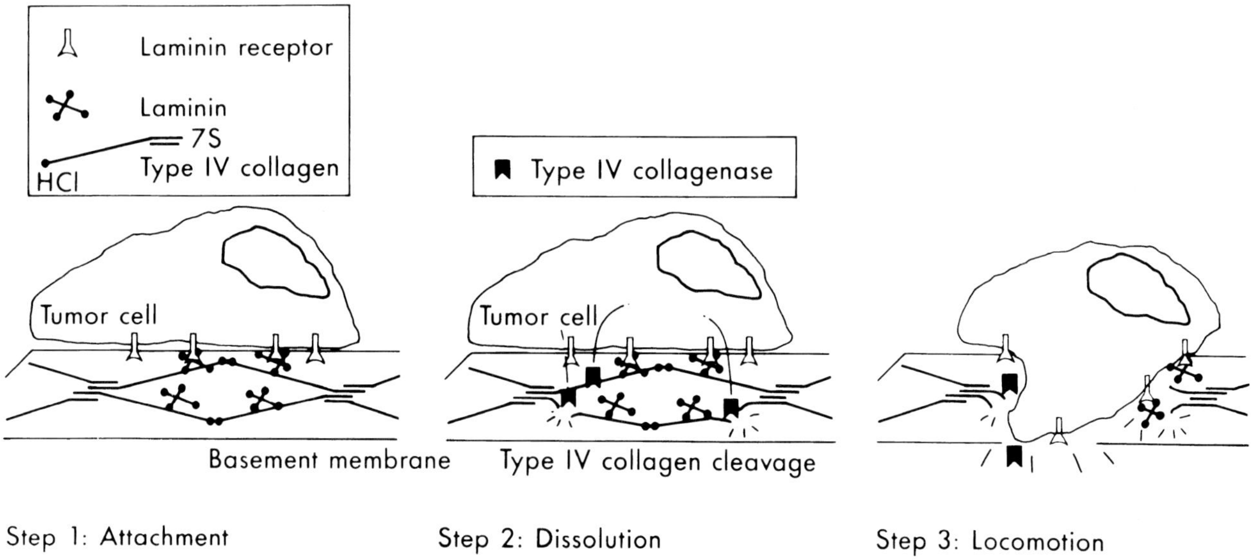

FIG. 4-2. A schematic representation of basement membrane invasion by a tumor cell, illustrating the three-step hypothesis. *Step 1,* tumor cell attachment to the matrix. *Step 2,* local degradation of the matrix by tumor cell-associated proteases. *Step 3,* tumor cell locomotion into the region of the matrix modified by proteolysis. (From Liotta LA. Tumor invasion and metastasis-role of extracellular matrix: Rhoads Memorial Award Lecture. Cancer Res 1986;46:1.)

migration.[46] They bind to cells through specific receptors.[47–50] The major fibronectin receptor on most cells is a noncovalent complex of two transmembrane glycoprotein subunits that is a member of the integrin family of heterodimers.[46] This fibronectin receptor originally was identified in human osteosarcoma cells.[51] Integrins recognize the arginine-glycine-aspartic acid sequence, which constitutes the recognition site of many adhesive proteins, including fibronectin, vitronectin, osteospontin, collagens, thrombospondin, fibrinogen, and von Willebrand's factor.[52] Increased expression of the fibronectin receptor was found by immunofluorescence in Rous sarcoma virus–induced tumors and after malignant transformation of fibroblasts in vitro.[53] Fibronectins also can be produced by some colorectal cancer cell lines, and the fibronectin-enriched microenvironment subsequently may alter the adherence and invasive potential of colon cancer cells, as suggested by Pujuguet and associates.[54] Kemperman and colleagues have shown that high levels of a specific integrin, a6b4, often are expressed by a metastatic mammary cell line and contribute to liver metastasis formation.[55] A β1-integrin also has been shown to contribute to the migration and invasion of pancreatic cancer cells in vitro.[56] Others have observed that downregulation of expression of the epithelium-specific cell adhesion molecule E-cadherin in squamous cell carcinomas of the head and neck is associated with tumor dedifferentiation and lymph node metastasis.[57] The downregulation of E-cadherin also has been shown in human esophageal cancer, and evidence suggests that it plays a role in aggressive thyroid carcinomas and colorectal cancer.[58–60] Finally, Mayer and associates showed a significant correlation between low E-cadherin expression and cellular dedifferentiation and disintegration of tissue architecture in patients with gastric carcinoma.[61] In addition, low E-cadherin expression was associated with tumor recurrence and death.

The second step, local degradation of the matrix, consists of the secretion of degradative enzymes that cause local lysis o the matrix. Higher levels of lytic enzymes are expressed by malignant tumors than by benign neoplasms or normal tissues.[1,22,25,62–70] Increased production of the cysteine proteinase cathepsin B has been observed in malignant breast tumors, but not in benign breast tumors or normal breast tissue.[71,72] Enhanced activity of cathepsin B appears to correlate with increased metastatic potential.[73,74] The role of the serine protease plasminogen activator in the process of invasion is not clear. Although increased production of this enzyme was observed in neoplastic transformation,[75,76] a consistent correlation between plasminogen activator production and malignant behavior in vivo could not be established in studies of murine melanoma cell lines with different invasive potential.[1,26,67,69] Some evidence suggests that protein kinase C may play a role in facilitating basement membrane invasion by tumor cells, and that this activity may be neutralized by plasminogen activator inhibitor.[77] In addition, specific isoforms of protein kinase C (PKCβ1) have been shown to induce maximal invasion of gastric cancer cells, and this effect appears to be dependent on localization of the protein within the cell.[78] Schwartz and colleagues have demonstrated inhibition of gastric invasion using protein kinase C inhibitors.[79]

The four major groups of connective tissue proteins are collagen, elastin, glycoproteins, and proteoglycans. Collagen is an important component because it functions as structural scaffolding for the other matrix components.[69] Type IV collagen is an important structural protein of basement membranes and is chemically and genetically different from types I and III stromal collagens and type II cartilage collagen.[1] Liotta and colleagues found that tumor cells could cause degradation of noncollagenous and collagenous components of the basement membrane.[31,80] The same investigators observed a strong correlation between increased production of collagenase IV and the potential of murine tumor cells to metastasize spontaneously.[69,81] In a paper by Zucker and associates, MMP-9 (a type IV collagenase) was found to be increased in the plasma of patients with colorectal and breast cancers, compared with control patients and 179 patients with lung cancer, genitourinary tract cancer, or lymphoma or leukemia.[82] The clinical significance of these findings needs further investigation. In another study, the expression of type IV collagenase in gastric carcinoma was found to be significantly higher in intestinal and atypical carcinomas compared with diffuse carcinomas.[83] In addition, collagenase IV expression was correlated significantly with lymphatic invasion and aneuploidy.[83] In a related in vivo experiment, high levels of Mr 92,000 progelatinase (a type IV collagenase) in rat sera were associated with disseminated metastatic adenocarcinoma in rats injected with 13762NF mammary carcinoma.[84] Again, the prognostic significance of these findings remains to be determined.

In addition to collagenase IV and cathepsin B, much work has focused on the exploration of various degradative enzymes and their relation to metastases. For instance, using a human prostate tumor cell line (DU-145), Powell and colleagues transfected tumor cells with matrilysin, a matrix metalloproteinase (MMP-7). Vector-only transfected cells caused invasion in only 1 of 9 mice (11%), compared with 12 of 18 (66%) mice in matrilysin-transfected tumor cells, suggesting a functional role for matrilysin in the initial invasion of prostate cancer.[85] In contrast, Martin and associates were able to confer resistance to antigen-induced tumor growth in vivo by transfecting mice with tissue inhibitors of metalloproteinases.[86] In addition to enzymes playing a role in the degradation and subsequent metastasis of human carcinomas, there also is evidence that certain inhibitors may play a role in the promotion of tumor growth. For instance, Shirasuna and associates showed that adenoid cystic carcinoma cells produced an extracellular matrix rich in plasminogen activator inhibitor type 1, which may help stabilize extracellular matrix components of tumor origin and promote the growth of carcinoma cells.[87] In a separate experiment, investigators showed that human macrophage inflammatory protein 1a upregulates matrix metalloproteinases and plasminogen activator production, and may modulate metastases through these channels.[88] Montgomery and colleagues showed that overexpression of tissue inhibitor metalloproteinases-2 inhibited growth and invasion in a human melanoma cell line.[89] Expression of plasminogen activator inhibitor type 2 by a sarcoma cell line has been shown to inhibit protein degradation and invasion in vitro,[90] supporting the contention that invasion is governed by a balance of matrix enzymes.

The third step of invasion is locomotion of the tumor cells into the matrix, which has been proteolytically modified during the previous step.[13] This may be accomplished through chemotactic or autocrine motility factors. It has been shown that various factors, including collagen peptides, formyl peptides, some connective tissue components, and component-derived materials, can act as chemoattractants in vitro.[13,91] Liotta and colleagues found that the human melanoma cell line A2058 produces, in culture, a factor that stimulates markedly its own motility and possesses both chemotactic and chemokinetic properties.[92]

TRANSPORT AND DISPERSAL OF TUMOR CELLS

After the tumor penetrates blood and lymphatic channels, cells are released and carried away, or they may grow locally and release tumor emboli later.[1] A common misconception is that the lymphatic and vascular systems are completely separate from each other and that some tumors disseminate through the lymphatics, whereas others spread through the bloodstream. However, it has been demonstrated experimentally that many connections exist between the lymphatic and vascular systems that allow the passage of tumor cells.[1,93–95] The presence of tumor cells in the blood circulation is not synonymous with metastasis. Most tumor cells entering the circulation are destroyed rapidly.[10,12] Turbulence in the bloodstream appears to play a significant role in the elimination of tumor cells from the circulation. The aggregation of tumor cells with each other or with blood cells such as lymphocytes and platelets may contribute to their protection and survival in the circulation.[96–98]

ENTRAPMENT OF TUMOR CELLS

Entrapment of tumor cells in the lymph nodes or capillaries of distant organs is an essential step in the metastatic process. In the lymphatic circulation, the tumor cells may be arrested in the first nodal basin they encounter, or they may traverse or bypass it to be arrested in more distant lymph nodes.[94] The usual site of initial arrest of tumor cells and growth of lymph node metastases is the subcapsular sinus.[21,99] Evidence regarding the role of the regional lymph nodes as potential filters for tumor cells is contradictory.[76,93] Clarification of this controversial issue will have significant clinical impact in regard to prophylactic removal of the regional lymph nodes.

Entrapment of tumor cells in the microvasculature of distant organs is a factor of paramount importance in the formation of hematogenous metastases. Mechanical cell entrapment in the capillary bed alone does not suffice to produce metastases.[100–102] Interactions of the tumor cells with the vascular endothelium play an important role in the formation of metastatic colonies.[1] Adherence of the tumor cells to endothelial cells and the subendothelial matrix appears to be essential in this step of the metastatic process.[102–104] Platelets facilitate the attachment of tumor cells to the capillary basement membrane.[98,105,106] Fibronectin, laminin, and type IV collagen are the basement membrane elements involved in tumor cell attachment.[47,91] It has been observed that preincubation of BL6 melanoma cells with whole laminin (injected through the tail vein of C57 black mice) enhances retention of tumor cells and promotes metastasis formation in the lung.[42] The role of cell attachment in the site specificity of metastases has been studied thoroughly[100,107–111] and is discussed later in this chapter. Fibrin deposition around tumor cells has been observed and postulated to contribute to the protection of tumor cells from host defense forces.[112–116]

The observation of an association between malignant tumors and coagulation first was made by Trousseau more than a century ago.[117] Abundant clinical and laboratory observations regarding this association were made in the 1970s.[118–125] Although fibrin has been demonstrated in some experimental metastasis models,[126–128] its exact role in tumor cell arrest and metastasis has not been established conclusively.[1,112]

EXTRAVASATION AND GROWTH OF METASTATIC COLONIES

To enter the parenchyma of an organ and give rise to the growth of metastatic colonies, the cells arrested in the microvasculature must extravasate following steps similar to those of invasion.[2,129] The tumor cells can grow and destroy the vessel, or migrate and follow leukocytes.[1,2] Retraction of the vascular endothelium after contact with the tumor cells exposes subendothelial tissues, which interact with the tumor cells.[130] Involvement of platelets at this step of the metastatic process seems probable.[131] Thrombi adherent to vascular endothelium and composed of tumor cells surrounded by platelets have been observed in experimental metastasis models.[132,133] Tumor cell–induced platelet aggregation in vitro has been well documented.[134–139] Pancreatic cancer cells have been shown to convert prothrombin to thrombin in a factor 5–dependent mechanism, and to activate factor 10 directly.[140] This ability to activate the coagulation system may play a role in the metastasis of pancreatic carcinoma, or contribute to the high incidence of thrombosis in this disease. A platelet-derived vascular permeability factor may contribute to easier passage of the tumor cells through the capillary wall.[141] In addition, platelets produce growth factors, such as platelet-derived growth factor and transforming growth factor-β, that contribute to tumor cell proliferation.[142] There is evidence that interleukin-1 may play a role in inducing the growth of metastatic lesions, and that this augmented growth can be inhibited with an interleukin-1 receptor antagonist.[143] Kobrin and associates also have shown that fibroblast growth factor may contribute to aberrant autocrine and paracrine pathways in pancreatic cancer.[144]

After extravasation into the organ parenchyma, the tumor cells must survive the immune forces of the host to establish metastatic colonies. Vascularization of the metastatic colonies is vital for their continuing growth. Work by Nicolson and colleagues suggests that tumor cell mitogens produced by organ-derived endothelial cells may play a role in supporting vascularization and promoting tumor growth.[145]

METASTATIC PATTERNS AND ORGAN SPECIFICITY

More than a century ago, Stephen Paget, based on autopsy observations of many patients with breast cancer, concluded that the pattern of metastasis was not random, but depended on the capacity of specific organs to support the growth of the metastasizing tumor cells.[146] His metaphor, "When a plant goes to seed, its seeds are carried in all directions but they can only live and grow if they fall on congenial soil," became known as the *seed and soil hypothesis*. This theory dominated the scientific thinking about metastasis for several decades, until Ewing attempted to explain site specificity based solely on anatomic considerations related to blood circulation.[147] However, this mechanical theory is unable to justify why organs with abundant blood flow, such as the spleen, heart, and skeletal muscles, are uncommon targets for metastatic dissemination.[93–95] In addition, observations from autopsies of patients who underwent peritoneovenous shunts for palliation of malignant ascites showed that metastases did not develop in all of them.[148,149] Some of the patients were completely free of metastases after long periods of survival, whereas others had small asymptomatic metastatic lesions. In some patients, inert tumor cells were identified in organ tissues by tumor markers without growing metastases. Even though hematogenous metastases were formed in some patients, they had not developed in the organ of the first capillary bed, but in more distant organs.[148,149] Because a peritoneovenous shunt is, in essence, a direct injection of tumor cells into the circulation, the mechanical theory is unable to explain reasonably the metastatic growth patterns observed in these studies.

The validity of the seed and soil hypothesis has been supported by several experimental studies. Intraarterial and subcutaneous injections of lung-colonizing tumor cells in mice with neonatal tissues transplanted in the thighs produced metastatic lesions in both the in situ and transplanted lungs, but not in other organs.[150,151] B16 melanoma cells intravenously injected in mice produced metastatic colonies in the in situ lungs and in subcutaneous or intramuscular implants of pulmonary or ovarian tissue, but not in implanted renal tissue or at the site of surgical trauma.[152] Significant differences in immediate tumor cell arrest between lung and kidney implants were not found in this study after the injection of ^{125}I-5-iodo-2-deoxyuridine–labeled cells, indicating that tumor growth in the implanted lung tissue was not caused by increased initial arrest of tumor cells.[152] A murine reticulum cell sarcoma, M5076, was found to metastasize preferentially to the intraabdominal viscera, specifically to the liver, spleen, kidney, and ovaries.[153] This pattern of metastasis was not influenced by the site of tumor cell injection. Further, intravenous injection of radiolabeled cells showed that they were arrested rapidly in the lungs, retained for 3 to 4 days, and then released, recirculated, and arrested in the liver, where they gave rise to metastatic colonies.[153] All these studies indicate that single mechanical arrest of tumor cells in an organ is not sufficient for the production of clinically significant metastases, but that the tumor cell properties and the microenvironment of the target organ are important elements in the growth of metastatic tumors.

Selection of tumor cells with high metastatic capacity and preference for specific organ colonization has been accomplished using both animal and human tumors. Lung-,[154] brain-,[155] and liver-colonizing[156] variants of B16 melanoma were selected. Cell lines and clones with enhanced spontaneous metastatic capacity to lymph nodes and lung were established from spontaneous lymph node and lung metastases that were formed after subcutaneous implantation of the rat 13762 mammary adenocarcinoma into the mammary fat pad of rats.[157] The introduction of the nude mouse in metastasis research enabled investigators to select metastatic variants from human tumors. Using this model, Morikawa and colleagues isolated cells with liver-metastasizing potential from heterogenous primary human colon carcinomas.[158] After four in vivo selection cycles, these cells produced lines with high metastatic efficiency. The metastatic capacity of the human carcinoma cells increased with each successive selection cycle. Another important observation in this study was that a comparable number of radiolabeled cells with low and light metastatic potential were arrested in the liver shortly after injection into the spleen. Differences were observed 24 hours after injection, and at 72 hours only highly metastatic cells survived in the liver. These findings provide further support for the hypothesis that metastasis is not the result of simple mechanical entrapment of cancer cells in the target organ. These authors have selected a highly metastatic cell line from the human pancreatic carcinoma cell line COLO 357 in the nude mouse.[159] This line was established after five passages of the fast-growing variant (FG) of COLO 357 through the nude mouse liver and produced extensive hepatic metastases in 100%

TABLE 4-1. *Metastatic potential of cell lines derived from a human pancreatic carcinoma*

Tumor cell lines	No. of animals	No. of mice with hepatic metastases (%)	No. of mice with pulmonary metastases (%)
FG	14	9 (64)	6 (43)
L3.1	12	9 (75)	4 (40)
L3.2	11	8 (73)	5 (45)
L3.3	12	10 (83)	4 (33)
L3.4	10	8 (80)	3 (30)
L3.5	11	11 (100)	1 (9)

(From Vezeridis MP, Tzanakakis GN, Metiner PA, Doremus CM, Tibbetts LM, Calabresi P. In vivo selection of a highly metastatic cell line from a human pancreatic carcinoma in the nude mouse. Cancer 1992;69(8):2062)

of the experimental animals when injected into the spleen. Although the incidence of hepatic metastases increased with each sequential passage, the incidence of pulmonary metastases decreased from 43% for FG to 9% for L3.5 (Table 4-1). In addition, the L3.5 line showed aggressive growth, with almost complete replacement of the hepatic parenchyma (Fig. 4-3) in one-third the mean time required for the development of macroscopic liver metastases after the injection of FG cells into the spleen. The selection of tumor cell lines with high metastatic efficiency and site preference provided the necessary tools for the study of tumor cell properties, host-related factors, and their respective roles in the survival and growth of metastatic colonies in different organs and tissues.

A prerequisite for the establishment of metastases in a specific organ is adherence of the tumor cells to the microvasculature of the target organ. The availability of vascular endothelial cell cultures enabled investigators to study tumor cell adhesiveness and its correlation with metastasis.[104,111,160–162] Korach and associates evaluated 11 cloned cell lines derived from a rat rhabdomyosarcoma for metastatic potential and attachment kinetics to confluent pig endothelial cell monolayers grown in vitro.[161] They observed that all 6 highly colonizing lines had high attachment rates, whereas the 4 or 5 lines with low colonizing capacity had low attachment rates to endothelial monolayers in vitro. Auerbach and colleagues compared the rate and extent of adherence of various murine tumor cells, including sarcoma, glioma, teratoma, hepatoma, bladder carcinoma, endothelioma, mammary adenocarcinoma, and lymphoma, to microvascular endothelial cells from the ovary, brain, lung, and liver, and to large-vessel endothelia from the thoracic duct and dorsal aorta.[104] They found that tumor cells differ in both adhesive propensity and adhesive preference for different endothelial cells, and that some of the adhesive preferences correlate with the known in vivo metastatic behavior of the tumors. Nicolson found that B16 melanoma sublines with high lung or brain colonization efficiency had significantly higher rates of adherence to murine lung or brain microvessel endothelial cells, respectively, and that sublines of the RAW 117 murine lymphoma with high liver or lung colonization efficiency adhered at higher rates to murine liver sinusoidal endothelial cells or lung microvessel endothelial cells, respectively.[162] Binding of the tumor cells to subendothelial basement membrane also may play an important role in the site specificity of metastases. Kramer and colleagues found that the metastatic cell lines B16-F1 (murine) and HS939 (human) melanoma adhered rapidly to extracellular matrix, whereas they attached slowly to endothelial cell monolayers.[163] Doerr and colleagues tested three human hepatoma, two human, and one rat mammary carcinoma cell line for clonal growth on tissue-specific biomatrices, and found that the tissue specificity in clonal growth of these lines correlated with their organ site specificity for metastasis in nude mice.[164]

The role of tumor cell adhesion to other cellular components of the target organ parenchyma in the site specificity of metastasis also has been studied during the last decade. Roos and colleagues found that tumor cells with preferential metastatic capacity to the liver adhere preferentially to liver endothelial cells and hepatocytes.[165,166] Gjoen and colleagues observed that metastatic colon carcinoma cells preferentially bind to liver macrophages.[167] Experimental evidence suggests that the leukocyte function–associated antigen mediates the adhesion of lymphoma cells to hepatocytes.[168,169] The identification of other mediators of tumor cell adhesion in the liver needs further investigation.

The ability of the metastatic tumor cell to degrade extracellular matrix and connective tissue is an important prerequisite for metastasis. Metastatic cancer cells have the ability to produce various degradative enzymes.[74,81,170–173] Because the molecular

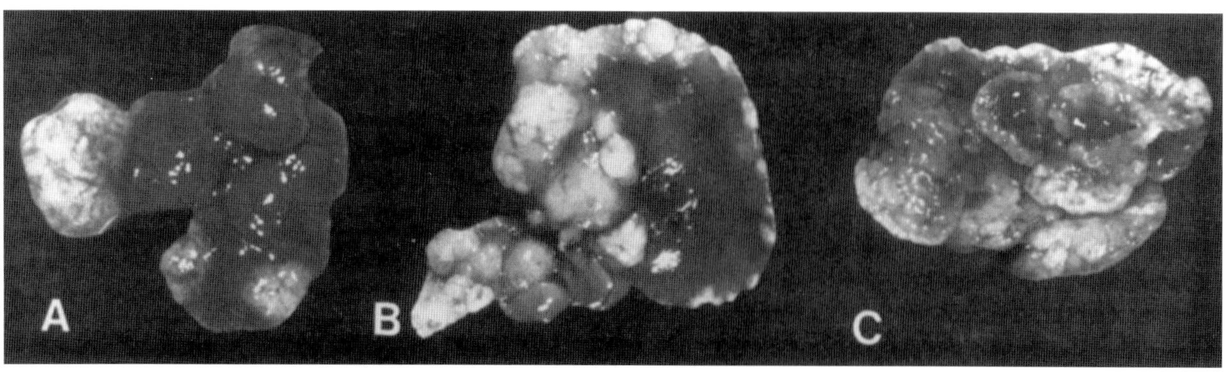

FIG. 4-3. Representative liver specimens from animals injected with **(A)** FG, **(B)** L3.3, and **(C)** L3.5 cells into the spleen. (From Vezeridis NP, Tzanakakis GN, Metiner PA, Doremus CM, Tibbetts LM, Calabresi P. In vivo selection of a highly metastatic cell line from a human pancreatic carcinoma in the nude mouse. Cancer 1992;69(8):2062.)

structure of the extracellular matrix is tissue specific,[102] the ability of cancer cells to produce specific degradative enzymes may be a decisive factor in their ability to form metastases in a particular tissue or organ. It is logical to assume that cancer cells producing elastase or type IV collagenase will be successful in metastasizing to organs with extracellular matrix rich in elastin or type IV collagen, such as the lung, and this hypothesis is supported by research findings.[102,170]

The influence of the organ environment on the growth of metastatic cancer cells also has been the focus of investigative interest during the last decade. Horak and associates studied the influence of microenvironment on tumor cell survival and behavior in vitro, using a spontaneous murine mammary carcinoma.[174] They observed that whereas the lungs and ovaries supported the survival of tumor cells, the liver and thyroid gland consistently decreased the survival of these cells. This observation was in agreement with the metastatic pattern of this tumor after the injection of tumor cells into the aortas of mice. Further, the effects on tumor cell survival were shown to result from soluble substances diffusing out of the organs. Nicolson and Dulski investigated murine B16 melanoma cell sublines selected in vivo for enhanced colonization of lung, brain, or ovary for survival and growth stimulation in vitro by soluble factors produced by suspensions of mouse lung, brain, liver, ovary, or kidney.[175] They found that the growth of lung-colonizing cells was stimulated by high concentrations of factors derived from other tissues. They also observed that liver tissue factors and high concentrations of kidney tissue factors inhibited cell growth. The B16 cell sublines tested had low liver and kidney colonization potential in vivo. The stimulation of cell growth was dose dependent. The findings from both these studies suggest that the site specificity of metastasis may be influenced by soluble organ-derived factors on the survival and growth of the tumor cells. Research has shown that basic fibroblast growth factor may play a role in promoting tumor growth in the metastatic colonies of melanoma and human pancreatic cancers.[176,177] Yamanaka and associates also showed a relation between the overexpression of acidic and basic fibroblast growth factors and advanced stage in human pancreatic cancer.[177]

Cavanaugh and Nicolson purified from porcine and rat lung–conditioned media a factor that preferentially promoted the growth of lung-metastasizing rat 13762NF mammary adenocarcinoma and murine B16 melanoma cell lines over their poorly metastasizing counterparts.[178] Other factors that may affect the growth of tumor cells in colonized organs are the cytostatic ability of specialized cells, such as the Kupffer cells of the liver, and exposure to specific elements of the immune system, such as natural killer (NK) cells and activated macrophages.[162]

Much work has been done examining the role of oncogenes and oncoproteins in predicting the aggressiveness and metastatic potential of primary tumors. Finkelstein and colleagues showed a higher incidence of K-*ras*-2 mutations in lymphogenous and hematogenous metastases compared with local recurrences.[179] Overall, 35% of primary colorectal cancers were mutated. Colorectal cancer with codon 12 aspartic acid substitutions, as the K-*ras*-2 mutation, accounted for most of the hematogenous deposits.[179] In another study, the expression of nm23 genes was evaluated in primary and liver metastases. Reduced expression of nm23 was a consistent finding in liver metastases, suggesting a possible role as a marker of metastatic progression in colorectal carcinoma.[180] These findings were confirmed by other investigators.[181] Although this work is promising, additional investigation is needed to clarify the role of oncogenes, and their protein products, in predicting metastases.

A century after Paget's initial observation, the seed and soil hypothesis has received considerable support from experimental studies. It has become increasingly evident that the formation and growth of metastases requires that tumor cells with metastatic potential reach organs in which their growth is enhanced or not inhibited by cellular or humoral components present in the new microenvironment.

ANGIOGENESIS AND METASTASIS

The role of angiogenesis in tumor growth is supported by experimental evidence.[182] Although observations regarding the rich vascularity of tumors date back to the 19th century,[183] the observation that tumors elicit the growth of new capillaries from the surrounding tissue was made in the 1940s with the use of the transparent chamber technique.[184] Using this technique, Greenblatt and Shubik demonstrated that capillary proliferation is induced even when the implanted tumor is separated from the vascular bed of the host by a millipore filter.[185] Subsequently, Folkman and colleagues isolated from the Walker 256 tumor a soluble factor capable of inducing neovascularization.[186] The fact that establishment of vascular supply is a prerequisite for the growth of a tumor to a size larger than 2 mm has been demonstrated by Folkman and Cotran.[187–189] This observation makes evident the role of angiogenesis in metastasis, because the primary tumor must grow beyond this size before the occurrence of metastases in most clinical cases. Further, the formation of clinically significant metastases results from the continued growth of neoplastic cells after their extravasation into the parenchyma of the distant organs, which requires neovascularization.

A strong correlation between angiogenesis and metastasis has been established by experimental and clinical studies. Liotta and associates observed that the appearance of tumor cells in the efferent circulation of mice with fibrosarcomas implanted in the thigh coincided with the neovascularization of the tumors, and that the number of released tumor cells and the number of pulmonary metastases correlated with the number of tumor vessels.[190] The architecture of the new tumor vessels differs considerably from the vasculature of normal tissues. The new tumor capillaries tend to be dilated, tortuous, and saccular, and they have a fragmented basement membrane that facilitates their penetration by tumor cells.[191,192] A classic clinical example of the relation between angiogenesis and metastasis is the natural history of malignant melanoma. Early, thin lesions confined to the epidermis are not vascularized and do not metastasize, whereas thicker lesions extending into the dermis acquire neovasculature and metastasize.[193] A quantitative relation between the intensity of angiogenesis and the probability of metastasis in cutaneous malignant melanoma has been reported.[194–196] Another study demonstrated a correlation between angiogenic activity and the incidence of metastases in patients with invasive breast carcinoma.[197]

Although the establishment of metastases requires the successful completion of several other steps, tumor angiogenesis is a necessary element of the metastatic cascade and represents a logical target for antimetastatic treatment.

EXPERIMENTAL MODELS FOR METASTASIS

The study of the pathogenesis of the metastatic process and the evaluation of antimetastatic interventions require the use of experimental models. Initially, experimental work used rodent models.[154,198] Tan and colleagues described a model of mesenteric lymph node and liver metastasis using orthotopic transplantation of the murine colon adenocarcinoma MCA-38 into the lymphoid follicle of the cecum in mice.[199] Metastatic models using human tumors are a relatively recent development. Although the athymic nude mouse model was introduced in cancer research in the late 1960s by Rygaard and Povlsen[200] and was used extensively in the study of other aspects of human tumor biology and response to chemotherapy,[201,202] its value in the study of metastasis was appreciated more fully during the last decade. The initial belief that malignant tumors rarely metastasize in nude mice[203–205] was altered after work by several investigators, using a variety of human tumors, established the fact that the nude mouse provides a useful in vivo model for the study of the biology and treatment of human cancer metastases.[206–211]

The nude mouse model has been used in the study of colorectal cancer metastasis. Giavazzi and colleagues studied the metastatic potential of human colon carcinoma cell lines from primary tumor, lymph node, and hepatic metastases using a model of tumor cell implantation into the spleen.[210] They observed that the implantation of cells derived from primary tumor and lymph node metastases produced few liver tumors after 90 days, whereas extensive liver tumors developed only 30 days after the injection of cells derived from hepatic metastases. These authors have used intrasplenic tumor cell inoculation to study the metastatic potential of human colon carcinoma cell lines.[212,213] The ten human colon adenocarcinoma cell lines exhibited substantial heterogeneity of potential for hepatic metastasis, with establishment of liver metastases ranging from 0% to 70% (see Fig. 4-3). The capacity of the cells to grow at the site of inoculation in the spleen and in the liver was associated with carcinoembryonic antigen production in the culture medium, levels of which ranged from undetectable to 5200 ng/mL.[213] The association of carcinoembryonic antigen production with the potential for hepatic metastasis is of great interest because the role of this tumor marker as a prognostic indicator is well established in the literature,[214,215] and because experimental evidence indicates that it has a biologic function related to tumorigenicity[216] and enhancement of hepatic metastases.[217] Further studies of the biologic function of carcinoembryonic antigen may reveal significant information related to the process of hepatic metastasis from colorectal carcinoma. These authors also have used intrasplenic injections to establish models of experimental metastasis from two human pancreatic carcinomas.[218,219] A good experimental model for hepatic metastasis is important because the liver is a common site of metastasis in patients with gastrointestinal carcinomas.

The site of tumor implantation is an important consideration in the development of a metastatic model. It is well known that human tumors rarely metastasize after subcutaneous or intramuscular implantation in nude mice.[1,211] Fidler found visceral metastases in only 1 of more than 200 mice with colorectal cancers implanted subcutaneously.[211] In contrast, other investigators observed that the implantation of colon cells into the spleens of nude mice resulted in the development of hepatic metastases in most of the animals.[210,212,213] Orthotopic implantation of human tumors in the nude mouse has generated considerable interest.[220–222] Orthotopic implantation of various human tumors resulted in the development of distant metastases much more frequently than did ectopic implantation.[222] This is clearly the case with human colon carcinomas, as demonstrated by Fidler.[222] Using a human pancreatic carcinoma, these authors developed a model of orthotopic transplantation of tumor fragments in the pancreas of the nude mouse, which produced metastases to the lymph nodes, liver, and lung[223] (Fig. 4-4). Fu and colleagues developed a metastatic model from colon cancer using orthotopic implantation of fragments of histologically intact patient specimens.[224] The use of tumor fragments instead of cell suspensions obviates the need for cell dissociation, which

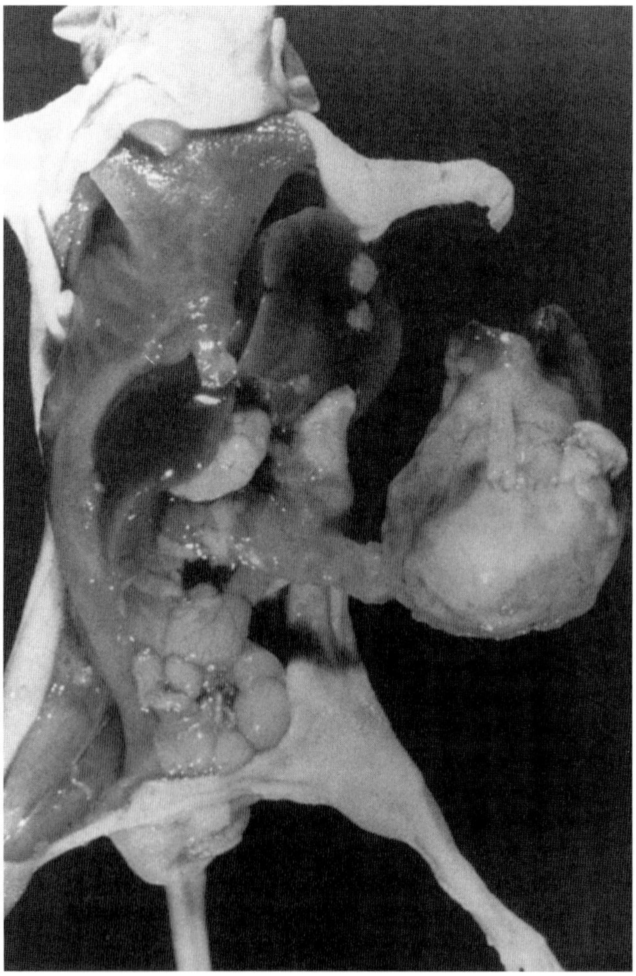

FIG. 4-4. Autopsy findings in a mouse transplanted with L3.3. Large growth at the site of the transplantation and metastatic nodules in the liver. (From Vezeridis MP, Doremus CM, Tibbetts LM, Tzanakakis G, Jackson BT. Invasion and metastasis following orthotopic transplantation of human pancreatic cancer in the nude mouse. Journal of Surgical Oncology, 1989;40:261.) See also color Figure 4-4.

may affect the biologic behavior of the tumor.[224] Further, it eliminates the possibility of direct injection of cells into the circulation, and enables the study of the entire metastatic process, including the initial step of invasion.[223] However, other orthotopic models using cancer cell implantation are adequate for studies of the biology and treatment of metastasis. Even the implantation of cells into the spleen, although it bypasses the initial step of invasion by introducing cells directly into the portal circulation, provides a good model for studying the subsequent steps of the metastatic process. An experimental model that is not perfect still may be suitable for the study of a particular aspect of a biologic process.

ANTIMETASTATIC STRATEGIES

Because most local tumors can be eradicated successfully with existing conventional treatment approaches, prevention of metastasis would equal a universal cancer cure, the dream of every clinician involved in the treatment of cancer. Although in theory, this appears to be simple and straightforward, in practice, the situation is much more complex. The most significant obstacle to prevention is the fact that in most patients with cancer, metastases already are established before the primary tumor is detected.[225] Effective treatment modalities for the eradication of established metastases are not available. Further, the diagnostic techniques that are available have severe limitations in detecting micrometastases. Totally successful antimetastatic therapy, in addition to the availability of effective antimetastatic agents, will require precise knowledge of the chronology of the metastatic process, the capability of detecting established metastases with absolute certainty, and the availability of treatments capable of eradicating established metastases (Table 4-2).

Although the overall value of preventing or inhibiting the establishment of new metastases is limited substantially by the fact that these prerequisites have not been met by current state-of-the-art interventions, antimetastatic strategies have the potential to benefit the subset of patients who are free of micrometastases at the time of diagnosis of the primary tumor. Because this subset cannot be defined clearly with available imaging techniques, patients without gross evidence of metastases should be considered candidates for trials evaluating antimetastatic strategies. The theoretic basis of preoperative antimetastatic therapy is supported by observations that surgical stress enhances the production and growth of tumor metastases.[226,227] This has been attributed to several factors, including discharge of tumor emboli into the blood during resection of the tumor,[228–230] impaired clearance of the circulating tumor emboli,[231] and immunosuppression.[232–234] In addition, experimental evidence suggests that some anesthetic agents enhance the production and accelerate the growth of spontaneous metastases.[235,236]

TABLE 4-2. *Prerequisites for successful antimetastatic therapy*

Precise knowledge of chronology of the process
Detection of all established metastases
Eradication of all established metastases
Availability of effective antimetastatic agents

(From Vezeridis MP. Biology of metastasis. In: Wanebo HJ, ed. Colorectal Cancer. St. Louis: Mosby-Year Book, 1992.)

Metastasis, as a multistep process, offers opportunities for intervention at various steps and through different mechanisms, because inhibition of the completion of any step leads to failure of the entire process. Inhibition of tumor angiogenesis has the potential to influence metastasis. Folkman and associates observed that the administration of heparin or a heparin fragment with cortisone to mice with reticulum cell sarcoma, Lewis lung carcinoma, or B16 melanoma produced a highly significant inhibition of pulmonary metastasis formation, with 4553 metastatic colonies found in the lungs of 73 control animals compared to only 3 of 39 treated animals.[237] The two pulmonary metastases found in the B16 melanoma–bearing mice were avascular and less than 0.1 mm in diameter. Other studies have demonstrated prevention of carcinomatosis and bloody ascites in rats with Walker 256 carcinoma implanted into the liver or peritoneal cavity by the angiogenesis inhibitor protamine,[238] and prevention of pulmonary metastases from Lewis lung carcinoma in mice by the angiostatic corticosteroids cortisone acetate and tetrahydro S in the presence of heparin.[239] Further knowledge regarding the biochemical and molecular mechanisms of angiogenesis and the development of new potent antiangiogenic agents undoubtedly will open new horizons for the use of antiangiogenesis as a strategy for the prevention of metastases.[240–244]

Modulation of tumor vascularity is another potential antimetastatic target. Razoxane (ICRF-159), given systemically, produces a significant inhibition of lung metastasis in mice with Lewis lung carcinoma implanted subcutaneously. Based on histologic studies of tumors from treated animals, the antimetastatic action of razoxane was attributed to alterations in the structure and integrity of the tumor vasculature, which reduced the entrance of cancer cells into the circulation.[245–247] In a clinical trial, patients with Dukes' C colorectal carcinoma who were treated with razoxane had a significantly lower incidence of hepatic metastasis and longer disease-free intervals compared with untreated control patients. However, there was no significant difference in the percentage of treated and control patients in whom metastases ultimately developed, and no beneficial effect was observed in any stage of the disease other than Dukes' C.[248] More clinical trials are needed for clarification of this issue.

The step of invasion constitutes another target of antimetastatic intervention. Inhibitors of proteolytic enzymes have been studied for their effect on the metastatic process. Trasylol, a protease inhibitor, was found to inhibit hematogenous metastases in rats after the treatment of tumor cells in vitro, without changing the viability and tumorigenicity of cells.[249] Another protease inhibitor, aprotinin, inhibited invasion by mammary carcinoma and significantly reduced pulmonary metastases in mice with Lewis lung carcinoma.[250] The sialyltransferase inhibitor, KI-8110, significantly reduced experimental lung metastases from colon adenocarcinoma in mice and increased the survival of the treated animals.[251] Intraperitoneal injection of the recombinant human tissue inhibitor or metalloproteinase, rTIMP, reduced by 83% the ability of a highly metastatic rat embryo cell line, transfected by c-H-*ras*-1, to colonize the lungs after intravenous injection in nude mice.[252] A tissue inhibitor of metalloproteinase, TIMP-2, was isolated from media conditioned with human melanoma or bovine aortic endothelial cells[253,254] and found to inhibit the invasion of a reconstituted basement membrane by human fibrosarcoma HT-1080 cells.[255] Transfection of invasive and metastatic rat cells with the complementary DNA for metalloproteinase inhibitor/tissue inhibitor of metalloproteinase 2 markedly reduced the in vivo growth rate and completely suppressed local tissue invasion after subcutaneous implantation, and partially suppressed the formation of lung colonies after intravenous injection in nude mice.[256]

Inhibition of adhesive interactions between cells and the extracellular matrix have been investigated as an antimetastatic intervention. The synthetic peptide Gly-Arg-Gly-Asp-Ser (GRGDS) inhibited dramatically the formation of pulmonary metastases in mice when concomitantly injected with B16-F10 melanoma cells. This phenomenon was dose dependent, unrelated to cytotoxicity or impairment of tumorigenicity, and attributed to inhibition of tumor cell retention in the lung.[257] The GRGDS peptide also inhibited lung colonization from intravenously injected murine fibrosarcoma cells when given immediately before the injection of tumor cells.[258] In another study, Humphries and colleagues showed that treatment with GRGDS significantly prolonged the survival time of mice injected intravenously with B16-F10 melanoma cells.[259] In this study, GRGDS was found to retain its full metastasis-inhibiting activity in thrombocytopenic mice or mice with platelet function impaired by acetylsalicylic acid. This finding minimizes the role of inhibition of platelet aggregation in the mechanism of antimetastatic action of the peptide that was suggested in a previous study.[258] In addition, GRGDS caused 86% inhibition of experimental metastases in NK cell–deficient mice, excluding the possibility of NK cell activity enhancement as part of the antimetastatic mechanism.[259] Inhibition of human amniotic basement membrane penetration by human melanoma and glioblastoma cells was caused by synthetic peptides containing the sequence Arg-Gly-Asp.[260] Polymerization of the Arg-Gly-Asp core sequence was found to augment the inhibition of pulmonary metastases in experimental and spontaneous metastasis models.[261]

Cell-surface alterations have been studied as antimetastatic approaches based on interference with cell–basement membrane interactions, important elements in the metastatic cascade. D-threo-1-phenyl-2-decanoylamino-3-morpholino-1-propanol, an inhibitor of glucosylceramide synthase, was found to inhibit experimental metastasis of murine Lewis lung carcinoma and to reduce laminin-mediated attachment and migration in vitro.[262] Treatment of tumor cells from three human colorectal cancer cell lines before their injection into the spleen of nude mice, with the inhibitor of sialic acid incorporation KI-8110, prevented liver colonization.[263] These interesting antimetastatic approaches merit further investigation.

Alteration of cell motility offers another antimetastatic target. Staurosporine, an inhibitor of protein kinase C, was found to inhibit the invasion of an artificial membrane by an invasive human bladder carcinoma cell line in a dose-dependent manner.[264] One study showed that staurosporine and other inhibitors of protein kinase C, such as MDL 27032 and H-7, inhibited cell adhesion and experimental metastasis of B16-F1 melanoma.[265] Kohn and Liotta demonstrated that the carboxyamide-amino-imidazole compound L651582 inhibited up to 60% of the autocrine motility factor-stimulated tumor cell motility and tumor cell adhesion to tissue culture plastic.[266] They also showed that this compound significantly prolonged the survival of nude mice with a heavy load of human ovarian cancer. Human trials with this interesting agent are under way. Isoai and associates purified from bovine liver the tumor invasion-inhibiting factor 2 (IIF-2),[267] which they subsequently synthesized.[268] The synthetic IIF-2 suppressed the chemotactic migration of highly metastatic B16 melanoma to fibronectin or laminin and invasion through Matrigel, a mixture of basement membrane components. IIF-2 did not inhibit type IV collagenase activity, cell proliferation, or binding to fibronectin and Matrigel. Concomitant injection of IIF-2 with B16-FE7 melanoma and Lewis lung carcinoma cells in mice significantly reduced lung colonization. The investigators interpreted these findings as suggesting that IIF-2 inhibits tumor invasion by impairing cell motility and inhibiting the migration of cells through the extracellular matrix after their arrest in the microvasculature of the lung.[268] Another promising anti-invasion approach is the use of monoclonal antibodies. The use of antiurokinase antibodies was shown to inhibit pulmonary metastases from a human epidermal carcinoma.[269]

The use of anticoagulant and antiplatelet strategies in metastasis was introduced in the 1960s when it was observed that warfarin sodium (Coumadin) treatment reduced the production of pulmonary metastases in the rat.[270] Subsequent studies confirmed this effect of anticoagulant and antiplatelet agents on experimental metastases.[134,271–275] Some studies showed an effect of aspirin or mopidamol (RA-233) on metastases from Lewis lung carcinoma in mice and V2 carcinoma in rabbits.[276,277] Research interest in agents that interfere in the metabolism of arachidonic acid, affecting platelet aggregation, was stimulated by a report from Honn and associates that showed a 75% reduction in pulmonary metastases and a 100% reduction in liver metastases from B16 amelanotic melanoma by prostacyclin.[278] Using ketoconazole, an inhibitor of thromboxane synthetase and 5-lipoxygenase, these authors observed a significant reduction in spontaneous pulmonary metastases from B16-F10 melanoma in mice.[279] In subsequent studies, significant inhibition of hepatic metastases from the human pancreatic adenocarcinoma, RWP-2, in nude mice by prostacyclin, ketoconazole, forskolin, verapamil, and indomethacin was shown.[280,281]

Two studies have reaffirmed the role of coagulation and platelets in metastasis. Nierodzik and associates treated seven different murine and human tumor cell lines with thrombin and found that thrombin treatment caused a 2- to 3-fold increase in the adhesion of five lines to platelets and a 10- to 156-fold increase in experimental pulmonary metastases from four of these lines.[282] Esumi and colleagues reported that recombinant desulfatohirudin, a highly specific inhibitor of thrombin, significantly inhibited experimental metastases from B16-F10 melanoma.[283]

Some clinical trials have been performed using anticoagulant or antiplatelet agents. In a randomized study, the Veterans Administration Cooperative Study Group showed that patients with small-cell carcinoma of the lung who were treated with warfarin had significantly improved survival compared with untreated control patients.[284] The results of another clinical study by the same group using mopidamol (RA-233) also have been reported.[285] In this study, RA-233 plus chemotherapy was compared with chemotherapy alone in 719 patients with advanced carcinomas of the lung and colon. Significantly prolonged survival was seen in patients who had non–small-cell lung cancer limited to one hemithorax and reduced mean plasma fibrinogen concentrations, whereas no survival differences were observed in other tumor categories.[285] More trials in patients with earlier stages of disease are needed to clarify this important issue. These authors have reported that the use of mopidamol in combination with dipyridamole strongly inhibits tumor cell–induced platelet aggregation and produces a 70% reduction in experimental hepatic metastases from the human pancreatic carcinoma, RWP-2, in nude mice.[286]

The role of immunotherapy in the prevention or eradication of established metastases has been studied in the last decade. There is convincing experimental evidence that lack of suppression of NK cell activity results in the enhancement of metastases.[287,288] There also is evidence that NK cells inhibit experimental metastases in vivo.[289,290] It has been demonstrated that the in vivo activation of macrophages with liposome-encapsulated muramyl peptides or lymphokines causes selective destruction of metastases.[291] One study showed that cytokine-activated murine vascular endothelial cells are capable of lysing murine melanoma and reticulum cell sarcoma cells.[292] Swainsonine, an indolizidine alkaloid, inhibited experimental metastasis of B16-F10 melanoma by a mechanism involving interleukin-2 production and augmentation of NK cell activity. This agent also inhibited spontaneous metastasis of B16-BL6 melanoma to the lung and M5076 reticulum sarcoma to the liver.[293,294]

Interleukin encapsulated in liposomes had an increased effect on pulmonary metastasis from MCA-106 murine sarcoma compared with free interleukin.[295] Another study showed a striking inhibition of hepatic metastases from human melanoma cells injected into the spleens of nude mice, by interleukin-2 in combination with cytotoxic T lymphocytes.[296]

Studies have investigated the effect of various dietary elements on metastasis. Combined dietary restriction of tyrosine and phenylalanine had a dramatic antimetastatic effect directed to spontaneous hematogenous metastasis from B16-BL6 melanoma and RT7-4bs hepatocarcinoma in mice.[297] Retinoids in the diet had an inhibitory effect on pulmonary metastases from a hamster melanoma in nude mice without inhibitory effects on primary invasiveness or growth rate.[298] In vitro studies with murine and human colon cancer cells showed that arginine was necessary for cell growth, and that an arginine-depleted diet inhibited the growth of hepatic metastases from a murine colorectal adenocarcinoma by 78%.[299] Recombinant growth hormone injections selectively supported growth and inhibited pulmonary metastases in rats with subcutaneous implants of PA-III prostate tumor receiving a standard-protein or an isocaloric, protein-depleted diet.[300]

Intensive investigation in these vital areas of cancer research is continuing and new avenues for antimetastatic intervention will be open in the future. Although it is highly unlikely that any one antimetastatic treatment will provide a universal cure for cancer as a single modality, successful antimetastatic approaches will be an important addition to the therapeutic armamentarium as part of multimodality treatment regimens.

REFERENCES

1. Fidler IJ, Balch CM. The biology of cancer metastasis and implications for therapy. Curr Probl Surg 1987;24:130.
2. Killion JJ, Fidler IJ. The biology of tumor metastasis. Semin Oncol 1989;16:106.
3. Fidler IJ, Hart IR. Biologic diversity in metastatic neoplasms: origins and implications. Science 1982;217:998.
4. Fidler IJ, Poste G. The cellular heterogeneity of malignant neoplasms: implications for adjuvant chemotherapy. Semin Oncol 1985;12:207.
5. Nicolson GL. Generation of phenotypic diversity and progression in metastatic tumors. Cancer Metastasis Rev 1984;3:25.
6. Schabel FM. Concepts for systemic treatment of micrometastasis. Cancer 1975;35:15.
7. Sugarbaker EV, Ketcham AS. Mechanisms and prevention of cancer dissemination: an overview. Semin Oncol 1977;4:19.
8. Sugarbaker EV. Cancer metastasis: a product of tumor-host interactions. Curr Probl Cancer 1979;3:1.
9. Fidler IJ. Tumor heterogeneity and the biology of cancer invasion and metastasis. Cancer Res 1978;38:2651.
10. Weiss L. A pathobiologic overview of metastasis. Semin Oncol 1977; 4:5.
11. Weiss L. Cancer cell traffic from the lungs to the liver. An example of metastatic inefficiency. Int J Cancer 1980;25:385.
12. Fidler IJ. Metastases: quantitative analysis of distribution and fate of tumor emboli labelled with 125I-5-iodo-2-deoxyuridine. J Natl Cancer Inst 1970;45:773.
13. Liotta LA. Overview of the biology of cancer invasion and metastases. In: Rosenberg SA, ed. Surgical treatment of metastatic cancer. Philadelphia: Lippincott, 1987:1.
14. Eaves G. The invasive growth of malignant tumors as a purely machanical process. J Pathol 1973;109:233.
15. Coman DR. Mechanisms responsible for the origin and distribution of blood-borne tumor metastases. Cancer Res 1953;13:397.
16. Laerum OD, Bjerkvig R, Steinsvag SK, et al. Invasiveness of primary brain tumors. Cancer Metastasis Rev 1984;3:223.
17. Gabbert H. Mechanisms of tumor invasion: evidence from in vivo observations. Cancer Metastasis Rev 1985;4:283.
18. Noguchi PD, Johnson JB, O'Donnell R, et al. Chick embryonic skin as a rapid organ culture assay for cellular neoplasia. Science 1978; 199:980.
19. Mareel MM. Invasion in vitro: methods of analysis. Cancer Metastasis Rev 1983;2:201.
20. Weiss L, Ward PM. Cell detachment and metastasis. Cancer Metastasis Rev 1983;2:111.
21. Carr I. Lymphatic metastasis. Cancer Metastasis Rev 1983;2:307.
22. Hart IR, Raz A, Fidler IJ. Effect of cytoskeleton-disrupting agents on the metastatic behavior of melanoma cells. J Natl Cancer Inst 1980; 64:891.
23. Gail MH, Boone CW. Density inhibition of motility in 3T3 fibroblasts and their SV40 transformation. Exp Cell Res 1971;64:156.
24. Gerham H, Katzin W, Cook RT. Mobility of cells from solid tumors. Int J Cancer 1978;21:309.
25. Strauli P, Haemmerli O. The role of cancer cell motility in invasion. Cancer Metastasis Rev 1984;3:127.
26. Hart IR. Selection and characterization of an invasive variant of the B16 melanoma. Am J Pathol 1979;97:587.
27. Raz A. Autocrine motility factor receptor in invasion (abstract). Clinical and Experimental Metastasis 1994;12:11.
28. Taraboletti G, Belotti D, Dejana E, Mantovani A, Giavazzi R. Endothelial cell migration and invasiveness are induced by a soluble factor produced by murine endothelioma cells transformed by polyoma virus middle T oncogene. Cancer Res 1993;53:3812.
29. Kikkawa Y, Umeda M, Miyazaki K. Autocrine and paracrine cell motility activities of ladsin secreted by gastric adenocarcinoma cell line STKM-1. (Abstract) Clin Exp Metastasis 1994;12:57.
30. Yabkowitz R, Mansfield PJ, Dixit VM, Suchard SJ. Motility of human carcinoma cells in response to thrombospondin: relationship to metastatic potential and thrombospondin structural domains. Cancer Res 1993;53:378.
31. Liotta LA, Kleinerman J, Catanzara P, et al. Degradation of basement membrane by murine tumor cells. J Natl Cancer Inst 1977;58:1427.
32. Liotta LA, Rao C, Barsky S. Tumor invasion and the extracellular matrix. Lab Invest 1983;49:633.
33. Siegal GP, Barsky SH, Terranova VP, et al. Stages of neoplastic transformation of human breast tissue as monitored by dissolution of basement membrane components. Invasion Metastasis 1981;1:54.
34. Albrechtsen R, Nielsen M, Wewer U, et al. Basement membrane changes in breast cancer detected by immunohistochemical staining for laminin. Cancer Res 1981;41:5076.

35. Ekblom P, Miettinen M, Rapola J, et al. Demonstration of laminin, a basement membrane glycoprotein in routinely processed formalin-fixed human tissues. Histochemistry 1982;75:301.
36. Van Cauwenberge D, Pierard GE, Foidard TM, et al. Immunohistochemical localization of laminin, type IV and type V collagen in basal cell carcinoma. Br J Dermatol 1983;108:163.
37. Rao CN, Marguilies IMK, Tralka TS, et al. Isolation of a subunit of laminin and its role in molecular structure and tumor cell attachment. J Biol Chem 1982;257:9740.
38. Rao CN, Barsky SH, Terranova VP, et al. Isolation of a tumor cell laminin receptor. Biochem Biophys Res Commun 1983;111:804.
39. Terranova VP, Rao CN, Kalebic T, et al. Laminin receptor on human breast carcinoma cells. Proc Natl Acad Sci USA 1983;80:844.
40. Malinoff H, Wicha MS. Isolation of a cell surface receptor protein for laminin from murine fibrosarcoma cells. J Cell Biol 1983;96:1475.
41. Wewer V, Liotta LA, Jaye M, et al. Altered levels of laminin receptor mRNA in various human carcinoma cells that have different abilities to bind laminin. Proc Natl Acad Sci USA 1986;83:7137.
42. Barsky SH, Rao CN, Williams JE, et al. Laminin molecular domains which alter metastasis in a murine model. J Clin Invest 1984;74:843.
43. Terranova VP, Liotta LA, Russo RG, et al. Role of laminin in the attachment and metastasis of murine tumor cells. Cancer Res 1982; 42:2265.
44. Jaskiewicz K, Chasen MR, Robson SC. Differential expression of extracellular matrix proteins and integrins in hepatocellular carcinoma and chronic liver disease. Anticancer Res 1993;13:2229.
45. Vacca A, Ribatti D, Roncali L, et al. Melanocyte tumor progression is associated with changes in angiogenesis and expression of the 67-kilodalton laminin receptor. Cancer 1993;72:455.
46. Akiyama SK, Larjava H, Yamada KM. Differences in the biosynthesis and localization of the fibronectin receptor in normal and transformed cultured human cells. Cancer Res 1990;50:1601.
47. Juliano RL. Membrane receptors for extracellular matrix macromolecules: relationship to cell adhesion and tumor metastasis. Biochimica et Biophysica Acta 1987;907:261.
48. Buck CA, Horwitz AF. Cell surface receptors for extracellular matrix molecules. Annu Rev Cell Biol 1987;3:179.
49. Hemler ME. Adhesive protein receptors on hematopoietic cells. Immunol Today 1988;9:109.
50. Hynes RO. Integrins: a family of cell surface receptors. Cell 1987; 48:549.
51. Pytela R, Pierschbacher MD, Ruoslahti E. Identification and isolation of a 140kd cell surface glycoprotein with properties expected of a fibronectin receptor. Cell 1985;40:191.
52. Ruoslahti E, Pierschbacher MD. New perspectives in cell adhesion: RGD and integrins. Science 1988;238:491.
53. Saga S, Chen WT, Yamada KM. Enhanced fibronectin receptor expression in Rous sarcoma virus induced tumors. Cancer Res 1988; 48:5510.
54. Pujuguet P, Hammann A, Moutet M, Martin F, Martin M. Deposition of cellular fibronectin by colorectal cancer cells and its regulation by extracellular matrix. (Abstract) Clin Exp Metastasis 1994;12:46.
55. Kemperman H, Wijnands Y, Rijk D, Roos E. The integrin a6b4 on TA3/Ha mammary carcinoma cells is involved in adhesion to hepatocytes. Cancer Res 1993;53:3611.
56. Rosendahl A, Erb D, Chalpoupka B, Kisker O, Weinel RJ. Contribution of b1-integrins to migration and invasion of pancreatic carcinoma cells. (Abstract) Clin Exp Metastasis 1994;12:45.
57. Schipper JH, Frixen UH, Behrens J, et al. E-cadherin expression in squamous cell carcinomas of head and neck: inverse correlation with tumor dedifferentiation and lymph node metastasis. Cancer Res 1991; 51:6328.
58. Kadowaki T, Shiozaki H, Inoue M, et al. E-cadherin and A-catenin expression in human esophageal cancer. Cancer Res 1994;54:291.
59. Brabant G, Hoang-Vu C, Cetin Y, et al. E-cadherin: a differentiation marker in thyroid malignancies. Cancer Res 1993;53:4987.
60. Kinsella AR, Green B, Lepts GC, Hill CL, Bowie G, Taylor BA. The role of the cell-adhesion molecule E-cadherin in large bowel tumour cell invasion and metastasis. Brit J Cancer 1993;67:904.
61. Mayer B, Johnson JP, Leitl F, et al. E-cadherin expression in primary and metastatic gastric cancer: down-regulation correlates with cellular dedifferentiation and glandular disintegration. Cancer Res 1993;53: 1690.
62. Bernacki RJ, Nicdbala MJ, Koryntnyk W. Glycosidases in cancer and invasion. Cancer Metastasis Rev 1985;4:81.
63. Dresden MH, Heilman SA, Schmidt JD. Collagenolytic enzymes in human neoplasms. Cancer Res 1972;32:993.
64. Strauch L. The role of collagenases in tumor invasion. In: Tarin D, ed. Tissue interactions in carcinogenesis. London: Academic Press, 1972:399.
65. Sylven B. Lysosomal enzyme activity in the interstitial fluid of solid mouse tumor transplants. Eur J Cancer 1968;4:463.
66. Jones PA, DeClerck YA. Extracellular matrix destruction by invasive tumor cells. Cancer Metastasis Rev 1982;1:289.
67. Liotta LA. Tumor invasion and metastases: role of the extracellular matrix. Rhoads memorial award lecture. Cancer Res 1986;46:1.
68. Tarin D. Investigations of the mechanisms of metastatic spread of naturally-occurring neoplasms. Cancer Metastasis Rev 1982;1:215.
69. Liotta LA, Thorgeirsson UP, Gabrisa S. Role of collagenases in tumor cell invasion. Cancer Metastasis Rev 1982;1:277.
70. Wooley DE. Collagenolytic mechanisms in tumor cell invasion. Cancer Metastasis Rev 1984;3:361.
71. Poole AR, Tiltman KJ, Recklies AD, et al. Differences in secretion of the proteinase cathepsin B at the edges of human breast carcinomas and firboadenomas. Nature 1978;273:545.
72. Recklies AD, Tiltman KJ, Stoker TAM, et al. Secretion of proteinases from malignant and nonmalignant human breast. Cancer Res 1980; 40:550.
73. Sloane BF, Dunn JR, Honn KV. Lysosomal cathepsin B: correlation with metastatic potential. Science 198;212:1151.
74. Sloan BF, Honn KV, Sadler JG, et al. Cathepsin B activity in B16 melanoma cells: a possible marker for metastatic potential. Cancer Res 1982;42:980.
75. Reich E. Tumor-associated fibrinolysis (abstract). Federation Proceedings 1973;32:2174.
76. Robbin RO. Plasminogen activator production as a possible biological marker for human neoplasia: some fundamental questions. In: Ruddon R, ed. Biological markers of neoplasis: basic and applied aspects. New York: Elsevier, 1978:421.
77. Kobayashi H, Moniwa N, Gotoh J, Sugimura M, Terao T. Role of activated protein C in facilitating basement membrane invasion by tumor cells. Cancer Res 1993;54:261.
78. Schwartz GK, Kiley SC, Dhupar SK, Kelsen D, Albino A. Protein kinase Cβ1 (PKCβ1) expression and localization: critical events in gastric cancer cell invasion? (Abstract) Clin Exp Metastasis 1994;12: 15.
79. Schwartz Gk, Jiang J, Kelsen D, Albino AP. Protein kinase C: a novel target for inhibiting gastric cancer cell invasion. J Natl Cancer Inst 1993;85:402.
80. Liotta LA, Abe S, Robey PG, et al. Preferential digestion of basement membrane collagen by an enzyme derived from a metastatic murine tumor. Proc Natl Acad Sci USA 1979;76:2268.
81. Liotta LA, Tryggvason K, Garbisa S, et al. Metastatic potential correlates with enzymatic degradation of basement membrane collagen. Nature 1980;284:67.
82. Zucker S, Lysik RM, Zarrabi MH, Moll U. Mr 92,000 type IV collagenase is increased in plasma of patients with colon cancer and breast cancer. Cancer Res 1993;53:140.
83. David L, Nesland JM, Holm R, Sobrinho-Simoes M. Expression of laminin, collagen IV, fibronectin and type IV collagenase in gastric carcinoma. Cancer 1994;73:518.
84. Nakajima M, Welch DR, Wynn DM, Tsuruo T, Nicolson GL. Serum and plasma Mr 92,000 progelatinase levels correlate with spontaneous metastasis of rat 13762NF mammary adenocarcinoma. Cancer Res 1993;53:5802.
85. Powell WC, Knox JD, Navre M, et al. Expression of the metalloproteinase matrilysin in DU-145 cells increases their invasive potential in severe combined immunodeficient mice. Cancer Res 1993;53:417.
86. Martin DC, Ruther U, Khokha R. Altered development of hepatocellular carcinoma in TIMP-1 transgenic mice. (Abstract) Clin Exp Metastasis 1994;12:12.
87. Shirasuna K, Saka M, Hayashido Y, Yoshioka H, Sugiura T, Matsuya T. Extracellular matrix production and degradation by adenoid cystic carcinoma cells: participation of plasminogen activator and its inhibitor in matrix degradation. Cancer Res 1993;53:147.
88. Johnatty RN, Rees RC, Taub DD. Effect of human MIP1a on the

production of matrix degrading enzymes by human T lymphocytes. (Abstract) Clin Exp Metastasis 1994;12:15.
89. Montgomery AMP, Mueller BM, Reisfeld RA, Taylor SM, DeClerck YA. Effect of tissue inhibitor of the matrix metalloproteinases-2 expression on the growth and spontaneous metastasis of a human melanoma cell line. Cancer Res 1993;54:5467.
90. Laug WE, Cao XR, Yu YB, Shimada H, Kruithof EK. Inhibition of invasion of HT1080 sarcoma cells expressing recombinant plasminogen activator inhibitor 2. Cancer Res 1993;53:6051.
91. McCarthy JB, Basara ML, Palm SL, et al. The role of cell adhesion proteins-laminin and fibronectin in the movement of malignant and metastatic cells. Cancer Metastasis Rev 1985;4:125.
92. Liotta LA, Mandler R, Murano G, et al. Tumor cell autocrine motility factor. Proc Natl Acad Sci USA 1986;83:3302.
93. del Regato JA. Pathways of metastatic spread of malignant tumors. Semin Oncol 1977;4:33.
94. Zeidman I, Buss JM. Experimental studies on the spread of cancer in the lymphatic system I: effectiveness of the lymph node as a barrier to the passage of embolic tumor cells. Cancer Res 1954;14:403.
95. Fisher B, Fisher ER. The interrelationship of hematogenous and lymphatic tumor cell dissemination. Surg Gynecol Obstet 1966;122:791.
96. Fidler IJ. The relationship of embolic homogeneity, number, size and viability to the incidence of experimental metastasis. Eur J Cancer 1973;9:223.
97. Fidler IJ, Bucana C. Mechanism of tumor cell resistance to lysis by syngeneic lymphocytes. Cancer Res 1977;37:3945.
98. Gasic GJ. Role of plasma platelets and endothelial cells in tumor metastasis. Cancer Metastasis Rev 1984;3:99.
99. del Regato JA. Pathophysiology of metastasis. In: Weiss L, Gilbert HA, eds. Pulmonary metastasis. Boston: Hall, 1978:104.
100. Hart IR. Seed and soil revisited: mechanisms of site-specific metastasis. Cancer Metastasis Rev 1982;1:5.
101. Tarin D. Clinical and experimental studies on the biology of metastasis. Biochem Biophys Acta 1985;780:227.
102. Zetter BR. The cellular basis of site-specific metastasis. N Engl J Med 1990;322:605.
103. Greene HSN, Harvey EK. The relationship between the dissemination of tumor cells and the distribution of metastasis. Cancer Res 1964; 24:799.
104. Auerbach R, Lu WC, Pardon E, et al. Specificity of adhesion between murine tumor cells and capillary endothelium: an in vitro correlate of preferential metastasis in vivo. Cancer Res 1987;47:1492.
105. Warren BA. Environment of the blood-borne tumor embolus adherent to vessel wall. J Med 1973;4:150.
106. Gasic GJ, Gasic TB, Galanti N, et al. Platelet tumor cell interaction in mice: the role in the spread of malignant disease. Int J Cancer 1973; 11:794.
107. Barsky SH, Rao CN, Williams JE, et al. Laminin molecular domains which alter metastasis in a murine model. J Clin Invest 1984;74:843.
108. Nicolson GL, Winkelhake JL. Organ specificity of blood-borne tumor metastasis determined by cell adhesion. Nature 1975;255:230.
109. Ruoslahti E. Fibronectin in cell adhesion and invasion. Cancer Metastasis Rev 1984;3:43.
110. McGuire EJ, Mascali JJ, Grady SR, et al. Involvement of cell-cell adhesion molecules in liver colonization by metastatic murine lymphoma/lymphosarcoma variants. Clin Exp Metastasis 1984;2:213.
111. Alby L, Auerbach R. Differential adhesion of tumor cells to capillary endothelial cells in vitro. Proc Natl Acad Sci USA 1984;81:5739.
112. Dvorak HF, Seneger DR, Dvorak AM. Fibrin as a component of the tumor stroma: origins and biological significance. Cancer Metastasis Rev 1983;2:44.
113. Cliffton EE, Agostino D. The effects of fibrin formation and alterations in the clotting mechanism on the development of metastatases. Vasc Dis 1965;2:43.
114. Sindelar WF, Tralka TS, Ketcham AS. Electron microscope observations on formation of pulmonary metastases. J Surg Res 1975;18:137.
115. Rickles F, Edwards R. Activation of blood coagulation in cancer: Trousseau's syndrome revisited. Blood 1983;62:14.
116. Gasic G, Tuszynski G, Gorelik E. Interaction of the hemostatic and immune system in the metastatic spread of tumor cells. Int Rev Exp Pathol 1986;29:173.
117. Trousseau A. Phlegmasia alba dolens. Clinique medicale de l'Hotel-Dieu de Paris. 3rd vol. London: New Sydenham Society, 1865:94.
118. Peck SD, Requam CW. Disseminated intravascular coagulation in cancer patients: supportive evidence. Cancer 1973;31:1114.
119. Ambrus JL, Ambrus CM, Pickren J, et al. Hematologic changes and thromboembolic complications in neoplastic disease and their relationship to metastasis. J Med 1975;6:433.
120. Sack GH, Levin J, Bell WR. Trousseau's syndrome and other manifestations of chronic disseminated coagulopathy in patients with neoplasms: clinical, pathophysiologic and therapeutic features. Medicine (Baltimore) 1977;56:1.
121. Rasche H, Dietrich M. Hemostatic abnormalities associated with malignant diseases. Eur J Cancer 1977;13:1053.
122. Lyman GH, Bettigole RE, Robson E, et al. Fibrinogen kinetics in patients with neoplastic disease. Cancer 1978;41:1113.
123. Zacharski LR, Henderson WG, Rickles FR, et al. Rationale and experimental design for the VA cooperative study of anti-coagulation (warfarin) in the treatment of cancer. Cancer 1979;44:732.
124. Donati MB, Poggi A. Malignancy and hemostasis. Br J Haematol 1980;44:173.
125. Edwards RL, Rickles FR, Gronlund M. Abnormalities of blood coagulation in patients with cancer. J Lab Clin Med 1981;98:917.
126. Wood S, Holyoke ED, Yardley JH. Mechanisms of metastasis production by blood-borne cancer cells. Can Cancer Conf 1967;4:167.
127. Chew EC, Wallace AC. Demonstration of fibrin in early stages of experimental metastases. Cancer Res 1976;36:1904.
128. Kinjo M. Lodgement and extravasation of tumor cells in blood-borne metastasis: an electron microscope study. Br J Cancer 1978;38:293.
129. Poste G, Fidler IJ. The pathogenesis of cancer metastasis. Nature 1979;283:139.
130. Weiss L. The biology of metastasis. In: McKenna RT, Murphy GP, eds. Fundamentals of surgical oncology. New York: McMillan, 1986: 6.
131. Mehta P. Potential role of platelets in the pathogenesis of tumor metastasis. Blood 1984;63:55.
132. Jones DS, Wallace AC, Fraser EF. Sequence of events in experimental metastasis of Walker 256 tumors: light, immunofluorescent and electron microscopic observations. J Natl Cancer Inst 1971;46:493.
133. Sindelar WF, Tralka TS, Ketcham AS. Electron microscopic observations on formation of pulmonary metastasis. J Surg Res 1975;18:137.
134. Gasic GJ, Gasic TB, Galanti N, et al. Platelet-tumor cell interactions in mice: the role of platelets in the spread of malignant disease. Int J Cancer 1973;11:704.
135. Gasic GJ, Boettiger D, Catalfanio JL, et al. Aggregation of platelets and cell membrane vesiculation by rat cells transformed in vitro by Rous sarcoma virus. Cancer Res 1978;38:2950.
136. Pearlstein E, Salk PL, Yogeeswaran G, et al. Correlation between spontaneous metastatic potential, platelet-aggregating activity of cell surface extracts, and cell surface extracts, and cell surface sialylation in 10 metastatic-variant derivatives of a rat renal sarcoma cell line. Proc Natl Acad Sci USA 1980;77:4336.
137. Honn KV, Cavanaugh P, Evans C, et al. Tumor-cell platelet aggregation induced by cathepsin B-like proteinase and inhibited by prostacyclin. Science 1982;217:540.
138. Tsuruo T, Kawabata H, Iida H, et al. Tumor-induced platelet aggregation and growth promoting factors as determinants for successful tumor metastasis. Clin Exp Metastasis 1986;4:25.
139. Gasic GJ, Tuszyuski GP, Gorelik E. Interaction of the hemostatic and immune systems in the metastatic spread of tumor cells. Int Rev Exp Pathol 1986;29:173.
140. Heinmoller E, Schropp T, Rosendahl A, Kisker O, Seitz R, Weinel RJ. Pancreatic carcinoma and the coagulation system. (Abstract) Clin Exp Metastasis 1994;12:50.
141. Nachman RL, Weksler B, Ferris B. Characterization of human platelet vascular permeability enhancing activity. J Clin Invest 1972;51:549.
142. Poggi A, Vicenzi E, Cioce V, et al. Platelet contribution to cancer cell growth and migration: the role of platelet growth factors. Hemostase 1988;18:18.
143. Chirivi RG, Garofalo A, Padura IM, Mantovani A, Giavazzi R. Interleukin 1 receptor antagonist inhibits the augmentation of metastasis induced by interleukin 1 or lipopolysaccharide in a human melanoma nude mouse system. Cancer Res 1993;53:5051.
144. Kobrin MS, Yamanaka Y, Friess H, Lopez ME, Kore M. Aberrant expression of type I fibroblast growth factor receptor in human pancreatic adenocarcinomas. Cancer Res 1993;53:4741.
145. Nicolson GL, Wakabayashi H, Hamada J, Jia L, Cavanaugh PG. The

role of organ microvessel endothelial cells in metastasis. (Abstract) Clin Exp Metastasis 1994;12:16.
146. Paget S. The distribution of secondary growth in cancer of the breast. Lancet 1989;1:571.
147. Ewing J. Neoplastic diseases: a treatise on tumors. Philadelphia: Saunders, 1928:77.
148. Tarin D, Price JE, Kettlewell MGW, et al. Clinicopathological observations on metastasis in man studied in patients treated with peritoneovenous shunts. BMJ 1984;288:749.
149. Tarin D, Price JE, Kettlewell MGW, et al. Mechanisms of human tumor metastasis studied in patients with peritoneovenous shunts. Cancer Res 1984;44:3584.
150. Kinsey DL. An experimental study of preferential metastasis. Cancer 1960;13:874.
151. Sugarbaker EV, Cohen AM, Ketcham AS. Do metastases metastasize? Ann Surg 1971;174:161.
152. Hart IR, Fidler IJ. Role of organ selectivity in the determination of metastatic patterns of B16 melanoma. Cancer Res 1980;40:2281.
153. Hart IR, Talmadge JE, Fidler IJ. Metastatic behavior of a murine reticulum cell sarcoma exhibiting organ-specific growth. Cancer Res 1981;41:1281.
154. Fidler IJ. Selection of successive tumor lines for metastasis. Nature 1973;242:148.
155. Brunson KW, Beattie G, Nicholson GL. Selection and altered properties of brain-colonizing metastatic melanoma. Nature 1978;272:543.
156. Tao T-W, Matter A, Vogel K, et al. Liver colonizing melanoma cells selected from B-16 melanoma. Int J Cancer 1979;23:854.
157. Neri A, Welch D, Kawaguchi T, et al. Development and biologic properties of malignant cell sublines and clones of a spontaneously metastasizing rat mammary adenocarcinoma. J Natl Cancer Inst 1982; 68:507.
158. Morikawa K, Walker SM, Jessup JM, et al. In vivo selection of highly metastatic cells from surgical specimens of different primary human colon carcinomas implanted into nude mice. Cancer Res 1988;48: 1943.
159. Vezeridis MP, Tzanakakis GN, Meitner PA, et al. In vivo selection of a highly metastatic cell line from a human pancreatic carcinoma in the nude mouse. Cancer 1992;69:2060.
160. Tao T-W, Johnson LK. Altered adhesiveness of tumor cell surface variants with reduced metastasizing capacity-reduced adhesiveness to vascular wall components in culture. Int J Cancer 1982;30:763.
161. Korach S, Poupon M-F, DuVilliard J-A, et al. Differential adhesiveness of rhabdomyosarcoma-derived cloned metastatic cell lines to vascular endothelial monolayers. Cancer Res 1986;46:3624.
162. Nicolson GL. Cancer metastasis: tumor cell and host organ properties important in metastasis to specific secondary sites. Biochem Biophys Acta 1988;948:175.
163. Kramer RH, Gonzalez R, Nicolson GL. Metastatic tumor cells adhere preferentially to the extracellular matrix underlying vascular endothelial cells. Int J Cancer 1980;26:639.
164. Doerr R, Zvibel I, Chinten D, et al. Clonal growth of tumors on tissue-specific biomatrices and correlation with organ specificity of metastases. Cancer Res 1989;49:384.
165. Roos E, Tulp A, Middelkoop OP, et al. Interactions between lymphoid tumor cells and isolated liver endothelial cells. J Natl Cancer Inst 1984;72:1173.
166. Roos E, Middelkoop OP, Van de Pavert IV. Adhesion of tumor cells to hepatocytes: different mechanisms for mammary carcinoma compared with lymphosarcoma cells. J Natl Cancer Inst 1984;73:963.
167. Gjoen T, Seljelid R, Kolset SO. Binding of metastatic colon carcinoma cells to liver macrophages. J Leukoc Biol 1989;45:362.
168. Roos E, Roossien FF. Involvement of leukocyte function-associated antigen-1 (LFA-1) in the invasion of hepatocyte cultures by lymphoma and T-cell hybridoma cells. J Cell Biol 1987;105:553.
169. Roossien FF, de Rijk D, Bikker A, et al. Involvement of LFA-1 in lymphoma invasion and metastasis demonstrated with LFA-1 deficient mutants. J Cell Biol 1989;108:1979.
170. Yusa T, Blood CH, Zetter BR. Tumor cell interactions with elastin: implications for pulmonary metastasis. Am Rev Respir Dis 1989;140: 1458.
171. Kao RT, Stern R. Elastases in human breast carcinoma cell lines. Cancer Res 1986;46:1355.
172. Zeydel M, Nakagawa S, Biempica L, et al. Collagenase and elastase production by mouse mammary adenocarcinoma primary cultures and cloned cells. Cancer Res 1986;46:6438.
173. Dano K, Andreasen PA, Grondahl-Hansen J, et al. Plasminogen activators, tissue degradation and cancer. Adv Cancer Res 1985;44:139.
174. Horak E, Darling DL, Tarin D. Analysis of organ-specific effects on metastatic tumor formation by studies in vitro. J Natl Cancer Inst 1986;76:913.
175. Nicolson GL, Dulski M. Organ specificity of metastatic tumor colonization is related to organ-selective growth properties of malignant cells. Int J Cancer 1986;38:289.
176. Blanckaert VD, Schelling ME, Elstad CA, Meadows GG. Differential growth factor production, secretion, and response by high and low metastatic variants of B16BL6 melanoma. Cancer Res 1993;53:4075.
177. Yamanaka Y, Friess H, Buchler M, et al. Overexpression of acidic and basic fibroblast growth factors in human pancreatic cancer correlates with advanced tumor stage. Cancer Res 1993;53:5289.
178. Cavanaugh PG, Nicolson GL. Purification and some properties of a lung-derived growth factor that differentially stimulates the growth of tumor cells metastatic to the lung. Cancer Res 1989;49:3928.
179. Finkelstein SD, Sayegh R, Christensen S, Swalsky PA. Genotypic classification of colorectal adenocarcinoma. Cancer 1993;71:3827.
180. Sisley K, Alcock H, Royds J, Rees RC. The evaluation of nm23 gene involvement as a potential predictor of metastasis in colorectal cancer. (Abstract) Clin Exp Metastasis 1994;12:30.
181. Lamb RF, Going JJ, Black DM, Pickford JR, Birnie GD. High frequency loss of heterozygosity (LOH) of nm23-H1 locus in metastatic colon tumours. (Abstract) Clin Exp Metastasis 1994;12:33.
182. Folkman J. What is the evidence that tumors are angiogenesis dependent? J Natl Cancer Inst 1990;82:4.
183. Shubik P. Vascularization of tumors: a review. J Cancer Res Clin Oncol 1982;103:211.
184. Algine GH, Chalkley HW, Legallais FY, et al. Vascular reactions of normal and malignant tissues in vivo. J Natl Cancer Inst 1945;6:73.
185. Greenblatt M, Shubik P. Tumor angiogenesis: transfilter diffusion stúdies in the hamster by transparent chamber technique. J Natl Cancer Inst 1968;41:111.
186. Folkman J, Merler E, Abernathy C, et al. Isolation of a tumor factor responsible for angiogenesis. J Exp Med 1971;133:275.
187. Folkman J. Tumor angiogenesis factor. Cancer Res 1974;34:2109.
188. Folkman J, Cotran RS. Relation of vascular proliferation to tumor growth. Int Rev Exp Pathol 1976;16:207.
189. Folkman J. Tumor angiogenesis. Adv Cancer Res 1985;43:175.
190. Liotta LA, Kleinerman J, Saidel GM. Quantitative relationships of intravascular tumor cells, tumor vessels and pulmonary metastases following tumor implantation. Cancer Res 1974;34:997.
191. Mahadevan V, Hart IR. Metastasis and angiogenesis. Reviews in Oncology 1990;3:97.
192. Nagy JA, Brown LF, Senger DR, et al. Pathogenesis of tumor stroma generation: a critical role for leaky blood vessels and fibrin deposition. Biochem Biophys Acta 1989;948:305.
193. Folkman J. What is the role of angiogenesis in metastasis from cutaneous melanoma? Eur J Cancer Clin Oncol 1987;23:361.
194. Srivastava A, Laidler P, Hughes LE, et al. Neovascularization in human cutaneous melanoma: a quantitative morphological and Doppler ultrasound study. Eur J Cancer Clin Oncol 1986;22:1205.
195. Srivastava A, Laidler P, Davies RP, et al. The prognostic signficance of tumor vascularity in intermediate thickness (0.76–4.0 mm thick) skin melanoma: a quantitative histologic study. Am J Pathol 1988; 133:419.
196. Herlyn M, Clark WH, Rodeck U, et al. Biology of tumor progression in human melanocytes. Lab Invest 1987;56:461.
197. Weidner N, Semple JP, Welch WR, et al. Tumor angiogenesis and metastasis: correlation in invasive breast carcinoma. N Engl J Med 1991;324:1.
198. Kripke ML, Gruys E, Fidler IJ. Metastatic heterogeneity of cells from an ultraviolet light-induced murine fibrosarcoma of recent origin. Cancer Res 1978;38:2962.
199. Tan MH, Holyoke ED, Goldrosen MH. Murine colon adenocarcinoma: syngeneic orthotopic transplantation and subsequent hepatic metastases. J Natl Cancer Inst 1977;59:1537.
200. Rygaard J, Povlsen CO. Heterotransplantation of human malignant tumor to nude mice. Acta Pathol Microbiol Scand Immunol (A) 1969; 77:758.
201. Giovanella BC, Stehlin JS, Shepard RC, et al. Correlation between

response to chemotherapy of human tumors in patients and nude mice. Cancer 1983;52:1146.
202. Taetle R, Jones OW, Honeysett M, et al. Use of nude mice xenografts as preclinical screens: characterization of xenograft-derived melanoma cell lines. Cancer 1987;60:1836.
203. Sharkey FE, Fogh J. Metastasis of human tumors in athymic nude mice. Int J Cancer 1980;24:733.
204. Fogh J, Orfeo T, Tiso J, et al. Twenty-three new human tumor lines established in nude mice. Exp Cell Biol 1980;48:229.
205. Sordat BC, Ueyama Y, Fogh J. Metastasis of tumor xenografts in the nude mouse. In: Fogh J, Giovanella BC, eds. The nude mouse in experimental and clinical research. 2nd vol. New York: Academic Press, 1982:95.
206. Hanna N, Fidler IJ. Expression of metastatic potential of allogenic and xenogenic neoplasms in young nude mice. Cancer Res 1981;41: 438.
207. Kyriazis AP, Kyriazis AA, McCombs WB, et al. Biological behavior of human malignant tumors grown in the nude mouse. Cancer Res 1981;41:3995.
208. Kozlowski JM, Fidler IJ, Campbell D, et al. Metastatic behavior of human cell lines grown in the nude mouse. Cancer Res 1984;44:3522.
209. Vezeridis MP, Turner MD, Kajiji SM, et al. Metastasis of human pancreatic cancer to liver in nude mice. Proc Am Assoc Cancer Res 1985;26:53.
210. Giavazzi R, Jessup MJ, Campbell DE, et al. Experimental nude mouse model of human colorectal cancer liver metastases. J Natl Cancer Inst 1986;77:1303.
211. Fidler IJ. Rationale and methods for the use of nude mice to study the biology and therapy of human cancer metastasis. Cancer Metastasis Rev 1986;5:29.
212. Vezeridis MP, Tibbetts LM, Doremus CM, et al. Differences in the potential for liver metastasis of seven human colon adenocarcinoma cell lines in a nude mouse model. Proc Am Assoc Cancer Res 1987; 28:80.
213. Tibbetts LM, Doremus CM, Tzanakakis GN, et al. Liver metastases with ten human colon carcinoma cell lines in nude mice and association with CEA production. Cancer 1993;71:315.
214. Wanebo HJ, Rao B, Pinsky CM, et al. Preoperative carcinoembryonic antigen level as a prognostic indicator in colorectal cancer. N Engl J Med 1978;299:448.
215. Sener SF, Imperato JP, Chmiel J, et al. The use of cancer registry data to study preoperative carcinoembryonic antigen level as an indicator of survival in colorectal cancer. CA Cancer J Clin 1989;39:50.
216. Jessup JM, Giavazzi R, Campbell D, et al. Growth potential of human colorectal carcinomas in nude mice: association with the preoperative serum concentration of carcinoembryonic antigen in patients. Cancer Res 1988;48:1689.
217. Hostetter RB, Augustus LB, Mankarious R, et al. Carcinoembryonic antigen as a selective enhancer of colorectal cancer metastasis. J Natl Cancer Inst 1990;82:380.
218. Vezeridis MP, Doremus GM, Tibbetts LM, et al. Experimental metastases from a human pancreatic adenocarcinoma in athymic mice. Surg Res Comm 1989;6:313.
219. Vezeridis MP, Meitner PA, Tibbetts LM, et al. Heterogeneity of potential for hematogenous metastasis in a human pancreatic carcinoma. J Surg Res 1990;48:51.
220. Fidler IJ. Critical factors in the biology of human cancer metastasis: twenty-eight G.H.A. Clowes Memorial Award Lecture. Cancer Res 1990;50:6130.
221. Fidler IJ. The biology of human cancer metastasis: 7th Jan Waldenstrom Lecture. Acta Oncol 1991;30:669.
222. Fidler IJ. Orthotopic implantation of human colon carcinomas into nude mice provides a valuable model for the biology and therapy of metastasis. Cancer Metastasis Rev 1991;10:229.
223. Vezeridis MP, Doremus CM, Tibbetts LM, et al. Invasion and metastasis following orthotopic transplantation of human pancreatic cancer in the nude mouse. J Surg Oncol 1989;40:261.
224. Fu X, Beterman JM, Monosov A, et al. Models of human metastatic colon cancer in nude mice orthotopically constructed by using histologically intact patient specimens. Proc Natl Acad Sci USA 1991;88: 9345.
225. Schabel FU. Concepts for systemic treatment of micrometastasis. Cancer 1975;35:15.
226. Tyzzer EE. Factors in the production and growth of tumor metastases. J Med Res 1913;28:309.
227. Lewis MR, Cole WH. Experimental increase of lung metastases after operative trauma (amputation of limb with tumor). Arch Surg 1958; 77:621.
228. Engell HC. Cancer cells in the circulating blood. Acta Chir Scand [Suppl] 1955;201:1.
229. Roberts S, Long L, Jonasson O, et al. The isolation of cancer cells from the blood stream during uterine curettage. Surg Gynecol Obstet 1960;111:3.
230. Liotta LA, Kleinerman J, Saidel GM. The significance of hematogenous tumor cell clumps in the metastatic process. Cancer Res 1976; 36:889.
231. Saba TM, Antikatzides TG. Decreased resistance to intravenous tumor-cell challenge during reticuloendothelial depression following surgery. Br J Cancer 1976;34:381.
232. Pollock RE, Lotzova E. Surgical-stress-related suppression of natural killer cell activity: a possible role in tumor metastasis. Nat Immun Cell Growth Regul 1987;6:269.
233. Uchida A, Kolb R, Micksche M. Generation of suppressor cells for natural killer activity in cancer patients after surgery. J Natl Cancer Inst 1982;68:735.
234. Yeager MP, Colacchio TA. Effect of morphine on growth of metastatic colon cancer in vivo. Arch Surg 1991;126:454.
235. Pollard M, Burleson CR, Luckett PH. Factors that modify the rate and extent of spontaneous metastases of prostate tumors in rats. In: Day SB, Myers WPL, Stansly P, Garattini S, Lewis MG, eds. Cancer invasion and metastasis: biologic mechanisms and therapy. New York: Raven Press, 1977:357.
236. Shapiro T, Jersky J, Katzav S, et al. Anesthetic drugs accelerate the progression of postoperative metastases of mouse tumors. J Clin Invest 1981;68:678.
237. Folkman J, Langer R, Linhardt RJ, et al. Angiogenesis inhibition and tumor regression caused by heparin fragment in the presence of cortisone. Science 1983;221:719.
238. Heuser LS, Taylor SH, Folkman J. Prevention of carcinomatosis and bloody malignant ascites in the rat by an inhibitor of angiogenesis. J Surg Res 1984;36:244.
239. Sakamoto N, Tanaka NG. Effect of angiostatic steroid with or without glucocorticoid activity on metastasis. Invasion Metastasis 1987;7:208.
240. Peterson HI. Tumor angiogenesis inhibition by prostaglandin synthetase inhibitors. Anticancer Res 1986;6:251.
241. Sidky YA, Borden EC. Inhibition of angiogenesis by interferons: effects on tumor and lymphocyte induced vascular responses. Cancer Res 1987;471:5155.
242. Tamargo RJ, Bok RA, Brem H. Angiogenesis inhibition by minocycline. Cancer Res 1991;51:672.
243. Ingber D, Fujita T, Kishimoto S, et al. Synthetic analogues of fumagilin that inhibit angiogenesis and suppress tumour growth. Nature 1990; 348:555.
244. Murata J, Saiki I, Makabe T, et al. Inhibition of tumor-induced angiogenesis by sulfated chitin derivatives. Cancer Res 1991;51:22.
245. Hellman K, Burrage K. Control of malignant metastases by ICRF-159. Nature 1969;224:273.
246. James SE, Salsbury AJ. Effect of 1,2-bis(3,5-dioxopiperazin-1-yl) propane on tumor blood vessels and its relationship to the antimetastatic effect in the Lewis lung carcinoma. Cancer Res 1974;34:839.
247. Salsbury AJ, Burrage K, Hellman K. Histological analysis of the antimetastatic effect of 1,2-bis (3,5-dioxopiperazin-1-yl) propane. Cancer Res 1974;34:843.
248. Hellman K, Gilbert J, Evans M, et al. Effect of razoxame on metastases from colorectal cancer. Clin Exp Metastasis 1987;5:3.
249. Stein-Werblowsky R. On the prevention of hematogenous tumor metastases in rats. The role of proteinase inhibitor "Trasylol." J Cancer Res Clin Oncol 1980;97:129.
250. Latner AL, Lonstaff E, Turner GA. Anti-tumor effect of aprotinin. Br J Cancer 1974;30:60.
251. Suda IK, Miyamoto Y, Toyoshima S, et al. Inhibition of experimental pulmonary metastasis of mouse colon adenocarcinoma 26 sublines by a sialic acid nucleotide conjugate having sialyltransferase inhibiting activity. Cancer Res 1986;46:858.
252. Alvarez OA, Carmichael DF, DeClerk YA. Inhibition of collagenolytic activity and metastasis of tumor cells by a recombinant human tissue inhibitor of metalloproteinases. J Natl Cancer Inst 1990;82:589.

253. Stetler-Stevenson WG, Krutzsch HC, Liotta LA. Tissue inhibitor of metalloproteinase (TIMP-2): a new member of the metalloproteinase inhibitor family. J Biol Chem 1989;264:17374.
254. DeClarck YA, Yean TD, Ratzkin BJ, et al. Purification and characterization of two related but distinct metalloproteinase inhibitors secreted by bovine aortic endothelial cells. J Biol Chem 1989;264:17445.
255. Albini A, Melchiori A, Santi L, et al. Tumor cell invasion inhibited by TIMP-2. J Natl Cancer Inst 1991;83:775.
256. DeClerck YA, Perez N, Shimada H, et al. Inhibition of invasion and metastasis in cells transfected with an inhibitor of metalloproteinases. Cancer Res 1992;52:701.
257. Humphries MJ, Olden K, Yamada KU. A synthetic peptide from fibronectin inhibits experimental metastasis of murine melanoma cells. Science 1986;233:467.
258. Ugen KE, Mabalingam M, Klein PA, et al. Inhibition of tumor cell-induced platelet aggregation and experimental tumor metastasis by the synthetic Gly-Arg-Gly-Asp-Ser peptide. J Natl Cancer Inst 1988; 80:1461.
259. Humphries MJ, Yamada KM, Olden K. Investigation of the biological effects of anti-cell adhesive synthetic peptides that inhibit experimental metastasis of B16-F10 murine melanoma cells. J Clin Invest 1988; 81:782.
260. Gehlsen K, Argraves WS, Pierschbacher MD, et al. Inhibition of in vitro tumor cell invasion by Arg-Gly-Asp-containing synthetic peptides. J Cell Biol 1988;106:925.
261. Saiki I, Iida J, Murata J, et al. Inhibition of the metastasis of murine malignant melanoma by synthetic polymeric peptides containing core sequences of cell-adhesive molecules. Cancer Res 1989;49:3815.
262. Inokuchi JI, Jimbo M, Momosaki K, et al. Inhibition of experimental metastasis of murine Lewis lung carcinoma by an inhibitor of glycosylceramide synthase and its possible mechanism of action. Cancer Res 1990;50:6731.
263. Wagner HE, Thomas P, Wolf BC, et al. Inhibition of sialic acid incorporation prevents hepatic metastases. Arch Surg 1990;125:351.
264. Schwartz GK, Redwood SM, Ohmura T, et al. Inhibition of invasion of invasive human bladder carcinoma cells by protein kinase C inhibitor staurosporine. J Natl Cancer Inst 1990;82;1753.
265. Dumont JA, Jones WD Jr, Bitonti AJ. Inhibition of experimental metastasis and cell adhesion of B16-F1 melanoma. Cancer Res 1992;52: 1195.
266. Kohn EC, Liotta LA. L651582: a novel antiproliferative and antimetastatic agent. J Natl Cancer Inst 1990;82:54.
267. Isoai A, Giga-Hama Y, Shinkai K, et al. Purification and characterization of tumor invasion-inhibiting factors. Jpn J Cancer Res 1990;81: 909.
268. Isoai A, Giga-Hama Y, Shinkai K, et al. Tumor invasion-inhibiting factor 2: primary structure and inhibitory effect on invasion in vitro and pulmonary metastasis of tumor cells. Cancer Res 1992;52:1422.
269. Ossowski L, Reich E. Antibodies to plasminogen activator inhibit human tumor metastasis. Cell 1983;35:611.
270. Agostino D, Clifton EE, Giralami A. Effect of prolonged coumadin treatment on the production of pulmonary metastases in the rat. Cancer 1966;19:284.
271. Hagmar B, Norby K. Evidence for effects of heparin on cell surfaces influencing experimental metastases. Int J Cancer 1970;5:72.
272. Kolenich JJ, Mansour EG, Flynn A. Hematological effects of aspirin. Lancet 1972;2:714.
273. Hover HC Jr, Ketcham AS. Techniques for inhibiting tumor metastases. Cancer 1975;35:5.
274. Mussoni L, Poggi A, DeGaestano G, et al. Effect of ditazole, an inhibitor of platelet aggregation on a metastasizing tumor in mice. Br J Cancer 1978;37:126.
275. Kohga S, Kinjo M, Tanaka K, et al. Effects of 5-(2-chlorobenzyl), 4,5,6,7-tetrahydrothieno [3,2-c] pyridine hydrochloride (tichlopidine), a platelet aggregation inhibitor, on blood borne metastasis. Cancer Res 1981;41:4710.
276. Wood S Jr, Hilgard P. Aspirin and tumor metastasis. Lancet 1972;2: 1416.
277. Hilgard P, Heller H, Schmidt CG. The influence of platelet aggregation inhibitors on metastasis formation in mice. Zeitschrift fur Krebsforschung 1976;86:243.
278. Honn KV, Cicone B, Skoff A. Prostacyclin: a potent antimetastatic agent. Science 1981;212:1270.
279. Nardone PA, Slotman GJ, Vezeridis MP. Ketoconazole: a thromboxane synthetase and 5-lipoxygenase inhibitor with antimetastatic activity in B16-F10 melanoma. J Surg Res 1988;44:425.
280. Tzanakakis GN, Agarwal KC, Vezeridis MP. Inhibition of hepatic metastasis from a human pancreatic adenocarcinoma (RWP-2) in the nude mouse by prostacyclin, forskolin and ketoconazole. Cancer 1990;65:446.
281. Tzanakakis GN, Agarwal KC, Veronikis DS, et al. Effects of antiplatelet agents alone or in combinations on platelet aggregation and on liver metastases from a human pancreatic adenocarcinoma in the nude mouse. J Surg Oncol 1991;48:45.
282. Nierodzik MLR, Kajumo F, Karpatkin S. Effect of thrombin treatment of tumor cells on adhesion of tumor cells to platelets in vitro and tumor metastasis in vivo. Cancer Res 1992;52:3267.
283. Esumi N, Fan D, Fidler IJ. Inhibition of murine melanoma experimental metastasis by recombinant desultatohirudin, a highly specific thrombin inhibitor. Cancer Res 1991;51:4549.
284. Zacharski LR, Henderson WG, Rickls FR, et al. Effect of warfarin anticoagulation on survival in carcinoma of the lung, colon, head and neck and prostate. Final report of VA Cooperative Study #75. Cancer 1984;53:2046.
285. Zacharski LR, Moritz TE, Baczek LA, et al. Effect of mopidamol on survival in carcinoma of the lung and colon: final report of Veterans Administration Cooperative Study No. 188. J Natl Cancer Inst 1988; 80:90.
286. Tzanakakis GN, Agarwal KC, Vezeridis MP. Prevention of human pancreatic cancer cell-induced hepatic metastasis in nude mice by dipyridamole and its analog RA-233. Cancer 1993;71:2466.
287. Hanna N. Expression of metastatic potential of tumor cells in young nude mice as correlated with low levels of natural killer cell mediated cytotoxicity. Int J Cancer 1980;26:675.
288. Hanna N, Fidler IJ. Relationship between metastatic potential and resistance to natural killer cell-mediated cytotoxicity in three murine tumor systems. J Natl Cancer Inst 1981;66:1183.
289. Hanna N, Burton RC. Definitive evidence that natural killer (NK) cells inhibit experimental tumor metastasis in vivo. J Immunol 1981; 127:1754,
290. Richie JP. Abrogation of hematogenous metastases in a murine model by natural killer cells. Surgery 1984;96:133.
291. Fidler IJ, Some S, Fogler WE, et al. Eradication of spontaneous metastases and activation of alveolar macrophages intravenous injection of liposomes containing muramyl dipeptide. Proc Natl Acad Sci USA 1981;78:1680.
292. Li L, Nicolson GL, Fidler IJ. Direct in vitro lysis of metastatic tumor cells by cytokine activated murine endothelial cells. Cancer Res 1991; 51:245.
293. Newton SA, White SL, Humphries MJ, et al. Swainsonine inhibition of spontaneous metastasis. J Natl Cancer Inst 1989;81:1024.
294. Humphries MJ, Matsumoto K, White SL, et al. Augmentation of murine natural killer cell activity by swainsonine, a new antimetastatic immunomodulator. Cancer Res 1988;48:1410.
295. Anderson RM, Katsanis E, Leonard AS, et al. IL-2 liposomes have increased local anti-tumor effects in mice with MCA-106 sarcoma pulmonary metastases. Cancer Res 1990;50:1853.
296. Crowley NJ, Vervaert CE, Seigler HF. Treatment of human melanoma hepatic metastases in nude mice with human cytotoxic T lymphocytes. Arch Surg 1991;126:433.
297. Abdallah RM, Starkey JR, Meadows GG. Dietary restriction of tyrosine and phenylalanine: inhibition of metastasis of three rodent tumors. J Natl Cancer Inst 1987;78:759.
298. Schleicher RL, Moon RC, Patel MK, et al. Influence of retinoids on growth and metastasis of hamster melanomas in athymic mice. Cancer Res 1988;48:1465.
299. Yeatman TJ, Riseley GL, Brunson ME. Depletion of dietary arginine inhibits growth of metastatic tumor. Arch Surg 1991;126:1376.
300. Torosian MH, Donoway RB. Growth hormone inhibits tumor metastasis. Cancer 1991;67:2280.

Surgery for Gastrointestinal Cancer: A Multidisciplinary Approach, edited by Harold J. Wanebo.
Lippincott-Raven Publishers, Philadelphia, © 1997.

CHAPTER 5

Genetics and Cancer of the Gastrointestinal Tract

Henry T. Lynch, Thomas Smyrk, and Jane Lynch

Anyone writing for a medical textbook faces the prospect of early obsolescence, but this chapter may be at particularly high risk, for two reasons. First, progress in molecular biology has been so rapid that we are still learning how to implement the new scientific knowledge. For example, the cloning of genes responsible for familial adenomatous polyposis (FAP) and hereditary nonpolyposis colorectal cancer (HNPCC) has helped clarify those conditions, but the newfound ability to identify asymptomatic carriers has raised unprecedented ethical, legal, and medical management issues. Our discussion of those issues, therefore, is necessarily preliminary. Second, progress in molecular biology will continue. It is likely that the genes for most forms of hereditary cancer will be identified within a decade of this writing. Many conditions now thought of as familial aggregations or geographic clustering will be shown to have a hereditary component. Some conditions thought to be hereditary may be proven to be chance aggregations or related to environmental exposure.

This chapter summarizes current thought about hereditary cancer of the gastrointestinal tract (Table 5-1). In the absence of a proven genetic basis for a cancer syndrome, the following descriptive terms are used:

Sporadic cancer: A cancer case with no family history of carcinoma for two generations, including siblings, offspring, parents, aunts and uncles, and both sets of grandparents.

Familial cancer: A cancer case with a history of cancer of that organ in one or more first- or second-degree relatives, in a setting that does not fit the hereditary cancer definition. Chance must always be considered in this setting. Common environmental factors may also explain familial clustering.

Hereditary cancer: A cancer case with a family history of cancer of that organ and, sometimes, syndrome-related cancers, with an incidence and distribution in the pedigree that is consistent with an autosomal dominant, highly penetrant cancer susceptibility factor. Other factors that support the hereditary cancer classification include frequent early age at onset, and an excess of synchronous and metachronous cancer.

These operational definitions are useful for descriptive purposes, providing that their limitations are understood. For example, an apparently sporadic cancer could represent a new germline mutation (and therefore be hereditary). Other potential sources of misclassification include incorrect family history, incomplete gene penetrance, incorrect paternity, or recessive inheritance from two parents who are heterozygous carriers of a deleterious gene when the cancer phenotype is expressed only in the homozygous state. As more deleterious genes are mapped and cloned, these problems will be minimized, but careful clinical observation will always be important, particularly with regard to the often-neglected family history.

A carefully compiled cancer family history is one of the most powerful and cost-effective components of a patient's medical workup. A registered nurse or other knowledgeable paramedical can be trained to gather this information. In most circumstances, a modified nuclear pedigree (Fig. 5-1) provides sufficient detail to suggest that familial or hereditary factors are operating. As seen in Figure 5-1, detailed cancer history must be compiled for all of the proband's first-degree relatives (siblings, progeny, and parents), as well as selected second-degree relatives (both sets of grandparents, aunts, and uncles). The second-degree relatives, being older and having passed through the cancer risk age, are often genetically informative because they are more likely to express the pertinent cancers if a hereditary cancer predisposition is present.

If a hereditary cancer syndrome is indicated by the family history, the physician will be able to extend appropriate cancer screening to all first-degree relatives of cancer patients. Unfortunately, even in disorders with a striking phenotype, such as the multiple adenomas of FAP, extension of such knowledge to at-risk relatives may not be accomplished in the clinical practice setting. Arvanitis and colleagues[1] have shown that the over-

Henry T. Lynch, Department of Preventive Medicine, Creighton University School of Medicine, 2500 California Plaza, Omaha, NE 68178

Thomas Smyrk, Clarkson Hospital, Department of Pathology, Omaha, NE 68178

Jane Lynch, Hereditary Cancer Institute, Creighton University School of Medicine, 2500 California Plaza, Omaha, NE 68178

TABLE 5-1. *Summary of current information about hereditary cancer of the gastrointestinal tract*

	Geographical/racial clustering	Familial aggregation	Hereditary syndromes	Disease/environmental associations
Esophagus	China; central Asia (Caspian littoral)	Yes[3–5]	Tylosis (rare)	Achalasia; Barrett's esophagus; congenital and aquired esophageal strictures; alcohol; cigarette smoking; epidermolysis bullosa; dyskeratosis congentia; adult-onset celiac disease; Fanconi's anemia
Stomach	Finland; Central America; South America	Yes[22,28]	FAP; HNPCC; gastric polyposis	Chronic gastritis; *Helicobacteri pylori* infection
Small bowel	None	Yes[33]	HNPCC (Lynch syndrome II); Peutz-Jeghers syndrome	
Colon	Urban areas of industrialized Western countries	Yes	FAP/HFAS; HNPCC; Juvenile polyposis; Peutz-Jeghers syndrome	Ulcerative colitis; Crohn's disease; common adenomatous colonic polyps
Liver	China; Japan; Thailand; Alaska (Alaskan natives)	Yes[63,68,69,71]	Hemochromatosis	Cirrhosis; hepatitis B virus infection
Gallbladder	Southwest American Indians	Yes[47–49]	None	Cholelithiasis
Pancreas	The Maori of New Zealand and Native Hawaiians	Yes[56]	HNPCC (Lynch syndrome II); von Hippel-Lindau disease; FAMMM syndrome; hereditary pancreatitis in single family with insulin-dependent diabetes mellitus	Diabetes mellitus; tropical calcific pancreatitis; chronic pancreatitis

FAP, familial adenomatous polyposis; HNPCC, hereditary nonpolyposis colorectal cancer; HFAS, hereditary flat adenoma syndrome; FAMMM, familial atypical multiple mole melanoma.

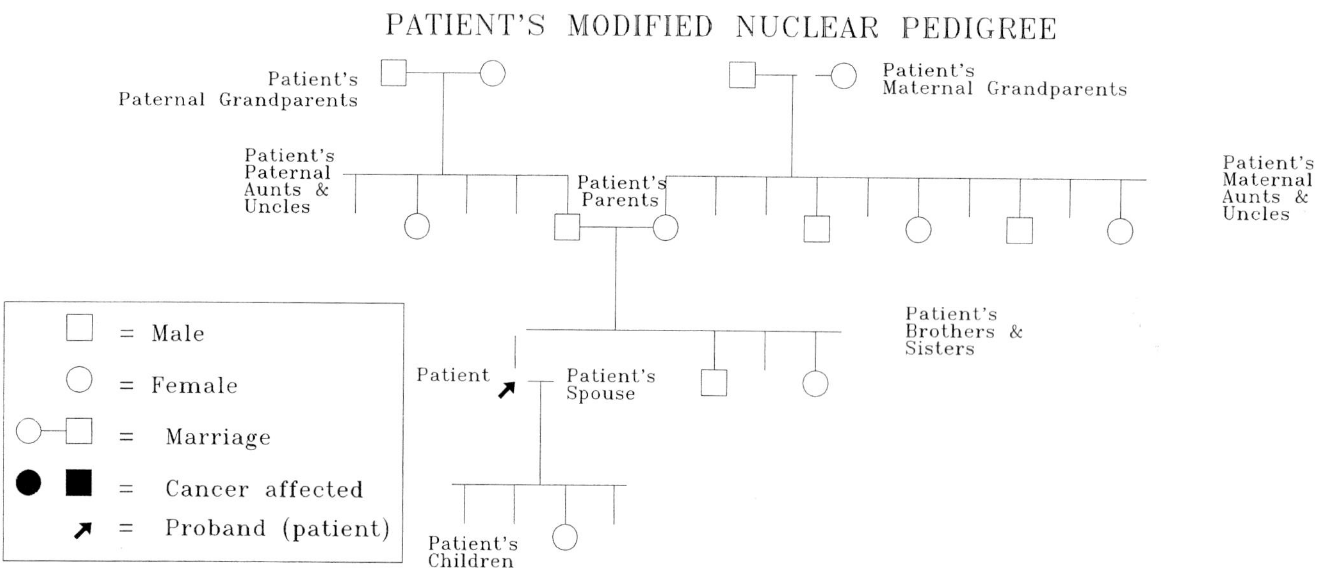

FIG. 5-1. Diagram of a modified nuclear pedigree. (Reproduced with permission from Lynch HT, Rozen P, Schuelke GS, Lynch JF. Hereditary colorectal cancer review: cedonic polyposis and nonpolyposis colonic cancer (Lynch syndrome I and II). Surv Dig Dis 1984;2:244.)

whelming majority of patients with FAP ultimately die of metastatic colorectal cancer (CRC), an unfortunate outcome that may be preventable by regular surveillance for high-risk patients and prophylactic colectomy when the FAP phenotype is identified.

ESOPHAGEAL CANCER

Squamous Carcinoma

Squamous carcinoma of the esophagus is renowned for the geographic variation of its incidence, with rates ranging from less than 10 per 100,000 in the West to as high as 245 per 100,000 in Linxian, China. No gastrointestinal tumor better illustrates the difficulty of separating genetic influences from environmental factors: what importance should be ascribed to a familial cluster of esophageal carcinoma in an area where the disease is endemic?

Numerous studies from high-risk areas have suggested that heredity does have some role, beginning with Pour and Ghadirian's[2] description of esophageal cancer in 13 of 19 people representing three generations of an Iranian family. In China, Ghadirian[3] found that 22.1% of esophageal cancer patients had a positive family history of this disorder, compared to 5.5% of control subjects. Similar familial aggregation has been observed in Kazakhstan in Central Asia, and in Iran, where Ghadirian[3] found a family history of esophageal cancer in 199 of 427 (47%) esophageal cancer patients of Turkoman descent.

Li and colleagues[4] performed a case–control study in Linxian, China, based on interviews with 1244 patients (758 men and 486 women) with cancer of the esophagus or gastric cardia and 1384 population-based control subjects (789 men, 525 women). Esophageal and proximal stomach cancer were more frequent (increased by 70%) among those patients whose parents had esophageal or gastric cancer. In contrast, the risk was only slightly increased among those patients whose spouses had such cancers. The authors concluded that "exposure early in life and/or genetic factors may be involved."

Carter and associates[5] attempted to determine the importance of genetic factors in esophageal cancer in high-incidence areas of northern China by performing segregation analysis on 221 high-risk families in the Yaocum Commune, Linxian, Henan Province of China. They found evidence of "autosomal recessive mendelian inheritance, with the alleged mendelian gene present at a frequency of 10%, causing 4% of this population to be predisposed to develop esophageal cancer. Large, unmeasured, residual familial factors, however, were also significant . . . . Both an autosomal recessive gene and unexplained environmental factors appear to be important in the etiology of esophageal cancer in the subpopulation studied." Possible environmental factors proposed by the authors were consumption of moldy foodstuffs, pickled vegetables, steaming hot gruel, and nitrosamines. In addition, nutritional deficiencies, fungal infections, and poor personal and oral hygiene may be contributing factors.

Outside of geographic high-risk areas, there is little known about the role of primary genetic factors in the etiology of esophageal carcinoma. The only documented example of hereditary esophageal cancer originally involved two families from Liverpool, England, who had a genodermatosis characterized by *late*-onset hyperkeratosis of the palms and soles (tylosis palmaris et plantaris). This dermatologic sign was originally found in 18 family members with carcinoma of the esophagus.[6] Follow-up of one of these families showed six new cases of esophageal cancer all occurring in individuals with tylosis.[7] The disorder is inherited as an autosomal dominant trait. The penetrance of carcinoma of the esophagus in patients with tylosis reaches 95% by age 63 years, with a mean age at diagnosis of 45 years.[8]

Marger and Marger[9] described the first American family with tylosis and esophageal carcinoma. As in the English families, the American family showed an autosomal dominant inheritance pattern for the paired association of tylosis and esophageal cancer.

In the United States and other countries of the Western industrialized world, risk factors associated with squamous carcinoma of the esophagus are low socioeconomic status, black race, cigarette smoking, and heavy alcohol consumption.[10]

Diseases associated with increased risk for squamous esophageal cancer include epidermolysis bullosa dystrophica (autosomal recessive), dyskeratosis congenita (possible sex linked), congenital and acquired esophageal strictures, achalasia, the adult-onset variety of celiac disease (autosomal dominant), and possibly Fanconi's anemia (autosomal recessive).[11]

In high-risk geographic areas or any of the high-risk situations listed previously, screening for esophageal dysplasia can be done with upper endoscopy. Dawsey and colleagues[12] studied a high-risk population in China and found that biopsy sampling of endoscopically abnormal areas (plaques, nodules, erosions) was effective in detecting severe dysplasia and early carcinoma. When severe dysplasia is found in a high-risk setting, consideration should be given to prophylactic esophagectomy with interposition of a segment of large bowel.[13]

Adenocarcinoma

Adenocarcinoma of the esophagus is essentially limited to patients with Barrett's esophagus, or columnar-lined lower esophagus. Barrett in 1950[14] described columnar-lined lower esophagus; he believed that it represented a congenitally short esophagus with intrathoracic stomach. It is now accepted that Barrett's esophagus is an acquired metaplasia, developing in about 10% of patients with protracted gastroesophageal reflux disease.

Barrett's esophagus is a premalignant condition. The incidence of malignancy in Barrett's esophagus is many times that of the general population, with estimates ranging from 1 in 52 patient years[15] to 1 in 411 patient years.[16] What factors determine which patients will go on to have malignancy in Barrett's esophagus? Fahmy and King[17] suggest that the occurrence of a white male predominance in Barrett's esophagus and in those who have adenocarcinoma of the esophagus is suggestive of a genetic influence. Their review of 300 patients with Barrett's esophagus revealed 45 with similar surnames. They recognized four families in that group that showed a strong familial expression of Barrett's esophagus. Others have also reported familial clustering of Barrett's esophagus.[18–21].

GASTRIC CARCINOMA

Gastric carcinoma is similar to esophageal carcinoma in that its incidence shows marked geographic variation. It is high in

Japan (160/100,000/y), Finland, and Chile, and much lower in the United States and the United Kingdom, where it has been declining during the past several decades and is now about 10/100,000/year. Gastric and esophageal carcinoma are also similar in that numerous familial aggregations of gastric cancer have been recorded in the literature, yet it is difficult to delineate specific genetic mechanisms that account for the inheritance of this disease. Interaction with common environmental exposures in families prone to gastric carcinoma is a confounding factor.[22]

The general consensus from the study of gastric cancer-prone families is that there is a threefold increased risk for gastric cancer among relatives of gastric cancer probands.[23–25] Studies of identical twins have shown a weak tendency for concordance of gastric cancer in monozygous as opposed to dizygous twins.[26,27]

Mecklin and coworkers[28] studied the clinical characteristics of gastric cancer among patients from Finland who were younger than 40 years of age. They noted a highly statistically significant ($P<0.001$) overrepresentation of gastric cancer among the parents of the index cases.

Palli and colleagues[29] studied 1016 gastric cancer patients and 1623 population-based control subjects who were interviewed as part of a multicenter study in Italy dealing with family history for gastric, esophageal, and colorectal cancer. They found an increased risk for gastric cancer when a sibling (odds ratio, 2.6) or parent (odds ratio, 1.7) had gastric cancer. The study was adjusted for potential confounders, including nutritional intake. They also found that adjusted cancer risk was higher among subjects with an affected mother as opposed to an affected father (odds ratios, 2.3 vs. 1.3). There was a further increase in cancer risk for those people reporting both parents (odds ratio, 3.0) or two or more siblings affected with gastric cancer (odds ratio, 8.5). Gastric cancer risk in association with a positive family history was found to be twice as great in residents of low-risk versus high-risk geographic areas.

The most celebrated gastric cancer family is that of Napoleon Bonaparte (reviewed by Sokoloff in 1938[30]). In his review, Sokoloff noted that Napoleon was obsessed by a fear of the "familial disease." Napoleon's father died of autopsy-confirmed gastric carcinoma, and Napoleon feared that he would also one day manifest this disease. He is said to have commented to Count Lobau, after a bout of chronic gastritis in 1806, that he "bore in himself the germ of premature death." He was constantly preoccupied with stomach cancer to the extent that he studied the anatomy of the stomach in cadavers brought to his palace for that purpose. Napoleon Bonaparte died in 1821 at 52 years of age. On his death bed at St. Helena, he gravely asserted "I am dying from the same disease as my father" and, in delirium and near death, he kept repeating, "pylorus . . . my father's pylorus." An autopsy showed findings consistent with gastric carcinoma, but there was no histologic verification.

We have reconstructed the pedigree of Napoleon Bonaparte's family based on Sokoloff's description (Fig. 5-2). Napoleon's father, Charles Bonaparte, died at age 39 years in 1785. The autopsy showed a large tumor in the pyloric portion of the stomach. Charles had complained of frequent vomiting, loss of weight, and pain in the epigastric region, and may well have been suffering from chronic gastritis. Napoleon had the same complaints.

Napoleon's mother, Letizia, is stated to have died of pneumo-

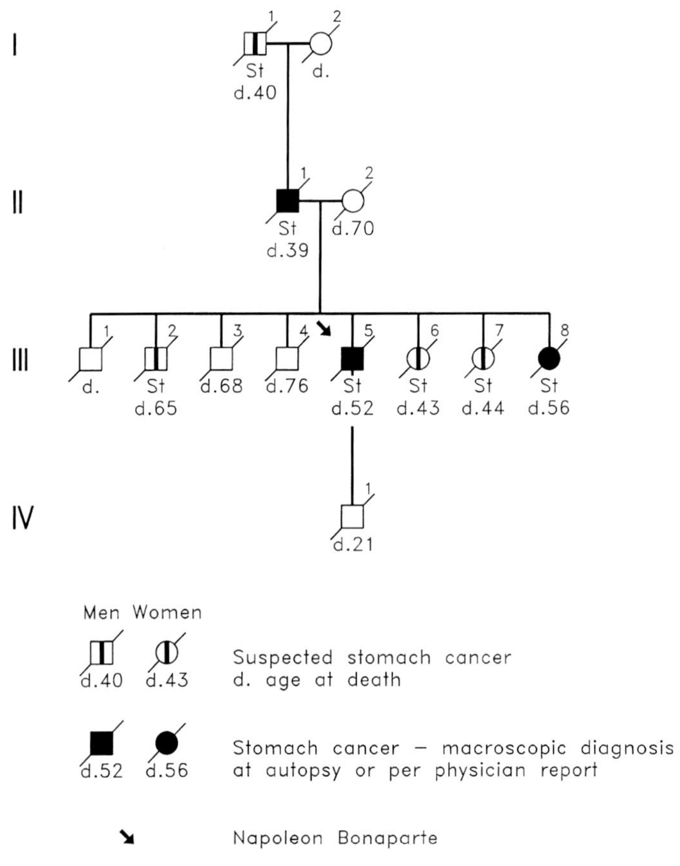

FIG. 5-2. Reconstructed pedigree of Napoleon Bonaparte.

nia at age 70 years. Napoleon's paternal grandfather, Charles Bonaparte, had "stomach disease" and may have died of stomach cancer at age 40 years. Napoleon's son, Napoleon II, died of pulmonary tuberculosis at 21 years of age.

Napoleon's sibship is of great interest. Two of his sisters, Elisa and Pauline, died at 43 and 44 years of age, respectively. Both of these sisters had a history suggesting "gastritis," and at death, stomach cancer was suspected. Another sister, Caroline, died at age 56 years and the diagnosis made by her physician was carcinoma of the stomach. Napoleon's brother, Joseph, also had a "gastric disturbance" but he died of a cerebral vascular accident. Another brother, Lucien, had gastric symptoms, and cancer of the stomach was suspected when he died at age 65 years. Two other brothers, Lewis and Jerome, died at older ages of conditions unrelated to cancer.

A most remarkable gastric cancer-prone family was described by Creagen and Fraumeni in 1973.[31] In this inbred kindred, gastric cancer was manifested in 12 people over four generations. The family resided in a rural county wherein mortality from gastric cancer was significantly increased compared to the surrounding area, but no specific environmental factors for gastric cancer could be identified. A battery of laboratory studies was performed on 16 family members. This revealed a high frequency "of cases with antibody to gastric parietal cells and cell-mediated immune defects. These observations suggest that mechanisms of autoimmunity and immunodeficiency, consistent with a genetic defect of T-lymphocytes, are involved in this family's susceptibility to stomach cancer."

Gastric carcinoma is a feature of several well established hereditary cancer syndromes. The tumor occurs in excess in Lynch syndrome II (HNPCC), as shown in an extended kindred reported by Cristofaro and colleagues in 1987 (Fig. 5-3).[32] Review of a large number of Lynch syndrome kindreds showed an increased risk of gastric carcinoma compared with age-specific cancer incidence rates.[33] It appears that gastric cancer was more common in earlier generations of Lynch syndrome kindreds, and that the declining incidence in the general population has been mirrored by a decline in familial cases (Lynch HT, personal observation).

Gastric cancer also occurs in excess in patients with FAP, at least in some parts of the world. Iwana and associates[34] reported an observed : expected ratio of 3 (2 to 7.7) for gastric cancer in Japanese FAP families. A review of patients with FAP in the Johns Hopkins registry,[35] however, did not reveal an increased relative risk for gastric cancer. Jagelman and colleagues[36] found gastric cancer in seven of 1255 FAP patients, compared to 10 patients with periampullary carcinoma and 29 with carcinoma elsewhere in the duodenum.

The difference between the Japanese experience, where gastric cancer predominates, and U.S. and English experience, where duodenal carcinoma is a more common complication of FAP, may reflect the differing incidence of gastric carcinoma in the general populations of the two societies.

The most common gastric manifestation of FAP is the fundic gland polyp. Domizio and coworkers[37] found fundic gland polyps in 44 of 102 FAP patients in a prospective screening program. These neoplastic lesions are also relatively common outside the FAP setting, where they constitute the second most common gastric polyp. They are typically small (<0.5 cm), sessile lesions in the gastric body. Histologically, there is cystic dilatation of glands; the cysts are lined by chief cells and parietal cells similar to those lining adjacent, nondilated glands (Fig. 5-4). Kinoshita and associates[38] found 26 patients with fundic gland polyps in 1388 gastrointestinal endoscopic evaluations, a prevalence of 1.9%. Fifteen patients (58%) had solitary fundic gland polyps. None of these patients had evidence of FAP.

There is a single report of familial aggregations of fundic gland polyps not associated with FAP. Tsuchikame and colleagues[39] described fundic gland polyposis in three related patients. The authors believed that theirs was the first documented example of multiple fundic gland polyps occurring in a family in the *absence* of polyposis coli. It is possible, however, that there might have been colonic flat adenomas present in this family. Flat adenomas are often subtle, and are seen predominantly in the right colon in the hereditary flat adenoma syndrome (HFAS), a disorder also characterized by a high frequency of fundic gland polyps[40] (see later discussion).

In addition to associations with FAP and HNPCC, a predisposition to gastric cancer may be inherited with a tendency to form hyperplastic polyps. Carneiro and colleagues[41] described a large pedigree characterized by an autosomal dominantly inherited predisposition to gastric polyposis coupled with a high incidence of gastric carcinoma. Two of the gastric carcinomas were of the diffuse type, one of which appeared to have originated from a hyperplastic polyp. Hyperplastic polyps were found in five of seven family members without carcinoma of the stomach. The remaining two individuals had marked foveolar hyperplasia. In addition, chronic atrophic gastritis (CAG) with complete intestinal metaplasia was observed in three of the patients. The authors concluded that "foveolar hyperplasia/hyperplastic polyps play a key role in the development of diffuse carcinomas in this inherited polyposis, confined to the stomach, with hyperplastic phenotype. The genetic and environmental mechanisms underlying this particular situation remain to be clarified."

A large subset of gastric cancers that arise in the sporadic setting are thought to do so by means of a series of precursor lesions that begins with chronic gastritis. Histologically recognizable points along the proposed pathway from normal to invasive carcinoma include CAG, CAG with intestinal metaplasia (CAG-IM), and CAG-IM with dysplasia.[42] The risk for subsequent carcinoma is low for patients with chronic gastritis alone (a common condition), but rises with the acquisition of atrophy, metaplasia, and dysplasia. In Finland, for example, carcinoma developed in 9% of patients with atrophic gastritis during long-term follow-up.[43] The presence of dysplasia confers higher risk, but the degree of risk and the time frame over which malignancy may develop are not clear. The cancers that develop in the setting of CAG-IM with dysplasia are usually of the "intestinal" type in the Laren classification. Intestinal-type tumors typically form well defined masses of gland-forming cells. The "diffuse" type, on the other hand, has an infiltrative growth pattern leading to diffuse thickening of the gastric wall. Histologically, diffuse carcinomas are poorly differentiated, often featuring signet cells.

The separation of gastric carcinoma into intestinal and diffuse types is very useful epidemiologically. Diffuse cancers have a low but relatively stable incidence in most parts of the world, whereas intestinal tumors account for a large but variable fraction of total gastric cancer. The proposed explanation for this phenomenon is that intestinal cancers are related to environmental exposures and diffuse cancers are related to host factors.

○ □ female or male without cancer
⊗ ⊠ gastrointestinal cancer, unconfirmed
colorectal cancer
gastric cancer
endometrial cancer
proband

multiple cancer sites
Cancer site and age at diagnosis
C = colon
E = endometrium
S = stomach
VC = vocal cords

? Sex unknown
B = born 19____
d = died - age

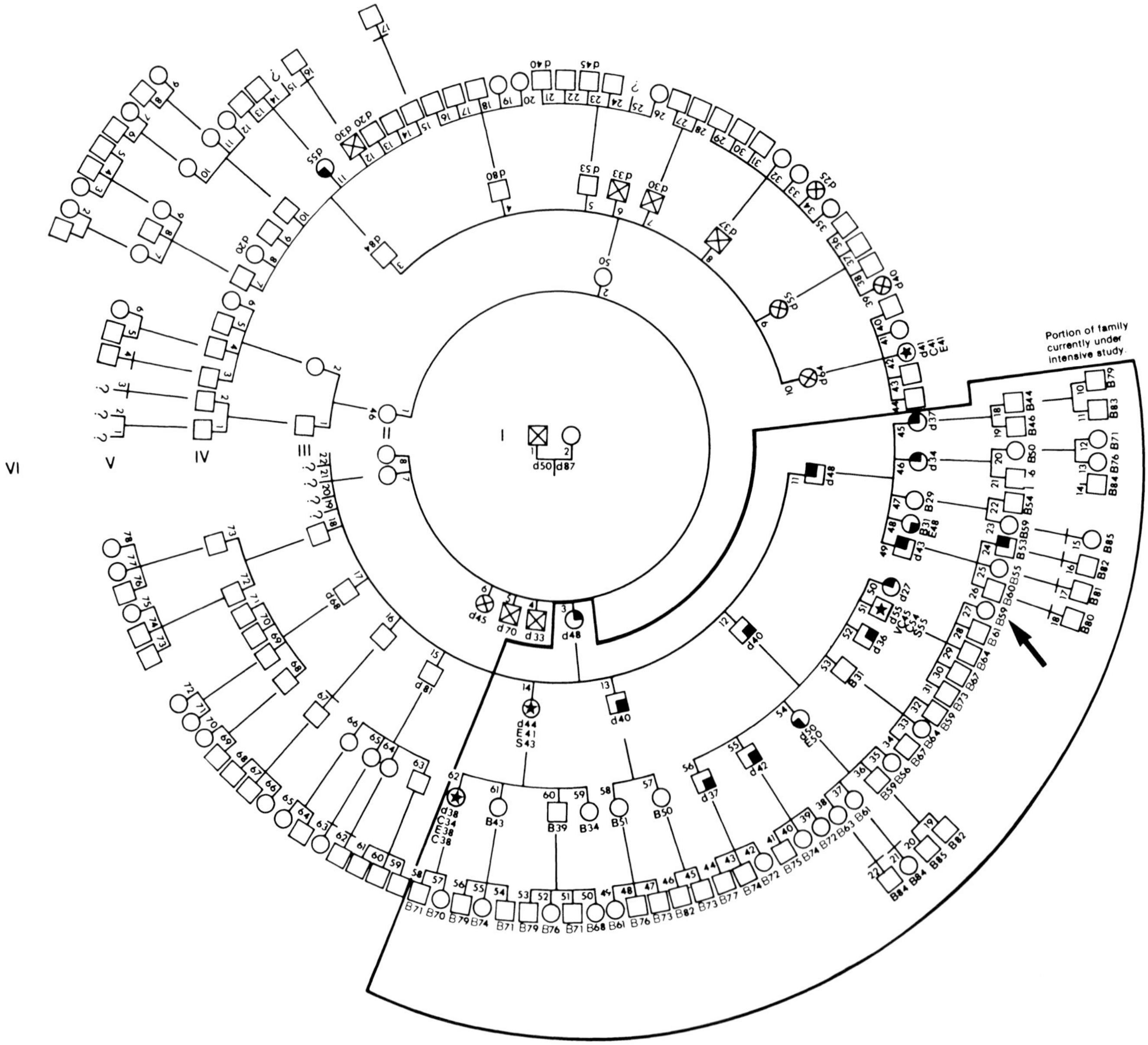

FIG. 5-3. Pedigree of a large hereditary nonpolyposis colorectal cancer Italian family containing numerous cases of gastric carcinoma. (Reproduced with permission from Cristofaro G, Lynch HT, Caruso ML, et al. New phenotypic aspects in a family with Lynch syndrome II. Cancer 1927;60:51.)

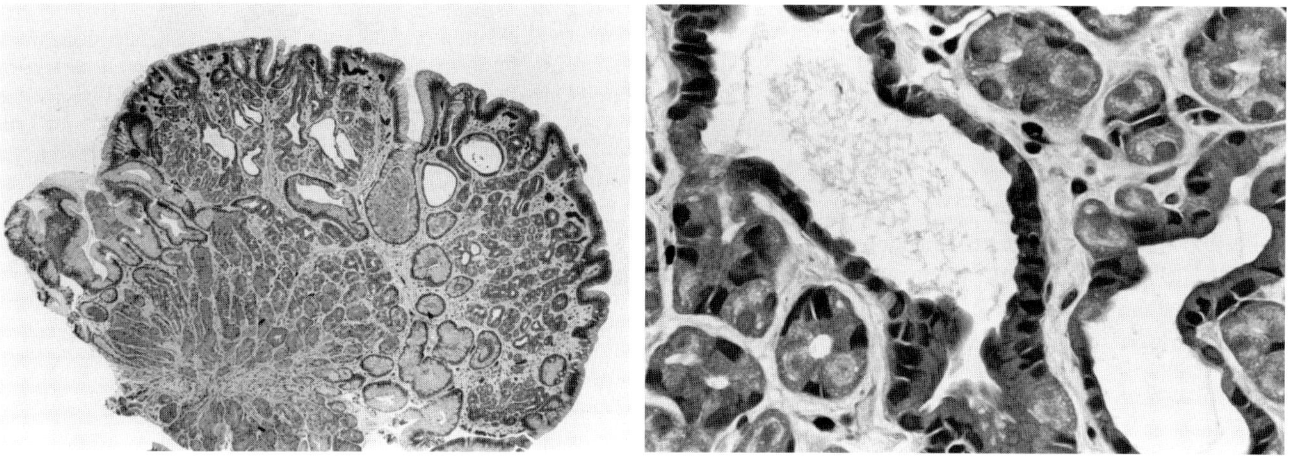

A B

FIG. 5-4. A, Fundic gland polyp. Scattered cysts in gastric body-type mucosa original magnification (×66). **B,** Fundic gland polyp. Cysts are lined by the same cell types that line the adjacent glands original magnification (×660).

Environmental risk factors for gastric carcinoma include diet (salted fish and meat and smoked foods), smoking and alcohol use, and infection with *Helicobacter pylori*. The decline in gastric cancer incidence in the United States over the past 50 years, probably reflecting a change in dietary habits, has been primarily a decline in the number of intestinal-type tumors. Diffuse gastric carcinoma has become relatively more common over the same time period.

This is not to say that heredity has no role in the development of intestinal-type gastric carcinoma. An illustration of the host's role in "environmental" cancers comes from our experience with gastric carcinoma in HNPCC. We predicted that the gastric cancers arising in this hereditary syndrome would more likely be of the diffuse type. The reverse turned out to be true, with all cancers reviewed showing intestinal features (Smtrk T, personal observation). This finding, combined with our observation that gastric carcinomas are less common in modern-day generations of HNPCC families than in earlier generations, is more typical of an environmental cancer than of one arising in a hereditary setting. Discoveries about the genetic defect in HNPCC may explain the apparent paradox, because it appears that HNPCC patients have defective DNA mismatch repair and are presumably more susceptible to environmental insults than the general population (see later discussion). It is likely that host susceptibility to other cancers related to environmental exposures is mediated by genetic factors yet to be discovered.

LYMPHOMA

Some types of gastrointestinal lymphoma show geographic variation in incidence. The best example is immunoproliferative small intestinal disease, previously known as Mediterranean lymphoma, which occurs predominantly in the Middle East.[44] Originally reported in Sephardic Jews, it is now recognized as a condition affecting young people of low socioeconomic status in developing countries. Genetic factors may play a role in the etiology of immunoproliferative small intestinal disease, because there is a preponderance of human leukocyte antigen (HLA)-AQ19 and HLA-12 in affected people.[45]

Three family members (a father and two adult daughters) with primary gastric lymphoma were described by Hayoz and colleagues.[46] The sisters had low-grade lymphoma of mucosa-associated lymphoid tissue. Their father manifested a high-grade form of later-onset gastric lymphoma. The lymphomas had been phenotypically characterized as of B-cell origin. The authors detected Epstein-Barr virus DNA by polymerase chain reaction in the biopsy specimen of the high-grade lymphoma. No chromosomal translocations were identified in either the low- or high-grade lymphomas.

Lymphoma is a complication of celiac disease. Lymphomas in this setting typically arise in the small intestine and typically show a T-cell phenotype. Because these lymphomas are associated with celiac disease, they show the geographic variation of that condition, being more common in northern Europeans.

GALLBLADDER CARCINOMA

The regional and racial hotbeds of carcinoma of the gallbladder are Latin America and the Native Americans of the southwestern United States, respectively.[47–49] Nelson and coworkers[48] reviewed medical records from the Fort Defiance Hospital, located on the Navajo Indian Reservation in northern Arizona, where about 95% of the patients are full-blooded Navajos. They found an inordinately high incidence of gallbladder disease, including a high rate of common duct stones and a high prevalence of gallbladder cancer (6% of patients undergoing laparotomy for gallbladder disease had cancer of the gallbladder). Reported prevalence rates for gallbladder cancer from other southwestern U.S. Native American tribes range from 3% to 3.8%.[50] Reichenbach[51] found the incidence of gallbladder and biliary tract cancer in Native Americans to be six times that of the non-Native American population, an observation based on a review of autopsy studies. Morris and colleagues[52] found an incidence of 5.1/100,000 in Native American men and 21.1 for Native American women.

The Native Americans of the southwestern United States are relatively homogeneous in that they have a fairly uniform dietary habit and are centrally located on reservations with similar environmental exposures. Their predilection to gallbladder cancer suggests host factor susceptibility wherein an underlying genetic predisposition is interacting with common environmental exposures. There are few studies of families with multiple members affected with gallbladder cancer. Garber and Shipley[53] observed carcinoma of the gallbladder in three members of a family of European ancestry. In their review of the literature, they found two additional families with multiple affected members.[54,55] The authors called attention to typhoid carrier status and unidentified carcinogens in the rubber industry as potential etiologic factors, in addition to gallstones.

Carcinoma of the gallbladder may be a component of hereditary syndromes. Wada and colleagues[56] described a 39-year-old patient with Peutz-Jeghers syndrome with hamartomatous polyps of the gallbladder and coexistent gallbladder carcinoma. Walsh and coworkers[57] reported multifocal dysplasia in the gallbladder in a woman from a family with the Gardner variant of FAP. The authors found seven additional reported cases of biliary neoplasia in FAP. Given the small numbers, chance must be considered as an explanation for these associations.

Among diseases associated with gallbladder cancer, the most consistent association is with gallstones[58]; it is estimated that 80% of patients with gallbladder cancer have gallstones, although less than 1% of those with known calculi will have gallbladder carcinoma.[59] It also appears that carcinoma of the gallbladder may be a rare complication of ulcerative colitis.[60]

CANCER OF THE LIVER

Hepatoblastoma

Hepatoblastoma is the most common primary hepatic tumor in children. Geographic clustering has not been reported. The tumors usually occur by age 3 years and they show a 2 : 1 male predominance. They are not associated with hepatitis B infection or cirrhosis.

There are rare reports of hepatoblastoma in patients with FAP; Li and associates[61] found 14 FAP kindreds in the literature with a hepatoblastoma. The tumor has also been described, albeit rarely, on a familial basis unassociated with FAP.[62]

About 5% of patients with hepatoblastoma have some associated congenital abnormality. Hepatoblastomas have been reported in patients with hemihypertrophy (autosomal recessive), Beckwith-Wiedemann syndrome (autosomal dominant), Sotos' syndrome (autosomal dominant), and Bannayan-Reilly-Rubalcaba syndrome (autosomal dominant), each of which has a hereditary etiology and is referred to as an overgrowth syndrome.[11]

Hepatocellular Carcinoma

Hepatocellular carcinoma (HCC) is one of the world's most common malignancies. Relatively uncommon in Europe and North America, HCC accounts for 20% to 40% of cancer deaths in parts of Asia and Africa. Alaskan natives also show a high incidence of the tumor. Boss and colleagues[63] studied HCC in an area of Alaska with high rates of hepatitis B virus (HBV) infection and an increased incidence of HCC. The incidence of HCC in Alaskan native men was four times that of the U.S. white population. Of 20 cases of HCC that had occurred in Alaskan natives from 1969 to 1981, all but 3 were in Eskimo men. The average age at diagnosis was 42 years. Five patients were younger than 23 years of age at the time of diagnosis, the youngest being 9 years of age. HCC occurs predominantly in adults, although it is the most common cause of pediatric hepatic malignancy in high-incidence areas.

Risk for HCC parallels the prevalence of HBV infection. Given the fact that there are over 200 million chronic hepatitis B carriers worldwide,[64] it might be expected that many examples of familial clustering of HCC will have circulating markers of HBV infection as a common etiologic factor. This has indeed been the case, as shown by the following examples.

Kaplan and Cole[65] described what they considered to be the first familial occurrence of HCC. They reported three male adult siblings, ages 64, 49, and 64 years, with histologically verified HCC. There were no cancers in the remainder of the family. Hagstrom and Baker[66] described HCC in three male siblings, ages 11, 22, and 31 years. There was no evidence of associated hepatic disease, and no other family members showed HCC. Denison and coworkers[67] reported two adult black male siblings with HCC, 31 and 37 years of age, both of whom had macronodular cirrhosis with features of subacute progressive viral hepatitis. Hepatitis-associated antigen was identified in the serum in one of the patients, but the death of the second had preceded the clinical use of this test.

Gilmore and associates[68] described a Chinese family studied after the death of one family member with HCC and hepatitis B surface antigenemia. One sibling had died of HCC 5 years earlier. The investigators traced three of the remaining six siblings and found evidence of prior or present HBV infection in all three, one of whom was also discovered to have HCC.

Lynch and colleagues[69] described a family in which histologically verified HCC was found in the mother and two of her four sons who were residents of an endemic area of Thailand. All of these people had evidence of HBV infection (Fig. 5-5).

Chang and colleagues[70] described two pairs of young brothers with histologically verified HCC, at ages 5 and 7 years in one family, and 7 and 9 years in the second family. In the first family, both affected children, their parents, and a younger sister were hepatitis B surface antigen (HBsAg) positive, whereas in the second family, both brothers, their mother, and maternal grandmother were HBsAg positive. The authors believed that the pattern of HBsAg suggested vertical transmission from mother to children, probably in the perinatal period. Given the early onset and almost simultaneous occurrence of HCC in these patients, the authors suggested that additional genetic or environmental factors must also be considered in the etiology of these cancers.

In an effort to sort out the interaction between hereditary and environmental factors, Shen and associates[71] performed a segregation analysis of HCC in 490 families who were sampled from a population-based epidemiologic survey of liver cancer in Qidong County, Jiangsu Province, China. Liability classes were defined by age, sex, and HBV infection status. The authors concluded that

> the maximum-likelihood model suggests that a recessive allele with population frequency .25 yields a lifetime risk . . . in the presence of both HBV infection and genetic suscepti-

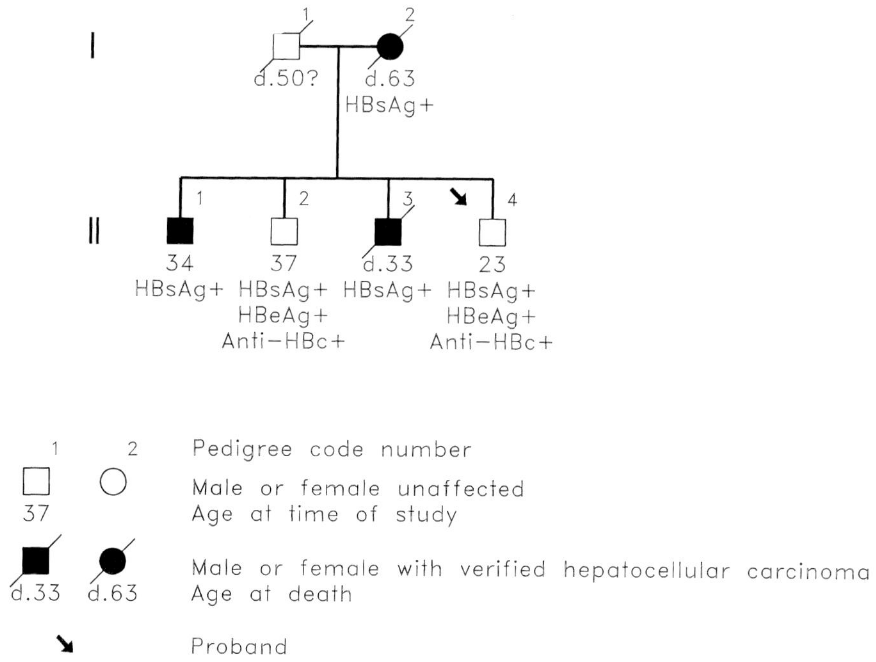

FIG. 5-5. Pedigree of family showing a mother and two sons with histologically verified hepatocellular carcinoma. All of these people, including the two cancer-free sons, had evidence of hepatitis B viral exposure. *HBeAg*, hepatitis B "e" antigen; *HBsAg*, hepatitis B surface antigen; *HBc*. (Reproduced with permission from Lynch HT, Srivatanskul P, Phornthutkul K, Lynch JF. Familial hepatocellular carcinoma in an endemic area of Thailand. Cancer Genet Cytogenet 1984;11:11.)

bility, of .84 for males and .46 for females. The model further predicts that, in the absence of genetic susceptibility, lifetime risk of primary hepatocellular carcinoma (PHC) is .09 for HBV-infected males and .01 for HBV-infected females and that, regardless of genotype, it is virtually zero for uninfected persons.

Hepatocellular carcinoma is not a component of any hereditary cancer syndrome. There are, however, a number of conditions other than chronic hepatitis B infection that are associated with increased risk for HCC. These include autosomal recessively inherited hemochromatosis in association with cirrhosis, α_1-antitrypsin deficiency with the zz phenotype, type I (autosomal recessive), and glycogen storage disease (autosomal recessive) due to deficiency of glucose-6-phosphatase.[11] Other disorders associated with HCC include glycogen storage disease type IV (autosomal recessive), which is associated with cirrhosis and HCC, and autosomal recessively inherited hereditary tyrosinemia, galactosemia (autosomal recessive), hereditary fructose intolerance (autosomal recessive), Wilson's disease (autosomal recessive), hepatic porphyrias and Fanconi's syndrome. In Fanconi's anemia (autosomal recessive), HCC may be secondary to treatment with androgens for pancytopenia.[72]

CANCER OF THE SMALL INTESTINE

Carcinoma of the small bowel is exceedingly rare. Approximately 1% of all malignancies of the intestine are located in the small bowel. Most of these are adenocarcinoma, but lymphoma, carcinoid tumor, and leiomyosarcoma also occur.

Adenocarcinoma of the small intestine does not show regional variation. No familial aggregations in the absence of a known hereditary syndrome have been described. A statistical excess of adenocarcinoma of the small intestine has been described in Lynch syndrome II[33] and in FAP.[73,74] Peutz-Jeghers syndrome also appears to confer increased risk for small bowel cancer (discussed later).

Other diseases associated with increased risk of small bowel malignancy include Crohn's disease and celiac disease. First-degree relatives of patients with Crohn's disease, usually those with chronic manifestations of the disease, have an excess of cancer of the small bowel.[75] Patients with the adult form of celiac disease show an increased risk for lymphoma of the small bowel and, to a lesser frequency, carcinoma of the small bowel.[76]

CARCINOID TUMORS

Carcinoid tumors of the gut arise from endocrine cells that are widely distributed throughout the gastrointestinal tract, from gastric cardia to anus. (Endocrine cells are much less common in the esophagus, accounting for the rarity of carcinoids there.) These lesions occur most commonly in the ileum (75% to 95% of gut carcinoids) and appendix (45%), with rectum, jejunum, stomach, and colon involved less often.

Several conditions are associated with carcinoid tumor. Carney and associates[77] described the syndrome of gastric carcinoids arising in atrophic nonantral mucosa. These patients often have pernicious anemia and are invariably hypergastrinemic. Two modern series have indicated that 25% to 50% of gastric carcinoids arise in this setting; such tumors are often multiple, usually small, and almost invariably indolent.[78,79]

Gastric carcinoids may also be a feature of multiple endocrine neoplasia (MEN type I).[80] Solcia and colleagues[81] described four patients with gastric argyrophil carcinoidosis arising in the oxyntic mucosa of patients with Zollinger-Ellison syndrome secondary to the gastrinomas of MEN type I. The stomach featured "multiple mucosal and submucosal carcinoids ... in combination with innumerable hyperplastic and dysplastic growths of argyrophil endocrine cells disseminated in the entire acidopeptic mucosa.'' The authors concluded that ''the genetic trait of the MEN syndrome has an important permissive role in the promotion of gastric carcinoids through the hypergastrinemia inherent in Zollinger-Ellison syndrome.''

Carcinoids are a rare complication of neurofibromatosis type I and are even more rarely present in von Hippel-Lindau disease.[80]

Carcinoid tumors of the lower gastrointestinal tract have been reported in association with celiac disease, Crohn's disease, and ulcerative colitis.[82–84]

Schimke[85] described several autosomal dominant pedigrees containing carcinoid tumors.

CANCER OF THE PANCREAS

There is less geographic variation in the incidence of pancreatic carcinoma than for other tumors of the gastrointestinal tract. The Maori of New Zealand and native Hawaiians are reported to have high rates of this disease.[86] Family history, on the other hand, does appear to be a significant risk factor. A population-based case–control study by Ghadirian and colleagues[87] found that 7.8% of patients with pancreatic cancer reported a positive family history of pancreatic cancer, versus 0.6% of control subjects. More detailed study of a subset of patients revealed no differences in environmental exposures between the two groups. Falk and coworkers[88] found that patients with pancreatic cancer were more likely than control subjects to report any cancer in a close relative (odds ratio, 1.86; 95% confidence interval, 1.42 to −2.44) and, most notably, pancreatic cancer in a close relative (odds ratio, 5.25; 95% confidence interval, 2.08 to 13.21).

Families have been described with multiple cases of pancreatic cancer. Ehrenthal and colleagues[89] reported pancreatic adenocarcinoma in women through three generations.

Lynch and coworkers[90–92] are studying some 35 extended families with multiple cases of pancreatic cancer and have identified a pattern of transmission that is consonant with an autosomal dominantly inherited factor in some of these families. Figures 5-6 and 5-7 depict several pedigrees of families prone to pancreatic cancer. The pancreatic cancers in families studied by us have been almost exclusively ductal adenocarcinomas. The survival rate has been poor, and the sex ratio shows a male predominance. All of these features are strikingly similar to pancreatic cancers in the general population,[91] which is expected to affect 26,300 people in 1996 (12,400 men and 13,900 women), and kill 27,800 (13,600 men and 14,200 women).[93] These dreadful statistics indicate that this disorder is invariably too far advanced for surgical cure at the time of its diagnosis. It would therefore seem prudent to identify high-risk people so that they might receive preferential attention to ensure earlier cancer diagnosis. Unfortunately, no serologic biomarker, such as CA 19-9, or screening modality, such as computed tomography scan of the abdomen, upper abdominal ultrasound, and endoscopic ultrasound of the pancreas, have resulted in earlier diagnosis.

Cigarette smoking is the environmental risk factor that has been most consistently associated with pancreatic cancer.[94,95] Coffee drinking was initially believed to be associated with an increased risk in some epidemiologic studies;[96,97] however, most other research has not corroborated this finding.[88] The role of alcohol in its etiology remains controversial.

There are several hereditary disorders that predispose to pancreatic cancer. These include hereditary pancreatitis (autosomal dominant),[98,99] multiple adenomatosis type I (autosomal dominant),[100] Lynch syndrome II (autosomal dominant),[101–103] von Hippel-Lindau disease (autosomal dominant),[104] a subset of the familial atypical multiple mole melanoma syndrome (autosomal dominant),[105,106] ataxia-telangiectasia (autosomal recessive),[107] and a single report of a family with autosomal dominant transmission of pancreatic cancer in concert with insulin-dependent diabetes mellitus and exocrine insufficiency.[108]

CANCER OF THE COLON

Regional variations in the incidence of colon cancer reflect societal behavior: colon cancer is more common in industrialized, Western countries and is probably related to dietary intake of fat (too much) and fiber (too little). It is likely, however, that heredity influences susceptibility to colon cancer in both low- and high-incidence areas. The best evidence for this assertion is provided by the work of Burt and colleagues[109] and Cannon-Albright and coworkers,[110] who described occasional adenomatous polyps and CRC in extended Utah pedigrees with an autosomal dominantly inherited mode of genetic transmission. The age of onset of CRC was comparable to general population expectations. There was no evidence of an increased occurrence of synchronous or metachronous CRC, nor was there an excess of extracolonic cancers.

Hereditary forms of CRC include the polyposis syndromes and the Lynch syndromes (HNPCC). These are summarized in Table 5-2.

Multiple Polyposis Syndromes

Familial Adenomatous Polyposis

Familial adenomatous polyposis (FAP), also known as adenomatous polyposis coli (APC), is the historical paradigm for hereditary CRC. This disease has taught clinicians more about the diagnosis and management of CRC than any other hereditary CRC disorder. The gene causing the disorder has been mapped to the long arm of chromosome 5.

Herrera and colleagues[111] provided the initial clue about the location of the abnormal gene when they identified a chromosomal deletion at the region of 5q in a child who had multiple congenital abnormalities, mental retardation, and multiple polyposis of the colon. Leppert and coworkers[112] and Bodmer and colleagues[113] almost immediately identified linkage of FAP to this same 5q locus. The gene has now been cloned and is termed *APC*. This is a large gene (>3,000,000 base pairs), and the sequences encoding the APC protein are separated into 15 pieces or exons. The APC protein is large and contains 2843 amino acids and 2 M2ss of 300 kd.

Bulow[114] traced the history of FAP to a report in 1861 by Luschka that ''may have been FAP.'' The first definite example of a patient with multiple colonic polyposis was published in 1881 by Sklifasowski.[115] The first ''familial'' example was that

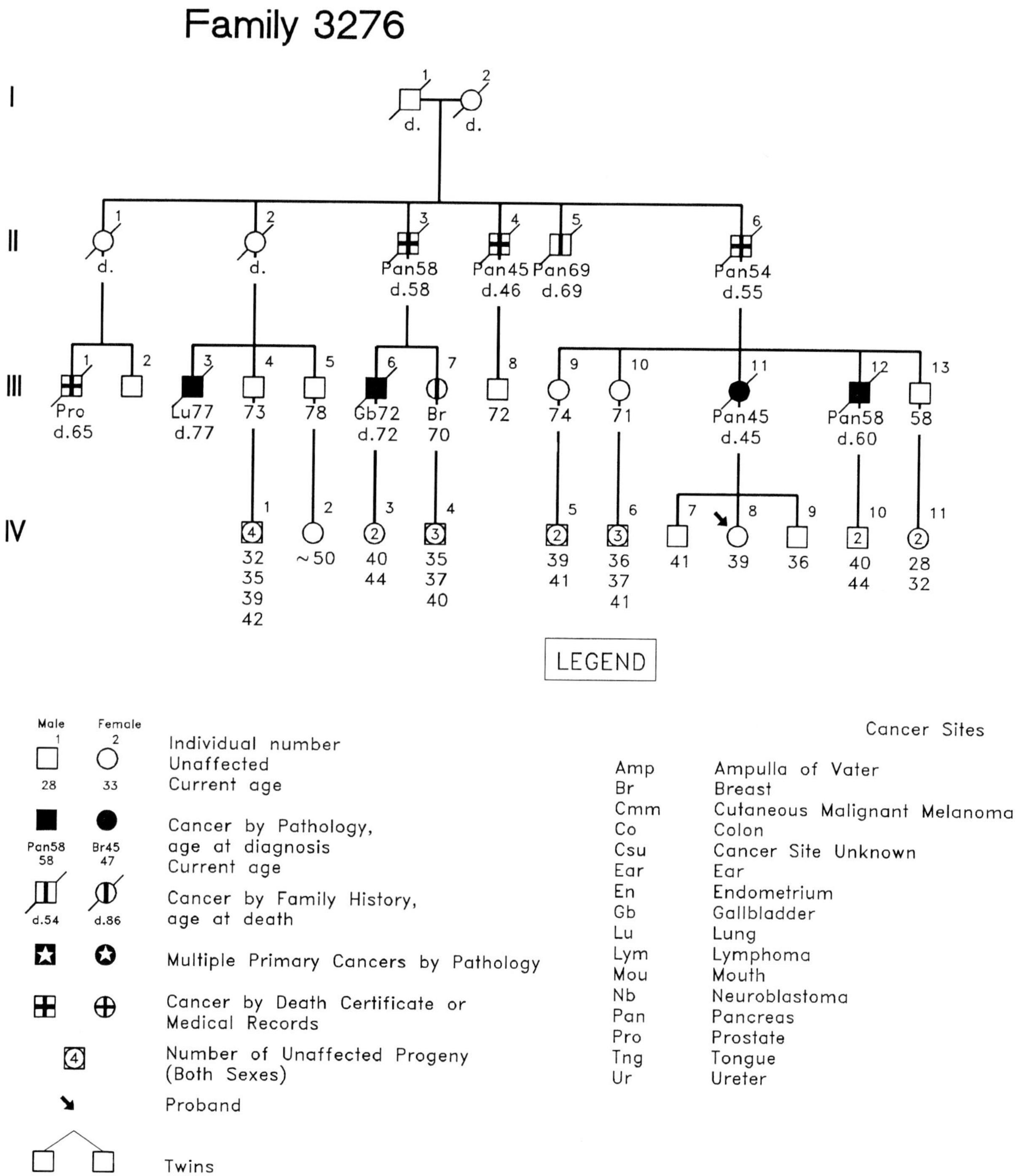

FIG. 5-6. Pedigree of a family in which six family members through two generations were affected with pancreatic cancer.

of a brother and sister with FAP reported by Cripps in 1882.[116] Examples of CRC occurring in patients with FAP were reported by Smith in 1887.[117] The idea of histologic progression from adenoma to adenocarcinoma was first elucidated by Handford in 1890. Finally, Lockhart-Mummery[118] was the first to express the concern that the hereditary factor was not for cancer per se, but for the presence of multiple adenomas.

Most affected patients have hundreds or thousands of adenomas carpeting the colon. The generally accepted lower limit for colonic adenomas in FAP is 100, but some patients may have fewer. Colonic adenomas are not the only manifestation of FAP. Specifically, Jagelman[74] accurately characterized the FAP phenotype as an inherited predisposition to aberrant growth. The phenotype of FAP is complex; indeed, its complexity has increased in direct proportion to the number and scope of investigations of FAP patients and their families. Some families consistently demonstrate extracolonic features such as osteomas, cutaneous signs (epidermoid cysts), and congenital hypertrophy

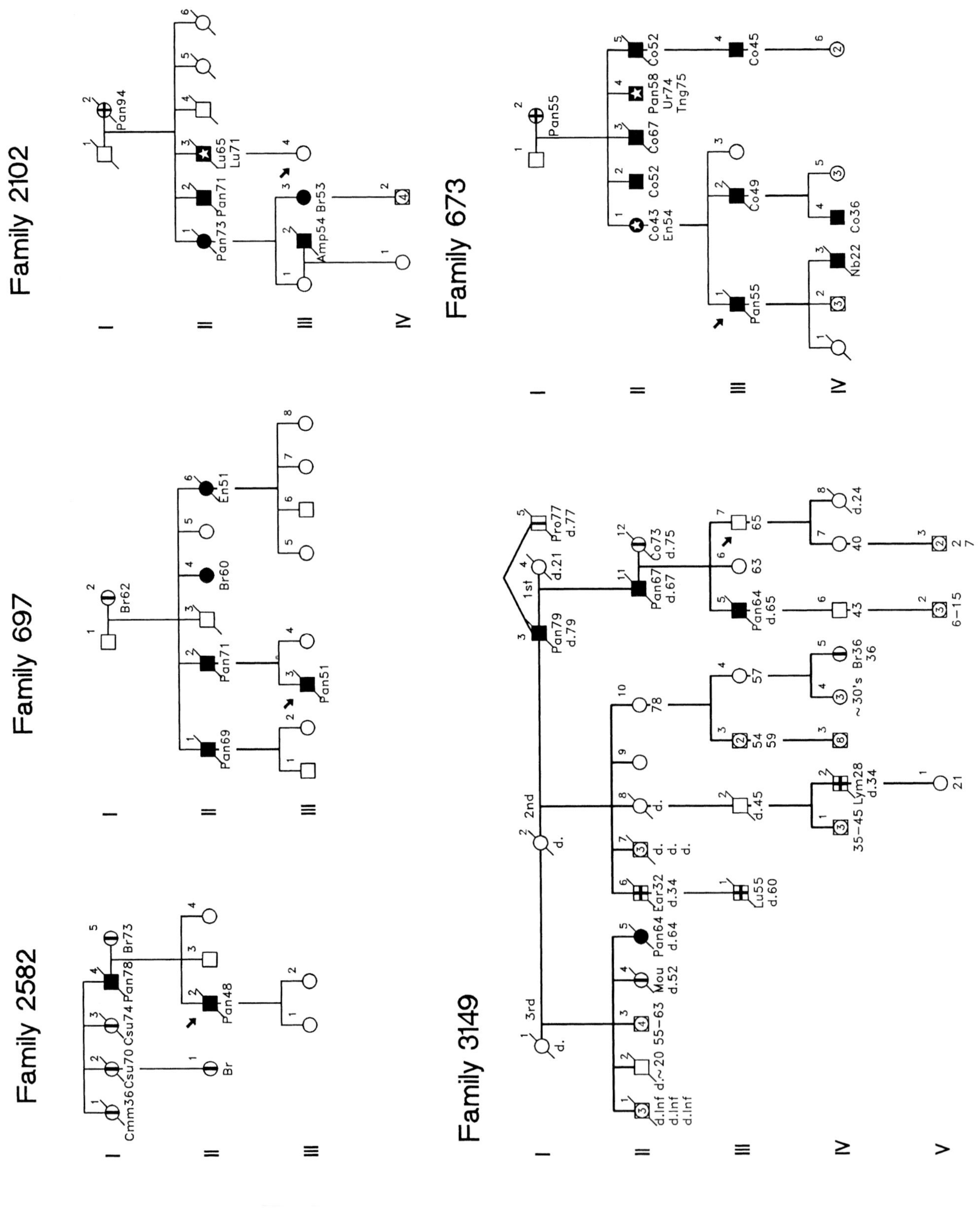

FIG. 5-7. Pedigrees of families in which pancreatic cancer occurs through two or three generations.

TABLE 5-2. *Hereditary forms of colorectal cancer*

Syndrome	Chromosome inheritance	Colon cancer risk	Colonic phenotype	Extracolonic phenotype
Familial adenomatous polyposis	5 q AD	High	Adenomas (100 to >1000); colorectal cancer	Periampullary adenoma and carcinoma; periampullary carcinoma most common cancers of stomach, small bowel, pancreas, thyroid (papillary histology), sarcomas, brain tumors. Desmoid tumors, particularly intraabdominal; congenital hypertrophy of retinal pigment epithelium
AFAP*	5q AD	High	Flat adenomas (1 to >100); right side > left; ordinary adenomas	Fundic gland polyps; adenomas of stomach and periampullary region; periampullary carcinoma
Hereditary nonpolyposis colorectal cancer	2p,3p AD	High	Occasional adenomas; may be larger, high-grade dysplasia	Carcinomas of endometrium, ovary, stomach, small bowel, pancreas, and transitional cell carcinoma of ureter and renal pelvis
Juvenile polyposis		Slight controversial	Juvenile polyps	Occasional juvenile polyps in small bowel and stomach. Rare gastric carcinoma.
Peutz-Jeghers syndrome	? AD	Slight	Hamartomatous polyps; small intestine > stomach, colon	Mucocutaneos melanin deposits; hamartomatous polyps (Peutz-Jeghers polyps) in stomach, small bowel, colon; carcinoma of duodenum; there may be an excess of cancer of other sites, but more research required

AD, autosomal dominant.
* Attenuated familial adenomatous polyposis.

of the retinal pigment epithelium (CHRPE). Families with these conditions were previously classified as Gardner's syndrome, but the descriptive subclassification probably is not valid because patients with this disorder have a defective gene at the same locus on chromosome 5q as patients with classic FAP.[112,113,119,120] Furthermore, when patients with FAP who lack Gardner's syndrome features are given panorex examinations, osteomas are frequently observed,[114,121] and careful ophthalmologic evaluation of the retinas often reveals CHRPE[122–125] in about 70% of FAP families. When CHRPE is observed in a family, it provides an excellent diagnostic clue, recognizable in childhood, to carriage of the abnormal gene. Olschwang and colleagues[126] noted that a range of phenotypic variation in the expression of CHRPE may be caused by different allelic manifestations of *APC* mutations.

The colon cancers of FAP are diagnosed at an average age of 39 years (cancer develops in virtually all FAP patients not given prophylactic colectomy). The site distribution is similar to that of the general population, with approximately 70% of cancers arising in the left colon. The histologic features do not differ from typical colon cancer.

Although cancer of the colon is the most noteworthy lesion in FAP, other cancers are integrally related to this hereditary disorder. Periampullary carcinoma is the most common extracolonic cancer in FAP. Other cancers reported in the setting of FAP include papillary thyroid carcinoma, sarcomas, brain tumors, hepatoblastoma, and cancers of the small bowel, stomach (particularly in Japan), and adrenal cortex.

Desmoid tumors pose a particularly difficult problem in FAP. Desmoids are benign fibrous tumors that do not metastasize but may be locally invasive. Rare in the general population, they are reported in 3.5% to 38% of patients with FAP, usually in those with previous abdominal surgery. The Roswell Park experience[127] illustrates the insidiously aggressive nature of desmoids in FAP. Twenty-one FAP patients with desmoids underwent a total of 60 operations related to their tumors. Nine patients underwent "curative" surgery; desmoids recurred in seven at a median of 61 months. Of those given curative or palliative resection, 47% had major postoperative morbidity. Long-term follow-up showed 5 patients alive without disease, 10 alive with disease, and 6 who died with disease.

Surveillance and Management

Management of patients at risk for FAP must, as in all forms of hereditary cancer, include genetic counseling (see subsequent section). Such counseling should begin early in life and must include, in addition to knowledge about the genetic risk, information about FAP's natural history. This is important, because patients must understand why they are being subjected to such rigorous surveillance so early in life. They must also be informed about the need for prophylactic colectomy should they manifest the polyposis phenotype.

We begin flexible sigmoidoscopic evaluation at about age 10 or 12 years. If available, molecular genetic screening can be done at that age.[128] However, we do not recommend doing molecular genetic presymptomatic screening in infancy and childhood because it could contribute to emotional disturbance of the child, and it could interfere with parental bonding. Furthermore, even when molecular genetic findings show that the patient has *not* inherited the deleterious gene, we still recommend baseline flexible sigmoidoscopy at about age 15 years, with repeat examinations every 2 to 3 years to 30 years of age, to protect against the small chance of a false-negative genetic test result. When the patient is found to be positive for the *APC* gene, we recommend that the screening be more intensive. When adenomas begin to appear, we recommend prophylactic subtotal colectomy with annual follow-up of the retained rectum. The option of a mucosectomy and the construction of an ileal pouch should also be considered. We also advise periodic upper endoscopy with visualization of the area at and surrounding the ampulla.

Genetic Counseling and Molecular Genetic Testing

Petersen and colleagues[128] discuss the presymptomatic direct detection of patients at risk for FAP using molecular genetic technology. The authors note that this approach, based on the cloning of the *APC* gene, has now enabled conclusive genetic testing for specific *APC* mutations in members of FAP families wherein the germline mutation has been characterized.

Petersen and colleagues performed presymptomatic molecular genetic diagnosis of FAP through direct detection of mutations in lymphocyte DNA from four families. Each of the families had a different mutation of the *APC* gene. They evaluated 27 progeny of FAP-affected parents, each of whom, based on the autosomal dominant mode of transmission of this disease, where at 50% risk. Of these people, 10 had already shown phenotypic aspects of FAP. Of the remaining 17 people, 2 had negative colonoscopic examinations at an early age and 9 had not had any prior colonic examinations. Six individuals from this particular group (54%) ''were found to carry their affected parent's mutation. No change in the conventional FAP colon screening regimen is recommended for these children. In contrast, when direct tests indicate that an individual does not have the FAP mutation, we recommend that screening be decreased. Reduction of uncertainty for at-risk FAP family members is an important benefit of genetic testing.''

It is likely that presymptomatic testing for FAP based on *APC* mutations will be available more widely for clinical application. Clearly, it is mandatory that physicians understand how to use this knowledge effectively.

Turcot's Syndrome

Turcot's syndrome is characterized by multiple adenomatous polyps of the colon in association with cerebral tumors. The eponym for the syndrome stems from a paper by Turcot and associates[129] describing two siblings who had an association of multiple adenomatous colonic polyps with cerebral tumors. Since that original report, a number of families showing the association of familial polyposis with central nervous system neoplasms have appeared in the literature, as reviewed by Jarvis and coworkers.[130]

Turcot's syndrome has been long thought to be a variant of FAP. More recently, Lasser and colleagues[131] described a family with patients showing typical Gardner's syndrome in which some members manifested multiple colonic polyps and neuroepithelial tumors consonant with Turcot's syndrome. The authors suggested that these findings were caused by pleiotropic mutations in the *APC* gene, based on linkage analysis showing highly suggestive evidence of linkage of the disease phenotype to the *APC* locus (linkage of disease score = 1.92). Clearly, the possibility must be considered that the neuroepithelial tumors in this family may have been part of the Gardner's syndrome variant of FAP and not truly the so-called Turcot's syndrome.

There may be multiple etiologies for Turcot's syndrome. Autosomal recessive inheritance may be one, as mentioned by Itoh and colleagues,[132,133] whereas linkage to the *APC* gene may be etiologic for other cases.[131] However, FAP is known for the variety of tumors that may develop, and certainly tumors of the central nervous system may be part of this cancer spectrum. We have also seen a family with the Gardner's syndrome type of FAP wherein an affected patient had a brain tumor in concert with multiple adenomatous colonic polyps (Lynch HT, personal observation).

Attenuated Familial Adenomatous Polyposis (AFAP)

This autosomal dominantly inherited syndrome is characterized by a predisposition to multiple colonic adenomas (usually <100), with proximal predominance and flat rather than polypoid growth.[90,134] The CRCs in this disorder are distributed randomly in the colon and have a later age of onset (~55 years) than those associated with FAP and the Lynch syndromes. HFAS is similar to FAP in that both syndromes feature colonic adenomas, have a high lifetime risk for CRC,[135] and are linked to the same chromosome 5q (*APC*) locus.[136,137] AFAP differs from FAP in that the colonic adenomas in AFAP are significantly fewer in number and are found more frequently in the *proximal* colon. Most of the adenomas in AFAP have the distinctive endoscopic and histologic features encompassed by the term ''flat adenoma.'' The criteria of Wolber and Owen[138] best characterize flat adenoma. They are:

1. A slightly elevated plaque of adenomatous mucosa not more than twice as thick as adjacent normal mucosa
2. Radial extension of adenomatous epithelium in superficial levels of adjacent mucosa
3. A lesion described by endoscopy as not pedunculated or exophytic

Figure 5-8 depicts the gross and microscopic features of flat adenoma.

The flat adenoma was originally described by Muto and colleagues,[139] who emphasized its tendency to harbor high-grade dysplasia. Subsequent studies from both Japan and North America[138,140] have found an increased incidence of high-grade dysplasia relative to polypoid adenomas of similar size.

Upper gastrointestinal findings in three of four kindreds we have described provided a new dimension to the clinicopathologic spectrum of AFAP and indicated an additional measure of phenotypic similarity to its FAP counterpart,[135] namely, the

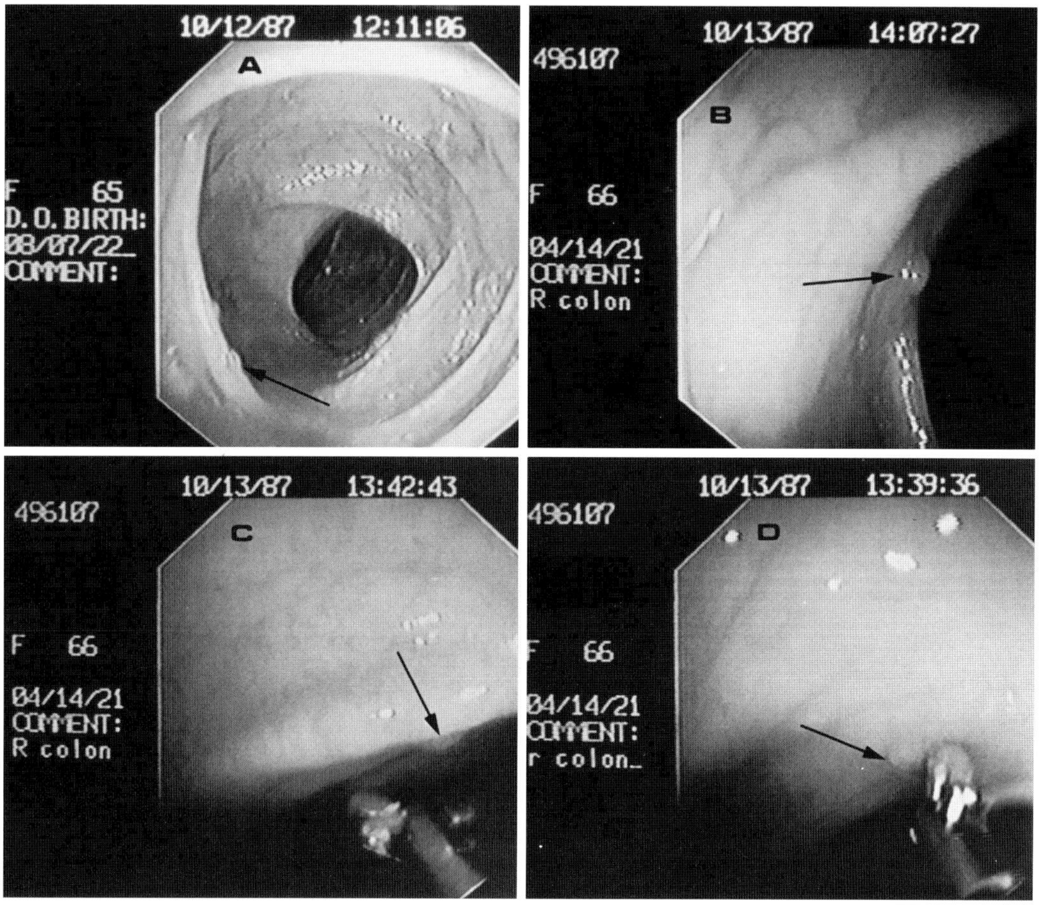

A

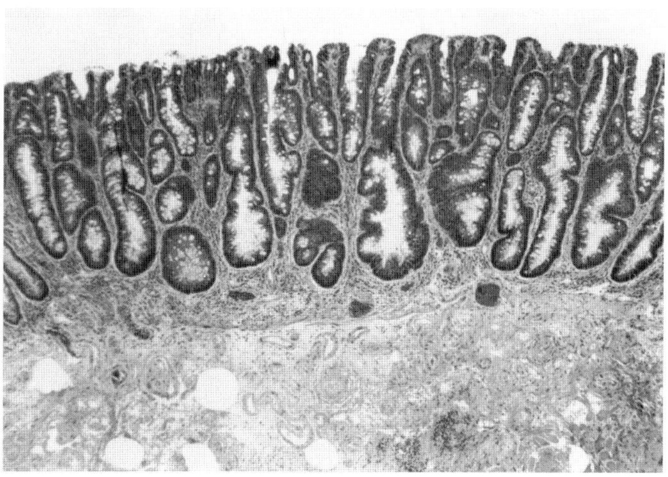

B

FIG. 5-8. A, Flat adenoma. Endoscopic views of small (<1 cm), flat lesions in the proximal colon. **(B).** Flat adenoma. Neoplastic tubules produce a slight mucosal thickening original magnification (×66).

presence of multiple flat adenomas. Figure 5-9 is a pedigree of one of our AFAP families. Fundic gland polyps have been discovered in more than half of patients examined, including three people who did not have colonic adenomas. This indicates that in some genetically at-risk patients, fundic gland polyps may precede the occurrence of colonic adenomas and may serve as a phenotypic marker for AFAP in the appropriate clinical setting. Other upper gastrointestinal manifestations of AFAP are gastric adenoma, periampullary adenoma, and periampullary carcinoma. The latter tumor has occurred in two patients under our care from unrelated AFAP families, leading us strongly to recommend upper endoscopic examination in patients deemed at risk for AFAP by family history.

Flat adenomas occur in the general population. Wolber and Owen[138] found that 8.5% of a large prospective series of colonic adenomas were flat; only 3 of 18 patients with flat adenoma had a family history of CRC. In our prospective study, 12% of patients undergoing colonoscopic examination who were not members of families with FAP or Lynch syndrome had polyps endoscopically and histologically consistent with flat ade-

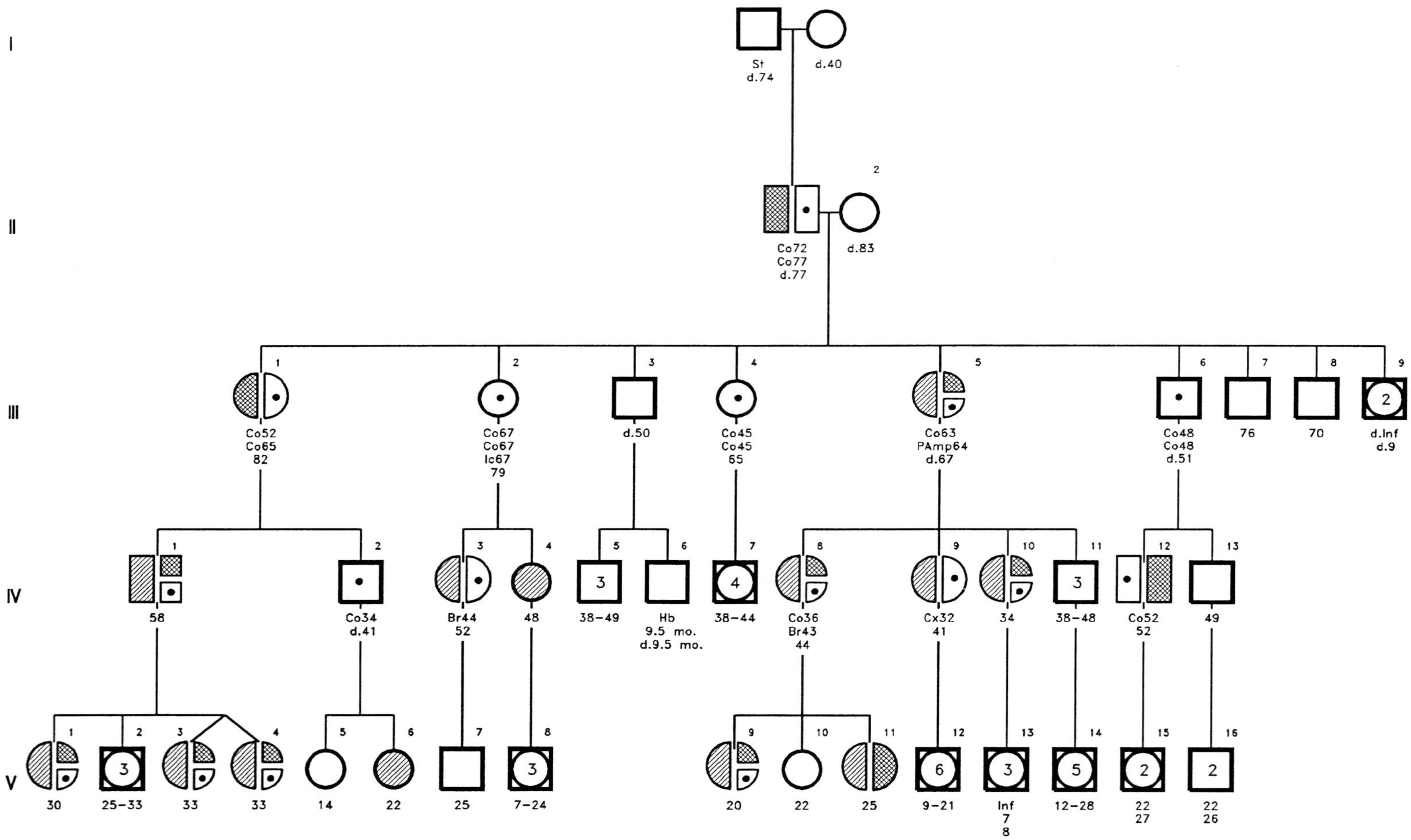

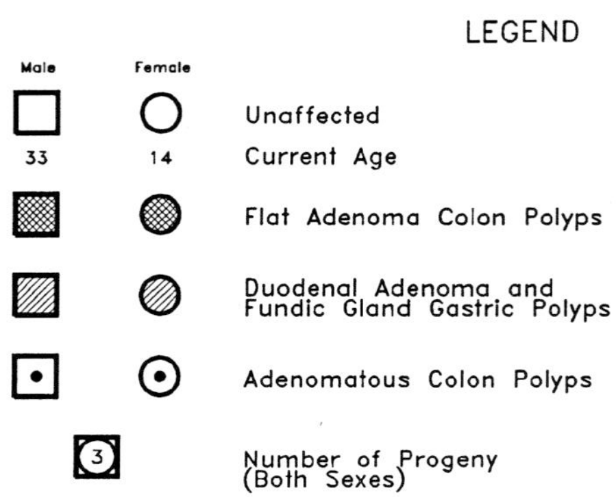

Cancer Site Abbreviations & Age at diagnosis

Br44	Breast
Co45	Colon
Cx32	Cervix
Hb	Hepatoblastoma
Ic67	Ileo Cecal
PAmp64	Periampullary
St	Stomach

FIG. 5-9. Updated pedigree of a family showing all of the characteristics of the hereditary flat adenoma syndrome. (Reproduced with permission from Lynch HT, Smyrk TC, Watson P, et al. Hereditary flat adenoma syndrome: a variant of familial adenomatous polyposis? Dis Colon Rectum 1992;35:411.)

noma.[141] None of the patients in our prospective series had more than one or two adenomas, in significant contrast to findings in families with AFAP. Hence, it is a constellation of findings that suggests AFAP, and not the presence of one or two flat adenomas, one or two fundic gland polyps, or any other single facet of the AFAP phenotype.

Finally, we have begun genetic counseling of patients from AFAP families based on germline mutation findings at the *APC* locus (Lynch and colleagues, in preparation).[142]

Peutz-Jeghers Syndrome

Peutz-Jeghers syndrome is an autosomal dominant hereditary disease characterized by hamartomatous polyps of the gastrointestinal tract and mucocutaneous melanin deposits. The condition is thought to be about one tenth as common as FAP.[109] Polyps are found most often in the small bowel, but are only slightly less common in the stomach and colon. The total number of polyps in any one person ranges from few to dozens. As hamartomas, Peutz-Jeghers polyps are composed of normal elements abnormally arranged. Thick bands of smooth muscle in an arborizing pattern provide a scaffold for mucosa indigenous to the site—that is, gastric mucosa covers gastric Peutz-Jeghers polyps, colonic mucosa covers colonic polyps, and so on. Figure 5-10 illustrates the histologic features of a Peutz-Jeghers polyp, juvenile retention polyp, and tubular adenoma.

Peutz-Jeghers syndrome carries an increased risk for carcinoma of several organs. Giardiello and colleagues[143] surveyed 31 patients with Peutz-Jeghers syndrome who were followed from 1973 to 1985. Cancer developed in 15 (48%) patients: gastrointestinal carcinoma in 4, extraintestinal carcinoma in 10, and multiple myeloma in 1. The cancers were diagnosed when the patients were relatively young, but after Peutz-Jeghers syndrome had been diagnosed (interval between diagnoses, 25 years; range, 1 to 64 years). The observed development of cancer in patients with Peutz-Jeghers syndrome was 18 times greater than expected in the general population ($P<0.0001$). A review of 72 patients with Peutz-Jeghers syndrome from St. Mark's Hospital[144] showed carcinoma in 16, a relative risk of 9. Foley and coworkers[145] reviewed 49 years' experience with the "Harrisburg family," which contains 12 affected family members, comprising the largest Peutz-Jeghers kindred reported. Two of the 12 had gastrointestinal malignancy, including 1 family member in whom a duodenal carcinoma developed in a hamartoma with adenomatous changes.

It is not clear whether gastrointestinal carcinomas arise in hamartomatous polyps or coincident adenomas. A 1987 review of nearly 500 Peutz-Jeghers polyps collected in the St. Mark's Hospital polyposis registry failed to discover any with dysplastic change.[146] Narita and associates[147] reported a patient with Peutz-Jeghers syndrome in whom 52 colonic polyps were resected endoscopically. Of these, 49 were hamartomatous and showed no dysplastic or carcinomatous changes. The other three polyps had adenomatous areas and foci of carcinoma.

We believe that patients with Peutz-Jeghers syndrome have an increased risk for carcinoma at several sites, including the gastrointestinal tract. Screening of patients at risk should begin in the second decade and should include fecal occult blood testing and flexible sigmoidoscopy. We advise surveillance of the upper and lower gastrointestinal tract every 3 to 5 years. Gastric, duodenal, and colonic polyps should be removed endoscopically. If surgical intervention is necessary, intraoperative endoscopy with polypectomy may prevent the development of a short bowel syndrome.

Familial Juvenile Polyposis

Juvenile polyps of the colon are a fairly common finding in childhood, occurring in as many as 1% of children. These hamartomatous polyps feature dilated crypts in an edematous, inflamed lamina propria (see Fig. 5-10*B*). In contrast to the Peutz-Jeghers polyp, the muscularis mucosae does not extend into the stalk or head of a juvenile polyp. Solitary juvenile polyps may cause bleeding, but are otherwise innocuous. One report from St. Mark's Hospital confirms that people with solitary juvenile polyps do not have an increased risk of CRC.[148]

Familial juvenile polyposis, conversely, may have significant colonic cancer consequences for affected patients. Unfortunately, the diagnosis may be difficult to establish, because affected patients may have only a few juvenile polyps and sporadic, innocuous juvenile polyps may be multiple. Only about half of all cases have a known family history, either because of low gene penetrance, asymptomatic affected relatives, or disease caused by a new mutation. The current working definition of juvenile polyposis, suggested by Jass and colleagues,[149] is as follows: more than five juvenile polyps in the colorectum; or juvenile polyps throughout the gastrointestinal tract; or any number of juvenile polyps with a family history of juvenile polyposis. Ruling out FAP is particularly difficult if biopsy samples are taken of only one or two polyps and they happen to contain dysplastic areas; therefore, if patients harbor multiple polyps, it is recommended that many polyps be sampled.

Familial juvenile polyposis has an autosomal dominant inheritance pattern. Symptoms usually begin in the first or second decade and include rectal bleeding, colicky abdominal pain, or, if gastric polyps are present, a protein-losing enteropathy. The colon is the site involved most often, with the number of polyps ranging from few to more than 100. Polyps may also be found in the stomach and occasionally in the small bowel. In rare instances, gastric juvenile polyposis occurs in the absence of small intestinal or colonic involvement.

Although typical hamartomatous juvenile polyps are not premalignant, the polyps of familial juvenile polyposis may contain areas of dysplasia and carcinoma. Jass has estimated that the cumulative lifetime risk of CRC in the syndrome is greater than 50%.[150] Murday and Slack[151] calculated a cumulative probability for CRC of 68% by age 60 years.

The management of familial juvenile polyposis is controversial. We favor consideration of prophylactic colectomy, given the estimates of high lifetime risk for CRC, but patients with few polyps might qualify for endoscopic surveillance with polypectomy. Juvenile polyposis limited to the stomach and small bowel may also be managed with surveillance and endoscopic polypectomy.

Inflammatory Bowel Disease

The risk for development of CRC is increased in patients who have had ulcerative colitis for more than 10 years. Estimates are that risk increases by 0.5% to 1% per year after the first decade of colitis.[152] The highest risk accrues to patients with pancolitis,

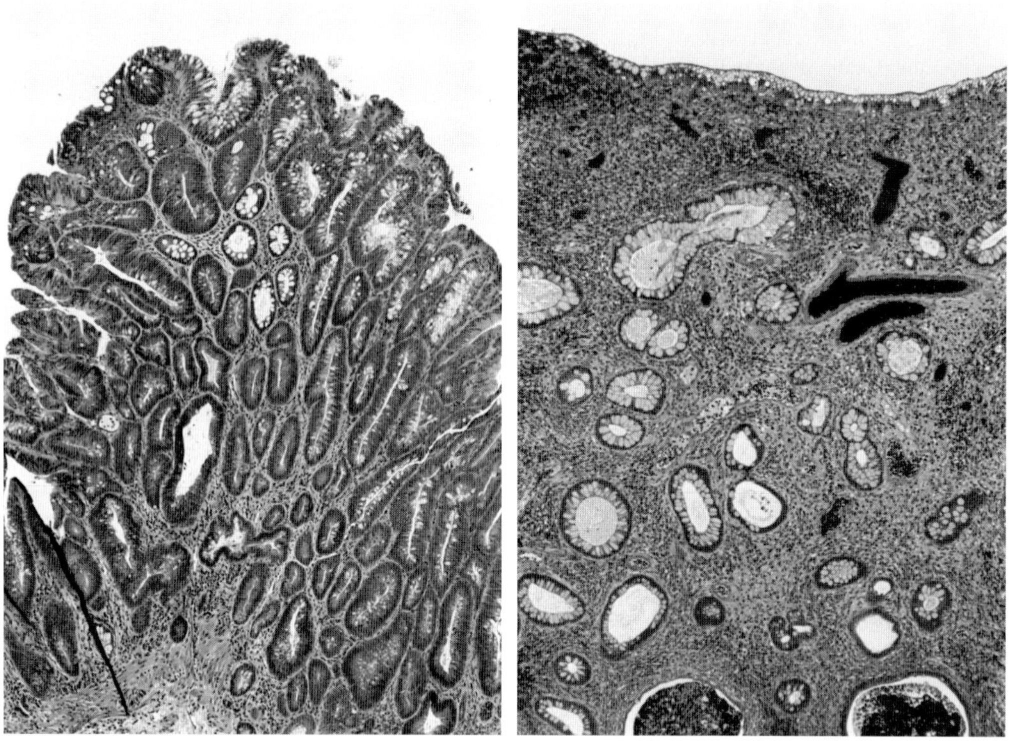

A B

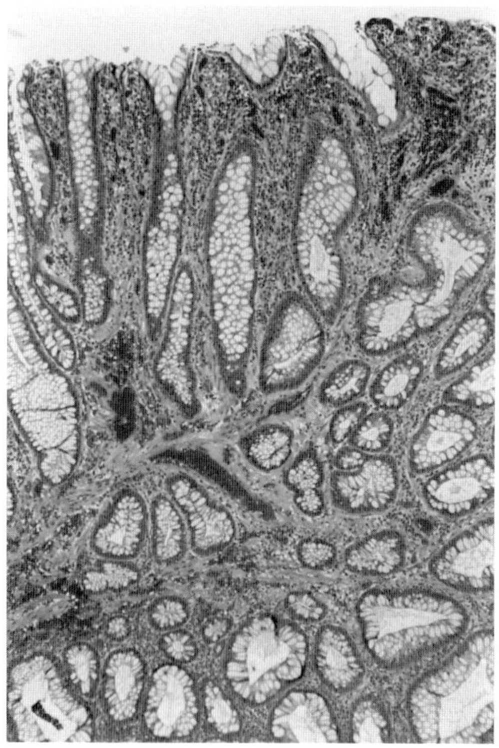

C

FIG. 5-10. A, Tubular adenoma. Neoplastic tubules form a polypoid mass. Tubules are lined by crowded cells with elongated nuclei. **B,** Juvenile retention polyp. Note dilated crypts in an expanded, inflamed lamina propria. There is no dysplasia. **C,** Peutz-Jegher's polyp. Branching smooth muscle forms a scafford for nonneoplastic colonic crypts original magnification, A–C, (×66).

or universal colitis. There is some evidence that those patients with associated primary sclerosing cholangitis are also at particularly high risk.[153] These high-risk subsets may be candidates for prophylactic proctocolectomy after their first decade of colitis. Alternatively, a surveillance program may be undertaken aimed at detecting high-grade dysplasia. However, the efficacy of surveillance in patients with ulcerative colitis remains controversial.[154]

Carcinoma of the colon also occurs in excess in patients with Crohn's disease.[155] CRC appears to occur in areas of stricture, fistulization, or intense inflammation. There also appears to be an association between regional enteritis and carcinoma of the small intestine, but this has been difficult to prove conclusively and to quantitate.

Endoscopic surveillance guidelines are not established for Crohn's disease. Hamilton[156] reviewed the subject of CRC in patients with Crohn's disease, and found a 4-fold to 20-fold increased risk of CRC compared with the general population. He described a series of 10 patients with Crohn's disease and CRC and compared these with 118 consecutive patients with CRC of the usual type. The patients with Crohn's disease were younger and they had a higher prevalence of mucinous carcinoma. Furthermore, Hamilton found dysplasia in all 10 patients, and all 10 resected carcinomas were adjacent to high-grade dysplasia. Because of these findings, he suggested that "surveillance should be considered for patients with clinically evident colorectal involvement by Crohn's disease or a bypassed segment of colorectum." More recently, Gillen and colleagues[157] found a fivefold increased risk for colon cancer in Crohn's disease patients. The risk was particularly high (18 ×) in patients with extensive colitis. We believe that it is prudent to apply ulcerative colitis-type surveillance to patients with extensive, longstanding Crohn's disease.

Rotter and Yang[158] reviewed the evidence in support of a genetic predisposition to inflammatory bowel disease. They characterized ulcerative colitis and Crohn's disease as "genetic diseases with complex non-mendelian patterns of inheritance." Evidence for an inherited predisposition includes familial aggregation, higher concordance in monozygotic versus dizygotic twins, the increased frequency of inflammatory bowel disease in several hereditary disorders, and the development of a genetically determined spontaneous mouse model of colitis.

Shanahan and associates[159] have explored the possibility that neutrophil autoantibodies found in association with ulcerative colitis may be a genetic marker of susceptibility. The authors observed an increased prevalence of neutrophil antibodies among not only the probands (68%, 26 to 38) but among their clinically unaffected family members (15.7%, 17 to 108), compared with control subjects (2.9%, 1 to 35) ($P<0.0001$ and $P<0.05$, respectively). The investigators concluded that their findings "are consistent with these antibodies being a potential marker of genetic susceptibility to ulcerative colitis and suggest the possibility of genetic heterogeneity within this disease."

The Lynch Syndromes

Hereditary nonpolyposis colorectal cancer, also referred to as Lynch syndromes I and II, poses a major public health problem. It is the most common hereditary cancer syndrome predisposing to CRC, accounting for as much as 10% of the total CRC burden. Its history is interesting. In 1895, Aldred Warthin, MD, pathologist at the University of Michigan Medical School at Ann Arbor, was told by his seamstress that she would die at an early age from cancer of the colon or female organs because "most of my family members die of these cancers." Just as she had predicted, she died at an early age of carcinoma of the endometrium. Her family, known as family G, was published by Warthin in 1913.[160] Warthin's colleagues Hauser and Weller[161] later extended the pedigree. The family was updated by Lynch and Krush in 1971[162] after their recognition in two kindreds of a cancer-prone syndrome that they called cancer family syndrome.[163] The syndrome was later referred to as HNPCC and more recently as Lynch syndromes I and II.[164] Family G was found to fulfill the criteria for Lynch syndrome II.[162]

Hereditary nonpolyposis colorectal cancer is inherited in an autosomal dominant pattern. Gene carriers have a very high risk for colon cancer, with an estimated lifetime penetrance of 85%. The cardinal features are *early* age of CRC onset (~44 years), *proximal* colonic predilection (~70%), and an excess of *synchronous* and *metachronous* CRC tumors (~45% 10 years after hemicolectomy or segmental resection). This is not a polyposis; patients appear to make adenomas at about the same rate as the rest of the population.

Hereditary nonpolyposis colorectal cancer is subdivided into Lynch syndrome I, in which malignancies are largely limited to the colon, and Lynch syndrome II, which shows all of the Lynch syndrome I features, but, as can be observed in Figures 5-11 and 5-12, has in addition an increased frequency of carcinoma of the endometrium,[165] transitional cell carcinoma of the ureter and renal pelvis,[92] and adenocarcinomas of the stomach,[32,166] small bowel,[167] ovary,[168] pancreas,[90] and biliary tract.[169] The subject of extracolonic cancers in the Lynch syndromes has been reviewed.[33]

Muir-Torre Syndrome

Muir-Torre syndrome and its initial association with Lynch syndrome II was first described by Lynch and colleagues.[170,171] The syndrome is characterized by cutaneous findings inclusive of multiple sebaceous adenomas, sebaceous carcinomas, and keratoacanthomas in association with visceral cancers, particularly those of the colon and endometrium. Other cancers have included transitional cell carcinoma of the ureter, renal pelvis, small bowel, stomach, and pancreas, malignant lesions that associate strongly with Lynch syndrome II. The prognosis of such patients in the original report by Muir and coworkers[172] and Torre[173] was highly favorable. This has been subsequently verified in Muir-Torre syndrome variants of Lynch syndrome II[170,171] and in a large series of Lynch syndrome patients seen throughout the world.[165]

Hall and associates[174] have described a five-generation family with at least two members manifesting the Muir-Torre phenotype. Many additional family members showed tumors consistent with Lynch syndrome II, including tumors of the gastrointestinal, gynecologic, and urological systems. Several of the affected subjects had multiple primary cancers. In addition, the prognosis appeared to be better than that found in the general population of cancer patients.

Differential Diagnosis

When considering a diagnosis of HNPCC, it is important to exclude FAP, HFAS, the hamartomatous polyposis syndromes (Peutz-Jeghers syndrome, familial juvenile polyposis syndrome), familial aggregations of CRC without criteria sufficient for hereditary CRC, the hereditary discrete polyp carcinoma problem, and familial chronic ulcerative colitis.[165,175] The distinction between FAP and HNPCC is usually easy, given the abundance of adenomas in the former and their paucity in the latter. However, the attenuated variant of FAP, which we have termed HFAS, may have very few adenomas. In these cases,

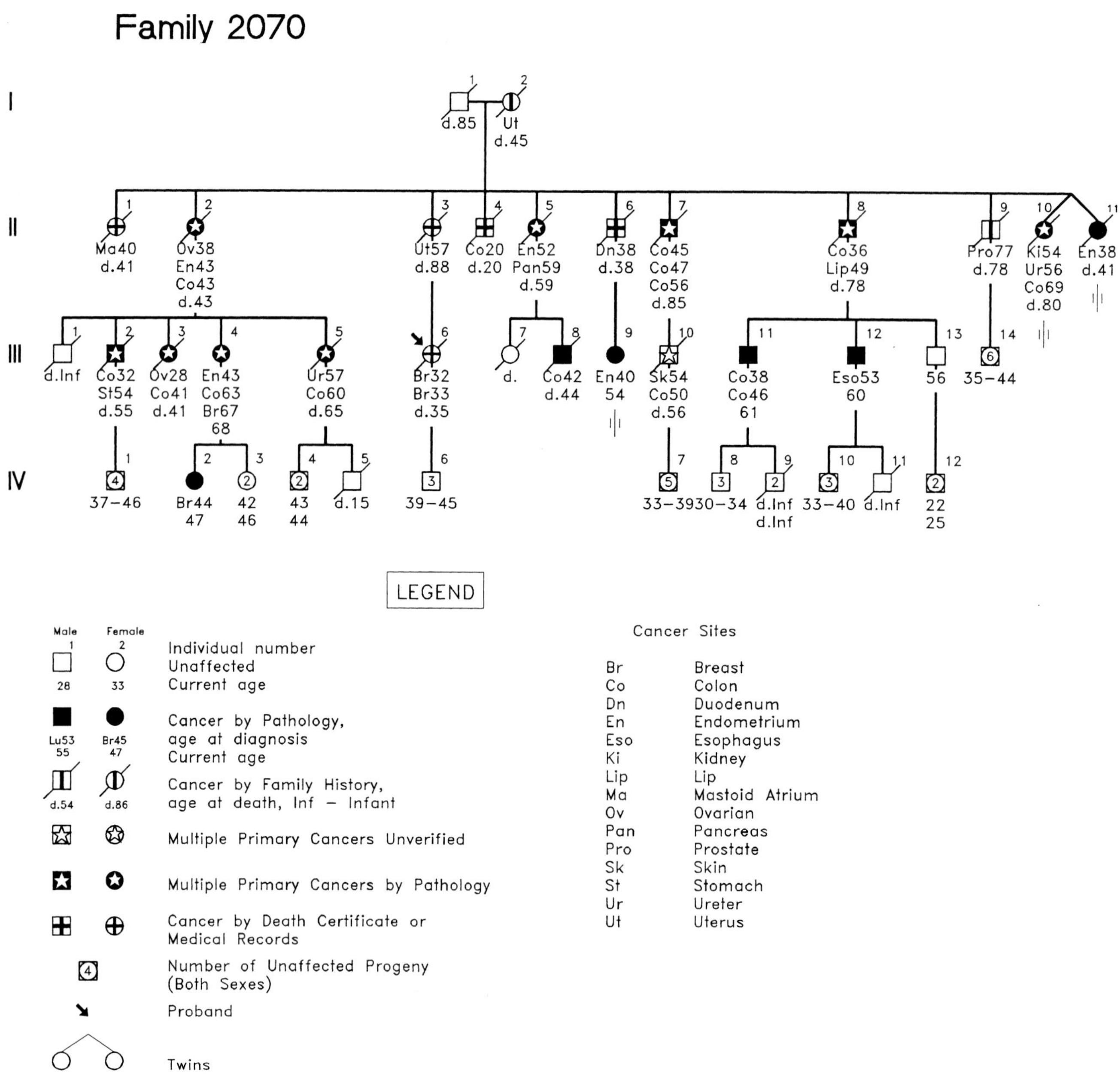

FIG. 5-11. Pedigree of a large Lynch syndrome II family illustrating extracolonic cancers, including ovarian, endometrial, and urologic tumors.

the presence of upper gastrointestinal lesions may be helpful because fundic gland polyps are a prominent feature of HFAS and are not seen in HNPCC. Periampullary adenomas and carcinomas may also occur in HFAS and are not typically a feature of HNPCC. The hamartomatous polyposes have distinctive pathologic features that should allow differentiation from HNPCC. The perennial problem of familial versus hereditary CRC will no doubt become less of a problem with advances in molecular biology.

The genetic basis for HNPCC has been proven by genetic linkage between cancer occurrences and chromosome 2p in some families and 3p in other families.[176,177] Mutations on either one of these two chromosomes account for 90% of all known HNPCC families. The defective genes appear to act by interfering with the cell's ability to repair DNA replication errors, so that mutations accumulate in very high numbers. The heavy mutational load was first suggested by the observation that most HNPCC and some sporadic CRCs showed variation in the electrophoretic mobility of $(CA)_n$ dinucleotide repeat fragments, a phenomenon described as microsatellite instability.[176,178–180] Parsons and colleagues[181] studied two CRC cell lines, one with microsatellite instability and one without it. The mutation rate of $(CA)_n$ repeats in the former was 100 times that of the latter. The unstable cells showed a defect in strand-specific mismatch repair that may have caused the high mutation rates. The repair defect affected an early step in the repair pathway. No defect in mismatch repair was observed in lymphoblastoid cells from an HNPCC family member with an unstable

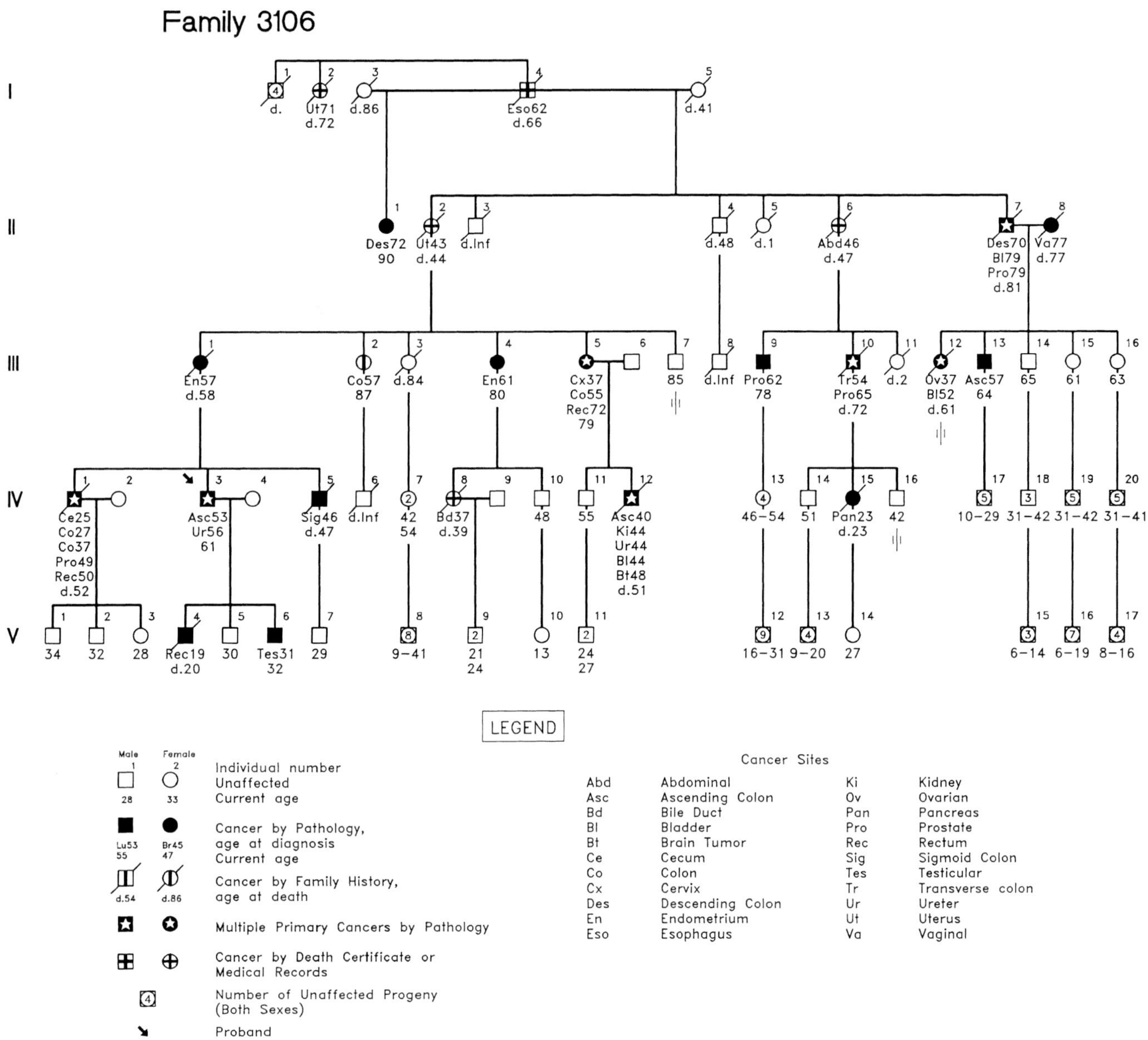

FIG. 5-12. Pedigree of an extended Lynch syndrome II family. Note the occurrence of pancreatic cancer at age 23 years in patient IV-15 and the multiple primary colonic cancers in patient IV-1.

tumor. The authors concluded that "a true mutator phenotype exists in a subset of tumor cells, the responsible defect is likely to cause transitions and transversions in addition to microsatellite alterations, and a biochemical basis for this phenotype has been identified."

The circle was completed with the localization of a DNA mismatch repair gene in the critical region of chromosome 2p by Leach and coworkers[182] and Fishel and colleagues[183] and the discovery of mutations in this gene in several HNPCC families. Subsequently, a second mismatch repair gene was found in the critical region of 3p, and mutations of that gene were found in the HNPCC families previously linked to chromosome 3p.[184,185]

The microsatellite instability that results from mutations in mismatch repair genes is referred to as replication error (RER +). Aaltonen and colleagues[178] found the RER + phenotype in 77% (10 of 13) of CRCs from HNPCC-affected patients, whereas 13% (6 of 46) of sporadic colon cancers were RER + . The RER + phenotype is not limited to colon cancer. Risinger and coworkers[186] studied endometrial carcinomas from Lynch syndrome II patients and compared them to sporadic occurrences of endometrial carcinoma. Microsatellite instability was found in 17% of sporadic endometrial carcinomas and in 75% of endometrial carcinomas from the Lynch syndrome II kindreds. It was therefore concluded that the HNPCC gene "is also involved in heritable and somatic forms of endometrial carcinoma."

A study of the incidence of microsatellite instability in more than 500 sporadic tumors of six differing types revealed the RER phenotype in 16.5% of 243 CRCs, 18% of 33 gastric carcinomas, and 22% of 18 endometrial carcinomas.[176,187] In contrast, no evidence of the RER phenotype was detected in cancers of the lung (N = 85), breast (N = 84), and testis (N = 86). The first three cancers are characteristic of the Lynch syndrome, whereas the latter three are not. These authors suggested that the cancers belonging to the Lynch syndrome tumor spectrum may have essential pathogenetic steps in common, including a tendency to multiple replication errors.

From the first descriptions of microsatellite instability, it has been apparent that sporadic RER + colon cancers are different from RER − tumors. Ionov and colleagues,[180] Thibodeau and associates,[179] Aaltonen and colleagues,[178] and Lothe and coworkers[187] all reported that RER + colon cancer were most often seen in the proximal colon. Poor histologic differentiation was also a consistent feature, as was, paradoxically, DNA diploidy. Kim and associates[188] confirmed the similarity between sporadic RER + colon cancers and the reported features of HNPCC with their prospective series of 137 cases of sporadic CRC stage II and III (Dukes' B and C). The 18 (13%) RER + cancers in the series were more likely to show right-sided location, exophytic growth pattern, large size, tendency for poorly differentiated histologic patterns, formation of extracellular mucins, and peritumoral Crohn's-like lymphoid reaction.

Hereditary nonpolyposis colorectal cancer is caused by an inherited germline mutation in DNA mismatch repair genes. Affected people are heterozygous for the defective gene and have normal repair activity, but cells at certain sites (proximal colon, endometrium, and so forth) are prone to acquire a mutation in the second allele, resulting in a "mutator phenotype." These cells accumulate mutations at a rate 100- to 1000-fold that of normal cells. In this setting, it is not surprising that malignancy eventually develops. One of the most interesting questions facing investigators is why the cancers of HNPCC are organ restricted. Certainly there are other organs (notably skin and lung) that are exposed to carcinogens that ought to be able to induce the mutator phenotype in cells heterozygous for defective mismatch repair. Yet lung cancers are unusual in HNPCC. Why? The answer will undoubtedly tell us much about carcinogenesis.

Finally, two *new* mutations have been identified in HNPCC, one at chromosome 2p (*PMS1*) and the second at chromosome 7 (*PMS2*).[189] These genes also play a role in DNA mismatch repair.

Management

As in all forms of hereditary cancer, genetic counseling is crucial to the management of the Lynch syndromes. We begin this counseling in the middle to late teenage years, depending on the patient's maturity. Because of the proximal predominance of colon cancer, we recommend that colonoscopy be initiated at age 25 years and that it be repeated every other year through age 35 years, and then annually thereafter. However, those people who show linkage to chromosome 2p or 3p should begin colonoscopy at age 20 years, to be repeated annually. In the case of women in kindreds with Lynch syndrome II, we recommend that they undergo endometrial aspiration biopsy and transvaginal ovarian ultrasound, Doppler color blood flow imagery of the ovaries, and CA 125 testing, beginning at age 25 years and repeated annually thereafter. The limitations of this screening must be emphasized to the patient.

Once CRC develops in a patient, we recommend subtotal colectomy because of the high risk for synchronous and metachronous CRCs. Women who present with CRC in Lynch syndrome II families, and who have completed their families, should be candidates for prophylactic total abdominal hysterectomy and bilateral salpingo-oophorectomy, to be performed at the time of their subtotal colectomy.

Finally, we recommend that patients with proven evidence of the germline mutation at 2p (*MSH2*) or 3p (*MLH1*) be given the option of prophylactic subtotal colectomy.

Genetic Counseling

The following description of our strategy for genetic counseling in the Lynch syndromes will serve as a model for all forms of hereditary cancer.

As a result of gene linkage in HNPCC,[176,177] followed by cloning of the *MUTS* homolog,[182,183] it will soon be possible to provide individual patients with a highly definitive genetic risk assessment, particularly once a simple blood test for this mutation becomes available. We will be able to tell our high-risk patients whether they have inherited the deleterious cancer-prone susceptibility gene, just as in the setting of FAP.[128]

Genetic counseling and management guidelines will need to be developed for the accurate use of results from blood testing (DNA) of these mutations. To do this, we need to learn more about the clinical implications of specific mutations. For example, families with the *MSH2* or the *MLH1* mutation can be compared to those without it, to see whether rates of extracolonic cancer differ between 2p-linked and 2p-unlinked HNPCC, or between 3p-linked[177] and 3p-unlinked families. This question is important when counseling patients relevant to the potential tumor spectrum in HNPCC. Questions as to whether environmental exposures make a difference in the cancer expression might be answered. Thus, genetic counselors may ultimately be able to provide information about the *avoidance* of certain environmental factors that could give rise to cancer of specific anatomic sites in HNPCC.

There are no established guidelines for genetic counseling in HNPCC using DNA to predict the patient's cancer susceptibility status. However, there is an emerging body of literature on genetic counseling dealing with a variety of noncancer hereditary disorders, such as phenylketonuria, coronary artery disease, diabetes mellitus, and Huntington's chorea, as well as cancer-prone disorders such as the MEN syndromes and FAP, to name a few, that have proven useful to clinicians. In the case of cancer, MEN types II and III[80,190] and FAP[128] have provided excellent contemporary examples of genetic counseling using biochemical markers of cancer risk (as in the case of pentagastrin-stimulated calcitonin in the MEN types II and III syndromes), and markers at chromosome 5q (in the case of FAP).[128] This experience will undoubtedly prove advantageous for the development of guidelines for counseling patients at risk for HNPCC.

Genetic counseling for any hereditary disorder must be based on highly accurate genetic risk information. The patient must be fully informed about his or her genetic risk. However, care must be taken to avoid unduly alarming the patient. It is imperative that the patient be thoroughly educated about the natural history of the cancer phenotype in HNPCC so that he or she can appreciate why the recommended surveillance measures are necessarily so rigorous. Without this knowledge, the patient's compliance may be compromised. The success of genetic counseling in HNPCC also depends on the patient's physician being knowledgeable, compassionate, and understanding about the cancer risk and natural history of HNPCC. Unfortunately, we have counseled many patients at risk for HNPCC, only to have their physicians tell them that they were too young to enter into a colonoscopy screening program and, furthermore, that cancer is predominantly an environmental disease, therefore "not to worry."

Education of patients from HNPCC families can be provided individually or in a group of as many as 15 or 20 family members. We have conducted group educational family counseling sessions followed by individual one-on-one genetic counseling. We were able to describe in detail the natural history of HNPCC and its genetic risk for these multiple family members. We encourage questions so as to be able to evaluate the level of their understanding, and thus reinforce the impact of the educational messages. This often allows individual family members to become more relaxed, to discuss matters among themselves in the group session, and to overcome inhibitions about asking pertinent questions. Family members often find that many of the questions asked by their relatives are representative of their own concerns.

The educational value of these sessions can be enhanced by providing written descriptive material about HNPCC in advance of the counseling sessions. In developing educational materials for these patients, we have taken great pains to present the material at the level of understanding for the average patient. Our educational brochure contains a drawing of a hypothetical pedigree so that the patient can appreciate the manner in which the cancer is transmitted through an HNPCC family. It contains descriptive material relevant to the age of onset, organs involved, including the excess of proximal colonic cancer, and the rationale for our specific surveillance and management recommendations. We also provide the patient with an accurate pedigree of his or her own family, depicting his or her position in the pedigree and its risk significance. This "take-home" material can be referred to from time to time by the patient. We also make this document, as well as the patient's pedigree (highlighting his or her position and its risk significance) available to the patient's family physician and encourage the physician to refer to it occasionally during patient visits. In addition, we provide the physician with a detailed letter explaining his or her patient's cancer genetic risk, the type of information we provided the patient with respect to the natural history of cancer in the family, and our surveillance and management recommendations. We believe this is essential so there will be no surprises when the patient visits his or her physician and discusses openly the concerns about differing facets of HNPCC's natural history, genetics, and management.

Individual Counseling

Counseling on an individual basis necessitates an empathic "listening ear" on the part of the counselor. During the counseling process, the anxieties and concerns of the patient must be listened to, interpreted, and addressed. There must be ample time allowed for the patient to ask questions and not feel the pressure of time. One or more additional counseling sessions may be required before the patient fully understands and indeed accepts the implications of his or her cancer risk and the need to enter into the appropriate surveillance program.

Lerman and colleagues[191,192] and Li and Fraumeni[193] have conducted extensive research on the psychological impact of cancer risk notification and adherence to breast cancer screening. This series of studies demonstrated that notification of high breast cancer risk can produce negative psychological consequences, including anxiety, traumatic stress symptoms, and impairment in daily functioning.[191–194] Moreover, such distress can impair adherence to breast cancer screening.[191,194] More recent work focuses on psychological issues in genetic testing for cancer susceptibility.[195–197] This subject has been recently reviewed by Lynch and coworkers.[198]

Extension of Genetic Counseling to All Available High-Risk Relatives

Once the HNPCC syndrome diagnosis has been established, it should become obligatory that cancer surveillance and management recommendations, within the context of genetic counseling, be extended to *all* available first-degree relatives of HNPCC-affected subjects. Unfortunately, this is not a common practice in the usual clinical practice setting. As already mentioned, Arvanitis and colleagues[1] have shown that even in such an obvious hereditary precancer disorder as FAP, where affected people can be easily identified through proctosigmoidoscopy, 59% of the FAP patients are not identified early, and, consequently, die of metastatic CRC. Clearly, this means that the message relevant to CRC risk among members of FAP families simply is not being adequately addressed. In HNPCC, where reliable premonitory physical signs of cancer risk are lacking, the problem will admittedly be more difficult to address. Nevertheless, the solution to this problem should become within grasp once a simple blood test for hMSH2 and hMLH1 becomes available. Much of the problem of neglect in providing high-risk family members with genetic counseling relates to shortcomings in the medical education of physicians. Typically, physicians are concerned primarily with the medical problems of individual patients who are under their care. They fail to focus attention on the disease risk in their patient's immediate relatives (who may be patients of other physicians); consequently, appropriate cancer control measures are not initiated.

Another problem is a presumed ethical concern about contacting high-risk collateral relatives and how such an effort might be construed by the medical community. This type of solicitation is disconcerting, and may unjustifiably be construed as an attempt at economic gain on the part of the physician.

Other barriers to effective genetic counseling and its cancer control benefit involve a patient's fear and denial, which, in turn, may have a negative impact on compliance. There may also be socioeconomic and educational problems. Health insurance carriers may not pay for screening procedures and high-risk patients might simply forego surveillance. The patient, based on past experiences of his or her relatives, may fear that if the insurance company is aware of the increased cancer risk, his or her policy or future policies may be denied. Some patients may fear that insurance carriers' knowledge of their own cancer risk will translate into similar problems for their siblings and children, and thus they may prefer to keep this information from the insurance company and in turn not request coverage for surveillance. We have witnessed many of these problems over the years.

DISCUSSION

We have attempted to describe the salient genetic, clinical, and societal features of hereditary cancer-prone disorders involving the gastrointestinal tract. Clearly, this is only a beginning. New hereditary disorders are likely to be described in the future, given the genetic heterogeneity that exists for most forms of cancer. In addition, the relationship between genotype and the phenotypic variation of many of these disorders will one day be more fully elucidated. For example, meticulous ophthalmologic and genetic studies have shown that the CHRPE phenotype in FAP is the result of a complex interaction between pigmentation and specific mutations in the *APC* gene.[126]

The linchpin for definitive etiologic determination in hereditary cancer will be the establishment of a molecular genetic diagnosis. This is already possible for most cases of FAP and the Lynch syndromes. Given the progress underway by the National Genome Project, it is probable that molecular genetic findings will one day characterize virtually all forms of hereditary gastrointestinal tract cancers.

Identifiable markers for dominantly inherited cancer susceptibility genes, such as the *APC* gene for FAP or *MSH2* and *MLH1* for the Lynch syndromes, enable the clinician to focus on relatives of affected people, either through gene linkage studies or, when available, testing for the germline mutation. Thus, molecular genetic technology enables the identification of a cancer risk that often is 100-fold greater than that of any known environmental carcinogenetic exposure. In addition, knowledge of molecular genetic status in FAP and Lynch syndrome patients will enhance research directed toward learning how environmental exposures interact with underlying genetic susceptibility for cancer expression. For example, putative cancer-preventive measures might be tested, such as dietary manipulations for prevention of colonic polyps in FAP and colon cancer (and other integral cancers) in the Lynch syndromes in patients who bear the respective cancer-prone genotypes.

The clinical application of cancer genetics will revolutionize the diagnosis and management of gastrointestinal tract cancer, just as advances in fiberoptics and endoscopy fostered dramatic changes in the previous decade. Physicians must become knowledgeable about cancer genetics and its many clinical and molecular genetic nuances, so that they can prudently use this knowledge for patient benefit. Genetic testing must now be used in the context of *families*, and not limited to *individuals*. Knowledge that a cancer syndrome exists effects interpersonal relationships within families, and creates societal concerns, particularly with respect to employability and health and life insurance. Physicians who deal with these families must gain new insights into genetic counseling.[199]

Malpractice lawyers are rapidly grasping the legal significance of cancer genetics. A new malpractice cottage industry is now emerging, in which malpractice lawyers may successfully obtain judgments against those physicians who have failed to act on genetic information, and may have denied their patient an opportunity for cancer prevention, early diagnosis, and appropriate management.

In the future, it will be mandatory that sufficient education be provided to physicians, insurance actuarials, medical directors of insurance companies, and even politicians, so that they can become more aware of the needs of patients at high genetic risk for cancer. These authorities must be shown the potential benefit of decreased morbidity and mortality through *early* cancer diagnosis and cancer *prevention* when genetic risk knowledge is used. Research demonstrating cost benefit advantage through early detection of people who are at inordinately high genetic risk for cancer of the gastrointestinal tract is desperately needed. Such findings should be useful to third-party carriers so that life and health insurance policies can be made available to high-risk patients that will cover surveillance, as well as management such as prophylactic surgery when indicated.

ACKNOWLEDGMENTS

Supported by grants from the Council for Tobacco Research, U.S.A., Inc. (#1297E); the Nebraska State Health Department Tobacco Grant; and the American Cancer Society (#EDT-84). The authors thank Suzanne Nord for technical assistance during preparation of the manuscript.

REFERENCES

1. Arvanitis ML, Jagelman DG, Fazio VN, Lavery IC, McGannon E. Mortality in patients with familial adenomatous polyposis. Dis Colon Rectum 1990;33:639.
2. Pour P, Ghadirian P. Familial cancer of the oesophagus in Iran. Cancer 1974;33:1649.
3. Ghadirian P. Familial history of esophageal cancer. Cancer 1985;56: 2112.
4. Li JY, Ershow AG, Chen ZJ, et al. A case-control study of cancer of the esophagus and gastric cardia in Linxian. Int J Cancer 1989;43: 755.
5. Carter CL, Hu N, Wu M, Lin W-Z, Murigande C, Bonney GE. Segregation analysis of esophageal cancer in 221 high-risk Chinese families. J Natl Cancer Inst 1992;84:771.
6. Howel-Evans W, McConnel RB, Clarke CA, Shepherd PM. Carcinoma of the oesophagus with keratosis palmaris et plantaris (tylosis). QJM 1958;27:413.
7. Harper PS, Harper RMJ, Howel-Evans W. Carcinoma of the oesophagus with tylosis. QJM 1970;155:317.
8. Shine I, Allison PR. Carcinoma of the oesophagus with tylosis. Lancet 1966;1:951.
9. Marger RS, Marger D. Carcinoma of the esophagus and tylosis: a lethal genetic combination. Cancer 1993;72:17.
10. Lynch HT, Ewers D, Krush AJ, Sharp EA, Swarz MJ. Esophageal cancer in a midwestern community. Am J Gastroenterol 1971;55:437.
11. Hodgson SV, Maher ER. A practical guide to human cancer genetics. New York: Cambridge University Press, 1993.
12. Dawsey SM, Wang GQ, Weinstein WM, et al. Squamous dysplasia and early esophageal cancer in the linxian region of China: distinctive endoscopic lesions. Gastroenterology 1993;105:1333.
13. Demeester TR, Johansson KE, Franze I, et al. Indications, surgical technique and long-term functional results of colon interposition or bypass. Ann Surg 1988;208:460.
14. Barrett NR. Chronic peptic ulcer of the oesophagus and "esophagitis." Br J Surg 1950;38:175.
15. Hameeteman W, Tytgat GN, Houthoff HJ, Vandentweet JG. Barrett's esophagus: development of dysplasia and adenocarcinoma. Gastroenterology 1989;96:1249.
16. Cameron AJ, Ott BJ, Payne WS. The incidence of adenocarcinoma in columnar-lined (Barrett's) esophagus. N Engl J Med 1985;313:857.

17. Fahmy N, King JF. Barrett's esophagus: an acquired condition with genetic predisposition. Am J Gastroenteral 1993;88:1262.
18. Prior A, Whorwell PJ. Familial Barrett's esophagus? Hepatogastroenterology 1986;33:86.
19. Gelfand MD. Barrett's esophagus in sexagenarian identical twins. J Clin Gastroenterol 1983;5:251.
20. Jochem VJ, Fuerst PA, Fromkes JJ. Familial Barrett's esophagus associated with adenocarcinoma. Gastroenterology 1992;102:1400.
21. Crabb DW, Berk MA, Hall TR, Conneally PM, Biegel AA, Lehman GA. Familial gastroesophageal reflux and development of Barrett's esophagus. Ann Intern Med 1985;103:52.
22. Graham S, Lilienfeld AM. Genetic studies of gastric cancer in humans: an appraisal. Cancer 1958;11:945.
23. Videbaek A, Mosbech J. The aetiology of gastric carcinoma elucidated by a study of 302 pedigrees. Acta Med Scand 1954;149:173.
24. Macklin MR. Inheritance of cancer of stomach and large intestine in man. J Natl Cancer Inst 1960;24:551.
25. Zanghivi G, Cannizo. Familial occurrence of gastric cancer in the two year experience of a population based registry. Cancer 1990;60:2047.
26. Goren PA. Genetic interpretation of studies on cancer in twins. Annals of Eugenics 1937–1938;8:219.
27. Lee FI. Carcinoma of the gastric antrum in identical twins. Postgrad Med J 1971;47:622.
28. Mecklin JP, Nordling S, Saario I. Carcinoma of the stomach and its heredity in young patients. Scand J Gastroenterol 1988;23:307.
29. Palli D, Galli M, Caporaso NE, et al. Family history and risk of stomach cancer in Italy. Cancer Epidemiol Biomarkers Prev 1994;3:15.
30. Sokoloff B. Predisposition to cancer in the Bonaparte family. Am J Surg 1938;40:673.
31. Creagen ET, Fraumeni JF. Familial gastric cancer and immunologic abnormalities. Cancer 1973;23:1325.
32. Cristofaro G, Lynch HT, Caruso ML, et al. New phenotypic aspects in a family with Lynch syndrome II. Cancer 1987;60:51.
33. Watson P, Lynch HT. Extracolonic cancer in hereditary nonpolyposis colorectal cancer. Cancer 1993;71,3:677.
34. Iwama T, Mishima Y, Utsunomiya J. The impact of familial adenomatous polyposis on the tumorigenesis and mortality at the several organs: its rational treatment. Ann Surg 1993;217:101.
35. Offerhaus, GJA, Giardiello FM, Drush AJ, et al. The risk of upper gastrointestinal cancer in familial adenomatous polyposis. Gastroenterology 1992;102:1980.
36. Jagelman DG, DeCosse JJ, Bussey HJR, the Leeds Castle Polyposis Group. Upper gastrointestinal cancer in familial polyposis coli. Lancet 1988;1:1149.
37. Domizio P, Talbert K, Spigelman AD, Williams CB, Phillips RNS. Upper gastrointestinal pathology in familial adenomatous polyposis: results from a prospective study of 102 patients. J Clin Pathol 1990; 43:738.
38. Kinoshita Y, Tojo M, Yano T, et al. The incidence of fundic gland polyps in patients without familial adenomatous polyposis. Gastrointest Endosc 1993;39:161.
39. Tsuchikame N, Tshimaru Y, Ohshima S. Takahashi M. Three familial cases of fundic gland polyposis without polyposis coli. Virchows Arch A Pathol Anat Histopathol 1993;422:337.
40. Lynch HT, Smyrk TC, Lanspa SJ, et al. Upper gastrointestinal manifestations in families with hereditary flat adenoma syndrome. Cancer 1992;71:2709.
41. Carneiro F, David L, Seruca R, Castedo S, Nesland JM, Sobrinho-Simoes M. Hyperplastic polyposis and diffuse carcinoma of the stomach: a study of a family. Cancer 1993;72:323.
42. Correa P, Shiao Y. Phenotypic and genotypic events in gastric carcinogenesis. Cancer Res 1994;54:1941S.
43. Siurala M, Lehtola J, Ihmaki P. Atrophic gastritis and its sequelae: results of 19–23 years follow-up examinations. Scand J Gastroenterol 1974;9:441.
44. Eidelman S, Parkins RA, Rubin CE. Abdominal lymphoma presenting as malabsorption: a clinicopathologic study of nine cases in Israel and review of the literature. Medicine 1966;45:111.
45. Haber DA, Mayer RJ. Primary gastrointestinal lymphoma. Semin Oncol 1988;2:154.
46. Hayoz D, Extermann M, Odermatt BF, Pugin P, Regamey C, Knecht H. Familial primary gastric lymphoma. Gut 1993;34:136.
47. Brown JE, Christensen C. Biliary tract disease among the Navajos. JAMA 1967;202:1050.
48. Nelson BD, Porvaznik J, Benfield JR. Gallbladder disease in southwestern American Indians. Arch Surg 1971;103:41.
49. Sampliner JE, O'Connell DJ. Biliary surgery in the southwestern American Indian. Arch Surg 1968;96:1.
50. Kravetz RE. Etiology of biliary tract disease in southwestern American Indians. Gastroenterology 1964;46:393.
51. Reichenbach DD. Autopsy incidence of diseases among southwestern American Indians. Arch Pathol 1967;84:81.
52. Morris DL, Buechley RW, Key CR, Morgan MV. Gallbladder disease and gallbladder cancer among American Indians in tricultural New Mexico. Cancer 1978;42:2472.
53. Garber JE, Shipley W. Carcinoma of the gallbladder in three members of a family. Cancer Genet Cytogenet 1989;39:141.
54. Trajber HJ, Szego T, DeCamargo AHS Jr, Mester M, Marujo WC, Roll S. Adenocarcinoma of the gallbladder in two siblings. Cancer 1982;50:1200.
55. Devor EJ, Buechley RW. Gallbladder cancer in Hispanic New Mexicans: II. familial occurrence in two northern New Mexico kindreds. Cancer Genet Cytogenet 1979;1:139.
56. Wada K, Tanada M, Yamaguchi K, Wada K. Carcinoma and polyps of the gallbladder associated with Peutz-Jeghers syndrome. Dig Dis Sci 1987;32:943.
57. Walsh N, Qizilbash A, Banersef R, Waugh GA. Biliary neoplasia in Gardner's syndrome. Arch Pathol Lab Med 1987;111:76.
58. Diehl AK. Epidemiology of gallbladder cancer: a synthesis of recent data. J Natl Cancer Inst 1980;65:522.
59. Lowenfels AB, Lindstrom CG, Conway MJ, Hastings PR. Gallstones and risk of gallbladder cancer. J Natl Cancer Inst 1985;75:77.
60. Joffe N, Antonioli DA. Primary carcinoma of the gallbladder associated with chronic inflammatory bowel disease. Clin Radiol 1981;32: 319.
61. Li FP, Thurber WA, Seddon J, Holmes GE. Hepatoblastoma in families with polyposis coli. JAMA 1987;257:2475.
62. Hartley AL, Birch JM, Kelsey AM, et al. Epidemiological and familial aspects of hepatoblastoma. Med Pediatr Oncol 1990a_:103.
63. Boss LP, Bender TR, Schreeder MT, Lanier AP, Harrison HH, Maynard JE. Hepatitis B testing in the families and villages of five young Eskimos with primary hepatocellular carcinoma. Am J Epidemiol 1981;114:95.
64. Gerin JL. Hepatitis B virus and primary hepatocellular carcinoma. Gastroenterology 1983;84:869.
65. Kaplan L, Cole SL. Fraternal primary hepatocellular carcinoma in three male siblings. Cancer 1968;22:142.
66. Hagstrom RM, Baker TD. Primary hepatocellular carcinoma in three male siblings. Cancer 1968;22;142.
67. Denison EK, Peters RL, Reynolds TB. Familial hepatoma with hepatitis-associated antigen. Ann Intern Med 1971;74:391.
68. Gilmore IT, Harrison JM, Parkins RA. Clustering of hepatitis B virus infection and hepatocellular carcinoma in a family. J R Soc Med 1981; 74:843.
69. Lynch HT, Srivatanskul P, Phornthutkul K, Lynch JF. Familial hepatocellular carcinoma in an endemic area of Thailand. Cancer Genet Cytogenet 1984;11:11.
70. Chang MH, Hsu HC, Lee CY, Chen DS, Lee CH, Lin KS. Fraternal hepatocellular carcinoma in young children in two families. Cancer 1984;53:1807.
71. Shen FM, Lee MK, Gong HM, Cai XQ, King MC. Complex segregation analysis of primary hepatocellular carcinoma in Chinese families: interaction of inherited susceptibility and hepatitis B viral infection. Am J Hum Genet 1991;49:88.
72. Mulvihill JJ, Ridolfi RL, Schultz FR, Borzy MS, Haughton PB. Hepatic adenoma in Fanconi anaemia treated with oxymethalone. Journal of Pediatrics 1975;87:122.
73. Lynch HT, Smyrk T, Watson P, et al. Hereditary colorectal cancer. Semin Oncol 1991;18:337.
74. Jagelman DG. Extracolonic manifestations of familial polyposis coli. Cancer Genet Cytogenet 1987;27:319.
75. Roth M-P, Petersen GM, McElree C, Vadheim CM, Panish JF, Rotter JI. Familial empiric risk estimates of inflammatory bowel disease in Ashkenazi Jews. Gastroenterology 1989;96:1016.
76. Holmes GKT, Dunn GI, Cocel R, Brookes VC. Adenocarcinoma of

the upper small bowel complicating coeliac disease. Gut 1980;21: 1010.
77. Carney JR, Vay L, Go W, et al. The syndrome of gastric argyrophil carcinoid tumors and nonantral gastric atrophy. Ann Intern Med 1983; 99:761.
78. Rindi G, Luinetti O, Cornaggia M, Capella C, Solcia E. Three subtypes of gastric argyrophil carcinoid and the gastric neuroendocrine carcinoma: a clinicopathologic study. Gastroenterology 1993;104:944.
79. Thomas RM, Baybick JH, Elsayed AM, Sobin LH. Gastric carcinoids: an immunohistochemical and clinicopathologic study of 104 patients. Cancer 1994;73:2053.
80. Anderson RJ, Lynch HT. Familial risk for neuroendocrine tumors. Curr Opin Oncol 1993;5:75.
81. Solcia E, Capella C, Fiocca R, Rindi G, Rosai J. Gastric argyrophil carcinoidosis in patients with Zollinger-Ellison syndrome due to type 1 multiple endocrine neoplasia: a newly recognized association. Am J Surg Pathol 1990;14:503.
82. Miller RR, Sumner HW. Argyrophilic cell hyperplasia and an atypical carcinoid tumor in chronic ulcerative colitis. Cancer 1982;50:2920.
83. Brown GA, Kollin J, Rajan PH. The coexistence of carcinoid tumor and Crohn's disease. J Clin Gastroenterol 1986;8:286.
84. Gardiner GW, Van Patter T, Murray D. Atypical carcinoid tumor of the small bowel complicating celiac disease. Cancer 1985;56:2715.
85. Schimke RN. Tumours of the neural crest system. In: Mulvihill JJ, Miller RW, Fraumeni JF, eds. The genetics of human cancer. Progress in cancer research and therapy series, vol 3. New York: Raven Press, 1977:170.
86. Miller AB. Epidemiology of gastrointestinal cancer. Compr Ther 1981;7:53.
87. Ghadirian P, Boyle P, Simard A, Baillargeon J. Reported family aggregation of pancreatic cancer within a population-based case-control study in the Francophone community in Montreal, Canada. Int J Pancreatol 1991;10:183.
88. Falk RT, William S, Pickle L, Fontham ET, Correa PT, Fraumeni JF. Lifestyle risk factors for pancreatic cancer in Louisiana: a case-control study. Am J Epidemiol 1988;128:324.
89. Ehrenthal D, Haeger L, Griffin T, Compton C. Familial pancreatic adenocarcinoma in three generations: a case report and a review of the literature. Cancer 1987;59:1661.
90. Lynch HT, Voorhees GJ, Lanspa SJ, McGreevy PS, Lynch JF. Pancreatic carcinoma and hereditary nonpolyposis colorectal cancer: a family study. Br J Cancer 1985;52:271.
91. Lynch HT, Boman BM, Lanspa SJ, Smyrk T, Lynch JF. Heritage of colonic polyps. In: Herrera L, ed. Familial adenomatous polyposis. New York: AR Liss 1991:9.
92. Lynch HT, Ens JA, Lynch JF. Lynch syndrome II and urologic manifestations. J Urol 1990;143:24.
93. Boring CC, Squires TS, Tong T, Montgomery S. Cancer statistics, 1994. CA Cancer J Clin 1994;44:7.
94. Auerbach O, Garfinkel L. Histologic changes in pancreas in relation to smoking and coffee-drinking habits. Dig Dis Sci 1986;31:1014.
95. Durbec JP, Chevillotte C, Bidart JM, Berthezene P, Sarles H. Diet, alcohol, tobacco, and risk of cancer of the pancreas: a case-control study. Br J Cancer 1983;43:463.
96. Macmahon B, Yen S, Trichopoulos D, Warren K, Hardi G. Coffee and cancer of the pancreas. N Engl J Med 1981;304:630.
97. Clavel F, Benhamou E, Auquier A, Tarayre M, Flamant R. Coffee, alcohol, smoking and cancer of the pancreas: a case control study. Int J Cancer 1989;43:17.
98. Castleman B. Case 25, case records of the Massachusetts General Hospital. N Engl J Med 1972;286:1353.
99. Davidson P, Costanza D, Swieconek JA, Harris JB. Hereditary pancreatitis: a kindred without gross aminoaciduria. Ann Intern Med 1968; 68:88.
100. Pipeleers-Marichal M, Somers G, Willems G, Foulis A, Imrie C, Bishop AE. Gastrinomas in the duodenum of patients with multiple endocrine neoplasia type 1 and the Zollinger-Ellison syndrome. N Engl J Med 1990;322:723.
101. Lynch HT, Kimberling W, Albano W, et al. Hereditary nonpolyposis colorectal cancer (Lynch syndromes I and II): parts I and II. Cancer 1985;56:934.
102. Lynch HT, Follett K, Shonka M, et al. Familial colon cancer in two high risk Nebraska counties. In: Magee PN, ed. Proceedings of the American Association for Cancer Research and American Society of Clinical Oncology. Baltimore, MD: Waverly Press, Inc, 1980:34.
103. Fitzgibbons RJ Jr, Lynch HT, Stanislav GV, et al. Recognition and treatment of patients with hereditary nonpolyposis colon cancer (Lynch syndromes I and II). Ann Surg 1987;206:289.
104. Fill WL, Lamiell JM, Polk NO. The radiographic manifestations of Von Hippel-Lindau disease. Radiology 1979;133:289.
105. Lynch HT, Fusaro RM. Pancreatic cancer and the familial atypical multiple mole melanoma (FAMMM) syndrome. Pancreas 1991;6:127.
106. Bergman W, Watson P, DeJong J, et al. Systemic cancer and the FAMMM syndrome. Br J Cancer 1990;61:932.
107. Swift M, Sholman L, Perry M, Chase C. Malignant neoplasms in the families of patients with ataxia telangiectasia. Cancer Res 1976;36: 209.
108. Burke W, Bennett RL, Schmidt R, Dellinger P, Evans JP. Autosomal dominant transmission of pancreatic cancer with diabetes and exocrine insufficiency in a large kindred [abstract]. Am J Hum Genet 1992; 51:A50.
109. Burt RW, Bishop DT, Cannon LA, Dowdle MA, Lee RE, Skolnick MH. Dominant inheritance of adenomatous colonic polyps and colorectal cancer. N Engl J Med 1985;312:1540.
110. Cannon-Albright AL, Skolnick MH, Bishop DT, Lee RS, Burt RW. Common inheritance of susceptibility to colonic adenomatous polyps and associated colorectal cancers. N Engl J Med 1988;319:533.
111. Herrera L, Kakati S, Gibas L, Pietrizak E, Sandberg AA. Gardner syndrome in a man with interstitial deletion of 5q. Am J Med Genet 1986;25:473.
112. Leppert M, Dobbs M, Scambler P, et al. The gene for familial polyposis coli maps to the long arm of chromosome 5. Science 1987;238: 1411.
113. Bodmer WF, Bailey CJ, Bodmer J, et al. Localization of the gene for familial adenomatous polyposis on chromosome 5. Nature 1987;328: 614.
114. Buluow S. Familial polyposis coli. Dan Med Bull 1987;34:1.
115. Sklifasowski NW. Polyadenoma tractus intestinalis. Vrach 1881;4: 55.
116. Cripps WH. Two cases of disseminated polyps of the rectum. Transactions of the Pathology Society of London 1882;33:165.
117. Smith T. Three cases of multiple polypi of the lower bowel occurring in one family. St Bartholomew's Hospital Report 1887;23:225.
118. Lockhart-Mummery P. Cancer and heredity. Lancet 1925;1::427.
119. Nakamura Y, Lathrop M, Leppert M, et al. Localization of the genetic defect in familial adenomatous polyposis within a small region of chromosome 5. Am J Hum Genet 1988;43:638.
120. Nishisho I, Nakamura Y, Miki Y, et al. Mutations on chromosome 5q21 in FAP and colorectal cancer patients. Science 1991;253:665.
121. Sondergaard J, Svendsen L, Witt I, Bulow S, Laritsen KB, Tetens G. Mandibular osteomas in the cancer family syndrome. Br J Cancer 1986;52:941.
122. Lewis RA, Crowder WE, Eierman LA, Nussbaum RL, Ferrell RE. The Gardner syndrome: significance of ocular features. Ophthalmology 1987;91:916.
123. Lyons LA, Lewis RA, Strong LC, Zuckerbrod S, Ferrell RE. A genetic study of Gardner's syndrome and congenital hypertrophy of the retinal pigment epithelium. Am J Hum Genet 1988;42:290.
124. Traboulsi EI, Krush AJ, Gardner EJ, et al. Prevalence and importance of pigmented ocular fundus lesions in Gardner's syndrome. N Engl J Med 1987;316:661.
125. Lynch HT, Priluck I, Fitzsimmons ML. Congenital hypertrophy of the retinal pigment epithelium (CHRPE) in non-Gardner's polyposis kindreds [letter]. Lancet 1987;2::333.
126. Olschwang S, Tiret A, Laurent-Puig P, Muleris M, Parc R, Thomas G. Restriction of ocular fundus lesions to a specific subgroup of APC mutations in adenomatous polyposis coli patients. Cell 1993;75:959.
127. Rodriguez-Bigas MA, Mahoney MC, Karakousis CP, Petrelli NJ. Desmoid tumors in patients with familial adenomatous polyposis. Cancer 1994;74:1270.
128. Petersen GM, Francomano C, Kinzler K, Nakamura Y. Presymptomatic direct detection of adenomatous polyposis coli (APC) gene mutations in familial adenomatous polyposis. Hum Genet 1993;91:307.
129. Turcot J, Despres J-P, St. Pierre F. Malignant tumors of the central nervous system associated with familial polyposis of the colon. Dis Colon Rectum 1959;2:465.
130. Jarvis L, Bathurst N, Mohan D, Beckly D. Turcot's syndrome: a review. Dis Colon Rectum 1988;31:907.
131. Lasser DM, DeVivo DC, Garvin J, and Wilhelmsen KC. Turcot's

syndrome: evidence for linkage to the adenomatous polyposis coli (APC) locus. Neurology 1994;44:1083.
132. Itoh H, Ohsato K. Turcot syndrome and its characteristic colonic manifestations. Dis Colon Rectum 1985;28:399.
133. Itoh H, Ohsato K, Tao T, Iida M, Watanabe H. Turcot's syndrome and its mode of inheritance. Gut 1979;20:414.
134. Lynch HT, Smyrk T, Lanspa SJ, et al. Flat adenomas in a colon cancer-prone kindred. J Natl Cancer Inst 1988;80:278.
135. Lynch HT, Smyrk TC, Watson P, et al. Hereditary flat adenoma syndrome: a variant of familial adenomatous polyposis? Dis Colon Rectum 1992;35:411.
136. Spirio L, Otterud B, Stauffer D, et al. Linkage of a variant or attenuated form of adenomatous polyposis coli to the adenomatous polyposis coli (APC) locus. Am J Hum Genet 1992;51:92.
137. Spiro L, Olschwang S, Groden J, et al. Alleles of the APC gene: an attenuated form of familial polyposis. Cell 1993;75:951.
138. Wolber RA, Owen DA. Flat adenoma of the colon. Hum Pathol 1991; 22:70.
139. Muto T, Kamiya J, Sawada T, et al. Small "flat adenoma" of the large bowel with special reference to its clinical pathologic features. Dis Colon Rectum 1985;28:847.
140. Adachi M, Muto T, Okinaga K, Morioka Y. Clinicopathologic features of the flat adenoma. Dis Colon Rectum 1991;34:981.
141. Lanspa SJ, Rouse J, Smyrk T, Watson P, Jenkins JX, Lynch HT. Epidemiologic characteristics of the flat adenoma of Muto: a prospective study. Dis Colon Rectum 1992;35:543.
142. Lynch HT, Smyrk T, Lynch J, Lanspa S, McGinn T, Cavalieri J. Genetic counseling in an extended attentuated familial adenomatous polyposis kindred. Am J Gastroenteral (in press).
143. Giardiello FM, Welso SB, Hamilton SR, et al. Increased risk of cancer in the Peutz-Jeghers syndrome. N Engl J Med 1987;316:1511.
144. Spigelman, AD, Murday V, Phillips RKS. Cancer and the Peutz-Jeghers syndrome. Gut 1989;30:1588.
145. Foley TR, McGarrity TJ, Abt AB, et al. Peutz-Jeghers syndrome: a clinicopathologic survey of the "Harrisburg family" with a 49 year follow-up. Gastroenterology 1988;95:1535.
146. Shepherd NA, Bussey HJR, Jas JR. Epithelial misplacement in Peutz-Jeghers polyps: a diagnostic pitfall. Am J Surg Pathol 1987;11:743.
147. Narita T, Eto, T, Ito T. Peutz-Jeghers syndrome with adenomas and adenocarcinomas in colonic polyps. Am J Surg Pathol 1987;11:16.
148. Nugent KP, Talbot IC, Hodgson SV, Phillips RKS. Solitary juvenile polyps: not a marker for subsequent malignancy. Gastroenterology 1993;105:698.
149. Jass JR, Williams GB, Bussey HJR, Morson BC. Juvenile polyposis: a precancerous condition. Histopathology 1988;13:619.
150. Jass JR. Pathology of polyposis syndromes with special reference to juvenile polyposis. In: Utsunomiya J, Lynch HT, eds. Hereditary colorectal cancer. Tokyo: Springer-Verlag, 1990:343.
151. Murday V, Slack J. Inherited disorders associated with colorectal cancer. Cancer Surv 1989;8:139.
152. Ransohoff DF. Colon cancer in ulcerative colitis. Gastroenterology 1988;94:1089.
153. Broome U, Lindberg B, Lofberg R. Primary sclerosing cholangitis in ulcerative colitis: a risk factor for the development of dysplasia and DNA aneuploidy? Gastroenterology 1992;102:1877.
154. Collins RH, Geldman M, Fordtran JS. Colon cancer, dysplasia, and surveillance in patients with ulcerative colitis. N Engl J Med 1987; 316:1654.
155. Glotzer, DJ. The risk of cancer in Crohn's disease. Gastroenterology 1985;89:438.
156. Hamilton SR. Colorectal carcinoma in patients with Crohn's disease. Gastroenterology 1985;89:398.
157. Gillen CD, Andrews HA, Prior P, Allan RN. Crohn's disease and colorectal cancer. Gut 1994;35:651.
158. Rotter JI, Yang H. Resolving the genetics of IBD: the challenge for the 90s. Progress in Inflammatory Bowel Disease 1993;14:1.
159. Shanahan F, Duerr RH, Rotter JI, et al. Neutrophil autoantibodies in ulcerative colitis: familial aggregation and genetic heterogeneity. Gastroenterology 1992;103:456.
160. Warthin AS. Heredity with reference to carcinoma. Arch Intern Med 1913;12:546.
161. Hauser IJ, Weller CV. A further report on the cancer family of Warthin. Am J Cancer 1936;27:434.
162. Lynch HT, Krush, AJ. Cancer family "G" revisited: 1895–1970. Cancer 1971;27:1505.
163. Lynch HT, Shaw MW, Magnuson CW, Larsen AL, Krush AJ. Hereditary factors in two large midwestern kindreds. Arch Intern Med 1966; 117:206.
164. Boland Cr, Troncale FJ. Familial colonic cancer without antecedent polyposis. Ann Intern Med 1984;100:700.
165. Lynch HT, Smyrk TC, Watson P, et al. Genetics, natural history, tumor spectrum, and pathology of hereditary nonpolyposis colorectal cancer: an updated review. Gastroenterology 1993;104:1535.
166. Boland CR. Cancer family syndrome: a case report and literature review. Am J Dig Dis 1978;23:25s.
167. Lynch HT, Smyrk TC, Lynch PM, et al. Adenocarcinoma of the small bowel in Lynch syndrome II. Cancer 1989;64:2178.
168. Lynch HT, Lynch PM. Tumor variation in the cancer family syndrome: ovarian cancer. Am J Surg 1979;138:439.
169. Mecklin J-P, Jarvinen HJ, Virolainen M. The association between cholangiocarcinoma and hereditary nonpolyposis colorectal carcinoma. Cancer 1992;69(5):1112.
170. Lynch HT, Lynch PM, Pester J & Fusaro RM. The cancer family syndrome: rare cutaneous phenotypic linkage of Torre's syndrome. Arch Intern Med 1981;141:607.
171. Lynch HT, Fusaro RM, Roberts L, Voorhees GJ, Lynch JF. Muir-Torre syndrome in several members of a family with a variant of the cancer family syndrome. Br J Dermatol 1985;113:295.
172. Muir EG Bell AJ, Barlow KA. Multiple primary carcinomata of the colon, duodenum, and larynx associated with kerato-acanthomata of the face. Br J Surg 1967;54:191.
173. Torre D. Multiple sebaceous tumours. Arch Dermatol 1968;98:549.
174. Hall NR, Williams MAT, Murday VA, Newton JA, Bishop DT. Muir-Torre syndrome: a variant of the cancer family syndrome. M Med Genet 1994;31:627.
175. Lynch HT, Watson P, Kriegler M, et al. Differential diagnosis of hereditary nonpolyposis colorectal cancer (Lynch syndrome I and Lynch syndrome II). Dis Colon Rectum 1988;31:372.
176. Peltomäki P, Aaltonen L, Sistonen P, et al. Genetic mapping of a locus predisposing to human colorectal cancer. Science 1993;260:810.
177. Lindblom A, Tannergard P, Werelius B, Nordenskjold M. Genetic mapping of a second locus predisposing to hereditary nonpolyposis colorectal cancer. Nature Genet 1993;5:279.
178. Aaltonen LA, Peltomäki P, Leach FS, et al. Clues to the pathogenesis of familial colorectal cancer. Science 1993;260:812.
179. Thibodeau SN, Bren G, Schaid D. Microsatellite instability in cancer of the proximal colon. Science 1993;260:816.
180. Ionov YM, Peinado A, Malkhosyan S, Shibata D, Perucho M. Ubiquitous somatic mutations in simple repeated sequences reveal a new mechanism for colonic carcinogenesis. Nature 1993;363:558.
181. Parsons R, Li G-M, Longley MJ, et al. Hypermutability and mismatch repair deficiency in RER + tumor cells. Cell 1993;75:1227.
182. Leach FS, Nicolaides NC, Papadopoulos N, et al. Mutations of a MutS homolog in hereditary non-polyposis colorectal cancer. Cell 1993;75: 1215.
183. Fishel R, Lescoe MK, Rao MRS, et al. The human mutator gene homolog MSH2 and its association with hereditary nonpolyposis colon cancer. Cell 1993;75:1027.
184. Papadopoulos N, Nicolaides NC, Wei Y-F, et al. Mutation of a mulL homolog in hereditary colon cancer. Science 1994;262:1625.
185. Bonner CE, Baker SM, Morrison PT, et al. Mutation in the DNA mismatch repair gene homologue hMLH1 is associated with hereditary non-polyposis colon cancer. Nature 1994;368:258.
186. Risinger JI, Berchuck A, Kohler MF, Watson P, Lynch HT, Boyd J. Genetic instability of microsatellites in endometrial carcinoma. Cancer Res 1993;53:5100.
187. Lothe RA, Peltomaki P, Meling GI, et al. Genomic instability in colorectal cancer: relationship to clinicopathological variables and family history. Cancer Res 1993;53:5849.
188. Kim, H, Jen J, Vogelstein B, Hamilton SR. Clinical and pathological characteristics of sporadic colorectal carcinomas with DNA replication errors in microsatellite sequences. Am J Pathol 1994;145:148.
189. Nicholaides NC, Papdopoulos N, Liu B, et al. Mutations of two PMS homologues in hereditary nonpolyposis colon cancer. Nature 1994; 371:75.
190. Chi DD, Toshima K, Donis-Keller H, Wells SA Jr. Predictive testing for multiple endocrine neoplasia type 2A (MEN 2A) based on the

detection of mutations in the RET protooncogene. Surgery 1994;116:124.
191. Lerman C, Daly M, Sands C, et al. Mammography adherence and psychological distress among women at risk for breast cancer. J Natl Cancer Inst 1993;85:1074.
192. Lerman C, Rimer B, Engstrom P. Cancer risk notification: psychological and ethical implications. J Clin Oncol 1991;9:1275.
193. Li FO, Fraumeni JF Jr. Predictive testing for inherited mutations in cancer-susceptibility genes. J Clin Oncol 1992;10:1203.
194. Lerman C, Rimer BK, Trock B, Balshem A, Engstrom PF. Factors associated with repeat adherence to breast cancer screening. Prev Med 1990;19:279.
195. Lerman C, Croyle R. Psychological issues in genetic testing for breast cancer susceptibility. Arch Intern Med 1994;154(6):609.
196. Croyle RT, Lerman C. Interest in genetic testing and colon cancer susceptibility: cognitive and emotional correlates. Prev Med 1993;22:284.
197. Daly M, Lerman C. Ovarian cancer risk counseling. Semin Oncol 1993;7:27.
198. Lynch HT, Lynch J, Conway T, Severin M. Psychological aspects of monitoring high risk women for breast cancer. Cancer 1994;74:1184.
199. Lynch HT, Watson P, Conway TA, et al. DNA screening for breast/ovarian cancer susceptibility based on linked markers. Arch Intern Med 1993;153:1979.

Surgery for Gastrointestinal Cancer: A Multidisciplinary Approach, edited by Harold J. Wanebo.
Lippincott-Raven Publishers, Philadelphia, © 1997.

CHAPTER 6

Monitoring After Resection of Upper and Lower Gastrointestinal Cancer

Paul H. Sugarbaker

The therapeutic effects of a cancer follow-up program depend on the postponement of serious morbidity or death as a result of this practice. Any adverse effects to the patient that the program avoids should be credited to the follow-up regimen. The therapeutic effects of a beneficial program depend on the advancement in time of diagnosis for this patient population, compared to patients managed by symptoms alone. If there are no earlier diagnoses, then the diagnostic activities constitute a liability. Additional tests and procedures are expensive and always carry some risk. Therefore, a reduction in morbidity or mortality brought about by the follow-up program must outweigh the costs and adverse effects of a program that results in earlier detection from patients' symptoms alone.

EVALUATION OF FOLLOW-UP

The success of the follow-up program depends on three variables: disease prevalence in the follow-up population, the characteristics of the screening procedures (their sensitivity and specificity), and the effectiveness of methods of treating the disease. The longer the preclinical phase, the earlier the diagnosis of additional disease, and the greater the likelihood of success of subsequent treatment, the more likely that follow-up will postpone death. The higher the sensitivity of the tests available (number of positive tests divided by number of patients with a disease), the greater the proportion of patients that may benefit. The greater the specificity (the number of patients without a positive test divided by the number of patients who do not have a disease process), the less likely that unnecessary risk will be incurred. The reliability of the follow-up plan reflects the ability of a series of tests to be consistent and give the same result time after time.

An important component of an effective follow-up plan is the difference in lead times. This means the difference between the times of diagnosis of recurrent disease in the intensively followed group and in a group that may be instructed concerning symptoms of recurrent disease but that is not subjected to a specific follow-up plan. Lead time is an estimate of the effectiveness of the follow-up program. The measure of the efficacy of follow-up would be demonstrated by a decreased mortality in the group subjected to a surveillance program compared to a group of patients left unfollowed. For follow-up programs to be successful, there must be a decrease in the overall morbidity and mortality of the targeted group.

The effectiveness of follow-up in terms of morbidity, mortality, and cost deserves special attention as the value of this component of health care is examined. Although patient reassurance is an accepted benefit, it is not enough to merit sustaining this expensive tradition in oncology. The lead time must substantially improve the outcome of the followed population. Because so few benefit from early detection and treatment of recurrent disease, this alone may not constitute sufficient value to recommend special follow-up. In addition to early detection and treatment of recurrent disease, surveillance for second primary colon cancers plus other malignancies, as well as general health maintenance may produce sufficient benefits to recommend continuing a balanced follow-up program for patients who undergo potentially curative (radical) resection of gastrointestinal malignancy.

COMPONENTS OF A FOLLOW-UP PROGRAM

An important question that must be answered before discussion about follow-up can proceed is, "Why perform follow-up in patients after a potentially curative resection of gastrointestinal cancer?" As listed in Table 6-1, several important concerns must be addressed for this diverse group of patients. Perhaps most important, surveillance for a second primary cancer must be pursued. This is crucial in colorectal cancer and early gastric cancer when a major portion of the cancer-prone organ remains in the patient after resection. For colorectal cancer, this can be performed through serial colonoscopic examination, through double-contrast barium enema examination, or through the staggered use of both examinations.

Director, Surgical Oncology, Washington Hospital Center, The Cancer Institute, 110 Irving Street, NW, Washington, DC 20010-2975

TABLE 6-1. *Components of follow-up programs after resection of gastrointestinal cancer*

A. Surveillance for second primary cancers in the gastrointestinal tract
B. Timely detection of recurrent disease combined with curative or palliative treatment
C. Health maintenance
D. Evaluation of the results of treatment

Second, timely detection of recurrent cancer combined with curative or palliative treatments should be instituted. Usually, this means additional surgery for these patients, but other treatments such as systemic chemotherapy, hepatic artery chemotherapy, or radiation therapy may be appropriate.

Health maintenance is a crucial part of the follow-up program. Treatment of chronic disease other than the gastrointestinal cancer in this patient population is mandatory as part of follow-up. There must be screening for other malignancies. Women who survive a colorectal cancer have two to three time the incidence of breast cancer as does the normal population. They also have a higher incidence of endometrial malignancy.[1] Men should be screened appropriately for prostate cancer. In this aged population, blood pressure monitoring, counseling regarding diet and nutrition, weight reduction, cigarette smoking, and other health maintenance activities are essential for a complete follow-up program. Also, time should be spent with the patients educating and reminding them as to the symptoms of recurrent gastrointestinal cancer. If possible, the patient and his or her family should participate in their own detection of recurrent disease.

Finally, follow-up allows an evaluation of the results of treatments. This may not be helpful to the patient in the short term, but it is in the best interest of a patient population over a long time period, as improvements in treatment are realized and feedback regarding methods of treatment and their quality-of-life considerations become possible. For the caregiver, evaluation of the results of treatment is a crucial aspect in oncology and must be pursued with diligence.

In our evaluation of follow-up programs for gastrointestinal cancer, three aspects are considered and given equal weight in assessing the value of this clinical activity. These are *surveillance* for second primary cancers in the gastrointestinal tract, *detection and treatment* of recurrent disease, and *health maintenance*.

SURVEILLANCE FOR SECOND PRIMARY COLON OR RECTAL CANCER

It has been well demonstrated that patients who survive one colon cancer are at increased risk for another large bowel cancer. Fortunately, through the use of colonoscopy or air contrast barium enema, patients who are kept polyp free are kept cancer free.[2–8] Shinya showed that regular colonoscopy after a colon cancer resection or after the removal of a malignant polyp would eliminate metachronous colon cancer in this population.[5] Patients who were not followed had a 10% incidence of additional malignancy in the bowel over a 5-year period. Few, if any oncologists would deny that surveillance for second primary gastrointestinal cancer is a necessary part of follow-up.

SELECTION OF GASTROINTESTINAL CANCER PATIENTS FOR COMPONENTS OF FOLLOW-UP

It is clear that there is a wide diversity of patients who have had a potentially curative resection for gastrointestinal cancer. Rational selection of patients for follow-up programs designed to fit a particular malignant disease will result in the most effective management. As shown in Table 6-2, not all gastrointestinal cancers have the same requirements for surveillance or for detection and treatment; however, all these groups of patients require health maintenance. Retroperitoneal and visceral sarcoma and pancreatic cancer are not usually followed in an attempt to find second primary cancers. Yet in retroperitoneal liposarcoma, surveillance may be indicated for the second primary cancers that do occur.[9]

The major differences in follow-up strategies concern detection and treatment of recurrent disease. Although surgery or regional chemotherapy may result in long-term survival in colorectal cancer, early gastric cancer, and appendix cancer and sarcoma, the natural history of most other abdominal and pelvic malignancies does not result in an isolated site of recurrent disease that can be completely surgically resected. Efforts to detect recurrent disease and to resect it will rarely be successful. Because there is such limited benefit in detection and treatment of recurrent gastric and pancreatic cancer, the major portion of this chapter on follow-up is devoted to an evaluation of follow-up of colorectal cancer patients.

TABLE 6-2. *Components of follow-up for selected gastrointestinal cancers*

	Surveillance for second primary	Detection and treatment of recurrence	Health maintenance
Large bowel	+	+	+
Early gastric	+	+	+
Retroperitoneal and visceral sarcoma	0	+	+
Gastric	+	0	+
Pancreatic	0	0	+
Appendix	0	0	+
Small bowel	0	0	+

+, indicated; 0, not indicated.

SELECTION OF COLORECTAL CANCER PATIENTS FOR INTENSIVE VERSUS RELAXED FOLLOW-UP

Much effort has been made to evaluate patients prognostically using preoperative testing to determine the precise anatomic setting of the primary cancer. Gross anatomic and histologic examination of the resected cancer specimen also provides accurate prognostic information. By the TMN classification, colorectal cancer can be separated into stages I through IV (Table 6-3). Patients with stage I cancer have approximately a 5% mortality as a result of colorectal disease, a prevalence that is unlikely to make detection and treatment of recurrent cancer worthwhile for this group of patients. Stage II patients have approximately a 30% recurrence rate, and stage III approximately a 70% recurrence rate. These two groups of patients are well suited for intensive follow-up programs to detect and further treat recurrence. Stage IV patients have known residual disease and should not be subjected to detection and treatment regimens unless these management plans are pursued within the context of a clinical trial.[10]

Patients can also be selected for follow-up on the basis of their general medical condition and fitness for additional treatment. Colorectal cancer patients who are candidates for further surgery merit intensive follow-up to detect and treat recurrent disease. The age of the patient by itself is not the crucial factor to be considered with regard to fitness for further surgical therapy. Rather, the patient's performance status and other disease states, as well as the difficulties encountered in the surgical treatment of the primary colon or rectal cancer, should be considered. Those patients who do not present a reasonable risk for further surgery should not be subjected to numerous diagnostic tests. This management plan would reveal disease requiring treatments that patients are not physically or mentally capable of receiving. Follow-up that incurs cost without benefit is to be avoided.

There are other factors in addition to the disease's histopathologic stage that can be used to identify patients at high risk for recurrence. Studies have shown that patients with an elevated postoperative carcinoembryonic antigen (CEA) blood test result were at great risk for recurrent disease.[11–17] If the postoperative baseline CEA is greater than five and there is no obvious cause for a noncancerous CEA elevation, such as cirrhosis, heavy smoking, or an inflammatory disease, patients must be considered at extremely high risk for recurrence. Also, patients who have an elevated preoperative CEA in addition to nodal positivity almost uniformly succumb to large bowel cancer. This represents a group of patients who should be considered to be at extremely high risk for recurrence.

To summarize Table 6-3, the surveillance program for second primary cancers should be pursued in all patients except those with stage IV disease. Health maintenance is required in all groups. However, only patients with stage II or III colorectal cancer who are fit for reoperative surgery should have intensive follow-up to detect and treat recurrent disease. By categorizing patients, the number that are subjected to an expensive "intensive" follow-up plan for detection and treatment is reduced. In addition, a more acceptable "relaxed" follow-up plan can be used for those patients unlikely to profit from surgery for recurrent disease.

SELECTION OF TEST TO BE USED IN FOLLOW-UP

Now that a group of patients who require an intensive follow-up plan and a group that requires a relaxed follow-up plan have been defined, what tests should be recommended for these two groups of patients?[18–38] Table 6-4 presents the menu of tests that have been used profitably in patients with large bowel cancer. Tests to be used in an intensive or a relaxed follow-up plan are indicated. In prospective clinical studies and in a consensus report, a symptom review plus physical examination combined with frequent serial tumor marker studies (CEA and cancer antigen [CA] 19-9) were recommended.[36] Laboratory tests are done as part of a health maintenance check, but liver function tests may also give some clues regarding recurrent disease in the liver or in bone. A chest radiograph may be recommended on a yearly basis to detect those few patients who may have isolated lung metastases that can be resected for long-term salvage. Unfortunately, the precise value of most of these tests has not been evaluated, so the clinician is forced to make a best guess in formulation of the optimal follow-up plan.

Other health maintenance tests such as prostate-specific antigen and digital rectal examination of the prostate are important in the man in this age group. Also, mammography and physical examination of the breast should be performed according to guidelines in women. A pelvic examination with cervical and endocervical cytology also is indicated.

Many tests listed in Table 6-4 may be indicated when the surveillance program suggests recurrent disease. Although a preoperative computed tomographic scan of the abdomen is recommended, it has not been shown to be of value in detecting recurrent disease before the patient's symptoms and serial tumor markers are manifest.[39–43] Computed tomography, when indi-

TABLE 6-3. *Indications for follow-up in patients with gastrointestinal cancer by TMN stage*

	Surveillance (all patients)	Detection and treatment: Surgically fit	Detection and treatment: Surgically unfit	Health maintenance (all patients)
Stage I	+	0	0	+
Stage II	+	+	0	+
Stage III	+	+	0	+
Stage IV	0	0	0	+

+, intensive follow-up indicated; 0, follow-up of little or no benefit.

TABLE 6-4. *Frequency of performance of indicated tests in intensive and relaxed follow-up plans*

		Intensive		Relaxed		
	Preoperative	Years 1–2	Years 3–5	Years 1–2	Years 3–5	After Year 5
Symptoms and physical examination	+	3 mo	3 mo	Yearly	Yearly	Yearly
Carcinoembryonic antigen, CA 19-9	+	3 mo	3 mo	0	0	0
Colonoscopy or contrast	+	Yearly	2 yearly	Yearly	2 yearly	3 yearly
Laboratory tests	+	Yearly	Yearly	Yearly	Yearly	Yearly
Chest radiograph	+	Yearly	Yearly	Yearly	Yearly	Yearly
*CT abdomen and pelvis	+	0	0	0	0	0
Prostate-specific antigen and rectal examination	+	2 yearly	2 yearly	2 yearly	2 yearly	2 yearly
Mammogram and breast check	+	2 yearly	2 yearly	2 yearly	2 yearly	2 yearly
Pelvic examination with cervical cytology	+	2 yearly	2 yearly	2 yearly	2 yearly	2 yearly
*CT chest	0	0	0	0	0	0
*MRI liver	0	0	0	0	0	0
*MRI pelvis	0	0	0	0	0	0
*Abdominal ultrasound	0	0	0	0	0	0
*Intrarectal ultrasound	+	0	0	0	0	0
*Oncoscint monoclonal antibody scan	0	0	0	0	0	0
*Laparoscopy	0	0	0	0	0	0
*Second look	0	0	0	0	0	0

+, indicated; 0, not indicated; CT, computed tomography; MRI, magnetic resonance imaging.
* Performed only for specific clinical indications in work up for suspect recurrent disease.

cated, should be of both abdomen and pelvis, with intravenous, oral, and intrarectal contrast. Occasionally, with a CEA rise but no obvious site of recurrent disease, the monoclonal antibody scan (Oncoscint) may be recommended. Laparoscopy and, in a few patients, second-look surgery may be necessary to diagnose the anatomic site of colorectal cancer recurrence and assess whether a surgical procedure can render the patient disease free.

BENEFITS OF INTENSIVE FOLLOW-UP PROGRAMS IN DETECTION AND TREATMENT OF RECURRENCE

The outcome of follow-up after potentially curative resection of large bowel cancer has been debated by numerous authors.[10,44–57] As discussed by August and Sugarbaker,[58] the number of patients who will benefit in the long term from early detection of recurrence and its aggressive treatment are few. One estimate is that 6% of patients will be salvaged.[58] The theoretical outcome of 100 patients with a potentially curative resection of colorectal cancer is shown in Figure 6-1. It should be obvious that the small number of patients salvaged would be difficult to detect in a controlled trial unless thousands of patients were entered and the data collection and analysis were flawless. In addition, a randomized trial of intensive follow-up with aggressive reoperation versus relaxed follow-up to show an improved survival in the two populations would be unlikely to show significant differences. When colorectal cancer recurs, the process can be expected to advance in an especially aggressive fashion. If one test is not positive, other tests or patient symptoms or signs should be expected to reveal recurrent cancer at approximately the same time. In other words, an extensive lead time for any one test, such as CEA, is unlikely to occur.

However, if all three components of a follow-up program (surveillance, detection and treatment, and health maintenance) are considered, the benefits from an expanded program seem considerably more significant. The positive effects from surveillance, detection and treatment, and health maintenance are estimated in Table 6-5, which assumes a 20% incidence of second primary malignancy in the half of the patients who survive their colorectal cancer. It also assumes 100% survival with further surgery or polypectomy to remove other large bowel tumors. This results in a salvage of 10 patients. The cost of this treatment is low because it is, for the most part, all outpatient management. Regarding detection and treatment, 50% of patients are assumed to have recurrence in this theoretic model, and approximately 30% will be candidates for reoperation. This may be resection of isolated liver metastases, resection of isolated lung metastases, resection of recurrent disease within the abdomen and pelvis, or treatment of low-volume peritoneal carcinomatosis. Of these 15 patients, approximately one third will be rendered disease free in the long term, for a total of 5 patients of the 100 salvaged by intensive follow-up and aggressive treatment of recurrent disease. Because these treatments involve sophisticated laboratory and radiologic tests, and because these patients will require approximately 30 reoperative inpatient procedures, the cost for this patient salvage is high.

Health maintenance would be used in the entire population of patients but would be operative only in those 50 patients who survive colon and rectal cancer. The incidence of another potentially fatal disease occurring is estimated to be 20% of the patients who survive. Half of these patients may be salvaged as a result of health maintenance, which constitutes a 5% salvage out of the entire group.

As can be seen in Table 6-5, approximately 20 patients of the original 100 are thought to have their lives prolonged as a direct result of the follow-up program and its three components, surveillance, detection and treatment of recurrent disease, and health maintenance. This number assumes that no single patient will be helped by more than one component of follow-up, surely a false assumption.

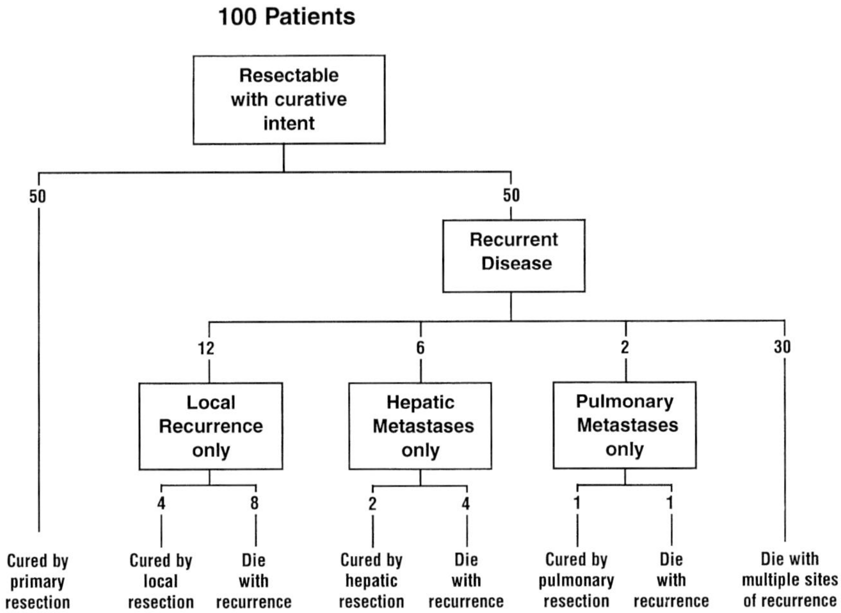

FIG. 6-1. Natural history of 100 patients treated for large bowel cancer. (From August DA, Ottow RT, Sugarbaker PH. Clinical perspective of human colorectal cancer metastasis. Cancer Metastasis Reviews 1984;3:303.

A positive effect stemming from differences in lead times has not been established by a controlled trial for the colorectal cancer patient population. Is it important to use an intensive follow-up plan with CEA testing and frequent visits to a physician to find recurrent disease at the earliest possible time? The difference in lead times is estimated to be 6 months in patients who had serial CEA blood tests and had a CEA elevation.[12,27] In these studies, approximately two thirds of the patients showed an elevation of CEA as the initial indicator of recurrent disease. The impact of CEA-detected recurrence in comparison to symptom-detected recurrence has not been determined. In all studies to date, both CEA blood tests and frequent visits to a physician were used, so it is impossible to determine the effect of one without the other.

However, intensive follow-up (which includes serial CEA assays) to detect and treat recurrent disease cannot be dismissed as unimportant in this patient population. If it is assumed that with optimized follow-up five patients live an additional 15 years as a result of this program, then 75 life-years are gained. This is assuming that the life of a colon cancer patient is increased from 60 to 85 years.[59] The cost per life-year may be estimated at $9000 (see Appendix 6-1).

LONG-TERM SURVIVAL OF PATIENTS WHO HAVE REOPERATIVE SURGERY

The salvage of approximately 30% of patients who undergo resection for isolated recurrent disease seems well established in the colorectal literature.[10] For liver metastases, lung metastases, recurrences within the abdomen and pelvis, and peritoneal carcinomatosis, a 30% long-term disease-free survival was reported with surgery and chemotherapy for recurrent disease; these data are reviewed in this volume. The prognostic features for selection of patients with liver metastases, lung metastases, locally recurrent cancer, and peritoneal carcinomatosis have also been presented. Not all patients with recurrent colorectal cancer profit from reoperative surgery, only selected ones.

It has been suggested that some surgeons are not capable of performing reoperative surgery for cancer with an acceptable morbidity and mortality.[60] A standard of practice may require the establishment of a core group of surgeons familiar with reoperative surgery and the diagnostic tests required to evaluate patients suspected of having recurrent disease. Liver resection, surgery for peritoneal carcinomatosis, and surgery for recurrent pelvic disease present difficult problems in management. They

TABLE 6-5. *Outcome of selective follow-up after potentially curative resection of large bowel cancer*

	Incidence* (%)	Salvage (%)	Patients	Costs
Surveillance	20	100	10	Low
Detection and treatment†	50	10	5‡	High
Health maintenance	20	50	5	Low
Totals	70	20	20	Acceptable

* Assumes 50% of patients have recurrence.
† Assumes the positive effect of "lead time" has been established for detection and treatment.
‡ Assumes five patients benefit from detection of recurrence and curative reoperative surgery. Each salvaged patient lives an additional 15 years (age 60–85 years), so that there is a gain of 75 life-years. The estimated cost is approximately $9,000/life-year. See Appendix 1 for details.

TABLE 6-6. *Appropriate settings for the different components of follow-up*

	Surveillance for second primary	Detection and treatment of recurrence	Health maintenance
Colorectal specialist or general surgeons's office	0	±	0
General medical physician	0	±	±
Nurse practitioner or physician's assistant	0	±	±
Endoscopy suite	+	0	0

+, indicated; ±, equivocal; 0, not indicated.

carry a high morbidity and mortality and limited patient salvage when carried out by the average general surgeon.

QUALITY CONTROL OF SURGERY FOR PRIMARY COLORECTAL CANCER

In some instances, reoperative surgery is successful because inadequate surgery was performed at the time of primary disease resection. If locally recurrent cancer can be curatively resected simply by a wider dissection of the large bowel, then inadequate prior surgery must be assumed. A reasonable expenditure of the health care dollar might be in training surgeons to perform the proper and reasonably extensive procedure with gentle handling of cancerous tissues for primary large bowel cancer.

PERSONNEL REQUIRED FOR OPTIMAL FOLLOW-UP

An important aspect of any follow-up program concerns the personnel responsible for its successful completion. Table 6-6 shows the possible locations and personnel for surveillance, detection and treatment, and health maintenance. The specialist is not well suited for completing all aspects of care unless a physician's assistant or nurse practitioner is available in the specialist's office for counseling the patient. The general practitioner's office is an ideal place for follow-up as long as this physician has been well versed in the signs and symptoms of recurrent cancer. It is assumed that this person can safely and accurately perform a straight sigmoidoscopic examination, which may be required as indicated in patients with low rectal anastomoses. The nurse practitioner or physician's assistant, if specially trained in the natural history of large bowel cancer and the signs and symptoms of recurrent disease, may see patients in follow-up. For total colonoscopy, the endoscopy suite must be used; if air contrast barium enema is used for surveillance, a radiology suite is required.

A complicating feature of this follow-up program is the need for adjuvant 5-fluorouracil chemotherapy in all patients with stage II and III colorectal cancer. For the first year, the medical oncologist must see these patients on a regular basis, and in many instances he or she may become the general practitioner who assumes continuing care for these patients. This assumes that the medical oncologist will take responsibility for all components of follow-up: surveillance for second primary disease, detection and treatment of recurrence, and health maintenance.

RATIONALE FOR MORE FREQUENT FOLLOW-UP IN POSTOPERATIVE YEARS 1 AND 2

The rationale for more frequent follow-up visits in the first 2 years after surgery comes from studies of time to recurrence for surgically treated large bowel cancer. Patients with large bowel cancer are most likely to have recurrence within the first 2 years.[61,62] Although some patients will develop recurrence in years 3 through 5 and even thereafter, they may have a less aggressive disease that is amenable to a less intensive follow-up program.

CRITERIA FOR EVALUATION OF A FOLLOW-UP PROGRAM

There are certain requirements that a follow-up program for patients with large bowel cancer must fulfill; these are itemized in Table 6-7. First, this program must optimize the patient's chance for long-term survival; however, it must not jeopardize the care that the patient receives for other cancers or other disease processes. The follow-up program must provide an acceptable cost–benefit ratio, whether this expense be to the patient, to a health maintenance organization, or an insurance company. Of course, the constraints of the follow-up plan must be acceptable to the patient, or he or she would not be expected to participate. It must also be acceptable to the physician; the colorectal specialist must not feel that he or she is deserting the patient or that the patient is being taken from his or her care. Data regarding the effectiveness of surgery, chemotherapy, and radiation therapy as treatment for primary disease must be accurately and critically accumulated. The follow-up program must reassure the patient, provide the patient with as accurate information as possible regarding colorectal cancer and health maintenance, and must provide for regular feedback from the patient to the health care provider. This means that the process must

TABLE 6-7. *Criteria for consensus development of a follow-up program in colorectal cancer*

Optimizes patient's chances for long-term survival of large bowel cancer
Acceptable cost–benefit analysis
Acceptable to the patient
Acceptable to the physician
Does little or no harm
Critically evaluates the effectiveness of treatment
Critically evaluates the patient's satisfaction with the health care system

critically evaluate itself as to the patient's concept of the effectiveness of treatment and the patient's satisfaction with the health care system.

It is unlikely that clinical trials in follow-up will be performed to guide the evolution of optimal programs. Rather, a consensus within the health care system, along with acceptance by patients, is more likely to determine the management plans that will be used.

FOLLOW-UP PROGRAMS FOR OTHER GASTROINTESTINAL CANCERS

The clinician may extrapolate from the model created for colorectal cancer to other selected gastrointestinal malignancies. Other cancers that may benefit from intensive follow-up include early and stage I gastric malignancy. In this disease process, there is a large postsurgical volume of cancer-prone epithelium remaining in the patient that requires surveillance. Also, detection and definitive treatment with subsequent total gastrectomy of recurrent disease may, in some instances, result in a surgical cure. Of course, health maintenance remains an important part of this therapy.

Patients with visceral sarcoma may have liver metastases. Early detection and liver resection salvages some of these patients. Also, patients with retroperitoneal sarcoma may often have local recurrence, especially if the initial surgeon did not pursue an extended and wide margin of resection. The lower the grade of malignancy, the more often the patient benefits by a detection and treatment program in follow-up.

Appendiceal malignancy is often a low-grade tumor characterized as pseudomyxoma peritonei. Detection of recurrent disease and definitive treatment using cytoreductive surgery and intraperitoneal chemotherapy has been of great benefit to this very small group of patients.[63,64] Patients with gastric or pancreatic cancer deserve health maintenance but do not profit from a surveillance program or a prevention and treatment follow-up strategy (see Table 6-2).

SUMMARY

Surveillance for a second primary cancer, detection and treatment of recurrent disease, and health maintenance are the essential components of follow-up in a patient population with potentially curative resection of a primary gastrointestinal cancer. The value of follow-up programs has been extensively studied in colorectal cancer. Of 100 patients with colorectal cancer in a follow-up program, approximately 20 should have prolonged life as a result of surveillance, detection and treatment, and health maintenance. Benefits may also occur with early gastric cancer and abdominal and pelvic sarcomas. In contrast, little, if any patient salvage is expected with surveillance or detection and treatment of resected stage II or III gastric cancer, pancreatic cancer, hepatoma, or cholangiocarcinoma. Detection of recurrent cancer and its treatment may be the most expensive and least effective part of the follow-up program. Lead time is minimal with intensive follow-up (including serial CEA blood tests) compared to the time of diagnosis based on symptoms of recurrent malignancy in an informed patient. Aggressive surgical management of selected patients with recurrent disease, with radiation therapy and chemotherapy when appropriate, will in the long term salvage the greatest number of patients and yield some palliative benefits. It is crucial that reoperative surgery be pursued by an experienced team familiar with this type of intervention. Comprehensive follow-up of colorectal cancer patients yields a high medical value in terms of its economic cost, and should continue to be pursued, made even more cost effective, and integrated into a complete management plan for all gastrointestinal cancers.

REFERENCES

1. Sugarbaker PH, Gundersson LL, Wittes RE. Colorectal cancer. In: DeVita VT Jr, Hellman S, Rosenberg SA, eds. Cancer: principles and practices of oncology, vol 1. 2nd ed. Philadelphia: JB Lippincott, 1985: 885.
2. Agnew CH, Cooley RN. Barium-enema study of postoperative recurrences of carcinoma of the colon. JAMA 1962;179:119.
3. Ekelund GR, Pihl B. Multiple carcinomas of the colon and rectum. Cancer 1974;33:1630.
4. Tornqvist A, Ekelund G, Leandoer L. Early diagnosis of metachronous colorectal carcinoma. Aust N Z J Surg 1981;51:442.
5. Shinya H. Neoplastic polypoid lesions. In: Shinya H, ed. Colonoscopy: diagnosis and treatment of colonic diseases. New York: Igaku-Shoin, 1982:161.
6. Buhler H, Seefeld U, Deyhle P, Buchmann P, Metzger U, Ammann R. Endoscopic follow-up after colorectal cancer surgery: early detection of local recurrences? Cancer 1984;54:791.
7. Larson GM, Bond SJ, Shallcross C, Mullins R, Polk HC. Colonoscopy after curative resection of colorectal cancer. Arch Surg 1986;121:535.
8. Chen YM, Ott DJ, Wolfman NT, Gelfand DW, Karsteadt N, Bechtold RE. Recurrent colorectal carcinoma: evaluation with barium enema examination and CT. Radiology 1987;163:307.
9. Fernandez-Trigo V, Sugarbaker PH. Sarcomas involving the abdominal and pelvic cavity. Tumori 1993;79:77.
10. American Joint Committee on Cancer. Manual for staging of cancer. 4th ed. Philadelphia: JB Lippincott, 1992.
11. McCartney WH, Hoffer PB. Carcinoembryonic antigen assay in hepatic metastases detection. JAMA 1976;236:1023.
12. Sugarbaker PH, Zamcheck N, Moore FD. Assessment of serial carcinoembryonic antigen (CEA) assay in postoperative detection of recurrent colorectal cancer. Cancer 1976;38:2310.
13. Finlay IG, McArdle CS. Role of carcinoembryonic antigen in detection of asymptomatic disseminated disease in colorectal carcinoma. Br Med J 1983;286:1242.
14. Carlsson U, Stewenius J, Ekelund G, Leandoer L, Nosslin B. Is CEA analysis of value in screening for recurrences after surgery for colorectal carcinoma? Dis Colon Rectum 1983;26:369.
15. Staab HJ, Anderer FA, Stumpf E, Hornung A, Fischer R, Kieninger G. Eighty-four potential second-look operations based on sequential carcinoembryonic antigen determinations and clinical investigations in patients with recurrent gastrointestinal cancer. Am J Surg 1985;149: 198.
16. Minton JP, Hoehn JL, Gerber DM, et al. Results of a 400-patient carcinoembryonic antigen second-look colorectal cancer study. Cancer 1985;55:1284.
17. Moertel CG, Fleming TR, Macdonald JS, Haller DG, Laurie JA, Tangen C. An evaluation of the carcinoembryonic antigen (CEA) test for monitoring patients with resected colon cancer. JAMA 1993;270: 943.
18. Ekman CA, Gustavson J, Henning A. Value of a follow-up study of recurrent carcinoma of the colon and rectum. Surg Gynecol Obstet 1977;145:895.
19. Hickey RC, Romsdahl MM, Johnson DE, et al. Recurrent cancer and metastases. World J Surg 1982;6:585.
20. Tornqvist A, Ekelund G, Leandoer L. The value of intensive follow-up after curative resection for colorectal carcinoma. Br J Surg 1982; 69:725.
21. Enker WE, Kramer RG. The follow-up of patients after definitive resections for large bowel cancer. World J Surg 1982;6:578.

22. Deveney KE, Way LW. Follow-up of patients with colorectal cancer. Am J Surg 1984;148:717.
23. Gianola FJ, Dwyer A, Jones AE, Sugarbaker PH. Prospective studies of laboratory and radiologic tests in the management of colon and rectal cancer patients: I. Dis Colon Rectum 1984;27:811.
24. Gail MH. The evaluation of serial marker measurements for monitoring patients at risk of recurrent cancer: application to colorectal cancer. In: Mastromari AJ, ed. The biology and treatment of colorectal cancer metastases. Amsterdam: Martinus Nijhoff, 1986:235.
25. Pugliese V, Aste H, Saccomanno S, Bruzzi P, Bonelli L, Santi L. Outcome of follow-up programs in patients previously resected for colorectal cancer. Tumori 1984;70:203.
26. Graffner H, Hultberg B, Johansson B, Moller T, Petersson BG. Detection of recurrent cancer of the colon and rectum. J Surg Oncol 1985; 28:156.
27. Sugarbaker PH, Gianola FJ, Dwyer A, Neuman NR. A simplified plan for follow-up of patients with colon and rectal cancer supported by prospective studies of laboratory and radiologic test results. Surgery 1987;102:79.
28. Barkin JS, Cohen ME, Flaxman M, et al. Value of a routine follow-up endoscopy program for the detection of recurrent colorectal carcinoma. Am J Gastroenterol 1988;88:1355.
29. Ovaska JT, Jarvinen HJ, Mecklin JP. The value of a follow-up program after radical surgery for colorectal carcinoma. Scand J Gastroenterol 1989;24:416.
30. Ovaska J, Jarvinen H, Kujari H, Perttila I, Mecklin JP. Follow-up of patients operated on for colorectal carcinoma. Am J Surg 1990;159: 593.
31. Fantini GA, DeCosse JJ. Surveillance strategies after resection of carcinoma of the colon and rectum. Surg Gynecol Obstet 1991;171:267.
32. Heine JA, Rothenberger DA. Cost-effective management of colon and rectal cancer. World J Surg 1991;15:597.
33. Kelly CJ, Daly JM. Colorectal cancer: principles of postoperative follow-up. Cancer 1992;70:1397.
34. Bohm B, Schwenk W, Hucke HP, Stock W. Does methodic long-term follow-up affect survival after curative resection of colorectal carcinoma? Dis Colon Rectum 1993;36:280.
35. Safi F, Link KH, Berger H. Is follow-up of colorectal cancer patients worthwhile? Dis Colon Rectum 1993;36:636.
36. Vernava AM, Longo WE, Virgo KS, Coplin MA, Wade TP, Johnson FE. Current follow-up strategies after resection of colon cancer: results of a survey of members of The American Society of Colon and Rectal Surgery. Dis Colon Rectum 1994;37:573.
37. Bruinvels DJ, Stiggelbout AM, Kievit J, van Houwelingen HC, Habbema DF, van de Velde CJH. Follow-up of patients with colorectal cancer: a meta-analysis. Ann Surg 1994;219:174.
38. Virgo KS, Wade TP, Longo WE, Coplin MA, Vernava AM, Johnson FE. Surveillance after curative colon cancer resection: practice patterns of surgical subspecialists. Ann Surg Oncol (Submitted for publication).
39. Zelas P, Haaga JR, Lavery IC, Fazio VW. The diagnosis by percutaneous biopsy with computed tomography of a recurrence of carcinoma of the rectum in the pelvis. Radiology 1980;151:525.
40. Shirkhoda A, Staab EV, Bunce LA, Herbst CA, McCartney WH. Computed tomography in recurrent or metastatic colon cancer: relation to rising serum carcinoembryonic antigen. J Comput Assist Tomogr 1984; 84:704.
41. Clark J, Bankoff M, Carter B, Smith TJ. The use of computerized tomography scan in the staging and follow-up study of carcinoma of the rectum. Surg Gynecol Obstet 1984;159:335.
42. Hollmann Von JP, Goebel N. Computertomographie (CT) und Sonographie (US) in der Rezidividiagnostik kolorektaler Tumoren. Fortschritt Rontgenstrahten 1985;143:665.
43. Krestin GP, Steinbrich W, Friedmann G. Recurrent rectal cancer: diagnosis with MR imaging versus CT. Radiology 1988;168:307.
44. Wangensteen OH. Cancer of the colon and rectum: with special reference to (1) earlier recognition of alimentary tract malignancy; (2) secondary delayed re-entry of the abdomen in patients exhibiting lymph node involvement; (3) subtotal primary excision of the colon; (4) operation in obstruction. Wis Med J 1949;48:591.
45. Bacon HE, Berkley JL. The rationale for re-resection of recurrent cancer of the colon and rectum. Dis Colon Rectum 1959;2:549.
46. Gilbertsen VA, Wangensteen OH. A summary of thirteen years' experience with the second look program. Surg Gynecol Obstet 1962;114: 438.
47. Griffen WO, Gilbertsen VA, Wangensteen OH. The second-look operation for abdominal malignancies. Monogr Natl Cancer Inst 1964;15: 267.
48. Curreri AR, Mackman S. Reoperation in carcinoma following resection and adjuvant chemotherapy. Surg Gynecol Obstet 1966;123:274.
49. Mackman S, Curreri AR, Ansfield FJ. Second-look operation for colon carcinoma after fluorouracil therapy. Arch Surg 1970;100:527.
50. Mackman S, Ansfield FJ, Ramirez G, Curreri AR. A second look at the second look operation in colonic cancer after the administration of fluorouracil. Am J Surg 1974;128:763.
51. Ellis H. Is a "second look operation" justified in suspected recurrences after abdominal cancer surgery. Br J Surg 1975;62:830.
52. Stearns MW. Diagnosis and management of recurrent pelvic malignancy following combined abdominoperineal resection. Dis Colon Rectum 1980;23:359.
53. Vassilopoulos PP, Yoon JM, Ledesma EJ, Mittelman A. Treatment of recurrence of adenocarcinoma of the colon and rectum at the anastomotic site. Surg Gynecol Obstet 1981;152:777.
54. Roseman JM, Minton JP. Aggressive surgery for management of recurrent intraabdominal carcinoma. J Surg Oncol 1983;23:107.
55. van Ooijen B, van der Burg MEL, Th. Planting AS, Siersema PD, Wiggers T. Surgical treatment or gastric drainage only for intestinal obstruction in patients with carcinoma of the ovary or peritoneal carcinomatosis of other origin. Surg Gynecol Obstet 1993;176:469.
56. Gwin JL, Hoffman JP, Eisenberg BL. Surgical management of nonhepatic intra-abdominal recurrence of carcinoma of the colon. Dis Colon Rectum 1993;36:540.
57. Averbach AM, Sugarbaker PH. Treatment for recurrent intraabdominal cancer with intestinal obstruction. Int Surg 1995;80:141.
58. August DA, Ottow RT, Sugarbaker PH. Clinical perspective of human colorectal cancer metastasis. Cancer Metastasis Rev 1984;3:303.
59. Stat Bite. Cost per life year gained for selected therapies. J Natl Cancer Inst 1992;84:1141.
60. Griffen WO Jr, Humphrey L, Sosin H. The prognosis and management of recurrent abdominal malignancies. Curr Probl Surg April 1969:1.
61. Polk HC, Spratt JS. Recurrent colorectal carcinoma: detection, treatment, and other considerations. Surgery 1971;69:9.
62. Polk HC, Spratt JS. Recurrent cancer of the colon. Surg Clin North Am 1983;63:151.
63. Sugarbaker PH, Jablonski KA. Prognostic features of 51 colorectal and 130 appendiceal cancer patients with peritoneal carcinomatosis treated by cytoreductive surgery and intraperitoneal chemotherapy. Ann Surg 1995;221:125.
64. Sugarbaker PH, Bowei Z, Banez Sese G, Shmookler B. Peritoneal carcinomatosis from appendiceal cancer: results in 69 patients treated by cytoreductive surgery and intraperitoneal chemotherapy. Dis Colon Rectum 1993;36:323.

APPENDIX 6-1.

Cost–Benefit Analysis of Follow-up With Reoperative Surgery in 100 Colorectal Cancer Patients

Assumptions

Two hundred patients will be managed 5 years. Half of these patients will qualify for intensive follow-up.

Fifty percent of the patients will have recurrence.

Mean time to recurrence is 18 months.

No patient who does not have recurrence will be operated on.

No patient will undergo more than 1 reoperation.

Charges for chemotherapy (80% of patients) and radiotherapy (15% of patients) are not included in costs for reoperative surgery.

Charges for health maintenance and surveillance are not included.

Charges for the dying process are not included (hospice or palliative surgery).

There are no surgical complications that require extended hospital stay, and no patients go on long-term parenteral feeding.

APPENDIX CHART 6-1

Expenses (in Dollars)

	Patient With Recurrence	Disease-Free Patient
Thirty percent of the patients with recurrence will be reoperated (15 patients) at a cost of $40,000 per patient	600,000	0
A single computed tomography scan of chest, abdomen, and pelvis is performed on the 30 patients with recurrence to help select patients for operation ($1500 per complete scan)	45,000	0
A surgical encounter occurs every 3 months for years 1 and 2 and every 6 months thereafter for years 3, 4, and 5	360	840
Carcinoembryonic antigen monitoring is every 3 months for years 1 and 2 and every 6 months for years 3, 4, and 5	180	420
A chest radiograph is obtained on a yearly basis ($75 per radiograph)	150	375
Routine hematologic and chemistry tests ($30 per visit)	180	420
Total expenses	645,870	2055

Thirty-three percent of reoperated patients will be cured (5 patients) and live on the average another 15 years (age 65–80 years; total of 75 life-years).

Approximate cost of detection and treatment, $9000 per life-year.

Surgery for Gastrointestinal Cancer: A Multidisciplinary Approach, edited by Harold J. Wanebo.
Lippincott-Raven Publishers, Philadelphia, © 1997.

CHAPTER 7

Clinical Use of Tumor Markers in Gastrointestinal Malignancies

Maureen Chung and Helena R. Chang

A tumor marker is a blood-borne substance found in excessive quantities or under abnormal conditions in patients with cancer.[1] Tumor markers can take the form of normal enzymes (neuron-specific enolase [NSE]), hormones (gastrin), tumor-associated glycoproteins (TAG), reexpression of oncofetal antigens (carcinoembryonic antigen [CEA] and α-fetoprotein [AFP]), or lipid-associated sialic acid antigens (CA 19-9). Tumor markers play multiple roles in oncologic surgery. Their obvious use is in the screening for carcinoma in asymptomatic subjects before clinical expression, thus affording treatment at an earlier stage. To date, no tumor marker has sufficient sensitivity (number of true-positive results) or specificity (number of true-negative results) to function in this manner. Other uses include the diagnosis of disease, the monitoring of disease progression or efficacy of treatment, the detection of disease recurrence, and treatment purposes.[2] This chapter outlines the use of tumor markers in the management of patients with a gastrointestinal malignancy.

ESOPHAGEAL AND GASTRIC CARCINOMAS

Esophageal neoplasms have no known specific tumor markers. Elevated levels of CEA, CA 19-9, and TAG have been detected for all adenocarcinomas of gastrointestinal origin, including the esophagogastric region. A new tumor marker for gastric carcinoma, CA 72-4, has been reported. Using a level of 5 U/mL as the cutoff, CA 72-4 has been shown to have a specificity of 91% and sensitivity of 68% in a cohort that included patients with gastric carcinoma, those with benign gastrointestinal diseases, and normal control subjects.[3] Levels of this marker correlate with disease stage and return to normal after curative surgery.[4] A correlation between CA 72-4 and CEA expression does not appear in gastric carcinoma.

Maureen Chung, Fellow in Surgery, Brown University School of Medicine, 825 Chalkstone Avenue, Providence, RI 02908
Helena R. Chang, Brown University, Roger Williams Medical Center, 825 Chalkstone Avenue, Providence, RI 02908

Adenocarcinoma of the stomach is frequently associated with elevated levels of CEA or CA 19-9. The relation between the expression of these antigens and prognosis or progression of disease is not clearly defined. Adenocarcinomas may express TAG 72, which is recognized by the B72.3 and CC49 antibodies. Patients with gastric carcinoma are known to have this antigen, and the level of expression correlates with stage of disease.[5] Radioimmunoguided surgery (RIGS) using the TAG antibody has been been successful in documenting lymphatic involvement at laparotomy in 80% of patients.[6]

COLORECTAL CARCINOMA

Carcinoembryonic Antigen

Two frequently used tumor markers in colorectal carcinoma are CEA and TAG 72. The CA 19-9 marker is used less frequently in managing patients with colorectal carcinoma. CEA was the first tumor marker described for colorectal carcinoma. Initially described in 1965 by Gold and colleagues,[7] CEA is an intracellular protein found in embryonic and fetal gut, pancreas, and liver, with decreased expression in the adult. It has been hypothesized that CEA functions by blocking terminal differentiation, allowing the proliferative potential to be maintained.[8]

Since the development of an assay to detect the expression of CEA,[9] much has been learned in terms of its clinical application[10] (Table 7-1). The use of CEA for screening of the general population is not indicated[11,12]; many other types of carcinoma may also be associated with CEA elevation. Elevated CEA is also seen in heavy smokers and in benign diseases of the gastrointestinal tract, including cirrhosis, pancreatitis, peptic ulcer disease, ulcerative colitis, intestinal polyps, and uremia.[13] Furthermore, CEA has been detected histochemically in benign colonic tissue.[14] In an Australian study of 2000 asymptomatic people, only 12.3% of patients with elevated CEA had colorectal carcinoma, and 25 patients with this neoplasm had normal levels of CEA. CEA screening in this population aided only two patients, or 0.001%.[12] In certain high-risk groups, CEA screening may

TABLE 7-1. *Clinical use of carcinoembryonic antigen in colorectal carcinoma*

Screening
No role
Prognosis
Level correlates with disease stage
Highest levels seen with visceral metastases
Follow-up
Should be done q 2 mo
Predates clinical recurrence by 6 mo
CEA-directed laparotomy → 50% resectable
Chemotherapy
Can be used to monitor response
Immunotherapy
Early work with anti-CEA monoclonal antibody encouraging

CEA, carcinoembryonic antigen.

play a role. In patients with Gardner's syndrome, a high-risk population for colorectal carcinoma, there is a small increase in CEA titer with the appearance of polyps and a return to normal baseline after polypectomy. CEA screening may aid in following these high-risk patients and help in the timing of their definitive surgery.[15]

Although CEA elevation cannot be used for screening, the degree of elevation may be used as a prognostic determinant. Wanebo and colleagues showed that the recurrence rate for Dukes' stage C lesions was higher in patients with elevated CEA (78% vs. 44%) and that the time to recurrence was significantly shorter in those patients with an elevated CEA (13 vs. 28 months).[16] Although CEA levels correlate with stage of disease, undifferentiated or poorly differentiated colorectal carcinomas often do not produce CEA, and a low serum CEA level can be misleading in these patients.[17]

Detection of CEA level has its greatest application in the follow-up of patients with colorectal carcinoma after definitive resection. In this select group of patients, CEA screening has a sensitivity of 89%.[18] The half-life of CEA is 4 to 5 days, so that after curative surgery, this marker returns to normal within weeks of resection.[19] CEA elevation predates clinical and radiologic detection of disease recurrence by approximately 6 months.[20] The increase in CEA is more often seen in patients with hepatic or pulmonary metastases and is less likely with local or pelvic recurrence.[21] Of patients undergoing a CEA-directed second-look laparotomy, 44% to 58% will be resectable,[22,23] with a 5-year survival after reexploration and resection of 31%.[24] Early exploration after CEA elevation is important because patients explored soon after the change in CEA is noted have a higher resectability rate.[25,26] The usefulness of CEA screening decreases with increasing length of follow-up, with sensitivity falling from 89% at 1 year to 60% at 5 years, with a similar decrease in specificity.[27] Patients with normal CEA levels at the time of initial diagnosis should also be followed with serial CEA titers. Zeng and associates found that 44% of patients with normal CEA levels at initial diagnosis had elevated levels at the time of their recurrence.[28] Finally, the degree of CEA elevation may correlate with site of recurrence. Low levels of elevation are more frequently associated with locoregional recurrence, whereas higher levels are seen with visceral metastases.[29]

Carcinoembryonic antigen levels may be used in determining the response to chemotherapy in patients with known disease. In a study of 47 patients with documented metastatic colorectal cancer, all patients with radiologically verified disease regression had a fall in CEA titer, whereas those with stable disease had little change in this value. Of the patients who failed to respond to chemotherapy, 74% showed a doubling in the CEA level.[30]

Studies have outlined the use of anti-CEA antibodies for immunotherapy. With use of anti-CEA monoclonal antibodies, survival in nude mice with colorectal carcinoma increased from 26 to 69 days.[31] Radiolabeled anti-CEA antibodies have also been used for the treatment of pulmonary metastases in animals, and preliminary results have been encouraging.[32] Because immunotherapy is most effective with microscopic disease,[33] its use is most likely to be in the adjuvant setting.

Tumor-Associated Glycoprotein 72 Antigen

The B72.3 and CC49 monoclonal antibodies recognize the TAG 72 antigen, a tumor-associated antigen that is present on the surface of adenocarcinomas. The B72.3 antibody was the first generation of antibodies to TAG 72, and CC49 is the second generation of antibodies.[34] TAG 72 is not detected in benign colonic polyps, with the exception of those with severe dysplasia.[35] These antibodies are most often used in the clinical setting of RIGS.

Use of radioactive isotopes coupled to the B72.3 monoclonal antibody permits both preoperative and intraoperative detection of metastatic sites of colorectal carcinoma. Oncoscint CR 103 is a radiolabeled antibody given to patients being evaluated for colorectal carcinoma, who are then scanned for presence of the isotope. In a study of 116 patients with colorectal carcinoma, the sensitivity for detecting the presence of carcinoma was 70% and the specificity was 90%. This method detected occult disease (ie, not apparent clinically or radiographically) in 12% of patients.[36] Its usefulness will probably lie in the evaluation of extrahepatic disease in patients with recurrent colorectal carcinoma after curative surgery. The side effects of monoclonal antibody administration are usually limited to allergic phenomena, including fever and itching.

The CC49 monoclonal antibody has gained its greatest popularity as part of the RIGS technique for the detection of occult metastases for colorectal carcinoma. Patients are injected with the isotope-labeled antibody 3 weeks before surgery. At exploration, the antibody is detected using a hand-held γ-counter. In patients undergoing exploration for primary colorectal carcinoma, RIGS was able to detect the presence of disease in all patients, and a major operation was aborted in 50% of patients because of RIGS-detected occult metastatic disease.[37] In patients being explored as part of a second-look procedure, RIGS was helpful in detecting extrahepatic metastatic disease, particularly lymph node involvement. The resection of these involved areas resulted in increased survival after resection. Martin and Carey have reported a 5-year survival of 0% in patients resected according to conventional techniques, compared to a 5-year survival of 60% for patients resected using RIGS as a guide to resection ($P = 0.0008$)[38] during the same time period. RIGS-related surgery will probably prove most helpful in evaluating lymph node involvement outside the usual field of resection, particularly those lymph nodes in the retroperitoneum and gastrohepatic ligament.[39]

Carcinoembryonic antigen and TAG 72 may play complementary roles in the evaluation of recurrence in patients with colorectal carcinoma. It is most likely that serial CEA evaluation will be the first-line diagnostic tool, followed by radiologic evaluation. This would then be followed by TAG 72-directed RIGS at exploration. Using this approach, RIGS detected 18% of recurrences missed by computed tomography scan and laparotomy.[40]

CA 19-9, another tumor marker, may be used as a prognostic indicator in patients with advanced colorectal carcinoma. High levels of CA 19-9 are associated with a shorter survival in this group of patients (13.5 vs. 30.1 months).[41]

Other Markers

A few tumor markers have more recently been studied experimentally and described in the literature. Colon-specific antigen-p is expressed in colorectal carcinoma. Using 10 U/mL as the cutoff, the sensitivity of this marker for colorectal carcinoma was 14%.[42] Despite its low sensitivity, it is very specific for colorectal carcinoma because it is not expressed in adenomas. The combination of this marker with CEA may be useful in evaluating patients with elevated CEA levels.

Monoclonal antibody 4D3 detects small intestinal mucin antigen in the serum of patients with colorectal carcinoma. The sensitivity of monoclonal antibody 4D3 assay in colorectal carcinoma increases with stage: in one study, 15% of patients with Dukes' stage A disease had elevated levels, whereas patients with Dukes' stage C and D lesions had levels of 32% and 75%, respectively.[43] Further testing of this antibody is needed to determine its specificity.

CA 195 is a tumor-associated antigen that shares an epitope with the Lewis A blood group. The specificity and sensitivity of CA 195 in colorectal carcinoma are 45% and 70%, respectively.[44] It is too early to indicate if CA 195 levels will be useful for the early detection of recurrent disease.[45]

EXOCRINE PANCREAS

Pancreatic carcinoma usually presents at an advanced stage because of the paucity and nonspecificity of symptoms.[46] Although a variety of markers are being evaluated in the diagnosis of adenocarcinoma of the pancreas, the tumor marker most closely associated with this disease is CA 19-9. Other markers, including CEA, CA 50, CA 242, and CA 494, also may prove to be clinically useful (Table 7-2).

CA 19-9

CA 19-9 is an antigen with an identical determinant to the sialylated Lewis A antigen.[47] The overall sensitivity of CA 19-9 for pancreatic carcinoma ranges between 71% and 95%.[48,49] There is no role for the screening of asymptomatic people with CA 19-9. In a prospective study of 866 patients,[50] 135 patients had an elevation in CA 19-9, but only 1 patient was diagnosed with pancreatic carcinoma. Most of the patients with false-positive results in this study had benign hepatobiliary disease with a correlation between CA 19-9 level and serum alkaline phosphatase.

In the patient who presents with weight loss or pain with a clinical suspicion of pancreatic carcinoma, early determination of CA 19-9 may lead to fewer tests and a more direct route to diagnosis of carcinoma. In a study by Richter and associates, the use of CA 19-9 levels, coupled with the use of abdominal ultrasound, resulted in 26% to 33% fewer tests needed for the diagnosis of pancreatic carcinoma.[51] The level of CA 19-9 in fluid aspirated from pancreatic cysts should be interpreted with caution because there may be low levels of both CEA and CA 19-9 in cystadenomas as well as cystadenocarcinomas.[52] Immunohistochemical localization of CA 19-9 can aid in the pathologic diagnosis of pancreatic carcinoma. In pancreatic carcinoma, the entire surface and cytoplasm of the cell is stained, with loss of polarity and staining of surrounding stroma. With atypia, the surrounding stroma is not stained. In normal cells, staining is restricted to the luminal surface. This technique may allow for the accurate diagnosis of pancreatic carcinoma in equivocal cases.[53]

The CA 19-9 level may be an indicator of surgical resectability and postoperative survival. In a study of 14 patients brought to surgery for pancreatic carcinoma, a CA 19-9 level less than 1000 U/mL correlated with resectability.[54] Postoperative CA 19-9 levels normalized in eight patients, and these patients survived longer than 18 months. The patients with elevated postoperative CA 19-9 levels all died within 12 months. It was also noted in this study that the elevation in CA 19-9 heralded clinical recurrence of disease by 1 to 7 months. This finding has been observed by other authors, with CA 19-9 elevation predating clinical recurrence by 1 to 10 months.[55]

Mucin Antigens

In addition to CA 19-9, a large group of mucin antigens are overexpressed in pancreatic carcinoma. This list includes CA 50, CA 242, CA 15-3, CA 494, Dupan-2, Ypan-1, and Span-1. CA 50 and CA 242 are sialylated carbohydrate antigens that

TABLE 7-2. *Tumor markers in pancreatic carcinoma*

Serum marker	Cutoff level	Sensitivity	Specificity	Remarks
CA19-9[48,49,97]	50 U/mL	71%–95%	88%	Increased with increased alkaline phosphatase
Carcinoembryonic antigen[98]	4.1 ng/mL	77%	83%	
CA 50[57,98]	137 U/mL	70%–77%	78%–84%	
CA 242[58,98]	21 U/mL	66%–88%	65%–81%	Not affected by increased bilirubin
CA 494[59]		90%	94%	Not affected by chronic pancreatitis

CA, cancer-associated antigen

are both situated on the same macromolecule as CA 19-9.[56] The sensitivities of CA 50 and CA 242 for pancreatic carcinoma are 70.6% and 66.2%, respectively, and their specificities are 77.9% and 64.7%, respectively.[57] The level of CA 242 correlates with tumor size and lymph node involvement, making this an attractive marker for clinical staging. The combination of these two markers results in a sensitivity of 75%. Early work with CA 242 indicates that in the face of benign hepatobiliary disease, CA 242 may be more specific than CA 50 or even CA 19-9.[58] Another similar marker, CA 494, is being evaluated. Its sensitivity is 90%, and when used in patients with chronic pancreatitis, its specificity is 94%.[59] CA 15-3 is being evaluated in the management of pancreatic cysts. Using a level of CA 15-3 greater than 30 U/mL as the cutoff in aspirated fluid, there is 100% sensitivity and specificity in differentiating mucinous cystadenocarcinomas from other mucinous cystic lesions.[60] Span-1 has a sensitivity and specificity for pancreatic carcinoma of 81.3% and 75.6%, respectively.[61] The false-positive results with this marker are often seen in patients with cirrhosis or chronic hepatitis. Further research is needed to determine the usefulness of these mucin antigens in the evaluation and treatment of patients with pancreatic carcinoma.

Other Pancreatic Tumor Markers

Other markers detected in the serum of patients with pancreatic carcinoma are mucin antigens, ribonuclease, and the leukocyte adherence inhibition test (gastrointestinal cancer antigen [GICA]). Ribonuclease is a potentially useful marker in the differentiation between pancreatic carcinoma and pancreatitis. The specificity of this marker, if patients with renal failure and necrotizing pancreatitis are excluded, is greater than 90%, with an accuracy of 85%.[62] There appears to be no correlation between ribonuclease level and stage of disease. Finally, leukocyte adherence inhibition testing with GICA yields abnormal results in 40% of patients with pancreatic carcinoma. The specificity of this test, however, approaches 94%, making it an attractive marker for differentiating chronic pancreatitis from pancreatic carcinoma.[63]

ENDOCRINE PANCREAS

When pathologic dysplasia of islet cells occurs, there is an excess of humoral products, particularly hormones. Before the identification and development of bioassays that could measure these hormones, islet cell neoplasms presented at a late stage and as part of a syndrome. The ability to measure serum hormonal levels has allowed for the earlier diagnosis of these neoplasms. The hormones secreted by the islet cells are insulin, gastrin, glucagon, vasoactive intestinal peptide, pancreatic peptide, and somatostatin.[64] In addition, because islet cells are derived from neural tissue, NSE, a marker of neural tissue, is also expressed in these neoplasms.

Endocrine pancreatic tumors can secrete more than one polypeptide. In immunohistochemistry staining, neoplastic cells can be stained positively for up to five peptides.[65] The functional status of islet cell tumors, in general, does not appear to affect prognosis or response to treatment. If the tumor is functional, however, there is a good correlation between hormonal level and clinical and radiologic response to treatment.[66]

Gastrin

Elevated levels of gastrin are seen in gastrinomas or the Zollinger-Ellison syndrome. An elevation in the fasting gastrin level, abnormally high basal acid output, a maximal acid output-to-basal acid output ratio greater than 0.6, or a significant increase in gastrin after calcium or secretin infusion form part of the biochemical diagnosis of this disease. Gastrin levels can be used for diagnosis, intraoperative localization of tumor, assessment of adequacy of surgery, follow-up for disease recurrence, or assessment of disease response to chemotherapy.

Secretin stimulates the release of gastrin into the peripheral circulation. The selective arterial secretin test can be used intraoperatively to localize a gastrinoma. Its use immediately before and after pancreaticoduodenectomy can aid in establishing the adequacy of surgical resection.[67] After curative resection, gastrin levels fall to normal within 24 hours,[68] with little or no change in levels for unsuccessful resections.[69] A persistent elevation in gastrin after "curative surgery" should prompt reexploration because unrecognized disease in lymph nodes may have been missed.[70] After surgery, serial gastrin levels should be obtained because an increase in gastrin level may indicate recurrence predating clinical or radiologic changes by up to 23 months.[70] In patients treated with chemotherapy, a fall in gastrin levels correlates with clinical response.[71]

Insulin, Glucagon, Somatostatin, and Pancreatic Peptide

The role of portal venous sampling of hormonal products for the localization of islet cell tumors is unclear. Norton and colleagues have reported a 75% success rate in localizing insulinomas with this modality.[72] A novel test using labeled somatostatin, however, may make venous sampling obsolete.[73] Most endocrine tumors possess high-affinity receptors for somatostatin. Using an indium-labeled analog, a preoperative scintigram may be used to localize cells with these receptors. This technique is sensitive for lesions greater than 1 cm in diameter. Obviously, this test does not detect receptor-negative lesions, which are seen in 40% of insulinomas.

As in gastrinomas, hormonal levels before and after surgery may be used to assess adequacy of resection and to detect early recurrence of disease. Care should be taken in interpreting postoperative glucagon levels because normal levels have been reported after noncurative surgery.[74] If glucagon levels are elevated with documented recurrence, however, they can be used to correlate with chemotherapeutic response.[75]

Neuron-Specific Enolase

Neuron-specific enolase is present in neural-derived tissue in the gastrointestinal tract. D'Alessandro and coworkers have shown that 92% of these neoplasms have elevated levels of NSE, and that there is no correlation between NSE level and functional status of the neoplasm.[76] A significantly increased level of NSE in malignant lesions is observed, with a fall after curative surgery.

CARCINOID TUMORS

Carcinoid tumors arise from the enterochromaffin cells in the crypts of Lieberkuhn and consist of pluripotential, neuroendocrine cells derived from the APUD (amine precursor uptake decarboxylase) line. Within the gastrointestinal tract, they most often originate in the appendix, but may also be found, in order of descending frequency, in the small intestine, rectum, and colon.[77] They can secrete multiple vasoactive substances, including bradykinin, serotonin, tachykinins, histamine, dopamine, and prostaglandins. Aside from the rare instance of leakage of vasoactive amines through the collateral retroperitoneal circulation,[78] these substances are not detected in the peripheral circulation in the absence of liver metastases. When these peptides are symptomatic, they give rise to the carcinoid syndrome.

The tumor markers most closely associated with the carcinoid syndrome are serotonin and 5-hydroxyindole acetic acid (5-HIAA), a major metabolite of serotonin. Twenty-four–hour urinary excretion of 5-HIAA is normally less than 9 mg. In the presence of carcinoid syndrome, these levels increase and are diagnostic of this clinical entity. Abnormal urinary levels of 5-HIAA may be seen with ingestion of bananas, tomatoes, pineapples, and phenothiazines. Normal urinary levels of 5-HIAA can be seen in one third of patients with carcinoid syndrome.[79] Platelet serotonin levels are thought to be more sensitive for carcinoid syndrome. Kema and associates have shown that of 30 patients with carcinoid syndrome, 10 had normal levels for both urinary 5-HIAA and platelet serotonin, 14 had elevated levels of both markers, and 6 had elevation only of platelet serotonin.[80]

BILIARY NEOPLASMS

The tumor markers associated with malignancies of the biliary tree are CEA and CA 19-9. The progression from benign to malignant biliary neoplasms involves little change in biliary concentration of these markers. In the case of the serum concentrations of these markers, however, there is a doubling in CEA levels and a 10-fold increase in CA 19-9 concentrations.[81] Although the levels of CEA and CA 19-9 are not proportional to clinical stage, there is a correlation between CA 19-9 levels and flow cytometric results. On immunohistochemistry, 100% of gallbladder carcinomas stain positive for CEA and 93% stain positive for CA 19-9. Because dysplastic epithelium does not stain positive for these markers, staining for these tumor markers may be helpful in differentiating borderline cases of gallbladder carcinoma from severe dysplasia.[82]

HEPATOCELLULAR CARCINOMA

α-Fetoprotein

α-Fetoprotein is the tumor marker most closely linked to hepatocellular carcinoma (HCC). Like CEA, it is an oncofetal antigen and is used not only for prenatal screening of neural tube defects, but for diagnosing hepatic neoplasms and germ cell malignancies in the adult. As with other tumor markers, screening of the general population for AFP is not recommended because of the inaccuracy of this marker and the low prevalence of HCC. In high-risk populations (cirrhotic patients) or in countries where this disease has a high prevalence (China), screening with AFP takes on greater importance. AFP screening in these populations, coupled with serial ultrasonography, has led to an earlier diagnosis of HCC, with the earlier form of the disease subcategorized as subclinical HCC (SHCC). Tang and coworkers have shown that screening of high-risk populations with serial AFP and ultrasound can diagnose SHCC, and that these patients have a higher resectability rate (50.7% for SHCC vs. 20.6% overall) and increased 5-year survival compared to patients diagnosed at the symptomatic stage.[83] Similar results have been reported in other studies of AFP screening mechanisms, with smaller tumor size, increased resectability, and improved survival in diagnosed patients.[84,85] The use of AFP screening must be coupled with serial ultrasonography, particularly in cirrhotic patients.[86] AFP levels are elevated in 25.6% of cirrhotic patients in the absence of HCC, with levels proportionally increased with Child's classification.[87] Very high levels of AFP in the absence of active liver dysfunction in a cirrhotic patient should alert the treating physician to the possibility of HCC.

Patients detected by AFP screening who undergo curative surgery have a better overall outcome than patients diagnosed at the symptomatic stage. Low preoperative AFP levels[88] and negative AFP levels within 2 months of curative surgery[89] are good prognostic signs. Total reliance on postoperative levels of AFP for the detection of recurrent disease should be avoided. Takayasu and colleagues have reported that in 48 cases of documented recurrent HCC after hepatectomy, 25% of patients had normal levels of AFP.[90] AFP levels may also be used to predict response to chemotherapy. Of patients treated with 5-fluorouracil and interferon-α, one third with low levels of AFP had a partial response to these drugs.[91]

Protein Induced by Vitamin K Absence

Protein induced by vitamin K absence (PIVKA-II), also known as DCP (des-γ-carboxyprothrombin), is produced by the malignant hepatocyte. Normal doses of vitamin K do not affect its level and it has been found to be a useful marker of HCC, particularly in the face of cirrhosis.[92] The sensitivity of PIVKA-II for HCC is only 48.2%, but the specificity of this marker in the presence of liver cirrhosis is 92.9%, and for chronic hepatitis the specificity is 96.9%.[93] Preliminary results indicate that PIVKA-II levels correlate with size of HCC and that the levels of this tumor marker fall after curative resection, suggesting a role for PIVKA-II in the postoperative management of these patients.[94] The combination of AFP and PIVKA-II screening has resulted in the earlier diagnosis of HCC in patients with cirrhosis.[95]

SQUAMOUS CELL CARCINOMA OF THE ANUS

There is an increased level of squamous cell carcinoma antigen in the serum of patients with anal epidermoid carcinoma.

Preliminary work indicates that this may be a useful marker in patients with this disease. A serum level of this marker greater than 2 ng/mL was seen more often in patients who had recurrence after treatment or had residual disease after initial therapy ($P = 0.0001$). The level of this marker at diagnosis also correlated with survival; patients with a normal level had a 5-year survival of 81%, whereas patients with an elevated level at diagnosis had a survival rate of 43%.[96]

CONCLUSION

No tumor markers are available for cancer screening. Although many tumor markers have been described, the three most useful ones clinically are CEA, CA 19-9, and AFP. In patients diagnosed with colorectal carcinoma, CEA is a useful marker for prognostic and surveillance purposes. CA 19-9 is clinically useful in the diagnosis of pancreatic carcinoma, and may be useful for follow-up of these patients. AFP has been useful in patients at high risk for HCC, especially when coupled with ultrasonography to screen high-risk populations. The clinical role of other tumor markers is still being evaluated.

REFERENCES

1. Torosian MH. The clinical usefulness and limitations of tumor markers. Surg Gynecol Obstet 1988;166:567.
2. Minton JP, Chevinsky AH. Present status of serum markers for the detection and monitoring of cancer. Resident and Staff Physician 1990; 36:53.
3. Martin-Perez E, Fernandez Arjona M, Baza B, et al. Determination of the tumor marker CA72-4 in gastric carcinoma. Rev Esp Enferm Apar Dig 1993;83:92.
4. Hamazoe R, Maeta M, Matsui T, Shibata S, Shiota S, Kaibara N. CA72-4 compared with carcinoembryonic antigen as a tumor marker for gastric cancer. Eur J Cancer 1992;28A:1351.
5. Filella X, Molina R, Jo J, Bedini JL, Joseph J, Ballests AM. Tumor associated glycoprotein-72 (TAG-72) levels in patients with non-malignant and malignant disease. Bull Cancer (Paris) 1992;79:271.
6. Martin EW, Mojzisik CM, Hinkle GH, et al. Radioimmunoguided surgery using monoclonal antibody. Am J Surg 1988;156:386.
7. Gold P, Johnson J, Freedman SO. Specific carcinoembryonic antigen of human digestive system. J Exp Med 1965;122:467.
8. Eidelman FJ, Fuks A, DeMarte L, Taheri M, Stanners CP. Human carcinoembryonic antigen, an intercellular adhesion molecule, blocks fusion and differentiation of rat myoblasts. J Cell Biol 1993;123:467.
9. Thomson DMP, Krupey J, Freedman SO, Gold P. The radioimmunoassay of circulating carcinoembryonic antigen of the human digestive system. Proc Natl Acad Sci USA 1969;64:161.
10. Torosian MH, Daly JM. An evaluation of the clinical usefulness of CEA in colorectal cancer. Oncology 1991;5:41.
11. Milburn Jessup J. Tumor markers: prognostic and therapeutic implications. In: Wanebo HJ, ed. Colorectal cancer. St. Louis: Mosby-Year Book, 1993:106.
12. Cullen KJ, Stevens DP, Frost MA, et al. Carcinoembryonic antigen (CEA), smoking and cancer in a longitudinal population study. Aust N Z J Med 1976;6:279.
13. Gordon PH. Malignant neoplasms of the colon. In: Gordon PH, Nivatsong S, eds. Principles and practice of surgery for the colon, rectum, and anus. St. Louis: Quality Medical Publishing, 1992:501.
14. Au FC, Stein B, Tang C. Carcinoembryonic antigen levels in colonic lesions. Br J Surg 1986;151:61.
15. Krush AJ, Zamcheck N, Lynch HT. CEA and genetics. Dis Colon Rectum 1983;26:404.
16. Wanebo HJ, Rao B, Pinsky CM, et al. Preoperative carcinoembryonic antigen level as a prognostic indicator in colorectal cancer. N Engl J Med 1978;299:448.
17. Steele G, Zamcheck N. The use of carcinoembryonic antigen in the clinical management of patients with colorectal cancer. Cancer Detect Prev 1985;8:421.
18. Attiyeh FF, Stearns M. Second-look laparotomy based on CEA elevations in colorectal cancer. Cancer 1981;47:2119.
19. Mai M, Takahashi Y. Prediction of recurrence of gastrointestinal cancer from standpoint of biological malignancies: tumor marker doubling time and its half life period line. Hum Cell 1993;6:82.
20. Carlsson U, Stewenius J, Ekelund G, Leandoer L, Nosslin B. Is CEA analysis of value in screening for recurrences after surgery for colorectal carcinoma? Dis Colon Rectum 1983:26:369.
21. Kilfoyle RG, Andersen CA. Carcinoembryonic antigen: its role in the management of colorectal cancer. Mil Med 1983;148:589.
22. Wanebo HJ, Stearns M, Schwartz MK. Use of CEA as an indicator of early recurrence and as a guide to a selected second-look procedure in patients with colorectal cancer. Ann Surg 1978;188:481.
23. Wanebo HJ, Llaneras M, Martin T, Kaiser D. Prospective monitoring trial for carcinoma of the colon and rectum after surgical resection. Surg Gynecol Obstet 1989;169:479.
24. Martin EW, Minton JP, Carey LC. CEA-directed second-look surgery in the asymptomatic patient after primary resection of colorectal carcinoma. Ann Surg 1985;202:310.
25. Minton JP, Martin EW. The use of serial CEA determinations to predict recurrence of colon cancer and when to do a second-look operation. Cancer 1978;42:1422.
26. Attiyeh FF, Stearns MW. Second look laparotomy based on CEA elevations in colorectal cancer. Cancer 1981;47:2119.
27. Denstman F, Rosen L, Khubchandani I, Sheets JA, Stasik JJ, Riether RD. Comparing predictive decision rules in postoperative CEA monitoring. Cancer 1986;58:2089.
28. Zeng Z, Cohen AM, Urmacher C. Usefulness of carcinoembryonic antigen monitoring despite normal preoperative values in node-positive colon cancer patients. Dis Colon Rectum 1993;36:1063.
29. Moertel CG, O'Fallon JR, Go VLW, O'Connell MJ, Thynne GS. The preoperative carcinoembryonic antigen test in the diagnosis, staging, and prognosis of colorectal cancer. Cancer 1986;58:603.
30. Mayer RJ, Garnick MB, Steele GD, Zamcheck N. Carcinoembryonic antigen (CEA) as a monitor of chemotherapy in disseminated colorectal cancer. Cancer 1978;42:1428.
31. Hyams DM, Esteban JM, Beatty BG, Wanek PM, Beatty JD. Prolongation of survival of nude mice bearing human colon cancer. Arch Surg 1989;124:175.
32. Blumenthal RD, Sahrkey RM, Haywood L, et al. Targeted therapy of athymic mice bearing GW-39 human colonic cancer micrometastases with ^{131}I-labeled monoclonal antibodies. Cancer Res 1992;52:6036.
33. Beatty JD. Immunotherapy of colorectal cancer. Cancer 1992;70:1425.
34. Muraro R, Kuroki M, Wunderlich D, et al. Generation and characterization of B72.3 second generation monoclonal antibody reactive with the tumor associated glycoprotein 72 antigen. Cancer Res 1988;48:4588.
35. Salem RR, Wolf BC, Sears HF, et al. Expression of colorectal carcinoma-associated antigens in colonic polyps. J Surg Res 1993;55:249.
36. Doerr RJ, Abdel-Nabi H, Krag D, Mitchell E. Radiolabeled antibody imaging in the management of colorectal cancer: results of a multicenter clinical study. Ann Surg 1991;214:118.
37. Nieroda CA, Mojzisik C, Sardi A, et al. The impact of radioimmunoguided surgery (RIGS) on surgical decision-making in colorectal cancer. Dis Colon Rectum 1989;32:927.
38. Martin EW, Carey LC. Second-look surgery for colorectal cancer: the second time around. Ann Surg 1991;214:321.
39. Arnold MW, Schneebaum S, Berens A, Mojzisik C, Hinkle G, Martin EW. Radioimmunoguided surgery challenges traditional decision making in patients with primary colorectal cancer. Surgery 1992;112:30.
40. Sardi A, Workman M, Mojzisik C, Hinkle G, Nieroda C, Martin EW. Intra-abdominal recurrence of colorectal cancer detected by radioimmunoguided surgery (RIGS system). Arch Surg 1989;124:55.
41. Kouri M, Nordling S, Kuusela P, Pyrhonen S. Poor prognosis associated with elevated serum CA19-9 level in advanced colorectal carcinoma, independent of DNA ploidy or SPF. Eur J Cancer 1993;29A:1691.
42. Pant KD, Shochat D, Nelson O, Goldenberg DM. Colon-specific antigen-p (CSAp): I. initial clinical evaluation as a marker for colorectal cancer. Cancer 1982;50:919.
43. Pinczower GD, Gianello RD, Williams RP, Preston BN, Preston H, Linnane AW. Monoclonal antibody 4D3 detects small intestinal mucin

antigen (SIMA) glycoprotein in the serum of patients with colorectal cancer. Int J Cancer 1993;54:391.
44. Kornek GV, Depisch D, Rosen HR, Temsch EM, Scheithauer W. Comparative analysis of CA72-4, CA195 and carcinoembryonic antigen in patients with gastrointestinal malignancies. J Cancer Res Clin Oncol 1992;118:318.
45. Verdi CJ, Ahmann FR, Schifman RB, Elvick AL, Ahmann ME, Marx PC. Comparative evaluation of serum CA 195 and carcinoembryonic antigen in metastatic carcinoma. Cancer 1993;71:3625.
46. Warshaw AL, Fernandez-del Castillo C. Pancreatic carcinoma. N Engl J Med 1992;326:455.
47. Magnani JL, Nilsson B, Brockhaus M, et al. A monoclonal antibody-defined antigen associated with gastrointestinal cancer is a ganglioside containing sialated lacto-N-fucopentaose II. J Biol Chem 1982;257: 14365.
48. Safi F, Roscher R, Beger HG. Tumor markers in pancreatic cancer: sensitivity and specificity of CA 19-9. Hepatogastroenterology 1989; 36:419.
49. Satake K, Kanazawa G, Kho I, Chung Y, Umeyama K. Evaluation of serum pancreatic enzymes, carbohydrate antigen 19.9 and CEA in various pancreatic diseases. Am J Gastroenterol 1985;80:630.
50. Frebourg T, Bercoff E, Manchon N, et al. The evaluation of CA 19.9 antigen level in the early detection of pancreatic cancer: a prospective study of 866 patients. Cancer 1988;62:2287.
51. Richter JM, Christensen MR, Rustgi AK, Silverstein MD. The clinical utility of the CA19-9 radioimmunoassay for the diagnosis of pancreatic cancer presenting as pain or weight loss: a cost-effective analysis. Arch Intern Med 1989;149:2292.
52. Sperti C, Cappellazzo F, Pasquali C, et al. Cystic neoplasms of the pancreas: problems in differential diagnosis. Am Surg 1993;59:740.
53. Ichihara T, Nagura H, Nakao A, Sakamoto J, Watanabe T, Takagi H. Immunohistochemical localization of CA19-9 and CEA in pancreatic carcinoma and associated diseases. Cancer 1988;61:324.
54. Glenn J, Steinberg WM, Kurtzman SH, Steinberg SM, Sindelar WF. Evaluation of the utility of a radioimmunoassay for serum CA 19-9 levels in patients before and after treatment of carcinoma of the pancreas. J Clin Oncol 1988;6:462.
55. Sperti C, Pasquali C, Catalini S, et al. CA 19-9 as a prognostic index after resection for pancreatic cancer. J Surg Oncol 1193;52:137.
56. Johansson C, Nilsson O, Baeckstrom D, Jansson EL, Lindholm L. Novel epitopes on the CA 50 carrying antigen: chemical and immunochemical studies. Tumour Biol 1991;12:159.
57. Rothlin MA, Joller H, Largiader F. CA 242 is a new tumor marker for pancreatic cancer. Cancer 1993;71:701.
58. Nilsson O, Johansson C, Glimelius B, et al. Sensitivity and specificity of CA242 in gastrointestinal cancer: a comparison with CEA, CA 50 and CA19-9. Br J Cancer 1992;65:215.
59. Friess H, Buchler M, Auerbach B, et al. CA 494 a new tumor marker for the diagnosis of pancreatic cancer. Int J Cancer 1993;53:759.
60. Rubin D, Warshaw AL, Southern JF, Pins M, Compton CC, Lewandrowski KB. Expression of CA15.3 in the cyst contents distinguishes benign from malignant pancreatic mucinous cystic neoplasms. Surgery 1994;115:52.
61. Kiriyama S, Hakayama T, Kondo T, et al. Usefulness of a new tumor marker, Span-1, for the diagnosis of pancreatic cancer. Cancer 1990; 65:1557.
62. Warshaw AL, Lee K-H, Wood W, Cohen AM. Sensitivity and specificity of serum ribonuclease in the diagnosis of pancreatic cancer. Am J Surg 1980;139:27.
63. Meduri F, Doni MG, Merenda R, et al. The role of the leukocyte adherence inhibition (LAI), CA 19-9, and tissue polypeptide antigen (TPA) tests in the diagnosis of pancreatic cancer. Cancer 1989;64:1103.
64. Freisen SR. Tumors of the endocrine pancreas. N Engl J Med 1982; 306:580.
65. Martensson H, Bottcher G, Sundler F, Nobin A. Localization and peptide content of endocrine pancreatic tumors. Ann Surg 1990;121:607.
66. Moertel CG, Hanley JA, Johnson LA. Streptozocin alone compared with streptozotocin plus fluorouracil in the treatment of advanced islet-cell carcinoma. N Engl J Med 1980;303:1189.
67. Imamura M, Takahashi K, Isobe Y, Hattori Y, Satomura K, Tobe T. Curative resection of multiple gastrinomas aided by selective arterial secretin test and intraoperative secretin test. Ann Surg 1989;210:710.
68. Deveney CW, Deveney KE, Stark D, Moss A, Stein S, Way LW. Resection of gastrinomas. Ann Surg 1983;198:546.
69. Malagelada J-R, Edis AJ, Adson MA, van Heerden JA, Go VLG. Medical and surgical options in the management of patients with gastrinoma. Gastroenterology 1983;84:1524.
70. Delcore R, Cheung LY, Friesen SR. Outcome of lymph node involvement in patients with Zollinger-Ellison syndrome. Ann Surg 1988;208: 291.
71. Norton JA, Sugarbaker PH, Doppman JL, et al. Aggressive resection of metastatic disease in selected patients with malignant gastrinoma. Ann Surg 1986;203:352.
72. Norton JA, Shawker TH, Doppman JL, et al. Localization and surgical treatment of occult insulinomas. Ann Surg 1990;212:615.
73. Weinel RJ, Neuhaus C, Stapp J, et al. Preoperative localization of gastrointestinal endocrine tumors using somatostatin-receptor scintigraphy. Ann Surg 1993;218:640.
74. Marynick SP, Fagadau WR, Duncan LA. Malignant glucagonoma syndrome: response to chemotherapy. Ann Intern Med 1980;93:453.
75. Prinz RA, Badrinath K, Banerji M, Sparagana M, Dorsch TR, Lawrence AM. Operative and chemotherapeutic management of malignant glucagon-producing tumors. Surgery 1981;90;713.
76. D'Alessandro M, Mariani P, Lomanto D, Carlei F, Lezoche E, Speranza V. Serum neuron-specific enolase in diagnosis and follow-up of gastrointestinal neuroendocrine tumors. Tumour Biol 1992;13:352.
77. Spread C, Berkel H, Jewell L, Jenkins H, Yakimets W. Colon carcinoid tumors: a population-based study. Dis Colon Rectum 1994;37:482.
78. Haq AU, Yook CR, Hiremath V, Kasimis BS. Carcinoid syndrome in the absence of liver metastasis: a case report and review of the literature. Med Pediatr Oncol 1992;20:221.
79. Beaton H, Homan W, Dineen P. Gastrointestinal carcinoids and the malignant carcinoid syndrome. Surg Gynecol Obstet 1981;152:268.
80. Kema IP, deVries EG, Schelling AM, Postmus PE, Muskiet FA. Improved diagnosis of carcinoid tumors by measurement of platelet serotonin. Clin Chem 1992;38:534.
81. Strom BL, Iliopoulos D, Atkinson B, et al. Pathophysiology of tumor progression in human gallbladder: flow cytometry, CEA, CA19-9 levels in bile and serum in different stages of gallbladder disease. J Natl Cancer Inst 1989;81:1575.
82. Yamaguchi K, Enjolji M. Carcinoma of the gallbladder: a clinicopathology of 103 patients and a newly proposed staging system. Cancer 1988; 62:1425.
83. Tang ZY, Yu YQ, Zhou XD, Yang BH, Ma ZC, Lin ZY. Subclinical hepatocellular carcinoma: an analysis of 391 patients. J Surg Oncol Suppl 1993;3:55.
84. Zhou XD, Tang ZY, Yu YQ, et al. Solitary minute hepatocellular carcinoma: a study of 14 patients. Cancer 1991;67:2855.
85. Lai CL, Lau JY, Wu PC, et al. Subclinical hepatocellular carcinoma in Hong Kong Chinese. Oncology 1992;49:347.
86. Imberti D, Fornari F, Sbolli G, Buscarini E, Squassante L, Buscarini L. Hepatocellular carcinoma in liver cirrhosis: a prospective study. Scand J Gastroenterol 1993;28:540.
87. Collazos J, Rodriguez J, deMiguel J. Serum alpha-fetoprotein in liver cirrhosis. Rev Clin Esp 1993;192:214.
88. Kakio T, Ito T, Sue K, Tanimizu M, Tsuji T. Survival simulation of hepatocellular carcinoma derived from follow-up studies of 450 patients. Acta Med Okayama 1993;47:339.
89. Zhang SP, Wang NJ. Clinical and pathological features of primary hepatocellular carcinoma in 26 patients survived over 10 years after operation. Chung Hua Ping Li Hsueh Tsa Chih 1992;21:290.
90. Takayasu K, Muramatsu Y, Moriyama N, et al. Clinical and radiologic assessments of the results of hepatectomy for small hepatocellular carcinoma and therapeutic arterial embolization for postoperative recurrence. Cancer 1989;64:1848.
91. Patt YZ, Yoffe B, Charnsangavej C, et al. Low serum alpha-fetoprotein level in patients with hepatocellular carcinoma as a predictor of response to 5-FU and interferon-alpha-2b. Cancer 1993;72:2574.
92. Takikawa Y, Suzuki K, Yamazaki K, et al. Plasma abnormal prothrombin (PIVKA-II): a new and reliable marker for the detection of hepatocellular carcinoma. J Gastroenterol Hepatol 1992;1:1.
93. Kasahara A, Hayashi N, Fusamoto H, et al. Clinical evaluation of plasma des-gamma-carboxy prothrombin as a marker protein of hepatocellular carcinoma in patients with tumors of various sizes. Dig Dis Sci 1993;38:2170.
94. Weitz IC, Liebman HA. Des-gamma-carboxy (abnormal) prothrombin and hepatocellular carcinoma: a critical review. Hepatology 1993;18: 990.

95. Tanikawa K. Early detection of hepatocellular carcinoma: high risk group and mass survey. Gan To Kagaku Ryoho 1993;20:864.
96. Goldman S, Svensson C, Bronnergard M, Glimelius B, Wallin G. Prognostic significance of serum concentration of squamous cell carcinoma antigen in anal epidermoid carcinoma. Int J Colorectal Dis 1993;8:988.
97. Parker N, Makin CA, Ching CK, et al. A new enzyme-linked lectin/mucin antibody sandwich assay (CAM 17.1/WGA) assessed in combination with CA 19-9 and peanut lectin binding assay for the diagnosis of pancreatic cancer. Cancer 1992;70:1062.
98. Pasanen PA, Eskelinen M, Partanen K, Pikkarainen P, Penttila I, Alhava E. Receiver operating characteristic (ROC) curve analysis of the tumor markers CEA, CA 50 and CA 242 in pancreatic cancer: results from a prospective study. Br J Cancer 1993;67:852.

Surgery for Gastrointestinal Cancer: A Multidisciplinary Approach, edited by Harold J. Wanebo.
Lippincott-Raven Publishers, Philadelphia, © 1997.

CHAPTER 8

Nutritional Support for the Patient With Gastrointestinal Cancer

Michael M. Meguid and Alessandro Laviano

EFFECT OF NUTRITION IN ETIOLOGY OF GASTROINTESTINAL CANCER

Based on available information, the National Academy of Sciences has formulated "Dietary Guidelines" with respect to diet, nutrition, and cancer risk. These guidelines are "consistent with good nutritional practices and likely to reduce the risk of cancer."[1] Similar recommendations were published by the American Cancer Society and the U.S. National Cancer Institute.[2,3] Fifty percent of deaths are from cancers related to dietary factors.[4] It is estimated that appropriate nutrition could reduce cancer deaths by an average of 35% of the present 150,000 deaths per year.[5]

The postulated mechanism by which the food in our diet influences the induction of neoplasms is conceptually a multievent process occurring over time, divided into three distinguishable sequences: "initiation" by a chemical of a normal cell to one with a monoclonal oncogene, containing damaged DNA,[6] 811"promotion" of the latter cell to a "preneoplastic" condition, and "progression" to form a clinically apparent, invasive cancer.[7,8] Dietary constituents, whether chemicals, nutrients, or xenobiotics (foreign compounds of no nutritional value requiring excretion by the body), can promote or inhibit carcinogenic factors,[9] as outlined in the schema given in Figure 8-1. Many chemicals known to produce cancer in experimental animals are introduced into the food chain from a variety of sources, and some of the more well documented ones are listed in Table 8-1.

To exert their carcinogenicity, most of these chemicals need to be metabolically activated to their reactive form by microsomal mixed-function oxidase enzyme systems (see Fig. 8-1). This activation requires multiple metabolic steps and leads to a product that binds with and damages DNA. If the cell divides while damaged, a mutation results. The critical genes affected by such changes may be cellular oncogenes. Carcinogens, including many drugs, insecticides, and xenobiotics, as well as dietary proteins and fats, can induce the activation of this enzyme system. After months to years, the altered cell may express different growth properties that either are unregulated or are affected by unknown or poorly understood biochemical events. The interactions of cells with a known carcinogen are influenced by a variety of nutrients; that is, the diet type may influence the occurrence, dosage, and duration of exposure to carcinogens.

A neoplastic cell, usually monoclonal in its early stages, develops into a tumor through sustained proliferation. Through several mechanisms, epigenetic promoters facilitate the proliferation of latent neoplastic cells to form tumors. Once neoplastic cells have proliferated to a number sufficient to insulate themselves from controlling influences, their further growth no longer depends on promoters. During the progressive growth of neoplasms, the cells may acquire new, permanently abnormal characteristics, resulting in further deviation from the normal, a process referred to as progression.

Conversely, the same microsomal mixed-function oxidase enzyme systems can be inhibited by a variety of drugs, such as steroids. They also contain enzymes that detoxify and inactivate ingested carcinogens—a process that leads to a decrease in carcinogenicity. Xenobiotics and dietary nutrients of both plant and animal origin can modify the effects of these enzymes by inducing the activity of these detoxifying systems, thereby directly participating in detoxification processes or inhibiting carcinogen binding to critical cellular macromolecules. Thus, dietary constituents may regulate activity of carcinogen-activating enzymes located in the cell's endoplasmic reticulum. Furthermore, a variety of cellular repair systems is available for repairing carcinogen-induced DNA damage and for excising DNA–carcinogen adducts. Dietary factors may play a role either by inhibition of the repair system or by xenobiotic induction of repair system activity.

Several dietary factors, such as retinoids, carotenoids, selenium, vitamin A, growth factors (protease inhibitors), and certain

Michael M. Meguid, Professor of Surgery, State University of New York, Health Science Center, 750 East Adams Street, Syracuse, NY 13210

Alessandro Laviano, Department of Clinical Medicine, Laboratory of Clinical Nutrition, viale dell-Universita, 37, 00185 Rome, Italy

STAGE OF CARCIOGENIC ACTIVITY	INITIATION			PROMOTION		PROGRESSION
	FOOD-BORNE CARCINOGEN v					
PROBABLE ACTION OF CARCINOGEN	ELECTROPHILIC --> REACTANT OR "FREE-RADICAL"	BINDING OF --> CARCINOGEN TO DNA/PROTEINS	ALTERATIONS IN --> DNA/PROTEINS CARCINOGEN-DAMAGED CELL	EXPRESSION--> IN ALTERED CELLULAR INFORMATION	GROWTH OF--> ALTERED CELLS BY PROLIFERATION PROMOTER	NEOPLASM--> METASTASIS
POSSIBLE SITES OF NUTRITIONAL INFLUENCE	o Detoxification of reactive carcinogenic compounds o Induction and inhibition of microsomal mixed-function oxidase enzyme systems	o Interference with binding to macro-molecules	o Modulation of DNA/protein damage repair	Induction & Inhbition by: o Specific dietary lipid factors o Tumor growth factors o Inhibition of tumor promoting action		o Influence of diet on tumor behavior e.g., lipids, proteins & hormones

FIG. 8-1. Aspects of the carcinogenic process that might be affected by nitrogen. (Reproduced with permission from Chen MC, Meguid MM, Surg Clin North Am 1986;66:931.) Postulated cancer prevention diets. A guide to food selections.

nutrient factors required by many cell lines, inhibit experimental tumor promotion. In fully formed tumors, dietary lipids, proteins, and hormones may affect growth by influencing tissue growth factors and hormones.

The daily diet should consist of a mixture of the four basic food groups, as listed in Table 8-2. Dietary sources rich in individual nutrients are listed in Table 8-3.

Dietary Risk Factors

Dietary factors appear to be implicated in a wide range of tumor types. Although tobacco is the single most important carcinogen to which the public is commonly exposed, the overall cancer risk attributable to diet may be greater because of diet's suspected role in so many different cancers.

TABLE 8-1. *Some food-borne carcinogens*

Source	Example
Naturally occurring	Mycotoxins Pyrrolizidine alkaloids
Contaminant	
Introduced before processing	DDT Trichloroethylene
Introduced during processing	Methylene chloride
Additive	Saccharin
Formed from food components	
Formed during processing	Nitrosamines Aryldiazonium compounds
Formed during preparation	Benzo(a)pyrene Heterocyclic amines
Formed in vivo	Nitrosamides/nitrosamines

Reproduced with permission from Williams GM. Food and cancer. Nutr Int 1985;1:49.

Esophageal Cancer

Exceptionally high rates of esophageal cancer occur in parts of Iran around the Caspian Sea, in parts of France and China, and in southern and eastern Africa. In the United States, black men in Washington, DC have the highest rates. Such regional variability suggests dietary factors in the etiology of esophageal cancer, given the immediate exposure of the esophagus to the contents of diet. Yet, no single common dietary factor has been identified. Alcohol plays a significant role in France and the United States,[10] but not in Iran or in other regions where the incidence of esophageal cancer is high. A diet deficient in fruits and vegetables may be the most common underlying feature, suggesting the role of vitamin A and C deficiency (see Table 8-3). Lower levels of both of these vitamins were seen among patients with esophageal cancer in the United States.

Other etiologic factors are the consumption of very hot beverages, use of millet grain containing asbestos-like silica fibers, mutagens and carcinogens formed during pickling of foods or production of alcoholic drinks, and deficiencies of other micronutrients such as riboflavin, zinc, and molybdenum.[11] Thus, it is likely that esophageal cancer has multiple etiologies, some of which are dietary.

Gastric Cancer

Until the early 1960s, gastric cancer was the leading cause of cancer death among men in the United States, but its rate

TABLE 8-2. *Constituents of a well balanced diet*

	Group			
	Fruit and vegetable	Meat	Grain	Milk
Number of servings per day	4	2	4	2
Foods/serving size	Salads Cooked vegetable, ½ c Canned fruit, ½ c Juices, ½ c Fresh fruit	2–3 oz of lean, cooked: Meat Poultry Fish Equal to 1 oz of meat: Egg, 1 Cooked dry beans, peas, lentils, ½ to ¾ c Peanut butter, 2 tbsp Nuts, ¼–½ c	Bread, 1 slice Cooked cereal, ½ c Cooked pasta, ½ c Rice, ½ c Grits, ½ c Dry cereal, ¾ c	Milk, 1 c Yogurt, 1 c

c, cup; oz, ounce; tbsp, tablespoon.

Reproduced with permission from Chen MC, Meguid MM. Postulated cancer prevention diets. A guide to food selections. Surg Clin North Am 1986;66:931.

TABLE 8-3. *Selected foods (in alphabetic order) rich in certain nutrients, and their postulated protective effect*

Vitamin A		Vitamin C		Fiber-rich foods	
High	Moderate	High	Moderate	High	Moderate
VEGETABLES					
Beet greens Broccoli Carrots Chard Chicory Collard greens Dandelion greens Kale Mustard greens Peppers, hot chili Pumpkin Spinach Sweet potatoes Tomatoes Turnip greens Winter squash	Asparagus Beets Brussel sprouts Corn Green beans Green peas Green peppers Lettuce Okra Romaine Snow peas Summer squash	Broccoli Collard greens Kale Parsley Peppers, green, hot chili Peppers, green, sweet Tomatoes Turnip greens Watercress	Asparagus Brussel sprouts Potato, white Cabbage Cauliflower Peas	Broccoli Brown rice Graham crackers Greens Lentils Oatmeal Popcorn Rye breads Shredded wheat cereal Whole-bran cereals Whole wheat Whole wheat pasta Winter squash	Beans Broccoli Cabbage Cauliflower Eggplant Parsnips Peas Potatoes Squash
FRUIT					
Apricots Cantaloupe Mangoes Nectarines Papayas Peaches	Watermelons	Cantaloupe Grapefruit Guava Lemons Limes Oranges Papayas Strawberries Tangerines	Apricots Bananas Blackberries Cherries Mangoes Peaches Pineapples Raspberries Watermelons	Apples Blackberries Figs, dried Pears Strawberries Tomatoes	Banana Cantaloupe Orange
POSTULATED PROTECTED ORGAN TISSUE					
Lung Gastric Esophagus		Gastric Esophagus		Colon Breast	

Reproduced with permission from Chen MC, Meguid MM. Postulated cancer prevention diets. A guide to food selections. Surg Clin North Am 1986;66:931.

has dramatically declined in parallel with the decline in use of food preservative processes (eg, smoking, salting, and pickling). These procedures are implicated as conducive to the formation of carcinogens and mutagens. In Japan, Chile, Iceland, and many developing nations in the southern hemisphere, the rates, although declining, remain high.

The hypothesis that dietary nitrate and nitrite support the formation of nitrosamines and nitrosamides has been studied extensively in animal models, and it is plausible that this is one mechanism of human gastric carcinogenesis.[12] Vitamin C inhibits this chemical process, and a combination of decreased consumption of nitrite and increased ingestion of fresh fruits and vegetables may account for the reduced incidence of gastric cancer. Epidemiologic studies have found increased risk associated with less frequent consumption of fruits, citrus fruits, and leafy green vegetables[13] (see Table 8-3).

Pancreatic Cancer

Although geographic distribution of pancreatic cancer in humans correlates with international differences in average coffee consumption, no association of coffee use with risk was shown in a prospective Norwegian study.[14] But, more recently, coffee consumption has been shown to be associated with an increased risk factor.[15] Despite this, the available data may be too inconsistent to be conclusive regarding the causal role of coffee consumption in the etiology of pancreatic cancer.

Colonic Cancer

High rates for cancer of the colon occur among populations characterized by high beef consumption, high fat intake, and low cereal consumption. Burkitt[16] hypothesized that diets high in fiber (see Table 8-3) protect against colonic cancer by increasing stool bulk and increasing colonic motility, thereby decreasing transit time. The combination of a high-fat, low-fiber diet appears to raise the risk.[17]

Patients with colorectal cancer have less frequent consumption of cruciferous vegetables, such as broccoli, cauliflower, and cabbage. This is consistent with animal data suggesting that this family of vegetables had specific anticarcinogenic activity.[18] Alcohol consumption has also been linked to cancer of the rectum.[19]

For the purpose of surgical awareness, the issue of the effect of malnutrition in the etiology of gastrointestinal cancer has been greatly simplified in this chapter by citing only salient human data. Despite these obvious limitations, some generalizations regarding common patterns of risk at different cancer sites may be possible. Although the nutrients and mechanisms may vary by site, the single most common underlying factor seems to be the lack or insufficient consumption of fruits and vegetables, which has been linked repeatedly to cancers of the esophagus. Specific cancer sites are linked to specific dietary exposures (eg, nitrates and gastric cancer, or fiber and colorectal cancer). Coffee has been studied in association with cancers of the pancreas. An association exists between dietary fat and risk for cancers of the colon, whereas alcohol is associated with cancers of the rectum. An awareness of these public health issues and subsequent behavioral modification, according to the information provided in Tables 8-2 and 8-3, will go a long way toward ameliorating the frequency of these types of cancer.

NUTRITIONAL SUPPORT IN PATIENTS WITH GASTROINTESTINAL CANCER

The uses of nutritional support, either as enteral or parenteral nutrition, in surgical practice was the subject of an extensive study and report by the Georgetown University Technology Assessment and Practice Guidelines Forum on the Evaluation of Total Parenteral Nutrition.[20–22] Their recommended practice guidelines as they relate to gastrointestinal cancer are closely adhered to in this chapter.

The primary indication for enteral or parenteral nutrition is to support the patient physiologically during an illness, to prevent malnutrition from occurring as a result of therapy, and to correct malnutrition that has occurred secondary to a disease state.[23,24] For definition and quantification of malnutrition, the reader is referred to Meguid and coworkers' review.[23] Thus, the presence of malnutrition, independent of the type of gastrointestinal cancer or its required treatment, along with the anticipation that a patient's nutritional status might deteriorate with surgery, should be the basis for the clinical decision to start nutritional support. There is little disagreement that for either the malnourished surgical patient or the surgical patient at high risk for development of malnutrition during treatment, perioperative or peritherapeutic nutritional support can correct deficits sufficiently to reduce the incidence of postoperative complications to that of well nourished patients undergoing similar operative procedures, and that these deficits can be corrected without additional significant risks arising from the treatment modality of nutritional support.

Frequency of Malnutrition in Patients With Gastrointestinal Cancer

Patients with upper gastrointestinal cancer are at high risk for malnutrition because the presence of malignant disease is often associated with reduced oral intake secondary to anorexia. Furthermore, a series of metabolic alterations leading to a catabolic state, probably initiated by cytokines, alters carbohydrate, fat, and protein metabolism, further contributing to the malnutrition. This adversely influences patient outcome. Also, cancer treatment (ie, extensive surgery, chemotherapy, and radiotherapy) frequently produces additional nutritional wasting in an already nutritionally compromised patient.

The frequency of malnutrition is related to disease site[25–27] (Table 8-4). As shown in Figure 8-2, approximately 60% to 65% of patients with pancreatic, esophageal, gastroduodenal, and abdominal carcinoma are malnourished. In contrast, of those patients presenting with colorectal, hepatobiliary, genitourinary–gynecologic, or retroperitoneal sarcomas, only 30% are malnourished. Thus, two of three patients who present with upper gastrointestinal cancer but only one of three presenting with lower gastrointestinal cancer are malnourished when first diagnosed and require serious nutritional support. This constitutes a reasonable and practical rule of thumb regarding the need for nutritional support when dealing with the patient with gastrointestinal cancer.

TABLE 8-4. *Literature references on incidence of malnutrition relative to gastrointestinal and other cancers*

Reference	Tumor type or site	Incidence of malnutrition
Issell BF, et al, 1978[28]	Lung (squamous cell)	50%
DeWys WD, et al, 1980[29]	Breast	36%
	Sarcoma	39%
	Colon	54%
	Prostate	56%
	Lung (small cell)	60%
	Lung	61%
	Pancreas	83%
	Gastric	83%
Samuels ML, et al, 1981[30]	Testicular cancer (stage III)	25%
Nixon DW, et al, 1981[31]	Colorectal cancer (metastatic)	60%
Popp MB, et al, 1981[32]	Diffuse lymphoma (advanced)	55%
Shamberger RC, et al, 1984[33]	Sarcoma	66%
Goodwin WJ, Torres J, 1984[34]	Head and neck cancer (advanced)	72%
Clamon GH, et al, 1985[35]	Lung (small cell)	~50%
Rickard KA, et al, 1985[36]	Neuroblastoma (advanced)	56%
Bashir Y, et al, 1990[37]	Bronchial carcinoma	66%
Larrea J, et al, 1992[38]	Esophagus	79%
	Rectum	40%
	Breast	9%
Tan YS, et al, 1992[39]	Gastrointestinal cancer	63%

Anorexia

During tumor growth, anorexia and reduced food intake are the major causes leading to development of malnutrition and eventually cachexia. Many hypotheses have been proposed, but consistent data in animals and humans indicate a key role for the hypothalamic serotonergic system in the development of cancer anorexia. As summarized schematically in Figure 8-3, catabolism of muscle during cancer growth occurs as the result of inadequate oral intake, low insulin concentrations, and increased interleukin-1 (IL-1) levels, which lead to gluconeogenesis, and increased plasma tryptophan concentrations. Increased availability of tryptophan, the precursor of serotonin, leads to increased cerebrospinal fluid tryptophan concentrations and increased serotonin synthesis in the hypothalamus, which results in the development of anorexia. The process is mediated by cytokines, particularly IL-1.[40,41] A close link exists between IL-1 and the hypothalamic serotonergic system: peripherally infused IL-1 increases brain tryptophan and serotonin concentrations, and intracerebrally infused IL-1 increases the neuronal

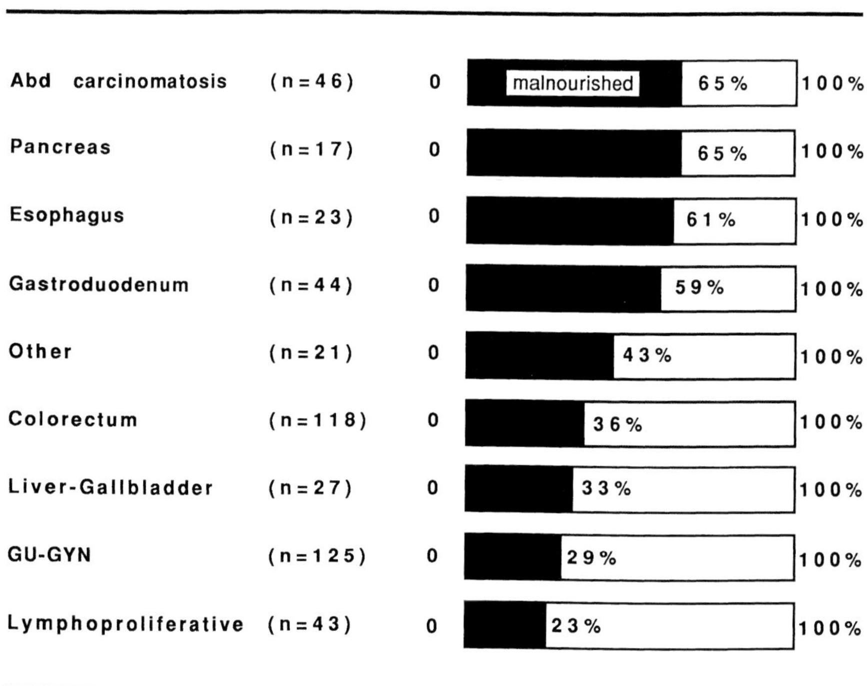

FIG. 8-2. Malnutrition in 464 patients after abdominal operation. GU-GYN, genitourinary-gynecologic.

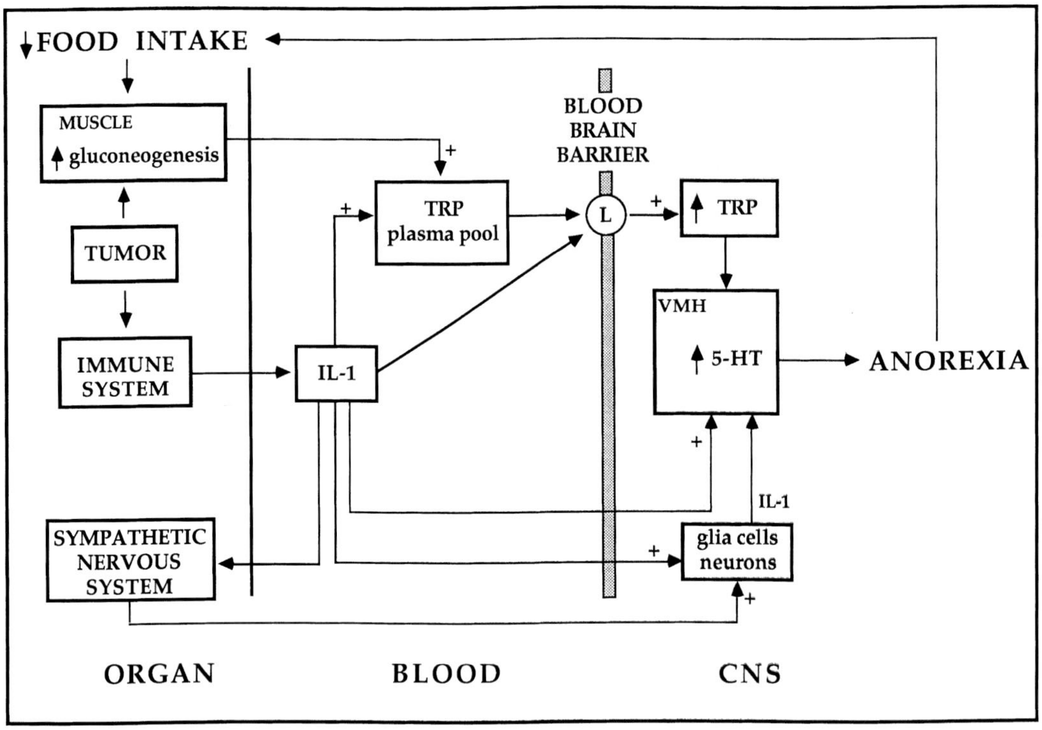

FIG. 8-3. Cytokine/serotonergic hypothesis of cancer anorexia. **CNS,** central nervous system; **5-HT,** 5-hydroxytryptamine; **IL-1,** interleukin-1; **TRP,** tryptophan; **VMH,** ventromedial nucleus of hypothalamus.

firing rate and release of serotonin. Based on our hypothesis (see Fig. 8-3),[42] it is likely that during tumor growth increased production/secretion of IL-1 occurs, which facilitates the supply of tryptophan to the brain. In addition, IL-1 acts on the hypothalamus itself to increase its neuronal activity and serotonin release. In other words, centrally acting IL-1 increases the hypothalamic neuronal firing rate and release of serotonin, whereas peripherally acting IL-1 supplies the hypothalamus with the precursor, tryptophan, to maintain the high rate of serotonin metabolism, leading to anorexia and diminished food intake and thereby reinforcing this vicious cycle (see Fig. 8-3).

Malnutrition and Its Relation to Increased Complications

Malnutrition has a deleterious effect on every major system in the body (Fig. 8-4), thereby affecting structure and function. Clearly, there is a link between deficient preoperative nutritional status and poor operative outcomes, such as gastrointestinal, septic, and nonseptic complications, including death, and prolonged hospital stay (Table 8-5). In the malnourished, the postoperative frequency of complications is higher.

Malnutrition affects postoperative gastrointestinal tract function, leading to a considerable delay in the resumption of normal oral intake. As demonstrated in Table 8-6, in the malnourished patient who has had an abdominal operation and who experiences no complication, the delay in resumption of normal oral intake is longer than in the well nourished counterpart who has had the same operation. And, because the frequency of complications is higher in the malnourished than in the well nourished patient undergoing similar operative procedures, the resumption of normal oral intake in the malnourished patient after a complication is delayed even further.[43]

Hypoproteinemia leads to delayed gastric emptying and prolonged ileus, a greater frequency of wound dehiscence, and an increased risk of wound infection—points repeatedly demonstrated in animal studies. Such studies reinforce repeated observations of higher frequencies of postoperative complications in hypoproteinemic surgical patients, an increased risk of sepsis in malnourished, burned children, and a decreased tolerance for

TABLE 8-5. *Frequency of postoperative complications according to nutritional status after intraabdominal surgery*

	Number of complications				
	Gastrointestinal	Septic	Nonseptic	Death	Total
Well nourished	16%	13%	21%	6%	36%
Malnourished	37%	34%	55%	20%	64%

Reproduced with permission from Meguid MM, Campos ACL, Meguid V, Debonis D, Terz JJ. IONIP: a criterion of surgical outcome and patient selection for perioperative nutritional support.

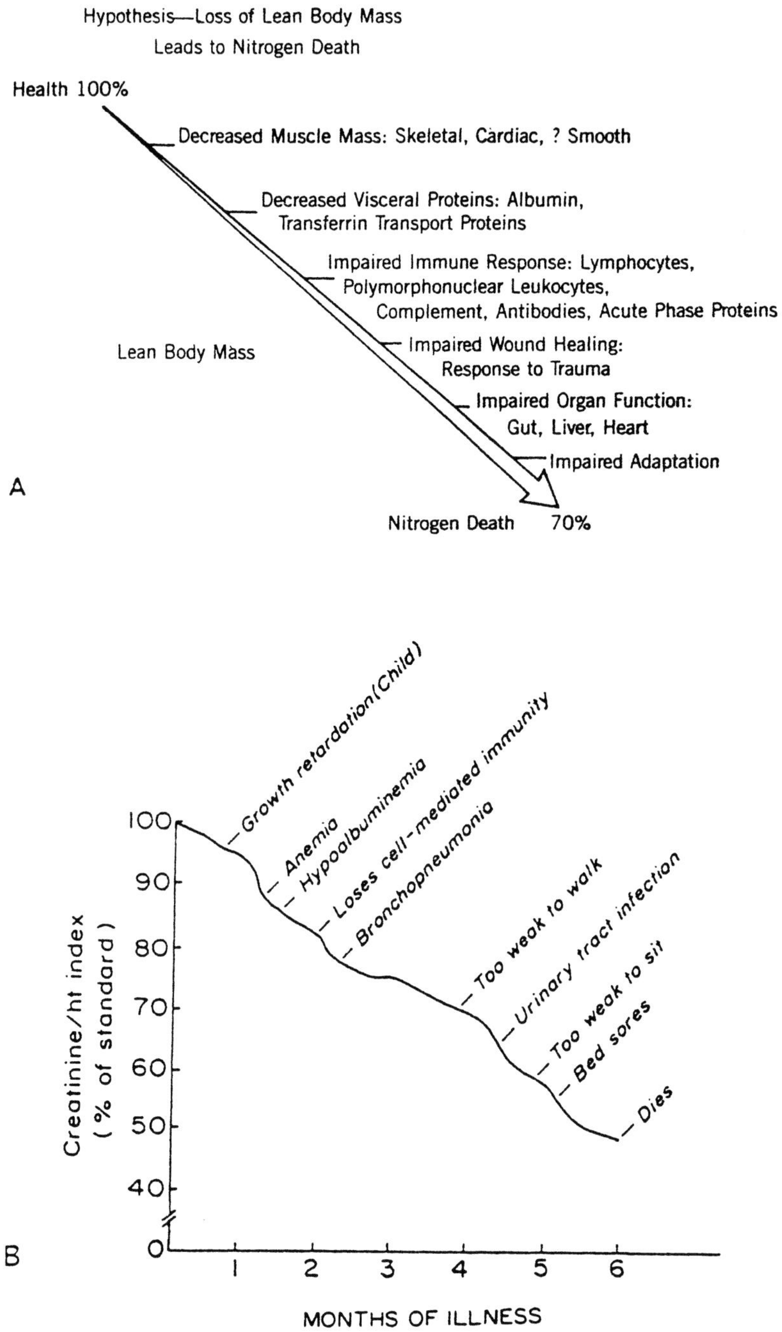

FIG. 8-4. A, Sequence of clinical and laboratory events in the natural history of starvation. (Reproduced with permission from Steffee WP. Malnutrition in hospitalized patients. JAMA 1980;244: 2630.) **B,** Creatinine–height index is a measure of skeletal muscle mass. (Reproduced with permission from Haymsfield SB, Bethel RA, Ansley JD, Nixon DW, Rudman D. Enteral hyperalimentation: an alternative to central venous hyperalimentation. Ann Intern Med 1979;90:63.)

hemorrhagic shock in a state of protein depletion, compared to well nourished control subjects.

Malnutrition also decreases skeletal muscle function and bulk, leading to reduced vital capacity and resting minute ventilation, and a significantly impaired hypoxic ventilatory response. The deterioration of respiratory muscle function leads to a higher frequency of postoperative bronchopneumonia and pulmonary sepsis, and an increased need for pulmonary intubation. Cardiac muscle mass also decreases, leading to a decreased force of cardiac contractility and an increased frequency of postoperative congestive cardiac failure and myocardial infarction. The decreased circulatory volume is associated with a greater frequency of postoperative cardiovascular accidents, and also leads to a fall in glomerular filtration rate, impaired renal function, and postoperative renal failure.

In malnourished patients, fibroblast activity is also reduced, with resultant delayed wound healing, failure of scar contracture, and increased postoperative frequency of wound dehiscence and enterocutaneous fistula formation. Furthermore, as most practicing surgeons intuitively know, more than one postoperative complication tends to develop in the malnourished patient, as shown in Table 8-7. Finally, the lack of adequate nutrient intake or starvation decreases the availability of amino acid precursors necessary for synthesis of brain neurotransmitters, leading to a state of mental dullness, depression, and apathy, as well as a sense of diminished self-motivation.

TABLE 8-6. *Number of days until resumption of oral intake* in 464 patients after abdominal surgery, according to nutritional status and complications*

	Well nourished patients		Malnourished patients	
Involved organ system	No complication	Complication	No complication	Complication
Abdominal carcinomatosis	8	32	22	33
Esophagus	7	18	30	40
Gastroduodenum	9	14	18	40
Pancreas	10	42†	15	29
Colorectum	8	12	19	19
Liver–gallbladder	6	13	11	62
Genitourinary/gynecologic		16	8	20
Lymphoproliferative	6	45†	8	21
Other	13†	10	32	42

* Normal intake is defined as eating 60% of estimated caloric needs.
† Median duration until normal oral intake resumption is disproportionately prolonged by one or more extreme instances.
Reproduced with permission from Meguid MM, Debonis D, Meguid V, Terz JJ. Nutritional support in cancer. Lancet 1983;2:230.

Nutritional Support Indications in Patients With Gastrointestinal Cancer

Whether parenteral or enteral nutrition stimulates tumor growth in humans remains unanswered.[44] This is, however, an irrelevant or impractical question in the context of providing nutritional support to a patient who is receiving active anticancer therapy! The general consensus is that in the absence of nutritional support, the tumor, which has an autonomous metabolism, will continue to grow at the expense of the patient's metabolic and nutritional status. Providing either parenteral or enteral nutrition merely ensures that the host remains nutritionally repleted to withstand surgical and adjuvant therapy.

Guidelines for the Use of Nutritional Support in Patients With Gastrointestinal Cancer

1. Parenteral or enteral nutrition is not *routinely* indicated in previously well nourished or mildly malnourished patients undergoing surgery, chemotherapy, or radiation therapy. Use total parenteral nutrition (TPN) for more severely malnourished patients and in those in whom severe gastrointestinal or treatment toxicities preclude adequate enteral intake for an anticipated 5 days or longer.
2. Patients who are candidates for TPN under the preceding criteria should receive TPN before or in conjunction with the start of therapy.
3. Nutritional support is seldom indicated in patients with advanced cancer associated with significant deterioration of performance status or those patients with disease documented to be unresponsive to chemotherapy or radiation therapy.
4. Nutritional support is not indicated in those patients who have evidence of terminal disease and are not candidates for further antitumor therapy.
5. Total parenteral nutrition is likely of benefit in those patients for whom treatment-associated toxicities preclude adequate oral or enteral intake, representing the dominant impediment to restoration of performance status. Such patients usually respond to antitumor therapy.
6. Nutritional support, either parenteral or enteral, may be of benefit in selected patients with malnutrition in whom the natural history of the underlying tumor is expected to permit a period of normal or near-normal performance status. Such patients usually are receiving antitumor therapy with reasonable expectation of response, or the natural history of the untreated tumor is of a protracted nature (eg, metastatic colon or ovarian cancer), where survival can be greater than 6 months.
7. Nutritional support is probably of no benefit in patients with severe malnutrition and rapidly progressive disease that has not responded to chemotherapy or radiation therapy.

Benefits of Nutritional Support in Patients With Gastrointestinal Cancer

Whenever possible, the gastrointestinal tract should be used. An alternative to TPN in patients who undergo esophageal, gastric, pancreaticobiliary, or colorectal procedures is enteral nutrition by means of an elemental diet delivered via a catheter jejunostomy placed at the time of operation. The rationale for this approach is that, although dysfunction of the stomach usually prevents oral or intragastric feeding after operation, the small bowel almost immediately regains its motility and absorbs nutrients, allowing the infusion of enteral nutrition into the proximal small bowel. An elemental diet seems ideal for postoperative feeding because it is predigested and it is almost totally absorbed.[45] In some patients, a nonelemental diet may also be effective, but it requires greater physician patience and nursing skill compared to the use of TPN.[46] When the use of postoperative TPN was compared to postoperative enteral nutrition in a series of randomized, prospective studies, both TPN and enteral nutrition were considered equally effective as methods of nutritional support.[47–51]

TABLE 8-7. *Summary and comparison of the type and number of postoperative complications and death in well nourished and malnourished patients after abdominal surgery*

Complication	Well nourished (n = 15)	Malnourished (n = 17)
Septicemia	+ *	+ * +
Pancreatitis	+	
Cardiopulmonary	+ +	+ + *+*+*+ +
Intraabdominal abscess		+ + +
Small bowel obstruction		+
Protracted ileus		+
Wound Infection	+ +	+ *
Wound dehiscence		+
Urinary tract infection		+
Total number of complications	6	16
Number with complications (%)	3 (20)†	10 (59)†
Number of deaths (%)	1 (7)‡	5 (29)‡

Multiple complications in individual patients are grouped in a box.

* Deaths.
† $P < 0.01$ (Fisher's exact test).
‡ $P = 0.23$ (Fisher's exact test) .

Reproduced with permission from Mughal M, Meguid MM. The effect of nutritional status on morbidity after elective surgery for benign gastrointestinal disease. JPEN J Parenter Enter Nutr 1987;11:140.

Total Parenteral Nutrition

The pooled analysis of 28 prospective, randomized, controlled trials of TPN use in patients with cancer reported in the English-language literature indicated a significant decrease in major complications, wound infection, and mortality from the use of TPN, compared to control subjects who received no significant amounts of nutrients.[52] TPN is used for supportive care in hospitalized cancer patients in whom it is anticipated that surgery, radiation therapy, or chemotherapy will produce or worsen malnutrition. Studies have shown that in the malnourished patient, the use of TPN may increase tolerance of or response to chemotherapy,[53] radiation therapy,[54] and surgery.[55] However, in cancer patients who are well nourished, reports suggest that the use of TPN is of no benefit and may be associated with higher incidence of infections.[56]

As shown in Figure 8-5, a stepwise linear regression analysis based on 464 patients undergoing abdominal surgery was developed by the principal author to analyze the relations between nutritional status, diagnosis, age, organ system involved with disease, and inadequate oral nutrient intake period (IONIP: defined as the number of days that has elapsed after operation until the patient is eating 60% of predicted caloric requirements[43]). From this analysis, three groups of patients were identified. Group 1 comprises high-risk gastrointestinal cancer patients in whom TPN should be started perioperatively, and includes those of any age who are malnourished and who have a diagnosis of carcinoma of the esophagus, the gastroduodenum, the liver–gallbladder, or the pancreas; an intraabdominal retroperitoneal sarcoma; or abdominal carcinomatosis. Group 2 consists of well nourished patients younger than 40 years of age and with primary carcinoma of any site or stage; usually they do not require TPN. Group 3 comprises well nourished patients older than 40 years of age or malnourished patients of all ages with malignancies of lymphoproliferative, genitourinary–gynecologic, or colorectal origin. Patients in this group need to be observed carefully, with the anticipation that IONIP will last from 5 to 10 days. If a complication occurs in patients in either groups 2 or 3, supportive TPN should be started without delay because IONIP is anticipated to be 10 days or longer, and adjuvant medical and radiation treatments further aggravate malnutrition.

Total parenteral nutrition is increasingly used in terminally ill cancer patients without clearly defined reasons.[57] To determine these reasons, 26 patients with limited life expectancy because of end-stage cancer were given TPN, and the validity of its use evaluated using the criteria of quality of life and ultimate outcome. Patients were divided into two groups according to use of TPN. In group 1 (n = 15; mean age 32 years), TPN was used as an adjunct to medical therapy. In group 2 (n = 11; mean age 56 years), TPN was used for in-hospital supportive care in terminally ill patients for whom no further antitumor therapy was made available. Nutritional status on admission; quality of life as assessed by extent of daily activities, pain, and ability to sustain oral intake; and ultimate treatment outcome were determined. The data are summarized in Table 8-8.

When TPN was given either as an adjunct to in-hospital aggressive therapy for cancer or as in-hospital supportive care, quality of life did not improve in most patients; nor did it influence ultimate outcome. These objective data thus raise the question of the validity of using TPN in terminally ill cancer patients. This practice of "last resort therapy" should be discouraged. Barring the cost factor, it is recognized that subjective physician reasons for giving TPN to terminally ill cancer patients exist, including ethical, religious, and emotional reasons.

Guidelines for the Use of Preoperative Nutritional Support in Gastrointestinal Cancer

1. Two to 3 days of TPN before operation does not improve surgical outcome, but improves physiologic criteria of function.

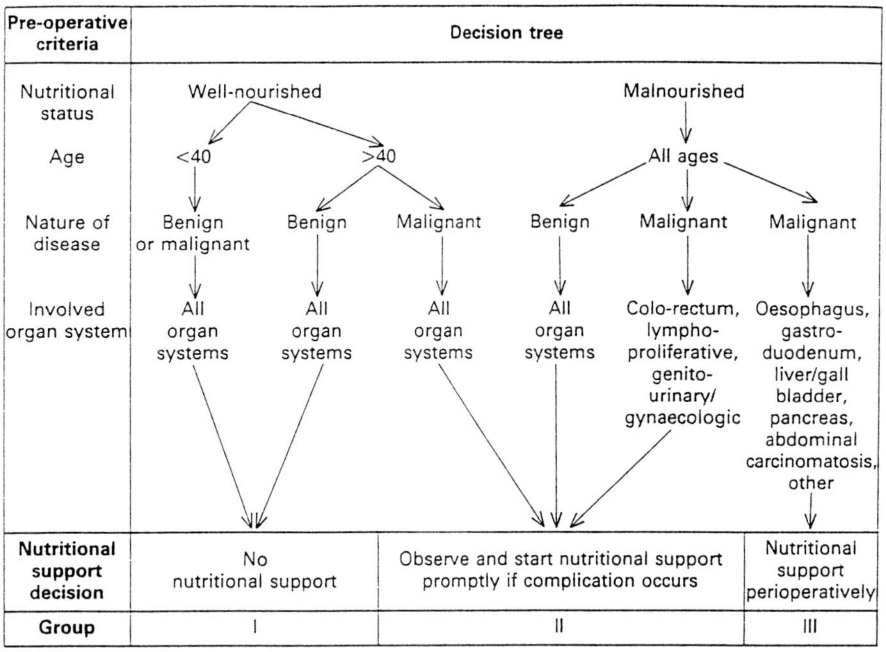

FIG. 8-5. Schema for assessing the need for nutritional support. Decision based on data showing relations between preoperative determined factors and inadequate oral nutrient intake period. (Reproduced with permission from Meguid MM, Campos ACL, Meguid V, Debonis D, Terz JJ. IONIP: a criterion of surgical outcome and patient selection for perioperative nutritional support. Br J Clin Pract 1988; 42:8.)

2. Postoperative surgical outcome is improved after 5 to 7 days of TPN.
3. A significant reduction in major postoperative complications and in mortality is achieved with 7 to 10 days of preoperative TPN.

The question whether preoperative TPN is of benefit in improving outcome has been repeatedly asked and extensively investigated because of its fundamental surgical interest. Table 8-9 summarizes the randomized, prospective trials that have been performed in patients with gastrointestinal disease to clarify the role of preoperative TPN in reducing postoperative morbidity and mortality.[25,26,56,58–60] Because a detailed analysis of these studies has been published,[61] only a few are presented here to support the thesis that malnourished patients benefit from preoperative TPN.

In a study from Germany, Muller and colleagues[27] assigned 125 patients with gastrointestinal carcinoma to receive either a regular hospital diet providing 2400 kcal/d, or preoperative TPN for 10 days. The incidence of malnutrition was 60% in both groups. On average, the control subjects lost 1 kg, whereas the study patients gained 2 kg, which was mostly extracellular fluid because serum albumin and total protein fell. As shown in Figure 8-6, the incidence of intraabdominal abscess, peritonitis, anastomotic leakage, and ileus was significantly reduced in the TPN group (19% vs. 11%, respectively). Although the cause of pneumonia in the control group was not stated, significantly more patients required ventilatory support compared with the TPN group. Operative mortality was significantly less in the TPN group (3% vs. 11%, respectively). Patients in the control group in whom postoperative complications developed were given TPN.

Bellantone and associates,[58] from Rome, Italy, studied 100 patients with a variety of gastrointestinal diseases undergoing resective operation who received either a standard hospital diet or preoperative TPN for at least 7 days. Only 33% of the patients in the study were considered malnourished. No relevant complication related to TPN was observed. The frequency of postoperative wound infection, bronchopneumonia, intraabdominal infection, or septicemia was similar in both groups. However, when only malnourished patients were considered, those who received preoperative TPN had a significantly lower incidence of postoperative sepsis (21% vs. 53.3%). In the subgroups of malnourished patients with gastric cancer, septic complications occurred in 100% of the patients in the control group but in only 16.7% of the study group. Postoperative mortality occurred

TABLE 8-8. *Quality of life and outcome in 26 terminally ill cancer patients receiving total parenteral nutrition*

	Nutritional status			Quality of life		
	Weight loss	Malnourished	Well nourished	Improved	Declined	Died
Group I* (n = 15)	−8.6 kg	11	4	2	6	7
Group II† (n = 11)	−21.0 kg	11	0	3	4	4

* Group I: young patients receiving medical therapy for advanced metastatic cancer.
† Group II: elderly patients receiving total parenteral nutrition and supportive care only for advanced metastatic cancer.

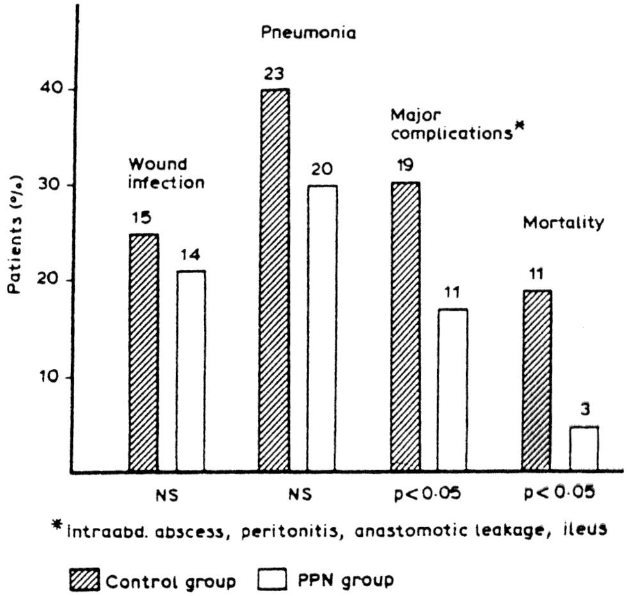

FIG. 8-6. Instances of major postoperative complications in patients who received preoperative parenteral nutrition (PPN), compared with control subjects. Numbers on top of columns refer to number of cases. (Reproduced with permission from Muller JM, Dienst C, Brenner U, Pichlmaier H. Preoperative parenteral feeding in patients with gastrointestinal carcinoma. Lancet 1982;1:68.)

in less than 5%, and was similar in both groups. This study supports the concept that when only malnourished patients are included in the study, the chances of demonstrating gross benefits from preoperative TPN are increased.

In a U.S. multicenter Veterans Affairs TPN study, 395 malnourished patients requiring laparotomy or noncardiac thoracotomy were randomly assigned to receive TPN for 7 to 15 days before and 3 days after surgery, or crystalloids and an oral diet.[56] The rates of major complications during the first 30 days after surgery in the two groups were similar. There was an increased rate of infectious complications in patients defined as either borderline or mildly malnourished, although in these patients, TPN had no demonstrable benefit. In contrast, severely malnourished patients receiving TPN had significantly fewer noninfectious complications versus controls (5% vs. 43%, respectively), with no concomitant increase in infectious complications. Data from this study indicate that the use of preoperative TPN in severely malnourished patients helps reduce postoperative complications.

The most recent study looking at the effects of perioperative nutritional support investigated the effects of at least 10 days of preoperative TPN or total enteral nutrition, both providing 150% of basal energy expenditure nonprotein energy, to reduce major postoperative complications and mortality in a homogeneous patient group with signs of depletion.[62] Fifty patients served as a depleted control group and 49 patients served as a nondepleted reference group and were operated on without delay.

Depleted control patients suffered significantly more septic complications than did patients in the nondepleted reference group. There was no significant difference, however, in septic complications between either of the nutritional support groups and the nondepleted control group. In high-risk patients, those with weight loss greater than 10% of body weight and over 500 mL of blood lost during operation, a significant decrease in major complications was observed as a result of nutritional support. It was concluded that preoperative nutritional support, in patients with severe depletion, resulted in a reduction in major complications to a degree that justifies its routine use in this selected group of patients.

Based on this international series of studies, it is concluded that 2 to 3 days of TPN before operation in malnourished patients with gastrointestinal cancer does not improve surgical outcome. An improvement in outcome is observed with 5 to 7 days of TPN, but only after 7 to 10 days of preoperative TPN in malnourished patients is a statistically significant reduction in major postoperative complications and mortality achieved.[61] Data clearly indicate that TPN is an effective treatment for preventing or treating the malnutrition accompanying neoplastic disease or resulting from antitumor therapy.

Guidelines for the Use of Postoperative Nutritional Support in Gastrointestinal Cancer

1. Improved nutritional status has not been uniformly demonstrated with postoperative TPN.
2. Give TPN when the anticipated period of postoperative functional starvation exceeds 5 days to preserve physiologic and nutritional status and to prevent further deterioration of physiologic function and nutritional status.
3. Total parenteral nutrition (TPN) reduces length of hospital stay.

After surgery, patients usually undergo a period of poor or inadequate oral intake (ie, a period of functional starvation). Most patients with adequate preoperative nutrition are able to tolerate a limited postoperative period of 3 to 5 days without nutrient intake with some loss in weight. The malnourished patient, however, is unable to withstand this type of controlled starvation, particularly if his or her procedure or diagnosis is associated with a recognized high complication rate and if a complication occurs. Hence, the decision to provide TPN immediately after surgery for supportive purposes, in the absence of conclusive contradictory data,[63–65] is usually based on clinical judgment alone. Table 8-10 summarizes the results from randomized, prospective studies concerning the role of parenteral or enteral nutrition in the postoperative period. These data have also been analyzed in detail,[61] and thus only a few examples are cited here.

To evaluate the effect of postoperative nutrition on reducing postoperative morbidity and mortality, Collins and associates[64] in the United Kingdom evaluated the use of intravenous amino acids alone in a group of patients, compared with a second group of patients receiving oral intake and a third group of patients receiving TPN. Patients had either abdominoperineal resection of the rectum or panproctocolectomy. Weight loss before operation ranged from 0% to 30%, and was equally distributed among the groups. Compared to the other postoperative treatments, TPN resulted in a significantly shorter period for

TABLE 8-9. *Summary of results from the use of preoperative total parenteral nutrition in patients undergoing abdominal surgery*

Year, author, type of study	No. of patients/ incidence of malnutrition	Diagnosis	Methods used for nutritional assessment	Composition of TPN solution*	Duration of pre-op TPN (d)	Complications (%)		Mortality (%)		Statistical significance	Change in nutritional status
						Controls	Study	Controls	Study		
1977 Holter and Fischer[25] (prospective randomized)	56 100%	Gastrointestinal cancer	Wt loss >4.5 kg in 2–3 mo	35 kcal/kg/d 0.2 g N/kg/d	3	19.2	13.3	7.7	6.6	NS	Serum albumin ↑ with TPN
Comments: Twenty-eight well nourished patients served as the control group. Of these patients, 7.1% had complications and none died (NS).											
1977 Moghissi, et al[26] (prospective sequential)	15 100%	Resectable esophageal carcinoma	Wt loss > 4–13 kg in 3–7 mo	35 kcal/kg/d 0.18–0.20 g N/kg/d + oral	5–7	?	?	?	?	—	Positive nitrogen balance with TPN. Controls remained negative. 9/10 patients gained wt with TPN; 4/5 patients lost wt (controls).
Comments: "Better" postoperative course with preoperative TPN.											
1979 Heatley, et al[60] (prospective, randomized)	74 ?	Esophageal or gastric cancer	Body weight Immune testing Nitrogen balance	40 kcal/kg/d 0.2 g N/kg/d + oral	7–10	83.3	35.9	22.2	15.4	NS	No change in body wt in both groups. Serum albumin ↓ in both groups. Urinary amino acid N output and immune testing similar in both groups.
Comments: For wound infections only: 30.5% of the control group vs. 7.7% of the study group ($P < 0.05$).											
1982 Muller, et al[27] (prospective, randomized)	127 60%	Gastrointestinal cancer	Weight loss Serum albumin Skin test	44 kcal/kg/d 0.24 g N/kg/d	10	19.0	11.0	11.0	3.0	$P < 0.05$	Wt gain with TPN; wt loss in controls. Serum albumin fell in both groups. Prealbumin, retinol-binding protein, transferrin rose with TPN and fell in controls. Positive skin tests ↑ with TPN, ↓ in controls.

Comments: No difference in incidence of postoperative wound infection and pneumonia.											
1988 Bellantone, et al[58] (prospective, randomized)	100 ?	Gastrointestinal diseases	Serum albumin Total lymphocyte count	30 kcal/kg/d (70% glucose/30% lipids) 0.2 g N/kg/d + oral	≥7	35.3	30.0	3.9	2.5	NS	Not stated.
Comments: When only malnourished patients were evaluated, 53.3% and 21% of the control and study groups, respectively, had complications ($P < 0.05$).											
1988 Smith and Hartemink[149] (prospective, randomized)	34 100%	Gastrointestinal diseases	PNI > 30%	50–60 kcal/kg/d 0.33–0.4 g N/kg/d	10	35.3	17.6	17.6	5.9	NS	Wt gain, ↑ triceps skinfold with TPN, ↑ immunologic state, improved PNI. Serum albumin and transferrin, NS.
Comments: In malnourished patients, TPN is justified when given preoperatively for 10 days.											
1988 Meguid, et al[43] (prospective, randomized)	66 100%	Gastrointestinal cancer	Wt loss > 10% in 2–3 mo Serum albumin Anthropometrics	40 ± 3 kcal/kg/d 0.3 ± 0.02 g N/kg/d + oral	6–12	56.0	31.3	0	3.0	NS	
Comments: Preoperative TPN end point determined by improvement in relaxation rate of adductor pollicis muscle, indicating decreased muscle fatiguability and improvement in stamina. Postoperative end point (eating 60% of preoperative estimated caloric requirements) reached by day 12 in control group, day 8 in TPN group.											
1989 Fan, et al[150] (prospective, randomized)	40 78%	Esophageal cancer	Wt loss > 10%	38.1 ± 5.5 kcal/kg/d 0.23 g N/kg/d + oral	14	75.0	85.0	30.0	30.0	NS	
Comments: Sample size not adequate to show difference. High incidence of catheter-related complications. Duration of hospital stay: TPN group 15 d; control group, 16 d. TPN group exhibited two types of changes in serum albumin concentrations. Those with decreased serum albumin concentrations associated with increased body weight had significantly higher incidence of postoperative pulmonary complications than group exhibiting increased serum albumin concentrations concomitant with increased body weight.											
1991 Veterans Affairs TPN Cooperative Study Group[56]	395 100%	Gastrointestinal and thoracic cancer and benign disease	Wt: 95% or less ideal body wt Serum albumin Serum prealbumin NRI†	1000 kcal above REE N = 1 g:150 kcal	7–15	Overall 24.6	25.5	10.5	13.4		Not stated.
						Infectious 6.4	14.4			$P < 0.20$	
						Noninfectious 22.2	16.7			$P < 0.20$	
						Severe malnutrition noninfectious 43.0	5.0			$P < 0.03$	
Comments: Use of preoperative TPN should be limited to patients who are severely malnourished unless there are other specific indications.											

TPN, total parenteral nutrition; PNI, prognostic nutritional index; REE, resting energy expenditure; NS, not significant.
* Estimated based on the information available in each study for a 60-kg person.

† Nutrition risk index $= 1.519 \times \text{albumin (g/L)} + 0.417 \times \frac{\text{Current wt}}{\text{Usual wt}} \times 100$

Modified from campos ACL, Meguid MM. A critical appraisal of the usefulness of perioperative nutritional support. Am J Clin Nutr 1992;55:117.

TABLE 8-10. *Summary of results from the use of parenteral or enteral nutrition in the postoperative period in prospective, randomized studies*

Year, author, type of study	Operations performed	No. of patients/ group	Nutritional support*	Duration of nutrition support	Methods of nutrition assessment	Results
1978 Collins, et al[64] (prospective, controlled)	Colorectal procedures	10 oral 10 TPN 10 AA	TPN = 36 kcal/kg/d 0.23 g N/kg/d AA = 0.23 g N/kg/d	Until "adequate" oral intake	Anthropometrics Total body nitrogen Total body potassium	Body wt ↓ oral and AA infusion Body wt ↑ TPN Total body potassium ↓ oral Total body nitrogen ↓ oral Skinfold thickness ↓ oral Hospital stay < TPN < oral or ↑ Wound healing: TPN better
Comments: AA infusion, only nutritional benefits; TPN infusion, clinical and nutritional benefits.						
1979 Preshaw, et al[65] (randomized, sequential)	Colorectal procedures	23 oral 24 TPN	TPN = 20–40 kcal/kg/d 0.16 g N/kg/d 0.9 g lipids/kg/d	24 h before until 5 d after operation	Body weight Total protein Serum albumin Total lymphocyte count	Nitrogen balance: TPN = positive, enteral nutrition = negative; anastomotic leak: 4/23 oral; 8/24 TPN (not significant)
Comments: Patients not malnourished. Explanation of increased number of fistulas in TPN group not provided.						
1983 Yamada, et al[63] (prospective, randomized)	Gastrectomy for advanced cancer	12 oral 11 TPN	TPN = 35 kcal/kg/d 0.11–0.13 g N/kg/d 0.9 g lipids/kg/d	18 d, starting 4 d after operation	Body weight Plasma proteins Serum albumin Delayed cutaneous hypersensitivity test Serum immunoglobulins	Body wt: TPN > oral Serum albumin: TPN > oral Phytohematogglutinin: TPN > oral Lymphocyte count/T cell/disease-free interval: TPN > oral Survival rate in noncurative resection: TPN > oral Postoperative complications: oral > TPN
Comments: Total 5-fluorouracil dose was greater in the TPN group because TPN provided patients with greater tolerance.						
1986 Askanazi, et al[66]	Radical cystectomy	22 TPN 15 D_5W	TPN = 1.3–1.6 predicted REE N = 0.3–0.4 g/kg	7 d until oral intake start	Length of hospital stay	Length of hospital stay: TPN = 17 d; D_5W = 24 d
1989 Woolfson and Smith[151] (prospective, randomized)	Esophagectomy Gastrectomy Cystectomy for cancer	62 TPN 60 control	TPN = 35 kcal/kg/d 1 g N/175 kcal non-N energy	6+ d starting 1 d after surgery	Plasma protein, serum albumin, retinol binding protein, thyroxin binding prealbumin, N balance	N balance: TPN = −5 g, control = −12 g Complications: 40% vs. 36% in TPN vs. controls Deaths: 8% and 0%, TPN vs. controls Catheter complications: 20% in TPN, 27% in controls. Time to discharge: 14 vs. 13 d, TPN vs. controls
Comments: Complication rate not lowered by TPN.						
1993 Sandstrom, et al[67] (prospective, randomized)	Gastroesophageal Hepatic Pancreatic Intestinal Vascular Urologic	150 TPN 150 glucose	TPN = 120% MEE 70% glucose 30% lipid Group glucose 250–300 g/h/d	15 d after operation	Anthropometrics, serum albumin, transferrin, retinol binding protein, N balance	Marginal nutritional benefits of TPN. Overall complications and deaths similar. Intolerance to TPN in 20% of cases.
Comments: Not all patients were malnourished on admission. Lack of benefit with systematic use of TPN after major operation.						

TPN, total parenteral nutrition; AA, amino acid solution; REE, resting energy expenditure; D_5W, 5% dextrose in water; MEE, measured energy expenditure.

* Estimated based on the information available in each study for a 60-kg person.

Modified from Campos ACL, Meguid MM. A critical appraisal of the usefulness of perioperative nutritional support. Am J Clin Nutr 1992; 55:117.

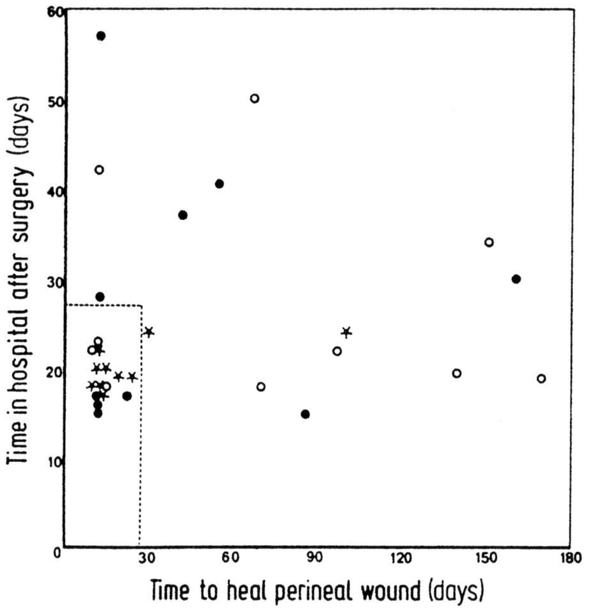

FIG. 8-7. Postoperative hospital stay and time taken for perineal wound healing in 30 patients. Patients at home with healed perineal wounds 4 weeks after surgery are enclosed by the broken line. Closed circles, controls; open circles, amino acid infusion; stars, intravenous hyperalimentation. (Reproduced with permission from Collins JP, Oxby CB, Hill GL. Intravenous amino acids and intravenous hyperalimentation as protein-sparing therapy after major surgery: a controlled clinical trial. Lancet 1978;1:788.)

perineal wound healing (Fig. 8-7), a decrease in the incidence of postoperative sepsis, and a shorter length of hospital stay.

In Japan, a group of patients undergoing gastrectomy for advanced gastric cancer and then given chemotherapy were studied by Yamada and colleagues.[63] Body weight, serum albumin, and total lymphocyte count were all improved by postoperative TPN compared with oral intake. Furthermore, the survival rate for noncurative resection and the disease-free interval were both greater in the group receiving TPN. In this study, TPN enabled the therapeutic dose of chemotherapy to be given, thereby explaining the prolonged disease-free interval.

In the United States, Askanazi and coworkers[66] randomized 35 patients undergoing radical cystectomy to receive either 5% dextrose solution plus electrolytes or TPN for 7 days after surgery until oral intake resumed. If the patients receiving 5% dextrose solution remained incapable of oral intake after 1 week, TPN was instituted. The group receiving immediate postoperative TPN had a median duration of hospitalization of 17 days, whereas the median duration for the group receiving 5% dextrose solution was 24 days (Fig. 8-8). Otherwise, no difference was noted in mortality or complications when the TPN group left the hospital. All other patient characteristics, such as age, sex, stage/grade of tumor, and extent of preoperative radiation therapy, were similar in the two groups. These results demonstrate that immediate postoperative institution of nutritional support reduced hospitalization time after radical cystectomy.

More recently, in Sweden Sandstrom and colleagues[67] published a study of 300 patients who had major abdominal surgery and who were randomized to receive either TPN or glucose starting on the first postoperative day and continuing for up to 15 days. The patients were studied regardless of their nutritional status. The percentage of malnourished patients was not stated. However, both groups had a low mean serum albumin concentration and weight loss on admission. Uncomplicated patients in both groups started to eat by the sixth to seventh postoperative day, confirming the data of Meguid and coworkers.[43] Patients on the glucose regimen who could not eat by the 15th postoperative day were given TPN, and patients who could not tolerate the standard TPN regimen received a modified formula. Several clinical, nutritional, physiologic, functional, and social variables were analyzed. At the end of the study, only marginal improvement in nutritional indices occurred with TPN. Overall complication rate and mortality were similar in both the TPN and glucose groups. The results of this study do not confirm general benefits of early and systematic postoperative nutrition to unselected patients, probably because most patients in both groups were able to eat within 8 to 9 days. However, TPN had a life-supporting role in patients receiving glucose who could not eat by the 15th postoperative day. About 20% of the patients randomized to receive TPN did not tolerate the metabolic and fluid burden associated with the TPN regimen used, and most patients in the TPN group presented with glycosuria without any history of diabetes, raising a question as to the validity of the type of TPN solutions used.

The studies of Collins and associates[64] and Yamada and colleagues[63] suggest that the use of TPN in the postoperative period significantly reduces complications and deaths after major abdominal surgery compared to oral intake. Askanazi and coworkers' study strongly suggests that TPN reduces postoperative length of hospital stay.[66] Only in the study of Sandstrom and colleagues[67] did the use of postoperative TPN not conclusively demonstrate the benefits sought by the investigators.

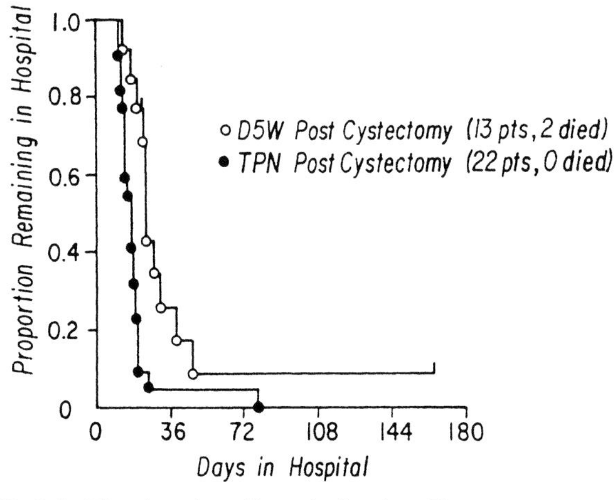

FIG. 8-8. The duration of hospitalization. The group receiving total parenteral nutrition (TPN) had a shorter median duration of hospitalization than the group receiving 5% dextrose in water (D5W) (17 vs. 24 days; $P < 0.002$). (Reproduced with permission from Askanazi J, Starker PM, Olsson C, Effect of immediate postoperative nutritional support on length of hospitalization. Ann Surg 1986;203:236.)

TABLE 8-11. *Usual electrolyte requirements during enteral or parenteral nutrition*

	Typical daily requirement	Forms used in total parenteral nutrition solutions
Sodium	70–100 mEq/d	Chloride, acetate, phosphate
Potassium	70–100 mEq/d	Chloride, acetate, phosphate
Magnesium	15–20 mEq/d	Sulfate
Calcium	10–20 mEq/d	Gluconate
Phosphate	20–30 mmol/d	Sodium, potassium

Reproduced with permission from Meguid MM, Campos ACL. Consensus in clinical nutrition. Cambridge: Cambridge University Press, 1994.

Nutrient Requirements of Patients With Gastrointestinal Cancer

Water and Electrolyte Requirements

A number of different schemes have been devised to calculate maintenance fluid needs, including ones using surface area (1500 mL/m^2/24 h), body weight (20 mL/kg/24 h), or caloric expenditure (1 mL/kcal/24 h). Water requirements based on caloric expenditure for calculating fluid needs is the most practical because 1 mL of water is needed for each calorie expended. Factors that significantly increase water and energy needs include fever, sepsis, burns, trauma, loss of gastrointestinal fluids, cardiac or pulmonary disease, and rapid body mass repletion after malnutrition. Additional fluid losses, such as external gastrointestinal losses and those due to high-output renal fistulas, must be accurately measured and analyzed for major electrolyte content, and the electrolyte content of the replacement fluids must be adjusted accordingly.

The usual daily requirements of electrolytes during enteral or parenteral nutrition are shown in Table 8-11. Withholding sodium, potassium, or phosphorus from TPN prevents retention of the remaining elements, including nitrogen, thereby making their inclusion essential.[68]

Energy and Nitrogen Needs

Energy derived from enteral or parenteral nutrients must include the caloric cost of several factors, including resting energy requirements (5% to 10% greater than basal requirement), increased energy requirements secondary to illness (stress factor), and energy requirements for physical activity (activity factor).

In clinical practice and in the absence of sophisticated techniques for measuring energy requirements, caloric needs to meet resting metabolic expenditure are calculated using the Harris-Benedict equations. These predictive equations are based on height (H), weight (W), age (A), and gender of normal adult men and women.

For men:

$$\text{RME (kcal/d)} = 66.4730 + 13.7516\,(W) + 5.0033\,(H) - 6.7550\,(A)$$

For women:

$$\text{RME (kcal/d)} = 655.095 + 9.563\,(W) + 1.8596\,(H) - 4.6756\,(A)$$

To calculate the patient's energy needs, the stress factor as outlined in Table 8-12 must be considered, whereas the activity factor is not always accounted for because, on admission to the hospital, activity decreases. A criticism of the Harris-Benedict method is that in some patients calorie requirements are somewhat overestimated, whereas in others they are underestimated. For practical purposes and in most cases, however, use of the Harris-Benedict equations is satisfactory. In the malnourished patient, current weight should be used in the Harris-Benedict equation to allow for additional energy required for rapid repletion. In contrast, ideal body weight should be used for slow repletion. If a thermodilution pulmonary artery catheter is in place for close monitoring of cardiac response to fluid resuscitation, it can be used to determine oxygen consumption, which is multiplied by the caloric value of oxygen (4.86 kcal/L at a nonprotein respiratory quotient of 0.85).

Maximum oxidation of infused glucose is approximately 55%. At higher infusion levels, carbon dioxide production is increased and fat synthesis is stimulated. Excessive exogenous glucose infusions embarrass both respiratory and hepatic functions in severely stressed patients. Studies comparing the protein-sparing effect of exogenous glucose and fat calories indicate that in injured and highly stressed patients, only glucose significantly suppresses gluconeogenesis.[69] Hence, parenteral glucose should constitute the major caloric source in TPN, whereas the rest of the caloric source should be from fat. Its use also meets the need for essential fatty acid requirements. Glucose and fat calories are interchangeable in most patients with gastrointestinal cancer. Thus, the addition of fat to glucose TPN, as in the currently used total nutrient admixture system, can achieve effective protein-sparing and anabolism.[70,71]

TABLE 8-12. *Adjustment of resting metabolic expenditure estimated by Harris-Benedict formula or kcal/kg method for changes imposed by various critical illnesses*

Patient	Stress factor
Well nourished, unstressed	1.0
Burned (before skin grafting)	
Normotensive	
0%–20% BSA	1.2–1.5
20%–40% BSA	1.5–2.0
>40% BSA	1.8–2.5
"Burn shock" (period of resuscitation)	0.5
Burned (after successful grafting)	1.0–1.3
Septic (acute phase)	
Normotensive	1.2–1.7
Hypotensive	0.5
Septic (recovery)	1.0
Multiple trauma (acute phase)	
Normotensive	1.1–1.5
Hypotensive	0.8–1.0
Multiple trauma (recovery)	1.0–1.2

BSA, burn surface area.

Modified from Schlichtig R, Ayres RC. Nutritional support of the critically ill. Chicago: Year Book Medical Publishers, 1988.

TABLE 8-13. *Usual recommendations for total parenteral nutrition*

Maintenance	Moderate stress*	Severe stress†
Caloric requirements		
25–30 kcal/kg/d	30–40 kcal/kg/d	40–45 kcal/kg/d
Protein requirements		
1.0–1.2 g/kg/d	1.3–1.4 g/kg/d	1.5–2.0 g/kg/d
Protein restricted:	0.5–0.8 g/kg/d	
Nonprotein calorie-to-nitrogen ratio		
(protein [g] − 6.25 = nitrogen [gm])		
200–300:1	150:1	<100:1

* Elective surgery, peritonitis, soft tissue trauma, malnutrition, renal failure, respiratory failure, pancreatitis, dialysis.

† Extensive burns, multiple long fractures, closed head injury, major sepsis, multiple trauma, multiple organ failure.

Protein calories are usually not included in calculations of daily caloric intake. Protein requirements as amino acids for intravenous feeding are the same as those for normal oral feeding (Table 8-13). Amino acids or protein hydrolysates administered enterally have an effect similar to that observed when given parenterally. It is recommended that 1.0 to 1.2 g/kg/d should be given for maintenance, 1.5 to 2.0 g/kg/d should be prescribed for repletion, and 2.0 to 2.5 g/kg/d given in patients with excess losses.

Calorie-to-Nitrogen Ratio

Using a TPN formula with a calorie : nitrogen ratio of 1 : 150, which provides 1.75 times the Harris-Benedict estimation of caloric expenditure, optimal nitrogen balance is produced in a large group of malnourished patients. Nitrogen balance studies[72] and tracer kinetics studies[73] show that receiving 35 to 40 kcal/kg/d and 0.2 to 0.3 g/kg/d of nitrogen leads to positive nitrogen balance in a large number of patients undergoing surgery for gastrointestinal cancer. This represents a calorie : nitrogen ratio ranging from 200 : 1 to 130 : 1.

Vitamins and Trace Elements

The recommended daily maintenance doses for vitamins and trace elements in parenteral requirements are at least as great as in the oral requirement, and are summarized in Table 8-14. Few data on their specific requirements for a variety of disease states, such as gastrointestinal cancer, exist for patients receiving TPN.

Techniques of Feeding the Patient With Gastrointestinal Cancer

In any given clinical situation, optimal perioperative feeding may be achieved by a combination of enteral and parenteral means. In the presence of a physiologically functional and dependable gastrointestinal tract, the use of the enteral route is desirable because of its numerous physiologic advantages. These include maintenance and stimulation of gut muscle mass, the hepatoenteral axis, brush border enzymes, and the barrier integrity and immunologic function of the gut.

Safe and Cost-Effective Use of Enteral and Parenteral Nutritional Support

The safety associated with the use of either enteral or parenteral nutrition is related to the existence of a nutrition support team and the use of standardized order forms. In the final report and statement of the Georgetown University Technology Assessment and Practice Guidelines Forum on the Evaluation of Total Parenteral Nutrition, published in 1990,[20–22] it was concluded that:

> . . . based on available data, it is recommended that the most safe and cost-effective care and delivery of nutritional support to patients in the hospital or home setting, either as TPN or using the enteral route, should be provided and supervised by knowledgeable health care professionals.

TABLE 8-14. *Recommended daily maintenance dose for vitamins and trace elements*

Element	Oral*	Intravenous†
Thiamine (B_1)	1.4 mg	3 mg/d
Riboflavin (B_2)	1.6 mg	3.6 mg/d
Nicotinic acid (niacin)	18 mg	40 mg/d
Pyridoxine (B_6)	2.2 mg	4 mg/d
Pantothenic acid	7 mg	15 mg/d
Folate	400 μg	400 μg/d
Vitamin B_{12}	3 μg	5 mg/d
Ascorbic acid	60 mg	100 mg/d
Vitamin A	1000 μg RE†	2500 IU/d
Vitamin D	5 μg	5 μg/d
Vitamin E	10 mg	50 mg/d
Vitamin K	NR§	10 mg/wk
Iron	2 mg	2 mg
Zinc‖	15 mg	4–10 mg¶
Copper	2–3 mg	0.5 mg
Chromium	0.05–0.2 mg	10–15 μg
Iodine	150 μg	150 μg
Fluorine	1.5–4 mg	0.4 mg
Manganese	2.3 mg	0.15–0.8 mg
Molybdenum	100 μg	100–200 μg
Selenium	20–50 μg	40–120 μg

* Committee on Dietary Allowances, 1980 and † Nutrition Advisory Group, 1979, Subcommittee on the 10th edition of the RDAs, Food and Nutrition Board Commission on Life Sciences, National Research Council. Recommended Dietary Allowances, 10th ed, Washington, DC: National Academy Press: 1989.

‡ Retinal equivalents: 1 μg RE = 1 μg retinol or 3.33 IU.

§ No recommendation.

‖ Patients with diarrhaea or ileostomies lose about 17 mg of zinc per liter of feces, but for patients with a high small bowel fistula, the losses are about 12 mg/L of fistula discharge.

¶ Multiplied by 2.5 if given as zinc sulfate. Because only 20% of orally administered zinc is absorbed, a further multiplication by 5 is required if given orally. Zinc levels in the blood reflect zinc ingestion rather than balance.

These are the essential goals of safety (the least mechanical, metabolic, and septic complications), improved quality of care and of cost-effective nutritional support, as best attained by utilization of a multi-disciplinary team approach of interested and appropriately-trained professionals.

Nutrition support teams have had the greatest impact in reducing all types of complications related to the delivery of nutrients to hospitalized patients. Before the advent of the nutrition support team, the average rates of mechanical, septic, and metabolic complications in one study were 33%, 21%, and 36%, respectively. After the team was instituted, these fell dramatically to 3.2%, 6.5%, and 3%, respectively. These representative data elegantly demonstrate the effectiveness and cost benefits of a nutrition support team.[74]

Techniques of Enteral Nutrition

Nasogastric

When the gastrointestinal tract is functioning but the patient will not or cannot eat, then tube feedings should be used. Patients with anorexia, nausea, oropharyngeal obstruction, or central nervous system disease can benefit from such tube feedings. Small, pliable nasogastric tubes are available and well tolerated by most patients. Despite this, the subjective distresses of nasogastric tube feeding in rank order include deprivation of tasting, drinking, and chewing of food; nasal soreness; rhinitis, sinusitis, and esophagitis; and mouth breathing. A distinct disadvantage of the nasogastric route is the concomitant increase in upper airway resistance, which interferes with ventilatory exchange, particularly in patients with chronic obstructive pulmonary disease. Under these circumstances, an alternate route, as outlined in the following sections, is best selected.

Pharyngostomy and Esophagostomy

Pharyngostomy or cervical esophagostomy (hypopharyngostomy) is indicated when a feeding tube in the nasopharynx is not tolerated or is contraindicated (eg, in borderline respiratory status), or when feedings in the hospital setting are necessary for prolonged periods. Either method is particularly useful in patients with prior subtotal gastrectomy or esophagogastrectomy; head and neck operations; and chronic obstructive pulmonary disease. The advantages of these procedures are that feeding can be provided by way of a stoma whose proximity to a potentially contaminated tracheotomy site does not pose a sepsis problem. Formal esophagostomy (mucosal incision below the cricopharyngeus) is usually performed in conjunction with head and neck procedures.[75] For long-term home enteral feeding, a permanent sinus can be created, allowing the feeding tube to be removed between meals.

Minor problems associated with the use of a pharyngostomy or esophagostomy include access site skin or soft tissue irritation, and accidental extubation because of excess length of the exteriorly placed tube. Major complications may include pulmonary aspiration due to vomiting from reflux esophagitis, stricture of the distal esophagus secondary to acid reflux around the tube, and arterial erosion with exsanguination, particularly in patients whose necks have been heavily irradiated.

Gastrostomy

In the patient undergoing gastrointestinal surgery, the advantages of a tube gastrostomy for feeding purposes include easy access to the stomach and bypassing more proximal esophageal mechanical, surgical, or functional obstructions.

Of the two basic types of gastrostomy, the first, the Stamm gastrostomy (G-tube), is intended for temporary use and the stoma tends to close promptly when the tube is removed.[76] The second is a permanent gastrostomy, in which a formal mucocutaneous ostomy is surgically fashioned (Depage-Janeway).[77] This procedure is more complex but has the advantage of not requiring the presence of a mechanical tube between feedings, and is indicated for permanent gastrostomy feedings. Some methods provide a valve within the gastrostomy[78] or interpose a reverse jejunal segment between the gastric ostium and the anterior abdominal wall to maintain gastrostomy continence.[79] Both types are useful for home enteral nutrition programs.[80]

Percutaneous Endoscopic Gastrostomy

A percutaneous endoscopic gastrostomy is indicated for patients requiring long-term enteral feeding who are considered poor risks for general anesthesia and laparotomy.[81] Contraindications to placement of a percutaneous endoscopic gastrostomy include ascites; morbid obesity; esophageal stricture, reflux, or obstruction; esophageal or gastric varices; and previous gastric surgery. Complication rates in reported series range from 7% to 10% and include abdominal wall infections, pericatheter leakage, pneumoperitoneum, intraabdominal extravasation, gastrocolic fistula, cutaneous stomal enlargement, and colonic or transcolonic placement.[82]

Jejunostomy

A tube jejunostomy is indicated when prolonged enteral nutritional support is anticipated, usually starting in the early postoperative period. The size of the catheter is usually relatively small (8 Fr), and its use is indicated when there is a proximal obstruction or fistula in the gastrointestinal tract, in the absence of a stomach, or when recovery of small bowel motility is anticipated long before recovery of gastric motility. The advantages of jejunostomy over gastrostomy are less stomal leakage and skin erosion; less gastric and pancreatic secretion because the stomach and duodenum are bypassed; less nausea, vomiting, and bloating compared to gastric or duodenal feeding, provided elemental diets are used; and reduced risk of pulmonary aspiration. As with nasoduodenal or nasojejunal feedings, a continuous infusion of isotonic formula is the optimal method of feeding with a jejunostomy.[83] A potential problem with intrajejunal feeding when polymeric diets are used is that there may be inadequate mixing of the nutrients with bile and pancreatic enzymes, resulting in incomplete digestion and, hence, malabsorption. This problem can be obviated by the use of an elemental diet. Surgeons have begun placing jejunostomy feeding tubes laparoscopically, and data on this technique and its complications are being collected.

Efficacy of Treatment

Most nutritional support plans encourage the use of the gastrointestinal tract whenever feasible, because it is a safe and effective route, and in general is cheaper than parenteral nutrition. The current generations of enteral diets are superior to current parenteral solutions because they contain glutamine, arginine, fish oils, nucleosides, and nucleotides. These nutrients have been shown to have beneficial physiologic effects in supporting gastrointestinal mucosal growth and function, important for critically ill patients in whom the gut mucosal barrier may become compromised.[84,85]

In cancer patients, enteral nutrition has been shown to increase body weight and lead to positive nitrogen balance, with suppression of protein catabolism.[86–88] In addition, some indices of immune function, such as complement factors and lymphocyte number, improved better with enteral nutrition compared with TPN.[89]

A few studies suggest that TPN is superior to enteral nutrition and that weight gain, nitrogen balance, and serum albumin are better restored in TPN compared with enteral nutrition.[27,90,91] Care must be taken when evaluating data of this type, because nutritional regimens were rarely homogeneous and oral diets often were not standardized. In addition, differences reported are often marginal and do not lead to improved treatment response rate or survival. Therefore, the indiscriminate use of TPN is not justified in malnourished cancer patients with a functional gastrointestinal tract, in whom perioperative enteral nutrition appears to be as effective as TPN in nutritional replenishment.

Experimental data suggest a selective indication for enteral nutrition in cancer patients receiving radiation therapy and chemotherapy.[92] Although oral diets may exacerbate the acute gastrointestinal side effects of radiation therapy, it has been reported that the use of elemental diets in dogs receiving abdominal radiation results in a significant protection of terminal ileum from mucosal damage, compared with a group of dogs receiving normal kennel rations.

Oral supplementation with glutamine may also further potentiate the beneficial effects of enteral nutrition. Glutamine is an essential nutrient for actively replicating cells. Tumors are major glutamine consumers and lead to host glutamine depletion, resulting in depressed host immune status and impaired mucosal integrity. Oral glutamine supplementation enhances the tumoricidal effectiveness of methotrexate and radiation therapy, while reducing morbidity and mortality.[93,94] It is likely that at least part of these effects results from the route of administration. In tumor-bearing animals, intestinal extraction of circulating glutamine across the basolateral membrane is diminished, whereas the uptake from gut lumen through the brush border is increased.[95] Accordingly, oral glutamine supplementation is preferable to parenteral administration because it supports host gastrointestinal cells without providing the tumor with an essential nutrient.[96] Studies addressing the effects of oral glutamine supplementation on morbidity, survival rate, and mortality of cancer patients receiving high-dose chemotherapy are underway.

Complications of Enteral Nutrition

Mechanical complications of nasogastric, pharyngostomy, and esophagostomy tubes fall into two broad categories: low-frequency–high-morbidity complications, and high-frequency–low-morbidity complications[97]; these are summarized in Table 8-15.

TABLE 8-15. *Mechanical complications of 255 feeding tubes*

Frequency	Complication	Morbidity High	Morbidity Low
Low	Carotid artery blowout	2	
	Acute abdomen	1	
	Aspiration	1	
	Tube intolerance → parenteral nutrition		6
	Malposition		3
	Cellulitis		1
	Cracked hub		1
High	Clogged tube		12
	Tube removed		120

Reproduced with permission from Butters M, Campos AC, Meguid MM. High frequency–low morbidity mechanical complications of tube feeding: a prospective study. Clin Nutr 1992;11:87.

Low-frequency–high-morbidity complications occur in less than 5% of patients. But, because of their dramatic nature and the notoriety they attract, many have been the subjects of single case reports, and they tend to overshadow the general usefulness of this route of feeding. They include injury along the nasogastric tube insertion site, arterial erosion, perforation of the gastrointestinal tract, and aspiration pneumonitis.

High-frequency–low-morbidity mechanical complications occur in more than 50% of patients[97,98] and consist mostly of dislodgement of feeding tubes. This complication can range from a minor annoyance to a major problem associated with impaired nutrient intake secondary to missed feedings, the extra time required and the problems and risks inherent in reinserting a tube after surgery, and the increased cost of supplies if a new tube is required. Replacement of a feeding tube is potentially a high-morbidity complication (eg, accidental removal of a gastrostomy or jejunostomy tube within 24 hours of operative placement, or of a nasogastric tube placed across a fresh esophageal anastomosis because in so doing one could disrupt the anastomosis).

Common problems related to gastrostomy use include discharge of gastric juice from the gastrostomy stoma site, which irritates the surrounding skin, and anastomotic leaks that may cause local infection, abscess formation, or peritonitis. Reported complication rates range from 6.5% to 15.7%, with mortality rates of 6.1% to 37%, reflecting the underlying condition of the patients considered for this procedure.[99,100]

Among the list of complications reported for jejunostomy use are free peritoneal leak, small bowel fistulization, small bowel obstruction, pneumonatosis intestinalis, and jejunal varices.[101]

The *metabolic complications* of enteral nutrition and their frequencies include fluid overload (31%), electrolyte imbalance (30%), hyperglycemia (30%), and uremia and dehydration (15%).[102] Symptoms of abdominal bloating, cramps, and diarrhea are related to high rates of feeding and to the high caloric density of the formula (ie, high fat content), although paralytic ileus and side effects of parasympathomimetic drugs must be excluded. Their frequency can be decreased when enteral feeds are administered on a continuous basis. Among the pathogenetic

(text continues on page 128)

SUNY Health Science Center
Syracuse

University Hospital

CONTINUOUS ENTERAL NUTRITION ORDER FORM

CHECK THE DESIRED ROUTE OF ADMINISTRATION AND FORMULA. FOLLOW THE SCHEDULE AS OUTLINED BELOW.

❑ **JEJUNOSTOMY** ❑ **NASODUODENAL** ❑ **NASOGASTRIC** ❑ **GASTROSTOMY**

PRODUCT	CALORIES/ml	PRODUCT	CALORIES/ml
❑ Advera	1.28	❑ NutriHep ◆	1.5
❑ ALITRAQ *	1.0	❑ Nutrivent/Pulmocare•	1.5
❑ Deliver 2.0 (Isocal HCN)	2.0	❑ Suplena	2.0
❑ Glucerna	1.0	❑ Sustacal Plus/Ensure Plus•	1.5
❑ Impact	1.0	❑ Ultracal	1.06
❑ Immun-Aid*	1.0	❑ Vivonex Plus*	1.0
❑ Isocal/Osmolite•	1.06		
❑ Isocal HN/Osmolite HN•	1.06		
❑ Lipisorb	1.35		
❑ Nepro	2.0		

* *Mixed and delivery by dietary*
◆ *Requires Approval of Nutrition Support Team*
• *Specific products interchanged based on product availability*

ADVANCEMENT SCHEDULE

1. Begin full strength at 25 ml/h.
2. Advance 10 ml/h q 6h as tolerated to goal of ______ ml/h.

ENTERAL NUTRITION ORDERS

1. **Pre-NG Feeding:** If small bore feeding tube is used, obtain chest x-ray to verify feeding tube in stomach.
2. **Nursing:**
   - Keep patient's head elevated at 30° at all times.
   - Give formula at room temperature, hang time 8h.
   - Check residual per nursing protocol.
   - q shift: check position of NG-tube, I/O, urine S/A or fingerstick glucose. (Call if fingerstick > 200).
   - q day: weight, cumulative I/O.
3. **Food and Nutritional Services:** Daily calorie count per dietitian.
4. **Lab Values: Day 1:** Nutrition Panel I and II
   Thereafter: q Tuesday: Nutrition Panel I and II
   Notify MD if glucose ≥ 200 mg/dl.
5. Problems of persistent nausea, diarrhea, and/or vomiting: contact a member of the Nutrition Support Team.

NUTRITION PANELS
I - Na, K, HCO_3, Cl, Glucose
II - ALP, creat, BUN, PO_4, Alb, Ca, Mg

MODULAR COMPONENTS (WHEN SPECIAL REQUIREMENTS ARE NEEDED)

Establish tolerance to designated enteral formula at goal rate before adding modular component. Select the desired modular component and follow the schedule below.

PRODUCT	CALORIES
❑ Polycose (CHO) *	23/Tbsp
❑ Promod (PRO) *	17/Tbsp
❑ Microlipid (FAT) *	4.5/ml
❑ MCT Oil (FAT) *	7.6/ml

1. Add __________ per 1000 ml enteral formula. If a second component: add __________ to above.
2. Mix thoroughly.
3. Run mixture at __________ ml/hr..
4. Follow enteral nutrition orders above.
5. Note osmotic effect that Polycose and Promod have on enteral prescription.
6. Establish tolerance to one modular component before addition of a second.

* *Mixed and delivered by dietary* • *Specific products interchanged based on product availability*

Noted by ______________________ **Signature** ______________________ **M.D.**

Print/Stamp Name ______________________ **M.D.**

Date __________ **Time** __________ **Date** __________ **Time** __________

40180 CLINICAL DATA SERVICES (4/94) G3.00

FIG. 8-9. Continuous enteral nutrition order form.

ENTERAL NUTRITION FORMULAS
(Analysis/1000 ml)

		Kcal/	gm/L			Non-Pro	mg/mEq/L		mg/L			mOsm/	ml for	Fiber	Indications
Formula	Form	ml	PRO	CHO	FAT	Kcal:gmN	Na	K	Ca	Mg	Phos	Kg H_2O	RDA	gm/L	for Use
Advera	Liquid	1.28	60	216	23	112:1	1046/45	2827/72	845	338	845	680	1515	8.9	Specialized nutrition for patients with HIV or AIDS
ALITRAQ	Powder	1.0	52.6	165	15.5	94:1	1000/44	1200/31	734	267	734	575	1500	---	Glutamine enriched for stressed patient with impaired GI function
Deliver 2.0/ Isocal HCN	Liquid	2.0	75	200	102	145:1	800/35	1690/43	1010	400	1010	640	1000	--	Very high calorie and nitrogen formula in limited fluid volume
Glucerna	Liquid	1.0	42	94	56	125:1	928/40	1561/40	704	282	704	375 Isotonic	1422	13.7	Formula for patient with diabetes or glucose intolerance
Immun-Aid	Powder	1.0	80	120	22	47:1	575/25	1055/27.8	500	200	500	460	2000	---	Formula for immuno-compromised patient. High in BCAA
Impact	Liquid	1.0	56	132	28	71:1	1100/48	1300/33	800	270	800	375 Isotonic	1500	---	Formula for immuno-compromised patient
Lipisorb	Liquid	1.35	57	161	57	125:1	1350/59	1690/43	850	340	850	630	1600	---	A readily absorbed fat blend with MCT to improve fat absorption
Nepro	Liquid	2.0	69.9	215.2	95.6	157:1	829/36.1	1057/27	1373	211	686	635	947	---	Moderate protein, calorically-dense product for patient requiring fluid and electrolyte restrictions
NutriHep	Liquid	1.5	40	290	21.2	209:1	320/14	1320/34	1000	400	1000	690	1000	--	High BCAA, low aromatic AA formula for patient with hepatic failure (encephalopathy)
Nutrivent or Pulmocare	Liquid Liquid	1.5 1.5	68 63	101 106	95 92	114:1 125:1	752/33 1310/57	2240/57 1902/49	1200 1057	600 423	1200 1057	450 490	1000 947	-- --	High fat formula for pulmonary disease; Nutrivent has omega-3 fatty acids and MCT
Osmolite or Isocal	Liquid Liquid	1.06 1.06	37 34	145 132	39 43	153:1 167:1	640/28 527/23	1020/26 1316/34	530 630	212 210	530 530	300 300 Isotonic	1887 1887	-- --	Isotonic formula
Osmolite HN or Isocal HN	Liquid Liquid	1.06 1.06	44 44	141 124	37 45	125:1 125:1	930/40 930/40	1570/40 1590/41	758 850	304 340	758 850	300 270 Isotonic	1321 1179	-- --	Isotonic formula with increased protein
Suplena	Liquid	2.0	30	255.2	95.6	392:1	783/34	1116/28.5	1385	211	728	600	947	---	Low in protein, fluid, PO_4, and electrolytes; high calorie for renal diet supplementation
Sustacal HC/ Sustacal Plus or Ensure Plus	Liquid Liquid	1.5 1.5	61 55	190 200	58 53	134:1 146:1	850/37 1141/50	1480/38 2113/54	850 706	340 283	850 706	650 690	1200 1420	--- --	High nitrogen formula for increased calories in limited fluid volume
Ultracal	Liquid	1.06	44	123	45	128:1	930/39.7	1610/41.7	850	340	850	310 Isotonic	1250	14.4	Isotonic formula with fiber (oat and soy)
Vivonex Plus	Powder	1.0	45	190	6.7	149:1	630/27	1070/27	557	222	557	650	1800	---	Elemental formula with glutamine

MODULAR COMPONENTS

			gm			mg/mEq		mg			mOsm/	ml for	Fiber	Indications
Formula	Form	Kcal	PRO	CHO	FAT	Na	K	Ca	Mg	Phos	Kg H_2O	RDA	gm/L	for Use
Polycose	Powder	23/tbsp	0	6/tbsp	0	110/4.8/ 100 gms	10/< 1/ 100 gms	30/100 gms	---	5/100 gms	40/tbsp	---	---	Carbohydrate source, glucose polymers
Promod	Powder	17/tbsp	3/tbsp	< 0.5/ tbsp	< 0.5/ tbsp	227/10/ 100 gms	985/25/ 100 gms	880/100 gms	---	660/100 gms	18/tbsp	---	---	Protein source (whey)
Microlipid	Liquid	4.5/ml	0	0	500/L	---	---	---	---	---	60	---	---	Long chain fat source that stays in suspension
MCT Oil	Liquid	7.6/ml	0	0	884/L	---	---	---	---	---	---	---	---	Medium chain triglycerides source

FIG. 8-9. *Continued.*

SUNY Health Science Center
Syracuse

University Hospital

INTERMITTENT ENTERAL NUTRITION
ORAL SUPPLEMENTATION ORDER FORM

CHECK THE DESIRED ROUTE OF ADMINISTRATION AND FORMULA. FOLLOW THE SCHEDULE AS OUTLINED BELOW.

(❑ **NASOGASTRIC** ❑ **GASTROSTOMY:** COMPLETE A 1 & 2 BELOW) ❑ **ORAL** (COMPLETE **B**)

A. 1. CHECK PRODUCT SELECTION FOR INTERMITTENT ADMINISTRATION

PRODUCT	CALORIES/ml	PRODUCT	CALORIES/ml
❑ Advera	1.28	❑ NutriHep ◆	1.5
❑ ALITRAQ *	1.0	❑ Nutrivent/Pulmocare•	1.5
❑ Deliver 2.0/Isocal HCN	2.0	❑ Suplena	2.0
❑ Glucerna	1.0	❑ Sustacal Plus/Ensure Plus•	1.5
❑ Impact	1.0	❑ Ultracal	1.06
❑ Immun-Aid*	1.0	❑ Vivonex Plus*	1.0
❑ Isocal/Osmolite•	1.0		
❑ Isocal HN/Osmolite HN•	1.06		
❑ Lipisorb	1.35		
❑ Nepro	2.0		

* MIXED AND DELIVERY BY DIETARY
◆ *REQUIRES APPROVAL OF NUTRITION SUPPORT TEAM*
• *SPECIFIC PRODUCTS INTERCHANGED BASED ON PRODUCT AVAILABILITY*

2. INTERMITTENT ENTERAL NUTRITION ORDERS

STAGE	AMOUNT OF FULL STRENGTH FORMULA	TIME
I	120 ml	06-10-14-18-22
II	240 ml	06-10-14-18-22
III	360 ml	06-10-14-18-22
IV	400 ml	06-10-14-18-22
V	480 ml	06-10-14-18-22

a. Advance one stage q 24h as tolerated until a final stage of (check one): ❑ Stage V or ❑ Stage _____ (specify) Maximum volume/feeding is 480 ml. If in 24h more formula is needed, additional bolus feedings can be provided. Indicate specific times when to administer the additional feedings. ______________________________

b. Flush tube **before** and **after** each feeding with 50 ml water.

c. Check position of NG feeding tube (if appropriate) per nursing protocol.

d. **Nursing:**
- During feeding and for 60 min. after, patient to sit upright at ≥ 45°, 90° preferred.
- Give formula at room temperature.
- Check residual. If > 100 ml, refeed 100 ml, discard rest and notify MD.
- Daily weight, I/O.

e. **Food and Nutritional Services:** Daily calorie count per dietitian.

f. **Lab Values:** Nutrition Panel-I q Tuesday

g. Call Nutrition Support Team for problems of persistent nausea, diarrhea and/or vomiting.

NUTRITION PANEL-I
Na, K, HCO_3, Cl, Glucose

B. ORAL SUPPLEMENTS : SELECT PRODUCT TYPE/FLAVOR AND ADMINISTRATION SCHEDULE

PRODUCT: FLAVORS AVAILABLE	CALORIES
❑ Sustacal Plus/Ensure Plus: Vanilla, Chocolate, Strawberry•	1.5/ml
❑ Fortified Pudding: Vanilla*	250/can
❑ Fortified Clear Liquid Drink: Punch *	136/8 oz serving
❑ Fortified Shake: Vanilla, Chocolate, Strawberry *	190/4 oz serving
❑ Nutrivent/Pulmocare: Vanilla•	1.5/ml
❑ Vivonex Plus: Variety of Flavor Packets *	10-15.5/packet

ADMINISTER PRODUCT:

With Meals:	❑ TID	❑ BID
Between Meals:	❑ TID	❑ BID
Evening Snack:		❑

* *MIXED AND DELIVERED BY DIETARY*
• *SPECIFIC PRODUCTS INTERCHANGED BASED IN PRODUCT AVAILABILITY*

Noted by ______________________ **Signature** ______________________ **M.D.**

Print/Stamp Name ______________________ **M.D.**

Date __________ **Time** __________ **Date** __________ **Time** __________

40175 CLINICAL DATA SERVICES (4/94) G3.00

FIG. 8-10. Bolus enteral nutrition oral supplementation order form.

ENTERAL NUTRITION FORMULAS
(Analysis/1000 ml)

Formula	Form	Kcal/ ml	gm/L PRO	CHO	FAT	Non-Pro Kcal:gmN	mg/mEq/L Na	K	mg/L Ca	Mg	Phos	mOsm/ Kg H_2O	ml for RDA	Fiber gm/L	Indications for Use
Advera	Liquid	1.28	60	216	23	112:1	1046/45	2827/72	845	338	845	680	1515	8.9	Specialized nutrition for patients with HIV or AIDS
ALITRAQ	Powder	1.0	52.6	165	15.5	94:1	1000/44	1200/31	734	267	734	575	1500	---	Glutamine enriched for stressed patient with impaired GI function
Deliver 2.0/ Isocal HCN	Liquid	2.0	75	200	102	145:1	800/35	1690/43	1010	400	1010	640	1000	--	Very high calorie and nitrogen formula in limited fluid volume
Glucerna	Liquid	1.0	42	94	56	125:1	928/40	1561/40	704	282	704	375 Isotonic	1422	13.7	Formula for patient with diabetes or glucose intolerance
Immun-Aid	Powder	1.0	80	120	22	47:1	575/25	1055/27.8	500	200	500	460	2000	---	Formula for immuno-compromised patient. High in BCAA
Impact	Liquid	1.0	56	132	28	71:1	1100/48	1300/33	800	270	800	375 Isotonic	1500	---	Formula for immuno-compromised patient
Lipisorb	Liquid	1.35	57	161	57	125:1	1350/59	1690/43	850	340	850	630	1600	---	A readily absorbed fat blend with MCT to improve fat absorption
Nepro	Liquid	2.0	69.9	215.2	95.6	157:1	829/36.1	1057/27	1373	211	686	635	947	---	Moderate protein, calorically-dense product for patient requiring fluid and electrolyte restrictions
NutriHep	Liquid	1.5	40	290	21.2	209:1	320/14	1320/34	1000	400	1000	690	1000	--	High BCAA, low aromatic AA formula for patient with hepatic failure (encephalopathy)
Nutrivent or Pulmocare	Liquid Liquid	1.5 1.5	68 63	101 106	95 92	114:1 125:1	752/33 1310/57	2240/57 1902/49	1200 1057	600 423	1200 1057	450 490	1000 947	-- --	High fat formula for pulmonary disease; Nutrivent has omega-3 fatty acids and MCT
Osmolite or Isocal	Liquid Liquid	1.06 1.06	37 34	145 132	39 43	153:1 167:1	640/28 527/23	1020/26 1316/34	530 630	212 210	530 530	300 300 Isotonic	1887 1887	-- --	Isotonic formula
Osmolite HN or Isocal HN	Liquid Liquid	1.06 1.06	44 44	141 124	37 45	125:1 125:1	930/40 930/40	1570/40 1590/41	758 850	304 340	758 850	300 270 Isotonic	1321 1179	-- --	Isotonic formula with increased protein
Suplena	Liquid	2.0	30	255.2	95.6	392:1	783/34	1116/28.5	1385	211	728	600	947	---	Low in protein, fluid, PO_4, and electrolytes; high calorie for renal diet supplementation
Sustacal HC/ Sustacal Plus or Ensure Plus	Liquid Liquid	1.5 1.5	61 55	190 200	58 53	134:1 146:1	850/37 1141/50	1480/38 2113/54	850 706	340 283	850 706	650 690	1200 1420	--- --	High nitrogen formula for increased calories in limited fluid volume
Ultracal	Liquid	1.06	44	123	45	128:1	930/39.7	1610/41.7	850	340	850	310 Isotonic	1250	14.4	Isotonic formula with fiber (oat and soy)
Vivonex Plus	Powder	1.0	45	190	6.7	149:1	630/27	1070/27	557	222	557	650	1800	---	Elemental formula with glutamine

ORAL SUPPLEMENTS

Formula	Form	Kcal	gm PRO	CHO	FAT	mg/mEq Na	K	mg Ca	Mg	Phos	mOsm/ Kg H_2O	ml for RDA	Fiber gm/L	Indications for Use
Fortified Clear Liquid Drink	Powdered Drink Mix 8 oz	136	8	30	< 1g	120/5.1	170/4.4	300	80	200	450	---	---	High calorie, high protein liquid supplement
Fortified Pudding (Ensure Pudding)	Pudding 5 oz can	250	6.8	34	9.7	240/10.2	330/8.5	200	68	200	---	---	---	High calorie, high protein liquid supplement appropriate for supraglottic diet
Fortified Shake	Liquid Shake Mix 4 oz	190	6	32	4	100/4.3	280/2.6	150	60	150	NA	800	---	High calorie, high protein liquid supplement

FIG. 8-10. *Continued.*

mechanisms of tube-feeding diarrhea are the use of contaminated tube feedings,[103] lactose intolerance, intolerance of high osmotic loads, inappropriate release of gastrointestinal polypeptide hormones, concomitant antibiotic therapy, the ingestion of laxatives, and hypoalbuminemia.[104] The use of pectin or mucilaginous hydrophilic colloid bulk laxatives (Metamucil) to promote a formed but soft stool[105] reduces the diarrhea associated with isotonic tube feedings.[106] A number of formulas containing nonviscous, water-insoluble fiber polysaccharides that are designed to bring the benefits of fiber to the hospitalized and chronically tube-fed patient, optimize normal bowel function. In certain patients, dietary fiber may be contraindicated.[107] Risk factors include quantity of fiber ingested, previous gastric surgery, organic stricture, concomitant illness or medications depressing bowel motility, and diabetic gastroparesis.[107,108] In these patients, tube feeding with fiber may not be tolerated and can contribute to fiber bezoars that might need to be surgically removed.[109]

Infectious complications are among the most commonly reported side effects of enteral tube feeding. Bacterial contamination of the enteral nutrient solution has been reported to occur in 30% to 90% of cases when open enteral feeding systems are used. This leads to diarrhea.[110] Other factors include the use of enteral powders requiring mixing[111] and the use of either sterile or tap water to dilute the formula.[112] A consequence of the diarrhea is its associated increased morbidity related to fluid and electrolyte losses. To minimize contamination of enteral nutrition solutions, it is recommended that a closed delivery system, a prepacked sterile enteral formula, and a sterile administration set be used.

Standardized Enteral Order Forms and Enteral Diet Selection

There are many instances in daily medical practice when the provision of enteral nutrition is suboptimal because the patient's caloric goals are not reached. The reasons for this primarily have to do with the user's lack of awareness of or familiarity with the patient's appropriate nutrient needs, the most suitable type or composition of enteral formulas, and their correct use in relation to a particular clinical setting.[113] By using the standardized enteral nutrition order forms, the number of days needed to meet a patient's caloric goal can be decreased, thereby achieving the desired nutrient goals and therapeutic benefits sooner.[114] The forms also serve as an educational tool for the house staff and consulting staff, and their use ensures a consistent level of care, as determined by nursing, nutritional, and metabolic standards.

For consistent and effective delivery of enteral nutrients, enteral nutrition order forms for the continuous (Fig. 8-9) and bolus (Fig. 8-10) delivery of enteral products are used. These order forms list the enteral formulary stocked by the hospital (which is reviewed yearly for necessary changes), as well as the advancement schedule of formulas based on osmolality, whether the feeding should be given continuously or intermittently, and standing orders to nursing and dietary staff for obtaining blood work to monitor tolerance. Such standardized forms ensure quality control in the care and delivery of enteral nutrition. Printed on the reverse side of these forms are representative cross sections of enteral products commercially available. In general, enteral nutrition formulas can be broadly classified into disease-specific diets, elemental diets, meal replacements, supplements, and modular components. The disease-specific diets address the metabolic needs of the stressed patient, or the patient with hepatic failure, diabetes, immune compromise, acute or chronic renal failure, or chronic obstructive pulmonary disease. Elemental diets are nonresidue balanced diets with protein components reduced to their basic elements. Meal replacement diets consist of balanced proportions of protein, carbohydrate, and fat with vitamins and electrolytes. Supplements contain protein, carbohydrate, and fat with particular emphasis on either protein or carbohydrates. Modular components contain only one component, and can be added to standard formulas to fortify a diet calorically or nitrogenously to meet the patient's particular metabolic needs.

In summary, enteral nutrition should be the mainstay of nutritional therapy of cancer patients and should be used in patients who have a functional gastrointestinal tract and can take in an adequate number of calories.

Venous Access for Total Parenteral Nutrition

Use of *peripheral vein cannulation* for TPN is contraindicated because the incidence of subcutaneous perivascular infiltration and mild to severe phlebitis were unacceptably high at 56% to 60% and 40%, respectively.

For *central venous cannulation*, two sites are most commonly used: the infraclavicular subclavian vein route and the supraclavicular internal jugular vein route. Both routes are popular and permit the delivery of hypertonic nutrient solutions in a dependable manner. The indication for use of either route is to provide nutrients for a period greater than 5 days, during which adequate nutrient intake to meet the patient's full nutrient requirements cannot be ensured. The benefits of TPN administered through these routes are legion and have been summarized.[23,24,115] They greatly outweigh the complications, which are disproportionately feared.

Right atrial catheters placed in either the superior or the inferior vena cava are a more versatile device for long-term venous access in patients requiring prolonged hospital nutrients, chemotherapy, blood products, and the frequent drawing of blood. These are the centrally placed Silastic Broviac and the longer Hickman catheters, which can have single, double, or even triple lumens. Numerous studies have shown that infectious complications are infrequent even in the immunocompromised patient, and that the multiple uses of the catheter resulting from its reliable venous access route greatly outweigh its potential complications.[116] Catheters should be meticulously cared for on a daily basis using an aseptic/antiseptic technique as outlined in a catheter maintenance protocol (Table 8-16).

TABLE 8-16. *Catheter maintenance protocol*

Cutdown site:	Dry sterile dressing until wound heals. Then no dressing.
Catheter exit site:	Daily skin cleansing with alcohol and 3% H_2O_2. Apply povidone–iodine (Betadine) on dry sterile dressing.
Catheter:	Heparin flush after blood sampling. Daily change. No millipore filter.

Reproduced with permission from Meguid MM, Eldar S, Wahba, A. The delivery of nutritional support. A potpourri of new devices and methods. Cancer 1985;55(Suppl 1):279. Cancer 1985;55:279.

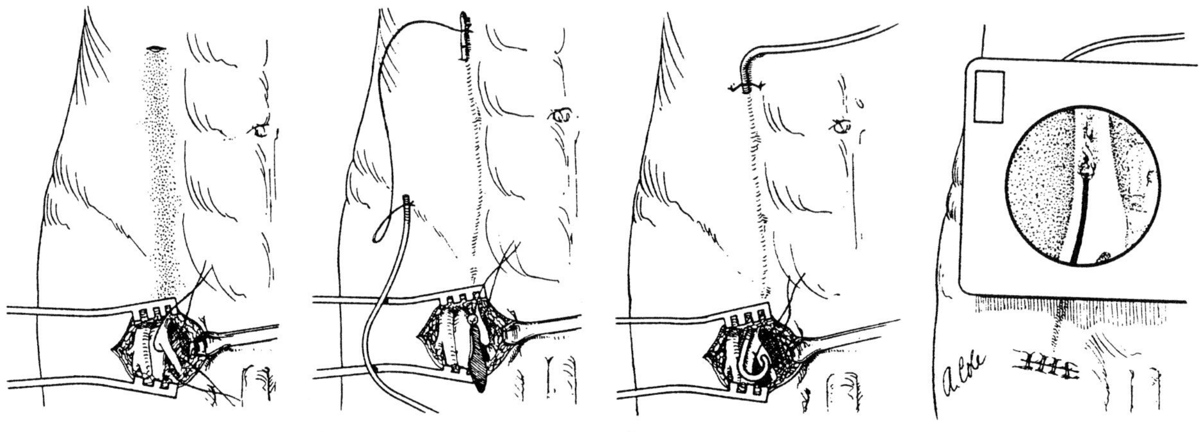

FIG. 8-11. Technique of cannulation of the inferior vena cava is shown. **A,** A tributary of the greater saphenous vein is isolated; **B,** a subcutaneous tunnel is made; **C,** the catheter is inserted through the venotomy; and **D,** the catheter is passed into the inferior vena cava under fluoroscopic visualization. (Reproduced with permission from Curtas S, Bonaventura M, Meguid MM. Cannulation of the inferior vena cava for long term central venous access: techniques and results. Surg Gynecol Obstet 1989; 168:121.)

Vascular access can often become problematic when continued nutritional support and other types of intravenous therapy are required during extended periods of hospitalization. Insertion of a central Silastic catheter with access sites on the upper torso may be contraindicated in some clinical conditions, including thrombosis of the subclavian vein; burns or trauma of the upper torso; the need for upper torso radiation therapy; median sternotomy with wound infection; or fresh tracheostomy. In such patients, insertion of a Silastic Hickman catheter for long-term use by way of a vein in the lower extremity is a rational alternative,[117] as illustrated in Figure 8-11.

An extension of the concept of immediate, continuous, and ad libitum access to the venous system is a subcutaneous implantable injection *port*. This is an alternative means of safe and reliable central venous access with improved patient convenience and cosmetic acceptability, although it is not recommended when frequent blood samples are needed because occlusion of the small-bore catheter is common (90%); this does not occur with the large-bore catheter, however. Ports are placed in the upper torso, using the same upper venous system as with subclavian or right atrial catheters. Single and double ports are available and are placed under either local or general anesthesia at surgery.

Complications of Central Venous Access

The complications of central venous access are summarized in Table 8-17, and fall broadly into three categories: mechanical, septic, and metabolic.

The rate of *mechanical complications* is inversely proportional to the skill and experience of the catheter inserter. The average frequencies of complications in 2050 patients were: mechanical, 6.7%; septic, 4.7%; and metabolic, 25.7%.[118–121] In a world review of 39,180 central venous catheters,[122] the most frequent mechanical complication experienced with successful insertion of a subclavian central venous catheter was malposition (6%), followed by arterial injury (1.4%), pneumohydrohemothorax (1.1%), vessel thrombosis (0.3%), thrombophlebitis (0.1%), and catheter embolism (0.1%). The death rate related to all these complications was 1.2%. The safest method of obtaining central venous access is by the internal jugular vein, although this is not the most widely used route.

Based on a number of studies,[123–125] patients with cancer, inflammatory bowel disease, pancreatitis, and sepsis are at high risk for subclavian thrombus formation because they have a deficiency of antithrombin III factor. To minimize the frequency of subclavian vein thrombosis, heparin is added to TPN solutions. In these patients, the vessel thrombosis rate was 52%; the addition of 6000 U/d of heparin to TPN, infused continuously, decreased the frequency of thrombosis. In patients with

(text continues on page 132)

TABLE 8-17. *Complications associated with the use of total parenteral nutrition*

Type of complication	Nature	Frequency
Mechanical	Catheter tip malposition	6%
	Arterial laceration	1.4%
	Pneumohydrohemothorax	1.1%
	Subclavian or superior vena cava thrombosis	0.3%
	Thrombophlebitis	0.1%
	Catheter embolism	0.1%
Septic	Catheter-related sepsis	7.4%
Metabolic		
Acute	Hyperglycemia/hypoglycemia	Avoidable
	Blood electrolyte abnormalities	
	Fluid overload	
	Hyperlipidemia	
Chronic	Metabolic bone disease	Rare
	Alterations in bile composition	
	Deterioration of liver function	

Modified from Meguid MM, Muscaritoli M. Current uses of total parenteral nutrition. Am Fam Physician 1993;47:383.

State University of New York
Health Science Center
Syracuse
University Hospital

PARENTERAL NUTRITION ORDER FORM

TPN: a 3 in 1 admixture bag for a 24 hour period — Orders must be sent to pharmacy by 1400 hours

ORDERS: CHECK ONE — Weight ______ Kg

☐ INDIVIDUALIZED		☐ STANDARDIZED	
______ gm/day	Amino Acids	50 g/l	1000 ml
______ gm/day ______ kcal/day	Carbohydrate (dextrose)	177 g/l 601 kcal/l	approx. 1
______ gm/day ______ kcal/day	Fat (lipid emulsion 20%) 500 ml supplies (100g) 1000 Kcal	40 g/l 400 kcal/l	kcal/ml

______ kcal/KG ______ gm/Prot./KG BAG NUMBER ______ INFUSION RATE ______ ml/hr for 24 HR

ADDITIVES

Amount Per 24 Hours		DAILY		ROUTINE		SPECIAL (Circle)	
		Sodium Chloride	mEq	Heparin	U/ml	Ascorbic Acid	500mg
Na	100mEq	Sodium Acetate*	mEq	Vitamin K_1	mg	Folic Acid	1mg
		Potassium Chloride	mEq	Regular Human Insulin	units	Selenium	120mcg
K	60-120mEq	Potassium Acetate*	mEq	Ranitidine	mg	Thiamine	100mg
PO_4	10-22mmol	Phosphate (as potassium salt) 1mmol phosphorus = 1.5mEq K)	mmol			Zinc	10mg
Mg	8-20mEq	Magnesium Sulfate	mEq				
Ca	10- 15mEq	Calcium Gluconate	mEq				
Vitamin (MVI-12)	10ml	MVI- 12	10ml				
Trace Elements(Conc.)	1ml	Trace Elements (Zn,Cu,Mn,Cr,Se)	1ml				
Molybdenum	25 mcg = 1ml	Molybdenum Elemental	25 mcg				

*Substitute acetate salts in hyperchloremic acidosis

LAB VALUES Date ______

Na	Cl	BUN	Gluc	Ca
				Mg
K	HCO_3	CRE		PO_4
				Alb
				Trig

TPN STANDING ORDERS:

Lab Values: DAY 1: Nutrition Panel I, II & III
DAY 2,3: Nutrition Panel I
Thereafter, q TUESDAY: Nutrition Panel I, II & III
Lab values: q FRIDAY: Nutrition Panel I & II

Nursing:
- Daily weights, cumulative I/O
  q SHIFT: I/O, fingerstick glucose, Notify MD if > 200 mg/dl
- Change catheter dressing q M ____ W ____ F ____ and pm ____
- Infuse daily TPN from 1900 to 1900 Hrs

DIETARY:
- Daily calorie counts during transitional feeding (tube feeding/po) or as per nutrition support team

NUTRITION PANELS:
PANEL I: Na, K, HCO_3, Cl, Glucose
PANEL II: ALP, Cre, BUN, PO_4, Alb, Ca, Mg
PANEL III: Chol, Trig

41230 Rev. 11/93

METHOD OF DISCONTINUING: CHECK ONE

☐ ROUTINE: When 60% of caloric requirements is provided by po diet or tube feeding, decrease TPN to 1/2 of current rate for one hour. Then discontinue TPN.

☐ PRE-OP AND ACUTE DISCONTINUATION: Infuse D10W at TPN rate through central catheter. If central catheter is removed, infuse D10W peripherally at TPN rate.

☐ FOR persistent fever of unkown etiology: a. draw isolator blood cultures from all ports of central catheter and also via peripheral route. b. discontinue TPN as above and remove central catheter if clinically indicated.

SIGNATURE MD	DATE	TIME
NOTE BY	DATE	TIME

CLINICAL DATA SERVICES G3.00

FIG. 8-12. Parenteral nutrition order form.

USUAL RECOMMENDATIONS

CALORIC REQUIREMENTS

Maintenance	Moderate Stress	Severe Stress
25 - 30 Kcal/kg/day	30 - 35 Kcal/kg/day	35 - 40 Kcal/kg/day
	Elective Surgery	Extensive Burns
	Peritonitis	Multiple Long Fractures
	Soft Tissue Trauma	Closed Head Injury
	Malnutrition	Major Sepsis
	Renal Failure	Multiple Trauma
	Respiratory Failure	Multiple Organ Failure
	Pancreatitis	
	Dialysis	

NON PROTEIN CALORIE TO NITROGEN RATIO

Maintenance	Moderate Stress	Severe Stress
200-300:1	150:1	<100:1

Protein (gm) ÷ 6.25 = Nitrogen (gm)

PROTEIN REQUIREMENTS

	(g/kg/day)
Protein restricted	0.5-0.8
Maintenance	1.0-1.2
Moderate stress	1.3-1.4
Severe stress	1.5-2.0

CHO-45-55%Kcal/day

Fat-30-40%Kcal/day

PROT ______________ **gm x 4.0 =** ______________ **Kcal**

CHO ______________ **gm x 3.4 =** ______________ **Kcal.**

FAT ______________ **gm x 10.0 =** ______________ **Kcal**

TOTAL (Kcal) ______________

FIG. 8-12. *Continued.*

normal levels of antithrombin III factor, the frequency of thrombosis is only 14%, and the addition of 1 U heparin/mL TPN formula appeared sufficient to prevent thrombosis.

In the United States, the average nationwide rate of *catheter sepsis* is 7.4%. The most effective method of diagnosis is the quantitative blood culture method for determining in situ sepsis. In all cases, when the catheter was incriminated by culture data, removal of the central venous catheter led to patient improvement. In no instance when the central venous catheter was deemed "innocent" did its removal lead to clinical improvement.[126] After removal for catheter-related sepsis, data now suggest that it is safe to reinsert a new sterile catheter in 12 hours.[127] In certain clinical situations (eg, critically ill patients for whom removal of the central venous catheter may not be a viable option), treating an established catheter-related sepsis episode with antibiotics can eradicate the catheter colonization, thereby prolonging the life and usefulness of the catheter.[128]

Because TPN can be regarded as a sophisticated form of fluid and electrolyte therapy, many of the reported *metabolic complications* have resulted from errors of omission. Thus, the complications due to an excess or deficit of electrolytes, vitamins, or trace elements are potentially avoidable, and therefore are not emphasized. The introduction of a safe and reliable fat source has obviated the metabolic complications derived from a glucose-based TPN,[129] including hyperglycemia, hypoglycemia, hyperosmolar syndromes, hypertriglyceridemia, abnormal lipid profiles, hyperinsulinemia, elevated epinephrine, elevation of liver function test results, hypercarbia,[130] essential fatty acid deficiencies, and venous thrombosis.

Standardized Total Parenteral Nutrition Order Form

Physicians, from consultant staff to house staff, differ greatly in their comfort levels in ordering parenteral solutions. To aid in delivery of a consistent level of nutritional support care, a parenteral nutrition order form is used (Fig. 8-12). This form is designed for ease of physician use, providing more precise guidelines for the prescription of TPN, including standard orders for the starting and stopping of TPN and for the comprehensive nursing and dietary care of the patient.

The form is based on the single delivery system of the total nutrient admixture concept,[131] and offers the following features:

1. A general-purpose, standard formula concentration (15 g glucose, 5 g amino acids, and 20 g lipids per 100 mL) or a space for individualized solutions
2. The average daily recommendations for electrolytes (Na, K, phosphate, Mg, Ca), vitamins, and trace elements (Zn, Cu, Mn, Cr, Se, Mo) in pediatric and adult dosages
3. The addition of heparin to prevent catheter thrombosis[125]
4. The addition of weekly vitamin K
5. The option to add insulin
6. Nursing and dietary orders to start and stop TPN
7. Laboratory tests for electrolytes, glucose, liver function, cholesterol, and triglycerides to monitor the patient's immediate and long-term tolerance of TPN.

The standardized form provides the additional benefit of acting as an educational tool,[132] because it provides not only prescription guidelines for the appropriate use of TPN, but reflects the philosophy of TPN. This approach is particularly useful for inexperienced house staff in providing nutritional support practice guidelines without compromising the quality of patient care.[133]

The standardized form with appropriate guidelines facilitates the ordering of TPN formulas and assists house staff in writing appropriate orders, leading to reduced prescription errors. In practice, this leads to a decrease in nonpatient-related nursing time and pharmacy time, and an overall reduction in the total cost of patient nutritional care because of less waste. In addition, the form is labor saving and decreases the need for refrigerator storage space.

Total Nutrient Admixture

The introduction of 3-L bags made of ethyl vinyl acetate has made the admixture of a fat emulsion to dextrose and amino acid possible. The advantages of this approach are numerous: cost savings during preparation, handling, and delivery; more uniform administration of a balanced solution containing the three macronutrients plus micronutrients over a 24-hour period, thus circumventing the metabolic disadvantages of a single energy-substrate system; less manipulation, and thus less risk of contamination; decreased lipid toxicity because of the greater dilution of the lipid emulsion and the longer duration of its infusion; ease of delivery and storage for patients on home TPN programs; the option of delivering nutritional support peripherally; and reduced long-term hepatic accumulation of triglycerides, attributed in part to glucose-based TPN.[131]

Types of Parenteral Formulations

Most patients are well served using a standard, general-purpose, mixed-fuel TPN formula. The selection of nutrient solutions for different catabolic states largely centers on the admixture of the major substrates—carbohydrate, fat, and protein. Sources of energy for patients undergoing surgical stress should include both carbohydrate and lipids. Glucose tolerance with TPN is optimal when 30% to 50% of the caloric source is delivered as fat,[129] because the maximum rate of glucose utilization is approximately 15 g/h in a variety of pathophysiologic conditions.[134]

The use of lipid in TPN is designed both to meet essential fatty acid needs and avoid the undesirable effects of glucose overloading. Based on several studies, it is recommended that only the minimal amount of glucose (50 to 150 g or about 2 g/kg/d) should be supplied, using lipids for the remaining caloric requirements[135,136] of the central nervous system, to prevent systemic acidosis and ketosis, reduce gluconeogenesis, and enhance mobilization of lipids. A comprehensive review of this subject has been published by Gilder.[137]

The use of branched-chain amino acid (BCAA)-enriched TPN continues to be controversial. A prospective, randomized, double-blind trial studying the effects of BCAA-enriched versus conventional TPN solutions in 23 hypercatabolic surgical patients showed that the group receiving a 45% BCAA-enriched TPN solution had improved nitrogen retention, elevation of absolute lymphocyte count, improved plasma transferrin levels, and reversal of anergy to skin test antigens in 60% of patients. However, no difference in morbidity or mortality was observed between the two groups. Under such circumstances, cost becomes the determinant factor in the use of BCAA-enriched solutions.

Total parenteral nutrition implies a decision to administer all the calories and nitrogen that a patient can effectively use. Examples of clinical conditions requiring modification of solutions are shown in the following section, given a hypothetical patient. As outlined in the section Nutrient Requirements of Patients With Gastrointestinal Cancer, once energy needs have been determined, TPN orders can be written.

How to Order Total Parenteral Nutrition

The selection of nutrient solutions for different catabolic states largely centers on the admixture of the major substrates (ie, protein, fat, and carbohydrate). An example of a hypothetical clinical condition requiring modification of the nutrient solution is given in the following case study.

CASE STUDY

A 48-year-old, well-nourished man is disease free after partial colectomy for a colonic cancer. However, he is hypoalbuminemic and septic from a small anastomotic leak. While the infection was being controlled, the patient was started on TPN. Energy needs based on the Harris-Benedict equation are: basal energy expenditure × 1.1 (activity factor) × 1.2 (injury factor = major surgery) = 1668 × 1.1 × 1.2 − 2201 kcal/d.

Formulation to be Used

As shown in Table 8-18, the stock TPN solution consists of 50 g/100 mL glucose, 20 g/100 mL fat, and 11 g/100 mL amino acids. However, there are a number of clinical conditions in which the standard formulation cannot be used, leading to modification of the TPN prescription. Some examples are given in Table 8-18.

Monitoring Use of Total Parenteral Nutrition in Surgical Practice

Table 8-19 summarizes the indices monitored to ensure safe use of TPN. Stringent TPN-related monitoring is required because mechanical, metabolic, and infectious complications may develop rapidly and can be life threatening.

Indications for Stopping Nutritional Support

An endpoint needs to be established as soon as TPN is initiated. This endpoint should be reviewed on a regular basis to ensure maximum benefit with least harm to the patient and should be revised as indicated by the patient's condition. Three clinical conditions dictate stopping nutritional support.

First, a life-threatening complication may develop that makes temporarily stopping nutritional support a prudent clinical decision. The complications that necessitate stopping TPN, at least temporarily, are confirmed sepsis or a severe metabolic complication such as hyperglycemia, nonketotic coma, or hyperammonemia. Sepsis must be suspected in any patient on TPN with fever, and its management with use of quantitative cultures was discussed earlier.

Second, the patient's underlying disease may have progressed to the terminal stage. In this situation, continuing aggressive medical support is inappropriate, and the decision to stop TPN becomes a difficult one because it implies that the chance of qualitative rehabilitation is negligible. Continuing TPN or enteral nutrition "just for the sake of doing something" is inappropriate because the costs of continuing treatment are too high. An appropriate interim course is to replace TPN or enteral nutrition with a hydration solution after discussion with the patient or family.

Further debate on this subject is provided in the Georgetown University Technology Assessment and Practice Guidelines Forum report[20–22]:

> One of the most significant aspects of the decision-making process involves the meaning of starvation and the symbolic and psychological significance of feeding to patients, family members, and care givers. Some clinicians claim that seriously debilitated patients seldom experience the symptoms of dehydration beyond a dry mouth and slight thirst [see references 138–145]; therefore, in their view, maintaining fluids and nourishment is not morally required in patient care. Other clinicians and ethicists argue for continued feeding and hydration for symbolic significance, for legal reasons, or for reasons of compassion or professional conscience.[139–141] Others regard nutrition and hydration as one form of treatment that may be initiated or withdrawn under the same conditions as any other medical treatment.[142–145] The ethical considerations of withdrawing treatment in the form of TPN have not been studied adequately and will need further discussion before the assessment of TPN can be completed.

The third clinical condition dictating cessation of nutritional support is when the rehabilitative endpoint for nutritional support has been met. For the patient in whom nutritional support is a critical step to full recovery, the theoretic moment for discontinuing supportive nutritional therapy is the point at which maximum benefit has been achieved at the least cost. There are no firm clinical or laboratory indices of optimal nutritional repletion, but Meguid and colleagues have recommended guidelines for establishing the point at which nutritional support can

TABLE 8-18. *Standard formulation and modified total parenteral nutrition prescriptions*

1. GENERAL-PURPOSE, MIXED-FUEL TPN

Nutrient ratio	kcal	g	mL	% Solution
50% Glucose	1102	324	648	15%
30% Fat	660	66	330	330 mL of 20% fat
20% Amino acid	439	107	973	5%
	2201 kcal		1951	
			150 (lytes)	
			2101 mL	

2. CHRONIC OBSTRUCTIVE PULMONARY DISEASE AND CYSTIC FIBROSIS

Decrease glucose and increase fat. Amino acids remain unchanged.

Nutrient ratio	kcal	g	mL	% Solution
20% Glucose	440	129	258	6.3%
60% Fat	1320	132	660	660 mL of 20% fat
20% Amino acid	440	107	972	5.2%
	2200 kcal		1890	
			150 (lytes)	
			2040 mL	

3. DIABETES

Increase fat and decrease glucose. Amino acids remain unchanged.

Nutrient ratio	kcal	g	mL	% Solution
30% Glucose	660	194	388	9.4%
50% Fat	1100	110	550	550 mL of 20% fat
20% Amino acid	440	107	972	5.2%
	2200 kcal		1910	
			150 (lytes)	
			2060 mL	

Concentrated stock solution = 70 g/100 mL glucose, 20 g/100 mL fat, 15 g/100 mL amino acid.

4. CONGESTIVE CARDIAC FAILURE

Decrease volume, increase concentration of nutrients.

Nutrient ratio	kcal	g	mL	% Solution
50% Glucose	1000	294	420	19.1%
34% Fat	680	68	340	340 mL of 20% fat
16% Amino acid	320	94	626	6.1%
	2000 kcal		1386	
			150 (lytes)	
			1536 mL	

5. ACUTE RENAL DISEASE

Concentrate solution, increase glucose and fat. Decrease amino acid concentration and decrease volume.

Nutrient ratio	kcal	g	mL	% Solution
50% Glucose	800	235	336	20.3%
35% Fat	560	56	280	280 mL of 20% fat
15% Amino acid	240	59	393	5.1%
	1600 kcal		1009	
			150 (lytes)	
			1159 mL	

6. HEPATIC DISEASE

Glucose and fat content remains unchanged. Decrease aromatic amino acids and increase branched-chain amino acids. Use Hepatamine with same nutrient concentrations as in acute renal disease. Volume will be increased because amino acid concentration in hepatamine is only 8 g/100 mL.

be discontinued based on their extensive study of 464 patients with malignancy of the gastrointestinal tract.[146] They found that the factors that influence when a patient can resume adequate food intake depend on nutritional status and the occurrence of complications. Similar findings were noted in patients after elective surgery for benign gastrointestinal disease.[147] Consequently, our practice has been to wait until a patient can eat 60% of his or her requirements, as demonstrated by objective calorie counts, before stopping TPN or distal enteral nutrition (ie, jejunal feeding). Thus, based on IONIP data, TPN is stopped when a patient can eat 60% of his or her estimated caloric requirements.

TABLE 8-19. *Monitoring the patient on total parenteral nutrition*

CLINICAL DATA CHECKED DAILY

Patient's sense of well-being: symptoms suggesting fluid overload, high or low blood glucose, electrolyte imbalance, and so forth
Patient's strength as judged by graded activity: getting out of bed, walking, stair climbing
Vital signs: temperature, blood pressure, pulse rate, and respiratory rate.
Fluid balance: weight. Fluid input (intravenous $\pm$ enteral) versus fluid output (eg, urine, stool, gastric suction)
Delivery equipment for total parenteral nutrition: composition of nutrient solution, tubing, pump, filter catheter, dressing (skin checked for local infection at time of dressing change)

LABORATORY DATA

Urine quantitative glucose

Blood glucose; Na^+, K^+, Cl^-, HCO_3^-; Blood urea nitrogen — Daily until patient is stable, then twice weekly*

Serum albumin, transferrin (or total iron binding capacity)*
Liver function studies
Serum creatinine
Ca^{2+}, PO_4, Mg^{2+}
Hemoglobin/hematocrit, white blood cell count

NH_3 and prothrombin time—baseline, then weekly
Micronutrient tests as indicated

* See total parenteral nutrition standing orders on the parenteral nutrition order form for ordering frequency.

Modified from Howard L, Meguid MM. Nutritional assessment in total parenteral nutrition. Clin Lab Med 1981;1:611. Clin Lab Med 1981; 1:611.

Home Nutritional Support

The guidelines for use of nutritional support in the home setting include the following:

1. Home TPN may improve the quality of life for the patient or decrease the costs compared with hospitalization, or both. Complications associated with home TPN are the result of long-term use, not of the setting.
2. The primary decision to initiate home TPN depends greatly on the clinical condition of the patient, particularly on the underlying disease, and on the available support system for maintaining care in the home.

Indications for Home Nutritional Support

The primary decision to initiate home nutritional support depends on the patient's primary diagnosis and clinical condition, and the available support system for maintaining care in the home. Home nutritional support may improve the patient's quality of life and decrease costs compared with hospitalization. The psychological, clinical, and economic benefits of home nutritional support[80] may explain why the number of home parenteral and enteral nutrition programs has increased by about 25% each year in the late 1980s and the early 1990s.[148]

A survey of 2968 patients with active cancer receiving home nutritional support (1672 home TPN, 1296 home enteral nutrition[148]) indicates that cancer represents the largest single diagnosis in patients starting home nutritional support. The mean survival time of cancer patients is 6 months after starting home parenteral and enteral nutrition, but 25% live beyond a year and 20% resume full oral nutrition. Although most patients with active cancer experience only partial rehabilitation, for those patients with longer survival, rehabilitation is more complete. The outcome is relatively better for children and for patients whose neoplasm is leukemia, lymphoma, or of the small bowel or liver. Adult patients with active cancer on home parenteral and enteral nutrition do not have a greater incidence of therapy-related readmissions than noncancer dysphagic patients receiving home nutritional support; however, their overall rehospitalization rate is much greater.

These objective data emphasize the growing role of home nutritional support in the optimal psychological, clinical, and cost-related treatment of patients with gastrointestinal cancer, provided that both patient and family assume the responsibility for learning the necessary techniques for a safe administration.

ACKNOWLEDGMENTS

Supported in part by grant DK43796 from the National Institutes of Diabetes and Digestive and Kidney Diseases, National Institutes of Health; a Hendricks Grant for Medical Research; and by grant CRG940731 from the North Atlantic Treaty Organization (NATO). Dr. Laviano is supported by grant AI93.00131.04 from the Italian National Research Council (CNR).

The authors thank Ms. Darlene Thompson for diligent editorial assistance.

REFERENCES

1. National Research Council, National Academy of Sciences. Diet, nutrition and cancer. Washington, DC: National Academy Press, 1982.
2. American Cancer Society. New York: American Cancer Society.
3. National Cancer Institute, Office of Cancer Communications. Bethesda, MD: National Cancer Institute.
4. Wynder EL, Gori GB. Contribution of the environment to cancer incidence: an epidemiological exercise. J Natl Cancer Inst 1977;58:825.
5. Doll R, Peto R. The causes of cancer: quantitative estimates of avoidable risks of cancer in the United States today. J Natl Cancer Inst 1981;66:1191.
6. Berenblum I. Carcinogenesis as a biological problem. Amsterdam: North American Elsevier, 1974.
7. Foulds L. Neoplastic development, vol 1. London: Academic Press, 1969.
8. Williams GM. Methods for evaluating chemical genotoxicity. Annu Rev Pharmacol Toxicol 1989;29.189.
9. Miller ED, Miller JA. Milestones in chemical carcinogenesis. Semin Oncol 1979;6:445.
10. Tuyns AJ, Pequignot G, Gignoux M, et al. Cancers of the digestive tract, alcohol and tobacco. Int J Cancer 1982;30:9.
11. Mettlin C. Epidemiologic findings relating diet to cancer of the esophagus. In: Reddy BS, Cohen LA, eds. Diet, nutrition and cancer: a critical evaluation. Boca Raton, FL: CRC Press, 1985.
12. Fraser P, Chilvers C, Beral V, et al. Nitrate and human cancer: a review of the evidence. Int J Epidemiol 1980;9:3.
13. Weisberger JH, Raineri R. Dietary factors and the etiology of gastric cancer. Cancer Res 1975;35:3469.

14. Heuch I, Kvale G, Jacobsen BK, et al. Use of alcohol, tobacco and coffee, and the risk of pancreatic cancer. Br J Cancer 1983;48:637.
15. MacMahon B, Yen S, Trichopoulos D, et al. Coffee and cancer of the pancreas. N Engl J Med 1981;304:630.
16. Burkitt DP. Epidemiology of cancer of the colon and rectum. Cancer 1971;28:3.
17. Dales LG, Friedman GD, Ury HK, et al. A case-control study of relationships of diet and other traits to colorectal cancer in American blacks. Am J Epidemiol 1979;109:132.
18. Graham S, Dayal H, Swanson M, et al. Diet in the epidemiology of cancer of the colon and rectum. J Natl Cancer Inst 1978;61:709.
19. Pollack ES, Nomura AMY, Heilbrun LK, et al. Prospective study of alcohol consumption and cancer. N Engl J Med 1984;10:617.
20. Final Report and Statement of the Technology Assessment and Practice Guidelines Forum. Evaluating total parenteral nutrition: part I. Nutrition 1990;6:313.
21. Final Report and Statement of the Technology Assessment and Practice Guidelines Forum. Evaluating total parenteral nutrition: part II. Nutrition 1990;6:391.
22. Final Report and Statement of the Technology Assessment and Practice Guidelines Forum. Evaluating total parenteral nutrition: part III. Nutrition 1990;6:475.
23. Meguid MM, Campos AC, Hammond WG. Nutrition support in surgical practice: current knowledge and research needs: part I. Am J Surg 1990;159:345.
24. Meguid MM, Campos AC, Hammond WG. Nutrition support in surgical practice: current knowledge and research needs: part II. Am J Surg 1990;159:427.
25. Holter AR, Fischer JE. The effects of perioperative hyperalimentation on complications in patients with carcinoma and weight loss. J Surg Res 1977;23:31.
26. Moghissi K, Hornshaw J, Teasdale PR, Dawes EA. Parenteral nutrition in carcinoma of the esophagus treated by surgery: nitrogen balance and clinical studies. Br J Surg 1977;64:125.
27. Muller JM, Dienst C, Brenner U, Pichlmaier H. Preoperative parenteral feeding in patients with gastrointestinal carcinoma. Lancet 1982; 1:68.
28. Issell BF, Valdivieso M, Zaren HA, et al. Protection against chemotherapy toxicity by IV hyperalimentation. Cancer Treat Rep 1978;62: 1139.
29. Dewys WD, Begg C, Lavin PT, et al. Prognostic effect of weight loss prior to chemotherapy in cancer patients: Eastern Cooperative Oncology Group. Am J Med 1980;69:491.
30. Samuels ML, Selig DE, Ogden S, Grant C, Brown B. IV hyperalimentation and chemotherapy for stage III testicular cancer: a randomized study. Cancer Treat Rep 1981;65:615.
31. Nixon DW, Moffitt S, Lawson DH, et al. Total parenteral nutrition as an adjunct to chemotherapy of metastatic colorectal cancer. Cancer Treat Rep 1981;65(Suppl 5):121.
32. Popp MB, Fisher RI, Wesley R, et al. A prospective randomized study of adjuvant parenteral nutrition in the treatment of advanced diffuse lymphoma: influence on survival. Surgery 1981;90:195.
33. Shamberger RC, Brennan MF, Goodgame JT Jr, et al. A prospective, randomized study of adjuvant parenteral nutrition in the treatment of sarcomas: results of metabolic and survival studies. Surgery 1984;96: 1.
34. Goodwin WJ, Torres J. The value of the prognostic nutritional index in the management of patients with advanced carcinoma of the head and neck. Head Neck Surg 1984;6:932.
35. Clamon GH, Feld R, Evans WK, et al. Effect of adjuvant central iv hyperalimentation on the survival and response to treatment of patients with small cell lung cancer: a randomized trial. Cancer Treat Rep 1985;69:167.
36. Rickard KA, Loghmani ES, Grosfeld JL, et al. Short- and long-term effectiveness of enteral and parenteral nutrition in reversing or preventing protein-energy malnutrition in advanced neuroblastoma: a prospective randomized study. Cancer 1985;56:2881.
37. Bashir Y, Graham TR, Torrance A, Gibson GJ, Corris PA. Nutritional state of patients with lung cancer undergoing thoracotomy. Thorax 1990;45:183.
38. Larrea J, Vega S, Martinez T, Torrent JM, Vega V, Nunez V. The nutritional status and immunological situation of cancer patients. Nutr Hosp 1992;7:178.
39. Tan YS, Nambiar R, Yo SL. Prevalence of protein calorie malnutrition in general surgical patients. Ann Acad Med Singapore 1992;21:334.
40. Yang Z-J, Koseki M, Meguid MM, Gleason JR, Debonis D. Synergistic effect of rhTNF-α and rhIL-1α in inducing anorexia in rats. Am J Physiol 1994;267:R1056.
41. Opara EI, Laviano A, Meguid MM, Yang Z-J. Correlation between food intake and CSF IL1α in anorectic tumour bearing rats. Neuroreport 1995;6:438.
42. Laviano A, Meguid MM, Yang Z-J, Gleason JR, Cangiano C, Rossi-Fanelli F. Cracking the riddle of cancer anorexia. Nutrition 1996 (in press).
43. Meguid MM, Campos ACL, Meguid V, Debonis D, Terz JJ. IONIP: a criterion of surgical outcome and patient selection for perioperative nutritional support. Br J Clin Pract 1988;42:8.
44. Rossi-Fanelli F, Franchi F, Mulier M, et al. Effect of energy substrate manipulation on tumor cell proliferation in parenterally fed cancer patients. Clin Nutr 1991;10:228.
45. Sagar S, Harland P, Shields R. Early postoperative feeding with elemental diet. Br Med J 1979;1:293.
46. Fick TE, van Rooyen W, Schattenkerk ME, Steller EP, Feenstra BWA, Bruining HA. A non-elemental versus an elemental diet for early postoperative enteral feeding by needle catheter jejunostomy. Clin Nutr 1986;5:105.
47. Yeung CK, Smith RD, Hill GL. Effect of an elemental diet on body composition: comparison with intravenous nutrition. Gastroenterology 1979;77:652.
48. Adams S, Dellinger EP, Wertz MJ, Oreskovich MR, Simonowitz D, Johansen K. Enteral versus parenteral nutritional support following laparotomy for trauma: a randomized prospective trial. J Trauma 1986; 26:882.
49. Bower RH, Talamini MA, Sax HC, Hamilton F, Fischer JE. Postoperative enteral nutrition: a randomized controlled trial. Arch Surg 1986; 121:1040.
50. Heylen AM, Lybeer MB, Penninck FM, Kerremans RP, Frost PG. Parenteral versus needle jejunostomy nutrition after total gastrectomy. Clin Nutr 1987;6:131.
51. Muggia-Sullam M, Bower RH, Murphy RF, Joffe SN, Fischer JE. Postoperative enteral versus parenteral nutritional support in gastrointestinal surgery: a matched prospective study. Am J Surg 1985;149: 106.
52. Klein S, Simes J, Blackburn GL. Total parenteral nutrition and cancer clinical trials. Cancer 1986;58:1378.
53. Torosian MH, Mullen JL, Miller EE, Zinsser KR, Stein TP, Buzby GP. Enhanced tumor response to cycle-specific chemotherapy by parenteral amino acid administration. JPEN J Parenter Enter Nutr 1983; 7:337.
54. Cheraskin E, Ringsdorf WM Jr, Hutchins K, Setyaamadja AT, Wideman GL. The effect of diet upon radiation response in cervical carcinoma of the uterus. Acta Cytol 1968;12:433.
55. Ford JH, Dudan RD, Bennett JS, Averett HE. Parenteral hyperalimentation in gynecologic oncology patients. Gynecol Oncol 1972;1:70.
56. Veterans Affairs Total Parenteral Nutrition Cooperative Study Group. Perioperative total parenteral nutrition in surgical patients. N Engl J Med 1991;325:525.
57. Meguid MM, Campos AC. The validity of using TPN in terminally ill cancer patients. Nutrition 1996 (in press).
58. Bellantone R, Doglietto GB, Bossola M, et al. Preoperative parenteral nutrition in the high risk surgical patient. JPEN J Parenter Enter Nutr 1988;12:195.
59. Detsky, AS, Jeejeebhoy KN. Cost-effectiveness of preoperative parenteral nutrition in patients undergoing major gastrointestinal surgery. JPEN J Parenter Enter Nutr 1984;8:632.
60. Heatley RV, Williams RHP, Lewis MH. Preoperative intravenous feeding: a controlled trial. Postgrad Med J 1979;55:541.
61. Campos ACL, Meguid MM. A critical appraisal of the usefulness of perioperative nutritional support. Am J Clin Nutr 1992;55:117.
62. Meijerink WJ, von Meyenfeldt MF, Rouflart MM, Soeters PB. Efficacy of perioperative nutritional support. Lancet 1992;340:187.
63. Yamada N, Koyama H, Hioki K, Yamada T, Yamamoto M. Effect of postoperative total parenteral nutrition as an adjunct to gastrectomy for advanced gastric carcinoma. Br J Surg 1983;70:267.
64. Collins JP, Oxby CB, Hill GL. Intravenous amino acids and intravenous hyperalimentation as protein-sparing therapy after major surgery: a controlled clinical trial. Lancet 1978;1:788.

65. Preshaw RM, Attisha RP, Hollingsworth WJ, Todd JD. Randomized sequential trial of parenteral nutrition in healing of colonic anastomoses in man. Can J Surg 1979;22:437.
66. Askanazi J, Starker PM, Olsson C, et al. Effect of immediate postoperative nutritional support on length of hospitalization. Ann Surg 1986; 203:236.
67. Sandstrom R, Drott C, Hyltander A, et al. The effect of postoperative intravenous feeding (TPN) on outcome following major surgery evaluated in a randomized study. Ann Surg 1993;217:185.
68. Rudman D, Millikan WJ, Richardson TJ, et al. Elemental balances during intravenous hyperalimentation of underweight adult subjects. J Clin Invest 1975;55:94.
69. Long JM, Wilmore DW, Mason, AD, et al. Effects of carbohydrate and fat intake on nitrogen excretion during total intravenous feeding. Ann Surg 1977;185:417.
70. Jeejeebhoy KN, Anderson GH, Nakhooda, AF, et al. Metabolic studies in total parenteral nutrition with lipid in man. J Clin Invest 1976;57: 125.
71. Macfie J, Smith RC, Hill GL. Glucose or fat as a nonprotein energy source?: a controlled clinical trial in gastroenterological patients requiring intravenous nutrition. Gastroenterology 1981;80:103.
72. Peters C, Fischer JE. Studies on calorie nitrogen ratio for total parenteral nutrition. Surg Gynecol Obstet 1980;151:1.
73. Sim AJW, Wolfe BM, Young VR, et al. Glucose promotes whole body protein synthesis from infused amino acids in fasting man. Lancet 1979;13:68.
74. Nehme AB. Nutritional support of the hospitalized patient: the team concept. JAMA 1980;243:1906.
75. Montgomery WW. Surgery of the upper respiratory system, vol 2. Philadelphia: Lea & Febiger, 1973.
76. Stamm M. Gastrostomy: a new method. Medical News 1894;54:324.
77. Depage A. Noveau proiede pour la gastrostmie. Journal de Chirurgie et Annales de la Societe Belge de Chirurgie 1901;1:715.
78. Spivack JL. Gastrostomy. In: Berk JE, ed. Developments in digestive diseases. Philadelphia: Lea & Febiger, 1980.
79. Lopez R, Suavez A, Santiago-Delpin EA. A reversed jejunal segment interposition as feeding gastrostomy. Arch Surg 1977;112:343.
80. Campos AC, Butters M, Meguid MM. Home enteral nutrition via gastrostomy in advanced head and neck cancer patients. Head Neck 1990;12:137.
81. Chung RS. Surgical treatment of morbid obesity. Nutr Int 1985;1:3.
82. Hull MA, Rawlings J, Murray FE, et al. Audit of outcome of long-term enteral nutrition by percutaneous endoscopic gastrostomy. Lancet 1993;341:869.
83. Widiss TL, Meguid MM. The enteral alternative: update. Contemp Surg 1981;19:75.
84. Tsujinaka T, Iijima S, Kido Y, et al. Role of nucleosides and nucleotide mixture in intestinal mucosal growth under total parenteral nutrition. Nutrition 1993;9:532.
85. Pastores SM, Kvetan V, Katz DP. Immunomodulatory effects and therapeutic potential of glutamine in the critically ill surgical patient. Nutrition 1994;10:385.
86. Bennegard K, Eden E, Ekman L, et al. Metabolic response of whole body and peripheral tissues to enteral nutrition in weight losing cancer and non-cancer patients. Gastroenterology 1983;85:92.
87. DeVries EGE, Mulder NH, Houwen B, et al. Enteral nutrition by nasogastric tube in adult patients treated with intensive chemotherapy for acute leukemia. Am J Clin Nutr 1982;35:1490.
88. Dresler CM, Jeevanandam M, Brennan MF. Metabolic efficacy of enteral feeding in malnourished cancer and non-cancer patients. Metabolism 1987;36:82.
89. Haffeejee, AA, Angorn IB. Nutritional status and non specific and humoral immune response in oesophageal carcinoma. Ann Surg 1979; 189:475.
90. Burt ME, Gorschboth CM, Brennan MF. A controlled prospective, randomized trial comparing the metabolic effects of enteral and parenteral nutrition in the cancer patient. Cancer 1982;49:1092.
91. Shanberger RC, Brennan MF, Goodgame JT, et al. A prospective randomized study of adjuvant parenteral nutrition in the treatment of sarcomas: results of metabolic and survival studies. Surgery 1984;96: 1.
92. McArdle, AH, Wittnich C, Freeman CR, et al. Elemental diets as prophylaxis against radiation injury. Arch Surg 1985;120:1026.
93. Souba WW, Klimberg VS, Copeland EM III. Glutamine nutrition in the management of radiation enteritis. JPEN J Parenter Enter Nutr 1990;14(Suppl 4):106S.
94. Klimberg VS, Nwokedi E, Hutchins LF, et al. Glutamine facilitates chemotherapy while reducing toxicity. JPEN J Parenter Enter Nutr 1992;16(Suppl 6):83S.
95. Salloum RM, Copeland EM III, Bland KI. Selective stimulation of brush border glutamine transport in the tumor-bearing rat. J Surg Res 1990;50:391.
96. Klimberg VS, Souba WW, Salloum RM, et al. Glutamine-enriched diets support muscle glutamine metabolism without stimulating tumor growth. J Surg Res 1990;48:319.
97. Butters M, Campos AC, Meguid MM. High frequency–low morbidity mechanical complications of tube feeding: a prospective study. Clin Nutr 1992;11:87.
98. Payne-James JJ, Rees RGP, Doherty J, Silk DBA. 7g weighed versus unweighted polyurethane nasoenteral tubes—spontaneous transpyloric passage and clinical performance: a controlled randomised trial. Clin Nutr 1990;9:102.
99. Meguid MM, Williams LF. The use of gastrostomy to correct malnutrition. Surg Gynecol Obstet 1979;149:27.
100. Shellito PC, Malt RA. Tube gastrostomy: techniques and complications. Ann Surg 1985;201:180.
101. Edington H, Zajko A, Reilly JJ. Jejunal variceal hemorrhage: an unusual complication of needle catheter jejunostomy. JPEN J Parenter Enter Nutr 1983;7:489.
102. Vanlandingham S, Simpson S, Daniel P, Newmark SR. Metabolic abnormalities in patients supported with enteral tube feeding. JPEN J Parenter Enter Nutr 1981;5:322.
103. Schreiner R, Eitzen H, Gfell M, et al. Environmental contamination of continuous drip feedings. Pediatrics 1979;63:232.
104. Silk DB.A. Fibre and enteral nutrition. Gut 30:246-264, 1989;
105. Frank AF, Greene CG. Successful use of a bulk laxative to control the diarrhea of tube feedings. Scand J Plast Reconstr Surg 1979;13: 193.
106. Zimmaro DM, Rolandelli RH, Koruda MJ, et al. Isotonic tube feeding formula induces liquid stool in normal subjects: reversal by pectin. JPEN J Parenter Enter Nutr 1989;13:117.
107. Emerson AP. Foods high in fiber and phytobezoar formation. J Am Diet Assoc 1987;12:1675.
108. Canivet B, Creisson G, Freychet P, Dageville X. Fibre, diabetes and risk of bezoar. Lancet 1980;2:862.
109. McIvor A, Meguid MM, Curtas S, et al. Intestinal obstruction from cecal bezoar: a complication of fiber-containing tube feedings. Nutrition 1990;6:115.
110. Flynn KT, Norton LC, Fisher RL. Enteral tube feeding: indications, practices and outcomes. Image J Nurs Sch 1987;19:16.
111. Freedland CP, Roller RD, Wolfe BM, Flynn NM. Microbial contamination of continuous drip feedings. JPEN J Parenter Enter Nutr 1989; 13:18.
112. Perez SK, Brandt K. Enteral feeding contamination: comparison of diluents and feeding bag usage. JPEN J Parenter Enter Nutr 1989;13: 306.
113. Abernathy GB, Heizer WD, Holcombe BJ, et al. Efficacy of tube feeding in supplying energy requirements of hospitalized patients. JPEN J Parenter Enter Nutr 1989;13:387.
114. Chapman G, Curtas S, Meguid MM. Standardized enteral orders attain caloric goals sooner: a prospective study. JPEN J Parenter Enter Nutr 1992;16:149.
115. Meguid MM, Muscaritoli M. Current uses of total parenteral nutrition. Am Fam Physician 1993;47:383.
116. Meguid MM, Akahoshi MP, Hill LR. Evaluation of the practice of using a hyperalimentation catheter for multiple purposes. Nutr Int 1986;2:45.
117. Curtas S, Bonaventura M, Meguid MM. Cannulation of the inferior vena cava for long term central venous access: techniques and results. Surg Gynecol Obstet 1989;168:121.
118. Padberg FT Jr, Ruggiero J, Blackburn GL, Bistrian BR. Central venous catheterization for parenteral nutrition. Ann Surg 1981;193:264.
119. Weinsier RL, Bacon J, Butterworth CE Jr. Central venous alimentation: a prospective study of the frequency of metabolic abnormalities among medical and surgical patients. JPEN J Parenter Enter Nutr 1982;6:421.
120. Jones KW, Seltzer MH, Slocum BA, et al. Parenteral nutrition compli-

cations in a voluntary hospital. JPEN J Parenter Enter Nutr 1984;8: 385.
121. Wolfe BM, Ryder MA, Hishikawa RA, et al. Complications of parenteral nutrition. Am J Surg 1986;152:93.
122. Burri C, Ahnefeld FW. The caval catheter. New York: Springer-Verlag, 1977.
123. Bailey MJ. Reduction of catheter-associated sepsis in parenteral nutrition using low-dose intravenous heparin. Br Med J 1979;1:1671.
124. Fabri PJ, Mirtallo JM, Ruberg RL, et al. Incidence and prevention of thrombosis of the subclavian vein during total parenteral nutrition. Surg Gynecol Obstet 1982;155:238.
125. Imperial J, Bistrian B, Bothe A, et al. Limitation of central vein thrombosis in total parenteral nutrition by continuous infusion of low-dose heparin. J Am Coll Nutr 1983;2:63.
126. Mosca R, Curtas S, Forbes B, Meguid MM. The benefits of isolator cultures in the management of suspected catheter sepsis. Surgery 1987;102:716.
127. Paston MJ, Meguid RA, Muscaritoli M, et al. Dynamics of central venous catheter-related sepsis in the rat. J Clin Microbiol 1993;31: 1652.
128. Douard MD, Arlet G, Leverger G, et al. Quantitative blood cultures for diagnosis and management of catheter-related sepsis in pediatric hematology and oncology patients. Intensive Care Med 1991;17:30.
129. Meguid MM, Akahoshi M, Jeffers S, et al. Amelioration of metabolic complications of conventional total parenteral nutrition. Arch Surg 1984;119:1294.
130. Askanazi J, Rosenbaum SH, Hyman, AL, et al. Effects of total parenteral nutrition on gas exchange and breathing patterns [abstract]. Crit Care Med 1979;7:125.
131. Campos, ACL, Paluzzi M, Meguid MM. The clinical use of total nutritional admixtures. Nutrition 1990;6:347.
132. Mitchell KA, Jones EA, Curtas S, Meguid MM. A standardized TPN order form reduces staff time and potential for error. Nutrition 1990; 6:457.
133. Fogel RS, O'Brien JM, Kay BG, et al. Try this simple TPN order form. Nursing 1987;17:58.
134. Burke JF, Wolfe RR, Ullany CJ, et al. Glucose requirements following burn injury. Ann Surg 1979;190:274.
135. Askanazi J, Carpentier YA, Elwyn DH, et al. Influence of total parenteral nutrition on fuel utilization in injury and sepsis. Ann Surg 1980; 191:40.
136. Nordenstrom J, Askanazi J, Elwyn DH, et al. Nitrogen balance during total nutrition. Ann Surg 1983;197:27.
137. Gilder H. Parenteral nourishment of patients undergoing surgical or traumatic stress. JPEN J Parenter Enter Nutr 1986;10:88.
138. Billings JA. Comfort measures for the terminally ill: is dehydration painful? J Am Geriatr Soc 1985;33:808.
139. Callahan D. On feeding the dying. Hastings Cent Rep 1983;13:22.
140. Meyers DW. Legal aspects of withdrawing nourishment from an incurably ill patient. Arch Intern Med 1985;145:125.
141. Seigler M, Weisbard, AJ. Against the emerging stream: should fluids and nutritional support be discontinued. Arch Intern Med 1985;145: 129.
142. Dresser RS, Boisaubin EV. Ethics, law and nutritional support. Arch Intern Med 1985;145:122.
143. Micetich KC, Steinecker PH, Thomasma DC. Are intravenous fluids morally required for a dying patient? Arch Intern Med 1983;143:975.
144. Wanzer SH, Adelstein SJ, Cranford RE, et al. The physician's responsibility toward hopelessly ill patients. N Engl J Med 1984;310:955.
145. Wanzer SH, Federman DD, Adelstein SJ, et al. The physician's responsibility toward hopelessly ill patients: a second look. N Engl J Med 320: 844-849, 1989;
146. Meguid MM, Debonis D, Meguid V, Terz JJ. Nutritional support in cancer. Lancet 1983;2:230.
147. Mughal M, Meguid MM. The effect of nutritional status on morbidity after elective surgery for benign gastrointestinal disease. JPEN J Parenter Enter Nutr 1987;11:140.
148. Howard L. Home parenteral and enteral nutrition in cancer patients. Cancer 1993;72(Suppl 11):3531.
149. Smith, RC, Hartemink R. Improvement of nutritional measures during preoperative parenteral nutrition in patients selected by the prognostic nutritional index: a randomized controlled trial. J Parenter Enteral Nutr 1988;12:687.
150. Fan ST, Lau WY, Wong KK, Chan YPM. Preoperative parenteral nutrition in patients with esophageal cancer: a prospective, randomised clinical trial. Clin Nutr 1989;8:23.
151. Woolfson AMJ, Smith JAR. Elective nutritional support after major surgery: a prospective randomised trial. Clin Nutr 1989;8:15.

Surgery for Gastrointestinal Cancer: A Multidisciplinary Approach, edited by Harold J. Wanebo.
Lippincott-Raven Publishers, Philadelphia, © 1997.

CHAPTER 9

Endoscopic Considerations in the Management of Gastrointestinal Malignancy

Hector R. Nava and Ryan F. Holbrook

HISTORY

From as early as 1795 to 1932, a variety of rigid endoscopic instruments were invented that were illuminated by candles, alcohol lamps, and eventually electric lights. These instruments were successful to a degree in viewing the rectum and esophagus, but were unsuccessful in viewing all but a small part of the stomach.[1]

The modern era of endoscopy began in 1932, when Schindler and Wolf designed and developed a semiflexible gastroscope using a series of convex lenses. In spite of a variety of improvements, this type of gastroscope remained inadequate to visualize large areas of the stomach, and for the esophagus separate instrumentation was required. These instruments also lacked channels for aspiration or biopsy. However, in recognition of his contributions to the progress of endoscopy, Schindler has been called "the father of the gastroscope."[2]

In 1950, Uji and the Olympus Corporation of Japan developed an intragastric camera incorporated at the top of a flexible tube that allowed photography of the gastric mucosa. The gastrocamera was quickly replaced in the United States by the flexible fiberoptic gastroscope, developed by Hirschowitz and colleagues, which was initially presented to the American Gastroscope Society in 1957. By 1970, the fiberoptic endoscope was sufficiently developed to allow complete evaluation of the esophagus, stomach, and duodenum, and included side-viewing as well as forward-viewing endoscopes. Developments followed that allowed the addition of channels for air insufflation and water irrigation, as well as open working channels for biopsy forceps, snares, cytology brushes, and other instruments of therapeutic endoscopy.[3–5]

With the development of fiberoptics came the development of a fiberoptic colonoscope by Overholt at the University of Michigan in 1967. In 1973, endoscopic polypectomy was first demonstrated to be a minimally invasive procedure, and has become the standard management for most polyps of the gastrointestinal tract. In 1983, the Welch-Allyn Company developed the video endoscope, which remains state-of-the-art instrumentation for endoscopy. With it, the entire endoscopic evaluation can be viewed on a television screen with excellent image resolution.[6,7]

DIAGNOSIS

Most of the time, the endoscopist has the benefit of a presumed diagnosis based on either a clinical history or a radiologic examination. However, when examining patients with benign symptoms or for screening, the endoscopist should be on the alert for the early endoscopic manifestations of cancer. Malignancy should be suspected when nodularity, rigidity, or ulceration is detected. On stenotic lesions, some of these changes may not be apparent if the stricture is significant or nearly complete. Infiltrating tumors tend to raise the mucosa at the proximal border, so the only tissue observed by the endoscopist is the normal mucosa, which does not reveal the true nature of the stenosis when biopsy samples are taken. In these cases, appropriate tissue for diagnosis may be obtained by taking blind brushings and biopsy samples inside the stricture. If endoscopic dilatations are being carried out, the brushings and biopsy samplings should be repeated after the endoscope is able to traverse the lumen. Even if the stenosis cannot be fully intubated with the endoscope, improved visibility within the lumen after dilatation may facilitate the biopsy procedure.

When frank ulcerations are present, the site with the highest yield of positive diagnoses is the junction between the ulcer and the normal mucosa. If possible, biopsy specimens should be taken from all four quadrants. The bed of the ulcer should not be sampled aimlessly because this often obtains necrotic, undiagnostic material. The best specimens are obtained by directing the biopsy forceps to areas of viable tissue and by stay-

Hector R. Nava, Vice Chairman, Surgical Oncology, Chief of Endoscopy and Research, State University of New York at Buffalo, Roswell Park Memorial Institute, Elm and Carlton Streets, Buffalo, NY 14263-0001

Ryan F. Holbrook, 910 West 5th Avenue, Suite 680, Spokane, WA 99204 ing away from the grossly necrotic ulcer bed. When sampling hard tissues, a close-range biopsy is better because this stabilizes the forceps so more force can be applied to the tissues, and the endoscopist can better monitor the targeted tissues selected for biopsy.

O'Donoghue and colleagues showed that with the combination of brushings with biopsy sampling, the diagnostic yield was 100%, compared with 87% when biopsy samples alone were considered.[8] A similar study by Cussó and associates[9] showed a 98% correct rate of diagnosis in esophageal malignancies, an improvement in the diagnostic yield of 20.8%, when cytology was added to biopsy.[9]

To ensure good preservation of biopsy and cytologic specimens, the material should be fixed immediately. Once the specimen has been separated from the suspected area, the instrument should be removed and the specimens fixed at once.

Common sense would dictate that brushings be taken before the biopsy samples because bleeding caused by the sampling procedure will have a negative impact on the quality of the cytologic specimens. Zargar and coworkers demonstrated that when brushings were taken first, the diagnostic accuracy was significantly higher than when biopsy specimens were taken first.[10]

In vivo staining has been used extensively in some centers, especially in east Asia, using Lugol, methylene blue, and indigo carmine for the delineation and detection of subtle mucosal changes that might be difficult to identify by plain endoscopy. With this technique, histologic sampling is directed with greater accuracy, increasing the yield of positive diagnoses.

Radiologic evaluation of the gastrointestinal tract before endoscopy is critical because it provides the endoscopist with clues as to the location and the nature of lesion. In strictures, it helps to delineate the length and tortuosity of the stricture and the potential for hazards below the stricture, and can identify unsuspected fistulization.

Endoscopy alone can be used to stage esophageal malignancies, differentiating early lesions arising on one wall of the esophagus from totally circumferential, obstructive lesions with a worse prognosis. In addition, evaluation of the entire length of the tumor gives additional information that correlates with staging, resectability, and even curability. In general, lesions less than 5 cm in length, without circumferential involvement, can be considered resectable and potentially curable, whereas lesions longer than 5 cm and those with circumferential involvement might be considered incurable by surgery alone. The latter patients might be candidates for neoadjuvant programs to attempt to reduce the bulk of the primary tumor before resection. In cancer of the proximal stomach and gastroesophageal junction, localization of the diaphragm by endoscopic means in relation to the tumor margins might help the surgeon to decide whether an operation can be done through a left thoracoabdominal incision as opposed to the Ivor Lewis approach (abdomen plus right chest).

Careful measurement of the tumor's proximal border helps to determine how high the esophagus needs to be transected to allow for an ample margin. In addition, careful measurements of the distal margin help to delineate how much stomach needs to be taken and how much can be preserved without compromising the margins. In particular, delineation of tumor involvement alongside the lesser curvature becomes a crucial factor as to the point of transection of the stomach in relation to the incisura angularis, or whether a total gastrectomy is required. Although endoscopy is not recommended for routine follow-up of patients with esophageal carcinoma after resection, it often is indicated when the patient manifests dysphagia. This dysphagia frequently is related to benign postoperative anastomotic stricture, especially if both proximal and distal margins were negative for tumor. On the other hand, patients with positive margins may have local recurrence secondary to tumor regrowth.

In cancer of the colon with nonobstructing tumor, total colonoscopy is indicated to rule out synchronous carcinomas or polyps, which may affect the extent of the resection.[11] After colon resection for carcinoma, periodic survey by total colonoscopy has also proven useful for the detection of local recurrences, metachronous carcinomas, and polyps.[12]

THERAPY FOR ESOPHAGEAL MALIGNANCY

Dilatation of an esophagus obstructed by a malignant process has been attempted for many years with various degrees of success. During the rigid endoscopy era, dilatations with soft-tipped metal bougies and with metal olives resulted in a high perforation rate and a dismal reputation for endoscopy-guided dilatation. With the introduction of flexible fiberoptic endoscopy, new instrumentation was developed that was adapted to the flexible fiberoptic system. The Savary system, consisting of a flexible tip attached to a semiflexible monofilament wire over which sequential, tapered-tip plastic bougies are threaded, has been successfully used for the temporary relief of malignant dysphagia.[13] With this technique, the endoscopist places the guidewire under visual control into the narrowed lumen. Some manipulation may be necessary to negotiate tortuous, irregular, and long strictures. With or without fluoroscopic control, with the wire left in place, the endoscopist advances the tapered bougies over the wire. The dilators range from 10 to 54 Fr in size. Although the classic method of dilatation in esophageal strictures has been to pass only three sequential dilators in one setting, we have found that maximum dilatation to 54 Fr can be accomplished in most cases of malignant strictures, with the exception of the most severely fibrotic strictures. During dilatation, if no resistance is met, we recommend skipping to the next higher size until some resistance is noticed. After that, we continue to dilate following the normal sequence, and we monitor for the presence of any blood on each dilator after removal. Once blood is noted on the dilator, the dilatation is concluded. The sharp back tip of the guidewire is threaded through the biopsy channel of the endoscope, which is protected with a polyvinyl catheter to facilitate the passage of the guidewire. Once the endoscope is armed over the guidewire, the instrument is advanced with a combination of blind and visually directed maneuvers back into the esophagus. When good visualization is obtained, the endoscope is directed through the malignant stricture until it is passed below the stenosis. On occasion, because of debris, blood, and mucus, as well as collapse of the tumor within the stricture, good visualization is not possible, but most of the time gentle manipulation of the endoscope, using insufflation, irrigation, and gentle rotation, and manipulation of the controls permits safe passage through the stricture. Once the stricture is passed, the guidewire is removed and the distal esophagus and the stomach are checked for any evidence of contusion or trauma from the dilators. The mucous and blood secretions usually are easily removed, and this clears the view significantly. The endoscopist withdraws back to the stricture, where measurements of the distal and proximal edges of the tumor are taken to determine the tumor's length and circumferential involvement.

Hydrostatic balloons have been developed that can be passed through the endoscope's biopsy channels provided they are 2.8 mm in diameter or larger. These balloons range from 5 to 18 mm and can generate pressures up to 60 lbs per square inch. The soft tip of the balloon is placed through the stricture under endoscopic visualization. Obstruction in or below the stricture is detected by the sensation of resistance to advance. Most of the time this can be overcome by gently manipulating the endoscopic controls, as well as by varying rotation to change the angle of approach to the stricture. Once the balloon is through the stricture, the endoscope and the balloon are pulled back to center the balloon on the tumor and to facilitate monitoring the inflation. During inflation there usually is significant discomfort, requiring administration of intravenous narcotics as part of the conscious sedation for the procedure. Although some endoscopists are hesitant to go to the larger dilator, in our experience using the 18-mm diameter, 8-cm long balloon, we have achieved a high degree of success in dilating and negotiating most malignant strictures, with a low incidence of perforation.[14] The balloon being larger than the tip of the standard endoscope allows us to use the "follow-the-balloon" technique, which simplifies the passage through somewhat difficult and tortuous strictures (see Chapter 22).

Ablation of obstructing esophageal tumors has been tried using different modalities, including laser, monopolar and bipolar electrofulguration, heater probe, alcohol injections, and photodynamic therapy. All these techniques meet with various degrees of success, but only Nd-YAG endoscopic laser therapy has been well accepted, and it has become standard therapy for obstructing esophageal tumors. Prospective, randomized studies of the different modalities have not been done, with the exception of a U.S./Canadian multicenter study of Nd-YAG laser and photodynamic therapy, in which no differences were found between the two modalities as to the rate of complications and the degree of palliation achieved.[15]

ENDOESOPHAGEAL PROSTHESES

As an alternative to endoscopic tumor ablation, a variety of endoesophageal prostheses have been designed. These include the modified Celestine prosthesis, the Atkinson tube, and the Wilson-Cook prosthesis. Most recently, self-expanding metal and mesh prostheses have been developed. All these prostheses are placed by endoscopic-assisted means and have met with various degrees of success. The Wilson-Cook, Atkinson, and Celestine prostheses are placed after aggressive dilatation of the tumor, and they share a similar design that includes a semirigid plastic wall with a proximal funnel that prevents the prosthesis from falling in, and a distal shoulder that helps to anchor the prosthesis from slipping up. They all come in different lengths, and some even in different diameters. The difficulty with prostheses is that because of the significant dilatation and force required to place them, their use has resulted in an increased frequency of complications (ie, perforation and bleeding). In addition, dislodgement of the prosthesis is common. Another drawback of the prosthesis is the rigidity of its wall and its inability to clear itself, which requires that patients consume a soft mechanical diet for the rest of their lives. An advantage of the prosthesis, on the other hand, is that once in place it does not require additional periodic treatments, achieving good and prolonged palliation in some patients.[16]

The primary indication for a prosthesis is a tracheoesophageal fistula that cannot be treated with endoscopic tumor ablation. Most of the prostheses offer only a moderate degree of success in blocking the fistula's tract.[17] A modified cuffed Wilson-Cook prosthesis has been developed that is designed to provide better occlusion of the fistula's tract by means of a self-inflating balloon.

In general, prostheses work better on lesions of the midesophagus. The gastroesophageal junction poses difficulties because of its angulation, and sometimes the end of the prosthesis is blocked by gastric mucosa. Prostheses in the cervical esophagus are difficult to place and maintain, and frequently are associated with a significant degree of discomfort; although the lumen might be widely patent, the disturbance to the swallowing mechanism prevents the prosthesis from achieving adequate palliation.

PERCUTANEOUS ENDOSCOPIC GASTROSTOMY

Percutaneous endoscopic gastrostomy (PEG) is frequently used to provide the patient with an avenue for nutrition beyond the obstructing esophageal malignancy. In a patient who is severely malnourished and with a diagnosis that does not make him or her a surgical candidate, placement of a PEG is recommended as soon as the obstructing esophageal tumor is traversed with the endoscope. Feeding into the gastrointestinal tract has many advantages over total parenteral nutrition. It is possible to provide home nutrition using the PEG tube until the patient is able to swallow on his or her own, or the PEG can be kept indefinitely as a tube or as a button for the rest of the patient's life. Patients with advanced carcinoma and significant weight loss who are extremely malnourished might have difficulty in healing. In placing a PEG, extreme caution must be taken in severely malnourished patients to avoid serious complications. Pull-through PEGs that rely on a balloon, T-bar, or other mechanisms of internal support to maintain the gastric wall against the parietal peritoneum do not provide even pressure around the PEG and can result in peritoneal leakage, which in this patient population might be fatal. A particularly difficult patient is the patient with ascites, which most authors believe is a contraindication to PEG because of the high rate of leaks and major complications. Our experience in these patients with pull-through PEG corroborates this.[18] We have begun using the Brown-Mueller T-fastener technique. With this method, the gastric wall is tacked down with four T-fasteners placed percutaneously under endoscopic guidance, and the PEG is placed in the center with the help of a series of dilators and further secured in place with a system consisting of a balloon inside and a supportive ring outside. Using this technique, we have almost completely eliminated major complications in this patient population, and these PEG tubes can be used confidently 24 hours after placement.[19]

An important but infrequently mentioned aspect of managing a patient with esophageal carcinoma is the observation that many of these patients have gastric emptying problems, especially when the primary tumor is locally advanced and has encroached on the vagi, in particular the right vagus, which carries the branch that innervates the pylorus. The gastric emptying difficulty is related to lack of relaxation of the pylorus, which in some cases becomes paralyzed in a contracted position. In addition, dismotility of the antrum plays an important role. The antrum normally contracts on average three times per minute, but in these patients there is an absence of contractions. If the clinician observes the area for a full minute during endoscopy, reduced motility as well as ineffective contractions can be detected. This condition is usually associated with large amounts of fluid, and food retention is observed by the endoscopist on entering the stomach. Further confirmation of the gastric emptying problem can be obtained by a technetium 99m sulfur colloid gastric emptying study. If gastric emptying difficulties are documented, these patients will not benefit from a patent esophagus or a gastrostomy tube, and will require placement of a feeding jejunostomy tube through the PEG.

In gastric cancer, histologic confirmation on the first endoscopic examination can pose some problems even in advanced cases. Even grossly malignant lesions do not yield a positive diagnosis on every biopsy taken. Awad and colleagues showed that in exophytic tumors, the positive yield per biopsy specimen was 47%, whereas in nonexophytic tumors the yield was only 17%.[20] In infiltrating tumors, Winawer and associates showed a diagnostic accuracy of only 50% for biopsy samplings plus brushings, compared with 92% in exophytic tumors.[21] The greater the number of biopsy specimens, the higher the rate of positive diagnosis. Graham and colleagues showed that the first biopsy sampling carries only a 70% positive diagnostic rate; however, when four biopsy samples are taken, the accuracy increases to 95%, and to 98.9% when seven specimens are obtained.[22] The addition of cytologic brushings further increases the accuracy, especially when specimens are obtained from areas that can be approached only tangentially.[23]

Early gastric carcinoma, first identified in Japan in the early 1960s, is now being identified with increased frequency in the United States.[24] For the endoscopist to detect early carcinoma, a complete and disciplined examination of the entire gastric mucosa is required, using a mechanically sound endoscope with good optics and illumination.

Endoscopic ultrasonography was introduced in the mid-1980s. This new technology permits sonographic examination of the hollow alimentary tract walls. Disruption of any of the five typical echo-delineated layers is readily detected, providing excellent correlation with the T-staging of the tumor, with an accuracy that ranges from 71% to 83%.[25,26] Regional lymph node metastases can also be detected by endoscopic ultrasonography. However, although this study reported an accuracy for lymph node metastasis of 87%, the accuracy dropped to 48% in inflammatory lymph nodes.[27] A newly introduced electronic ultrasound device will permit ultrasonically guided biopsy of extraluminal masses or lymph nodes. Prospective studies, however, will be necessary to determine the role of endoscopic ultrasonography in the staging and management of alimentary tract malignancy.

CONCLUSION

Flexible fiberoptic endoscopy, followed by video endoscopy, has made a tremendous impact on the diagnosis and management of gastrointestinal malignancy. Therapeutic endoscopy continues to expand with the introduction of new technology, as major surgical procedures are being replaced by outpatient endoscopic procedures. Flexible endoscopy will continue to expand its role in dealing successfully with cancer of the alimentary tract.

REFERENCES

1. Henning N, Berry LH. History of gastrointestinal endoscopy. In: Berry LH, ed. Gastrointestinal panendoscopy. 1st ed. Springfield, IL: Charles C Thomas, 1974:5.
2. Schindler R. Gastroscopy. New York: Hafner, 1966.
3. Morrissey JF, Tanaka Y, Thorsen WB. The relative value of the Olympus model 6T-5 gastrocamera and Olympus model GI-F gastrocamera fiberscope. Gastrointest Endosc 1968;15:197.
4. Hirschowitz BJ, Curtiss LE, Peters CW, Pollard HM. Demonstration of a new gastroscope: the "fiberscope." Gastroenterology 1958;35:50.
5. Uji T. Studies on photograph of gastric mucosa and its application (in Japanese). Tokyo Journal of Medical Science 1953;61:135.
6. Takemoto T, Noguchi T, Fuji T, Okita K. History of endoscopic diagnosis and treatment. Gann Monograph on Cancer Research 1990;37;3.
7. Fukuchi G, Hoshihara Y. New progress in endoscopic diagnosis by electronic endoscope. Gann Monograph on Cancer Research 1990;37:33.
8. O'Donoghue J, Waldron R, Gough D, et al. An analysis of the diagnostic accuracy of endoscopic biopsy and cytology in the detection of oesophageal malignancy. Eur J Surg Oncol 1992;18:332.
9. Cussṕ X, Mones-Xiol J, Vilardel F. Endoscopic etiology of cancer of the esophagus and cardia: a long term evaluation. Gastrointestinal Endoscopy 1989;35:321.
10. Zargar SA, Khuvoo MS, Jan GM, et al. Prospective comparison of the value of brushings before and after biopsy in the endoscopic diagnosis of gastrointestinal malignancy. Acta Cytol 1991;35:549.
11. Pagana TJ, Ledesma EJ, Mittelman A, Nava HR. The use of colonoscopy in the study of synchronous colorectal neoplasms. Cancer 1984; 53:356.
12. Nava HR, Pagana TJ. Postoperative surveillance of colorectal carcinoma. Cancer 1982;49:1043.
13. Dumon JFD, Meric B, Sivak MV, Fleisher D. A new method of esophageal dilatation using Savary-Gilliard bougies. Gastrointest Endosc 1985;31:379.
14. Holbrook RF, DeLeon R, Nava HR. Esophageal perforations secondary to dilatation of malignant esophageal strictures [abstract]. Accepted for presentation at the SAGES Scientific Session, Orlando, Florida, March 13 and 14, 1995.
15. Lightdale CJ, Heier SK, Marcon NE. Photodynamic therapy with pontine sodium versus thermal ablation therapy with Nd-YAG laser for palliation of esophageal cancer: a multicenter randomized trial. Gastrointestinal Endoscopy 1995;42:6.
16. Tytgat GN, den Hartog Jager FCA, Haver Kamp HJ. Positioning of a plastic prosthesis under fiberendoscopic control in the palliative treatment of cardio-esophageal cancer. Endoscopy 1976;8:180.
17. George R, Mesko TW, Nava HR. Malignant TEF: management by endoprosthesis [abstract]. Presented at the 96th Annual Meeting of the Eastern Division of the Canadian Association of Clinical Surgeons, Ottawa, Ontario, Canada, April 30–May 1, 1992.
18. Zera RT, Nava HR, Fischer J. Percutaneous endoscopic gastrostomy (PEG) in cancer patients. Surg Endosc 1993;7:304.
19. George R, Nava HR. T-fastener gastropexy for PEG: avoiding gastrostomy tube contamination of upper aerodigestive tumor by microorganisms [abstract]. Presented at the 96th Annual Meeting of the Eastern Division of the Canadian Association of Clinical Surgeons, Ottawa, Ontario, Canada, April 30–May 1, 1992.
20. Awad JA, Lee EY, Wang TC, et al. Effect of mucosal thickening near gastric carcinoma on the endoscopic diagnosis of malignancy. Dig Dis Sci 1990;35:317.
21. Winawer SJ, Posner G, Lightdale CJ. Endoscopic diagnosis of advanced gastric cancer: factors influencing yield. Gastroenterology 1975;69:1183.
22. Graham DY, Schwartz JT, Cain GD, et al. Prospective evaluation of

biopsy numbers in the diagnosis of esophageal and gastric carcinoma. Gastroenterology 1982;82:228.
23. Bemvenuti GA, Hattori K, Levin B, et al. Endoscopic sampling for tissue diagnosis in gastrointestinal malignancy. Gastrointest Endosc 1975;21:159.
24. Lehnert T, Sternberg SS, Sprossmann M, et al. Early gastric cancer. Am J Surg 1989;157:202.
25. Rosch T, Lorenz R, Zenker K, et al. Local staging and assessment of resectability in carcinoma of the esophagus, stomach and duodenum by endoscopic ultrasonography. Gastrointest Endosc 1992;38:460.
26. Saito N, Takeshita K, Nabu H, et al. The use of endoscopic ultrasound in determining the depth of cancer invasion in patients with gastric cancer. Surg Endosc 1991;5:14.
27. Tio TL, Coene PP, Luiken GJ, et al. Endosonography in the clinical staging of esophagogastric carcinoma. Gastrointest Endosc 1990; 36(Suppl 2):S2.

Surgery for Gastrointestinal Cancer: A Multidisciplinary Approach, edited by Harold J. Wanebo.
Lippincott-Raven Publishers, Philadelphia, © 1997.

CHAPTER 10

Laparoscopy in Gastrointestinal Malignancies

Alan T. Lefor, John L. Flowers, and Robert W. Bailey

Although cholecystectomy was performed only by "conventional" open surgical techniques as recently as 1987, it is now performed laparoscopically throughout the world. The ever-expanding scope of laparoscopic surgery now includes a variety of diagnostic, therapeutic, and palliative procedures of importance in the care of the cancer patient. The first laparoscopic procedure recorded in the literature was a gynecologic procedure performed in Russia by Ott in 1901.[1] Telescopes were rigid tubes through which only the operating surgeon could view the field. Laparoscopy was almost entirely limited to use as a diagnostic tool. It was not until the early 1980s, with the development of high-quality electronic video cameras, that the equipment necessary for today's advanced laparoscopic surgery became available.[2] These cameras allow the entire operating team access to the same view. It is certain that future developments will be forthcoming in the technologic aspects of laparoscopic surgery. It is of great importance that these issues be openly discussed and questions answered using the mechanism of prospective trials whenever possible.

Laparoscopic surgery has a number of applications in the care of the patient with gastrointestinal malignancies. Specific indications for the use of laparoscopy in the care of the cancer patient have not yet been established;[3] however, there are two principles that should guide the use of laparoscopy in the cancer patient. First, as with the use of laparoscopy in nonmalignant conditions, the procedure should not be undertaken simply because it can be performed laparoscopically. That is, the laparoscopic nature of a procedure should not alter the indications for its conduct. Second, when laparoscopy is used for diagnosis, staging, and treatment, the laparoscopic conduct of the procedure should compromise neither the nature of the procedure, nor the amount or source of the tissue obtained.

Alan T. Lefor, Assistant Professor of Surgery and Oncology, Department of Surgery, University of Maryland Cancer Center, 22 South Greene Street, Baltimore, MD 21201-1595

John L. Flowers, Assistant Professor of Surgery, Director, Center for Advances in Videoscopic Surgery, University of Maryland at Baltimore, 22 South Greene Street, Baltimore, MD 21201

Robert W. Bailey, Division Head of General Surgery, Greater Baltimore Medical Center, 6565 North Charles Street, Suite 315, Towson, MD 21204

Surgeons have been involved in the diagnosis, staging, treatment, and palliation of malignancies for centuries. Laparoscopy is assuming a role in each of these areas. Laparoscopy has a role in establishing the *diagnosis* of cancer in some situations by allowing biopsy samples to be taken of intraperitoneal and retroperitoneal masses and lymph nodes, as well as visceral lesions, and permitting the examination of abdominal contents under direct vision or with ultrasound probes. Laparoscopy is useful in the *staging* of established malignancies such as pancreatic cancer and esophageal cancer. Laparoscopy also has a role in the surgical *treatment* of a variety of malignancies, including gastric carcinoma, pancreatic cancer, and colon cancer. Laparoscopy may be the appropriate approach for the definitive therapy of these lesions, or may be a way to provide a palliative procedure such as a cholecystojejunostomy in a patient with unresectable carcinoma of the pancreas. Last, laparoscopy can play an important role in the *palliative care* of the cancer patient through procedures such as feeding tube placement or intestinal stoma creation.

PATIENT SELECTION

Patients who are not candidates for open diagnostic laparotomy also may not be suitable for a laparoscopic investigation. A thorough history and physical examination is always required as part of the preoperative evaluation, with attention to any coexisting medical illnesses that increase the risk of perioperative complications. Before they can give complete informed consent, all patients must be apprised of the potential complications related to the laparoscopic conduct of the operation, such as abdominal wall injury (hernia or hemorrhage), visceral injury, and complications of related to pneumoperitoneum, including subcutaneous emphysema, hypercarbia, pneumothorax, and CO_2 embolism. The possibility of conversion to an open procedure must be fully discussed with the patient.

Avoidance of perioperative complications is especially important in patients with malignancy, in view of their limited life expectancy, immunosuppression, and diminished physiologic reserve. One effective method of avoiding complications is avoidance of laparoscopic procedures in patients with absolute contraindications and careful patient selection in patients with relative contraindications to laparoscopic intervention. The only universally accepted absolute contraindication to laparoscopy is uncorrectable coagulopathy. Inability to tolerate general anesthesia may also be considered an absolute contraindication in most cases, because the degree of manipulation of tissue necessary to obtain a diagnosis or palliate unresectable disease usually precludes the sole use of local or regional anesthesia.

Relative contraindications to elective laparoscopy have traditionally included pregnancy, minor bleeding disorders, previous upper abdominal surgery, significant intestinal obstruction or distention, intraabdominal sepsis, and advanced cardiopulmonary disease.[4] Unfortunately, many patients with gastrointestinal malignancy requiring intraabdominal surgery possess relative contraindications because of the anatomic consequences of their diseases. Many patients have had extensive prior abdominal surgery. In patients without previous abdominal surgery, intraabdominal metastases or carcinomatosis may result in unsuspected adhesions between viscera and the abdominal wall, dense matting of bowel loops that prevent safe dissection, and small intestinal distention due to partial obstruction. Ascites may cause free small bowel loops to float, resulting in injury during insertion of the Verress needle or operating ports, or may prevent formation of an adequate pneumoperitoneum by occupying most of the available space in the peritoneal cavity. Prior radiation therapy may increase the friability of the intestinal wall and cause mesenteric fibrosis and shortening, resulting in bleeding during trivial manipulation and predisposing to tears and perforation.

Once in the operating room, the approach must be individualized. Extra care is necessary during creation of the pneumoperitoneum and insertion of operating ports. Open laparoscopy with the use of a modified Hassan cannula is frequently necessary. Diseased bowel must be handled with appropriate instruments, using great care. Preoperative colon preparation is useful in selected cases in which extensive mobilization and retroperitoneal dissection is anticipated. Careful closure of all port sites, including 5-mm puncture sites, is necessary in patients with ascites to prevent ascitic leak and the potential for infected ascites.

LAPAROSCOPY IN THE DIAGNOSIS OF CANCER

General Considerations

Patients often present with constitutional symptoms and undergo evaluation by imaging studies in the hope of identifying an underlying cause. The use of diagnostic laparoscopy in the evaluation of abdominal malignancies has been reported.[5] In this series of 25 patients with suspected malignancies, 17 (68%) had a positive study for cancer, but these investigators believed that subsequent patient management had been altered by the laparoscopic findings in all 25 (100%) patients.

Biopsy of Masses

Masses that are identified preoperatively are often amenable to laparoscopic biopsy. Accurate preoperative imaging studies, however, are essential to localize the mass before attempts at laparoscopic biopsy. Laparoscopic "fishing expeditions" may be less fruitful than such endeavors performed using conventional open techniques because of the lack of tactile sensation. A number of techniques are available for the biopsy of masses under laparoscopic guidance, including:

- Percutaneous insertion of a Tru-cut biopsy needle with direct puncture of the mass: this is easily performed under the direct vision afforded by the laparoscope. Careful placement of the needle entry site is important and is usually best done directly over the selected lesion, because the needle may not reach a lesion far from the entrance site.
- Wedge biopsy using the electrocautery: this method should be used cautiously to avoid destruction of the specimen with the electrocautery.
- Cup forceps biopsy: careful use of these forceps allows removal of adequate tissue for histopathologic examination while avoiding destruction of the specimen.

Whatever method is used, the surgeon must take great care to avoid losing the specimen. A retrieval bag may be useful for larger specimens that will not pass through a trocar sheath.

Liver Biopsy and Evaluation of Liver Tumors

Laparoscopy is extremely useful in the evaluation of liver lesions. It may be helpful in patients with liver lesions diagnosed by imaging studies, or in those with unknown hepatic lesions (see Table 10-1). Laparoscopic investigation of hepatic lesions can include inspection, palpation (with a probe), intraoperative ultrasound (discussed later), and directed biopsy.[3] Lesions that are located on the thin edge of the liver may be easily sampled using two applications of the linear stapler, avoiding destruction of the tissue, as shown in Figure 10-1.[6] This method is also useful in obtaining blind liver biopsy specimens when the specimens required are larger than those available with a Tru-cut needle.

Lymph Node Biopsy

The need for lymph node biopsy or sampling usually occurs as a result of one of three clinical situations. Abnormal nodes detected on preoperative imaging studies such as computed tomography (CT) scans or lymphangiography may require a targeted biopsy. Alternatively, suspect lymph nodes requiring histologic evaluation may be seen during the course of diagnostic laparoscopy. Specific dissection of discrete lymph node groups may also be necessary for staging of malignancies such as Hodgkin's lymphoma.

Essentially all major lymph node groups in the abdomen can be accessed using a laparoscopic approach. Specimens from lymph nodes in the celiac axis and portal, peripancreatic, mesenteric, periaortic, iliac, and pelvic regions can be obtained with varying degrees of technical difficulty. In cases where specific lymph nodes are identified preoperatively with imaging studies, it may be helpful to mark the area of dissection with clips and use intraoperative radiographs as a guide to ensure that the desired area has been evaluated. Biopsy of iliac and portal lymph nodes is fairly straightforward, with careful dissection

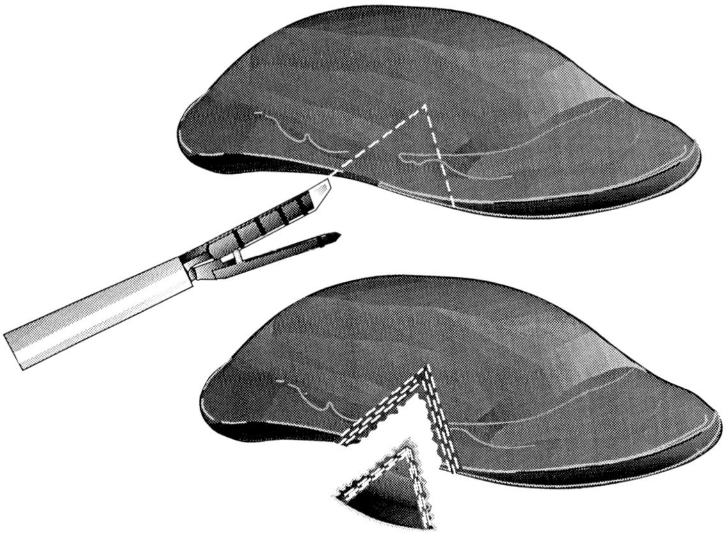

FIG. 10-1. Technique of liver biopsy with two applications of the linear stapler at approximately 90°, yielding a wedge of liver tissue from the thin edge of the liver. (Reprinted with permission from Lefor AT, Flowers JL. Laparoscopic wedge biopsy of the liver. J Am Coll Surg 1994;178:307.)

on the surface and lateral aspects of the corresponding vessels. Celiac axis and peripancreatic node specimens require entry into the lesser sac through either the lesser omentum or the gastrocolic ligament, and are moderately difficult to obtain. Mesenteric, periaortic, and pericaval lymph nodes are most difficult to sample, often requiring extensive mobilization of the colon and difficult retraction. However, all of these areas can be safely accessed by an experienced laparoscopic surgeon.

Laparoscopic Intracorporeal Ultrasound

One of the most important developments in the laparoscopic evaluation of malignancies is the laparoscopic ultrasound probe.[7] Intraoperative ultrasound was first described in 1958, and advancements in the technology have had a significant impact on the intraoperative management of a number of complex problems.[8] The essential equipment consists of a probe and a scanner connected by a cable. The laparoscopic application of these devices is limited by the size and location of the access ports used. The direct contact of the probe with the liver affords superior resolution compared to that obtained with transabdominal ultrasound imaging. A wide variety of probes is becoming available for laparoscopic examinations, including flexible or rigid tips, linear or circular arrays, and the capacity for multiple scanning frequencies (eg, 5 and 7.5 MHz).

Examination of the liver begins with the right lobe. Screening is usually performed starting from the lateral to the medial aspect, and then from medial to lateral. The screening area of the transducer must be known; currently used probes have an area of about 3.8 cm. Therefore, the transducer is withdrawn a distance slightly less than the screening area to ensure adequate examination. The smaller size of the left lobe makes it easier to examine.

When searching for lymphadenopathy, it is critical to adapt the technique to the specific area being studied, ensuring good acoustic contact between the probe and the tissue. Saline solution may be instilled to aid in this process.[7] Doppler techniques are useful to identify blood vessels that aid in the identification of lymph nodes.

The ability to examine the biliary tree with laparoscopic intracorporeal ultrasound (LICU) has been described.[9] This report establishes the accuracy of this technique compared to cholangiography in determining common duct size and presence of choledocholithiasis. The use of LICU in 176 patients has been reported.[10] In this series, 145 patients underwent laparoscopic cholecystectomy, and 31 patients underwent staging laparoscopy with examination of the liver. From these preliminary studies, it appears that LICU has potential in the intraoperative evaluation of patients with malignancies. It is also clear that the value of this procedure is limited by operator skill, and therefore it is important to gain experience with this technique whenever possible. Newer probes under development will permit biopsy of deep lesions under ultrasound guidance, allowing the biopsy needle to pass directly through the probe. Combined with technologic advances in probe design, an experienced operator will be able to gain important information that will affect patient management.

LAPAROSCOPY IN THE STAGING OF GASTROINTESTINAL MALIGNANCIES

General Considerations

The use of laparoscopy to stage accurately a wide variety of intraabdominal malignancies is a relatively recent application of this methodology. Perhaps the most important benefit of laparoscopic staging is the *exclusion of patients with unresectable disease from further invasive procedures.*

It is, however, difficult to assess the utility of this approach. Table 10-1 lists the indications for laparoscopic diagnosis and staging at the University of Dundee. The results of laparoscopy performed on the basis of these indications were analyzed by a 2-year prospective evaluation, and the following parameters assessed: diagnostic yield, management benefit, and management disadvantage.[3] The results of this trial showed a 90% diagnostic yield. The authors concluded that management was affected in 30% of patients by the performance of a laparoscopic staging procedure. There were only two cases (4%) in which

TABLE 10-1. *University of Dundee indications for laparoscopic diagnosis and staging of patients with malignancies*

All patients with tumors that present at an advanced stage
All patients with mass lesions detected by diagnostic imaging
Patients with ascites and negative cytologic findings
All patients with hepatic lesions detected by imaging studies
All patients with unexplained weight loss
Some patients with lymphomas

Adapted from Cuschieri A. Diagnosis and staging of tumors by laparoscopy. Seminars in Laparoscopic Surgery 1994;1:3.

laparoscopy failed to identify disease that signaled unresectability: a missed hepatic lesion in segment eight, and portal vein involvement by a tumor of the head of the pancreas.

Laparoscopy is extremely accurate for the identification of peritoneal disease, which is often missed by standard noninvasive imaging studies such as CT scanning, ultrasonography, and magnetic resonance imaging.[11] Lesions that are only a few millimeters in size can be sampled for biopsy with extreme accuracy. Liver and peritoneal disease is often found in patients with negative CT scans, supporting the use of laparoscopy to identify these lesions.[11] A representative laparoscopic view of such lesions is shown in Figure 10-2.

A series of 162 patients with a variety of malignancies, including 98 patients with hepatic lesions and 64 patients with nonhepatic intraabdominal malignancy, underwent laparoscopic staging.[12] All of these patients were thought to be resectable for cure based on a number of preoperative imaging studies. Biopsies were performed in 37% of cases. In 36% of cases, laparoscopy yielded information that prevented unnecessary laparotomy because of the identification of lesions that were unresectable. Conversely, 12% of patients who had laparoscopic findings suggesting resectability were found at laparotomy to be unresectable. Sites missed included positive lymph nodes, hepatic vein involvement, and missed peritoneal metastases. This study supports the use of laparoscopy to prevent unnecessary laparotomy in those patients who will not benefit from resection.

Ascites

Intraabdominal malignancies commonly present with ascites, which is exudative in nature. Paracentesis is carried out initially. Laparoscopic examination is not necessary if cytologic examination demonstrates malignancy. However, if the cytologic study is negative for malignancy, laparoscopy offers an excellent way to make a diagnosis. Preoperative CT scan may help direct the exploration. Patients with CT scans that suggest ovarian disease are brought to open laparotomy because this is necessary for definitive staging in cases of ovarian cancer.

Laparoscopy is facilitated in patients with tense ascites by repeated paracentesis begun 24 hours before surgery.[13] In a series of 47 patients with ascites, laparoscopy revealed carcinomatosis in 22, ovarian cancer in 11, and 3 patients each with mesothelioma, hepatoma, and hepatic myelofibrosis, 2 patients with pancreatic cancer, and 1 patient with squamous cancer, chronic lymphatic leukemia, breast cancer, and lymphoma.[13] The accuracy of laparoscopy in the evaluation of malignant disease presenting as ascites was been reported in this series as 100%.[13]

Esophageal Cancer

Early laparoscopic studies of the staging of esophageal cancer were usually characterized by little manipulation of the abdominal contents to identify disease, and were commonly limited to observation of the parietal peritoneal surfaces. A prospective trial was undertaken to compare the accuracy in diagnosing intraabdominal metastatic disease by scintigraphy, ultrasound scanning, and laparoscopy.[14] Of the 50 patients studied, 23 had esophageal carcinoma, 14 had gastric carcinoma, and 13 had suspected intraabdominal metastatic spread from other lesions. The accuracy of identification of metastatic disease was determined by laparoscopic biopsy, laparotomy, and autopsy. The overall accuracy was 72% for scintigraphy, 75% for ultrasound, and 96% for laparoscopy. Thirteen patients without hepatic metastatic disease had nodal or peritoneal disease diagnosed only by laparoscopy. This study demonstrates the value of laparos-

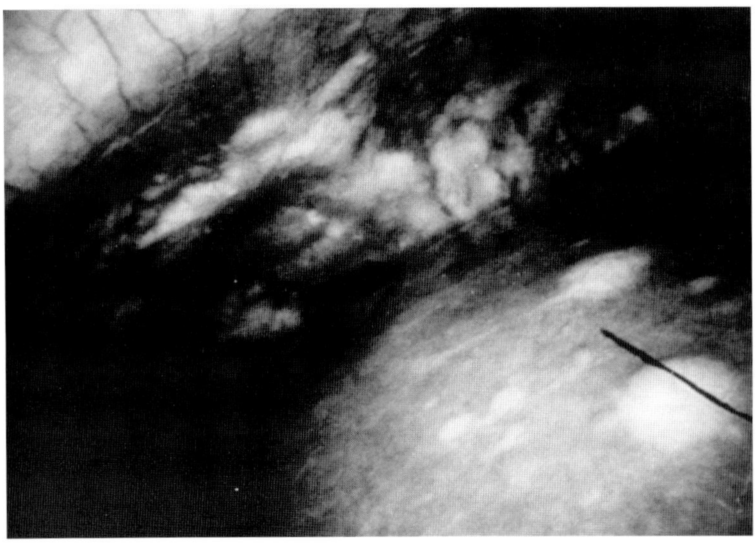

FIG. 10-2. Laparoscopic examination of the peritoneal cavity allows identification of small lesions on peritoneal surface such as those seen here, which are unlikely to be visualized on preoperative imaging studies. (Reprinted with permission from Lefor AT. Laparoscopic surgery for cancer. PPO Updates 1995;9(7):5.)

copy, and its ability to obviate the need for laparotomy in patients with lesions not resectable for cure.

In another study, 369 patients with carcinoma of the esophagus and cardia of the stomach underwent laparoscopy, revealing single or multiple intraabdominal metastases in 52 patients (14%).[15] This study suggested that intraabdominal metastases become more common as the location of the primary tumor becomes more distal, being greatest in lesions of the cardia. More recent data suggest that abdominal lymph node metastases may be present despite the location of the primary tumor.[16]

The sensitivity, specificity, and accuracy of laparoscopy, ultrasound, and abdominal CT scan were compared in 90 patients with biopsy-proven carcinoma of the esophagus or gastric cardia.[17] Laparoscopy was found to be significantly more sensitive and more accurate ($P<0.05$) than either ultrasound or abdominal CT scanning in diagnosing hepatic disease. Peritoneal disease was not identified by ultrasound or CT scan, but laparoscopy identified it in eight of nine (89%) of cases. Lymph node metastases were identified most accurately by laparoscopy, although the difference between laparoscopy and CT scanning failed to achieve statistical significance. These authors concluded that laparoscopy offers an accurate, reliable, and safe method of preoperative assessment in patients with carcinoma of the esophagus.

Thoracoscopic lymph node staging has been shown to provide accurate preresection staging of thoracic node status.[18,19] The staging accuracy of thoracoscopy has been validated in a trial comparing thoracoscopy to noninvasive staging techniques. This study found greater accuracy with thoracoscopic staging.[20] More recently, routine laparoscopic lymph node assessment in patients with carcinoma of the esophagus has been combined with thoracoscopic lymph node staging. Laparoscopic evaluation of intraabdominal disease was correct in 17 of 18 patients (94%) in a prospective trial.[16] Laparoscopy failed to identify a positive lymph node in 1 one 18 patients (6%). Three patients were downstaged as a result of laparoscopic evaluation of intraabdominal lymph nodes. Six of 18 (33%) patients had unsuspected celiac lymph node involvement at laparoscopy. Lymph nodes near the diaphragm may be difficult to evaluate without extensive dissection. Laparoscopic staging can also be combined with placement of an enteral feeding tube during the same procedure in patients with impending esophageal obstruction.

These studies establish the value of laparoscopic evaluation in patients with carcinoma of the esophagus. This approach has low morbidity and can correctly identify intraabdominal disease with a high level of accuracy. Its utility will be further established with ongoing prospective trials.

Hepatic Tumors

The accurate evaluation of the liver is a critical component of tumor staging for many malignancies of interest to the surgeon, because the presence of metastatic disease in the liver often obviates the need for major resections. Radiologic imaging alone is imperfect. In one series, 63 of 150 (42%) patients with colorectal carcinoma were found to have unresectable disease at laparotomy after an imaging evaluation demonstrated resectable lesions.[21] This demonstrates one of the major benefits of laparoscopic staging, the ability to exclude from laparotomy those patients with unresectable lesions in a way that minimizes postoperative pain and hospitalization.

An important tool in the management of hepatic lesions is intraoperative hepatic ultrasonography. In a study of 30 patients undergoing planned hepatic resection and 32 patients undergoing laparotomy with resection of a gastrointestinal primary malignancy, intraoperative ultrasonography was compared with CT angioportography.[22] Of the 30 patients slated to undergo hepatic resection, the procedure was changed or guided by the ultrasonographic result in 20 cases (67%). Of the 32 patients undergoing resection of their primary tumor, 5 (16%) had the stage of their disease altered based on the results of intraoperative ultrasonography.

Having demonstrated the value of laparoscopy and intraoperative ultrasonography, combining the two procedures is a natural extension of the technology. In a study of 50 patients undergoing laparoscopic evaluation of hepatic tumors, laparoscopic ultrasonography was performed in 43 patients.[23] Laparoscopy alone demonstrated that lesions shown to be resectable by preoperative imaging studies were unresectable in 23 (46%) patients. Hepatic lesions not visible by laparoscopic examination alone were identified by laparoscopic ultrasonography in 14 patients. Furthermore, the use of laparoscopic ultrasonography provided staging information in addition to that gained by laparoscopy in 18 (42%) patients.

It is clear that the usefulness of the information gained through laparoscopic ultrasonography is highly dependent on the skill of the operator, and thus continued practice with this technology is important. The ultimate value of this imaging modality will be determined by continued prospective evaluation. It appears that laparoscopic ultrasonography has the potential to avoid unnecessary laparotomy in a substantial proportion of patients with hepatic lesions.

Pancreatic Cancer

Laparoscopy has been used in the staging of patients with carcinoma of the pancreas for some time. An early report describes the experience with 23 patients with pancreatic cancer.[24] This study was carried out before the widespread use of abdominal CT scan and the advent of high-quality optics for laparoscopy. This report emphasized the utility of biopsy under direct vision.

In a report of 40 patients with carcinoma of the pancreas, Warshaw and coworkers found 26 patients without evidence of metastatic disease, and 14 patients with metastatic disease that precluded a curative resection.[25] Laparoscopy was performed as the final study before laparotomy only if the imaging studies were negative for metastatic disease. The negative findings at laparoscopy were confirmed in 23 of 26 patients at laparotomy. The positive laparoscopic findings in 14 of 40 patients altered the therapeutic course of all 14 patients. Findings in these patients were single, small (1- to 2-mm) nodules in the liver (n = 6), peritoneal surfaces (n = 7), and omentum (n = 1), all of which were verified histologically. The three instances of false-negative findings resulted from incomplete examination of the liver (n = 2) and the presence of a central liver lesion (n = 1). The overall accuracy was 93%, and with negative findings, 88%.

Another application of laparoscopy in the staging of patients with carcinoma of the pancreas is the ability to obtain specimens for cytologic examination. In 40 patients with lesions that were resectable according to the results of preoperative imaging studies, peritoneal washings were obtained (27 at laparoscopy and 13 at laparotomy).[26] Malignant cells were found in 12 (30%) of the specimens. Liver metastases were seen in six patients, all of whom had negative cytologic findings. Positive cytologic results were found in 6 of 8 patients who had previously undergone needle biopsy, and in 6 of 32 patients who had not, suggesting that intraperitoneal spread may be enhanced by needle biopsy. Laparoscopy is described as an excellent method to obtain cytologic washings, which may be of importance in the evaluation of patients with carcinoma of the pancreas.

The ability of laparoscopy to detect metastatic disease not otherwise identified has been reported by others.[27] The use of laparoscopy and laparoscopic ultrasonography has been described in the evaluation of 40 consecutive patients thought to have a resectable pancreatic lesion.[28] Resectability was confirmed in 12 patients with negative laparoscopic examinations, for a sensitivity of 100%. Occult metastatic disease was identified in 14 patients, including liver lesions (n = 10), peritoneal surfaces (n = 8), and hilar lymphadenopathy (n = 2). Laparoscopy failed to demonstrate metastatic disease in three patients. As for predicting resectability, laparoscopy alone failed to identify the 12 patients with locoregional tumor unresectability, with an overall specificity of only 50%. However, the combined use of laparoscopy and laparoscopic ultrasonography resulted in a sensitivity of 92%, a specificity of 88%, and an accuracy of 89%.

The use of laparoscopy or combined laparoscopy and laparoscopic ultrasonography appears to be most helpful in the identification of lesions that suggest unresectability in patients with negative imaging studies. The prospective evaluation of these techniques is essential to define fully the ultimate role for these techniques.

LAPAROSCOPY AND TREATMENT OF GASTROINTESTINAL MALIGNANCIES

Laparoscopic approaches have been used to treat a wide variety of malignancies. Many of these techniques were applied with a curative intent, although some were conducted as palliative procedures. In this section, the various tumor sites that have been treated with laparoscopic techniques are reviewed.

Gastric Cancer

The application of laparoscopic techniques to gastric resection has been made possible by the rapid advances in stapling technology in the early 1990s. The first laparoscopic gastric resection using a Billroth II reconstruction performed intraabdominally was reported in 1992.[29] Since that time, the same group has continued to apply laparoscopic surgical techniques to gastric surgery.[30] In this series of 16 patients, all were operated on for benign disease, although two patients had foci of cancer found at the time of histologic examination. These two patients later underwent open lymphadenectomy.

Laparoscopic gastric resection remains a technically demanding procedure, with precise identification of anatomic structures essential to its successful completion. The surgeon stands between the patients' legs with the patient in modified lithotomy position. Monitors are placed superiorly, similar to the configuration used for laparoscopic cholecystectomy. Localization of lesions is facilitated by the use of intraoperative flexible endoscopy. The initial dissection includes mobilization of the greater curvature. The first portion of the duodenum is mobilized and transected with the GIA stapling device (US Surgical, Norwalk, CT). The lesser curvature of the stomach is then mobilized, and control of the vascular structures obtained. The stomach is then transected and a gastrojejunostomy performed with the GIA stapling device.

The inability to perform extensive lymphadenectomy at this time may limit the applicability of laparoscopic gastric resection to malignancies, but it is clear that advances in technology may make this possible.

Colon Cancer

Carcinoma of the colon is a common disease in the United States, making it potentially attractive for treatment with a laparoscopic approach. There is great interest in determining whether the benefits of laparoscopic surgery (shorter hospitalization, less pain, earlier return to normal activity) can be extended to patients with colon cancer without compromising the fundamental principles of oncologic surgery. Traditional colectomy is a well established surgical procedure requiring adequate margins of resection, complete excision of lymph node-bearing tissue, and thorough evaluation of the entire peritoneal cavity as fundamental components of the operation. Laparoscopic colon resection is clearly an ''advanced'' procedure requiring more training, experience, and time to complete than open colectomy.[31]

The principles of laparoscopic colon resection, however, are similar to those applied to open colon resection. Inspection of the peritoneal cavity and mobilization of the colon are carried out under laparoscopic guidance. The anastomosis is usually performed extracorporeally or transanally using conventional techniques, making the technique of laparoscopic colon resection less difficult to learn. Thus, the term ''laparoscopic assisted colectomy'' is often applied to this procedure. The use of animal models has facilitated the testing of some of these techniques and may be an important educational tool.[32] Intracorporeal anastomotic techniques may also be used, but remain a greater technical challenge.

Accepted indications for laparoscopic colon resection include segmental resections for diverticular disease, polyps, rectal prolapse, and intestinal volvulus.[33] The indications for use of laparoscopic resection in the management of colonic malignancies remains undefined at this time, and it should be carried out only in the setting of a prospective trial.[33–35] It is reasonable to perform laparoscopic resection of colonic malignancies with synchronous hepatic or pulmonary metastases as a palliative procedure. When performed appropriately, a laparoscopic colon resection for cancer should include the following components: resection of tumor in the bowel wall and adjacent soft tissues, resection of an adequate margin of normal bowel, and an adequate lymph node resection with associated vascular pedicle.[32]

The preoperative factors affecting suitability for laparoscopic colonic surgery are similar to those in other laparoscopic procedures. Patients should undergo a routine mechanical and antibiotic bowel preparation. Intraoperative positioning of the patient and trocars is critical in laparoscopic colon resections, although a variety of trocar placements may be used successfully. Poor trocar placement can prevent the successful completion of a laparoscopic colon resection. A Foley catheter and nasogastric tube are placed in every patient before the start of surgery. In general, the surgeon and assistant stand on the side opposite the bowel to be resected. Although some prefer the dorsolithotomy position,[36] others prefer the patient in supine position.[33] The dorsolithotomy position has two potential advantages. First, intraoperative colonoscopy, facilitated by the use of low stirrups, may be necessary for localizing the lesion in the operating room. Second, a recently described technique demonstrates the utility of the colonoscope in dissecting the hepatic and splenic flexures.[37] The 0° or 30° laparoscope may be used for these procedures.

In general, for a left hemicolectomy, two right-sided and one left-sided ports are used, in addition to the umbilical camera port (Fig. 10-3). The abdomen is explored thoroughly, with special attention to the liver, just as in open surgical approaches. Ports are best placed as they are needed, allowing for flexibility, rather than using a static pattern that places all ports synchronously.[34] After mobilizing the right colon along the avascular lateral plane, an incision is made in the periumbilical region and the bowel brought extracorporeally. The bowel is resected

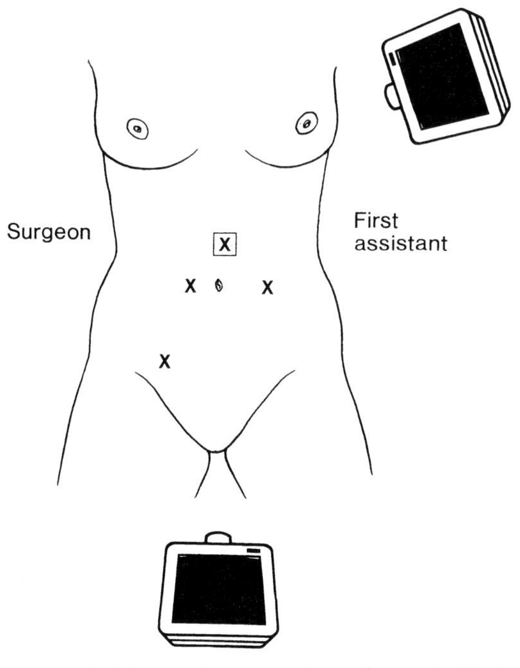

FIG. 10-3. A left hemicoloectomy is performed with the surgeon and first assistant standing on the patient's right side, allowing medial mobilization of the left colon. The laparoscope is placed through the left upper quadrant port (indicated by the "X" with a square around it) while a Babcock clamp is placed through the left-sided port, placed over the left colon. The surgeon operates through the right and infraumbilical port. The specimen is removed through an incision made around the left-sided port. (Reprinted with permission from Ota D. Laparoscopic management of colon cancer. Seminars in Laparoscopic Surgery 1994;1:18.)

and replaced in the abdominal cavity. A canine model has demonstrated the feasibility of an adequate right hemicolectomy for the treatment of cancer with an intracorporeal stapled anastomosis.[32] A wide range of colonic resections has been performed laparoscopically, including left colon resections, abdominoperineal resections, and sigmoid colectomies.

The safety and efficacy of laparoscopic colectomy has been studied retrospectively. In a series of 51 laparoscopic colon resections, 24 patients underwent operation for cancer.[38] Most of these were performed using intracorporeal anastomoses, but 14% were converted to laparoscopic assisted cases, and 8% were converted to open procedures. This series included right, transverse, left, low anterior, and abdominoperineal colon resections. Operative time averaged 2.6 hours and hospitalization averaged 4.6 days. Complications were reported in 8% of patients.

In another series, 66 patients underwent attempted laparoscopic colon resections, with a conversion rate to open colectomy in 41%.[39] Major morbidity was reported in 24% of patients, with no mortality. Length of hospitalization, hospital cost, and lymph node harvest were compared with patients who underwent open colon resection. Mean postoperative hospital stay was significantly less in patients with laparoscopic sigmoid and right colectomies than for those patients converted to open operation or those who underwent conventional open techniques. Total hospital cost for patients undergoing conventional open right hemicolectomy was less than that for the converted group, but more than those having a laparoscopic resection. Lymph node harvest was comparable in all three groups. These authors conclude that laparoscopic colectomy can be performed with acceptable morbidity and mortality, but that there is no definite cost savings. This series represents the initial laparoscopic experience of a group of experienced colon and rectal surgeons.

Laparoscopic colon resection was performed in 80 patients and compared to a control group of 53 patients undergoing conventional open colectomy by the same group of surgeons.[40] Analysis included complications, rate of conversion, length of procedure, duration of postoperative ileus, hospital stay, hospital cost, and adequacy of the specimen obtained. Operations were converted to open procedures in 23% of patients, which decreased to 15% in the second half of the series. The length of procedure was greater in those undergoing laparoscopic resection (mean, 221 minutes) than in those undergoing open colectomy (mean, 183 minutes). Operating room and total hospital charges were also greater in those patients undergoing laparoscopic resection compared with those having open colectomy. Patients having a laparoscopic colectomy had an average postoperative stay of 5.2 days, compared with 7.8 days for those having open colectomies. The pathology specimens were of similar quality in all groups. This study further validates that laparoscopic colectomy can be performed safely with shorter hospitalization, but at higher overall cost. Perhaps with greater experience operating times will decrease, as was suggested by this study.

The use of laparoscopic resection of the colon for the treatment of malignancies is under study. The American Society of Colon and Rectal Surgeons does not currently endorse the application of laparoscopic technology to cure carcinoma.[34] The studies detailed previously have shown that laparoscopic colon resection is safe and feasible, and obtains pathologic specimens similar to those obtained with open surgery. Although it is tempting to obtain the same benefits of decreased hospitalization and recovery for patients undergoing colon resection as have been shown in patients undergoing cholecystectomy through the use of laparoscopy, there is no conclusive evidence at this time to demonstrate that this is uniformly the case. We must also consider the issue of compromised cancer control and complications in this discussion.[35] Cancer control issues include extent of lymph node resection, port site recurrences, and adequacy of intraperitoneal staging in the absence of tactile sensation. The series reviewed earlier suggest that a lymph node resection similar to that in open surgery is possible. The issue of port site metastases is discussed later, but rates from 0% to 3.2% have been reported, compared to less than than 1% in open colon resection.[41] The problem with many of the anecdotal reports in the literature is that the overall denominator is not known, and only through a prospective trial can these issues be adequately studied. The 1-year port site recurrence rate has been reported at less than 1% in the first 252 patients in the registry of the American Society of Colon and Rectal Surgeons.[42]

An attempt to evaluate some of the parameters of response to colon resection in an experimental model has been reported.[43] Two groups of 10 pigs each underwent colon resection, one group using open techniques and one group undergoing laparoscopic colon resection. T-cell immune function as assayed by delayed-type hypersensitivity testing was better preserved after laparoscopic than after open colon resection.

At the present time, laparoscopic colon resections should not be carried out for the attempted cure of malignancies outside of carefully controlled prospective trials. Although laparoscopic surgery has the potential to save hospitalization time and recovery time, such savings must not be made at the expense of overall survival. The prospective trial underway at many centers throughout the United States, funded by the National Institutes of Health, should address the issues of cancer control, costs, and quality of life.[35]

Hepatic Tumors

Although the use of laparoscopy in the staging of hepatic lesions, either primary or metastatic, has become fairly widespread, laparoscopic treatment of hepatic malignancies is rarely performed. This is a result of the technical difficulty of this procedure as well as the scarcity of patients with lesions amenable to laparoscopic resection. The laparoscopic treatment of hepatic lesions has been reported. A benign liver cyst was fenestrated under laparoscopic guidance, and effective therapy was provided for a benign condition while avoiding the potential morbidity of a laparotomy.[44]

Although there are a number of techniques available for liver resection, the ultrasonic dissector is preferred by some. A randomized, prospective trial has shown that a laparoscopic version of this device is effective in laparoscopic cholecystectomy.[45] It is natural that this device may be used for hepatic resection. An animal trial was reported demonstrating hepatic resection on pigs using the ultrasonic dissector.[46] The ultrasonic dissector was effective in dissecting the intraparenchymal structures, including vascular structures. A single case of a left lateral segmentectomy in a human performed laparoscopically has been reported.[47] With improved instrumentation becoming available, perhaps more hepatic resections will be performed laparoscopically.

Another application of laparoscopic technology to the treatment of liver lesions is cryotherapy. Cryosurgery has been shown effective in the treatment of some hepatic malignancies.[48] Ultrasound monitoring of this procedure is essential. With the advent of laparoscopic ultrasound probes and cryotherapy probes, it may be possible to perform cryotherapy of hepatic lesions. However, anatomic limitations may prevent the use of this technology because of limited exposure of certain lesions.

Pancreatic Cancer

Resection with the intent to cure is possible in only about 10% to 20% of patients who present with carcinoma of the pancreas, and 5-year survival rates are only about 3%.[49] It is heartening that several more recent series have reported 5-year survival rates as high as 20%. Patients with pathologically negative lymph nodes have an even higher survival rate.[50] Many of the patients who are not resectable for cure often require surgical palliation. Laparoscopic surgery has the potential to provide this palliation while minimizing postoperative pain and length of hospital stay, both especially important considerations in patients with limited life expectancy.

The laparoscopic resection of pancreatic tumors is technically feasible, but unlikely to become widely practiced. Gagner and Pomp reported performing a pylorus-preserving pancreaticoduodenectomy in a patient with chronic pancreatitis and pancreas divisum.[51] Reconstruction was performed with a gastrojejunostomy, hepaticojejunostomy, and pancreaticojejunostomy. The patient's postoperative course was complicated by delayed gastric emptying, and he was discharged on the 30th postoperative day.

The use of laparoscopy in the staging of patients with carcinoma of the pancreas was discussed extensively earlier. In addition, laparoscopic techniques may be useful for palliative surgical procedures. Unfortunately, palliative therapy is all that is indicated for many patients. It is possible to palliate the three symptoms of this disease—biliary obstruction, gastrointestinal obstruction, and pain—using laparoscopic techniques. As many as 57% of patients who present with pancreatic cancer undergo palliative surgery.[49]

A particularly attractive concept is to stage patients using laparoscopic techniques, and then perform palliative bypass surgery at the same time using a laparoscopic approach in patients found to have unresectable disease.[52,53] Nonoperative palliation of obstructive jaundice using an endoscopically placed stent has been shown to be effective compared to surgical palliation, and also is associated with lower complication rates.[50]

Palliation for obstructive jaundice may be performed nonoperatively using an endoprosthesis, or may be carried out using a number of bypass procedures that can be performed laparoscopically. The simplest technique is cholecystojejunostomy, which has been described using both sutured and stapled techniques.[54] Choledochoduodenal or choledochojejunal anastomoses may also be fashioned laparoscopically.[54] The biliary bypass is then combined with a gastroenterostomy, performed at the surgeon's discretion. Similarly, the celiac plexus may be injected under laparoscopic guidance to provide pain relief.[55]

Such a combined approach was used by Mouiel in 12 patients with excellent results.[54]

By combining a staging procedure with the appropriate palliative procedures using laparoscopic techniques, it may be possible to minimize a patient's hospitalization and provide palliation identical to that afforded by an open procedure.

Gallbladder Cancer

Although it is rare, the presence of a gallbladder malignancy is a possibility that must always be kept in mind by the laparoscopic surgeon while performing a laparoscopic cholecystectomy. This disease, most common in older women, is the fifth most common malignancy of the gastrointestinal tract and is associated with a dismal prognosis.[56] It is estimated that carcinoma will be present in 1% of all cholecystectomy specimens.[56] Although laparoscopic cholecystectomy is the procedure of choice for patients with symptomatic cholelithiasis, the presence of gallbladder carcinoma remains a contraindication to the laparoscopic conduct of this procedure.[57,58] Preoperative diagnosis of this disease is difficult because the sensitivity for ultrasonography in early cases is only about 20%. In view of the difficulty of making a preoperative diagnosis, it is not surprising that the diagnosis is often made only after histologic examination of the surgical specimen.

The optimal treatment for this rare disease remains elusive. In a large retrospective study of 724 patients from a number of European centers, although only 4% of patients presented with Tis lesions, these were the only patients with any hope of long-term survival.[59] Prognosis in stages T1 and T2 was markedly worse, although there are no data to support the use of extended surgical resections in these patients. Furthermore, others have shown that the use of adjuvant chemotherapy or radiation therapy does not significantly affect survival.[60]

The treatment of patients suspected of having carcinoma of the gallbladder preoperatively should include a definitive procedure performed through conventional open surgical techniques as the initial procedure. Clinical data from 10 patients with laparoscopically discovered gallbladder carcinoma have been reported.[61] All 10 patients were thought to have resectable disease based on preoperative studies and intraoperative findings. The interval to exploration at the referral center was 14 to 74 days, with a median of 30 days. Gross intraperitoneal dissemination was found in four patients. These investigators conclude that patients in whom gallbladder carcinoma is suspected on visual examination of the gallbladder during attempted laparoscopic cholecystectomy should be converted immediately to an open procedure, or the procedure should be terminated and the patient referred for definitive therapy. During the conduct of a laparoscopic cholecystectomy, any evidence of the presence of a carcinoma is cause for conversion to an open procedure. Routine examination of the specimen with frozen section if suspect areas are present should also be carried out, with conversion to an open procedure if positive for malignancy.[57]

In summary, any patient with a lesion that is preoperatively suspect for malignancy should undergo cholecystectomy by a conventional open cholecystectomy. If the diagnosis is suspected during a laparoscopic cholecystectomy, frozen sections are obtained and the procedure converted to an open cholecystectomy if histologic analysis demonstrates malignancy. If the diagnosis is made only after laparoscopic cholecystectomy, then the port sites should be excised.[62]

Spleen

Although the spleen rarely harbors primary or secondary tumors in the human, the surgical oncologist is often called on to perform a splenectomy for hematologic diseases. The spleen is well within the reach of the laparoscopic surgeon, and the benefits of laparoscopic surgery include shortened hospitalization and decreased postoperative pain. A number of series in the literature report laparoscopic removal of the spleen.[63–71] These have been performed for a number of indications, including staging of Hodgkin's lymphoma, idiopathic thrombocytopenia purpura (ITP), thrombotic thrombocytopenia purpura, acquired immunodeficiency syndrome-related thrombocytopenia, hereditary spherocytosis, autoimmune hemolytic anemia, leukemia, and splenic abscess.

The laparoscopic conduct of this procedure should not alter the indications for operation. Once the decision to perform a splenectomy has been made, laparoscopic splenectomy may offer the patient some advantages in terms of decreased postoperative hospitalization and recovery time. Splenectomy was commonly performed for the staging of lymphomas in the past, and one series demonstrated a significant increase in splenectomies performed for this reason over the time period 1963 to 1982, compared to 1946 to 1962.[72] However, more recent trends show that splenectomies are now being performed more often for cytopenic/anemic diseases, and fewer for Hodgkin's disease.[73] The consequences of splenectomy are poorly understood at an immunologic level, but it is clear that the spleen plays a major role in a wide range of immune responses.[74] Patients should receive a preoperative pneumococcal vaccine to help avoid the infectious complications of the asplenic state.[75,76]

The preoperative embolization of the splenic artery has been used in the management of patients with massive splenomegaly as an adjunct to surgery.[77] Although this measure has been adopted by some surgeons performing laparoscopic splenectomy,[64,70] this measure has not been adopted at the University of Maryland. The patient can be positioned in several ways for this laparoscopic splenectomy, with some groups preferring a right lateral decubitus position.[78] In the series from the University of Maryland, 61 patients were brought to the operating room for laparoscopic splenectomy, and 51 procedures (84%) were successfully completed.[63] The remaining 16% underwent conversion to open splenectomy, usually for bleeding. Laparoscopic splenectomy has become the standard method for splenectomy in patients with hematologic diseases at the University of Maryland. Conversion rates in other series have been reported as 2 of 22 (9%)[64] and 3 of 13 (19%).[68] The details of the technique have been adequately described elsewhere.[63] Five 12-mm trocars are inserted as shown in Figure 10-4, and the entire procedure is performed with a 30° laparoscope. Briefly, dissection begins at the lower pole of the spleen with the division of the small vessels. The hilum is then identified and isolated. The hilar vessels are divided en masse with a linear stapling device, as shown in Figure 10-5. Dissection continues cephalad with division of the short gastric vessels, using a linear stapler. The ligamentous attachments of the spleen are divided last to aid in supporting the organ. Removal of the spleen is facilitated by

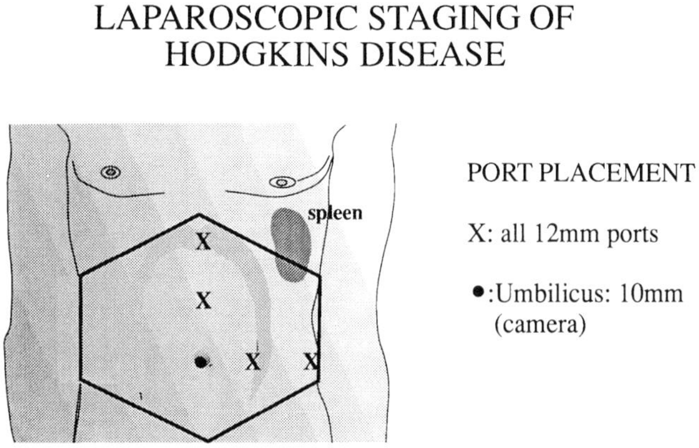

FIG. 10-4. Laparoscopic splenectomy is accomplished with five ports placed as shown here. (Reprinted with permission from Lefor AT, Flowers JL, Heyman M. Laparoscopic staging of Hodgkin's disease. Surg Oncol 1993;2:217.)

placing it in a bag. A midline port site can be enlarged slightly, allowing digital morselization of the spleen and removal. Alternatively, the midline site can be enlarged to a few centimeters, allowing removal of the spleen intact, an important consideration in patients with malignancy for whom careful examination of the tissue is critical. Other approaches have been advocated, including full mobilization of the spleen before dissection of the hilum.[71] However, in the University of Maryland series, it has been shown that maintaining the ligamentous attachments of the spleen assists in exposure of the vascular structures.

It is important to make a thorough search for accessory splenic tissue, identified in 10% of the patients in the University of Maryland series. Accessory spleens are identified in up to 18% of patients undergoing splenectomy.[79] The magnification afforded by the laparoscope may aid in this task. In a series of 100 patients undergoing splenectomy for ITP, 13 patients had a poor response to splenectomy, with 5 of them requiring accessory splenectomy.[79] None of the patients in the University of Maryland series has relapsed with ITP, but longer follow-up may be required to address this issue definitively. A positive response in 18 of 22 (82%) patients with ITP was observed. It is difficult to predict who will respond to splenectomy, with no predictive factors being identified even in large series of patients with ITP.[80]

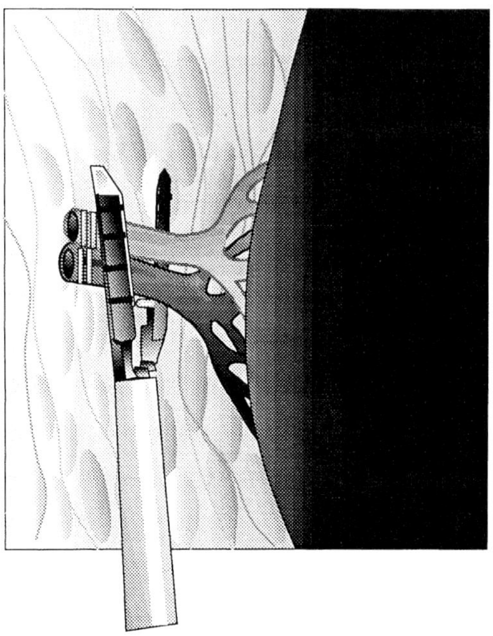

FIG. 10-5. The hilum of the spleen is isolated and divided by a single application of the linear stapler, as shown in this diagram. (Reprinted with permission from Lefor AT, Flowers JL, Heyman M. Laparoscopic staging of Hodgkin's disease. Surg Oncol 1993;2:217.)

Mean blood loss in the University of Maryland series is 475 mL for laparoscopic splenectomy and 1250 mL for those converted to open splenectomy. Transfusion was necessary in 5 of the 51 patients (10%). Mean operative time was 2.3 hours (range, 1.5 to 4.5 hours) for laparoscopic splenectomy. Postoperative nasogastric suction has not been used in these patients, with no obvious deleterious effects. Most patients tolerate liquids the day after surgery and are discharged on the second postoperative day, with a mean hospital stay of 2.7 days in 51 patients. Postoperative complications have included wound infections, a pleural effusion, and recurrent arrhythmias, but there have been no instances of postoperative hemorrhage or subphrenic abscess in the patients successfully undergoing laparoscopic splenectomy at the University of Maryland.

Although laparoscopic splenectomy is a technically demanding procedure, it offers the patient the potential for decreased postoperative pain and hospitalization with more rapid return to normal activities of living. Further prospective data will be needed to confirm these observations. Surgical alternatives to splenectomy have been offered as a way to reduce the incidence of postoperative infections, such as partial splenectomy.[81] These procedures may also prove amenable to laparoscopic techniques in the future.

Port Site Metastases

One of the most important concerns expressed regarding the laparoscopic conduct of procedures for the treatment of cancer relates to the problem of tumor dissemination. Several reports describe tumor implants at trocar sites after laparoscopic cholecystectomy in patients harboring unsuspected carcinoma of the gallbladder.[57,82–85] A number of case reports describe tumor implants at port sites, even when the tumor-bearing specimen may not have been near that port.[86–91] In one early report, tumor recurred not only at the site of specimen extraction, but also at a separate trocar site.[82] These investigators suggest reexcision of trocar sites or irradiation of these sites in patients ultimately found to have carcinoma of the gallbladder after laparoscopic cholecystectomy. There are several possible mechanisms for this process, but the mechanism is probably related to operative technique.[92]

Metastatic wound implants after open tumor resection are well reported. In one series of 1603 open resections for colon cancer, there were 11 cases of wound recurrence, for an incidence of 0.7%.[93] There is concern, however, that there may be something related to port sites in laparoscopic procedures that enhances tumor growth. The case of a patient with an unsuspected carcinoma undergoing a laparoscopic cholecystectomy that was converted to open surgery for technical reasons, with metastases developing at ports sites but not at the laparotomy incision, supports this concept.[83]

The following are some possible suggested mechanisms of tumor dissemination to port sites:

- There may be increased shedding of tumor cells after instrumentation and manipulation. The surgeon should avoid grasping the organ near the tumor if at all possible.[88]
- Tumor cells may be carried by instruments to distant port sites.
- The extraction of a tumor may coat the sides of the wound with tumor cells, although this does not explain appearance of port site metastases at other sites. The use of extraction sacks may diminish the likelihood of this possibility.[88]
- Exfoliated tumor cells may be carried in the carbon dioxide gas as the pneumoperitoneum is released, which then lodge on the sides of the wound.[94] This may occur through small leaks that are present throughout the procedure, perhaps explaining the appearance of lesions at ports sites distant to that used for tumor removal.
- There may be an immunologic effect of the pneumoperitoneum that permits local tumor growth. This may be mediated by a number of factors, including altered cytokine levels.[95]

An early case report of a port site lesion described a metastasis appearing within 8 days of the laparoscopic exploration.[89] The period between the laparoscopic procedure and the appearance of port site metastases varies widely, from 7 days to 10 months.[88] One problem in evaluating this issue is the lack of knowledge regarding the true incidence. Although there are many case reports in the literature, the denominator (the total number of cases performed) is unknown as yet. These concerns underscore the need for carefully controlled, prospective clinical trials to determine the true incidence of these complications.

Experimental studies to investigate this phenomenon are beginning to appear. Significant alterations in tumor necrosis factor levels were observed in animals undergoing abdominal insufflation, compared to those undergoing laparotomy.[95] In another study, mice received intradermal inoculation of tumor and then underwent either laparotomy or insufflation of the abdomen.[96] At the end of the study period, tumors in those animals that had undergone laparotomy showed significantly more growth than in animals that had undergone insufflation alone. These authors suggest that laparotomy is more immunosuppressive than insufflation, and recommend continued investigation of laparoscopic treatment of malignancies. A more recent study demonstrated that laparoscopic cholecystectomy results in a much lower postoperative hepatic catabolic stress response compared to that observed after open surgical techniques.[97] Further investigation of the effects of laparoscopy on cytokine levels may yield information to explain some of the clinical observations that have been made in the treatment of cancer patients.

In an effort to determine the incidence of port site recurrences in the clinical application of laparoscopy, Ramos and coworkers used a survey to obtain data from physicians who performed laparoscopic colon resections for malignancies, and received 208 of 252 (83%) surveys.[42] Three cases of port or extraction site tumor recurrences were identified, of which two also had associated diffuse peritoneal carcinomatosis. All three of these patients had T_x, N_{1-3}, M_0 lesions, and the authors concluded that the recurrence of tumor in the ports site was more a manifestation of dissemination of disease than of a novel site for recurrent tumor.

The other major concern with laparoscopic treatment of cancer is the adequacy of resection possible using available instrumentation, particularly regarding margins, completeness of lymphadenectomy, and understaging as a result of the loss of palpation. Answers to these questions will be obtained only from careful prospective trials, some of which are now ongoing in the United States. Clearly, the potential for cure should not be compromised for the sake of using a technologic advance and the possibility of a shorter hospital stay. Until data are available from these prospective trials, laparoscopic tumor resections, particularly colonic resections, should be performed only under hospital protocol approval, with adequate informed consent.[92]

LAPAROSCOPY IN THE PALLIATIVE CARE OF THE CANCER PATIENT

Although we often seek to diagnose, stage, and treat patients with malignancy, surgical intervention in some cancer patients is limited to palliative care. Laparoscopic procedures may be an important tool in the surgeon's armamentarium, especially because such procedures can benefit the patient in terms of decreased postoperative pain and length of hospital stay.

Feeding Tube Placement

Enteral feedings are preferable to parenteral feedings in patients who can tolerate them, yet not all patients with cancer are able to take in enough calories by mouth, necessitating placement of a feeding tube. Open surgical gastrostomy is most often performed in the United States by the method of Stamm.[98] This was the only method available until 1980, when percutaneous endoscopic gastrostomy (PEG) was developed.[99] However, placement of a PEG requires upper endoscopy, which is not possible in all patients. Furthermore, the use of a PEG tube, which necessitates pulling the tube through the tumor-bearing area, has been reported to result in implantation of the tumor at the PEG site in three cases.[100] In this subset, including patients with head and neck tumors, Zenker's diverticula, and large hiatal hernias, open surgical gastrostomy remains the preferred method of enteral access.

The technique for laparoscopic gastrostomy was originally described in 1990.[101] Several techniques are now available, either purely laparoscopic, or hybrids of endoscopic and laparoscopic techniques. Briefly, after obtaining a pneumoperitoneum with the camera near the umbilicus, a 5-mm port is placed over the stomach. The stomach is grasped with an atraumatic grasper and a PEG kit used to place the feeding tube. T-fasteners are used to create a four-point support, and an introducer needle is placed through the 5-mm port site. A guidewire is passed and the gastrostomy tube placed using a modified Seldinger technique.

Although formal laparotomy is not needed, the stomach is directly visualized using this technique. A retrospective review has established the usefulness of this technique.[99] In this study, 32 patients who underwent laparoscopic gastrostomy and 37 patients who underwent open gastrostomy were reviewed. The underlying illnesses and contraindications to PEG placement were similar in both groups. Operative time was significantly greater in the open gastrostomy group (62 ± 19 minutes) compared to the laparoscopic gastrostomy group (38 ± 7 minutes). Complication rates were 11% in the open group and 6% in the laparoscopic group. These investigators concluded that laparoscopic gastrostomy is a safe and effective alternative procedure in patients unable to undergo placement of a PEG.

Laparoscopic placement of jejunostomy tubes has also been described.[102] Four ports are used, with the camera at the umbilicus and three 5-mm ports used for operating. Identification of the proximal jejunum at the ligament of Treitz is the most important component of this procedure. A loop of bowel about 20 cm from the ligament of Treitz is brought to the abdominal wall without tension, using graspers. A small (3-cm) midline incision is made and a loop of bowel exteriorized through this incision. The feeding tube is then placed into the loop in a standard Witzel fashion, using conventional instrumentation. The jejunal loop is then replaced in the abdominal cavity and the tube secured. The fascia is closed in the usual fashion. With further improvements in laparoscopic instrumentation, this procedure may soon be performed entirely intracorporeally.

Laparoscopic conduct of these procedures may be associated with shorter hospitalization and decreased postoperative pain, as well as fewer complications. All of these may significantly improve the quality of life of the cancer patient. Furthermore, laparoscopic placement allows a more complete examination of the peritoneal cavity than would be possible through the small incision often used to place feeding tubes.

Laparoscopic Colostomy and Ileostomy

Decompression of the intestinal tract may be an important procedure in the cancer patient, especially in those with carcinomatosis and resulting intestinal obstruction. The importance of colonic decompression in patients with obstructing carcinomas of the colon has been described.[103] The initial presentation of carcinoma of the colon is obstruction in 15% to 21% of patients, most commonly in the left colon. Five-year survival rates in these patients are significantly less than those in patients without obstruction. The common presentation of this common disease underscores the importance of procedures that may decrease postoperative pain, incidence of ileus, and recovery time.

Laparoscopic creation of a loop colostomy has been described.[104] In this technique, after mobilizing the sigmoid colon, a drain is passed through its mesentery and is used to extract

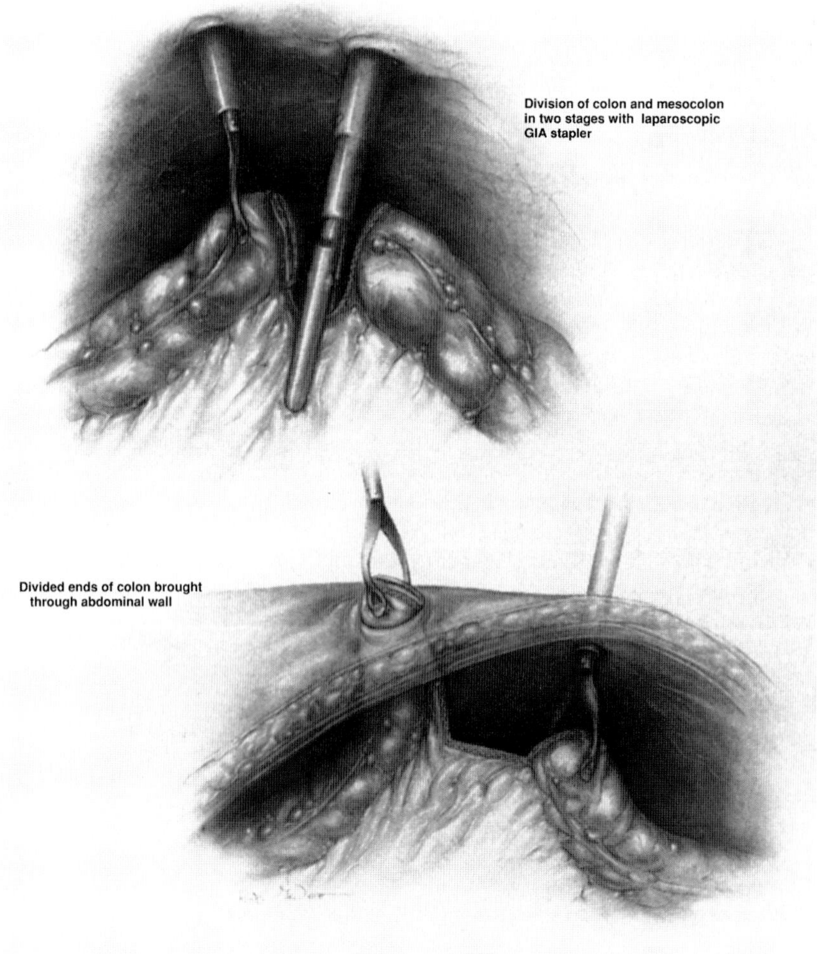

FIG. 10-6. An end colostomy and mucous fistula can be fashioned using laparoscopic instrumentation by placing two trocars in the area of the bowel to be divided. The bowel is grasped and divided using a linear stapler. Both ends are then brought out through separate sites and matured to the skin. (Reprinted with permission from Lyerly HK, Mault JR. Laparoscopic ileostomy and colostomy. Ann Surg 1994;219:317.)

the colon through a special 3.5-cm trocar placed in the left lower quadrant. The need for a special trocar as well as creation of the stoma while maintaining pneumoperitoneum make this a difficult technique.

A more recent modification of this procedure has been described; it is associated with decreased postoperative pain and ileus, and with a rapid recovery.[105] This technique calls for creation of the stoma site in the desired area after mobilizing the intestine. The peritoneum at the stoma site is left intact, and a trocar is placed directly through this site. A grasper is then used to extract the intestine through the stoma site, which occludes the opening and allows recreation of the pneumoperitoneum. Alternatively, a stapling device can be introduced to divide the bowel and mesentery, allowing creation of an end stoma (Fig. 10-6).

Although small laparotomy incisions may be used for the creation of intestinal stomas, the presence of metastatic disease or peritoneal implants may make such procedures difficult to perform. Use of a laparoscopic approach results in discharge from the hospital within 24 to 48 hours of surgery, as well as permitting the inspection of the abdominal cavity for other lesions. In one study, 17 of 19 (89%) patients were successfully diverted using laparoscopic techniques.[92] The remaining two patients had extensive adhesive disease that could not be managed laparoscopically, and required conversion to open laparotomy. Other procedures such as laparoscopic gastrostomy may also be carried out as needed.

THE FUTURE OF LAPAROSCOPY IN THE CARE OF THE CANCER PATIENT

There are a number of developments that will benefit the conduct of all laparoscopic surgical procedures, including those carried out for malignancy. The exciting technology now under development will soon be in the operating room. Cuschieri has pointed out that we need to "see better, feel better, increase the precision of maneuverability and handling, reduce contamination, facilitate specimen extraction and bring order to the present ergonomic chaos in our operating rooms."[106] New developments in the technology of imaging are being applied to laparoscopic surgery. Although head-mounted displays have been tested, they are probably less than optimal for the laparoscopic surgeon because of the isolation they create. Although current three-dimensional imaging systems are not without their limitations, new systems may provide a true improvement in tissue visualization. Continued improvement in instrumentation will certainly be an important part of the evolution of laparoscopic surgery. Access devices allowing insertion of the surgeon's hand into the abdomen while maintaining pneumoperitoneum will be made available, allowing palpation of tissue at the time of laparoscopy. New methods of tissue extraction include a sleeve system and an extracorporeal pneumoperitoneal access bubble.[106] Both of these systems provide potential advantages, especially for the removal of large tumor specimens.

Training of surgeons in these newly emerging techniques remains a complicated problem. Because hospitals decide what procedures may be performed by surgeons, criteria for training and furnishing credentials must be developed.[107] The Society of American Gastrointestinal Endoscopic Surgeons has suggested criteria for training and credentialling. The cost considerations of these procedures will also have to be considered, especially in the present climate of increased pressure to reduce costs. It remains to be shown whether some advanced laparoscopic procedures result in a true cost savings when the increased cost of instrumentation and operating room time are factored into the total expenses incurred. This will have to be carefully studied prospectively. The differential between true costs and hospital charges must also be considered.

The surgeon has traditionally been involved in the diagnosis, staging, treatment, and palliation of patients with malignancies. Laparoscopy is rapidly becoming an important tool in each of these areas of the care of the cancer patient. The ultimate application of laparoscopic techniques depends on the imagination of surgical investigators as well as careful analyses of risks and benefits. There may be uses of this technology that, over time, prove not to be ultimately advantageous to the patient compared to traditional open surgical techniques. Only through the conduct of carefully controlled studies will the facts be elucidated, allowing this methodology to be used where it will benefit the patient and avoided where it will not.

REFERENCES

1. Gunning JE. The history of laparoscopy. J Reprod Med 1974;12:223.
2. Zucker KA. The role of laparoscopy in malignant disease. Principles and Practices of Oncology Updates 1993;7(11):1.
3. Cuschieri A. Diagnosis and staging of tumors by laparoscopy. Seminars in Laparoscopic Surgery 1994;1:3.
4. Greene FL, Bianco JE. Laparoscopy's growing role in abdominal tumor diagnosis. Contemporary Oncology January 1994:14.
5. Easter DW, Cuschieri A, Nathanson LK, Lavalle-Jones M. The utility of diagnostic laparoscopy for abdominal disorders. Arch Surg 1992; 127:379.
6. Lefor AT, Flowers JL. Laparoscopic wedge biopsy of the liver. J Am Coll Surg 1994;178:307.
7. Jakimowicz J. Laparoscopic intraoperative ultrasonography, equipment, and technique. Seminars in Laparoscopic Surgery 1994;1:52.
8. Machi J, Sigel B. Intraoperative ultrasonography. Radiol Clin North Am 1992;30:1085.
9. Stiegmann GV, McIntyre RC, Pearlman NW. Laparoscopic intracorporeal ultrasound. Surg Endosc 1994;8:167.
10. Jakimowicz J. Review: intraoperative ultrasonography during minimal access surgery. J R Coll Surg Edinb 1993;38:231.
11. Lightdale CJ. Laparoscopy for cancer staging. Endoscopy 1992;24: 682.
12. Hemming AW, Nagy AG, Scudamore CH, Edelman K. Laparoscopic staging of intraabdominal malignancy. Surg Endosc 1995;9:325.
13. Salky BA. Laparoscopic staging of intraabdominal malignancy. In: Paterson-Brown S, Garden J, eds. Principles and practice of surgical laparoscopy. Philadelphia: WB Saunders, 1994:432.
14. Shandall A, Johnson C. Laparoscopy or scanning in oesophageal and gastric carcinoma. Br J Surg 1986;72:449.
15. Dagnini G, Caldironi MW, Marin G, Buzzaccarini O, Tremolada C, Ruol A. Laparoscopy in abdominal staging of esophageal carcinoma. Gastrointest Endosc 1986;32:400.
16. Krasna MJ, Flowers JL, McLaughlin JL, Attar S. Combined thoracoscopic and laparoscopic staging of esophageal cancer [abstract]. Proceedings of the American Association of Thoracic Surgeons 1995.
17. Watt I, Stewart I, Anderson D, Bell G, Anderson JR. Laparoscopy, ultrasound and computed tomography in cancer of the oesophagus and gastric cardia: a prospective comparison for detecting intra-abdominal metastases. Br J Surg 1989;76:1036.
18. Fiocco M, Krasna MJ. Thoracoscopic lymph node dissection in the staging of esophageal carcinoma. J Laparoendosc Surgery 1992;2: 111.
19. Krasna MJ, McLaughlin JS. Thoracoscopic lymph node staging for esophageal cancer. Ann Thorac Surg 1993;56:671.
20. Belani CP, White CS, Slawson R, et al. Value of minimally invasive

thoracoscopy versus non-invasive staging techniques in esophageal cancer. Proceedings of the American Society of Clinical Oncolog 1994.
21. Babineau TJ, Lewis WD, Jenkins RL, Bleday R, Steele GD. Role of staging laparoscopy in the treatment of hepatic malignancy. Am J Surg 1994;167:151.
22. Solomon MJ, Stephen MS, Gallinger S, White GH. Does intraoperative hepatic ultrasonography change surgical decision making during liver resection. Am J Surg 1994;168:307.
23. John TG, Greig JD, Crosbie JL, Miles WF, Garden OJ. Superior staging of liver tumors with laparoscopy and laparoscopic ultrasound. Ann Surg 1994;220:711.
24. Cuschieri A, Hall AW, Clark J. Value of laparoscopy in the diagnosis and management of pancreatic carcinoma. Gut 1978;19:672.
25. Warshaw AL, Tepper JE, Shipley WU. Laparoscopy in the staging and planning of therapy for pancreatic cancer. Am J Surg 1986;151:76.
26. Warshaw AL. Implications of peritoneal cytology for staging of early pancreatic cancer. Am J Surg 1991;161:26.
27. Nishizaki T, Matsumata T, Adachi E, Sugimachi K. Laparoscopy preferable to imaging procedures in detecting metastases of a pancreas carcinoma to the liver. Surg Endosc 1994;8:1340.
28. John TG, Greig JD, Carter DC, Garden OJ. Carcinoma of the pancreatic head and periampullary region. Ann Surg 1995;221:156.
29. Goh PMY, Tekant Y, Kum CK. Totally intraabdominal laparoscopic Billroth II gastrectomy. Surg Endosc 1992;6:160.
30. Goh P. Laparoscopic Billroth II gastrectomy. Seminars in Laparoscopic Surgery 1994;1:171.
31. Dean PA, Beart RW, Nelson H, Elftmann TD, Schlinkert RT. Laparoscopic assisted segmental colectomy: early Mayo clinic experience. Mayo Clin Proc 1994;69:834.
32. Böhm B, Milsom JW, Kitago K, Brand M, Stolfi VM, Fazio VW. Use of laparoscopic techniques in oncologic right colectomy in a canine model. Ann Surg Oncol 1995;2:6.
33. Elftmann TD, Nelson H, Ota DM, Pemberton JH, Beart RW. Laparoscopic assisted segmental colectomy: surgical techniques. Mayo Clin Proc 1994;69:825.
34. Cohen SM, Wexner SD. Laparoscopic right hemicolectomy. Surgical Rounds 1994;17:627.
35. Ota DM. Laparoscopic colectomy for cancer: a favorable opinion. Ann Surg Oncol 1995;2:3.
36. Jager RM, Ballantyne GH, Fleshman JW, Franklin ME. The technical nuances in laparoscopic colorectal surgery. Contemporary Surgery 1994;45:355.
37. Reissman P, Teoh TA, Piccirillo M, Nogueras JJ, Wexner SD. Colonoscopic assisted laparoscopic colectomy. Surg Endosc 1994;8:1352.
38. Phillips EH, Franklin M, Carroll BJ, Fallas MJ, Ramos R, Rosenthal D. Laparoscopic colectomy. Ann Surg 1992;216:703.
39. Falk PM, Beart RW, Wexner SD, et al. Laparoscopic colectomy: a critical appraisal. Dis Colon Rectum 1993;36:28.
40. Hoffman GC, Baker JW, Fitchett CW, Vansant JH. Laparoscopic assisted colectomy: initial experience. Ann Surg 1994;219:732.
41. Berman IR. Laparoscopic colectomy for cancer: some cause for pause. Ann Surg Oncol 1995;2:1.
42. Ramos JM, Gupta S, Anthone GJ, Ortega AF, Simons AJ, Beart RW. Laparoscopy and colon cancer: is the port site at risk? Arch Surg 1994;129:897.
43. Bessler M, Whelan RL, Halverson A, Treat MR, Nowygrod R. Is immune function better preserved after laparoscopic versus open colon resection. Surg Endosc 1994;8:881.
44. Tate JJ, Lau WY, Li AK. Transhepatic fenestration of liver cyst: a further application of laparoscopic surgery. Aust N Z J Surg 1994;64:264.
45. Payne HH. Ultrasonic dissector. Surg Endosc 1994;8:416.
46. Baer HU, Metzger A, Barras JP, Mettler D, Wheatley AM, Czerniak A. Laparoscopic liver resection in the large white pig: a comparison between waterjet dissector and ultrasound dissector. Endosc Surg Allied Technol 1994;2:189.
47. Azagra JS, ed. Proceedings of the First International Congress, European Association of Surgical Sciences, Ischia, Italy, 1994.
48. Ravikumar TS, Kane R, Cady B, Jerkins R, Clouse M, Steele G Jr. A 5-year study of cryosurgery in the treatment of liver tumors. Arch Surg 1991;126:1520.
49. Neuberger TJ, Wade TP, Swope TJ, Virgo KS, Johnson FE. Palliative operations for pancreatic cancer in the hospitals of the US Department of Veterans Affairs from 1987 to 1991. Am J Surg 1993;166:632.
50. Lillemoe KD. Current management of pancreatic carcinoma. Ann Surg 1995;221:133.
51. Gagner M, Pomp A. Laparoscopic pylorus-preserving pancreaticoduodenectomy. Surg Endosc 1994;8:408.
52. Shima SM, Banting SB, Cuschieri A. Laparoscopy in the management of pancreatic cancer. Br J Surg 1992;79:317.
53. Hawasli A. Laparoscopic cholecysto-jejunostomy for obstructing pancreatic cancer. J Laparoendosc Surg 1992;1:351.
54. Mouiel J. Palliative laparoscopic surgery for abdominal malignancies. Seminars in Laparoscopic Surgery 1994;1:26.
55. Lillemoe KD, Cameron JL, Kaufman HS, Yeo CJ, Pitt HA, Sauter PK. Chemical splanchnicectomy in patients with unresectable pancreatic cancer. Ann Surg 1993;217:447.
56. Abi-Rached B, Neugut AJ. Diagnostic and management issues in gallbladder carcinoma. Oncology 1995;9:19.
57. Copher JC, Rogers JJ, Dalton ML. Trocar site metastasis following laparoscopic cholecystectomy for unsuspected carcinoma of the gallbladder. Surg Endosc 1995;9:348.
58. Targarona EM, Pons MJ, Viella P, Trias M. Unsuspected carcinoma of the gallbladder: a laparoscopic dilemma. Surg Endosc 1994;8:211.
59. Cubertafond P, Gainant A, Cucchiaro G. Surgical treatment of 724 carcinomas of the gallbladder. Ann Surg 1994;219:275.
60. Sariego J, Aharonian A, Byrd M, Matsumoto T, Kerstein M. Adenocarcinoma of the gallbladder. Contemporary Surgery 1994;44:91.
61. Fong Y, Brennan MF, Turnbull A, Coit DG, Blumgart LH. Gallbladder cancer discovered during laparoscopic surgery. Arch Surg 1993;128:1054.
62. Ferzli GS, Daou R. Laparoscopic cholecystectomy and gallbladder cancer. Surg Endosc 1994;8:1357.
63. Flowers JL, Lefor AT, Steers JA, Heyman M, Graham SM, Imbembo AL. Laparoscopic splenectomy in patients with hematologic diseases. Annals of Surgery 1996 (in press).
64. Poulin EC, Thibault C, Mamazza J. Laparoscopic splenectomy. Surg Endosc 1995;9:172.
65. Lefor AT, Melvin WS, Bailey RW, Flowers JL. Laparoscopic splenectomy in the management of immune thrombocytopenia purpura. Surgery 1993;114:613.
66. Tulman S, Holcomb GW, Karamanoukian HL, Reynhout J. Pediatric laparoscopic splenectomy. J Pediatr Surg 1993;28:689.
67. Schlinkert RT, Braich TA. Laparoscopic assisted splenectomy for treatment of presumed immune thrombocytopenia purpura: initial results. Mayo Clin Proc 1994;69:422.
68. Phillips EH, Carroll BJ, Fallas MJ. Laparoscopic splenectomy. Surg Endosc 1994;8:931.
69. Carroll BJ, Phillips EH, Semer CJ, Fallas M, Morgenstern L. Laparoscopic splenectomy. Surg Endosc 1992;6:183.
70. Poulin E, Thibault C, Mamazza J, Girotti M, Côté G, Renaud A. Laparoscopic splenectomy: clinical experience and the role of preoperative splenic artery embolization. Surg Laparosc Endosc 1993;2:248.
71. Cadiere GB, Verroken R, Himpens J, Bruyns J, Efira M, De Wit S. Operative strategy in laparoscopic splenectomy. J Am Coll Surg 1994;179:668.
72. Wilhelm MC, Jones RE, McGehee R, Mitchener JS, Sandusky WR, Hess CE. Splenectomy in hematologic disorders. Ann Surg 1988;207:581.
73. Marble KR, Deckers PJ, Kern KA. Changing role of splenectomy for hematologic disease. J Surg Oncol 1993;52:169.
74. Llende M, Santiago-Delpin EA, Lavergne J. Immunobiological consequences of splenectomy. J Surg Res 1986;40:85.
75. Weintraub LR. Splenectomy: who, when and why. Hosp Pract June 1994:27.
76. Dawson AA, Jones PF, King DJ. Splenectomy in the management of haematologic disease. Br J Surg 1987;74:353.
77. Fujitani RM, Johs SM, Cobb SR, Mehringer CM, White RA, Klein SR. Preoperative splenic artery occlusion as an adjunct for high risk splenectomy. Am Surg 1988;54:602.
78. Hashizume M, Sugimachi K, Kitano S, et al. Laparoscopic splenectomy. Am J Surg 1994;167:611.
79. Akwari OE, Itani KMF, Coleman RE, Rosse WF. Splenectomy for primary and recurrent immune thrombocytopenia purpura. Ann Surg 1987;206:529.

80. Coon WW. Splenectomy for idiopathic thrombocytopenic purpura. Surg Gynecol Obstet 1987;164:225.
81. Hoekstra HJ, Tamminga RYJ, Timens W. Partial splenectomy in children: an alternative for splenectomy in the pathologic staging of Hodgkin's disease. Ann Surg Oncol 1994;1:480.
82. Pezet D, Fondrinier E, Rotman N, et al. Parietal seeding of carcinoma of the gallbladder after laparoscopic cholecystectomy. Br J Surg 1992; 79:230.
83. Jacobi CA, Keller H, Monig S, Said S. Implantation metastasis of unsuspected gallbladder carcinoma after laparoscopy. Surg Endosc 1995;9:351.
84. Clair DG, Lautz DB, Brooks DC. Rapid development of umbilical metastases after laparoscopic cholecystectomy for unsuspected gallbladder carcinoma. Surgery 1993;113:355.
85. Weiss SM, Wengert PA, Harkavy SE. Incisional recurrence of gallbladder cancer after laparoscopic cholecystectomy. Gastrointest Endosc 1994;40:244.
86. Cava A, Roman J, Quintela AG, Martin F, Aramburo P. Subcutaneous metastasis following laparoscopy in gastric adenocarcinoma. Eur J Surg Oncol 1990;16:63.
87. O'Rourke N, Price PM, Kelly S, Sikora K. Tumor inoculation during laparoscopy. Lancet 1993;342.
88. Nduka CC, Monson JRT, Menzies N, Darzi A. Abdominal wall metastases following laparoscopy. Br J Surg 1994;81:648.
89. Stockdale AD, Pocock TJ. Abdominal wall metastasis following laparoscopy. Eur J Surg Oncol 1985;11:373.
90. Walsh DCA, Wattchow DA, Wilson TG. Subcutaneous metastases after laparoscopic resection of malignancy. Aust N Z J Surg 1993; 63:563.
91. Fusco MA, Paluzzi MW. Abdominal wall recurrence after laparoscopic assisted colectomy for adenocarcinoma of the colon. Dis Colon Rectum 1993;36:858.
92. Ota DM. Laparoscopic management of colon cancer. Seminars in Laparoscopic Surgery 1994;1:18.
93. Hughes ESR, McDermott FT, Polglase AL, Johnson WR. Tumor recurrence in the abdominal wall scar tissue after large-bowel cancer surgery. Dis Colon Rectum 1983;26:571.
94. Birkett DH. Spilled cells, spilled clips, spilled stones: new problems or old challenges. Surg Endosc 1995;9:269.
95. Bessler M, Allendorf JDF, Chao JD, et al. Permissive tumor growth after laparotomy versus laparoscopy is associated with altered TNF levels. Surg Forum 1994;45:486.
96. Allendorf JDF, Bessler M, Kayton ML, Whelan RL, Treat MR, Nowygrod R. Tumor growth after laparotomy or laparoscopy. Surg Endosc 1995;9:49.
97. Gleruo H, Heindorff H, Flyvbjerg A, Jensen SL, Vilstrup H. Elective laparoscopic cholecystectomy nearly abolishes the postoperative hepatic catabolic stress response. Ann Surg 1995;221:214.
98. Grant JP. Comparison of percutaneous endoscopic gastrostomy with Stamm gastrostomy. Ann Surg 1988;207:598.
99. Murayama K, Schneider PD, Thompson JS. Laparoscopic gastrostomy: a safe method for obtaining enteral access. J Surg Res 1995; 58:1.
100. Lee DS, Mohit-Tabatabai MA, Rush BF, Levine C. Stomal seeding of head and neck cancer by percutaneous endoscopic gastrostomy tube placement. Ann Surg Oncol 1995;2:170.
101. Edelman DS, Unger SW. Laparoscopic Gastrostomy. Surg Gynecol Obstet 1992;174:401.
102. Ota DM, Evans DB, Mansfield PF. Placement of a feeding jejunostomy. In: Ballantyne GH, Leahy PF, Modlin IM, eds. Laparoscopic surgery. Philadelphia: WB Saunders, 1993:467.
103. Leitman IM, Sullivan JD, Brams D, DeCosse JJ. Multivariate analysis of morbidity and mortality from the initial surgical management of obstructing carcinoma of the colon. Surg Gynecol Obstet 1992;174: 513.
104. Lange V, Meyer G, Shardey HM, Schildberg MD. Laparoscopic creation of a loop colostomy. J Laparoendosc Surg 1991;1:307.
105. Lyerly HK, Mault JR. Laparoscopic ileostomy and colostomy. Ann Surg 1994;219:317.
106. Cuschieri A. Whither minimal access surgery: tribulations and expectations. Am J Surg 1995;169:9.
107. Soper NJ, Blunt LM, Kerbl K. Laparoscopic general surgery. N Engl J Med 1994;330:409.

Surgery for Gastrointestinal Cancer: A Multidisciplinary Approach, edited by Harold J. Wanebo.
Lippincott-Raven Publishers, Philadelphia, © 1997.

CHAPTER 11

Imaging Strategies for the Diagnosis, Staging, and Follow-up of Gastrointestinal Malignancies

Robert A. Kane, Jonathan B. Kruskal, and Steven Eustace

The goal of imaging in patients with gastrointestinal malignancies is accurately to diagnose and stage tumors preoperatively to facilitate treatment stratification. This chapter discusses innovations in imaging technology that are of practical importance to physicians managing patients with gastrointestinal malignancies. The advantages and disadvantages of the various cross-sectional techniques are emphasized, and the relative sensitivities and shortcomings of these techniques discussed, with reference to specific tumors of the hollow-lumen and solid abdominal organs.

When imaging patients with known or suspected gastrointestinal malignancies, the imaging technique selected must, where possible, identify the primary lesion and detect evidence for local, regional, or even distant spread. Cross-sectional technologies, including computed tomography (CT), ultrasound (US), and magnetic resonance imaging (MRI), play a role in both the primary diagnosis and evaluation for metastatic disease. By providing reformatted images of major vessels, CT or MR angiography and US with color flow can identify the presence of thrombus arising from or adjacent to a tumor, and can demonstrate tumor invasion of major vessels. These data are of crucial practical importance to the surgeon planning the resection, and frequently serve to modify the selected surgical approach.

Bowel lumen contrast opacification, such as occurs with the upper gastrointestinal tract study or barium enema, provides information about the primary lesion but cannot be relied on for detection of extraluminal disease. Certainly, these luminal contrast techniques are able to identify evidence for serosal involvement or drop metastases, but they are neither sensitive nor specific for these purposes. Endoluminal US (ELUS), when performed properly by an experienced operator, can be useful for determining the depth of bowel wall penetration by tumors in the esophagus, stomach, and rectum. ELUS, however, is not reliable beyond the bowel wall, and although it may detect enlarged lymph nodes, is not sensitive for detecting the presence of tumor in these nodes. Intraoperative US (IOUS), using specially designed transducers, is the most sensitive imaging technique for detecting liver metastases and for evaluating the pancreas. This technique is being used more and more frequently during surgery in patients with colorectal carcinoma, both for staging purposes and for guiding segmental resections. IOUS is also being used to guide surgeons during cryoablation of liver tumors. It is also expected that laparoscopic ultrasound (LUS) will be used more frequently for both the diagnosis and staging of abdominal malignancies. With this technique, high-resolution images of the liver, pancreas, and biliary system can be obtained and biopsy guidance provided.

In the past 5 years, several innovative imaging advances have been made to facilitate both the diagnosis and staging of gastrointestinal malignancies. These have included technical improvements in MRI, which previously played a rather limited role in abdominal imaging, largely because of motion artifacts resulting from peristalsis and the lack of bowel lumen contrast-enhancing agents suitable for use with MRI. Software and other technical improvements, including the use of surface receiving coils placed over the regions or organs of interest, allow a more rapid data acquisition, further reducing motion artifact and improving the signal-to-noise ratio. For imaging of tumors in solid abdominal organs, MRI as it is currently performed has not fully justified its use over CT. MR cholangiopancreatography is being used to image the extrahepatic bile and pancreatic ducts. This noninvasive technique is much easier to perform than endoscopic retrograde cholangiopancreatography (ERCP), requires no contrast material administration, and has none of the complications associated with ERCP, such as pancreatitis or biliary sepsis. CT cholangiography, in which imaging of the bile ducts is enhanced by the rapid biliary excretion of intravenously administered contrast agents, remains experimental.

Magnetic resonance angiography, which can provide three-dimensional images of the hepatic vasculature and major ab-

Robert A. Kane, Department of Radiological Sciences, New England Deaconess Hospital, One Deaconess Road, Boston, MA 02215

Jonathan B. Kruskal, Department of Radiological Sciences, New England Deaconess Hospital, One Deaconess Road, Boston, MA 02215

Steven Eustace, Department of Radiological Sciences, New England Deaconess Hospital, One Deaconess Road, Boston, MA 02215 dominal vessels, has the advantage of not requiring administration of intravenous contrast material. CT angiography, on the other hand, which does require rapid bolus contrast administration, also provides three-dimensional images of the principal abdominal and hepatic vessels, and has been greatly facilitated by the development of spiral CT scanning, whereby scanning data are acquired volumetrically and two- or three-dimensional images are reformatted from the stored data in any required plane. The latest-generation electron-beam CT scanners are being used clinically in a few centers; initial results suggest that the extremely rapid acquisition of data that occurs with this technique may permit evaluation of small vessel patency and tumor vascularity. The use of three-dimensional workstations has allowed images to be reformatted in any plane or dimension from volumetrically acquired CT data. From this, virtual colonoscopy has developed, whereby images of the entire lumen of the colon are recreated from the CT data and can be viewed at any site or from any angle within the lumen.

THE ESOPHAGUS

Squamous cell carcinoma and adenocarcinoma of the esophagus account for approximately 2% of the total yearly deaths due to malignancies in the United States. Almost 10,000 cases are documented annually in the United States. Squamous cell tumors are observed throughout the esophagus, whereas adenocarcinomas occur more distally at or near the gastroesophageal junction, or in the mid- to distal esophagus, at a site of columnar metaplasia occurring in Barrett's esophagus.

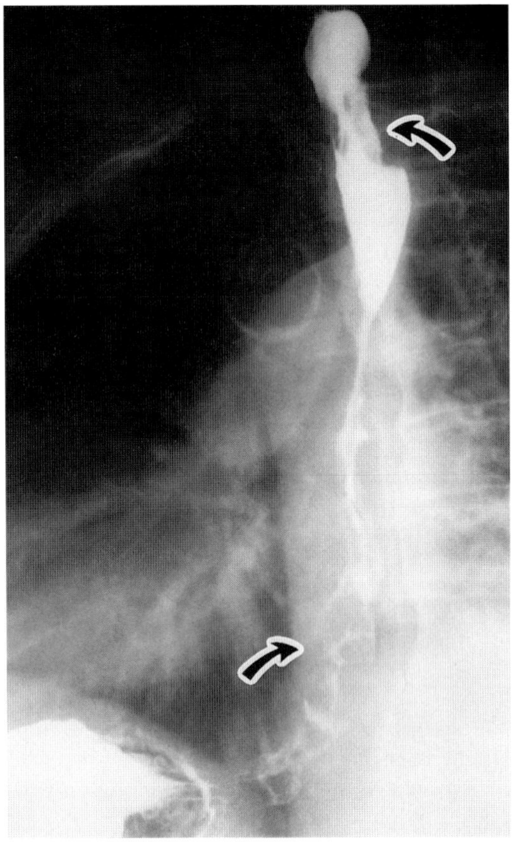

FIG. 11-1. Synchronous primary adenocarcinomas of the esophagus. A single double-contrast image of the entire esophagus demonstrates two large polypoid intraluminal masses *(arrows)* in the esophagus, both of which were adenocarcinoma.

Diagnosis and Staging

Esophagoscopy and single- or double-contrast barium swallow studies are the most useful diagnostic modalities for evaluating the esophageal mucosa and lumen. Although the contrast examination provides an accurate demonstration of the proximal and distal extent of the disease, and of luminal narrowing, endoscopy permits a diagnostic biopsy sample to be taken at the time of the study. None of the studies provides information as to the extent of tumor infiltration or extraesophageal disease, and thus should not be used for staging purposes. Esophageal carcinoma may manifest as a focal or diffuse mucosal irregularity, a polypoidal endoluminal protrusion, or as an eccentric or annular constricting lesion (Fig. 11-1). Squamous cell carcinoma or adenocarcinoma comprise most esophageal cancers. However, rarer tumors do exist, some of which may arise in the submucosal layer of the esophageal wall, such as the aggressive spindle cell tumor or carcinosarcoma, which tends to arise in the middle third of the esophagus as a large, bulky, polypoid mass. Asymmetric luminal narrowing should be seen with barium contrast studies, but these rare tumors are usually best evaluated and staged with cross-sectional imaging studies such as CT scanning.

Development of improved and more radical surgical techniques, chemotherapy protocols, and radiation therapy regimens has led to a greater need for accurate esophageal tumor staging. Current methods of esophageal tumor staging are based on the TNM system.[1] Unlike previous classifications, the TNM system emphasizes the depth of tumor invasion into or through the esophageal wall rather than tumor size or the degree of circumferential luminal involvement. Accurate tumor staging is crucial for stratifying patients into specific treatment protocols. Any imaging technique used for staging esophageal tumors must be able accurately to determine the depth of tumor extension into the esophageal wall, determine whether there is extension beyond the esophageal wall or any direct invasion into adjacent vital structures, detect the presence or absence of infiltration into adjacent lymph nodes, and detect the presence or absence of local or distant metastases. For staging purposes, oncologists need to know whether the tumor extends into or through the submucosa, the muscularis propria, or into adjacent structures. To complicate matters somewhat, separate staging systems have been described for CT and ELUS studies. However, because current treatment protocols used by most oncologists rely on the TNM system, it is best if imaging modalities attempt to provide clinically useful information appropriate for TNM staging. To do this optimally, a thorough knowledge of pathways of early nodal spread is essential; these pathways also depend on the location of the primary tumor.

Patients with esophageal tumors that are restricted to the superficial layers of the esophageal wall at the time of initial diagnosis have a significantly better long-term survival (40% 5-year survival) than those in whom the tumor has extended beyond the esophageal wall (4% 5-year survival).[2,3] Obviously, tumor grade and histology and type of treatment will influence these survival statistics. Patients in whom no lymph node spread is detected have a 5-year survival of 42%, versus 3% for node-positive patients.[2,3] Approximately 75% of patients are reported to have local lymph node metastases at the time of initial presentation. Although imaging studies such as ELUS or CT scanning may detect the presence of enlarged lymph nodes, these techniques are insensitive for predicting the presence of tumor in these lymph nodes. False-positive interpretations may result from nodes that are enlarged because of an infectious or inflammatory etiology, an unrelated disorder the patient may have, or because of radiation or even medications the patients may have taken. Whereas esophagoscopy and contrast studies are unable to evaluate the depth of tumor invasion, CT and, more recently, ELUS have provided the most widely accepted and used methods of staging, each with its own advantages and disadvantages.

Computed Tomography

Computed tomography facilitates the identification of tumor penetration through the esophageal wall by visualizing disruption of the periesophageal fat plane (Fig. 11-2). The images of the esophageal lumen may be improved by using a barium paste. Intravenous contrast material helps to differentiate between blood vessels and lymph nodes adjacent to the esophagus. In the elderly or malnourished patient population, as is frequently observed in patients with advanced esophageal cancer, this fat plane may not be apparent, and staging with CT scanning then becomes unreliable. This may result in overestimation of the depth of tumor invasion. Because extraesophageal tumor spread significantly affects staging and subsequent treatment, it becomes crucial to determine accurately whether spread has occurred. Under normal circumstances, however, the periesophageal fat plane is absent or indistinct in the mid-esophagus at the level of the carina and left atrium. The presence of tumor invasion is then determined at this level if, in addition to direct contact with these structures, there is compression or displacement of the carina or left atrium. These imaging characteristics have a positive predictive value of 83% for tumor invasion at this level.[4,5] The determination of aortic invasion demands that in addition to loss of the fat plane at that level, there is greater than 90° of direct contact between the tumor and the aorta; a positive predictive value of 70% to 95% has been described for this imaging feature. CT scanning becomes less reliable for staging purposes when tumors arise at or near the gastroesophageal junction. In this region, collapsed mucosa in a nondistended stomach, the presence of a sliding hiatus hernia, prolapsed gastric folds, or the obliquity of the gastroesophageal mucosal junction in an axial plane may simulate a mass. CT, unlike US,

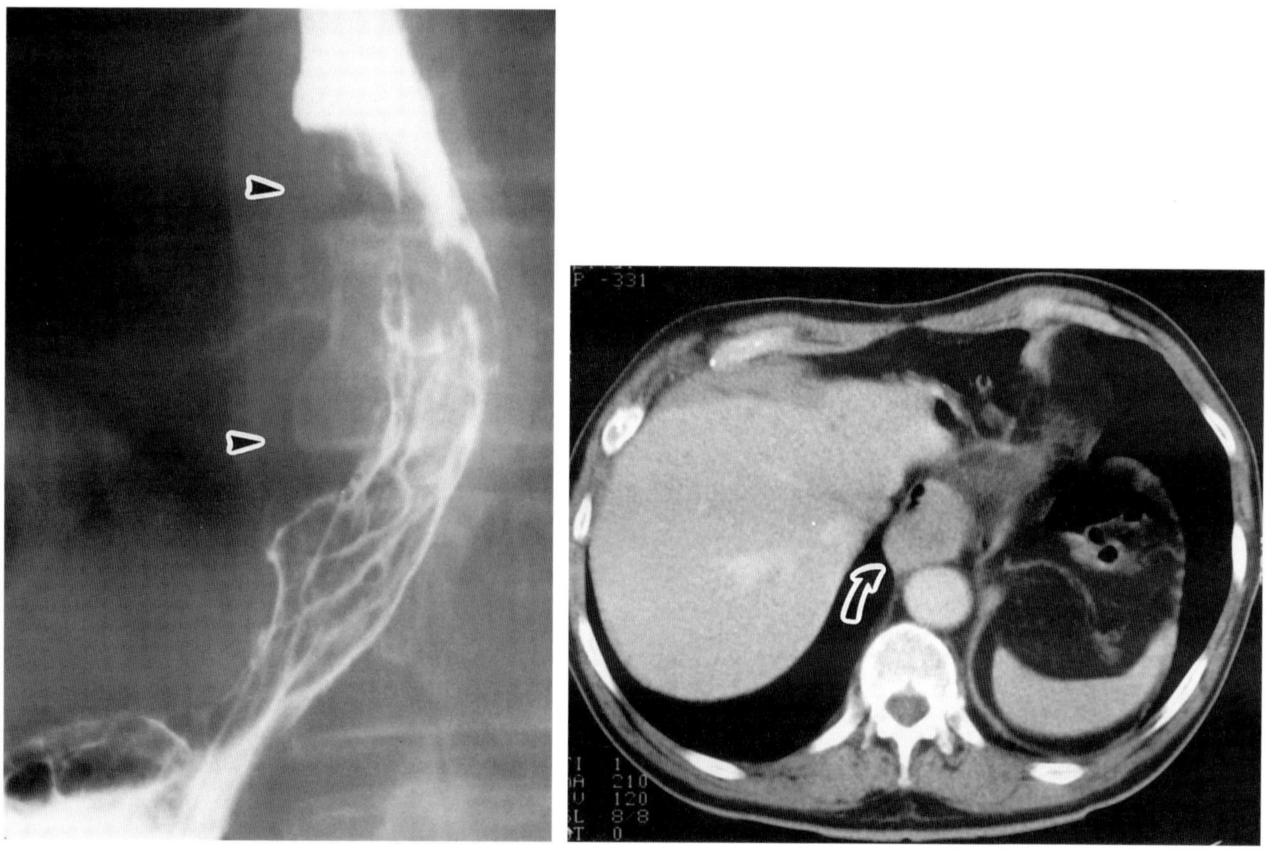

A B

FIG. 11-2. Adenocarcinoma of the esophagus. A single image obtained during a double-contrast upper gastrointestinal examination **(A)** demonstrates a large polypoid mass in the distal esophagus *(arrowheads)* that does not extend into the stomach. A single axial computed tomography image of the same tumor **(B)** demonstrates extensive narrowing of the esophageal lumen by the tumor *(arrow)*, with a well defined fat plane between the tumor and the adjacent aorta.

does not enable visualization of the precise depth of tumor invasion into the esophageal wall, but merely determines the presence or absence of tumor extension beyond the esophageal lumen both locally and distally, such as into the liver, and may identify the presence of enlarged periesophageal lymph nodes.[6–9]

Computed tomography is not sensitive for determining the presence or absence of lymph node invasion. This point will be reiterated several times during discussion of the role of most imaging techniques in imaging the various organs of the gastrointestinal tract. When lymph nodes of 6 mm or less in maximum diameter are considered normal and nodes with a maximum short axis diameter greater than 10 mm are considered abnormal, CT is reported to have an accuracy of between 57% and 61% for predicting the presence of nodal invasion by the tumor.[7–10] This unfortunately leaves a rather large gray area in which numerous false-positive nodes may be identified. Lymph nodes that contain tumor may not be enlarged, and enlarged nodes may result from an infectious or inflammatory etiology. This low accuracy rate for predicting nodal invasion results largely from the 30% of nodes that, when considered to be of normal size, are subsequently shown to be infiltrated by tumor. Furthermore, with esophageal cancer spreading preferentially to certain perigastric nodal chains, it is important to know that CT scanning is particularly poor at detecting left gastric nodal enlargement and tumor infiltration.

Computed tomography is effective for the detection of liver metastases, with a reported sensitivity between 67% and 75%.[11,12] Detection of liver metastases is improved by the use of intravenous contrast material and is markedly improved by direct enhancement of the portal vein, which is achieved with the administration of contrast into the superior mesenteric artery, a technique known as CT arterial portography. This method, which has a reported sensitivity of up to 95%, relies on the liver metastases and adjacent parenchyma having a different blood supply; liver metastases may receive a predominantly hepatic arterial supply, whereas normal liver parenchyma receives a predominantly portal venous blood supply.[11,12] CT is particularly poor at detecting peritoneal deposits, which may go undetected despite being present in abundance. Secondary features such as ascites and hepatic subcapsular deposits may only suggest the presence of peritoneal spread.

Endoluminal Sonography

Tumor staging using high-frequency (7.5 to 12 MHz) transducers passed through an endoscope is rapidly gaining popularity. Using ELUS, it is possible to visualize five alternating hyperechoic and hypoechoic layers of the esophageal wall (Fig. 11-3). Under normal circumstances, the interface between the probe and the balloon is hyperechoic, that between the mucosa and muscularis mucosa is hypoechoic, the submucosa is hyperechoic, the muscularis propria is hypoechoic, and the interface between muscle wall and mediastinal fat is hyperechoic. Distortion of this laminated pattern facilitates assessment of the degree of penetration by tumor with an accuracy of between 59% and 92%, when subsequently compared with resected specimens.[13–18] The diagnosis of direct infiltration into adjacent structures by ELUS has a reported accuracy of 89% to 94%.[13–18] The development of mechanical radial catheter transducers in-

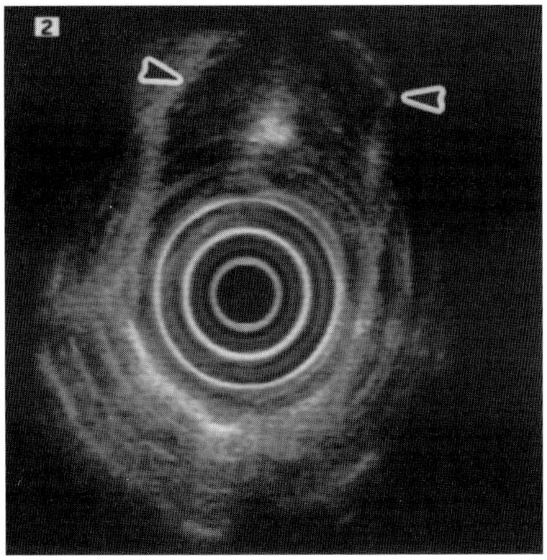

FIG. 11-3. Esophageal adenocarcinoma. An endoscopic ultrasound image demonstrates a large esophageal adenocarcinoma *(arrowheads)* extending through the esophageal wall.

troduced through the biopsy channel of a gastroscope has enabled staging of tight stenotic lesions and lesions at the gastroesophageal junction, sites often inadequately assessed at CT.[19] False-positive determination of the extent of tumor depth may occur when the tumor has ulcerated, with large villous-type tumors, after tumor biopsy, or when the tumor induces a desmoplastic response in the adjacent tissue layers. In these situations, the US images may suggest invasion to a greater depth than has occurred, emphasizing the importance of careful real-time imaging.

Sonographic evaluation of lymph node invasion is impaired by the relatively limited field of view afforded by this modality. Nevertheless, accuracy figures for the presence of lymph node metastases in the mediastinum of between 69% and 88% have been reported.[20] Unlike CT, it is the shape and echo character of the node rather than its size that is used to define the presence or absence of malignancy. Some authors believe that nodes that have been infiltrated by tumor cells are usually hypoechoic and have clearly defined margins, whereas "benign" nodes are usually hyperechoic and have indistinct margins.[20] The hyperechogenicity results from fat normally found within the hilum of a node. Tumor invasion replaces this fat, which may result in loss of the expected echotexture. Nonetheless, inflamed or infected nodes may demonstrate similar features. Unlike CT, ELUS is accurate in staging disease in certain areas below the diaphragm, especially when used to evaluate spread into the stomach wall and the presence of enlarged lymph nodes along the lesser curvature of the stomach.[20]

Magnetic Resonance Imaging

The role of MRI in staging esophageal carcinoma is still being evaluated. There is a wide variation in the T1 and T2 measurements of the normal and abnormal esophagus, and these signal characteristics cannot be used to make histologic diagnosis in a patient with esophageal wall thickening.[21] MRI is poor at defining depth of tumor penetration. Tracheobronchial and aortic invasion may be difficult to diagnose, with a large number of indeterminate results. The accuracy of MRI for detecting mediastinal invasion is only 40% to 50%.[21] MRI may also miss tumor in lymph nodes that are not enlarged, although the identification of T2 signal hyperintensity within lymph node parenchyma may indicate tumor infiltration. Similarly, susceptibility to movement degradation may obscure nodes within the abdomen, particularly near the stomach, where peristalsis further degrades image quality. Technical improvements, including faster imaging sequences, endoluminal MR contrast agents, and improved soft tissue resolution, may overcome these limitations to imaging the esophagus. MRI is reported to be more accurate in the evaluation of liver metastases than CT, but this may depend on the specific type of CT scan performed, the resolution of the MR scanner being used, and the imaging skills and interests of the radiologist interpreting the study.[21] The obliteration of tissue planes surrounding the esophagus after surgery makes the interpretation of CT scans difficult and unreliable. ELUS, on the other hand, may detect recurrence even without mucosal involvement, particularly recurrence at or near the site of anastomosis.[22]

Palliation of unresectable tumors may be achieved by repeated dilatation, surgical or endoscopic insertion of an endoprosthesis, irradiation, laser surgery, or bypass surgery. Endoscopic insertion of plastic tubes requires general anesthesia, and perforation, food impaction, and dislocation of the tube are well recognized complications. Many of these complications may be overcome by fluoroscopically guided placement of self-expanding metallic stents. Treatment of dysphagia by insertion of a metal stent was first proposed in 1983 by Frimberger,[23] and has been subsequently used and modified by several workers. Ideally, a stent should have an adequate lumen, an efficient radial force, and a length sufficient to cover elongated strictures. Cwikiel and coworkers[24] have described successful placement of self-expanding Nitinol stents in 40 patients with fluoroscopic guidance. Nitinol, an alloy of nickel and titanium, has thermal and shape memory, as well as superelastic behavior similar to rubber. Encasement in gelatin allows marked compression of the stent and hence the use of a relatively small delivery system for stent placement. Resorbtion of gelatin leads to self-expansion of the stent. Such stents have greater longitudinal flexibility and expand to provide a greater lumen than plastic tubes.

Summary

Conventional diagnosis of esophageal tumors follows either endoscopic evaluation or a barium swallow. Staging decisions dictating operability of a lesion require either ELUS or CT evaluation. ELUS is more accurate than CT scanning at assessing the depth of tumor infiltration (ELUS 92%, CT 60%) and the presence of nodal metastases (ELUS 88%, CT 74%), whereas CT is more accurate than ELUS for detecting the presence of distant metastases (ELUS 70%, CT 90%). A suggested diagnostic algorithm is to use CT to determine operability and then use ELUS to assess the depth of tumor invasion and hence the prognosis. Endoscopic ultrasound is the best method of detecting local tumor recurrence. CT is better at detecting distant metastases. Fluoroscopically placed, self-expanding metallic stents are an attractive alternative treatment for patients with inoperable tumors.

THE STOMACH

Gastric carcinoma has traditionally had the grim reputation of late presentation associated with advanced disease, a low rate of resectability, and a 5-year survival rate of between 5% and 10%.[25] Since 1930, there have been consistent reports of a declining incidence in Europe and the United States, and overall survival rates reported from Japan have shown dramatic improvement.[25] The occurrence and patterns of presentation of gastric carcinoma vary considerably throughout the world, with a peak incidence in Japan and Chile and a lower incidence in the United States. Radiologic imaging plays a valuable role in both the initial diagnosis of the disease and in staging local disease and detecting distant spread. Moreover, endoluminal contrast and cross-sectional imaging studies play a vital role in patient follow-up, in evaluating the surgical anastomosis for complications such as leaks, strictures, intussusception, and blind loop syndromes, and in the detection of local disease recurrence or metastases.

Diagnosis and Staging

The double-contrast barium study represents the radiologic diagnostic method of choice for gastric carcinoma. Early forms of this disease, which are frequently detected in Japan, where large population screening programs are undertaken, are often subtle and may produce only minor mucosal irregularities or even be missed at barium examination. In patients presenting with advanced gastric cancer, the prominent imaging features that may be identified, such as lack of gastric distensibility or a linitis plastica appearance, result from tumor infiltration through or along the submucosal layer. The tumor growth may have variable patterns and the appearance may be circumferential, infiltrative, ulcerating, mass-like, or even fungating (Fig. 11-4). Despite significant technical advances in endoscopy and double-contrast barium studies that permit earlier detection of gastric tumors, more than 25% of patients who undergo surgical exploration receive palliative treatment only because advanced disease or extension of tumor beyond the confines of the stomach is discovered at the time of surgery.[26] Even though adenocarcinoma is the most common primary gastric malignancy, lymphoma of the stomach does occur and has a variable imaging appearance, from massive fold thickening (Fig. 11-5) to nodularity, mural infiltration, and ulceration.

The major radiologic advance in the diagnosis, treatment, and management of gastric carcinoma relates to improved methods of staging, similar to what has been described with esophageal carcinoma. Staging of gastric cancer is based on the TNM classification, reported by Kennedy in 1970, in which it was clearly demonstrated that patient survival correlated with the depth of tumor invasion at the time of initial diagnosis.[27] Like esophageal carcinoma, accurate staging of gastric tumors involves a thorough evaluation of the extent of tumor invasion of the stomach wall, the presence or absence of enlarged local perigastric or distant lymph nodes, and the presence or absence of local or distant metastases, particularly in the liver, peripancreatic region, the lesser sac, or the mesentery.

For staging purposes, several anatomic regions should be specifically evaluated with CT scanning. Initial lymphatic

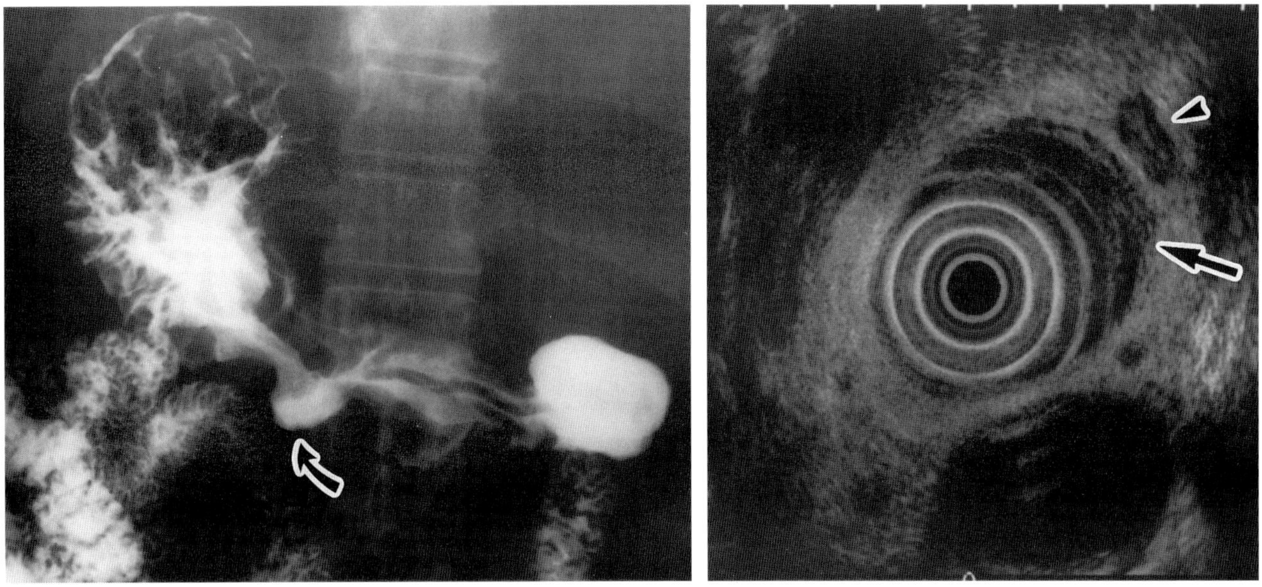

A B

FIG. 11-4. Adenocarcinoma of the stomach. A large circumferential carcinoma is present in the body of the stomach **(A)** with an excavated ulcer crater *(curved arrow)* along the greater curvature ulcer of the stomach. Endoscopic ultrasound of the stomach **(B)** demonstrates the tumor extending through the stomach wall *(arrow)* with an enlarged perigastric lymph node *(arrowhead).*

spread occurs into the perigastric nodes, followed by spread to the paraaortic, hepatoduodenal, retropancreatic, and mesenteric nodes. Spread may occur along the gastrocolic, gastrohepatic, and hepatoduodenal peritoneal ligaments; hematogenous spread is most frequent to the liver, followed by the adrenal glands, ovaries, and bone. Peritoneal seeding may result in thickening of the rectal wall (Blumer's shelf; Fig. 11-6) or periumbilical nodes. An enlarged left supraclavicular (Virchow) node is a poor prognostic sign. Metastases are not infrequent to the stomach, and may arise from breast or lung cancer, melanoma, or Kaposi's sarcoma (Fig. 11-7).

Both CT and ELUS represent favored methods for tumor staging. Endoscopic US probes with frequencies ranging from 7 to 12 MHz have greatly improved the local staging of gastric tumors by being able to detect depth of tumor invasion and local spread beyond the muscularis propria layer.[20] In addition,

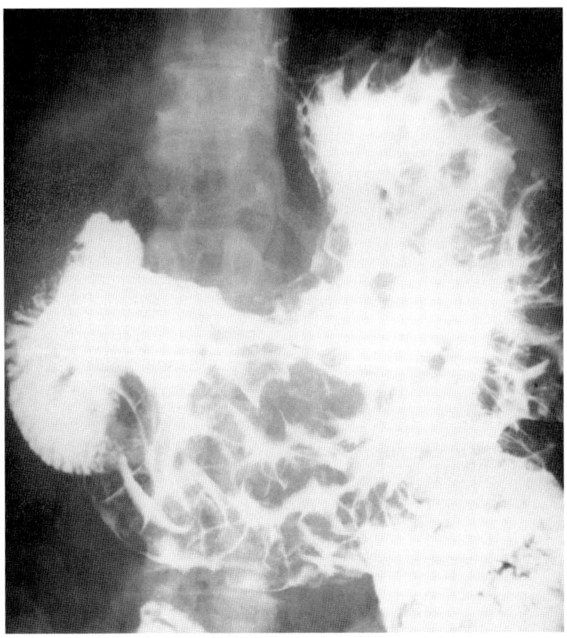

FIG. 11-5. Gastric lymphoma. Massive thickening of the gastric folds is present in this patient with lymphoma that involved both the stomach and several segments of small bowel.

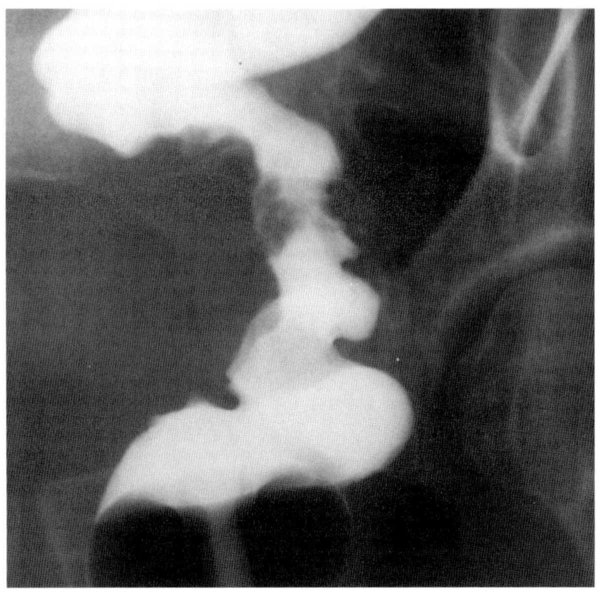

FIG. 11-6. Gastric drop metastases to the rectum. Circumferential mural irregularities are present in this persistently narrowed rectum that resulted from drop metastases from gastric adenocarcinoma.

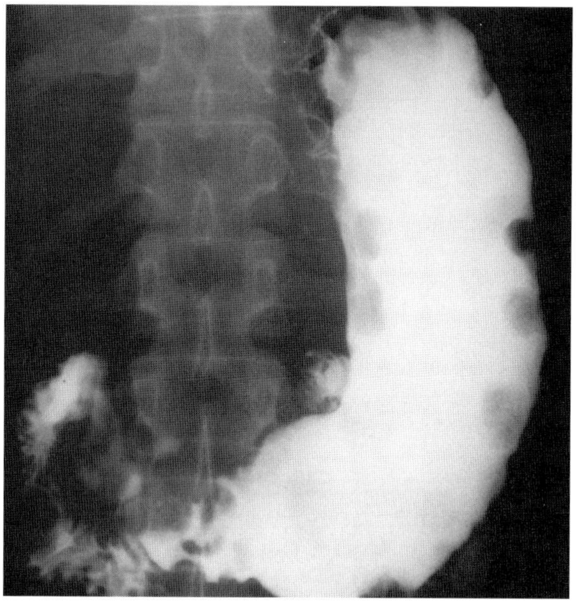

FIG. 11-7. Metastatic Kaposi's sarcoma to the stomach. Multiple submucosal nodules are demonstrated throughout the stomach in this patient.

the development of mechanical radial catheter transducers passed through the biopsy channel of a gastroscope has enabled staging at sites of narrowing such as produced by gastroesophageal and ampullopancreatic carcinomas; these have decreased the frequency of incomplete examination at ELUS.[20] Accurate determination of tumor infiltration depends on the experience of the operator, who should be aware of the technical factors that may result in overstaging of the tumor. US may detect the presence of enlarged perigastric lymph nodes, but is not sensitive for predicting whether tumor invasion has occurred into these nodes. Loss of the central echogenic zone of a lymph node, which normally results from hilar fat, may suggest the presence of tumor invasion, but this measure of the presence of malignancy remains operator dependent and rather insensitive.

The extent of gastric wall invasion correlates strongly with patient survival.[27] As was discussed in the section on evaluation of esophageal disease, endoscopic US, when properly performed, permits visualization of five discrete layers in the stomach wall. This technique may be enhanced by filling the stomach with water and suctioning off any excess gas or air bubbles. Furthermore, an understanding of the physics of US, including optimizing the gain settings, the depth of field, the focal zones, and the time–gain compensation curve, also helps to improve image quality for better evaluation of the extent of disease. The depth of tumor penetration may be assessed by identifying focal mucosal disruption, manifest as local change in echo texture. Endoscopic US has a reported sensitivity of 92% in detecting tumor invasion when comparison is made with resected specimens.[28]

Ultrasound enables differentiation of nodes from vessels or bowel loops by real-time imaging. Using unsubstantiated criteria for lymph node involvement such as lymph node shape, where round nodes are often found to be infiltrated by tumor, and where elongated nodes are usually uninvolved, and echotexture (hypoechogenicity suggests tumor infiltration, hyperechogenicity suggests benignity), an assessment of tumor invasion of lymph nodes may be made with a reported specificity of approximately 78%.[26] These remain very controversial criteria. Nodal size is a less reliable criterion because inflamed or infected nodes also are enlarged, and early tumor invasion may not cause node enlargement.[26] Surgeons not only should be familiar with the criteria for nodal involvement used in their Department of Radiology, but must be cognizant of the fact that no current imaging modality is completely sensitive for predicting lymph node involvement. Usually, histologic examination is required for a definitive diagnosis to be made.

In a patient with gastric carcinoma, endoscopic US, when properly performed, may allow visualization of the lateral segment of the left lobe of the liver, and both the celiac and left gastric lymph nodes, especially if these are enlarged. This technique, however, does not allow visualization of the right lobe and medial segment of the left lobe of the liver, and is therefore not useful for detection of distant metastatic disease. Similarly, endoscopic US cannot evaluate the retroperitoneum and the nodal chains, where gastric cancer is known to spread early in the course of metastasis.

Computed Tomography

Computed tomography scanning enables the identification of gastric wall thickening (Fig. 11-8) in a properly gas-distended stomach. In an underdistended stomach, particularly if no oral contrast material has been administered, the gastric rugae frequently simulate wall thickening. CT is particularly unreliable when the stomach is not distended or where bowel lumen becomes compressed, such as at the esophageal hiatus,[28,29] but is more reliable if the stomach is distended with air and fluid, using water and effervescent granules. CT imaging can be performed in the same way an upper gastrointestinal study is performed, by acquiring images of the patient in various oblique positions after ingestion of oral contrast agents and granules for gas distention. CT relies on an increase in nodal size to predict nodal infiltration by tumor.[29,30] This has been shown to be of low predictive value (48%).[29] CT enables visualization of the entire abdomen and chest and is therefore superior to US as a method for determining regional and distant metastases. CT plays a useful role in detecting local and distant spread, particularly in identifying enlarged lymph nodes or liver metastases. In our experience and in that of others,[31] contrast-enhanced CT scans are as sensitive as MRI for detecting liver metastases. Peritoneal seeding is poorly visualized, but should be suspected in the presence of ascitic fluid.

Magnetic Resonance Imaging

Currently, MRI plays little or no role in evaluating the presence and extent of gastric carcinoma. MRI is unable to determine the extent of tumor infiltration, or to identify lymph node invasion. The theoretic development of endoluminal coils, placed through a nasogastric tube, may overcome these limitations. The role of MRI in the staging of gastric carcinoma is still unclear. Peristalsis and air in the stomach lumen result in image degradation. Technical improvements in abdominal MRI have included faster image acquisition and the use of oral MR

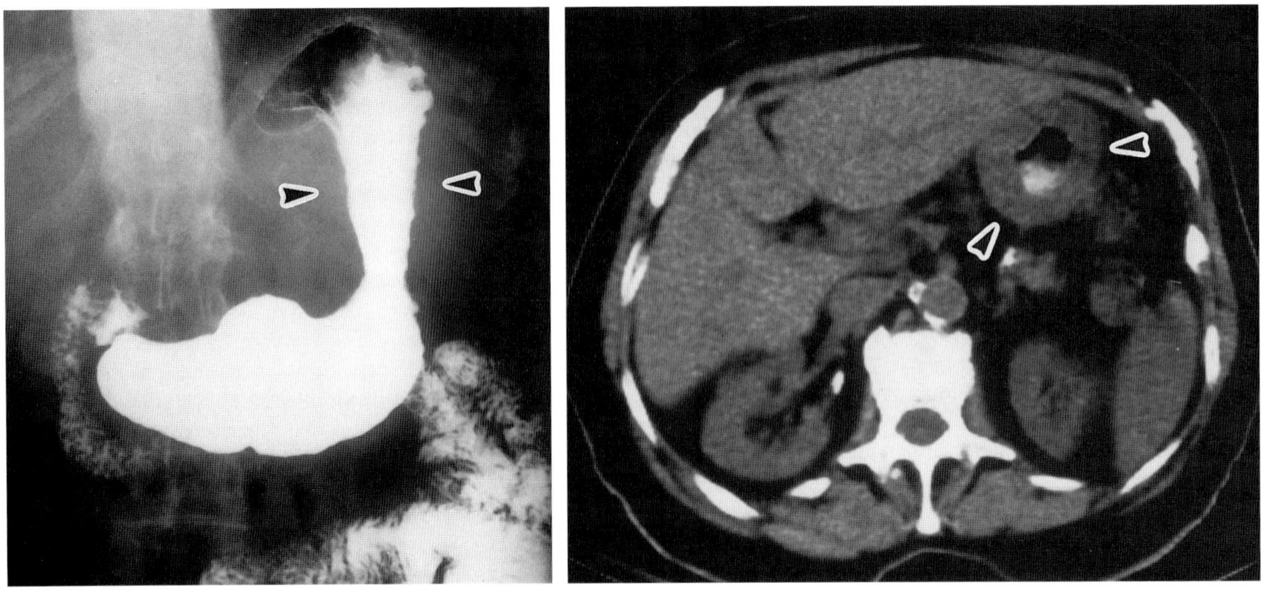

A B

FIG. 11-8. Infiltrating adenocarconima of the stomach. Images from an upper gastrointestinal series **(A)** and a computed tomography scan **(B)** demonstrate lack of distensibility and massive gastric wall thickening *(arrowheads)* in a patient with gastric adenocarcinoma. Submucosal spread of tumor produces this linitus plastica appearance.

contrast agents. Although these have resulted in improved imaging of upper abdominal tumors, MRI cannot currently be recommended above CT or ELUS for staging purposes. MRI does play a role in the detection of liver metastases, where it is useful for differentiating between liver metastases and vascular hemangiomas. Much research is underway in MR contrast agents for lymphography; it is hoped that MRI will be able to play a role in detecting tumor infiltration of lymph nodes, but this is not currently available in a clinical setting.

Summary

Double-contrast barium study and endoscopy are the methods of choice for diagnosing gastric carcinoma. CT is the method

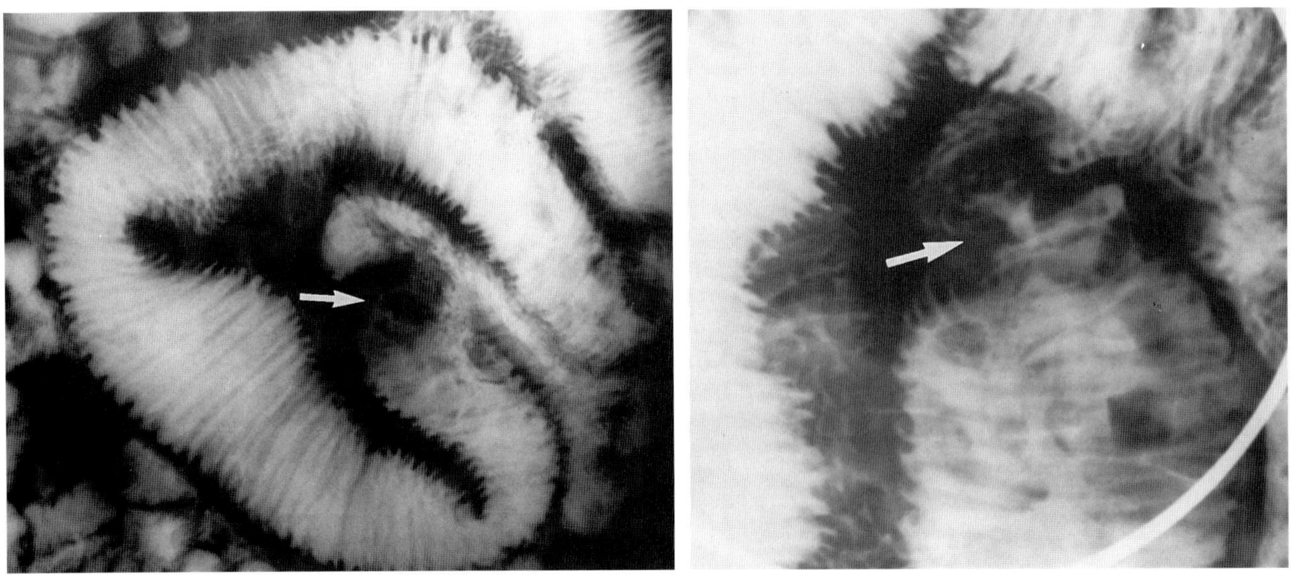

A B

FIG. 11-9. Adenocarcinoma of the jejunum. A small bowel series **(A)** demonstrates dilatation of the barium-filled proximal small bowel extending to a point of irregular narrowing in the mid-jejunum *(arrow)*. This dilatation resulted from a circumferential primary adenocarcinoma of the jejunum (**B,** *arrow)*.

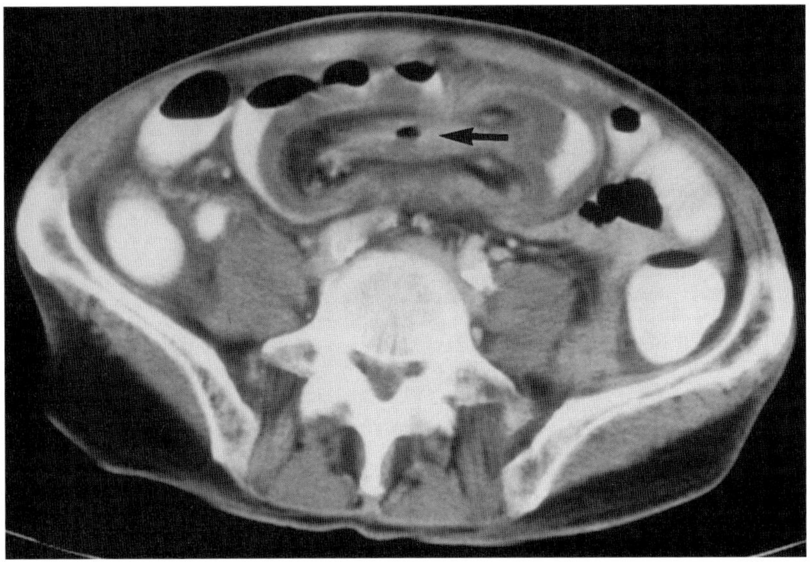

FIG. 11-10. Small bowel lymphoma with ileocolic intussusception. A typical computed tomographic scan appearance of ileocolic intussusception with mesenteric fat and contrast material *(straight arrow)* present within the lumen of the intussuscipiens.

of choice for detecting extragastric spread of tumor and for determining resectability, whereas ELUS enables accurate local staging.

THE SMALL BOWEL

Benign and malignant tumors of the small bowel are rare, representing 1.7% to 6.5% of all gastrointestinal tract neoplasms. The rarity of small bowel tumors is thought to reflect in part high levels of IgA, the paucity of bacterial proliferation at this site, and an alkaline environment. Adenocarcinoma occurs more frequently in the jejunum (Fig. 11-9) than in the ileum, almost as often as in the duodenum. Most jejunal tumors are found in the first 30 cm beyond the ligament of Treitz. Adenocarcinomas may be multiple, and it is then necessary to distinguish these from metastases. The diagnosis is often not made before surgical intervention or autopsy because most tumors produce vague symptoms, and the diagnosis of this rare condition is therefore often not considered. The disease is usually advanced in patients presenting with symptoms of complications such as bleeding, obstruction, or perforation. In adults presenting with small bowel intussusception (Fig. 11-10), a primary small bowel tumor, including lymphoma of the small bowel, must be excluded. Adenomas are the most common benign neoplasm (23% of all small bowel tumors),[32] followed by spindle cell tumors or leiomyomas, and then by lipomas. Malignant tumors include adenocarcinoma, lymphoma, leiomyosarcoma, and carcinoid. Although most of these tumors have no distinguishing imaging features, carcinoid tumors and lipomas arising in the small bowel do have pathognomonic imaging characteristics that allow them to be diagnosed prospectively on imaging studies.

Primary small bowel carcinoid, often arising in the terminal ileum, may appear as a small, slightly lobulated soft tissue mass that may contain central calcifications[33] (Fig. 11-11). A radiat-

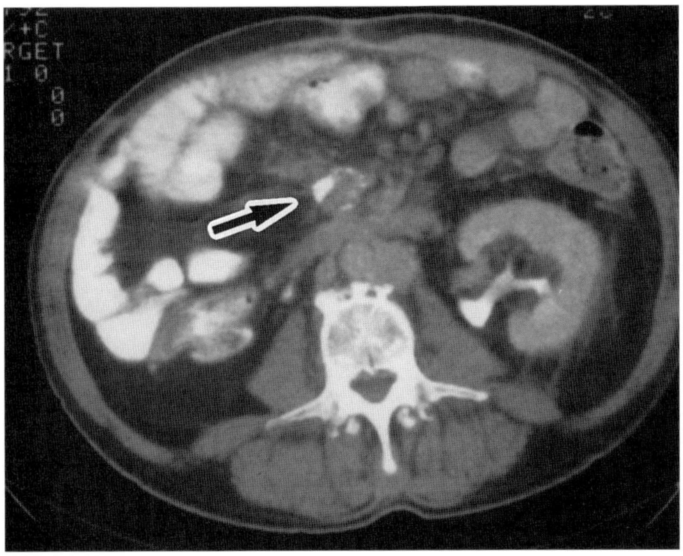

FIG. 11-11. Carcinoid tumor of the small bowel. A computed tomography scan demonstrates an irregular calcified soft tissue mass in the mid-abdomen *(arrow)* with infiltration of the adjacent mesenteric fat and retraction of adjacent loops of bowel.

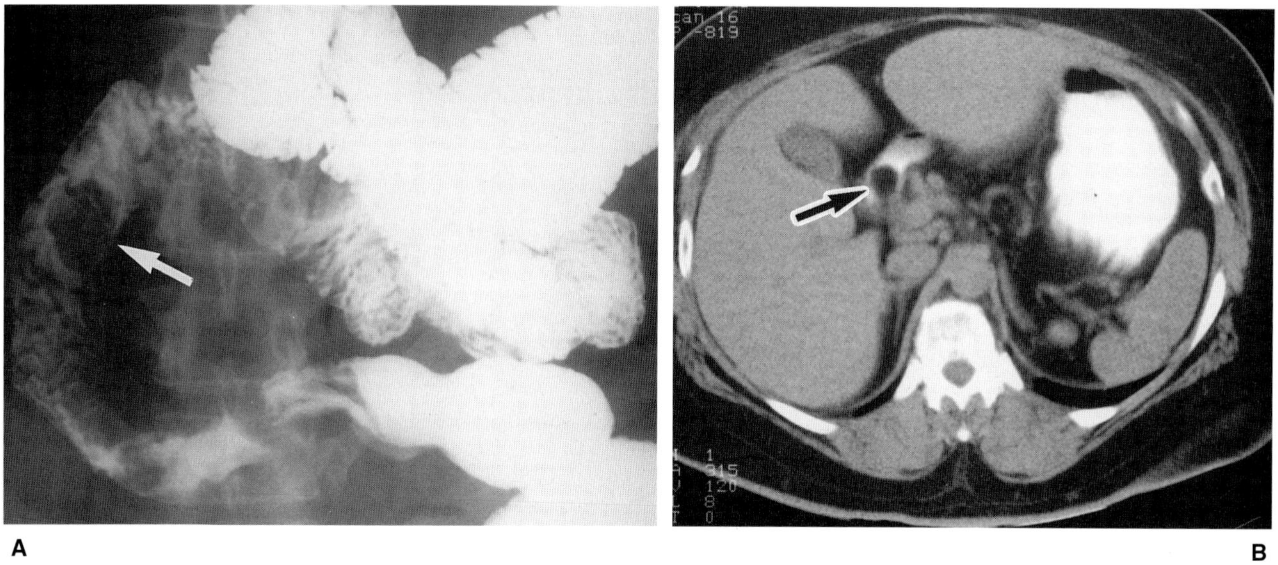

FIG. 11-12. Duodenal lipoma. A well circumscribed intraluminal filling defect *(arrow)* is present in the descending duodenum **(A)**. A duodenal mass with a density similar to fat *(arrow)* is easily demonstrated on a computed tomography scan **(B)**.

ing soft tissue pattern extends from the periphery of the tumor into the adjacent mesenteric fat, displacing and and even appearing to invade adjacent small bowel loops. This desmoplastic response causes sharp angulation of small bowel loops in the vicinity of the tumor. These features are uncommon with carcinoid tumors arising in other parts of the gastrointestinal tract.

Lipomas occur throughout the gastrointestinal tract and on barium studies typically demonstrate sharply defined, often mobile intraluminal sessile or pedunculated defects that change shape with compression. Thin-section CT scanning can confirm the presence of a lipoma by demonstrating an intraluminal lesion with homogeneous low or fat density (−30 to −100 Hounsfield units; water = 0)(Fig. 11-12).[33]

Diagnosis and Staging

Diagnosis of most benign and malignant small bowel tumors is notoriously difficult because the resulting radiologic signs may be subtle or indeed absent. Imaging features resulting from the tumor, such as liver metastases, regional lymphadenopathy, intussusception, or an adjacent desmoplastic reaction may suggest the diagnosis but are seldom diagnostic.

The small bowel barium study is the diagnostic method of choice to detect the presence of small bowel tumors. The accuracy of the examination largely depends on the interest of the radiologist and the method of examination. The barium follow-through method has a detection rate of between 50% to 70%. By careful enteroclysis technique, however, a correct diagnosis of small bowel cancer can be made in approximately 85% of cases. Enteroclysis has been considered particularly useful for demonstrating ileal tumors, with the follow-through examination adequate for the more proximal bowel.[34] Retrograde small bowel studies are performed by filling the entire colon and refluxing back into the terminal ileum. This is a useful technique for detecting tumors in the distal ileum (Fig. 11-13).

The typical image of primary adenocarcinoma of the small intestine is one of circumferential or asymmetric luminal narrowing producing strictures or indentation of the barium column (see Fig. 11-9). Other useful signs include polypoid mucosal defects, mucosal ulceration within the confines of the small bowel lumen or beyond the lumen (Fig. 11-14), and an irregular filling defect in the presence of small bowel intussusception (see Fig. 11-10). Nevertheless, subtle mucosal abnormalities frequently go undetected on barium studies and lesions may be obscured by overlying bowel loops or gas. Similarly, extension of the tumor beyond bowel wall can be inferred only by identifying displacement of adjacent bowel loops. CT scanning plays a useful role in this regard, easily detecting extraluminal spread of disease, mesenteric invasion, and regional adenopathy. Metastases not infrequently occur to the small bowel, particularly from breast and lung cancer, melanoma, or Kaposi's sarcoma. Drop metastases from the stomach, pancreas, and colon also occur, initially invading the serosal surface of the colon (Fig. 11-15).

Many limitations of the small bowel barium study may be overcome by filling the small bowel with barium in a controlled manner, using a small bowel enema technique or enteroclysis. By this technique, dilute barium is introduced by controlled yet rapid injection or infusion through a Maglinte catheter, which is advanced to the distal duodenum and secured in position with an inflatable balloon near the tip. This permits the entire small bowel to be distended with dilute contrast material, effectively providing a double-contrast appearance. The transit of dilute barium through small bowel is then continuously monitored by fluoroscopic screening and recorded by intermittent compression spot films (see Fig. 11-5).[35]

Computed Tomography

Computed tomography is commonly used as a screening test in patients with vague abdominal symptoms. Evaluation of the

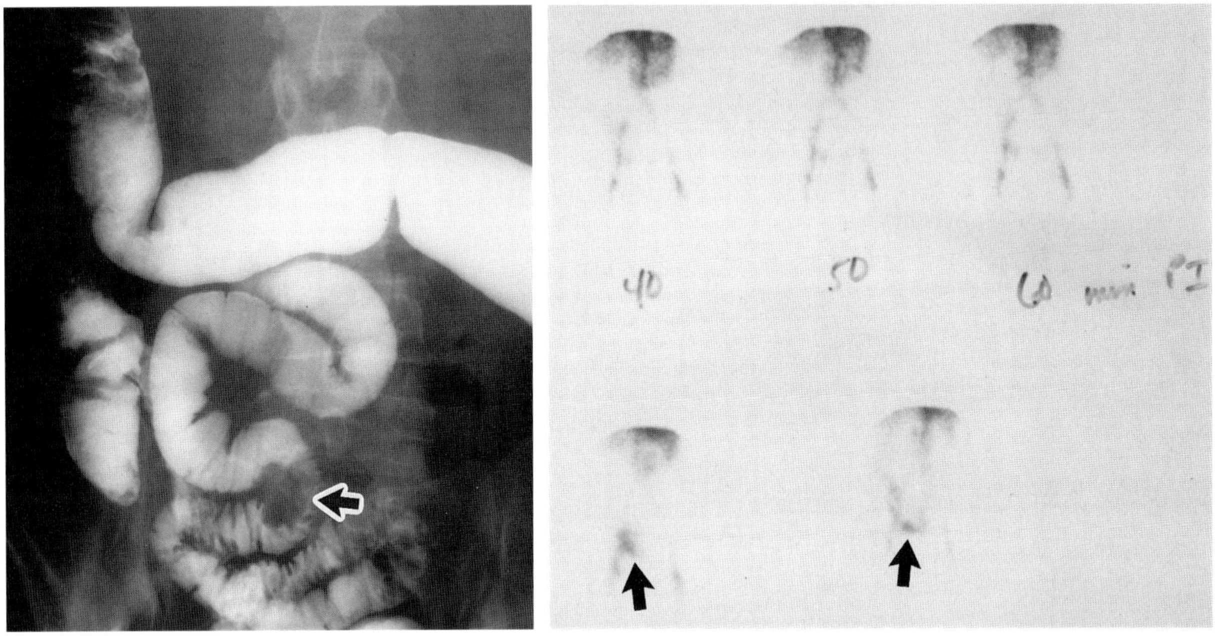

A B

FIG. 11-13. Carcinoid tumor of the terminal ileum. A retrograde small bowel study **(A)** performed by instilling barium into the colon and refluxing into the terminal ileum demonstrates an irregular intraluminal filling *(arrow)* defect in the distal ileum. A tagged red blood cell bleeding study **(B)** demonstrates a focal area of increasing radioactivity in the right lower quadrant *(arrows)* consistent with a bleeding site.

small bowel requires attention to fine detail and should be undertaken only with uniform opacification of all small bowel segments. Using this technique, bowel wall thickness greater than 3 mm and mesenteric lymph nodes greater than 4 mm are considered abnormal. A wall thickness of greater than 1.5 cm has a reported likelihood of resulting from malignancy in as many as 85% of cases.[32]

Conventional barium examinations remain superior to CT for evaluating intraluminal and mucosal disease,[33] but CT is far more accurate for evaluating the intramural and extraintestinal components, including involvement of the mesentery, peritoneal cavity, retroperitoneum, and solid organs.[33] Routine CT examinations usually result in inadequate evaluation of most primary gastrointestinal lesions unless specific techniques aimed at improving resolution are used. Common pitfalls that occur in CT of the small bowel result from inadequate contrast filling of the bowel lumen or incomplete intestinal distention. As Balthazar has described,[33] empty collapsed or fluid-filled bowel loops can present as a soft tissue mass mimicking a mesenteric tumor. The hallmark of malignant lesions on CT include eccentric or asymmetric thickening of the bowel wall, the irregular and lobulated inner and outer contour, or the focal soft tissue mass usually measuring greater than 2 cm from the luminal to serosal surface.[33] Associated features include abrupt transitions, luminal narrowing, and sometimes a spiculated outer contour. The diagnosis may be confirmed by the presence of regional adenopathy or liver metastases.[33]

Computed tomography can reliably establish the presence of intussusception (see Fig. 11-10) by demonstrating a characteristic target appearance that results from mesenteric fat invaginating into the lumen of the intussuscipiens.

Computed tomographic identification of a fatty density mass within the bowel wall is typical of a lipoma.[36] Leiomyomas and leiomyosarcomas are often bulky,[37] grow eccentrically, may cavitate, and are sometimes calcified. Lymphoma tends to produce uniform bowel wall thickening of greater than 2 cm and, although often circumferential, may produce aneurysmal dilatation of the lumen.[38] Adenocarcinomas tend to occur within proximal segments of the small bowel (see Fig. 11-9) and present as solitary soft tissue masses causing luminal narrowing and obstruction[39] (see Fig. 11-6). Carcinoid tumors tend to occur distally, favoring the distal ileum. Small-sized tumors are associated with an extensive cicatricial reaction, displacement of adjacent bowel loops, and soft tissue strands within the mesentery.[40]

Angiography

Angiography, often used to evaluate an occult source of small bowel hemorrhage, may determine the size and extent of the tumors and their anatomic location before surgical resection. Differentiation of benign and malignant tumors is not consistently possible. A dense capillary stain and enlarged feeding arteries and draining veins are the most common findings (see Fig. 11-7). These findings are not specific, but are most commonly identified in intestinal leiomyomas.[41] A similar pattern may be identified in small bowel neurogenic tumors, especially in von Recklinghausen's disease.[42] Carcinoid tumors show a stellate pattern as a result of the presence of associated retracted loops of mesentery. A large size, in excess of 5 cm, and a lobulated or irregular contour are reported to be strongly suggestive of malignancy.

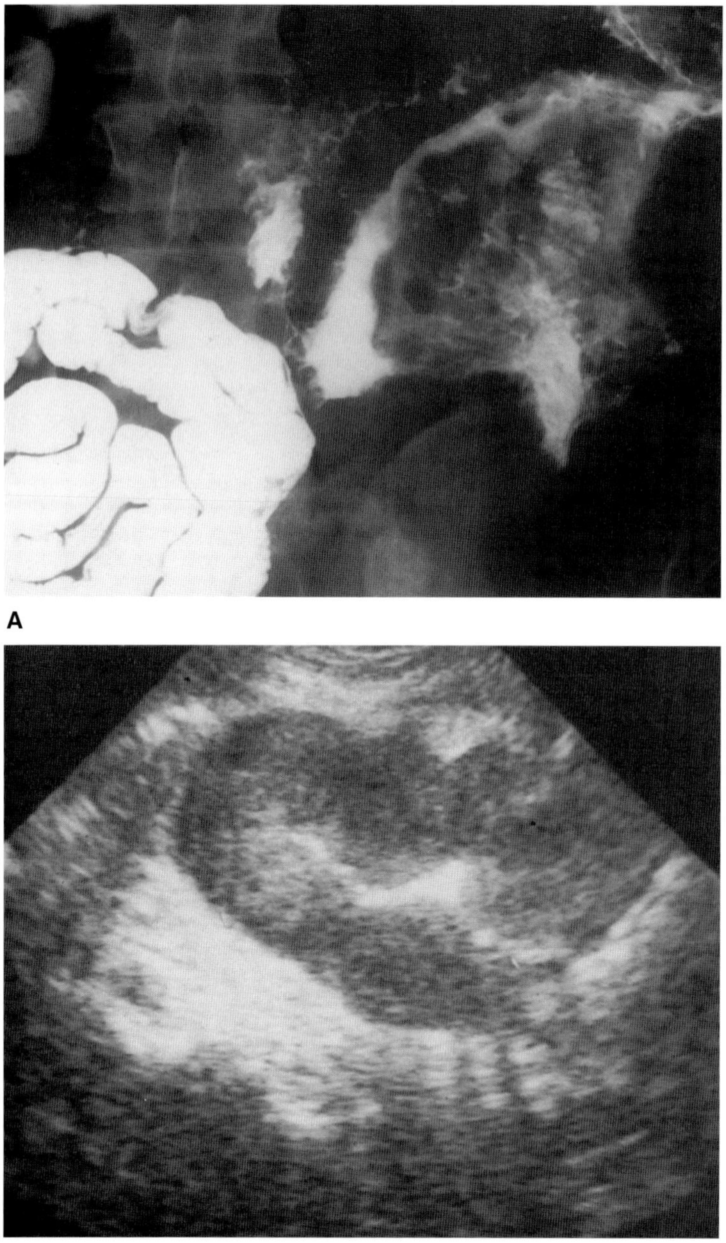

A

B

FIG. 11-14. Melanosarcoma of the small bowel. A large ulcerating small bowel mass **(A)** is present, displacing adjacent loops of bowel and extending well beyond the expected confines of the small bowel lumen. Ultrasound of the mass **(B)** demonstrates the pseudokidney sign, with the tumor having a similar appearance to a kidney.

Transabdominal Ultrasound

Several attempts have been made to characterize and identify small bowel tumors with transabdominal US facilitated by bowel lumen water loading. Like CT, transabdominal US enables not only identification of mural and intraluminal masses but the determination of extraluminal tumor extension.[43] Sonography, routinely limited by gas within overlying loops, may be successfully performed after water loading. In such a way, lymphoma is seen as a homogeneous, poorly echogenic or echo-poor region expanding the wall, leiomyosarcoma is typically seen as an extraluminal bulky mass (similar to the CT appearance), and adenocarcinoma presents as an intraluminal isoechoic mass. Lipoma expectedly manifests as a uniform hyperechoic mass surrounded by hypoechoic bowel wall, producing a "bull's eye" appearance.[36] In the setting of mechanical small bowel obstruction, hyperactive dilated small bowel loops may be traced using US to a transition point, which may be used to search for a tumor or intussusception.

Scintigraphy

Tagged red cell studies may be used to detect sources of occult hemorrhage and thus detect occult adenocarcinoma, leiomyosarcoma, or neuroendocrine tumors (see Fig. 11-13). These studies, however, are not sensitive, and false-positive results may arise from areas of inflammation and intussusception, the presence of heterotopic gastric mucosa, or even a Meckel's diverticulum containing gastric mucosa.

The determination of local tumor extension currently is not

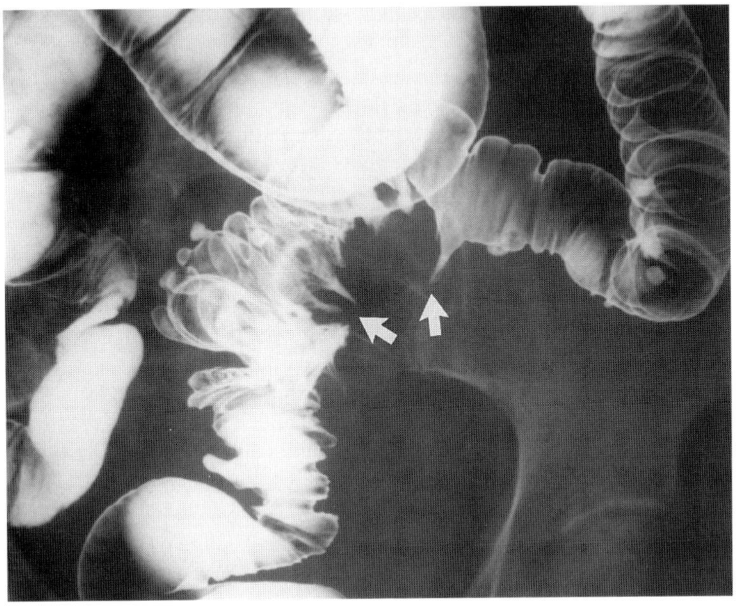

FIG. 11-15. Breast metastases to the sigmoid colon. Serosal implants resulting from metastatic disease have a spiculated appearance *(arrow)*.

possible and staging therefore essentially involves the determination of distant spread beyond the bowel wall, best achieved by CT. CT enables not only the recognition of disease within the abdomen, but the visualization of disease within the chest. US may complement CT in the evaluation of liver disease. Similarly, some studies have suggested that MRI may be of even greater value in determining the presence or absence of liver metastases in these patients. Angiography may be helpful in patients with metastatic carcinoid tumor.

Summary

Despite extensive development and refinement of diagnostic and staging methods of tumors of both the upper and lower gastrointestinal tract, imaging methods for the diagnosis and staging of small bowel tumors remain varied but individually limited. At the time of writing, barium studies remain the most important radiologic examination of the small bowel, with the dedicated small bowel barium enema or enteroclysis study being the diagnostic method of choice for these tumors. CT is the best method for staging and follow-up.

COLORECTAL CANCER

Each year, 155,000 new cases of colorectal cancer are diagnosed in the United States, making it the second most common tumor in both men and women. Survival in these patients is directly related to the stage of disease at the time of initial diagnosis. There are three accepted staging methods; the conventional system, or Dukes' classification, has been abandoned in many centers and replaced by the more detailed TNM classification, which takes account of additional data provided by newer imaging modalities, such as ELUS or rectal US, which can provide useful information about the depth of tumor invasion into the bowel wall. A third, less commonly used classification was developed for purposes of CT staging. Imaging studies in patients with colorectal cancer involve making the initial diagnosis, excluding synchronous colonic lesions (found in up to 5% of patients with one known lesion), and accurately staging the disease. Imaging also plays a vital role in the detection of potentially treatable recurrent disease after surgical resection. In addition, imaging is required for evaluating the surgical anastomoses, excluding the more common complications of the primary tumor, and detecting complications that may arise after surgery, such as staple line leaks, tumor recurrence, and problems related to stomas. More recently, US guidance has been used during cryoablation of hepatic colorectal cancer metastases.[44]

Diagnosis and Staging

The main choice to be made in investigating patients for colon cancer is whether to use barium enema (Figs. 11-16 and 11-17; see Fig. 11-15) or colonoscopy. Major factors that must be considered are safety, completeness, cost, sensitivity, and patient preference.[45] The reported perforation rates for enema and colonoscopy are approximately 1 in 5000 and 1 in 500 to 1000, respectively. Barium enema reaches the cecum in 99% of patients, and colonoscopy in 55% to 95%, with a wide spectrum operator. The cost for colonoscopy varies from 2 to 10 times that of barium enema. Colonoscopy by experts should detect 95% of cancers, but 5% of examinations fail to reach the cecum. High-quality barium enemas are as sensitive as or slightly more sensitive than colonoscopy, but significant tumors are missed by both techniques. We believe that flexible sigmoidoscopy should be the initial examination. If this demonstrates a polyp (15% of patients), colonoscopy should follow. If the results of sigmoidoscopy are negative, barium enema should follow.[45] Patients with adenomas should have a colonoscopy to remove them and should not have a barium enema. Patients without adenomas should have a double-contrast barium enema because it is cheaper and safer and is as accurate for detecting cancer, although it is slightly less sensitive for detecting significant polyps in the sigmoid colon. Most barium misses are in the sigmoid colon (up to 90% in some series), whereas colonoscopic misses tend to be in the proximal ascending colon through failure to reach the lesion.

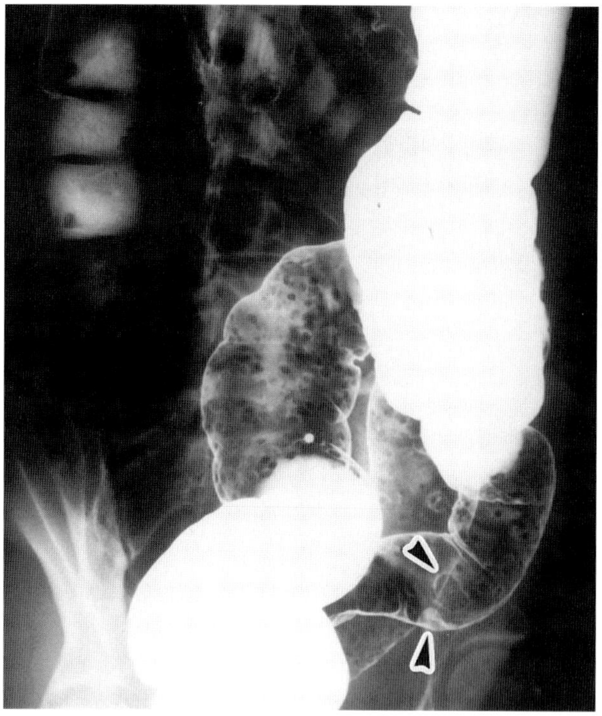

FIG. 11-16. Adenocarcinoma developing in familial adenomatous polyposis syndrome. Multiple mucosal polyps carpet the colonic walls in this patient with familial polyposis syndrome. Two larger polyps *(arrowheads)* in the sigmoid colon contained adenocarcinoma.

Of patients with polyps somewhere in the colon, only 10% have polyps exclusively in the ascending colon.[45] This finding is in accord with the facts that one third of adenomas occur proximal to the splenic flexure[46] and that two thirds of right-sided polyps have an associated left-sided lesion.[47] Thus, 90% of patients with colon polyps have a polyp in the descending colon within reach of the 60-cm flexible sigmoidoscope.

Although colonoscopy and double-contrast barium enema are the diagnostic modalities of choice for detecting tumors of the colon, ELUS, CT, and MRI using endorectal coils have been successfully used in the diagnosis of colonic, rectal, and low sigmoid tumors. CT in patients after adequate bowel preparation may be an alternative to barium enema as a diagnostic tool in the elderly, debilitated patient in whom inability to retain barium represents a significant problem.[48]

The barium enema is a simple, safe, and highly effective examination of the colon when performed and interpreted properly[49] (see Fig. 11-16). In the current era of cost containment and more vigorous screening for colon cancer, the role of the barium enema in diagnosing neoplasia is being promoted more aggressively.[50] The importance of a clean colon cannot be overemphasized; it has been estimated that 10% to 40% of colon cancers are missed on the initial barium examination, mainly because of poor colon preparation.[51,52] The reported average false-positive rate for colonic polyps has been about 8%.[51] Both single- and double-contrast examinations have sensitivities of about 90% to 95% for detecting polyps 1 cm or larger.[53–55] However, for polyps less than 1 cm in size, the double-contrast barium enema is more sensitive (88% vs. 72%).[53,54] The chance that polyps less than 1 cm in diameter contain invasive carcinoma is only 1%; the much higher prevalence of malignancy for larger polyps warrants their accurate detection.[52,56] At barium

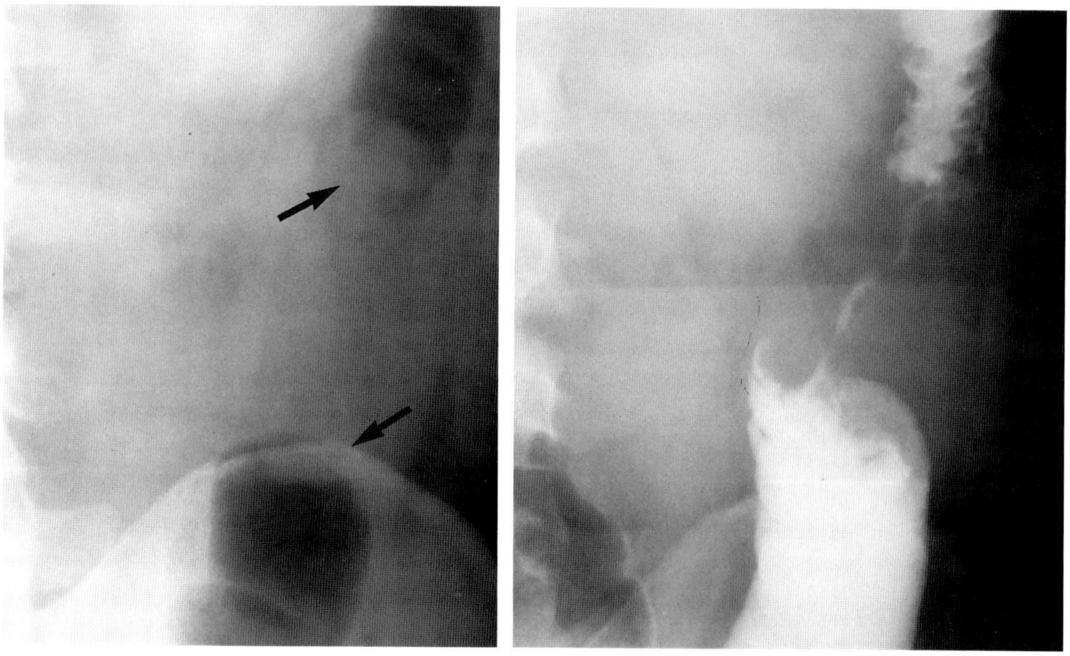

A B

FIG. 11-17. Carcinoma of the descending colon. A plain film of the abdomen **(A)** demonstrates a soft tissue mass in the left lower quadrant with a sharp cutoff of the air column in the descending colon *(arrow)*. A single-contrast barium enema **(B)** confirms the presence of a circumferential obstructing tumor at this site.

enema, colon tumors may present as intraluminal polypoidal defects (see Fig. 11-17), annular constricting lesions, ulcerating masses, or as diffusely infiltrated bowel wall. The accepted quality control standard for barium enemas dictates that if 80% to 90% of polyps 1 cm or larger be detected.[49] Difficulties may occur when evaluating patients with familial polyposis syndromes (see Fig. 11-16). The enema is also a useful modality for detecting serosal metastases to the colon or rectum (see Fig. 11-15).

Endoluminal US, MRI using endorectal coils, and CT have all been used to provide accurate assessment of the depth of tumor penetration of bowel wall, to identify lymph node invasion, and to detect distant metastases.

Endorectal Ultrasound

Both nonoptic rigid US (rigid rectal probes) and endoscopic transcolorectal endosonography probes have been used. Probes operating at a 7- to 10-MHz frequency have an axial resolution of 0.2 mm. In addition, a small catheter echoprobe (7 MHz with an axial resolution of 0.5 mm) introduced through the biopsy channel of a large-caliber endoscope can be used to assess a severely stenotic tumor mass.[57] By filling the air-filled lumen with an attached water balloon, intimate contact may be achieved with adjacent mucosa, enabling clear visualization of the colonic wall. Rigid transrectal probes may be used to assess rectal tumors, and the echocolonoscope may be used to visualize more proximal tumors, including those of the right colon.

Both nonoptic and endoscopic transcolorectal endosonography are accurate methods of assessing the depth of carcinomatous infiltration, compared to study of histologic sections from resection specimens[58] (Fig. 11-18). Accuracy of transrectal US staging of rectal tumors has varied from 72% to 97%,[58] with a lower sensitivity for detecting lymph node involvement. Although overstaging may occur in T2 carcinomas because endoscopic US is unable to distinguish inflammation from true tumor infiltration, understaging may occur in T3 carcinoma as a result of local tissue damage after low anterior resection or laser photocoagulation therapy.[59]

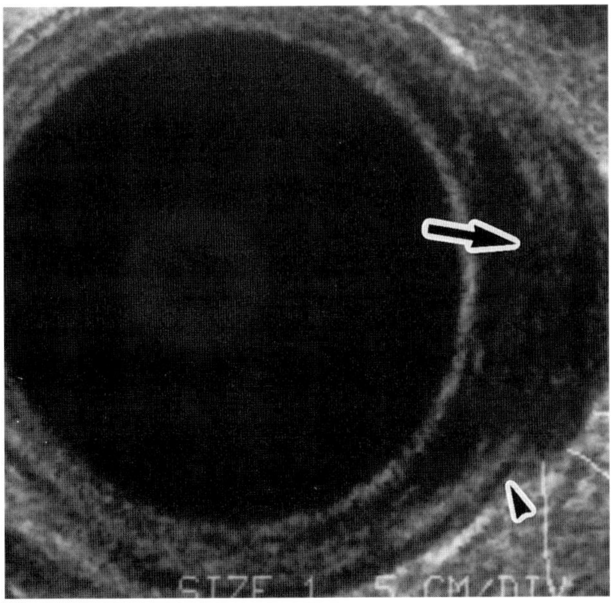

FIG. 11-18. Stage T3 rectal carcinoma. An endorectal ultrasound study demonstrates a stage T3 rectal carcinoma *(arrow)* extending into and beyond the muscularis propria layer *(arrowhead)*, into the perirectal space.

The accuracy of endoscopic US in enabling correct positive and negative diagnoses of regional lymph node metastases in rectal carcinoma was 72% in one study using a nonoptic instrument, and 67% in another study using a echocolonoscope to stage colonic tumors.[60] The overall prevalence of lymph node metastases is related to the depth of tumor invasion: 11% in T1, 20% in T2, 53% in T3, and 60% in T4.[60] Transhepatic sonography using a 3- to 5-MHz probe is a sensitive technique for detecting hepatic metastases and intraabdominal adenopathy, competitive with CT and MRI, but less sensitive for detecting lymphadenopathy.

Computed Tomography

Early reports suggested that CT was an excellent method for staging colorectal carcinoma because of its cross-sectional anatomic capability and its ability to detect metastases.[61] A negative pelvic CT examination does not imply an absence of spread beyond the rectal wall into the perirectal space; on the other hand, detection of spread beyond the rectal wall is highly indicative of advanced disease. In effect, CT examination is unable to differentiate T2 and T3 tumors[62,63] (Fig. 11-19). Tumor infiltration of nodes is detected on the basis of increased nodal size; nodes larger than 1 cm in size are considered pathologic. CT is thus limited by an inability to detect infiltrated lymph nodes of normal size. Some authors now consider that the identification of any lymphadenopathy suggests nodal metastases because perirectal and colonic nodes are not usually visible on abdominal CT scans[63] (see Fig. 11-19). CT both understages (9%) and overstages (44%) colon cancer, with only approximately 47% of cases being correctly staged.[63] Based on these data, Freeny and colleagues[63] recommend no role for CT in the routine staging of colorectal cancer. CT is particularly valuable as a modality to detect liver metastases, with its sensitivity increasing with the use of intravenous contrast and spiral technique, and with direct injection of contrast to the celiac and mesenteric vessels at the time of CT, so-called CT arterioportography.[64] CT arterioportography is the most sensitive (95%) modality for detection; hepatic metastases, because they are supplied by branches of the hepatic artery, are hypoperfused after superior mesenteric injection, unlike normal hepatic parenchyma, and are identified as hypodense, unenhanced nodules or foci.[64]

Magnetic Resonance Imaging

The development and use of endorectal coils has facilitated the use of MRI of colonic, and particularly rectal tumors.[65,66] MRI may provide correct evidence of tumor invasion using dedicated, high-resolution endorectal coils (see Fig. 11-12). In one in vitro study, high-resolution MRI provided accurate detection and determination of the depth of tumor invasion. Such information is not provided by standard pelvic coils. MRI is

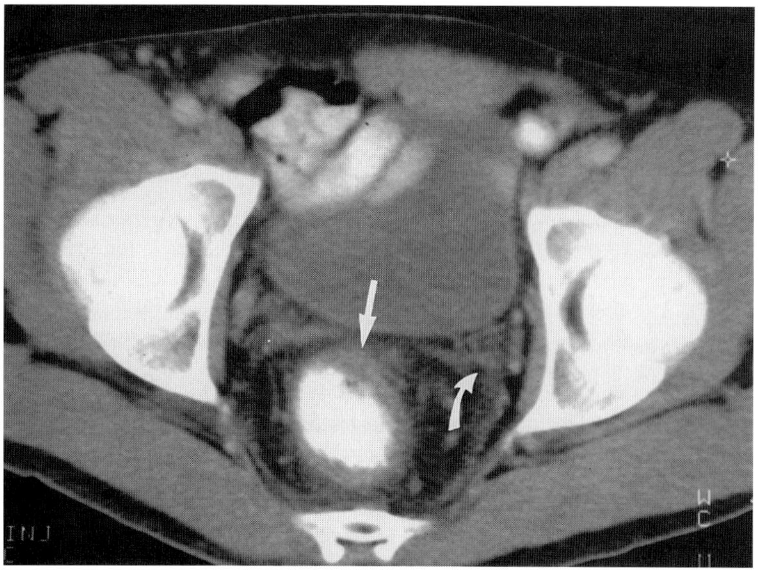

FIG. 11-19. Carcinoma of the rectum. A circumferential rectal carcinoma characterized by rectal wall thickening *(straight arrow)* is demonstrated on this computed tomography image with invasion into perirectal fossa and pelvic lymphadenopathy *(curved arrow).*

unable to determine lymph node infiltration on the basis of signal characteristics alone. Both CT and MRI use nodal size as the determinant of tumor infiltration.[65] MRI has not yet reliably permitted the differentiation of benign from malignant masses in the pelvis after abdominoperitoneal resection of a rectal carcinoma. MRI is valuable in the detection of liver metastases and may afford even greater sensitivity than CT.[61] Despite technical improvements in MRI and CT, transrectal US remains the best modality for evaluating depth of tumor penetration into the rectal wall.

Primary malignancies also occur in the appendix, the most common being carcinoid tumors, which are usually found incidentally in resected specimens. Tumors of the appendix, such as the less common mucinous cystadenocarcinoma, may obstruct the appendiceal lumen, resulting in acute appendicitis or even an appendiceal mucocele (Fig. 11-20). Cecal tumors may also obstruct the appendiceal lumen.

Detection of Tumor Recurrence

Colonoscopy and barium enema are the modalities of choice to detect recurrent tumor in patients who have undergone an anterior resection and bowel anastomosis. CT and MRI are of particular value in patients who have undergone abdominoperineal resection in whom colonoscopy and barium enema cannot be performed.[67] CT is the method of choice to evaluate the presence or absence of local tumor recurrence, affording not only visualization of the resection site but an evaluation of the liver.[65] Tumor recurrence is suggested at CT if there is invasion of adjacent structures, an increase in size, heterogeneity of the contents of the mass, asymmetry, or associated lymphadenopathy. CT is unable to differentiate between tumor recurrence and postoperative fibrosis.[65] After abdominoperineal resection, tumor recurrence is indicated by invasion of surrounding structures, enlarged lymph nodes, or a rounded soft tissue mass. If

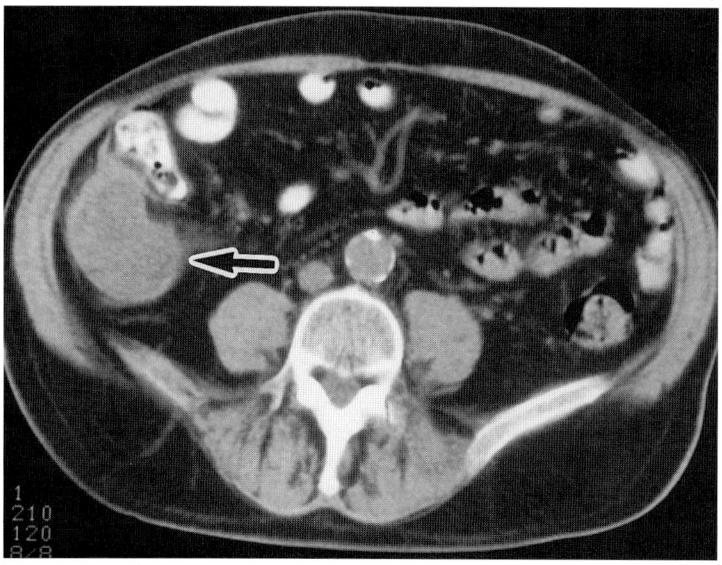

FIG. 11-20. Appendiceal mucinous cystadenocarcinoma. The cystadenocarcinoma has obstructed the appendiceal lumen, resulting in the formation of an appendiceal mucocele *(arrow).*

the scan is equivocal, needle biopsy should be performed to make or confirm the diagnosis. MRI may differentiate recurrence and fibrosis in some cases, with tumor recurrence producing greater signal on T2-weighted images than postoperative fibrosis, but this feature is not specific.[65]

Evaluation of tumor recurrence with ELUS allows early detection of recurrence at the resection site; however, in many cases normal tissue planes have been disrupted by the surgery and it is not possible to distinguish between changes related to surgery, postoperative fibrosis, and recurrent tumor. Both US and CT may guide a definitive diagnostic biopsy procedure.[59]

Scintigraphy represents an experimental alternative to invasive diagnostic biopsy. Positron emission tomography after intravenous injections of ^{18}F-fluorodeoxyglucose may demonstrate actively metabolizing tissue and thus differentiate tumor from scar.[68] Monoclonal antibody imaging using ^{111}In-labeled compounds and single photon emission computed tomography imaging may be helpful not only in detecting recurrence but in preoperative staging. Immunoscintigraphy has been shown to be effective when used to detect pelvic recurrence (74%, vs. 57% for CT), particularly because normal-sized nodes with tumor involvement that cannot be identified at CT will often be hot at immunoscintigraphy.[69] Although CT is more effective than immunoscintigraphy at detecting tumor recurrence in the liver, immunoscintigraphy is more sensitive at detecting recurrence in the extrahepatic abdomen (66% vs. 34%).[69]

Summary

Double-contrast barium enema and colonoscopy are the preferred methods to diagnose colorectal carcinoma. As Stevenson has suggested,[45] the use of barium enema as the routine initial imaging investigation subjects those 15% to 20% of patients with polyps to unnecessary double procedures, and misses many important lesions in the sigmoid colon that could easily have been seen with the flexible sigmoidoscope. ELUS enables accurate determination of local tumor invasion and lymph node infiltration. CT enables evaluation of possible liver metastases. In vitro studies suggest that MRI with high-resolution endorectal coils may enable determination of local tumor infiltration as well as the evaluation of distant spread to the liver. CT and, more recently, immunoscintigraphy represent the favored modalities to detect tumor recurrence. Once cancer has been diagnosed, imaging for staging does not seem to offer very great benefit to patients. Follow-up for early detection of metastatic disease has not been helpful because no effective treatment is available. The possibility of effective chemotherapy and local treatment of small liver metastases may alter the relevance of sophisticated imaging techniques for the detection of small metastases, especially in the liver.[45]

PANCREATIC TUMORS

Despite technical advances in cross-sectional imaging of the pancreas, the overall impact on patient survival has been minimal.[70] With currently available means of detection, pancreatic adenocarcinoma remains the neoplasm least likely to be confined to the organ of origin at the time of diagnosis.[71] At the time of diagnosis, 65% of patients have advanced local disease or distant metastases, 21% have localized disease with regional lymph node spread, and only 14% have tumor confined to the pancreas.[72] This reflects the lack of a distinct capsule around the gland, which allows rapid infiltration of tumor into the peripancreatic tissues. A clinically useful imaging study should not only evaluate local tumor growth but should search for evidence of extraglandular metastases, which most commonly occur in the liver, regional lymph nodes, peritoneum, and lungs. Differences in biologic behavior have been demonstrated between pancreatic tumors that invade the portal vein or retroperitoneum, and those that spread to regional lymph nodes or beyond the pancreatic capsule.[73] Also, patient survival may be improved when tumors smaller than 2 cm are detected.[74] For these reasons, imaging procedures must not only be able to determine size and location of tumors, but must accurately determine or exclude the presence and extent of extrapancreatic spread.

Diagnosis and Staging

Of the variety of imaging techniques available for imaging the pancreas, dynamic bolus-enhanced incremental CT and US remain the most sensitive.[73] Megibow has demonstrated that dynamic intravenous contrast material enhancement permits visualization of small pancreatic lesions, an assessment of peripancreatic arterial and venous patency or invasion, and maximum visibility and detectability of hepatic metastases.[70] Using this technique, lesions were equally well identified in the head (94%) and body/tail (96%) of the pancreas.[70] Ward and colleagues[75] have depicted the spectrum of CT appearances of pancreatic carcinoma. After contrast enhancement, the tumor mass is most commonly hypodense (78%)[70] compared with surrounding parenchyma (Fig. 11-21). Hyperdense tumors are unusual and often represent islet cell or acinar cell tumors.[75] Cystic lesions of the pancreas are either serous or mucinous cystadenomas or adenocarcinomas. Contrast enhancement also allows the diffuse forms of pancreatic carcinoma to be identified.[76] Megibow[70] has described secondary radiologic findings resulting from the primary tumor mass, which include atrophy of the gland proximal to the mass and dilatation of the proximal pancreatic duct and, possibly, biliary tree. In one report, endoscopic US of the pancreas was shown to be more accurate than dynamic CT and MRI in the diagnosis of pancreatic tumors, especially for tumors less than 3 cm in size.[77] The efficacy of endoscopic US remains extremely user dependent, and it cannot be recommended ahead of CT or transcutaneous US for evaluation of pancreatic tumors.

Survival and resectability may correlate with tumor size, which, when considered in isolation, is not a major indicator of prognosis.[78,79]

A thorough preoperative evaluation of pancreatic tumors requires a search for both local and distant metastatic disease. Because peripancreatic extension of tumor has important prognostic and therapeutic implications,[70] vessels and lymph nodes should specifically be evaluated. Cross-sectional imaging depicts lymphadenopathy, which may be the result of reactive hyperplasia. Nonenlarged nodes may harbor occult tumor.[70] A rich network of intraglandular lymphatics drain to five peripancreatic groups before passing to nodes in the porta hepatis and groups surrounding the proximal celiac and superior mesenteric arteries. Spread finally reaches paraaortic and distal superior

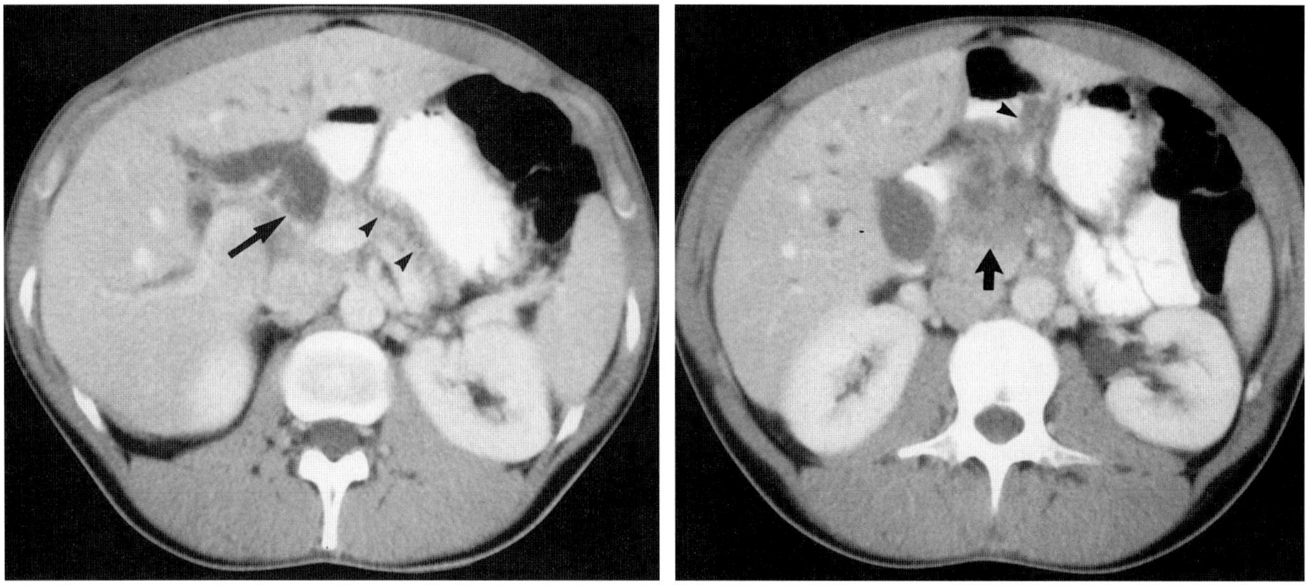

A B

FIG. 11-21. Pancreatic carcinoma. **A,** Computed tomography slice demonstrating double duct dilatation of the common bile duct *(arrow)* and pancreatic duct *(arrowheads)*. **B,** Hypodense irregular mass in pancreatic head *(arrow)*, invading the stomach wall *(arrowhead)*.

mesenteric groups.[80] Lymph node involvement in patients with tumors less than 2 cm in size decreased 1-year survival from 89% to 59%.[81] Porta hepatis nodes may result in obstructive jaundice, even if the primary tumor is located in the pancreatic tail. Similarly, nonpancreatic tumors may metastasize to the porta hepatis and peripancreatic nodes, simulating an advanced pancreatic malignancy.

The presence of vascular encasement or invasion has significant therapeutic and prognostic implications. Venous extension is usually by direct contiguous growth, as opposed to arterial encasement, which results from tumor extension in the periarterial lymphatics.[70] CT and MRI can both depict perivascular adventitial changes not demonstrable as encasement with angiography.[70] A negative dynamic enhanced CT scan effectively precludes further angiographic evaluation.[82] Venous obstruction, most commonly of the splenic vein, may be recognized by the presence of collateral veins in predictable locations[83] (Fig. 11-22). Periarterial thickening with loss of periarterial fat[84] is not specific for pancreatic carcinoma, and has been described in chronic pancreatitis[85] and metastases to peripancreatic lymph nodes.[86]

Distant metastases most frequently (15% to 25%) occur in

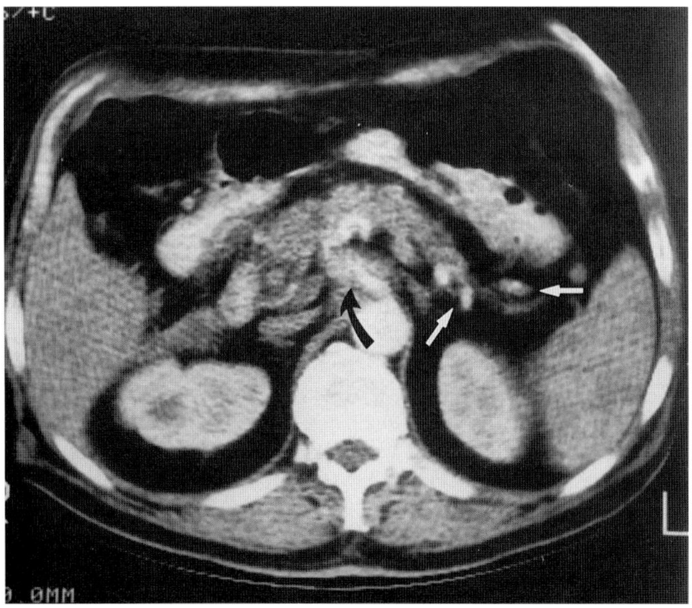

FIG. 11-22. Inoperable pancreatic cancer invading the celiac axis *(curved arrow)* and occluding the splenic vein, leading to varices *(arrows)*.

the liver and peritoneal cavity,[87] often invading the serosal layer near the cecum and sigmoid colon. Numerous adjacent organs, such as stomach and duodenum, may be involved by contiguous tumor invasion, and the appropriate fluoroscopic studies should be performed based on the clinical and cross-sectional findings.

Ultrasound examination of the pancreas performed transcutaneously or intraoperatively remains to a large extent operator dependent. With careful attention to detail, lesions larger than 1 cm with an echotexture different from adjacent parenchyma should be identified. IOUS is particularly useful for evaluating extrapancreatic tumor spread and peripancreatic vessel encasement or invasion (Fig. 11-23).

Despite technical advances, MRI cannot challenge CT as the primary imaging modality for pancreatic lesions.[70,88–90] This has been in part the result of phase and respiratory artifacts and limited spatial and contrast resolution.[89] As a result, the soft tissue resolution that has made MRI effective in studying other organ systems has not been fully realized for imaging the pancreas.[89] The development of specific contrast materials and improvements in fat saturation and fast spin-echo sequences should improve signal derived from the pancreas. Fat-suppressed spin-echo imaging reduces respiratory-induced phase artifact, improves the dynamic range of intraabdominal signal intensities, and renders the pancreas relatively higher in signal intensity than surrounding organs and tissue.[91,92]

Magnetic resonance cholangiopancreatography is being used with increasing frequency as a noninvasive alternative to ERCP.[93] This technique has not quite achieved the spatial resolution afforded by contrast-enhanced radiography, but does yield an impressive amount of diagnostic information for a noninvasive technique (Fig. 11-24). Motion degradation remains a major limiting factor to imaging the intrahepatic bile ducts, but the ability to image extrahepatic ducts without having to administer contrast material makes the technique worth considering. Moreover, sedation and anesthesia are avoided. Data sets can be acquired in such a way as to permit three-dimensional reconstruction and viewing in multiple planes. The technique has difficulty depicting minor ductal narrowing, which is of questionable importance anyway.[93] It is also important to realize that the ductal system is not selectively displayed; what is displayed is any and all fluid with signal characteristics similar to those of bile. Thus, blood, proteinaceous debris, or calculi may lead to focal nonvisualization of the ducts.[93]

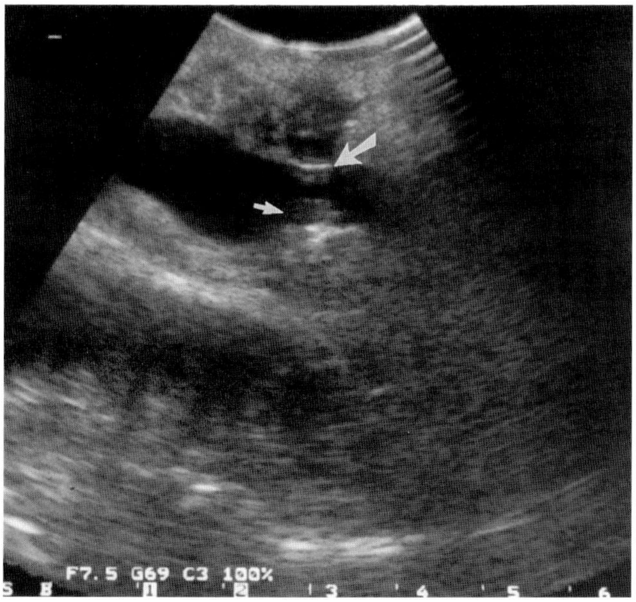

FIG. 11-23. Intraoperative ultrasound demonstrating invasion and intraluminal growth of pancreatic cancer in the superior mesenteric vein *(arrows)*.

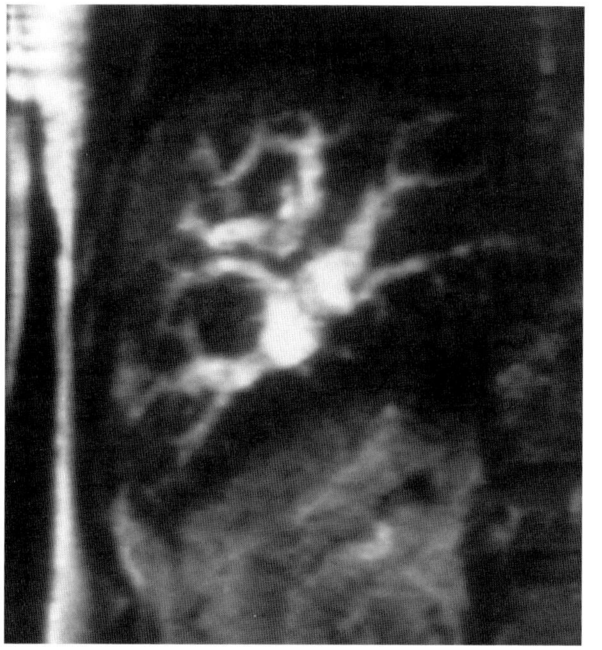

FIG. 11-24. Intrahepatic bile duct dilatation from a Klatzkin tumor. A reformatted three-dimensional magnetic resonance cholangiogram demonstrates diffuse intrahepatic bile duct dilatation resulting from obstruction at the confluence of the left and right hepatic veins.

Several studies have prospectively compared the roles of CT, MRI, and modalities such as angiography and ERCP in predicting resectability of pancreatic tumors.[88,89,94] Warshaw and associates[94] showed no added benefit of using MRI in addition to CT; the combined findings of CT and angiography showed that more than 87% of pancreatic head tumors were unresectable because of vascular encasement, but neither modality sufficed alone. With multiple modalities, 90% of unresectable tumors were identified. Semelka and coworkers[89] showed that lesions involving the biliary system were diagnosed with ERCP with a higher level of confidence than with MRI and CT (Fig. 11-25). CT was limited when the disease processes were not contour-deforming. They suggested that MRI may be useful when clinical history and CT findings are discordant.

Nonductal Pancreatic Tumors

Although ductal adenocarcinoma accounts for 95% of the malignant tumors of the pancreas, a variety of stromal tumors with more favorable prognoses also occur in the pancreas. Solid lesions in and adjacent to the pancreas may represent focal pancreatitis (usually chronic), acinar cell tumors, lymphoma,

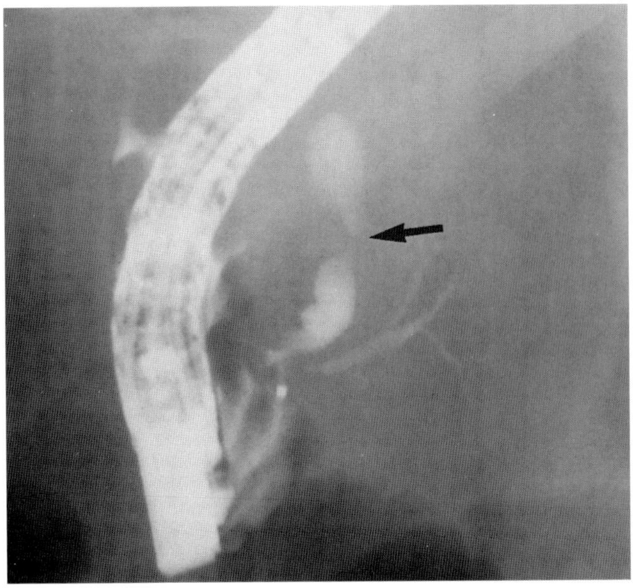

FIG. 11-25. Endoscopic retrograde cholangiopancreatography demonstrating malignant stricture *(arrow)* of common bile duct secondary to small pancreatic carcinoma.

metastases, invasion by tumor in lymph nodes in the hepatoduodenal ligament, and intraparenchymal lymph node enlargement. These are all extremely difficult to differentiate on imaging studies, and often require pathologic confirmation. *Periampullary tumors* resemble pancreatic head carcinoma and may cause obstruction of both the distal common bile duct and the pancreatic duct. Of the nonductal pancreatic neoplasms, islet cell tumors are frequently hypervascular, which permits good visualization of the enhancing tumor adjacent to moderately enhancing normal pancreatic tissue on dynamic contrast-enhanced images.[90] Because insulinomas are frequently functional, patients tend to present early when tumors are small (<2 cm).[95] Insulinomas are most commonly benign (90%)[95] and are frequently hypervascular. The small size at initial presentation combined with a rich vascular supply partially explains the superior ability of conventional angiography over CT in depicting these tumors[96] (Fig. 11-26). Because MRI is more sensitive to gadolinium enhancement than CT is to iodine enhancement, vascular tumors such as insulinomas should be more conspicuous on contrast-enhanced MR than contrast-enhanced CT images.[97] IOUS of the pancreas, however, remains the best modality for detecting these small pancreatic tumors. Approximately 50% of gastrinomas are malignant and tend to occur in the pancreatic head[95]; unlike ductal adenocarcinomas, they are hyperintense on T2-weighted MRI and do not enhance as intensely as insulinomas after contrast administration. Both the primary tumor and hepatic metastases may show ring enhancement.

Microcystic (or serous) cystadenoma is a benign tumor occurring in older patients, with an increased incidence in von Hippel-Lindau disease.[98] These possess multiple small cysts that range in size from 0.1 to 2 cm (Fig. 11-27). The tumor frequently has a characteristic central scar, and although it may extend well beyond the confines of the pancreas, it does not invade adjacent organs.[90] Macrocystic (or mucinous) cystadenocarcinoma is malignant or possesses malignant potential and occurs more frequently in women.[90] Tumors tend to be large, multiloculated, and encapsulated, with large, irregular cystic

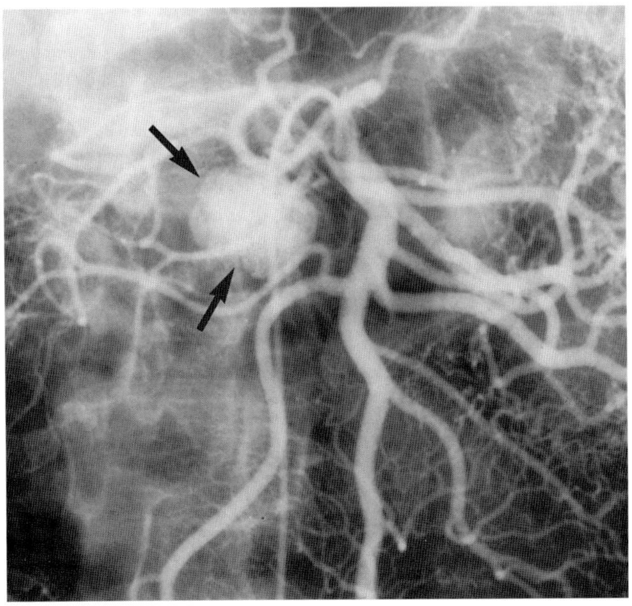

FIG. 11-26. Superior mesenteric arteriogram demonstrating a dense hypervascular blush *(arrows)* in an insulinoma.

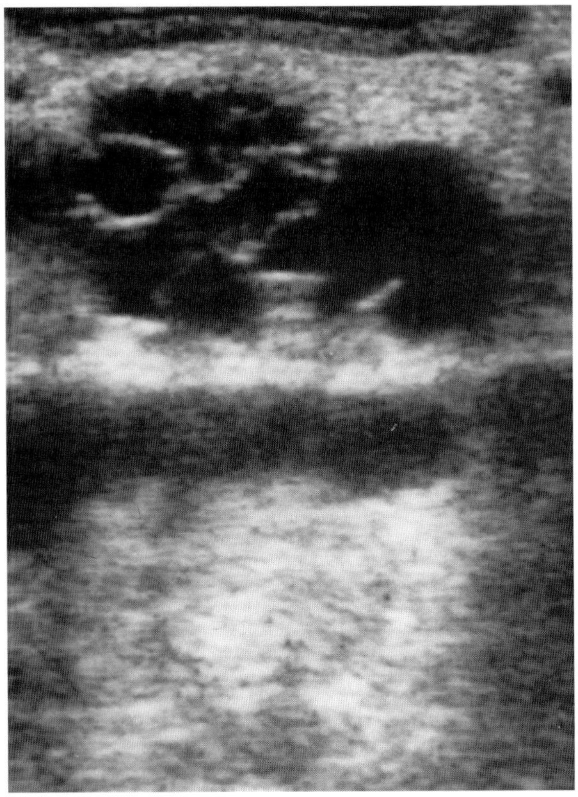

FIG. 11-27. Intraoperative ultrasound demonstrating a microcystic adenoma of the pancreas, with the larger cyst measuring 1.8 cm.

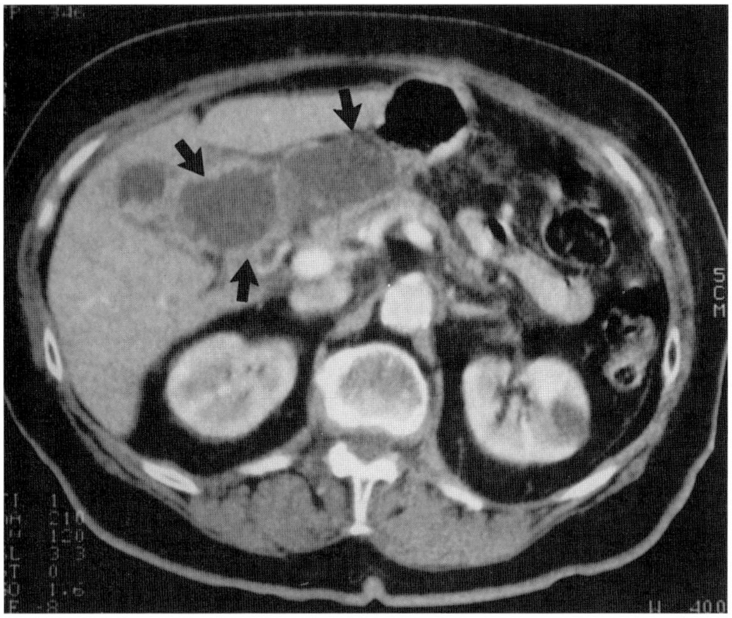

FIG. 11-28. Computed tomography scan demonstrating a large mucinous cystadenocarcinoma of the pancreas *(arrows)* with individual cysts measuring up to 4 cm in diameter.

spaces surrounding thickened septa,[99] and occur most commonly in the pancreatic body or tail (Fig. 11-28). The solid and papillary epithelial neoplasm is a rare tumor with low-grade malignant potential occurring most commonly in women aged 20 to 30 years. Non-Hodgkin's lymphoma may involve the peripancreatic or intrapancreatic lymph nodes, or may involve the pancreas directly. No distinguishing imaging characteristics exist. Metastases to the pancreas occur most commonly from the gastrointestinal tract, kidney, breast, lung, prostate, and melanoma.

As Semelka and Ascher have suggested,[90] CT should remain the first-line imaging modality when evaluating pancreatic tumors. MRI, endoscopic US, and angiography may be helpful if a patient has a clinical history or biochemical profile suspect for a pancreatic malignancy and CT or US findings are equivocal, or if distinction between focal pancreatitis and a malignancy needs to be made with equivocal CT and US findings. MRI and US can be valuable staging techniques in patients in whom an optimal dynamic contrast-enhanced CT cannot be obtained, although angiography is indicated primarily to provide the surgeon with a vascular road map before resection, or to evaluate patients in whom CT is equivocal.[100]

Malignant Biliary Obstruction

The long-term prognosis in patients with malignant biliary obstruction remains poor, despite advances in diagnosis and treatment.[101] Only 5% to 20% of patients with malignant biliary obstruction have surgically resectable tumors at the time of diagnosis.[31] Several authors have advocated the use of preoperative angiography to determine resectability of pancreatic and periampullary tumors, claiming that CT alone is not sufficiently accurate for this purpose.[101] However, although certain CT findings are less reliable for determining resectability, the accuracy of thin-section CT compares favorably with angiography for assessing resectability.[101] Endoscopic cholangiography provides little information as to the extraluminal extent of pancreatic or ampullary disease, but is helpful in that biopsy samples or brushings can be obtained, or even stent placement can be performed for palliative purposes. Similarly, with the increasing use of percutaneous or endoscopic stenting, accurate noninvasive staging of tumors is necessary because most patients with unresectable tumors can be treated nonoperatively, with no adverse effect on survival rates.[101]

Percutaneous Biopsy of the Pancreas

Both CT and US can be used for percutaneous biopsy of the pancreas.[102] These diagnostic procedures are routinely performed to confirm the diagnosis of ductal adenocarcinoma. Because most pancreatic adenocarcinomas are unresectable at the time of diagnosis, a successful percutaneous biopsy often obviates the need for surgical exploration.[102] Accuracy is higher with lesions larger than 3 cm, especially if 16- to 19-gauge needles are used and lesions are in the body or tail.[102] US has a higher reported accuracy (67% to 97%)[103] than CT (50% to 94%).[104] Needle passage through the gastrointestinal tract, including the colon, seldom causes complications, with cited complication rates ranging from 3% to 6.7%.[105]

Follow-up of Pancreatic Malignancies

After tumor resection, the anatomic distortion caused by procedures such as a Whipple procedure makes pancreatic tumor recurrence difficult to determine. A thorough understanding of the various surgical anastomoses is essential before attempting image interpretation. Bowel loops should be well opacified with water-soluble oral contrast materials because the afferent loops tend to reside in the porta hepatis and may be misinterpreted as a soft tissue mass resembling abscess, lymphadenopathy, or tumor recurrence. Coombs and associates[106] have demonstrated the most frequent site of recurrence to be the liver, which should therefore be incorporated into the imaging field for any follow-up studies. Tumor recurrence may result in obstruction to the afferent loop with or without intrahepatic bile duct dilatation.

GALLBLADDER AND BILIARY SYSTEM

Diagnosis and Staging

Carcinoma of the gallbladder is usually advanced at the time of clinical presentation. The tumor may appear as focal or diffuse gallbladder wall thickening (which may be indistinguishable from cholecystitis), an intraluminal papillary mass, or a solid mass occupying the gallbladder fossa (Fig. 11-29). Malignant neoplasms of the gallbladder include primary adenocarcinoma, sarcomas, and metastases, most commonly from melanoma. Seventy-five to 90% of primary adenocarcinomas of the gallbladder are associated with gallstones, and carcinoma will develop in 25% of porcelain gallbladders. Not all solid lesions of the gallbladder represent adenocarcinoma. Possibilities other than gallbladder carcinoma include the nonneoplastic tumors such as inflammatory polyps and the hyperplastic cholecystoses (cholesterolosis and adenomyomatosis), and benign neoplasms such as adenomas and mesenchymal and granular cell tumors.

Ultrasound or dynamic, contrast-enhanced, thin-section CT scanning remain the cornerstones for evaluation of gallbladder disease, with US remaining the investigation of choice.[107] US is able to evaluate and measure gallbladder wall thickness and intraluminal mass lesions, and determine the presence of intrahepatic or extrahepatic bile duct dilatation. A thorough evaluation should include a search for spread into the liver, the subhepatic space, adjacent bowel, bile ducts, and regional lymphatics, as well as distant hematogenous metastases. Biliary scintigraphy simply determines patency of the intrahepatic bile and cystic duct. Mild mucosal thickening is an early but rare finding in gallbladder carcinoma, and more than 50% of early cancers demonstrate no intraluminal protrusion.[107] MRI provides no advantage over CT for evaluating gallbladder disease, and is less helpful when evaluating local spread. MR cholangiography is still experimental and requires extensive clinical evaluation. CT contrast agents designed to opacify the biliary system are not being used in the United States.

Cholangiocarcinoma may develop in an intrahepatic or extrahepatic sites and present either with biliary ductal dilatation or with features similar to hepatocellular carcinoma. Eighty-four percent involve the common hepatic duct or its bifurcation[108] (Fig. 11-30). The pattern of growth may be infiltrative, nodular, or papillary, and the associated desmoplastic response accounts for the frequent false-negative biopsy rate.[108] As Burrell and colleagues have suggested,[108] the primary role of the radiologist is to define the proximal extent of the tumor and to predict resectability by evaluating local and distant spread. Predisposing conditions such as primary sclerosing cholangitis, ulcerative colitis, and choledochal cysts should be searched for.[108] Also, the extent, if any, of intrahepatic spread should be defined using dynamic contrast-enhanced CT as a guide to surgeons contemplating segmental hepatic resections.[108,109] False-positive results may occur with lymphadenopathy due to hyperplasia rather than tumor invasion. The bile ducts are best evaluated with US (down to the head of the pancreas, where artifacts from bowel gas limit resolution) or endoscopy. An advantage of endoscopy is that malignant biliary obstructions can be treated palliatively by using endostents, sphincterotomy, and brachytherapy. When successful cannulation of the duct is not possible, combined percutaneous and endoscopic procedures help to

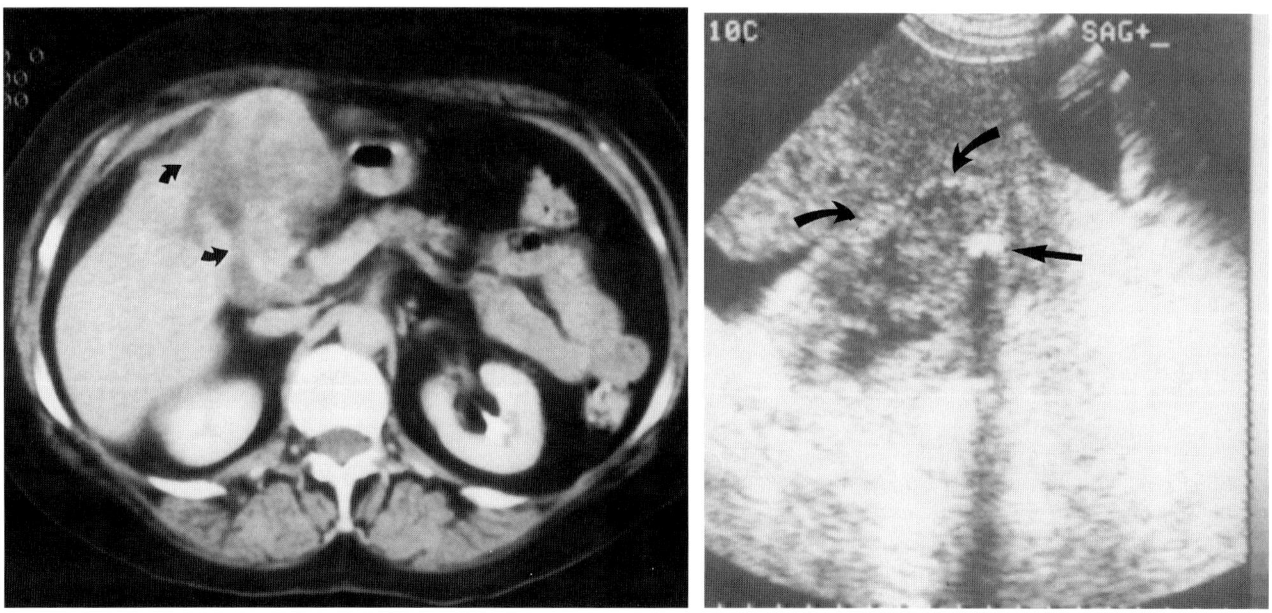

A B

FIG. 11-29. Gallbladder carcinoma. **A,** Large mass on computed tomography obliterating the gallbladder and invading the adjacent liver *(arrows).* **B,** Polypoid intraluminal gallbladder cancer *(curved arrows)* without hepatic invasion. Note the gallstone *(straight arrow)* engulfed by the mass.

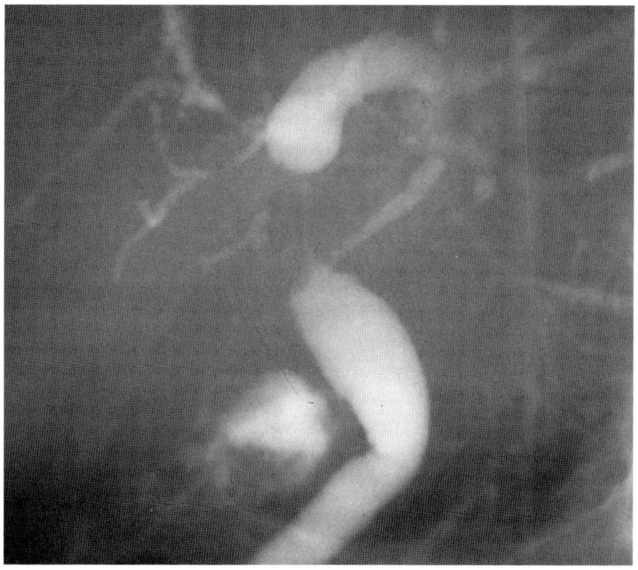

FIG. 11-30. Endoscopic retrograde cholangiopancreatography demonstrating malignant stricture of the common hepatic and right hepatic ducts secondary to cholangiocarcinoma.

overcome mechanical problems such as a large mass or tight stenosis.[108] Dynamic, contrast-enhanced, thin-section CT is useful for evaluating and excluding extraductal spread of tumor, lymphadenopathy, hepatic or pancreatic invasion, and distant peritoneal metastases.[101] The addition of angiography to the examination of patients with potentially resectable lesions is not justified when high-quality CT examinations are performed.[101] Endosonography has been reported to be helpful in the staging of and differentiating between pancreatic and ampullary carcinomas.[109] Cross-sectional imaging with MRI or cholangiography provides no advantage over CT.

THE LIVER

A large variety of diagnostic modalities are available for imaging the liver, including US, CT, MRI, nuclear medicine scans, and angiography. Angiography as a diagnostic tool has been almost completely replaced by the cross-sectional imaging modalities. Similarly, nuclear medicine scans are no longer used for diagnostic screening, but have an important role in functional evaluation of certain liver lesions, such as hemangiomas and focal nodular hyperplasia.[110] Conventional technetium sulfur colloid liver scans are less accurate than US and CT scans, particularly for lesions less than 2 to 3 cm in diameter.[111] Neither monoclonal antibody imaging nor positron emission tomography scanning has proven useful in detection, localization, or characterization of liver tumors.

Consequently, US, CT, and MRI are the primary imaging modalities for detection and characterization of liver lesions, and the information that is obtained with all three may be redundant but is often complementary. The primacy of one technique over another and the order of imaging may vary from one institution to another, depending on local expertise and equipment. In this chapter, an attempt is made to provide an overview of the relative roles of the three modalities and a rationale for efficient use of these techniques.

Hepatic Anatomy

The most extensive and complete segmentation of the liver is based on the Couinaud system of dividing the liver into eight segments based on vertical divisions following the hepatic veins and horizontal divisions following the branches of the portal structures.[112] These vascular structures, as well as the ligaments and fissures of the liver, can be equally well demonstrated by US, CT, and MRI. However, the horizontal planes are somewhat difficult to characterize fully on transverse cross-sectional imaging. In our practice, a simpler scheme of segmental classification is used (Fig. 11-31), dividing the left lobe into lateral and medial segments separated by the left hepatic vein, undivided left portal vein, and ligamentum teres. The right lobe is separated into anterior and posterior segments, using the right hepatic vein and bifurcation of the right portal vein as landmarks. The right lobe is separated from the medial segment of the left lobe by the middle hepatic vein and a plane between the gallbladder fossa and inferior vena cava.

The caudate lobe is deep within the liver and extends from the caudate process of the right lobe in a leftward direction toward or across the spine. The anterior margin of the caudate lobe is defined by the fissure for the ligamentum venosum, a remnant of the sinus venosus in the fetus.[113]

The portal venous and arterial blood supply can be well demonstrated by all three cross-sectional modalities, as can the hepatic venous drainage. The normal bile ducts are best seen in their extrahepatic location from the liver hilus to the head of the pancreas and duodenal sweep, but current state-of-the-art imaging may show portions of the central intrahepatic bile ducts

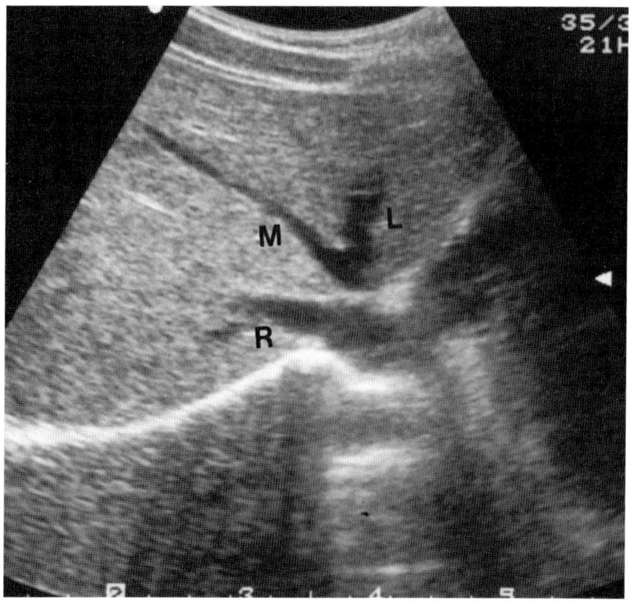

FIG. 11-31. Hepatic vein confluence with the inferior vena cava. The left (L) and middle (M) hepatic veins have a common trunk, whereas the right (R) hepatic vein has its own separate origin.

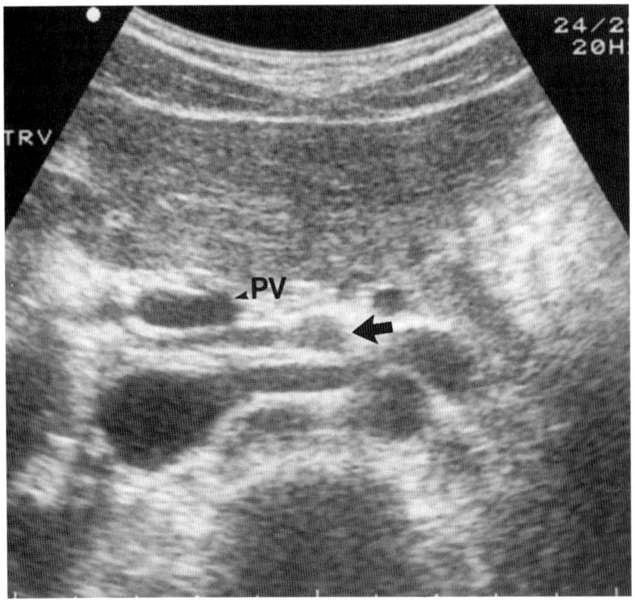

FIG. 11-32. Replaced right hepatic artery is seen arising from the superior mesenteric artery *(arrow)*, coursing posterior to the main portal vein (PV) into the liver hilus.

as a normal finding. However, these are extremely small and of lesser caliber than the adjacent portal venous branches. Anomalous vascular supply can be frequently detected by US as well as by rapid-sequence spiral CT and MR angiography, although routine CT and MRI may not demonstrate these anomalies as well. An accessory or replaced right hepatic artery is the most common, being found in 12% to 25% of all patients. This arises from the superior mesenteric artery, passes posterior to the main portal vein, and subsequently into the porta hepatis (Fig. 11-32). Accessory or replaced left hepatic artery occurs in approximately 10% to 12% of patients, arising from the left gastric artery and passing through the fissure for the ligamentum venosum into the left lobe along the undivided left portal vein.[114]

The branching pattern of the hepatic veins at the confluence with the inferior vena cava is quite variable. The three major veins may arise separately, but frequently the left and middle hepatic veins share a common trunk (see Fig. 11-31). Occasionally all three hepatic veins share a common trunk, and also, rarely, there may be a fourth hepatic vein arising at the confluence. More commonly, in about 5% of patients, an accessory inferior right hepatic vein is seen arising laterally from the inferior vena cava, several centimeters distal to the hepatic vein confluence.

Imaging Strategies for the Liver

The controversy over which cross-sectional imaging method is superior in detection of primary and secondary liver neoplasms is still unresolved. In the United States, most of the debate has ranged between CT and MRI. Those in favor of CT argue that it is preferable because of its ability to image both liver and the peritoneum and retroperitoneum to assess for both intrahepatic and extrahepatic disease, and hence offers a more complete examination than US or MRI.[115,116] MRI advocates claim similar sensitivity to CT plus the ability to discriminate cysts and hemangiomas from metastatic or primary tumors.[117] Our own experience has been similar to reports from Europe and Japan, in that US has been fully competitive with CT and MRI in liver tumor detection.[118,119]

Thus, the choice of the initial imaging method for evaluation of liver tumors is best individualized, based on the experience, expertise, and type of imaging equipment available at the institution. There are several points that most investigators would agree on; one is that the continuously evolving technology makes prospective comparative trials difficult because major technology advances may occur during the trial or subsequently as the results are being presented, written, and published. Consequently, definitive statements are difficult to make based on evaluation of the literature. A second point of universal agreement is that combinations of two or more modalities will obviously result in higher detection rates than any single modality, although at a greater expense to the health care system.

Third, most authors would agree that CT arterial portography is the single most effective nonsurgical method of liver lesion detection. This is an invasive and expensive procedure, however, requiring angiographic catheterization of the superior mesenteric artery, transfer of the patient from angiography to the CT table, and injection of contrast material with subsequent rapid scanning during the portal venous phase. Many authors also advocate delayed CT imaging several hours after the initial CT portogram.[61] This combined study can therefore be quite expensive, involving arteriographic charges, CT charges, and some time spent in a day care or observation unit after removal of the catheter. However, if the information derived is sufficient to avoid unnecessary surgery, by virtue of finding sufficient additional lesions in the liver to make a patient inoperable, then the cost of this study may still be justifiable.

The fourth point of agreement among investigators of liver imaging techniques is that all techniques perform poorly in the detection of extrahepatic disease, particularly in patients with primary colorectal cancers. Even combinations of multiple cross-sectional imaging techniques frequently fail to demonstrate metastatic lymphadenopathy in the abdomen, and all methods routinely fail to demonstrate peritoneal seeding and surface metastases on the liver until these reach a very large volume.[120] The maximal detection of liver tumors is accomplished by surgical exploration, inspection, and palpation, in combination with the use of IOUS.[121–123] Multiple series have consistently shown IOUS to be the most powerful liver imaging technique, demonstrating 96% to 98% of all detectable liver lesions, down to a size as small as 3 to 5 mm in diameter. The information obtained from IOUS frequently alters surgical management, and consequently we advocate routine use IOUS during all surgical procedures fo᷊ potential resection of liver tumors.[123]

Because of the poor performance of preoperative imaging modalities in detection of extrahepatic disease, our surgeons have begun to use laparoscopy as a method to evaluate the abdomen for the presence of peritoneal seeding and metastatic lymphadenopathy, thereby attempting to avoid unnecessary laparotomy in patients who would be deemed inoperable by virtue of their extrahepatic disease. We have begun using laparoscopic US of the liver during these sessions. Specially designed laparoscopic US probes can fit through a 10-mm port, and preliminary results suggest the same potential for detecting additional liver lesions as has been experienced with IOUS. Laparoscopic US is technically more challenging and somewhat more time consuming, and further studies are necessary to define its proper place in the diagnostic armamentarium, but early results show promise for the accurate detection of liver tumors.[124] The combination of laparoscopy for evaluation of extrahepatic disease and laparoscopic US for assessment of intrahepatic disease has the potential to decrease substantially the number of unnecessary laparotomies in patients who are ultimately unresectable, thereby reducing costs to the health care system as well as enhancing patient care by earlier discharge and less morbidity.

Primary Hepatic Tumors

Worldwide, hepatocellular carcinoma is the most common liver tumor, usually arising on a background of chronic hepatitis B as well as in association with dietary carcinogens such aflatoxin. The incidence in the United States is much lower than worldwide, but it is still much more common than other primary hepatic cancers. In the United States, hepatomas most often arise in the setting of alcoholic cirrhosis. Many of these patients have advanced Laennec's cirrhosis with extensive scarring, regeneration, and nodularity, both microscopic and macroscopic. This makes imaging of the liver notoriously difficult, and multiple studies have shown rather poor lesion detection rates, generally ranging from 60% to 80% for US, CT, and MRI.[116,125,126] Even CT arterial portography was regarded as relatively insensitive in the detection of primary liver tumors.[127] Hepatocellular carcinoma has a wide spectrum of appearances, ranging from discrete, solitary, and well defined nodules to multifocal, multicentric nodules or even a diffuse infiltrating appearance, which can be very difficult to detect when superimposed on a background of diffuse chronic liver disease.[110] When the tumor presents as a large solitary mass, careful imaging may disclose small satellite nodules that are more frequently seen in the background of chronic liver disease. The rare fibrolamellar hepatoma, which arises on a background of normal liver, seldom shows satellitosis (Fig. 11-33). Fibrolamellar hepatomas frequently have a central scar,[128] but central scarring is a common feature of focal nodular hyperplasia and hemangiomas, and has even been reported in primary hepatic lymphoma. Hepatocellular carcinoma has a peculiar propensity to invade the portal vein, which may occur in up to 25% of patients with advanced hepatoma (Fig. 11-34). These tumors also invade the hepatic vein, although less frequently, and can indeed extend into the inferior vena cava and right atrium. It is rare for other primary or secondary liver tumors to exhibit venous invasion, although we have seen this with cholangiocarcinoma and gastrointestinal metastases. These are so rare, however, that the presence of a tumor with venous invasion is almost conclusive evidence for a histologic determination of hepatoma. Calcification within hepatomas is said to occur in 15% to 20%, but this is probably

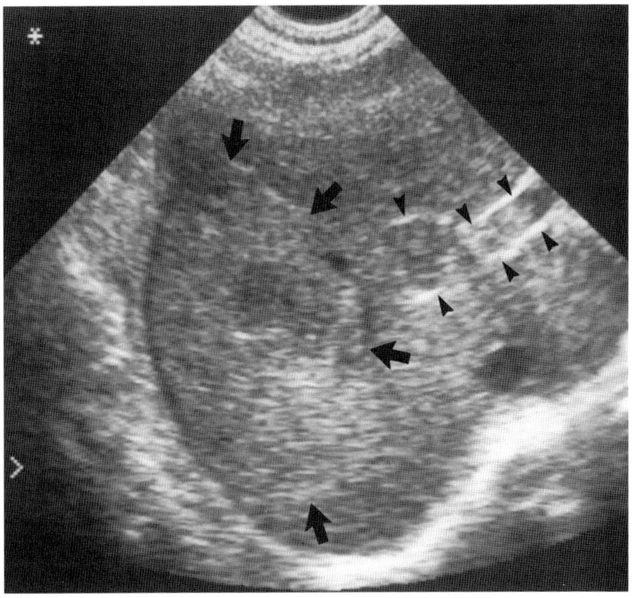

FIG. 11-34. Hepatoma causing a parenchymal liver mass *(arrows)* and invasion of the right and main portal veins *(arrowheads)*.

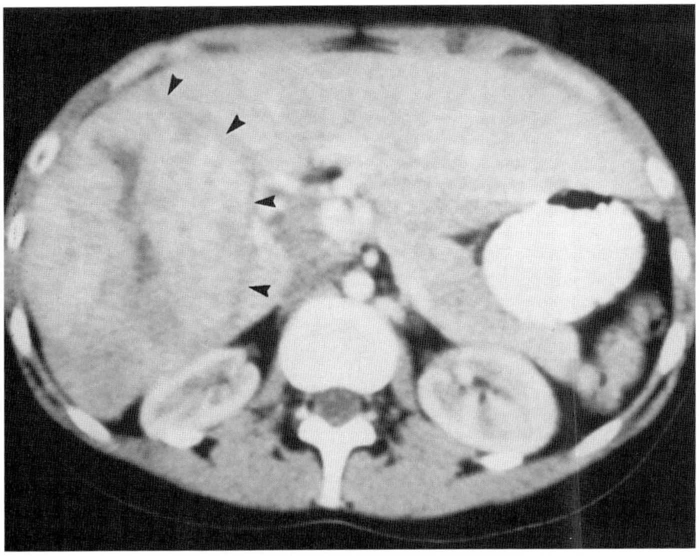

FIG. 11-33. Fibrolamellar hepatoma with a large central scar *(arrowheads)*.

no longer accurate because lesions are being detected at an earlier stage, particularly with the intensive surveillance programs in patients at risk.

Apart from the propensity of fibrolamellar hepatoma to show a central scar, there is no consistently predictable appearance of hepatocellular carcinoma on US, CT, or MRI. Lesions may have low, intermediate, or high echogenicity, low or high attenuation on CT, and variable enhancement after contrast administration. The lesions are typically of low signal intensity on T1-weighted MRI, and of high intensity on T2-weighted images, sometimes showing a "nodule-in-nodule" appearance. This appearance is considered highly suggestive of hepatoma, but is seen only in approximately one third of cases.[126]

Cholangiocarcinoma is seen with approximately one tenth the frequency of hepatoma. Although many of these tumors arise extrahepatically in the common duct, intrahepatic cholangiocarcinomas also occur, both centrally at the bifurcation of the common hepatic duct into right and left ducts, as well as peripherally in the liver. Several preexisting clinical conditions are associated with increased risk for development of cholangiocarcinoma. These include choledochal cyst, Caroli's disease, Oriental cholangiohepatitis, prior Thorotrast administration, and inflammatory bowel disease with sclerosing cholangitis.

The central cholangiocarcinoma, the so-called Klatzkin tumor, usually presents early because of the development of ductal obstruction and jaundice. This tumor is very scirrhous, and a discrete mass may be difficult to visualize by any of the cross-sectional modalities (Fig. 11-35). Often the only manifestations recognizable are the presence of dilated peripheral bile ducts in the liver. When a mass is visualized in association with a Klatzkin tumor, it usually shows increased echogenicity on US and low attenuation on CT with minimal contrast enhancement; rarely, there is invasion of the portal vein.[129]

Peripheral intrahepatic cholangiocarcinoma tends to present as a large, focal, solitary mass, often showing areas of necrosis and calcification. The appearance and behavior are more similar to those of large focal hepatocellular carcinoma. The lesions tend to be of mixed to increased echogenicity, and decreased density on CT with variable contrast enhancement. Central scarring has been described in this tumor as well as in fibrolamellar hepatoma,[130,131] but this finding can also be seen in benign tumors such as focal nodular hyperplasia and hemangioma.[132]

Hepatoblastoma is almost completely a malignancy of the pediatric age group and is, in fact, the most common hepatic tumor in children. These usually present as large, heterogeneous masses with normal to increased echogenicity, calcifications, and often cystic areas of necrosis. The tumors are usually of low density on CT with enhancement, particularly peripherally, and the MRI appearance typical of most tumors is low signal intensity on T1-weighted images and high signal intensity on T2. Although these tumors may "mature" into benign entities in children, the rare occurrence of hepatoblastoma in adults is usually a highly malignant condition.

Angiosarcomas may arise in the liver but are extremely rare, with most of them seen in patients with prior exposure to Thorotrast (secondary to particulate radiation from thorium dioxide) or in patients with other toxic exposures such as arsenic or polyvinylchloride. These lesions may also involve the spleen, peritoneal surfaces, and lymph nodes. Angiosarcomas are highly malignant but have no specific sonographic, CT, or MRI features. Other tumors in the liver associated with Thorotrast administration include hepatocellular carcinoma and cholangiocarcinoma.

Primary hepatic lymphoma is also a rare tumor but may present as a large, solitary hepatic mass without distinguishing features. Although secondary involvement of the liver by lymphoma almost invariably presents with hypoechoic masses (Fig. 11-36), the large solitary lymphomas show variable echogenicity. A central scar has been reported in hepatic lymphomas, as well as in many other hepatic tumors.

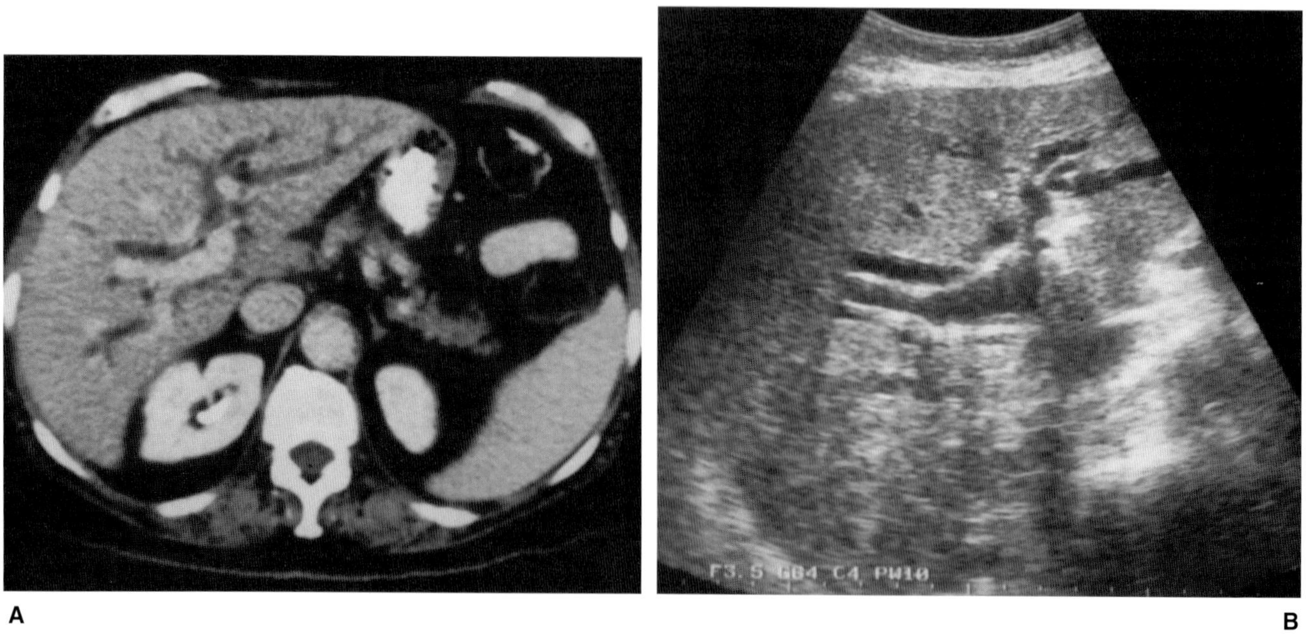

A B

FIG. 11-35. Klatzkin tumor. Computed tomography **(A)** and ultrasound **(B)** scans show intrahepatic bile duct dilatation up to the confluence, but no extrahepatic bile duct dilitation. Neither study defines a discrete mass, as frequently occurs with Klatzkin tumor.

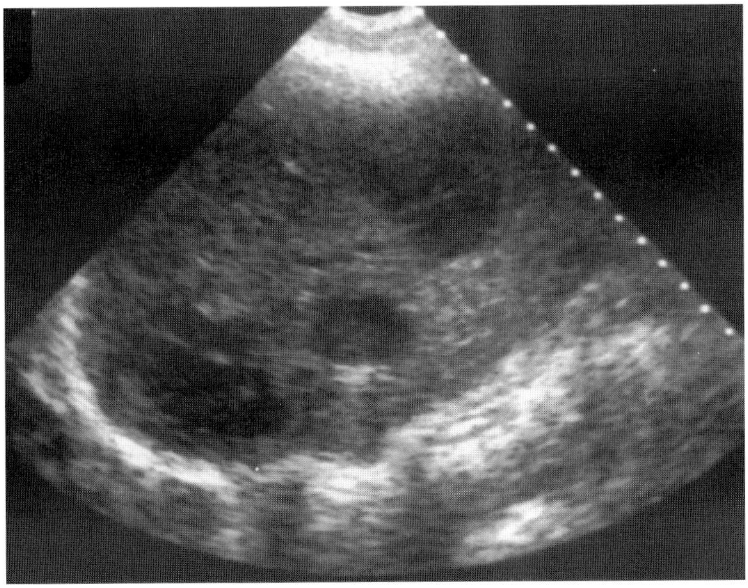

FIG. 11-36. Hepatic lymphoma. Multiple liver masses show the typical hypoechoic appearance characteristic of lymphoma.

Metastatic Liver Tumors

In North America, metastatic tumors in the liver are much more common than primary hepatic tumors. Metastatic disease in the liver is most often nodular and can be unifocal or multifocal; less frequently, an infiltrating diffuse form is seen. Metastases arising from the gastrointestinal tract are typically focal in nature, as are neuroendocrine metastases and those arising from most sarcomas, melanoma, renal cell carcinoma, and nasopharyngeal carcinomas. Primary carcinomas of the lung and breast may present with either focal or infiltrative forms of metastatic disease. Similarly, a lymphoma with secondary involvement of the liver may present as either focal or diffuse involvement, but leukemic involvement of the liver is nearly always in the diffuse infiltrative form.

Although there are no definitive appearances on MRI, CT, or US to allow histologic characterization of liver metastases, there are certain fairly consistent features. A mass with a hypoechoic rim on US has a very high probability of being a malignant lesion, either primary or secondary. This is most notable in metastases from the gastrointestinal tract, particularly colorectal metastases, which often show a bull's eye pattern, with increased echogenicity centrally surrounded by a hypoechoic rim of tumor[133] (Fig. 11-37). Mucin-producing gastrointestinal tract tumors may in fact show calcification within the central portion of the tumor. The bull's eye pattern is not all-inclusive, however, because some colorectal metastases may appear as hyperechoic masses or hypoechoic nodules. The latter pattern seems to be more associated with undifferentiated colorectal metastases. Most metastatic lesions are hypodense on CT and show variable enhancement patterns after administration of intravenous contrast, with some of the variability being related to timing of the scans relative to the administration of contrast.[134] Gastrointestinal tract metastases show rim enhancement, whereas neuroendocrine, renal cell, and sarcomatous metastases are often diffusely hypervascular. Hypervascular metastases tend to show increased echogenicity on US.

On MRI, metastases appear hypointense on T1-weighted images and exhibit increased signal intensity on T2-weighted images. The hypervascular tumors tend to be the most intense on T2 sequences. A halo of increased intensity is seen at times on T2-weighted images, making the metastasis appear larger on T2 than on T1 sequences. There is controversy over whether this halo represents tumor versus edema in the surrounding liver,[135,136] but for surgical and oncologic planning it is best to assume that the halo represents tumor. Another feature seen on MRI is wedge-shaped areas of increased signal intensity on T2-weighted images, extending to the liver capsule peripheral to the tumor. This appearance results from obstruction of portal branches and may be a subtle sign of metastatic disease.[137]

A few metastatic lesions have highly characteristic appear-

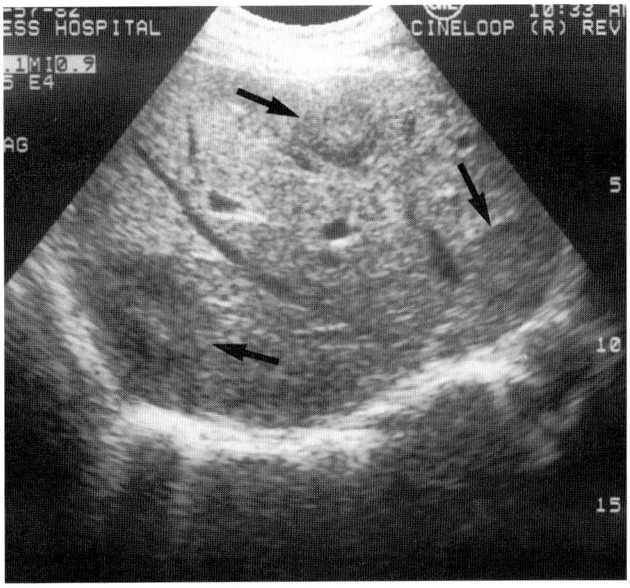

FIG. 11-37. Bull's-eye pattern of hepatic metastases *(arrows)* typically seen with metastatic adenocarcinoma from gastrointestinal tract origin, especially colorectal cancer.

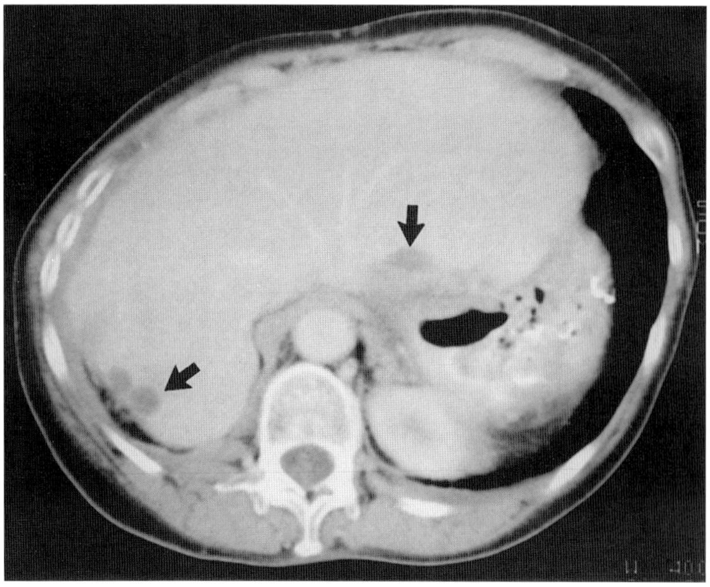

FIG. 11-38. Cystic ovarian metastases present as low-density, subcapsular or surface liver lesions on computed tomography scan *(arrows)*.

ances that may provide clues to their histologic identity. Focal hepatic lymphoma as a secondary manifestation is characteristically hypoechoic on US images (see Fig. 11-36). Mucin-producing carcinomas of the gastrointestinal tract typically show calcification in their liver metastases, a finding which is also seen in metastatic medullary carcinoma of the thyroid. Although any hypervascular metastasis may outgrow its blood supply and undergo necrosis with cystic degeneration, the overall appearance still usually suggests a primarily solid lesion containing areas of liquefaction. Ovarian metastases, however, show a characteristic appearance, with the lesion being predominantly cystic and frequently involving the surface of the liver rather than the deep hepatic parenchyma (Fig. 11-38). No other tumor exhibits this type of behavior.

Despite these somewhat characteristic appearances, most liver metastases have few distinguishing features. Percutaneous fine-needle or core biopsy under guidance with CT or US is the most expeditious method of obtaining cytologic or histologic identification and confirmation of metastases. If the differential diagnosis includes possibility of primary liver tumor or lymphoma, core biopsies are preferred because histologic characteristics may be necessary confidently to identify the tumor type. For most metastatic lesions, however, fine-needle sampling and cytologic analysis may be as good as core biopsy for diagnosis.

Pitfalls in Liver Imaging

There are many benign conditions causing focal hepatic masses that must be discriminated from malignant lesions. Hepatic cysts are seen in at least 5% of the population, and may be single or multiple. Most of these probably arise from biliary duct epithelium. These are readily recognizable, having razor-sharp, smooth margins with the adjacent hepatic parenchyma. Septations and indentations are common. On US, cysts are hypoechoic to anechoic and there is increased transmission of sound through the lesion. On CT scanning, cysts are homogeneous and of lower density, in the range of 0 to 15 Hounsfield units, similar to the density of water. There is no enhancement on administration of contrast material. On MRI, cysts are of low intensity on T1-weighted and very high intensity on T2-weighted scans, showing behavior similar to water or bile. Complicated cysts with hemorrhage or infection may prove troublesome in that the echogenicity may increase, CT density may increase, and MRI signal intensity may be variable depending on the amount and nature of hemoglobin.[138]

The most common benign tumor of the liver is the cavernous hemangioma, with estimates of occurrence ranging from 3% to 7% of the general population. These lesions may be single or multiple and are most frequent in the right lobe, but may be seen anywhere within the liver. The US appearance shows a characteristic lesion with homogeneous increased echogenicity and sharp, well circumscribed, smooth margins (Fig. 11-39A). Larger hemangiomas may show posterior acoustic enhancement and hypoechoic spaces within the lesion corresponding to venous lakes or dilated vascular sinuses.[139]

On CT, hemangiomas are hypodense, sharply circumscribed lesions on noncontrast studies and show a characteristic enhancement pattern after injection of contrast material, with slow enhancement over several minutes, beginning at the periphery and proceeding into the center of the lesion. Delayed scans from 5 to 20 minutes after injection typically show homogeneous enhancement equal to or greater than that of the surrounding liver parenchyma.[140] On MRI, hemangiomas show a pattern similar to that of hepatic cysts—that is, sharply circumscribed, smooth-margined, low-intensity lesions on T1-weighted images, and high intensity on T2 (see Fig. 11-39B). Typically, the intensity on T2-weighted sequences increases progressively from first to second to third echoes, but this is also the behavior of simple cysts, and the distinction between cyst and hemangioma cannot be made by MRI.

There are many atypical hemangiomas that do not conform to the classic descriptions, however. Central scarring is a common feature within hemangiomas, and if present, the scar shows lesser echogenicity than the surrounding hemangioma, increased CT density, and lack of enhancement after intravenous contrast material administration. The central scar may show low or high signal on CT. There are also some rare hemangiomas that are diffusely hypoechoic on US, and these lesions are typi-

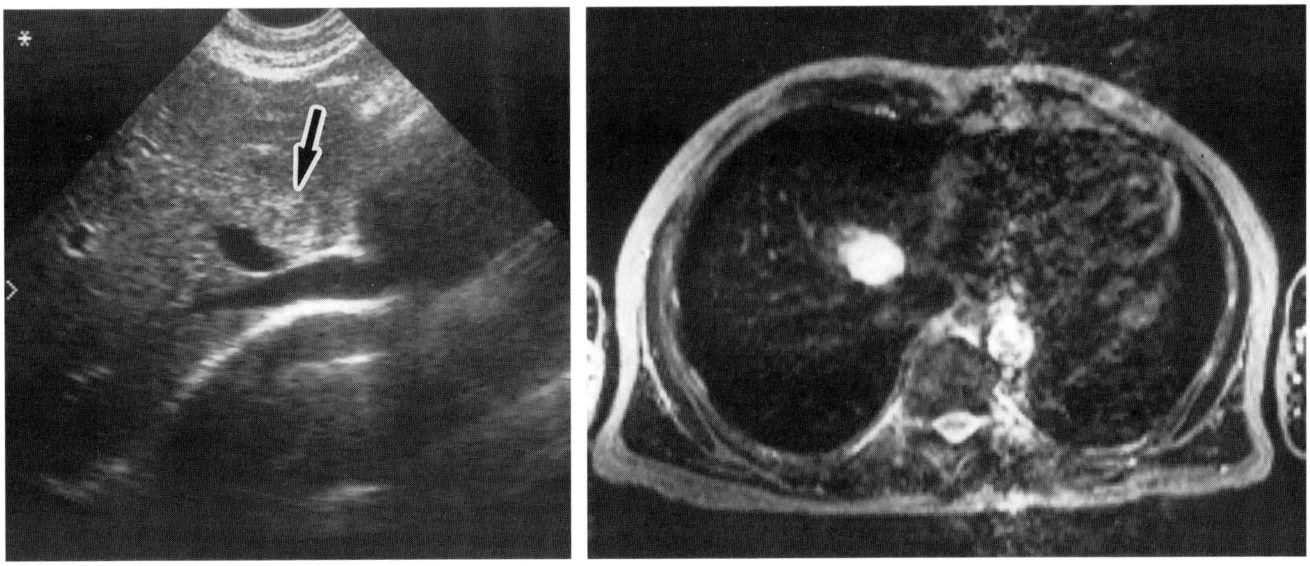

A B

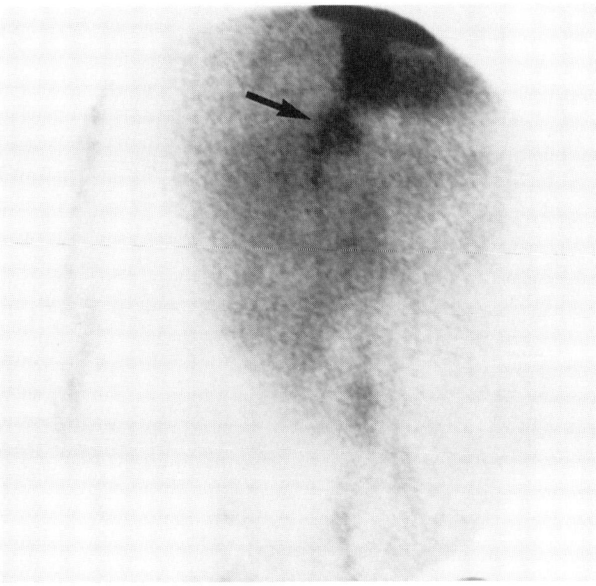

C

FIG. 11-39. Hemangioma. **A,** Ultrasound shows hyperechoic mass *(arrow)* near the right hepatic vein. **B,** The lesion shows marked hyperintensity on heavily T2-weighted magnetic resonance imaging scan (lightbulb sign). **C,** Sixty-minute tagged red cell radionuclide scan shows persistent activity within the lesion *(arrow)*, thereby confirming hemangioma.

cally seen in patients with diffuse, fatty livers in which the liver parenchyma shows an overall increase in echogenicity, thereby making the hemangioma relatively hypoechoic.

The single most specific test for hemangioma is the radionuclide-tagged red cell scan. In this test, radiolabeled red blood cells are administered intravenously. Rapid-sequence images are obtained during the early angiographic phase, and subsequent delayed images at 30 and 60 minutes are obtained. The hemangiomas show diminished activity on the early angiographic phase and prolonged activity on the delayed images, with the persistent activity being much greater than in the surrounding liver parenchyma (see Fig. 11-39C). This test is the most specific, with virtually no false-positive results, even in atypical hemangiomas. The only limitation for tagged red cell scanning is size, with lesions much smaller and 2 to 3 cm being below the resolution limits for this test. The addition of tomographic (single photon emission CT) scanning increases the accuracy for smaller lesions.[141]

Other benign liver tumors include hepatic adenomas and focal nodular hyperplasia, both of which have variable appearances on all cross-sectional imaging modalities. These are usually unifocal, but multiple lesions have been described. In glycogen storage disease in particular, multiple hepatic adenomas or hepatomas have been reported. There are no completely characteristic findings in either of these two lesions. Central scarring is common in focal nodular hyperplasia, but is seen in many other hepatic tumors, including hepatomas and hemangiomas. There is one feature of focal nodular hyperplasia that is characteristic. Because of the presence of reticuloendothelial cells within the tumor, approximately 50% of focal nodular hyperplasia lesions take up sufficient technetium-labeled sulfur colloid to show either isointense or hyperintense activity compared with the surrounding normal liver parenchyma. This feature is rarely seen in adenomas, and is virtually unheard of in malignant hepatic tumors.[142]

Hepatic lipomas are rare benign tumors that appear highly

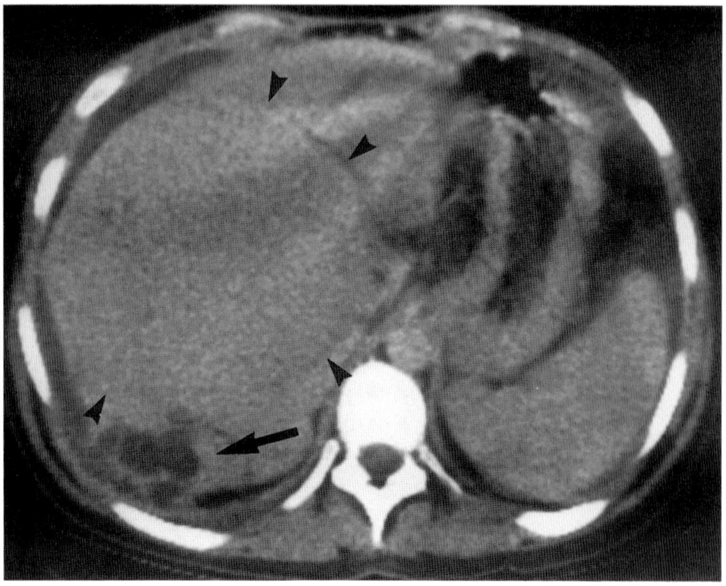

FIG. 11-40. Giant regenerative macronodule. Pretransplant computed tomography scan demonstrates large solid mass *(arrowheads)* in the right lobe causing obstruction of peripheral right lobe bile ducts *(arrow)*.

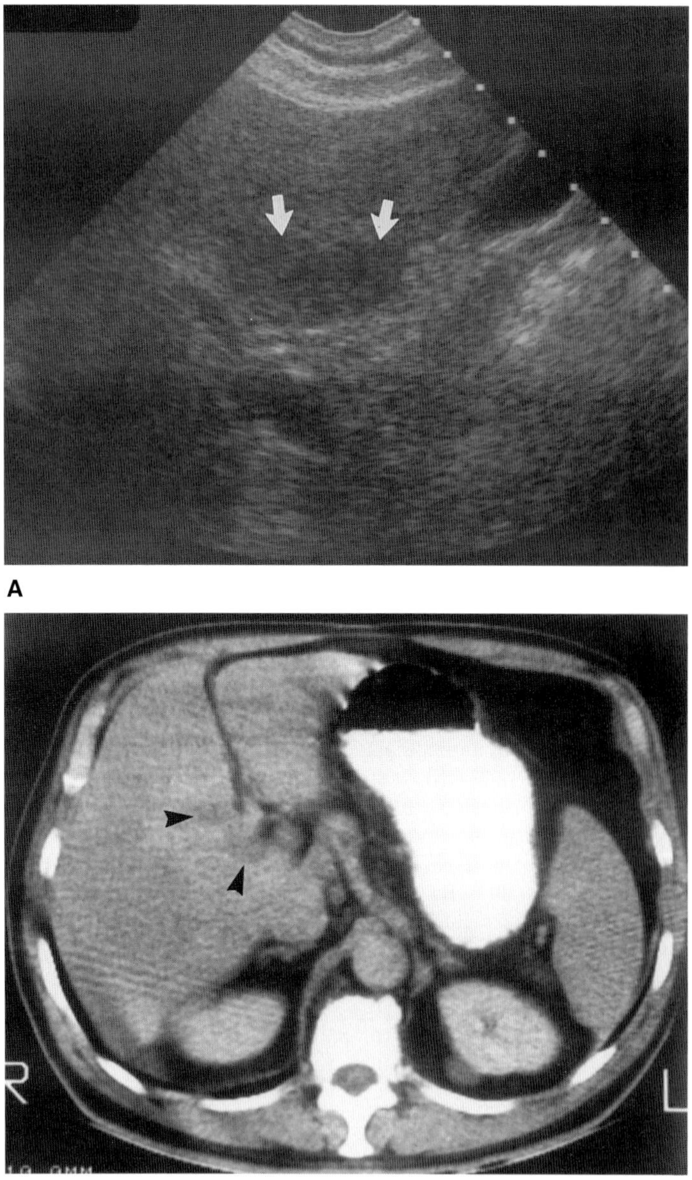

FIG. 11-41. Fatty liver with focal sparing. **A,** Ultrasound demonstrates an oval hypoechoic "lesion" adjacent to porta hepatitis *(arrows)*. The remaining liver shows increased echogenicity due to fatty infiltration. **B,** computed tomography scan shows hyperdense island of sparing *(arrowheads)* in the same location.

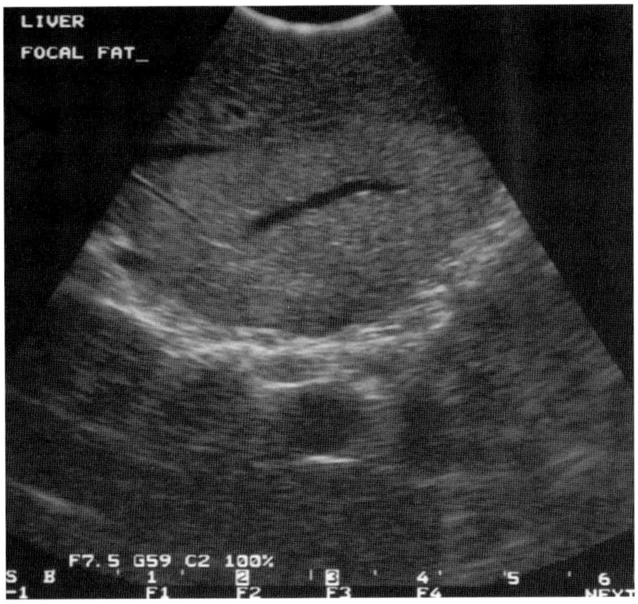

FIG. 11-42. Focal fat. Ultrasound shows oval area of increased echogenicity near the porta hepatis, with a vessel coursing unaffected through this pseudolesion.

echogenic on US, similar to the appearance of hemangioma. However, on CT, the fat in a lipoma results in lowered attenuation in the lesion, with densities in the fat range of −30 to −100 Hounsfield units.

Certain diffuse hepatic parenchymal changes may result in pseudomasses that can simulate the appearance of a neoplasm. In patients with cirrhosis, the liver often has a nodular texture because of reparative attempts that form regenerative nodules. These are typically smaller than 5 mm in size and are not readily visualized, but occasionally giant regenerative macronodules can occur that can form large, easily detectable masses and even cause biliary obstruction (Fig. 11-40). These regenerative macronodules can simulate the appearance of a hepatoma arising on a background of cirrhosis. These macronodules typically are very homogeneous on US and CT, and the radionuclide sulfur colloid scan shows uptake of colloid within the lesion similar to that of the surrounding hepatic parenchyma, thereby allowing differentiation from hepatoma, which would be universally cold on sulfur colloid scan.[128]

Fatty infiltration of the liver may occur on a background of diffuse liver disease or may be seen in association with diabetes, hyperalimentation, and obesity. This results in a diffuse increase in the echogenicity of the liver and a diffuse decrease in the density of the liver on CT. Frequently, there are islands of focal sparing from the diffuse fatty infiltration that appear as hypoechoic masses on US and hyperdense masses on CT (Fig. 11-41). These pseudolesions often have a flat or geographic contour rather than the typical spherical shape that is seen with tumors, and their location also shows predictable patterns, being situated near the porta hepatis, the main left and right portal veins, and the bare area of the liver adjacent to the gallbladder.[143] Occasionally the situation may be reversed, with the same typical sites showing areas of focal fatty infiltration while the remainder of the liver is normal. Normal hepatic vasculature can be seen to pass through these focal areas without compression or alteration of its course, which may provide a clue as to the nature of these pseudolesions (Fig. 11-42). When the pseudolesions of focal fat and focal sparing are in typical locations and show the characteristic US and CT appearances, biopsy may not be necessary. However, if there is high clinical suspicion for hepatoma or metastatic disease, or if the location of these focal pseudolesions is atypical, image-guided biopsy often is required to establish a definitive diagnosis.

CONCLUSIONS

There are many imaging modalities available to evaluate malignancies in the gastrointestinal tract. These various modalities often provide complementary and additional information, but on many other occasions, the information is redundant. In this age of economic constraints on health care use, it is imperative to develop cost-effective strategies for diagnostic evaluation.

Unfortunately, in most cases, the experience described in the literature does not identify single modalities that consistently provide all or nearly all the necessary information. There is even considerable controversy in most instances over proper sequencing of successive examinations. This is unfortunate, but reflects the reality of constantly evolving technologies, variations in availability of state-of-the-art equipment, as well as variability in the interest, experience, and expertise of the diagnostic imaging personnel.

Consequently, in our opinion, the only solution readily available is to establish local algorithms for diagnostic workup and follow-up of gastrointestinal malignancies based on the unique characteristics of each institution. Ideally, this should be done with collaboration between the clinicians and radiologists. Such a partnership should lead to optimal choices for appropriate and cost-effective workups, thereby enhancing patient care without undue cost to the health care system.

REFERENCES

1. Beahrs OH, Henson DE, Hutter RVP, Myers MH, eds. Manual for staging of cancer. American Joint Committee on Cancer. 3rd ed. Philadelphia: JB Lippincott, 1988:63.
2. Younghusband JD, Aluwihare APR. Carcinoma of the oesophagus: factors affecting survival. Br J Surg 1970;57:422.
3. Mandard AM, Marnay J, Gignoux M, et al. Cancer of the oesophagus and associated lesions: detailed pathological study of 100 esophagectomy specimens. Hum Pathol 1984;15:660.
4. Marx MV, Balfe DN. Computed tomography of the esophagus. Semin Ultrasound CT MR 1987;8:316.
5. Inculet RI, Keller SM, Dwyer A, Roth JA. Evaluation of noninvasive tests for the preoperative staging of carcinoma of the esophagus: a prospective study. Ann Thorac Surg 1985;40:561.
6. Lefor AT, Merino MM, Steinberg SM, et al. Computed tomographic projection of extraluminal spread and prognostic implications of lesion width in esophageal carcinoma. Cancer 1988;62:1287.
7. Quint LE, Glazer GM, Orringer MB, Gross BH. Esophageal carcinoma: CT findings. Radiology 1985;155:171.
8. Thompson WM, Halvorsen RA, Foster WL, Williford ME, Postlethwait RW, Korobkin M. Computed tomography for staging esophageal and gastroesophageal cancer: reevaluation. Am J Roentgenol 1983;141:951.
9. Picus D, Balfe DM, Koehler RE, Roper CL, Owen JW. Computed tomography in the staging of esophageal carcinoma. Radiology 1983;146:33.

10. Glazer GM, Gross BH, Quint LE, Francis IR, Bookstein FL, Orringer MB. Normal mediastinal lymph nodes: number and size according to the American Thoracic Society Mapping. Am J Roentgenol 1985; 144:261.
11. Heiken JP, Weymen PJ, Lee JK, et al. Detection of focal hepatic masses: prospective evaluation with CT, delayed CT, CT during arterial portography, and MR imaging. Radiology 1989;171:47.
12. Bernardino M, Erwin B, Steinberg H, Baumgartner B, Torres W, Gedgaudas-McClees R. Delayed hepatic CT scanning: increased confidence and improved detection of hepatic metastases. Radiology 1986;159:71.
13. Botet JF, Lightdale C. Pictorial essay: endoscopic sonography of the gastrointestinal tract. Am J Roentgenol 1991;156:63.
14. Tio TL, Cohen P, Coene PP, Uddin J, den Hartog Jager FCA, Tytgat GN. Endosonography and computed tomography of esophageal carcinoma: preoperative classification compared to the new (1984) TNM system. Gastroenterology 1989;96:1478.
15. Rice TW, Boyce GA, Sivak MV. Esophageal ultrasound and the preoperative staging of carcinoma of the esophagus. J Thorac Cardiovasc Surg 1991;101:536.
16. Vilgrain V, Mompoint D, Palazzo L, et al. Staging of esophageal carcinoma: comparison of results with endoscopic sonography and CT. Am J Roentgenol 1990;155:277.
17. Rosch T, Classen M. A new ultrasound probe for endosonographic imaging of the upper GI tract: preliminary observations. Endoscopy 1990;22:41.
18. Botet J, Lightdale C, Zauber A, Gerdes H, Urmacher C, Brennan M. Preoperative staging of esophageal cancer: comparison of endoscopic US and dynamic CT. Radiology 1991;181:419.
19. Tio TL, Tytgat GNJ, Cikot RJLM, Houthoff HJ, Sars PRA. Ampullopancreatic carcinoma: preoperative TNM classification with endosonography. Radiology 1990;175:455.
20. Sugimachi K, Ohno S, Fujishima H, Kuwano H, Mori M, Misawa T. Endoscopic ultrasonographic detection of carcinomatous invasion and of lymph nodes in the thoracic esophagus. Surgery 1990;107:366.
21. Petrillo R, Balzarini L, Bidoli P, et al. Esophageal squamous cell carcinoma: MRI evaluation of mediastinum. Gastrointest Radiol 1990; 15:275
22. Lightdale CJ, Botet JK, Kelsen DP, Turnbull AD, Brennan MF. Diagnosis of recurrent upper gastrointestinal cancer at the surgical anastomosis by endoscopic ultrasound. Gastrointest Endosc 1989;35:407.
23. Frimberger E. Expanding spiral: a new type of prosthesis for the palliative treatment of malignant esophageal stenoses. Endoscopy 1983;15:213.
24. Cwikiel W, Stridbeck H, Tranberg K, et al. Malignant esophageal strictures: treatment with a self-expanding Nitinol stent. Radiology 1993;187:661.
25. Kruskal JB, McCully RB, Madden MV, Dent DM. Gastric carcinoma: a current clinical profile. S Afr Med J 1986;70:7.
26. Botet J, Lightdale C, Zauber A, et al. Preoperative staging of gastric cancer: comparison of endoscopic US and dynamic CT. Radiology 1991;181:426.
27. Sobin LH, Hermanek P, Hutter RVP. TNM classification of malignant tumors: a comparison between the new (1987) and old editions. Cancer 1988;6:2310.
28. Tio TL, den Hartog Jager FCA, Tytgat GNJ. The role of endoscopic ultrasonography in assessing local resectability of esophagogastric malignancies: accuracy, pitfalls, and predictability. Scand J Gastroenterol 1986;21(Suppl 123):78.
29. Dehn TC, Reznek RH, Nockler IB, White FE. The pre-operative assessment of advanced gastric cancer by computed tomography. Br J Surg 1984;71:413.
30. Halvorsen RA, Thompson WM. Computed tomographic staging of gastrointestinal malignancies: I. esophagus and stomach. Invest Radiol 1987;22:2.
31. Kruskal JB, Kane RA. Correlative imaging of malignant liver tumors. Semin Ultrasound CT MR 1992;13:336.
32. Laurent F, Raynaud M, Biset JM, Boisserie-Lacroix M, Grelet P, Drouillard J. Diagnosis and categorization of small bowel neoplasms: role of computed tomography. Gastrointest Radiol 1991;16:115.
33. Balthazar EJ. CT of the gastrointestinal tract: principles and interpretation. Am J Roentgenol 1991;156:23.
34. Herlinger H, Maglinte DDT. Tumors of the small intestine. In: Herlinger H, Maglinte DDT, eds. Clinical radiology of the small intestine. Philadelphia: WB Saunders, 1989:399.
35. Herlinger H. A modified technique for the double contrast small bowel enema. Gastrointest Radiol 1978;3:201.
36. Eustace S, Murray J, O'Connell D. Sonographic diagnosis of lipoma induced intussusception. J Clin Ultrasound 1993;21:472.
37. Megibow AJ, Balthazar EJ, Hulnich DH, Naidich DP, Bosniak MA. CT evaluation of gastrointestinal leiomyomas and leiomyosarcomas. Am J Roentgenol 1985;144:727.
38. Megibow AG, Balthazar EJ, Hulnick, Naidich DP, Bosniak MA. Computed tomography of gastrointestinal lymphoma. Am J Roentgenol 1983;141:541.
39. Dudiak KM, Johnson CD, Stephens DH. Primary tumours of the small intestine: CT evaluation. Am J Roentgenol 1989;152:995.
40. Farah MC, Hasan Jafri SZ, Schwab RE, et al. Duodenal neoplasms: role of CT. Radiology 1987;162:839.
41. Valls C, Sancho C, Bechini J, Dominguez J, Montana X. Intestinal leiomyomas: angiographic imaging. Gastrointest Radiol 1992;17:220.
42. Vujic I, Sbrocchi RD, Stanley JH. Angiographic demonstration of gastrointestinal neurofibromas in von Recklinghausen's disease. Gastrointest Radiol 1983;8:283.
43. Bin W, Jianguo L, Baowei D. The sonographic appearances of small bowel tumours. Clin Radiol 1992;46:30.
44. Kane RA, Hughes LA, Cua EJ, Steele GD, Jenkins RL, Cady B. The impact of intraoperative ultrasonography on surgery for liver neoplasms. J Ultrasound Med 1994;13:1.
45. Stevenson G. Medical imaging in the prevention, diagnosis, and management of colon cancer. Advances in Gastrointestinal Radiology 1991;1:1.
46. Williams CB, Macrae FA, Bartram CI. A prospective study of diagnostic methods in adenoma follow up. Endoscopy 1982;143:74.
47. Leinicke J, Dodds W, Hogan W, et al. Comparisons of colonoscopy and roentgenography for detecting polypoid lesions of the colon. Gastrointest Radiol 1977;2:125.
48. Day JJ, Freeman AH, Coni NK, Dixon A. Barium enema or computed tomography for the frail elderly patient? Clin Radiol 1993;48:48.
49. Ott DJ, Gelfand DW. How to improve the efficacy of the barium enema examination. Am J Roentgenol 1993;160:491.
50. Gelfand DW, Laufer I, eds. Colon cancer: diagnosis in an era of cost containment. Reston, VA: American College of Radiology, 1990.
51. Ott DJ. Radiographic efficacy. In: Ott DJ, Wu WC, eds. Polypoid disease of the colon. Baltimore: Urban & Schwarzenberg, 1986:99.
52. Rice RP. Lowering death rates from colorectal cancer: challenge for the 1990s. Radiology 1990;176:297.
53. Gelfand DW, Chen YM, Ott DJ. Detection of colonic polyps on single-contrast barium enema study: emphasis on the elderly. Radiology 1987;164:333.
54. Ott DJ, Chen YM, Gelfand DW, Wu WC, Munitz HA. Single-contrast vs double-contrast barium enema in the detection of colonic polyps. Am J Roentgenol 1986;146:993.
55. Ott DJ, Gelfand DW, Wu WC, Kerr RM. Sensitivity of double-contrast barium enema: emphasis on polyp detection. Am J Roentgenol 1980;135:327.
56. Ott DJ, Gelfand DW, Wu WC, Munitz HA, Chen YM. How important is radiographic detection of diminutive polyps of the colon? Am J Roentgenol 1986;146:875.
57. Tio TL, Coene PP, van Delden OM, Tytgat GN. Colorectal carcinoma: preoperative TNM classification with endosonography. Radiology 1991;179:165.
58. Wang KY, Kimmey MB, Nyberg DA, et al. Colorectal neoplasms: accuracy of US in demonstrating the depth of invasion. Radiology 1987;165:827.
59. Glaser F, Schlag P, Herfarth C. Endorectal ultrasonography for the assessment of invasion of rectal tumours and lymph node involvement. Br J Surg 1990;77:883.
60. Rifkin MD, Ehrlich SM, Marks G. Staging of rectal carcinoma: prospective comparison of endorectal US and CT. Radiology 1989;170: 319.
61. Heiken JP, Weymen PJ, Lee JK, et al. Detection of focal hepatic masses: prospective evaluation with CT, delayed CT, CT during arterial portography and MR imaging. Radiology 1989;171:47.
62. Balthazar EJ, Megibow AJ, Hulnick D, Naidich DP. Carcinoma of the colon: detection and preoperative staging by CT. Am J Roentgenol 1988;150:301.

63. Freeny PC, Marks WM, Ryan JA, Bolen JW. Colorectal carcinoma evaluation with CT: preoperative staging and detection of postoperative recurrence. Radiology 1986;158:347.
64. Soyer P, Levesque M, Elias D, et al. Detection of liver metastases from colorectal cancer: comparison of intraoperative US and CT during arterial portography. Radiology 1992;183:541.
65. Krestin GP, Steinbrech W, Friedmann G. Recurrent rectal cancer: diagnosis with MR imaging versus CT. Radiology 1988;168:307.
66. Ebner F, Kressel HY, Mintz MC, et al. Tumour recurrence versus fibrosis in the female pelvis: differentiation with MR imaging at 1.5T. Radiology 1988;166:333.
67. deLange EE, Fechner RE, Wanebo HJ. Suspected recurrent rectosigmoid carcinoma after abdominoperineal resection: MR imaging and histopathological findings. Radiology 1989;170:323.
68. Strauss LG, Clorius JH, Schlag P, et al. Recurrence of colorectal tumours: PET evaluation. Radiology 1989;170:329.
69. Collier BD, Abdel-Nabi H, Doerr R, et al. Immunoscintigraphy performed with ^{111}In-labeled CYT-103 in the management of colorectal cancer: comparison with CT. Radiology 1992;185:179.
70. Megibow AJ. Pancreatic adenocarcinoma: designing the examination to evaluate the clinical questions. Radiology 1992;183:297.
71. Cutler SJ, Myers MH, White PL. Who are we imaging and why? CA Cancer J Clin 1976;37:421.
72. Luetmer PH, Stephens DH, Ward EM. Chronic pancreatitis: reassessment with current CT. Radiology 1989;171:353.
73. Manabe T, Ohshio G, Baba N, Tobe T. Factors influencing prognosis and indications for curative pancreatectomy for ductal adenocarcinoma of the head of the pancreas. Int J Pancreatol 1990;7:187.
74. Ishikawa O, Ohhigashi H, Sasaki Y, et al. Practical usefulness of lymphatic and connective tissue clearance for the carcinoma of the pancreatic head. Ann Surg 1988;208:215.
75. Ward EM, Stephens DH, Sheedy PF. Computed tomographic characteristics of pancreatic carcinoma: an analysis of 100 cases. Radiographics 1983;3:547.
76. Wittenberg J, Simeone JE, Ferrucci JT, et al. Non-focal enhancement in pancreatic carcinoma. Radiology 1982;144:131.
77. Muller MF, Meyenberger C, Bertschinger P, Schaer R, Marincek B. Pancreatic tumors: evaluation with endoscopic US, CT and MR imaging. Radiology 1994;190:745.
78. Connolly MM, Dawson PJ, Michelassi F, Moossa AR, Lowenstein F. Survival in 1001 patients with carcinoma of the pancreas. Ann Surg 1987;206:366.
79. Mannell A, vanHeerden JA, Weiland LH, Ilstrup DM. Factors influencing survival after resection of ductal adenocarcinoma of the pancreas. Ann Surg 1991;203:403.
80. Fortner JG. Regional pancreatectomy for cancer of the pancreatic ampulla with other related sites: tumor staging and results. Ann Surg 1984;199:418.
81. Tsuchiya R, Oribe T, Noda T. Size of the tumor and other factors influencing prognosis of the head of the pancreas. Gastroenterol 1985; 80:459.
82. Freeny PC, Marks WM, Ryan JA, Traverso LW. Pancreatic ductal adenocarcinoma: diagnosis and staging with dynamic CT. Radiology 1988;166:125.
83. Marn CS, Glazer GM, Williams DM, Francis IR. CT angiographic correlation of collateral venous pathways in isolated splenic vein occlusion: new observations. Radiology 1990;175:375.
84. Megibow AJ, Bosniak MA, Ambos MA, Beranbaum ER. Thickening of the celiac axis and/or superior mesenteric artery: a sign of pancreatic carcinoma on computed tomography. Radiology 1982;144:131.
85. Luetmer PH, Stephens DH, Fischer AP. Obliteration of periarterial retropancreatic fat on CT in pancreatitis: an exception to the rule. Am J Roentgenol 1989;153:63.
86. Baker ME, Cohan RH, Nadel SN, Leder RA, Dunnick NR. Obliteration of the fat surrounding the celiac axis and superior mesenteric arteries is not a specific CT finding of carcinoma of the pancreas. Am J Roentgenol 1990;155:991.
87. Howard JM, Jordan GL. Cancer of the pancreas. Curr Probl Cancer 1977;2:5.
88. Steiner E, Stark DD, Hahn PF, et al. Imaging of pancreatic neoplasms: comparison of MR and CT. Am J Roentgenol 1989;152:487.
89. Semelka RC, Kroeker MA, Shoenut JP, Kroeker R, Yaffe CS, Macflikier AB. Pancreatic disease: prospective comparison of CT, ERCP, and 1.5-T MR imaging with dynamic gadolinium enhancement and fat suppression. Radiology 1991;181:785.
90. Semelka RC, Ascher SM. MR imaging of the pancreas. Radiology 1993;188:593.
91. Semelka RC, Chew W, Hricak H, Tomei E, Higgins CB. Fat-saturation MR imaging of the upper abdomen. Am J Roentgenol 1990;155: 1111.
92. Mitchell DG, Vinitski S, Saponaro S, Tasciyan T, Burk DL, Rifkin MD. Liver and pancreas: improved spin-echo T1 contrast by shorter echo time and fat suppression at 1.5T. Radiology 1991;178:67.
93. Outwater EK, Gordon SJ. Imaging the pancreatic and biliary ducts with MR. Radiology 1994;192:19.
94. Warshaw AL, Zhuo-yun G, Wittenberg J, et al. Preoperative staging and assessment of resectability of pancreatic cancer. Arch Surg 1990; 125:230.
95. Mozell E, Stenzel P, Woltering EA, Rosch J, O'Doriso TM. Functional endocrine tumors of the pancreas: clinical presentation, diagnosis and treatment. Curr Probl Surg 1990;27:304.
96. Galiber AK, Reading CC, Charboneau JW, et al. Localization of pancreatic insulinoma: comparison of pre- and intraoperative US with CT and angiography. Radiology 1988;166:405.
97. Semelka RC, Cummings M, Shoenut JP, Yaffe CS, Kroeker MA, Greenberg HM. Islet cell tumors: comparison of dynamic contrast-enhanced CT and MR imaging with dynamic gadolinium enhancement and fat suppression. Radiology 1993;186:799.
98. Itai Y, Moss AA, Ohtomo K. Computed tomography of cystadenoma and cystadenocarcinoma of the pancreas. Radiology 1982;145:419.
99. Compagno J, Oertel JE. Mucinous cystic neoplasms of the pancreas with overt and latent malignancy: a clinicopathologic study of 41 cases. Am J Clin Pathol 1978;69:573.
100. Nghiem HV, Freeny PC. Radiologic staging of pancreatic adenocarcinoma. Radiol Clin North Am 1994;32:71.
101. Gulliver DJ, Baker ME, Cheng CA, Meyers WC, Pappas TN. Malignant biliary obstruction: efficacy of thin-section dynamic CT in determining resectability. Am J Roentgenol 1992;159:503.
102. Brandt KR, Charboneau JW, Stephens DH, Welch TJ, Goellner JR. CT- and US-guided biopsy of the pancreas. Radiology 1993;187:99.
103. Hall-Craggs MA, Lees WR. Fine-needle aspiration biopsy: pancreatic and biliary tumors. Am J Roentgenol 1986;147:166.
104. Del Maschio A, Vanzulli A, Sironi S, et al. Pancreatic cancer versus chronic pancreatitis: diagnosis with CA 19-9 assessment, US, CT and CT-guided fine-needle biopsy. Radiology 1991;178:95.
105. Smith E. Complications of percutaneous abdominal fine-needle biopsy. Radiology 1991;178:253.
106. Coombs RJ, Zeiss J, Howard JM, Thomford NR, Merrick HW. CT of the abdomen after the Whipple procedure: value in depicting postoperative anatomy, surgical complications and tumor recurrence. Am J Roentgenol 1990;154:1011.
107. Tsuchiya Y. Early carcinoma of the gallbladder: macroscopic features and US findings. Radiology 1991;179:171.
108. Burrell MI, Zeman RK, Simeone JF, et al. The biliary tract: Imaging for the 1990s. Am J Roentgenol 1991;157:223.
109. Tio TL, Tytgat GN, Cikot RJ, Houthoff HJ, Sars PR. Ampullopancreatic carcinoma: preoperative TNM classification with endosonography. Radiology 1990;175:455.
110. Kruskal JB, Kane RA. Correlative imaging of malignant liver tumors. Semin Ultrasound CT MR 1992;13:336.
111. Alderson PO, Adams DF, McNeil BJ, et al. Computed tomography, ultrasound, and scintigraphy of the liver in patients with colon or breast carcinoma: a prospective comparison. Radiology 1983;149: 225.
112. Couinaud C, LeFoie M. Etudes anatomiques et chirureicales. Paris: Masson, 1957.
113. Kane RA. Sonographic anatomy of the liver. Semin Ultrasound 1981; 2:190.
114. Michels NA. Blood supply to the upper abdominal organs with a descriptive atlas. Philadelphia: JB Lippincott, 1955.
115. Harned II RK, Chezmar JL, Nelson RC. Imaging of patients with potentially resectable hepatic neoplasms. Am J Roentgenol 1992;159: 1191.
116. Miller WJ, Federle MP, Campbell WL. Diagnosis and staging of hepatocellular carcinoma: comparison of CT and sonography in 36 liver transplantation patients. Am J Roentgenol 1991;157:303.

117. Ferrucci JT. Liver tumor imaging: current concepts. Am J Roentgenol 1990;155:473.
118. Clarke MP, Kane RA, Steele GD, et al. Prospective comparison of preoperative imaging and intraoperative ultrasonography in the detection of liver tumors. Surgery 1989;106:849.
119. Kane RA, Longmaid HE, Costello P, et al. Non-invasive imaging in patients with hepatic masses: a prospective comparison of ultrasound, CT and MR imaging [abstract]. Am J Roentgenol 1993;160 (suppl 4):133.
120. Sugarbaker PH. Surgical decision making for large bowel cancer metastatic to the liver. Radiology 1990;174:621.
121. Machi J, Isomoto H, Kurohji T, et al. Accuracy of intraoperative ultrasonography in diagnosing liver metastases from colorectal cancer: evaluation with postoperative follow-up results. World J Surg 1991;15:551.
122. Soyer P, Levesque M, Elias D, et al. Detection of liver metastases from colorectal cancer: comparison of intraoperative US and CT during arterial portography. Radiology 1992;183:541.
123. Kane RA, Hughes LA, Cua EJ, Steele GD, Jenkins RL, Cady B. The impact of intraoperative ultrasonography on surgery for liver neoplasms. J Ultrasound Med 1994;13:1.
124. Kane RA, Roizental M, Kruskal JB, et al. Preliminary investigation of liver and biliary imaging with a dedicated laparoscopic ultrasound system [abstract]. Radiology 1994;193(p):287.
125. Miller WJ, Baron RL, Dodd GD, Federle MP. Malignancies in patients with cirrhosis: CT sensitivity and specificity in 200 consecutive transplant patients. Radiology 1994; 193:645.
126. Winter TC, Takayasu K, Muramatsu Y, et al. Early advanced hepatocellular carcinoma: evaluation of CT and MR appearance with pathologic correlation. Radiology 1994;192:379.
127. Soyer P, Bluemke DA, Hruban RH, Sitamann JV, Fishman EK. Primary malignant neoplasms of the liver: detection with helical CT during arterial portography. Radiology 1994;192:389.
128. Kane RA, Curatolo P, Khettry U. "Scar sign" on computed tomography and sonography in fibrolamellar hepatocellular carcinoma. J Comput Assist Tomogr 1987;11:27.
129. Thorsen MK, Quiroz R, Lawson TL, et al. Primary biliary carcinoma: CT evaluation. Radiology 1984;152:479.
130. Friedman AC, Lichtenstein JE, Goodman Z, et al. Fibrolamellar hepatocellular carcinoma. Radiology 1985;157:583.
131. Hamrick-Turner J, Abbitt PL, Ros PR. Intrahepatic cholangiocarcinoma: MR appearance. Am J Roentgenol 1992;158:77.
132. Rummeny E, Weissleder R, Sironi S, et al. Central scars in primary liver tumors. Radiology 1989;171:323.
133. Green B, Bree RL, Goldstein HM, Stanley C. Gray scale ultrasound evaluation of hepatic neoplasms: patterns and correlations. Radiology 1977;124:203.
134. Burgener FA, Hamlin DJ. Contrast enhancement of focal hepatic lesions on CT: effect of size and histology. Am J Roentgenol 1983; 140:297.
135. Lee MJ, Saini S, Compton CC, et al. MR demonstration of edema adjacent to a liver metastasis: pathologic correlation. Am J Roentgenol 1991;157:499.
136. Outwater E, Tomaszewski JE, Daly JM, et al. Hepatic colorectal metastases: correlation of MR imaging and pathologic appearance. Radiology 1991;180:327.
137. Itai Y, Ohtomo K, Kokubo T, et al. Segmental intensity differences in the liver on MR images: a sign of intrahepatic portal flow stoppage. Radiology 1988;167:17.
138. Stark DD, Moss AA, Goldberg HI. Nuclear magnetic resonance of the liver, spleen, and pancreas. Cardiovasc Intervent Radiol 1986;8: 329.
139. Taboury J, Porcel A, Tubiana J-M, Monnier J-P. Cavernous hemangiomas of the liver studied by ultrasound: enhancement posterior to a hyperechoic mass as a sign of hypervascularity. Radiology 1983;149: 781.
140. Freeny PC, Vimont TR, Barnett DC. Cavernous hemangioma of the liver: ultrasonography, arteriography, and computed tomography. Radiology 1979;132:143.
141. Rabinowitz SA, McKusick KA, Strauss HW. ^{99m}Tc red blood cell scintigraphy in evaluating focal liver lesions. Am J Roentgenol 1984; 143:63.
142. Sandler MA, Petrocelli RD, Marks DS, Lopez R. Ultrasonic features and radionuclide correlation in liver cell adenoma and focal nodular hyperplasia. Radiology 1980;135:393.
143. Scott WW, Sanders RC, Siegelman SS. Irregular fatty infiltration of the liver: diagnostic dilemmas. Am J Roentgenol 1980;135:67.

Surgery for Gastrointestinal Cancer: A Multidisciplinary Approach, edited by Harold J. Wanebo.
Lippincott-Raven Publishers, Philadelphia, © 1997.

CHAPTER 12

Pathology of Upper Gastrointestinal Cancer

Special Problems and Considerations

Grant N. Stemmermann and Amy Noffsinger

Gastrointestinal neoplasms challenge the highest skills of the surgeon and pathologist. Accuracy in the diagnosis of precursor lesions affects patient screening, management, and prognosis. This, in turn, depends on adequate sampling of sites most likely to contain early cancers and their precursors, and on the ability of the pathologist to identify dysplastic lesions that have a high potential for malignancy. Estimates of the probability of disease-free survival after resection of an invasive cancer depend on the extent of the resection and an accurate appraisal of the tumor stage. This chapter focuses on those aspects of the diagnosis and treatment of upper gastrointestinal cancer that are most likely to be influenced by the interaction of the pathologist and the clinician.

ESOPHAGUS

Squamous cell carcinoma (SCC) is a common tumor worldwide, but shows wide regional variation in incidence and causal associations. Heavy alcohol and cigarette consumption are characteristic risk factors in Western Europe and North America.[1] These habits are more frequently encountered in men; as a result, the male : female incidence ratio exceeds 4 : 1 in these areas. The risk of SCC increases exponentially with increasing alcohol consumption and linearly with increasing cigarette use, attaining a relative risk of 155 in men who consume 12 g of alcohol and 30 g of tobacco per day.[2] Diets deficient in protective antioxidants, combined with the consumption of carcinogens in poorly preserved foods, have been implicated in the generation of SCC in central Asia and China.[1] In these areas, this cancer may be the most common cause of death.

Squamous cell carcinoma is diagnosed at a late stage in most Western countries, presenting with lesions resembling those shown in Figures 12-1 and 12-2. The application of cytologic screening programs in high-risk areas of China has resulted in the discovery of in situ and early SCC in the majority of cases.[3] Replication of the Chinese experience in Western society will require screening of high-risk people, in many of whom self-destructive behavior discourages adequate health surveillance. The prevailing pattern of late-stage diagnoses might be corrected if cytologic screening for SCC were included in alcohol abuse programs.

Data from the Surveillance, Epidemiology, and End Results (SEER) program[4] indicate that long-term survival with SCC was only 8.9% in patients diagnosed in the years 1983 to 1987. Localized esophageal cancer had a 20.5% 5-year survival rate, but only 25% of cancers were diagnosed at this stage. It is possible that more extensive lymph node resections, as advocated by Japanese surgeons,[5] might increase survival in patients with localized tumors, if only because such resections will discover and therefore reclassify patients with unsuspected lymph node disease.

Adenocarcinoma

Adenocarcinoma of the esophagus is most common in white men in Western Europe and North America. This tumor shares many epidemiologic features with cancer of the cardia of the stomach. Indeed, it is often difficult to determine whether a cancer is derived from the esophagus or the stomach (Fig. 12-3). The development of esophageal adenocarcinoma is preceded by the development of Barrett's change in the distal esophagus. This form of metaplasia may have the attributes of gastric, small intestinal, or colonic mucosa. The metaplastic epithelium may become dysplastic. Increasing degrees of dysplasia incur an increasing risk for development of adenocarcinoma,[6–8] as shown in Figures 12-4 and 12-5.

The distribution of localized, regional, distant, and unstaged adenocarcinoma of the esophagus is similar to that found with SCC, and the long-term prognosis is equally grim. It is important that men older than 50 years of age who have significant reflux esophagitis be screened to discover the presence and

Grant N. Stemmermann, Department of Pathology, University of Cincinnati, School of Medicine, Cincinnati, OH 45267
Amy Noffsinger, Department of Pathology, University of Cincinnati, School of Medicine, Cincinnati, OH 45267

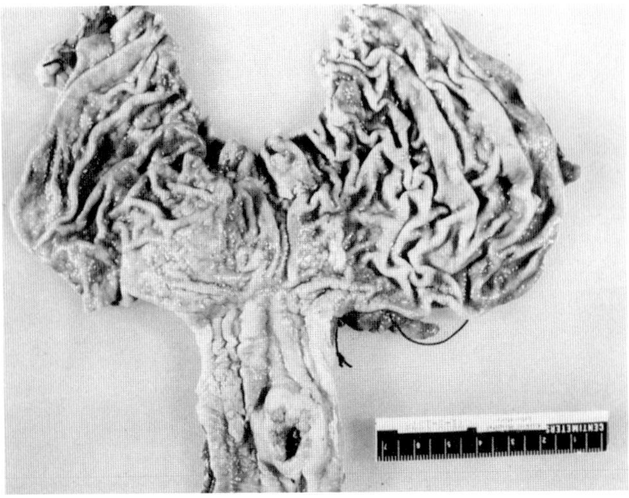

FIG. 12-1. A centrally ulcerated, stratified squamous cancer of the distal esophagus.

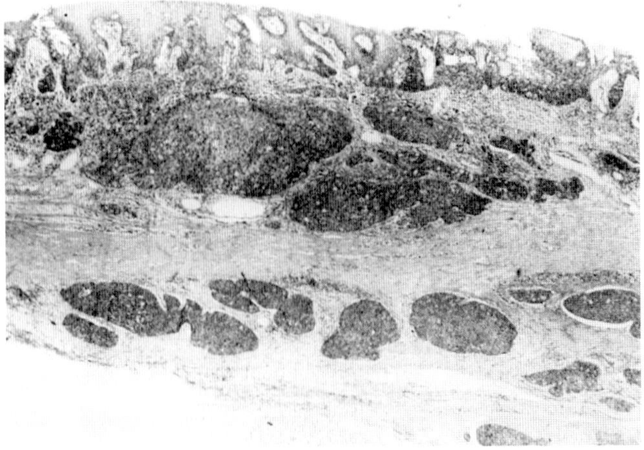

FIG. 12-2. Transmural extension of stratified squamous cancer. Esophageal cancer is usually diagnosed at this stage in the United States. (Hematoxylin & eosin stain; original magnification ×5.)

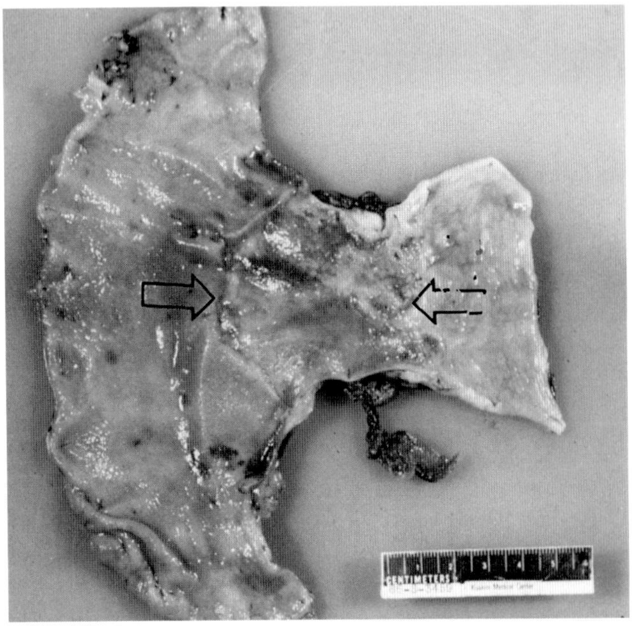

FIG. 12-3. A flat, slightly depressed adenocarcinoma at the cardioesophageal junction. The tumor margins are marked by arrows. It is obviously difficult to assign a primary site to this tumor. In this case, the tumor was classified as esophageal because the extent of esophageal involvement was greater than that of the gastric component.

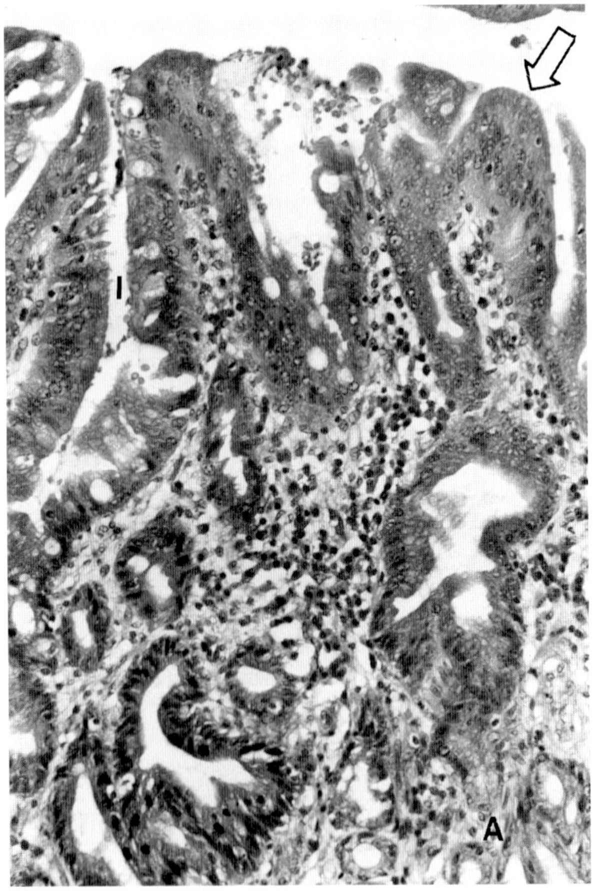

FIG. 12-4. Barrett's cancer in distal esophagus. Intestinal glands with goblet cells (I) and antral glands (A) are shown. The loss of nuclear polarity and distorted nucleocytoplasmic ratio in some superficial cells justifies the designation of moderate atypia *(arrow)*. (Hematoxylin & eosin stain, original magnification ×60.)

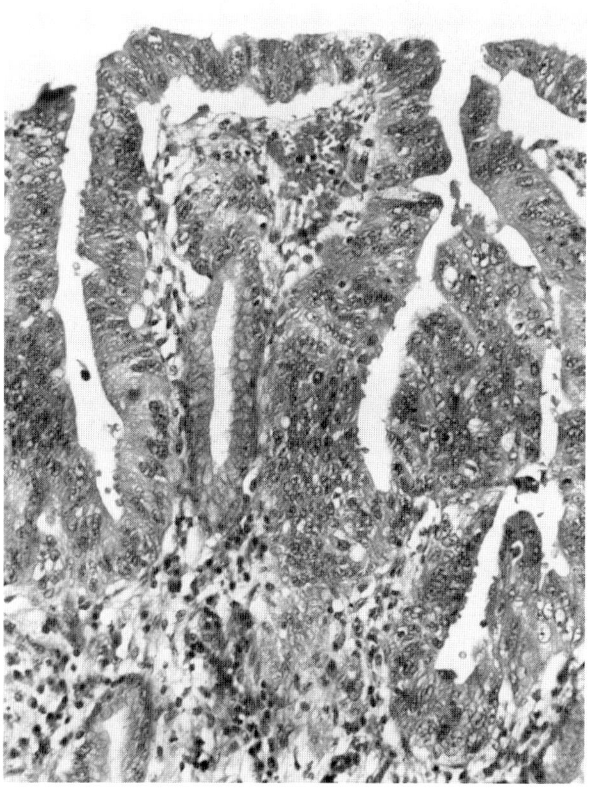

FIG. 12-5. Barrett's change. Nuclear enlargement, with pleomorphic cells showing papillary folding and loss of mucus production, constitute severe degree of dysplasia. (Hematoxylin & eosin stain, original magnification ×60.)

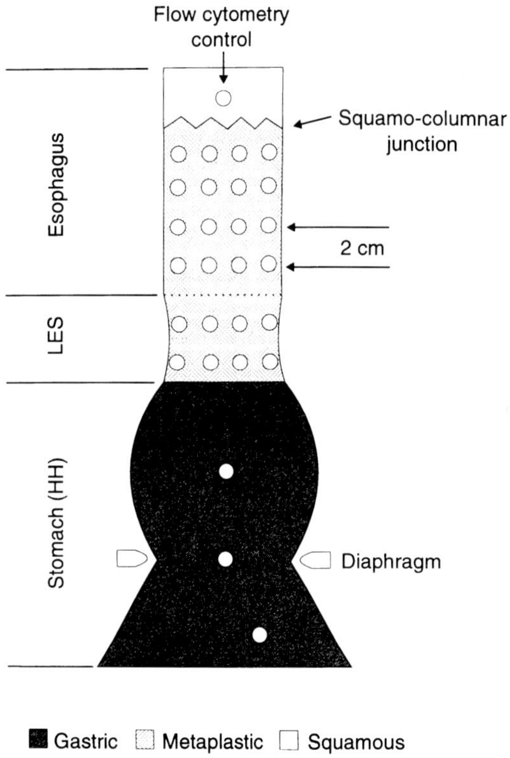

FIG. 12-6. Diagram showing preferred sites of biopsies of the distal esophagus and proximal stomach, to be used in assessing the presence and extent of Barrett's changes, and the degree of atypia in the metaplastic mucosa. *LES,* lower esophageal sphincter. (Courtesy of Dr. R. Haggitt, University of Washington Medical Center, Seattle, WA.)

extent of Barrett's change. Those patients with mild or no dysplasia should be followed at 3-year intervals, whereas those with dysplasia should be treated surgically. The optimal pattern of biopsy procedures necessary to rule out the presence of severe dysplasia is shown in Figure 12-6.

STOMACH

Adenocarcinoma

The three parts of the stomach—cardia, corpus, and pyloric antrum—give rise to tumors showing distinct epidemiologic,

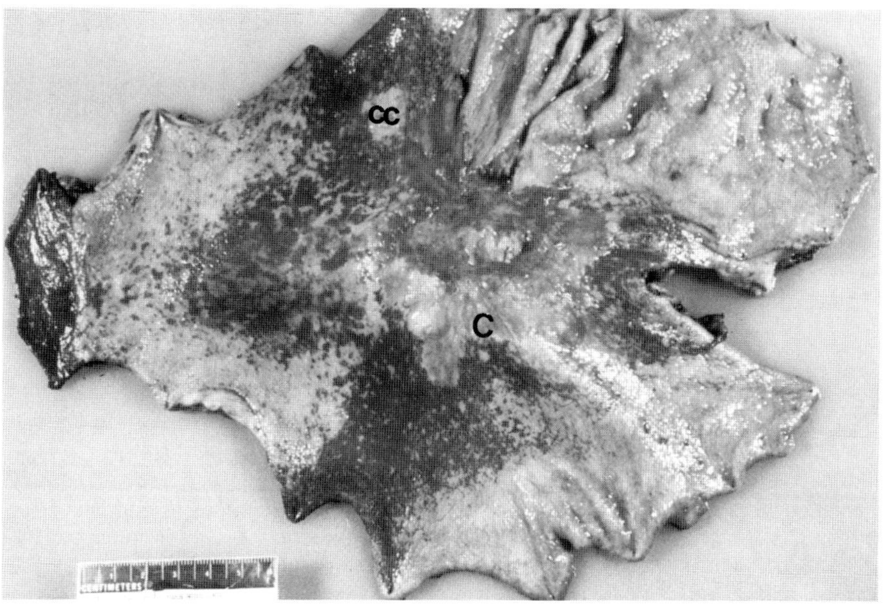

FIG. 12-7. A cancer (C) is present at the incisura on the lesser curvature of this subtotally resected stomach. A stain for alkaline phosphatase is positive in the duodenal cuff, along the lesser curvature at the junction of the corpus and antrum. The normal stomach mucosa is unstained, as is the cancer and a second multicentric cancer on the anterior wall (CC).

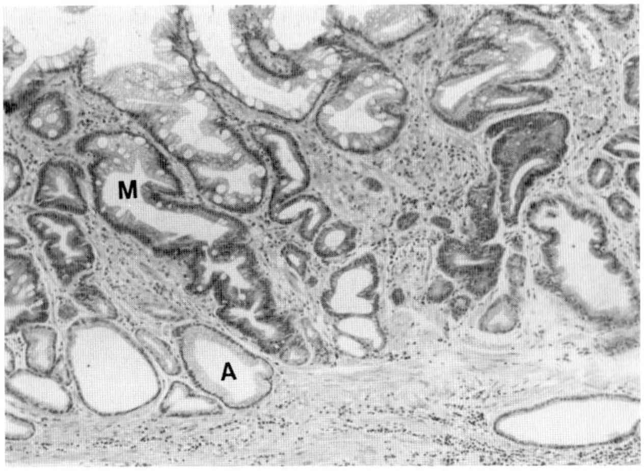

FIG. 12-8. Intestinal metaplasia of the antrum. The intestinalized glands (M) are lined by goblet and absorption cells. Antral glands (A) persist in the deepest portion of the antrum and are occasionally cystic. (Hematoxylin & eosin stain; original magnification ×40.)

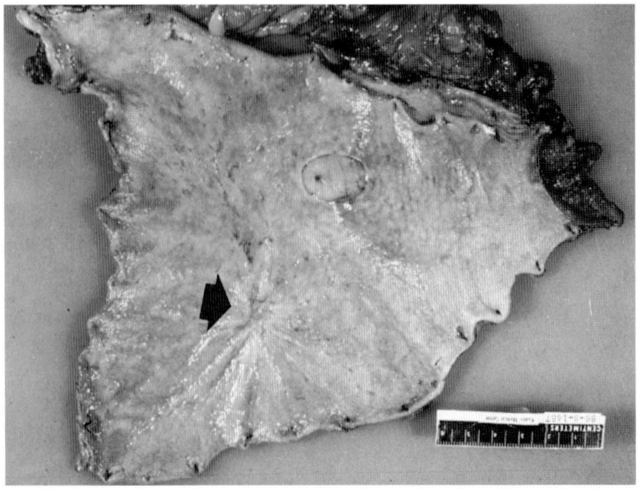

FIG. 12-10. A small diffuse cancer *(arrow)* is present on the anterior wall of the corpus of the nonintestinalized stomach. The center of the tumor is slightly depressed and the edge slightly elevated. Such tumors cannot be palpated externally if they are not fixed to the muscularis propria.

morphologic, and behavioral characteristics. Antral cancer predominates in populations exposed to the combined effects of poor nutrition and *Helicobacter pylori* infection.[9,10] Superficial gastritis and intestinal metaplasia precede its development (Figs. 12-7 and 12-8). These tumors may be well or poorly differentiated, but usually form recognizable glands (Fig. 12-9). The so-called intestinal-type carcinoma of Lauren[11] falls into this category. Antral tumors occur more frequently in men than women and are most common after 60 years of age. They commonly metastasize to the liver, where they form discrete masses. The risk of acquiring this tumor is inversely related to the maximum acid output and directly related to the antibody level against *H pylori*.[10] The serum pepsinogen group I is a good surrogate marker for the maximum acid output,[12] and a level below 25 ng/dL, combined with evidence of *H pylori* infection, identifies people who should be considered for endoscopic surveillance at 5-year intervals.

Cancers may develop in the nonatrophic corpus in association with superficial gastritis due to *H pylori* infection. These tumors are frequently composed of signet ring cells and show a diffuse growth pattern (Figs. 12-10 through 12-12). Late forms of this tumor spread diffusely through the abdominal cavity and do not form discrete liver metastases. They correspond to the diffuse-type stomach cancer in Lauren's classification.[12] Most of the stomach cancers in patients younger than 50 years of age fall into this category. They may present as Krukenberg tumors of the ovary. Early stages of this tumor may be so inconspicuous that they cannot be seen by the endoscopist or palpated by the

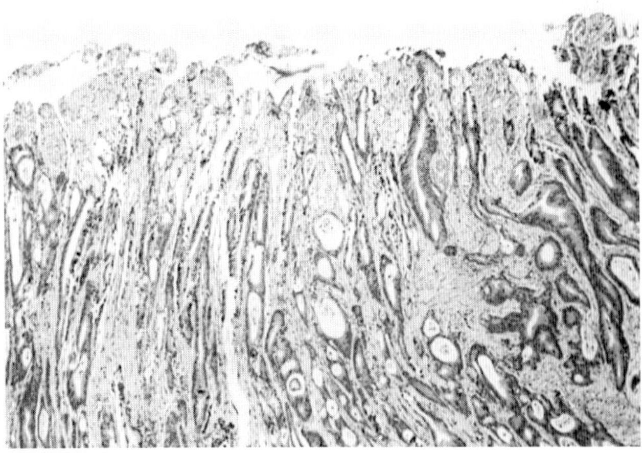

FIG. 12-9. Intestinal-type carcinoma, stomach. The term derives from the recognizable glands formed by the tumor, rather than its similarity to the small or large intestine. (Hematoxylin & eosin stain; original magnification ×40.)

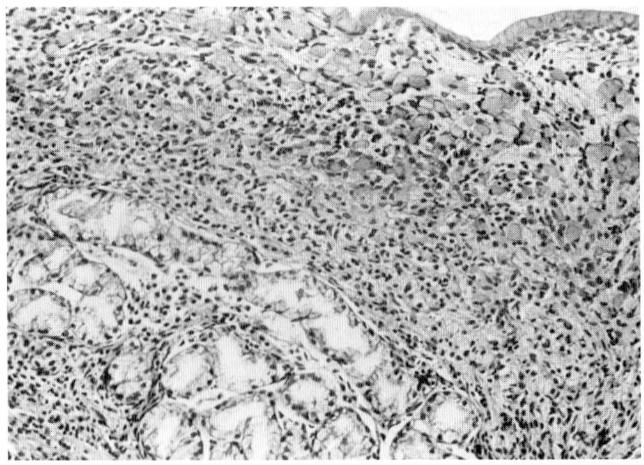

FIG. 12-11. The typical histologic pattern of an early diffuse tumor is characterized by replacement of the neck region of the gastric glands by formless aggregates of signet ring cells. The normal surface epithelium and the deeper portions of the glands persist. (Hematoxylin & eosin stain; original magnification ×40.)

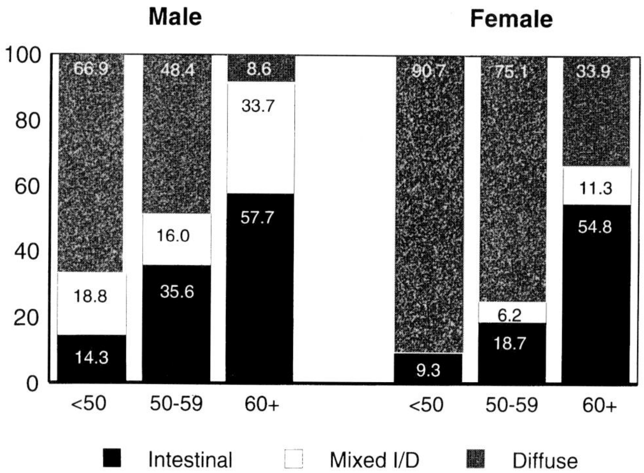

FIG. 12-12. The percentage distribution of diffuse and intestinal gastric cancers as a function of sex and age. Women are more likely to have diffuse cancers than men at early age levels, and are less likely to have mixed tumors.

surgeon. Such occult tumors are occasionally found in random biopsy samples of the stomach in younger patients with *H pylori* gastritis. The relative proportion of diffuse and intestinal tumors in the two sexes and at different ages is shown in Figure 12-12.

Cancer of the atrophic corpus may complicate autoimmune gastritis (pernicious anemia). Affected patients—usually women—show antral and intestinal metaplasia of the oxyntic mucosa. The decrease in acid production results in a rise in the pH of the stomach contents to levels approaching normality. Bacteria growing in the milieu may produce genotoxic products. This form of gastritis is associated with hyperplasia of the antral cells that produce gastrin (Fig. 12-13). The resulting increase in gastrin production has a trophic effect on the oxyntic mucosa

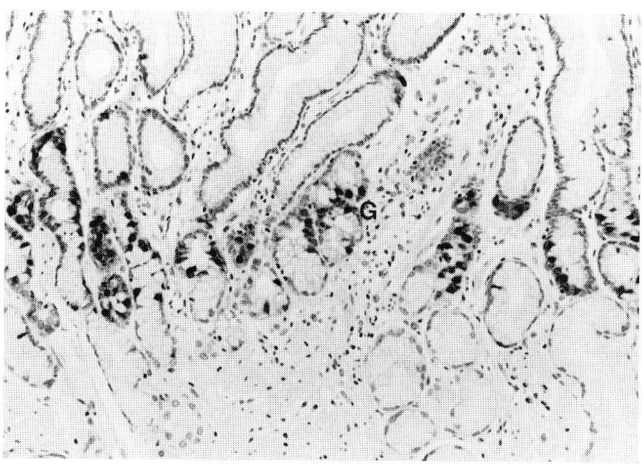

FIG. 12-13. Antral mucosa in patient with pernicious anemia. The antral mucosa is not affected by the inflammation that affects the oxyntic mucosa, but this immunohistochemical stain illustrates the conspicuous hyperplasia of the gastrin-producing cells (G) that develops in response to prolonged achlorhydria. (Hematoxylin & eosin stain; original magnification ×60.)

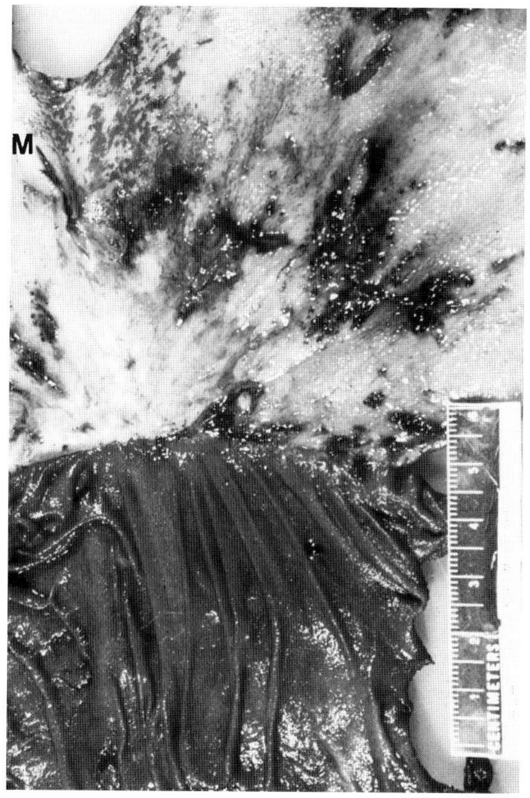

FIG. 12-14. Gross appearance of gastrojejunal anastomosis. The jejunal mucosa is uniformly stained for the presence of alkaline phosphatase. The residual gastric pouch shows patchy intestinal metaplasia (M). The mucosa is hemorrhagic, but otherwise unremarkable.

and its endocrine cells. The increased cell turnover that results from autoimmune destruction of gastric epithelium results in an increase in the number of cells in the S phase of the mitotic cycle, when they are most vulnerable to genotoxic agents. The trophic effect of gastrin on transformed cells increases their malignant potential.

Finally, cancer of the cardia arises in three distinct settings. First, it can arise in the residual stomach after subtotal gastrectomy for benign disease.[13] The increased risk does not appear until 20 years after surgery, but increases progressively thereafter. The risk is higher in women than men and is higher after gastrojejunostomy than after gastroduodenostomy. The tumors develop in a mucosa showing severe reflux gastritis, and may be very difficult to identify endoscopically (Figs. 12-14 and 12-15). Second, cancer of the cardia may occur among members of families affected by the hereditary nonpolyposis cancer syndrome,[14] as shown in Figures 12-16 and 12-17. Adenomatous polyps and cancer of the cardia may also occur in patients with familial polyposis who have escaped colorectal cancer as a result of prophylactic colectomy.[15] Third, as noted earlier, cancer of the cardia may also develop in the stomach of white men who are subject to the same risk factors that have been associated with adenocarcinoma of the distal esophagus.[16] This cancer is not related to *H pylori* infection.[10] Its rates have been stable or rising since 1940 in Western Europe and North America. This trend contrasts with that of cancer of the antrum, which has shown a dramatic decline in these areas.

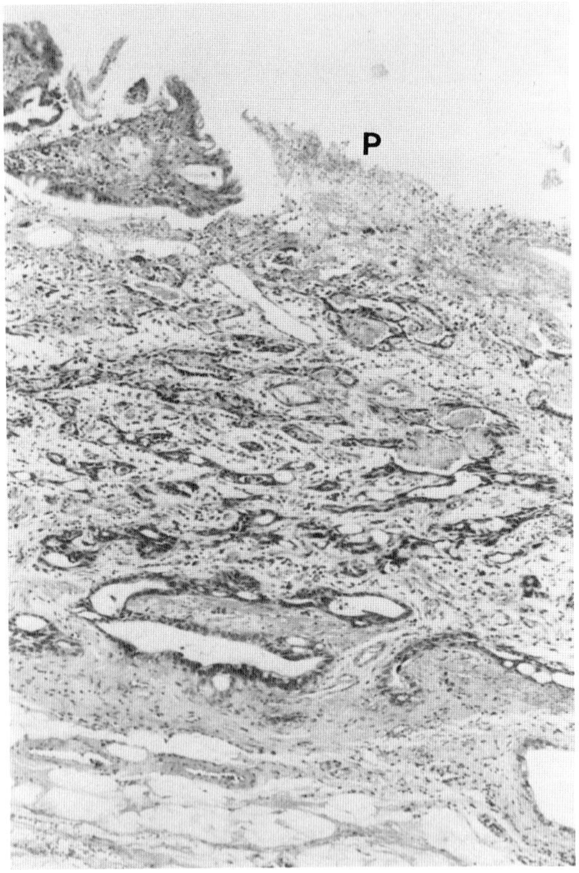

FIG. 12-15. Microscopic detail of mucosa form gastric pouch shown in Figure 12-14. The pyogenic membrane (P) on the surface marks the hemorrhagic areas seen in the gross specimen and covers groups of pleomorphic, anastomosing carcinomatous glands. (Hematoxylin & eosin stain; original magnification ×40.

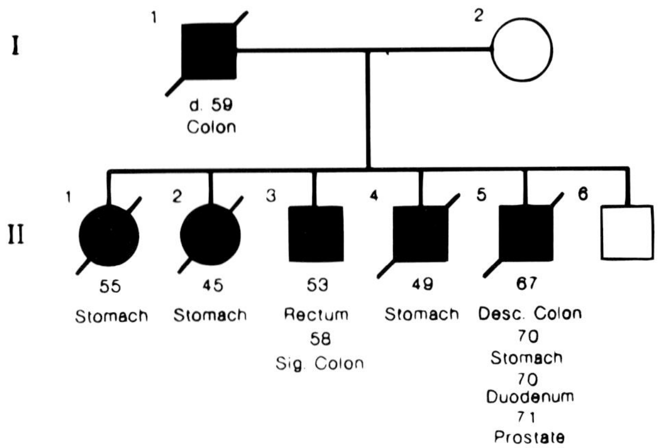

FIG. 12-17. The kindred of the patient whose stomach is illustrated in FIgure 12-16. The patient is number II 5. He had prior cancer of the descending colon and synchronous cancer of the duodenum.

It is reasonable to screen patients endoscopically for gastric cancer if they fall into one of the high-risk groups described earlier. The examination need not be more frequent than every 3 years because Japanese studies indicate that the median interval from the diagnosis of early cancer to dissemination is 37 months.[17] Patients in, or migrants from, countries at high risk for antral cancer (Japan, Korea, northeast China, Latin America, and Eastern Europe) should be screened if they give evidence of *H pylori* infection or have a pepsinogen group I level below 25 ng/dL. Their initial examination should include biopsies of any observed lesion and programmed biopsies from six sites in the stomach, as shown in Figure 12-18. It is important that each of these biopsy specimens be labeled as to site of origin, and sent to the pathologist in separate containers. This allows the examiner to estimate the surface area of chronic gastritis, a

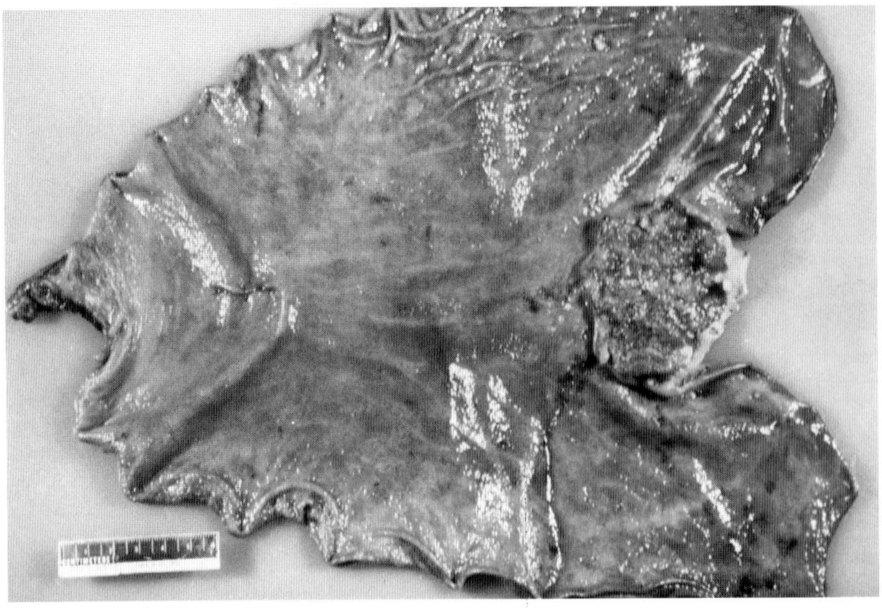

FIG. 12-16. Carcinoma of the cardia in a patient with familial gastric cancer. The tumor arises in a stomach free of intestinal metaplasia as determined by absence of alkaline phosphatase. The nonneoplastic mucosa showed no evidence of atrophy or inflammation.

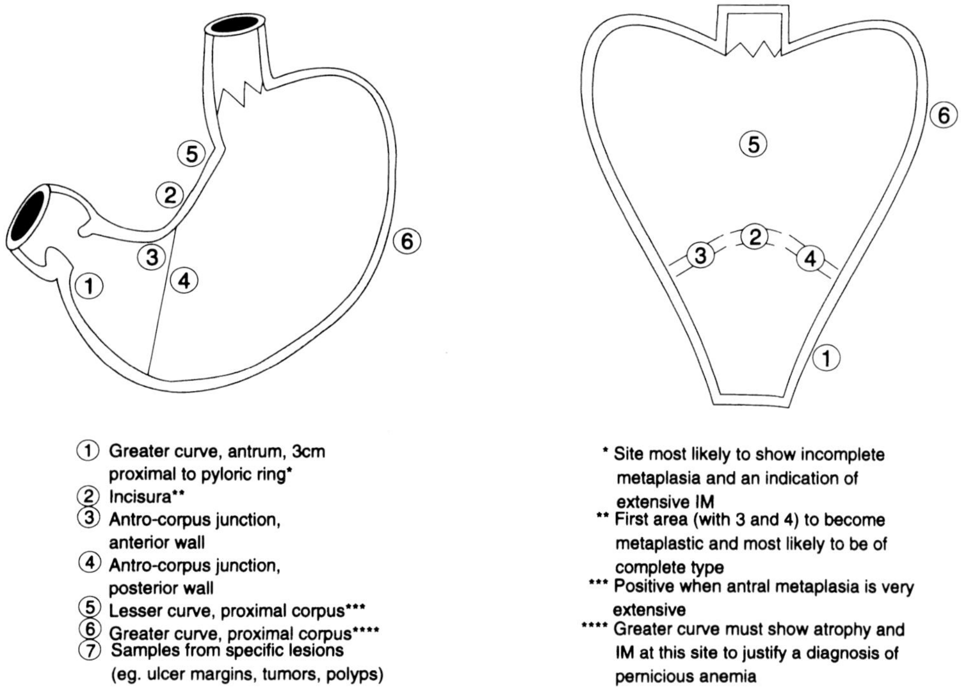

FIG. 12-18. Diagram showing recommended biopsy sites in a screening endoscopy. IM, intestinal metaplasia.

factor that is significantly and directly related to the risk of gastric cancer.[18] A diagnosis of pernicious anemia cannot be made unless the mucosa of the proximal greater curvature is affected by the process. An unlabeled biopsy specimen from this site could easily be mistaken for pyloric antrum because of the antral metaplasia that is characteristic of this condition. Finally, the precise localization of each biopsy specimen is especially important if one of the programmed biopsy samples contains a cancer that was unapparent to the endoscopist. Such a tumor will be just as difficult for the surgeon to identify and remove, and for the pathologist to find in the resected specimen.

Long-term survival after resection for gastric carcinoma is stage dependent, but shows wide international variation, with Japanese patients showing better stage-for-stage survival than patients in the United States.[19–23] This difference has been explained on the basis of ethnic differences in host–tumor relationships, or on the basis of the more radical lymph node resections that are standard procedures in Japan. A technical rather than a biologic basis for the difference is supported by a study that compared Japanese patients in Hawaii who were treated by conventional American methods with Japanese patients treated in Tokyo.[24] The radically treated Tokyo Japanese showed better stage-stratified survival than those in Hawaii, a difference that was statistically significant ($P = 0.0001$) in patients with stage III cancers. Lymphadenectomy-related stage migration or differing therapeutic efficacy could explain the survival differences in these two groups of Japanese patients. A biologic contribution to better Japanese survival is supported by stage-stratified survival differences among Japanese Americans when they are compared with U.S. whites in the SEER registries.[25] The overall relative 5-year survival of Japanese Americans in this study was 27%, compared to 15% for U.S. whites. This study found the greatest differences in survival in patients with stage I and II cancers. The Japanese 5-year survival was 92% and 69% for these stages, respectively, whereas the corresponding U.S. white rates were 66% and 44%.

Accurate staging of cancer in a resected specimen will follow if surgeon and pathologist make a cooperative effort to do so. The yield of lymph nodes that the pathologist can harvest from the specimen can be increased if the surgeon injects India ink into the perigastric tissues, as shown in Figure 12-19.[26] Radical lymph node dissection, if carried out according to Japanese protocols, requires that the source of all resected nodes be clearly identified. The fresh, unopened stomach should be sent to the laboratory as soon as it has been resected. After frozen sections have established disease-free margins, samples of fresh

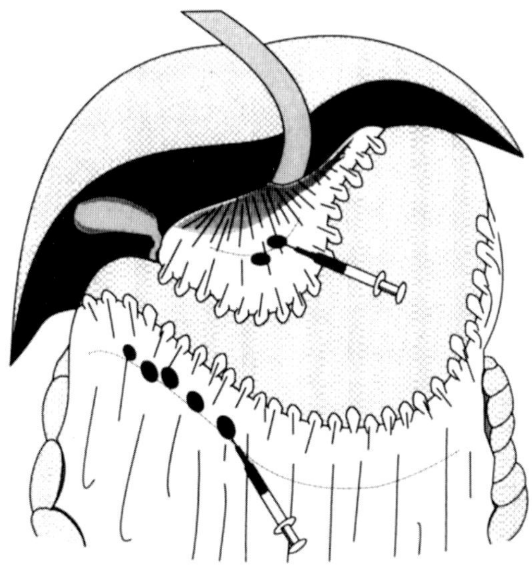

FIG. 12-19. Diagram showing technique used to highlight lymphatic drainage with India ink before resection. (Adapted from Maruyama K, Okabayoshi K, Kinoshita T. Progressin gastric surgery in Japan and its limit in radicality. World J Surg 1987:11;8.

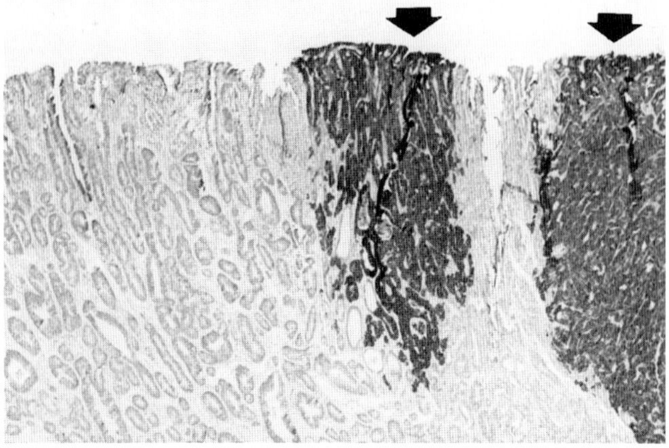

FIG. 12-20. This section is from a fairly well differentiated intestinal-type cancer that has not penetrated the submucosa. A single, 3-mm lymph node adjacent to the tumor contained a microscopic focus of metastatic cancer. Immunohistochemical stains identify two small clones *(arrows)* of cancer cells that are strongly labeled by antibody against epithelial growth factor receptor. (Original magnification ×40.)

tumor may be removed for flow cytometry or placed in frozen storage for molecular biology studies. After being opened along the greater curvature, the specimen should be pinned to a cork or paraffin plate and floated upside-down in a pan of buffered formaldehyde for at least 12 hours. The outer limits of the tumor are more easily defined in the fixed specimen, and small, unsuspected multicentric tumors may now come to light, especially if the specimen has been stained to demonstrate alkaline phosphatase. Alkaline phosphatase is normally not present in the stomach, and its presence signals areas of intestinal metaplasia while leaving cancerous mucosa unstained,[27] as shown in Figure 12-7. The pathologist should harvest as many nodes as possible from the greater and lesser curvatures, separately identifying those less than or more than 3 cm from the tumor. The

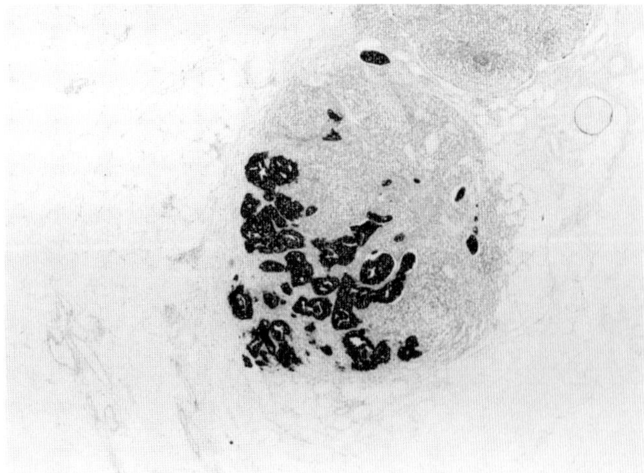

FIG. 12-21. The single lymph node metastasis from this tumor is strongly labeled for epithelial growth factor receptor, suggesting that it is derived from a subpopulation of similar cells in the primary tumor. (Original magnification ×20.)

tumor, or tumors, should be precisely located within the stomach. Future reviewers will appreciate a diagram or gross photograph that demonstrates this location.

The accuracy of estimates of the risk of recurrence may be improved if TNM staging is supplemented by immunohistochemistry. There is now good evidence that some gastric tumor markers, such as epithelial growth factor receptor (Figs. 12-20 and 12-21), predict high risk of recurrence,[28] and cytokeratin stains may highlight unapparent micrometastases in regional lymph nodes. It is time for these procedures to move from the research laboratories into the service sector.

Lymphoma

Gastric lymphoma accounts for approximately 50% of gastrointestinal lymphomas.[29] It differs from lymphomas at other gastrointestinal sites in three respects: high male : female ratio, better 5-year survival, and close association with *H pylori* infection.[30,31] It is possible that some gastric lymphomas are not actually neoplasms, but result from an exuberant, clonal B-cell response to *H pylori* infection. This concept is supported by the observation that some tumors resolve after appropriate antibiotic therapy.[32] High-grade gastric lymphomas with the potential for systemic spread do occur in populations with a high frequency of *H pylori* infection.[33] Pseudolymphoma must be distinguished from the real thing to avoid an unnecessary gastric resection. The tests that make this distinction include identification of *H pylori* infection (see Figs. 12-20 and 12-21), a therapeutic trial of antibiotics, and careful pathologic examination of the tumor. The pathologic study demands scrupulous management of biopsy specimens. Some tissue should be fixed immediately in B-5 fixative, and an equal amount of fresh tissue should be set aside for immunohistochemical cell typing.

CONCLUSION

It is apparent that the surgeon and the pathologist must interact if they are to extract the most reliable information from biopsy or resection specimens. The pathologist should receive biopsy specimens that are clearly identified as to their point of origin and fresh, unopened resection specimens that are delivered to the laboratory as soon as possible after they have been removed. The surgeon should receive a report that includes all of the information necessary to stage the tumor according to the guidelines of the American College of Surgeons. The laboratory should also be able to provide a menu of immunohistochemical markers to supplement these criteria. Finally, special procedures that may improve survival predictions, including wide, programmed lymph node dissections for esophageal and gastric cancer, require joint planning by surgeons and pathologists to manage properly the additional study material that these procedures generate.

REFERENCES

1. Day NE, Munoz N. Esophagus. In: Schottenfeld D, Fraumeni J, eds. Cancer epidemiology. 1st ed. Philadelphia: WB Saunders, 1982:556.
2. Tuyns AJ, Pequinot G, Jensen OM. Le cancer de l'oesophage en Ille-

et-Villiare en fonction des niveaux de consummation de l'acool et de tabac. Bull Cancer 1977;64:45.

3. Li JY. Epidemiology of esophageal cancer in China. Monogr Natl Cancer Inst 1982;63:113.
4. Miller BA, Riles LAG, Hankey BF, Kosary CL, Edwards BK, eds. Cancer statistics review 1973–1989. National Cancer Institute Publication No. 92-2789. Bethesda, MD: National Cancer Institute, 1992:VIII-6.
5. Baba M, Aikou T, Yoshinaka H, et al. Long term results of esophagectomy with three-field lymphadenectomy for carcinoma of the thoracic esophagus. Ann Surg 1993;219:310.
6. Wu G, Beer DG, Moore JH, et al. Sucrase-isomaltose gene expression in Barrett's esophagus and adenocarcinoma. Gastroenterology 1993; 105:837.
7. Westerveld BD, Pals G, Bosma A, et al. Gastric proteases in Barrett's esophagus. Gastroenterology 1987;93:744.
8. Rabinovitch PS, Reid BJ, Haggit RC, Norwood TH, Rubin CE. Progression to cancer in Barrett's esophagus with genomic instability. Lab Invest 1988;60:65.
9. Correa P. A tumor model for gastric carcinogenesis. Cancer Res 1988; 48:3554.
10. Stemmermann GN. The role of *H. pylori* in the etiology of gastric cancer. In: Devita V, Hellman S, Rosenberg SA, eds. Cancer prevention. Philadelphia: JB Lippincott, 1991:1.
11. Lauren T. The two histologic main types of gastric carcinoma: diffuse and so-called intestinal type carcinoma. Acta Pathol Microbiol Scand 1965;64:31.
12. Samloff IM, Secrist DM, Passaro E. Serum pepsinogen I levels and their relation to gastric acid secretion in patients with and without ulcer. Gastroenterology 1976;70:309.
13. Lundegard G, Adami HO, Helmick C, Zack M, Meirick D. Stomach cancer after partial gastrectomy for benign ulcer disease. N Engl J Med 1988;319:195.
14. Lynch H, Smyrk TC, Watson P, et al. Genetics, natural history, tumor spectrum and pathology of hereditary non polyposis cancer syndrome. Gastroenterology 1990;104:1535.
15. Spigelman AD Williams CB, Talbot IC, et al. Upper gastrointestinal cancer in patients with familial adenomatous polyposis. Lancet 1989; 1:783.
16. Wong H, Antonioli DA, Goldman H. Comparative features of gastric and esophageal adenocarcinomas. Hum Pathol 1986;17:482.
17. Tsukuma H, Mishima T, Oshim A. Prospective study of "early" gastric cancer. Int J Cancer 1983;31:421.
18. Kato,I, Tominaga S, Ito Y, et al. A prospective study of atrophic gastritis and stomach cancer risk. Jpn J Cancer Res 1992;83:1137.
19. Bearhs OH, Myers MH. Manual for staging of cancer. Philadelphia: JB Lippincott, 1988.
20. Wanebo H, Kennedy BJ, Chmiel J, et al. Cancer of the stomach: a patient care study by the American College of Surgeons. Ann Surg 1993;218:583.
21. Maruyama K. Surgical treatment and results of gastric cancer. Tokyo: National Cancer Press, 1987.
22. Miwa K. Evaluation of TNM classification of stomach cancer and a proposal for its rational stage grouping. Jpn J Clin Oncol 1984;14:385.
23. Nakajima T, Nishi M, Kajitani T. Improvement of treatment of gastric cancer with surgery and chemotherapy. Semin Surg Oncol 1991;7:365.
24. Hundahl S, Stemmermann GN, Oishi A. Racial factors cannot explain superior Japanese outcomes in stomach cancer. Arch Surg 1996;131: 170.
25. Young JL, Ries LJ, Pollack ES. Cancer patient survival among ethnic groups in the United States. J Natl Cancer Inst 1984;73:341.
26. Maruyama K, Okabayashi K, Kinoshita T. Progress in gastric surgery in Japan and its limits in radicality. World J Surg 1987;11:418.
27. Stemmermann GN, Hayashi T. Intestinal metaplasia of the gastric mucosa: a gross and microscopic study of its distribution in various disease states. J Natl Cancer Inst 1968;41:627.
28. Yasui W, Hata J, Yokozaki Y, et al. Interaction of epithelial growth factor and its receptor in progression of gastric cancer. Int J Cancer 1988;41:211.
29. Otter R, Bieger R, Kluin PM, et al. Primary gastrointestinal non-Hodgkin's lymphoma in a population based registry. Br J Cancer 1989;60: 745.
30. Wotherspoon AC, Ortiz-Hidalgo C, Falzon MR, Isaacsen PG. *Helicobacter pylori* and primary B-cell lymphoma. Lancet 1991;338:1175.
31. Parsonnet J, Friedman GD, Vandersteen DP, et al. *Helicobacter pylori* infection and the risk of gastric carcinoma. N Engl J Med 1991;325: 1127.
32. Wotherspoon AC, Doglioni C, Diss TC, et al. Regression of low grade primary lymphoma of mucosa associated lymphoid tissue after eradication of *Helicobacter pylori* infection. Lancet 1993;342:575.
33. Parsonnet J, Hansen S, Rodriguez L, et al. *Helicobacter pylori* and gastric lymphoma. N Engl J Med 1994;330:1267.

PART II

Esophageal Cancer

Surgery for Gastrointestinal Cancer: A Multidisciplinary Approach, edited by Harold J. Wanebo.
Lippincott-Raven Publishers, Philadelphia, © 1997.

CHAPTER 13

Endosonographic Evaluation of the Patient With Esophageal Carcinoma

Staging Considerations

Jacques Van Dam

The prognosis for patients with carcinoma of the esophagus remains poor despite aggressive combination therapies and radical surgical resection.[1–3] Attempts to improve the survival of patients with esophageal carcinoma have been confounded by the lack of effective therapeutic options in the later stages of the disease and an inability to identify patients accurately in the early stages. Ultrasound technology is a powerful diagnostic technique when applied to medical practice. Endoscopic ultrasonography combines the access of endoscopy with the diagnostic versatility of ultrasonography to offer perhaps the most noteworthy advance in gastrointestinal endoscopy since the early 1980s. This novel technique affords close-proximity imaging of the gastrointestinal tract and provides detailed images of the esophageal wall and its adjacent structures.[4] Therefore, endosonography is ideally suited for staging esophageal cancers.

Endosonography images the gastrointestinal tract wall as a five-layered structure of differing echogenicities (alternating hyperechoic and hypoechoic layers), although some high-frequency ultrasound transducers may image additional layers.[5,6] The endosonographically imaged layers correspond in general with mural histology (Table 13-1). Cystic structures are readily identified by endosonography, both in the esophagus and elsewhere in the gastrointestinal tract.[7–9] The thickness of the layers of the normal gastrointestinal tract is not an exact measure of histologic thickness because the endoscopic ultrasound images are a measure of time and not simply distance. Ultrasonographic thickness represents the time required for an ultrasonic pulse emitted by a transducer to travel to and return from a reflective tissue interface, rather than the actual distance between tissue and transducer. Time (t) is related to distance (d) by the equation d = vt, where v is the velocity of sound in the tissue being imaged. Moreover, sound-wave velocity varies with the acoustic impedance of each portion of the gastrointestinal tract wall. Interpretation of endosonographic images therefore requires an understanding of the physical characteristics of ultrasound as well as a knowledge of three-dimensional anatomy.

The approach to tumor staging is not a fixed science, but rather a dynamic process. Historically, as more was learned about the natural history of specific cancers, and as new technologies became available to diagnose and treat tumors, the classification and staging of cancer was amended to take advantage of such modern advances (eg, the various modifications of the Dukes' classification for staging colorectal cancer). Based on this premise, the American Joint Committee on Cancer and the International Union Against Cancer (UICC; Union Internationale Contre le Cancer) agreed in 1987 on a uniform classification system of malignancy, including esophageal cancer.[10–13] The result of this collaboration was the formulation of the new TNM classification, in which *T* refers to depth of penetration of the primary tumor into, or through the gastrointestinal tract wall, *N* refers to the status of regional lymph nodes with regard to malignant involvement, and *M* refers to the presence or absence of distant metastases (Table 13-2). The depth of tumor penetration and the existence of lymph node metastases are the most important factors for determining the prognosis and mode of treatment for patients with esophageal carcinoma.[14] Involvement of nonregional lymph nodes (eg, malignant involvement of celiac axis lymph nodes in patients with esophageal carcinoma) is considered metastatic disease (M1). Once classified, tumors are staged at all anatomic locations from stage 0 (best prognosis) to stage IV (poorest prognosis; Table 13-3).

ENDOSONOGRAPHIC EVALUATION OF DEPTH OF TUMOR PENETRATION (T STAGE)

Endosonography is highly accurate and superior to computed tomographic (CT) scan for the preoperative staging of esopha-

Jacques Van Dam: Brigham and Women's Hospital, 75 Francis Street, Boston, MA 02115

TABLE 13-1. *Correlation between echogenicity and esophageal mural morphology*

Mural component	Echogenicity
Superficial mucosa	Hyperechoic
Deep mucosa	Hypoechoic
Submucosa and acoustic interface between the submucosa and muscularis propria	Hyperechoic
Muscularis propria	Hypoechoic
Adventitia	Hyperechoic

geal carcinoma (Figs. 13-1 through 13-4; Tables 13-4 and 13-5).[15–22] However, endosonography is not a substitute for CT scan but rather a useful adjunct for the preoperative staging of esophageal cancer. There is a learning curve for the endosonographic staging of esophageal tumors, as noted by Rice and colleagues.[23,24] The accuracy for preoperative T staging in their first 28 cases was 59%, but improved to 81% in the next 52 patients evaluated.[23,24] Endosonography is accurate in identifying the early stages of disease and in detecting advanced, nonresectable esophageal carcinoma, although there is considerable interobserver variation.[25,26] The most difficult assessment is for T2 tumors, for which the accuracy is poorest.[22] Assessment of vascular involvement in patients with esophageal cancer has important implications regarding the approach to therapy. Compared with CT scan, endosonography provides a more sensitive and reliable determination of local vascular involvement.[27] The differentiation of mucosal and submucosal disease in early esophageal cancer (T1) is problematic and has led to overstaging in some cases. Endosonographic evaluation of patients with superficial esophageal carcinoma has demonstrated an overall accuracy of 72% for T staging.[28]

The addition of high-resolution ultrasound probes for staging esophageal carcinoma has provided mixed results.[29,30] The ultrasound probes contain transducers with frequencies of up to (and sometimes more than) 15 to 20 MHz. These instruments may provided highly detailed images of superficial carcinomas, but lack the ability to image deeply into the tissue adjacent to the esophagus and thus usually are incapable of assessing regional lymph node metastases.[29] On average, 20-MHz probes penetrate no deeper than 2 cm.[29] In addition, orientation when imaging from the stomach (to assess for celiac axis lymphadenopathy) may be problematic.[30]

TABLE 13-2. *American Joint Committee on Cancer (AJCC)/International Union Against Cancer (UICC) classification of esophageal cancer*

PRIMARY TUMOR (T)

- TX Primary tumor cannot be assessed
- T0 No evidence of primary tumor
- Tis Carcinoma in situ
- T1 Tumor invades lamina propria or submucosa
- T2 Tumor invades muscularis propria
- T3 Tumor invades adventitia
- T4 Tumor invades adjacent structures

REGIONAL LYMPH NODES (N)

- NX Regional lymph nodes cannot be assessed
- N0 No regional lymph node metastasis
- N1 Regional lymph node metastasis

DISTANT METASTASIS (M)

- MX Presence of distant metastasis cannot be assessed
- M0 No distant metastasis
- M1 Distant metastasis

From Beahrs OH, Henson DE, Hutter RVP, et al, eds. Manual for Staging of Cancer, 4th ed. American Joint Committee on Cancer. Philadelphia: JB Lippincott, 1988.

TABLE 13-3. *AJCC/UICC staging of esophageal cancer*

STAGE GROUPING			
Stage 0	Tis	N0	M0
Stage I	T1	N0	M0
Stage IIA	T2	N0	M0
	T3	N0	M0
Stage IIB	T1	N1	M0
	T2	N1	M0
Stage III	T3	N1	M0
	T4	Any N	M0
Stage IV	Any T	Any N	M1

From Beahrs OH, Henson DE, Hutter RVP, et al, eds. Manual for Staging of Cancer, 4th ed. American Joint Committee on Cancer. Philadelphia: JB Lippincott, 1988.

ENDOSONOGRAPHIC EVALUATION OF LYMPH NODE METASTASES (N STAGE)

The endosonographic assessment of lymph node metastases has been shown to be more accurate than CT scan (Tables 13-6 and 13-7). However, the precise differentiation of malignant from benign lymph nodes remains problematic. Unlike CT scan, which can determine only lymph node size, endoscopic ultrasonography provides additional information, including lymph node shape, border characteristics, and central echogenicity[31] (Fig. 13-5). However, micrometastases, readily detectable by histologic evaluation, may not produce endosonographically detectable changes, leading to understaging, and large-sized, inflammatory lymph nodes may be incorrectly classified as metastatic and therefore overstaged. Attempts to classify lymph nodes by specific endosonographic features have improved the accuracy of lymph node classification but are cumbersome, subjective, and have not yet been widely studied.[32,33] Heintz and colleagues used computer-supported B-mode analysis (ProgramMicroscale; Digithurst, Nuremberg, Germany) to evaluate lymph node characteristics in vitro on resected specimens of patients with esophageal and gastric carcinoma.[34] However, subjective evaluation or computer analysis did not reliably distinguish benign from malignant lymph nodes.[34] Catalano and associates developed a system of analysis in which four endosonographic characteristics of lymph nodes (size, shape, border demarcation, and central echo pattern) were evaluated[32] (see Fig. 13-5). Sensitivity and specificity were 89.1% and 91.7%, respectively, when such stringent criteria were used. The four criteria were demonstrated to be additive in their ability to predict lymph node metastases, and when all four criteria were present, accuracy in predicting lymph node metastases was reportedly 100%.[32]

However, all four criteria were observed in regional lymph nodes only in a minority of cases. An association between depth

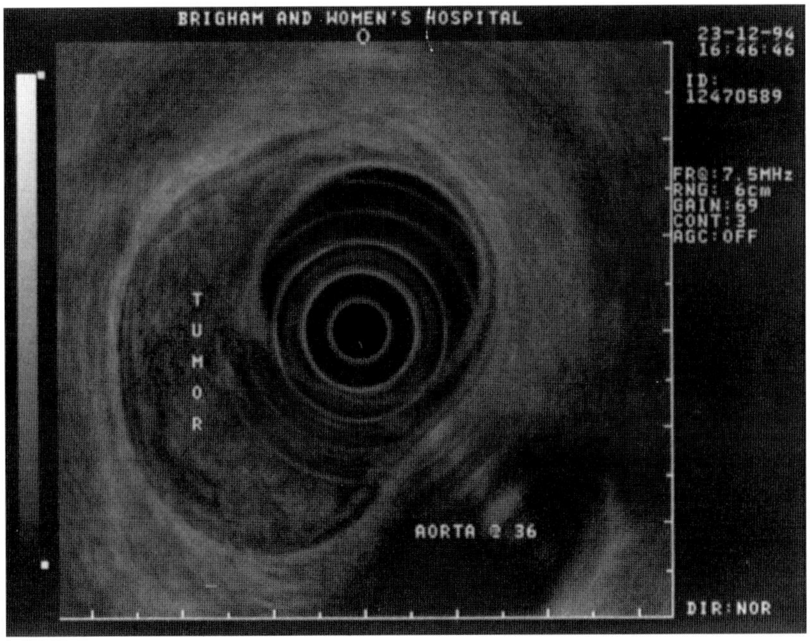

FIG. 13-1. Endosonograph of a patient with esophageal cancer. The echoendoscope produces artifactual concentric rings noted in the center of image. The anechoic area surrounding the ultrasound transducer is created by a water balloon placed over the transducer to provide acoustic coupling with the tumor. The water balloon is displaced anteriorly by the bulky tumor. The tumor is noted on the left of the endosonograph and is relatively hypoechoic. The aorta is noted in the bottom right of the endosonograph. The orientation of the image is similar to that of a chest CT scan in which the spine would appear posteriorly (at the bottom of the image).

of tumor penetration (T stage) and lymph node metastasis (N stage) may aid in reliably predicting lymph node metastases. In a review of the association between T stage and N stage for 103 patients with surgically resected specimens of esophageal carcinoma, lymph node involvement, given as a percentage, increased with the depth of tumor penetration as follows: Tis (n = 4) N1 (0%); T1 (n = 14) N1 (14.3%); T2 (n = 18) N1 (33.3%); T3 (n = 60) N1 (73.3%); T4 (n = 7) N1 (85.7%).[35] Similarly, in their series of over 400 cases, Dittler and coworkers reviewed the accuracy of endosonography for assessing lymph node metastases and noted that the incidence of lymph node metastases increased with advancing T stage (T1: 4%; T2: 52%; T3: 82%; T4: 91%).[36] Therefore, tumor involvement of lymph nodes increases with advancing T stage, and this may be one of the most sensitive indicators of lymph node metastases.[35,36] Metastatic lymph nodes located in the region of the celiac axis indicate metastatic disease (M1) for patients with esophageal cancer (Fig. 13-6).

Endoscopic ultrasonography is not equivalent to histologic assessment of sampled tissue, however, and the knowledge that lymph node involvement with tumor increases with depth of tumor penetration provides only an indirect or statistical advantage in determining tumor stage. Newer, more direct approaches to regional lymph node evaluation include endoscopic ultrasound-guided fine-needle aspiration of suspected lymph nodes. The Pentax/Hitachi FG-32UA ultrasound endoscope (Pentax

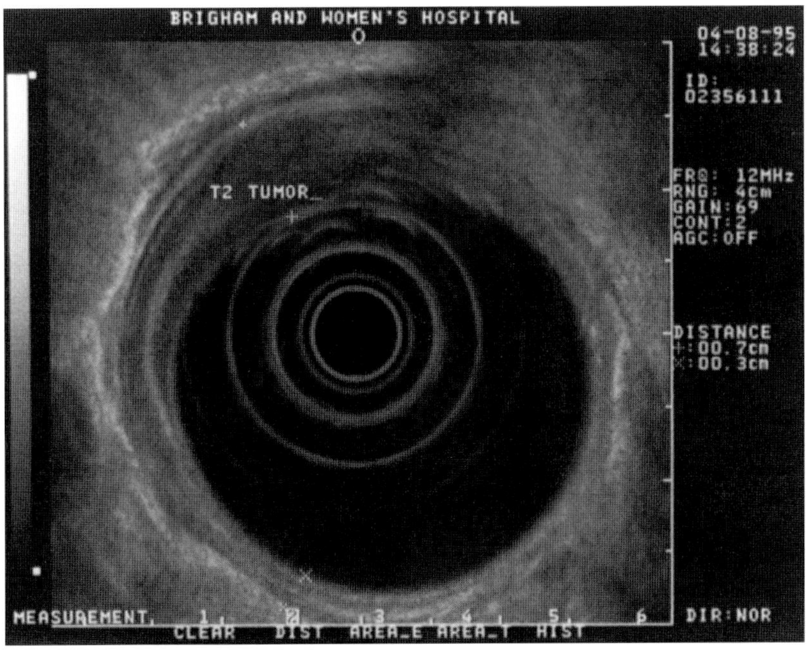

FIG. 13-2. Endosonograph of a patient with a T2 adenocarcinoma of the esophagus. The normal five layers of the esophageal wall may be seen at the bottom of the image. The wall thickness measures 3 mm. The tumor is noted in the "11 o'clock" position and penetrates 7 mm into the muscularis propria but does not penetrate the adventitia.

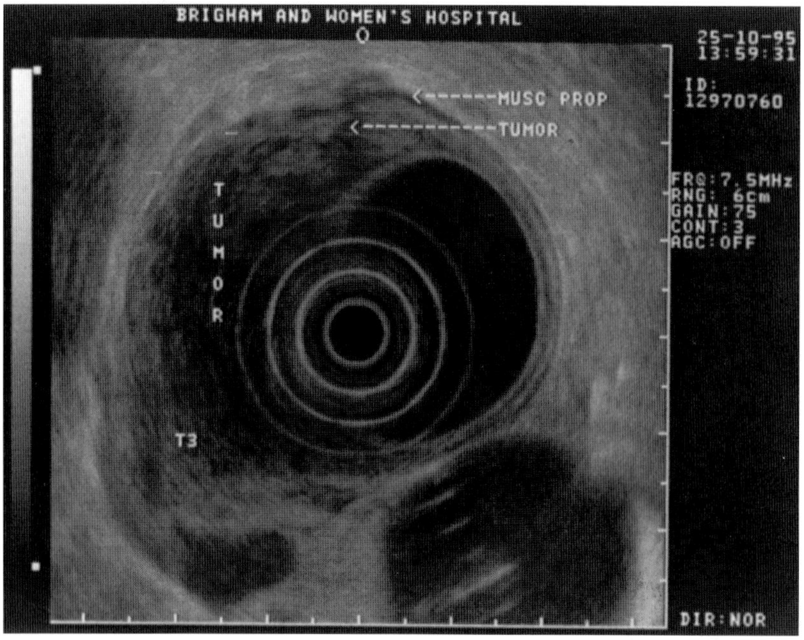

FIG. 13-3. Endosonograph of a patient with a T3 esophageal cancer. The normal-appearing five layers of the esophageal wall may be seen on the right side of the image. The fourth hypoechoic layer, the muscularis propria, is labeled. On the left side of the image, the tumor is observed penetrating beyond the adventita (T3). The aorta is the round, hypoechoic structure located at "5 o'clock" on the image.

Precision Instruments, Orangeburg, New York) is designed to permit ultrasound scanning parallel to the long axis of the insertion tube and, thereby, ultrasound-guided tissue sampling. Preliminary reports using this system are promising, and the safety and efficacy of this exciting new technology require additional study.[37,38] Wegener and colleagues reported the use of endoscopic ultrasound-guided fine-needle aspiration for mass lesions in the dorsal mediastinum in nine patients.[38] The size of the lesion on CT scan or endoscopic ultrasound was less than 2 cm in four patients. Endoscopic ultrasound-guided fine-needle aspiration revealed malignancy in seven of the nine patients, benign lymph node enlargement in one, and a dystrophic thyroid gland in one. Thus, endoscopic ultrasound-guided fine-needle aspiration may provide enhanced sensitivity and specificity for the assessment of periesophageal mass lesions.

The most accurate and effective approach to esophageal tumor staging is the combination of endosonography and CT scan. Using this approach, CT scan should be performed first to detect distant metastases (M stage). If no distant metastases are detected, endosonography should be performed to determine depth of tumor penetration and the presence of regional lymph adenopathy (T, N stages). The role of regional lymph node assessment by thoracoscopy is under investigation, and preliminary results are promising.[39] The relative safety and efficacy of this invasive technique are the focus of intense investigation. The relative merits of thoracoscopy versus endoscopic ultra-

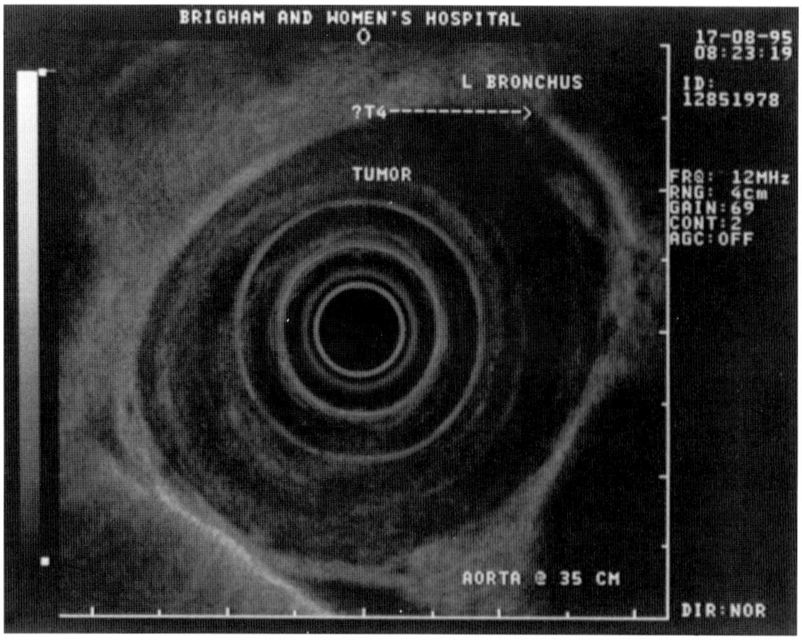

FIG. 13-4. Endosonograph of a patient with esophageal cancer. At high frequency scanning (12 MHz), enhanced resolution imaging is obtained. The tumor is observed immediately adjacent to the left bronchus suggesting tumor involvement of the adjacent structure (T4).

TABLE 13-4. *Preoperative endosonographic assessment of T-Stage**

Accuracy	Number of patients	Reference
59%	28	Rice et al., 1991[23]
75%	28	Yoshikane et al., 1994[28]
77%	82	Soquet et al., 1992[18]
79%	63	Kallimanis, et al., 1995[51]
82%	45	Fok et al., 1992[69]
85%	739	Souquet et al., 1994[22]
86%	63	Grimm et al., 1993[70]
86%	167	Dittler et al., 1994[44]
90%	67	Grimm et al., 1992[71]

* Compared with histopathological staging of the resected specimen.

sound have not yet been determined, and the results of trials comparing the two techniques are anticipated. The addition of endoscopic ultrasound-guided fine-needle aspiration has revolutionized the endoscopic assessment of regional lymph nodes for patients with esophageal cancer. However, more studies carefully assessing the safety and efficacy of the technique are required.

ENDOSONOGRAPHIC EVALUATION OF THE PATIENT WITH ESOPHAGEAL CANCER AFTER MEDICAL–SURGICAL THERAPY

Despite improved surgical technique and preoperative and postoperative adjuvant therapy, recurrence of disease remains the most common cause of mortality in patients with esophageal cancer. Methods for patient surveillance after surgery or adjuvant therapy include patient history (eg, dysphagia, weight loss), upper gastrointestinal contrast radiograph (barium swallow), endoscopy with biopsy, and CT scan. Endosonography has been used with variable success to detect residual tumor infiltration after medical treatment of esophageal cancer in the absence of endoscopic lesions.[40–44] Nousbaum and colleagues studied 34 patients with inoperable esophageal cancer using endosonography and CT scan before medical treatment. In this study, patients were considered inoperable because of distant metastasis (50%), poor general condition (42%), or concurrent cancer (8%). Ten patients receiving chemotherapy and radiation therapy had a complete resolution of endoscopically detectable tumor, including endoscopic biopsy specimens negative for residual tumor. Combination therapy consisted of chemotherapy (three cycles of fluorouracil 800 mg/m^2 per day for 5 days, and cisplatinum 70 mg/m^2 per day on day 2 of the cycle) and radiation therapy (three cycles of 3 Gy daily for 5 days). When endosonography suggested the persistence of tumor infiltration in patients who were endoscopically negative and biopsy negative for tumor, local tumor recurrence or distant metastases appeared within a few months. Alternatively, when endosonography failed to detect residual tumor in these patients, no tumor recurrence or progression was observed within 8 months, suggesting that endosonography is superior to endoscopy with biopsy and CT scan for assessing response of esophageal cancer to medical therapy.[42]

In contrast, Dittler and coworkers examined 25 patients with T3 esophageal or gastroesophageal junction carcinomas who received either three to six cycles of chemotherapy (etoposide-doxorubicin-cisplatin or cisplatin-leucovorin-etoposide-fluorouracil) or combined chemotherapy-radiation therapy (fluorouracil and 30 to 60 Gy).[41] All patients underwent endosonographic staging before and after medical therapy, followed by surgical resection. In all cases but one (T4), restaging resulted in the tumor being classified once again as a T3 tumor. However, histopathologic examination of the resected specimen after therapy and restaging revealed T0 (no tumor cells) in 2 cases, T1 in 1 case, T2 in 12 cases, T3 in 7 cases, and T4 in 3 cases. Dittler and coworkers concluded that endosonographic restaging of esophageal cancers was not a reliable predictor of tumor response to combination chemotherapy-radiation therapy.[41] Similarly, Catalano and associates,[40] and Souquet and colleagues,[18] and others[43,44] independently demonstrated that endosonographic surveillance after surgery with or without adjuvant chemotherapy-radiation therapy was limited by imaging artifact.[18,40] Specifically, interpretation of endosonographic imaging was impeded by hypoechoic esophageal wall thickening that was the result of either surgical artifact in the region of the anastomosis or benign inflammation or fibrosis.[18,40] Thus, endosonography appears to be sensitive but relatively nonspecific in detecting anastomotic recurrence of esophageal cancer.

TABLE 13-5. *Endosonography compared with CT scan for preoperative T-staging of esophageal carcinoma*

Accuracy EUS	Accuracy CT	Number of patients	Reference
76%	49%	41	Hordijk et al., 1993[49]
82%	50%	28	Kalantzis et al., 1992[72]
89%	59%	74	Tio et al., 1989[20]

ENDOSONOGRAPHY IN PATIENTS WITH HIGH-GRADE MALIGNANT STRICTURES

Most patients with esophageal carcinoma present late in the course of their disease. The relative elasticity of the esophagus and its anatomic location within the chest, free of restricting adjacent organs or bony structures, allows for significant tumor growth before the onset of symptoms. Thus, patients often remain relatively free of symptoms until the tumor has grown to a relatively advanced stage, at which time it may produce dysphagia, odynophagia, weight loss, or bleeding. Patients with high-grade malignant strictures represent a subgroup of up to 20% to 44% of patients with esophageal carcinoma (Table 13-8).[18,20,23,45–50] In a study of 79 patients with esophageal carcinoma who underwent preoperative staging using endoscopic ultrasonography, 21% patients (26.6%) presented with high-grade malignant stricture defined as a tumor obstruction precluding passage of an echoendoscope without prior dilatation.[48] Nineteen of the 21 patients (91%) had stage III or IV disease as determined by histopathologic assessment of the surgical specimen. Patients with high-grade malignant stricture were significantly more likely to have a relatively advanced stage of disease (stage III and IV; $P < 0.05$) compared with patients presenting with less severe malignant strictures and subse-

TABLE 13-6. *Preoperative endosonographic assessment of lymph node metastases*

Sensitivity	Specificity	Accuracy	Number of patients	Reference
70%	70%	70%	28	Rice et al., 1991[23]
58%	85%	72%	28	Yoshikane et al., 1994[28]
75%	70%	73%	167	Dittler et al., 1994[44]
		79%	739	Soquet et al., 1994[22]
90%	72%	83%	47	Grimm et al., 1992[71]
90%	77%	86%	63	Grimm et al., 1993[70]

quently found to have a relatively earlier stage of disease (stage 0, I, or II). The approximate percentages of patients in each stage reported in this study were similar when a larger number of patients were included in the series.[50] Attempts to stage esophageal tumors from the region proximal to a stenosis (incomplete staging) have poor overall accuracy, usually less than 50%.[48–50] Thus, the presence of malignant strictures severe enough to prevent passage of the echoendoscope would appear to represent an important prognostic factor.

A single, subsequent retrospective study suggested that esophageal dilatation before endoscopic ultrasound staging of patients with esophageal cancer was safe.[51] Kallimanis and associates reported a 0% perforation rate and suggested that morbidity should be low if care was taken in dilating patients with high-grade malignant strictures sufficiently to pass the echoendoscope.[51] Additional reports, however, have supported and the initial suggestion that aggressive dilatation may result in esophageal perforation.[52] Thus, most endosonographers now suggest that esophageal dilatation to achieve passage of the echoendoscope for staging is not warranted and poses a risk of esophageal perforation that outweighs the benefit of staging.[47,48,50,52,53]

The high-frequency (20 MHz) ultrasound probe is an alternative method for the endosonographic evaluation of patients with high-grade malignant strictures. In one study of such patients evaluated using the endosonographic probe, 13 of 14 patients were staged preoperatively as having at least a T2 tumor when the cancer was demonstrated to penetrate through the muscularis propria.[54] In a similar study, Grimm and colleagues used a wire-guided endosonographic probe (7.5-MHz transducer; 7.9-mm outer diameter) to evaluate 11 patients with high-grade malignant strictures.[55] The results demonstrated the probe to be safe and useful in that the tumor, esophageal wall layers, and regional lymph nodes could be visualized in all patients with no complications reported.[55] Follow-up studies by Grimm in a larger number of patients with malignant high-grade esophageal stenosis (n = 27) demonstrated all patient to have either a T3 or T4 tumor (63% or 37%, respectively).[56] In another study, Souquet and coworkers successfully used the "mini-probe" in 10 of 11 patients in whom preoperative endosonography using the dedicated echoendoscope could not be completed because of stenosing tumors.[18] However, in this report, the limited depth of penetration provided by the high-frequency ultrasound probe precluded correct classification of many periesophageal lymph nodes.[18] Continued refinement of ultrasound probes, including the development of nonoptical linear array probes,[57] may eventually yield a tool capable of reliably staging tumors not evaluable by dedicated echoendoscopes.

TABLE 13-7. *Endosonography compared with CT scan for preoperative N-staging of esophageal carcinoma*

Accuracy EUS	Accuracy CT	Number of patients	Reference
72%	46%	28	Kalantzis et al., 1992[72]
74%	58%	82	Soquet et al., 1992[18]
80%	51%	74	Tio et al., 1989[20]

IMPACT OF ENDOSONOGRAPHIC EVALUATION OF PATIENTS WITH ESOPHAGEAL CARCINOMA

Endosonography has an impact on the clinical management of patients with esophageal carcinoma by providing accurate pretherapeutic staging information, aiding in the prognosis of patients presenting with variable stages of the disease, and aiding in posttreatment evaluation. Accurate preoperative staging of esophageal cancer is useful only if the results of such staging have an impact on treatment.[58] When surgery is considered the only therapeutic modality, patients benefit from endosonographic evaluation only when the results of such evaluation demonstrate advanced disease, and surgery is thereby avoided.[59] When palliation is the only treatment modality under consideration, the role of endoscopic ultrasonography is limited.[22]

Endoscopic ultrasonography has been shown to predict accurately the outcome of patients undergoing surgery for cancer of the esophagus or gastroesophageal junction.[59] In a prospective analysis of 86 patients who underwent preoperative staging using endoscopic ultrasonography, patients with no endosonographic evidence for regional lymph node metastases, N0 (n = 17), had a median survival of 28 months, whereas patients who were endosonographically determined to have lymph node metastases, N1 (n = 60), had a median survival of 10 months, and patients in whom celiac axis lymph nodes metastases were detected by endosonography, M1 (n = 13), had a median survival of 3 months.[59] This study showed that the outcome for patients with esophageal or gastroesophageal junction cancer is strongly related to the results of endosonographic staging. Endoscopic ultrasound may also be used to evaluate patients with cancer metastatic to the esophagus, although its role in such patients has been less well characterized.[60]

ENDOSONOGRAPHIC EVALUATION OF THE PATIENT WITH BARRETT'S ESOPHAGUS

Barrett's esophagus is a condition in which the normal squamous epithelial lining of the esophagus is replaced by metaplastic columnar epithelium. Esophageal cancer is 30 to 40 times

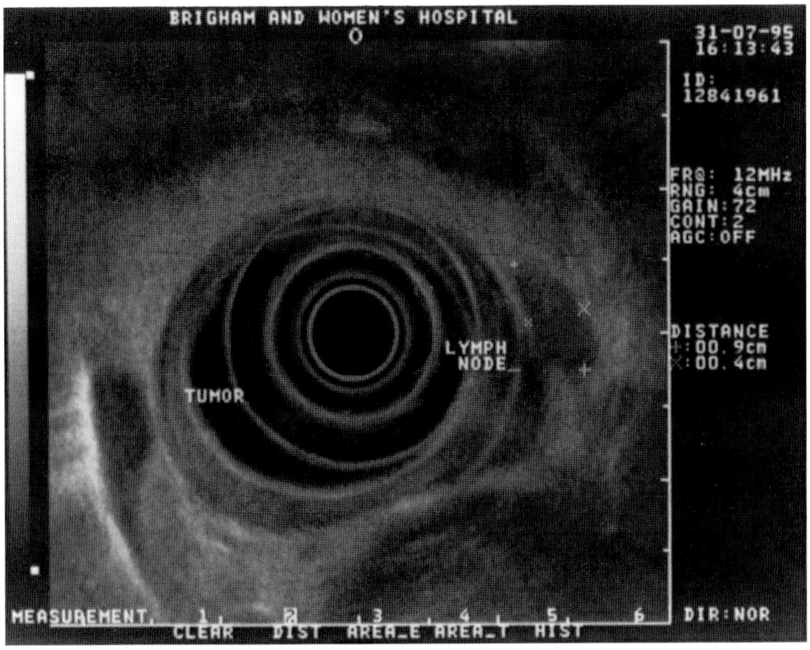

FIG. 13-5. Endosonograph of a regional lymph node in a patient with esophageal cancer. The lymph node is small (less than 1 cm), elongated, not hypoechoic, with an indistinct "fuzzy" border. These four endosonographic criteria suggest benignity.

more likely to develop in patients with Barrett's esophagus than in the general population.[61] There is compelling evidence to suggest that esophageal carcinoma develops in patients with Barrett's esophagus through a premalignant stage of dysplasia.[62,63] The time course for the progression of high-grade dysplasia to carcinoma is unknown, but unsuspected carcinoma has been found in 33% to 38% of resected specimens when esophagectomy is performed for Barrett's esophagus and high-grade dysplasia.[61,64–66] The goal of endoscopic surveillance of Barrett's esophagus is to detect neoplastic lesions by endoscopic biopsy that may not be apparent by gross endoscopic inspection. High-grade dysplasia and adenocarcinoma in Barrett's esophagus have been detected in endoscopically normal-appearing mucosa.[67] There currently is no consensus regarding the optimum management of patients with Barrett's esophagus and high-grade dysplasia because the natural history of the metaplasia-dysplasia-carcinoma sequence is variable.

Because endoscopic ultrasound obtains high-resolution images of the esophageal wall, it has been suggested that endosonography may be useful in detecting early carcinoma in patients with Barrett's esophagus and high-grade dysplasia.[62] To date, only a limited number of patients with Barrett's esophagus have been endosonographically assessed. Dancygier and Classen reported the results of four patients with Barrett's esophagus eval-

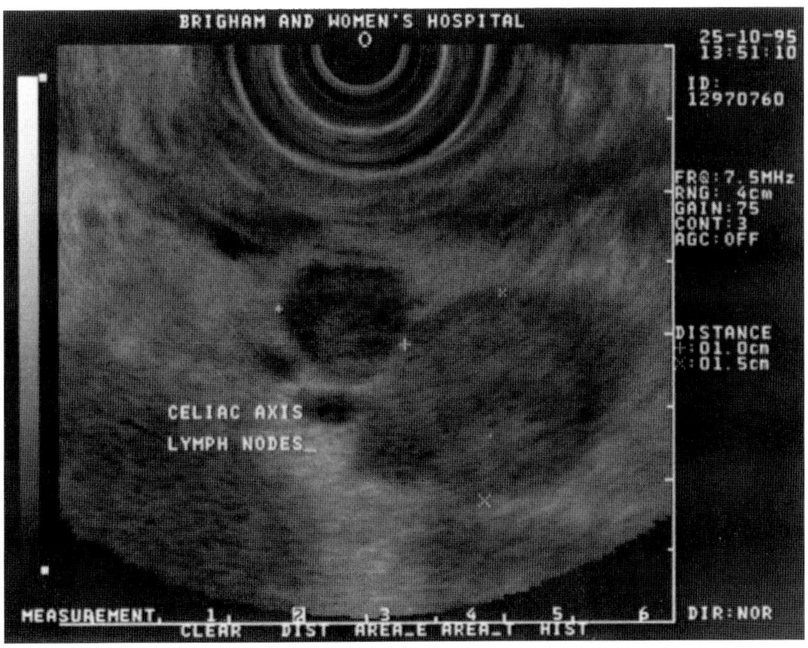

FIG. 13-6. Two large (1.0 and 1.5 cm, respectively) round lymph nodes in the region of the celiac axis. Celiac lymphadenopathy indicates metastatic disease (M1) in patients with cancer of the cervical esophagus.

TABLE 13-8. *Percent of patients presenting with high grade malignant strictures precluding passage of the echoendoscope*

Percent	Total number of patients	Reference
21.0%	28	Rice et al., 1991[23]
21.0%	67	Grimm et al., 1992[71]
25.0%	204	Catalano, et al., 1995[50]
26.0%	74	Tio et al., 1989[20]
26.6%	79	Van Dam et al., 1993[48]
28.5%	28	Kalantzis et al., 1992[72]
30.0%	253	Dittler et al., 1994[44]
31.6%	63	Grimm et al., 1993[70]
36.0%	89	Fok et al., 1992[69]
36.4%	41	Hordijk et al., 1993[49]
37.5%	38	Dancygier and Classen, 1989[46]
44.0%	82	Soquet et al., 1992[18]
62.0%	63	Kallimanis et al., 1995[51]

uated endosonographically and noted that in one such patient, endosonography identified focal thickening that on biopsy demonstrated only dysplasia, but at surgery proved to be a small carcinoma.[46]

Falk and coworkers used endosonography prospectively to evaluate nine patients with Barrett's esophagus and high-grade dysplasia who subsequently underwent esophagectomy.[68] Preoperative endoscopy and biopsy revealed high-grade dysplasia without evidence of carcinoma in all patients. Preoperative endosonography was compared with the histopathologic diagnosis of the resected specimen in all cases. After surgery, three of the nine patients were found to have intramucosal carcinoma, defined as carcinoma extending beyond the basement membrane into the lamina propria or the muscularis mucosae, but not beyond. Preoperative endosonography detected tumor in only one of these patients, but overstaged the tumor as invasive carcinoma (T2, N0). In two of the six patients with no detectable tumor by histological evaluation, endosonography predicted invasive carcinoma (T2, N0).[68] Overstaging of patients with Barrett's esophagus was attributed to mucosal nodularity, a finding that has been noted in the presence or absence of dysplasia in other, similar studies.[66,69] This study therefore demonstrated that endosonography does not consistently predict the presence of intramucosal carcinoma in patients with Barrett's esophagus and high-grade dysplasia.[68]

REFERENCES

1. Coia LR, Engstrom PF, Paul A. Nonsurgical management of esophageal cancer: report of a study of combined radiotherapy and chemotherapy. J Clin Oncol 1987;5:1783.
2. Earlam R, Cunha-Menlo J. Oesophageal squamous cell carcinoma: a critical review. Br J Surg 1980;67:381.
3. Kelsen D, Bains M, Hilaris B, Martini N. combined modality therapy of esophageal cancer. Semin Oncol 1984;11:168.
4. Paracher VK, Meroni E, Spinelli P. Anatomy of the thoracic duct: an endosonographic study. Gastrointest Endosc 1995;42:188.
5. Tanaka Y, Yasuda K, Aibe T, Fuji T, Kawai K. Anatomical and pathological aspects in ultrasonic endoscopy for GI tract. Scand J Gastroenterol 1984;19(Suppl 94):43.
6. Tio TL, Tytgat GNJ. Endoscopic ultrasonography of normal and pathologic upper gastrointestinal wall structure: comparison of studies in vivo and in vitro with histology. Scand J Gastroenterol 1986;21(Suppl 123):27.
7. Van Dam J, Rice TW, Sivak MV Jr. Endoscopic ultrasonography and endoscopically-guided needle aspiration for the diagnosis of upper gastrointestinal tract foregut cysts. Am J Gastroenterol 1992;87:762.
8. Van Dam J, Zuccaro G Jr, Sivak MV Jr. Endosonographic diagnosis of a submucosal gastric cyst. J Ultrasound Med 1992;11:61.
9. Ferrari AP Jr, Van Dam J, Carr-Locke DL. Endoscopic needle aspiration of a gastric duplication cyst. Endoscopy 1995;27:270.
10. Beahrs OH, Henson DE, Hutter RVP, Myers MH, eds (American Joint Committee on Cancer). Manual for staging cancer. 4th ed. Philadelphia: JB Lippincott, 1988:57.
11. Hutter RVP. At last—worldwide agreement on the staging of cancer. Arch Surg 1987;122:1235.
12. International Union Against Cancer. TNM classification of malignant tumors. 4th ed. Berlin: Springer-Verlag, 1987:40.
13. Sobin LH, Hermanek P, Hutter RVP. TNM classification of malignant tumors: a comparison between the new (1987) and the old editions. Cancer 1988;61:2310.
14. Skinner DB, Ferguson MK, Soriano A, Little AG, Staszak VM. Selection of operation for esophageal cancer based on staging. Arch Surg 1986;204:391.
15. Botet JF, Lightdale CJ, Zauber AG, Gerdes H, Urmacher C, Brennan MF. Preoperative staging of esophageal cancer: comparison of endoscopic US and dynamic CT. Radiology 1991;181:419.
16. Grimm H, Sollano J, Hamper K, Noar M, Soehendra N. Endoscopic ultrasound (EUS) of esophagogastric cancer: a new requirement for preoperative staging [abstract]? Gastrointest Endosc 1988;34:176.
17. Lightdale CJ, Botet JF: Esophageal carcinoma. Pre-operative staging and evaluation of anastomotic recurrence. Gastrointest Endosc 1990; 36:S11.
18. Souquet JC, Napoleon B, Pujol B, Valette PJ, Chollet R, Lambert R. Endosonography-guided treatment of esophageal carcinoma. Endoscopy 1992;24:(Suppl 1)324.
19. Tio TL, Coene PPLO, Schouwink MH, Tytgat GNJ. Esophagogastric carcinoma: preoperative TNM classification with endosonography. Radiology 1989;173:411.
20. Tio TL, Cohen P, Coene PP, Udding J, Den Hartog Jager FCA, Tytgat GNJ. Endosonography and computed tomography of esophageal carcinoma: preoperative classification compared to the new (1987) TNM system. Gastroenterology 1989;96:1478.
21. Ziegler K, Sanft C, Semsch B, Friedrich M, Gregor M, Riecken EO. Endosonography is superior to computed tomography in staging tumors of the esophagus and cardia [abstract]. Gastroenterology 1988;94:517.
22. Souquet JC, Napoléon B, Pujol B, et al. Endoscopic ultrasonography in the preoperative staging of esophageal cancer. Endoscopy 1994;26: 764.
23. Rice TW, Boyce GA, Sivak MV Jr. Esophageal ultrasound and the preoperative staging of carcinoma of the esophagus. J Thorac Cardiovasc Surg 1991;101:536.
24. Rice TW. Esophageal ultrasound in the preoperative staging of esophageal carcinoma: the Cleveland Clinic Experience. Presented at Endoscopic Ultrasonography: A Tutorial, March 21–22, 1991, Cleveland, Ohio.
25. Catalano MF, Sivak MV Jr, Bedford RA, et al. Observer variation and reproducibility of endoscopic ultrasonography. Gastrointest Endosc 1995;41:115.
26. Tio TL, Den Hartog Jager FCA, Tytgat GNJ. The role of endoscopic ultrasonography in assessing local resectability of oesophagogastric malignancies. Scand J Gastroenterol 1986;21(Suppl 123):78.
27. Ginsberg GG, Al-Kawas FH, Nguyen CC, et al. Endoscopic ultrasound evaluation of vascular involvement in esophageal cancer: a comparison with computed tomography [abstract]. Gastrointest Endosc 1993;39: 276.
28. Yoshikane H, Tsukamoto Y, Niwa Y, et al. Superficial esophageal carcinoma: evaluation by endoscopic ultrasonography. Am J Gastroenterol 1994;89:702.
29. McLoughlin RF, Cooperberg PL, Mathieson JR, Stordy SN, Halparin LS. High resolution endoluminal ultrasonography in the staging of esophageal carcinoma. J Ultrasound Med 1995;14:725.
30. Fockens P, van Dullemen HM, Tytgat GNJ. Endosonography of stenotic esophageal carcinomas: preliminary experience with an ultrathin, balloon-fitted ultrasound probe in four patients. Gastrointest Endosc 1994;40:226.

31. Grimm H, Hamper K, Binmoeller KF, Soehendra N. Enlarged lymph nodes: malignant or not? Endoscopy 1992;24(Suppl 1):320.
32. Catalano MF, Sivak MV Jr, Rice T, Gragg LA, Van Dam J. Endosonographic features predictive of lymph node metastasis. Gastrointest Endosc 1994;40:442.
33. Vassallo P, Wernecke K, Roos N, Peters PE. Differentiation of benign from malignant superficial lymphadenopathy: the role of high-resolution US. Radiology 1992;183:215.
34. Heintz A, Mildenberger P, Georg M, Braunstein S, Junginger Th. Endoscopic ultrasonography in the diagnosis of regional lymph nodes in esophageal and gastric cancer: results of studies in vitro. Endoscopy 1993;25:231.
35. Catalano MF, Sivak MV Jr, Rice TW, Bedford R, Van Dam J. Depth of tumor invasion of esophageal carcinoma (ECA) is predictive of lymph node metastasis: role of endoscopic ultrasonography (EUS) [abstract]. Am J Gastroenterol 1992;87:1245.
36. Dittler HJ, Rosch T, Lorenz R, Siewert JR, Classen M. Failure of endoscopic ultrasonography to differentiate malignant from benign lymph nodes in esophagogastric cancer [abstract]. Gastrointest Endosc 1992;38:240.
37. Wiersema MJ, Kochman ML, Chak A, Cramer HM, Kesler KA. Real-time endoscopic ultrasound-guided fine-needle aspiration of a mediastinal lymph node. Gastrointest Endosc 1993;39:429.
38. Wegener M, Adamek RJ, Sedmann B, Pfaffenbach B. Endosonographically guided fine-needle aspiration puncture of paraesophagogastric mass lesions: preliminary results. Endoscopy 1994;26:586.
39. Krasna MJ, McLaughlin JS. Thoracoscopic lymph node staging for esophageal cancer. Ann Thorac Surg 1993;56:671.
40. Catalano MF, Van Dam J, Sivak MV Jr, van Stolk RU, Rice TW. Postoperative screening for recurrence of esophageal carcinoma (ECA) by endoscopic ultrasonography (EUS) [abstract]. Am J Gastroenterol 1992;87:1245.
41. Dittler HJ, Rösch T, Fink U, Siewert JR, Classen M. Endosonographic re-staging of carcinoma of the esophagus and cardia following radio- and chemotherapy [abstract]. Gastrointest Endosc 1992;38:61.
42. Nousbaum JB, Robaszkiewicz M, Cauvin JM, Calament G, Gouerou H. Endosonography can detect residual tumour infiltration after medical treatment of oesophageal cancer in the absence of endoscopic lesions. Gut 1992;33:1459.
43. Hordijk ML, Kok TC, Wilson JHP, Mulder AH. Assessment of response of esophageal carcinoma to induction chemotherapy. Endoscopy 1993;25:592.
44. Dittler HJ, Fink U, Siewert GR. Response to chemotherapy in esophageal cancer. Endoscopy 1994;26:769.
45. Bown SG, Hawes R, Matthewson K, et al. Endoscopic laser palliation for advanced malignant dysphagia. Gut 1987;28:799.
46. Dancygier H, Classen M. Endoscopic ultrasonography in esophageal diseases. Gastrointest Endosc 1989;35:220.
47. Dittler HJ, Siewert JR. Role of endoscopic ultrasonography in esophageal carcinoma. Endoscopy 1993;25:156.
48. Van Dam J, Rice TW, Catalano MF, Kirby T, Sivak MV Jr. High-grade malignant stricture is predictive of esophageal tumor stage: risks of endosonographic evaluation. Cancer 1993;71:2910.
49. Hordijk ML, Zander H, van Blankenstein M, Tilanus HW. Influence of tumor stenosis on the accuracy of endosonography in preoperative T staging of esophageal cancer. Endoscopy 1993;25:171.
50. Catalano MF, Van Dam J, Sivak MV Jr. Malignant esophageal strictures: staging accuracy of endoscopic ultrasonography. Gastrointest Endosc 1995;41:535.
51. Kallimanis GE, Gupta PK, Al-Kawas FH, Tio LT, Benjamin SB, Bertagnolli ME. Endoscopic ultrasound for staging cancer, with or without dilation, is clinically important and safe. Gastrointest Endosc 1995;41:540.
52. Binmoeller KF, Seifert H, Seitz U, Izbicki JR, Kida M, Soehendra N. Ultrasonic esophagoprobe for TNM staging of highly stenosing esophageal carcinoma. Gastrointest Endosc 1995;41:547.
53. Roubein LD. Endoscopic ultrasonography and the malignant esophageal stricture: implications and complications. Gastrointest Endosc 1995;41:613.
54. Nesje LB, Odegaard S, Matre K, Svanes K, Viste A, Kimmey MB. Evaluation of oesophageal stenotic lesions using a 20 MHz linear transendoscopic ultrasound system [abstract]. Endoscopy 1992;24:655.
55. Grimm H, Binmoeller KF, Soehendra N. Ultrasonic esophagoprobe (prototype I) for endosonographic staging of esophageal cancer [abstract]. Endoscopy 1992;24:652.
56. Grimm H. Endoscopic ultrasonography with the ultrasonic esophagoprobe. Endoscopy 1994;26:818.
57. Glover JR, Sargeant IR, Bown SG, Lees WR. Non-optic endosonography in advanced carcinoma of the esophagus. Gastrointest Endosc 1994;40:194.
58. Siewert JR, Dittler HJ. Esophageal carcinoma: impact of staging on treatment. Endoscopy 1993;25:28.
59. Hiele M, Lerut A, Schurmans P, et al. Endoscopic ultrasound accurately predicts outcome in patients undergoing surgery for esophageal or esophagogastric junction carcinoma [abstract]. Gastrointest Endosc 1992;38:286.
60. Varanasi RV, Saltzman JR, Krims P, Crimaldi A, Colby J. Breast carcinoma metastatic to the esophagus: clinicopathological and management features of four cases, and literature review. Am J Gastroenterol 1995;90:1495.
61. Spechler SJ, Goyal RK: Barrett's esophagus. N Engl J Med 1986;315:362.
62. Hameetman W, Tytgat GNJ, Houthoff HJ, Van Den Tweel JG. Barrett's esophagus: development of dysplasia and adenocarcinoma. Gastroenterology 1989;96:1249.
63. Reid BJ, Blount PL, Rubin CE, Levine DS, Haggitt RC, Rabinovitch PS. Flow-cytometric and histological progression to malignancy in barrett's esophagus: prospective endoscopic surveillance of a cohort. Gastroenterology 1992;102:1212.
64. Altorki NK, Sunagawa M, Little AG, Skinner DB. High-grade dysplasia in the columnar-lined esophagus. Am J Surg 1991;161:97.
65. Falk GW, Rice TW, Achkar E, Petras RE. High grade dysplasia in Barrett's esophagus is associated with early cancer [abstract]. Gastroenterology 1992;102:355.
66. Palley SL, Samplinger RE, Garewal HS. Editorial: management of high-grade dysplasia in Barrett's esophagus. J Clin Gastroenterol 1989;11:369.
67. Reid BJ, Weinstein WM, Lewin KJ, et al. Endoscopic biopsy can detect high-grade dysplasia or early adenocarcinoma in Barrett's esophagus without grossly recognizable neoplastic lesions. Gastroenterology 1988;94:81.
68. Falk GW, Catalano MF, Sivak MV Jr, Rice TW, Van Dam J. Endosonography in the evaluation of patients with Barrett's esophagus and high-grade dysplasia. Gastrointest Endosc 1994;40:207.
69. Fok M, Cheng SWK, Wong J. Endosonography in patient selection for surgical treatment of esophageal carcinoma. World J Surg 1992;16:1098.
70. Grimm H, Binmoeller KF, Hamper K, Koch J, Henne-Bruns D, Soehendra N. Endosonography for preoperative locoregional staging of esophageal and gastric cancer. Endoscopy 1993;25:224.
71. Grimm H, Binmoeller KF, Hamper K, Soehendra N. Accuracy of endoscopic ultrasound (EUS) in preoperative staging of esophageal carcinoma [abstract]. Endoscopy 1992;24:652.
72. Kalantzis N, Kallimanis G, Laoudi F, Papavasiliou E, Gabriel G. Endoscopic ultrasonography and computed tomography in preoperative (TNM) classification of oesophageal carcinoma [abstract]. Endoscopy 1992;24:653.

Surgery for Gastrointestinal Cancer: A Multidisciplinary Approach, edited by Harold J. Wanebo.
Lippincott-Raven Publishers, Philadelphia, © 1997.

CHAPTER 14

Transthoracic Resection for Carcinoma of the Thoracic Esophagus and Cardia

F. Henry Ellis, Jr.

Esophagogastrectomy remains the preferred treatment for patients with carcinoma of the esophagus and cardia whose general condition permits and who do not have metastatic disease. Lesions of the cardia are included in this discussion because their treatment and the results thereof are the same as for lesions of the lower thoracic esophagus. Because cell type does not alter the results of therapy, adenocarcinomas in Barrett's esophagus, which now comprise at least 30% of all intrathoracic esophageal malignancies, are also included. Unfortunately, palliation of the progressive effects of disabling dysphagia resulting from these lesions remains the chief goal of the therapy, because long-term survival after resection remains suboptimal. The use of neoadjuvant therapy (see Chap. 17) and radical "en bloc" resection (see Chap. 16) are under study in an effort to improve long-term results. Although the transhiatal approach has its advocates (see Chap. 15), standard transthoracic resection remains the most commonly used approach for the surgical treatment of this disease, and thus the results of its use are the standard to which other therapeutic approaches must be compared.

The surgical approach for transthoracic resection of malignant lesions of the esophagus and cardia is controversial. Although historically a left thoracotomy was the usual approach used for resection of most cancers of the thoracic esophagus, today there are those who prefer a combined abdominal and right thoracic approach (Ivor Lewis)[1] or a transhiatal approach. I prefer to individualize the approach to the specific location of the tumor.[2] Thus, for lesions of the lower thoracic esophagus and cardia, a left thoracotomy is preferred. For lesions requiring an anastomosis at or near the aortic arch, an Ivor Lewis approach is used. The transhiatal approach is particularly useful for lesions at any location if clinical evaluation, including computer-assisted imaging of the tumor or intraesophageal ultrasonography, suggests that the cancer is confined to the esophageal wall and does not involve adjacent structures. It is also appropriate for patients with adenocarcinoma in Barrett's esophagus to ensure complete removal of all the abnormal mucosa, which may extend proximal to the growth for a considerable distance. In this chapter, only the techniques of esophagogastrectomy and esophagogastrostomy through a left thoracotomy and by a combined laparotomy and right thoracotomy (Ivor Lewis) are discussed.

The stomach remains the ideal esophageal substitute. Only if previous operations on the stomach have made it unsuitable should other portions of the gastrointestinal tract be used for this purpose. A feeding jejunostomy is considered by some to be an essential part of the surgical treatment of carcinoma of the esophagus and cardia.[3] However, a prospective, randomized study comparing the results in patients receiving enteral feedings by jejunostomy with the results of those fed by conventional measures revealed no statistically convincing evidence of the superiority of the former, although, to be sure, enteral jejunostomy feedings better fulfill the nutritional and caloric requirements of the postesophagogastrectomy patient.[4] In my opinion, the use of a feeding jejunostomy should be individualized, and one should not be used after every esophagogastrectomy.

HISTORICAL COMMENTS

The surgical approach to carcinoma of the esophagus has a long and fascinating history. By the latter part of the 19th century, largely through the work of Billroth[5] and Czerny,[6] lesions of the cervical esophagus became amenable to surgical resection. Not until 1913, however, was complete resection of the intrathoracic esophagus accomplished successfully by Franz Torek of New York City, although direct gastrointestinal continuity was never reestablished in his patient.[7] Subsequently, many transthoracic esophageal resections and reconstructions were attempted, but without success. The first successful transthoracic resection of a cancer of the cardia was reported by Zaaijer in 1913 using a preliminary thoracoplasty.[8] By 1933, however, the Japanese surgeon Ohsawa had resected 51 carcinomas of the cardia and 50 carcinomas of the esophagus through a left thoracotomy with a primary intrathoracic anastomosis,[9]

Deaconess Hospital, Harvard Medical School, Suite 2C, 110 Francis Street, Boston, MA 02215.

a feat first performed successfully in the United States by Marshall at the Lahey Clinic in 1937,[10] 1 year before the operation performed by Adams and Phemister,[11] who usually are given priority for this advance. Subsequently, this approach was perfected by Richard Sweet of the Massachusetts General Hospital, leading to his reports of large numbers of patients with carcinoma of the thoracic esophagus treated by transthoracic resection through a left thoracotomy. By 1954, he had performed an esophagogastrectomy through a left thoracotomy in 300 of 450 patients with carcinoma of the esophagus.[12] Although his operative mortality of 25% for middle thoracic esophageal lesions was high, in the later years of his study, it was only 7% for lesions at the lower end of the esophagus. The 5-year survival of patients leaving the hospital after surviving resection was a commendable 17%. Although Sweet championed the left thoracic approach, the combined abdominal and right thoracic approach described by Lewis in 1946[1] has been preferred by others. These are the two approaches most commonly used for resection of thoracic esophageal malignancies.

TRANSTHORACIC ESOPHAGOGASTRECTOMY

Patient Preparation

Patient preparation for standard transthoracic esophagogastrectomy is neither complicated nor prolonged. Complicated scanning techniques are rarely necessary, although they may enable more accurate preoperative staging of the lesion. How-

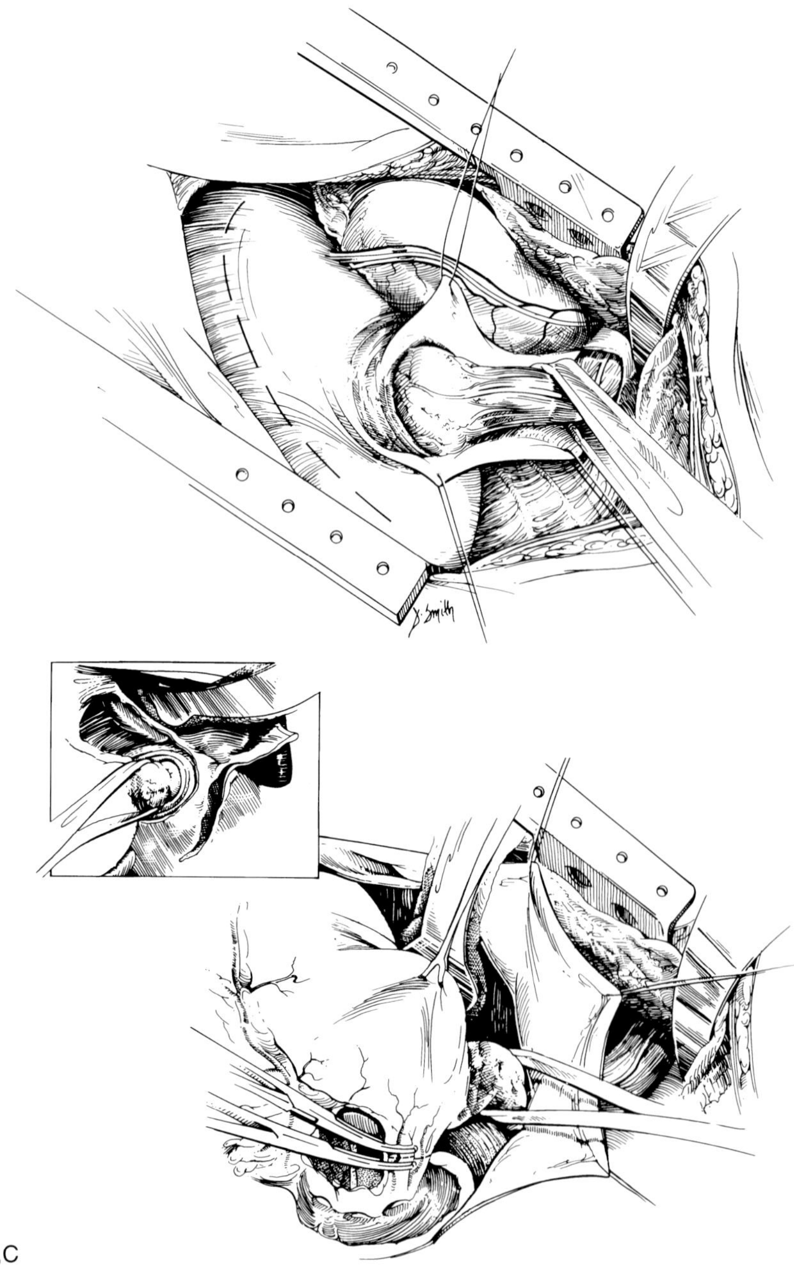

A

B,C

FIG. 14-1. Transthoracic exposure of distal esophagus and cardia. **(A)** The mediastinal pleura has been opened and the esophagus mobilized proximal to the tumor. The dashed line indicates the site of the diaphragmatic incision. **(B)** After cephalad retraction of the diaphragmatic flap, the upper abdomen is exposed and the distal esophagus and tumor are mobilized and elevated with an encircling Penrose drain. **(C)** Ligation and division of short gastric vessels.

ever, because they rarely accurately determine resectability, their routine use is open to question. Patients in experimental neoadjuvant protocols are exceptions, however, to this view. Attention to the cardiorespiratory system is essential. Tobacco smoking must be discontinued for at least 1 week before surgery. Pulmonary function studies are justified in heavy smokers and patients with clinical evidence of impaired respiratory function. Preoperative preparation with bronchodilators may improve pulmonary function in some patients with chronic obstructive pulmonary disease. An abnormal electrocardiogram in a patient with symptoms suggestive of angina requires consultation with a cardiologist, who may recommend a preoperative thallium exercise tolerance test or special monitoring during the operation. Unless the patient has marked inanition and weight loss of 20% of normal body weight or more, which is now rare in the United States, preoperative hyperalimentation to improve the nutritional status of the patient is rarely indicated. Esophageal obstruction is common in patients with carcinoma of the esophagus or cardia, so the esophagus should be lavaged the night before and the morning of operation to prevent aspiration of retained material during induction of anesthesia.

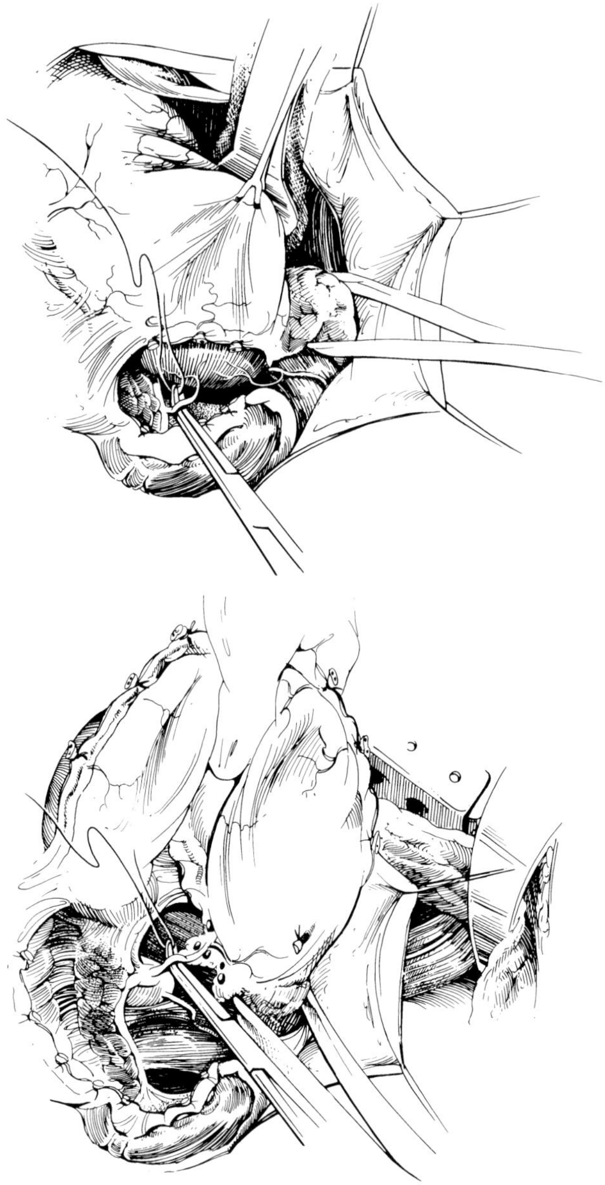

FIG. 14-2. (A) After elevation of the stomach, the posterior gastric artery arising from the splenic artery is doubly ligated and divided, as is a branch from the left inferior phrenic artery. **(B)** Further elevation of the stomach allows identification, ligation, and division of the left gastric artery at its origin from the celiac axis. The right gastroepiploic artery is preserved. (Reproduced with permission from Ellis FH Jr. Carcinoma of the esophagus and cardia. In: Ritchie WP Jr, Steele GD Jr, Dean RH, eds. General surgery. Philadelphia: JB Lippincott, 1995:91.)

Surgical Technique

The Left Thoracic Approach

Exposure for esophagogastrectomy for lesions involving the esophagogastric junction or lower esophagus is best obtained through a left thoracotomy. A thoracoabdominal incision provides slightly greater exposure, but prolongs the operative procedure unnecessarily and may lead to an unstable costal arch or chondritis with a chronically draining sinus. The left thorax is entered through the bed of the nonresected eighth rib, the angle of which may require division to provide better exposure. The mediastinal pleura is opened to permit the esophagus to be mobilized proximal to the growth and encircled with a Penrose drain to provide traction (Fig. 14-1*A*). The diaphragm is opened using a semilunar incision near the costal arch, which provides better exposure than does a radial incision through the diaphragmatic crural noose, and preserves the nerve supply to most of the diaphragm. This approach creates a flap of diaphragm that, when elevated and retracted cephalad, results in excellent exposure of the left upper abdomen (Figs. 14-1*B*and *C*). Resectability is determined and the procedure is continued with dissection of the growth from the esophageal hiatus. In cases of cancer of the cardia, this maneuver often must include resection of diaphragmatic muscle as well. The gastrohepatic omentum is ligated and divided. Mobilization is continued by division of the short gastric vessels with preservation of the right gastroepiploic artery (Fig. 14-1*C*). If the spleen or tail of the pancreas are involved, these also can be removed.

After mobilization of the upper portion of the greater curvature of the stomach, the posterior gastric vessels are exposed. The posterior gastric artery arising from the splenic artery and a recurrent branch of the left inferior phrenic artery are identified, and both are ligated and divided (Fig. 14-2*A*). Dissection then is continued along the greater curvature of the stomach, with care taken to separate the transverse mesocolon from the omentum so as to separate the middle colic artery from the right gastroepiploic artery. Preservation of the latter vessel is essential to provide adequate blood supply to the stomach, because only it and the right gastric artery will remain after resection. Attention then is drawn to the origin of the left gastric artery as it arises from the celiac axis. Care is taken to include in the resected specimen all the nodes and node-bearing tissue along this vessel. The artery is clamped, doubly ligated with heavy nonabsorbable suture material, and divided, the distal

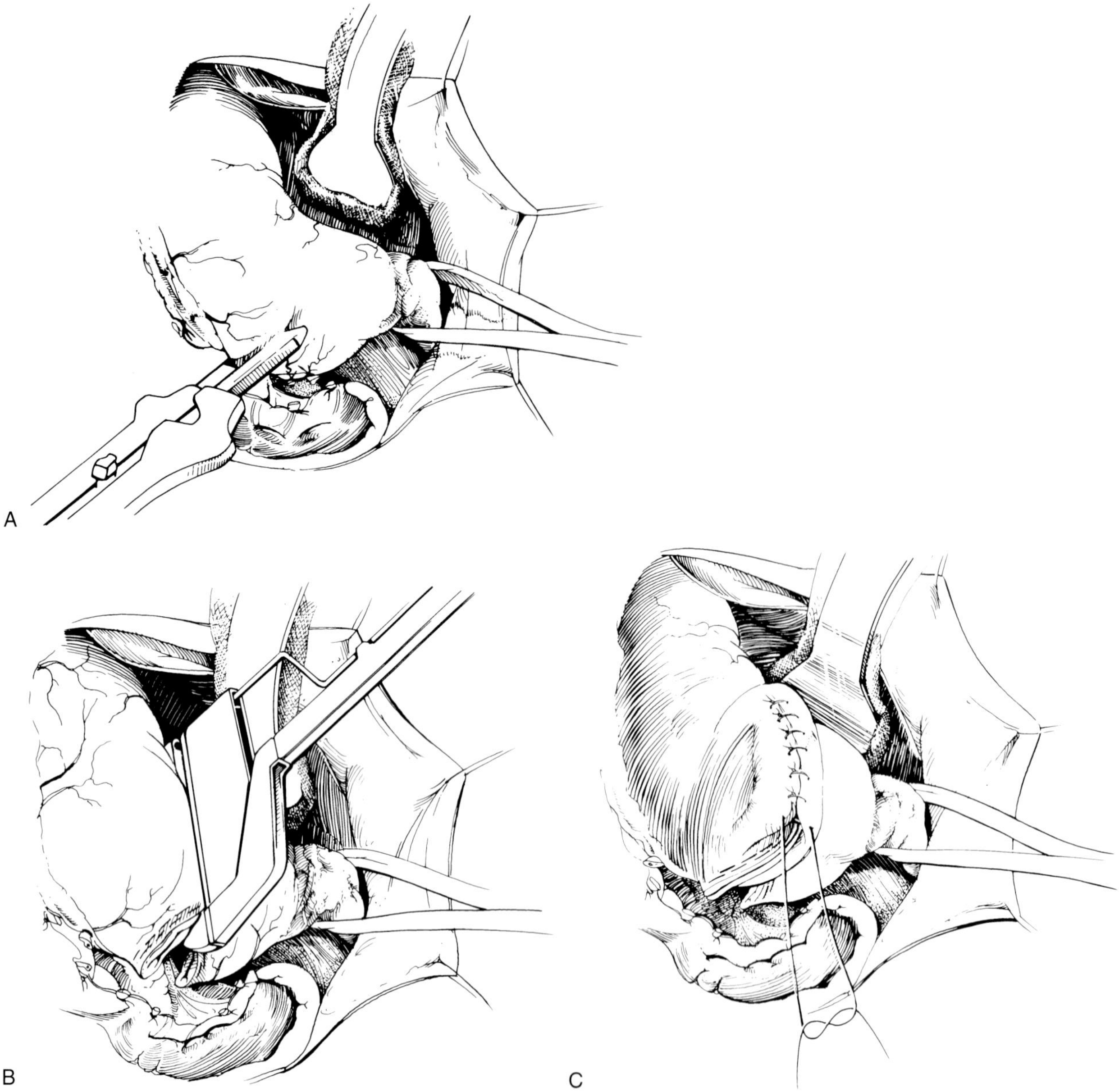

FIG. 14-3. Preparation of the stomach for esophagogastrostomy. **(A)** The GIA stapler is placed at right angles to the greater curvature of the stomach. **(B)** The TA-90 stapler is placed tangentially along the lesser curvature of the stomach to include in the resected specimen the nodes in the region of the ligated left gastric artery. (C) Interrupted nonabsorbable sutures cover the stapled suture line. (Reproduced with permission from Ellis FH Jr. Carcinoma of the esophagus and cardia. In: Ritchie WP Jr, Steele GD Jr, Dean RH, eds. General surgery. Philadelphia: JB Lippincott, 1995:91.)

end being ligated with a catgut suture that is cut long to identify it for subsequent pathologic examination (Fig. 14-2*B*).

The amount of stomach to be resected is determined; this is greater for carcinomas of the cardia than for those of the distal esophagus. The GIA stapling device (Ethicon, Summit, NJ) is placed at right angles to the greater curvature, well below the growth, and the stomach is divided partially (Fig. 14-3*A*). The point of division of the gastric lesser curvature is then identified below the point of the ligated left gastric artery, and a TA-90 stapler (U.S. Surgical Co., Norwalk, CT) is applied tangentially and activated, thus partially transforming the gastric remnant into a tubular structure (Fig. 14-3*B*). The stapled edges are oversewn with interrupted nonabsorbable sutures (Fig. 14-3*C*).

The divided bowel is freed completely from the hiatus and withdrawn into the thorax, followed by the prepared distal stomach. The hiatus is dilated manually to avoid postoperative constriction. A site at least 5 cm above the palpable limits of the tumor is selected, where an end-to-side anastomosis between the esophagus and stomach is carried out. When the resection site is less than 5 cm beyond the growth, a local recurrence rate of more than twice that if the anastomosis is between 5 and 10 cm proximal to the lesion has been reported.[13] A hand-sewn,

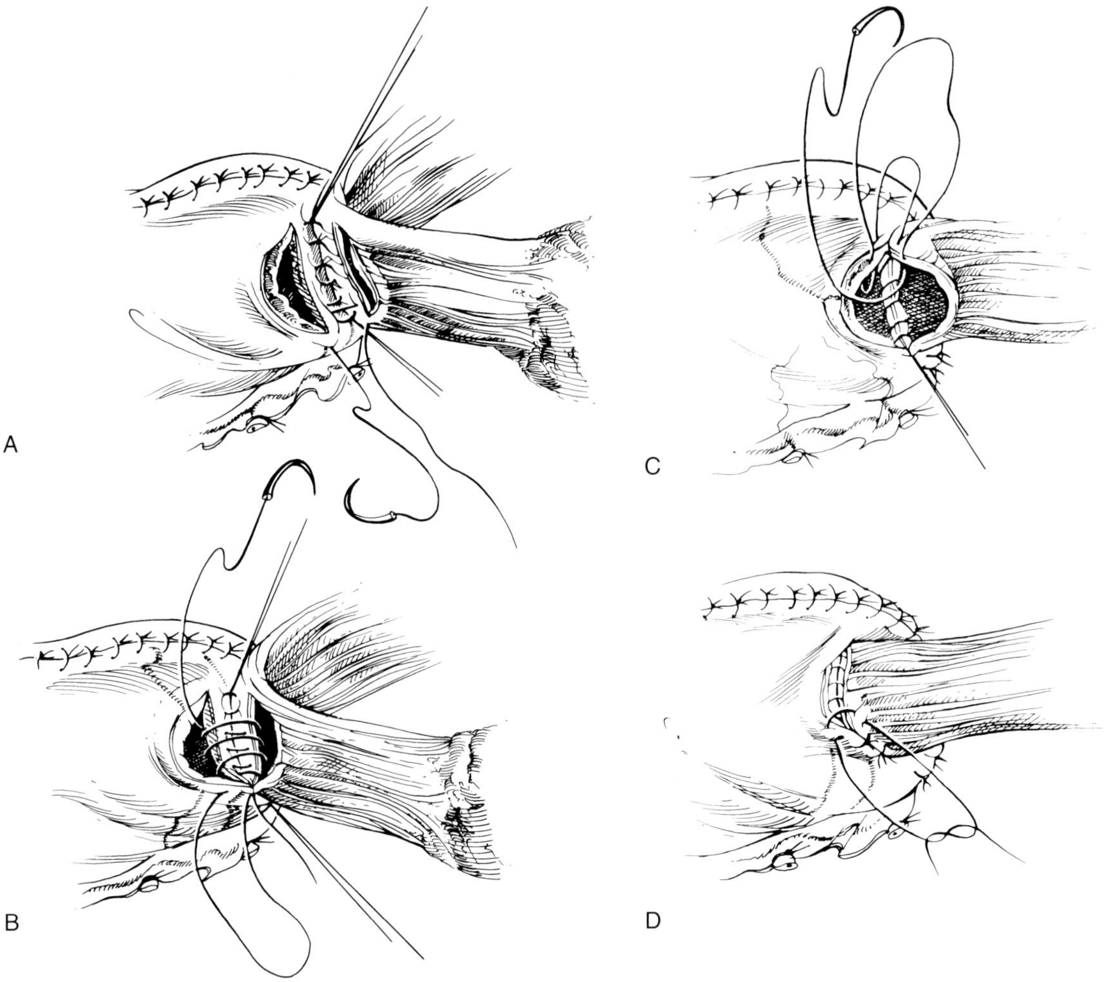

FIG. 14-4. **(A)** After the stomach has been advanced through the manually widened hiatus into the posterior mediastinum, interrupted nonabsorbable sutures are placed between the stomach and esophagus, and transverse incisions are made in these organs in preparation for completion of the posterior suture line. **(B)** Completion of the posterior suture line with a through-and-through fine catgut continuous suture. **(C)** Commencement of the anterior mucosal closure with a continuous fine catgut suture. **(D)** Completion of the anastomosis with interrupted nonabsorbable sutures in the gastric serosa and the esophageal muscle. (Reproduced with permission from Ellis FH Jr. Carcinoma of the esophagus and cardia. In: Ritchie WP Jr, Steele GD Jr, Dean RH, eds. General surgery. Philadelphia: JB Lippincott, 1995:91.)

two-layer anastomosis is used rather than a stapled esophagogastrostomy. The anastomosis is performed without clamps, both to avoid tension as well as to maintain an adequate blood supply to the anastomotic site. The posterior anastomotic layer is begun with interrupted nonabsorbable sutures; the stomach and esophagus are opened by incisions made into the two organs (Fig. 14-4*A*); and the posterior anastomosis proceeds using a continuous 3-0 catgut suture passed through the entire thickness of the bowel wall (Fig. 14-4*A* and *B*). After the posterior layer is completed, the esophagus is transsected, care being taken to prevent retraction of the mucosa. The anterior mucosal layer is approximated by continuing the posteriorly completed continuous catgut suture, now passed to the outside of the bowel (Fig. 14-4*C*). The final external layer of the anterior anastomosis is completed using interrupted nonabsorbable sutures for the seromuscular layer (Fig. 14-4*D*), and the anastomosis is complete (Fig. 14-5).

To prevent postoperative gastric distention, a nasogastric tube is passed transnasally by the anesthesiologist across the anastomosis and into the intrathoracic stomach. The diaphragm is closed with interrupted figure-of-eight nonabsorbable sutures and the chest is closed in layers, with an intercostal tube placed for postoperative drainage.

The Ivor Lewis Procedure

The Ivor Lewis procedure facilitates the performance of a high intrathoracic esophagogastrectomy and esophagogastrostomy in the region of the aortic arch or above because, after division of the azygos vein, there is no impediment to its performance, as there would be in a left thoracotomy because of the presence of the left-sided aortic arch. The abdominal portion of the operation is initiated through an upper midline incision,

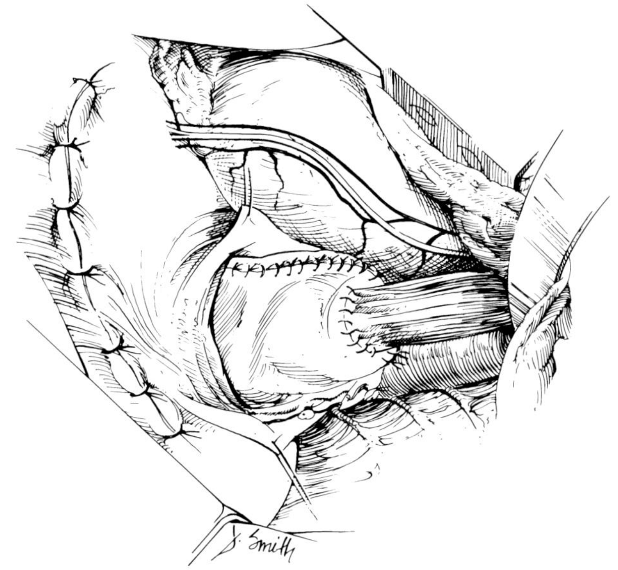

FIG. 14.5. Completed intrathoracic esophagogastrostomy and closure of diaphragmatic incision. (Reproduced with permission from Ellis FH Jr. Carcinoma of the esophagus and cardia. In: Ritchie WP Jr, Steele GD Jr, Dean RH, eds. General surgery. Philadelphia: JB Lippincott, 1995:91.)

skirting to the left of the umbilicus and extending slightly below it. The abdomen is explored thoroughly. The presence of an isolated liver metastasis does not preclude resection, however, because restoration of the swallowing mechanism is one of the main goals of the operation. Only if tumor invasion of adjacent structures prevents safe performance of the resection is the operation abandoned.

The left lobe of the liver is mobilized, permitting exposure of the esophagogastric junctional area. The phrenoesophageal ligament is incised and the esophagus is encircled with a Penrose drain after division of the gastrohepatic omentum (Fig. 14-6*A*). Mobilization of the gastric fundus is facilitated by supporting the spleen with a moist pack placed behind it. The stomach is separated from the greater omentum by entrance into the lesser sac. A suitable spot along the greater curvature of the stomach is selected and division of the short gastric vessels proceeds in a cephalad direction (Fig. 14-6*B*). Mobilization of the gastric fundus is completed by ligation and division of the posterior gastric vessels, as already described (Fig. 14-6*C*).

The greater curvature of the stomach is mobilized distally, separating the mesocolon from the omentum to identify the middle colic and right gastroepiploic vessels, which are preserved carefully (Fig. 14-7*A*), permitting separation of the greater omentum from the stomach until the duodenum is reached. The performance of a gastric drainage procedure is controversial, but an extramucosal pyloromyotomy may facilitate postoperative gastric emptying (Fig. 14-7*B*). Further mobilization is provided by incising the posterior abdominal peritoneum to permit mobilization of the duodenum. The origin of the left gastric artery is exposed easily after these maneuvers, and is clamped, doubly ligated with nonabsorbable sutures, and divided (Fig. 14-7*C*). After widening the esophageal hiatus manually and ensuring that the stomach has been mobilized completely, the abdomen is closed using through-and-through, nonabsorbable, figure-of-eight interrupted sutures and staples in the skin.

The patient then is repositioned and draped for a right thoracotomy entering the right chest through the bed of the nonresected sixth rib. It usually is necessary to divide the sixth rib posterior to its angle to provide better exposure. The mediastinal pleura is opened and the malignant neoplasm identified. The azygos vein is ligated and divided and the esophagus is encircled proximal and distal to the growth, using two Penrose drains to encircle normal esophagus on each side of the growth, thus facilitating its mobilization and elevation (Fig. 14-8). These maneuvers permit wide excision of tissues surrounding the growth, including a portion of the mediastinal pleura. It may be necessary to establish a subadventitial line of cleavage along the aorta to remove the growth completely. Care must be taken to avoid injury to the thoracic duct. If it is injured, the duct should be ligated low in the thorax near its point of entry into the thorax from the abdomen. The inferior pulmonary ligament is divided, permitting complete mobilization of the distal intrathoracic esophagus. The stomach then is advanced into the thorax, care being taken to avoid rotating it inadvertently during this maneuver. Once the stomach has been elevated into the thorax, a TA-90 stapler is positioned tangentially along the lesser gastric curvature to include in the resected specimen the fatty, node-bearing tissue along the divided left gastric artery (Fig. 14-9*A*). The stapler is activated and the stapled stomach is oversewn with interrupted nonabsorbable sutures (Fig. 14-9*B*).

A site on the proximal esophagus well cephalad to the palpable margins of the growth is selected. The uppermost portion of the fundus of the stomach is laid in the mediastinum to permit the performance of an end-to-side esophagogastrostomy without tension, by the technique already described (Fig. 14-10). Occasionally, examination of frozen sections of the proximal margin of the resected esophagus may reveal submucosal spread or a skip area of esophageal involvement by cancer, necessitating further resection of the proximal esophagus. In these cases, the final anastomosis may have to be performed in the neck. This can be accomplished after closing the thorax, repositioning the patient, and exposing the cervical esophagus through a left cervical incision.

The intrathoracic stomach must maintain its mediastinal position to avoid excessive postoperative prolapse of this organ into the right thorax, with resulting torsion leading to impaired gastric emptying. This can be insured by suturing the posterior aspect of the stomach to the mediastinal pleura posterolaterally, and its medial anterior wall anteromedially to the divided pleura in the region of the inferior pulmonary ligament (see Fig. 14-10). Insertion of a nasogastric tube and closure of the thorax concludes the operation.

Postoperative Care

Although attention to the technical details of the performance of the operation are essential if postoperative complications are to be minimized, no less important is the careful postoperative management of these patients. Hyperalimentation, if it was required before surgery, should of course be continued. If a feeding jejunostomy tube was placed at the time of resection, enteral feedings are begun in the recovery room after completion of

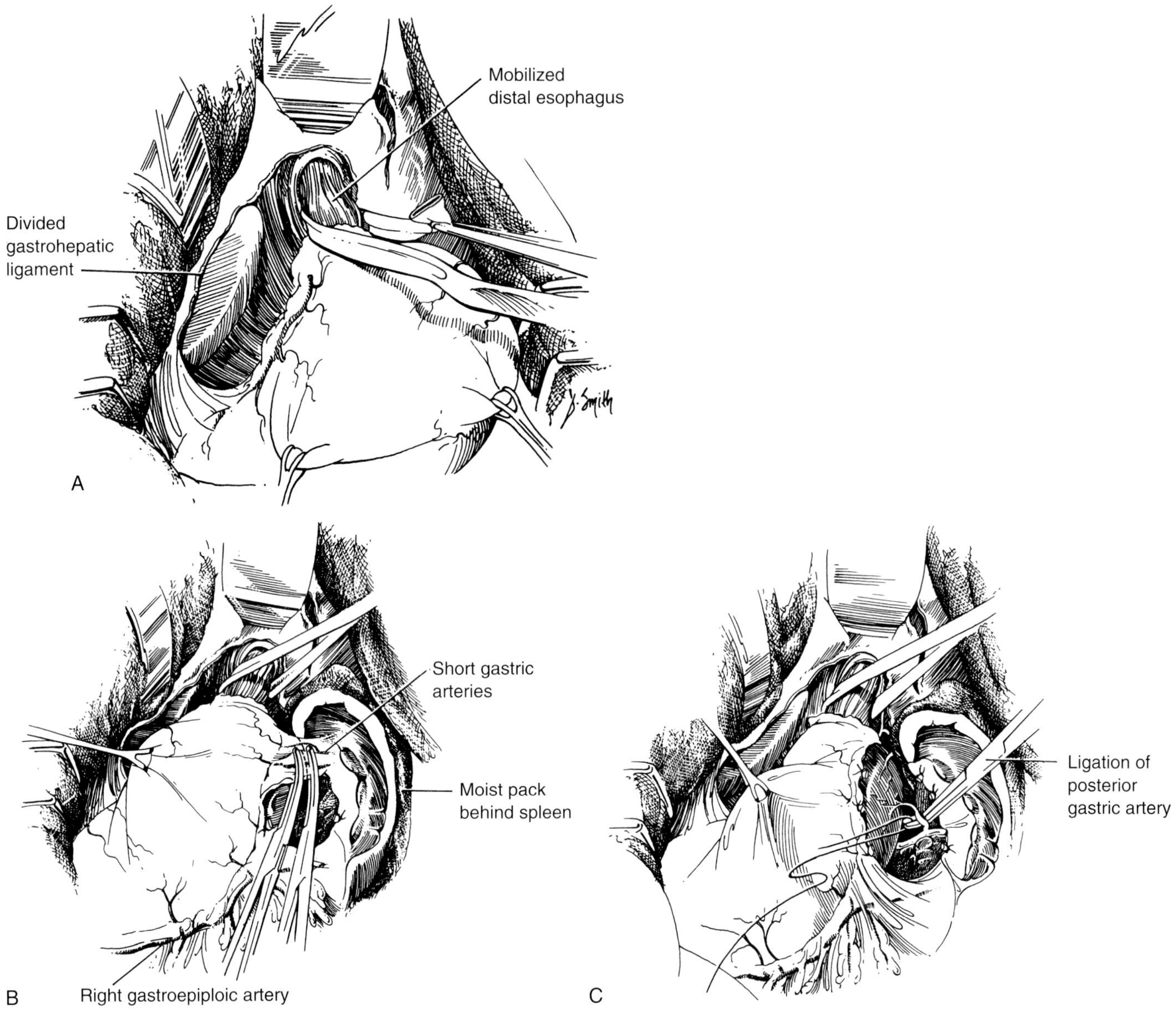

FIG. 14-6. Transabdominal mobilization of the stomach. **(A)** The phrenoesophageal membrane and gastrohepatic omentum have been divided and the distal esophagus mobilized and encircled with a Penrose drain. **(B)** Division of short gastric vessels. **(C)** Ligation of the posterior gastric artery arising from the splenic artery in preparation for its division to permit mobilization of the posterior wall of the stomach. (Reproduced with permission from Ellis FH Jr. Carcinoma of the esophagus and cardia. In: Ritchie WP Jr, Steele GD Jr, Dean RH, eds. General surgery. Philadelphia: JB Lippincott, 1995:91.)

the procedure, using either a full-strength elemental or polymeric diet (Vivonex TEN, Sandoz Nutrition, Minneapolis, MN; Formula 9119, Ross Laboratories, Columbus, OH) at 10 mL/h. The enteral feeding infusion rate is increased gradually by 10 mL/h every 12 to 24 hours until the patient's nutritional needs are met. For those patients not receiving enteral jejunostomy feedings, conventional intravenous fluid and electrolyte replacement is provided, oral feedings being delayed until the fourth or fifth postoperative day, at which time a contrast radiographic study of the anastomotic site ensures its integrity. Oral liquids are then cautiously administered before proceeding to a more advanced diet. Only after an oral diet is tolerated are the intercostal and nasogastric tubes removed. The use of a broad-spectrum antibiotic such as cefazolin for the first 24 to 48 hours, or until the chest tube is removed, is also recommended to minimize postoperative wound infections, empyema, or mediastinitis from a small contained anastomotic leak. Careful attention to the respiratory status of these patients is also required throughout the postoperative period to minimize postoperative respiratory complications.

Patients with an uncomplicated postoperative course are usually discharged within 10 days of the operation, taking multiple small feedings. Antireflux measures help to minimize late problems related to gastroesophageal reflux. Recumbency should be delayed for several hours after eating to avoid regurgitation, and the head of the patient's bed should be elevated 6 to 8

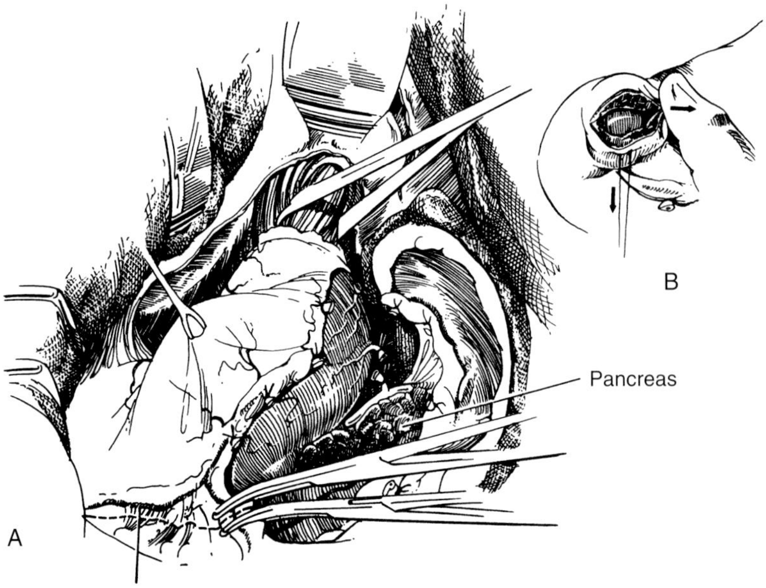

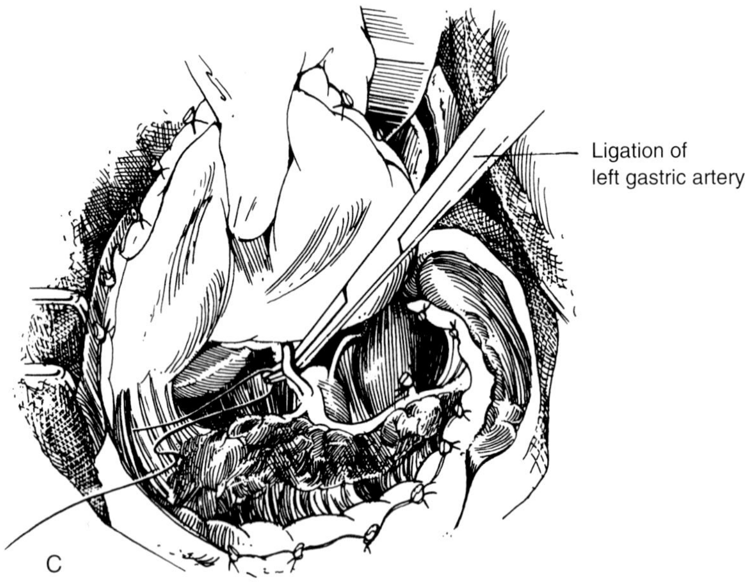

FIG. 14-7. Continuation of gastric mobilization. **(A)** Clamping and division of omental branches of the right gastroepiploic artery, which is preserved. The dotted line indicates the continued direction of this mobilization. **(B)** An extramucosal pyloromyotomy has been completed. (C) Ligation of the left gastric artery at its origin from the celiac axis in preparation for its division. (Reproduced with permission from Ellis FH Jr. Carcinoma of the esophagus and cardia. In: Ritchie WP Jr, Steele GD Jr, Dean RH, eds. General surgery. Philadelphia: JB Lippincott, 1995: 91.)

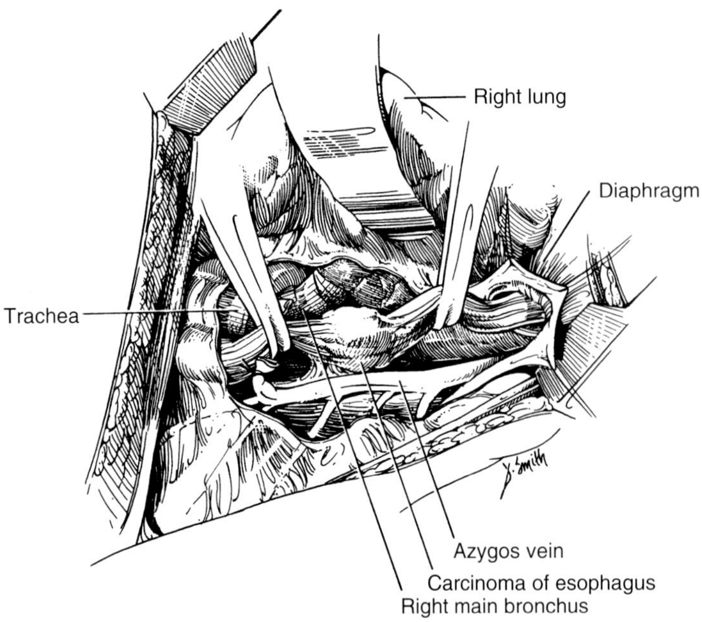

FIG. 14-8. Right transthoracic exposure of the thoracic esophagus. Mobilization of the esophagus after division of the azygos vein and placement of encircling Penrose drain on each side of the tumor. (Reproduced with permission from Ellis FH Jr. Carcinoma of the esophagus and cardia. In: Ritchie WP Jr, Steele GD Jr, Dean RH, eds. General surgery. Philadelphia: JB Lippincott, 1995:91.)

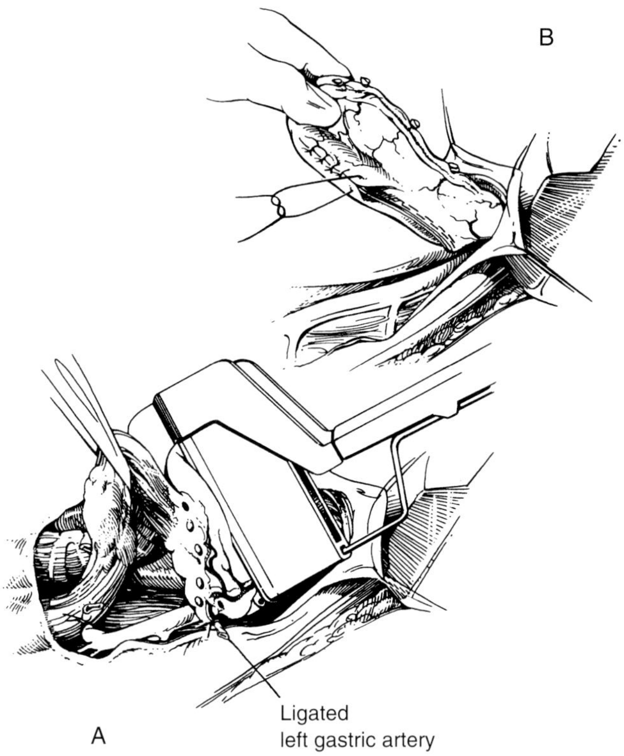

FIG. 14-9. (A) Placement of the TA-90 stapler across the stomach tangentially to include the divided left gastric artery and accompanying lymph nodes. **(B)** The stapled lesser curvature suture line is oversewn with interrupted nonabsorbable sutures. (Reproduced with permission from Ellis FH Jr. Carcinoma of the esophagus and cardia. In: Ritchie WP Jr, Steele GD Jr, Dean RH, eds. General surgery. Philadelphia: JB Lippincott, 1995:91.)

inches for similar reasons. The use of H_2 blockers or a proton pump inhibitor to minimize acid secretion and a prokinetic drug to enhance gastric emptying may also be advisable.

Results

The reported results of surgery for carcinoma of the esophagus and cardia vary greatly depending on the time frame encompassed by the reporting surgeons. Earlam and Cunha-Melo reviewed the surgical literature on squamous cell carcinoma of the esophagus during the 25-year period from 1953 to 1978, which included data on 83,783 patients.[14] Only 58% of the patients were considered operable, of whom two thirds underwent resection. The hospital mortality rate after resection was 29%. The 5-year survival rate adjusted for hospital mortality was 18%, representing only 4% of all patients analyzed. A more recent review by Müller and colleagues involved an analysis of all papers, which included at least a summary in a Western European language, published during the decade from 1980 to 1989.[15] They did not report operability rates because many of the reports contained no information on this point, but 56% were considered to have operable disease and underwent resection. The average hospital mortality rate after resection was 13%, less than half of what had been reported in the earlier report by Earlam and Cunha-Melo,[14] and the 5-year survival rate was 20%. Thus, the main advances in surgical therapy observed during this more recent decade included a higher resectability rate, a marked reduction in postoperative hospital mortality, and an improved 5-year survival rate. In their opinion, neither more radical operations nor neoadjuvant therapy were successful in improving long-term results. It is important, therefore, to base therapeutic recommendations on current rather than historical data concerning management of this disease.

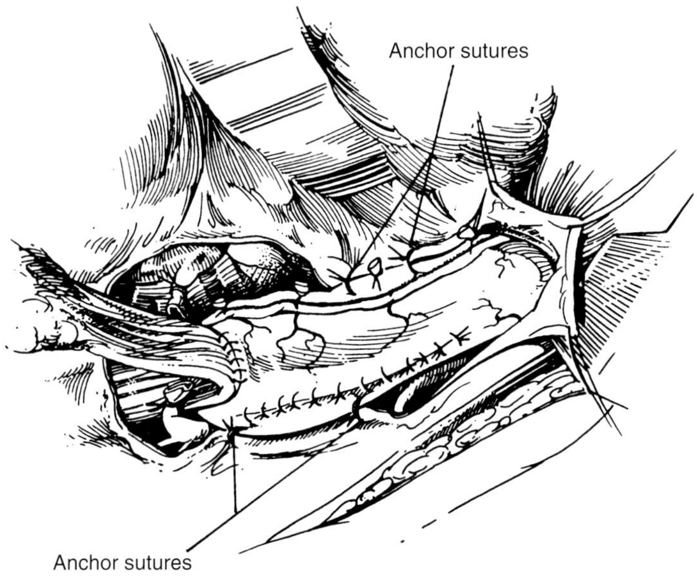

FIG. 14-10. The posterior row of the anastomosis is performed with interrupted nonabsorbable sutures. The gastric tube is fixed in the mediastinum anteromedially to the pleura of the divided inferior pulmonary ligament and posterolaterally to the parietal pleura of the chest wall to prevent torsion or intrathoracic prolapse of the stomach. (Reproduced with permission from Ellis FH Jr. Carcinoma of the esophagus and cardia. In: Ritchie WP Jr, Steele GD Jr, Dean RH, eds. General surgery. Philadelphia: JB Lippincott, 1995:91.)

TABLE 14-1. *Transthoracic esophagogastrectomy for carcinoma of the esophagus: reported results*

Author	Year	Country	Operability (%)	# Surgical cases	Resectability (%)*	Mortality (%)		Complications (%)		5-y Survival (%)
						30-day	Hospital	Major	Overall	
Bertelsen et al[16]	1985	Denmark	82	298	63.4		24			14.8
Hennessy and O'Connell[17]	1986	Ireland	NS	230	87	17.5	22			19.5
Galandiuk et al[18]	1986	United States	70.6	168	50		7.1		72.6	15.4†
Bluett et al[19]	1987	United States	46.3	144	72	10			41	14
Wong[20]	1987	Hong Kong	75	284	81.7	6.9	18.5		45	24.4‡
King et al[21]	1987	United States	NS	100	NS	3		27		22.8
Lu et al[22]	1987	China	78.9	1306	78.5		4.9			20.9
Mathisen et al[23]	1988	United States	NS	104	NS	2.9		15		§
Ellis[24]	1989	United States	82.3	310	88.7	2.2	4.4	14.5	24.7	20.8
Griffin et al[25]	1989	England	NS	202	NS		10.4			28
Page et al[26]	1990	England	NS	115	NS	8.7		15.6		22.1‡
Katlic et al[27]	1990	United States	58.6	261	63.5		21.5		40.1	21.9‖
Lund et al[28]	1990	Denmark	93.5	657	78	19			33	9¶
Law et al[29]	1992	Hong Kong	80	500	81.6	4.8	16.5		82.7	15
Nakadi et al[30]	1993	Belgium	47	187	89.8	5.9			35	34.2†
Salama & Leong[31]	1993	England	77.8	133	73.6		10.2			17.3
Rahamin & Cham[32]	1993	England	NS	298	NS	10	23			23

* Percentage of patients who underwent operation.
† Curative resection.
‡ Three-year survival.
§ 33.2% for squamous cell carcinoma, 7.7% for adenocrcinoma.
‖ Last decade of study.
¶ Unresected patients included.
NB, not stated.

Listed in Table 14-1 are data obtained from selected reports published from 1985 to 1993 inclusive from various parts of the world, some of which concern only esophageal cancers, whereas others also include both carcinoma of the esophagus and carcinoma of the cardia. Only papers reporting on 100 or more patients that included a detailed analysis of pertinent data are listed. In so far as possible, these reports are restricted to transthoracic procedures with an intrathoracic anastomosis using the stomach as an esophageal substitute. Excluded are transhiatal resections, radical "en bloc" and "three-field" procedures, as well as multitudinous reports on the results of various neoadjuvant modalities, topics that are reviewed in subsequent chapters. Not all of the reports include all patients with cancer of the esophagus and cardia encountered at the institution involved, so that operability figures are not always available. Some reports concern only patients having resections, so that resectability rates in these instances are unavailable. Operative mortality data are reported variously by different authors, so it is not always clear whether the data refer to 30-day mortality or overall hospital mortality rates. Only a few reports included both figures. Five-year survival data were also reported differently in the reports, some using the actuarial method, and others used an adjusted actuarial figure excluding hospital deaths and late deaths not due to cancer. Those reports based on curative resection only are so indicated in the table, as are figures related to survival rates at less than 5 years or to data restricted only to a recent sample of the patient population under review.

Operability rates varied tremendously in these reports, from 46.3% to 82.3%, with a median of 77.8%. The resectability rates varied from 50% to 89.8%, with a median of 78%. Thirty-day and overall hospital mortality rates also varied, with a median 30-day mortality of 5.9% and a median overall hospital mortality rate of 16.5%. The chief causes of postoperative mortality reported in these publications were either pulmonary in nature or of cardiovascular origin. Sepsis was also frequently mentioned, often as the result of an anastomotic leak. The overall complication rate, exclusive of hospital deaths, varied from 24.7% to 82.7%, with a median of 40%. Again, respiratory complications predominated, including atelectasis, bronchopneumonia, and empyema. Other causes were cardiac arrhythmias, wound and urinary tract infections, "contained" leaks, thoracic duct injury, and impaired gastric emptying, either early or late. The main late complication was anastomotic stricture, usually benign, but sometimes malignant. The median 5-year survival rate was 20.8%.

Thus, data from this more recent, highly selected group of reports indicate improvements in operability and resectability rates comparable to those reported in the extensive literature review of Müller and associates,[15] with a reduction in operative mortality. The 5-year survival rate of patients surviving resection, however, has undergone little change over the years. However, if one considers the entire patient population involved, more esophageal cancer patients now are available for long-term survival after resection because of higher operability and resectability rates and a lower hospital mortality rate. This is further borne out by a study comparing the overall survival of esophageal cancer patients during three different time intervals, two from the Mayo Clinic and one from the Lahey Clinic, total-

TABLE 14-2. *Carcinoma of the esophagus and cardia, January 1970–July 1994*

	Percentage of patients		
Operations (422)*			
Resections (379)	91.1		
30-day mortality		2.4	4.0
Hospital mortality		1.6	
Exploratory (43)	8.9		
Mortality		11.6	
Complications†			
Major	13.1		
Minor	12.6		
Five-year survival‡			
Overall	20.8		
Curative	23.3		
Stage I	50.8		
Stage IIA	37.5		
Stage IIB	16.2		
Stage III	13.6		
Stage IV	0.0		

* Number of procedures in parentheses.
† Based on patients operated on before 1990.
‡ Based on patients operated on before 1988.

ing 2027 patients.[24] The overall 5-year survival rate, including unresected patients, nearly quadrupled from 4% to 15% during this period, not because of any improvement in surgical technique or surgical care, but because of an increase in operability and resectability rates with a decrease in operative mortality.

Whether there are advantages or disadvantages to the transhiatal compared to the transthoracic approach is not answered by this analysis. Although I prefer to individualize the approach, using the transhiatal method for appropriate cases, others have condemned it as being an inadequate cancer operation.[33] This controversy is discussed in greater detail in Chapter 15, but as yet a comparison of the two approaches has failed to show that the transhiatal approach is safer than the transthoracic approach, or that it is a less effective cancer operation.[34]

Because of the wide variation in reported results, it is important to review one's own personal experience in determining therapy. From January 1970 to July 1994, 422 patients with cancer of the esophagus or cardia underwent operation on my service, a period during which the operability rate was 82% (Table 14-2). Three hundred seventy-nine of these patients underwent resection, for a resectability rate of 91.1%. Nine patients (2.4%) died within 30 days of operation, and six more patients failed to leave the hospital, for an overall hospital mortality rate of 4%. Major postoperative complications occurred in 13.1%. Satisfactory palliation of dysphagia was achieved in 80%. The overall adjusted actuarial 5-year survival rate after "curative" resections, calculated on the basis of patients operated on before 1988, was 23.3%. These data differ from the median values depicted in Table 14-2 by demonstrating a higher resectability rate and lower 30-day and hospital mortality rates. The 5-year adjusted actuarial survival rates, however, are similar.

As in other series, the importance of stage on survival was clearly evident, with no patients in stage IV surviving 5 years, and more that three times as many patients in stage I surviving 5 years than in stage III. In another study, the beneficial effect of early diagnosis was clearly demonstrated by comparing the results of resection of adenocarcinoma in patients with Barrett's esophagus whose lesion was detected under surveillance, with the results in those in whom the diagnosis was made only after symptoms developed (62% 5-year survival rate, compared to 20%).[35] It is tempting to conclude from these findings that improvement in long-term survival after resection of carcinoma of the esophagus or cardia will depend on early diagnosis rather than on more radical operations or the use of neoadjuvant therapy. Time will tell whether this view is correct. Until then, results of standard transthoracic resection for carcinoma of the esophagus and cardia remain the gold standard for comparison with alternative therapeutic modalities.

REFERENCES

1. Lewis I. The surgical treatment of carcinoma of the esophagus with special reference to a new operation for growths of the middle third. Br J Surg 1946;34:18.
2. Ellis FH Jr. Esophagogastrectomy for carcinoma: technical considerations based on anatomic location of lesion. Surg Clin North Am 1980; 60:265.
3. Gerndt SJ, Orringer MB. Tube jejunostomy as an adjunct to esophagectomy. Surgery 1994;115:164.
4. Swails WS, Babineau TT, Ellis FH Jr, et al. The role of enteral jejunostomy feeding after esophagogastrectomy: a prospective randomized study. Dis of Esoph 1995;8:193.
5. Billroth T: Ueber die Resection des Oesophagus. Arch Klin Chir 1871; 13:65.
6. Czerny. Neue Operationen. Zentralbl Chir 1877;4:433.
7. Torek F. The first successful case of resection of the thoracic portion of the oesophagus for carcinoma. Surg Gynecol Obstet 1913;16:614.
8. Zaaijer JH. Erfolgreiche transpleurale Resektion eines Cardiocarcinoms. Beitr Klin Chir 1913;83:419.
9. Ohsawa T. The surgery of the esophagus. Arch Jpn Chir 1933;10:605.
10. Marshall SF. Carcinoma of the esophagus: successful resection of lower end of esophagus with re-establishment of esophageal gastric continuity. Surg Clin North Am 1938;18:643.
11. Adams WE, Phemister IB. Carcinoma of lower thoracic esophagus: report of successful resection and esophagogastrostomy. J Thorac Cardiovasc Surg 1938;9:621.
12. Sweet RH. Late results of surgical treatment of carcinoma of the esophagus. JAMA 1954;155:422.
13. Tam PC, Cheung HC, Ma L, et al. Local recurrences after subtotal esophagectomy for squamous cell carcinoma. Ann Surg 1987;205:189.
14. Earlam R, Cunha-Melo JR. Oesophageal squamous cell carcinoma: I. a critical review of surgery. Br J Surg 1980;67:31.
15. Müller JM, Erasmi H, Stelzner M, Zieren U, Pichlmaier H. Surgical therapy of oesophageal carcinoma. Br J Surg 1990;77:845.
16. Bertelsen S, Aasted A, Vejlsted H. Surgical treatment for malignant lesions of the distal part of the esophagus and the esophagogastric junction. World J Surg 1985;9:633.
17. Hennessy TPJ, O'Connell R. Carcinoma of the hypopharynx, esophagus and cardia. Surg Gynecol Obstet 1986;162:243.
18. Galanduik S, Hermann RE, Gassman JJ, Cosgrove DM. Cancer of the esophagus: the Cleveland experience. Am Surg 1986;203:101.
19. Bluett MK, Sawyers JL, Healy D. Esophageal carcinoma: improved quality of survival with resection. Ann Surg 1987;53:126.
20. Wong J. Esophageal resection for cancer: the rationale of current practice. Am J Surg 1987;153:18.
21. King MR, Pairolero PC, Trastek VF, Payne WS, Bernatz PE. Ivor Lewis esophagogastrectomy for carcinoma of the esophagus: early and late functional results. Ann Thorac Surg 1987;44:119.
22. Lu YK, Li YM, Gu YZ. Cancer of esophagus and esophagogastric junction: analysis of results of 1,025 resections after 5 to 20 years. Ann Thorac Surg 1987;43:176.
23. Mathisen DJ, Grillo HC, Wilkins EW Jr, Moncure AC, Hilgenberg AD. Transthoracic esophagectomy: a safe approach to carcinoma of the esophagus. Ann Thorac Surg 1988;45:137.
24. Ellis FH Jr. Treatment of carcinoma of the esophagus or cardia. Mayo Clin Proc 1989;64:945.

25. Griffin S, Desai J, Charlton M, Townsend E, Fountain SW. Facts influencing mortality and morbidity following oesophageal resection. Eur J Cardiothorac Surg 1989;3:419.
26. Page RD, Khalil JF, Whyte RI, Kaplan DK, Donnelly RJ. Esophagogastrectomy via left thoracophrenectomy. Ann Thorac Surg 1990;49:763.
27. Katlic MR, Wilkins EW Jr, Grillo HC. Three decades of treatment of esophageal squamous carcinoma at the Massachusetts General Hospital. J Thorac Cardiovasc Surg 1990;99:929.
28. Lund O, Kimose HH, Aagaard MT, Hasenkam JM, Erlandsen M. Risk stratification and long-term results after surgical treatment of carcinoma of the thoracic esophagus and cardia: a 25 year retrospective study. J Thorac Cardiovasc Surg 1990;99:200.
29. Law SL, Fok M, Cheng SWK, Wong J. A comparison of outcome after resection for squamous cell carcinomas of the esophagus and cardia. Surg Gynecol Obstet 1992;175:107.
30. Nakadi I, Houben J-J, Gay F, Closset J, Gelin M, Lambilliothe JP. Does esophagectomy cure a resectable esophageal cancer? World J Surg 1993;17:760.
31. Salama FD, Leong YP. Resection for carcinoma of the esophagus. J R Coll Surg Edinb 1993;34:97.
32. Rahamin J, Cham CW. Oesophagogastrectomy for carcinoma of the esophagus and cardia. Br J Surg 1993;80:1305.
33. Hagen JA, Peters JH, DeMeester TR. Superiority of extended en bloc esophagogastrectomy for carcinoma of the lower esophagus and cardia. J Thorac Cardiovasc Surg 1993;106:850.
34. Streitz JM Jr. Comparison of transhiatal and transthoracic esophagogastrectomy. Semin Thorac Cardiovasc Surg 1992;4:300.
35. Streitz JM Jr, Andrews CW Jr, Ellis FH Jr. Endoscopic surveillance of Barrett's esophagus: does it help? J Thorac Cardiovasc Surg 1993;105:383.

Surgery for Gastrointestinal Cancer: A Multidisciplinary Approach, edited by Harold J. Wanebo.
Lippincott-Raven Publishers, Philadelphia, © 1997.

CHAPTER 15

Transhiatal Esophagectomy for Carcinoma of the Thoracic Esophagus

John S. Bolton and George M. Fuhrman

HISTORY

Before the development of endotracheal anesthesia, there were a few intrepid attempts to attack surgically carcinoma of the thoracic esophagus by an extrathoracic approach. Denk[1] in 1913 developed an experimental technique for transmediastinal esophagectomy without thoracotomy using a vein stripper to avulse the esophagus, and suggested this approach as a technique for resecting esophageal carcinoma. Esophagectomy without thoracotomy was successfully accomplished for the first time by Grey-Turner and Durh in 1933.[2] After the development of endotracheal positive-pressure ventilation, transthoracic, transpleural esophagectomy was introduced by Adams and Phemister in 1938,[3] and transthoracic esophagectomy (TTE) became the standard surgical approach to esophageal carcinoma for the next 40 years. Kirk, in 1974,[4] and Orringer and Sloan in 1978[5] reintroduced the transhiatal technique for resection of carcinoma of the thoracic esophagus in an attempt to avoid the high incidence of pulmonary complications and the highly morbid intrathoracic anastomotic leak seen after transthoracic resection. Subsequent to these publications, several large series have demonstrated the feasibility and widespread applicability of transhiatal resection for carcinoma of the thoracic esophagus.[6–10]

INDICATIONS

Transhiatal esophageal resection may be used for carcinoma of any segment of the thoracic esophagus. Transhiatal resection is indicated for all histologic types of esophageal cancer, including squamous carcinoma and adenocarcinoma, the latter rising rapidly in incidence in the United States.[11] For the purposes of this discussion, carcinoma of the cardia of the stomach that grossly involves the lower esophagus is included, because the development of an adequate proximal margin for this lesion almost invariably requires resection of a significant portion of the thoracic esophagus. Bulky, mid-esophageal cancers, densely adherent to the membranous portion of the trachea, left mainstem bronchus, or descending aorta are uncommon, but when encountered, are problematic. This situation can be suspected on preoperative computed tomography (CT) scan; when this situation is encountered, preoperative chemotherapy and radiation therapy may be indicated, and if a good response to therapy is achieved, transhiatal resection can be carried out.

In most situations, transhiatal resection and transthoracic resection represent two alternative routes of access to accomplish a similar objective, and the lower incidence of severe cardiopulmonary complications and avoidance of a potentially morbid intrathoracic anastomotic leak with the transhiatal resection make it preferable. This is particularly true in patients who are at higher operative risk because of cardiopulmonary comorbidity or advanced age. Transhiatal esophagectomy (THE) is also particularly well suited for patients with severe dysplasia or intramucosal carcinoma discovered during a surveillance program for Barrett's columnar-lined lower esophagus, in whom there is no rationale for wide mediastinal lymph node dissection and in whom minimizing perioperative morbidity and mortality is of paramount importance.

With the transhiatal technique, wide radial (circumferential) margins for lower esophageal cancers and resection of lower periesophageal, left gastric, and celiac nodes are technically feasible; however, systematic resection of mid-mediastinal lymph nodes (levels 4 and 7)[12] is not possible. The inclusion of these nodes in the resection has not been proven to be of therapeutic benefit. If desired for staging purposes, these lymph nodes can be obtained using a thoracoscopic technique.[13]

PREOPERATIVE STUDIES/PREPARATION

A careful review of prior gastric or duodenal ulcer disease or prior gastric surgical procedures is necessary, because the presence of these might preclude use of a gastric reconstruction. Thorough history and physical examination with particular attention to cardiopulmonary comorbidity and any other poten-

John S. Bolton: Ochsner Medical Institutions, 1514 Jefferson Highway, New Orleans, LA 70121
George M. Fuhrman: Ochsner Medical Institutions, 1514 Jefferson Highway, New Orleans, LA 70121

TABLE 15-1. *American Society of Anesthesiologists (ASA) risk classification*

I	A normal healthy patient
II	A patient with a mild-to-moderate systemic disease
III	A patient with a severe systemic disease that limits activity, but is not incapacitating
IV	A patient with an incapacitating systemic disease that is a constant threat to life
V	A moribund patient not expected to survive 24 hours with or without an operation

tially life-threatening comorbidity should be carried out, as well as a review of performance status and assignment of American Society of Anesthesiologists (ASA) risk status (Table 15-1).[14] Although other preoperative risk classifications are available,[15] ASA status has been validated as a significant predictor of risk for major thoracic and upper abdominal surgery.[16] In addition, the ASA risk classification has the advantage of emphasizing the worst (most likely to be life-threatening) comorbidity, and includes implicitly an assessment of performance status. In evaluating cardiopulmonary status, pulmonary function tests are routinely done in all patients with a history of smoking and those older than 65 years of age. Cardiac evaluation is based on clinical symptoms, signs, and performance status; if clinical evidence of ischemic symptoms or rhythm disturbances exists, cardiac evaluation should be exhaustive.

Essential preoperative diagnostic studies include upper gastrointestinal endoscopy, noting the upper limit of the cancer and the upper limit of Barrett's metaplasia (if present). The distal extent of tumor should also be noted, especially if the stomach is involved, and the rest of the stomach and duodenum should be carefully examined to rule out other neoplasms or the presence of major deformity from chronic peptic ulcer disease.

Computed tomography scan of the chest and abdomen is the best, albeit not perfect, imaging study and should be done to assess resectability, feasibility of resection by THE, and stage of the neoplasm. Liver or lung metastases preclude any attempt at resection of the primary tumor, given the short life expectancy in this situation. In the absence of distant metastasis, local invasion in the mid-mediastinum is usually the critical factor in deciding whether resection by THE is possible. The important areas to assess on CT are the trachea and left mainstem bronchus, aorta, pericardium, and diaphragm. Several generally accepted criteria—not absolutely accurate but at least predicting for a potentially difficult THE and for radial margin involvement in the surgical specimen—are:

1. Bowing or anterior displacement of the membranous portion of the trachea or left mainstem bronchus, or projection of tumor into the lumen of the trachea[17–19] (Fig. 15-1)
2. Close approximation of the tumor (with loss of the normal fat plane) to the aorta around greater than 90° of its circumference[17–19] (Fig. 15-2)
3. Loss of the fat plane between the tumor and the pericardium (this fat plane must be present above and below the tumor for this sign to be valid) and anterior displacement of the left atrium[17,18]
4. Encirclement of the diaphragm crura[17]

Of these, involvement of the tracheobronchial tree is the most common, and when present, increases the risk of laceration

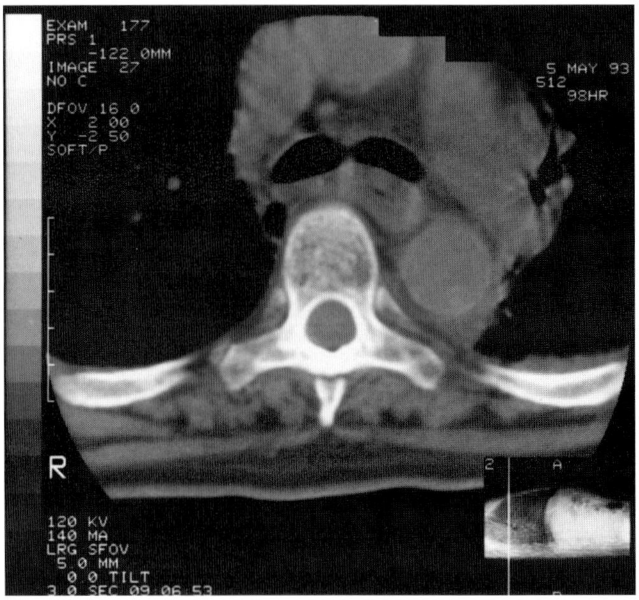

FIG. 15-1. Bowing and anterior displacement of the membranous portion of the left mainstem bronchus by carcinoma of the midthoracic esophagus.

of the membranous portion of the trachea during THE. When involvement of the tracheobronchial tree is suspected on CT scan, bronchoscopy should be carried out. In the absence of bronchoscopic evidence of tracheobronchial involvement, resection should be attempted, because CT scan evidence of tracheobronchial involvement is not 100% reliable. A trial THE dissection can be attempted, but the surgeon should have a low threshold for conversion to transthoracic resection if adherence to the tracheobronchial tree is confirmed at surgery.

Involvement of the aorta or pericardium is rare (less than 3% of esophageal cancers[20]), and CT scan is not very reliable at

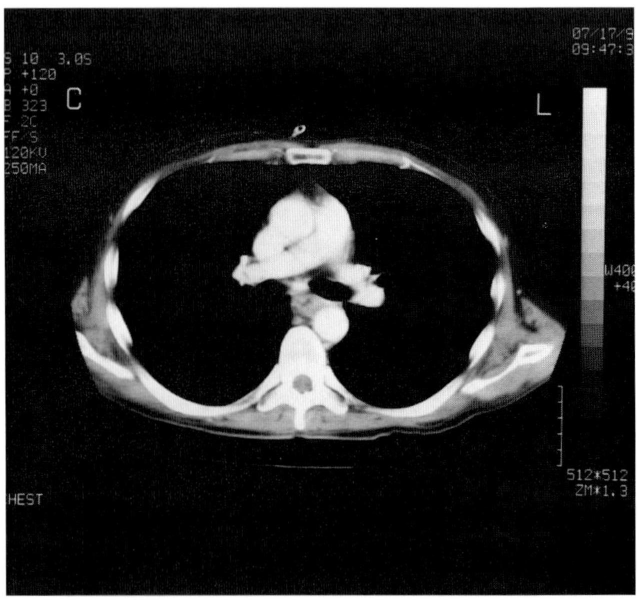

FIG. 15-2. Close approximation of esophageal carcinoma to the descending thoracic aorta.

differentiating mere proximity from actual invasion of these structures. Trial dissection by the transhiatal route is indicated and is feasible in most cases. Diaphragmatic involvement may be present with bulky tumors of the lower esophagus or esophagogastric junction, but this rarely presents major difficulty in performing THE.

When suspicion of local mediastinal invasion is high (particularly of the membranous portion of the trachea or left mainstem bronchus), preoperative chemotherapy and radiation therapy should be considered, in the hope of reducing tumor size and facilitating resection. Preoperative concern with regard to radial margin involvement does not preclude THE, because in the face of proximity to the tracheobronchial tree or the aorta, wide margins are not obtainable by any currently available surgical technique, including TTE. In these cases, it is assumed that resection will be palliative unless the patient has a good response to preoperative chemotherapy and radiation therapy.

Computed tomography scan is not a precise staging tool because it cannot differentiate level of invasion of the esophageal wall with accuracy, and it underestimates lymph node involvement.[21] This inaccuracy in staging does not change surgical management, however.

Preoperative preparation includes smoking cessation and institution of bronchopulmonary toilet in patients who are actively smoking or who have a history of bronchitis. Nutrition is carefully assessed; in general, preoperative parenteral nutrition is not indicated unless the patient has lost more than 10% of body weight in the preceding 2 months or has severe hypoalbuminemia. For patients undergoing elective resection (such as patients in a Barrett's surveillance program found to have severe dysplasia, carcinoma in situ, or intramucosal carcinoma) who have a sedentary lifestyle, a 3-week preoperative exercise program can improve performance status and physical reserve. In patients presenting with dysphagia secondary to advanced, obstructing lesions, this is not an option.

Preoperative colonoscopy is done if preexisting gastric or duodenal disease, prior gastric surgery, or extensive involvement of the upper stomach by tumor indicates the likely need for colon interposition. If colon interposition is anticipated, mesenteric angiography is done in patients older than the age of 65 years, or with a history of peripheral vascular disease or prior aortic surgery. Mechanical bowel preparation with osmotic cathartics, use of a sequential compression device to prevent deep venous thrombosis, perioperative antibiotics (cephalosporin), and type and cross-match for two units of packed red blood cells are routinely performed.

Preoperative chemotherapy, radiation therapy, or both are not used routinely. Although a number of small, phase II studies have suggested improvement in survival with the use of neoadjuvant programs using chemotherapy only,[22,23] or chemotherapy and radiation therapy,[24–28] this has not been the case in all series.[29–32] Furthermore, the small number of patients included in most of these reports creates wide confidence intervals in the statistical analysis of response rates and disease-free survival. In addition, the many pitfalls in the use of historical controls as a background against which results of neoadjuvant studies are compared, including the introduction of better preoperative staging techniques and better diagnostic techniques leading to earlier diagnosis of esophageal adenocarcinoma in Barrett's surveillance programs, makes the evidence for survival benefit in neoadjuvant therapy programs less than convincing. Furthermore, the available randomized, phase III studies comparing preoperative chemotherapy[32] or chemotherapy/radiation therapy[33–35] to surgical resection alone have not shown survival benefit with the addition of preoperative therapy. Because these neoadjuvant programs can add significant treatment toxicity,[31,36,37] and because their use may increase operative mortality if radiation therapy, bleomycin, or mitomycin are components of the preoperative treatment program owing to an increased risk of postoperative pulmonary failure,[38–41] we are in agreement with Kelsen and colleagues, who concluded that "outside of carefully designed clinical trials, surgery alone or radiation alone remain standard therapy."[32]

Selected patients with marginally resectable or locally unresectable tumors (which are usually located in the mid-thoracic esophagus) as predicted by preoperative CT scan are recommended for preoperative cytoreductive therapy. In this situation, combined chemotherapy and radiation therapy are used, because combined therapy programs have been shown to provide better local response rates and pathologic complete response rates[24,25,27] than do programs using chemotherapy[23,31,42] or radiation therapy[43] only. Available evidence indicates that squamous carcinoma and adenocarcinoma of the esophagus respond at similar rates to preoperative programs using 5-fluorouracil, cisplatin, and radiation therapy, with objective response rates of 50% to 70%[24,25] and pathologic complete response rates of 15% to 40%[24,25,28–30] with radiation therapy doses up to 50 Gy. Although concern has been raised about the possibility of higher operative mortality with the use of radiation therapy before TTE,[44] operative mortality experience with transhiatal resection after preoperative combined modality therapy has been favorable,[27,28] with the exception of one reported series.[45] Because at least 40% of patients have recurrent or persistent carcinoma with dysphagia despite chemotherapy and radiation therapy, and because restoration of swallowing is the main goal of palliation, we consider chemotherapy and radiation therapy to be *preoperative* therapy, and carry out resection 6 weeks after completion of therapy unless metastatic disease has developed in the meantime.

OPERATIVE TECHNIQUE

After induction of general endotracheal anesthesia, bronchoscopy is carried out if the tumor is approximating the trachea or left mainstem bronchus on preoperative CT scan. A double-lumen endotracheal tube is not routinely used, except when a bulky mid-esophageal tumor or the use of preoperative radiation therapy suggest the likelihood of a difficult transhiatal dissection and the possible need for transthoracic conversion. The patient is placed in the supine position, a shoulder roll is inserted, the neck is flexed, and the head is extended and turned to the right. Sterile skin preparation and draping is carried out from the chin to the pubis, preparing the chest widely to a point posterior to the mid-axillary line to provide access for chest tube placement. The left neck must be kept free of intravenous line placement because this will be the site of access to the proximal esophagus.

Abdominal access is provided by an upper midline incision that is carried over the lower end of the sternum with excision of the xiphoid process. The abdomen is explored for metastatic disease, paying particular attention to the liver, peritoneal surfaces, and regional lymph nodes. Mobilization of the stomach begins along the greater curvature, staying outside of and carefully

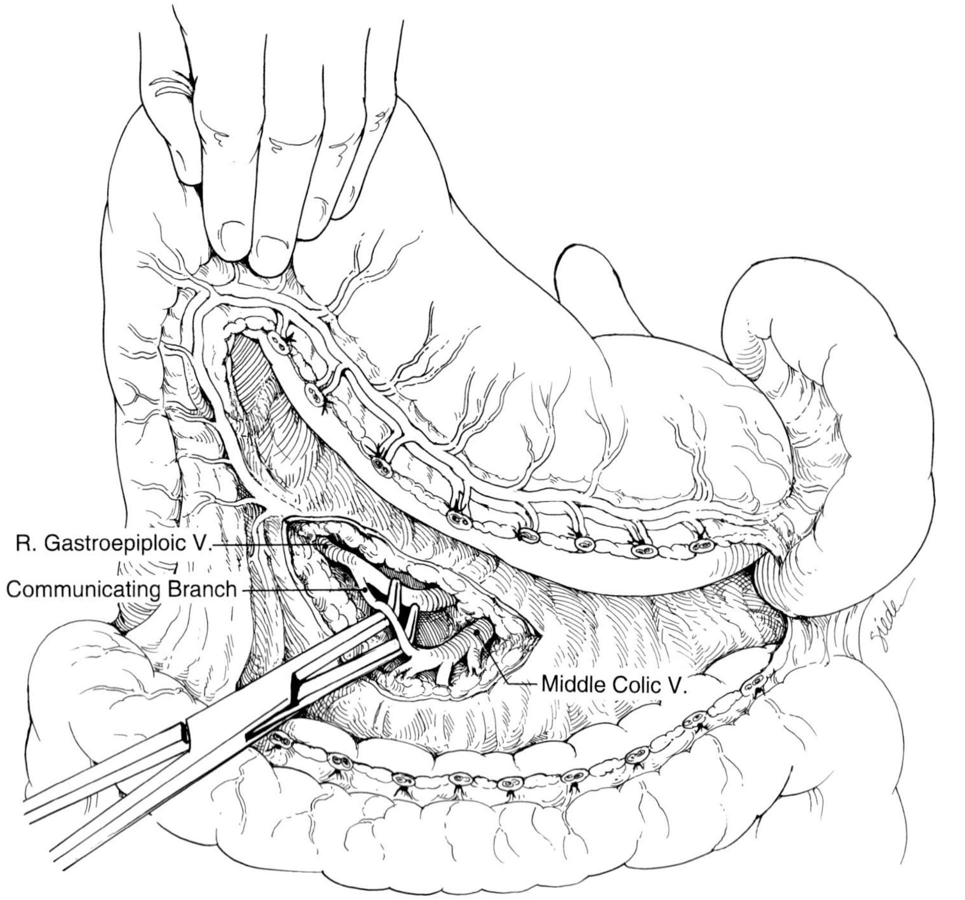

FIG. 15-3. Communicating branch from the middle colic vein to the right gastroepiploic vein, which must be ligated and divided to permit full mobilization of the stomach.

preserving the right gastroepiploic arcade, which is the major blood supply for the gastric interposition. Branches of the right gastroepiploic vessels to the greater omentum are divided between fine (3-0) silk ligatures, avoiding ''bunching'' of the intervening mesentery so as not to restrict the mobility of the greater curve or crimp the right gastroepiploic vessels. As the dissection proceeds distally, posterior adhesions from the antrum to the mesocolon and the anterior surface of the pancreas are freed. There is often a communicating branch from the middle colic vein that joins the right gastroepiploic vein at its base, just before it enters the superior mesenteric vein (Fig. 15-3). This branch must be sought and carefully divided; otherwise it may be torn away at its junction with the right gastroepiploic vein when the gastric interposition is delivered to the neck. Distal mobilization is completed with a Kocher maneuver to mobilize the duodenum and head of the pancreas. A pyloromyotomy or pyloroplasty is performed; if pyloroplasty is chosen, this should be only 1 cm in length so as not to restrict gastric length.

Proximal mobilization of the greater curvature of the stomach proceeds with division of the short gastric and posterior gastric vessels, aided by a mechanical ''upper hand'' retractor. Splenectomy is performed only if the primary tumor involves the spleen or if the splenic hilar nodes are involved.

The stomach is then lifted anteriorly and superiorly, exposing and placing on stretch the left gastric vessels. During retraction on the stomach, care must be taken to avoid injury to the right gastroepiploic vessels. The proximal hepatic lymph nodes and left gastric lymph nodes are mobilized and the left gastric artery is taken at its origin from the celiac axis. The stomach is then retracted inferiorly, the lesser omentum is widely mobilized (preserving the right gastric artery and vein), and the celiac lymph nodes are mobilized. The peritoneum overlying the hiatus is opened, sweeping all nodal and soft tissue down onto the specimen. Mobilization of the stomach is now complete.

If the tumor is located at the gastroesophageal junction or the terminal esophagus and is bulky, involvement of the crus of the diaphragm, pericardium, or the lower mediastinal pleura may be present. In these cases, a cuff of the right or left crus, or both, can be sacrificed as necessary to provide an adequate radial margin (Fig. 15-4). If the diaphragmatic crura are not involved, the right and left crus can simply be split using the cautery to permit wide exposure to the posterior mediastinum. By the use of a mechanical retractor to elevate the lower end of the sternum and the costal margins, and deep manual retractors (Deaver) to open the diaphragmatic hiatus, excellent exposure to the posterior mediastinum is provided. Under direct vision, a packet including the pericardium anteriorly, the right and left mediastinal pleura laterally, and all posterior tissue down to the aorta can be developed around a bulky lower esophageal tumor. Once the dissection has extended for several centimeters beyond the upper margin of the tumor, the dissection is shifted to a plane just outside the esophageal wall, mobilizing the esophagus from the periesophageal soft tissues. Usually, the avascular plane anterior to the esophagus is bluntly developed as a first step, and then a similar plane is developed by blunt finger dissection posteriorly. Then, under direct vision, the lateral ''stalks'' are

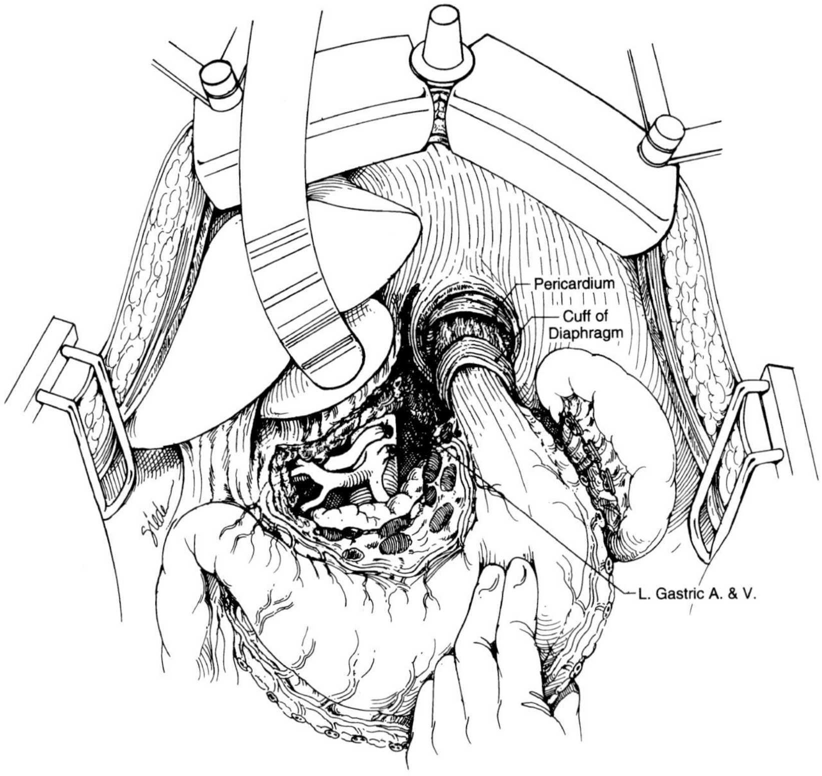

FIG. 15-4. A cuff of the right and left crus of the diaphragm, and if necessary, the posterior pericardium, can be resected en bloc with the esophagus to provide an adequate radial margin for a carcinoma of the distal esophagus.

first clipped and then divided. In this manner, dissection proceeds from the hiatus to the level of the carina. The periesophageal lymph nodes (level 8 mediastinal lymph nodes) are removed en bloc with the specimen.

Once the transhiatal dissection has reached the level of the carina, dissection is interrupted until the cervical mobilization has advanced well into the superior mediastinum. If desired, a second surgeon can be used for this portion of the procedure to shorten the operative time. An incision is made parallel to the anterior border of the left sternocleidomastoid muscle from the mid-neck to the suprasternal notch. The sternocleidomastoid muscle and the carotid artery and internal jugular vein are mobilized laterally, dividing the middle thyroid vein, and also dividing the omohyoid muscle and the inferior thyroid artery if necessary to increase exposure. The esophagus is encircled low in the neck, identifying the left recurrent laryngeal nerve and gently keeping it in contact with the trachea as it is mobilized away from the esophagus. As the esophagus is encircled, dissection is kept in immediate contact with the esophageal wall to avoid injury to the right recurrent laryngeal nerve in the lower neck; the nerve will not be harmed as long as the periesophageal tissue is not included in the mobilization of the esophagus.

Blunt finger dissection then proceeds down the esophagus into the superior mediastinum. Injury to the left recurrent laryngeal nerve, the membranous portion of the trachea, the azygos vein, and the thoracic duct is avoided by maintaining the dissection in direct contact with the esophageal wall, brushing the surrounding soft tissue away from the esophagus. As the carina is reached from the cervical dissection, upward traction is applied to the cervical esophagus by a Penrose drain while downward traction is applied to the gastroesophageal junction by a second Penrose drain encircling the gastroesophageal junction. The operating surgeon then simultaneously continues the transhiatal dissection upward and the cervical dissection downward until the upper and lower dissections meet (Fig. 15-5), first in the midline anteriorly, next in the midline posteriorly, and the remaining lateral attachments are bluntly torn away, maintaining the plane of dissection in close contact with the esophageal wall and, insofar as possible, pushing the surrounding soft tissue away from the esophagus so as to confine the shearing force close to the esophageal wall. At this point, the esophagus is completely free of its mediastinal attachments.

For mid-esophageal cancers, a decision must be made about the feasibility of resection by the transhiatal approach based on the preoperative CT findings and a trial dissection by the transhiatal route. In most cases, transhiatal resection is possible; however, the surgeon should not hesitate to convert to a transthoracic approach if a bulky tumor adherent to the membranous portion of the trachea or the aorta is encountered. The major reason for conversion in these cases is to ensure operative safety, not to enhance the surgical margin, because the proximity of the tumor to a critical structure constrains the margin regardless of the operative approach. If the chest CT scan is carefully reviewed before surgery, intraoperative conversion to transthoracic resection should seldom be necessary. Preoperative radiation therapy may induce mediastinal fibrosis and adherence of the esophagus to surrounding mediastinal tissue, although the degree of this reaction varies considerably from one patient to another. A trial transhiatal dissection is warranted in every case, with conversion to a transthoracic approach if the periesophageal fibrosis is severe. In our experience, conversion to a transthoracic approach, for any cause, has been necessary in only 5% of patients in whom an initial transhiatal dissection has been attempted.

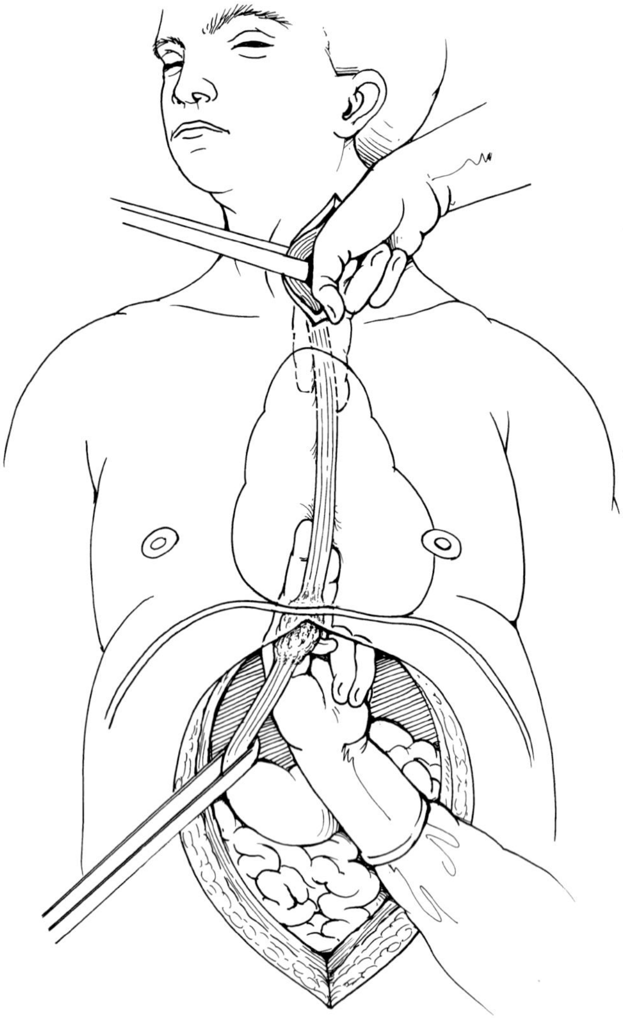

FIG. 15-5. Simultaneous transhiatal and transcervical dissection of the mediastinal portion of the esophagus.

Arterial hypotension is frequently encountered during the blunt mediastinal dissection, and the patient's blood pressure should be continuously monitored by the surgeon and the anesthesiologist during this time. It is often necessary for the surgeon to work for brief periods of approximately 30 seconds during the deeper portions of the mediastinal dissection and then allow a 30- to 60-second period for the patient's blood pressure to recover before continuing the dissection. If the patient's blood pressure is particularly labile or takes more than a few seconds to return to normal on cessation of the mediastinal dissection, hypovolemia may be present and additional intravenous fluid should be given. During the typical transhiatal mediastinal dissection, blood loss is limited to 500 mL or less; rapid and persisting bleeding may indicate a tear of the azygos vein or of an esophageal artery as it arises from the aorta, and requires conversion to transthoracic exposure for delineation and control of the bleeding site.

When injury to the membranous portion of the distal trachea or the proximal left mainstem bronchus is incurred during mobilization of the esophagus, right thoracotomy is required for exposure and repair. Either primary closure or closure with a pericardial patch can be used, depending on the extent of the defect in the membranous trachea. If necessary, the repair can be bolstered by a vascularized intercostal muscle flap and, if a significant postoperative air leak develops, this can be managed by the temporary use of high-frequency jet ventilation or bilateral bronchial intubation.

After the esophagus has been freed completely from its mediastinal attachments, the anesthesiologist is instructed to withdraw the nasogastric tube and the upper thoracic esophagus is pulled into the neck and divided with the gastrointestinal anastomosis stapler. Provided that an adequate proximal margin is ensured, several centimeters of the upper thoracic esophagus should be preserved because this facilitates the subsequent esophagogastric anastomosis and may also enhance postoperative swallowing.[46] A Penrose drain is sutured to the lower end of the transected esophagus, and the thoracic esophagus is then extracted from the mediastinum and delivered into the abdominal cavity and onto the anterior chest wall. Using four to six applications of the gastrointestinal anastomosis stapler (4.8-mm staple length), a gastric tube is created based on the greater curvature of the stomach and the right gastroepiploic vessels, thereby excising the cardia, lesser curvature of the stomach, and the attached left gastric, hepatic, and celiac lymph nodes (Fig. 15-6). By excising the lesser curvature of the stomach, several centimeters of additional length is gained for the gastric interposate. While the specimen is being examined by the pathologist for adequacy of proximal and distal margins using frozen sections, the gastrointestinal anastomosis staple line is oversewn with interrupted 3-0 silk suture.

If any doubt exists as to the viability of the proximal gastric stump, this can be assessed by intravenous fluorescein injection and use of the Wood lamp. A Penrose drain is then affixed to the proximal gastric stump with a 2-0 silk suture and the gastric interposate is delivered to the neck, taking care to avoid torsion. In most instances there is a generous redundancy in gastric length such that a length of gastric interposate can be delivered into the neck that allows for a comfortable anastomosis at or above the skin level (Fig. 15-7). Anastomosis is done in a single layer of interrupted 3-0 silk or Vicryl suture, and the redundant stomach is then pulled back down into the chest so that the anastomosis lies at or slightly below the level of the thoracic inlet (Fig. 15-8). If there is any evidence of constriction by the thoracic inlet, the head of the left clavicle and left portion of the manubrium can be resected; however, this is rarely necessary. The prepyloric antrum is then hitched to the diaphragmatic hiatus with several 3-0 silk seromuscular sutures to prevent undue tension on the anastomosis.

For tumors in the proximal thoracic esophagus, additional exposure can be obtained if necessary by an upper sternal split, as advocated by Orringer[47] and by Kirk.[48] This technique is also useful in cases where gastric length is impaired by scarring caused by prior hiatal hernia surgery or gastrostomy placement, or by the need to resect more than the upper third of the stomach due to tumor involvement. In these situations, if the tumor does not involve the upper thoracic esophagus, 6 to 8 cm of proximal thoracic esophagus can be preserved and the anastomosis can be performed in the upper mediastinum through an upper mediastinal split, with division of the left innominate vein if necessary to facilitate exposure.

If the cardia and fundus of the stomach are extensively involved, adequate distal stomach to reach the neck may not be present after resection of the tumor. In these cases, left colon in-

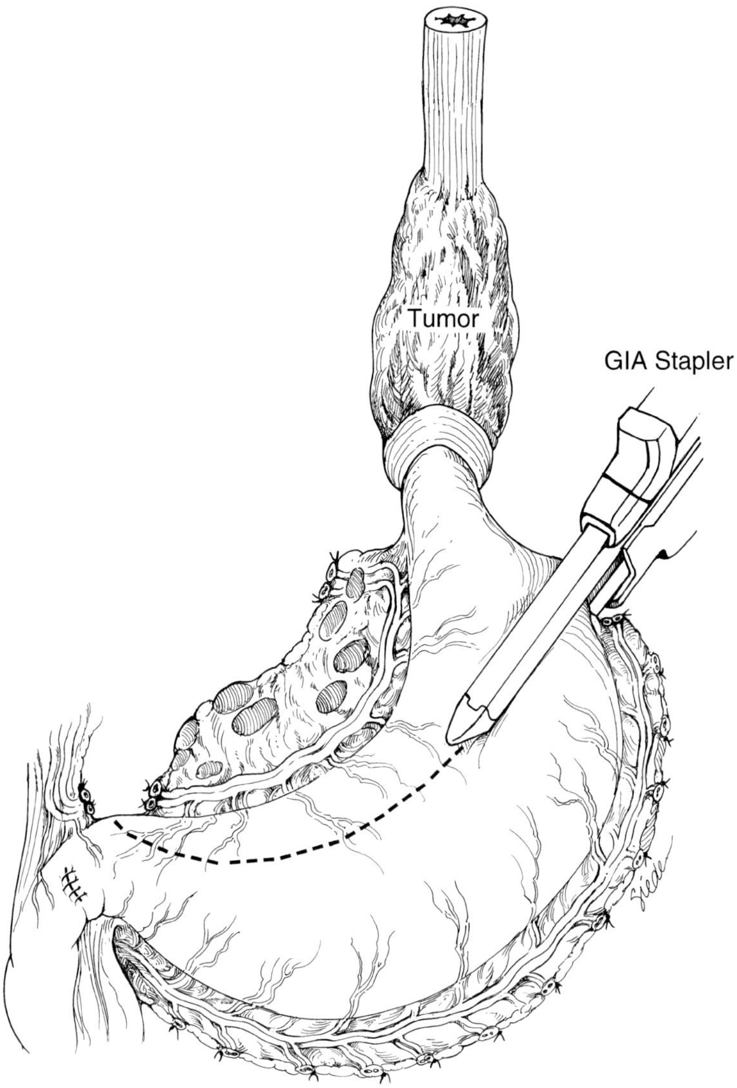

FIG. 15-6. The GIA stapler is used to create a gastric tube, based on the greater curvature of the stomach and the right gastroepiploic vessels, thereby completing resection of the esophagus, cardia and lesser curve of the stomach, and attached lymph nodes.

terposition is done, using the technique of DeMeester and colleagues.[49] Preoperative upper gastrointestinal endoscopy and CT scan are the keys to identifying these cases before surgery, thus ensuring adequate preoperative study and preparation of the colon.

The esophagogastric anastomosis is drained by two closed suction drains brought out through the left neck. If an anastomotic leak develops, it is imperative that it be well controlled by means of a cervical drain to prevent mediastinal or pleural suppuration. Before abdominal closure, a feeding jejunostomy tube is placed. Abdominal and cervical wound closure is performed in the routine fashion, and chest tubes are placed if required by entry into either the right or left pleura during the mediastinal dissection.

POSTOPERATIVE CARE

The patient is extubated as soon as possible after surgery, and postoperative care follows the routine for any major upper gastrointestinal operation. Nasogastric suction is maintained until bowel function resumes, at which time a liquid diet is initiated and advanced to solid feedings as tolerated, with the patient instructed to masticate thoroughly before swallowing. The anastomotic drains are not removed until the 10th postoperative day, and if purulent drainage develops, a water-soluble contrast swallow is obtained to document the extent of the anastomotic fistula. Provided the anastomotic leakage is well controlled, systemic sepsis will not ensue and the resultant fistula will be a self-limited and relatively benign complication. If the contrast swallow reveals no perianastomotic abscess and the stomach empties readily, the cervical drains can be incrementally advanced beginning on the 10th postoperative day and the fistula will close over the next 5 to 7 days as the drains are progressively advanced. If cellulitis or suppuration of the soft tissue of the neck develops at any time, further drain advancement should be delayed, the patient should be placed on NPO status, and intravenous broad-spectrum antibiotics should be administered until the inflammation subsides.

OPERATIVE RESULTS

Reported operative mortality rates with THE have ranged from 0% to 25%[6–10,44,50–63] (Table 15-2), reflecting variations

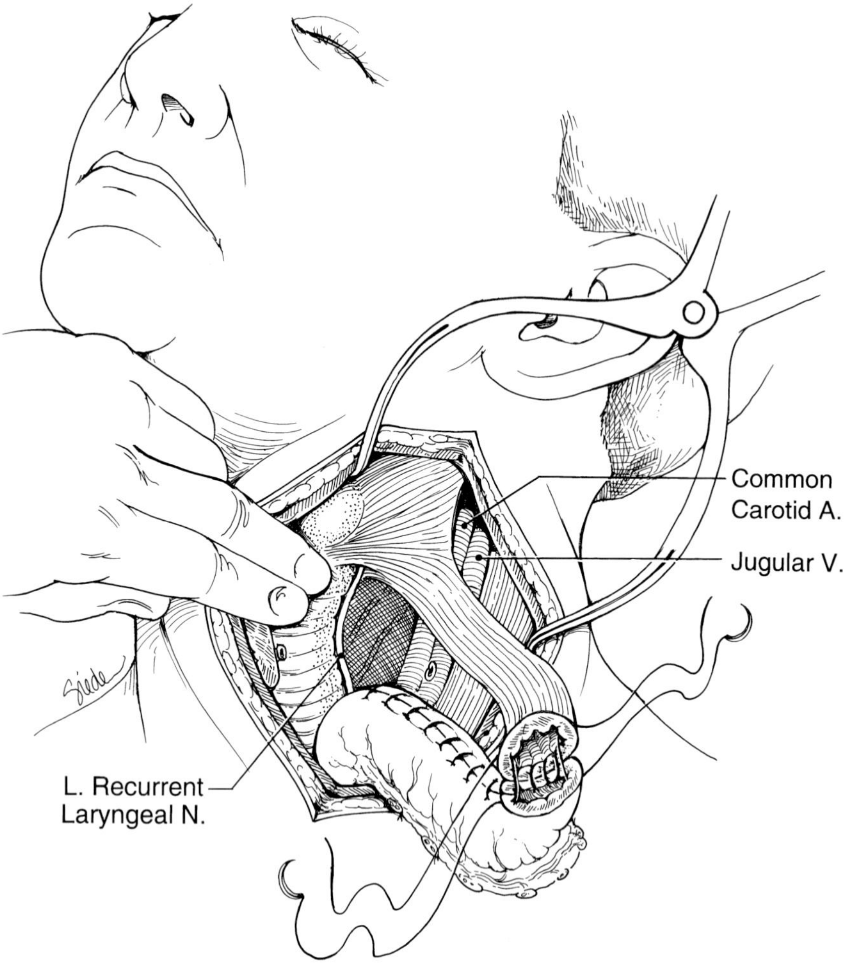

FIG. 15-7. Completing the cervical esophagogastrostomy.

in patient selection and operative experience. With proper patient selection and operative technique, operative mortality should be 5% or less, and the series reporting high operative mortality rates have either included an extremely morbid patient population[52,60] or have been a reflection of operative inexperience.[44] It cannot be overemphasized that patients who have advanced metastatic disease or extremely morbid coexisting illnesses (ASA risk status IV) are not candidates for esophageal resection by any means.

The operative mortality of THE can be compared to the historical mortality rates reported for TTE, including a 17% mortality rate reported by Postlethwait in a collected series from 16 institutions with extensive experience in esophageal cancer resection,[64] a 15% mortality rate reported by Cukingnan and Carey[65] in a collected series from 14 experienced esophageal surgeons, and a 29% mortality rate reported by Earlam and Cunha-Melo[66] in a collected review of 83,783 cases collected from the world literature between 1960 and 1980. In most series, pulmonary complications and intrathoracic anastomotic leaks account for most of the postoperative deaths. However, historical comparisons fail to control for the many improvements in anesthesia, antibiotics, and critical care that have occurred over the past several decades. A number of retrospective, nonrandomized, comparative studies have compared relatively concurrent surgical experiences with THE and TTE, performed by the same surgeons at a single institution. In several of these studies, there was a clear selection bias, with poorer-risk patients who were not considered candidates for transthoracic resection undergoing THE.[52,54,58,67] Among these nonrandomized, comparative studies, operative mortality for the two procedures is similar,[44,52,54–59,68] with several authors concluding that THE is the preferable procedure because of a lower risk of pulmonary complications[9,58,68] or because THE was useful in extending the indications for resection to poor-risk patients,[54,58] whereas several authors concluded that, in the absence of a significantly lower operative mortality for THE, transthoracic resection should remain the treatment of choice.[55,57]

Conspicuously lacking in most of these nonrandomized, comparative studies is an objective assessment of preoperative risk status, to determine the extent to which sicker patients were selectively treated by THE. The one study that included this analysis demonstrated a statistically significant bias toward selecting THE for patients who were ASA III or IV status before surgery. Despite this finding, this study revealed a significantly lower operative mortality for THE, with most of the operative deaths in the TTE group occurring among patients older than 65 years of age who were ASA III or IV (43% mortality in this subgroup).[67] One small, prospective, randomized study[50] compared THE and TTE in 67 patients undergoing esophagectomy for squamous carcinoma of the esophagus and found no

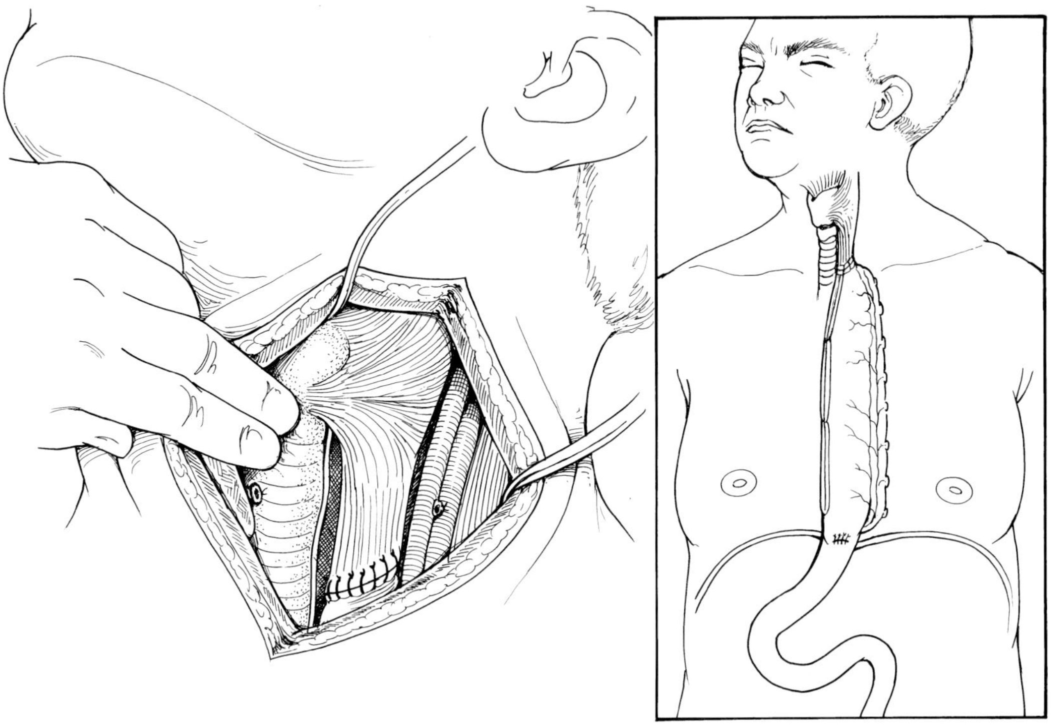

FIG. 15-8. Redundant stomach is pulled back down into the chest; the anastomosis lies at or slightly below the level of the thoracic inlet.

difference in operative mortality between the two procedures; patients who were 70 years of age or older, who had chronic cardiac, pulmonary, renal, or liver insufficiency, or who had Karnofsky performance status of 60 or less were excluded from this trial, and operative mortality was low for both THE (6%) and TTE (8.6%). Thus, it is likely that for younger, low-risk patients, operative mortality will be low for either procedure providing that the surgeon is experienced in esophageal resection. However, in the elderly or high-risk patient, THE may offer a significantly safer alternative to transthoracic resection.

TABLE 15-2. *Reported operative mortality rates for transhiatal resection of esophageal carcinoma*

Author	No. of cases	Operative mortality (%)
Goldminc[50]	32	6
Gotley[51]	54	11
Fok[52]	38	18
Bolton[53]	48	0
Pac[9]	118	6.7
Tilanus[10]	141	5
Orringer[6]	417	5
Hankins[54]	26	8
Giuli[44]	80	17
Shahian[55]	30	13
Moon[56]	63	13
Jauch[57]	49	16
Makëla[58]	43	9
Steiger[59]	21	10
Hambraeus[60]	26	25
Sabanathan[61]	24	0
Baker[62]	20	0
Terz[63]	36	8.3
Barbier[7]	50	2
Finley[8]	82	2.4
TOTAL	1398	7.5

Intraoperative injury to the left recurrent laryngeal nerve during THE has been reported in 3% to 16% of patients undergoing THE,[6,9,10,50,52,54,55,57–59,67] and was temporary in about half of the reported cases.[6,9] The risk of recurrent laryngeal nerve paresis after THE appears to be higher than after TTE in some series,[9,10] and the same in others.[50,55] The presence of this complication significantly increases the risk of pulmonary complications in the early postoperative period by interfering with normal glottic closure during swallowing and coughing. The incidence of nerve injury can be reduced by identifying and preserving the nerve during mobilization of the cervical esophagus and by avoiding the use of mechanical retraction in the left tracheoesophageal groove.[68] In the absence of recurrent laryngeal nerve injury, pulmonary complications after THE are relatively low[9,10,58,68]; this is one of the major advantages of avoiding transthoracic resection. Pneumothorax occurs in most transhiatal resections and is treated by chest tube drainage; this should not be considered a significant complication of the transhiatal approach.

To minimize the risk of postoperative cardiac or cerebrovascular complications, prolonged intraoperative hypotension must be avoided during the mediastinal dissection phase of THE, by the measures discussed in the section on Operative Technique.

Chylothorax or chyloperitoneum has occurred in 2% of our series of esophageal carcinoma resections. When the chylous drainage persistently exceeds 1500 mL/d, early reoperation to secure the chyle leak is advisable; prolonged, high-volume chyle fistula presents a formidable metabolic and nutritional challenge and has a high mortality rate.

The risk of anastomotic leak appears to be higher after THE than for intrathoracic esophagogastric anastomosis; although the reported incidence varies from 4%[51] to 39%,[57] most series report a leak rate of 10% to 20%. The increased leak rate appears to be the result of a more tenuous blood supply to the proximal gastric stump owing to the longer gastric interposate and, in some instances, to a "blow-out" of the anastomosis during vigorous coughing in the postoperative period. Provided that the anastomosis is adequately drained, this complication is self-limited and not life threatening, in contradistinction to the less frequently seen intrathoracic leak seen with transthoracic esophagectomy, which is associated with significant morbidity and a mortality rate of as high as 69%.[69] If an anastomotic leak becomes apparent after THE, the measures discussed in the Postoperative Care section should be adopted.

An additional advantage of THE is the low postoperative incidence of problematic gastroesophageal reflux. Several series suggest that this occurs in only 0% to 5%[6–9] of patients after THE, compared with 14% to 23% of patients with an intrathoracic anastomosis.[70] Anastomotic recurrence of cancer also appears to be infrequent after THE owing to the extensive longitudinal margins obtained for cancer of the lower and mid-thoracic esophagus. Anastomotic recurrences have been reported in 0% to 13%[7–9,56] of patients undergoing THE, compared with 14% to 22% of patients undergoing TTE.[9,56] After THE, the ability to swallow a regular diet is maintained permanently by more than 90% of patients,[6–8,56] and a modified Visick score of 1 or 2 is attained in 94% of patients at 1-year follow-up.[71]

Anastomotic stricture requiring dilatation occurs in 20% to 40% of patients after THE[10,51,58,67]; this incidence appears to be similar to that seen after TTE with intrathoracic anastomosis, and is higher if a stapled anastomotic technique is used.[72] Most strictures become symptomatic within the first 3 months after surgery. Periodic dilatation under endoscopic guidance, using either balloon dilators or Savary dilators, is begun as soon as the patient experiences progressive symptoms of dysphagia. A series of three to five dilatations is usually required. These strictures respond to dilatation in most cases, and dense strictures requiring regular anastomotic dilatation, daily self-dilatation, or anastomotic revision occur in less than 5% of patients.[6] Late strictures, presenting more than a year after surgery, are usually caused by recurrent carcinoma.

DISEASE-RELATED SURVIVAL

In the single, prospective, randomized trial comparing THE with TTE, and in all of the multiple, nonrandomized, comparative studies except one, survival after THE is identical to that after TTE (Table 15-3). In the single study in which patients resected by THE had a significantly worse long-term survival, reported by Fok and associates,[52] the survival analysis included deaths from all causes, and it is clear that the THE group had a higher incidence of comorbid conditions, including pulmonary tuberculosis in 24%. For both procedures, survival strongly depends on tumor stage in all reported series. Because esophageal cancer in the United States is at least stage III at clinical presentation in greater than 80% of patients undergoing esophagectomy,[6,9,54,70] overall 5-year survival in most series of resected esophageal cancer is in the range of 10% to 15%.[56] In more recent years, early detection of adenocarcinoma of the esophagus has become more prevalent through the use of endoscopic surveillance programs for patients found to have Barrett's metaplastic epithelium during evaluation for gastroesophageal reflux symptoms, or as a serendipitous finding during upper gastrointestinal endoscopy for other upper gastrointestinal complaints. The 5-year survival for stage I esophageal adenocarcinoma appears to be at least 90%[73] after surgical resection, and THE is an ideal procedure for this favorable patient group.

Mediastinal lymph node staging—especially for levels 4 and

TABLE 15-3. *Long-term survival: comparison of THE and TTE*

Author		2 yr.	3 yr.	5 yr.	Median survival time	
Goldminc[50]*	THE	47%	32%			
(67 pts.)	TTE	41%	17%			NS†
Bolton[53]	THE	40%				
(55 pts.)	TTE	22%				NS
Pac[9]	THE	30%	30%	13%		
(238 pts.)	TTE	35%	26%	10%		NS
Fok[52]	THE	20%	15%		6.3 mos.	
(210 pts.)	TTE	32%	27%		11.3 mos.	p = .048
Goldfaden[68]	THE		22%			
(72 pts.)	TTE		20%			NS
Hankins[54]	THE	24%	24%		12.3 mos.	
(78 pts.)	TTE	19%	11%		9.8 mos.	NS
Shahian[55]	THE				12.6 mos.	
(95 pts.)	TTE				14.1 mos.	NS
Moon[56]	THE	37%	24%	12%		
(88 pts.)	TTE	41%	16%	16%		NS
Jauch[57]	THE		25%			
(86 pts.)	TTE		22%			NS

* prospective randomized study
† NS = Not significant

7 lymph nodes—cannot be systematically carried out during THE; therefore, pathologic understaging may occur with this procedure. Because there is no evidence that wide mediastinal lymph node clearance is therapeutic, and because no effective postoperative adjuvant therapy program exists, the inability of THE to provide mediastinal lymph node clearance is currently not an argument against the use of THE.

SUMMARY

Transhiatal esophagectomy for carcinoma of the thoracic esophagus and gastroesophageal junction is an attractive alternative to transthoracic resection, offering similar disease-related survival and a lower postoperative morbidity and mortality rate, especially for elderly patients and patients at high operative risk (ASA risk status III or IV). Adequate patient selection and careful attention to operative technique are necessary to maximize end results. Long-term survival depends on tumor stage. An increasing number of patients with stage 0 and stage I esophageal cancer are being seen as a result of the efforts of surveillance programs for Barrett's esophageal metaplasia; long-term survival for this group of patients after THE is greater than 90%. Most patients, however, present with stage III esophageal cancer. These patients can be effectively palliated with THE, but 5-year survival is poor (15%), and improved survival for these patients depends on the development of more effective adjuvant systemic chemotherapy.

REFERENCES

1. Denk W. Zur Radikaloperation des Oesophaguskarzinous. Langenbecks Arch Klin Chir 1913;40:1065.
2. Turner GG, Durh MS. Excision of the thoracic esophagus for carcinoma, with construction of an extra-thoracic gullet. Lancet 1933;2:1315.
3. Adams WE, Phemister DB. Carcinoma of the lower thoracic esophagus: report of a successful resection and esophagogastrostomy. J Thorac Surg 1937;7:621.
4. Kirk RM. Palliative resection of oesophageal carcinoma without formal thoracotomy. Br J Surg 1974;61:689.
5. Orringer MB, Sloan H. Esophagectomy without thoracotomy. J Thorac Cardiovasc Surg 1978;76:643.
6. Orringer MB, Marshall B, Stirling MC. Transhiatal esophagectomy for benign and malignant disease. J Thorac Cardiovasc Surg 1993;105:265.
7. Barbier PA, Becker CD, Wagner HE. Esophageal carcinoma: patient selection for transhiatal esophagectomy. A prospective analysis of 50 consecutive cases. World J Surg 1988;12:263.
8. Finley RJ, Inculet RI. The results of esophagogastrectomy without thoracotomy for adenocarcinoma of the esophagogastric junction. Ann Surg 1989;210:535.
9. Pac M, Basoglu A, Kocak H, et al. Transhiatal versus transthoracic esophagectomy for esophageal cancer. J Thorac Cardiovasc Surg 1993;106:205.
10. Tilanus HW, Hop WC, Langenhorst BL, Lauschot JJ. Esophagectomy with or without thoracotomy: is there any difference? J Thorac Cardiovasc Surg 1993;105:898.
11. Blot EJ, Devesa SS, Kneler RW, Fraumeni JF. Rising incidence of adenocarcinoma of the esophagus and gastric cardia. JAMA 1991;265:1287.
12. Beahrs O, Henson D, Hutter R, Kennedy B, eds. Manual for staging of cancer. 4th ed. Philadelphia: JB Lippincott, 1992:122.
13. Collard JM, Lengele B, Otte JB, Kestens PJ. En bloc and standard esophagectomies by thoracoscopy. Ann Thorac Surg 1993;56:675.
14. American Society of Anesthesiologists. New classification of physical status. Anesthesiology 1963;24:111.
15. Gagner M. Value of preoperative physiologic assessment in outcome of patients undergoing major surgical procedure. Surg Clin North Am 1991;71:1141.
16. Vacanti CJ, Van Houten RI, Hill RC. A statistical analysis of the relationship of physical status to postoperative mortality in 68,388 cases. Anesth Analg 1970;49:564.
17. Overhagen H, Lameris JS, Berger MY, et al. CT assessment of resectability prior to transhiatal esophagectomy for esophageal/gastroesophageal junction carcinoma. J Comput Assist Tomogr 1993;17:367.
18. Takashima S, Takeuchi N, Shiozaki H, et al. Carcinoma of the esophagus: CT vs. MRI imaging in determining resectability. AJR Am J Roentgenol 1991;156:297.
19. Picus D, Balfe DM, Koehler RE, Roper CL, Owen JW. Computed tomography in the staging of esophageal carcinoma. Radiology 1983;146:433.
20. Postlethwait RW. Surgery of the esophagus. 2nd ed. Norwalk, CT: Appleton-Century-Crofts, 1986:369.
21. Vilgrain V, Mompoint D, Palazzo L, et al. Staging of esophageal carcinoma: comparison of results with endoscopic sonography and CT. AJR Am J Roentgenol 1990;155:277.
22. Wright C, Mathisen D, Wain J, et al. Adenocarcinoma of the esophagus: results of a pilot study on neoadjuvant chemotherapy with surgical resection. Proceedings of the American Society of Clinical Oncology 1994;13:221.
23. Carey RW, Hilgenberg AD, Wilkens EW, et al. Long-term follow-up of neoadjuvant chemotherapy with 5-fluorouracil and cisplatin with surgical resection and possible postoperative radiotherapy and/or chemotherapy in squamous cell carcinoma of the esophagus. Cancer Invest 1993;11:99.
24. Forastiere AA, Heitmiller R, Lee DJ, Abrams R, Zahurak M. A four week intensive preoperative chemo-radiation program for locoregional cancer of the esophagus. Proceedings of the American Society of Clinical Oncology 1994;13:195.
25. Adelstein DJ, Rice TW, Tefft M, et al. Concurrent chemotherapy and hyperfractionated radiotherapy followed by surgical resection for esophageal carcinoma. Proceedings of the American Society of Clinical Oncology 1994;13:206.
26. Pruitt D, Ajlouni M, Lewis J, Doyle T, Machuta S. Adenocarcinoma of the gastroesophageal junction: a multimodality treatment approach using preoperative radiation therapy combined with 5-FU and cisplatin. Proceedings of the American Society of Clinical Oncology 1994;13:222.
27. Orringer MB. Multimodality therapy for esophageal carcinoma: update. Chest 1993;103:4065.
28. Stewart JR, Hoff SJ, Johnson DH, et al. Improved survival with neoadjuvant therapy and resection for adenocarcinoma of the esophagus. Ann Surg 1993;218:571.
29. Seitz JF, Giovannini M, Padaut-Cesana J, et al. Concomitant chemoradiation therapy as palliative or neoadjuvant treatment of adenocarcinoma of the esophagus and gastroesophageal junction. Proceedings of the American Society of Clinical Oncology 1992;11:172.
30. Bedenne L, Seitz JF, Milan C, et al. Pre-operative radiotherapy and chemotherapy in epidermoid oesophageal cancers: results of a phase II multicentric trial by the French Foundation for Carcinology of the Digestive Tract. Proceedings of the American Society of Clinical Oncology 1993;12:199.
31. Ajani JA, Roth JA, Ryan MB, et al. Intensive preoperative chemotherapy with colony-stimulating factor for resectable adenocarcinoma of the esophagus or gastroesophageal junction. J Clin Oncol 1993;11:22.
32. Kelsen DP, Minsky B, Smith M, et al. Preoperative therapy for esophageal cancer: a randomized comparison of chemotherapy versus radiation therapy. J Clin Oncol 1990;8:1352-61.
33. Roth JA, Pass HI, Flanagan MM, et al. Randomized clinical trial of preoperative and postoperative adjuvant chemotherapy with cisplatin, vindesine, and bleomycin for carcinoma of the esophagus. J Thorac Cardiovasc Surg 1988;96:242.
34. Orringer M, Turrisi A, Whyte R, Natale R, Iannettoni M, Forastiere A. A randomized trial comparing transhiatal esophagectomy (THE) to preoperative concurrent chemoradiation (CT/XRT) followed by esophagectomy in locoregional esophageal carcinoma. Proceedings of the American Society of Clinical Oncology 1995;14:199.
35. Le Prise E, Etienne PL, Meunier B, et al. A randomized study of chemotherapy, radiation therapy, and surgery versus surgery for localized squamous cell carcinoma of the esophagus. Cancer 1994;73:1779.

36. Petruska P, Naunheim K, Roy T, et al. Preoperative chemo-radiation for esophageal carcinoma. Proceedings of the American Society of Clinical Oncology 1992;11:182.
37. Poplin E, Kraut M, Herskovic A, Kincie J, Stiger Z, Vaitkevicius VK. Chemo-radiotherapy of esophageal carcinoma. Proceedings of the American Society of Clinical Oncology 1992;11:191.
38. Kukla L, Lad T, McGuire W, Thomas P. Multimodality therapy of squamous carcinoma of the esophagus. (Abstract) Proceedings of the American Society of Clinical Oncology American Association for Cancer Research 1981;22:449.
39. Franklin R, Steiger Z, Vaishampayan G, et al. Combined modality therapy for esophageal squamous cell carcinoma of the esophagus with chemotherapy, radiotherapy, and surgical therapy. J Thorac Cardiovasc Surg 1981;82:713.
40. Leichmann L, Steiger Z, Seydel L. Combined preoperative chemotherapy and radiation for cancer of esophagus. Semin Oncol 1984;11:75.
41. Adelstein D, Snow N, Sharan V, et al. Post-operative respiratory failure after pre-operative chemotherapy and mediastinal radiation therapy for esophageal cancer. Proceedings of the American Society of Clinical Oncology 1984;3:135.
42. Hoffman P, Vokes E, Ferguson M, Haraf D, Krishnasamy S, English C. Induction chemotherapy, surgery, and concomitant chemo-radiotherapy for carcinoma of the esophagus. Proceedings of the American Society of Clinical Oncology 1992;11:193.
43. Gignoux M. Roussel A, Paillot B, et al. The value of preoperative radiotherapy in esophageal cancer: results of a study of the EORTC. World J Surg 1987;11:426.
44. Giuli R, Saudo Garnier H. Diagnostic, therapeutic, and prognostic features of cancers of the esophagus: results of the international prospective study conducted by the OESO group (790 pts). Surgery 1986;99: 614.
45. Tribble CG, Flanagan TL, Christensen CP, Daniel TM, Kron IL. The influence of preoperative radiation therapy on morbidity and mortality for transhiatal esophagectomy. Am Surg 1991;57:716.
46. Jehle EC, Maier G, Becker HD. Functional outcome following esophagectomy for esophageal cancer. Digestive Disease Week Abstracts 1993;128.
47. Orringer MB. Partial median sternotomy: anterior approach to the upper thoracic esophagus. J Thorac Cardiovasc Surg 1984;87:124.
48. Kirk RM. Partial and complete sternotomy for blunt oesophagectomy. Br J Surg 1987;74:685.
49. DeMeester TR, Johansson KE, Franze I, et al. Indications, surgical technique, and long term functional results of colon interposition or bypass. Ann Surg 1988;208:460.
50. Goldminc M, Maddern G, LaPrise E, Meunier B, Campion JP, Launois B. Oesophagectomy by a transhiatal approach or thoracotomy: a prospective randomized trial. Br J Surg 1993;80:367.
51. Gotley DC, Beard J, Cooper MJ, Britton DC, Williamson RC. Abdominocervical (transhiatal) oesophagectomy in the management of oesophageal carcinoma. Br J Surg 1990;77:815.
52. Fok M, Siu KF, Wong J. A comparison of transhiatal and transthoracic resection for carcinoma of the thoracic esophagus. Am J Surg 1989; 158:414.
53. Bolton JS, Ochsner JL, Abdoh AA. Surgical management of esophageal cancer: a decade of change. Ann Surg 1994;219:475.
54. Hankins JR, Attar S, Coughlin TR, et al. Carcinoma of the esophagus: a comparison of the results of transhiatal versus transthoracic resection. Ann Thorac Surg 1989;47:700.
55. Shahian M, Neptune WB, Ellis FH, Watkins E. Transthoracic versus extrathoracic esophagectomy: mortality, morbidity and long term survival. Ann Thorac Surg 1986;41:234.
56. Moon MR, Schulte WJ, Haasler GB, Condon RE. Transhiatal and transthoracic esophagectomy for adenocarcinoma of the esophagus. Arch Surg 1992;127:951.
57. Jauch KW, Bacha EA, Denecke H, Anthuber M, Schildberg FW. Esophageal carcinoma: prognostic features and comparison between blunt transhiatal dissection and transthoracic resection. Eur J Surg Oncol 1992;18:553.
58. Makëla J, Laitinen S, Kairaluoma MI. A comparison of transthoracic and transhiatal resection for thoracic esophageal carcinoma: observations of 30 years. Ann Chir Gynaecol 1991;80:340.
59. Steiger Z, Wilson RF. Comparison of the results of esophagectomy with and without a thoracotomy. Surg Gynecol Obstet 1981;153:653.
60. Hambraeus GM, Walther BS. Oesophagectomy without thoracotomy: experiences from 30 cases. Scand J Thorac Cardiovasc Surg 1988;22: 215.
61. Sabanathan S, Hashimi H, Pradhan GN. Transhiatal oesophagectomy in the management of carcinoma of the thoracic oesophagus. J R Coll Surg Edinb 1988;33:192.
62. Baker JW, Schechter GL. Management of panesophageal cancer by blunt resection without thoracotomy and reconstruction of the stomach. Ann Surg 1986;203:491.
63. Terz JJ, Beatty JD, Kokal WA, Wagman LD. Transhiatal esophagectomy. Am J Surg 1987;154:42.
64. Postlethwait RW. Complications and deaths after operations for esophageal carcinoma. J Thorac Cardiovasc Surg 1983;85:827.
65. Cukingnan RA, Carey JS. Carcinoma of the esophagus. Ann Thorac Surg 1978;26:274.
66. Earlam R, Cunha-Melo JR. Oesophageal squamous cell carcinoma: a critical review of surgery. Br J Surg 1980;67:381.
67. Bolton JS, Sardi A, Bowen JC, Ellis JK. Transhiatal and transthoracic esophagectomy: a comparative study. J Surg Oncol 1992;51:249.
68. Goldfaden D, Orringer MB, Appelman HD, Kalish R. Adenocarcinoma of the distal esophagus and gastric cardia: comparison of results of transhiatal esophagectomy and thoracoabdominal esophagogastrectomy. J Thorac Cardiovasc Surg 1986;91:242.
69. Müller JM, Erasmi H, Stelzner M, Zieren U, Pichlmaier H. Surgical therapy of oesophageal carcinoma. Br J Surg 1990;77:845.
70. King RM, Pairolero PC, Trastek VF, Payne WS, Bernatz PE. Ivor Lewis esophagogastrectomy for carcinoma of the esophagus: early and late functional results. Ann Thorac Surg 1987;44:119.
71. DeLeyn P, Coosemans W, Lerut T. Early and late functional results in patients with intrathoracic gastric replacement after oesophagectomy for carcinoma. Eur J Cardiothorac Surg 1992;6:79.
72. Lam TC, Fok M, Cheng SW, Wong J. Anastomotic complications after esophagectomy for cancer: a comparison of neck and chest anastomoses. J Thorac Cardiovasc Surg 1992;104:395.
73. Rusch V, Levine D, Haggitt R, Reid B. The management of high grade dysplasia and early cancer in Barrett's esophagus. Cancer 1994;74: 1225.

Surgery for Gastrointestinal Cancer: A Multidisciplinary Approach, edited by Harold J. Wanebo.
Lippincott-Raven Publishers, Philadelphia, © 1997.

CHAPTER 16

Radical Esophagectomy

Leonard Girardi and Nassar Altorki

The earliest historical records describing syndromes of dysphagia were recovered in the northern provinces of the Chinese mainland. The "hard of swallowing" disease instilled intense fear in the local population because of its debilitating and inevitably fatal course. Almost 20 centuries later, carcinoma of the esophagus remains an equally deadly disease with dismal survival rates. Pessimism regarding the outcome of surgical therapy was reinforced by a report published in 1980 by Earlam and Cunha-Melo[1] summarizing the world literature to date. The resectability rate for over 80,000 collected cases was 39%, and the overall 5-year survival rate for resected patients was a mere 10%, obtained at the expense of a formidable 25% operative mortality rate. However, significant strides have been accomplished since that publication in both operative techniques and perioperative care, such that Earlam and Cunha-Melo's report should be considered of historical interest rather than a representation of the current state of the art. Indeed, the worldwide mortality of esophagectomy has been more than halved since the mid-1980s, and in many esophageal centers an operative mortality in the 5% to 10% range is a standard achievement.[2] The same period also witnessed an important drive to refine the TNM staging system for esophageal carcinoma (Table 16-1). A new TNM staging system was adopted in 1985 that stressed wall penetration rather than tumor length as an important determinant of survival. Collaborative international research is ongoing to define further the nebulous "N" descriptor, which currently does not permit substaging based on the number and location of nodes involved with metastatic cancer, both seemingly important determinants of survival.

Nonetheless, despite improved perioperative surgical outcomes and refinements in the staging system, a combination of factors has stymied a major improvement in overall survival rates. Primarily, most patients present with advanced-stage disease at the time of diagnosis, such that curative intervention may not be possible. Early detection of esophageal cancer in eastern Asia through mass screening programs has resulted in impressive cure rates after surgical resection. Despite earlier attempts to portray the disease in eastern Asia as biologically different from its Western counterpart, no scientific evidence, including factors related to growth rate, tumorigenicity, and oncogene or growth factor expression, has yet emerged to support that proposition.[3,4] Indeed, survival rates in the 80% to 90% range have been reported by Western investigators after surgical resection of early adenocarcinoma of the esophagus/cardia.[5] Clearly, esophageal carcinoma is no less curable than any of the other common malignancies if detected and treated at an early stage. The use of combination chemotherapy or radiation therapy in a neoadjuvant manner has resulted in variable response rates and has not generally resulted in improved survival. The demonstration of possible survival benefit in a small subset of patients treated by preoperative cisplatinum, vindesine, and bleomycin has been reported, but awaits confirmation by further studies.[6] An intergroup study, in progress at the time of writing, randomizes patients to chemotherapy followed by surgical resection versus surgery alone, and may further elucidate the role of preoperative chemotherapy.

Surgical resection remains the standard of therapy for patients with esophageal carcinoma, but controversy persists regarding the extent of resection. Adopting the view that most patients with esophageal carcinoma have metastatic disease at the time of diagnosis, some surgeons advocate a limited resection whereby the tumor-bearing esophagus is extirpated without an attempt at complete mediastinal and abdominal lymph node dissection.[7,8] Others have attempted to extend the principles of en bloc resection practiced for other malignancies of the gastrointestinal tract to esophageal carcinoma, hoping to garner the modest but definite improvement in survival rates seen in other malignancies with these surgical techniques. Logan proposed an en bloc resection for carcinoma of the lower esophagus and cardia and achieved an overall 16% 5-year survival rate, which remains among the best obtained.[9] The procedure was not adopted by others primarily because of the 21% operative mortality. Skinner modified Logan's approach for carcinoma of the cardia and lower esophagus and extended its use to tumors of the middle and cervical esophagus.[10] The operative mortality in his series was 11%, with an impressive 3-year survival rate of 24%. En bloc resection is, however, a technically demanding procedure associated with a significant learning curve, and is thus practiced only in a few esophageal centers worldwide.

Nasser Altorki: The New York Hospital—Cornell University Medical College, 525 East 68th Street, New York, NY 10021

TABLE 16-1. *TNM staging system for esophageal carcinoma*

PRIMARY TUMOR	
TX	Primary tumor cannot be assessed
TO	No evidence of primary tumor
Tis	Carcinoma in situ
T1	Tumor invades lamina propria or submucosa
T2	Tumor invades muscularis propria
T3	Tumor invades adventitia
T4	Tumor invades adjacent structures
LYMPH NODE	
NX	Regional nodes cannot be assessed
TO	No regional lymph node metastasis
N1	Regional lymph node metastasis
DISTANT METASTASIS	
MO	No distant metastasis
M1	Distant metastasis (including positive celiac nodes)

CONCEPT

The deep location of the esophagus within the narrow confines of the mediastinum and its proximity to other vital structures has precluded the application of the principles of ''en bloc'' resection to the surgical management of esophageal cancer. In addition, although the pathways of lymphatic drainage of organs such as the colon are easily defined by their mesentery, the adult esophagus lacks a well defined mesentery. Furthermore, an extensive plexus of lymphatics drains the esophagus throughout its course from the neck to the upper abdomen. Embryologically, however, the distal half of the fetal esophagus is suspended by a dorsal mesentery that determines its vascular supply and lymphatic drainage.[11] The remnants of the fetal mesoesophagus are represented in the adult by the lymphovascular tissue wedged between the esophagus and the prevertebral fascia, containing the azygos vein, the thoracic duct, and their tributaries. Laterally and anteriorly, the esophagus is abutted by the two pleural surfaces and the pericardium, which should be construed as serosal equivalents. An en bloc esophagectomy would therefore include the tumor-bearing esophagus within a wide envelope of tissue that includes both pleural surfaces laterally, the pericardium anteriorly, and all lymphatic and vascular tissue between the esophagus and the prevertebral fascia, as well as a thorough mediastinal and abdominal lymphadenectomy (Fig. 16-1). The gastrointestinal tract is then divided 10 cm on either side of the tumor. The presence of nodal metastasis beyond the limits of the proposed resection signals incurability by the en bloc technique, and a more limited resection is advocated.

RATIONALE

Advocates of en bloc esophagectomy, authors included, propose that cure by extended surgical resection is possible in the presence of limited nodal metastasis. A multivariate analysis of several prognostic factors that may define ''potentially curable cancer of the esophagus'' was reported in 1982.[12] The gross and histopathologic features of the neoplasm were analyzed in 91 resected specimens. The extent of mural penetration and the presence or absence of nodal metastasis emerged as the only significant determinants of long-term survival. Among patients with positive nodes, a survival benefit was noted in those with less than five nodal metastasis treated by en bloc resection. A more recent report on 100 patients treated by en bloc resection showed that patients with negative nodes and partial wall penetration had a 70% and a 55% disease-free survival at 3 and 5 years, respectively.[13] Patients with partial wall penetration and one to four positive nodes had a 5-year survival of 29%. These results strongly suggest that nodal metastasis is not uniformly predictive of occult disseminated disease. More recent evidence has lent support to the notion that cure may be possible in patients with limited nodal spread treated by aggressive surgical resection. Kato and associates reported an overall 5-year survival of 33.6% in 59 patients with positive nodes treated by esophagectomy with abdominal mediastinal and bilateral cervical lymphadenectomy.[14] Furthermore, patients with one, two, three, and four positive nodes had 5-year survival rates of 74%, 34%, 27%, and 22%, respectively. Based on these observations, we propose en bloc esophagectomy for patients with potentially curable esophageal cancer, defined as those in whom partial (T1/T2) wall penetration and in some cases full wall penetration (T3) is associated with no identifiable nodal metastasis (clinical N0) or less than four positive nodes. Patients with extensive

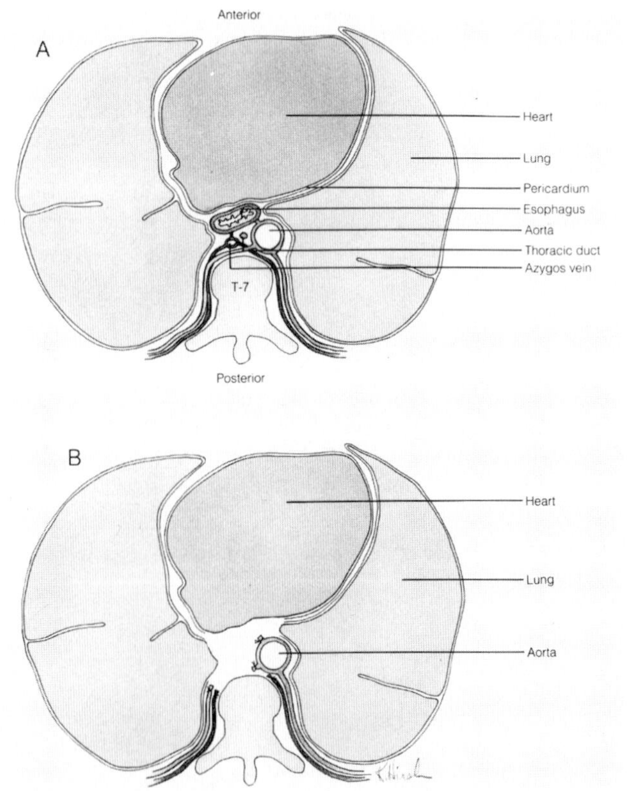

FIG. 16-1. The esophagus is resected within an envelope of adjoining tissue, including both pleural surfaces, pericardia and the mesoesophagus.

nodal metastasis or celiac nodal spread identified before surgery by endoscopic ultrasonography or during intraoperative staging maneuvers are either treated nonoperatively or subjected to less extensive resection, if clinically indicated.

PREOPERATIVE WORKUP AND STAGING

Once a diagnosis of esophageal carcinoma is established, a staging workup is initiated to determine the extent of the disease. Our staging protocol includes computed tomography and endoscopic ultrasonography to evaluate malignant mural penetration, nodal status, as well as the presence or absence of distant metastasis. Radionuclide bone scans are performed when indicated by clinical or biochemical criteria. Bronchoscopy is performed routinely for tumors of the cervical, upper, and midthoracic esophagus. The general condition of the patient and his or her ability to tolerate major surgery are carefully evaluated. Nutritionally depleted patients are hyperalimented for at least 10 to 14 days before surgery through a surgically placed feeding jejunostomy. Pulmonary function testing is routinely performed and patients with forced expiratory volumes less than 1.5 L in 1 second are not considered candidates for en bloc esophagectomy. A careful cardiac evaluation is performed, up to and including cardiac catheterization if necessary. Although no absolute upper limit for age is established, we generally avoid en bloc resection in patients older than 75 years of age. Patients eligible for surgical resection are then begun on a mechanical bowel preparation for 3 days should a colon segment by necessary for esophageal reconstruction. Over the last several years, the entire preoperative workup and staging has been done on an outpatient basis, and patients are admitted to the hospital on the day of the planned procedure.

SURGICAL APPROACH

The goal of en bloc resection is total removal of the digestive tract for 10 cm on either side of the tumor, along with an upper abdominal lymphadenectomy and posterior mediastinectomy. The choice of the surgical approach is dictated by the location of the tumor and its distance from the pulsations of the arch of the aorta observed at preoperative esophagoscopy. Tumors located at the cardia or 10 cm distal to the aortic arch are approached through a left thoracotomy. This approach provides excellent exposure for radical dissection of the lower mediastinum, the hiatal tunnel, and the upper abdomen. Tumors of the middle and upper thoracic esophagus and potentially curable tumors located less than 10 cm from the aortic arch are approached through a right thoracotomy. This approach allows excellent exposure of the trachea and mainstem bronchi. A laparotomy is performed to accomplish the abdominal part of the operation. Carcinomas of the cervical or cervicothoracic esophagus are approached through a generous cervical collar incision with or without a partial sternotomy. A simultaneous laparotomy is done to prepare the esophageal substitute.

Resection of Lower-Third Tumors

The patient is placed in a straight left lateral thoracotomy position. The thorax is entered through the sixth interspace. The costal margin is not divided. The left hemithorax is explored to detect unsuspected metastases. Dissection begins 10 cm proximal to the tumor by isolating the esophagus and submitting a periesophageal node for frozen section examination. The presence of metastatic carcinoma signals incurability, and the procedure is converted to a standard resection. The diaphragm is incised peripherally in a semilunar fashion from the back of the sternum anteriorly to the spleen posteriorly. A peripheral incision allows for a more secure closure and avoids injury to the phrenic nerve or denervation of a significant portion of the left hemidiaphragm. The abdomen is rapidly explored to exclude metastatic disease. The area of the tumor is then carefully evaluated for mobility and extent of nodal disease, particularly for involvement of the celiac lymph nodes. The omentum is detached from the colon in the avascular plane, carefully preserving the right gastroepiploic vessels. Mobilization of the colon is continued to the left splenic flexure and down the left paracolic gutter in case a segment of left colon is necessary for esophageal reconstruction. Dissection then proceeds along the superior border of the pancreas and the splenic artery, sweeping all retroperitoneal lymphatics and areolar tissue toward the esophageal hiatus. The left gastric artery is exposed at its origin from the celiac axis and divided. The coronary vein is similarly treated. Using the electrocautery, a 1-inch cuff of diaphragmatic muscle is resected circumferentially around the esophagus. This nicely exposes the distal descending thoracic aorta. The thoracic duct is identified, doubly ligated, and divided as it passes through the aortic hiatus. The two ascending lumbar veins are also divided as they join to form the azygos vein. The lesser omentum is divided, thus completing the abdominal part of the operation. The posterior mediastinectomy begins by incising the mediastinal pleura overlying the aorta from the aortic arch to the esophageal hiatus. Dissection proceeds along the aortic adventitia, dividing all esophageal and bronchoesophageal vessels. Further dissection proceeds dorsally onto the vertebral bodies. The prevertebral dissection proceeds cephalad from the distal thoracic aorta previously exposed at the hiatus to a point 10 cm proximal to the tumor. Systematically, all intercostal vessels to the right of the aorta as well as all lymphatics are carefully ligated and divided. This frees the azygos vein and thoracic duct, which are retained with specimens and are again divided at the proximal end of the dissection. The intercostal vessels are again ligated as they reflect off the vertebral bodies onto the right pleura, and the latter is incised along the entire length of the dissection, thus entering the right hemithorax and completing the posterior dissection. Anteriorly, the left inferior pulmonary ligament is incised close to the lung and dissection proceeds along the back of the hilum of the left lung and onto the subcarinal space. The pericardium is incised and entered on the surface of the inferior pulmonary vein, and the incision is carried distally along the pleuropericardial reflection to the diaphragm. Working from within the pericardial cavity, the surgeon carries the incision to the right side and emerges into the right chest behind the right inferior pulmonary vein. The pericardial incision is then carried caudally to the diaphragm. Dissection continues along the back of the hilum of the left lung to clear all lymphatic and areolar tissue toward the subcarinal space, which is thoroughly dissected to expose the carina and the right mainstem bronchus. Dissection at this point is carried to the wall of the esophagus, which is visualized for the first time during the procedure. The right and left vagus nerves

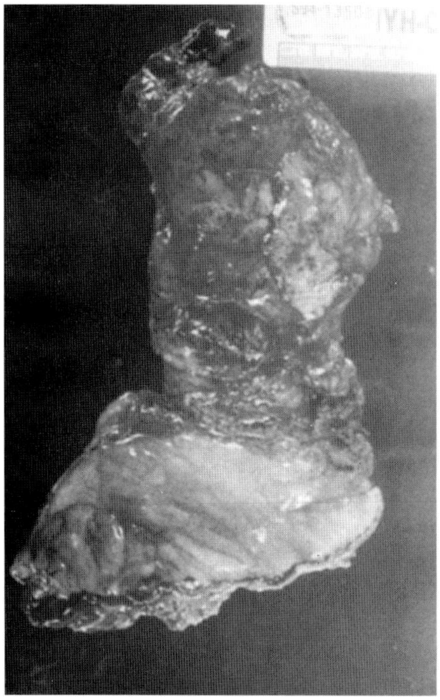

FIG. 16-2. An en bloc resection of a lower esophageal tumor. The esophagus is not visible, but is contained in an envelope of adjoining mediastinal tissue.

are divided, preserving the left recurrent laryngeal nerve. Finally, the entire specimen is lifted out of the mediastinum to expose the right inferior pulmonary ligament, which is divided flush with the right lung, thus completing the dissection (Fig. 16-2). The digestive tract is divided 10 cm on either side of the tumor. A frozen-section examination of the esophageal margin is always performed. Reconstruction is either performed in the subaortic position or, alternatively, the esophagus is dissected underneath the aortic arch and into the neck. The esophageal substitute is then passed under the aortic arch, and both the esophageal stump and the substitute are gently positioned in the prevertebral cervical space in preparation for a cervical anastomosis performed through a separate cervical incision. A subtotal esophagectomy is preferred for most cases of squamous cell carcinoma, a tumor that is notorious for multicentricity and extensive submucosal spread.[15] For carcinoma of the cardia or Barrett's adenocarcinoma, reconstruction is accomplished in the mediastinum or the neck. However, the presence of residual columnar metaplasia or carcinoma in situ at the margin should prompt a subtotal esophagectomy and a cervical anastomosis. The diaphragm is reattached, and the esophageal substitute is sutured to the edges of the hiatus. The chest incision is closed with bilateral pleural drainage.

Our choice of esophageal substitute is dictated by the stage of the disease and the general condition of the patient. The stomach is more frequently used for reconstruction, except in relatively young patients with early-stage disease, in whom an isoperistaltic segment of left colon is preferred, because approximately one third of patients reconstructed by an intrathoracic esophagogastrostomy have significant reflux-related complications like stricture or bleeding. In addition, we believe that patients with associated Barrett's esophagus probably are more likely to reacquire columnar metaplasia after an esophagogastric anastomosis. Regardless of the esophageal substitute, the anastomosis is performed using a single-layer technique of 4-0 or 5-0 monofilament suture material.

En Bloc Resection Through Right Thoracotomy

Tumors of the mid-thoracic esophagus and those arising above the tracheal carina are usually approached through a right thoracotomy. The incision provides excellent exposure of the tracheal bifurcation and is a safer approach to tumors intimately related to the aortic arch. The chest is entered through the fifth interspace, and lymph nodes located 10 cm on either side of the tumor are excised and submitted for frozen-section examination. If intraoperative staging suggests that the tumor is favorable, an en bloc esophagectomy is performed (Fig. 16-3). The pleura is incised along the anterior surface of the vertebral bodies from the thoracic inlet to the esophageal hiatus. The intercostal vessel and lymphatics are sequentially ligated and divided, thus exposing the prevertebral fascia and reflecting the azygos vein and thoracic duct anteriorly. Dissection proceeds anterior to the aorta, dividing its esophageal and bronchoesophageal branches. The contralateral pleura is widely opened along the entire length of the dissection. The thoracic duct is doubly ligated, and divided in the lower thorax and superiorly where it crosses the esophagus. Anteriorly, the tracheoesophageal plane is developed, with care taken to identify and preserve the left recurrent laryngeal nerve unless it is involved by tumor. The azygos vein is next divided flush with its caval junction, and

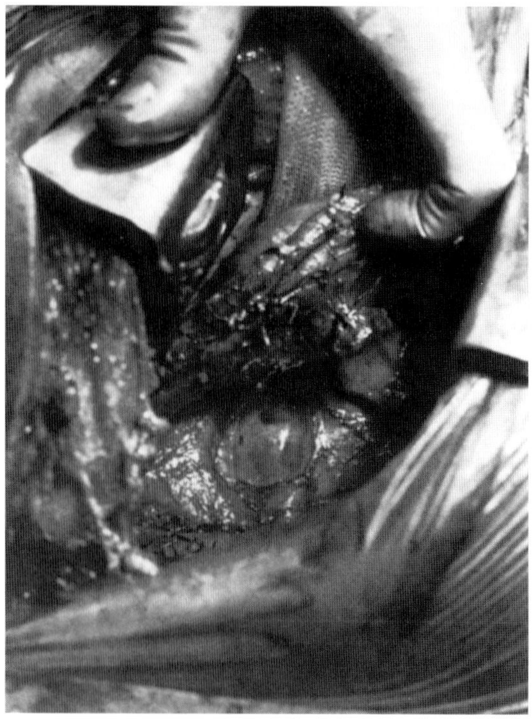

FIG. 16-3. En bloc resection through a right thoracotomy. Specimen with azygos vein and thoracic duct retracted to expose tracheal bifurcation and excised portion of pericardium.

dissection proceeds caudally along the right mainstem bronchus to clear all lymphatics from the subcarinal space. A window of pericardium between the pulmonary veins is excised en bloc with the tumor, and the right inferior pulmonary ligament is divided flush with the lung parenchyma, as is the left pulmonary ligament. We have extended the lymph node dissection in the superior mediastinum to include the right and left paratracheal nodes as well as the right recurrent chain of nodes along the right recurrent laryngeal nerve. Clearly, particular care is exercised to avoid injury to either nerves. The mobilized en bloc specimen is left in situ and the chest is closed and drained. The patient is repositioned for a simultaneous laparotomy and neck incision. The abdominal portion of the en bloc procedure is performed as previously described. The mobilized specimen is delivered into the abdomen after the esophagus is severed in the neck. The esophageal substitute is advanced to the neck, usually in the orthotopic position, and a cervical reconstruction is performed.

Tumors of the Cervical Esophagus

These tumors are usually approached through a generous cervical collar incision. Additional exposure, when necessary, is obtained through a partial upper sternotomy. A bilateral modified neck dissection is performed carefully to preserve both recurrent nerves. Tumors close to the cricopharyngeus junction require a laryngectomy as well. If a total thyroidectomy is necessary, then the parathyroid glands are preserved and autotransplanted. The intrathoracic esophagus is mobilized bluntly through both incisions, and the esophageal substitute is advanced to the hypopharynx or higher for reconstruction.

POSTOPERATIVE CARE

Patients are cared for after surgery in the intensive care unit, where they usually are maintained on mechanical ventilatory support for 24 to 48 hours. Fluid infusions are titrated to maintain a urine output of 1 mL/kg/h, but aggressive overhydration is avoided because of a propensity for increased extravascular lung water after resection of the thoracic duct and extensive mediastinal lymphadenectomy. All drainage tubes are removed by the third or fifth postoperative day. Once the integrity of the anastomosis is confirmed by a barium swallow, patients are gradually advanced to a regular diet and are usually discharged home by the 10th postoperative day.

RESULTS

Between January, 1988 and June, 1994, 75 patients underwent resection for carcinoma of the thoracic esophagus. Among 30 patients resected by the en bloc technique, there was 1 hospital death (3.4%) secondary to a massive pulmonary embolus. At least one complication occurred in 30% of patients. Morbidity rate was not significantly different between patients undergoing en bloc resection and those resected by more standard techniques. Actuarial 5-year survival was 63% after en bloc resection, compared with a 20% 5-year survival in patients receiving a standard resection. This survival benefit is only partially explained by patient selection because at least 50% of

TABLE 16-2. *Five-year survival rates after 2- and 3-field dissection according to pTNM staging*

	Less extensive 2-field dissection		Extensive 3-field dissection	
pTNM stage	n	5-year survival rates	n	5-year survival rates
O	4	100%	4	75.0%**
I	26	69.2 ± 9.1%	35	94.1 ± 5.7%
IIA	71	47.9 ± 5.9%	39	82.5 ± 6.6%
IIB	43	46.5 ± 7.6%	27	57.3 ± 14.1%
III	96	27.1 ± 4.5%	69	55.8 ± 6.6%
IV-pN*	36	11.1 ± 5.2%	99	28.0 ± 5.4%

* Stage IV due to pN factor.
** One patient died of non-malignant disease.

patients in the en bloc group had nodal metastasis. Similar results have been reported by other investigators. Collard and associates reported on 65 patients with esophageal carcinoma resected by an en bloc technique with a 2.4% hospital mortality.[16] Long-term survival was determined by the extent of wall penetration of the primary tumor into the esophageal wall and by the presence or absence of extrathoracic nodal metastases. In their series, the difference between N1 and N2 disease was not determined by the number of involved nodes, as originally proposed by Skinner, but rather by whether the nodes were intrathoracic (N1) or extrathoracic (N2). Survival of patients without nodal metastases was 58% at 3 years. Patients with intrathoracic nodal spread had a 3-year survival of 32%, regardless of the degree of mural penetration. In an earlier report, DeMeester and colleagues reported an operative mortality of 7% after en bloc resection of carcinoma of the lower esophageal and cardia.[17] The actuarial survival rates were 76%, 66%, and 53% at 1, 2, and 5 years, respectively. A more recent report from the same group compared long-term outcome after esophageal resection for carcinoma of the distal esophagus and cardia in three groups of patients defined by preoperative and intraoperative staging.[18] Group 3 patients received a palliative operation because of the presence of extensive disease. Patients in groups 1 and 2 had apparently limited disease and underwent en bloc resection (group 1, n = 30) or transhiatal resection (group 2, n = 16) based on their ability to withstand transthoracic resection. Overall survival was significantly better after en bloc resection than after transhiatal resection (41% versus 14%, $P <$ 0.001). Specifically, patients resected by the en bloc technique had superior survival to patients at comparable stages (41% versus 21%) subjected to transhiatal resection. Patients with early lesions defined as intramural tumors (T1 or T2) associated with less than five positive nodes had a 75% survival after en bloc resection, compared with 20% for transhiatal resections. Survival of patients with advanced lesions, comprising transmural tumors associated with five or more positive nodes, was significantly better after en bloc than transhiatal resection (27% versus 9%). Lerut and colleagues reported their experience with 232 patients undergoing resection for carcinoma of the esophagus, excluding those in the cervical esophagus and those located at the gastroesophageal junction.[19] One hundred twenty-nine patients received a curative resection, defined as clearance of all gross tumor. Fifty-four patients in the curative resection group were treated with a radical resection (en bloc). Hospital mortality was 7.4% for the curative radical (en bloc) group and 10.6% for the curative nonradical group. No differences in survival were found between adenocarcinoma and squamous carcinoma, nor by the location of tumor in the esophagus. Survival was significantly better in patients treated by curative radical (en bloc) resection versus those receiving a curative nonradical resection (48.5% versus 41%, $P < 0.002$). This survival advantage was especially evident in patients with nodal metastases rather than those with negative nodes. The survival advantage was apparent even when only stage III and IV patients treated with curative intent were compared. The 5-year survival rates were 22% versus 13% in favor of en bloc resections ($P < 0.05$). Significantly, 5-year survival for patients with stage I disease was 90%, indicating that early lesions are as curable as any other early-stage cancer.

REFERENCES

1. Earlam R, Cunha-Melo JR. Oesophageal squamous cell carcinoma: I. a critical review of surgery. Br J Surg 1980;67:381.
2. Muller JM, Erasmi H, Stelzner M, et al: Surgical therapy of oesophageal carcinoma. Br J Surg 1990;77:845–857.
3. Park JG, Frucht H, LaRocca RV, et al. Characteristics of cell lines established from human gastric carcinoma. Cancer Res 1990;50:2773.
4. Rodriguez E, Rao PH, Ladanyi M, Altorki NA, et al. 11p-13–15 is a specific region of chromosomal rearrangement in gastric and esophageal adenocarcinomas. Cancer Res 1990;50:6410.
5. Lerut T, Coosemans W, Van Raemdock D, et al. Surgical treatment of Barrett's carcinoma: correlations between morphologic findings and prognosis. J Thorac Cardiovasc Surg 1994;107:1059.
6. Roth JA, Putnam JB Jr, Lichter AS, et al. Cancer of the esophagus. In: Devita VT Jr, Hellman S, Rosenberg SA, eds. Cancer: principles and practice of oncology. Philadelphia: JB Lippincott, 1993:776.
7. Orringer MB. Ten-year survival after esophagectomy for carcinoma: surgical triumph or biologic variation? Chest 1989;96:970.
8. Ellis F, Gibb P, Watkins E. Esophagogastrectomy: a safe widely applicable, and expeditious form of palliation for patients with carcinoma of the esophagus and cardia. Ann Surg 1983;198:531.
9. Logan A. The surgical treatment of carcinoma of the esophagus and cardia. J Thorac Cardiovasc Surg 1963;46:150.
10. Skinner DB. En-bloc resection for neoplasms of the esophagus and cardia. J Thorac Cardiovasc Surg 1983;85:59.
11. Arey LB. Developmental anatomy: a textbook and laboratory manual of embryology. Philadelphia: WB Saunders, 1954.
12. Skinner DB, Dowalatshahi KD, DeMeester TR. Potentially curable cancer of the esophagus. Cancer 1982;50:2571.
13. Altorki NA, Skinner DB. En bloc esophagectomy: the first 100 patients. Hepatogastroenterology 1990;37:360.
14. Kato H, Tachimori Y, Watanabe H, et al. Lymph node metastasis in thoracic esophageal carcinoma. J Surg Oncol 1991;48:106.
15. Mandard AM, Marnay J, Gignoux M, et al. Cancer of the esophagus and associated lesions: detailed pathologic study of 100 esophagectomy specimens. Hum Pathol 1984;15:660.
16. Collard JM, Otte JB, Reynaert M, et al. Feasibility and effectiveness of en bloc resection of the esophagus for esophageal cancer: results of a prospective study. Int Surg 1991;76:209.
17. DeMeester TR, Zaninotto G, Johansson KE, et al. Selective therapeutic approach to cancer of the lower esophagus and cardia. J Thorac Cardiovasc Surg 1988;95:42.
18. Hagen JA, Peters JH, DeMeester TR. Superiority of extended en bloc esophagogastrectomy for carcinoma of the lower esophagus and cardia. J Thorac Cardiovasc Surg 1993;106:805.
19. Lerut T, De Lyn P, Coosemans W, et al. Surgical strategies in esophageal carcinoma with emphasis on radical lymphadenectomy. Ann Surg 1992;216:583.

Surgery for Gastrointestinal Cancer: A Multidisciplinary Approach, edited by Harold J. Wanebo.
Lippincott-Raven Publishers, Philadelphia, © 1997.

CHAPTER 17

Carcinoma of the Esophagus

Combined Modality Treatment of Esophageal Cancers

David Paul Kelsen

Esophageal cancers are virulent tumors with a grim prognosis. Although in the past surgical resection was considered the only potentially curative treatment, combined modality therapy with radiation and chemotherapy for esophageal cancers has become a promising nonoperative approach. Because of the high distant failure rates as well as the substantial risk of local recurrence when any single treatment modality is used, multimodality therapy has been widely studied. Because surgery as initial treatment is frequently unsuccessful as a result of inability to effect curative resection of the primary tumor, neoadjuvant or primary chemotherapy is an attractive option for potentially providing increased local control as well as destroying distant metastases in both the operative and nonoperative setting.

FAILURE PATTERN

Knowledge of the potential failure pattern (sites of recurrent disease) is important in planning therapy for patients who have apparently localized cancers at the time of diagnosis. Tumors that have a high local failure rate but a low incidence of distant metastases (eg, low-grade sarcomas, or endometrial carcinoma) may best be treated by aggressive resection with or without the use of radiation therapy. On the other hand, in a disease in which there is a high likelihood of distant failure regardless of whether local recurrence is seen, systemic therapy early in the treatment plan is rational. The failure patterns for esophageal cancer have been assessed in two ways, either by site of clinical progression (which has obvious drawbacks), or at autopsy (Table 17-1).

Several autopsy studies have been performed in patients with esophageal cancer (no second-look operation studies are available).[1–4] The median duration from diagnosis to death in two of these studies[2,3] was short (4 and 6.4 months, respectively). In this situation, as opposed to tumors with a more indolent natural history (eg, breast cancer), the extent of tumor found at autopsy was probably a reasonable reflection of cancer involvement at the time of diagnosis. In esophageal cancer autopsy series, some patients had only local disease, and others only distant metastases. However, in most, postmortem examinations revealed both local and systemic disseminated malignancy. These four studies suggest that in patients (whether Western or Asian) who present after weeks to months of symptoms, esophageal cancer is a disseminated disease at the time of diagnosis.

Because local failure rates are substantial despite definitive regional treatment, because many patients with newly diagnosed esophageal cancer cannot undergo potentially curative resections, and because the risk of systemic metastases is high, neoadjuvant (preoperative) therapy is an attractive concept.

EXPERIMENTAL RATIONALE FOR NEOADJUVANT THERAPY

Several laboratory models have been used to study the effect on survival of the timing of chemotherapy for solid tumors in relation to surgery. In one study, Fisher and colleagues, using a mouse model, found that resection of the primary tumor caused a marked increase in the labeling index of metastasis compared to animals in which the primary tumor was left in place.[5] Survival was also shorter in the resection group. In a second study, Fisher and colleagues investigated the timing of chemotherapy, given either before or after resection.[6] In this model, survival was best when chemotherapy was given before operation, mimicking the neoadjuvant approach. Similar results have been reported by other investigators.[7–9]

Muggia and Gill summarized practical and some theoretic considerations involving neoadjuvant chemotherapy.[10] Impor-

David P. Kelsen: Chief, Gastrointestinal Oncology Service, Department of Medicine, Mount Sloan-Kettering Cancer Center, Professor of Medicine Cornell University Medical College.

TABLE 17-1. *Sites of metastases esophageal cancer failure pattern: autopsy data*

	Anderson and Ladd[2]*	Bosch et al[3]	Mandard et al[4]†
Patient number	79	82	111
Local only (%)	9	27	—
Distant only (%)	2	7	—
Local + distant (%)	82	50	75
Sites of disease (%)			
Local	91	77	61
Lung	52	20	31
Liver	47	28	23
Lymph nodes	73	61	74
Adrenal	20	12	9
Trachea–bronchus	17	33	16

* Autopsy performed a median of 4 months from diagnosis.
† Autopsy performed a median of 6.3 months from diagnosis.

Modified from Kelsen D, Atiq OT. Therapy of upper gastrointestinal tract cancers. In: Haskell CM, ed. Current problems in cancer. Boston: Mosby-Year Book, 1991:239.

tant points favoring use of primary chemotherapy include its potential ability to induce early tumor regression or reduce tumor bulk, leading to improved local control; the possibility of using more conservative local measures; and, finally, the ability prospectively to identify patients before surgery (or before radiation therapy) who respond to chemotherapy and who might therefore benefit from additional postoperative treatment. Potential drawbacks of preoperative therapy include the possibility that systemic therapy may allow emergence of a resistant clone, and that there will be delays in effective local control measures, with the risk of tumor spread. After chemotherapy, if a major response occurs, the surgeon may be uncertain as to the proper extent of resection. An additional possibility is that some patients responding to chemotherapy (with palliation of their symptoms) might refuse standard local measures of surgery or radiation.

Another positive factor in favor of neoadjuvant treatment is early therapy of established but subclinical distant metastases as well as the primary tumor. Usually, neoadjuvant treatment is given when the patient is best able to tolerate potential toxicities. Because most chemotherapy combinations have substantial potential side effects, the appropriate identification of high-risk patients to receive neoadjuvant therapy is important.

CHOOSING THE APPROPRIATE PATIENT FOR NEOADJUVANT TREATMENT

As with most solid tumors, the stage of an esophageal cancer has been highly correlated with survival. High-risk patients have tumor that are stage T3–4NanyM0 (patients with M1 disease are, with currently available therapy, incurable with rare exceptions). Currently, definitive staging is performed postoperatively, after pathologic evaluation of the resected specimen, or after intraoperative staging of unresectable disease. Patients with, for example, T3N0 disease have at least a 50% chance of death within 5 years of operation.[11] The presence of nodal metastasis is an even more ominous finding. *Pretreatment*, noninvasive identification of high-risk patients would allow use of neoadjuvant approaches in the population at greatest risk if treated with conventional therapy. Routine staging with computed tomography scan or magnetic resonance imaging of the abdomen and chest are not highly accurate for determining depth of tumor invasion (T stage) or for assessing regional nodal involvement (N stage). Endoscopic ultrasonography has been demonstrated to be highly accurate in assessment of T stage in the newly diagnosed patient, but is less useful in assessing nodal involvement. In a prospective comparison of dynamic computed tomography scanning versus endoscopic ultrasonography for gastric and esophageal cancers, Lightdale and colleagues demonstrated that endoscopic ultrasonography was significantly better for assessing T and N stages.[12] Tio and coworkers reported similar results.[13] Investigators at Memorial Sloan-Kettering Cancer Center have shown that, in gastric cancer, stage by preoperative endoscopic ultrasonography is highly correlated with outcome as indicated by disease-free survival.[14]

Four neoadjuvant approaches have been studied in patients with apparently localized esophageal cancers: preoperative radiation therapy followed by a planned surgical procedure, preoperative chemotherapy followed by an operation, a combination of chemotherapy and concurrent radiation followed by surgery, or chemotherapy with radiation (no operative procedure). Pilot trials involving small groups of patients suggested potential advantages for all of these approaches. More recently, random assignment trials have strongly supported all preoperative treatment approaches for chemotherapy and radiation therapy in patients with epidermoid carcinoma.

RADIATION BEFORE SURGERY

The major advantage (in theory) of radiation therapy before a planned surgical procedure is the potential to increase resection rates and decrease local failure. However, radiation therapy is, like surgery itself, a treatment of localized disease; it does not address the risk of systemic failure.

Three prospective, randomized studies involving radiation therapy alone before an operation have been reported. Launois and colleagues treated 124 patients with either 40 Gy given over 8 to 12 treatment fractions followed by surgery, or surgery alone.[15] There were no significant differences in operability, resectability, treatment-related mortality, or average or long-term survival (4.5 months in radiation therapy–surgery, vs. 8.2 months for surgery alone), with 9.5% and 11.5%, respectively, alive at 5 years.

In a similar study, the European Organization for Research and Treatment of Cancer treated 208 patients with either 33 Gy of radiation given in 8 to 12 treatment fractions, or with surgery alone.[16] There were no significant differences in any important parameter. Finally, Wang and associates treated 360 patients with 40 Gy before surgery or with surgery alone. An update of this Chinese trial indicated no survival benefit with preoperative radiation therapy.[17] Thus, at present, there are no data indicating that neoadjuvant radiation alone before surgery is of benefit, even in increasing potentially curative resection rates.

NEOADJUVANT CHEMOTHERAPY PLUS RADIATION THERAPY FOLLOWED BY SURGERY

The use of concurrent chemotherapy plus radiation therapy followed by surgery has been studied primarily in phase II trials, although one phase III study is underway (Table 17-2). In gen-

TABLE 17-2. *Esophageal cancer preoperative chemotherapy–radiation therapy phase II trials*

Study	Regimen/radiation dose	Patient no.	Operable (%)	Resectable (%)	Operative mortality (%)	Major response/pathologic complete response (%)	Median survival (mo)	5-Year survival
Franklin[40]	FU–mitomycin C/3000 cGy	30	76	76	13	NS/20	18*	30*†
Leichman[41]	FU–CDDP/3000 cGy	21	90	71	27	NS/24	18	NS
SWOG[18]	FU–CDDP/3000 cGy	106	63	49	11	NS/17	12	16†
RTOG[42]	FU–CDDP/3000 cGy	41	66	66	4	NS/20	13	8†
Forastiere[20]	FU–VLB–CDDP/ 3750–4500 cGy	43‡	95	91	2	42/24	29	34
Urba[22]	FU/4900 cGy	24§	79	79	4	41/8	11	33

FU, 5-fluorouracil; *CDDP,* cisplatin; *VLB,* vinblastine; *NS,* not stated.
* Completely resected patients only.
† Three-year survival.
‡ Adenocarcinoma and epidermoid carcinoma patients.
§ Adenocarcinoma only.

Ilson DH, Kelsen DP. Combined modality therapy in the treatment of esophageal cancer (review) Semin Oncol 1994. 1994;21:493.

eral, nonrandomized trials using concurrent chemotherapy and radiation followed by attempted resection have provided disappointing results. A large-scale study was performed by the Southwest Oncology Group (SWOG) and the Radiation Therapy Oncology Group (RTOG), based on pilot trials from Wayne State University Hospital.[18,19] A total of 154 evaluable patients (SWOG, n = 113; RTOG, n = 41) received cisplatin and a 5-fluorouracil infusion plus 30 Gy of concurrent radiation therapy; all were operable at the beginning of therapy. In the SWOG portion of the study, the operability rate was 63.6%; 53% of patients had resectable disease, including 13% of patients who had gross residual tumor left behind. The median duration of survival was 1 year. Sixteen percent and 7.5% (SWOG and RTOG, respectively) of patients were alive at 3 years. These results are similar to those seen with surgery alone. However, the use of concurrent chemotherapy plus radiation therapy followed by surgery is still undergoing study using a different operative technique (transhiatal esophagectomy). At the University of Michigan, Orringer and colleagues reported the preliminary results of a phase II trial of cisplatin, vinblastine, and 5-fluorouracil plus 4500 cGy of radiation.[20,21] Although resection rates were high and early survival data encouraging, toxicity in the phase II trial was substantial, with 80% of patients having severe myelosuppression; the treatment plan required 3 weeks of continuous hospitalization. In a follow-up study, a random-assignment trial comparing this regimen with surgery alone is underway at the University of Michigan. In a different phase II study, the same group used a different schedule of radiation therapy (350 cGy in 14 fractions) plus 5-fluorouracil by continuous infusion.[22] Twenty-four patients were treated. Although response was seen in 41% of patients, toxicity was substantial, including three deaths (12.5%). Because the median survival was 11 months (no improvement over historical controls), the authors concluded that combining radiation therapy and chemotherapy before surgery was still an investigational approach.

NEOADJUVANT CHEMOTHERAPY BEFORE SURGERY

The results of phase II studies involving the use of chemotherapy alone before surgery have been reviewed in detail (Table 17-3).[23] Overall, major objective regressions are seen in 40% to 55% of patients, with 3% to 10% of patients having complete remissions. Only a few small-scale phase III trials have been reported to date. Roth and colleagues randomly assigned patients to surgery only or to cisplatin–vindesine–bleomycin chemotherapy followed by exploration.[24] There was a total of 39 patients in the study. No differences between the two groups were seen in resection rates, operative morbidity (which was less for the chemotherapy arm), or operative mortality. The chemotherapy response rate, assessed before surgery, was 47%. Although there were no differences in overall survival, a subgroup analysis demonstrated that patients responding to preoperative chemotherapy had a substantial improvement in median survival compared to those undergoing surgery only (>20 months versus 8.6 months, $P = 0.05$). However, because of the small number of patients in the study, and because it was an unplanned (retrospective) analysis, definitive conclusions cannot be made.

Kelsen and associates compared two preoperative techniques for patients: preoperative radiation therapy versus preoperative chemotherapy.[25] The study was limited to patients with epidermoid cancer. A high dose of radiation (5500 cGy delivered by multifield techniques) was compared to a cisplatin–vindesine–bleomycin chemotherapy regimen. A total of 96 patients were treated. Both techniques (chemotherapy and radiation therapy) were equally effective in inducing major objective responses (chemotherapy, 55%, radiation therapy, 64%). Operability and resectability rates were also similar (operability: chemotherapy, 75%, radiation therapy, 77%; resection: chemotherapy, 58%, radiation therapy, 65%), whereas treatment-related mortality was slightly less for the chemotherapy arm. Because the study design allowed a postoperative crossover, and

TABLE 17-3. *Esophageal cancer preoperative chemotherapy therapy phase II/III trials*

Study	Regimen	Patient no.	Operable (%)	Resectable (%)	Operative mortality (%)	Major response/ pathologic complete response (%)	Median survival (mo)	5-Year survival
PHASE II TRIALS								
Coonley[43]	CDDP–BL	34	100	76	11	17/0	10	6
Kelsen[44]	CDDP–BL–VDS	34	100	82	5.6	53/3	16	17.5
Kelsen[45]	CDDP–M–VDS	14	93	86	7	NS/7	8	NS
Forastiere[46]	CCDP–M–VLB	27*	86	86	0	44/3*	14	21†
Kies[47]	CDDP–FU	25	54	38	0	42/0	17.8	17
Hilgenberg[48]	CDDP–FU	35	89	77	4	57/7	NS	54‡
PHASE III TRIALS								
Roth[49]	CDDP–BL–VDS	17	89	35§	12	47/6	9	25†‖
	Surgery	19	95	21§	0	—	9	5†‖
Schlag[50]	CDDP–FU	29	83	71	21	47/NS	8	NS
	Surgery	40	100	77	12	—	9	NS
Nygaard[27]	CDDP–BL	50	82	58	15	NS	NS	3†
	Surgery	41	93	69	13	—	NS	9†
	Radiation (3500 cGy)	48	75	54	11	NS	NS	21†
	Radiation/CDDP–BL	47	72	66	24	NS	NS	17†

CDDP, cisplatin; *BL,* bleomycin; *VDS,* vindesine; *M,* mitoguazone; *VLB,* vinblastine; *FU,* 5-fluorouracil; *NS,* not stated.

* Trial treated adenocarcinoma and epidermoid carcinoma. Response proportion represents the pooled adenocarcinoma and epidermoid carcinoma patients.

† Three-year actuarial survival.

‡ Actuarial survival at 3.5 years.

§ Curative resection.

‖ Not statistically significant.

Ilson DH, Kelsen DP. Combined modality therapy in the treatment of esophageal cancer (review). Semin Oncol. 1994; 21:493.

because most patients received both chemotherapy and radiation with only the sequence varying, it was not possible to assess the impact on long-term survival of chemotherapy or radiation therapy alone. The long-term survival rate was approximately 20%. The conclusion of the study was that, because chemotherapy was as effective at causing regression of local regional disease as radiation therapy, but allowed simultaneous treatment of systemic micrometastases, it was logical to pursue chemotherapy in combined modality regimens, as opposed to preoperative radiation. In a study reported only in abstract form, Schlag and associates[26] assigned patients to receive surgery alone, or surgery after three cycles of preoperative chemotherapy using fluorouracil and cisplatin. Toxicity was substantial, and no improvement in survival was noted in this small-scale trial. More recently, Nygaard and coworkers[27] performed a four-arm study in which patients underwent operation alone, chemotherapy with cisplatin and bleomycin followed by operation, radiation before operation, or radiation and concurrent chemotherapy before operation. Again, no significant survival advantage was seen for the chemotherapy followed by surgery arm. All of these trials, however, had limited power because of the small number of patients entered. A large-scale intergroup trial is underway in the United States, and a similar trial is underway in Great Britain. The current Intergroup trial is discussed later.

A NONOPERATIVE APPROACH TO LOCAL-REGIONAL DISEASE: CHEMOTHERAPY PLUS RADIATION THERAPY

Two approaches using chemotherapy plus radiation therapy without operation have been studied. The first involves chemotherapy (usually for one or two cycles) followed by definitive radiation therapy (usually 50 to 60 Gy). The second involves concurrent chemotherapy and radiation therapy. Although most of these trials were small, single-arm, phase II pilot studies, several important prospective, randomized studies have been reported.

Chemotherapy Plus Concurrent Radiation

The first studies combining chemotherapy with concurrent radiation were performed in the 1970s. For example, Kolaric and colleagues performed a series of small-scale trials in which patients with inoperable but localized tumors received either chemotherapy alone or chemotherapy and radiation.[28–32] The agents they studied included bleomycin, adriamycin, and a combination of the two. In each trial, the response rate to combined modality therapy was superior to that of chemotherapy alone. However, only a slight increase in survival was noted. A larger

Eastern Cooperative Oncology Group (ECOG) phase III trial compared bleomycin with concurrent radiation versus radiation alone. There was no difference in survival outcome, which is not surprising considering the limited antineoplastic activity of bleomycin when used as a single agent.[33] However, more recent studies using multidrug regimens of either mitomycin C plus 5-fluorouracil or cisplatin plus 5-fluorouracil are more promising.[34–36]

An Intergroup trial involving RTOG and SWOG tested the hypothesis that the use of cisplatin and 5-fluorouracil plus concurrent radiation (61 patients) would be superior to radiation alone (60 patients).[37] Even though the dose of radiation given in the combined modality arm (5000 cGy) was less than that for patients receiving radiation alone (6400 cGy), a survival advantage was seen for patients given chemotherapy plus radiation (median survival of 12.5 vs. 8.9 months). More important, at 2 years, 38% of the chemotherapy plus radiation therapy patients were alive, versus 10% of the radiation therapy only patients. Although the substantial toxicity for patients receiving chemotherapy plus radiation was described as tolerable, close to two thirds of patients receiving combined modality therapy had severe or life-threatening toxicities. In this study, two additional cycles of chemotherapy after completion of radiation were planned; approximately half (54%) the patients received both additional postradiation courses. Data on the failure pattern were less detailed. The local failure rate at 1 year was 62% for radiation therapy only, and 44% for combined treatment. Herskovic and coworkers, in a follow-up study, assigned patients to the investigational arm alone. In a preliminary analysis, survival was almost identical to that of chemotherapy plus radiation therapy patients in the initial study, supporting the beneficial effects of combined modality therapy. Toxicity data were not reported in detail. In both studies, most of the patients had epidermoid carcinomas.[38]

The ECOG has reported in abstract the results of a second trial of systemic therapy (using mitomycin plus 5-fluorouracil) plus concurrent radiation versus radiation alone.[39] In the trial, the study design allowed patients, at the discretion of the attending physician, to undergo surgery after completion of chemotherapy and 40 Gy of radiation or 40 Gy of radiation alone. Because surgery was performed in a nonrandomized fashion, interpretation of the data is more difficult. In the preliminary report, a survival advantage was noted for the chemotherapy–radiation therapy arm. Taken together, the data from these two trials strongly suggest that chemotherapy and concurrent radiation is superior to radiation alone, at least for patients with epidermoid carcinoma of the esophagus.

Chemotherapy Followed by Radiation Therapy

Less extensive data are available on the use of induction chemotherapy followed by radiation therapy, either alone or with concurrent chemotherapy. Although several phase II trials have been performed, and have demonstrated tolerance, no random assignment trials are yet available. The rationale for giving neoadjuvant chemotherapy before chemotherapy plus radiation therapy first would again be to reduce tumor bulk in the area to be irradiated and address the systemic failure pattern. At present, a prospective phase II trial of neoadjuvant chemotherapy followed by concurrent chemotherapy plus radiation therapy is underway by RTOG and ECOG.

THE CURRENT U.S. INTERGROUP TRIALS

Two different approaches to neoadjuvant therapy of esophageal cancer are under study using the Intergroup method. A large-scale Intergroup Trial (including RTOG, SWOG, Cancer and Acute Leukemia Group B, ECOG, and North Central Cancer Treatment Group) is underway addressing the issue of whether preoperative and postoperative adjuvant chemotherapy improves outcome for patients with operable esophageal cancers. This study, Intergroup Trial 013, continues to accrue patients, with over 280 patients entered. The study design calls for three cycles of cisplatin and 5-fluorouracil given at once-monthly intervals. After surgery, resected patients receive two additional cycles of chemotherapy. Patients randomly assigned to standard therapy undergo surgery alone.

In the second Intergroup phase III trial, the increasing evidence that concurrent chemotherapy plus radiation is superior to radiation alone has led to a study testing the order of treatment and total radiation dose. The survival advantage for concurrent radiation therapy plus cisplatin–5-fluorouracil in the RTOG study is very encouraging; preliminary data for the ECOG are supportive. The second Intergroup trial compares concurrent chemotherapy plus radiation using 5040 Gy versus chemotherapy at a higher dose of 6480 cGy. There are no random-assignment trials comparing best local-regional therapy (ie, surgery vs. radiation [with or without neoadjuvant chemotherapy]).

In conclusion, the use of neoadjuvant chemotherapy followed by definitive treatment of the primary lesion using surgery or radiation is a promising approach to esophageal cancer. The potential ability to control systemic disease while decreasing local failure gives us the chance to improve disease-free and overall survival. For concurrent chemotherapy and radiation therapy, tolerance has been established and initial reports indicate improved outcome as measured by survival with evidence of decreased local failure rates.

Future advances will require the development of increasingly effective systemic therapy; the identification of paclitaxel as an active agent in both epidermoid carcinoma and adenocarcinoma is encouraging. More data on the difference in outcome for adenocarcinoma (which currently is seen in half of all newly diagnosed patients) are forthcoming. For now, use of chemotherapy plus surgery should be considered investigational. Enough data have been amassed to support the use of concurrent chemotherapy and radiation therapy in clinical practice for patients with epidermoid carcinoma of the esophagus; for adenocarcinoma, less data are available.

ACKNOWLEDGMENT

The author gratefully acknowledges the expert assistance of Ann Riley-Martin in the preparation of the manuscript.

REFERENCES

1. Chan KW, Chan EY, Chan CW. Carcinoma of the esophagus: an autopsy study of 231 cases. Pathology 1986;18:400.
2. Anderson I, Ladd T. Autopsy findings in squamous cell carcinoma of the esophagus. Cancer 1982;50:1587.
3. Bosch A, Frias Z, Caldwell W, et al. Autopsy findings in carcinoma of the esophagus. Acta Radiol Oncol 1979;18:103.

4. Mandard AM, Chasle J, Marnay J, et al. Autopsy findings in 111 cases of esophageal cancer. Cancer 1981;48:329.
5. Gunduz N, Fisher B, Saffer E. Effect of surgical removal on the growth and kinetics of residual tumor. Cancer Res 1979;39:1361.
6. Fisher B, Gunduz N, Saffer EA. Influence of the interval between primary tumor removal and chemotherapy on kinetics and growth of metastases. Cancer Res 1983;43:1488.
7. Schatten WE. An experimental study of postoperative tumor metastases: I. growth of pulmonary metastases following total removal of primary leg tumor. Cancer 1958;11:455.
8. Simpson-Herren L, Sanford AH, Holmquist JP. Effects of surgery on the cell kinetics of residual tumor. Cancer Treat Rep 1976;60:1749.
9. Pendegrast WJ Jr, Drake WP, Mardiney MR Jr. A proper sequence for the treatment of B16 melanoma: chemotherapy, surgery and immunotherapy. J Natl Cancer Inst 1976;57:539.
10. Muggia FM, Gill I. Primary chemotherapy. In: DeVita VT Jr, Hellman S, Rosenberg SA, eds. Cancer: principles and practice of oncology updates. 3rd ed. Philadelphia: JB Lippincott, 1990:1.
11. Kelsen D. Adjuvant therapy of upper gastrointestinal tract cancers. Semin Oncol 1991;18:543.
12. Lightdale C, Botet J, Brennan M, et al. Endoscopic ultrasonography compared to computerized tomography for preoperative staging of gastric cancer. Gastrointest Endosc 1989;35:154.
13. Tio TL, Coene PP, Luiken GJ, Tytgat GN. Endosonography in the clinical staging of esophagogastric carcinoma. Gastrointest Endosc 1990;36:S2.
14. Smith JW, Brennan MF, Botet JF, Gerdes H, Lightdale CJ. Preoperative endoscopic ultrasound can predict the risk of recurrence after operation for gastric carcinoma. J Clin Oncol 1993;11:2380.
15. Launois B, Delarue D, Campion JP, Kerbaol M. Preoperative radiotherapy for carcinoma of the esophagus. Surg Gynecol Obstet 1981;153: 690.
16. Gignoux M, Roussel A, Paillot B, et al. The value of preoperative radiotherapy in esophageal cancer: results of a study of the E.O.R.T.C. World J Surg 1987;11:426.
17. Wang LJ, Huang GJ, et al. Combined preoperative irradiation and surgery versus surgery alone for carcinoma of the midthoracic esophagus: a prospective randomized study in 360 patients [abstract]. In: the Fourth World Congress of the International Society for Diseases of the Esophagus, Rennes, France, 1989:63.
18. Poplin E, Fleming T, Leichman L, et al. Combined therapies for squamous-cell carcinoma of the esophagus: a Southwest Oncology Group Study (SWOG-8037). J Clin Oncol 1987;5:622.
19. Andersen AP, Berdal P, Edsmyr F, et al. Irradiation, chemotherapy and surgery in esophageal cancer: a randomized clinical study. The first Scandinavian trial in esophageal cancer. Radiother Oncol 1984; 2:179.
20. Forastiere AA, Orringer MB, Perez-Tamayo C, et al. Concurrent chemotherapy and radiation therapy followed by transhiatal esophagectomy for local-regional cancer of the esophagus. J Clin Oncol 1990; 8:119.
21. Orringer MB, Forastiere AA, Perez-Tamayo C, Urba S, Takasugi BJ, Bromberg J. Chemotherapy and radiation therapy before transhiatal esophagectomy for esophageal carcinoma [see comments]. Ann Thorac Surg 1990;49:348.
22. Urba SG, Orringer MB, Perez-Tamayo C, Bromberg J, Forastiere A. Concurrent preoperative chemotherapy and radiation therapy in localized esophageal adenocarcinoma. Cancer 1992;69:285.
23. Kelsen DP, Bains M, Burt M. Neoadjuvant chemotherapy and surgery of cancer of the esophagus. Semin Surg Oncol 1990;6:268.
24. Roth JA, Pass HI, Flanagan MM, Graeber GM, Rosenberg JC, Steinberg S. Randomized clinical trial of preoperative and postoperative adjuvant chemotherapy with cisplatin, vindesine, and bleomycin for carcinoma of the esophagus. J Thorac Cardiovasc Surg 1988;96: 242.
25. Kelsen DP, Minsky B, Smith M, et al. Preoperative therapy for esophageal cancer: a randomized comparison of chemotherapy versus radiation therapy. J Clin Oncol 1990;8:1352.
26. Schlag P, Herrmann R, Raeth V, et al. Preoperative chemotherapy in esophageal cancer. A phase II study. Acta Oncologica 1988;27:811.
27. Nygaard K, Hagen S, Hansen HS, et al. Pre-operative radiotherapy prolongs survival in operable esophageal carcinoma: a randomized, multicenter study of pre-operative radiotherapy and chemotherapy: the second Scandinavian trial in esophageal cancer. World J Surg 1992; 16:1104.
28. Kolaric K, Maricic Z, Dujmovic I, et al. Therapy of advanced esophageal cancer with bleomycin, irradiation and combination bleomycin and irradiation. Tumori 1976;62:255.
29. Kolaric K, Maricic Z, Roth A, Dujmovic I. Chemotherapy versus chemoradiotherapy in inoperable esophageal cancer: results of three controlled studies. Oncology 1980;37(Suppl 1):77.
30. Kolaric K, Maricic Z, Roth A, Dujmovic I. Bleomycin infusions combined with radiotherapy in the treatment of inoperable esophageal cancer. Tumori 1980;66:615.
31. Kolaric K, Maricic Z, Roth A, Dujmovic I. Combination of bleomycin and adriamycin with and without radiation on the treatment of inoperable esophageal cancer: a randomized study. Cancer 1980;45:2265.
32. Kolaric K, Maricic Z, Roth A, et al. Adriamycin alone and in combination with radiotherapy in the treatment of inoperable esophageal cancer. Tumori 1977;63:485.
33. Earle JD, Gelber RD, Moertel CG, Hahn RG. A controlled evaluation of combined radiation and bleomycin therapy for squamous cell carcinoma of the esophagus. Int J Radiat Oncol Biol Phys 1980;6:821.
34. Coia LR, Engstrom PF, Paul A. Nonsurgical management of esophageal cancer: report of a study of combined radiotherapy and chemotherapy. J Clin Oncol 1987;5:1783.
35. Keane TJ, Harwood AR, Elhakim T, et al. Radical radiation therapy with 5-fluorouracil infusion and mitomycin C for oesophageal squamous carcinoma. Radiother Oncol 1985;4:205.
36. John M, Flam M, Wittlinger P, Mowry PA. Inoperable esophageal carcinoma: results of aggressive synchronous radiotherapy and chemotherapy: a pilot study. Am J Clin Oncol 1987;10:310.
37. Herskovic A, Martz K, Al-Sarraf M, et al. Combined chemotherapy and radiotherapy compared with radiotherapy alone in patients with cancer of the esophagus [see comments]. N Engl J Med 1992;326: 1593.
38. Al-Sarraf M, Martz K, Herskovic A, et al. Superiority of chemo-radiotherapy in patients with esophageal cancer. Final report of an intergroup randomized and confirmed study. Proc ASCO 1996;15:464.
39. Sischy B, Ryan L, Haller D, et al. Interim report of EST 1282 phase III protocol for the evaluation of combined modalities in the treatment of patients with carcinoma of the esophagus, stage I and II [abstract]. Proceedings of the American Society for Clinical Oncology 1990;9: 105.
40. Franklin R, Steiger Z, Vaishampayan G, et al. Combined modality therapy for esophageal squamous cell carcinoma. Cancer 1983;51: 1062.
41. Leichman L, Steiger Z, Seydel HG, et al. Preoperative chemotherapy and radiation therapy for patients with cancer of the esophagus: a potentially curative approach. J Clin Oncol 1984;2:75.
42. Seydel HG, Leichman L, Byhardt R, et al. Preoperative radiation and chemotherapy for localized squamous cell carcinoma of the esophagus. A RTOG Study. Int J Radiat Oncol Biol Phys 1988;14:33.
43. Coonley CJ, Bains M, Hilaris B, et al. Cisplatin and bleomycin in the treatment of esophageal carcinoma. A final report. Cancer 1984;54: 2351.
44. Kelsen D, Hilaris B, Coonley C, et al. Cisplatin, vindesine, and bleomycin chemotherapy of local-regional and advanced esophageal carcinoma. Am J Med 1983;75:645.
45. Kelsen DP, Fein R, Coonley C, et al. Cisplatin, vindesine, and mitoguazone in the treatment of esophageal cancer. Cancer Treat Rep 1986; 70:255.
46. Forastiere AA, Gennis M, Orringer MB, et al. Cisplatin, vinblastine, and mitoguazone chemotherapy for epidermoid and adenocarcinoma of the esophagus. J Clin Oncol 1987;5:1143.
47. Kies MS, Rosen ST, Tsang TK, et al. Cisplatin and 5-fluorouracil in the primary management of squamous esophageal cancer. Cancer 1987; 60:2156.
48. Hilgenberg AD, Carey RW, Wilkins EW Jr, et al. Preoperative chemotherapy, surgical resection, and selective postoperative therapy for squamous cell carcinoma of the esophagus. Ann Thorac Surg 1988; 45:357.
49. Roth JA, Pass HI, Flanagan MM, et al. Randomized clinical trial of preoperative and postoperative adjuvant chemotherapy with cisplatin, vindesine, and bleomycin for carcinoma of the esophagus. J Thorac Cardiovasc Surg 1988;96:242.
50. Schlag P, Herrmann R, Raeth V, et al. Preoperative chemotherapy in esophageal cancer. A phase II study. Acta Oncologica 1988;27:811.

Surgery for Gastrointestinal Cancer: A Multidisciplinary Approach, edited by Harold J. Wanebo.
Lippincott-Raven Publishers, Philadelphia, © 1997.

CHAPTER 18

Esophageal Cancer: The Japanese Experience

Hiroshi Akiyama, Masahiko Tsurumaru, and Harushi Udagawa

DETECTION OF CARCINOMA OF THE ESOPHAGUS

One of the essential factors in improving survival in carcinoma of the esophagus is its early detection. In high-incidence areas, mass screening testing is important. On the other hand, in low-incidence areas, mass examination is not cost effective, and esophageal cancers are usually detected on routine medical examination or during investigation of other unrelated conditions. In early carcinoma of the esophagus, 57% of patients are asymptomatic.[1] Pain and soreness are occasional symptoms of early cancer of the esophagus. These were seen in 22% of our patients with this disease; dysphagia or a feeling of dysphagia was found in 14% of early cases. We advise that even minor complaints be taken into consideration, and that a thorough investigation be done.

Tumor type, its extent, and the degree of pliability of the esophageal wall correlate with the severity of symptoms. For example, a polypoid tumor, even though large in size, may cause few symptoms and no dysphagia whatsoever. On the other hand, a small, scirrhous circumferential carcinoma would soon result in severe dysphagia. Although the main symptom of carcinoma of the esophagus is dysphagia, there is no direct correlation between duration or severity of dysphagia and tumor stage, resectability, or prognosis. Therefore, a widespread campaign needs to be instituted stressing the need for early detection, annual routine individual check-ups, and incidental examination of the esophagus concomitantly with examination for other diseases.

ADVANCES IN DIAGNOSTIC MEASURES

Since the mid-1980s, there have been extensive advances in the detection and accurate diagnosis of early cancer of the esophagus. Composite examinations with endoscopy, radiography, ultrasonography, and endoscopic ultrasonography are extensively carried out.[2–6] Accurate and precise diagnosis of the depth of tumor invasion is required for deciding on the surgical and or other therapeutic strategy.

In endoscopy, common mucosal findings of early esophageal cancer include unevenness or roughness, irregularity, redness or faded color, and shading of the mucosal vascular network. When these changes are found, further endoscopic investigation with vital staining techniques using iodine and toluidine blue (tolonium chloride) is carried out. This examination is mandatory for more precise diagnosis of extent and depth of tumor invasion, and assessment of the presence of multifocal or concomitant intraepithelial cancers. The Japanese Society for Esophageal Diseases[7] has typed superficial cancers of the esophagus based on endoscopic findings, as shown in Table 18-1. Figure 18-1*A* shows the endoscopic finding of the slightly depressed type (0-IIc) of intraepithelial cancer of the esophagus. The margin of the lesion is well demonstrated with clear demarcation by iodine vital staining (Fig. 18-1*B*). The lesion was removed by endoscopic mucosal resection and was proven to be confined within the epithelium (Fig. 18-1*C*).

Double-contrast radiography, as described by Shirakabe and colleagues,[4] is also important in the early diagnosis of esophageal cancer, as in the examination of early cancer of the stomach. It was stated that there were no difficulties in differentiating mucosal cancers from submucosal cancers.[4] Differentiation between epithelial and muscularis mucosae cancer is not easy with an en face view. Irregularity of the esophageal wall in both en face and profile views, and interpretation of the irregularity of the mucosal pattern, are key points in the radiologic detection of early esophageal cancer.

The use of high-frequency endoscopic ultrasonography (Fujinon, Tokyo, Japan; linear, 20 MHz) has made it possible to assess the finer structures of the esophageal wall.[6] Figure 18-2 is an endoscopic echogram of superficial cancer of the esophagus showing the depth of submucosal tumor invasion.

For advanced cancer of the esophagus, assessing the presence of local invasion to surrounding important organs, with or without malignant fistulas or distant vascular metastases, is an important part of the diagnosis. The phenomenon of abnormality of the esophageal axis in locally advanced tumor with invasion

Hiroshi Akiyama: Toranomon Hospital Department of Surgery, 2-2-2, Toranomon Minato-Ku, Tokyo, 105, Japan.
Masahiko Tsurumaru: Toranomon Hospital Department of Surgery, 2-2-2, Toranomon Minato-Ku, Tokyo, 105, Japan.
Harushi Udagawa: Toranomon Hospital Department of Surgery, 2-2-2, Toranomon Minato-Ku, Tokyo, 105, Japan.

TABLE 18-1. *Types of carcinoma of the esophagus based on endoscopic findings*

Type	Description
0	Superficial
0-I	Superficial and protruding
0-II	Superficial and flat
0-IIa	Slightly elevated
0-IIb	Flat
0-IIc	Slightly depressed
0-III	Superficial and distinctly depressed
1	Protruding
2	Ulcerative and localized
3	Ulcerative and infiltrative
4	Diffusely infiltrative
5	Unclassifiable

Japanese Society for Esophageal Diseases. Guidelines for the clinical and pathologic studies on carcinoma of the esophagus. 8th ed. Tokyo: Kanehara & Co., Ltd., 1992.

to the surrounding fixed organs, as described by Akiyama and colleagues,[8] is one of the conventional findings in late cancer of the esophagus. This finding is well demonstrated by computed tomography, magnetic resonance imaging, or endoscopic ultrasonography.

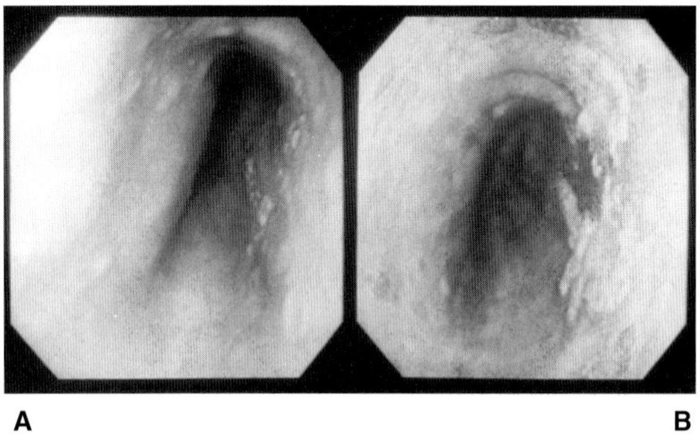

A B

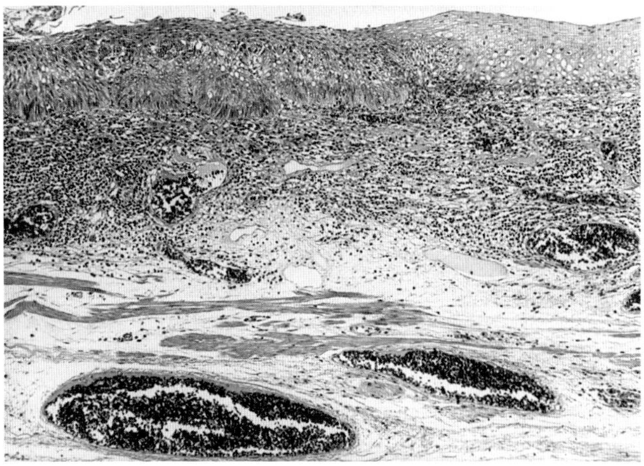

C

FIG. 18-1. (A) Endoscopic finding of slightly depressed type (0-IIc) of intraepithelial cancer of the esophagus. **(B)** Margin of cancer is well demarcated by iodine vital staining. See also Color Figures 18-1**A** and **(C).** Endoscopically resected specimen shows the lesion to be confined to the epithelium. HE × 18.

The biologic malignancy[1,9,10] of the tumor is even more important in assessing advancement and prognosis in cancer of the esophagus. For example, a patient with a high-malignancy submucosal tumor, even without dysphagia, could already be nonresectable, not because of local condition, but because of advanced lymphatic or vascular spread, whereas a patient with tumor invading the adventitia could be cured if the tumor is of low malignant grade.

STAGING

Cancer of the esophagus was first included in the TNM classification in 1968. With increasing analysis of patients and improvement in the quality of diagnosis, revision of the third edition became necessary. Thus, a proposal for a new TNM classification was made in 1985 by the Japanese Committee for Registration of Esophageal Carcinoma. This was based on analysis of 3681 patients registered in Japan during the period between 1969 to 1978. With acceptance of this proposal by the International Union Against Cancer (UICC), a new TNM classification was published by the UICC in 1987.[11] The data from the Japanese patients, which became the basis of the revised TNM classification, were reported by Iizuka.[12]

Many important revisions were made in the fourth edition of the TNM classification. Regarding the demarcation level, the lower border of the thoracic vertebra was changed to the tracheal bifurcation; the T classification criteria of length of tumor and invasion to surrounding structures was changed to the depth of tumor invasion; and the range of N for thoracic lesions was changed from mediastinal to mediastinal and abdominal nodes.

Even in this revision, the cervical and celiac lymph nodes were not included as regional nodes for the thoracic esophagus. The definition of regional and distant lymph nodes is often vague. Far from being rare, metastases to the cervical and celiac nodes are rather common in cancers not only of the upper, but also middle and lower thoracic esophagus. Moreover, patients with metastatic nodes in the cervical and celiac region sometimes can be cured. Therefore, inclusion of cervical and celiac lymph node metastases and blood-borne organ metastases into the single category of M—distant metastases—seems inappropriate. Therefore, it is proposed that cervical and celiac nodes should be classified as part of the N category. The following parts of this chapter are based on this philosophy, and stage IV disease due to the pN factor (ie, metastases to the cervical or celiac lymph nodes) is called stage IV-N. The prognosis of patients with stage IV disease due to organ metastases (stage IV-M) is considered separately.

SURGICAL STRATEGY AND TECHNIQUES

The depth of tumor invasion is clearly related to the frequency of lymph node metastases (Fig. 18-3). The studies were based on histologic examination of all nodes dissected from the patients who underwent complete collothoracoabdominal (three-field) lymph node dissection.[1,13–15]

Endoscopic Mucosal Resection and Esophagectomy Without Thoracotomy

No nodal metastases were found in patients with intraepithelial and lamina propria mucosae cancers, although there is a theoretic

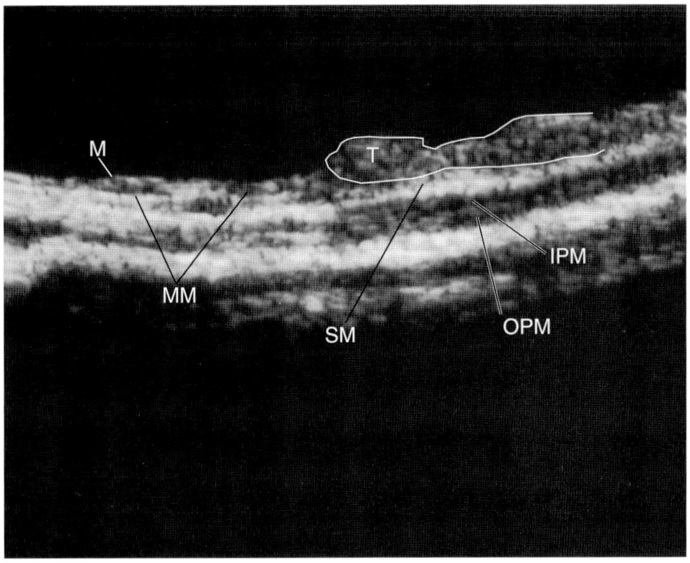

FIG. 18-2. Endoscopic sonogram of superficial cancer of the esophagus. Thin hypoechoic layer, which is suspected to be closely related to muscularis mucosae, is disrupted by the tumor. Hyperechoic layer of submucosa under the tumor is slightly thinned but continuous. Slight invasion of the tumor into the submucosal layer was histologically proven. *T*, tumor; *M*, mucosa (epithelium); *MM*, muscularis mucosae; *SM*, submucosa; *IPM*, inner circular proper muscle layer; *OPM*, outer longitudinal proper muscle layer.

risk of lymphatic spread in the latter type. Therefore, endoscopic mucosal resection[16] is recommended for intraepithelial and lamina propria mucosae cancers. However, metastases were occasionally found in patients with muscularis mucosae cancer. Therefore, for muscularis mucosae cancers, the indications for endoscopic mucosal resection remain controversial.

In the past,[17] before anesthesia had been developed adequately, the main purpose of exploring the technique of esophagectomy without thoracotomy as a serious alternative in surgery for carcinoma of the esophagus was to avoid the necessity for thoracotomy. However, because it was carried out blind, it was thought to be dangerous, and the procedure did not gain acceptance for many years except in cases of malignancy of the hypopharynx or cervical esophagus. In these circumstances, the thoracic esophagus was more or less normal, and extraction without thoracotomy was therefore performed with relative ease. In more recent years, this technique has been revived.[18–20] It is also used for removal of malignancies located in the mediastinum.[21] However, esophagectomy without thoracotomy may not be appropriate for cancers with possible adventitial invasion or mediastinal nodal metastases. The following indications are thought to be appropriate for esophagectomy without thoracotomy: epithelial or lamina propria mucosae cancers (too large or too numerous for endoscopic resection, or those with field carcinogenesis; see Fig. 18-3); advanced cancers in patients with risk factors; and palliative resection.

Thoracoscopic esophagectomy may be useful for benign lesions of the esophagus. However, when its aim is only a simple

Depth of Tumor Invasion (no. of patient with positive nodes / no. of patient)		Frequency of lymph node metastasis (0–100%)	Surgical strategy
ep	(0/5)	0%	Endoscopic resection For wide or multiple (field carcinogenetic) cancers, esophagectomy without thoracotomy may be chosen.
lpm	(0/2)	0%	
mm	(1/6)	16.7%	For mm cancers, 2-field (TA) dissection may also be chosen.
sm	(27/51)	52.9%	3-field (CTA) dissection
mp	(18/25)	72.0%	
$a_{1\sim2}$	(107/129)	82.9%	
a_3	(9/11)	81.8%	For a*3 cancers, local resection should be RO**
Total	(162/229)	70.7%	

FIG. 18-3. Surgical strategy in relation to the depth of tumor invasion and frequency of lymph node metastases. *Tumor invasion to adjacent organs; **no residual tumor; *ep*, epithelium; *lpm*, lamina propria mucosae; *mm*, muscularis mucosae; *sm*, submucosa; *mp*, muscularis propria; *a*, adventitia; *TA*, thoracoabdominal; *CTA*, collothoracoabdominal.

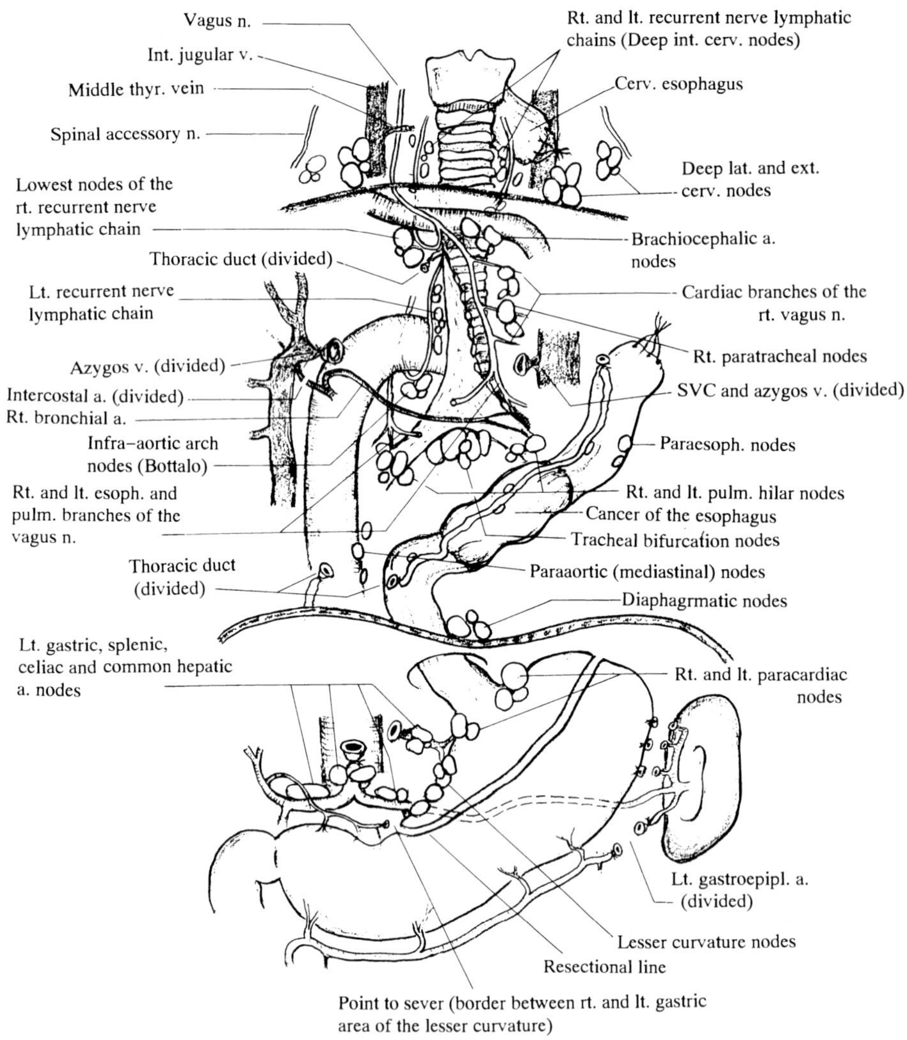

FIG. 18-4. Extent of esophageal and gastric resection and systematic radical lymph node dissection. Extent of extensive three-field dissection is shown. In two-field dissection, no cervical dissection is carried out. *a*, artery; *n*, nerve; *v*, vein.

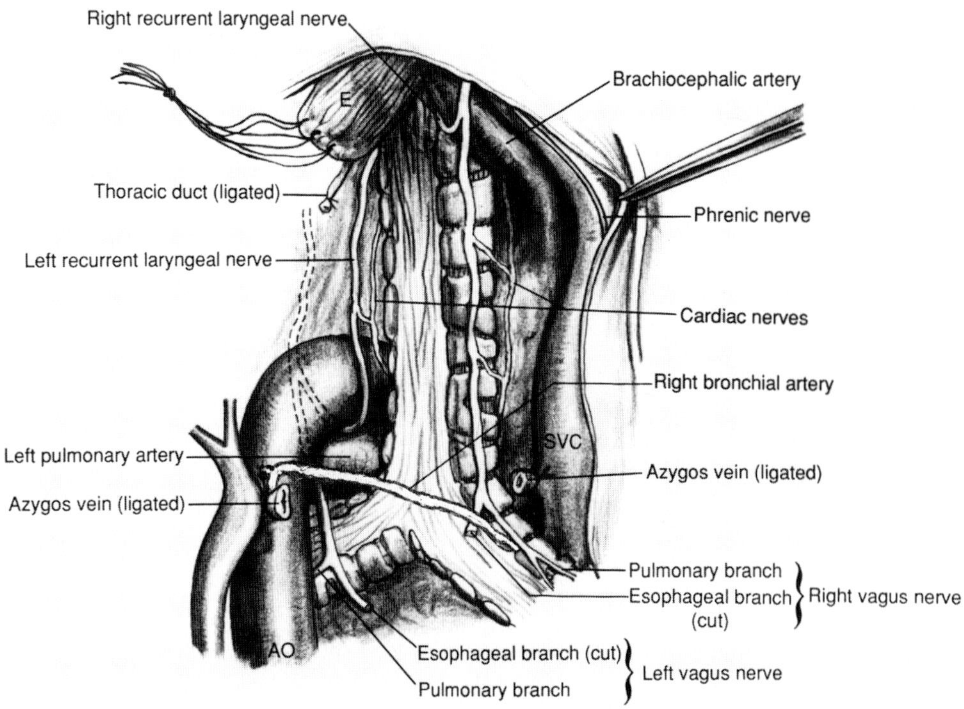

FIG. 18-5. Completion of superior mediastinal dissection.

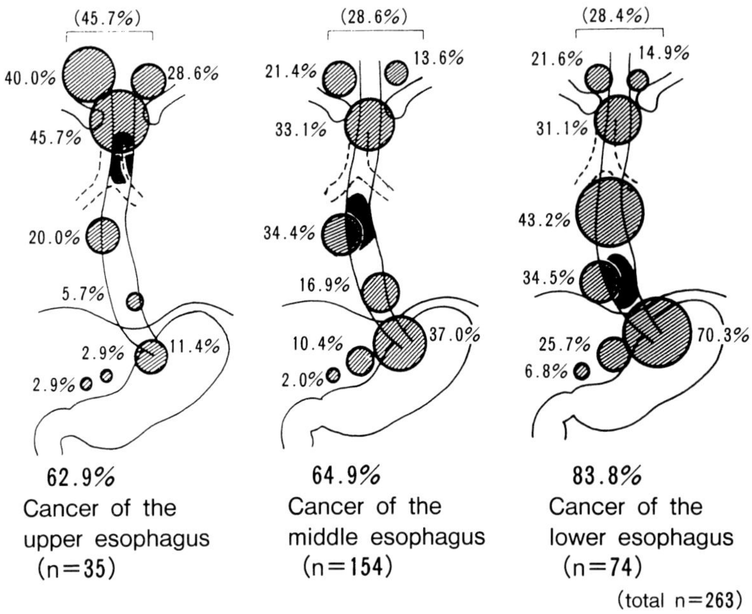

FIG. 18-6. Frequency of lymph node dissection according to tumor location.

esophagectomy, and when cervical and abdominal incisions are already made, conventional esophagectomy without thoracotomy is superior because of the simplicity and quickness with which it may be undertaken. It is hoped some degree of nodal dissection will soon become possible using this technique, thus minimizing operative risks.

Systematic Lymph Node Dissection

Once cancer has invaded the submucosa, the frequency of nodal involvement suddenly increases to 52.9%, a finding that correlates well with the presence of a well developed lymphatic network in the submucosal layer. Therefore, submucosal or deeper cancer should be treated by systematic lymph node dissection.[1,13–15,22]

For collothoracoabdominal lymph node dissection, or three-field dissection (Fig. 18-4), a right thoracotomy through the fourth intercostal space, laparotomy through an upper midline incision, and a collar incision in the lower neck are routinely used. Both resections and reconstruction of the esophagus are carried out in one stage. After the mediastinal dissection is completed through a right thoracotomy, the patient is turned from the left lateral to the supine position, and the abdominal and cervical procedures are performed simultaneously by two surgical teams. In patients with advanced cancer of the upper thoracic esophagus, upper median sternotomy maybe added to achieve more complete dissection of the cervicothoracic region.

The cervicothoracic region is the most important area because tumor spreads there most frequently. The right and left recurrent laryngeal nerve lymphatic chains were the most frequent sites of metastasis. In almost half (45.6%) of the patients, metastases

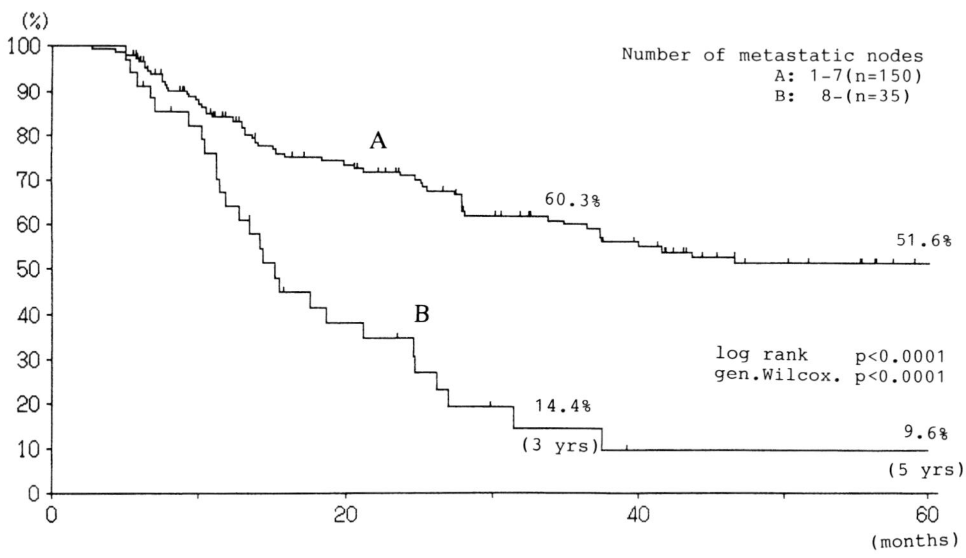

FIG. 18-7. Number of positive nodes most significantly dividing the outcome into favorable and unfavorable (three-field dissection). One to seven positive nodes (curve A) were associated with a more favorable outcome, eight or more positive nodes (curve B) with an unfavorable one.

TABLE 18-2. *Five-year survival rates after two- and three-field dissection according to pTNM staging*

	Less extensive, two-field dissection		Extensive three-field dissection	
pTNM stage	n	5-Year survival rates	n	5-Year survival rates
O	4	100%	4	75.0%†
I	26	69.2% ± 9.1%	35	94.1% ± 5.7%
IIA	71	47.9% ± 5.9%	39	82.5% ± 6.6%
IIB	43	46.5% ± 7.6%	27	57.3% ± 14.1%
III	96	27.1% ± 4.5%	69	55.8% ± 6.6%
IV-pN*	36	11.1% ± 5.2%	99	28.0% ± 5.4%

* Stage IV disease due to pN factor.
† One patient died of nonmalignant disease.

were found in the cervical and superior mediastinal region, emphasizing that cancer of the thoracic esophagus frequently metastasizes to these lymph nodes. Furthermore, the cervicothoracic region is the most difficult region to manage surgically; it is anatomically complex, including the trachea, the brachiocephalic artery, the superior vena cava with its draining small branches, the vagus nerves with its vulnerable cardiac branches, and the right and left recurrent laryngeal nerves. Cardiac nerves of the right side are also carefully preserved.[1,6,13,14] The extent of dissection and status of completion of superior mediastinal dissection are shown in Figure 18-5. Frequency of lymph nodes metastases according to tumor location is shown in Figure 18-6. Although there was a clear correlation between the anatomic location of the tumor and the sites of metastases, lymphatic spread was widely seen regardless of the location of the primary lesion.

RESULTS

Number of Metastatic Nodes and Prognosis for Cure

One of the best indicators for prognosis after radical lymphadenectomy is the number of lymph nodes involved. There may be a critical number of metastasized lymph nodes beyond which the prognosis is unfavorable. As shown in Figure 18-7, the critical number of metastatic nodes that most significantly indicated a more favorable prognosis, even by radical three-field lymph node dissection, was between one and seven, whereas eight or more indicated an unfavorable prognosis ($P < 0.0001$). The latter implies the upper limit of involved nodes for cure even by radical resection.

Comparison of Prognosis According to the Extent of Nodal Dissection and pTNM Staging

Five-year survival rates after two-field mediastinal and abdominal dissection[22] and three-field cervical, mediastinal, and abdominal dissection[1,13–15] according to pTNM classification, are shown in Table 18-2. The number of patients with stage IV-pN disease (stage IV due to histopathologically proven nodal metastases, but not due to other distant or organ metastases) in the extensive three-field dissection group is larger than that in the less extensive two-field dissection group because of downstaging or stage migration. For example, positive cervical nodes in stage IV-pN patients in the two-field dissection group comprised only those found by preoperative examination or by detection of metastases-containing suspect nodes at operation. Consequently, the results are somewhat statistically deviated. In stage III (Fig. 18-8) and IV-pN disease, survival rates significantly improved after extensive dissection.

Overall Survival

The 5-year survival rates for patients with all depths of cancer invasion after extensive three-field and less extensive two-field dissections were 55.0% and 38.3%, respectively. However, because patients with mucosal cancer rarely have nodal metastases, it is fair to exclude patients with mucosal cancers from the series, to study the effect of nodal dissection. With the exclusion

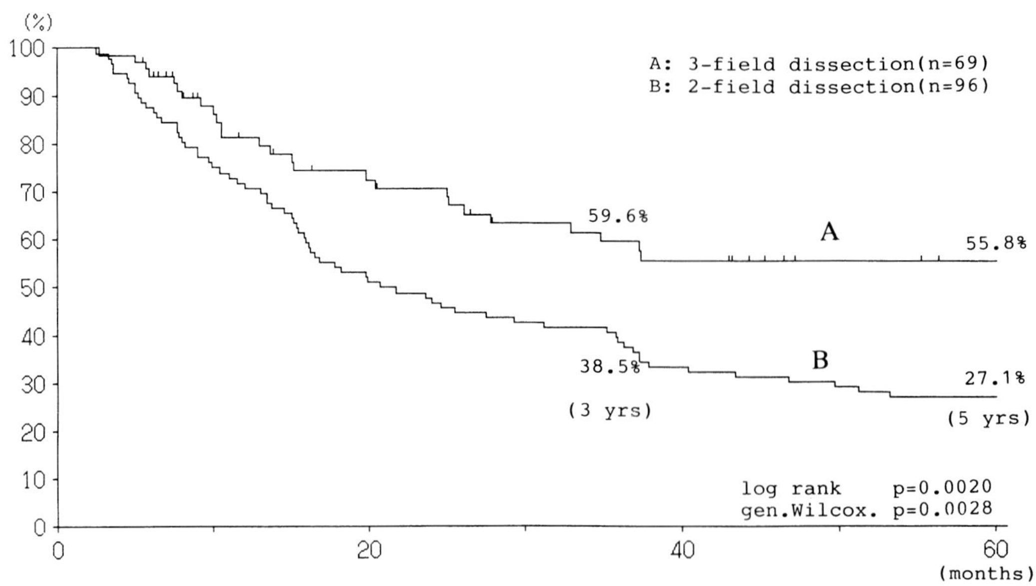

FIG. 18-8. Comparison of survival curves after two- and three-field dissections (pTNM stage III).

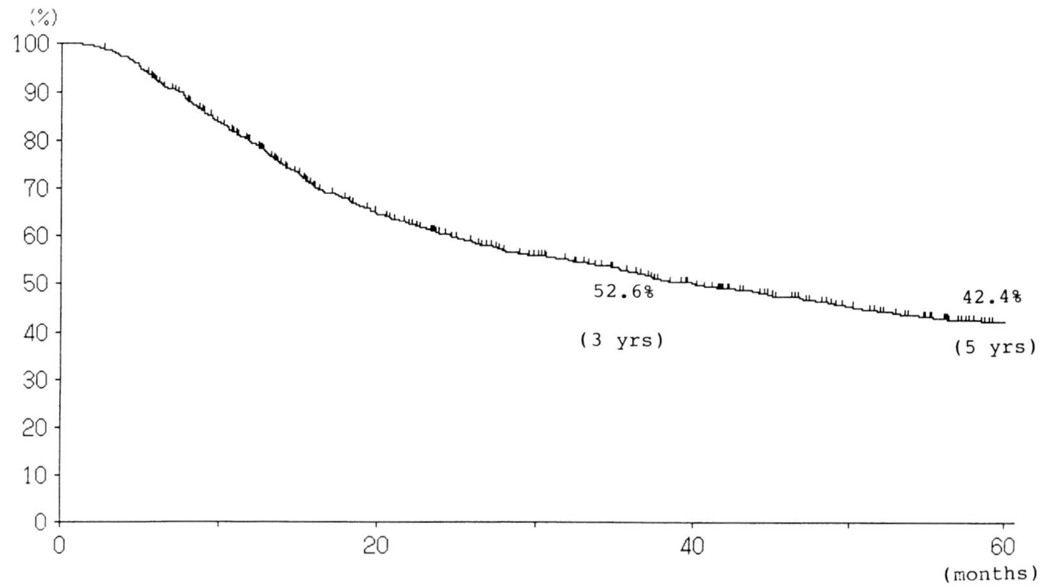

FIG. 18-9. Overall survival after all types of resection.

of mucosal cancers, the 5-year survival rates after less extensive and extensive dissections were 37.1% and 52.2%, respectively. The results are significantly better in the radical lymphadenectomy group. Long-term results after all resections, including those undergoing curative and palliative resection, and esophagectomy without thoracotomy, but excluding patients with endoscopic local mucosal resections and cases with operative and hospital deaths, are shown in Figure 18-9. The 3- and 5-year survival rates were 52.6% and 42.4%, respectively.

NEOADJUVANT TREATMENT

The use of adjuvant therapy for this disease has attracted increasing attention, since the introduction of cis-diaminedichloroplatinum (CDDP) and new types of combination chemotherapy.[22] The most common combination was two courses of CDDP and 5-fluorouracil, in which the CDDP dose was 100 mg/m^2 and the 5-fluorouracil dose was 1000 mg/m^2 on days 1 to 4. Adjuvant radiation therapy consisted of a total dose of 40 Gy of linear accelerator irradiation delivered in 20 fractions over 4 weeks. The Japanese n-factor and a-factor status of the patients was also investigated to clarify differences of background that are not considered so meticulously by TNM staging. The most uniform subgroup of patients, the pTNM stage IV-N patients, showed the clearest differences in survival between the different types of adjuvant therapy. Among the patients in pTNM stage IV-N, those given chemotherapy survived significantly longer than those who received no adjuvant therapy (Fig. 18-10).

Surgery is no more than a form of local therapy, like radiation therapy, and it is not by itself a sufficient treatment for disease that has spread beyond a certain region. It seems logical that the

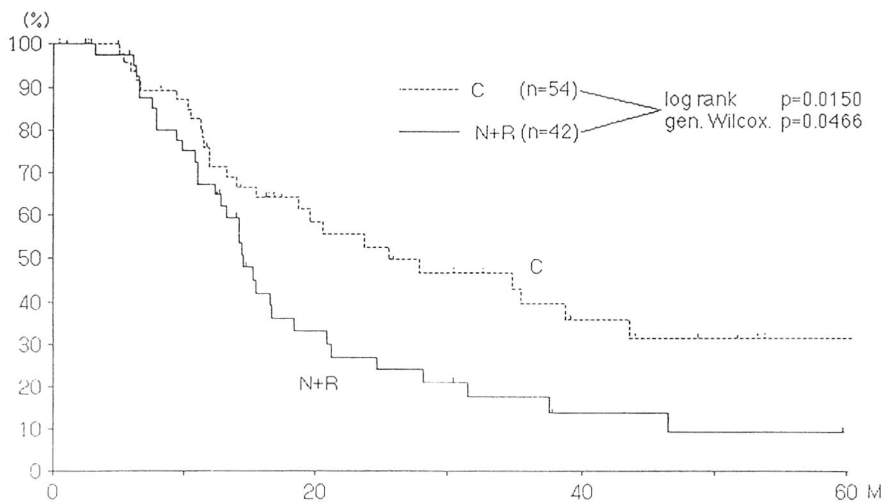

FIG. 18-10. Survival curves for pTNM IV-N patients with and without adjuvant chemotherapy. *C*, adjuvant chemotherapy; *N+R*, no adjuvant chemotherapy, but adjuvant radiation therapy.

combination of surgery and systemic adjuvant therapy should be more effective than the combination of surgery and another local treatment (eg, radiation therapy), although the latter regimen would be more effective for the local control of disease.

REFERENCES

1. Akiyama H. Surgery for cancer of the esophagus. Baltimore: Williams & Wilkins, 1990.
2. Endo M, Takeshita K, Yoshida M. How we can diagnose the early stage of esophageal cancer: endoscopic diagnosis. Endoscopy 1986; 18(Suppl 3):11.
3. Ide H, Nogami A, Hanashi T, et al. A clinical study on prognosis of submucosal esophageal cancer. Stomach and Intestine 1990;25:1067.
4. Shirakabe H, Yamaki G, Fukuchi S, et al. Discussion on what to do for clinical classification of early esophageal carcinoma. Stomach and Intestine 1990;25:1087.
5. Udagawa H, Watanabe G, Tsurumaru M, et al. Significance of ultrasound as preoperative examination for esophageal carcinoma. In: Wagai T, Fukuda M, eds. Ultrasound in medicine and biology. Amsterdam, New York, Oxford: Excerpta Medica 1988:167.
6. Akiyama H. Esophageal cancer: toward improved results. Komei Nakayama Prize. Tokyo: Nakayama Institute of Cancer Research, 1992.
7. Japanese Society for Esophageal Diseases. Guidelines for the clinical and pathologic studies on carcinoma of the esophagus. 8th ed. Tokyo: Kanehara & Co., Ltd., 1992.
8. Akiyama H, Kogure T, Itai Y. The esophageal axis and its relationship to the resectability of carcinoma of the esophagus. Ann Surg 1972; 176:30.
9. Inokuchi K. Milestones along the road to improvement of results in the treatment of squamous cell carcinoma of the esophagus. In: Sato T, Iizuka T, eds. Color atlas of surgical anatomy for esophageal cancer. Tokyo, Berlin: Springer-Verlag, 1992:1.
10. Akiyama H, Tsurumaru M, Ono Y, et al. Background of lymph node dissection for squamous cell carcinoma of the esophagus. In: Sato T, Iizuka T, eds. Color atlas of surgical anatomy for esophageal cancer. Tokyo, Berlin: Springer-Verlag, 1992:9.
11. International Union Against Cancer, Committee on TNM Classification. TNM classification of malignant tumors. 4th ed. Berlin: Springer-Verlag, 1987:40.
12. Iizuka T. The fourth edition of the UICC TNM classification of esophageal carcinoma and its relevance for comparison of international data. In: Sato T, Iizuka T, eds. Color atlas of surgical anatomy for esophageal cancer. Tokyo, Berlin: Springer-Verlag, 1992:117.
13. Akiyama H, Tsurumaru M, Udagawa H, Kajiyama Y. Systematic lymph node dissection for esophageal cancer-effective or not? Diseases of the Esophagus 1994;7:2.
14. Akiyama H, Tsurumaru M, Udagawa H, Kajiyama Y. Radical lymph node dissection for cancer of the thoracic esophagus. Ann Surg 1994; 220:364.
15. Tsurumaru M, Akiyama H, Udagawa H, Ono Y, et al. Cervical-thoracic-abdominal lymph node dissection for intrathoracic esophageal carcinoma. In: Diseases of the esophagus, vol 1. Malignant disease. Mount Kisco, NY: Futura, 1990:187.
16. Makuuchi H, Machimura T, Mizutani G, et al. Endoscopic mucosal resection for early carcinomas of the esophagus. UICC Kyoto International Symposium, March, 1993.
17. Denk W. Zur Radikaloperation des Oesophaguskarzinomas. Zentralbl Chir 1913;40:1065.
18. Akiyama H, Hiyama M, Miyazono H. Total esophageal reconstruction after extraction of the esophagus. Ann Surg 1975;182:547.
19. LeQuesne LP, Ranger D. Pharyngolaryngectomy with immediate pharyngogastric anastomosis. Br J Surg 1966;53:105.
20. Kirk RM. Palliative resection of oesophageal carcinoma without formal thoracotomy. Br J Surg 1974;61:689.
21. Orringer MB. Transhiatal esophagectomy without thoracotomy for carcinoma of the thoracic esophagus. Ann Surg 1984;200:282.
22. Akiyama H, Tsurumaru M, Kawamura T, et al. Principles of surgical treatment for carcinoma of the esophagus. Ann Surg 1981;194:438.

Surgery for Gastrointestinal Cancer: A Multidisciplinary Approach, edited by Harold J. Wanebo.
Lippincott-Raven Publishers, Philadelphia, © 1997.

CHAPTER 19

Radiation Therapy in the Treatment of Esophageal and Gastric Cancer

Bruce D. Minsky and Theodore L. Phillips

ESOPHAGEAL CANCER

There are a number of approaches to the use of radiation therapy in the treatment of esophageal cancer. These include radiation therapy in the adjuvant setting (preoperative or postoperative) or as a primary treatment modality (alone or in conjunction with chemotherapy). In general, the results of external beam radiation therapy alone in the treatment of esophageal cancer have been as discouraging as those with surgery. Depending on the series, the median survival is usually less than 1 year, and 5-year survival rates range from 2% to 20%.

Although the overall results of surgery and radiation therapy are similar, the patient population selected for treatment with each modality is quite different. First, patients with poor prognoses are commonly selected for treatment with radiation therapy. These include patients who are not surgical candidates because of medical contraindications or locally advanced or metastatic disease. Second, nonoperative series report results based on clinically staged patients, whereas surgical series report results based on pathologically staged patients. Pathologic staging has the advantage of excluding some patients with metastatic disease. Third, because many patients treated with radiation therapy alone are approached in a palliative rather than potentially curative fashion, the doses and techniques of radiation therapy are commonly suboptimal. Despite these adverse selection factors, the use of radiation therapy does offer a defined cure rate as well as significant impact on the palliation of dysphagia.

Much of the discussion in this chapter focuses on the results of randomized trials. In settings in which randomized trials are not available, selected nonrandomized trials are discussed.

Bruce D. Minsky, Associate Professor of Radiation Oncology, Cornell University Medical College, Memorial Sloan Kettering Cancer Center, 1275 York Avenue, New York, NY 10021.

Theodore L. Phillips, Professor and Chairman, University of California, San Francisco, 1855 Folsom Street, San Francisco, CA 94103.

Primary Radiation Therapy Alone

External Beam

Many series have reported results of external beam radiation therapy alone for esophageal carcinoma. Most series include patients with unfavorable features such as clinical T4 lesions, positive lymph nodes, and unresectable disease. For example, in the series by De-Ren, 184 of the 678 patients had stage IV disease.[1]

The use of radiation therapy in the potentially curative setting requires doses of at least 50 Gy at 1.8 to 2.0 Gy/fraction. Given the large size of many unresectable esophageal cancers, doses in the range of 60 Gy or greater are probably required. The results of selected series of radiation therapy alone are seen in Table 19-1.[1–3] Overall, the 5-year survival for patients with carcinoma of the esophagus treated with radiation therapy alone is approximately 10%.

External Beam Plus Intraluminal Brachytherapy

Intraluminal brachytherapy has been used in a variety of settings for esophageal cancer.[4] It can be delivered by high-dose or low-dose rate.[5] Although there are technical differences between the two dose rates, there are no clear therapeutic advantages. Briefly, a radioactive source is placed intraluminally by bronchoscopy or a nasogastric tube.

The major limitation of brachytherapy is the effective treatment distance. The primary isotope is ^{192}Ir, which can effectively treat to a distance of 1 cm from the source. Therefore, if any portion of the tumor is more than 1 cm away, it will receive a suboptimal radiation dose.

In the curative setting, the best approach is to add brachytherapy as a boost (10 to 20 Gy) after external beam radiation (50 to 60 Gy). The limited nonrandomized data suggest that outcome may be improved when brachytherapy is added to external beam. This approach is being prospectively examined by the Radiation Therapy Oncology Group (RTOG 92-07). In the pal-

TABLE 19-1. *Radiation therapy alone for esophageal carcinoma: selected trials*

Series	Histology	Clinical stage	Total number	5-Year survival (%)
De-Ren[1]	Various	II	177	22
		III	501	28
		<5 cm	59	25
		5 cm	115	25
		>5 cm	504	6
		Total*	678	8
Newaishy, et al[2]	Squamous	"Inoperable"	444	9
Okawa, et al[3]	Squamous	T1	47	18
		T2	147	10
		T3	94	3
		Total	288	9
		I	43	20
		II	130	10
		III	92	3
		IV	23	0

* Includes 184 patients with stage IV disease.

liative setting, it is used to improve swallowing. The effectiveness of intraluminal brachytherapy in this setting is controversial.

Adjuvant Radiation Therapy

Rationale

The rationale for adjuvant therapy in clinically resectable esophageal cancer is based on the patterns of failure after potentially curative surgery. Unfortunately, few surgical series report patterns of failure data. The incidences of local–regional failure in the surgical control arms of the preoperative radiation therapy randomized trials conducted by Mei and colleagues[6] and Gignoux and associates[7] were 12% and 67%, respectively. The local–regional failure rate in the surgical control arm from the postoperative radiation therapy randomized trial by Teniere and colleagues[8] was 35% for patients with negative local–regional lymph nodes and 38% for patients with positive local–regional lymph nodes. Therefore, although most patients with esophageal cancer die of distant metastases, the incidence of local–regional failure after surgery alone in patients with clinically resectable disease is high enough to support the use of adjuvant radiation therapy.

Preoperative Radiation Therapy

Rationale

Theoretic advantages of preoperative radiation therapy in the treatment of esophageal cancer include biologic (decreased tumor seeding and increased radiosensitivity due to more oxygenated cells), physical (increased resectability), and dosimetric (patients who undergo a gastric pull-up or intestinal interposition are not limited to the postoperative dose of 45 to 50 cGy) factors.

Results

There are six randomized trials of preoperative radiation therapy for esophageal cancer[6,7,9–12] (Table 19-2). The series by Launois and colleagues,[9] Gignoux and coworkers,[7] and Nygaard and colleagues[12] are limited to patients with squamous cell carcinoma. Patients with both squamous cell carcinoma and adenocarcinoma are included in the series by Arnott and associates.[10] The series by Huang and colleagues[11] and Mei and coworkers[6] do not mention histologic type.

Overall, there were no differences in resectability rates between patients who underwent preoperative radiation therapy compared with surgery alone. Local–regional failure rates were reported in only two of the six series. Mei and colleagues[6] reported no difference in local–regional failure; however, Gignoux and associates[7] reported a significant decrease in local–regional failure (46% vs. 67%) in patients who received preoperative radiation therapy compared with surgery alone.

Two of the six series reported an improvement in survival with preoperative radiation therapy. The series from Nygaard and associates was a four-arm trial in which patients were randomized preoperatively to chemotherapy (two cycles of cis-

TABLE 19-2. *Preoperative radiation therapy for esophageal carcinoma: randomized trials*

Series	Histology	Total number	Total dose (cGy)	Fraction size (cGy)	Resectable (%)		Local failure (%)		5-Year survival (%)	
					Surgery	RT	Surgery	RT	Surgery	RT
Mei, et al[6]	NA	206	4000	NA	85	93	12	13	30	35
Gignoux, et al[7]	Squamous	229	3300	330	58	47	67	46*	8	10
Launois, et al[9]	Squamous	109	4000	NA	70	76	NA	NA	10	10
Arnott, et al[10]	Squamous and adenocarcinoma	176	2000	200	NA	NA	NA	NA	17	9
Huang, et al[11]	NA	160	4000	200	90	92	NA	NA	25	46‡
Nygaard, et al[12]	Squamous	186	3500†	175	NA	NA	NA	NA	5	18 (3-y)*

* $P = 0.009$.
† With or without chemotherapy.
‡ Statistical analysis not performed.
NA, not available; *RT*, radiation therapy.

platin/bleomycin), radiation therapy, combined modality therapy, or surgery alone.[12] Patients who received preoperative radiation therapy (with or without chemotherapy) had a significant improvement in overall 3-year survival (18% versus 5%, $P = 0.009$). The 48 patients who received preoperative radiation therapy alone had a 20% 3-year survival, although this did not reach statistical significance. A similar improvement in survival was reported by Huang and coworkers (46% versus 25%).[11] However, a statistical analysis was not performed.

There are many criticisms of the preoperative randomized trials. For example, none used conventional doses of radiation therapy, and none allowed an adequate radiation therapy–surgery interval (4 to 5 weeks). As is discussed later, these unconventional techniques preclude an accurate assessment of radiation-related morbidity.

In summary, because only two of the six series reported local–regional failure rates, it is difficult to draw firm conclusions regarding the influence of preoperative radiation therapy on the incidence of local–regional failure. Regarding the impact on survival, two series report an improvement (one in which 50% of the patients received chemotherapy). However, four of the six series report no advantage in overall survival. Nonrandomized trials conducted by Yadava and colleagues[13] and Sugimachi and associates[14] also report no survival benefit. Based on the available randomized, albeit poorly designed, trials, adjuvant preoperative radiation therapy does not appear to decrease local–regional failure or improve survival.

Postoperative Radiation Therapy

Rationale

The primary advantage of adjuvant postoperative radiation therapy is more accurate case selection. Patients with pathologic T1–2N0M0 disease and those with metastatic disease can be excluded from treatment. The major disadvantage is dosimetric, because patients who undergo a gastric pull-up or intestinal interposition are limited to 45 to 50 Gy.

Results

There are many encouraging nonrandomized reports of postoperative radiation therapy in the treatment of esophageal cancer. For example, Kasai and colleagues report an 88% 5-year survival in node-negative patients who received postoperative radiation therapy.[15] There are only two randomized trials of postoperative radiation therapy (Table 19-3). The discussion is limited to patients treated in the adjuvant setting (complete resection and negative margins with or without local–regional lymph nodes).

Teniere and colleagues[8] reported results of 221 patients with squamous cell carcinoma randomized to surgery alone versus postoperative radiation therapy (45 to 55 Gy at 1.8 Gy/fraction). The minimum follow-up was 3 years. For the total patient group, the addition of postoperative radiation therapy had no significant impact on survival.

The series by Fok and associates[16] included patients with both squamous cell carcinoma and adenocarcinoma. It should be emphasized that patients with both curative and palliative resections were included in this series. Although the total dose of radiation therapy was conventional, the dose per fraction (3.5 Gy/fraction) was unconventional. There was no significant improvement in median survival, local failure, or distant failure with the addition of postoperative radiation therapy.

Postoperative radiation therapy is commonly recommended for patients with positive local–regional lymph nodes. Although the data from Teniere and colleagues[8] support the use of postoperative radiation therapy for local–regional control, the benefit was limited to patients with negative lymph nodes (postoperative radiation therapy, 10% local failure; vs. surgery alone, 35% local failure). There was no significant benefit for patients with positive nodes.

In summary, although adjuvant postoperative radiation therapy may decrease local–regional failure in node-negative patients, it has no impact on overall survival.

Preoperative Plus Postoperative Versus Postoperative Radiation Therapy

An alternative approach to adjuvant therapy is preoperative plus postoperative radiation therapy. Iizuka and associates[17] compared this approach to patients who received postoperative radiation therapy alone. There was no surgical control arm. In their trial, 364 patients with histologically diverse tumors were randomized to preoperative plus postoperative radiation therapy (30 Gy followed by surgery followed by postoperative radiation therapy up to 54 Gy) versus postoperative radiation therapy alone (50 Gy). Limiting the analysis to the 207 eligible patients, there was a significant improvement in 4-year survival (33% versus 20%) as well as median survival (22 months versus 13 months) in patients who received postoperative radiation therapy compared with preoperative plus postoperative radiation

TABLE 19-3. *Postoperative radiation therapy for esophageal carcinoma: randomized trials*

Series	Number	Local failure (%) LN+	LN−	Overall	Distant failure (%)	Median disease-free survival	Overall survival (%)	
Teniere, et al[8]								
Radiation	119	30	10*	NA	NA	NA	85	19
Surgery	102	38	35	NA	NA	NA	70	19
Fok, et al[16]								
Radiation	30	NA	NA	10	40	15 mo	NA	NA
Surgery	30	NA	NA	13	30	21 mo	NA	NA

* Statistically significant.
LN+, lymph node positive; *LN−*, lymph node negative; *NA*, not available.

therapy. The major criticisms of this trial are that only 207 of 364 randomized patients were eligible for analysis, and that a higher percentage of patients who received preoperative plus postoperative radiation therapy had primary tumors greater than 7 cm in size (56% versus 39%).

Combined Modality Therapy for Esophageal Cancer

Given the limited success of radiation therapy when used as either a single modality or in the adjuvant setting (preoperative or postoperative), a number of investigators have explored the use of systemic chemotherapy in conjunction with radiation therapy. There are good reasons for combining systemic chemotherapy with radiation therapy for the treatment of esophageal cancer. These include an objective response rate of 40% to 60% in patients with metastatic disease, the observation that most patients with esophageal cancer die of distant metastasis, and some of the active chemotherapeutic agents in esophageal cancer (ie, 5-fluorouracil [5-FU], cisplatin, mitomycin C) are radiation sensitizers.

In a randomized trial from Memorial Sloan-Kettering Cancer Center, 96 patients with clinically resectable squamous cell carcinoma of the esophagus were randomized to either preoperative radiation therapy (55 Gy) or preoperative chemotherapy (5-FU and cisplatin).[18] There were no significant differences in the resectability rates, overall objective response rates, and local failure rates between the two preoperative therapies. Because there was a postoperative cross-over, it was not possible to compare the survival rates. The overall survival for both arms was 20% at 5 years, and the median survival was 10 to 12 months. Based on this trial, the Intergroup trial, Eastern Cooperative Oncology Group (ECOG) PE-289/RTOG 91-12, of neoadjuvant chemotherapy followed by concurrent chemotherapy and radiation therapy was designed.

Preoperative Combined Modality Therapy

In general, there are two approaches to preoperative combined modality therapy. Patients either have a planned operation (Table 19-4) or, for a variety of reasons, are selected to undergo an operation (Table 19-5). It is important to analyze the data from these two approaches separately because the selection factors for surgery may have an impact on the results.

There is one randomized trial of preoperative combined modality therapy versus surgery alone.[19] The combined modality segment was sequential rather than concurrent. Patients first received 5-FU/cisplatin followed by 20 Gy in 10 fractions, followed by additional 5-FU/cisplatin. A total of 86 patients with squamous cell carcinoma of the esophagus were randomized. There was no difference in survival (47% at 1 year). Because the preoperative combined modality therapy was not concurrent, the dose of radiation was not conventional, and the follow-up was short, these data should be interpreted with caution.

The results of selected nonrandomized series in which patients undergo planned preoperative combined modality therapy followed by a planned operation are presented in Table 19-5. Initial studies from Leichman and colleagues from Wayne State University report the results of 21 patients with squamous cell carcinoma.[20] Patients received 30 Gy at 2.0 Gy/fraction with two cycles of concurrent 5-FU and cisplatin. If there was residual tumor in the specimen, patients received an additional 20 Gy after surgery. Of the 21, 19 underwent an operation. The pathologic complete response rate was 37% and the median survival was 18 months. The operative mortality was 27%. In addition to the substantial mortality, 48% of patients required hyperalimentation during the preoperative therapy.

Although the morbidity and mortality rates were high, the complete response rates were encouraging, and this pilot trial was expanded to a Southwest Oncology Group trial (SWOG 80-37). The results were reported by Poplin and coworkers in 1987.[21] A total of 113 patients with squamous cell carcinoma underwent the preoperative therapy designed by Leichman and associates. Of the 113, only 71 underwent surgery. The pathologic complete response rate was 16% and the operative mortality was 11%. Despite a 3-year actuarial survival rate of 16%, all patients were dead of disease by 4 years.

At the University of Michigan, two separate series have been reported. Urba and colleagues reported the results of 24 patients with adenocarcinoma of the esophagus who underwent preoper-

TABLE 19-4. *Planned preoperative combined modality therapy for esophageal carcinoma: selected trials*

Series	Number	Histology	Number undergoing surgery	Operative mortality (%)	Pathologic complete response (%)	Survival
Le Prise, et al[19]	39	Squamous	35	11	9	47% 1-y
Leichman, et al[20] (Wayne State)	21	Squamous	19	27	37	18 mo (median)
Poplin, et al[21] (Southwest Oncology Group)	113	Squamous	71	11	16	12 mo (median) 16% 3-y (All dead of disease at 4 y)
Urba, et al[22] (Michigan)	24	Adenocarcinoma	19	16	10	11 mo (median)
Forastiere, et al[23,24] (Michigan)	43	Squamous and adenocarcinoma	39	2	27	29 mo (median) 46% 3-y
Naunheim, et al[25]	47	Squamous and adenocarcinoma	39	5	21	23 mo (median) 40% 3-y
Stewart, et al[26]	24	Adenocarcinoma	23	0	25	76% 2-y

TABLE 19-5. *Preoperative combined modality therapy with or without surgery for esophageal carcinoma: selected nonrandomized trials*

Series	Number	Failure (%)		Median survival (mo)		
		Local	Distant	Adenocarcinoma	Squamous	All
Gill, et al[27]						
Surgery	46	25	36	14	36	NA
No surgery	36	17	12	15	26	NA
Kavanagh, et al[28]*						
Surgery	72	24	39	NA	NA	9†
No surgery	71	44	38	NA	NA	15‡

* Results limited to the 103 of 143 patients who had no clinical evidence of metastatic disease at the time of preoperative assessment.
† All dead of disease by 5 years.
‡ All dead of disease by 3.5 years.
NA, not available.

ative continuous-infusion 5-FU and concurrent radiation therapy followed by a transhiatal esophagectomy.[22] Although patients received 49 Gy, it was delivered at 3.5 Gy/fraction. The pathologic complete response rate was 11% and the median survival was only 11 months. The operative mortality was 16%. The large radiation fraction sizes may have contributed to the morbidity and mortality reported in this series.

In a separate series from the University of Michigan, Forastiere and colleagues reported a group of 39 patients with both squamous cell cancer and adenocarcinoma who received preoperative 5-FU, vinblastine, cisplatin, and concurrent radiation therapy.[23,24] Radiation therapy was delivered with either large fractions (2.5 Gy) or with hyperfractionation (150 cGy twice daily). Patients received the therapy on an inpatient basis for 21 days. After the preoperative therapy, a transhiatal esophagectomy was performed. The pathologic complete response rate was 27%, the 3-year actuarial survival rate was 46%, and the operative mortality was only 2%. A randomized trial of this approach is being performed at the University of Michigan.

It is unclear whether the addition of surgery after combined modality therapy is of benefit (see Table 19-5). In a nonrandomized trial by Gill and associates, patients received two cycles of 5-FU, cisplatin, and radiation therapy.[27] Patients who were either treated palliatively or were medically inoperable were excluded from surgery. Therefore, the patients with better prognoses were selected for surgery. Although the differences were not statistically significant, the local failure and distant failure rates were higher in the patients who underwent surgery compared with those who did not undergo surgery.

A similar trial was reported by Kavanagh and associates.[28] Patients received 44 to 46 Gy plus chemotherapy with either etoposide, 5-FU, cisplatin, or carboplatin. After reevaluation, those who were potentially operable underwent surgery and, if they had positive margins, received postoperative radiation therapy. Patients who were either medically or technically inoperable also received additional radiation therapy, to a total dose of 60 to 64 Gy. The patients who underwent surgery had a lower local failure rate (44% vs. 24%), but there was no difference in distant failure or median survival. However, regardless of the type of treatment, all patients were dead of disease within 3.5 to 5 years.

Radiation Therapy Alone Versus Combined Modality Therapy

There are four randomized trials comparing radiation therapy alone with combined modality therapy[12,29–31] (Table 19-6). Unfortunately, in three of the four trials, inadequate doses of systemic chemotherapy were delivered. For example, in the small trial from Araujo and colleagues,[29] patients received only one cycle of 5-FU, mitomycin-C, and bleomycin. In the European Organization for Research and Treatment of Cancer trial reported by Roussel and associates, subcutaneous methotrexate was used.[31] In the Scandinavian trial reported by Nygaard and coworkers, patients received inadequate doses of chemotherapy (cisplatin 20 mg/m^2 and bleomycin 10 mg/m^2, for a maximum of two cycles).[12]

The only trial that was designed to deliver adequate doses of systemic chemotherapy with concurrent radiation therapy was reported by Herskovic and colleagues, from RTOG (RTOG 85-01).[30] In this trial, patients received four cycles of 5-FU (1000 mg/m^2 $\times$ 4 days) and cisplatin (75 mg/m^2, day 1). Radiation therapy (50 Gy) was given concurrently with chemotherapy beginning on day 1. A higher dose of radiation (64 Gy) was used in the radiation therapy control arm. At 2 years, patients who received combined modality therapy had a significant improvement in survival (38% versus 10%) as well as a significant decrease in local failure (44% versus 65%) and distant failure (12% versus 26%). With longer follow-up, the 3-year actuarial survival of patients who received combined modality therapy was 31%. There were no 3-year survivors in the radiation therapy control arm.[32]

A similar randomized trial of radiation therapy alone versus combined modality therapy (EST-1282) was performed by ECOG.[33] However, because patients had the option of surgery after 40 Gy, the results are more difficult to interpret. An interim analysis revealed a significant improvement in median survival (14.9 months versus 9 months) in patients who received combined modality therapy. Final results of this trial are pending.

Based on the positive results from the RTOG 85-01 trial, the conventional nonoperative treatment for esophageal carcinoma, in the United States, is combined modality therapy rather than radiation therapy alone. An Intergroup trial (ECOG PE-289/ RTOG 91-12) was activated to determine if there is an advan-

TABLE 19-6. *Randomized trials of radiation therapy versus combined modality therapy for esophageal cancer*

Series	Number	Complete response (%)	Survival (%)	Failure (%) Local	Failure (%) Distant
Nygaard, et al (Scandinavia)[12]					
Radiation therapy	51	NA	6 (3-y)	NA	NA
Combined modality	46	NA	0	NA	NA
Araujo, et al (National Cancer Institute Brazil)[29]					
Radiation therapy	31	58	6 (5-y)	84	23
Combined modality	28	75	16	61	32
Herskovic, et al (Radiation Therapy Oncology Group)[30]					
Radiation therapy	60	NA	10 (2-y)*	65	26
Combined modality	61	NA	38	44*	12*
Roussel, et al (European Organization for Research and Treatment of Cancer)[31]					
Radiation therapy	69	NA	6 (3-y)	NA	NA
Combined modality	75	NA	12	NA	NA

* Statistically significant.
NA, not available.

tage with neoadjuvant chemotherapy as well as higher doses of radiation therapy. In this phase II trial, patients with squamous cell carcinoma received three cycles of neoadjuvant 5-FU and cisplatin followed by two additional cycles of 5-FU and cisplatin and concurrent radiation therapy (64.8 Gy). Results are pending at this time. The replacement phase III Intergroup trial (RTOG 9405) will test whether intensification of the radiation dose from 50 to 64.8 Gy in the combined modality arm of RTOG 8501 is of benefit.

There are a number of single-arm trials of combined modality therapy alone for esophageal cancer[34–37] (Table 19-7). The trial reported by Coia and associates is the only combined modality therapy trial in which patients with clinical early-stage esophageal cancer (stages I and II) were treated and analyzed separately.[35] Patients received 5-FU, mitomycin C, and 60 Gy. Combining clinical stages I and II, the local failure rate was 25%, the 5-year actuarial survival rate was 30%, and the 5-year actuarial local relapse-free survival rate was 70%.

Similar to the other cancer therapies, combined modality therapy is associated with acute toxicity. In a separate toxicity analysis from Coia and associates, an additional 33 patients with stage III and IV disease were included.[35] For the total group of 90 patients, the incidence of grade III toxicity was 22% and that of grade IV toxicity was 6%. There was no treatment-related mortality. A similar increase in toxicity was noted in the RTOG 85-01 trial. Compared with radiation therapy alone, the use of combined modality therapy was associated with a higher incidence of grade III toxicity (44% versus 25%) and grade IV toxicity (20% versus 3%). There was one treatment-related death in the combined modality arm.

Adenocarcinoma Versus Squamous Cell Carcinoma

Given the increasing incidence of adenocarcinoma of the esophagus compared with squamous cell carcinoma, treatment results need to be examined with regard to histologic type. In the series by Coia and associates,[35] patients with adenocarcinoma had improved survival compared with squamous cell carcinoma. In contrast, Gill and colleagues[27] and Forastiere and colleagues[23,24] reported that patients with squamous cell carcinoma had an improved survival compared with adenocarci-

TABLE 19-7. *Combined modality therapy alone for esophageal cancer: selected trials*

Series	Stage	Number	Histology	Local failure (%)	Actuarial survival (%) Overall	Actuarial survival (%) Local relapse free
John, et al[34]	I–III	30	Squamous and adenocarcinoma	27	29 (2-y)	NA
Coia, et al[35]	I	13	Both	26	73 (5-y)	100 (5-y)
	II	44	Both	45	20	59
	All	16	Adenocarcinoma	NA	38	71
	All	39	Squamous	NA	27	58
	Total	57	Both	25	30	70
Izquierdo, et al[36]	"Unresectable"	25	Squamous	NA	8 (4-y) 8 mo (median)	NA
Seitz, et al[37]	I–III	35	Squamous	NA	21 (2-y)	NA

NA, not available.

noma. Naunheim and associates reported no survival difference with different histologic types.[25] Until randomized trials are performed in which patients are stratified, the impact of histologic type cannot be adequately assessed.

Morbidity of Radiation Therapy

The morbidity of radiation therapy is a function of dose, technique, and whether the patient received chemotherapy or underwent surgery. There are limited toxicity data in patients who received radiation therapy in the adjuvant setting. The preoperative adjuvant radiation therapy trials used unconventional radiation doses and techniques, thereby making the data difficult to interpret.

The best-documented acute radiation-related morbidity data are from the control arm of RTOG 85-01.[30,32] In this arm, 60 patients received radiation therapy alone, to a dose of 64 Gy. The incidence of acute grade III toxicity was 25% and grade IV toxicity was 3%. There were no treatment-related deaths.

Likewise, there are few reports of long-term radiation-related morbidity. In general, patients who received radiation therapy alone have a 30% to 60% incidence of esophageal stricture. However, almost half of the strictures are associated with a local recurrence. The incidence of grade III + pneumonitis or pericarditis is 5%. If appropriate radiation techniques are used, spinal cord myelitis should not occur.

Conclusions and Recommendations

Because of selection bias, it is difficult to determine what the best treatment is for esophageal cancer. Although there are design flaws in all of the trials of adjuvant radiation therapy for esophageal cancer, there is no clear survival advantage when radiation therapy is delivered in the adjuvant setting (preoperative or postoperative). Preoperative plus postoperative radiation therapy does not appear to have an advantage compared with postoperative radiotherapy alone. When radiation therapy is used as a primary modality, the most favorable results are seen when it is combined with adequate doses of systemic chemotherapy. National trials are in progress that are examining the effectiveness of neoadjuvant chemotherapy and higher doses of radiation therapy (ECOG PE-289/RTOG 91-12 and RTOG 94-05), as well as the role of surgery after combined modality therapy.

GASTRIC CANCER

Radiation therapy has been used as both an adjuvant and as a primary modality in the treatment of gastric cancer. The adjuvant setting is limited to patients in whom a potentially curative operation has been performed. Radiation as a primary therapy has been used in patients after an incomplete (noncurative) resection. This section examines the results of radiation therapy with or without chemotherapy in the treatment of adenocarcinoma of the stomach. Other histologic types such as sarcomas and lymphomas are discussed in other chapters.

Radiation Therapy in the Adjuvant Setting

Rationale

The rationale for radiation therapy in the adjuvant setting is based on patterns of failure after potentially curative surgery. These failure patterns have been examined both by clinical methods[38] and in a reoperation series from the University of Minnesota.[39]

As with other gastrointestinal malignancies, the incidence of local–regional failure increases with increasing penetration of the tumor through the muscle wall as well as with the presence of lymph node metastasis. Depending on the method used for analysis, the incidence of local failure as a component of failure after potentially curative surgery varies from 38% to 67% (Table 19-8). The clinical method of assessing failure relies on physical examination, radiography, and, in some patients, the operative findings. In contrast, the reoperation method uses a planned second-look operation at least every 6 months. This method offers the most accurate appraisal of the anatomic distribution of failure. The failure sites documented in the reoperation series from the University of Minnesota as well as superimposed radiation fields covering these failure sites are shown in Figure 19-1. Even in patients in whom a complete resection is performed, local–regional failure is a significant problem. Therefore, it is reasonable to investigate the use of adjuvant radiation therapy.

Results

There are few data examining the role of postoperative radiation therapy with or without chemotherapy after a "curative"

TABLE 19-8. *Patterns of failure after potentially curative surgery in gastric cancer*

	Cumulative incidence of failure (%)*	
	Clinical[38]	Reoperation[39]
FAILURE SITE		
Total local–regional	38	67
Gastric bed	21	54
Abdominal scar		5
Anastomosis	25	26
Nodes	8	42
Peritoneal seeding	23	41
Local		19
Diffuse		22
Distant	52	22
LOCAL FAILURE BY TNM STAGE		
T1N0	0	
T1–2N0	19	
T3N0	50	
T4N0	40	
T1–2N1–2	24	
T3N1–2	36	
T4N1–2	56	

* Local failure as a component of failure.

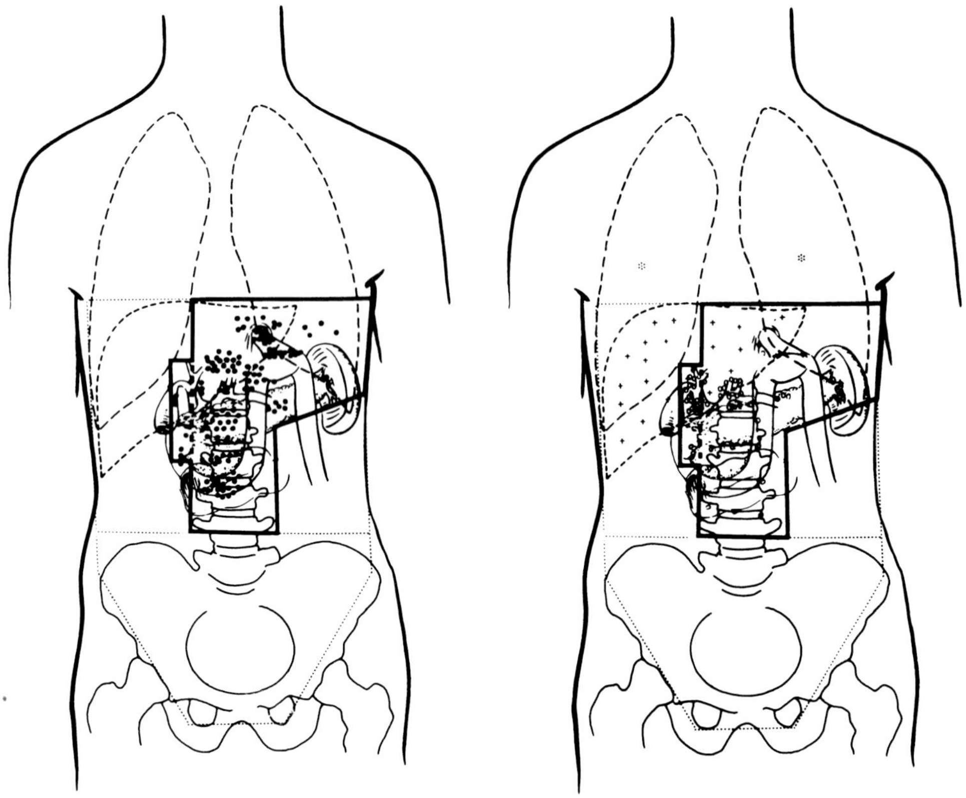

FIG. 19-1. Patterns of failure in 82 evaluable patients in the University of Minnesota reoperation series for gastric cancer. The superimposed radiation fields cover the areas of lymph node drainage, gastric remnant anastomosis, duodenal stump, and gastric bed structures. (Modified from Gunderson LL, Sosin H. Adenocarcinoma of the stomach: areas of failure in a reoperation series (second or symptomatic looks). Clinicopathologic correlation and implications for adjuvant therapy. Int J Radiat Oncol Biol Phys 1982;8:1.)

resection. The only randomized data are a subset analysis of a randomized trial by Dent and colleagues[40] (Table 19-9). Virtually all of the other randomized as well as nonrandomized trials of postoperative radiation or radiation plus chemotherapy include patients with residual disease.

In the series from Dent and colleagues, 142 patients with a variety of stages of gastric cancer were randomized postoperatively to two separate treatment programs, depending on stage. ''Division I'' included patients without metastatic disease. Limiting the analysis to the 30 patients with local–regional disease who underwent a potentially curative resection, the combination of radiation plus chemotherapy had a negative impact on 2-year survival compared with surgery alone. This difference did not reach statistical significance.

Based on the high incidence of local–regional failure as well as the moderate response rate with the combination of radiation plus 5-FU-based chemotherapy in the advanced setting, a pilot study was performed at the Mayo Clinic/North Central Cancer Treatment Group in which patients with locally unresectable gastric cancer received 4500 cGy plus concurrent 5-FU and leucovorin. Based on these pilot data, a phase III Intergroup trial (INT 0116) has been activated. After a potentially curative resection of gastric cancer, patients are randomized to either observation alone or postoperative combined modality therapy consisting of 45 Gy and concurrent 5-FU/leucovorin. This Intergroup trial is one of the few in which 5-FU-based chemotherapy is delivered as a systemic therapy (monthly cycles).

Most trials of combined modality therapy did not use systemic levels of 5-FU-based chemotherapy. In general, 3 to 5 days of bolus 5-FU (350 to 500 mg/m^2 bolus) was delivered during the first and sometimes the last 3 days of the radiation therapy. It must be emphasized that with this schedule, 5-FU is designed as a radiation sensitizer rather than as a systemic therapy. Until the results of the Intergroup 0116 trial are available, the role of postoperative radiation therapy with or without chemotherapy in the adjuvant setting remains investigational. However, in selected cases in which treatment is recommended, given the in vitro and in vivo evidence of 5-FU radiosensitization of radiation,[46] most investigators would agree to add 5-FU-based chemotherapy to radiation.

Radiation Therapy After ''Noncurative'' Surgery

Randomized Trials

As discussed earlier, most trials examining the role of radiation therapy (with or without chemotherapy) in gastric cancer include patients who have not undergone potentially curative surgery. The seminal trial examining the role of postoperative combined modality therapy in gastric cancer was reported by Moertel and coworkers in 1969.[41] Patients with advanced gastric cancers were randomized to 40 Gy postoperatively or 40 Gy plus 5-FU as a radiation sensitizer. As seen in Table 19-9, there was a significant improvement in survival with the combination of radiation plus 5-FU. This improvement with combined modality therapy is consistent with the results obtained in other gastrointestinal sites, such as esophageal, rectal, and pancreatic cancer, in which the combination of radiation therapy plus concurrent chemotherapy is superior to radiation therapy alone.

TABLE 19-9. *External beam radiation therapy with or without chemotherapy for gastric cancer: selected randomized trials*

Series	% "Curative" resections (%)	Number	Treatment	Survival	Local failure (%)
Dent, et al[40]†	43	35	20 Gy chemotherapy	30% 2-y	
	48	31	Surgery	40% 2-y	
Subset analysis					
	100	15	20 Gy + chemotherapy	38% 2-y	
	100	15	Surgery	60% 2-y	
Moertel, et al[41]	0	25	35–40 Gy + chemotherapy	13 mo (mean)*	
			Surgery	6 mo (mean)*	
Schein, et al	0		50 Gy	6% 4-y*	
(GITSG 8274)[42]	0		50 Gy + chemotherapy	18% 4-y*	
GITSG[43]	0	50	Chemotherapy	11% 3-y	
	0	45	43.2 Gy + chemotherapy	7% 3-y	
Moertel, et al[44]	NA	23	Surgery	4% 5-y*	
	NA	39	37.5 Gy + chemotherapy	23% 5-y*	
Subset analysis					
		29	(Accepted Rx)	20% 5-y	39
		10	(Refused Rx)	30% 5-y	
		33	Either surgery or refused Rx		54
Allum, et al[45]	15	138	Chemotherapy	27% 5-y	12
		153	45–50 Gy	20% 5-y	8*
		145	Surgery	24% 5-y	22*

* Statistically significant difference.
† "Division I" only (T1–3N1–2M0).
GITSG, Gastrointestinal Tumor Study Group; *NA,* not available; *Rx,* treatment consisting of combined chemotherapy plus radiation.

The other randomized trials in Table 19-9 also include patients with unresectable or residual disease. Furthermore, none of the trials delivered adequate doses of radiation to control residual disease. In general, after a compete resection and negative margins, 45 to 50 Gy is recommended. Patients with residual disease require at least 60 Gy.

In the study from the British Stomach Cancer Group by Allum and colleagues,[45] there was a significant decrease in local recurrence in patients who received postoperative radiation therapy versus surgery alone (8% versus 22%). There was no improvement in survival with postoperative radiation. The chemotherapy, however, was not delivered concurrently with the radiation.

The Gastrointestinal Tumor Study Group (GITSG) performed two consecutive trials comparing combined radiation plus chemotherapy versus radiation alone in patients with locally unresectable gastric cancer. In the first GITSG study from Schein and colleagues, almost 25% of patients who received the combined modality therapy either died or deteriorated within the first 10 weeks.[42] However, with further follow-up, there was a significant improvement in 4-year survival (18% vs. 6%) with combined radiation plus chemotherapy compared with chemotherapy alone.

Because of the early high morbidity and mortality with this trial, the GITSG made four modifications to the protocol. In the replacement trial, patients received chemotherapy before receiving combined modality therapy, doxorubicin was added, a rigorous review of surgical entry criteria was performed, and radiation therapy was delivered as continuous rather than split course.[43] Patients were randomized to either postoperative chemotherapy alone (5-FU/methyl-lomustine/doxorubicin) versus combined modality therapy. The incidence of grade III + toxicity varied from 52% to 59%. In contrast with the first GITSG trial, there was no difference in survival.

In 1984, Moertel and coworkers reported the results of a subsequent randomized trial from the Mayo Clinic of postoperative radiation (37.5 Gy) plus 5-FU versus surgery alone.[44] Although there was a significant improvement in survival in those patients who received postoperative radiation plus chemotherapy versus surgery alone (23% versus 4%), this improvement may have been because of the 10 patients who were randomized to receive postoperative treatment and refused. The 5-year survival of those 10 patients who refused radiation plus chemotherapy was higher compared with the remaining 29 who were randomized to the treatment arm and accepted treatment (30% versus 20%). There was a decrease in local–regional failure in those who received postoperative combined modality therapy versus those who were randomized to surgery alone or refused postoperative combined modality treatment (39% versus 54%). These data illustrate the problems with interpretation of studies that allow prerandomization.

Nonrandomized Trials

The results of selected nonrandomized trials of postoperative radiation therapy with or without chemotherapy are given in Table 19-10. Despite the fact that only 50% to 75% of the patients underwent potentially curative surgery, the overall 4- to 5-year survival rates are approximately 25%.[47,48] Similar to the randomized trials, these trials also included patients with unresectable or residual disease.

TABLE 19-10. *External beam with or without chemotherapy for gastric cancer: selected nonrandomized trials*

Series	Curative resections (%)	Number	Treatment	Survival	Local failure (%)
Slot, et al[47]	74	57	30–50 Gy + chemotherapy	26% 5-y	21
Caudry, et al[48]	51	45	40–50 Gy ± chemotherapy	23% 4-y	NA

NA, not available.

In summary, the randomized data comparing postoperative radiation plus chemotherapy versus chemotherapy or surgery in patients with locally unresectable disease are conflicting. The conflicting results may be explained by suboptimal doses of chemotherapy and radiation, as well as by the selection of patients with poor prognoses and unresectable disease. As with radiation in the adjuvant setting, the use of postoperative radiation with or without chemotherapy in patients with locally unresectable disease remains investigational.

Intraoperative Radiation Therapy

An alternative method of delivering radiation therapy is intraoperative radiation. The theoretic benefit of this approach lies in the ability to deliver a more intensive dose of radiation to the tumor bed while excluding the surrounding normal tissues from the high-dose field. The results of selected trials of intraoperative radiation (with or without external beam) are given in Table 19-11. A small randomized trial was reported from the National Cancer Institute.[49] Patients with grossly resected stage III/IV disease were randomized to receive 20 Gy intraoperative electron beam versus 50 Gy postoperative external beam radiation. The mean time to local failure was significantly improved in the intraoperative radiation arm (21 vs. 8 months). The postoperative complication rate was lower (40% vs. 72%) and the median survival was higher (21 vs. 10 months) with intraoperative radiation. However, none of these differences reached statistical significance.

Takahashi and Abe randomized patients based on their day of hospital admission to surgery plus intraoperative radiation (28 to 35 Gy) versus surgery alone.[50,51] There was an improvement in survival with surgery plus intraoperative radiation, although it was limited to patients with stage III and IV disease. Although the results are impressive, the unusual randomization method and the failure to stratify patients by prognostic factors are problematic. Furthermore, the more extensive surgical staging and possibly earlier presentation of gastric cancer in Japan make it difficult to compare these with data from other countries.

In the phase II trial reported by Calvo and associates, patients received 15 Gy intraoperative radiation followed by 40 to 46 Gy external beam radiation after surgery.[52] 5-FU-based chemotherapy was delivered with a variety of techniques. With a median follow-up of 22 months and a maximum follow-up of 71 months, the overall survival was 39%. Severe late complications included 13% gastrointestinal bleed, 13% vertebral body collapse, and 19% enteritis. The higher complication rates noted in this series may have been related to the combination of external beam plus intraoperative radiation.

In summary, the limited data suggest that intraoperative radiation may be beneficial in selected patients with gastric cancer. The optimal method by which to combine it with surgery and external beam radiation has yet to be determined. Intraoperative radiation therapy remains investigational.

Palliative Radiation Therapy

In the palliative setting, radiation therapy does provide symptomatic relief of symptoms such as bleeding, obstruction, and pain in approximately 50% to 75% of patients.[53] Patients with

TABLE 19-11. *Intraoperative with or without postoperative external beam radiation therapy for gastric cancer: selected series*

Series	IORT (Gy)	External beam (Gy)	5-FU	Severe complications	Survival: Stage	Survival: Number	Survival: IORT	Survival: 5-Year	Local control
Sindelar and Kinsella[49]	20	None	No	40%	Median 21 mo				Mean 21 mo* to local failure
Takahashi and Abe[50,51]	28–35	None	No	NA	I	24	Yes	87%	NA
						43	No	93%	
					II	20	Yes	84%	
						11	No	62%	
					III	30	Yes	62%	
						38	No	37%	
					IV	27	Yes	15%	
						18	No	0%	
Calvo, et al[52]	15	40–46	Yes	13% Gastrointestinal 13% Bone 19% Bowel	39% with maximum follow-up of 71 mo (median 22-mo follow-up)				100% for primary cancers with residual disease

* Versus 8 mo with 50-Gy external beam ($P = 0.02$).
IORT, intraoperative radiation therapy; *NA,* not available.

favorable prognostic factors such as a high performance status, microscopic compared with gross residual disease, and who receive 5-FU-based chemotherapy tend to have a higher response rate. Overall, the median duration of palliation is 4 to 18 months.[53–55]

Conclusions and Recommendations

The incidence of local–regional failure after potentially curative surgery in gastric cancer is high enough to consider adjuvant therapy. The role of radiation therapy with or without chemotherapy in the adjuvant setting remains unclear. The ongoing phase III Intergroup trial of adjuvant radiation plus chemotherapy versus surgery alone will address this issue. Almost all the series examining the role of postoperative treatment in gastric cancer include patients who have microscopic or gross residual disease, thereby making the data difficult to interpret. In the setting of locally unresectable or residual disease, postoperative radiation therapy and 5-FU-based chemotherapy may decrease local–regional failure and improve survival; however, this still cannot be considered the standard of care. In those cases in which patients are selected to receive radiation therapy, it is reasonable to add 5-FU-based chemotherapy, at least as a radiation sensitizer. Intraoperative radiation therapy appears promising, but remains investigational. In the palliative setting, radiation therapy offers symptomatic relief in most patients.

REFERENCES

1. De-Ren S. Ten-year follow-up of esophageal cancer treated by radical radiation therapy: analysis of 869 patients. Int J Radiat Oncol Biol Phys 1989;16:329.
2. Newaishy GA, Read GA, Duncan W, et al. Results of radical radiotherapy of squamous cell carcinoma of the esophagus. Clin Radiol 1982; 33:347.
3. Okawa T, Kita M, Tanaka M, et al. Results of radiotherapy for inoperable locally advanced esophageal cancer. Int J Radiat Oncol Biol Phys 1989;17:49.
4. Armstrong JG. High dose rate remote afterloading brachytherapy for lung and esophageal cancer. Semin Radiat Oncol 1993;4:270.
5. Caspers RJL, Zwinderman AH, Griffioen G, et al. Combined external beam and low dose rate intraluminal radiotherapy in oesophageal cancer. Radiother Oncol 1993;27:7.
6. Mei W, Xian-Zhi G, Weibo Y, et al. Randomized clinical trial on the combination of preoperative irradiation and surgery in the treatment of esophageal carcinoma: report on 206 patients. Int J Radiat Oncol Biol Phys 1989;16:325.
7. Gignoux M, Roussel A, Paillot B, et al. The value of preoperative radiotherapy in esophageal cancer: results of a study of the E.O.R.T.C.. World J Surg 1987;11:426.
8. Teniere P, Hay J, Fingerhut A, et al. Postoperative radiation therapy does not increase survival after curative resection for squamous cell carcinoma of the middle and lower esophagus as shown by a multicenter controlled trial. Surg Gynecol Obstet 1991;173:123.
9. Launois B, Delarue D, Campion JP, et al. Preoperative radiotherapy for carcinoma of the esophagus. Surg Gynecol Obstet 1981;153:690.
10. Arnott SJ, Duncan W, Kerr GR, et al. Low dose preoperative radiotherapy for carcinoma of the oesophagus: results of a randomized clinical trial. Radiother Oncol 1993;24:108.
11. Huang GJ, Gu XZ, Wang LJ, et al. Combined preoperative irradiation and surgery for esophageal carcinoma. In: Delarue NC, ed. International trends in general thoracic surgery. St. Louis: CV Mosby, 1988:315.
12. Nygaard K, Hagen S, Hansen HS, et al. Pre-operative radiotherapy prolongs survival in operable esophageal carcinoma: a randomized, multicenter study of pre-operative radiotherapy and chemotherapy. The second Scandinavian trial in esophageal cancer. World J Surg 1992; 16:1104.
13. Yadava OP, Hodge AJ, Matz LR, et al. Esophageal malignancies: is preoperative radiotherapy the way to go? Ann Thorac Surg 1991;51: 189.
14. Sugimachi K, Matsufuji H, Kai H, et al. Preoperative irradiation for carcinoma of the esophagus. Surg Gynecol Obstet 1986;162:174.
15. Kasai M, Mori S, Watanabe T. Follow-up results after resection of thoracic esophageal carcinoma. World J Surg 1978;2:543.
16. Fok M, Sham JST, Choy D, et al. Postoperative radiotherapy for carcinoma of the esophagus: a prospective, randomized controlled trial. Surgery 1993;113:138.
17. Iizuka T, Ide H, Kakegawa T, et al. Preoperative radioactive therapy for esophageal carcinoma: randomized evaluation trial in eight institutions. Chest 1988;93:1054.
18. Kelsen DP, Minsky BD, Smith M, et al. Preoperative therapy for esophageal cancer: a randomized comparison of chemotherapy vs. radiation therapy. J Clin Oncol 1990;8:1352.
19. Le Prise E, Etienne PL, Meunier B, et al. A randomized study of chemotherapy, radiation therapy, and surgery versus surgery for localized squamous cell carcinoma of the esophagus. Cancer 1994;73:1779.
20. Leichman L, Steiger Z, Seydel HG, et al. Preoperative chemotherapy and radiation therapy for patients with cancer of the esophagus: a potentially curative approach. J Clin Oncol 1984;2:75.
21. Poplin E, Fleming T, Leichman L, et al. Combined therapies for squamous-cell carcinoma of the esophagus: a Southwest Oncology Group Study (SWOG-8037). J Clin Oncol 1987;5:622.
22. Urba SG, Orringer MB, Perez-Tamayo C, et al. Concurrent preoperative chemotherapy and radiation therapy in localized esophageal adenocarcinoma. Cancer 1992;69:285.
23. Forastiere A. Treatment of localregional esophageal cancer. Semin Oncol 1992;19:57.
24. Forastiere A, Orringer MB, Perez-Tamayo C, et al. Concurrent chemotherapy and radiation therapy followed by transhiatal esophagectomy for local-regional cancer of the esophagus. J Clin Oncol 1990;8:119.
25. Naunheim KS, Petruska PJ, Roy TS, et al. Preoperative chemotherapy and radiotherapy for esophageal carcinoma. J Thorac Cardiovasc Surg 1992;5:887.
26. Stewart JR, Hoff SJ, Johnson DH, et al. Improved survival with neoadjuvant therapy and resection for adenocarcinoma of the esophagus. Ann Surg 1993;218:571.
27. Gill PG, Denham JW, Jamieson GG, et al. Patterns of treatment failure and prognostic factors associated with the treatment of esophageal carcinoma with chemotherapy and radiotherapy either as sole treatment of followed by surgery. J Clin Oncol 1992;10:1037.
28. Kavanagh B, Anscher M, Leopold K, et al. Patterns of failure following combined modality therapy for esophageal cancer, 1984–1990. Int J Radiat Oncol Biol Phys 1992;24:633.
29. Araujo CMM, Souhami L, Gil RA, et al. A randomized trial comparing radiation therapy versus concomitant radiation therapy and chemotherapy in carcinoma of the thoracic esophagus. Cancer 1991;67:2258.
30. Herskovic A, Martz L, Al-Sarraf M, et al. Combined chemotherapy and radiotherapy compared with radiotherapy alone in patients with cancer of the esophagus. N Engl J Med 1992;326:1593.
31. Roussel A, Jacob JH, Jung GM, et al. Controlled clinical trial for the treatment of patients with inoperable esophageal carcinoma: a study of the EORTC Gastrointestinal Tract Cancer Cooperative Group. In: Schlag P, Hohenberger P, Metzger U, eds. Recent results in cancer research. Berlin: Springer-Verlag, 1988:21.
32. Al-Sarraf M, Pajak T, Herskovic A, et al. Progress report of combined chemo-radiotherapy (CT-RT) vs. radiotherapy (RT) alone in patients with esophageal cancer: an intergroup study [abstract]. Proc ASCO 1993;12:197.
33. Sischy B, Ryan L, Haller D, et al. Interim report of EST 1282 phase III protocol for the evaluation of combined modalities in the treatment of patients with carcinoma of the esophagus [abstract]. Proc ASCO 1990;9:10.
34. John MJ, Flam M, Ager Mowry PA, et al. Radiotherapy alone and chemoradiation for nonmetastatic esophageal carcinoma. Cancer 1989; 63:2397.
35. Coia LR, Engstrom PF, Paul AR, et al. Long-term results of infusional 5-FU, mitomycin-C, and radiation as primary management of esophageal cancer. Int J Radiat Oncol Biol Phys 1991;20:29.
36. Izquierdo MA, Marcuello E, Gomez de Segura G, et al. Unresectable

nonmetastatic squamous cell carcinoma of the esophagus managed by sequential chemotherapy (cisplatin and bleomycin) and radiation therapy. Cancer 1993;71:287.
37. Seitz JF, Giovannini M, Padaut-Cesana J, et al. Inoperable nonmetastatic squamous cell carcinoma of the esophagus managed by concomitant chemotherapy (5-fluorouracil and cisplatin) and radiation therapy. Cancer 1990;66:214.
38. Landry J, Tepper JE, Wood WC, et al. Patterns of failure following curative resection of gastric cancer. Int J Radiat Oncol Biol Phys 1990; 19:1357.
39. Gunderson LL, Sosin H. Adenocarcinoma of the stomach: areas of failure in a reoperation series (second or symptomatic looks). Clinicopathologic correlation and implications for adjuvant therapy. Int J Radiat Oncol Biol Phys 1982;8:1.
40. Dent DM, Werner ID, Novis B, et al. Prospective randomized trial of combined oncological therapy for gastric carcinoma. Cancer 1979;44: 385.
41. Moertel CG, Childs DS, Reitemeier RJ, et al. Combined 5-fluorouracil and supervoltage radiation therapy of locally unresectable gastrointestinal carcinoma. Lancet 1969;1:865.
42. Schein PS, Smith FP, Woolley PV, et al. Current management of advanced and locally unresectable gastric carcinoma. Cancer 1982;50: 2590.
43. Gastrointestinal Tumor Study Group. The concept of locally advanced gastric cancer: effect of treatment on outcome. Cancer 1990;66:2324.
44. Moertel CG, Childs DS, O'Fallon JR, et al. Combined 5-fluorouracil and radiation therapy as a surgical adjuvant for poor prognosis gastric carcinoma. J Clin Oncol 1984;2:1249.
45. Allum W, Hallissey MT, Ward LC, et al. A controlled, prospective randomized trial of adjuvant chemotherapy or radiotherapy in resectable gastric cancer: interim report. Br J Cancer 1989;60:739.
46. Lawrence TS, Maybaum J. Fluoropyrimidines as radiation sensitizers. Semin Radiat Oncol 1993;3:20.
47. Slot A, Meerwaldt JH, van Putten WLJ, et al. Adjuvant postoperative radiotherapy for gastric carcinoma with poor prognostic signs. Radiother Oncol 1989;16:269.
48. Caudry M, Escarmant P, Maire JP, et al. Radiotherapy of gastric cancer with a three field combination: feasibility, tolerance, and survival. Int J Radiat Oncol Biol Phys 1987;13:1821.
49. Sindelar WF, Kinsella TJ. Randomized trial of resection and intraoperative radiotherapy in locally advanced gastric cancer [abstract]. Proc ASCO 1987;6:91.
50. Abe M. Intraoperative radiation therapy for gastric cancer. In: Dobelbower RR, Abe M, eds. Intraoperative radiation therapy. Boca Raton, FL: CRC Press, 1991:166.
51. Takahashi T, Abe M. Intra-operative radiotherapy for carcinoma of the stomach. Eur J Surg Oncol 1986;12:247.
52. Calvo FA, Aristu JJ, Azinovic I, et al. Intraoperative and external radiotherapy in resected gastric cancer: updated report of a phase II trial. Int J Radiat Oncol Biol Phys 1992;24:729.
53. Falkson G, Van Eden EB, Sandison AG. A controlled clinical trial of fluorouracil plus imidazole carboxamide dimethyl triazeno plus vincristine plus bis-chloroethyl plus radiotherapy in stomach cancer. Med Pediatr Oncol 1976;2:111.
54. Klaassen DJ, MacIntyre JM, Catton GE, et al. Treatment of locally unresectable cancer of the stomach and pancreas: a randomized comparison of 5-fluorouracil alone with radiation plus concurrent and maintenance 5-fluorouracil: an Eastern Cooperative Oncology Group study. J Clin Oncol 1985;3:373.
55. Mantell BS. Radiotherapy for dysphagia due to gastric carcinoma. Br J Surg 1982;69:69.

Surgery for Gastrointestinal Cancer: A Multidisciplinary Approach, edited by Harold J. Wanebo.
Lippincott-Raven Publishers, Philadelphia, © 1997.

CHAPTER 20

Palliation of Bronchoesophageal Fistula, Obstruction, and Other Complications

Gordon F. Murray and Alexander Vasilakis

Paper #5. Willy Meyer, M.D., New York, "Extrathoracic and Intrathoracic Esophagoplasty in Connection With Resection of the Thoracic Portion of the Esophagus for Carcinoma" . . . No Discussion

AMA Minutes, 1913

The most disappointing facet of Dr. Willy Meyer's presentation at the Annual Meeting of the American Medical Association on June 18, 1913, in Minneapolis, Minnesota, was that no one had shown any interest. His paper, entitled "Extrathoracic and Intrathoracic Esophagoplasty in Connection with Resection of the Thoracic Portion of the Esophagus for Carcinoma,"[1] presented a clear and concise review of the then available and suggested methods of treatment. Dr. Meyer's determined response to indifference was to initiate a forum that, in time, developed into the first society for thoracic surgery in the world. Nearly fourscore years after the founding of the American Association for Thoracic Surgery, the challenge of effective palliation of complicated esophageal carcinoma remains daunting. Cure becomes an elusive goal, and the primary consideration in treating patients with advanced disease should be a focus on attaining effective palliation.[2] Attaining symptomatic relief can be difficult. The palliative treatment of complicated esophageal carcinoma has included dilatation, intubation, enteric bypass, and esophagogastrectomy. Careful definition of the extent of disease before the selection of treatment may avoid inappropriately staged regimens and unnecessary operative risks, and may identify favorable candidates for aggressive excisional therapy.[3] The establishment of esophagogastric continuity, restoration of effective swallowing, and avoidance of aspiration are the goals of any chosen therapy.

Gordon F. Murray, Professor and Chairman, Department of Surgery, West Virginia University School of Medicine, Morgantown, WV 26506-9238.

Alexander Vasilakis, Assistant Professor of Surgery, West Virginia University School of Medicine, Morgantown, WV 26506-9238.

ESOPHAGEAL OBSTRUCTION

Esophageal carcinoma most often presents initially with dysphagia.[4] Unfortunately, symptoms seldom appear until the tumor involves most of the esophageal circumference, and the tumor burden is extensive. Severe weight loss and debilitation characterize the patient with advanced esophageal carcinoma. Pain, sialorrhea, and regurgitation may also be present. Pulmonary injury secondary to aspiration is often apparent on the initial chest roentgenogram. In most cases, symptoms prompt the clinician to recommend a contrast esophogram and an endoscopy with biopsy.[5] The lesion is characterized by ragged narrowing of the lumen (Fig. 20-1). This irregular appearance strongly suggests a malignant lesion, but the diagnosis must be confirmed by subsequent esophagoscopy and biopsy.

Palliative Resection

Resection of the tumor mass, if possible, offers the best palliation and is the procedure of choice.[2] Although long-term survival is usually not achieved, symptomatic relief and improved quality of life have been reported in many series.[6] Surgical resection of the tumor with reestablishment of gastrointestinal continuity by means of an esophagogastric anastomosis is the most widely used surgical procedure for attempted palliation of obstructing esophageal carcinoma. In the case of small lower esophageal lesions, this may be done through a left thoracotomy with an incision in the diaphragm. Other investigators have advocated a transhiatal exposure through separate midline abdominal and cervical incision. Our approach to the esophagogastrectomy is that advocated by Ivor Lewis,[7] which combines a midline abdominal incision with a separate right thoracotomy. Palliative resection for carcinoma of the upper esophagus deserves special scrutiny, because irradiation or intubation offers a reasonable alternative to incomplete resection. In contrast to lower esophageal tumors, recognition of nonresectable lesions in the cervical or thoracic esophagus is often delayed until late in the procedure, when thoracotomy is undertaken.

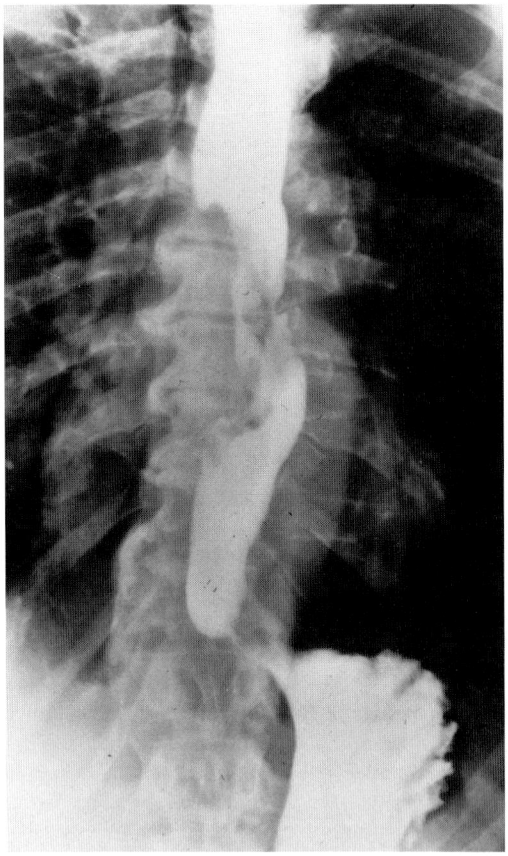

FIG. 20-1. Barium esophogram detailing a nearly obstructing carcinoma of the mid-esophagus.

In the past, the 30-day mortality for esophagogastrectomy has been as high as 27% to 40%.[8] However, in more recent years, the operative mortality associated with resection has been 6% or less.[9] Morbidity is also minimal, and the incidence of anastomotic leak has progressively decreased. Palliation with resection has achieved a success rate of 80% or more, and most patients are able to eat a normal diet.

Mean survival for resected patients with obstructing carcinoma, however, rarely exceeds a year,[3] and long-term survival is in general low (<15%).[10] Further, the large number of serious complications reported in some series[8] has discouraged wide acceptance of resection as an effective palliative procedure.

Gastrostomy

Simple reliance on gastrostomy as therapy defines the nihilistic extreme. Gastrostomy provides little relief for patients with obstructing esophageal carcinoma. Although it does offer a means of administering calories to patients, gastrostomy alone does not provide the ability to swallow or address the morbidity related to aspiration. The creation of a gastrostomy in these patients provides neither demonstrable improvement in nutritional status nor improved survival.[11,12]

Esophageal Dilatation

The simplest approach to the management of esophageal obstruction is mechanical dilatation. This procedure traditionally has been performed with soft-tipped dilators,[13] or, more recently, with inflatable, low-compliance balloons.[14] Mercury-filled Maloney bougies can be used as dilators in an antegrade fashion if the obstruction will permit (Fig. 20-2). If the obstruction can be traversed, guided dilators over a string or wire such as the Savary or Eder-Puestow types can be used. The risk of perforation of the esophagus with manual dilatation is generally below 10%, except in those cases in which the esophagus has been previously irradiated. Excellent results have been obtained using an inflatable, low-compliance balloon.[14,15] Balloon dilatation of very tight esophageal strictures has resulted in a considerable reduction in the perforation rate by taking advantage of evenly distributed stationary radial forces within the stricture.[15] Advantages of this technique include the precise endoscopic placement of the uninflated balloon within the stricture or radiographic placement over a soft guidewire. This avoids traction on the esophagus and minimizes the development of shear forces associated with traditional bougienage, lowering the risk of perforation. In addition, the inflatable balloon permits the surgeon to control the timing and force of dilation.[15] Once the diameter of the esophagus is reduced below 12 mm, conventional mercury-weighted bougies become ineffective because of the loss of the longitudinal stiffness of the dilator. Eder-Peustow dilators have been used effectively to dilate advanced esophageal strictures in the past; however, the snowplow effect of the dilator with the creation of extreme longitudinal shear forces can lead to an increased risk of perforation. With all methods, gradual dilation of the esophagus over several sessions is safest. The disadvantage of esophageal dilatation is that its benefits are brief. In some instances, relief from dysphagia may last only hours. Esophageal dilatation is most effective when used as a therapeutic adjunct during the placement of an intraluminal esophageal stent.

Esophageal Intubation

Esophageal intubation with an intraluminal stent is attractive in that it has the theoretic advantage of meeting all of the goals of palliative therapy by maintaining a functional lumen past the obstruction. Early attempts at placing these devices required a laparotomy with oral insertion of the stent and positioning primarily by means of traction through a gastrotomy. The complication rates for these early pull-through procedures were unacceptably high.

Advances in the field of endoscopy have allowed the placement of intraluminal stents almost exclusively by the pulsion method, primarily through the esophagoscope.[16–29] The results with a variety of devices have been reported. Most of the devices bear the names of their developers and are made of a variety of materials, primarily rubber, plastic, and metal (Fig. 20-3). Although most esophageal intubations are successful as a result of improved endoscopic techniques, avoidance of laparotomy, and newer devices, the morbidity and mortality of esophageal intubation have been reported to be as high as 10% to 25%.[21,29] The key to the successful management of patients undergoing esophageal intubation is the avoidance of complications. Perforation and stent migration are the most frequent hazards, with an incidence as high as 25% for each.[16–23,29] Other complications include hemorrhage, pressure necrosis, stent obstruction, and fistula formation.[29]

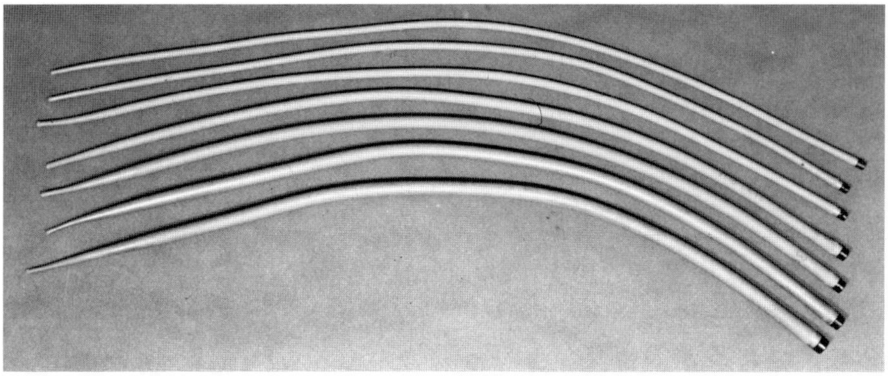

FIG. 20-2. Several sizes of weighted mercury-filled bougies.

The incidence of perforation, hemorrhage, and fistula formation is directly related to the extent of esophageal dilatation required before the placement of the stents. Both pulsion or traction methods require prior dilatation of the malignant stricture. Basic stent designs have a minimal outer diameter of 15 mm, and aggressive dilatation often is required before stent placement. Malignant esophageal tissue can be resistant to mechanical dilatation, so the process of creating a sufficiently dilated lumen should be gradual, using two or more treatments spread over several days before attempting to place the stent.

Stent designs have continued to evolve, with the expansile metal stent the most recent development.[24–28] Placement of these devices requires endoscopic guidance over metal guidewires and positioning under fluoroscopic control. The expandable stents have an initial diameter of 3 mm and then expand to 15 mm, effectively forcing the site of obstruction open (Fig. 20-4). The resulting snug fit apparently reduces the incidence of stent migration. These devices require less esophageal dilatation before placement and therefore have lower complication rates compared with standard plastic prostheses. The smaller initial diameter also allows placement under monitored anesthesia care rather than general anesthesia, which is often required for standard intubation. This advantage further reduces the risk of the procedure. With the use of the expansile metal stent, the risks of perforation, migration, hemorrhage, and death from esophageal intubation have been reduced to less than 5%.[27,28]

Food impaction of any esophageal stent is a problem that can be overcome by adequate patient education and compliance with an established nutritional program. Food should be thoroughly chewed before swallowing. Some foods should be avoided, such as vegetable and fruit skins, nontoasted bread, and tough meats. Plenty of fluid should accompany food ingestion to enhance movement of food through the stent lumen.

New designs in esophageal stents have led to easier and more reliable placement with a reduction in complication rates. The most successful design is the expansile metal stent. Successful placement of an esophageal stent can reliably improve dysphagia, allow control of secretions, avoid aspiration, and improve the quality of the remaining short life of these patients.

Laser Therapy

Laser ablation of the obstructing tumor mass is possible using the neodymium:yttrium–aluminum garnet laser.[30–37] A conventional endoscope is used to deliver laser energy through a fiberoptic bundle, and photocoagulation and vaporization of the obstructing tissue creates a channel through the mass. A combination of forceful dilatation and laser vaporization of the tumor allows progressive recanalization of the esophageal lumen.

There are two approaches to laser irradiation for treating esophageal obstruction. The prograde approach uses a laser fiber that is passed repeatedly through the obstruction. This gradually opens a channel that is eventually enlarged to permit adequate swallowing. In the retrograde approach, the fiberoptic delivery port is first advanced beyond the obstruction without irradiating the tissue. Subsequently, it is repeatedly retracted through the mass, irradiating the obstructing tissue on its way out, finally creating an adequate channel. This retrograde approach is faster and has been associated with shorter hospitalization times.[34]

The most distressing disadvantage of laser ablation is early recurrence of the obstruction. The tumors are often so bulky that successful canalization requires multiple treatments with the laser, sometimes only a few days apart. There is also the ever-present danger of perforation caused by misguided laser

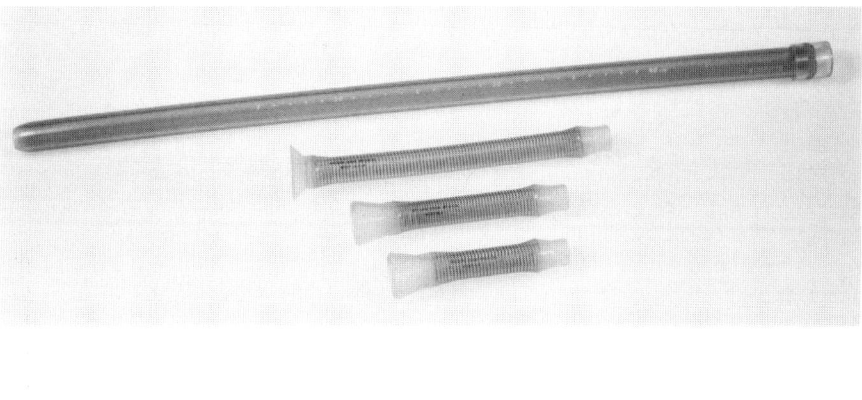

FIG. 20-3. Several sizes of guided dilators.

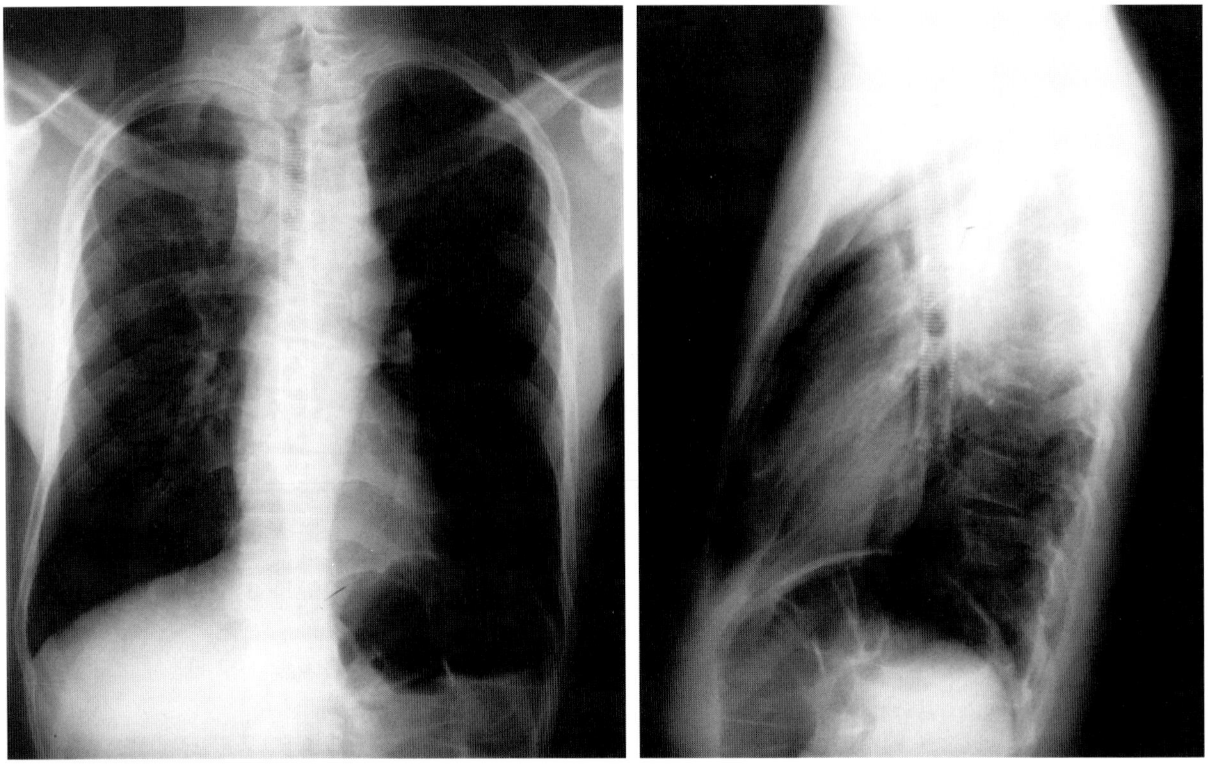

FIG. 20-4. Posteroanterior *(left)* and lateral *(right)* chest roentgenograms demonstrating a spiral wire-supported esophageal endoprosthesis in place.

radiation. Perforation or hemorrhage occurs in 5% to 10% of cases. The laser unit itself is costly, and is not widely available.[30–36] Bipolar electrocoagulation therapy of obstructing esophageal tumors has been reported to be at least as effective in establishing an esophageal lumen as laser ablation. This method offers a less expensive alternative to laser ablation while achieving similar success rates.[38]

Laser photocoagulation therapy and bipolar electrocoagulation of esophageal obstructions offer no clear palliative advantages over conventional dilatation or esophageal intubation therapies. Use of the laser has not been accompanied by a decrease in procedural complications or an improved survival rate. When used in conjunction with the placement of an esophageal stent, it may have a benefit when an adequate channel can be opened immediately rather than after several conventional dilatations.[36] With this alternative, immediate palliation can be obtained, allowing the patient to use the oral route for alimentation and providing a way to control secretions and avoid aspiration. The best results of laser ablation can be expected from an experienced endoscopist with the skill to apply this powerful modality safely.

Radiation Therapy

Radiation therapy is another treatment consideration in patients with obstructing carcinomas of the esophagus that are inoperable.[39–43] Despite the fact that many regimens have been developed, radiation therapy has not appreciably altered the natural history of esophageal carcinoma. Relief of dysphagia, however, can be expected in 60% to 70% of patients until recurrent tumor further compromises the patient. The limitations of radiation therapy include poor local and regional control of the tumor for any reasonable length of time before the rapid recurrence of symptoms. In addition, the maximal dose of radiation is finite and cannot be administered after a treatment of 6000 to 6600 cGy has been delivered without a marked increase in the incidence of radiation-related complications. Frequent complications include radiation pneumonitis and postradiation stricture. Constrictive pericarditis, hemorrhage, radiation myelitis, and esophagorespiratory fistula have been reported, but are less common. Radiation therapy tends to be more effective in cervical or upper thoracic esophageal tumors. Five-year survivors have been reported; however, they comprise less than 10% of patients in all series.

Variable tumor regression and relief of dysphagia have been reported in series studying the effects of multimodality protocols combining chemotherapy and radiation therapy,[44] or chemotherapy, radiation therapy, and surgery.[45] It is not uncommon for the patients in these protocols to have complete relief of dysphagia, to the point of being able to resume oral alimentation before esophagectomy. The potentiating effects of the combination of chemotherapeutic agents and simultaneous radiation therapy to the tumor are still under investigation. A survival benefit has been reported in small groups of patients with localized tumors with concurrent cisplatin-based chemotherapy and radiation therapy, at the expense of increased side effects. There is no evidence that palliation of unresectable tumors of the esophagus by combinations of chemotherapy and radiation therapy is superior to any other methods already mentioned.

Fundal Bypass

Fundal bypass of obstructing, unresectable distal esophageal tumors has been described.[46] Mobilization of the fundus of the stomach in selected cases may result in an adequate conduit to reach into the thorax through a separate incision in the left diaphragm. A side-to-side anastomosis of the fundus and esophagus bypasses the obstruction and provides an open route for oral alimentation. On rare occasions, this option may be elected in the right chest in the conduct of an attempted Ivor Lewis resection.[7]

ESOPHAGORESPIRATORY FISTULA

Malignant esophagorespiratory fistula is a particularly disastrous consequence of esophageal cancer.[47–54] About 5% to 15% of all patients with esophageal carcinoma ultimately experience this complication. The most common site of occurrence is between the mid-esophagus and the left mainstem bronchus. Less often, the right mainstem bronchus (Fig. 20-5), trachea (Fig. 20-6), or the lung are involved. In the latter circumstance, the condition may masquerade as a recurring pneumonitis or lung abscess. Although the fistula may be present at the time of the original diagnosis of malignancy, frequently it occurs after radiation therapy for inoperable recurrent disease. Once the complication occurs, the surgeon is immediately faced with two disease processes that are potentially and invariably fatal: esophageal carcinoma and pulmonary sepsis. All untreated patients eventually die from pulmonary sepsis. Even when treated, nearly 90% of patients are dead within 6 months.[48] However, the need for adequate treatment planning is emphasized by the fact that all untreated patients die miserably from lung soilage, and the disease is confined to the thorax in as many as half of the patients. Successful palliation hinges on early interruption of pulmonary soilage and restoration of functional integrity to both the respiratory and digestive tracts. Esophageal intubation bridging the fistula area,[55–58] surgical diversion,[59,60] esophageal exclusion,[61–69] and esophageal resection[70,71] are treatment options that should be considered.

The therapeutic challenge is made more formidable by associated malnutrition and pulmonary complications. Patients with malignant esophagorespiratory fistula present in a dehydrated, debilitated, anemic, and anergic state. Aggressive nutritional support and management of pulmonary sepsis are the cornerstones of all therapy. Nutritional supplementation begun before definitive therapy has been instituted has been associated with a significant reduction of wound infection and postoperative complications. Ideally, the nutritional support is begun before the patient has lost more than 10% of body weight. Enteral nutrition delivered through access to the small intestine is acceptable and avoids the hazards and added cost of parenteral nutrition. An aggressive program of pulmonary hygiene and broad-spectrum intravenous antibiotics should be instituted soon after presentation to limit the lung injury related to persistent contamination.

Radiation Therapy

When a malignant esophagorespiratory fistula occurs de novo, it may be controlled, in rare instances, by radiation therapy.[72] More commonly, esophagorespiratory fistulas are reported as a consequence of radiation therapy, and opportunity for healing is negligible. Yamada and coworkers[72] and Burt and colleagues[47] have reported that radiation therapy provides temporary relief of esophagorespiratory fistulas. The mechanism for temporary relief is thought to be the transient soft tissue swelling secondary to the inflammatory response caused by the radiation. Once the total dose of radiation therapy has been given, the inflammation subsides, allowing the fistula to reopen and pulmonary soilage to resume. Overall, those patients receiving radiation therapy have a prolonged survival compared with those who receive supportive care; however, death by pulmonary sepsis intervenes in most patients. Radiation therapy is effectively used in controlling local disease after exclusion of the fistula by intubation or bypass.[73] Such treatment may provide effective pain relief and often extends survival.

External Diversion

Simple diversion of saliva by a cervical esophagostomy with a feeding jejunostomy may prolong survival by a few weeks.

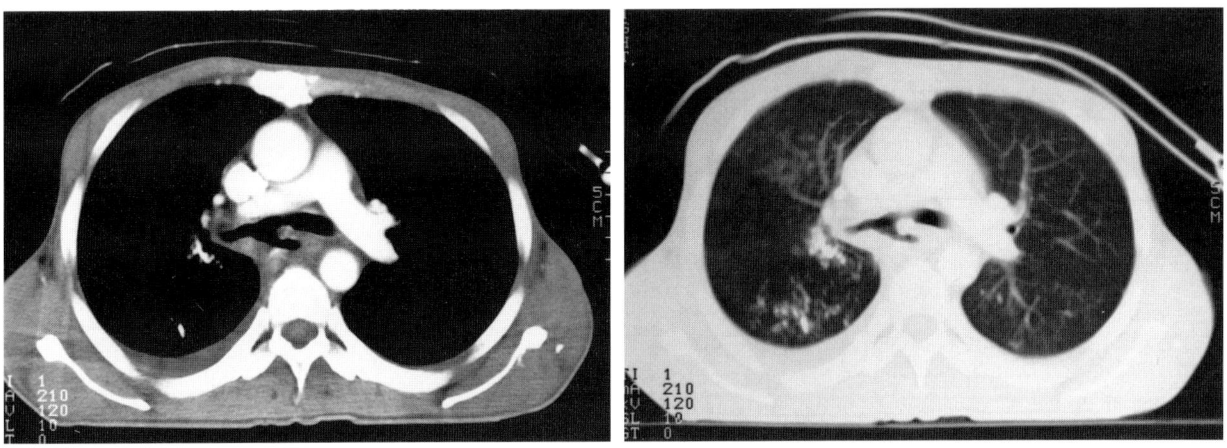

FIG. 20-5. Sequential computed tomography scans through the chest revealing a communication between the esophagus on the right mainstem bronchus.

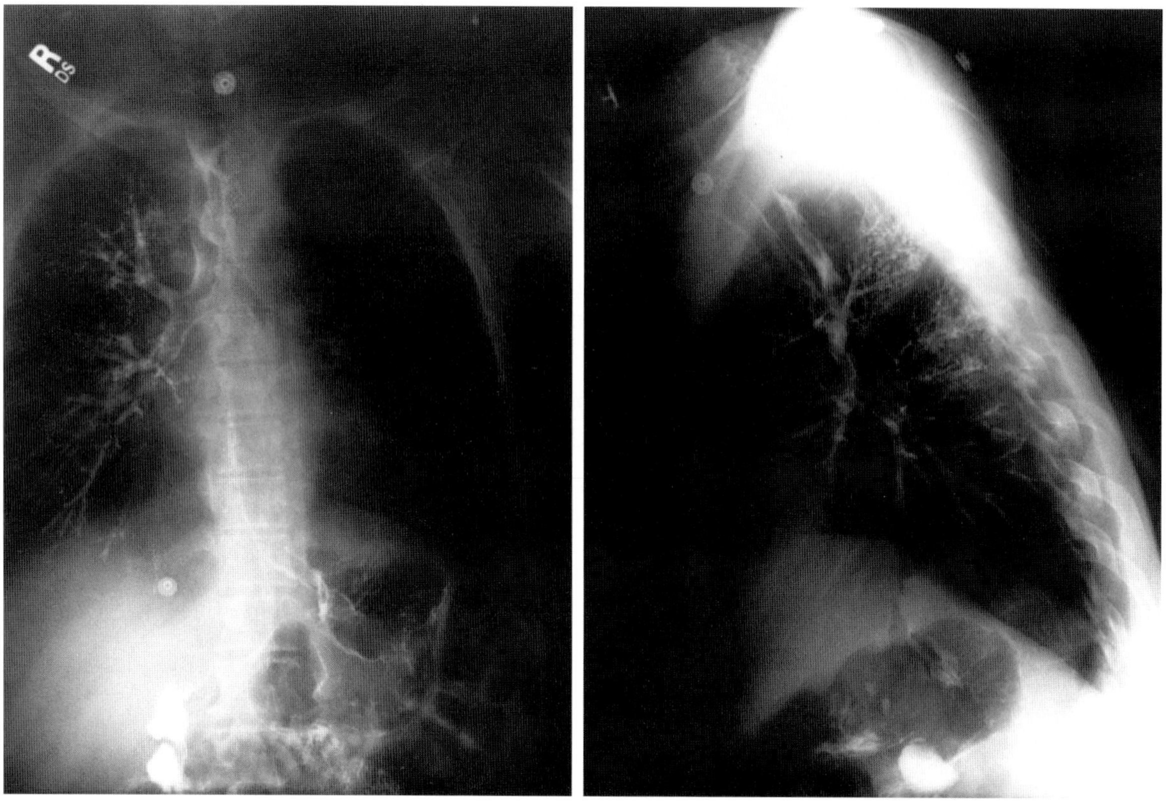

FIG. 20-6. Posteroanterior *(left)* and lateral *(right)* contrast studies revealing a tracheoesophageal fistula.

However, this effort alone provides no hope or dignity to the patient, who still cannot swallow. Division of the cervical esophagus, cervical esophagostomy, and gastrostomy prevent sepsis from ongoing aspiration of swallowed oral secretions and permit use of an extracorporeal gastric tube, developed by Akiyama and Hiyama.[62] This approach, providing modest palliation, may be the maximum effort the patient will tolerate. Such external diversion for patients with an esophagorespiratory fistula is usually reserved for the most debilitated patients.[59]

Esophageal Intubation

The goal of effective operative palliation must always be weighed against operative risk in patients with a life expectancy of only a few months. In many cases, esophageal intubation becomes the treatment of choice. An accurately placed endoprosthesis may achieve satisfactory palliation for a limited amount of time by sealing the fistula and relieving the distal obstruction associated with the carcinoma. This approach seems most applicable in elderly or debilitated patients whose general condition precludes more extensive operative procedures. An esophageal endoprosthesis is also useful in patients in whom an esophagorespiratory fistula develops as a consequence of radiation therapy used to treat the primary esophageal malignancy. In the presence of esophagorespiratory fistula, most methods of intubation have a relatively high initial mortality (about 25%) and are often complicated by tube migration, hemorrhage, sepsis, and aspiration. Less often, survivors enjoy a reasonably comfortable existence with a diet of thick liquids and freedom from aspiration.

Esophageal Exclusion and Bypass

In suitable patients, esophageal exclusion and bypass affords the best palliation. If possible, restoration of gastrointestinal continuity should be accomplished at the time of the esophageal exclusion. The stomach, with its rich blood supply, has been identified as the most reliable conduit for esophageal bypass. Use of colon or jejunal bypass conduits is reserved for instances in which gastric transposition is not an option. Gastric tubes using the greater curvature of the stomach have been used as reversed[61] or isoperistaltic[64] conduits. The entire stomach in the retrosternal position has also been used successfully to bypass unresectable esophageal carcinoma.[63] After appropriate mobilization of the entire stomach or creation of a greater curvature tube, a substernal tunnel is created. The neck is explored and the cervical esophagus is isolated. The gastric conduit is brought into the neck and a cervical esophagogastric anastomosis is performed. At the time of bypass, the body of the esophagus is divided and secured at both ends. It is less certain whether drainage of the totally excluded esophageal segment is necessary. It has been reported that secretions from the excluded esophagus are not excessive and are usually cleared through the esophagorespiratory fistula by vigorous coughing.[63] We prefer to decompress the distal esophagus into a Roux-en-Y jejunal limb to drain the excluded esophageal segment and diminish symptoms of aspiration. If both the proximal and distal esophagus are sutured closed, a proximal catheter esophagostomy vent should be provided to prevent disruption of the excluded esophageal segment in the early postoperative period. This precaution is especially important if the patient requires prolonged positive-pressure ventilation.

Significant anastomotic complications occur after esophageal exclusion and bypass procedures, and are often associated with prior radiation therapy. In our experience, the risk of cervical anastomotic leaks is exceedingly high with tubed gastric reconstruction. Frequently, with an anastomotic leak, the excluded proximal esophagus reopens, leading to disastrous consequences due to recurring aspiration. The complication rates for esophageal exclusion and bypass have been reported to be as high as 30% to 50%,[66,69] which emphasizes the fact that the risk–benefit ratio of any proposed operative intervention for advanced esophageal carcinoma must be carefully determined in each individual case. Quality-of-life issues are a strong consideration in this subgroup of patients with very limited survival. Those patients referred after prompt diagnosis of malignancy or rapid detection of an esophagorespiratory communication are patients who benefit the most from esophageal exclusion and bypass. Aggressive operative reconstruction should be avoided in patients presenting with advanced sepsis and malnutrition from their malignancy.

Esophageal Resection

The principles of excision and repair applied so effectively to acquired benign esophagorespiratory fistula usually are not appropriate for the malignant defect. Although pneumonectomy and total esophagectomy have been advocated for intrathoracic malignant esophagobronchial fistulas, we have never undertaken the procedure, anticipating excessive mortality and little hope for cure. Malignant tracheoesophageal fistula occurring in the cervical area is an exception.[70] Total laryngectomy, tracheostomy (mediastinal), esophagectomy, and pharyngogastrostomy may provide the desired palliation. Transhiatal esophagectomy greatly facilitates the performance of this challenging procedure.

OTHER COMPLICATIONS

Aortoesophageal fistula is usually a complication of the erosion of a thoracic aortic aneurysm into the esophagus. Only 15% of cases arise from a primary esophageal neoplasm eroding into the aorta.[74] The typical patient presents with Chiari's triad of mid-thoracic pain, sentinel hemorrhage, and subsequent rapid, fatal exsanguination. Esophagoscopy, revealing a small bleeding sinus, or a thoracic aortic angiogram are equally effective in making a presumptive diagnosis when there is a reasonable index of suspicion. Immediate thoracotomy is mandated. Initial control of the aorta is followed by resection of the area of malignant infiltration. Establishing distal circulation with an aortoaortic jump graft or extraanatomic bypass are both acceptable approaches. The esophagus is concurrently diverted and excluded with definitive reconstruction undertaken at an interval. Establishment of appropriate intestinal access facilitates alimentation until swallowing can be resumed.

REFERENCES

1. Meyer W. Extrathoracic and intrathoracic esophagoplasty in connection with resection of the thoracic portion of the esophagus for carcinoma. JAMA 1914;62:100.
2. Keagy BA, Murray GF, Starek PJK, Battaglini JW, Lores ME, Wilcox BR. Esophagogastrectomy as palliative treatment for esophageal carcinoma: results obtained in the setting of a thoracic surgery residency program. Ann Thorac Surg 1984;38:611.
3. Murray GF, Wilcox BR, Starek PJK. The assessment of operability of esophageal carcinoma. Ann Thorac Surg 1977;23:393.
4. Ellis FH, Gibb SP. Esophagogastrectomy for carcinoma: current hospital mortality and morbidity rates. Ann Surg 1979;190:699.
5. Bruni HC, Nelson RS. Cancer of the esophagus and cardia: diagnosis evaluation in 113 cases. J Thorac Cardiovasc Surg 1975;70:367.
6. Cukingnan RA, Carey JS. Carcinoma of the esophagus (collective review). Ann Thorac Surg 1978;26:274.
7. Lewis I. The surgical treatment of carcinoma of the oesophagus: with special reference to a new operation for growths of the middle third. Br J Surg 1946;34:18.
8. Postlethwait RW. Complications and deaths after operations for esophageal carcinoma. J Thorac Cardiovasc Surg 1983;85:827.
9. Ellis FH, Gibb SP, Watkins E Jr. Esophagogastrectomy: a safe, widely applicable and expeditious form of palliation for patients with carcinoma of the esophagus and cardia. Ann Surg 1983;198:531.
10. Hankins JR, Cole FN, Atlar S, McLanghlin JS. Carcinoma of the esophagus: experience with a philosophy for palliation. Ann Thorac Surg 1977;23:400.
11. King TC, Zimmermann JM. Gastrostomies in patients with incurable cancer. Am Surg 1965;31:251.
12. Connar RG, Sealy RC. Gastrostomies and their complications. Ann Surg 1956;143:245.
13. Aste H, Munizzi F, Martines H, Pugliese V. Esophageal dilation in malignant dysphagia. Cancer 1985;56:2713.
14. Taub S, Rodan BA, Bean WJ, Koerner RS, Mullin DM, Feng TS. Balloon dilatation of esophageal strictures. Am J Gastroenterol 1986; 81:14.
15. Dawson SL, Mueller PR, Ferrucci JT Jr, et al. Severe esophageal strictures: indications for balloon catheter dilatation. Radiology 1984;153: 631.
16. Mackler SA, Mayer RM. Palliation of esophageal obstruction due to carcinoma with a permanent tube. J Thorac Cardiovasc Surg 1954;28: 431.
17. Mousseau M, LeForestier J, Barbin J, Hardy M. Place de l'intubation a demeure dans le traitement palliatif du cancer de l'esophage. Arch Mal Appar Digest 1956;45:208.
18. Celestin LR. Permanent intubation in inoperable cancer of the oesophagus and cardia. Ann R Coll Surg Engl 1959;25:165.
19. den Hartog Jager FCA, Bartelsman JF, Tytgat GN. Palliative treatment of obstructing esophagogastric malignancy by endoscopic positioning of a plastic prosthesis. Gastroenterology 1979;77:1008.
20. Angorn IB. Intubation in the treatment of carcinoma of the esophagus. World J Surg 1981;5:535.
21. Unruh HW, Pagliero KM. Pulsion intubation versus traction intubation for obstructing carcinomas of the esophagus. Ann Thorac Surg 1985; 40:337.
22. van den Brand-Gradel V, den Hartog Jager FC, Tytgat GN. Palliative intubation of malignant esophagogastric obstruction. J Clin Gastroenterol 1987;9:290.
23. Loizou LA, Rampton D, Bown SG. Treatment of malignant strictures of the cervical esophagus by endoscopic intubation using modified endoprostheses. Gastrointest Endosc 1992;38:158.
24. Bethge N, Knyrim K, Wagner HJ, Starck E, Pausch J, Kleist DV. Self-expanding metal stents for palliation of malignant esophageal obstruction: a pilot study of eight patients. Endoscopy 1992;24:411.
25. Neuhaus H, Hoffmann W, Dittler HJ, Niedermeyer HP, Classen M. Implantation of self-expanding esophageal metal stents for palliation of malignant dysphagia. Endoscopy 1992;24:405.
26. Schaer J, Katon RM, Ivancev K, Uchida B, Rosch J, Binmoeller K. Treatment of malignant esophageal obstruction with silicone-coated metallic self-expanding stents. Gastrointest Endosc 1992;38:7.
27. Knyrim K, Wagner HJ, Bethge N, Keymling M, Vakil N. A controlled trial of an expansile metal stent for palliation of esophageal obstruction due to inoperable cancer. N Engl J Med 1993;329:1302.

28. Boyce HW Jr. Stents for palliation of dysphagia due to esophageal cancer. N Engl J Med 1993;329:1345.
29. Merandi SF, Quinn SF, Clark RA. Complications of esophageal prostheses: roentgenologic manifestation. South Med J 1989;82:1365.
30. Goldberg SJ, King KH. Endoscopic Nd:YAG laser coagulation as palliative therapy for obstructing esophageal carcinoma. Am J Gastroenterol 1986;81:629.
31. Pietrafitta JJ, Dwyer RM. New laser technique for the treatment of malignant esophageal obstruction. J Surg Oncol 1987;35:157.
32. Pietrafitta JJ, Carstens MH, Dwyer RM. Endoscopic laser therapy for the treatment of malignant esophageal obstruction. Lasers Surg Med 1987;7:487.
33. Murray FE, Bowers GJ, Birkett DH, Cave DR. Palliative laser therapy of advanced esophageal carcinoma: an alternative perspective. Am J Gastroenterol 1998;83:816.
34. Pietrafitta JJ, Bowers GJ, Dwyer RM. Prograde versus retrograde endoscopic laser therapy for the treatment of malignant esophageal obstruction: a comparison of techniques. Lasers Surg Med 1988;8:288.
35. Moon BC, Woolfson IK, Mercer CD. Neodymium:yttrium-aluminum-garnet laser vaporization for palliation of obstructing esophageal carcinoma [and discussion]. J Thorac Cardiovasc Surg 1989;98:11.
36. Wetstein L, Brenner A. Management of unresectable malignant esophageal obstruction. Mil Med 1990;155:324.
37. Sankar MY, Joffe SN. Endoscopic contact Nd:YAG laser resectional vaporization (ECLRV) and esophageal dilatation (ED) in advanced malignant obstruction of the esophagus. Am Surg 1991;57:259.
38. Johnston JH, Fleischer D, Petrini J, Nord HJ. Palliative bipolar electrocoagulation therapy of obstructing esophageal cancer. Gastrointest Endosc 1987;33:349.
39. Earlam R, Cunha-Melo Jr. Oesophageal squamous cell carcinoma: II. a critical review of radiotherapy. Br J Surg 1982;69:457.
40. Pearson JG. Value of radiation therapy. JAMA 1974b3-7:181.
41. Pearson JG. The value of radiotherapy in managing squamous oesophageal cancer. Br J Surg 1971;58:794.
42. Ellis FH Jr, Salzman FA. Carcinoma of the esophagus: surgery vs. radiotherapy. Postgrad Med 1977;61:167.
43. Herskovic A, Martz K, Al-Sarraf M, et al. Combined chemotherapy and radiotherapy compared with radiotherapy alone in patients with cancer of the esophagus. N Engl J Med 1992;326:1593.
44. Steiger Z, Franklin R, Wilson RF, et al. Eradication and palliation of squamous cell carcinoma of the esophagus with chemotherapy, radiotherapy, and surgical therapy. J Thorac Cardiovasc Surg 1981;82:713.
45. Brown SG. Palliation of malignant dysphagia: surgery, radiotherapy, laser, intubation alone or in combination. Gut 1991;32:841.
46. Popovsky J. Esophagogastrostomy in continuity for carcinoma of the esophagus: its use for unresectable tumors of the lower third of the esophagus and cardia. Arch Surg 1980;115:637.
47. Burt M, Diehl W, Martini N, et al. Malignant esophagorespiratory fistula management options and survival. Ann Thorac Surg 1991;52:1222.
48. Gschossmann JM, Bonner JA, Foote RL, Shaw EG, Martenson JA. Su J. Malignant tracheoesophageal fistula in patients with esophageal cancer. Cancer 1993;72:1513.
49. Koval JC, Curley RM. Bronchoesophageal fistula in small cell lung cancer [letter]. Chest 1990;98:512.
50. Lewis JE, Murray RE. Pulmonary sequestration with bronchoesophageal fistula. J Pediatr Surg 1968;3:575.
51. Steiger Z, Wilson RF, Leichman L, Franklin R, Dindogru A, Kinzie J. Management of malignant bronchoesophageal fistulas. Surg Gynecol Obstet 1983;157:201.
52. Little AG, Ferguson MK, DeMeester TR, Hoffman PC, Skinner DB. Esophageal carcinoma with respiratory tract fistula. Cancer 1984;53:1322.
53. Symbas PN, Mckeown PP, Hatcher CR Jr, Vlasis SE. Tracheoesophageal fistula from carcinoma of the esophagus. Ann Thorac Surg 1984;38:382.
54. Duranceau A, Jamieson GG. Malignant tracheoesophageal fistula. Ann Thorac Surg 1984;37:346.
55. Buess G, Schellong H, Kometz B, Grubner R, Junginger TH. A modified prosthesis for the treatment of malignant esophagotracheal fistula. Cancer 1988;61:1679.
56. Hordijk ML, Dees J, van Blankenstein M. The management of malignant esophagorespiratory fistulas with a cuffed prosthesis. Endoscopy 1990;22:241.
57. Smith JL, Michaletz PA, Tabibian N, Schwartz JT, Graham DY. Improved palliation of a respiratory esophageal fistula with a cuffed esophageal prosthesis. Am J Gastroenterol 1987;82:1175.
58. Ghazi A, Nussbaum M. A new approach to the management of malignant esophageal obstruction and esophagorespiratory fistula. Ann Thorac Surg 1986;41:531.
59. Schreiber H, Pories WJ. External diversion for palliative treatment of malignant tracheoesophageal or bronchoesophageal fistulas. Am J Surg 1976;131:775.
60. Skinner DB, Demeester TR. Permanent extracorporeal esophagogastric tube for esophageal replacement. Ann Thorac Surg 1976;22:107.
61. Heimlich HJ. Esophagoplasty with reversed gastric tube. Am J Surg 1972;123:80.
62. Akiyama H, Hiyama M. A simple esophageal bypass operation by the high gastric division. Surgery 1974;75:674.
63. Orringer MB, Sloan H. Substernal gastric bypass of the excluded thoracic esophagus for palliation of esophageal carcinoma. J Thorac Cardiovasc Surg 1975;70:836.
64. Postlethwait RW. Technique for isoperistaltic gastric tube for esophageal bypass. Ann Surg 1979;189:673.
65. Robinson JC, Isa SS, Spees EK, Rogers EL, Gadacz TR. Substernal gastric bypass for palliation of esophageal carcinoma: rationale and technique. Surgery 1982;91:305.
66. Conlan AA, Nicolaou N, Hammond CA, Pool R, de Nobrega C, Mistry BD. Retrosternal gastric bypass for inoperable esophageal cancer: a report of 71 patients. Ann Thorac Surg 1983;36:396.
67. Ong GB, Lam KH, Lim STK, Wong J. Jejunal loop bypass and fundoplication for malignant esophagobronchial fistula. Surg Gynecol Obstet 1982;154:165.
68. Campion JP, Bourdelat D, Launois B. Surgical treatment of malignant esophagotracheal fistulas. Am J Surg 1983;146:641.
69. Orringer MB. Substernal gastric bypass of the excluded esophagus: results of an ill-advised operation. Surgery 1984;96:467.
70. Ginsberg RJ, Cooper JD. Esophageal fistula. World J Surg 1983;7:455.
71. Ong GB, Lam KH, Wong J, Lim TK. Factors influencing morbidity and mortality in esophageal carcinoma. J Thorac Cardiovasc Surg 1978;76:745.
72. Yamada S, Takai Y, Ogawa Y, Kakuto Y, Sakamoto K. Radiotherapy for malignant fistula to other tract. Cancer 1989;64:1026.
73. Judd DR, Codd J. Palliation for malignant esophagorespiratory fistula. J Thorac Cardiovasc Surg 1967;54:751.
74. Carter R, Mulder GA, Snyder EN Jr, Brewer LA III. Aortoesophageal fistula. Am J Surg 1978;136:26.

Surgery for Gastrointestinal Cancer: A Multidisciplinary Approach, edited by Harold J. Wanebo.
Lippincott-Raven Publishers, Philadelphia, © 1997.

CHAPTER 21

Barrett's Esophagus–Adenocarcinoma of the Esophagus

J. C. Rosenberg and David Fromm

Norman Barrett's name has become firmly established as the eponym of a condition he discussed in a review of the literature on esophagitis. In this paper, published in 1950, he erroneously characterized the condition that currently bears his name as a congenitally short esophagus that pulled a tubular stomach up into the mediastinum.[1] Allison had been doing seminal work in the area of esophagitis during this period, and in 1953 correctly pointed out that the mucosa of the esophagus could occasionally be similar to that of the stomach.[2,3] He first used the eponym, "Barrett's ulcer," generously giving credit to his English colleague for making the distinction between peptic ulcers of the esophagus and the superficial erosions of reflux esophagitis. Allison further noted that there appeared to be a relation between the occurrence of gastric mucosa lining the esophagus and reflux esophagitis associated with hiatal hernia. One of the patients described in his paper of 1953 was reported to have an esophageal carcinoma, "arising in, and confined to, the abnormal segment." This prescient article was not given due consideration by Barrett, who subsequently concluded, in 1957, thatgastric mucosa was present in the esophagus as a "result of a failure of the embryonic lining of the gullet to achieve normal maturity."[4] Eventually it became clear that the columnar-lined esophagus was an acquired condition, related to reflux esophagitis, and that it had a predilection to develop into an adenocarcinoma. The rarity of this clinical presentation 40 years ago contrasts sharply with the situation today. The incidence of adenocarcinoma of the esophagus in white men has doubled from the early 1970s to the late 1980s, and the increase in rates of esophageal adenocarcinoma during this latter decade have been on the order of 5% to 10% per year.[5,6] Most can be shown to have arisen in a Barrett's esophagus.

The association of adenocarcinoma of the esophagus with hiatal hernias was commented on as early as 1870.[7] Adler, in a series of studies of hiatal hernia and adenocarcinoma of the esophagus extending from 1959 to 1963, concluded that the replacement of the squamous cell epithelium of the esophagus by columnar cells could be the origin of an adenocarcinoma of the esophagus.[8,9] This columnar epithelium has the potential to undergo dysplastic changes and malignant transformation.

MORPHOLOGY OF BARRETT'S ESOPHAGUS

Gross Anatomy

The squamocolumnar junction (sometimes referred to as the Z-line or ora serrata) is normally located at the junction of the stomach with the esophagus. Based on the studies that identify the esophagus by virtue of the presence of the lower esophageal sphincter, many patients will have columnar epithelium extending orad into the esophagus.[10] It is thus critical, in deciding whether Barrett's esophagus is present, to determine where the gastroesophageal junction is located and how far craniad the columnar epithelium extends before it is considered abnormal. Because the distal esophageal sphincter is not an anatomic structure, other anatomic landmarks are used to identify where the squamocolumnar junction should be. These include the site of the peritoneal reflection, the diaphragmatic hiatus, and the termination of the characteristic tubular appearance of the esophagus.

It has been recommended that the glandular epithelium should extend more than 2 to 3 cm orad from the gastroesophageal junction to make a diagnosis of Barrett's esophagus.[11–13] Histologic confirmation of the gastroesophageal junction can be obtained by noting the most distal location of the submucosal esophageal glands and the change in orientation of the layers of the muscularis propria.

The distribution of the glandular mucosa within the esopha-

This paper is adapted from an article that originally appeared in the February, 1993 update to *Cancer Prevention*, edited by Vincent T. DeVita, Samuel Hellman, and Steven A. Rosenberg, copyright JB Lippincott Co.

J.C. Rosenberg, Professor of Surgery, Wayne State University, Chief of Surgery, Hutzel Hospital, 4707 St. Antoine, Detroit, MI 48201-1498.

David Fromm, Penberthy Professor of Surgery, Wayne State University, Chief of Surgery, Hutzel Hospital, 4707 St. Antoine, Detroit, MI 48201-1498.

gus can either be circumferential, with tongues of columnar epithelium extending cephalad in an irregular fashion, or patchy with finger-like projections of glandular mucosa surrounded by squamous epithelium. The length of esophagus involved by this metaplastic change can vary from a few centimeters to almost the entire esophagus. In contrast, islands of columnar epithelium in the proximal esophagus are thought to represent remnants of embryonic gastric epithelium. During embryonic development, the entire esophagus is lined with columnar epithelium. Embryologic rests are usually located just below the cricopharyngeus and have been encountered in 4% to 10% of patients undergoing esophagoscopy.

Endoscopic Findings

The location of the squamocolumnar junction should be about 40 cm from the incisors, at the same level as the esophageal sphincter, which can be recognized as a circumferential mucosal rosette that can be opened by insufflation of air. The pinchcock action of the crura at the esophageal hiatus can be localized by having the patient take deep breaths, and if the patient has a hiatal hernia, it can be recognized by the presence of a nontubular hernia pouch that contains rugal folds that slide back and forth across the diaphragmatic hiatus as air is insufflated into the esophagus. The proximal margin of the gastric folds is the best landmark for the end of the esophagus and the beginning of the stomach.[14]

The most characteristic feature of the metaplastic esophageal epithelium is the color change that takes place between the squamous epithelium of the normal esophagus and the Barrett's mucosa. The former is a pale pink-gray, whereas the latter has a richer pink, velvety appearance. Congestion of the friable mucosa, linear erosions covered with pseudomembranes, a large, deep ulcer, and stricture formation are other suggestive features. Staining of the esophageal mucosa with toluidine blue at the time of endoscopy may aid in identifying columnar epithelium. Iodine (Lugol's solution) reacts with the glycogen of the squamous epithelium, staining it dark, and does not affect the columnar epithelium.[15] However, these measures are not sufficiently helpful or reliable to merit routine use. The measurement of transmural electrical potential differences (columnar epithelium has a higher negative charge than squamous epithelium)[16] also has not been widely adopted as a means of identifying Barrett's mucosa.[17]

Histologic Characteristics

There are three groupings of columnar cells in Barrett's esophagus.[18,19] One is similar to the gastric glands of the fundus and body of the stomach, and is referred to as *gastric–fundic epithelium*. The surface of this type of epithelium is covered with mucous cells and is pitted, as is the mucosa in the fundus and body of the stomach. The deeper glandular tissue contains chief and parietal cells as well as mucous cells. The appearance resembles a form of atrophic mucosa that might be found in the fundus and body of the stomach. A second type of epithelium seen in Barrett's esophagus resembles the epithelium seen in the cardia, and is referred to as *junctional-type epithelium*. The third kind of mucosa present in Barrett's esophagus is characteristic of the small and large intestine and contains large numbers of goblet cells, and is referred to as *specialized columnar-type epithelium*.

The cardia, fundus, and antrum of the stomach normally contain mucus-secreting cells that are distinctively different from the classic goblet cells of the intestine. Goblet cells are found in the stomach only under pathologic conditions. The mucous cells normally found in the stomach stain positively for neutral mucin with periodic acid-Schiff reagent, but stain negatively for acid mucopolysaccharide with reagents such as alcian blue.[20] In contrast to the mucous cells of the stomach, goblet cells stain positively for acid mucopolysaccharide with alcian blue. This type of epithelium has been called intestinal metaplastic epithelium. It is further characterized by irregularly sized and shaped villous projections.[21] Paneth and enterochromaffin cells such as occur in the small intestine may also be present in the specialized type of columnar epithelium. Mature, functioning absorptive cells, characterized by the presence of the specialized apical striated border, are not frequently seen in this form of Barrett's mucosa.[22–24]

The content and organization of the various forms of columnar epithelium found in Barrett's esophagus vary. A single type of Barrett's epithelium may be present, or any combination of the three types. The specialized columnar type occurs most often and is most frequently associated with malignant transformation, similar to its counterpart in the stomach. There is a tendency for the different forms of epithelium to be confined to zones within the mucosa. Intestinal metaplastic (specialized) epithelium usually occurs adjacent to the proximal squamous mucosa, whereas the other forms tend to be found more distally. The interface between these zones is indistinct and irregular. Chronic inflammatory changes and mononuclear cell infiltrates are common to all forms of Barrett's esophagus. Many esophagi involved with Barrett's esophagus may have a doubling or thickening of the smooth muscle layer, with some fibrosis.[25,26]

FUNCTIONAL CONSIDERATIONS

The lower esophageal sphincter is defective in 93% of patients with Barrett's esophagus, which is in contrast to 46% among patients with uncomplicated esophagitis and 4% among control subjects.[27,28] The mean amplitude of contractions in the distal esophagus is also significantly reduced in the presence of Barrett's esophagus. pH monitoring shows much greater esophageal acid and alkaline exposure in patients with columnar epithelium than in patients with esophagitis alone.[28]

Mucin secretion by Barrett's epithelium differs from that of normal gastric mucosa.[29–31] Normal gastric mucosa is characterized by neutral mucin, but acid mucins of the sulfomucin type are found in most cases of Barrett's esophagus. Submucosal esophageal glands and goblet cells of the colon are rich in sulfomucins, whereas the goblet cells of the small intestine contain only sialomucins. Among the columnar cells found in the metaplastic mucosa, the colonic type of goblet cells containing sulfomucins are most frequently associated with esophageal adenocarcinomas.

Fundic-type epithelium in the esophagus can in some instances secrete acid, particularly when stimulated by histamine.[32–34] Pepsin elaboration may also take place, as evidenced by the finding of acid proteases (pepsinogen isoenzymes) in the gastric–fundic type of metaplastic columnar epithelium.[35–38] However, it is unlikely that the volume of acid–peptic factors would be sufficient to produce ulceration.

Hormonal production can also occur. Immunohistochemical evidence of gastrin, bombesin, substance P, somatostatin, and serotonin synthesis has been demonstrated in Barrett's esophagus.[39] Gastrin and somatostatin are most frequently identified in the cancers, whereas somatostatin and serotonin predominate in nonmalignant tissue. Although disaccharidase activity is normally located in brush borders of intestinal cells, this activity is deficient or absent in Barrett's mucosa.[40]

ETIOLOGY AND PATHOGENESIS

Congenital Persistence of the Columnar-Lined Esophagus

A congenital origin of Barrett's mucosa would be consistent with the embryologic development of the esophagus, which is a tube of columnar cells during early embryonic life. This solid tube subsequently develops a lumen that becomes lined with ciliated columnar cells at the 40-mm fetal stage. During the 14th to 17th weeks of embryonic life, squamous cells appear in the middle third of the esophagus and spread craniad and caudad, gradually lining the entire lumen of the esophagus by the seventh month of gestation. The cervical esophagus is the last area to change from columnar to squamous epithelium.[41,42] If this process is arrested during fetal life, segments of the esophagus could remain lined with glandular epithelium rather than squamous epithelium. Alternatively, patches of fundic gastric mucosa in the esophagus might represent heterotopic deposits of displaced embryonic tissue, such as occasionally occurs in a Meckel's diverticulum.[41] Functioning heterotopic gastric mucosa in the cervical esophagus has been reported in up to 10% of children and adults.[43–46] However, these patients are not included among those referred to as having a Barrett's esophagus, and are infrequently symptomatic. About 6% may complain of dysphagia, and stricture formation and carcinoma occur rarely. The frequency of reflux esophagitis and Barrett's esophagus in these patients is the same as in a population of patients without gastric mucosa in the cervical esophagus.[44] Furthermore, the specialized type of epithelium found in Barrett's esophagus characterized by goblet cells does not occur in the patches of gastric mucosa found in the cervical esophagus, and these lesions do not have the same malignant potential that the columnar-lined lower esophagus has.

Acquired Origin of Columnar-Lined Lower Esophagus: Association With Reflux Esophagitis

In 1960, Goldman and Beckman proposed that Barrett's epithelium is most likely acquired in response to esophageal injury.[47] Similar observations from other investigators have strengthened this hypothesis.[9,48–50] Most clinical and experimental studies of the pathology of reflux esophagitis do not reveal replacement of the squamous cell mucosa of the esophagus by columnar epithelium,[51–54] as might be expected based on the fourfold to fivefold more rapid turnover of columnar cells compared with squamous cells. However, a few studies have shown this to happen under certain conditions.[55–57]

The prevalence of Barrett's esophagus at endoscopy among patients with reflux esophagitis ranges from 2.5% to 23.8%, with a mean of about 10%.[13] A 21-fold greater prevalence was found in an extensive autopsy series compared to a concurrent endoscopic series.[58] The prevalence of Barrett's esophagus increases with age, reaching a plateau in the seventh decade. Half the maximum prevalence is reached by age 40 years, which is the estimated median age of development.[59] This is consistent with an acquired rather than a congenital etiology. Furthermore, conditions predisposing to reflux esophagitis are also associated with Barrett's esophagus, and these patients are also at increased risk for development of adenocarcinoma of the esophagus; these conditions include scleroderma (wherein one third of patients have been found to have Barrett's esophagus),[60,61] the aftermath of esophagogastrectomy (in one series half the patients had glandular epithelium in the distal esophagus after this operation),[62] Zollinger-Ellison syndrome,[63] and patients with achalasia who have had an esophagomyotomy.[64,65]

Patients with reflux esophagitis and a columnar cell-lined lower esophagus have been shown to have a significantly greater esophageal acid exposure with poorer clearance and a higher acid output than patients who have reflux esophagitis and a squamous cell lining.[27,28,66] All of these studies have had their critics,[67,68] and there is no consistent relation allowing prediction of which patients with reflux esophagitis will go on to have Barrett's esophagus. The possibility that regurgitation of alkaline secretions into the esophagus may play a role in the pathogenesis of Barrett's esophagus has also been considered.[69,70] It is known that biliary and pancreatic secretions can cause esophagitis,[71] and it appears that patients with duodenogastric reflux and Barrett's esophagus have more problems than those who do not experience regurgitation of alkaline secretions into the stomach and esophagus.[70] It is also known that a glandular lining can develop in the distal esophagus after a total gastrectomy,[72] indicating that incompetence of the lower esophageal sphincter and acid–peptic digestion are not the only requirements for the development of a Barrett's esophagus.

Barrett's esophagus has been reported to develop in both adults and children receiving chemotherapy.[73,74] In a carefully conducted study, 63% of 16 women whose esophagus was normal by esophagoscopy before chemotherapy had a columnar cell-lined lower esophagus 6 months after receiving methotrexate, 5-fluorouracil, and cyclophosphamide.[73] It was postulated that the drugs induced mucosal erosions and ulcerations with reepithelialization by undifferentiated stem cells that developed into a typical Barrett's mucosa. The possibility that gastroesophageal reflux plays a role in the pathogenesis of Barrett's esophagus cannot be excluded.

Many series of Barrett's esophagus with and without complicating adenocarcinoma include a high percentage of patients with a history of smoking and alcohol consumption.[11,75] However, not all studies confirm this,[76,77] and a comparative study of patients with various malignancies of the esophagus and stomach, with and without Barrett's esophagus, only showed a significant relationship between cigarettes, alcohol, and squamous cell carcinoma of the esophagus.[78] *Helicobacter pylori* has been found in some specimens of Barrett's mucosa, but it is not likely that it plays a causative role in the development of Barrett's esophagus.[79]

Genetic Factors

Two observations suggest a possible genetic predisposition to the development of Barrett's esophagus. The first is a consistent finding in many series of patients with Barrett's esophagus, with and without adenocarcinomas, that this condition rarely occurs in nonwhites.[76,80–85] Second, there are several reports of familial Barrett's esophagus, one of which suggested an autosomal dominant inheritance pattern with nearly complete penetrance.[76,86,87] It is not clear whether the genetic association is related to reflux esophagitis per se or the development of metaplasia. Harle and associates[76] stated that their experience with twins in whom adenocarcinoma developed within months of each other gave credence to a congenital basis for Barrett's esophagus rather than an acquired one, because one of the twins had a long history of reflux esophagitis and the other did not.

Twenty-one of 23 patients with nonmalignant variants of Barrett's esophagus were white in the University of Chicago series, as were all of the 20 patients with malignant Barrett's esophagus. In contrast, their overall patient population and their patients with squamous cell carcinoma of the esophagus were approximately one-third African American.[76] In the Detroit metropolitan area, the ratio of blacks to whites with squamous cell carcinoma is approximately 4 to 1. That ratio is reversed when patients with adenocarcinoma are reviewed.[83] At the Baltimore Veterans Administration Medical Center, 36% of white patients with esophageal cancer had adenocarcinoma of the esophagus, compared with only 2.4% of black patients with cancer of the esophagus.[80]

Although there are those who continue to believe that some forms of Barrett's esophagus could be of congenital origin,[88,89] the evidence for this is weak. Nor does it appear that the columnar cells represent an overgrowth of epithelium from the stomach or submucosal glands of the esophagus into an esophagus denuded of a mucosa by erosive esophagitis. As has been pointed out, Barrett's mucosa and these other glandular tissues are histologically different. The many studies of Barrett's mucosa, clinical and experimental, morphologic and functional, and its capacity to undergo dysplastic changes and neoplastic transformation, suggest that it arises from cells that have undergone a genetic transformation, the nature of which is unclear.

DIAGNOSIS AND MANAGEMENT OF BARRETT'S ESOPHAGUS

Approximately 80% of patients with Barrett's esophagus are male, most often white, and 40 years of age or older. Children up to 15 years of age have also been found to have Barrett's esophagus.[13] Other than esophagoscopy and biopsy, there are no clinical tests or signs or symptoms of reflux esophagitis that can distinguish between patients with and without this complication. Furthermore, it appears that patients who have the metaplastic columnar epithelium have fewer symptoms than those who do not.[27,28] Radiographic studies have a low diagnostic specificity and sensitivity, but suspicion can be high when the classic picture of a stricture and ulceration is present.

The generally accepted average prevalence rate of Barrett's esophagus found endoscopically among patients with reflux symptoms is 10%. To establish the diagnosis, biopsy specimens should be obtained using a large (3.5-mm) forceps beginning 3 cm above the gastroesophageal junction and again every 2 cm from each quadrant until passing the squamocolumnar junction.[90] Two to four specimens at each level are necessary to obtain a complete histopathologic picture and to detect areas of dysplasia and in situ carcinoma.[91] Areas of high-grade dysplasia and carcinoma can be patchy.

Management of Patients Without Dysplasia

Patients with Barrett's esophagus who show no signs of dysplasia on systematic biopsy of the involved esophagus are treated no differently than other patients with reflux esophagitis, except for surveillance endoscopy when they are asymptomatic. Symptomatic patients must be monitored very closely and biopsied periodically (see below) to prevent an underlying carcinoma from being overlooked. An antireflux procedure is indicated when medical therapy cannot control disabling symptoms or if a significant complication of reflux esophagitis supervenes. Regression of the metaplastic epithelium has been reported only in a small number of patients undergoing operative or nonoperative therapy.[89,92–94] In a review of 159 patients who had an antireflux procedure, 3% demonstrated complete regression, and 8% had partial regression.[13] Thus, neither operative nor nonoperative treatment of reflux esophagitis significantly limits the progress of Barrett's esophagus or protects the patient from development of an adenocarcinoma.[95]

RISK OF ADENOCARCINOMA DEVELOPING IN BARRETT'S ESOPHAGUS AND RECOMMENDATIONS FOR SCREENING PATIENTS WITHOUT DYSPLASIA

It has been suggested that the risk of esophageal cancer in patients with Barrett's esophagus is about 30- to 40-fold greater than that in the general population.[96] However, the incidence of malignancy (the percentage of patients with Barrett's esophagus in whom adenocarcinoma develops over a given period of time) is a more reliable indicator of the risk than the prevalence of cancer. The latter does not consider the time span over which the cancers develop, and is usually reported as the percentage of patients newly diagnosed with Barrett's esophagus (ie, those who were found to have a coexisting carcinoma). The Working Party on Barrett's Esophagus, reporting to the World Congress of Gastroenterology in 1990, made the additional suggestion of requiring that the risk be estimated on patients with Barrett's esophagus who undergo endoscopic surveillance.[90] Using the measurement of the number of cancers found per patient-years of follow-up, and following these guidelines, they found estimates of 1/175,[82] 1/56,[97] and 1/52[98] in the literature. One series reporting a lower incidence of cancer in their patients with Barrett's esophagus (1/441) relied on information obtained from historical sources rather than from endoscopic surveillance. In Australia, an incidence 61 times the age-adjusted incidence of esophageal carcinoma was found (ie, 1/96 patient-years). A more recent review expanded the data base on which estimates of the incidence of adenocarcinoma in patients with Barrett's esophagus could be determined[99] and supported the view that it could be as high as 125 times greater than in the general population.[98]

Early estimates of the prevalence of carcinoma in patients with Barrett's esophagus put this figure at 10% (ie, among 1225 patients undergoing esophagoscopy with a clinical diagnosis of reflux esophagitis, 140 had Barrett's esophagus and 12 had adenocarcinoma).[100] Among 241 patients with Barrett's esophagus seen at the Lahey Clinic, 27% presented with adenocarcinoma,[99] a figure close to the 25% prevalence reported by the group from the University of Western Ontario.[76] Another study of the prevalence of Barrett's esophagus in patients with adenocarcinoma of the esophagus and esophagogastric junction from Johns Hopkins Hospital, based on extensive histopathologic examination of 61 surgically resected specimens, found metaplastic columnar epithelium in the esophagus in 64% of patients.[101] Before surgery, only 38% of the patients had been known to have Barrett's esophagus. A previous publication from the same institution had reported that the overall prevalence of Barrett's esophagus in patients undergoing esophagoscopy and biopsy for evaluation of symptoms compatible with gastroesophageal reflux was 8%. Their yearly prevalence of Barrett's esophagus ranged from 4% to 14%.[102] They postulated that Barrett's esophagus was "underrecognized" by pathologists and endoscopists who examine the esophagus in a routine manner.

There are some striking differences in the interpretations given to the incidence and prevalence figures. Haggitt considered the possibility that adenocarcinoma in Barrett's esophagus represented a "new epidemic,"[103] citing the data published by Blot and associates that showed that over the past two decades the incidence of adenocarcinoma of the esophagus and gastric cardia increased at a rate exceeding that of any other cancer.[104] Spechler estimated an incidence of 500 cancers per 100,000 Barrett's esophagus patients per year,[105] a figure equivalent to the incidence of lung cancer in older white men and greater than the incidence of esophageal cancer in the high-risk areas of China, where mass surveillance programs for cancer of the esophagus have been shown to result in improved survival after surgery.[106] Conversely, other authors have questioned whether the benefits of frequent endoscopy and biopsy are worth the effort and expense of such a large undertaking.[107–110] It is argued that there is no evidence that routine surveillance will increase survival of patients with carcinoma in Barrett's esophagus, and urged that surveillance be confined to patients who are at greater risk for development of cancer, such as those with dysplasia or those who will be candidates for operative therapy.

Specific recommendations have been made by the group at the Cleveland Clinic after reviewing their experience with this problem. They reported an incidence of adenocarcinoma in Barrett's esophagus of 0.64% per year and estimated that the cost of yearly endoscopic surveillance would be $62,000, with 78 lost work days to discover one cancer during the follow-up period.[111] They concluded that biannual examinations made better sense. The Working Party on Barrett's Esophagus also recommended that patients without dysplasia should have thorough histologic sampling at approximately 18- to 24-month intervals, with more frequent follow-up if dysplasia developed.[90] The American Society for Gastrointestinal Endoscopy recommend "periodic" endoscopic examinations with multiple brushings and biopsy samplings, but were not precise as to how frequently they should be done.[112] Others endorse frequent and close endoscopic surveillance of all patients with Barrett's esophagus, but also are often reluctant to provide precise recommendations because there are no good data to support a specific frequency.[11,76,100,108,113,114]

Management of Patients With Dysplasia in Barrett's Esophagus

Tytgat's review of the incidence of cancer in esophageal columnar metaplasia (his term for Barrett's esophagus) stressed the fact that adenocarcinoma "does not appear to arise de novo but rather to evolve through a series of progressively worsening dysplastic changes in the columnar epithelium."[115] It is Ried's view, based on studies that he and his colleagues have carried out, and from a review of the literature, that "patients appear to progress from Barrett's specialized metaplasia to abnormalities in the indefinite/low-grade dysplasia range, to high-grade dysplasia and eventually to carcinoma."[116] "Specialized metaplasia" refers to the intestinal-type goblet and columnar cells seen in Barrett's esophagus. It has been suggested that dysplasia is significantly greater in patients with Barrett's esophagus of 8 cm or greater.[117]

Dysplasia is defined as unequivocal neoplastic alterations in the appearance and organization of the columnar cells, without evidence of invasiveness. It can be further subdivided into low-grade and high-grade varieties. Low-grade dysplasia may be difficult to differentiate from hyperplastic changes secondary to inflammation and includes those diagnoses that can be characterized as indeterminate or indefinite.[118] High-grade dysplasia is present when there is gross distortion of the glands, with cells crowded together and containing hyperchromatic nuclei with large nucleoli. High-grade dysplasia includes examples of in situ carcinoma.[24,98,118–122] Intramucosal carcinoma is considered "early carcinoma." It is diagnosed when there is invasion of sheets of malignant cells into the lamina propria of the mucosa but not extending through the muscularis mucosa. Submucosal extension of the cancer has also been referred to as early carcinoma.[118,119] These two entities should not be confused with dysplasia.

In a study of 81 patients with Barrett's esophagus followed with endoscopic biopsy for a total of 289 patient-years, dysplasia developed in 28%.[123] Of 10 patients with low-grade dysplasia on the initial endoscopy, 1 progressed to adenocarcinoma in 4.3 years, 2 regressed after 3 to 5 years, and 7 remained the same for 1.5 to 7 years. Low-grade dysplasia developed in 10 additional patients during the period of surveillance. Thus, patients with low-grade dysplasia require closer surveillance than patients who do not have dysplasia. They should have repeat biopsies every 6 to 24 months.[116]

It is widely accepted that the pathologic diagnosis of the various forms of dysplasia on biopsy is difficult. Rigorous adherence to the guidelines suggested for performing biopsies on patients with Barrett's esophagus should be adhered to to be sure that the involved mucosa is adequately sampled.[90,112] It is also important that pathologists experienced in the diagnosis of gastrointestinal malignancies be relied on to diagnose dysplasia.

Although there is unanimous agreement that high-grade dysplasia is an ominous marker for the development of invasive cancer, there is little agreement about what to recommended once a diagnosis of high-grade dysplasia is made. A number of groups recommend esophagectomy for high-grade dysplasia, even though the data supporting this are somewhat anecdotal.[121,122,124,125] In one series of five patients who had high-grade dysplasia and underwent esophagectomy, three superficially invasive cancers were found.[122] This group also found that 93% of 43 esophagectomy specimens resected for Barrett's carcinoma had high-grade dysplasia.[122] In another report, three of eight patients with dysplasia were found to have invasive cancer after an esophagectomy was performed.[124] The Lahey Clinic group followed 176 patients for a total of 497 patient-years. Five patients were found to have adenocarcinoma 1, 2, 2, 4, and 10 years after the initial diagnosis of Barrett's esophagus. In all five, high-grade dysplasia had developed before invasive carcinoma was detected.[99] The Mayo Clinic has the largest series of esophagectomies for high-grade dysplasia.[125] A total of 50% of 18 patients had invasive carcinoma. Overall 5-year survival was 66.7%.

Another approach is to follow patients with high-grade dysplasia very closely "and recommend surgery only when unquestionable proof of malignancy has been obtained . . . because it is unknown if and when high-grade dysplasia will progress to carcinoma in an individual patient and because the risks of surgical resection are substantial."[98] The group making this recommendation base their view on data similar to those presented by those who recommend esophagectomy—namely, five of eight patients with high-grade dysplasia in whom invasive carcinoma developed after a follow-up of 1.5 to 10 years. Three patients underwent surgery; one died after surgery. All three cancers were found not to have penetrated the muscularis propria, and the excised lymph nodes were negative for tumor. Advocates of the nonoperative approach also point out that in some patients with high-grade dysplasia the condition may remain stable for years without becoming invasive, and in others it may even regress.[16,126] Ried recommends medical treatment to diminish reflux and repeat biopsy in 3 months, in the hope that the high-grade dysplasia will regress.[116] It is his contention that systematic endoscopic biopsies can detect early carcinoma before it becomes advanced and unresectable. Palley and colleagues recommend repeat biopsy within 1 month before considering esophagectomy, presumably to be sure of the diagnosis before undertaking the operation.[127]

From the preceding review of this problem, it is obvious that more reliable information is required to formulate a sound recommendation regarding what to do for patients with high-grade dysplasia. Until more precise markers of malignancy are developed, the dilemma of what to do about the malignant potential of Barrett's esophagus will remain unresolved. The preponderant view at present is to recommend esophagectomy for high-grade dysplasia.

MARKERS OF MALIGNANCY OTHER THAN DYSPLASIA

Because flow cytometry can be used to quantitate DNA content of nuclei and also determine the fraction of cells in the synthetic (S) phase or mitotic (G2) phase of the cell cycle, it has been used to determine if the malignant potential of Barrett's mucosa can be predicted. Most Barrett's adenocarcinomas are aneuploid (>70%). Dysplasia, in the absence of cancer, is present in approximately 44% of patients with aneuploidy.[128] Because aneuploidy is found more frequently than dysplasia in patients with Barrett's esophagus, and because some cancers may be diploid with normal G2/tetraploid fractions,[129] this modality is not sufficiently reliable for diagnostic purposes. However, determination of aneuploidy and increased G2/tetraploid cell populations may be useful in following patients with dysplasia.[129]

Flow cytometric studies have also produced insights into the pathogenesis of malignancy in Barrett's metaplasia. The presence of aneuploidy and increased G2 tetraploid content in metaplastic, dysplastic, and malignant forms of Barrett's esophagus suggest that these cells have an acquired genomic instability that is related to the process of carcinogenesis.[129] Cytogenetically abnormal clones have been detected in Barrett's mucosa that have been shown to progress to high-grade dysplasia and adenocarcinoma, lending credence to the theory that cancer develops by a multistep pathway of clonal evolution.[130]

The most frequently mutated gene in human cancer is one that can inhibit tumor growth, the tumor suppressor gene *P53*, located on the short arm of chromosome 17 (17p).[131] Mutations of this gene can be detected by analysis of cellular DNA or by detecting expression of the abnormal protein that is coded for by the mutated *P53*. Deletions in 17p may also be a manifestation of *P53* mutation. In one study, nonmalignant Barrett's esophagus expressed normal *P53*, whereas 42% of patients with malignant Barrett's esophagus had mutated *P53*.[132] Another group found 17p allelic depletions in 92% of 13 aneuploid Barrett's carcinomas. A total of 67% also had *P53* protein overexpression.[133] In another study, abnormal *P53* expression was found in 5% of patients with Barrett's metaplasia negative for dysplasia, 15% of patients with low-grade dysplasia, 45% of patients with high-grade dysplasia, and 53% of patients with Barrett's carcinoma.[134]

Mucin histochemistry has also been investigated as a predictor of malignancy. The mucin synthesized by the goblet cells of the specialized intestinal metaplastic cells of Barrett's mucosa is the same as that from the goblet cells of the colon, that is, a sulfated acid mucin that is foreign to the mucosa of the stomach, and that elaborates neutral mucins.[29–31] The detection of sulfated acid mucins in one study did not appear to be a sensitive or specific predictor of malignancy.[135] There are not sufficient data to be able to say whether depleted sialomucins in dysplastic Barrett's mucosa can be used as a predictor of malignant transformation.[30]

Flow cytometry has also been used to analyze for growth-regulatory peptides (epidermal growth factor and transforming growth factor-α) and their receptors in Barrett's esophagus and carcinoma. They may be increased in these instances, but the clinical utility of this finding remains to be established.[136] Mutations of the three *RAS* genes have not been detected under similar situations.[137]

Ornithine decarboxylase, an enzyme of polyamine biosynthesis, has been shown to be increased in Barrett's epithelium without concomitant increases in the polyamines putrescine, spermidine, and spermine. In these experiments, inhibitors of ornithine decarboxylase also inhibited the in vitro growth of Barrett's metaplastic epithelium.[138]

EXTRAESOPHAGEAL MALIGNANCIES, GASTROESOPHAGEAL CANCER, AND BARRETT'S ESOPHAGUS

Contradictory reports regarding the frequency of multiple malignancies in patients with cancer in Barrett's esophagus are irreconcilable. Among 115 patients followed over a 10-year period, 28 malignancies occurred in 25 patients.[82] Fifteen were head and neck and lung cancers that may have been related to the high rate of cigarette smokers (85%) and alcohol abusers (76%) in this series. However, five patients had colon cancer, and others have reported even higher frequencies of colon cancer in patients with Barrett's esophagus. A review of the problem concluded that a relation between cancer in Barrett's esophagus and colon cancer remains to be proved.[90] The same may be said for the occurrence of squamous cell carcinoma in Barrett's esophagus. A total of 16 such cases have been reported in the literature.[139] These anecdotal reports of a high frequency of synchronous and metachronous multiple cancers in Barrett's esophagus require confirmation by a controlled statistical study.

During the same period of time that the number of esophageal adenocarcinomas arising from the metaplastic epithelium of Barrett's esophagus has increased, there has been an increase in the number of cancers involving the cardia and gastroesophageal junction. Cancers arising from the proximal stomach have clinical and pathologic characteristics that are different from those of the distal stomach, but are similar to those of the adenocarcinomas arising in Barrett's esophagus.[24,140–143] It is possible that many of the gastroesophageal adenocarcinomas arise from what has been referred to as "short segment Barrett's esophagus."[90] This designation refers to the presence of acid-mucin–containing goblet cells (ie, staining positive with alcian blue) that define the specialized intestinal metaplastic epithelium thought to be the cell type in Barrett's esophagus that has the capacity to become cancerous. Although the distal 3 cm of the esophagus may contain glandular mucosal cells normally found in the stomach, the specialized metaplastic intestinal columnar cells are considered abnormal (ie, pathologic) when they are present anywhere in the area of the gastroesophageal junction.[90,98,144] Because of the similarities between the gastroesophageal and esophageal carcinomas, they are being treated the same way, and many series have lumped the two together when discussing the results of therapy.

MANAGEMENT OF ADENOCARCINOMA IN BARRETT'S ESOPHAGUS

Attempts at chemoprevention using 13-*cis*-retinoic acid showed little promise in one preliminary study, which also suggested α-difluoromethylornithine, an irreversible inhibitor of ornithine decarboxylase, as a potential chemopreventive agent.[145]

Current approaches to the staging and treatment of patients with adenocarcinoma do not differ from those that have been in vogue since the 1980s in treating squamous cell carcinoma. Accurate clinical staging continues to be difficult, with great dependence being placed on endoultrasonography and computed tomography of the chest and upper abdomen. Accurate pathologic staging after esophageal resection depends on the removal of the relevant draining lymph nodes at the time of esophagectomy to determine if they are involved. The regional lymph nodes of the intrathoracic esophagus include those in the mediastinal and perigastric areas, excluding the celiac nodes that are considered distant metastases if they are involved.[146]

Stage I cancer is invasive cancer confined to the mucosa or submucosa without lymph node involvement. Stage II is divided into lymph node negative (IIA) and lymph node positive (IIB). Stage IIA includes tumors that invade the adventitia (T3); stage IIB does not. T3 tumors with lymph node involvement are considered stage III, along with tumors that invade adjacent organs, regardless of lymph node involvement. Stage IV is any cancer with distant metastases. When this staging system was applied to 94 patients with squamous cell carcinoma who survived a curative resection, no differences in 5-year survival were found between stages IIA, IIB, and II (about 20%).[147] Conversely, a larger study from Japan did show differences among these three stages,[148] indicating that additional refinements in the staging system for cancer of the esophagus may be necessary.

Until the early 1980s, esophagectomy alone was the mainstay of therapy for adenocarcinoma of the esophagus. The multimodality protocols for squamous cell carcinoma that use adjuvant chemotherapy and radiation therapy to control micrometastatic disease and improve local control are now also being used to treat adenocarcinoma of the esophagus. Like squamous cell carcinoma of the esophagus, adenocarcinoma of the esophagus has proved to be a tumor that is not easily cured by surgery alone or by multimodality therapy.

Up until the 1980s, publications on the results of surgery consisted of case reports or reviews of the literature with a collection of several patients from the authors' experience. A study published in 1974 compared an experience with 18 patients who had esophagectomy for adenocarcinoma (11 of whom had adenocarcinoma of the esophagogastric junction) with an experience with more than 200 patients with squamous cell carcinoma. It was concluded that "the prognosis for adenocarcinoma of the esophagus is as poor as, and probably worse than, that for epidermoid carcinoma."[149] However, experience with adenocarcinoma of the esophagus was still limited. As of 1975, the total number of cases reported in the literature was only 57.[150] By 1983, the largest series of patients with adenocarcinoma of Barrett's esophagus reported from a single center still consisted of no more than 20 patients and, again, the results of surgical therapy were no better than those reported for squamous cell carcinoma.[11,151] Up until the 1990s there were many similar reports, presenting a variable amount of data and varying lengths of follow-up. In 1991, the Lahey Clinic published their series of 60 esophagectomies for Barrett's cancer, with a hospital mortality rate of 3.3%.[85] Overall adjusted survival curves calculated by the Kaplan-Meier method resulted in a 23.7% 5-year survival that was not statistically significantly different from their results with adenocarcinoma of the cardia (22.4%) and squamous cell carcinoma of the esophagus (17.3%). In this series, stage was a significant independent predictor of survival. The 3-year survival for stage I disease was 85.7%; it was 53.6% for stage IIA and 0% for stage IV. There were insufficient numbers in the other stages to generate meaningful data.

In a series from Munich, of 106 resected patients with cancer in Barrett's esophagus, the 30-day mortality rate was 5.4%.[152] Among the 36.3% of patients with T1 and T2 primaries, the mortality rate was 2.6%. Patients with T3 and T4 primaries had a mortality rate of 11.7%. Again, "the 5-year survival rates of all patients with Barrett's carcinomas were not significantly different from the series of squamous cell carcinomas (Barrett's carcinoma: 5-year survival rate 29%; squamous cell carcinoma: 5-year survival rate 25%)."[152] Furthermore, no difference in prognosis was found between these patients and those with cancers of the cardia. The one encouraging finding was the close to 75% 4-year actuarial survival of 21 patients with adenocarcinomas confined to the mucosa and submucosa. Moon and colleagues found no difference in morbidity and survival between transhiatal and transthoracic esophagectomy for adenocarcinoma of the esophagus in their series of 93 patients.[153] They also obtained an 86% overall 5-year survival in 14 patients with stage I and II disease, a finding that would relate to the previous discussion in this chapter on the topic of screening patients with Barrett's esophagus for early carcinoma.

Probably because of the similarity in behavior between adenocarcinoma and squamous cell carcinoma of the esophagus, many clinical therapeutic trials include patients with either lesion in their series. An example of this is the report by Herskovic and coworkers of the prospective, controlled, randomized study carried out by the Radiation Therapy Oncology Group.[154] The median survival was 8.9 months in the patients treated with radiation alone, compared with 12.5 months in the patients treated with concurrent cisplatin and 5-fluorouracil. This difference remained significant when controlled for the 12.4% of patients who had adenocarcinoma. In a randomized study of postoperative radiation versus surgery alone, 20% of the patients had adenocarcinoma.[155] Their response was the same as that of the patients with squamous cell carcinoma; no benefit was seen in any of the groups of patients.

An ongoing prospective, controlled, randomized trial of surgery alone versus preoperative chemotherapy conducted by the Radiation Therapy Oncology Group has also entered patients with both squamous cell carcinoma and adenocarcinoma. More than half of the patients entered into this study have had adenocarcinoma of the esophagus. The results of this study have not yet been reported. It is scientifically conducted trials such as these that will determine the best treatment for adenocarcinoma arising in Barrett's esophagus.

REFERENCES

1. Barrett N. Chronic peptic ulcer of the oesophagus and oesophagitis. Br J Surg 1950;38:175.
2. Allison PR. Peptic ulcer of the oesophagus. Thorax 1948;3:419.
3. Allison PR, Johnston AS. The oesophagus lined with gastric mucous membrane. Thorax 1953;8:87.
4. Barrett N. The lower esophagus lined by columnar epithelium. Surgery 1957;41:881.
5. Blot WJ, Devesa SS, Kneller RW, Fraumeni JF. Rising incidence of adenocarcinoma of the esophagus and gastric cardia. JAMA 1991; 265:1287, and 1993;270:1320.
6. Yang PC, Davis S. Incidence of cancer of the esophagus in the US by histologic type. Cancer 1988;61:612.
7. Smithers DW. The association of cancer of the stomach and oesophagus with herniation at the oesophageal hiatus of the diaphragm. Br J Radiol 1955;28:554.
8. Adler RH, Rodriguez J. The association of hiatus hernia and gastroesophageal malignancy. J Thorac Surg 1959;37:553.
9. Adler RH. The lower esophagus lined by columnar epithelium: its association with hiatal hernia, ulcer, stricture and tumor. J Thorac Cardiovasc Surg 1963;45:13.
10. Goyal RK, Clancy JJ, Spiro HM. Lower esophageal ring. N Engl J Med 1970;282:1298.
11. Skinner DB, Walther BC, Riddell RH, et al. Barrett's esophagus: comparison of benign and malignant cases. Ann Surg 1983;198:554.
12. Winters C, Spurling TJ, Chobanian SJ, et al. Barrett's esophagus: a prevalent, occult complication of gastroesophageal reflux disease. Gastroenterology 1987;92:118.
13. Phillips RW, Wong RKH. Barrett's esophagus: natural history, incidence, etiology and complications. Gastroenterol Clin North Am 1991;20:791.
14. McClave SA, Boyce HW, Gottfried MR. Early diagnosis of columnar-lined esophagus: a new endoscopic diagnostic criterion. Gastrointest Endosc 1987;33:413.
15. Burbige EJ, Radigan JI. Characteristics of the columnar-cell lined (Barrett's) esophagus. Gastrointest Endosc 1979;25:133.
16. Kinard HB, Jones JD, Orlando RC, et al. Esophageal potential difference measurement as an indicator of mucosal disease. Gastroenterology 1979;76:1169.
17. Herlihy KJ, Orlando RC, Bryson JC, et al. Barrett's esophagus: clinical endoscopic, histologic, manometric and electrical potential difference characteristics. Gastroenterology 1984;86:436.
18. Trier J. Morphology of the epithelium of the distal esophagus in patients with midesophageal peptic strictures. Gastroenterology 1970; 58:444.
19. Paull A, Trier J, Dalton D, et al. The histologic spectrum of Barrett's esophagus. N Engl J Med 1976;295:476.
20. Ham AW, Leeson TS. Histology. 4th ed. Philadelphia: JB Lippincott, 1961.
21. Mangla JC. Barrett's esophagus: an old identity rediscovered. J Clin Gastroenterol 1981;3:347.
22. Gottfried MR, McClave SA, Boyce HW. Incomplete intestinal metaplasia in the diagnosis of columnar lined esophagus (Barrett's esophagus). Am J Clin Pathol 1989;92:741.
23. Rothery GA, Patterson JE, Stoddard CJ, et al. Histological and histochemical changes in the columnar lined (Barrett's) esophagus. Gut 1986;27:1062.
24. Thompson JJ, Zinsser KR, Enterline HT. Barrett's metaplasia and adenocarcinoma of the esophagus and gastroesophageal junction. Hum Pathol 1983;14:42.
25. Takubo K, Sasajima K, Yamashita K, et al. Double muscularis mucosae in Barrett's esophagus. Hum Pathol 1991;22:1158.
26. Rubio CA, Aberg B. Further studies on the musculo-fibrous anomaly of the Barrett's mucosa in esophageal carcinomas. Pathol Res Pract 1991;187:1009.
27. Iascone C, DeMeester TR, Little AG, et al. Barrett's esophagus: functional assessment proposed pathogenesis, and surgical therapy. Arch Surg 1983;118:543.
28. Stein HJ, Hoeft S, DeMeester TR. Reflux and motility pattern in Barrett's esophagus. Diseases of the Esophagus 1992;5:21.
29. Jass JR. Mucin histochemistry of the columnar epithelium of the oesophagus: a retrospective study. J Clin Pathol 1981;34:866.
30. Lapertosa G, Baracchini P, Fulcheri E, et al. Mucin histochemical analysis in the interpretation of Barrett's esophagus: results of a multicenter study. Am J Clin Pathol 1992;98:61.
31. Chajfec G, Schnell T, Sontag S. Barrett's esophagus: a preneoplastic disorder. Am J Clin Pathol 1992;98:5.
32. Hershfield NB, Lind JF, Hildes JA, et al. Secretory function of Barrett's epithelium. 1965;Gut 6:535.
33. Heitmann P, Strauszer T, Sapunar J, et al. Lower esophagus lined with columnar epithelium: morphological and physiological correlation. Gastroenterology 1967;53:611.
34. Ustach TJ, Lobon F, Shuster MM. Demonstration of acid secretion from esophageal mucosa in Barrett's ulcer. Gastrointest Endosc 1969; 16:98.
35. Mangla JC, Kim YM, Guarasci G, et al. Pepsinogens in epithelium of Barrett's esophagus. Gastroenterology 1973;65:949.
36. Mangla JC, Schenk EA, Desbaillets L, et al. Pepsin secretion, pepsinogen and gastrin in Barrett esophagus. Gastroenterology 1976;70:669.
37. Mangla JC, Camp R, Dalton D. Agar gel electrophoretic patterns of pepsinogen zymogens in Barrett esophagus. Biochem Med 1980;24: 39.
38. Pals G, Ericksson AW, Pronk JC, et al. Differential expression of pepsinogen isozymogens in a patient with Barrett esophagus. Clin Genet 1988;34:90.
39. Banner B, Memoli VA, Warren WH, et al. Carcinoma with multidirectional differentiation arising in Barrett's esophagus. Ultrastruct Pathol 1983;4:205.
40. Berenson MM, Herbot JJ, Freston JW. Enzyme and ultrastructural characteristics of esophageal columnar epithelium. Dig Dis 1974;19: 895.
41. Ming SC. Tumors of the esophagus and stomach. In: Atlas of tumor pathology, second series, fascicle 7. Washington, DC: Armed Forces Institute of Pathology.

42. Johns BAE. Developmental changes in the oesophageal epithelium in man. J Anat 1952;86:431.
43. Variend S, Howat AJ. Upper esophageal gastric heterotopia: a prospective necropsy study in children. J Clin Pathol 1988;41:742.
44. Borhan-Manesh F, Farnum JB. Incidence of heterotopic gastric mucosa in the upper esophagus. Gut 1991;32:968.
45. Hamilton JW, Thune RG, Morrissey JF. Symptomatic ectopic gastric epithelium in the cervical esophagus: demonstration of acid production with Congo red. Dig Dis Sci 1986;31:337.
46. Jabbari M, Goresky CA, Lough J, et al. The inlet patch: heterotopic gastric mucosa in the upper esophagus. Gastroenterology 1985;89: 352.
47. Goldman MC, Beckman RC. Barrett syndrome: case report with discussion about concepts of pathogenesis. Gastroenterology 1960;39: 104.
48. Hayward J. The treatment of fibrous stricture of the oesophagus associated with hiatal hernia. Thorax 1961;16:45.
49. Mossberg SM. The columnar-lined esophagus (Barrett's syndrome: an acquired condition?) Gastroenterology 1966;50:671.
50. Naef AP, Savary M. Conservative operations for peptic esophagitis with stenosis in columnar-lined lower esophagus. Ann Thorac Surg 1972;13:543.
51. Ingram PR, Keswani RK, Muller WH. A correlative histopathologic study of experimental surgical reflux esophagitis. Surg Gynecol Obstet 1960;111:403.
52. Helsingen N. Short esophagus: a sequel of reflux oesophagitis: experimental observations in gastrectomized rats. Acta Chir Scand 1961; 120:327.
53. Ismail-Beigi F, Horton PF, Pope CE. Histological consequences of gastroesophageal reflux in man. Gastroenterology 1970;58:163.
54. Hennessy TPJ, Edlich RF, Buchin RJ, et al. Influence of gastroesophageal incompetence on regeneration of esophageal mucosa. Arch Surg 1968;97:105.
55. Behar J, Sheaban DG, Biancani P, et al. Medical and surgical management of reflux esophagitis: a 38-month report on a prospective clinical trial. N Engl J Med 1975;293:263.
56. Bremner CG, Lynch VP, Ellis FH. Barrett's esophagus: congenital or acquired? An experimental study of esophageal mucosal regeneration in the dog. Surgery 1970;68:209.
57. Gillen P, Keeling P, Byrne PJ, et al. Experimental columnar metaplasia in the canine oesophagus. Br J Surg 1988;75:113.
58. Cameron AJ, Zinsmeister AR, Ballard DJ, et al. Prevalence of columnar-line (Barrett's) esophagus: comparison of population-based clinical and autopsy findings. Gastroenterology 1990;99:918.
59. Cameron A, Lowboy CT. Barrett's esophagus: age, prevalence and extent of columnar epithelium. Gastroenterology 1992;103:1241.
60. Halpert RD, Laufer I, Thompson JJ, et al. Adenocarcinoma of the esophagus in patients with scleroderma. AJR Am J Roentgenol 1983; 140:927.
61. Katzka DA, Reynolds JC, Saul SH, et al. Barrett's metaplasia and adenocarcinoma of the esophagus in scleroderma. Am J Med 1987; 82:46.
62. Hamilton SR, Yardley JH. Regeneration of cardiac type mucosa and acquisition of Barrett mucosa after esophagogastrostomy. Gastroenterology 1977;72:669.
63. Karl TR, Pindick F, Sicular A. Zollinger-Ellison syndrome with esophagitis and Barrett's mucosa. Am J Gastroenterol 1983;78:611.
64. Sprung DJ, Gibb SP. Barrett's esophagus in a patient with achalasia. Am J Gastroenterol 1985;80:330.
65. Agha FP, Jeren DF. Barrett's esophagus complicating achalasia after esophagomyotomy. J Clin Gastroenterol 1987;9:232.
66. Mulholland MW, Reid BJ, Levin DS. Elevated gastric acid secretion in patient's with Barrett's metaplastic epithelium. Dig Dis Sci 1989; 34:1229.
67. Parrilla P, Martinez de Haro LF, Aguayo JL, et al. Evaluation of the magnitude of gastro-esophageal reflux in Barrett's esophagus. Gut 1990;31:946.
68. Richter JE. Barrett's esophagus: too much acid, alkali or both? Gastroenterology 1990;98:798.
69. Waring JP, Legrand J, Chinichian A, et al. Duodenogastric reflux in patients with Barrett's esophagus. Dig Dis Sci 1990;35:759.
70. Atwood SE, DeMeester TR, Bremner CG, et al. Alkaline gastroesophageal reflux: implications in the development of complications in Barrett's columnar-lined lower esophagus. Surgery 1989;106:764.
71. Gillison EW, deCastro VAM, Nyhus LM, et al. The significance of bile in reflux esophagitis. Surg Gynecol Obstet 1972;134:419.
72. Tada T, Suzuki T, Iwafuchi M, et al. Adenocarcinoma arising in Barrett's esophagus after total gastrectomy. Am J Gastroenterol 1990;85: 1503.
73. Sartori S, Nielson I, Indelli M, et al. Barrett esophagus after chemotherapy with cyclophosphamide, methotrexate, and 5-fluorouracil (CMF): an iatrogenic injury? Ann Intern Med 1991;114:210.
74. Dahms BB. Barrett's esophagus in three children after antileukemia chemotherapy. Cancer 1987;60:2896.
75. Kalish RJ, Clancy PE, Orringer MB, et al. Clinical epidemiologic and morphologic comparison between adenocarcinoma arising in Barrett's esophageal mucosa and in the gastric cardia. Gastroenterology 1984; 86:461.
76. Harle IA, Finely RJ, Belsheim M, et al. Management of adenocarcinoma in a columnar-lined esophagus. Ann Thorac Surg 1985;40:330.
77. Levi F, Ollyo JB, LaVecchia C, et al. The consumption of tobacco, alcohol and the risk of adenocarcinoma in Barrett's esophagus. Int J Cancer 1990;45:852.
78. Gray JR, Coldman AJ, MacDonald WC. Cigarette and alcohol use in patients with adenocarcinoma of the gastric cardia or lower esophagus. Cancer 1992;69:2227.
79. Iascone C, Stipa S. Pathogenesis of Barrett's esophagus (BE). Diseases of the Esophagus 1992;5:13.
80. Rogers EL, Goldkind L, Goldkind SF. Increasing frequency of esophageal cancer among black veterans. Cancer 1982;49:610.
81. Smith RRL, Hamilton SR, Boitnott JK, et al. The spectrum of carcinoma arising in Barrett's esophagus: a clinicopathologic study of 26 patients. Am J Surg Pathol 1984;8:563.
82. Spechler SJ, Robbins AH, Rubins HB, et al. Adenocarcinoma and Barrett's esophagus: an overrated risk? Gastroenterology 1984;87: 927.
83. Rosenberg JC, Budev H, Edwards RC, et al. Analysis of adenocarcinoma in Barrett's esophagus utilizing a staging system. Cancer 1985; 55:1353.
84. Sanfey H, Hamilton SR, Smith RRK, et al. Carcinoma arising in Barrett's esophagus. Surg Gynecol Obstet 1985;161:570.
85. Streitz JM, Ellis FH, Gibb SP, et al. Adenocarcinoma in Barrett's esophagus: a clinicopathologic study of 65 cases. Ann Surg 1991; 213:122.
86. Jochem VJ, Fuerst PA, Fromkes JJ. Familial Barrett's esophagus associated with adenocarcinoma. Gastroenterology 1992;102:1400.
87. Crabb DW, Berk MA, Hall TR, et al. Familial gastroesophageal reflux and development of Barrett's esophagus. Ann Intern Med 1985;103: 52.
88. Ransom JM, Patel GK, Clift SA, et al. Extended and limited types of Barrett's esophagus in the adult. Ann Thorac Surg 1982;33:19.
89. Brand DL, Ylvisaker JT, Gelfand M, et al. Regression of columnar esophageal (Barrett's) epithelium after anti-reflux surgery. N Engl J Med 1980;302:844.
90. Dent J, Bremner CG, Collen MJ, et al. Working party report to the World Congress of Gastroenterology, Sydney 1990. J Gastreoenterol Hepatol 1991;6:1.
91. Katz PO, Castell DO. Barrett's esophagus: today's dilemma. Diseases of the Esophagus 1990;3:55.
92. Wesdorp ICE, Bartelsman J, Schipper MEI, et al. Effect of long-term treatment with cimetidine and antacids in Barrett's oesophagus. Gut 1981;22:724.
93. Saltzman M, Barwick K, McCullum RW. Progression of cimetidine-treated reflux esophagitis to a Barrett's stricture. Dig Dis Sci 1982; 27:181.
94. Cheu HW, Grosfeld JL, Heifetz SA, et al. Persistence of Barrett's esophagus in children after antireflux surgery: influence on follow-up care. J Pediatr Surg 1992;27:260.
95. Hamilton SR, Hutcheon DF, Ravich WJ, et al. Adenocarcinoma in Barrett's esophagus after elimination of gastroesophageal reflux. Gastroenterology 1984;86:356.
96. Spechler SJ, Goyal RK. Barrett's esophagus. N Engl J Med 1986; 315:362.
97. Robertson CS, Mayberry JF, Nicholson DA, et al. Value of endoscopic surveillance in the detection of neoplastic change in Barrett's esophagus. Br J Surg 1988;75:760.
98. Hamecteman W, Tygat GNJ, Houthoff HJ, et al. Barrett's esophagus:

development of dysplasia and adenocarcinoma. Gastroenterology 1989;96:1249.
99. Williamson WA, Ellis FH, Gibb SP, et al. Barrett's esophagus: prevalence and incidence of adenocarcinoma. Arch Intern Med 1991;151: 2212.
100. Naef AP, Savary M, Ozello L. Columnar-lined lower esophagus: report on 140 cases of Barrett's esophagus with 12 adenocarcinomas. J Thorac Cardiovasc Surg 1975;70:826.
101. Hamilton SR, Smith RL, Cameron JL. Prevalence and characteristics of Barrett's esophagus in patients with adenocarcinoma of the esophagus or esophagogastric junction. Hum Pathol 1988;19:942.
102. Sarr MG, Hamilton S, Marrone GC, et al. Barrett's esophagus: its prevalence and association with adenocarcinoma in patients with symptoms of gastroesophageal reflux. Am J Surg 1985;149:187.
103. Haggitt RC. Adenocarcinoma in Barrett's esophagus: a new epidemic? Human Pathol 1992;23:475.
104. Blot WJ, Denesa SS, Kneller RW, et al. Rising incidence of adenocarcinoma of the esophagus and gastric cardia. JAMA 1991;265:1287.
105. Spechler SJ. Endoscopic surveillance for patients with Barrett's esophagus: does the cancer risk justify the practice? Ann Intern Med 1987;106:902.
106. Huang GJ, Wu YK. Carcinoma of the esophagus and cardia. New York: Springer-Verlag, 1984.
107. Margulis AR, Shapiro HA. Barrett's esophagus. Radiology 1984;150: 602.
108. Sampliner RE. Does Barrett's esophagus need to be detected? Arch Intern Med 1986;146:43.
109. van der Veen AH, Dees J, Blankenstein JD, et al. Adenocarcinoma in Barrett's oesophagus: an overrated risk. Gut 1989;30:14.
110. Collins BJ, Abott M, Thomas RJS, et al. Clinical profile in Barrett's esophagus: who should be screened for cancer? Hepatogastroenterology 1991;38:341.
111. Achkar E, Carey W. The cost of surveillance for adenocarcinoma complicating Barrett's esophagus. Am J Gastroenterol 1988;83:291.
112. The role of endoscopy, in the surveillance of premalignant conditions of the upper gastrointestinal tract: guidelines for clinical application. Gastrointest Endosc 1988;34(Suppl):18.
113. Atkinson M. Barrett's oesophagus: to screen or not to screen? Gut 1989;30:2.
114. Skinner DB. The columnar-lined esophagus and adenocarcinoma. Ann Thorac Surg 1985;401:321.
115. Tytgat GNJ. Incidence of cancer in esophageal columnar metaplasia (Barrett's esophagus). Diseases of the Esophagus 1992;5:29.
116. Ried BJ. Barrett's esophagus and esophageal adenocarcinoma. Gastroenterol Clin North Am 1991;20:817.
117. Iftikhar SY, James PO, Steele RJC, et al. Length of Barrett's esophagus: an important factor in the development of dysplasia and adenocarcinoma Gut 1992;33:1155.
118. Ried BJ, Haggitt RC, Rubin CE, et al. Observer variation in the diagnosis of dysplasia in Barrett's esophagus. Hum Pathol 1988;19:166.
119. Ried BJ, Weinstein WM, Lewin KJ, et al. Endoscopic biopsy can detect high-grade dysphasia or early adenocarcinoma in Barrett's esophagus without grossly recognizable neoplastic lesions. Gastroenterology 1988;94:81.
120. Schmidt HG, Riddell RH, Walther B, et al. Dysplasia in Barrett's esophagus. J Cancer Res Clin Oncol 1985;110:145.
121. Lee RG. Dysplasia in Barrett's esophagus: a clinicopathologic study of 6 patients. Am J Surg Pathol 1985;9:845.
122. Hamilton SR, Smith RL. The relationship between columnar epithelial dysphasia and invasive adenocarcinoma arising in Barrett's esophagus. Am J Clin Pathol 1987;87:301.
123. Altorki NK, Sunagawa M, Little AG, et al. High-grade dysplasia in the columnar-lined esophagus. Am J Surg 1991;161:97.
124. Miros M, Kerlin P, Walker N. Only patients with dysplasia progress to adenocarcinoma in Barrett's esophagus. Gut 1991;32:1441.
125. Pera M, Trastek VF, Carpenter HA, et al. Barrett's esophagus with high-grade dysplasia: an indication for esophagectomy? Ann Thorac Surg 1992;54:199.
126. Burke AP, Sobin LH, Shekitka KM, et al. Dysplasia of the stomach and Barrett's esophagus: a follow-up study. Mod Pathol 1991;4:336.
127. Palley SL, Sampliner RE, Garewal HS. Management of high-grade dysplasia in Barrett's esophagus. J Clin Gastroenterol 1989;11:369.
128. Garewal HS, Sampliner RE, Fennerty MB. Flow cytometry in Barrett's esophagus: what have we learned so far? Dig Dis Sci 1991;36: 548.
129. Ried BJ, Blount PL, Rubin CE, et al. Flow-cytometry and histological progression to malignancy in Barrett's esophagus: prospective endoscopic surveillance of cohort. Gastroenterology 1992;102:1212.
130. Rashind WH, Norwood T, Levine DS, et al. Persistent clonal areas and clonal expansion in Barrett's esophagus. Cancer Res 1992;52: 2946.
131. Roth J. Molecular surgery for cancer. Arch Surg 1992;127:1298.
132. Casson AG, Mukhopadhyay T, Cleary KR, et al. p 53 gene mutations in Barrett's epithelium and esophageal cancer. Cancer Res 1991;51: 4495.
133. Blount PL, Ramel S, Raskind WH, et al. 17p Allelic deletions and p53 protein overexpression in Barrett's adenocarcinoma. Cancer Res 1991;51:5482.
134. Ramel S, Reid BJ, Sanchez CA, et al. Evaluation of p 53 protein expression in Barrett's esophagus by two-parameter flow cytometry. Gastroenterology 1992;102:1220.
135. Haggitt RC, Reid BJ, Rabinovitch PS, et al. Correlation between mucin histochemistry, flow cytometry and histologic diagnosis for predicting increased cancer risk. Am J Pathol 1988;131:53.
136. Jankowski J, Hopwood D, Wormsley KG. Flow-cytometric analysis of growth regulatory peptides and their receptors in Barrett's oesophagus and oesophageal adenocarcinoma. Scand J Gastroenterol 1992; 27:147.
137. Hollstein MC, Smits AM, Galiava C, et al. Amplification of epidermal growth factor receptor gene but no evidence of ras mutations in primary human esophageal cancers. Cancer Res 1988;48:5119.
138. Garewal HS, Gerner EW, Sampliner RE, et al. Ornithine decarboxylase and polyamine levels in columnar upper gastrointestinal mucosae in patients with Barrett's esophagus. Cancer Res 1988;48:3288.
139. Paraf F, Flejou JF, Potet F, et al. Esophageal squamous carcinoma in five patients with Barrett's esophagus. Am J Gastroenterol 1992;87: 746.
140. Antonioli DA, Goldman H. Changes in the location and type of gastric adenocarcinoma. Cancer 1982;50:775.
141. Wang HH, Antonioli DA, Goldman H. Comparative features of esophageal and gastric adenocarcinomas: recent changes on type and frequency. Hum Pathol 1986;17:482.
142. Kalish RJ, Clancy PE, Orringer MB, et al. Clinical, epidemiologic and morphologic comparison between adenocarcinomas arising in Barrett's esophageal mucosa and in gastric cardia. Gastroenterology 1984;86:461.
143. MacDonald WC, McDonald JB. Adenocarcinoma of the esophagus and/or gastric cardia. Cancer 1987;60:1094.
144. Gottfried MR, McClave SA, Boyce HW. Incomplete intestinal metaplasia in the diagnosis of columnar lined esophagus (Barrett's esophagus). Am J Clin Pathol 1989;92:741.
145. Garewal HS, Samliner RE, Fennerty MB. Chemopreventive studies in Barrett's esophagus: a model of premalignant lesion for esophageal adenocarcinoma. Monogr Natl Cancer Inst 1992;13:51.
146. Beahrs OH, Henson DE, Hutter RVP, et al. Manual for staging of cancer. 3rd ed. Philadelphia: JB Lippincott, 1988.
147. Hermanek P, Husemann B, Hohenberger W. The new TNM classification and stage grouping of intrathoracic oesophageal carcinoma. Diseases of the Esophagus 1991;4:77.
148. Japanese Committee for Registration of Esophageal Carcinoma Cases. Parameters linked to ten-year survival in Japan in resected cases of esophageal carcinoma. Chest 1989;96:1005.
149. Hankins JR, Cole FN, Attar S, et al. Adenocarcinoma involving the esophagus. J Thorac Cardiovasc Surg 1974;68:148.
150. Poleynard GD, Marty AT, Birnbaum WB, et al. Adenocarcinoma in the columnar-lined (Barrett) esophagus. Arch Surg 1977;112:997.
151. Witt TR, Bains MS, Zaman MB, et al. Adenocarcinoma in Barrett's esophagus. J Thorac Cardiovasc Surg 1983;85:337.
152. Siewert JR, Hoelscher AH, Bollschweiler E. Surgical therapy of cancer in Barrett's esophagus. Diseases of the Esophagus 1992;5:57.
153. Moon MR, Schulte WJ, Hoasler GB, et al. Transhiatal and transthoracic esophagectomy for adenocarcinoma of the esophagus. Arch Surg 1992;127:951.
154. Herskovic A, Martz K, Al-Sarraf M, et al. Combined chemotherapy and radiotherapy compared with radiotherapy alone in patients with cancer of the esophagus. N Engl J Med 1992;326:1593.
155. Fok M, Sham JST, Choy D, et al. Postoperative radiotherapy for carcinoma of the esophagus: a prospective randomized controlled study. Surgery 1993;113:138.

Surgery for Gastrointestinal Cancer: A Multidisciplinary Approach, edited by Harold J. Wanebo.
Lippincott-Raven Publishers, Philadelphia, © 1997.

CHAPTER 22

Endoscopic Laser Therapy for Obstructing Gastroesophageal Malignancy

Hector R. Nava and Ralph George

As fiberoptic technology was developed for use in the gastrointestinal tract, it was a natural step to combine fiberoptic systems with evolving laser technology. The endoscopic application of the argon laser for the coagulation of gastrointestinal bleeding in humans was first reported by Dwyer and colleagues in 1975.[1] Fleischer and associates first reported the endoscopic application of the neodymium-doped, yttrium–aluminum garnet (Nd:YAG) laser for the palliation of malignant esophageal obstruction in humans.[2]

Although a variety of lasers have been used for tumor ablation, the Nd:YAG laser has properties that are especially suited to this purpose. This chapter addresses our experience and that published in the literature.

ND:YAG LASER PHYSICS

The Nd:YAG solid laser has an invisible wavelength of 1060 nm and requires a second, low-power visible laser (ie, helium–neon) for aiming. It is not absorbed by water, permitting undiminished transmission through a water-containing flexible optic fiber, and is not absorbed by hemoglobin, allowing for tissue penetration of up to 5 to 7 mm. Superficial tumor can be vaporized, and deeper damage consists of carbonization and coagulation. At power settings from 50 to 100 W and pulses between 0.5 and 2.0 seconds, large amounts of tumor can be treated in a short time, making this laser ideal for the rapid debulking of large, obstructing esophageal tumors.

INDICATIONS

Squamous carcinomas and adenocarcinomas of the esophagus often present at an advanced stage. The goal in these patients is effective palliation in terms of normal deglutition. Over the last decade, a number of modalities have been used to achieve this. None is fully effective and all have their disadvantages. Long-term relief in these patients often requires a combination of modalities, both thermal and prosthetic, to maintain esophageal patency for the duration of their lives.

Initial palliation of unresectable, obstructing endoluminal esophageal tumor is the most common indication for Nd:YAG therapy of esophageal cancer. Most authors agree that in this circumstance laser therapy results in rapid and safe swallowing when used as first-line therapy for endoluminal tumor.[3–5] With some exceptions, better-quality swallowing is provided[6,7] and fewer complications occur[8,9] than would be the case with an endoluminal prosthesis.

Although both thermal coagulation with cautery[10] and chemical necrolysis[11] can be effective in the setting of malignant obstruction, neither modality offers the unique combination of coagulation and vaporization that the laser provides; nor, in many cases, do they provide luminal patency after a single treatment sitting, as laser does when used in a retrograde fashion.[12]

Unresectable disease is not the only indication for laser therapy. With improved chemotherapeutic regimens, many patients are now enrolled in neoadjuvant protocols of combination chemotherapy that often include radiation therapy.[13] Early and initial tumor ablation relieves obstruction and allows patients to participate in such trials while maintaining deglutition. Although bleeding is more commonly associated with gastric and colorectal malignancies, laser coagulation can effectively control hemorrhage, which may at times be the only indication for the ablation of esophageal cancer.[14]

Endoscopic laser can be used to maintain the patency of a previously inserted endoprosthesis whose ends may become overgrown with progressive tumor. Several authors have reported success in this scenario, effectively prolonging the usefulness of the prosthesis.[15,16]

The final group in whom esophageal laser therapy is indicated comprises those with an anastomotic recurrence after esophagogastrectomy.[17] The recurrence is usually in a short, straight segment, and detected early because these patients are

Hector R. Nava, Chief of Endoscopy/Associate Chief of Surgical Oncology, G.I. Endoscopy Unit, Roswell Park Cancer Institute, Elm and Carlton Streets, Buffalo, NY 14263.

Ralph George: Department of Surgery, St. Clare's Mercy Hospital, 154 LeMarchant Road, St. Johns, Newfoundland, Canada A1C-588.

followed closely, which makes these obstructions amenable to laser treatment.

CONTRAINDICATIONS

Contraindications are few. Even in patients with poor performance status, endoscopic relief of their malignant dysphagia, although not without risk, represents one of the least invasive means of effective palliation.

An absolute contraindication is the presence of tracheoesophageal or esophagobronchial fistula. In this instance, our preferred method of management is placement of an endoluminal prosthesis, thus achieving luminal patency and occluding the fistula to prevent aspiration.[18]

Relative contraindications include patients with extraluminal or submucosal tumor. In these cases, normal tissue must be ablated and treatment is often painful, technically difficult, and associated with a higher complication rate.[19] This group is probably best managed by endoluminal intubation.[20]

Rapidly growing tumors that require repeated laser sessions to maintain patency can often be better managed by intubation techniques, and the same may apply to very long stenotic lesions that would require multiple, tedious laser sessions.[6]

Some tumors of the gastroesophageal junction have a long horizontal segment. These can be difficult to treat by any method, and good function may not follow, even with successful recannulation.[21] Although laser therapy can be attempted in such patients, they represent a group who may ultimately require an alternative means of nutritional support.

Proximal lesions are often difficult to treat by laser therapy[22,23] because the upper esophageal sphincter makes positioning of the endoscope difficult. Unfortunately, these patients also tend to do poorly with an endoprosthesis. Brunstaud and colleagues, in one of the largest series of laser-treated cases, warned that even when luminal patency is achieved through cervical lesions, the functional results are often poor.[24] This is a group of patients who may ultimately require alternative interventions, such as percutaneous endoscopic gastrostomy tube placement, to maintain adequate nutrition.

EVALUATION

Pretreatment endoscopy allows for cytologic brushing and biopsy procedures to be performed, confirming the diagnosis of malignancy and allowing assessment of the proximal margin. Lesions in the upper esophagus undergo routine bronchoscopy, evaluating the membranous trachea and mainstem bronchi for transmural involvement. The relation of the tumor to the tracheobronchial tree is also assessed by barium swallow and computed tomography. Bulky ulcerated tumor or established fistulas affecting the respiratory tree are usually easy to diagnose. Early manifestations of airway involvement may be suggested by subtle mucosal changes detected at bronchoscopy, such as discoloration, nodularity, or friability of the respiratory mucosal surface. Compression of the trachea or bronchus without mucosal changes does not indicate impending fistulization, and some of these patients can have effective laser debulking if care is taken to avoid treating tumor along the anterior esophageal wall.

A barium swallow is always performed and kept on display in the endoscopy suite during the procedure. The swallow demonstrates the length and tortuosity of the lumen, serving as a road map through the lesion during therapy. The barium study may also demonstrate the existence of a fistula to the respiratory tree, which is a contraindication to laser therapy. In patients who require urgent endoscopy, retained barium may make endoscopic evaluation impossible, and in these cases a gastrograffin study is preferred. The transparent gastrograffin can be evacuated through the endoscope suction channel, and any residue does not impair visibility.

Finally, computed tomography of the mediastinal structures is helpful in defining the thickness of the esophageal wall and the proximity of related structures, suggesting areas to be concentrated on or avoided during the laser treatment.[25]

Routine investigations and general assessment are conducted and include electrocardiogram, complete blood count, and coagulation profile. These results may alter the level of monitoring or anesthetic approach to a particular patient.

TECHNIQUE

Initial reports, including Fleischer and colleagues' original papers, described a technique of antegrade treatment.[2,26] By this method the proximal margin was treated, beginning centrally and delivering the therapy in concentric rings. As the proximal margin cleared, the endoscope was passed more distally. Typically, this method required several sittings to work through a lengthy tumor, and coagulated or charred tissue would have to be debrided to clear the distal view.

In 1986 and 1987, Pietrafitta and Dwyer reported a retrograde approach,[27,28] combining laser therapy with pretreatment dilatation, allowing the endoscope to be passed through the tumor. Therapy could then be initiated in a retrograde fashion with improved visualization, and often completed at a single setting. The retrograde method is now the preferred approach, with equivalent success but significantly fewer treatments required compared with the antegrade technique.[12]

Our preference is also for the retrograde procedure. Patients are pretreated with an antisialogogue, given topical pharyngeal anesthesia, and then sedated as the endoscope is passed orally with the patient in the left lateral decubitus position. Patients are routinely monitored with pulse oximetry and an automated blood pressure cuff. Patients with significant comorbid conditions may have more aggressive monitoring, and patients with especially difficult lesions may on occasion be treated under general anesthesia.

Once the proximal margin of the tumor is visualized, our preference is to dilate the lesion with a hydrostatic balloon (TTS; Microvasive Co., Watertown, MA), 18 mm in diameter when inflated and 8 cm in length. Dilation is monitored endoscopically as the balloon is inflated to its maximum pressure of 35 pounds per square inch, and held in position for 2 minutes. We have developed a technique of ''chasing the balloon'' to facilitate traversing the stricture. Before deflation, the endoscope is brought into contact with the balloon. As the balloon is deflated, it is gently nudged forward by careful manipulation and steady pressure, including rotation of the scope. The soft tip of the balloon follows the esophageal lumen, quickly guiding the endoscope through a stricture that might otherwise be obscured by postdilatation bleeding and debris. Longer neoplasms may require sequential dilations. When the tumor has been negotiated, the now deflated balloon is drawn back into the biopsy channel and removed.

Long, tortuous, and fibrotic malignancies may not be amenable to balloon dilatation. In this circumstance, an endoscopically placed guidewire is passed and fluoroscopically monitored dilatation with Savary dilators is performed.[30] After passage of a 45-Fr (or larger) dilator, the endoscope can usually be passed with the guidewire fed through the biopsy channel as the endoscope is advanced. The tumor can then be passed under direct vision as the endoscope follows the guidewire to the distal margin of the cancer, with the assurance that the endoscope will not create a false channel. A polyethylene catheter placed in the biopsy channel allows for retrograde feeding of the guidewire.

Protective eyewear is worn by everyone in the endoscopy suite, including the patient. The quartz conducting fiber is passed through the biopsy channel, and must be visible just beyond the tip so as not to damage the endoscope when the laser is fired. With the fiber in view, the laser is turned on. Initial settings vary between users. Most set the pulse time between 0.5 and 2.0 seconds, and the power from 50 to 100 W. Endoscopes with large biopsy or double channels facilitate the evacuation of smoke secretions. The tumor is treated preferably in a retrograde fashion, with the endoscopist firing the laser using a foot pedal. As much as possible, the treatment should be directed along the axis of the esophageal lumen to prevent overpenetration and perforation. This is especially important with thin-walled lesions or in the vicinity of adjacent structures such as the aortic arch or left mainstem bronchus. It is wise to mark the margins of the lesion with a line of coagulation. It this is not carefully done at the beginning of the procedure, the edematous reaction in adjacent tissue may make it difficult to determine the boundary of the tumor. The endoscopist must remain oriented to position at all times and remain cognizant of surrounding structures as the treatment proceeds. The interaction of the laser with the tissue is observed and controlled to produce the desired affect of coagulation, carbonization, or vaporization by altering the distance from the quartz tip to the target, and changing the laser settings.

The fiber tip will become hot and must be kept off the surrounding tissue to prevent it from being covered with coagulum. Any debris that accumulates on the tip will lead to overheating and damage the fiber (and possibly the endoscope itself) and may have to be removed to clean carbon debris. Smoke needs to be suctioned intermittently to maintain a clear field of view.

Patient discomfort can result from the perception of heat, which may necessitate a short respite as the tissue cools, or moving the treatment to a different area. Coaxially delivered CO_2, which cools and clears the quartz fiber tip, can lead to uncomfortable gastric distention. If this occurs, the endoscope can be passed on to the stomach after turning off the laser and withdrawing the fiber from the biopsy channel. The suction channel can then be used to decompress the stomach before returning to the treatment.

In most instances, the lumen can be opened in a single treatment session, typically using an average of 7000 to 8000 J of energy, depending on the length of the tumor.

RESULTS

Laser treatments are usually successful in achieving luminal patency. In 308 patients, Spinelli and colleagues report patency in 94% of patients but improved swallowing in only 74%. The report draws the distinction between technical success, which is nearly always possible, and a functional success that can be limited by tumor site, particularly for lesions in the proximal esophagus.[30] Similarly, Mellow and Pinkas reported a 97% technical success, but defined functional success as the ability to maintain adequate caloric intake by mouth alone. This degree of functional success was achieved in 70% of patients, and poor performance status at accession correlated with poor functional outcome.[31]

Eckhauser found some measure of improvement in all patients, but less improvement in those treated with cervical lesions,[14] and Schwesinger and Chumley found an improvement in performance status in most patients who underwent laser therapy.[32]

Although it is intended as palliative therapy, several authors have suggested that improved survival can occur as a result of laser treatment of malignant dysphagia. This may be a result only of the improved nutritional intake the therapy affords the patient. Case–control studies by Karlin and associates[33] and Siegal and coworkers[34] demonstrated significantly prolonged survival in patients palliated by laser therapy, and Hahl and colleagues found improved survival at 1 year for patients managed by laser treatment compared to those who had endoluminal intubation.[9]

It is generally thought that the quality of swallowing is superior after laser therapy compared with the insertion of a luminal prosthesis. Although this conclusion is somewhat controversial, it has been supported by a randomized trial.[7] The clear advantage of the laser over intubation techniques lies in its significantly lower complication rate.[7–9,35]

The disadvantage of laser palliation is the recurrence of dysphagia as the tumor regrows. Sargeant and colleagues found that retreatment was required approximately every 5 weeks to maintain adequate deglutition.[36] Likewise, Brown and coworkers reported 18 of 34 patients with advanced disease having recurrent dysphagia within a mean of 6 weeks.[37] Most authors agree that without any other concurrent therapy, the malignant dysphagia is likely to recur and may require retreatment as often as every 4 to 8 weeks.[38,39] More frequent retreatment suggests a rapid tumor regrowth and would be an indication to consider intubation as an alternative therapy.

Efforts have been made to improve the dysphagia-free interval between laser treatments. External beam radiation therapy after laser ablation improved the interval between dilatations to a mean of 13 weeks in patients receiving 30 Gy to the area of the tumor. In this report by Sargeant and colleagues, higher doses of external beam radiation were associated with less effective palliation than the 30-Gy dose.[36]

Other authors have combined endoscopic laser therapy with brachytherapy. Using iridium 192 endocavitary afterloading treatment with prior laser recanalization of the esophageal lumen, Bader and associates reported that 77% of 48 patients experienced permanent relief of dysphagia, with a mean survival of 5.9 months.[40] Randomized trials have not demonstrated as dramatic a benefit. Sander and colleagues randomized 39 patients to laser alone or laser plus afterloading treatment with iridium 192. All patients experienced restenosis, but an improvement in the dysphagia-free interval was demonstrated for the patients with squamous cell primaries.[41] Harper and coworkers found that laser therapy combined with combination chemotherapy was associated with fewer laser treatments per month compared with laser treatment alone.[42] The results of these trials suggest than an impact on the dysphagia-free interval can be achieved with the addition of adjuvant chemotherapy or radiation.

COMPLICATIONS

Laser therapy has been associated with a procedure-related mortality in the range of 0% to 4%,[32,43] and a morbidity of 2% to 10%.[23,43–45] In a large collected series of 1184 patients, the overall complication rate was 4.9%. The common morbidities were perforation in 2.1%, fistulization in 0.8%, hemorrhage in 0.7%, and sepsis in 0.6%. Procedure-related mortality in the same series was 1%.[46]

With this degree of procedure safety, some authors are reporting that upward of 40% of their patients can be treated on an outpatient basis.[23,32] At present, we admit all patients who are receiving their first treatment, and any patients with extensive disease, for posttherapy observation. Some patients experience a transitory increase in dysphagia as a result of tumor sloughing and edema in the treated area, and may require 24 hours of intravenous fluid support until they are able to resume oral intake. Previously treated patients who return with partial obstruction can be treated in a single sitting on an outpatient basis.

Transient bacteremia is documented to occur with laser therapy, and patients with valvular heart disease or prosthetic joints should receive antibiotic prophylaxis.[47]

Benign pneumoperitoneum has been described after laser treatment. The condition requires no intervention and is thought to be a result of the insufflated coaxially delivered CO_2 that cools and clears the quartz conducting fiber tip during the laser therapy.[48]

Stricture secondary to fibrosis in the treated area is a potential long-term complication, usually managed with dilatation.[49]

CONCLUSION

Ablation with the Nd:YAG laser has become the procedure of choice for the initial relief of malignant esophageal dysphagia, with the unique properties of this laser, permitting both coagulation and vaporization of tissue, facilitate the therapy. Combining the treatment with dilatation and treating the tumor in a retrograde fashion can often achieve recanalization in a single treatment session. Because the technique requires only mild sedation, it can be performed with a short hospital stay or in some cases as an outpatient procedure.

Technical success in achieving a patent lumen is accomplished in upward of 90% of patients, and solid food can be consumed by 80% of patients after treatment. Mortality and morbidity rates are in the range of 1% and 5%, respectively, in the largest collective series of laser therapy. The complication rate of laser therapy is consistently lower than that for endoluminal intubation procedures, and the procedure seems to result in a better quality of swallowing. Dysphagia has a tendency to recur, and patients may need therapy as often as monthly to maintain good patency. The addition of adjuvant radiation therapy (external beam or intracavitary) or chemotherapy seems to significantly prolong the dysphagia-free interval.

The presence of an associated tracheoesophageal fistula or rapidly growing tumor requiring frequent ablation are indications for endoprosthetic intubation. The ultimate care of these patients with advanced esophageal cancer may require a combination of techniques and modalities to keep them free of dysphagia and provide them with optimal nutrition, resulting in significant improvement in quality of life.

REFERENCES

1. Dwyer RM, Haberback BJ, Bass J, et al. Laser induced hemostasis in the canine stomach. JAMA 1975;231:486.
2. Fleischer D, Kessler F, Hayes O. Endoscopic Nd-YAG laser therapy for carcinoma of the esophagus: a new palliative approach. Am J Surg 1982;143:280.
3. Goldberg SJ, King KH. Endoscopic Nd-YAG laser coagulation as palliative therapy for obstructing esophageal carcinoma. Am J Gastroenterol 1968;81:629.
4. Buset M, Dunham F, Baize M, de Toeuf J, Cremer M. Nd-YAG laser, a new palliative alternative in the management of esophageal cancer. Endoscopy 1983;15:353.
5. Cello JP, Gerstenberger PD, Wright T, Melnick J, Meiselman MS. Endoscopic neodymium-YAG laser palliation of nonresectable esophageal malignancy. Ann Intern Med 1985;102:610.
6. Alderson D, Wright PD. Laser recanalization vs. endoscopic intubation in the palliation of malignant dysphagia. Br J Surg 1990;77:1151.
7. Carter R, Smith JS, Anderson JR. Laser recanalization vs. endoscopic intubation in the palliation of malignant dysphagia: a randomized prospective study. Br J Surg 1992;79:1167.
8. Buset M, des Marez B, Baize M, et al. Palliative endoscopic management of obstructive esophagogastric cancer: laser or prosthesis? Gastrointest Endosc 1987;33:357.
9. Hahl J, Salo J, Ovaska J, Haapiainen R, Kalima T, Schroder T. Comparison of endoscopic Nd-YAG laser therapy and oesophageal tube in palliation of oesophagogastric malignancy. Scand J Gastroenterol 1991; 26:103.
10. Nava HR, Schuh ME, Nambisan R, Clark JL, Douglass HO Jr. Endoscopic ablation of esophageal malignancies with the neodymium-YAG laser and electrofulguration. Arch Surg 1989;124:225.
11. Angelini G, Pasini AF, Ederle A, Castagnini A, Talamini G, Bulighin G. Nd-YAG laser vs. polidocanol injection for palliation of esophageal malignancy: a prospective, randomized Study. Gastrointest Endosc 1991;37:607.
12. Pietrafitta JJ, Bowers GJ, Dwyer RM. Prograde vs. retrograde endoscopic laser therapy for the treatment of malignant esophageal obstruction: a comparison of techniques. Lasers Surg Med 1988;8:288.
13. Trillet V, Montbarbon X, de Laroche G, Lambert R, Gerard JP. Combination 5-fluorouracil-cisplatin before laser and radiotherapy in 47 patients with inoperable epidermoid carcinoma of the esophagus. Collog INSERM 1986;137:661.
14. Eckhauser ML. Palliative therapy of upper gastrointestinal malignancies using the Nd-YAG laser. Am Surg 1990;56:158.
15. Techini P, Breda B, Abrescia F, et al. Nd-YAG laser disobstruction of esophageal endoprostheses occluded by neoplastic development in the palliative treatment of esophageal cancer [in Italian]. Chir Ital 1986; 38:44.
16. Sargeant IR, Loizou LA, Tulloch M, Thorpe S, Brown SG. Recanalization of tube overgrowth: a useful new indication for laser in palliation of malignant dysphagia. Gastrointest Endosc 1992;38:165.
17. Brennan FN, McCarthy JH, Laurence BH. Endoscopic Nd-YAG laser therapy for palliation of upper gastrointestinal malignancy. Med J Aust 1990;152:27.
18. George RL, Mesko TW, Nava HR. Malignant tracheoesophageal fistula: management by endoprosthesis [abstract]. Proceedings of the Annual Meeting of the Society of Surgical Oncology 1993;46:P11.
19. Fleischer D. Endoscopic laser therapy for carcinoma of the esophagus. Endoscopy Review 1984;1:37.
20. Urschel JD, Cockburn JS, Foote AV. Palliation of oesophageal cancer: endoscopic intubation and laser therapy. Postgrad Med J 1991;67:414.
21. Fleischer D, Sivak MV Jr. Endoscopic Nd-YAG laser therapy as pallia-

tion for esophagogastric cancer: parameters affecting initial outcome. Gastroenterology 1985;89:827.
22. Merono E, Martin de Argila C, Garcia-Plaza A. The palliative treatment of esophageal tumors with the laser (Nd-YAG): the results of an initial experience [in Spanish]. Rev Clin Esp 1993;192:365.
23. Lightdale CJ, Zimbalist E, Winawer SJ. Outpatient management of esophageal cancer with endoscopic Nd-YAG laser. Am J Gastroenterol 1987;82:46.
24. Brunetaud JM, Maunoury V, Cochelard D, Boniface B, Cortot A, Paris JC. Parameters affecting laser palliation in patients with advanced digestive cancers. Lasers in Surgery and Medicine 1989:9:169.
25. Caroline DF, Krevsky B, Friedman AC, Lev-Toaff AS, Radecki PD. Endoscopic laser therapy for carcinoma involving the esophagus: the value of pretreatment computed tomography. Am J Gastroenterol 1988; 83:908.
26. Fleischer D, Kessler F. Endoscopic Nd-YAG laser therapy for carcinoma of the esophagus: a new form of palliative treatment. Gastroenterology 1983;85:600.
27. Pietrafitta JJ, Dwyer RM. Endoscopic laser therapy of malignant esophageal obstruction. Arch Surg 1986;121:395.
28. Pietrafitta J, Dwyer RM. New laser technique for the treatment of malignant esophageal obstruction. J Surg Oncol 1987;35:157.
29. Dumon JF, Meric B, Sivak MV, Fleischer D. A new method of esophageal dilation using Savary-Gilliard bougies. Gastrointest Endosc 1985; 31:379.
30. Spinelli P, Dal Fante M, Mancini A. Endoscopic palliation of malignancies of the upper gastrointestinal tract using Nd-YAG laser: results and survival in 308 treated patients. Lasers Surg Med 1991;11:550.
31. Mellow MH, Pinkas H. Endoscopic laser therapy for malignancies affecting the esophagus and gastroesophageal junction: analysis of technical and functional efficacy. Arch Intern Med 1985;145:1443.
32. Schwesinger WH, Chumley DL. Laser palliation for gastrointestinal malignancy. Am Surg 1988;54:100.
33. Karlin DA, Fisher FS, Krevsky B. Prolonged survival and effective palliation in patients with squamous cell carcinoma of the esophagus following endoscopic laser therapy. Cancer 1987;59:1969.
34. Siegel HI, Laskin KJ, Dabezies MA, Fisher RS, Krevsky B. The effect of endoscopic laser therapy on survival in patients with squamous cell carcinoma of the esophagus: further experience. J Clin Gastroenterol 1991;13:142.
35. Paolucci V, Henne T, Schmidt-Matthiesen A. Endoscopic palliative tube and laser therapy in advanced cancer of the esophagus and cardia [in German]. Chirurg 1990;61:43.
36. Sargeant IR, Loizou LA, Tobias JS, Blackman G, Thorpe S, Bown SG. Radiation enhancement of laser palliation for malignant dysphagia: a pilot study. Gut 1992;33:1597.
37. Brown SG, Hawes R, Matthewson K, et al. Endoscopic laser palliation for advanced malignant dysphagia. Gut 1987;28:799.
38. Krasner N, Barr H, Skidmore C, Morris AL. Palliative laser therapy for malignant dysphagia. Gut 1987;28:792.
39. Rutgeerts P, Vantrappen G, Broeckaert L, et al. Palliative Nd-YAG laser therapy for cancer of the esophagus and gastroesophageal junction: impact on the quality of remaining life. Gastrointest Endosc 1988; 34:87.
40. Bader M, Dittler HJ, Ultsch B, Ries G, Siewert JR. Palliative treatment of malignant stenoses of the upper gastrointestinal tract using a combination of laser and afterloading therapy. Endoscopy 1986;18(Suppl 1): 27.
41. Sander R, Hagenmueller F, Sander C, Riess G, Classen M. Laser vs. laser plus afterloading with iridium-192 in the palliative treatment of malignant stenosis of the esophagus: a prospective, randomized and controlled study. Gastrointest Endosc 1991;37:433.
42. Harper PG, Highley M, Houston S, et al. Significant palliation of advanced gastric/esophageal adenocarcinoma (g-o/0) with laser endoscopy and combination chemotherapy [abstract]. Proceedings of the Annual Meeting of the Society of Surgical Oncology 1992;11:A472.
43. Loizou LA, Grigg D, Atkinson M, Robertson C, Bown SG. A prospective comparison of laser therapy and intubation in endoscopic palliation for malignant dysphagia [see comments]. Gastroenterology 1991;100: 1303.
44. Wolf EL, Frager J, Brandt LJ, Frager DH, Bernstein LH, Beneventano TC. Radiographic appearance of the esophagus and stomach after laser treatment of obstructing carcinoma. AJR Am J Roentgenol 1986;146: 519.
45. Naveau S, Chiesa A, Poynard T, Chaput JC. Endoscopic Nd-YAG laser therapy as palliative treatment for esophageal and cardial cancer: parameters affecting long-term outcome [see comments]. Dig Dis Sci 1990;35:294.
46. Ell C, Riemann J, Lux G, Demling L. Palliative laser treatment of malignant stenoses in the upper gastrointestinal tract. Endoscopy 1986; 18(Suppl 1):21.
47. Kohler B, Riemann JF. Incidence of bacteremia after endoscopic laser treatment of stenosing processes in the upper gastrointestinal tract. Am J Gastroenterol 1987;82:1026.
48. Brooks PT, Troop AC, Barr H, Krasner N. Massive pneumoperitoneum following laser therapy of inoperable oesophageal carcinoma. Clin Radiol 1988;39:305.
49. Bown SG. Endoscopic laser therapy for oesophageal cancer. Endoscopy 1986;18(Suppl 3):26.

PART III

Gastric Cancer

Surgery for Gastrointestinal Cancer: A Multidisciplinary Approach, edited by Harold J. Wanebo.
Lippincott-Raven Publishers, Philadelphia, © 1997.

CHAPTER 23

Gastric Cancer Staging and Natural History

B. J. Kennedy

As of 1996, gastric carcinoma was estimated to be the 13th most common and the 10th most deadly cancer in the United States.[1] With approximately 22,800 new cases and 14,000 deaths in 1996, there has been a steady decline in the incidence of gastric cancer to the current lower rate since 1930, when it was the most deadly type of cancer, causing 38% of cancer deaths in the United States. This decrease has not been the result of any planned health promotion or major change in treatment intervention. Despite this decrease in gastric cancer, there is a suggestion that the location of the cancers has shifted from the antral portion of the stomach to the proximal stomach and gastroesophageal junction.

The decreased rate of gastric cancers has not been noted in many countries, including Japan, Chile, Korea, and China, among others. Japan has the highest incidence and the highest mortality. After World War II, there was an increase in mortality, but mortality declined after 1950. Japan's rapidly increasing aged population may result in a slowing down of the rate of decline because the disease is related in part to aging.

Gastric cancer occurs approximately twice as often in men than women and in both sexes the incidence increases with advancing age. One of the reasons for the decline in mortality rates in Japan in the past years has been the result of mass screening. The high incidence of this disease has made screening programs reasonable and cost effective. Such is not the case in the United States.

NATURAL HISTORY AND DIAGNOSIS

Causative Factors

Many risk factors have been reported worldwide and have been found to differ depending on specific lifestyles and regions. Hence, dietary factors, protective factors, environmental conditions, cultural background, social and economic factors, transportation, storage of foods, education, familial factors, race, age, and sex all have been correlated with the incidence of gastric cancer. As some of these factors change, such as dietary habits, the incidences of this disease continues to change.

Division of Medical Oncology, Medical School, University of Minnesota, University Hospital and Clinic, Box 286, 420 Delaware Street SE, Minneapolis, MN 55455

Databases

In the United States, three major databases have been studied in determining incidence, survival, and other factors relating to malignant diseases. These include the Surveillance Epidemiology End Results (SEER) of the National Cancer Institute, the patient care studies by the Commission on Cancer of the American College of Surgeons, based on tumor registries, and the more recent National Cancer Data Base, also conducted by the American College of Surgeons, with continuing update of the data entered through cancer registries. The SEER program collects date about cancer from nine population-based cancer registries, covering about 10% of the U.S. population. The American College of Surgeons programs are representative of cancer throughout the United States and reflect a broad, community-based sampling of the cancer problem.

Patterns of Spread

Gastric cancers usually arise as a localized tumor. They can spread by local extension to involve adjacent normal structures, and the disease can be extended by local invasion, lymphatic spread, or hematogenous dissemination. The rationale for treatment is based on the site of the tumor and the method of extension. Local extension occurs through the length of the stomach, either toward the duodenum or the esophagus. Deep invasion erodes through the submucosa muscularis and gastric serosa. Distal metastases are most common in the liver. Peritoneal metastases may be widely disseminated, including to the ovaries (Kurkenberg's tumor) and rectal shelf (Blumer's tumor). The pattern of spread has been the foundation for the development of the staging systems.

Signs and Symptoms

In the United States, early gastric cancer is seldom detected, in contrast to the results of Japanese screening, where more

TABLE 23-1. *Incidence of symptoms in American College of Surgeons Patterns of Care study of 18,265 patients*

Symptom	Incidence
Weight loss	61.6%
Abdominal pain	51.6%
Nausea	34.3%
Dysphagia	26.1%
Melena	20.2%

Wanebo HJ, Kennedy BJ, Chmiel J, Steele G Jr, Winchester D, Osteen R. Cancer of the stomach: a patient case study by the American College of Surgeons. Ann Surg 1993;218:583.

than half of patients are of the earliest stage. These results are obtained with the use of frequent endoscopy with ultrasonography as well as double-contrast radiography of the stomach. In U.S. studies, a combination of symptoms may occur, none of which is specifically diagnostic of gastric cancer[2] (Table 23-1). Weight loss often indicates more advanced disease, and patients with weight loss have a significantly shorter survival than those without weight loss. Dysphagia may indicate a cancer in the cardia or gastroesophageal junction. Vomiting is more consistent with an antral carcinoma obstructing the pylorus. Physical examination cannot detect an early carcinoma. An epigastric mass, enlarged liver, ascites, jaundice, or palpable supraclavicular lymph nodes indicate extensive and incurable disease.

Diagnosis

When gastric cancer is suspected, upper endoscopy is a preferred procedure because a biopsy can also be performed in the same setting. Combined with ultrasonography, an accurate determination of the depth of invasion of the primary tumor (pT) stage can be made. The computed tomography scan is more valuable for evaluating the extent of lymph node involvement as well as metastases to the liver, adrenals, and ovaries. There is no specific serum tumor marker for gastric cancer. However, carcinoembryonic antigen levels are frequently elevated in patients with extensive disease and may be used as a marker in monitoring the progress during treatment.

Screening

The high incidence of gastric cancer in Japan, Chile, China, and Korea has made screening programs for gastric cancer reasonable and cost effective. As a result of these screened populations, the Japanese data demonstrate that approximately 50% of the newly diagnosed patients have early gastric cancer. The significance of such screening programs is obvious in view of the very high cure rate with surgical treatment of early gastric cancer. In the United States, the incidence of gastric cancer is too low to warrant a routine screening program. Hence, less than 8% of gastric cancers are limited to the mucosa or submucosa, the earliest stage.

STAGING

The TNM system for classification of cancers is the principal method for determining the extent of disease, selection of treatment, and prognosis, and provides a reliable means for reporting treatment results. Through a series of international meetings, the TNM system has become unified.

History

The first classification for stomach cancer was made in 1966 by the Union Internationale Contre le Cancer (UICC). Because of technical advances, this was revised in 1968. The American Joint Committee on Cancer (AJCC) developed a staging system based on the description of the degree of penetration of the stomach wall by the primary tumor at the time of initial diagnosis.[3] Using data from SEER, the prognostic significance of depth of tumor invasion was confirmed.[4] A striking feature was the importance of age in the survival of patients. In Japan, 64% of patients with curative resections were younger than 60 years of age,[5] compared with 28% in the SEER data. Meetings between the AJCC and the Japanese Cancer Committee led to the development of a unified staging system. There would be only two types of staging, clinical and pathologic, and removal of the primary tumor for pathologic staging was no longer a requirement. In May, 1985, the UICC accepted the unified staging system.[6,7] In 1988, publications of the UICC and AJCC contained the same staging classification for gastric cancer. The 1992 fourth edition of the AJCC's *Manual for Staging of Cancer* continued to accept this staging classification.[8]

Principles of Classification

The classification defines the extent of disease in terms of, first, the primary tumor (pT), expressed in terms of the degree of penetration by the cancer through the stomach wall; second, the regional lymph nodes (N), which are the perigastric lymph nodes and lymph nodes along the left gastric common hepatic, splenic, and celiac arteries; and third, distant metastases (M). The description of the primary lesion is similar for the clinical (cT) and pathologic classification (pT).

The prognosis of gastric cancers depends on the extent of penetration of the wall by the tumor and involvement of adjacent organs. Although size and histologic type have not been found to be as useful in estimating prognosis, the tumors in the gastroesophageal junction appear to have a poorer prognosis than those located elsewhere.

Rules for Classification

Clinical staging (cTNM) is based on evidence acquired before definitive treatment is instituted. It includes physical examination, imaging, endoscopy, biopsy, and other clinical findings.

Pathologic staging depends on data acquired clinically plus results of surgical exploration and examination of the resected stomach or biopsy specimen. Pathologic assessment of the regional lymph nodes entails removal of the nodes sufficient to validate the absence of metastases and evaluate the highest pN category.

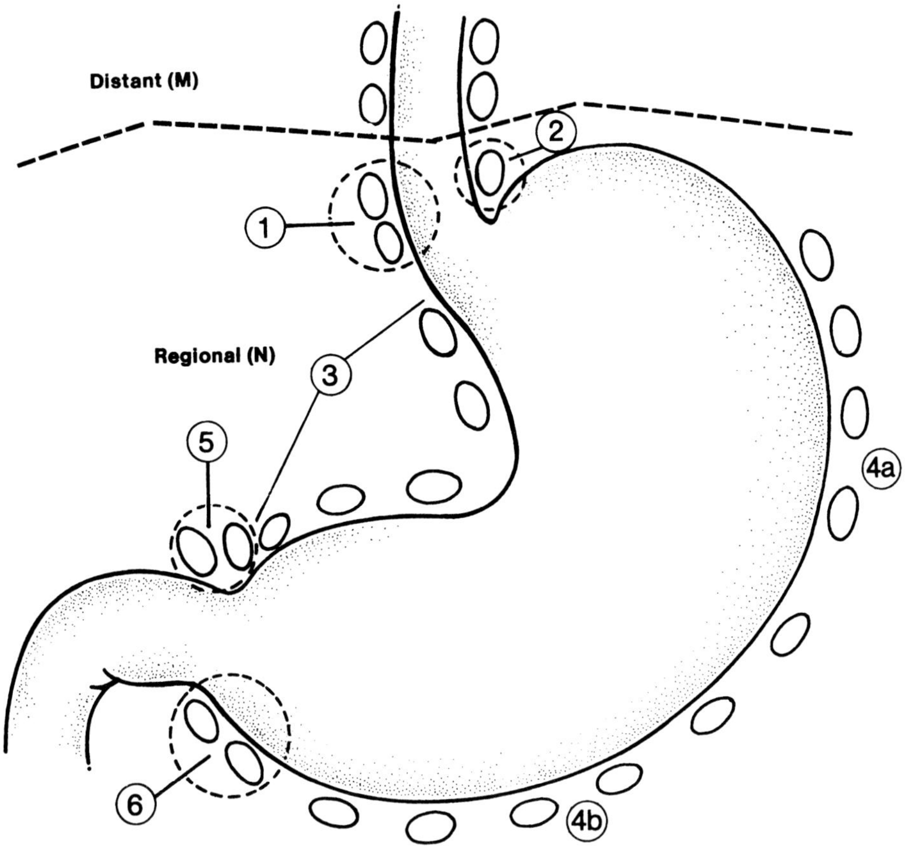

FIG. 23-1. Perigastric regional lymph nodes along the lesser (1, 3, 5) and greater (2, 4a, 4b, 6) curvatures. (Reproduced with permission from American Joint Committee on Cancer. Stomach. In: Beahrs OH, Henson DE, Hutter RVP, Kennedy BJ, eds. Manual for staging of cancer. 4th ed. Philadelphia: JB Lippincott, 1992:63.)

Definitions of T, N, and M

Primary Tumor (T)

The principal factor is the degree of penetration of the stomach wall by carcinoma.

TX: Primary tumor cannot be assessed
T0: No evidence of primary tumor
Tis: Carcinoma in situ—intraepithelial tumor without invasion of the lamina propria
T1: Tumor invades lamina propria or submucosa
T2: Tumor invades the muscularis propria or the subserosa*
T3: Tumor penetrates the serosa (visceral peritoneum) without invasion of adjacent structures†‡
T4: Tumor invades adjacent structures†‡

Regional Lymph Nodes (N)

The principal factor is the distance of metastatic nodes from the primary tumor. The regional lymph nodes are the perigastric nodes along the lesser (1, 3, 5) and greater (2, 4a, 4b, 6) curvatures (Fig. 23-1) and the nodes located along the left gastric (7) and common hepatic (8), splenic (10,11), and celiac arteries (9) (Fig. 23-2). Involvement of other intraabdominal lymph nodes, such as the hepatoduodenal (12), retropancreatic, mesenteric, and paraaortic, is classified as distant metastasis.

The numeric order corresponds to the proposals of the Japanese Research Society for Gastric Cancer Study in Surgery and Pathology.[9]

NX: Regional lymph node(s) cannot be assessed
N0: No regional lymph node metastasis
N1: Metastasis in perigastric lymph node(s) within 3 cm of the edge of the primary tumor
N2: Metastasis in perigastric lymph node(s) more than 3 cm from the edge of the primary tumor, or in lymph nodes along the left gastric, common hepatic, splenic, or celiac arteries

Distant Metastasis (M)

MX: Presence of distant metastasis cannot be assessed
M0: No distant metastasis
M1: Distant metastasis

TNM Stage Grouping

Classification of T, N, and M provides a system of precise description of the anatomic extent of the disease. Each T, N,

* A tumor may penetrate the muscularis propria with extension into the gastrocolic or gastrohepatic ligaments or into the greater or lesser omentum without perforation of the visceral peritoneum covering these structures. In this case, the tumor is classified T2. If there is perforation of the visceral peritoneum covering the gastric ligaments or omenta, the tumor should be classified T3.

† The adjacent structures of the stomach are the spleen, transverse colon, liver, diaphragm, pancreas, abdominal wall, adrenal gland, kidney, small intestine, and retroperitoneum.

‡ Intramural extension to the duodenum or esophagus is classified by the depth of greatest invasion in any of these sites, including the stomach.

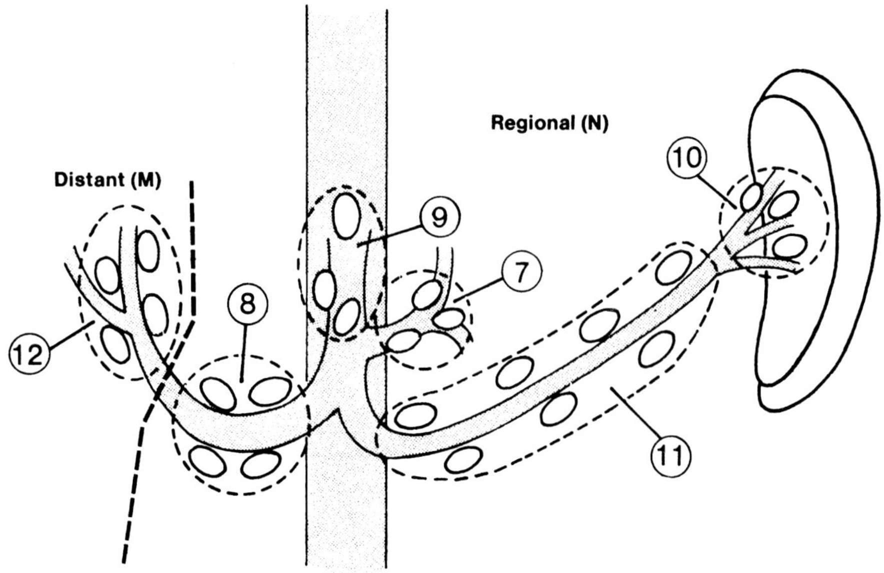

FIG. 23-2. Perigastric regional lymph nodes along the left gastric (7), common hepatic (8), splenic (10, 11), and celiac (9) arteries. (Reproduced with permission from American Joint Committee on Cancer. Stomach. In: Beahrs OH, Henson DE, Hutter RVP, Kennedy BJ, eds. Manual for staging of cancer. 4th ed. Philadelphia: JB Lippincott, 1992:63.)

and M has several categories. By condensing these categories, a system of TNM stage groupings is established. These stage groupings (0 to IV) provide a means for determining prognosis as a result of treatments rendered. Comparison of the results of treatments can thus be made.

Stage Grouping	
Stage 0	Tis N0 M0
Stage IA	T1 N0 M0
Stage IB	T1 N1 M0
	T2 N0 M0
Stage II T1 N1 M0	T2 N1 M0
	T3 N0 M0
Stage IIIA	T2 N2 M0
	T3 N1 M0
	T4 N0 M0
Stage IIIB	T3 N2 M0
	T4 N1 M0
Stage IV	T4 N2 M0
	Any T Any N M1

Survival

The Commission on Cancer of the American College of Surgeons analyzed data from over 700 tumor registries on 18,365 patients with gastric cancer. These data represented the study of patients diagnosed in 1982 and 1987. The study showed that gastric cancer is a disease of aging, with 48% of the men and 58% of the women older than 70 years of age. In comparing the 18,365 patients from the United States to Japanese reports, it is apparent that in the United States patients present with more advanced stages (66% stage III and IV) than the Japanese (52%). As a result of more advanced cancers, the overall survival of all patients with gastric cancer is poorer in the United States (14%) than in Japan (45.4%). The survival of patients according to stage demonstrated the reliability of the current staging system (Fig. 23-3). There has been a trend toward a higher survival rate in the United States. The 11% 5-year survival from 1960 to 1963 has increased to 18% in the 1983 to 1990 era ($P = 0.05$).[1]

The overall 5-year survival rate for resected patients in the Japanese series was 56.3%, versus 19% in the American College of Surgeons' report[2,10] (Table 23-2). The 5-year survival rate in the subgroups was 59% for stage IA, 44% for stage IB, 15% for stage IIIA, and 9% for stage IIIB.

Japanese surgeons conduct a more aggressive node dissection and more careful pathologic staging; the superior Japanese survival rates may reflect this practice. In the United States, patients may have been deemed to have less disease than what truly existed (understaged). The American College of Surgeons series probably represents the status of gastric cancer management overall in the United States. The Japanese data represent a careful coordination of major centers in Japan. Hence, comparison with the high Japanese standard is an incentive for surgeons and pathologists in the United States to carefully stage

TABLE 23-2. *Comparison of gastric cancer results as recorded by the American College of Surgeons (ACS) study and selected Japanese hospitals*

	Incidence (%)		Resected patient survival (%)	
	Japan	ACS study	Japan	ACS study
No. of patients	15,589	18,365	12,535	10,237
Stage I	33.7	17.1	95.6	50.0
Stage II	14.5	16.9	70.1	29.0
Stage III	28.7	35.5	36.3	13.0
Stage IV	23.1	30.5	23.1	3.0
Overall survival	45.4%	14%	56.3%	19%

Data from Wanebo HJ, Kennedy BJ, Chmiel J, Steele G Jr, Winchester D, Osteen R. Cancer of the stomach: a patient case study by the American College of Surgeons. Ann Surg 1993;218:583; and Maruyama K, Okaboyashi K, Kinoshita T. Progress in gastric cancer surgery and its limits of radicality. World J Surg 1987;11:418.

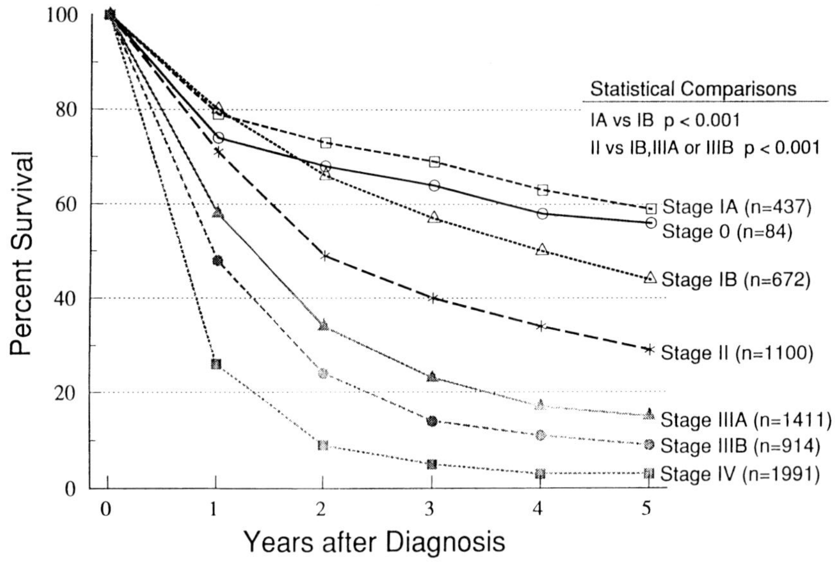

FIG. 23-3. Overall 5-year survival rates according to pathologic stage of 6609 patients diagnosed in 1982. (Reproduced with permission from American Joint Committee on Cancer. Stomach. In: Beahrs OH, Henson DE, Hutter RVP, Kennedy BJ, eds. Manual for staging of cancer. 4th ed. Philadelphia: JB Lippincott, 1992:63.)

pathologically the gastric cancer and consider more aggressive surgical intervention.

The classification of gastric cancer for purposes of staging allows the physician to select appropriate treatment and compare results of treatment on a regional, national, and international basis more confidently.[11]

REFERENCES

1. Parker SL, Tong T, Bolden S, Wingo PA. Cancer statistics 1996. CA Cancer J Clin 1996;46:5.
2. Wanebo HJ, Kennedy BJ, Chmiel J, Steele G Jr, Winchester D, Osteen R. Cancer of the stomach: a patient case study by the American College of Surgeons. Ann Surg 1993;218:583.
3. Kennedy BJ. TNM classification for stomach cancer. Cancer 1970;26: 971.
4. Curtis RE, Kennedy BJ, Myers MH, Hankey BF. Evaluations of AJC stomach cancer staging: an analysis of 1275 SEER patients. Semin Oncol 1985;12:21.
5. Miwa K. Evaluations of the TNM classification of stomach cancer for its rational stage grouping. Jpn J Clin Oncol 1984;14:385.
6. Kennedy BJ. Evolution of the international gastric cancer staging classifications. Scand J Gastroenterol 1987;22(Suppl 133):8.
7. Kennedy BJ. The unified international gastric cancer staging classification. Scand J Gastroenterol 1987;22(Suppl 133):11.
8. American Joint Committee on Cancer. Stomach. In: Beahrs OH, Henson DE, Hutter RVP, Kennedy BJ, eds. Manual for staging of cancer. 4th ed. Philadelphia: JB Lippincott, 1992:63.
9. Japanese Research Society for Gastric Cancer. The general rules for the gastric cancer study in surgery and pathology. Japanese Journal of Surgery 1982;11:127.
10. Maruyama K, Okaboyashi K, Kinoshita T. Progress in gastric cancer surgery and its limits of radicality. World J Surg 1987;11:418.
11. Kennedy, BJ. Staging of gastric cancer. In: Nishi M, Ichikawa H, Nakajima T, Maruyama K, Tahara E, eds. Gastric cancer. Tokyo: Springer-Verlag, 1993:102.

Surgery for Gastrointestinal Cancer: A Multidisciplinary Approach, edited by Harold J. Wanebo.
Lippincott-Raven Publishers, Philadelphia, © 1997.

CHAPTER 24

Operative Strategies

J. Rüdiger Siewert, Knut Böttcher, and Hubert J. Stein

AIMS OF SURGERY

The aim of any surgical approach to gastric carcinoma should be a complete resection with no residual tumor left behind at the end of the operation. This situation corresponds to the R0 category of the International Union Against Cancer (UICC), namely, a curative resection.[1] Complete tumor resection by this definition comprises the following:

Primary tumor: no residual tumor at the oral and aboral resection margins and the tumor bed

Lymphatic drainage: as a minimal requirement, no residual tumor in the peripheral or border lymph nodes (relative R0 resection).

To improve a patient's prognosis, the tumor must be removed with an adequate safety margin. The extent of this safety margin depends on the growth pattern of the tumor (ie, the Laurén classification). Gastric carcinoma with a "diffuse type" growth pattern requires a larger oral and aboral safety margin compared with tumors with an "intestinal type" growth pattern. This is also true for the tumor bed, the "third dimension" of the resection.

A safety margin should also be respected in the area of the lymphatic drainage. This means that the number of removed lymph nodes must exceed the number of obviously invaded nodes seen on routine examination, if the prognosis of the patient is to be improved by the surgical procedure. By multivariate analysis, the ratio of invaded to removed lymph nodes (the so-called "lymph node ratio") is a dominant independent prognostic factor.[2] A lymph node ratio below 0.2—that is, less than 20% of removed nodes invaded by tumor—is required to improve the prognosis in gastric carcinoma. Lymph node resection of this extent is justified by the high prevalence of the so-called microinvolvement in the lymph nodes of tumors staged as N0 on routine examination. This extensive resection defines the *absolute R0 resection*. Surgical procedures that do not lead to complete tumor resection will not improve the patient's prognosis, and must be considered *palliative resections*.

An extensive preoperative diagnostic assessment and staging are required to define the tumor situation and tailor the therapeutic concept to the individual patient.

BASIC INFORMATION REQUIRED FOR SURGICAL DECISION MAKING

Epidemiology

There are marked differences in the epidemiology of gastric carcinoma between the Western and Eastern hemispheres[3]:

- In the West, tumors located in the proximal stomach and cardia are increasing in prevalence, whereas in the East, tumors located in the distal stomach predominate (Fig. 24-1).
- Patients with gastric cancer in the West are about 10 to 15 years older than patients in the East.
- In Japan, gastric carcinoma is increasingly diagnosed at the stage of "early cancer." The prevalence of early gastric cancer is now at around 40% to 45% in Japanese series. In contrast, the diagnosis of an "early cancer" in the West remains a rather rare situation, with a prevalence of early gastric cancer of around 10% to 15%.
- In the East, tumors of Borrmann types I and II predominate.

Grading and Tumor Growth Pattern

Because of interobserver errors, information regarding *tumor grading* cannot reliably be used. Consequently, the tumor grade is only of limited therapeutic value. A grade III or IV tumor may, however, respond favorably to chemotherapy.

In contrast, information regarding the *growth pattern* of the tumor (Laurén classification[4]) is of major therapeutic relevance because it determines the extent of luminal resection. Although

J. Rüdiger Siewert, Professor of Surgery, Department of Surgery, Klinikum rechts der Isar, Technische Universität München, Ismaningerstr. 22, D-81675 München, Germany

Knut Böttcher, Department of Surgery, Klinikum rechts der Isar, Technische Universität München, Ismaningerstr. 22, D-81675 München, Germany

Hubert J. Stein, Department of Surgery, Klinikum rechts der Isar, Technische Universität München, Ismaningerstr. 22, D-81675 München, Germany

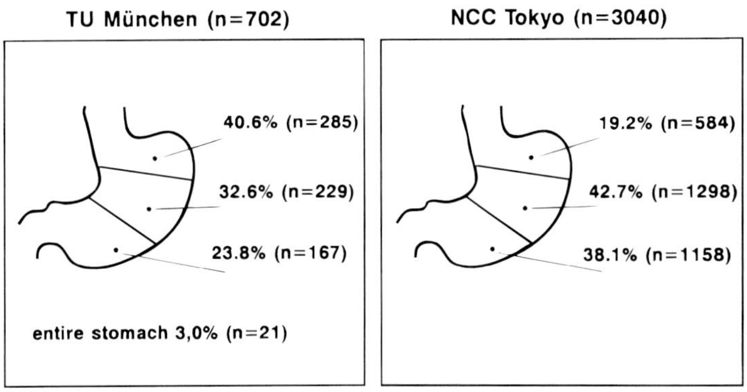

FIG. 24-1. Epidemiologic localization of gastric cancer.

a safety margin of 3 cm appears sufficient in patients with an intestinal-type growth pattern, a safety margin of 5 to 6 cm is required for tumors with nonintestinal-type growth to achieve complete tumor removal. Intestinal-type tumors are more common in the proximal third of the stomach, are detected at an earlier stage, and lymph node metastases are less common. An R0 resection can therefore more often be achieved in patients with intestinal-type tumors (Fig. 24-2). If the growth pattern of the tumor is included in the decision regarding the extent of resection, the Laurén classification is not an independent prognostic factor.

Rules of Tumor Progression

There is a good correlation between the depth of wall penetration of the primary tumor and the extent of lymph node metastases. Lymphatic vessels of the stomach reach only to the submucosa. Consequently, a tumor can metastasize to the lymph nodes only after invasion of the submucosa. This is reflected in the clinical situation: lymph node metastases are extremely rare (<5%) in patients with a tumor limited to the mucosa (pT1A). In patients with tumor invading the submucosa (pT1B), the prevalence of lymph node metastases increases to 20%. With increasing depth of tumor penetration, the prevalence of lymph node metastases increases further (Fig. 24-3). Lymph node skipping is extremely rare (<2%).

Tumor infiltration of the serosa (pT3) is associated with a high prevalence of free tumor cells in the peritoneal cavity. The probability of peritoneal carcinosis increases accordingly in this situation. Diffuse-type tumors cause peritoneal carcinosis more often than intestinal-type tumors.

The probability of distant metastases is primarily determined by the degree of vascular invasion of the primary tumor. Distant metastases occur most often by the portal vein (ie, hepatic metastases predominate).

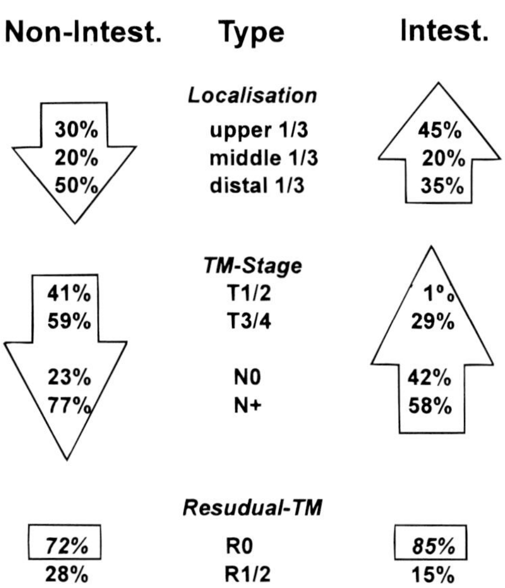

FIG. 24-2. Types of tumor growth in gastric cancer.

Lymphatic Drainage

The lymphatic drainage of the stomach follows the anatomy of the larger vessels. The embryonic stomach is initially located strictly in the center of the yolk sac and rotates during embryogenesis. Blood vessels and the lymphatic vessels originating from the centrally located celiac axis follow this rotation. This explains why the lymphatic drainage of the stomach is directed toward the celiac trunk. The classification of the Japanese Research Society for Gastric Cancer takes this anatomic situation into account.[5] The lymph nodes located of and parallel to the greater and lesser curvature (lymph node stations 1 to 6) are combined into compartment I. The central lymph nodes along the large vessels and toward the celiac axis (lymph node stations 7 to 12) are combined into compartment II. Lymphatic metastases beyond the celiac axis are considered systemic metastases. This is reflected in the UICC TNM classification, which considers the prognosis of patients with lymph node metastases in compartment III similar to the prognosis with distant organ metastases (M_{Lymph}).

Extraperitoneal gastric tumors located at the cardia, the posterior wall of the proximal fundus, and tumors that grow beyond the pylorus are exempt from these rules of lymph node metastasis. These tumors have a direct extraperitoneal lymphatic drainage toward the left and right paraaortic nodes.

Special Aspects of Proximal-Third Gastric Cancer

For a number of reasons, this subgroup of gastric carcinoma must be considered a separate entity.

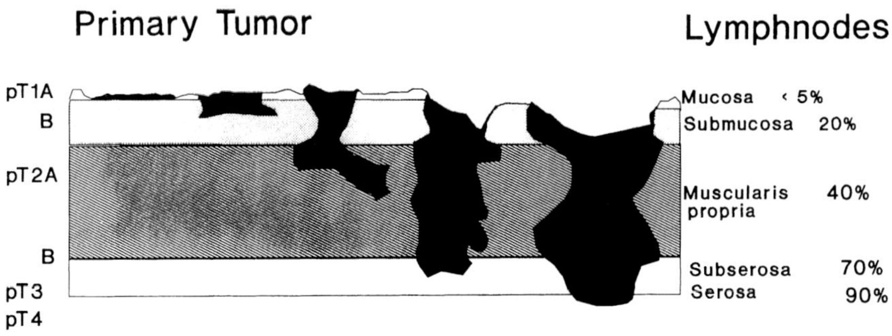

FIG. 24-3. Depth of tumor penetration and prevalence of lymph node metastases in gastric cancer.

Definition

Carcinoma of the proximal gastric third frequently cannot be differentiated from true carcinoma of the cardia. In addition, these tumors must be distinguished from adenocarcinoma of the distal esophagus (Barrett's carcinoma). Our experience shows that these three tumor entities can be best discriminated based on the location of the tumor center.[6] The diagnosis of a Barrett's carcinoma is usually easy, because the accompanying columnar-type epithelium can be documented in 75% to 85% of patients. At least 50% of the tumor mass must be located in the tubular esophagus to classify a tumor as Barrett's carcinoma. To classify a tumor as proximal gastric carcinoma, the tumor center must be aboral of the anatomic cardia. Tumors whose center is located within 2 cm oral or aboral of the anatomic cardia represent true carcinomas of the cardia (Fig. 24-4).

With regard to therapy, it is only necessary definitely to differentiate Barrett's carcinoma from the other two entities. This is because a Barrett's carcinoma must be treated as esophageal cancer, whereas the therapeutic principles are similar for true carcinoma of the cardia and tumors of the proximal gastric third.[7]

Anatomy

A portion of the gastric fundus (posterior wall, lesser curvature, greater curvature) is located extraperitoneally. These areas as well as the anatomic cardia have a direct extraperitoneal lymphatic drainage toward the left renal hilus and the left adrenal gland. This must be taken into account when performing a surgical resection (Fig. 24-5).

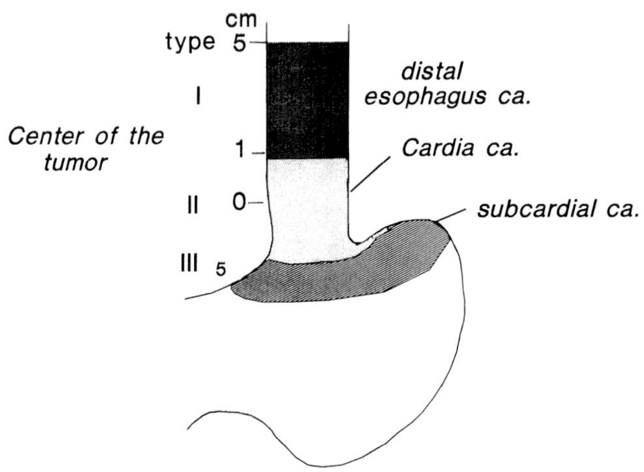

FIG. 24-4. Definition of cancer of the cardia in relation to cancers of the distal esophagus and subcardia (proximal stomach). (Siewert JR, Hölscher AH, Becker K, Gössner W. Kardiakarzinom: Verscheiner therapeutisch relevantan Klassifikation. Chirurg 1987;58:25.)

T Classification

The T classification of tumors located in the proximal gastric third is difficult. Compared with tumors at other locations, tumors of the proximal third frequently infiltrate an area of the gastric wall that is not covered by a serosal lining. Because these tumors do not reach the serosa, they cannot be classified as T3 tumors by the UICC system, and remain T2 tumors regardless of the true depth of infiltration. This situation leads to a down-staging and the erroneous assumption of a poor prognosis for tumors in a proximal location. In a recent analysis,[7] we showed that the prognosis of proximal tumors—when classified according to the true depth of infiltration—is not different from that of more distally located tumors (Table 24-1).

N Classification

The N category in the UICC classification is another area of concern. Because of their relatively frequent extraperitoneal

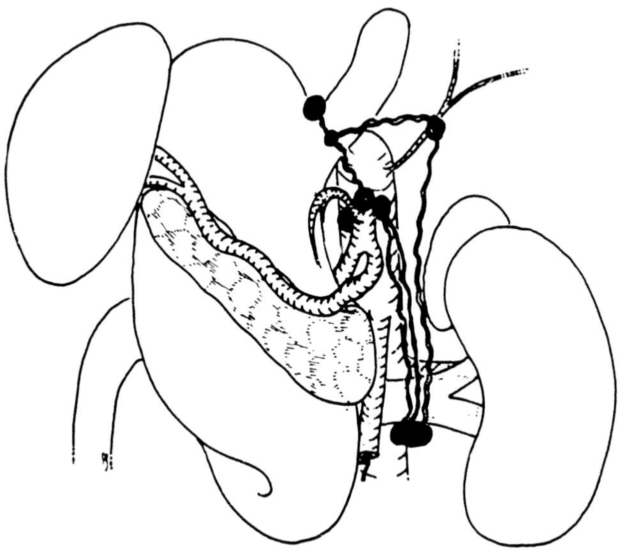

FIG. 24-5. Extraperitoneal lymphatic drainage of relevance in cardial and subcardial gastric cancer. (Sarrazin R, Pissas A, Dyon JF, Bouchet Y. Lymphatic drainage of the stomach. Anat Clin 1980;2:95.)

TABLE 24-1. *Gastric cancer in the proximal versus middle/distal third: prognosis according to UICC stage after modification*

Stage		No. of patients	Median survival (mo)	5-Year survival (%)	*P*-value
IA	p	20	—	92	0.70
	md	75	—	86	
IB	p	16	—	59	0.62
	md	21	—	64	
II	p	34	71.3	74	0.62
	md	39	—	54	
IIIA	p	46	23.9	27	0.28
	md	49	23.8	30	
IIIB	p	48	11.8	14	0.06
	md	40	21.5	17	
IV	p	34	15.5	15	0.41
	md	44	8.3	11	

UICC, International Union Against Cancer; *P*, proximal third; *md*, middle distal third.

From Siewert JR, Böttcher K, Stein HJ, Roder JD, Busch R. The problem of proximal third gastric cancer. World J Surg 1995;19:523.

location, tumors of the proximal third often metastasize directly to the retroperitoneum. It is unclear whether these lymph node metastases should be classified as N1 or N3 (M_{Lymph}). Until there is a clear definition, the clinician therefore should differentiate only between N0 and N + categories. The situation is similar in esophageal and cardia carcinoma.

Gender

The male gender is much more frequently involved if the tumor is located in the proximal third of the stomach.

PREOPERATIVE STAGING AS A PRECONDITION FOR SURGICAL DECISION MAKING

Preoperative staging plays an important role in the diagnostic work-up of patients with gastric carcinoma. Preoperative staging not only allows a tailored surgical approach, but permits identification of patients who will not benefit from primary surgical therapy. The primary aim of preoperative staging is to define the tumor stage (TNM). Additional relevant prognostic factors should also be assessed and included in the process of therapeutic decision making. The accuracy of preoperative staging has gained significantly with the introduction of endoluminal ultrasonography, surgical laparoscopy, and the Maruyama computer program.[8–11]

Endoscopic ultrasound allows prediction of the T category with an accuracy of 85%, although its accuracy regarding the N category is only about 65% to 75%.[8]

Surgical laparoscopy permits a definitive statement regarding peritoneal carcinosis and also enables a reassessment of the endosonographic T category with the use of direct laparoscopic ultrasonography. In addition, biopsy sampling of various lymph nodes (including those at the celiac axis) can be

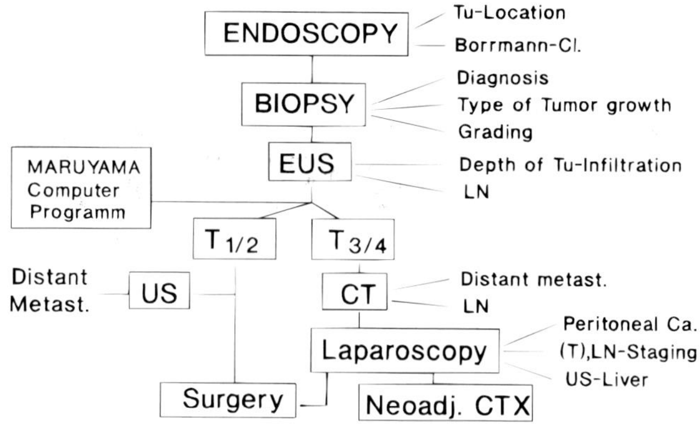

FIG. 24-6. Diagnostic procedure in gastric cancer. *EUS*, endoscopic ultrasound; *LN*, lymph node; *CT*, computed tomography; *US*, ultrasound; *CTX*, chemotherapy.

performed. This markedly increases the accuracy of endoluminal ultrasonography in the preoperative staging of the N category. Finally, liver metastases can be excluded or proven by means of laparoscopic ultrasound and biopsy.[9]

The preoperative staging of gastric carcinoma, in contrast to other tumors, can be performed with the help of a validated and well established *computer program*.[10,11]

Our current diagnostic approach to gastric carcinoma based on preoperative staging is given in Figure 24-6. This approach allows the identification of a group of patients with locally advanced gastric carcinoma who may benefit from preoperative chemotherapy.[12]

SURGICAL INDICATIONS

With the help of the previously outlined staging modalities, the tumor stage can be predicted with an accuracy of 80% to 85%. The indications for surgical therapy should be guided by the tumor stage and the chances of achieving complete tumor removal with the surgical procedure. Patient-dependent risk factors should also be considered. Because of standardization, gastric resections can, however, also be performed safely in patients with increased surgical risk.

The indication for a surgical procedure is given when complete tumor removal can be anticipated with surgical resection. Whether preoperative or postoperative adjuvant therapy can improve the results of surgery in this situation is unclear at present. If, based on preoperative staging, complete tumor removal is not anticipated with surgical resection, a down-staging of the tumor by preoperative chemotherapy should be considered.[12]

Based on pretherapeutic staging, three basic situations of therapeutic relevance have to be differentiated:

1. Gastric carcinoma *stage IA and the so-called mucosa carcinoma*: This subgroup of of patients with early gastric carcinoma can be cured by local excision because the probability of lymphatic metastasis is far below 5% in these tumors. Such limited surgery may be performed endoscopically or laparoscopically.[13,14] On the other hand, even with the aid of endoscopic ultrasonography it is not possible to determine definitively whether the tumor is limited to the mu-

cosa. An excision of the entire gastric wall should therefore always be preferred in these patients to obtain a specimen that permits a histologic diagnosis of "mucosa carcinoma."

2. The second group includes *tumor stages IB (submucosa carcinoma), II, and IIIA*. Lymph node metastases can be expected in a high percentage of these patients. Based on the published data, this group of patients receives most benefit from radical surgery, in particular from systematic lymphadenectomy.[15–17] In this group of patients, it is possible to achieve an R0 resection in the area of the primary tumor as well as the lymphatic drainage when adequate surgical techniques are applied.
3. The third group encompasses locally advanced gastric tumors that may already have distant metastases (*tumor stages IIIB and IV*). In this situation, a complete tumor removal usually cannot be achieved by surgical resection. Rather, microscopic or macroscopic residual tumor remains in situ at the end of the surgical resection. The procedure is only of palliative character, and cannot improve the patient's prognosis. Consequently, neoadjuvant therapeutic modalities are being investigated in this group of patients.[12]

In summary, primary surgical resection and lymphadenectomy are indicated for tumor stages IB, II, and IIIA. Neoadjuvant therapeutic modalities should be used before surgery in patients with tumor stages IIIB und IV. Alternatively, a palliative surgical procedures can be applied in these patients. These precepts are valid for gastric carcinoma at any location.

CHOICE OF PROCEDURE

The selection of surgical procedure in patients with gastric carcinoma (Fig. 24-7) should be adjusted primarily to the location of the tumor. Based on the recommendations of the UICC, but also those of the Japanese Research Society for Gastric Cancer, the stomach is divided into thirds. Although the borders between these thirds are not exactly defined, this definition has proven useful in determining the extent of resection.

The growth pattern of the tumor is another factor that determines the extent of the resection. Infiltrative growing tumors (diffuse type) have to be differentiated from noninfiltrative growing tumors (intestinal type). As outlined above, the growth pattern defines the necessary minimum safety margin.

The expected location of lymph node metastases is the final parameter to be considered when selecting the extent of the extraluminal resection. The probability of lymph node metastases in relation to the tumor stage has been defined by the Japanese Research Society for Gastric Cancer and in the work of Maruyama and colleagues.[5,18]

Distal-Third Gastric Carcinoma

Depending on the growth pattern, a subtotal (intestinal-type carcinoma) or a total (diffuse-type carcinoma) gastrectomy should be performed. As with gastric carcinoma at other locations, a D2 lymph node dissection is the method of choice. In patients with very distal tumors, the lymph node dissection has to be extended to include lymph node stations 12 (hepatoduodenal ligament nodes), 13 (retroduodenal nodes), and 16 (right paraaortic nodes).

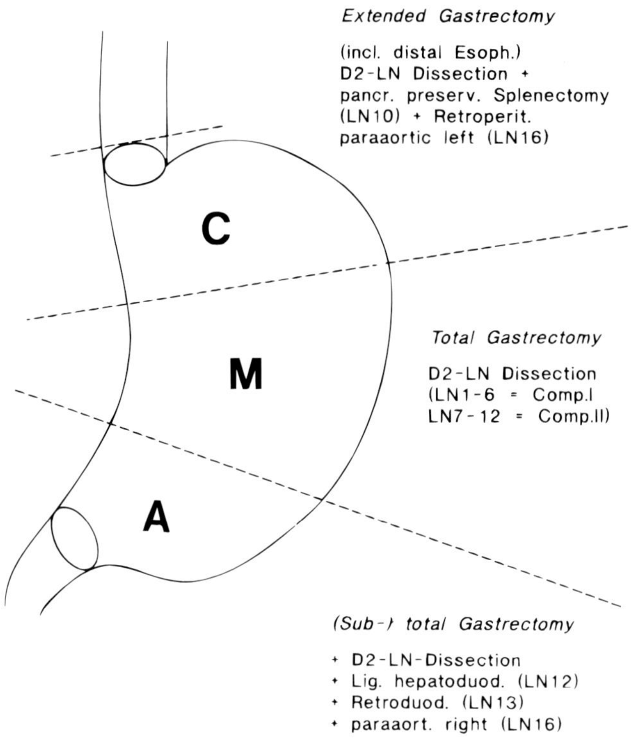

FIG. 24-7. Choice of surgical procedure in gastric cancer. *C,* cardia; *M,* middle third; *A,* anterior third.

Middle-Third Gastric Carcinoma

These tumors always require a total gastrectomy and a D2 lymph node dissection. The D2 resection encompasses lymph node stations 1 to 6 (compartment I) and 7 to 11 (compartment II).

Proximal-Third Gastric Carcinoma

These tumors usually require an extended gastrectomy, including the distal esophagus. To determine the extent of the distal esophagectomy with certainty, we recommend an intraoperative frozen section of the oral resection margin. For proximal-third carcinoma, a D2 lymph node dissection is also the standard procedure. In addition, a lymphadenectomy of lymph node stations 11 and 12 must be performed. This is best accomplished through a pancreas-preserving splenectomy.[19,20] A retroperitoneal paraaortic lymphadenectomy (lymph node station 16) is essential to account for the retroperitoneal lymphatic drainage from the posterior wall of the fundus or cardia toward the left adrenal gland and the hilus of the kidney (see Fig. 24-5).

TECHNIQUE

Lymphadenectomy

The removal of lymph node stations 1 to 6 along the greater and lesser curvature comprises the D1 lymph node dissection. Currently, however, a D2 lymph node dissection is considered

TABLE 24-2. *Recommendations for the pathologic–anatomic evaluation of surgical specimen*

Exact localization of tumor
Histologic tumor diagnosis according to the World Health Organization classification
T category
Tumor grading (G)
Safety margins (R) in cm/mm
Number of resected lymph nodes
Number of involved lymp nodes and their localization (N category)
Ratio of removed to involved lymph nodes (lymph node ratio)
M category (if possible)
Associated changes in nontumor tissue

standard therapy (lymph node stations 7 to 11 in addition to stations 1 to 6). For tumors in the middle third, this rule is valid without exception. For tumors in the proximal or distal third of the stomach, a D2 lymph node dissection and removal of additional lymph node stations depending on the location of the tumor is indicated (D3 or D4 dissection).

In Western countries, lymphadenectomy is performed in the so-called ''en-bloc technique,'' that is, the lymphatic tissue is removed en bloc from the periphery to the center. All lymph nodes are attached to the specimen and the pathologist is able to identify the anatomic location of the nodes, dissect and count the nodes, and perform histopathologic evaluation of tumor invasion. Only an en bloc specimen allows assessment of all the essential prognostic parameters (Table 24-2). In the East, the lymph nodes are dissected individually and classified according to their anatomic location by the surgeon.

Subtotal Gastrectomy

The luminal extent of the resection with a subtotal gastrectomy comprises about 80% of the stomach. At the lesser curvature, the resection should reach up to about 2 cm below the anatomic cardia. At the greater curvature, the resection has to go beyond the right and left gastroepiploic arteries. The small remaining fundus is fed through the short gastric vessels from the splenic hilus.

Because subtotal gastrectomy is only performed for tumors located in the distal third, the resection has to be extended as far as possible beyond the pylorus. In any case, the dissection of the duodenum should be extended beyond the border of the gastroduodenal artery into the extraperitoneal space. The duodenal stump can be closed with a stapler. Closure of the remaining proximal stomach can also be performed with staplers. This prevents contamination of the situs (Fig. 24-8*A*).

Extraluminal resection and lymphadenectomy must be as radical as with a total gastrectomy. Limitations exist only with respect to lymph node station 2 (left of the cardia). At the lesser curvature, lymph node station 1 has to be included in the lymphadenectomy. To perform the lymphadenectomy in the correct layer (ie, the adventitia of the arteries), dissection should be started along the gastroduodenal artery, which has already been dissected for closure of the duodenal stump (Fig. 24-8*B*). From there it is easy to find the correct dissection layer to the common hepatic artery, which is the starting point for the lymphadenectomy. Toward the periphery, lymphadenectomy should be continued beyond the bifurcation of the hepatic artery. The right gastric artery should be ligated at its origin. In addition to lymph nodes in compartments I and II, a lymphadenectomy of lymph node station 13 and of the right paraaortic and paracaval nodes (lymph node station 16) should always be performed with a subtotal gastrectomy. This requires a sufficient mobilization of the duodenum according to Kocher. Lymph node station 13 represents the border lymph node toward the periphery. This lymph node is marked and pulled through the foramen of Winslow behind the hepatoduodenal ligament. The surgeon's left index finger is then inserted into the foramen of Winslow to push the portal vein cephalad and anteriorly toward the surgeon. Further dissection of the lymph nodes can be continued on the adventitia of the

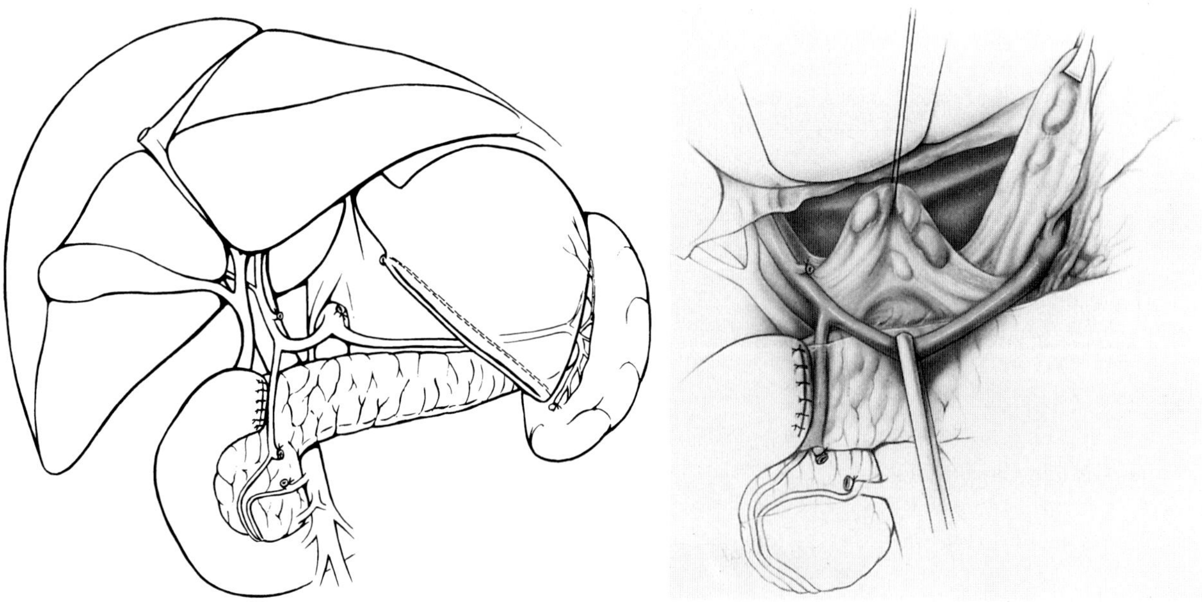

A B

FIG. 24-8. (A) Extent of resection in subtotal gastrectomy. **(B)** Start of lymph node dissection along the gastroduodenal artery and the common hepatic artery.

portal vein. Medially, the left gastric artery is ligated and severed at its origin. The left gastric vein is similarly ligated and cut. The posterior dissection is continued to the diaphragmatic crura, and the left and right phrenic arteries are ligated.

After severing the vagus nerve, the entire lymphatic and fatty tissue can be pulled aborally. Further dissection along the lesser curvature is performed using a vagotomy technique: the anterior and posterior sheaths of the hepatogastric ligament are divided step by step. This allows complete removal of the lymph nodes along the lesser curvature (Fig. 24-9).

The resection of lymph node station 11 is performed at the upper border of the pancreas toward the splenic hilus. This lymph node station should be dissected with great care, because a splenectomy would compromise the blood supply of the gastric stump. Resection of the greater omentum is obligatory.

Before reconstruction of the intestinal passage, the lesser curvature of the gastric stump and the resection line are oversewn with interrupted sutures. Only a small portion of the resection line toward the greater curvature is used for the anastomosis. Reconstruction of alimentary tract continuity can be performed with a retrocolic or antecolic jejunal loop, with the gastroenterostomy in an isoperistaltic direction (oralis partialis). A side-to-side jejunojejunostomy (according to Braun) is recommended (Fig. 24-10).

Analyses of the quality of life and patient satisfaction after total and subtotal gastrectomy have shown that symptoms and objective signs of alkaline reflux into the esophagus are common sequelae of this reconstruction.[21,22] Consequently, we have modified the reconstruction to a Roux-en-Y configuration.

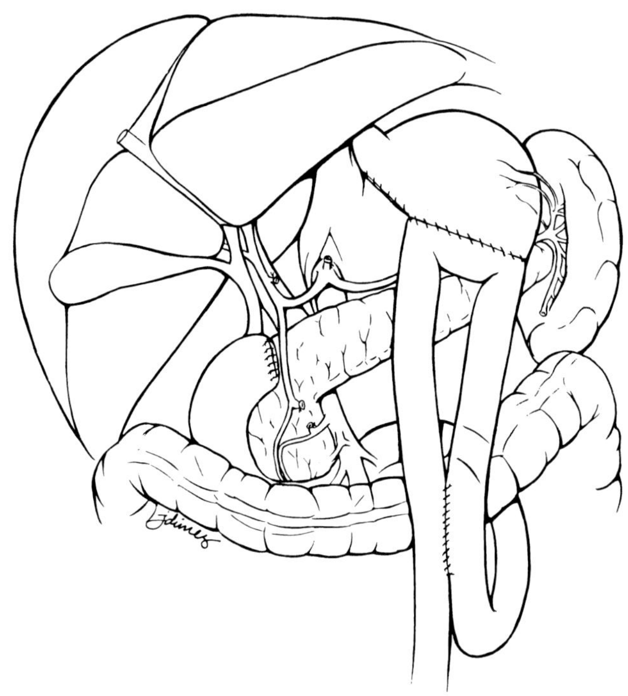

FIG. 24-10. Reconstruction after subtotal gastrectomy.

Total Gastrectomy

A total gastrectomy is always performed together with a systematic lymphadenectomy of compartments I and II. As discussed earlier, an extension of the lymph node dissection may be indicated, depending on the location of the tumor.

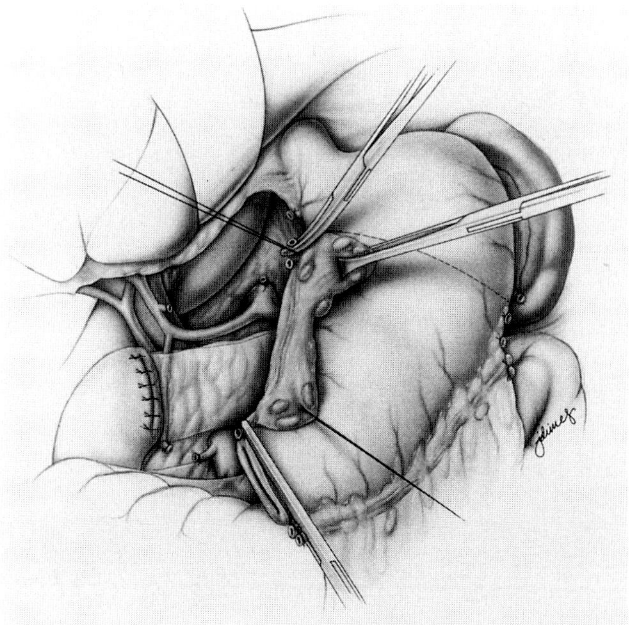

FIG. 24-9. Lymph node dissection along the lesser curvature in subtotal gastrectomy.

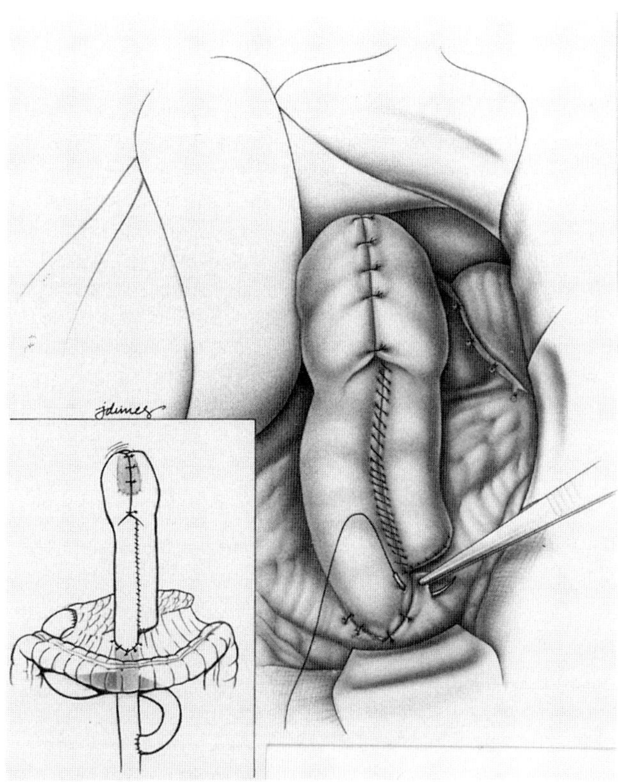

FIG. 24-11. Reconstruction after total gastrectomy with pouch formation and jejunoplication.

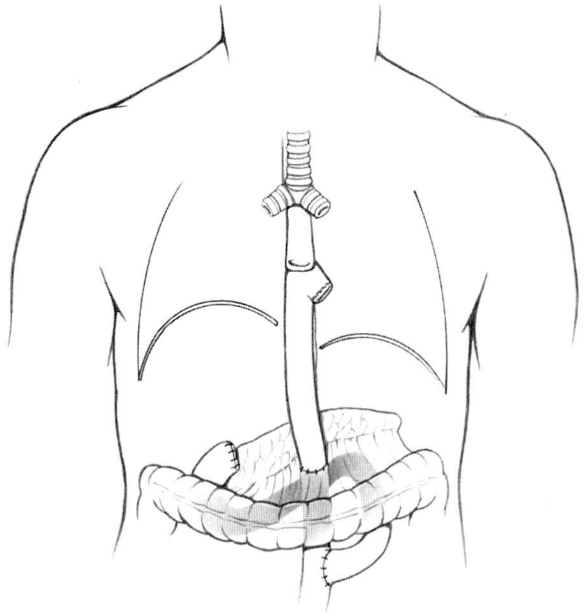

FIG. 24-12. Orally extended total gastrectomy: reconstruction with esophagojejunostomy and Roux-en-Y insertion of the ascending loop.

Analyses of quality of life after total gastrectomy support reconstruction using a pouch. Because the advantages conferred by pouch reconstruction are significant only in the long term, the patient's prognosis must be taken into account when considering the type of reconstruction. If the prognosis is good, a pouch must be recommended (Fig. 24-11). If the prognosis is poor, the easiest reconstruction (Roux-en-Y esophagojejunostomy) should be performed (Fig. 24-12).

For construction of a pouch, a side-to-side anastomosis over a distance of 10 to 15 cm between the ascending and descending portion of the first jejunal loop is usually sufficient (the Hunt-Rodino pouch). A jejunoplication can be added to the pouch.[23,24] Whether a Roux-en-Y biliary diversion should be added to the pouch to avoid alkaline reflux into the pouch and the distal esophagus is a matter of controversy.

The esophagointestinal anastomosis can be easily performed with a circular stapler. In controlled studies, this type of reconstruction has been shown to be superior to a manual anastomosis.[25]

Extended Gastrectomy

The gastrectomy can be extended toward various portions of the distal esophagus; toward a splenectomy, including a complete dissection of the lymph node stations 10 and 11 (pancreas-preserving splenectomy); or toward the right side with a resection of the head of the pancreas.

Orally Extended Total Gastrectomy

The extent of resection of the distal esophagus depends on the individual tumor situation. An essential prerequisite for resection of the distal esophagus is a wide splitting of the esophageal hiatus that opens the posterior mediastinum. This allows an unhampered dissection of the distal esophagus, including the surrounding lymphatic and fatty tissue and the periesophageal lymph nodes (the so-called transhiatal partial esophagectomy). Generous splitting of the hiatus allows resection of the esophagus almost up to the level of the azygos vein. After the resection margins have been defined—if necessary with the help of frozen sections—the esophagus is transected distal to a purse-string clamp. Before any further manipulations, the head of the circular stapler is introduced into the oral portion of the esophagus and the purse-string suture is tied. Only then is the specimen removed.

From a technical and functional point of view, the construction of a pouch in this situation does not make sense because the pouch is located partially within the chest and cannot function as a reservoir. The reconstruction is performed end-to-side with an esophagojejunostomy and distal implantation of the ascending loop in the Roux-en-Y technique. The distance between the esophagointestinal anastomosis and the end-to-side anastomosis should be at least 40 to 50 cm. The anastomosis between the esophagus and the jejunum is performed in the so-called Krückstock technique, namely, the circular stapler is introduced through the severed jejunum into the descending loop, and the thorn is advanced and then connected with the head of the stapler. A rich blood supply to the jejunal loop is the essential prerequisite for a safe anastomosis. To ensure a sufficient blood supply, it is absolutely necessary to assess the vascularization of the jejunum using diaphanoscopy and identify a suitable loop. If these steps are followed, anastomotic leakage is rare. The redundant part of the interposed jejunal loop is closed with a linear stapler (see Fig. 24-12).

Left-Sided Extension of the Gastrectomy

Whenever possible, a resection of the tail of the pancreas should be avoided, because this is followed by septic complica-

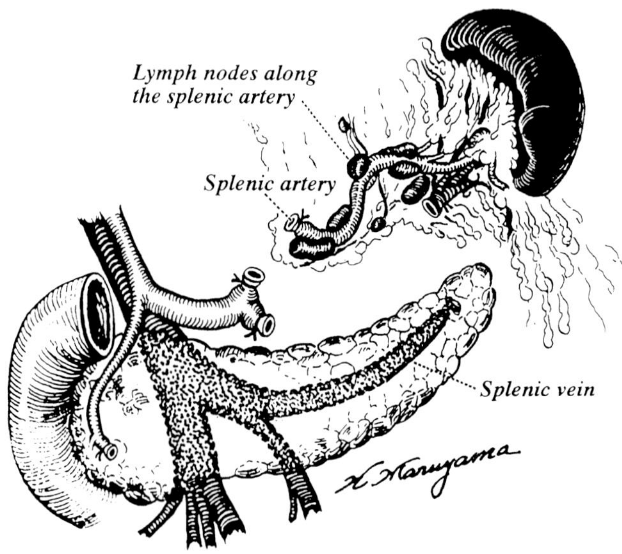

FIG. 24-13. Pancreas-preserving splenectomy and lymph node dissection according to Maruyama. (Maruyama K. A new dissection technique of superior pancreatic lymph nodes, pancreas preserving radical gastrectomy. Japanese Journal of Gastroenterologic Surgery 1979;12:961.)

tions in 20% to 25% of patients (pancreatic fistulas and abscesses). The only indication for resection of the pancreatic tail is direct invasion of a posterior wall tumor into the pancreas. A pancreas-preserving splenectomy and lymphadenectomy should be performed in all other situations (Fig. 24-13). For this purpose, the splenic artery and vein can be isolated, ligated, and cut to the left of the aorta. The entire vascular and lymphatic bundle can then be dissected from the superior border of the pancreas. The blood supply to the pancreatic tail is maintained through retropancreatic and intrapancreatic vessels.[19] The dissection is continued to the splenic hilum and includes the splenectomy. These lymphatics, including the spleen, are removed en bloc with the gastric specimen. At the end of this dissection, the tail of the pancreas is mobilized and can easily be turned to the right to allow easy removal of left paraaortic lymph nodes in the retroperitoneal triangle between the aorta, hilus of the left kidney and left adrenal gland, and diaphragm, respectively. The adrenal gland may be removed. The reconstruction after this procedure is the same as the reconstruction after total gastrectomy.

Left Upper Abdominal Evisceration

This procedure corresponds to the left-sided extension of the gastrectomy, including left-sided pancreatic resection and occasionally resection of the left colonic flexure as well. A left-sided adrenalectomy is obligatory. This procedure is indicated only if an absolute R0 resection can be achieved (Fig. 24-14).

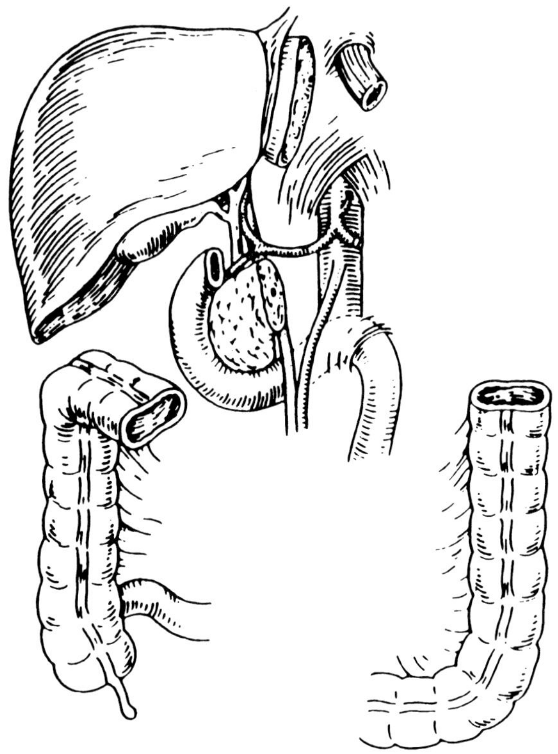

FIG. 24-14. Left upper abdominal evisceration. (Nishi M, Ohta K, Nakajima T. Combined resection. In: Nishim, Ichika H, Nokajima T, Maruyama K, Tahara E, eds. Gastric cancer Berlin: Springer-Verlag, 1993:306.)

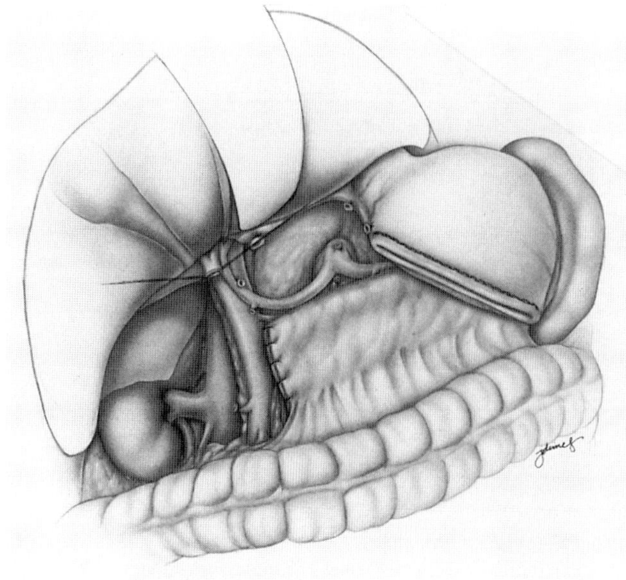

FIG. 24-15. Right-sided extension of gastrectomy (according to the Whipple operation).

Right-Sided Extension of the Gastrectomy

A resection of the head of the pancreas as an extension of a total or subtotal gastrectomy is rarely indicated. If lymph node metastases have developed in this region or the tumor has directly invaded the head of the pancreas, such extensive resections improve the prognosis only in exceptional situations. The procedure is indicated only if an absolute R0 resection can be achieved. The surgical technique corresponds to the Whipple operation (Fig. 24-15).

MORBIDITY AND MORTALITY

Early Postoperative Complications

Early postoperative complications can result from leakage of the anastomoses. In this respect, an esophagointestinal anastomosis is more critical than a gastroenterostomy. Leakages of the duodenal stump are rare in gastric cancer surgery. The lymphadenectomy may cause lymphatic fistulas, or a pancreatic fistula, if the pancreatic capsule has been injured (Table 24-3). All these situations eventually lead to an infection of the surgical situs and must be considered as septic complications. Revisional surgery is, however, rarely needed. Adequate drainage usually is sufficient to manage the complication. Fluid collections can safely be localized and drained using computed tomography. In rare situations a septic focus may, however, result in arosion of a large vessel and intraabdominal bleeding. This situation obviously requires immediate surgical revision.

The mortality of the described procedures for gastric carcinoma is well below 5% in specialized centers, and is directly related to the extent of the resection (see Table 24-3).

TABLE 24-3. *Postoperative morbidity and mortality according to the extent of resection*

Extent of resection	Leakage rate (%)	Abscess rate (%)	Complication rate (%)	Mortality (%)
Subtotal gastrectomy				
GGCS (n = 382)	2.9	1.6	19.9	6.0*
NSCT (n = 282)	—	—	30.1	11.0†
TUM (n = 188)	1.1	2.7	17.5	4.2†
Total gastrectomy				
GGCS (n = 787)	7.2	5.5	30.0	4.4*
NSCT (n = 350)	—	—	38.3	7.7†
TUM (n = 307)	4.8	3.8	22.8	5.2†
Extended total gastrectomy				
GGCS (n = 389)	12.3	4.9	38.0	5.7*
TUM (n = 334)	7.8	7.5	32.9	6.9†

* 30-Day mortality.
† Hospital mortality.
GGCS, German Gastric Cancer Study; *NSCT*, Norge Stomach Cancer Trial; *TUM*, Technische Universität München.

From Roder JD, Böttcher K, Siewert JR, Busch R, Hermanek P, Meyer HJ, and the German Gastric Cancer Study Group. Prognostic factors in gastric carcinoma. Cancer 1993;72:2089 [GGCS]; Viste A, Haugstvedt T, Eide GE, et al. Postoperative complications and mortality after surgery for gastric cancer. Ann Surg 1988;207:7 [NSCT], and Böttcher K, Becker K, Busch R, Roder JD, Siewert JR. Prognosefaktoren beim Magenkarzinom: Ergebnisse einer uni- und multivariaten Analyse. Chirurg 1992;63:656 [TUM].

Late Complications

With the introduction of the Roux-en-Y biliary diversion, alkaline reflux esophagitis has disappeared as a late complication of gastrectomy. Dumping seems to be less common after total gastrectomy compared with subtotal resections. Dumping can be very annoying to the patient, but the symptoms can usually be managed with conservative therapy.

The role of food passage through the duodenum remains controversial. Based on laboratory data, a duodenal passage certainly has advantages (ie, improved resorption of glucose, iron, and calcium). These advantages, however, obviously do not translate into an improved quality of life and are therefore of no clinical relevance.[26]

The need for frequent, small meals after total gastrectomy can be improved markedly with the construction of a pouch, which allows the patient to eat a normal number of normal-volume meals.

Gastrectomy is always followed by pancreatocybal asynchrony, which may lead to disturbances in food resorption. Substitution of pancreatic enzymes is therefore necessary after gastrectomy. Vitamin B_{12} must also be substituted after gastrectomy.

Analyses of the quality of life after gastrectomy show that most patients adapt to the altered situation. The body weight of patients after gastrectomy remains, however, usually about 10% to 15% below the calculated ideal body weight. Among all patients who had a gastrectomy, those with a pouch reconstruction have the best quality of life, followed by those with a subtotal gastrectomy. The quality of life is worst in patients with simple esophagojejunostomy and Roux-en-Y diversion, particularly if the anastomosis is located within the chest. Because of the increasing prevalence of proximal-third tumors in the West, the latter type of reconstruction will unfortunately be more commonly required. Esophagoduodenostomy or simple esophagojejunostomy without Roux-en-Y biliary diversion have been abandoned by most counts as reconstructive procedures, and their use can no longer be recommended.

Postoperative complications are also of prognostic importance. Multivariate analyses have shown that postoperative complications have an independent negative impact on the long-

TABLE 24-4. *Risk factors for postoperative morbidity in surgery of gastric cancer*

Independent factor	Chi^2-value	*P*-value
Concomitant diseases	26.74	0.0001
Type of resection	24.85	0.0001
Experience of surgical department	20.08	0.0001
Age	4.58	0.032

From Böttcher K, Siewert JR, Roder JD, Busch R, Hermanek P, Meyer HJ, für die Deutsche Magencarcinom-Studiengruppe (GGCS '92). Risiko der chirurgischen Therapie des Magencarcinoms in Deutschland: Ergebnisse der Deutschen Magencarcinom-Studie 1992. Chirug 1994;65:298.

TABLE 24-5. *Risk factors for postoperative mortality in surgery of gastric cancer*

Independent factor	Chi^2-value	*P*-value
Karnofsky index	32.06	0.0001
Concomitant diseases	24.20	0.0001
Lymph node metastases	11.16	0.001
Tumor diameter	10.96	0.001
Experience of surgical department	10.45	0.001
Age	4.97	0.026

From Böttcher K, Siewert JR, Roder JD, Busch R, Hermanek P, Meyer HJ, für die Deutsche Magencarcinom-Studiengruppe (GGCS '92). Risiko der chirurgischen Therapie des Magencarcinoms in Deutschland: Ergebnisse der Deutschen Magencarcinom-Studie 1992. Chirug 1994;65:298.

term survival of patients with gastric cancer.[2] This cannot be explained by a higher postoperative mortality, but appears to result from a modulation of the immune system.

The general status of the patient (Karnofsky index), the presence of accompanying diseases, and the experience of the surgeon and the institution have been identified in multivariate analyses as independent risk factors for postoperative morbidity and mortality. These data should affect choices with regard to the surgeons and institutions who treat patients with gastric carcinoma, and the selection of patients for resection (Tables 24-4 and 24-5).

PREOPERATIVE CHEMOTHERAPY

In phase II studies, preoperative chemotherapy has been shown to be beneficial for patients with locally advanced gastric carcinoma.[12] An exact staging is prerequisite for preoperative chemotherapy (see section on Preoperative Staging).

The surgical therapy of patients with gastric carcinoma who had preoperative chemotherapy is not different from the surgical approach to patients who did not have preoperative therapy. Chemotherapy may induce a fibrous scarring of perigastric and gastric structures. This does not, however, increase the difficulty or risk of the surgical procedure. Also, the risk of postoperative bleeding or infection is not increased after chemotherapy.

An analysis of prognostic factors (Table 24-6) shows that the nodal status and consequently lymphadenectomy persist as the leading predictors of survival after preoperative chemotherapy. In other words, the extent of resection must not be reduced after preoperative chemotherapy. Rather, a systematic lymph node dissection of compartments I and II, similar to that in patients who have a primary resection, is also mandatory after chemotherapy. The luminal extent of resection in this situation depends on the primary tumor *before* chemotherapy. Even if there has been a complete remission with chemotherapy, the extent of the resection must be based on tumor location and size before neoadjuvant therapy. The same is true for the extent of the lymphadenectomy.

Studies clearly show that preoperative chemotherapy does not increase the postoperative morbidity or mortality. However, septic complications tend to have a prolonged course after preoperative chemotherapy.[27,28]

TABLE 24-6. *Prognostic factors after neoadjuvant chemotherapy: univariate and multivariate analyses*

	Significance (*P*-value)	
Prognostic factor	Univariate	Multivariate
Lymph node ratio	0.0002	0.001
Sex	0.008	0.03
Mucositis	0.012	NS
Nausea	0.0015	NS
pN category	0.02	NS
pUICC stage	0.02	NS
Response after neoadjuvant chemotherapy	0.03	NS

VICC, International Union Against Cancer.

TABLE 24-7. *Prognostic factors in gastric carcinoma: literature survey*

Prognostic factors	Reference no.
Preoperative risk factors	2
Sex	29
Borrmann classification	29, 30
Tumor diameter	2, 30, 31
Depth of tumor invasion (pT)	2, 16, 17, 29–33
Tumor grading	34
Lymphatic and vascular invasion	29, 35, 36
Tumor cell dissociation at the invasion front	37
DNA ploidy	29, 38, 39
Nodal state (pN)	2, 30–33, 40
Number of resected lymph nodes, lymph node ratio	2, 17, 31
Lymph node dissection	16, 29–31, 41
Distant metastases (pM)	2, 30, 31
Splenectomy	16
Residual tumor (R)	2, 17, 31
Postoperative complications	2

LONG-TERM RESULTS

Prognostic Factors

The published literature contains a number of studies assessing prognostic factors in patients with gastric carcinoma (Table 24-7). In these studies, a complete tumor resection (R0 resection) and nodal status are the leading predictors of survival. From a surgical point of view, the lymph node ratio (ie, ratio of invaded to removed nodes) is an additional important independent prognostic factor. The implication is that only a radical lymph node dissection can improve this ratio, which corresponds to the hypothetic prognostic factor of Shiu and colleagues.[42]

Five-Year Survival Rates

The 5-year survival rates show marked differences between patients from the East and West, particularly for patients with stage II and IIIA gastric carcinoma (Fig. 24-16). Although the 5- year survival for patients with stage II or IIIA gastric carcinoma in the United states is around 30% and 15%, respectively, these numbers are 45% and 30% in Germany, and 75% and 60% in Japan. Because epidemiologic differences cannot account for the differences in survival between Germany and the Unites States, the superior survival rates in Germany are most likely the result of the more radical surgical approach and adequate lymphadenectomy, which is routinely performed in most German institutions but not in the United States.

The differences between the Japanese results and those from the United States and Germany may reflect an even more radical surgical approach to gastric carcinoma in Japan. Epidemiologic and other factors must, however, also be taken into account when survival rates from Japanese centers are assessed. The distribution of the tumor, the age of the patients, and the growth pattern of the tumor differ markedly between Japanese and

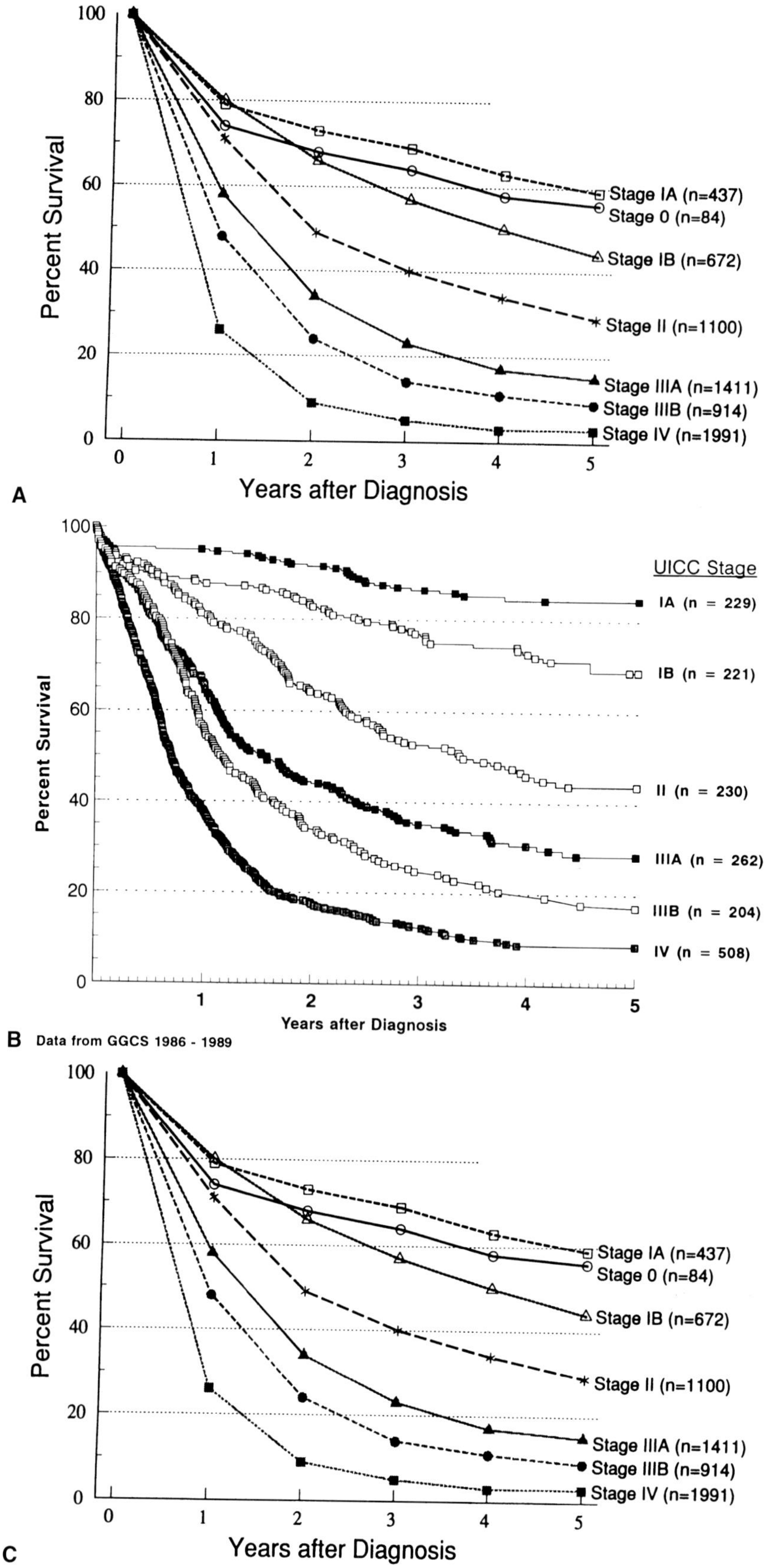

FIG. 24-16. Five-year survival rates for resected gastric cancer. **(A)** Data from the United States (Wanebo HJ, Kennedy BJ, Chmiel J, Steele G Jr, Winchester D, Osteen R. Cancer of the stomach: a patient care study by the American College of Surgeons. Ann Surg 1993;218:583.) **(B)** Data from the German Gastric Cancer Study. (Roder JD, Böttcher K, Siewert JR, Busch R, Hermanek P, Meyer HJ, and the German Gastric Cancer Study Group. Prognostic factors in gastric carcinoma. Cancer 1993;72:2089. **(C)** Collected data from the National Cancer Center Tokyo.

Western series (see section on Basic Information Required for Surgical Decision Making). Furthermore, postoperative chemotherapy is standard procedure in patients with stage II or III gastric carcinoma in Japan, whereas this is rarely performed in Germany or the United States. Finally, survival curves from Japanese centers usually only show tumor-related deaths, and the postoperative mortality or deaths from other reasons are not included. This is in sharp contrast to survival curves from Western centers, which include all deaths during the follow-up period. These factors prohibit a direct stage-by-stage comparison of survival rates between Eastern and Western series. After adjustment for epidemiologic differences, however, the prognosis of patients with gastric carcinoma in Japan and Germany is similar.[3] Nevertheless, the Japanese experience and results have to be considered the current standard for the treatment of gastric carcinoma.

Studies have identified a final prognostic factor. The experience of the individual surgeon and his or her institution directly influences the prognosis of the patient.[43] This is because a higher rate of R0 resections, a larger number of removed lymph nodes (ie, more radical lymphadenectomy), and a lower rate of postoperative complications are seen in experienced centers. These data support the concentration of treatment of gastric carcinoma at experienced institutions.

REFERENCES

1. Hermanek P, Sobin LH. Union Internationale Contre le Cancer: TNM classification of malignant tumors. 4th ed. Berlin: Springer-Verlag, 1992.
2. Roder JD, Böttcher K, Siewert JR, Busch R, Hermanek P, Meyer HJ, the German Gastric Cancer Study Group. Prognostic factors in gastric carcinoma. Cancer 1993;72:2089.
3. Bollschweiler E, Böttcher K, Hölscher AH, et al. Is the prognosis for Japanese and German patients with gastric cancer really different? Cancer 1993;71:2918.
4. Laurén P. The two histologic main types of gastric carcinoma: diffuse and so-called intestinal-type carcinoma. Acta Pathol Microbiol Scand 1965;64:31.
5. Japanese Research Society for Gastric Cancer. The general rules for the gastric cancer study in surgery and pathology. Japanese Journal of Surgery 1981;11:127.
6. Siewert JR, Hölscher AH, Becker K, Gössner W. Kardiakarzinom: Versuch einer therapeutisch relevanten Klassifikation. Chirurg 1987; 58:25.
7. Siewert JR, Böttcher K, Stein HJ, Roder JD, Busch R. The problem of proximal third gastric cancer. World J Surg 1995;19:523.
8. Dittler HJ, Siewert JR. Role of endoscopic ultrasonography in gastric carcinoma. Endoscopy 1993;25:162.
9. Siewert JR, Feussner H. Derzeitiger Stellenwert der Laparoskopie in der onkologischen Chirurgie. Dtsch Med Wochenschr 1994;114:1518.
10. Kampshöer GHM, Maruyama K, van de Velde CJH, Sasako M, Kinoshita T, Okabayashi K. Computer analysis in making preoperative decisions: a rational approach to lymph node dissection in gastric cancer patients. Br J Surg 1989;76:905.
11. Bollschweiler E, Böttcher K, Hölscher AH, et al. Preoperative assessment of lymph node metastases in patients with gastric cancer: evaluation of the Maruyama computer program. Br J Surg 1992;79:156.
12. Fink U, Stein HJ, Schuhmacher C, Wilke HJ. Neoadjuvant chemotherapy: an update. World J Surg 1995;19:509.
13. Hiki Y, Sakakibara Y, Mieno H, Shimao H, Kobayashi N, Katada N. Endoscopic treatment of gastric cancer. Surg Endosc 1991;5:11.
14. Ohgami M, Kumai K, Wakabayashi G, Otani Y, Katajima M. Innovative treatment for early gastric cancer, laparoscopic wedge resection of the stomach using the lesion-lifting method [in Japanese]. Stomach and Intestine 1993;28:1461.
15. Siewert JR, Böttcher K, Roder JD, Busch R, Hermanek P, Meyer HJ, the German Gastric Cancer Study Group. Prognostic relevance of systematic lymph node dissection in gastric carcinoma. Br J Surg 1993; 80:1015.
16. Shiu MH, Moore E, Sanders M, et al. Influence of the extent of resection on survival after curative treatment of gastric carcinoma: a retrospective multivariate analysis. Arch Surg 1987;122:1347.
17. Jaehne J, Meyer HJ, Maschek H, Geerlings H, Bruns E, Pichlmayr R. Lymphadenectomy in gastric carcinoma: a prospective and prognostic study. Arch Surg 1992;127:290.
18. Maruyama K, Guvén P, Okabayashi K, Sasako M, Kinoshita T. Lymph node metastases of gastric cancer: general pattern in 1931 patients. Ann Surg 1989;210:596.
19. Maruyama K. A new dissection technique of superior pancreatic lymph nodes, pancreas preserving radical gastrectomy. Japanese Journal of Gastroenterological Surgery 1979;12:961.
20. Maruyama K, Okabayashi K, Kinoshita T. Progress in gastric cancer surgery in Japan and its limits of radicality. World J Surg 1987;11: 418.
21. Buhl K, Lehnert T, Schlag P, Herfarth C. Reconstruction after gastrectomy and quality of life. World J Surg 1995;19:558.
22. Roder JD, Herschbach P, Henrich G, Nagel M, Böttcher K, Siewert JR. Lebensqualität nach totaler Gastrektomie wegen Magenkarzinom. Dtsch Med Wochenschr 1992;117:241.
23. Siewert JR, Schattenmann G. Esophagojejunoplication. In: Herfarth C, Schlag P, eds. Gastric cancer. Berlin: Springer-Verlag, 1979:272.
24. Herfarth C, Schlag P, Buhl K. Surgical procedures for gastric substitution. World J Surg 1987;11:689.
25. Siewert JR, Böttcher K. Ösophagojejunoplikatio in Stapler- Technik: Ergebnisse einer kontrollierten Studie. Langenbecks Arch Chir 1992; 377:186.
26. Siewert JR, Schattenmann G, Ebert R. Importance of the duodenal passage following gastrectomy. In: Herfarth C, Schlag P, eds. Gastric cancer. Berlin: Springer-Verlag, 1979:272.
27. Fink U, Schuhmacher C, Stein, HJ, et al. Preoperative chemotherapy for stage III/IV gastric carcinoma: feasibility, response, and outcome after surgical resection. Br J Surg 1995;82:1248.
28. Fink U, Schuhmacher C, Böttcher K, et al. Neoadjuvant chemotherapy with etoposide/Adriamycin and cisplatin (EAP) in locally advanced gastric carcinoma. In: Salmon SE, ed. Adjuvant therapy of cancer VII. Philadelphia: JB Lippincott, 1993:272.
29. Korenaga D, Haraguchi M, Okamura T, Baba H, Saito A, Sugimachi K. DNA ploidy and tumor invasion in human gastric cancer: histopathologic differentiation. Arch Surg 1989;124:314.
30. Maruyama K. The most important prognostic factors for gastric cancer patients: a study using univariate and multivariate analyses. Scand J Gastroenterol 1987;22(Suppl 133):63.
31. Böttcher K, Becker K, Busch R, Roder JD, Siewert JR. Prognosefaktoren beim Magenkarzinom: Ergebnisse einer uni- und multivariaten Analyse. Chirurg 1992;63:656.
32. Baba H, Korenaga D, Okamura T, Saito A, Sugimachi K. Prognostic factors in gastric cancer with serosal invasion: univariate and multivariate analyses. Arch Surg 1989;124:1061.
33. Bozzetti F, Bonfanti G, Morabito A, et al. A multifactorial approach for the prognosis of patients with carcinoma of the stomach after curative resection. Surg Gynecol Obstet 1986;162:229.
34. Nishi M, Ohta K, Nakajima T. Combined resection. In: Nishi M, Ichikawa H, Nakajima T, Maruyama K, Tahara E, eds. Gastric cancer. Berlin–Heidelberg–New York: Springer-Verlag, 1993:306.
35. Gabbert HE, Meier S, Gerharz CD, Hommel G. Incidence and prognostic significance of vascular invasion in 529 gastric cancer patients. Int J Cancer 1991;49:203.
36. Noguchi Y. Blood vessel invasion in gastric carcinoma. Surgery 1990; 107:140.
37. Gabbert HE, Meier S, Gerharz CD, Hommel G. Neue histomorphologische Prognoseparameter beim Magencarcinom. Chirurg 1992;63:647.
38. Sasaki K, Takahashi M. Flow cytometric DNA measurement of gastric cancers: clinico-pathological implication of DNA ploidy. Pathol Res Pract 1989;184:561.
39. Yonemura Y, Suggiyama K, Fujimura T, et al. Correlation of DNA ploidy and proliferative activity in human gastric cancer. Cancer 1988; 62:1497.

40. Msika S, Chastang C, Houry S, Lacaine F, Huguier M. Lymph node involvement as the only prognostic factor in curative resected gastric carcinoma: a multivariate analysis. World J Surg 1989;13:118.
41. Akoh JA, Macintyre IMC. Improving survival in gastric cancer: review of 5-year survival rates in English language publications from 1970. Br J Surg 1992;79:293.
42. Shiu MH, Perrotti M, Brennan MF. Adenocarcinoma of the stomach: a multivariate analysis of clinical, pathologic and treatment factors. Hepatogastroenterology 1989;36:7.
43. Böttcher K, Siewert JR, Roder JD, Busch R, Hermanek P, Meyer HJ, für die Deutsche Magencarcinom-Studiengruppe (GGCS '92). Risiko der chirurgischen Therapie des Magencarcinoms in Deutschland: Ergebnisse der Deutschen Magencarcinom-Studie 1992. Chirurg 1994; 65:298.

Surgery for Gastrointestinal Cancer: A Multidisciplinary Approach, edited by Harold J. Wanebo.
Lippincott-Raven Publishers, Philadelphia, © 1997.

CHAPTER 25

Optimum Resection With Lymph Node Dissection for Gastric Cancer

Keiichi Maruyama, Mitsuru Sasako, Taira Kinoshita, Takeshi Sano, and Hitoshi Katai

THE RESULTS OF THERAPY FOR GASTRIC CANCER IN THE UNITED STATES AND JAPAN

Table 25-1 shows 5-year survival rates for patients with gastric cancer treated in the United States, Germany, and Japan. The overall 5-year survival rate was 17.5% in the data base of the American College of Surgeons,[1] compared with 63.6% in the data base of the Japanese Nationwide Registry.[2] The proportion of early cancer was apparently higher in the Japanese series, which might account for the higher overall survival rate. However, the 5-year survival rates in each stage still were different in the two countries: 100% versus 59% in stage Ia; 90% versus 44% in stage Ib; 72% versus 29% in stage II; 48% versus 15% in stage IIIa; and 29% versus 9% in stage IIIb. The German results were in between, but closer to the Japanese results.[3]

What are the possible factors responsible for the difference? It has been documented that patient backgrounds and tumor types are different in Japan and the Western countries. Japanese patients are about 10 years younger and have lower proportions of proximal tumors and diffuse-type carcinomas compared with Western patients.[4,5] Although these factors may have contributed to the better treatment results in the Japanese series, the difference seems to be too large for this to be the only explanation. These authors believe that the most important factor is different surgical strategy, particularly in regard to lymph node (LN) dissection.[6,7]

K. Maruyama: Head of Department of Surgical Oncology, National Cancer Center Hospital, 5-1-1, Tsukiji, Chou-ku, Tokyo, 104 Japan

M. Sasako: Department of Surgical Oncology, National Cancer Center Hospital, 5-1-1, Tsukiji, Chou-ku, Tokyo, Japan

T. Kinoshita: Department of Surgical Oncology, National Cancer Center Hospital, 5-1-1, Tsukiji, Chou-ku, Tokyo, Japan

T. Sano: Department of Surgical Oncology, National Cancer Center Hospital, 5-1-1, Tsukiji, Chou-ku, Tokyo, Japan

H. Katai: Department of Surgical Oncology, National Cancer Center Hospital, 5-1-1, Tsukiji, Chou-ku, Tokyo, Japan.

In this chapter, the basic aspects and surgical procedures of lymphadenectomy are discussed.

REGIONAL LYMPH NODES OF THE STOMACH

By the TNM classification of the International Union Against Cancer (UICC), the regional LNs of the stomach include the perigastric nodes and the nodes along the left gastric, common hepatic, splenic, and celiac arteries. Metastasis to the regional LNs is classified as N1 or N2[8] (Fig. 25-1). The involvement of nodes other than these is regarded as distant metastasis.

The Japanese classification of gastric carcinoma uses a different system, which may appear more complicated but covers a wider area than the TNM classification[9] (Fig. 25-2). In the Japanese classification, the regional nodes are numbered from 1 to 16 according to their anatomic site. They are termed N1, N2, N3, or N4 according to the location and extension of the primary tumor (Fig. 25-3).

Because the TNM classification was established on the basis of the simplified Japanese classification, the nodal states described using these systems are comparable, if not identical, insofar as N0, N1, and N2 are concerned. For further details of LN classification, please refer to the English translation of the Japanese classification system.[10]

LYMPHATIC CHANNELS FROM THE STOMACH

The classification of regional LNs was established on the basis of surgical, anatomic, pathologic, and lymphographic studies. Hagiwara and colleagues clearly demonstrated the lymphatic channels by operative lymphography. They used fine, activated carbon particles in polyvinylpyrrolidone solution as a contrast medium.[11]

When 0.5 mL of this solution is injected into the subserosal space of the posterior wall of the distal third of the stomach, it quickly stains the lymphatic channels and regional nodes draining from the injection site (Fig. 25-4). The stained perigas-

TABLE 25-1. *Treatment results of gastric cancer patients in the United States, Germany, and Japan*

	USA	Germany	Japan
Organization	ACS	GGCS	JRSGC
No. of Hospitals	>700	19	141
Period	1982	1986–89	1979–82
No. of Patients	6,609	1,654	17,884
Lost to follow-up	—	0.8%	3.5%
5-Year Survival rate	KM	CSR	RSR
All cases	17.5%	36.5%	63.6%
Stage Ia	59%	85.2%	100.0%
Ib	44%	69.2%	89.9%
II	29%	43.7%	71.7%
IIIa	15%	28.6%	47.8%
IIIb	9%	17.7%	28.8%
IV	3%	8.7%	11.5%

ACS, the American College of Surgeons[1]; GGCS, the German Gastric Cancer Study Group[3]; JRSGC, The Japanese Research Society for Gastric Cancer[2]; KM, survival rate by Kaplan-Meier; CSR, cumulative survival rate; RSR, relative survival rate or age and sex-adjusted survival rate.

tric nodes near the injection site (numbers 3, 4, 5, and 6) are classified as N1. The stained nodes along the upper border of the pancreas (numbers 7, 8, 9, and 11) are classified as N2. The paraaortic nodes are numbered 16 and are classified as N4. Other stained nodes are classified as N3. This technique demonstrates five major lymphatic channels from the injection point: channels along the right gastroepiploic, superior mesenteric, left gastric, and splenic arteries, and a channel crossing the anterior surface of the pancreas. All the channels eventually flow into the paraaortic nodes.

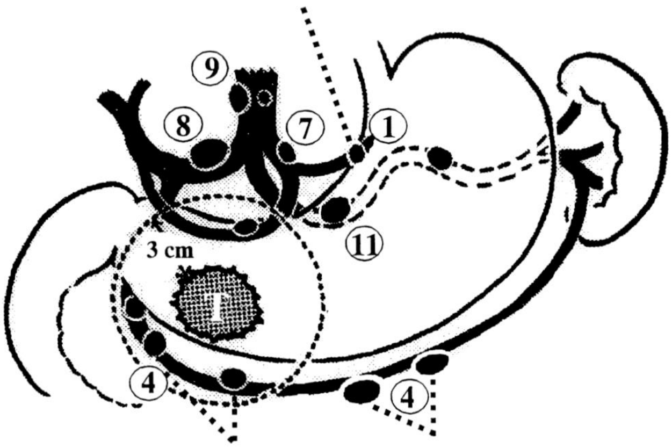

FIG. 25-1. Regional LN of the stomach, TNM classification. Metastasis in perigastric LNs within 3 cm of the edge of the primary tumor is classified as N1. N2 means metastasis in perigastric nodes more than 3 cm from the edge of the primary tumor or in LNs along the left gastric, common hepatic, splenic, or celiac arteries. Involvement of other intra-abdominal LNs such as the hepatoduodenal, retropancreatic, mesenteric, and paraaortic is classified as distant metastasis. (Hermanek P, Sovin LH. UICC TNM classification of malignant tumors, 4th ed. Berlin: Springer Verlag, 1987:43.)

TABLE 25-2. *5-year survival rate by systematic (D2/D3) and non-systematic (D0/D1) LN dissection (excluding M1)*

	Systematic (D2/D3)		Non-systematic (D0/D1)	
	Patients	5-YSR	Patients	5-YSR
Total	3,242	*71.1%	470	66.6%
Stage I	1,667	*91.8%	370	82.7%
Stage II	477	*72.8%	34	63.6%
Stage III	829	*46.2%	47	22.2%
Stage IV	269	3.0%	19	6.1%

*$P < 0.05$. 5-YSR, cumulative 5 year survival rate, National Cancer Center, 1969–1988.

Retrospective analysis of survivals by degree of LN dissection showed significantly better 5-YSR in the systematic lymphadenectomy group than the non-systematic group in Stage I, II and III (TNM Classification). D2 means complete removal of N1 and N2, and D3 means complete removal of N1, N2 and N3.

When the contrast solution is injected at the posterior surface of the middle third of the stomach (Fig. 25-5), it stains the lymphatic channels and nodes in a different sequence. Nodes 1, 3, 4, 5 and 6 are classified as N1, and nodes 7, 8, 9, 10, and 11 are classified as N2.

Figure 25-6 shows the lymphatic channels and nodes stained after injection into the proximal third of the stomach. Nodes 1, 2, 3, and 4 are classified as N1, and nodes 7, 8, 9, 10, and 11 are classified as N2. The contrast solution flows into the channels along the posterior gastric, left subphrenic, and left gastric arteries. It also flows into the paraaortic nodes.

RATIONAL LYMPHADENECTOMY FOR GASTRIC CANCER

Studies of the lymphatic channels of the stomach have demonstrated possible pathways of tumor spread and suggested the range of rational lymphadenectomy. The LNs along these channels have a high incidence of metastasis (Fig. 25-7) and should be removed.

Another essential consideration is whether a patient with LN

TABLE 25-3. *Surgical complications in Dutch trial comparing D1 versus D2 gastrectomy (80 hospitals in 5 years [1989–1993])*

	D1	D2
Number of patients	513	483
Hospital deaths	6.4%	9.9%
Complications	25.0%	37.9%
Hospital stay	17.9 days	22.3 days
Patients/year/hospital	1.3	1.2

A prospective randomized trial to compare D1 versus D2 gastrectomy was organized in the Netherlands.[14] Total of 996 patients were treated at 80-member hospitals in the 5-year period from 1989 to 1993. That means a hospital treated an average of only 2.5 patients a year; 1.3 patients by D1 and 1.2 patients by D2. The number is not enough to master a new surgical procedure, and this situation will be a major reason of high mortality and morbidity.

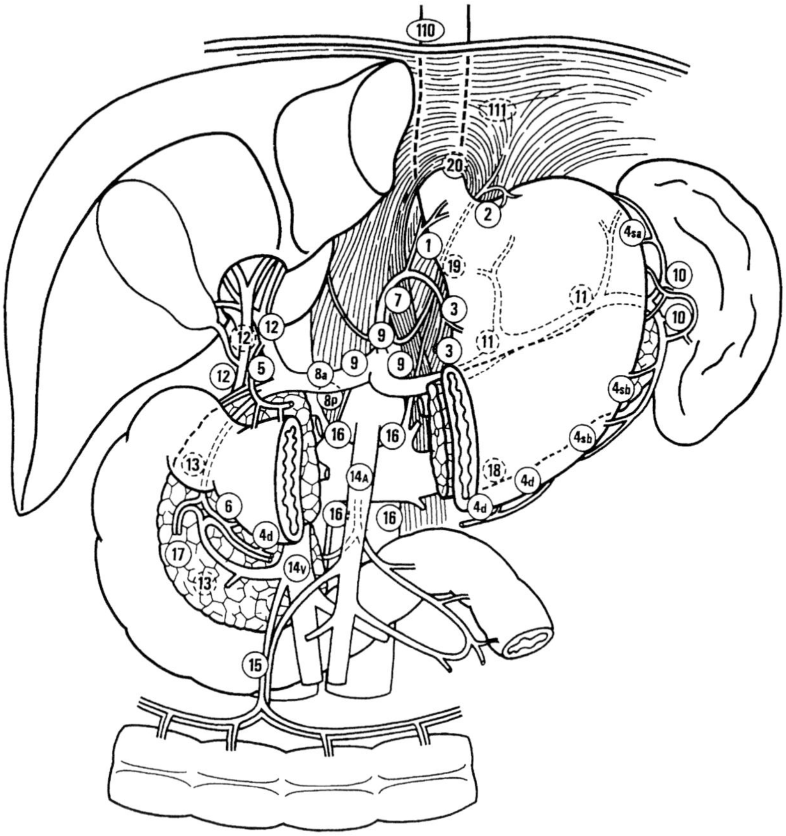

FIG. 25-2. Regional LN of the stomach, Japanese classification. Japanese N classification covers a wider area than in the TNM system, including LNs along the hepatoduodenal ligament, behind the pancreas, at the root of the mesenterium, and at the para-aortic area. All these nodes are numbered from No. 1 to No. 16.[9,10]

metastasis is likely to survive if the positive LNs are removed.[7,12] If the probability of survival is high, the nodes should be dissected. This can be evaluated by examining the survival rate of patients with positive nodes in each nodal station. As shown in Figure 25-7, the nodes classified as N1 and N2 are associated with high 5-year survival rates.[7]

Complete clearance of nodes N1 and N2 is termed *D2 dissection* or *systematic LN dissection* in the Japanese manual, and is the standard procedure for curative surgery for gastric cancer. *D3 dissection* indicates complete removal of nodes N1, N2, and N3, and is termed *extended LN dissection. D1 dissection* means that node N1 is removed completely, but node N2 is not. *D0 dissection* indicates incomplete clearance of node N1.

D2 dissection was termed *R2 dissection* until 1993.[9] However, the letter "R" is used to refer to residual tumor in the TNM classification. To avoid confusion, the Japanese Research Society for Gastric Cancer selected the letter "D" to describe the degree of LN dissection.[10]

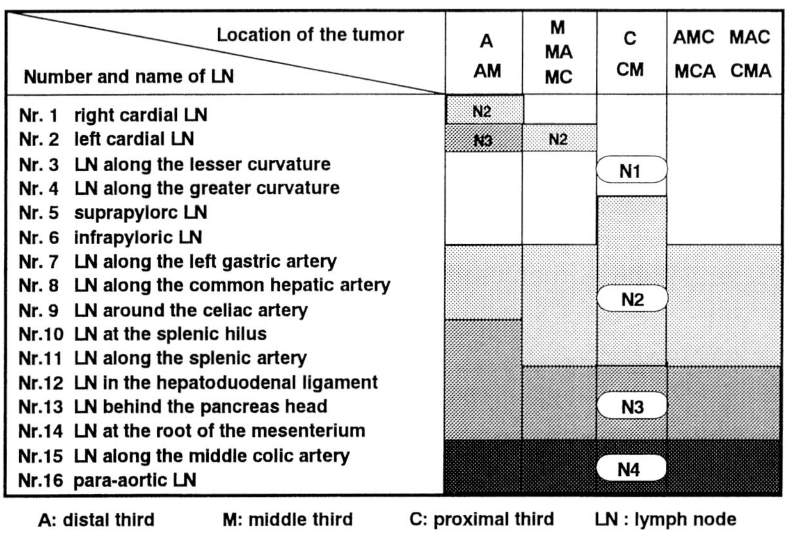

FIG. 25-3. N Classification in Japanese manual. The 16 core nodes are anatomically defined, nominated, and numbered. Furthermore, they are grouped into N1, N2, N3, and N4, according to the location and extension of the primary tumor.[9,10]

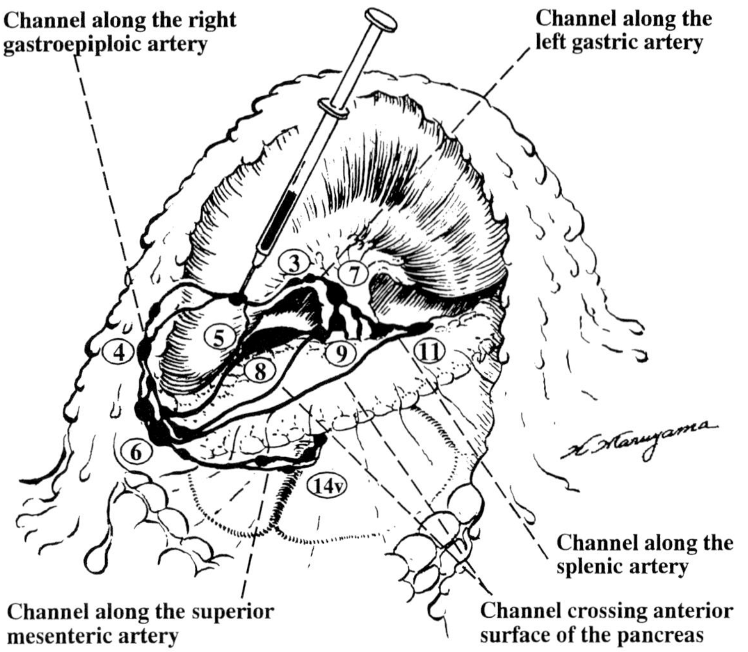

FIG. 25-4. Lymphatic channels from distal third of the stomach. A stream runs along the right gastroepiploic artery and arrives at LN No. 6. Then it branches off in two directions; the channel along the superior mesenteric artery and the channel crossing the anterior surface of the pancreas. The other stream runs along the left gastric artery and arrives at the LN stations Nos. 8, 9, and 11.

EFFECTIVENESS OF SYSTEMATIC LYMPH NODE DISSECTION

In these authors' retrograde analysis, the overall 5-year survival rate after D2 and D3 gastrectomy (63.8%) was significantly higher than after D1 (41.2%) or D0 (20.3%) dissection (Fig. 25-8). As shown in Table 25-2, this superiority of D2 and D3 dissection over D0 and D1 dissection was significant in stage I, II, and III tumors. In the German Gastric Carcinoma Study, Siewert and associates reported that radical lymphadenectomy significantly improved the survival rate in patients with stage II and IIIa tumors.[13]

A multivariate analysis of patients with gastric cancer treated in these authors' hospital showed that the most important prognostic factor was depth of tumor invasion, followed by LN metastasis and distant metastasis (Fig. 25-9). The degree of LN dissection was the fourth most important prognostic factor.

Although LN dissection provides local disease control for gastric cancer, extended lymphadenectomy may have no survival benefit for patients with peritoneal disease or distant me-

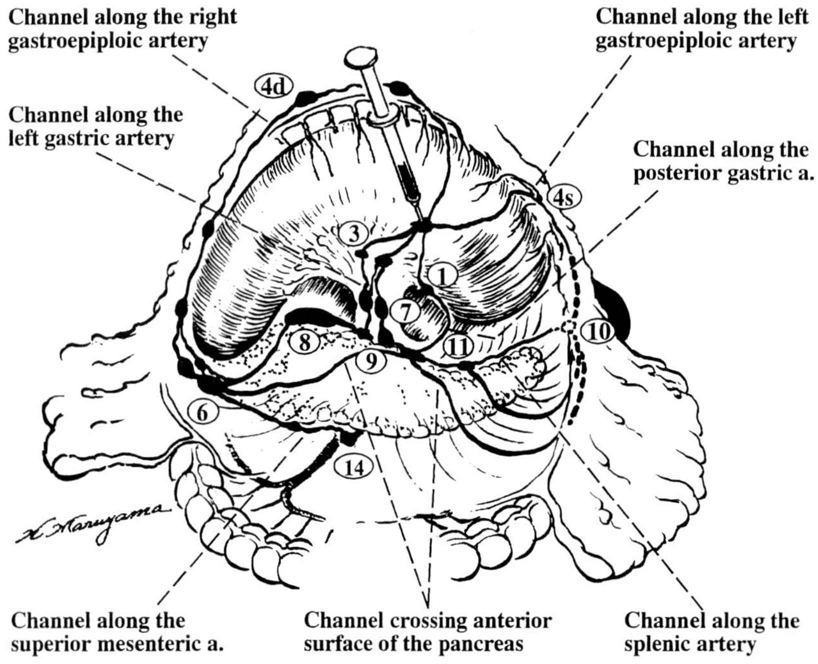

FIG. 25-5. Lymphatic channels from the middle third of the stomach. Right side lymphatic streams flow in the same channels from the distal third of the stomach. The other streams run along the left gastroepiploic artery, the splenic artery, and the posterior gastric artery, and arrive finally at the LN stations Nos. 11, 9, and 8.

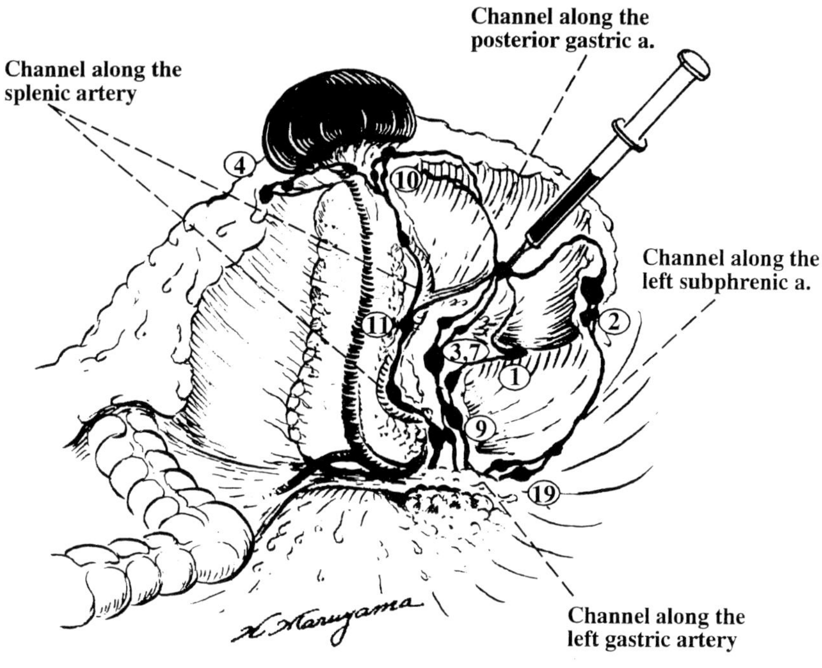

FIG. 25-6. Lymphatic channels from upper third of the stomach. From the upper third of the stomach, the lymphatic streams flow in all directions. The first stream runs towards the greater curvature and splenic hilus, then flows in the channel along the splenic artery. The second flows along the posterior gastric artery, then joins the channel along the splenic artery. The third stream is directed to the LN Nos. 1 and 3, then runs along the left gastric artery. All these streams finally arrive at the LNs Nos. 11 and 9. The last stream arrives at the LN No. 2, and flows directly into the para-aortic LN passing the channel along the left subphrenic artery.

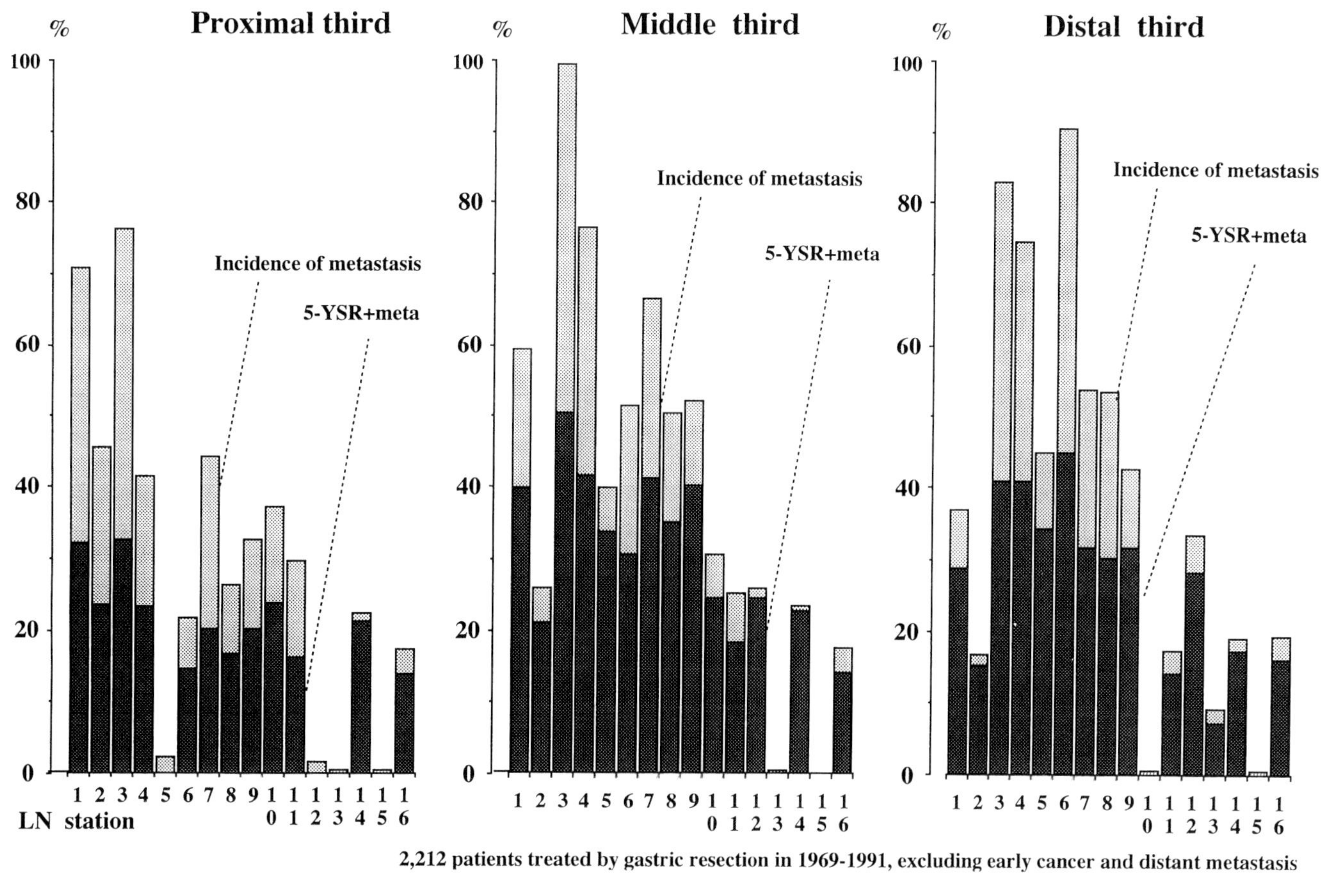

FIG. 25-7. Incidence of metastasis at each LN station and 5-YSR of the patients with positive nodes. The data were different by location of the primary tumor. For example, in case of middle-third cancer, this graph shows that the incidence of metastasis at the LN No. 9 (LN around the celiac artery) was 12%, and the 5-YSR was 41% if the node-positive patients were treated by systematic LN dissection. 5-YSR + meta, 5-year survival rate of patients with the metastatic nodes.

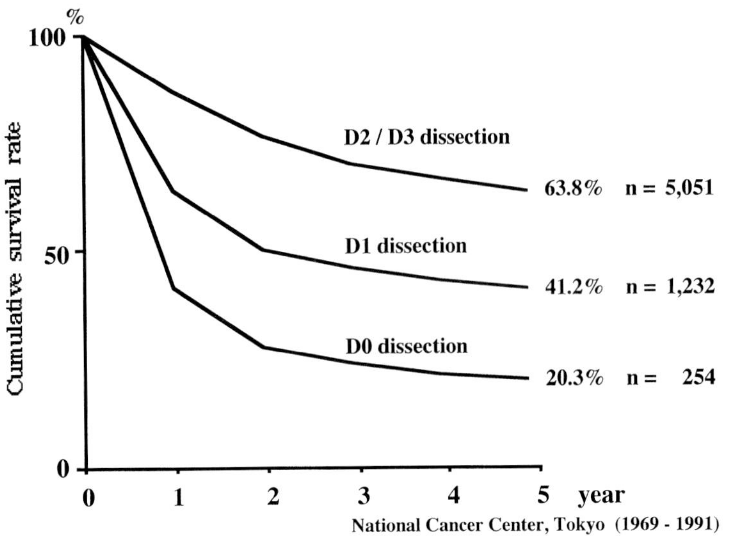

FIG. 25-8. Survival rates by degree of LN dissection. As the D2 and more LN dissection have been standard surgical procedures in the National Cancer Center, most patients belong to the D2/D3 group. The D2/D3 group showed significantly better survival from the D1 and D0 groups, which have more conservative or insufficient lymphadenectomy.

tastases. Therefore, it is important to select patients in whom LN dissection is potentially beneficial.

MORBIDITY AND MORTALITY AFTER SYSTEMATIC LYMPHADENECTOMY

The surgical procedure for systematic lymphadenectomy is not simple.[12] It should only be performed by or under the supervision of specialized surgeons. D2 dissection usually takes 3 hours for distal gastrectomy and 4 hours for total gastrectomy. The mortality rate was low in the series by these authors from 1982 to 1991. There were 7 surgical deaths among 1895 patients who underwent D2 and D3 dissection. The mortality rate was 0.4%, similar to the 0.5% rate (3 of 574 patients) associated with D0 and D1 dissection. The Japanese Nationwide Registry from 1979 to 1982 reported a surgical mortality rate of 1.7% in 17,884 patients, most of whom were treated by D2 gastrectomy.[2]

Astonishingly high morbidity and mortality rates associated with D2 lymphadenectomy have been reported from European multicenter trials. From the Netherlands, Bonenkamp and colleagues reported a postoperative mortality rate of 9.9% in the D2 group, and concluded that D2 dissection should not be used as standard therapy for Western patients[14] (Table 25-3). A high mortality rate also was reported from the British Medical Research Counsel (MRC) trial.[15]

Possible explanations for this contrast between Japanese and Western trials have been the topic of extensive discussion.[16] Several factors have been considered, including differences in patient characteristics and perioperative management strategies. Sue-Ling and associates pointed out that, in the Dutch trial, one member hospital treated an average of only 1.2 patients per year using D2 gastrectomy. They stressed that this number is too low to allow for mastery of a new surgical procedure.[17] Based on his experience in the German trial, Siewert believed the Dutch results were caused by surgical inexperience and unnecessary resection of the distal pancreas (personal communication, May 1995).

Precise knowledge, careful observation and assessment, and fine technique are essential for LN dissection. A teaching sys-

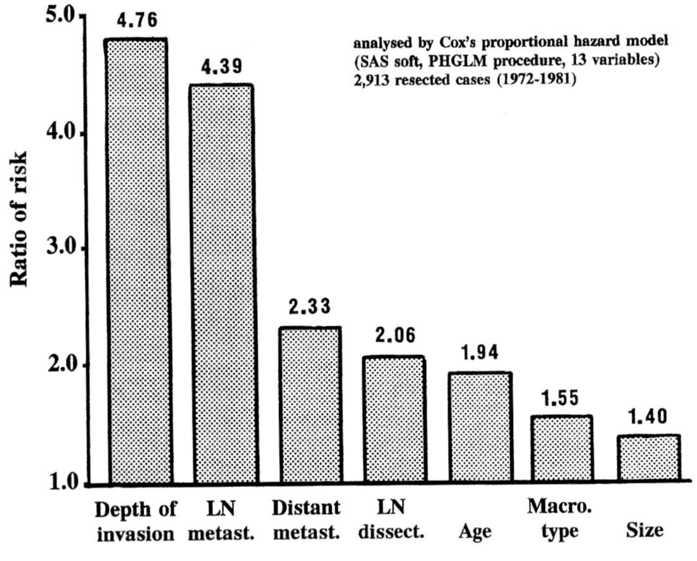

FIG. 25-9. Most important prognostic factors for patients with gastric cancer. Depth of invasion was accepted as the most important prognostic factor by the highest ratio of risk in multivariate analysis. LN metastasis and distant metastasis were the second and the third factors, and all these factors are already fixed at the beginning of treatment. However, the forth important prognostic factor was degree of LN dissection, a treatment factor. It means that patient prognosis can be improved primarily by this surgical treatment.

tem should be established to ensure effective and safe lymphadenectomy.

CONCLUSION

These authors believe that lymphadenectomy is worthwhile when the following criteria are satisfied: there is a significant chance of metastasis in the target nodes, survival can be expected after dissection of the involved nodes, and the technique is safe enough not to increase operative mortality. D2 gastrectomy for gastric cancer without peritoneal or distant metastasis satisfies these conditions.

Systematic LN dissection requires specialized training and may be associated with higher morbidity, but is beneficial for many patients with gastric cancer.

REFERENCES

1. Wanebo HJ, Kennedy BJ, Chmiel J, et al. Cancer of the stomach: a patient care study by the American College of Surgeons. Ann Surg 1993;218:583.
2. Japanese Research Society for Gastric Cancer. Treatment results of gastric carcinoma in Japan: 39th report of nationwide registry in 1979-82. Tokyo: National Cancer Center Press, 1995.
3. Roder JD, Boettcher K, Siewert JR. Results of the German Gastric Cancer Study: multivariate analysis of potentially prognostic factors in 1654 resected patients. In: Nishi M, Sugano H, Takahashi T, eds. International Gastric Cancer Congress. Bologna: Monduzzi Editore, 1995:47.
4. Fielding JWL. Gastric cancer: different diseases. Br J Surg 1989;76: 1227.
5. Bollschweiler E, Maruyama K, Siewert JR, et al. Is the prognosis for Japanese and German patients with gastric cancer really different? Cancer 1993;71:2918.
6. McCulloch P. Personal review: extended lymphadenectomy for gastric cancer. GI Cancer 1995;1:105.
7. Maruyama K, Sasako M, Kinoshita T, et al. Effectiveness of systematic lymph node dissection in gastric cancer surgery. In: Nishi M, Ichikawa H, Nakajima T, Maruyama K, Tahara E, eds. Gastric cancer. Tokyo: Springer-Verlag, 1993:293.
8. Hermanek P, Sovin LH. UICC TNM classification of malignant tumours. 4th ed. Berlin: Springer-Verlag, 1987:43.
9. Japanese Research Society for Gastric Cancer. The general rule for gastric cancer study in surgery and pathology. Japanese Journal of Surgery 1981;11:127.
10. Japanese Research Society for Gastric Cancer. Japanese classification of gastric carcinoma. 1st English ed. Tokyo: Kanehara, 1995.
11. Hagiwara A, Takahashi S, Sawai K, et al. Lymph nodal vital staining with newer carbon particle suspensions compared with India ink: experimental and clinical observations. Lymphology 1992;25:84.
12. Maruyama K. Surgical treatment and end results of gastric cancer. Tokyo: National Cancer Center Press, 1985.
13. Siewert JR, Böttcher K, Roder JD, and the German Gastric Carcinoma Study Group. Prognostic relevance of systematic LN dissection in gastric carcinoma. Br J Surg 1993;80:1015.
14. Bonenkamp J, Songun I, van de Velde CJH, et al. Randomized comparison of morbidity after D1 and D2 dissection for gastric cancer in 996 Dutch patients. Lancet 1995;345:745.
15. Fayers P, Cuschieri A, and Co-operative Group of Gastric Surgery. Postoperative morbidity and morality in a randomized controlled trial comparing R1 and R2 resections: the UK experience. In: Nishi M, Sugano H, Takahashi T, eds. International Gastric Cancer Congress. Bologna: Monduzzi Editore, 1995:43.
16. Sue-Ling HM, McCulloch P, Guadagni S, et al. D1 versus D2 dissection for gastric cancer. Lancet 1995;345:1515.
17. Sue-Ling HM, Johnston D, Martin IG, et al. Gastric cancer: a curable disease in Britain. BMJ 1993;307:591.

Surgery for Gastrointestinal Cancer: A Multidisciplinary Approach, edited by Harold J. Wanebo.
Lippincott-Raven Publishers, Philadelphia, © 1997.

CHAPTER 26

Selective Gastric Resection and Lymphadenectomy

Chew-Wun Wu

Despite a decrease in incidence since the early decades of this century, adenocarcinoma of the stomach remains a significant health problem throughout the world.[1] In Taiwan, a recent official report showed that cancer of the stomach ranked third in death rate of 10 leading sites of malignant neoplasms.[2]

Although surgical resection offers the only prospect of cure, the outcome is dismal. Studies from Japan have suggested an improved survival in patients who underwent radical lymph node dissection in curative resection of gastric adenocarcinoma.[3,4] Our findings also support that contention (Fig. 26-1). Nevertheless, the validity of these results is questioned because the Japanese and our data have been obtained through retrospective analysis. Efficacy of radical lymph node dissection can be determined only by prospective, randomized clinical trials. Work along these lines is currently in progress in the United Kingdom, The Netherlands, and Taiwan.

JAPANESE GENERAL RULES FOR GASTRIC CANCER STUDY

The Japanese Research Society for Gastric Cancer has published general rules for the gastric cancer study in surgery and pathology.[5] Based on the location of the cancer, tumors are described as A for antrum (lower-third stomach), M for midbody (middle-third stomach), C for cardia (upper-third stomach), D for duodenum, and E for esophagus. If the lesion extends from one area to the other, multiple-letter codes are used, with the primary involved portions listed first, followed by the less involved portion(s). For instance, when the lesion arises in the antrum and extends into the middle third, it is coded "AM."

The lymph nodes around the stomach are numbered from 1 to 16 (Fig. 26-2). These lymph nodes are classified into four groups (n1 to n4; Table 26-1). This grouping refers to the anatomic location as it relates to the primary tumor, and is not related to the order of possibility of metastasis, as in primary, secondary, tertiary, and quaternary lymph nodes. We have used this system in the series reported here. In the TNM classification,[6] N1 and N2 are defined as regional lymph nodes, whereas N3 and N4 are distant metastases. This deviation in staging needs to be recognized when interpreting study results.

RELATION OF LYMPH NODE METASTASES TO DEPTH OF CANCER INVASION

We find, as have others, that there is a significant correlation between lymph node metastasis and depth of cancer invasion.[7–9] Lymph node metastasis in patients with early gastric cancer (defined as cancer invasion limited to mucosa and submucosa) is confined to n2, whereas in patients with tumor invasion beyond the submucosa (advanced cancer), metastasis to n3 or n4 is not rare (Table 26-2). The depth of invasion can be evaluated with some degree of accuracy preoperatively by endoscopic sonography or transabdominal ultrasonography with the fluid-filled stomach technique (Fig. 26-3).

STRATEGY FOR SELECTION OF OPERATIVE MODALITIES

Radical resection of gastric cancer requires a complete removal of the primary tumor combined with a sufficiently wide dissection of lymph nodes. Resection may need to be combined with removal of involved adjacent organs.

The presence of microscopic spread around the gross margin of a gastric cancer is common. For the complete removal of the primary tumor, a margin of 3 cm is required for superficial and well defined tumors, and of 5 cm for ill-defined tumors. The well defined tumors are of the polypoid or fungating type (Borrmann type I)[10] and circumscribed excavating type (Borrmann type II). The ill-defined tumors are of the ulcerated and infiltrating type (Borrmann type III) and diffusely thickened type (Borrmann type IV). The surgeon must examine the re-

Professor of Surgery, School of Medicine, National Yang-Ming University, Chief, Section of General Surgery, Department of Surgery, Veterans Hospital-Taipei, Republic of China.

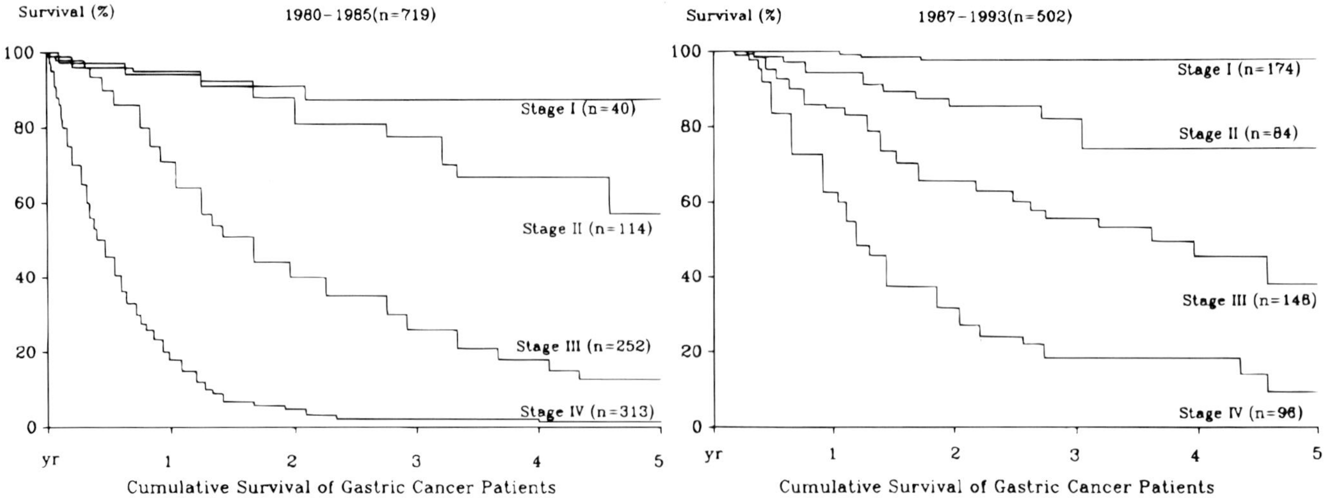

FIG. 26-1. Five-year survival rates in patients with gastric cancer in two different periods.

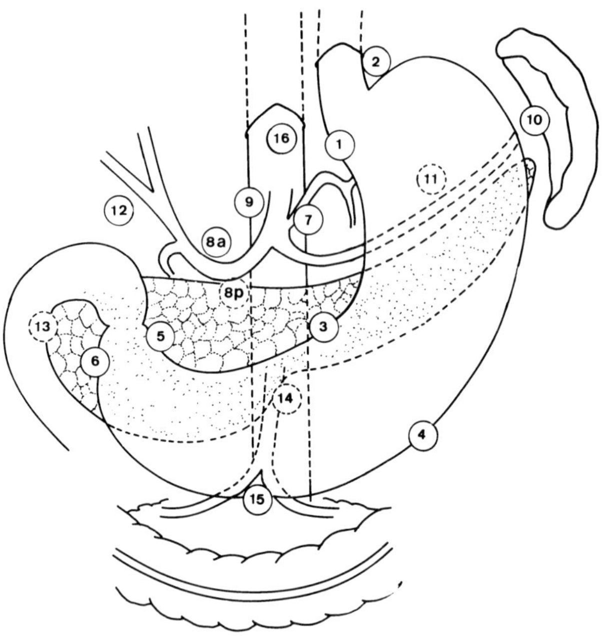

FIG. 26-2. Designation of regional lymph nodes of stomach according to Japanese rules for the gastric cancer study. *1,* right paracardial; *2,* left paracardial; *3,* lesser curvature; *4,* greater curvature; *5,* suprapyloric; *6,* infrapyloric; *7,* left gastric artery; *8a,* above common hepatic artery; *8p,* behind common hepatic artery; *9,* celiac axis; *10,* splenic hilum; *11,* splenic artery; *12,* hepatoduodenal ligament; *12a,* hepatic artery; *12b,* common bile duct; *12p,* behind portal vein; *13,* retropancreatic head; *14,* mesenteric root; *15,* middle colic artery; *16,* para-aortic. (From Japanese Research Society for Gastric Cancer. The general rules for the gastric cancer study in surgery and pathology. 12th ed. Tokyo: Kanahara Shuppan, 1993.)

moved stomach to ensure an adequate margin before reconstruction. A routine frozen section confirmation of adequate tissue margins may avoid reoperation and reresection when a delayed permanent microscopic analysis demonstrates unsuspected positive margins.

For adjacent organs involved by cancer through direct extension, such as the lower third of the esophagus, the body and tail of the pancreas, a portion of the liver, the transverse colon, the duodenum, and the head of the pancreas, a procedure for resection of the involved organs should be included, preferably in an en bloc dissection.

The lymph node metastatic pattern varies with different locations of the primary tumor within the stomach.[4,7–9] For sufficiently wide dissection of lymph nodes, an understanding of lymphatic spread as it relates to location of the primary tumor is of practical import, because the status of the lymphatics can be determined with confidence only after the resection has been completed.

TABLE 26-1. *Grouping and lymph node designation used in the Japanese rules for the gastric cancer study*

	Location of main tumor		
Group	Upper-third stomach	Middle-third stomach	Lower-third stomach
n1	1, 2, 3, 4	1, 3, 4, 5, 6	3, 4, 5, 6
n2	5, 6, 7, 8a, 9, 10, 11	2, 7, 8a, 9, 10, 11	1, 7, 8a, 9
n3	8p, 12, 13, 14	8p, 12, 13, 14	8p, 2, 10, 11, 12, 13, 14
n4	16	16	16

The numbers indicate the lymph node designation (see Fig. 26-1).

Data from Japanese Research Society for Gastric Cancer. The general rules for the gastric cancer study in surgery and pathology. 12th ed. Tokyo: Kanahara Shuppan, 1993.

TABLE 26-2. *Positive correlation of depth of cancer invasion and extent of lymph node metastasis**

Depth of cancer invasion	No. of patients	Percentage of patients with lymph node metastasis, by grade of lymph node metastasis				
		n0	n1	n2	n3	n4
Mucosa	75	96	1	3	0	0
Submucosa	59	78	12	10	0	0
Muscularis	100	49	28	16	5	2
Serosa	233	22	25	34	12	9
Adjacent structures	35	11	31	29	17	11
Total	502	44	21	22	8	5

* Japanese rules for the Gastric Cancer Study.

SELECTION OF LYMPHADENECTOMY ACCORDING TO LOCATION OF GASTRIC CANCER

Adenocarcinoma of the Lower Third of the Stomach (Antrum)

A radical distal subtotal gastrectomy is the standard procedure for adenocarcinoma arising in the antrum.[11] The pancreatic head, hepatoduodenal ligament, mesocolon, and duodenum are organs adjacent to and have lymphatic communication with the distal stomach. Therefore, advanced cancer in the lower third of the stomach has a high incidence of metastasis to the hepatoduodenal ligament (no. 12), retropancreatic (no. 13), and superior mesenteric vein (no. 14v) lymph nodes.[8] In contrast, there was no lymph node metastasis at the splenic hilum (no. 10; Table 26-3).[8] An extended lymphadenectomy includes lymph nodes of the n1 and n2 groups, and resection of the hepatoduodenal ligament, retropancreatic, and superior mesenteric vein nodes may be recommended (Fig. 26-4). In lymph node metastasis along the splenic artery (no. 11) or over the right paracardia (no. 1), proved by frozen-section biopsy, combined organ (en bloc) resection to facilitate node dissection by a hemipancreaticosplenectomy or a total gastrectomy should be considered.[11] Also, duodenal invasion by gastric cancer is not rare. In the current series, 10.8% of all patients with cancer in the lower third of the stomach had duodenal involvement. At least 3 cm of the first portion of the duodenum must be resected.

The incidence of lymph node metastases in early cancer of the lower-third stomach was 16.4%. The extent of nodal metastasis was confined to n2, especially involving the left gastric artery (no. 7) and common hepatic artery (no. 8a) nodes. A conservative lymphadenectomy, including lymph nodes of the n1 group and those along the left gastric artery, common hepatic artery, and celiac axis, is recommended.

Adenocarcinoma of the Middle Third of the Stomach (Midbody)

When the tumor is located at the mid-stomach, a total or distal subtotal gastrectomy is decided by the distance between the cardia and the tumor. A tumor arising in this location is prone to metastasize to nearly all of the lymph node groups adjacent to the stomach (Table 26-4). For advanced cancer, when tumors grow in an upward direction, lymph nodes along the splenic artery and in the splenic hilum are also frequently involved.[9,12] The high frequency of lymph node metastases along the splenic artery and splenic hilum is an important surgical consideration, especially when the tumor involves the upper stomach.

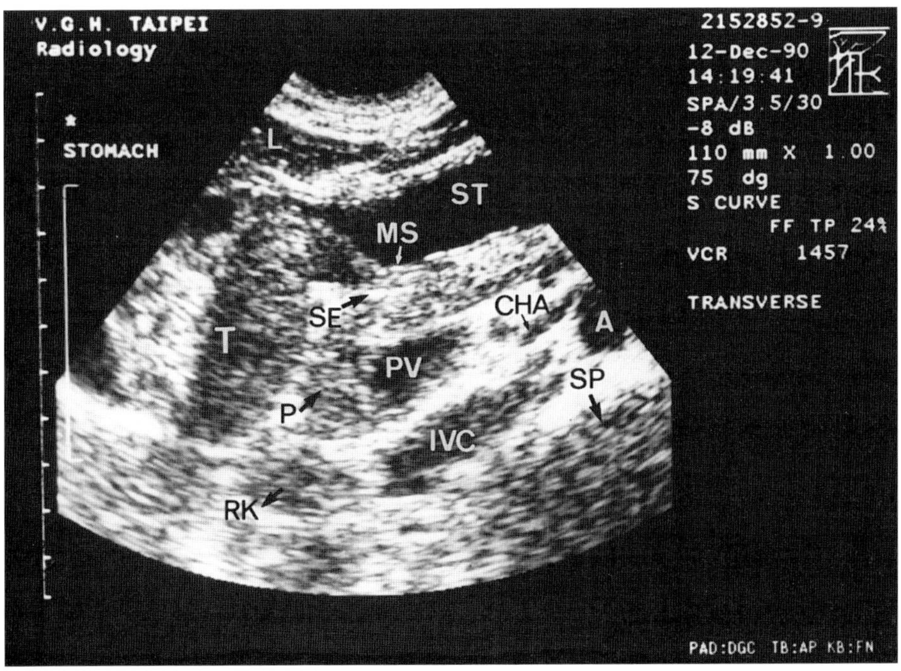

FIG. 26-3. Invasion of stomach cancer to the stomach wall serosa is demonstrated by a transabdominal ultrasonogram with the fluid-filled stomach technique. *ST,* stomach; *L,* liver; *P,* pancreas; *RT,* right kidney; *T,* tumor; *MS,* mucosal surface; *SE,* serosa; *PV,* portal vein; *IVC,* inferior vena cava; *A,* aorta; *CHA,* common hepatic artery; *SP,* splenic artery. (Courtesy of Dr. Jen-I Huang, Taipei, Republic of China.)

TABLE 26-3. *The extent and frequency (%) of lymph node metastases from adenocarcinomas of the lower third of the stomach*

Group	Lymph node designations	Early cancer	Advanced cancer: Antrum and duodenum	Advanced cancer: Antrum	Advanced cancer: Antrum and midbody	Advanced cancer: Antrum, midbody, and duodenum
n1	3	1.6	50.0	33.3	59.3	50.0
	4	4.9	37.5	32.1	43.0	37.5
	5	1.6	31.3	28.2	23.3	25.0
	6	8.2	68.8	55.1	53.5	62.5
n2	1	0	0	2.6	4.7	37.5
	7	3.3	31.3	24.4	22.1	28.6
	8a	4.9	43.8	16.7	23.3	50.0
	9	0	6.3	6.4	4.7	25.0
n3	2	0	0	0	2.3	0
	8p	0	6.3	1.3	3.5	25.0
	10	0	0	0	0	0
	11	0	6.3	1.3	8.1	12.5
	12	0	12.5	10.3	10.5	25.0
	13	0	12.5	2.6	8.1	25.0
	14	0	12.5	2.6	2.3	0
n4	16	0	6.3	3.8	5.8	25.0
Cases		61	16	78	86	8

The incidence of lymph node metastases in early cancer of the middle stomach was 9.4%. The extent of nodal metastasis was confined to n2, especially involving the left gastric artery (no. 7) and common hepatic artery (no. 8a) nodes. A lymphadenectomy encompassing the n1 group and numbers 7, 8, and 9 is indicated.

Adenocarcinoma of the Upper Third of the Stomach (Cardia)

When advanced cancer is located in the proximal stomach, a total gastrectomy with splenectomy and pancreatic tail resection is the procedure most commonly performed. We prefer a total gastrectomy rather than proximal subtotal gastrectomy, because patients may easily suffer bile reflux esophagitis after proximal gastrectomy. Advanced cancer of the upper third of the stomach frequently metastasizes to lymph nodes at the splenic artery (no. 11) and splenic hilum (no. 10), but rarely to the hepatoduodenal ligaments and mesenteric root (Table 26-5). Therefore, a hemipancreaticosplenectomy to facilitate the lymph node dissection of numbers 10 and 11 is highly recommended. When the tumor invades the esophagus by more than 1 cm, lymph node metastasis in the thorax may occur, and thoracotomy with lymph node dissection around the paraesophagus (no. 110) and supradiaphragm (no. 112) should be considered.

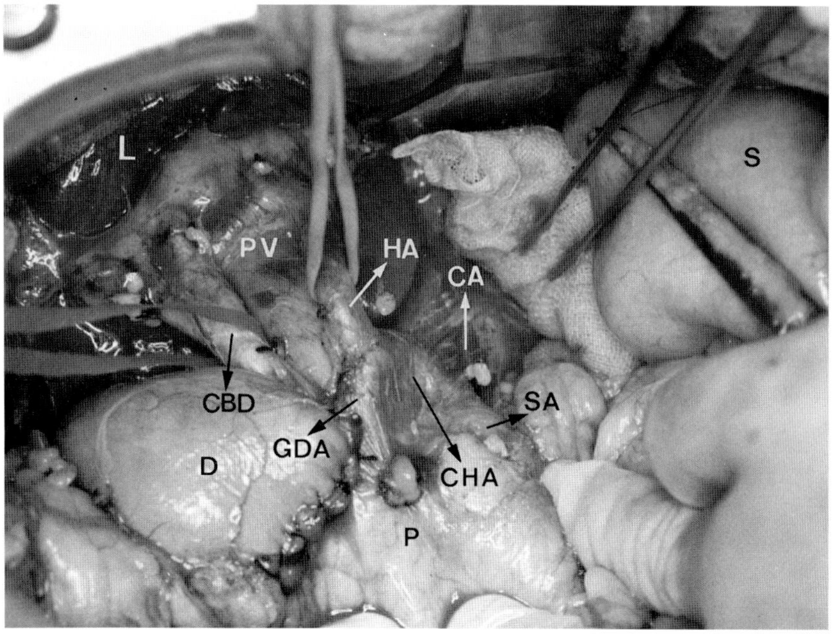

FIG. 26-4. Skeletonizing of the elements of the hepatoduodenal ligament and the celiac axis. *D,* duodenum; *P,* pancreas; *S,* remnant stomach; *L,* liver; *CBD,* common bile duct; *PV,* portal vein; *HA,* hepatic artery; *CHA,* common hepatic artery; *CA,* celic axis with ligated left gastric artery; *GDA,* gastroduodenal artery; *SA,* splenic artery.

TABLE 26-4. *The extent and frequency (%) of lymph node metastases for adenocarcinoma of the middle third of the stomach*

Group	Lymph node designations	Early cancer	Advanced cancer: Middle and lower thirds	Advanced cancer: Middle third	Advanced cancer: Middle and upper thirds
n1	1	0	9.8	5.6	20.0
	3	3.8	53.7	33.3	65.0
	4	0	46.3	11.1	30.0
	5	3.8	24.4	8.3	10.0
	6	0	36.6	5.6	15.0
n2	2	0	2.4	0	10.0
	7	3.8	24.4	19.4	45.0
	8a	1.9	29.3	2.8	5.0
	9	0	9.8	2.8	5.0
	10	0	0	2.8	10.0
	11	0	12.2	5.6	10.0
n3	8p	0	4.9	0	5.0
	12	0	4.9	2.8	5.0
	13	0	0	0	10.0
	14	0	4.9	0	0
n4	16	0	7.3	2.8	5.0
Cases		53	41	36	20

The rate of lymph node metastasis for early cancer of the cardia is 5%. Most commonly, a total gastrectomy with n1 and n2 nodal resection (confined to nos. 7, 8, 9, and 11) is the extent of surgery needed. No splenectomy is necessary. The spleen is an important organ in host immunity against cancer,[13] and it should be preserved during gastric cancer surgery unless lymph node metastasis is suspected in the splenic hilum.

Adenocarcinoma of the Entire Stomach

Adenocarcinoma occupying the entire stomach wall (n = 35) obviously demonstrated more extensive and higher lymph node metastatic rates in n1, n2, n3, and n4. The lymph node dissection should be much more aggressive and encompassing.

Paraaortic Lymph Node

Patients with paraaortic lymph node (n4) metastases have a poor prognosis. However, Yonemura and colleagues[14] reported a 5-year survival rate of 20% by extending the dissection to remove the paraaortic lymph nodes (R4) lying above and below the left renal vein. With the extended dissection, these authors

TABLE 26-5. *The extent and frequency (%) of lymph node metastases from adenocarcinomas of the upper third of the stomach*

Group	Lymph node designations	Early cancer	Advanced Cancer: Cardia and midbody	Advanced Cancer: Cardia	Advanced Cancer: Cardia and exophagus*	Advanced Cancer: Cardia, midbody, and esophagus*
n1	1	5.0	27.3	21.1	26.7	66.7
	2	0	9.1	10.5	26.7	66.7
	3	0	63.6	42.1	60.0	100.0
	4	0	45.5	10.5	33.3	33.3
n2	5	0	9.1	0	13.3	33.3
	6	0	9.1	0	20.0	0
	7	0	27.3	21.1	46.7	66.7
	8a	0	9.1	0	0	33.3
	9	0	9.1	5.3	6.7	33.3
	10	0	27.3	5.3	20.0	33.3
	11	0	36.4	15.8	26.7	33.3
n3	8p	0	0	0	0	0
	12	0	0	0	0	0
	13	0	9.1	0	0	0
	14	0	0	0	0	0
n4	16	0	9.1	0	13.3	0
Cases		20	11	19	15	3

* When tumor involved the esophagus, metastases extended to lymph nodes around the paraesophagus (17.6%) and supradiaphragm (12.5%).

report a longest survival of 52 months, and a 4-year cumulative survival of only 6.3% (n = 26). The value of R4 gastrectomy deserves further evaluation.

TECHNICAL CONSIDERATIONS

The stomach is approached through a right upper oblique abdominal incision. If a total gastrectomy is contemplated, a vertical upper midline incision is added. This approach affords wide exposure of the upper abdomen along the longitudinal axis of the stomach. After exploring the abdominal cavity to rule out distant metastasis, the extent and location of the tumor is evaluated and the scope of the radical gastrectomy is planned. Lavage with 100 mL normal saline is performed to provide a specimen for cytologic testing. Waterproof pads are applied to the abdominal incision to prevent potential bacterial contamination or the deposition of cancer cells.

The radical gastrectomy commences with detaching the greater omentum from the transverse colon. The duodenum is mobilized and the anterior surface of the pancreas and the mesocolon is dissected off the head of the pancreas and the transverse colon. Then the infrapyloric lymph nodes (no. 6) are removed, with division of the right gastroepiploic artery and vein at their origin. The dissection continues to include the lymph nodes around the superior mesenteric vein (no. 14). Next, the lesser omentum is divided from the underside of the liver, so that good exposure is provided for dissection of the lymph nodes in the hepatoduodenal ligament (no. 12) and retropancreatic head (no. 13). This can best be achieved by pulling the gastroduodenum downward. The duodenum is divided distal to the pylorus and the stomach and omentum are retracted upward and toward the left, which simplifies the isolation and division of the right gastric artery (no. 5). The pancreas is now exposed, and dissection of the anterior capsule of the pancreas can be continued to include the lymph nodes along the common hepatic artery (no. 8a) and those near the celiac axis (no. 9). The lymph node-bearing fatty tissue is dissected until the left gastric artery (no. 7) is divided and double-ligated at its origin (see Fig. 26-4). If the lymph nodes behind the common hepatic artery (no. 8p) are suspected to harbor metastases, they can be removed after isolation and traction of the artery. The lymph nodes along the splenic artery (no. 11) are now exposed and can be readily dissected. At this point, if a distal pancreaticosplenectomy is planned to facilitate the removal of lymph nodes along the splenic artery (no. 11) and splenic hilum (no. 10), the splenic artery is isolated and divided at its origin. The proximal peritoneal attachments of the stomach and distal esophagus are incised. If a subtotal gastrectomy is planned, lymph nodes of the right cardia (no. 1) are dissected, including division of the vagus nerve. The proximal extent of (subtotal or total) resection of the stomach is then determined. After removal of the specimen, the surgeon should inspect and assess whether adequate tumor-free margins have been obtained. The specimen consists of stomach and perigastric lymph nodes (nos. 3 and 4 after subtotal gastrectomy, or nos. 1 through 4 after total gastrectomy).

The continuity of the gastrointestinal tract is reconstructed by a Billroth I or Billroth II anastomosis for a subtotal gastrectomy, depending on the extent of resection. End-to-side esophagojejunostomy is the procedure after total gastrectomy.

TABLE 26-6. *Morbidity and mortality for 502 patients after radical gastrectomy for gastric cancer*

	Morbidity	Mortality
Anastomotic leakage	25 (5.0%)	2 (0.4%)
Abdominal abscess	22 (4.4%)	5 (1.0%)
Chylous leakage	22 (4.4%)	0
Pulmonary infection	9 (1.9%)	0
Diabetes mellitus	7 (1.4%)	0
Wound infection	4 (0.8%)	0
Urinary infection	3 (0.6%)	0
Stroke	3 (0.6%)	1 (0.2%)
Bleeding	3 (0.6%)	0
Pancreatic fistula	2 (0.4%)	1 (0.2%)
Pancreatitis	2 (0.4%)	0
Cholecystitis	2 (0.4%)	0
Fungemia	1 (0.2%)	1 (0.2%)
Asphyxia	1 (0.2%)	1 (0.2%)
Anesthetic mishap	1 (0.2%)	1 (0.2%)
Pulmonary emboli	1 (0.2%)	1 (0.2%)
Ileus	1 (0.2%)	1 (0.2%)
Totals	100 (19.9%)	14 (2.8%)

Some patients had more than one compilcation.

PERIOPERATIVE MORBIDITY AND MORTALITY

In the present series, the overall morbidity rate was 19.9%, and the mortality rate was 2.8%. The most frequent morbidities were anastomotic leakage (5.0%), abdominal abscess (4.4%), chylous leakage (4.4%), and pulmonary infection (1.9%; Table 26-6). Diabetes mellitus developed in 40% (6 of 15) of patients who underwent a subtotal (about 70%) distal pancreatic resection, whereas only 1 of 85 patients who underwent a hemipancreatectomy had this complication. Most occurrences of anastomotic leakage were minor in extent. There were only two patients who died of anastomotic leakage, one from esophagojejunostomy and the other from a Billroth I anastomosis. In total, there were two patients with Billroth I anastomotic leakage, and one was successfully treated by gastrojejunal disruption.[15] The procedure of lymph node dissection creates large raw areas in the peritoneal surface with subsequent accumulation of a large amount of serosanguineous discharge. If the discharge is not adequately drained, abscess formation may follow. Fortunately, this was largely controlled by a close continuous irrigation device.[16] Chylous leakage and pancreatitis were handled conservatively, but one of the two patients with pancreatic fistula died.[17] Three patients had episodes of stroke, and one died. The other five patients died because of systemic fungemia due to total parenteral nutrition for malnutrition, asphyxia due to aspiration of gastric contents, dislodgement of endotracheal tube during transportation from operating room to recovery room, pulmonary emboli due to deep vein thrombosis of the leg, and intestinal perforation due to stool impaction in the cecum, respectively.

LONG-TERM RESULTS

Lymph node metastases were observed in 56.0% of 502 cases. The cumulative survival rates for n0, n1, n2, and n3 disease were 91.9% (n = 222), 54.7% (n = 104), 25.8% (n = 112), and 15.7% (n = 38), respectively. The overall 5-year cumulative survival rate was 58.9%. For patients with stage I (TNM classification) cancers, the 5-year cumulative survival rate was 97.5%; stage II, 74.4%; stage III, 37.9%; and stage IV, 9.2% (see Fig. 26-1). The survival results in this study parallel those reported by others[3,16] for radical lymphadenectomy.

REFERENCES

1. Correa P. Human gastric carcinogenesis: a multistep and multi- factorial process. First American Cancer Award Lecture on cancer epidemiology and prevention. Cancer Res 1992;52:6733.
2. Department of Health. Executive Yuan. Death rate of ten leading sites of malignant neoplasm. Taiwan area. 1992.
3. Kodoma Y, Sugimachi K, Soejima K, Matsusaka T, Inokuchi K. Evaluation of extensive lymph node dissection for carcinoma of the stomach. World J Surg 1981;5:241.
4. de Aretxabala X, Konishi K, Yonemura Y, et al. Node dissection in gastric cancer. Br J Surg 1987;74:770.
5. Japanese Research Society for Gastric Cancer. The general rules for the gastric cancer study in surgery and pathology. 12th ed. Tokyo: Kanahara Shuppan, 1993.
6. Hermanek P, Sobin LH. TNM classification of malignant tumors. Geneva: International Union Against Cancer, 1992:45.
7. Maruyama K, Gunvén P, Okabayashi K, Sasako M, Kinoshita T. Lymph node metastases of gastric cancer: general pattern in 1931 patients. Ann Surg 1989;210:596.
8. Wu CW, Hsieh MC, Lo SS, Tsay SH, Lui WY, P'eng FK. Lymph node metastasis from carcinoma of the distal one-third of the stomach. Cancer 1994;73:2059.
9. Wu CW, Hsieh MC, Tsay SH, Lui WY, P'eng FK. Adenocarcinoma of midstomach: clinical and pathoanatomic relation to lymph node metastases. J Clin Gastroenterol 1994;19:259.
10. Borrmann R. Geschmulste des Magens und Duodenums. In: Henke F, Lubarsch O, eds. Handbuch der speziellen pathologischen Anatomie und Histologie, vol IV/I. Berlin: Springer-Verlag, 1926:865.
11. Wu CW, Hsieh MC, Lo SS, Lui WY, P'eng FK. Results of curative gastrectomy for distal third gastric carcinoma. J Am Coll Surg 1996 (in press).
12. Shiu MH, Papacristou DN, Kosloff C, Eliopoulos G. Selection of operative procedure for adenocarcinoma of the midstomach. Ann Surg 1980; 192:730.
13. Wu CW, Chi CW, Ho CK, et al. Effect of arginase on splenic killer cell activity in patients with gastric cancer. Dig Dis Sci 1994;39:1107.
14. Yonemura Y, Katayama K, Kamata T, et al. Surgical treatment of advanced gastric cancer with metastasis in para-aortic lymph node. Int Surg 1991;76:222.
15. Wu CW, Kung SP, Hsieh MJ, Lui WY, P'eng FK. Gastrojejunal disconnection in the presence of purulent peritonitis as an alternative approach in gastroduodenal operations. Surg Gynecol Obstet 1993;177:188.
16. Wu CW, Chen Y, Hsieh MJ, Lui WY, P'eng FK. Use of a modified Foley catheter for continuous irrigation of intra-abdominal abscess. Br J Surg 1992;79:1296.
17. Wu CW, Hsieh MJ, Lo SS, et al. Morbidity and mortality after radical gastrectomy for patients with carcinoma of the stomach. J Am Coll Surg 1995;181:26.
18. Macintyre JMC, Akoh JA. Improving survival in gastric cancer: review of operative mortality in English language publications from 1970. Br J Surg 1991;78:773.

Surgery for Gastrointestinal Cancer: A Multidisciplinary Approach, edited by Harold J. Wanebo.
Lippincott-Raven Publishers, Philadelphia, © 1997.

CHAPTER 27

Early Gastric Cancer

Michio Sowa

Early gastric cancer is defined as gastric cancer in which cancer cell infiltration is restricted to the lamina propria mucosae or submucosal layers.[1] Its rate of detection has been substantially increased as a result of advances in endoscopic diagnosis, which have also contributed to the marked improvement in the overall outcome of surgery for gastric cancer and, accordingly, a marked reduction in the mortality of this malignant disease.

If gastric cancer is detected in the early stage, the chance of curative resection is large.[2–4] Although it is true that no special surgical skill is required for resection of early gastric cancer, surgeons must refrain from a nonaggressive approach to the treatment of early gastric cancer. It is of vital importance to select a surgical method appropriate to each individual case, making use of clinical findings, gross type of lesion, histopathologic findings, and findings regarding lymph node metastasis. This chapter deals principally with the gross findings and metastatic nodal involvement in early gastric cancer.

THE DESIGNATION AND FREQUENCY OF EARLY GASTRIC CANCER

In the general rules formulated by the Japanese Research Society for Gastric Cancer,[5] the term "early gastric cancer" does not appear in the classification by gross type, but is referred to as "superficial gastric cancer," the designation emphasizing depth of invasion. Japanese clinicians usually use the term "early gastric cancer." As reported by Johansen,[6] it has also been called superficial carcinoma (Friesen, 1962), surface carcinoma (Mason, 1967), Fruhkarzinom (Wiendl, Piger, and colleagues, 1971), oberflachlicher Schleimhautkarcinome (Verse, 1903, 1908), and le cancer de l'estomac au debut or precoce (Gutmann and Bertrand, 1938).[6]

Thus, early gastric cancer has long been a focus of clinical investigation. However, the previous designations, which were assigned before 1970, were derived from postmortem examinations and, notably, at that time early gastric cancer was found in no more than 10% of gastric cancer patients. Since 1970, it has been detected clinically with increasing frequency because of progress in the technique and increased use of endoscopy. In Japan, the incidence of gastric cancer has been comparatively high, with high rates of detection of around 30% reported by Japanese investigators.[7–9] The 2033 patients operated on for gastric cancer at our clinic included 716 (35.4%) with early gastric cancer. As shown in Table 27-1, the rate of detection of early gastric cancer was as high as 46.2% during 1990 to 1992. This high rate has been attributed to two factors: first, improvements in diagnostic techniques, including radiology, endoscopy, biopsy, and cytology; and second, the popularization of mass screening examinations of the stomach with complete physical examination. The mass screening examination system, which has been well developed in Japan, is considered a particularly important contributory factor.

CLINICOPATHOLOGIC FEATURES OF EARLY GASTRIC CANCER

Accurate diagnosis of early gastric cancer should be established with reference to its gross type, histologic morphology, superficial extension, depth of invasion, and extent of metastasis. Early gastric cancer should be distinguished from advanced gastric cancer, to which Borrmann's classification is applicable. According to the general rules of the Japanese Research Society for Gastric Cancer, early gastric cancer comes under type 0. This classification system gives priority to macroscopic findings, especially the morphology of the mucosal surface, and takes no account of other characteristics, including etiology.

Gross Type

At the 4th Meeting of the Society for Gastrointestinal Endoscopy of Japan (1962), early gastric cancer was defined as malignancy restricted to the mucosa or submucosa of the stomach and classified into type I, type II (including subsets), and type III (Fig. 27-1):

Type I (protruded type): Evident tumorous protrusion is present.
Type II (superficial type): No evident protrusion or depression is present. This type is divided into three subsets, as follows:

First Department of Surgery, Osaka City University, Medical School, 1-5-7 Asahi-machi, Abeno-ku, Osaka, 545 Japan.

TABLE 27-1. *Resected gastric cancer patients according to depth of invasion of the gastric wall: Data from First Department of Surgery, Osaka City University Hospital, 1975–1992**

m	sm	pm	ss	se	si, sei
1975–1979 (n = 465)					
59 (12.7%)	62 (13.3%)	58 (12.5%)	60 (12.9%)	186 (40.0%)	40 (8.6%)
1980–1984 (n = 564)					
80 (14.2%)	96 (17.0%)	73 (12.9%)	35 (6.2%)	264 (46.9%)	16 (2.8%)
1985–1989 (n = 613)					
123 (20.1%)	120 (19.6%)	69 (11.3%)	30 (4.9%)	222 (36.1%)	49 (8.0%)
1990–1992 (n = 381)					
97 (25.5%)	79 (20.7%)	49 (12.9%)	26 (6.8%)	117 (30.7%)	13 (3.4%)

* Classification of tumor invasion depth according to the Japanese Research Society for Gastric Cancer.[5]
m, mucosal neoplastic involvement; *sm,* submucosal neoplastic involvement; pm, muscle layer neoplastic involvement; se, serosal neoplastic involvement; sel, neoplastic involvement with direct infiltration of other organ beyond serosa.

IIa (slightly protruded): This subset features only slight protrusion.
IIb (flat): This subset features neither protrusion nor depression on the normal mucosal surface.
IIc (slightly depressed): this subset features easily discernible depression.
Type III (excavated type): A prominent excavation in the gastric mucosal surface is present.

Notably, a distinction is drawn between type I and type IIa according to the following criteria: a lesion with a protrusion that is more than twice as high as the normal mucosal width is classified as type I, and a lesion with a lesser degree of protrusion as type IIa. In addition, early gastric cancer often has complex morphologic features, for example, a combination of shallow and deep depression (type IIc + III) or a shallow depression and a slight protrusion (type IIc + IIa). The first Roman numeral indicates the predominant pattern.

Age Distribution

The depressed type (IIc or IIc + III) is prevalent in the group of patients 50 years of age or younger, and the protruded type (I or IIa) is more common in the older age group.[10–12] In our series, patients 60 years of age or older and those younger than 50 years of age tended to have protruded lesions and depressed lesions, respectively. These findings were compatible with those of other authors.

Depth of Invasion

In general, the frequency of detection of early gastric cancer restricted within the lamina propria mucosae (m cancer) is similar to that of lesions that have invaded the submucosal layer (sm cancer). However, sm cancer is apt to be prevalent in the IIa + IIc group, and m cancer to be so in the IIa, IIc, or IIb group. A review of the Japanese literature revealed similar trends.[12] More recently, it has become possible to detect even minute lesions, and thus the percentage of m cancer cases in the population as a whole with types IIa or IIc early gastric cancer is especially high.

Histopathologic Type

Controversy persists concerning the histopathologic type of early gastric cancer. Some authors have reported that undiffer-

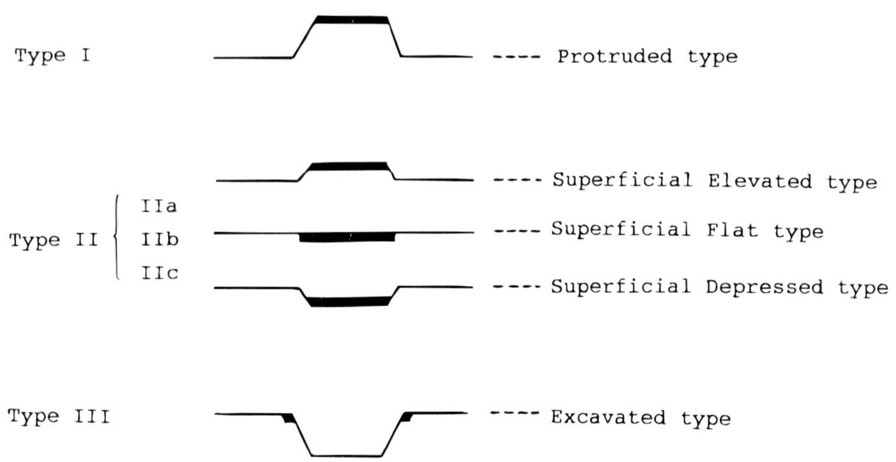

FIG. 27-1. Macroscopic classification of early gastric cancer, as defined by the Japan Society for Gastroenterological Endoscopy in 1962.

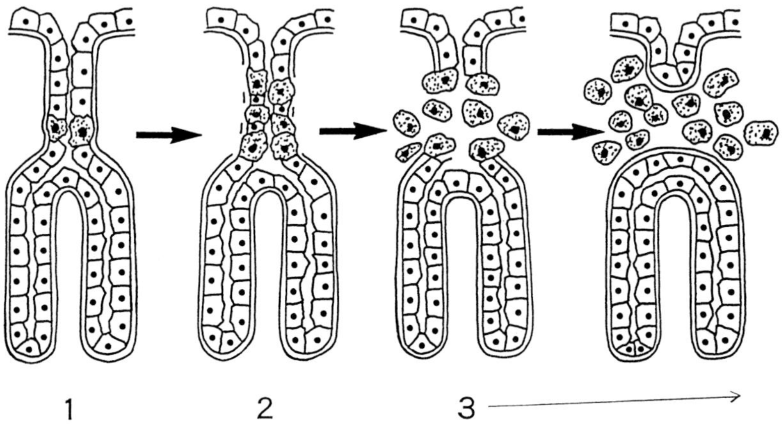

FIG. 27-2. Histogenesis of an undifferentiated gastric carcinoma. (1) Birth of cancer cells at the cervical part of a gland. (2) Destruction of the basal membranes. (3) The cervical structures are broken down and cancer cells proliferate dispersively without forming a ductular structure. (Reproduced with permission from Nakamura K. Natural history of gastric carcinoma [in Japanese]. I to Cho [Stomach and Intestine] 1992;27:11.)

entiated carcinomas (por, sig, and muc) are prevalent, whereas others have reported that differentiated carcinomas (pap, tub1, and tub2) predominate. At our clinic, differentiated carcinomas were found significantly more often in the protruded group than in the depressed group (IIc, IIc + III, or III + IIc).

Ohta and colleagues[8] reported that differentiated carcinomas accounted for 87.8% of protruded-type cases of early gastric cancer, and undifferentiated carcinomas for 66.3% of depressed-type cases. In the population we studied, differentiated carcinomas accounted for 83.3% of protruded lesions and undifferentiated carcinomas for 57.1% of depressed lesions.

Most type I and IIa carcinomas displayed localized growth and many type IIc, IIc + III, and III showed infiltrative growth. The former carcinomas develop into Borrmann type I or II malignancies (mostly differentiated carcinomas), and the latter into Borrmann type II or IV malignancies, unless treatment is administered.

Oncogenesis and Pathology

Histopathologically, most type I and IIa lesions are classified as papillary or tubular adenocarcinomas. Signet ring cell carcinomas are rare in this group. Many type IIc and IIc + III lesions are classified as poorly differentiated adenocarcinomas containing signet ring cells.

As the lesions progress, they grow and proliferate, assuming a variety of forms. If they are left untreated, they form metastatic foci in many parts of the body and finally prove fatal.

In view of this natural history of gastric cancer, study of the histogenesis and morphology of gastric cancer is important. In general, the gastric mucosa present in the stomach can be divided into two categories: the gastric mucosa proper (pyloric gland, fundic [oxyntic] gland, and cardiac gland), and the intestinal metaplastic mucosa. Cell division occurs in the cervical (neck) portion of the gastric gland or the lower portion of the intestinal metaplastic gland. In these locations, cell division is always in progress and epithelial cells are renewed incessantly.[13]

If mutation occurs during this process of cell division in the gastric mucosa, mutants will, in the process of oncogenesis, begin proliferating through repeated cell division. It is unquestionable, therefore, that the cervical portion of the gastric gland and the lower portion of the intestinal metaplastic gland can be the origin of gastric cancer cells. Cancer cells born in the cervical portion of the gastric gland exist separately, without forming tubular structures in the nearby lamina propria mucosae. These cells develop into an undifferentiated carcinoma (Fig. 27-2). On the other hand, those born in the lower portion of the intestinal metaplastic gland, which form tubules, develop into a differentiated carcinoma (Fig. 27-3).

Why do undifferentiated carcinoma cells fail to maintain tu-

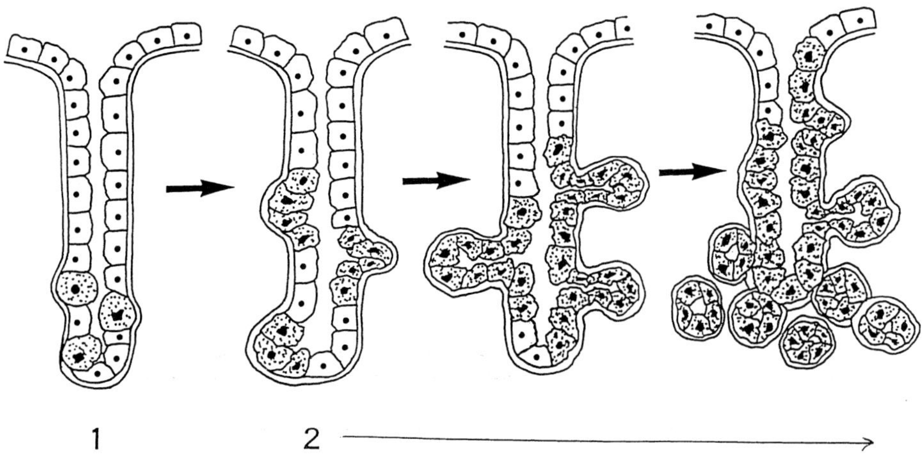

FIG. 27-3. Histogenesis of a differentiated gastric carcinoma. (1) Birth of cancer cells at the lower part of a gland. (2) While maintaining the basal membranes, the cells grow and form a ductular structure. Finally, they proliferate like a tree shooting out buds. (Reproduced with permission from Nakamura K. Natural history of gastric carcinoma [in Japanese]. I to Cho [Stomach and Intestine] 1992;27:11.)

TABLE 27-2. *Gross type and incidence of lymph node metastasis in early gastric cancer: Data from First Department of Surgery, Osaka City University Hospital, 1975–1992*

Gross type	n0 n (%)		n1 n (%)		n2 n (%)		n3 n (%)	Total n (%)	
PROTRUDED OR ELEVATED									
I(IIa)	41		8		2			51	
IIa (I)	67	186 (83.8)	5	24 (10.8)		12 (5.4)		72	222 (100)
IIa IIc	78		11		10			99	
FLAT									
IIb	8	(100)						8	(100)
DEPRESSED OR EXCAVATED									
IIc	334		27		7		1 (0.2)	369	
IIc III	129	471 (89.4)	16	45 (8.5)	2	10 (1.9)		147	527 (100)
III IIc	8		2		1			11	
Total (%)	665	(87.9)	69	(9.1)	22	(2.9)	1 (0.1)	757	(100)
					92	(12.1)			

n0, no lymph node metastasis; *n2,* metastasis to group 2 lymph nodes; *n1,* metastasis to group 1 lymph nodes; *n3,* metastasis to group 3 lymph nodes.

bular structures? The answer is that, in comparison with differentiated carcinoma cells, they have little ability to construct the basal membrane that is essential for maintenance of the tubular structures. The morphologic difference between differentiated and undifferentiated carcinomas is probably related to a corresponding difference at the molecular level. In this context, Tahara[14] showed that the formation of the basal membrane depended on the expression of E-cadherin on the cell surface.

Lymph Node Metastasis

In our literature review, we found that the incidence of metastatic nodal involvement in early gastric cancer was 13.8% on the average.[15] The percentages of m cancer and sm cancer cases in the early gastric cancer population studied by us were 0.8% and 22.9%, respectively; this difference in percentage was remarkable. The corresponding average values reported by other authors[16,17] were 4.4% and 22.8%. After reviewing the Japanese literature, Sakita and coworkers[12] reported similar values (4% and 18.9%, respectively). When classified by location according to the general rules of the Japanese Research Society for Gastric Cancer,[5] the incidences of metastasis to regional lymph nodes of groups n1, n2, and n3 were 9.1%, 2.9%, and 0.1%, respectively, in our series (Table 27-2). Similar values (8.7%, 2.8%, 1.2%, and 0.6% for n1, n2, n3, and n4, respectively) have been reported by other investigators.[17] Therefore, careful surveillance of regional lymph nodes is considered important in the management of patients with early gastric cancer. The question of why m cancer is able to metastasize to lymph nodes is of some interest to us. Our series included five cases (0.6%) of m cancer with metastatic nodal involvement. Each featured depressed-type lesions commonly measuring 30 mm in maximum diameter, as well as an ulcer scar in the center of the tumor focus (Table 27-3).

The gross type and size of early gastric cancer tumors are thought to be the most important factors regulating the likelihood of metastatic nodal involvement. In our series, protruded lesions were more likely to metastasize than depressed ones. The frequency of lymph node metastasis was considerably higher (21.2%) in the IIa + IIc group than in the IIa and I groups. It has been reported that protruded lesions metastasize nearly twice as often as depressed lesions. In sum, then, among protruded lesions, those classified as sm (by depth of invasion) and IIa + IIc (by gross type) had the greatest tendency toward development of remote metastases.

TABLE 27-3. *Clinical and histologic characteristics of early gastric cancer and pattern of lymph node metastasis: invading no deeper than the lamma propria mucasae: Data from First Department of Surgery, Osaka City University Hospital, 1975–1992*

Case	Age	Sex	Gross type	Location	Size (cm)	Histology	Lymph node metastasis†
1	41	M	IIc	M	3.5 × 3.0	por	1/31 (no. 1)
2	55	M	IIc + III	A	3.0 × 2.0	sig	1/19 (no. 6)
3	53	M	IIc	M	4.6 × 2.6	tub_2	1/25 (no. 3)
4	38	F	IIc	CM	10.0 × 7.0	por	1/36 (no. 3)
5	30	F	IIc	M	1.2 × 1.2	sig	1/56 (no. 3)

† Given as number of metastatic nodes/number of resected nodes, with the lymph node station in parentheses. *por,* poorly differentiated adenocarcinoma; *sig,* signet ring cell carcinoma; tub_2, moderately differentiated tubular adenocarcinoma.

TABLE 27-4. *Size of lesion and incidence of lymph node metastasis in early gastric cancer: Data from First Department of Surgery, Osaka City University Hospital, 1975–1992*

Size (mm)	N0 n (%)		n1 n (%)		n2 n (%)		n3 n (%)	Total n (%)	
1–10	73		2		6			75	
11–20	204	446 (91.4)	17	31 (6.3)	5	11 (2.3)	—	227	488 (100)
21–30	169		12					186	
31–40	105		8		4			117	
41–50	57	219 (81.4)	12	38 (14.1)	2	11 (4.1)	1 (0.4)	71	269 (100)
51	57		18		5			81	
Total n(%)	665	(87.8)	69	(9.2)	22	(2.9)	1 (0.1)	757	(100)
					92 (12.1)				

n0, no lymph node metastasis; *n1,* metastasis to group 1 lymph nodes; *n2,* metastasis to group 2 lymph nodes; *n3,* metastasis to group 3 lymph nodes.

Early gastric carcinomas not more than 10 mm in maximum diameter rarely metastasize to regional lymph nodes. However, large ones measuring 30 mm or more in maximum diameter feature a high risk of lymph node metastasis. Most important, lymph node metastases were observed in 30% of cases with lesions exceeding 50 mm in maximum diameter, and remote nodes were involved in some of these cases (Table 27-4). Therefore, particular caution must be exercised in the surgical treatment of early gastric cancer of the superficial spreading type.

PROGNOSIS AND RECURRENCE

Sano and colleagues[17] suggested a detailed explanation for the recurrence of early gastric cancer. It is true that the overall results of surgery for gastric cancer have been much improved, in particular because it has become possible to detect it at an early stage. However, even early gastric cancer proves fatal to some patients, and the biologic activity of this type of cancer may show individual variation.

It has been shown that depth of invasion and nodal metastasis are factors affecting the prognosis of gastric cancer. We have also reported that the prognosis of early gastric cancer is poor in the group of patients with lymph node metastases. The gross type of early gastric cancer also seems to have some effect on prognosis, because sm cancer and lymph node metastasis are prevalent in the IIa + IIc group. We previously reported[16] that the 5- and 10-year rates of survival after resection for early gastric cancer were 96% and 92%, respectively, in the group with m cancer; 92.2% and 86.7% in the group with sm cancer; 97.6% and 93.2% in the group with protruded-type cancer; 94.3% and 90.7% in the group with depressed-type cancer; and 89.6% and 76.7% in the group with type IIa + IIc cancer. Prognosis was very poor in the last group. These findings suggest that type IIa + IIc gastric cancer probably differs in biologic activity from the other types, and that the poor prognosis of type IIa + IIc gastric cancer results from the prevalence of sm cancer and lymph node metastasis.

Study of the DNA ploidy pattern of early gastric cancer, which is related to the tumor's degree of malignancy, is thus of great importance.[18,19] Our previous studies[20] demonstrated that most type IIa + IIc gastric carcinomas showed an aneuploid pattern. Hirayama and associates[21] stated that the expression of epidermal growth factor and transforming growth factor would be "suggestive [of] the presence of" malignancy in early gastric cancer. Consequently, not only clinicopathologic examination but molecular biologic study is considered essential for characterization of factors influencing the prognosis of early gastric cancer.

Since resection of early gastric cancer has become feasible, the number of long-term postoperative survivors of this disease has increased. These survivors, however, face the risk of development of cancer of another organ or multiple organs. In some of our patients, heterochronic multiple cancer involving the colon, lung, breast, or thyroid gland developed after surgery for early gastric cancer.[19] Sano and colleagues[17] also encountered 48 cases of multiple cancer. In their patients, the colon was the most common site for multiple cancer. They stressed the importance of periodic examinations of various organs after surgery for early gastric cancer.

The most frequent type of recurrence of early gastric cancer is hematogenous metastasis to the liver followed by lymphatic peritoneal dissemination. In affected patients, recurrent undifferentiated lesions often develop in the peritoneum.

SPECIAL FORMS OF EARLY GASTRIC CANCER

Early gastric cancer usually grows in two directions: horizontally within the mucous membrane, and vertically into the deeper layers. However, some lesions spread superficially within the mucosa, and feature virtually no deep invasion (superficial spreading or SUPER type), whereas others have a strong tendency to invade deeply (penetrating or PEN type).

SUPER Type

As stated, the SUPER type of early gastric cancer spreads superficially, eventually covering a wide portion of the mucous membrane, but does not penetrate into the deeper layers. It was designated the superficial type of carcinoma by Stout.[22]

of gastric cancer remains to be elucidated. In Japan, SUPER-type gastric carcinoma is defined as an m or sm carcinoma that covers an area of 25 cm^4 or more, as estimated by multiplying the longest diameter by that perpendicular to it.[23] SUPER-type early gastric cancer is predominant in women, especially those who are young.[23,24] Among lesions of this type, those macroscopically classified as depressed (poorly differentiated) carcinomas and protruded (well differentiated) carcinomas are located in regions M (middle stomach) and A (antrum), respectively.

The proportion of SUPER-type cases in the population with early gastric cancer varies rather widely (8% to 21%) in reports.[24–26] SUPER-type lesions are, at any rate, not rare. When classified by depth of invasion, sm cancer is more frequent in this type (68%) than in the entire group of patients with early gastric cancer (48%).[26] Yasui and colleagues[23] and Kumagai and associates[26] reported that sm carcinomas accounted for as many as 85% of protruded lesions of SUPER-type and 67% of depressed lesions. Whatever the case may be, the depth of invasion of sm cancer usually is slight. Metastatic nodal involvement with the SUPER type is two to six times as frequent as metastasis in the entire group of patients with early gastric cancer.[23,26] Furthermore, SUPER-type cases are positive for lymphatic invasion (ly) factors with comparatively high frequency.

PEN Type

Inoguchi and colleagues[27] and Okamura and coworkers[28] defined PEN-type early gastric carcinomas as those measuring 4 cm or less in maximum diameter and invading the submucosa extensively and deeply. According to the definition proposed by Hirayama and associates,[21] lesions included in the PEN type have spread to include 100 mm^2 of the mucosa and are deeply invasive in the submucosa (sm2 or sm3). They reported that PEN-type early gastric carcinomas were recognized as relatively small lesions of type IIa + IIc macroscopically and as well differentiated adenocarcinomas histologically. In their series, many such lesions metastasized through the vascular system, often resulting in liver involvement. The 5-year survival of their patients with PEN-type lesions was 65%, which was somewhat lower than that of patients with SUPER-type lesions.

Hirayama and colleagues[21] reported that the middle portion of the stomach was the site of predilection for both well and poorly differentiated lesions of the PEN type. They gave a detailed description of the PEN type, as follows. Macroscopically, many PEN-type lesions are of the depressed type. They display an infiltrative pattern of growth, and hematogenous metastasis occurs frequently. Poorly differentiated lesions of this type are predominant in female patients in their fifth or sixth decades. The location of the tumor focus is commonly mucosa with fundus glands, and the lesions are highly infiltrative.

These observations raise the possibility that poorly differentiated PEN-type early gastric cancer is a precursor of linitis plastica. This appears to be consistent with our finding that a poorly differentiated type IIc early gastric cancer lesion occasionally advances to linitis plastica.

Molecular biologic studies of the proliferative activity of cancer cells have demonstrated that epidermal growth factor and transforming growth factor-β are less activated in SUPER-type than in PEN-type gastric carcinoma.[24] However, more extensive and intensive studies must be performed to clarify the precise role of these growth factors.

EARLY CANCER OF THE GASTRIC REMNANT

Cancer of the remnant stomach has been studied with increasing interest. Clinically, however, it has often been detected only at an advanced stage,[29] so that satisfactory therapeutic results have rarely been obtained.[30] In spite of this, the probability of detecting this malignancy at an early stage is gradually increasing in parallel with progress in endoscopic examination.

Unfortunately, however, these lesions are usually detected only after disease has become advanced, and the number of reports describing early cancer of the remnant stomach is relatively small.[31]

Gastric remnant cancer has only rarely been detected after surgery for early gastric cancer. For example, the rate of detection was only 1.5% (9/585) in our series of cases of early gastric cancer.[32]

Gastric remnant cancer may develop after gastrectomy for either a benign or a malignant lesion, as we previously reported. A tumor of the former category in the region of the anastomosis is often detected after a Billroth II resection. A tumor of the latter category usually appears in the gastric remnant rather than in the region of the anastomosis, and it usually takes the form of a protruding lesion.

In 1993, we reviewed 124 cases of early cancer of the remnant stomach reported in Japan, including those we encountered ourselves.[33] In 51% of the cases reviewed, patients were symptomless when lesions were detected at periodic or mass screening examination. This finding suggests the importance of close follow-up of gastrectomized patients.

The length of time between first and second surgery was more than 10 years in the malignant group. In the entire population reviewed, lesions were more often found in site C (nonsutured portion) than in site A (stump) or site B (anastomosed portion). However, in the benign group or Billroth II group, site B was most often involved.[33,34]

In Europe and the United States, many authors[35–38] have studied mucosal dysplasia of the gastric remnant.

Experimental findings in animals have suggested that reflux of duodenal fluid containing bile into the stomach is responsible for oncogenesis in the remnant stomach.[39–42]

On the basis of histopathologic findings, DNA histograms,[43] and measurements of ornithine decarboxylase activity,[44,45] we showed that the proliferative activity of mucosal epithelial cells in anastomosed portions of remnant stomachs was increased in patients who underwent Billroth II resection.

The finding that tumor development in site B is frequent after Billroth II resection suggests that cancer is induced in this portion because of long-standing stimulation after Billroth II resection in the benign group. On the other hand, site C was often involved in the malignant group. This clinical evidence suggests that malignancies were new lesions in the gastric remnant.

It is of considerable interest that the protruded-type lesions were prevalent in both the benign group and the malignant group. However, the reason for this remains obscure.

These observations can be summarized as follows: the risk of carcinogenesis in the gastric remnant is high after gastrectomy for malignancy, and even after gastrectomy for a benign lesion, localized cancer may develop in the region of the anastomosis, which is chronically exposed to nonphysiologic stimuli.

Finally, the percentage of advanced cases in the population with gastric remnant cancer after surgery for early gastric cancer was very high, and, overall, therapeutic results have been quite discouraging. We therefore once again emphasize the importance of periodic follow-up in patients who have undergone surgery for early gastric cancer.

SURGERY FOR EARLY GASTRIC CANCER

In Japan, new developments in and increased use of diagnostic techniques have improved overall results of therapy for gastric cancer. However, the postoperative course of patients operated on for advanced gastric cancer is discouraging, even when multidisciplinary treatment, including radiation therapy and chemotherapy, is performed concomitantly. The principal cause of death in these patients is cancer recurrence. Recurrent nodal metastasis results from lack of detection of metastatic lymph nodes or insufficient removal of metastatic lymph nodes at first operation. With a view to preventing recurrence, extended surgery, including removal of distant regional lymph nodes, began to be performed in the 1980s.[46]

Early gastric cancer, however, is rarely associated with lymph node metastasis. A reasonable inference, therefore, is that the standard surgical treatment for early gastric cancer should be gastrectomy with removal of n2 nodes (D2 operation). Removal of group n3 nodes may also be required in selected cases.

Results of Surgery for Early Gastric Cancer

Subgastrectomy with removal of n2 nodes (D2 resection) was performed by Ohta and colleagues as a standard operation. Their 5-year survival rates after gastrectomy for early gastric cancer surpassed 90%; they therefore considered early gastric cancer a completely curable disease, provided it was detected and treated at an early stage.[10]

Great technical advances in endoscopic examination of the stomach have also been achieved, enabling the discovery of minute gastric tumors of 10 mm or less in maximum diameter. At present, surgical intervention is not always considered the rational treatment for early gastric cancer, because it may negatively affect patient quality of life. Therefore, reduced surgery and endoscopically guided resection for early gastric cancer have drawn increasing clinical attention.

The Definition and Problem of Reduced Surgery

Reduced surgery for early gastric cancer is defined as that featuring a minimal extent of resection, and therefore is less invasive to the patient than major gastrectomy, It attempts to preserve organ function, while achieving complete cure. However, it is actually quite difficult to determine the appropriate extent of gastrectomy and lymph node removal (D1 or D2). It is also difficult to ascertain the depth of a lesion and the degree of expansion of the tumor focus, and to detect all metastatic nodes before or during surgery.

Depth of invasion is an important factor regulating lymph node metastasis. Submucosal cancer carries a clearly higher risk for lymph node metastasis than does m cancer. Because surgical treatment is expected to achieve complete cure of early gastric cancer, the use of reduced resection must be avoided unless the possibility of metastatic nodal involvement can be totally excluded.[47] The risk of such metastasis also increases as the area occupied by the lesion increases in excess of 2 cm in diameter; therefore, tumor area also must be considered when selecting reduced surgery. Many authors[22,23] have reported that SUPER-type lesions measuring 5 cm or more in diameter metastasize to lymph nodes and invade the submucosa with a high degree of frequency, and have advised that decisions concerning reduced surgery for early gastric cancer should be made with great caution.

Reduced Surgery for Early Gastric Cancer

Attempts have been made to minimize the extent of resection for m early stage cancer, which rarely metastasizes to regional lymph nodes, not only to achieve cure, but to preserve organ function and improve patient quality of life.

Reduction in the Extent of Gastrectomy

Total or subtotal gastrectomy is being replaced by two-thirds gastrectomy, cardiectomy, or pylorus-preserving gastrectomy. By reducing the range of resection in this fashion, the patient is relieved of symptoms related to a small stomach, and can enjoy eating.

Reduction of Lymph Node Dissection

Attempts have also been made to reduce the extent of lymph node removal by substituting D1 + α (selective lymph nodes among n2) for D2. Clinicopathologic studies of gastric cancer have demonstrated that the incidence of lymph node metastasis in early gastric cancer is 2% to 5% among patients with m cancer and 10% to 20% among patients with sm cancer. It has also been shown that group n2 nodes are involved in less than 5% of patients with early gastric cancer. Among those positive nodes of group n2, nodes 7 and 8a (forward upper nodes of the common hepatic arterial stem) are often involved. Therefore, these two nodes should be specifically targeted in D2, and removal of all group n2 nodes is unnecessary. In sum, the procedure of choice is considered to be D1 with removal of nodes 7, 8a, and 9 in region C, or D1 with removal of nodes 7, 8a, 9, and 12 in region A.[48–51]

Preservation of the Greater and Lesser Omenta and the Omental Bursa

Cancer cells have probably disseminated in advanced gastric cancer that has invaded the serosa. In this type of patient with advanced disease, resection of both omenta, permitting simultaneous removal of the regional lymph nodes, is indicated. Bursectomy also should be performed in the event that the serosa of the posterior wall has been invaded. Early gastric cancer, however, does not necessitate such a broad extent of resection.[48–50,52]

Ohara and colleagues[48] proposed that reduced surgery be selected if all the following criteria are fulfilled: first, diagnosis as m cancer has been established by preoperative fluoroscopy, endoscopy, and endoscopically guided ultrasonography; second, the lesion is found to be stage I (no serosal invasion, no peritoneal metastasis, no lower metastasis, no lymph node metastasis) at laparotomy; and third, the lesion is not palpable as a hard nodule or mass. Hardness on palpation is considered a useful criterion for exclusion because ulceration in the focal site—which is often observed in either sm or m cancer that has metastasized to the lymph nodes—is hard on palpation. However, a protruded m cancer lesion is also hard on palpation. This being the case, more significance should be assigned to the depth of a lesion than to its hardness in preoperative examination. Mucosal cancer cases account for more than 80% of patients with type IIa or IIc lesions, and more than half of those with type IIa + IIc lesions have sm cancer. This complex type is difficult to diagnose preoperatively, is apt to metastasize, and reduced surgery for it is contraindicated.

Function-Preserving Surgery for Early Gastric Cancer

Pylorus-Preserving Gastrectomy

This surgical procedure has been used for treatment of gastric ulcer and other benign lesions.[51] It has drawn increasing attention as a possible treatment for gastric cancer, as well. The pyloric sphincter plays an important role in storage, mixing, and excretion of ingested food. It also prevents reflux of duodenal fluid into the stomach. The objectives of pylorus-preserving gastrectomy are to prevent the dumping syndrome and to maintain the functions of digestion and absorption. Dissection is performed at the pyloric antrum just 1.5 cm oral to the pyloric ring (Fig. 27-4). If the distance from the pyloric ring is greater than 1.5 cm, the motor function of the remnant pyloric antrum is abnormally increased, resulting in disturbance of food passage. If, however, it is smaller, the sphincter function becomes insufficient, as pointed out by Nakatani and associates.[53] They considered the following to be criteria for selection of pylorus-preserving gastrectomy: early gastric cancer; lesion located in region M or the proximal part of region A; protruding lesion 2.0 cm or less in diameter or depressed lesion 1.0 cm or less in diameter; and a distance from the anal edge of the lesion to the pyloric ring more than 45 mm (or that to the edge of dissection, 30 mm).

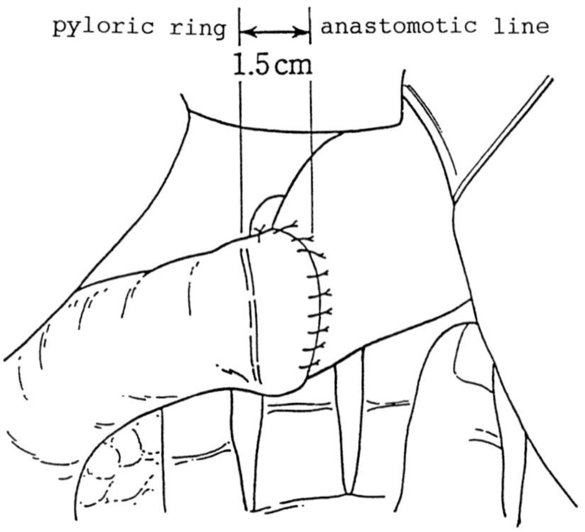

FIG. 27-4. Pylorus-preserving gastrectomy.

Vagus Nerve-Preserving Gastrectomy

This resection, which is also a reduced operative procedure for early gastric cancer, was originated by Miwa and coworkers.[54] It is considered useful for the treatment of selected patients with early gastric cancer. In this procedure, even though the hepatic and peritoneal branches of the vagus nerve are preserved, proper lymph node removal can be performed (Fig. 27-5).

Preservation of the Hepatic Branch

After dissociation of the lesser omentum, the stomach is pulled in a left-lower direction and then one or two cord-like ramifications derived from the frontal vagal stem are confirmed and fixed with tape. The frontal gastric branch of the vagus nerve running toward the stomach is then dissected. Detachment is carried out from the dissected portion to the line of gastric incision, including the right cardiac lymph nodes.

Preservation of the Peritoneal Branch

With the caudate lobe of the liver pulled upward with a hook, the stomach is pulled down slightly and the peritoneum that covers the abdominal portion of the esophagus and the right crus of the diaphragm is dissected. Next, the fingers are inserted along the posterior wall of the pars abdominalis to identify the posterior vagal stem. When this part of the nerve has been taped, it is possible to identify the posterior gastric branch and the peritoneal branch. With the tape gradually being slid downward, the posterior gastric branch is dissected to identify the peritoneal ganglion connected to the peritoneal branch.

The hepatic and peritoneal branches of the vagus nerve can be preserved if reduced gastrectomy is performed using the previously described methods. It is important to preserve these two branches. Sacrifice of the celiac nerve plexus ganglion is prohibited. Metastatic involvement of nodes 7 or 8 is a contraindication to this type of reduced surgery.

In summary, however, reduced gastrectomy to preserve the pylorus and vagus nerve (especially the hepatic and celiac branches) is thought to be of considerable value in the treatment of patients with early gastric cancer.

Advances in Endoscopic Surgery for Early Gastric Cancer

Endoscopic surgery for early gastric cancer was tried for the first time in 1969 by Tsuneoka and colleagues,[55] who performed

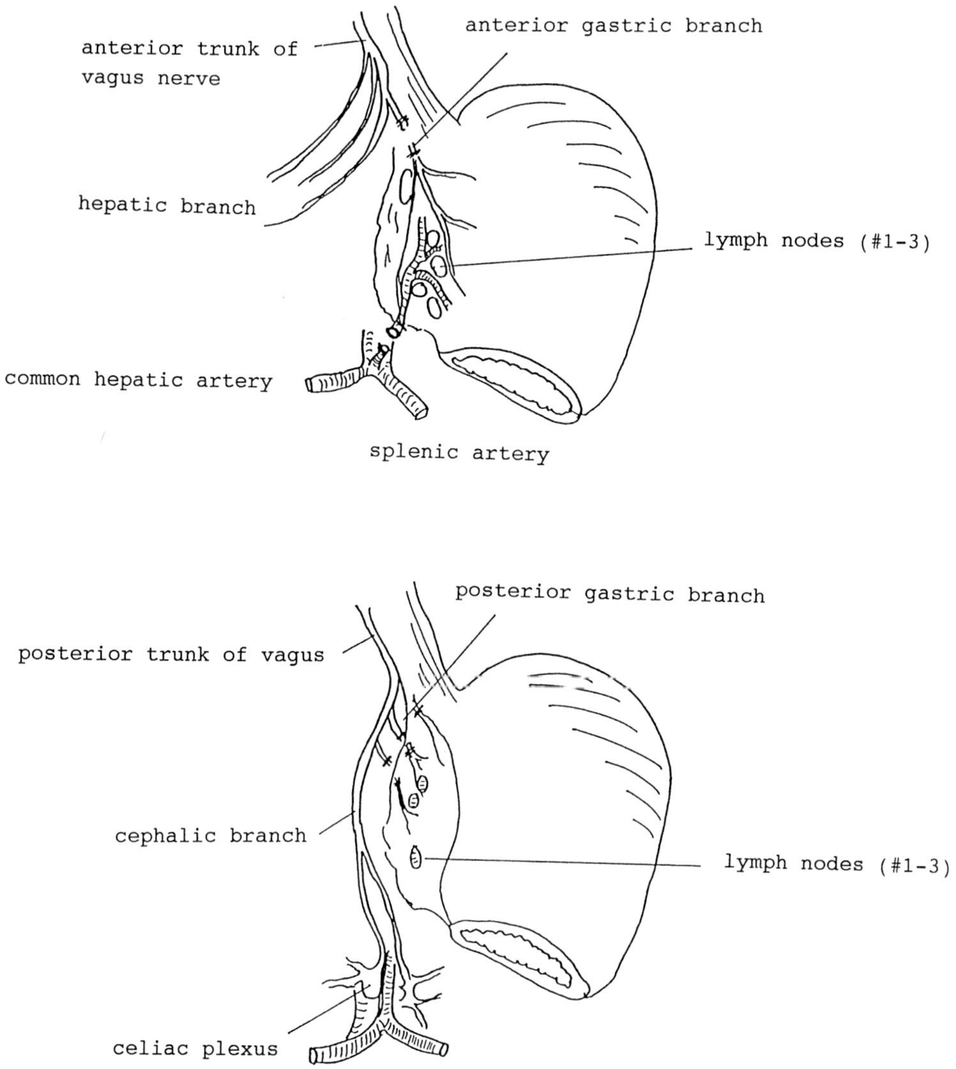

FIG. 27-5. Vagal nerve supply to the stomach.

endoscopic polypectomy on a protruded-type gastric tumor. The utility of gastric endoscopy has been greatly augmented since it became possible to use the laser with it.[56–59] The laser most commonly used in endoscopy is the Nd:YAG laser, which achieves stable and sufficient vaporization without the risk of perforation.[56] Almost simultaneously with laser endoscopy, certain procedures for endoscopic resection (mucosal resection) were devised: endoscopic double-snare polypectomy[60,61] (1980), endoscopic resection with local injection of high-saline epinephrine[62] (1983), and strip biopsy.[63–65] These procedures offer two remarkable advantages over laser endoscopy: the apparatus required is inexpensive, and tissue specimens can be obtained. For these reasons, they are frequently used in the treatment of early gastric cancer.

Indications for Radical Endoscopic Surgery for Early Gastric Cancer

The absence of lymph node metastasis is a prerequisite for radical endoscopic treatment of early gastric cancer. In Japan, however, it has been well established over years of surgical and pathologic experience that there are some types of early gastric cancer that rarely metastasize to regional lymph nodes. At present, radical endoscopic surgery is performed for such lesions.

Characteristics of Endoscopic Surgery

Endoscopic Resection

There are two methods of endoscopic resection: double-snare polypectomy for protruded lesions, and mucosal resection for flat or depressed lesions. Both of these methods use high-frequency electric current. More details regarding these two methods of endoscopic resection are given in the following (Fig. 27-6).

Endoscopic Double-Snare Polypectomy

This type of resection is indicated for pedunculate type I early gastric cancer.[61,65] Patients with this lesion are free of

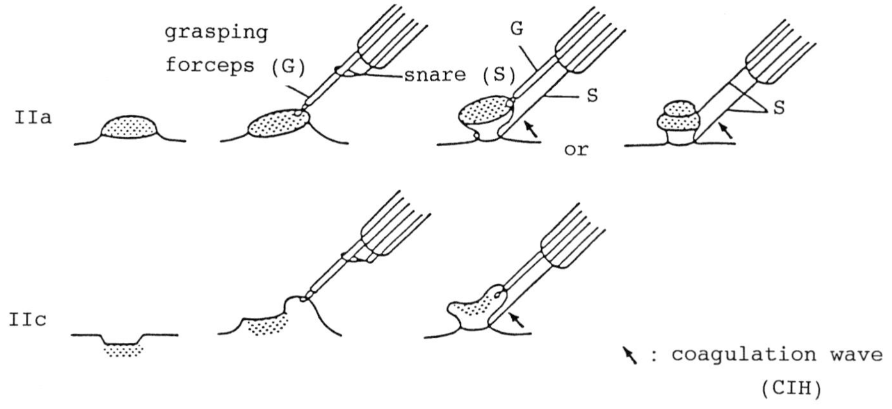

FIG. 27-6. Endoscopic resection. (Takekoshi T, Takagi K, Kato T. Radical endoscopic treatment of early gastric cancer. Gann Monograph on Cancer Research 1990;37:111.)

metastatic nodal involvement. Therefore, complete cure can be achieved with this method, and affected patients should undergo laparotomy.

Endoscopic Mucosal Resection

In 1973, Ottejan and coworkers[63] developed big-particle biopsy (or snare biopsy). In addition, Tada and colleagues[64,65] devised the jumbo biopsy, which they called the strip biopsy, for the purpose of obtaining large tissue samples measuring 1 to 2 cm in diameter. They applied this technique to radical endoscopic surgery for slightly protruded or depressed early gastric carcinomas as well as flat lesions. Under endoscopic guidance, physiologic saline is injected focally into the submucosa to induce swelling, and the swollen tissue then is excised using the standard polypectomy method.

In 1983, Hirao and coworkers[62] invented endoscopic resection with local injection of high-saline epinephrine. In this method, the area to be resected is first demarcated with markings drawn endoscopically. Swelling is induced in the demarcated region by injection of hypertonic saline and epinephrine. Next, an incision is made in the surrounding mucosa using a high-frequency knife, and tumor tissue is detached toward the tumor. Finally, the tissue is removed by strangulation with snare clamps.

This method is useful for radical resection of minute or small early gastric tumors. One of its merits is that postoperative tissue sampling from the treated region can be performed to confirm complete removal. Lesions less than 2.0 cm in diameter are generally considered indications for this type of treatment.

Endoscopic Laser Surgery

A variety of lasers are used in endoscopically guided radical laser surgery. The most frequently used is the Nd:YAG laser. Two methods are available for laser irradiation, the contact method and the noncontact method. A consistent depth of penetration of laser energy in tissue is obtained with the former method, which is therefore considered the method of choice.

The Future of Endoscopic Resection for Early Gastric Cancer

According to a report from the institution where endoscopic surgery has been performed with the greatest frequency, the frequency of detection of early gastric cancer has increased year by year, and patients with early gastric cancer now account for approximately half of all patients with gastric cancer. Early gastric cancer for which endoscopic surgery is indicated also has increased in frequency, and the proportion of such cases in the population of all cases of early gastric cancer has risen to 27%.[66]

In the early period of its clinical use, before 1981, endoscopic resection was performed on not more than half of all applicable cases. In 1988, however, endoscopic resection was performed in as many as 85% of such cases. Accordingly, the frequency of endoscopic resection in the population with early gastric cancer greatly increased, from 2.5% to 5% in the initial period to 22% in 1988.[67] In the future, opportunities for use of this safe method of surgical treatment will no doubt increase further, because mass screening examination of the stomach will continue to increase in frequency, and because further advances in diagnostic technique can be expected. The prognosis of patients undergoing this form of treatment is very good.

As mentioned earlier, gastrectomy cannot be performed effectively unless the depth of invasion and extent of vascular involvement have been accurately determined in advance. It is therefore advisable to perform focal endoscopic resection before reduced gastrectomy, and also before endoscopic laser sur-

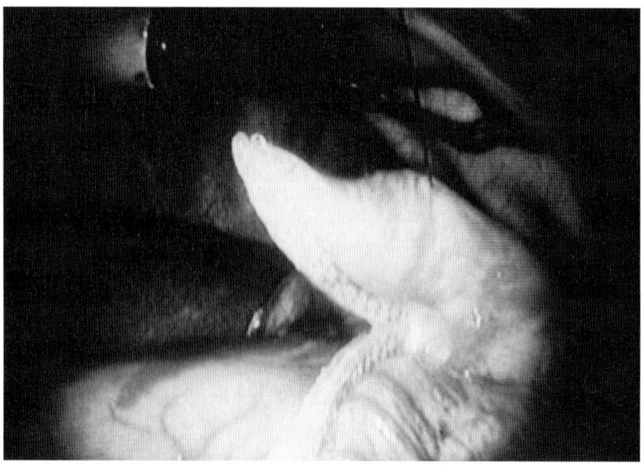

FIG. 27-7. Laparoscopic surgical procedure. Tumor focus is lifted and the gastric wall is then resected together with the tumor by endoscopic gastrointestinal stapler.

gery. Laser cauterization should be performed only after the depth of invasion and extent of vascular involvement have been ascertained.

The instruments and techniques used for laparoscopic surgery have also undergone improvement. In our clinic, we have begun performing laparoscopic resection for early gastric cancer. As shown in Figure 27-7, after it has been located endoscopically, the tumor focus is lifted and then the gastric wall is resected together with the tumor by endoscopic gastrointestinal stapler. Using this procedure, the lesion can be totally resected with certainty, and postoperative bleeding from the surgical wound is minimal. This type of surgery ensures that histopathologic examination of lesions can be performed. Its outcome has so far been favorable. To sum up, it is no exaggeration to say that endoscopic resection, properly applied, is a safe and excellent radical treatment for early gastric cancer.

CONCLUSIONS

In the past, standard gastrectomy with D2 resection (removal of group n2 lymph nodes) was performed for all cases of early gastric cancer without exception, and no other methods were seriously considered. More recently, however, the modes of progression and metastasis of early gastric cancer as well as its biologic characteristics have been clarified. Now, a variety of procedures, including gastrectomy, pylorus-preserving gastrectomy, and endoscopic resection can be performed as appropriate for individual patients with a high degree of safety. These procedures are less invasive than major surgery, and patient quality of life can be expected to be improved by organ preservation. If, however, cancer cells remain in situ after such procedures, local recurrence is possible. Therefore, procedures should be performed only in those cases in which their use is clearly indicated.

Endoscopic resection for early gastric cancer will grow in popularity because it enables the detection of minute lesions. However, surgeons must perform it only after obtaining well informed consent from patients, and must honor patient decisions to the fullest possible extent. The times when treatment was left entirely to the judgment of the surgeon are over. We have entered a period in which the use of endoscopic surgery for early gastric cancer is spreading, to the great benefit of patients afflicted with this disease.

REFERENCES

1. Murakami T. Early cancer of the stomach. World J Surg 1979;3:685.
2. Sowa M, Kato Y, Yoshino H. Early gastric carcinoma: clinicopathological analysis of 448 cases from 20 years' experience. Osaka City Med J 1987;33:137.
3. Green PHR, O'Toole KM, Slonim D, et al. Increasing incidence and excellent survival of patients with early gastric cancer: experience in a United States medical center. Am J Med 1988;85:658.
4. Itoh H, Oohata Y, Nakamura K, et al. Complete ten-year postgastrectomy follow-up of early gastric cancer. Am J Surg 1989;153:14.
5. Japanese Research Society for Gastric Cancer. Japanese classification of gastric carcinoma. First English edition. Kanehara: Tokyo, 1995.
6. Johansen AA. Early gastric cancer. Curr Top Pathol 1976;63:1.
7. Kidokoro T. Frequency of resection, metastasis and five years survival rate of early gastric carcinoma in a surgical clinic. In: Murakami T, ed. Early gastric cancer. Baltimore–London–Tokyo: University Park Press, 1971:45.
8. Ohta H, Takagi K, Ohashi I, et al. Studies of the 1000 cases of early gastric cancer: with special reference to macroscopic classification [in Japanese with English abstract]. Japanese Journal of Gastroenterological Surgery 1981;14:1399.
9. Sano T, Kobori O, Muto T. Lymph node metastasis from early gastric cancer: endoscopic resection of tumor. Br J Surg 1992;79:241.
10. Ohta H, Seki M, Takagi K. Clinical study of 2000 operative cases of early gastric cancer: a comparison between each 1000 cases for the first and latter halves [in Japanese with English abstract]. Journal of the Japanese Society of Clinical Surgeons 1990;51:1404.
11. Yamagiwa H. Pathological study of histogenesis and development of gastric carcinoma [in Japanese]. Japanese Journal of Cancer Clinics 1969;15:970.
12. Sakita T. Early gastric cancer registry statistics in Japan [in Japanese]. Gastroenterol Endosc 1983;25:317.
13. Nakamura K. Natural history of gastric carcinoma [in Japanese]. I to Cho (Stomach and Intestine) 1992;27:11.
14. Tahara E. Molecular mechanism of stomach carcinogenesis. J Cancer Res Clin Oncol 1993;119:1.
15. Sowa M, Kato Y, Nishimura M, et al. Surgical approach to early gastric cancer with lymph node metastasis. World J Surg 1989;13:630.
16. Sowa M, Umeyama K. A clinicopathological study of early gastric carcinoma: with reference to these macroscopic types in the lesion [in Japanese with English abstract]. Journal of the Japanese Surgical Society 1986;87:1185.
17. Sano T, Sasako M, Kinoshita T, et al. Recurrence of early gastric cancer. Cancer 1993;72:3174.
18. Sowa M, Chung YS, Nishimura M, et al. An immunohistological study of gastric cancer: with special reference to the expression of carbohydrate antigens and nuclear DNA ploidy patterns. Eur J Surg Oncol 1989;15:307.
19. Sowa M, Yoshino H, Kato Y, et al. Early carcinoma of the stomach: cytometric DNA pattern and macroscopic type in relation to clinical characteristics [in Japanese]. Geka Chiryou (Surgical Treatment) 1986; 55:810.
20. Sowa M, Yoshino H, Kato Y, et al. An analysis of the DNA ploidy patterns of gastric cancer. Cancer 1988;62:1325.
21. Hirayama D, Fujimori T, Arao M, et al. Clinicopathological and immunohistochemical study of penetrating and superficial spreading type of early gastric cancers [in Japanese with English abstract]. Japanese Journal of Gastroenterology 1990;87:2434.
22. Stout AP. Superficial spreading type of carcinoma of the stomach. Arch Surg 1942;44:651.
23. Yasui A, Hirase Y, Miyake M. Pathology of superficial type of gastric cancer. I to Cho (Stomach and Intestine) 1973;8:1305.
24. Sekiguchi R, Asada Y, Hayashi K, et al. Clinicopathological evaluation of endoscopic diagnosis in superficial spreading type of early gastric cancer [in Japanese with English abstract]. Progress in Digestive Endoscopy 1988;33:138.
25. Honda T, Takeshita K, Tani M, et al. Clinicopathological and endoscopic evaluation of the superficial spreading type of early gastric cancer [in Japanese with English abstract]. Progress in Digestive Endoscopy 1990;36:203.
26. Kumagai K, Gonda H, Urabe M, et al. Clinicopathological study of superficial spreading type of early carcinoma of the stomach [in Japanese]. Japanese Journal of Gastroenterological Surgery 1982;15:453.
27. Inoguchi K, Furusawa M, Sowjima K, et al. Clinicopathological analysis of early carcinoma of the stomach: superficial spreading type and penetrating growth type [in Japanese with English abstract]. Japanese Journal of Cancer Clinics 1967;13:1017.
28. Okamura T, Sugimachi K, Korenaga D. Penetrating growth type of early gastric carcinoma [in Japanese]. Sohgo Rynsho (Clinical All-Round) 1988;37:29.
29. Sowa M, Kato Y, Ohkita M. Carcinoma of the remnant stomach [in Japanese]. Japanese Journal of Gastroenterological Surgery 1984;17: 15.
30. Kidokoro T. Long-term results of resected cancer for the remnant stomach in Japan [in Japanese]. Journal of the Japanese Society for Cancer Therapy 1982;17:2029.
31. The 13th Japanese Research Society for Gastric Cancer. Studies on the relapse after surgery for early gastric cancer [in Japanese]. Journal of the Japanese Society of Clinical Surgeons 1982;7:141.
32. Sowa M, Koto Y, Onoda N, et al. Early cancer of the gastric remnant:

with special emphasis on the importance of follow-up of gastrectomized patients. Hepatogastroenterology 1992;39:400.
33. Sowa M, Onoda N, Nakanishi I, et al. Early stage carcinoma of the gastric remnant in Japan. Anticancer Res 1993;13:1835.
34. Sowa M, Koto Y, Umeyama K. Cancer of remnant stomach following gastric surgery for benign conditions. Osaka City Med J 1989;35:21.
35. Schrumpt E, Standoos J, Myren A, et al. Mucosal changes in the gastric stump 20–25 years after partial gastrectomy. Lancet 1977;2:467.
36. Geboes K, Rutgeerts P, Broeckart L, et al. Histologic appearance of endoscopic gastric mucosal biopsies 10–20 years after partial gastrectomy. Ann Surg 1980;192:179.
37. Mortensen NJMC, Thomas WEG, Jones SM. Endoscopic screening for premalignant changes 25 years after gastrectomy: results of a five-year prospective study. Br J Surg 1984;71:363.
38. Johan G, Offenhans A, Stadt J, et al. The mucosa of the gastric remnant harboring malignancy: histological findings in the biopsy specimens of 504 asymptomatic patients 15 to 46 years after partial gastrectomy with emphasis on nonmalignant lesions. Cancer 1989;64:698.
39. Kondo K, Kikuchi M, Yokoyama I, et al. Histological studies concerning the development of gastric stump carcinoma by endoscopic mucosal biopsies [in Japanese with English abstract]. Japanese Journal of Cancer Clinics 1987;33:651.
40. Langhans P, Heger RA, Hohenstein J, et al. Operation-sequel carcinoma: an experimental study. Hepatogastroenterology 1981;28:34.
41. Miwa K, Kamata T, Hasegawa H, et al. Gastric surgery and cancer risk [in Japanese]. Digestive Surgery 1990;13:1505.
42. Kaibara N, Nishidoi H, Koga S, et al. Experimental and clinical studies on the development of carcinoma of the remnant stomach [in Japanese with English abstract]. I to Cho (Stomach and Intestine) 1982;17:1359.
43. Sowa M, Chung YS, Fujimoto Y, et al. A histologic study of endoscopic biopsies of the gastric remnant mucosa following subtotal gastrectomy, with special reference to changes of the stomal mucosa. Digestive Endoscopy 1990;2:169.
44. Sowa M, Nakanishi K, Chung YS, et al. Ornithine decarboxylase activity of the mucosa of the gastric remnant using endoscopic biopsy specimen: comparison between B-I and B-II. Digestive Endoscopy 1991;3:201.
45. Nakanishi I, Sowa M, Otani S. Ornithine decarboxylase activity in the mucosa of gastric remnant following gastric surgery. Cancer Epidemiol Biomarkers Prev 1993;2:569.
46. Nishi M, Tsuchiya S, Ishihara S. The change of treatment for the gastric cancer [in Japanese]. Japanese Journal of Cancer of the Digestive Organs 1991;1:453.
47. Sowa M, Ohkita H, Nitta M, et al. Evaluation of clinicopathological analysis of the early gastric cancer. World J Surg 1981;5:717.
48. Ohara T. Rational view of reduced radical gastrectomy for early gastric cancers [in Japanese with English abstract]. Japanese Journal of Gastroenterological Surgery 1991;24:167.
49. Kumagai K, Yasui A, Nishida Y, et al. Possibility of performing a modified operation on the depressed type early gastric carcinoma [in Japanese with English abstract]. Japanese Journal of Cancer Clinics 1989;35:677.
50. Yoshikawa T, Kitamura M, Arai K, et al. Lymph node metastasis of early gastric cancer and lymph node dissection [in Japanese with English abstract]. Japanese Journal of Surgery 1988;18:1506.
51. Maki T, Shiratori T, Hatatuku T, et al. Pylorus preserving gastrectomy as an improved operation for gastric cancer [in Japanese]. Surgery 1967;61:83.
52. Sakakibara N, Urabe M. Rational standard operation for early gastric cancer [in Japanese]. Gastroenterological Surgery 1988;11:195.
53. Nakatani K, Watanabe A, Sawada H, et al. Pylorus preserving gastrectomy for early gastric cancer: preliminary report [in Japanese]. Japanese Journal of Surgery 1991;6:763.
54. Miwa K, Kinami S, Matsumoto H, et al. Quality of life in patients after nerve-saving extended lymph adenectomy for gastric cancer [in English proceeding]. Journal of the Japanese Society for Cancer Therapy 1994;19:98.
55. Tsuneoka K, Uchida T. Fibergastroscopic polypectomy with snare method and its significance developed in our department: polyp resection and recovery instruments [in Japanese with English abstract]. Gastroenterol Endosc 1969;11:174.
56. Oguro Y. Indication and limitation of endoscopic treatment for early gastric cancer [in Japanese with English abstract]. Igaku no Ayumi 1989;151:17.
57. Takemoto T, Okazaki Y, Otani T, et al. Palliative laser therapy. Endoscopy 1987;19:12.
58. Tajiri H, Oguro Y. Laser endoscopic treatment for upper gastrointestinal cancers. Gann Monograph on Cancer Research 1990;37:101.
59. Okazaki Y, Oshita Y, Otani T, et al. Present status of endoscopic therapy for gastric cancer mainly by laser irradiation [in Japanese with English abstract]. I to Cho (Stomach and Intestine) 1984;19:885.
60. Takekoshi K, Takagi A, Fujii A, et al. The treatment of early gastric cancer by endoscopic double snare polypectomy (EDSP) [in Japanese with English abstract]. Japanese Journal of Cancer Clinics 1986;32:1185.
61. Takekoshi T, Takagi K, Kato T. Radical endoscopic treatment of early gastric cancer. Gann Monograph on Cancer Research 1990;37:111.
62. Hirao M, Kobayashi T, Haseda S, et al. Endoscopic resection of early gastric carcinomas and other gastric lesions with malignant potential [in Japanese with English abstract]. Gastroenterol Endosc 1983;25:1942.
63. Ottenjann R, Lux G, Henke M, et al. Big particle biopsy. Endoscopy 1973;5:139.
64. Tada M, Karita M, Yanai H, et al. Evaluation of endoscopic strip biopsy therapeutically used for early gastric cancer [in Japanese with English abstract]. I to Cho (Stomach and Intestine) 1988;23:373.
65. Tada M, Shimata M, Murakami F, et al. Development of the strip-off biopsy [in Japanese with English abstract]. Gastroenterol Endosc 1984;26:833.
66. Ottenjann R, Lux G, Henke M, Strauch M. Big particle biopsy. Endoscopy 1973;5:139.
67. Takekoshi T, Fujii A, Baba Y, et al. Radical endoscopic resection of early gastric cancer [in Japanese]. Gastroenterological Surgery 1991;14:829.

Surgery for Gastrointestinal Cancer: A Multidisciplinary Approach, edited by Harold J. Wanebo.
Lippincott-Raven Publishers, Philadelphia, © 1997.

CHAPTER 28

Adjuvant Therapy of Stomach Cancer: Clinical Trial Results

Judy L. Smith, Russell E. Luke, III, and Harold O. Douglass, Jr.

Gastric cancer remains a major cause of cancer death despite a significant decrease in its incidence since the 1950s. Surgery remains the only potentially curative therapeutic option, yet the overall results from surgery alone remain poor. Thirteen thousand deaths from gastric cancer will occur annually in the United States, with many more in areas where the disease is endemic (eg, Japan, Korea). Five-year survival for all patients presenting with gastric cancer is approximately 10%.

One third of all patients with gastric cancer present with disease that is amenable to surgical resection for cure; the remainder are candidates for palliative therapy. The proportion of potentially resectable gastric malignancies has increased over the latter half of this century as a result of earlier diagnosis, improved surgical techniques, and enhanced perioperative care. Investigation of adjuvant therapies has been vigorous during this period, but no significant improvement in cure rates has resulted. Adjuvant therapies have not demonstrably altered patient survival after resection in gastric cancer, yet much can be learned from a review of adjuvant trials. A review of completed trials can offer suggestions as to the direction future surgical adjuvant programs in gastric cancer should follow.

To understand surgical adjuvant research, the patterns of dissemination and failure after surgery in gastric cancer must be clarified. Gastric cancer has four distinct patterns of spread. Direct extension of the malignancy can occur once the tumor grows through the wall of the stomach. This may occur frequently and early in the course of the disease.[1,2] Peritoneal dissemination also may occur once transmural growth of the malignancy has occurred, or may be the result of intraoperative contamination (eg, transection of the viscus with "positive" margins). Lymphatic spread through the numerous lymphatic channels is common in gastric cancer. There are abundant lymphatics in the submucosal and subserosal layers of the gastric wall and in the submucosal plexus of the distal esophagus, which lead to an extensive and varied pattern of lymph node involvement. In addition to the lesser and greater curvature lymphatics usually removed, the celiac, porta hepatis, subpyloric, gastroduodenal, splenic, suprapancreatic, retropancreaticoduodenal, periesophageal, superior mesenteric, and periaortic lymph nodes are at risk. At times, these lymph nodes may contain metastatic cancer when the perigastric nodes do not. Hematogenous spread is primarily through the portal venous system to the liver. In some patients, dissemination may bypass the portal system and metastases may be found in the bone, lung, brain, or other distant sites. In these situations, lymph node metastases can usually be identified, suggesting that the initial shedding of cancer cells was by way of the lymphatic circulation. Transperitoneal dissemination to the surface of the liver, the ovaries, and other pelvic organs, and to other intraperitoneal sites occurs in 30% to 50% of patients.

Surgical therapy is effective in small, early-stage malignancies as a technique to control locoregional disease. Radical lymphadenectomy improves survival in patients with early lymphatic spread. Locoregional recurrence remains a significant problem in up to 30% of all patients, but more extensive lymphadenectomy is believed to remove a number of these sites of relapse. Adjuvant therapies used to prevent or treat locoregional disease include external beam radiation therapy, intraoperative radiation therapy (IORT), and intranodal chemotherapy. Intraperitoneal therapies attempt to control direct peritoneal dissemination. Systemic chemotherapy and immunotherapy adjuvant studies attempt to improve survival by decreasing hematogenous dissemination.

RADIATION THERAPY

Gunderson and Sosin, in 1982, reported that 88% of patients reviewed had a locoregional component of failure after potentially curable surgery.[1] This frequency of recurrence may be

Judy L. Smith, Surgical Oncology, State University of New York at Buffalo, Roswell Park Cancer Institute, Elm and Carlton Streets, Buffalo, NY 14263.

Russell E. Luke, III, Surgical Oncology, State University of New York at Buffalo, Roswell Park Cancer Institute, Elm and Carlton Streets, Buffalo, NY 14263.

Harold O. Douglass, Surgical Oncology, Roswell Park Cancer Institute, Elm and Carlton Streets, Buffalo, NY 14263.

TABLE 28-1. *Kyoto University nonrandomized trial of surgery and IORT: 5-year survival rates in gastric cancer patients*

	Gastrectomy alone		Gastrectomy plus IORT (2800–4000 cGy)	
Extent of tumor	No. of patients	5-Year survival	No. of patients	5-Year survival
Mucosa	43	93%	20	87%
Muscularis	11	62%	18	77%
Local nodes	38	37%	19	45%
Through serosa	18	0%	27	20%

IORT, intraoperative radiation therapy.
Sindelar WF. Intraoperative radiotherapy in carcinoma of the stomach and pancreas. Recent Results Cancer Res 1988;110:226.

reduced by radical lymphadenectomy, but it still identifies a significant feature of gastric cancer that contributes to both morbidity and mortality.

Moertel and colleagues, in 1984, randomized 62 patients to either no postoperative therapy or postoperative 5-fluorouracil (5-FU) and external beam radiation therapy (3750 cGy). The 5-year survival rate in the 23 control patients was 4%. In the 29 patients who received chemotherapy plus radiation therapy, the 5-year survival was 23%. This appeared to be a significant difference, but follow-up of the 10 patients randomized to chemotherapy plus radiation therapy who refused treatment revealed a 5-year survival rate of 30%. These 10 patients negated any potentially significant results,[3] emphasizing the importance of evaluating the survival of all patients entered into a study.

The European Organization for Research and Treatment of Cancer (EORTC) evaluated postoperative external beam radiation therapy plus chemotherapy in 1989.[4] Using historic control subjects, 115 patients were randomized to four treatment arms:

A. 30 patients were given postoperative radiation therapy with 5550 cGy.
B. 30 patients were given radiation therapy and a short course of 5-FU.
C. 26 patients were given radiation therapy and an extended course of 5-FU.
D. 29 patients were given radiation with short and long course of 5-FU.

When adjusted for stage, there were no significant differences in survival among groups or in comparison to historic control subjects.

To improve the cure rate of gastric cancer after resection, Abe and coworkers used IORT to control locoregional disease. They effectively demonstrated that IORT could safely be delivered without significant complications and with improvement in local control.[6–9] Patients treated at Kyoto University were assigned to IORT or surgery alone according to the day of the week on which they were explored. IORT appeared to improve survival in patients with regional lymph node spread or tumors that had penetrated the serosa[5] (Table 28-1). Although some degree of bias may have influenced which day of the week patients underwent gastric resection, a better method of randomization was not physically feasible.

Sindelar and associates, in 1983, published results of a randomized study comparing IORT to external beam radiation therapy in 41 patients.[10] No surgical control group was included. A slight improvement in local control was demonstrated, but there was no significant difference in survival. Similar results were noted in the National Cancer Institute trial published in 1988 comparing surgery (with external beam radiation therapy in select patients) to surgery and IORT.[5]

One problem with radiation therapy as a surgical adjuvant is that it is, like surgery, a local treatment. Its use implies that surgical resection was regionally incomplete. Conceptually, it is reasonable to expect that the combination of a local and a systemic treatment would be more effective than two local treatments.

CHEMOTHERAPY

Adjuvant trials in gastric cancer using chemotherapy began as early as 1957. Despite years of research, no therapeutic agent or regimen has uniformly been shown to increase the survival of patients with gastric cancer. A review of the significant controlled, randomized studies demonstrates this fact.

The Veterans Administration Surgical Oncology Group (VASOG) conducted two trials in the 1960s and one that began in 1974. All were controlled and randomized. Thiotepa, floxuridine, and the combination of 5-FU and semustine (methyl-CCNU [MeCCNU]) were compared to surgery alone (Table 28-2). No difference in survival was seen between any adjuvant group and its randomized surgical control group.[11]

In 1976, Fujimoto and colleagues published results of a study from Chiba University comparing surgery alone to surgery plus

TABLE 28-2. *Veterans Administration Surgical Oncology Group controlled, randomized trials of chemotherapy: 5-year survival rates in gastric cancer patients*

	No. of patients/5-year survival		
Chemotherapy	Control arm	Treatment arm	Significance
Thiotepa	250/20%	195/28%	NS
Floxuridine	241/15%	217/17%	NS
5-Fluorouracil and semustine	156/38.9%	156/37.8%	NS

NS, not significant.
Data from Higgens GA, Amadeo JH, Smith DE, Humphrey DW, Keehn RJ. Efficacy of prolonged intermittent therapy with combined 5-FU and methyl-CCNU following resection for gastric carcinoma. Cancer 1983;52:1105.

TABLE 28-3. *Results of studies of intravenous and intraperitoneal chemotherapy in gastric cancer patients*

Trial no.	Groups	No. of patients
Trial I (1959–1961)	1. Control	107
	2. Intraoperative IP MMC with postoperative IV MMC	129
	3. Intraoperative IP thiotepa with postoperative IV thiotepa	123
Trial II (1961–1963)	1. Control	95
	2. Intraoperative IP, lower-dose MMC with postoperative IV MMC	95
	3. Intraoperative IP, lower-dose thiotepa	95
Trial III (1964–1966)	1. Control	139
	2. Intraoperative IP MMC Postoperative I.V. MMC	141*
	3. Intraoperative IP cyclophosphamide and chromomycin AS	155
Trial IV (1966–1969)	1. Control	195
	2. Intraoperative IP and IV MMC with postoperative MM IV push for 1 day	186*
Trial V (1969–1971)	1. Control	210
	2. Intraoperative IP and IV MMC with postoperative IV MMC	191
	3. Intraoperative and postoperative 5-FU IV	195*
Trial VI (1972–1975)	1. Control	171
	2. MMC intraoperative IP with postoperative 5-FU and MMC IV	144
	3. MMC IV on day of surgery with postoperative 5-FU	145*

* Positive groups identified; see text.

IP, intraperitoneal; *IV,* intravenous; *MMC,* mitomycin C; *5-FU,* 5-fluorouracil.

Data from Kimura T, Koyama Y. Preventive chemotherapy after radical operations in stomach cancer. Advances in Medical Oncology, Research and Education 1979;9:255.

intravenous 5-FU and a long-term oral fluorouracil analog (futraful). There were 120 patients in the control group and 129 received postoperative therapy. A significant improvement in the treatment group was demonstrated ($P < 0.005$).[12]

Kimura and Koyama reported on adjuvant trials performed in Japan in 1979.[13] Patients (N = 2516) were evaluated from 1959 to 1979 in six separate trials using intravenous and intraperitoneal chemotherapy (Table 28-3). Results from these six studies suggested an improvement in survival of patients with stage III gastric cancer who received postoperative 5-FU (trial V, group 3). The evaluation of the sixth trial revealed an improvement in survival in group 3 patients with moderately differentiated tumors. Advanced-stage patients in trial III, group 2, treated with mitomycin C (MMC), had improved survival. In trial IV, group 2 had relatively high survivals. Total doses of more than 0.6 mg/kg of MMC were necessary to achieve the effect.

Nakajima and colleagues also found MMC to be effective as an adjuvant in some stages of gastric cancer.[14] In a trial published in 1978 of surgery alone versus surgery and postoperative intravenous MMC, no difference in survival at 5 and 10 years was found overall. A significant improvement was identified in the subgroup of patients with moderately advanced lymph node involvement and those in whom serosal penetration was found. In this more advanced group, improvement in survival persisted at 10 years. Patients with cancers at either very early or much later stages treated with adjuvant MMC did not benefit from this program.

The Gastrointestinal Tumor Study Group (GITSG) evaluated 142 patients randomized to receive MeCCNU and 5-FU or observation after curative resection for gastric adenocarcinoma. Results published in 1982 revealed a statistically significant difference in the 5-year survival of the treated group of 71 patients (43%) compared with the control group (27%; $P < 0.03$).[15] A 10-year update noted the continuing survival advantage among the patients who had received chemotherapy.[13] This conflicts with the previously discussed results of the VASOG, as well as with a study by the Eastern Cooperative Oncology Group. The latter study compared survivals of patients receiving postoperative adjuvant 5-FU and MeCCNU with those treated by surgery alone and found no significant difference in survival between the two groups (control arm, 89 patients, 42% 5-year survival, vs. treatment arm, 91 patients, 37% 5-year survival).[16] This study also identified significant toxicity with the adjuvant treatment.

In 1988, Bonfanti and associates published additional studies using 5-FU and MeCCNU. In a three-arm trial, they compared surgery alone (69 patients) to 5-FU plus MeCCNU (75 patients), to 5-FU, MeCCNU, and levamisole (69 patients). There was no significant enhancement of survival with either treatment regime compared with the concurrent control group.[17]

Alcobendas and Estape and coworkers evaluated the adjuvant use of MMC. An initial evaluation suggested that the therapy may be useful compared to surgery alone. Ten-year follow-up showed a continued statistically significant survival advantage for the patients who received MMC ($P < 0.001$).[18,19]

Jakesz and colleagues used MMC, 5-FU, and cytosine arabinoside (Ara C) in 53 patients as adjuvant therapy. Compared with 34 control patients (randomized), no survival benefit could be identified.[20] Allum and coworkers used a similar regimen in a three-arm trial comparing surgery alone to 5-FU and MMC or 5-FU, MMC, and radiation therapy. No survival advantage was seen in either treatment group.[21] They also used 5-FU, doxorubicin, and MMC as a postsurgical adjuvant and compared this regimen to surgery and surgery plus radiation therapy. Once more, a survival advantage could not be identified.[22]

Coombes and associates, in 1990, published results of an adjuvant trial using postoperative 5-FU, doxorubicin, and MMC, but could identify no significant difference between treatment and surgery alone.[23] Krook and colleagues evaluated

5-FU plus doxorubicin in a controlled fashion and saw similar results—no difference in survival.[24]

The results of the EORTC study on 5-FU, doxorubicin, and MMC adjuvant chemotherapy were reported at the Society of Surgical Oncology meeting.[25] Three hundred fourteen patients were randomized to surgery or adjuvant therapy with 5-FU, adriamycin, and MMC. At a median follow-up, treated patients had a slight advantage in time to progression but no overall survival benefit.

In summary, 8 of the 21 prospective, randomized, controlled trials discussed here showed a survival advantage for adjuvant therapy in patients with gastric adenocarcinoma. Six of these are from Japan. The GITSG trial using 5-FU and MeCCNU was not confirmed by two similar studies and will not be repeated because of the carcinogenic risk of the nitrosourea. The trial by Alcobendas and colleagues using high-dose MMC remains unconfirmed, probably because of the severe hematologic toxicity expected at this dose of MMC. The Chiba University data with 5-FU and oral FT-207 (futraful) and the work by Kimura's and Nakajima's groups have also not been duplicated in the West.

In Japan, surgical adjuvant therapy often starts in the operating room with MMC given intravenously or as a diluted solution into the peritoneal cavity. As soon as the patient is able to ingest fluids orally, treatment with a fluorinated pyrimidine is instituted, usually as a daily dose taken by mouth. Administration of a cell cycle-specific antimetabolite on a daily basis reflects a common sense approach to the management of solid tumors whose doubling times average 40 to 60 days. Administration of chemotherapy within an hour of resection of the cancer may be a more effective approach to the control of those cells inevitably liberated during the manipulation and resection of the cancer.

As traditionally administered in the United States—as bolus courses of toxic doses of drugs initiated 4 to 6 weeks or more after surgery—the Western approach to surgical adjuvant treatment misses both of the logical concepts that form the foundation for surgical adjuvant therapy in Japan. Western concepts of surgical adjuvant therapy are based on treatment programs for advanced metastatic disease; this may not be appropriate for treatment of patients after cancer resection. Bolus courses of therapy may be appropriate for neoadjuvant (preoperative) treatment programs, when bulky tumor is present. A therapeutic randomized test of these treatment concepts has never been performed.

The principal problem with the Western surgical adjuvant approach relates to the division of labor and the fact that treatment tends to depend on patient rotation through the various oncologic disciplines rather than being truly multidisciplinary. When a patient has recovered from surgery, the surgeon may forward the patient to the radiation or medical oncologist, or turn the patient back to the internist or primary practitioner for consideration for further referral. True multidisciplinary therapy involves the development of a complete treatment team at the time of diagnosis to optimize treatment, reduce unnecessary delays, and possibly enhance the duration and quality of patient survival.

CHEMOIMMUNOTHERAPY

With the development of immunotherapeutic agents, there has been great interest in evaluation of adjuvant immunotherapeutic treatment of gastric cancer, particularly in Japan and Korea. The results of randomized, controlled trials are intriguing.

Yamamura and colleagues, in 1986, compared surgery alone (43 patients) to surgery plus 5-FU and MMC, with (39 patients) or without (40 patients) the addition of a streptococcal extract, OK 432. There was no significant survival difference between the patients in the surgical control group and those in the chemotherapy plus surgery group. There was a significant survival advantage with chemoimmunotherapeutic adjuvant treatment.[26] Ochiai and coworkers evaluated 39 patients receiving MMC, 5-FU, Ara C, and bacille Calmette-Guerin (BCG) cell wall extract immunotherapy to 35 patients receiving chemotherapy and 24 patients treated by surgery alone. A significant survival advantage was seen with chemoimmunotherapy among those patients whose surgery was not thought to be curative. No survival difference was seen for those who had curative surgery.[27]

In 1988, Kim published results of a trial using picibanil (a *Nocardia* extract) and chemotherapy (MeCCNU and futraful or 5-FU, MMC, Ara C, and futraful) versus surgery alone. A significant advantage was seen ($P < 0.05$) in the treatment arm (74 patients) compared with surgical control subjects (64 patients).[28] In 1991, additional trials were published by Kim. A three-arm trial of surgery alone versus chemotherapy (MMC, 5-FU, oral 5-FU) with or without picibanil was performed. Patient entry was weighted toward chemoimmunotherapy plus surgery. Five-year survival was significantly prolonged with the addition of immunotherapy ($P < 0.05$). Survival in the control group (94 patients) was 24.4% at 5 years. In the chemotherapy group (77 patients), there was a 29.8% 5-year survival rate, whereas in the chemoimmunotherapy group (159 patients), a 45.3% 5-year survival was noted.[29]

Similar data have been elicited using OK 432.[30] Surgery alone (64 patients, 23.4% 5-year survival) was compared to surgery plus OK 432 plus MMC, 5-FU, and Ara C (74 patients, 44.6% 5-year survival). The survival advantage was significant ($P < 0.05$). The second phase of this study compared surgery alone to surgery plus MMC, and 5-FU with a third group receiving surgery, chemotherapy, plus OK 432. There was no significant survival difference seen between the chemotherapy and control arms. The group receiving chemoimmunotherapy with OK 432 had a significantly greater 5-year survival (45.3% for chemoimmunotherapy, versus 29.8% and 23.4% for the surgery plus chemotherapy and surgery alone arms, respectively). OK 432 was also found to be effective in prolonging survival of patients with stage II to IV gastric cancer after curative surgery by the Kyoto Research Group for Digestive Surgery in 1992.[31]

Hattori and coworkers found a survival advantage at 3 years with chemoimmunotherapy with MMC and PSK (a protein-bound polysaccharide extract from the mycelium of Coriolus versicolor Quel) and FT-207 (a 5-FU derivative) after gastrectomy in a small group of patients.[32]

Overall, the work of these few investigators confirms the previous data that suggest no benefit for adjuvant chemotherapy, and suggests great promise for immunochemotherapy in the adjuvant setting in gastric cancer.

With the exception of the use of levamisole in colorectal cancer, immunochemotherapy has not been successful in Western trials. Why the success in Japan and Korea? Most U.S. trials have used BCG, BCG extracts, or extracts of corynebacteria. Perhaps these were inappropriate agents (although BCG appears beneficial when injected into the bladder in patients with superficial bladder tumors).

Immunotherapeutic agents used in Japan and Korea are different and usually have never been seriously tested in the United States. Only a relative of OK 432, a *Streptococcus pyogenes* extract, has been tested in the United States: Coley's toxins did cause occasional histologically documented complete regression of advanced inoperable cancers, usually sarcomas.[33]

INTRAPERITONEAL CHEMOTHERAPY

Intraperitoneal chemotherapy provides a method of administration of adjuvant therapy that may reach peritoneal metastases and intraperitoneal lymph nodes more effectively than intravenous therapies.

The first trial of intraperitoneal therapy was begun in 1957 by Longmire. A 10-year follow-up was published in 1971 by Dixon and colleagues.[34] The initial trial compared 89 surgical control subjects to 82 patients randomized to treatment with intraperitoneal, intraportal, and intravenous thiotepa. The second phase compared 183 placebo control subjects to 177 patients randomized to intraperitoneal and intravenous thiotepa. There were no significant survival differences at 5 or 10 years.[34]

Schiessel and colleagues, in 1989, published a controlled trial of intraperitoneal cisplatin and found no significant improvement in survival.[35] Takahashi and associates compared 424 patients receiving intranodal or intraperitoneal MMC on activated carbon particles to historical control subjects and found a survival advantage for treatment. The carbon particles were identified in 70% of regional lymph nodes containing metastatic disease.[36]

Kimura and coworkers' data, already discussed (see Table 28-3), showed an improvement in survival in two groups of patients receiving intraperitoneal and intravenous chemotherapy.[13] Fujimura and colleagues used hyperthermic peritoneal perfusion with MMC and cisplatin in patients with peritoneal tumor dissemination and saw survival advantages.[37] Koga and associates used a similar technique with MMC alone as prophylaxis and saw a trend toward improvement in the treated group.[38]

Leichman and colleagues published preliminary results of a phase II trial in 1992. Thirty-eight patients were treated with preoperative 5-FU, leucovorin, and cisplatin. Postoperative treatment included intraperitoneal floxuridine and cisplatin with intravenous sodium thiosulfate. The preliminary report noted preoperative tumor shrinkage in 45% of patients, as measured by computed tomography scan, a 38% remission when evaluated by endoscopy, and an 8% complete response by pathologic evaluation of the resected specimen.[39]

Intraperitoneal chemotherapy is safe and feasible, and may play a role in the adjuvant treatment of gastric cancer in an attempt to decrease peritoneal recurrence.

Further, intraperitoneal chemotherapy exposes free-floating intraperitoneal tumor cells, and cells spilled into the peritoneal cavity during resection, to high concentrations of the chemotherapeutic agents, and transperitoneal absorption of the drugs provides concentrations of drug in the portal circulation and liver at least equivalent to those resulting from bolus intravenous injection. The total dose of drug to which other organs are exposed (the "area under the pharmacokinetic curve") is similar whether the drugs are administered intravenously or into the peritoneal cavity. If chemotherapeutic agents can be administered into the peritoneal cavity in a particulate form (eg, adsorbed to charcoal particles or as liposomes), more of the therapeutic agent may reach retroperitoneal lymph nodes, another relative tumor sanctuary from intravenous chemotherapy.

NEOADJUVANT THERAPY

Neoadjuvant therapy can be used to decrease the tumor burden before resection, or to attempt to improve the prognosis of patients with resectable but late-stage cancers. Initial work by Wilke and colleagues using preoperative etoposide, doxorubicin, and cisplatin demonstrated an ability to down-stage disease in at least 44% of patients with advanced gastric cancers[40] and appeared to prolong survival. Later investigation by Ajani and coworkers[41] failed to duplicate these results. Kelsen and associates noted severe toxicity with this regimen.[42] Kiyabu and colleagues, in 1992, used preoperative 5-FU, leucovorin, and cisplatin in 25 patients. Pathologic evaluation revealed 1 complete response, 4 subtotal responses, 4 partial responses, and 16 patients with no response.[43] Ajani and coworkers, using etoposide, 5-FU, and cisplatin, also found a 24% clinical response rate, but there were no complete responders.[44]

There have been no published randomized trials of neoadjuvant chemotherapy. Leichman's group at the University of Southern California is accruing patients to such a study. Early data suggest that intraperitoneal and neoadjuvant therapies may have an important role in future studies.

PROBLEMS

A metaanalysis of 11 randomized trials published since 1980 was performed by Hermans and coworkers.[45] These authors concluded that postoperative chemotherapy should not be considered a standard therapy in gastric cancer.[45] This conclusion appears obvious, but obscures important information. Numerous problems are encountered when statistically combining trials of published adjuvant therapy of gastric cancer data (or of any published material, for that matter). These include differences in eligibility, differences in staging, differences in the reporting of results, and uncertainty with regard to the management and outcomes of canceled and ineligible patients.

Trials performed in Japan, many not reviewed in this discussion, have several factors that may preclude comparison to those performed elsewhere. Japanese surgeons perform extended resections and stage patients based on the stringent criteria of the Japanese Research Society for Gastric Cancer.[46] Because of early screening and the aggressive early use of endoscopy, the stage of patients diagnosed with gastric cancer is usually lower, and a longer survival is seen overall. Although this may indicate a difference in tumor biology, it far more likely represents the benefit of early screening and more aggressive surgery. Chemotherapy is usually different as well, with an emphasis on MMC and 5-FU given early and sequentially. Chemotherapy is usually given soon after surgery, and frequently begins in the operating room or within 7 days after surgery. A review by Douglass

TABLE 28-4. *Survey of adjuvant chemotherapy trials in gastric cancer*

	Positive trials (N = 16)	Negative trials (N = 17)
Performed in Japan	14	5
Used mitomycin C	14	6
Therapy started or continued postoperatively	2	8
Systemic therapy on day of surgery	9	0
Preoperative chemotherapy	4	1
Used fluorinate and pyrimidine	11	10
Intraperitoneal chemotherapy	4	1

Data from Douglass HO. Adjuvant therapy of gastric cancer: have we made any progress? Ann Oncol 1994;5(Suppl 3):49.

evaluated the characteristics of 33 trials[47] (Table 28-4). Most of the positive trials were performed in Japan and used MMC or and fluorinated pyrimidines, or both.[47]

OVERVIEW

No standard adjuvant therapy has been shown to improve survival after surgical resection of gastric adenocarcinoma, and future studies should be based on the data that have been accumulated to date. A number of lessons can be derived from published studies that should guide future treatment programs:

1. Trials should include two or three courses of high doses of MMC, with cytokines such as granulocyte–macrophage colony-stimulating factor to ameliorate toxicity.
2. A critical evaluation of the immunologic adjuvants that appear to be beneficial in Japanese and Korean trials should be undertaken in the United States.
3. Intraperitoneal chemotherapy with either a fat-soluble or particulate agent should be used to treat microscopic peritoneal disease and be incorporated into retroperitoneal lymphatics, where concentrations of intravenously injected drugs are miniscule.
4. Preoperative and intraoperative chemotherapy with a prolonged postoperative component is probably more effective than therapy begun 4 to 6 weeks after surgery. Treatment should be initiated before surgery, or, at the latest, while the patient is in the operating room and before the incision has been closed. IORT may deserve a placebo-controlled trial.
5. Postoperative treatment should include a fluoridinated pyrimidine, perhaps administered orally, taken daily for an extended period.
6. Trials should continue to have a surgery control group with stringent and uniform staging and surgical quality-control criteria. There is no evidence that any available adjuvant treatment can compensate for less than a complete and thorough resection of the cancer and its surrounding lymph nodes.

REFERENCES

1. Gunderson LL, Sosin H. Adenocarcinoma of the stomach: areas of failure in a re-operation series (second or symptomatic look). Clinicopathologic correlation and implications for adjuvant therapy. Int J Radiat Oncol Biol Phys 1982;8:1.
2. Dockerty MB. Pathologic aspects of primary malignant neoplasms of the stomach. In: Remine WH, Preistly JT, Berkson J, eds. Cancer of the stomach. Philadelphia: WB Saunders, 1964:173.
3. Moertel CG, Childs DS, O'Fallon JR, Holbrook MA, Schutt AJ, Reitemeier RJ. Combined 5-fluorouracil and radiation therapy as a surgical adjuvant for poor prognosis gastric carcinoma. J Clin Oncol 1984;2:1249.
4. Bleiberg H, Goffin JC, Dalesio O, et al. Adjuvant radiotherapy and chemotherapy in resectable gastric cancer: a randomized trial of the gastro-intestinal tract cancer cooperative group of the EORTC. Eur J Surg Oncol 1989;15:535.
5. Sindelar WF. Intraoperative radiotherapy in carcinoma of the stomach and pancreas. Recent Results Cancer Res 1988;110:226.
6. Abe M, Yabumoto E, Takahashi M, Tobe T, Mori K. Intraoperative radiotherapy of gastric cancer. Cancer 1984;34:2034.
7. Abe M, Takahashi M, Yabumoto E, et al. Techniques, indications and results of intraoperative radiotherapy of advanced cancers. Ther Rad 1975;116:693.
8. Tobe T, Hikasa Y, Matsuda S, Kaneko I, Mori K, Abe M. Treatment of gastric cancer with combined surgery and intraoperative radiotherapy. World J Surg 1979;3:715.
9. Abe M, Takahashi M, Yabumoto E, Adachi H, Yoshii M, Mori K. Clinical experiences with intraoperative radiotherapy of locally advanced cancers. Cancer 1980;45:40.
10. Sindelar WF, Kinsella TJ, Tepper JE, et al. Randomized trial of intraoperative radiotherapy in carcinoma of the stomach. Am J Surg 1993;165:178.
11. Higgens GA, Amadeo JH, Smith DE, Humphrey EW, Keehn RJ. Efficacy of prolonged intermittent therapy with combined 5-FU and methyl-CCNU following resection for gastric carcinoma. Cancer 1983;52:1105.
12. Fujimoto S, Akao T, Itoh B, et al. Protracted oral chemotherapy with fluorinated pyrimidines as an adjuvant to surgical treatment for stomach cancer. Ann Surg 1976;185:462.
13. Kimura T, Koyama Y. Preventive chemotherapy after radical operations in stomach cancer. Advances in Medical Oncology, Research and Education 1979;9:255.
14. Nakajima T, Fukami A, Kajitani OT. Long-term follow-up study of gastric cancer patients treated with surgery and adjuvant chemotherapy with mitomycin C. Int J Clin Pharmacol 1978,5:209.
15. The Gastrointestinal Tumor Study Group. Controlled trial of adjuvant chemotherapy following curative resection for gastric cancer. Cancer 1982;49:1116.
16. Engstrom PF, Lavin PT, Douglass HO, Brunner KW. Postoperative adjuvant 5-fluorouracil plus methyl-CCNU therapy for gastric cancer patients. Cancer 1985;55:1868.
17. Bonfanti G, Gennari L, Bozzetti F. Adjuvant treatments following curative resection for gastric cancer: the Italian Gastrointestinal Tumor Study Group. Br J Surg 1988;75:1100.
18. Alcobendas F, Milla A, Estape J, et al. Mitomycin C as an adjuvant in resected gastric cancer. Ann Surg 1983;198:13.
19. Estape J, Grau JJ, Alcobendas F, et al. Mitomycin C as an adjuvant treatment to resected gastric cancer: a ten year follow-up. Ann Surg 1991;219.
20. Jakesz R, Dittrich C, Funovics J, et al. The effect of adjuvant chemotherapy in gastric carcinoma is dependent on tumor histology: 5-year results of a prospective randomized trial. Recent Results Cancer Res 1988;110:44.
21. Allum WH, Hallissey MT, Kelly KA. Adjuvant chemotherapy in operable gastric cancer: 5-year follow-up of first British Stomach Cancer Group trial. Lancet 1989;1:571.
22. Allum WH, Hallissey MT, Ward LC, et al. A controlled, prospective, randomized trial of adjuvant chemotherapy or radiotherapy in resectable gastric cancer: interim report. Br J Cancer 1989;60:739.
23. Coombes RC, Schein PS, Chilvers CED, et al. A randomized trial comparing adjuvant fluorouracil, doxorubicin, and mitomycin with no treatment in operable gastric cancer. J Clin Oncol 1990;8:1362.

24. Krook JE, O'Connell MJ, Wieand HS, et al. A prospective, randomized evaluation of intensive-course 5-fluorouracil plus doxorubicin as surgical adjuvant chemotherapy for resected gastric cancer. Cancer 1991; 67:2454.
25. Lise M, Nitti D, Marchet A, et al. Prognostic factors in resectable gastric cancer: results of EORTC study no 40813 on FAM adjuvant chemotherapy. 4th Annual Cancer Symposium of the Society of Surgical Oncology, 1994.
26. Yamamura Y, Nishimura M, Sakamoto J, et al. A randomized controlled trial of surgical adjuvant therapy with mitomycin C, 5-fluorouracil and OK-432 in patients with gastric cancer. Gan To Tagaku Ryoho 1986;13:2134.
27. Ochiai T, Sato H, Hayashi R, et al. Postoperative adjuvant immunotherapy of gastric cancer with BCG-cell wall skeleton: three to six year follow up of a randomized clinical trial. Cancer Immunol Immunother 1983;14:167.
28. Kim JP. Immunochemosurgery as a new approach to reasonable treatment of advanced cancer. Ann Acad Med Singapore 1988;17:48.
29. Kim JP. Immunochemosurgery (postoperative immunochemotherapy) as reasonable treatment of stage III gastric carcinoma. Onkologie 1991; 14:148.
30. Kim JP, Kwon OJ, Oh ST, Yang HK. Results of surgery on 6589 gastric cancer patients and immunochemosurgery as the best treatment of advanced gastric cancer. Ann Surg 1992;216:269.
31. Kyoto Research Group for Digestive Surgery. A comprehensive multi-institutional study on postoperative adjuvant immunotherapy with oral streptococcal preparation OK-432 for patients after gastric cancer surgery. Ann Surg 1992;7:44.
32. Hattori T, Niimoto M, Koh T, et al. Post-operative long-term adjuvant immunochemotherapy with mitomycin-C, PSK and FT-207 in gastric cancer patients. Japanese Journal of Surgery 1979;9:110.
33. Nauts HC. The beneficial effects of bacterial infections on host resistance to cancer: end results in 449 cases. Cancer Research Institute Monograph no. 8. 2nd ed. New York: Cancer Research Institute, 1980.
34. Dixon WJ, Longmire WP, Holden WD. Use of triethylenethiophosphoramide as an adjuvant to the surgical treatment of gastric and colorectal carcinoma: ten year follow-up. Ann Surg 1971;173:26.
35. Schiessel R, Funovics J, Schick B, et al. Adjuvant intraperitoneal cisplatin therapy in patients with operated gastric carcinoma: results of a randomized trial. Acta Med Austriaca 1989;16:68.
36. Takahashi T, Hagiwara A, Sawai K, Kondo S, Yamaguchi T. Intensive intraoperative local chemotherapy for lymph node and peritoneal metastases in gastric cancer. Onkologie 1991;14:152.
37. Fujimura T, Yonemura Y, Fushida S, et al. Continuous hyperthermic peritoneal perfusion for the treatment of peritoneal dissemination in gastric cancers and subsequent second-look operation. Cancer 1990; 65:65.
38. Koga S, Hamazoe R, Maeta M, Shimizu N, Murakami A, Murakama A. Prophylactic therapy for peritoneal recurrence of gastric cancer by continuous hyperthermic peritoneal perfusion with mitomycin C. Cancer 1988;61:232.
39. Leichman L, Silberman H, Leichman CG, et al. Preoperative systemic chemotherapy followed by adjuvant postoperative intraperitoneal therapy for gastric cancer: a University of Southern California Pilot Program. J Clin Oncol 1992;10:1933.
40. Wilke H, Preusser P, Fink U, et al. Neoadjuvant chemotherapy with etoposide/adriamycin/cisplatin (EAP) in locally advanced gastric cancer. Proceedings of the American Society of Clinical Oncologists 1988; 7:100.
41. Ajani JA, Mayer RJ, Ota DM, et al. Preoperative and postoperative chemotherapy (CT) for patients with potentially resectable gastric carcinoma. Proceedings of the American Society of Clinical Oncologists 1992;11:265.
42. Kelsen D, Atiq OT, Saltz L, et al. FAMTX versus etoposide, doxorubicin, and cisplatin: a random assignment trial in gastric cancer. J Clin Oncol 1992;10:541.
43. Kiyabu M, Leichman L, Chandrasoma P. Effects of preoperative chemotherapy on gastric adenocarcinomas. Cancer 1992;70:2239.
44. Ajani JA, Ota DM, Jessup JM, et al. Resectable gastric carcinoma: an evaluation of preoperative and postoperative chemotherapy. Cancer 1991;68:1501.
45. Hermans J, Bonenkamp JJ, Boon MC, et al. Adjuvant therapy after curative resection for gastric cancer: meta-analysis of randomized trials. J Clin Oncol 1993;11:1441.
46. Yoshikawa K. Chemotherapy of stomach carcinoma as an adjuvant to surgery: a review. Jpn J Clin Oncol 1981;11(Suppl):281.
47. Douglass HO. Adjuvant therapy of gastric cancer: have we made any progress? Ann Oncol 1994:5(Suppl 3):49.

Surgery for Gastrointestinal Cancer: A Multidisciplinary Approach, edited by Harold J. Wanebo.
Lippincott-Raven Publishers, Philadelphia, © 1997.

CHAPTER 29

Surgical Palliation of Gastric Cancer

Russell E. White and Michael P. Vezeridis

Despite a generally decreasing incidence of gastric cancer worldwide, the proportion of patients presenting with advanced cancers has remained relatively high.[1–3] Between 30% and 80% of patients are found to have stage IV gastric cancer at the time of diagnosis, with an estimated 5-year survival of 3%.[4,5] One fourth of all patients are deemed inoperable at the time of diagnosis.[6] Furthermore, at the time of operative exploration, only 30% to 50% of patients are found to be candidates for curative resection.[7–10] There are notable exceptions to this pattern. In Japan, for instance, where the incidence of gastric cancer is considerably higher, 30% of all cases are found to have superficial lesions at diagnosis, and overall 5-year survival is greater than 50%.[6,11] However, in Western countries, more than half of all patients with gastric cancer are found to be incurable, and the goal in these patients becomes effective palliation.

Webster's defines palliation as an action intended "to moderate the intensity of: to ease without curing." Effective palliation clearly involves relief of symptoms. The most common symptoms associated with gastric cancer are abdominal pain and weight loss. Other symptoms include nausea and vomiting, weakness, gastrointestinal bleeding, and dysphagia, particularly in proximal gastric cancers (Table 29-1).

The qualities of acceptable palliation are listed in Table 29-2. When evaluating various forms of palliative therapy, achievement of these qualities must be considered. Increased survival time is a somewhat controversial goal in palliation. However, it can readily be stated that therapy that decreases life expectancy is certainly not, in general, acceptable palliation, whereas therapy that relieves symptoms and increases expected survival time (without curing) fulfills the goals of palliation.

The principal determinants of incurability, and therefore consideration of palliation, are the presence of malignant ascites or distant metastases, tumor unresectability , or the presence of carcinomatosis (Table 29-3). Although the first two of these four characteristics may often be determined before surgery, the last two are usually discovered at operation. Large tumor size or direct extension into neighboring organs should not be considered synonymous with unresectability. Although noninvasive imaging techniques have improved dramatically since the early 1980s, surgical exploration remains the only avenue to evaluate resectability fully. Laparoscopy may prove to be of value in this area, but it appears likely that even this modality will not obviate the need for complete, open surgical exploration in many cases.

Russel E. White: 4 Pickett Lane, Greenfield, MA 01301
Michael P. Vezeridis: Associate Professor of Surgery, Division of Surgical Oncology, Brown University, 825 Chalkstone Avenue, Providence, RI 02908

OPERATIVE PALLIATION

Operative palliation may be broken down into the following categories: alimentary tract intubation for feeding or decompression; gastroenteric anastomosis (bypass); and resection. Resection may be further subdivided into partial gastrectomy, total gastrectomy, and extended resection that involves resection of contiguous, involved organs. Major areas of controversy include when, if ever, intubation for feeding purposes only, without further surgical intervention, should be performed; whether resectional palliation provides better quality of life compared with bypass without increased morbidity and mortality; and whether total gastrectomy or extended resection should be performed for palliation.

In evaluating the literature that compares different surgical modalities, the surgeon must bear in mind that virtually all studies are retrospective and nonrandomized in nature because of the heterogeneous nature of the patient population and pursuant ethical difficulties in randomizing all patients with incurable gastric cancer into different treatment groups. An obvious difficulty rises in comparing degree of palliation between different treatment groups. Although some authors have tried to quantify this measure, most report palliation in very subjective terms, which may in fact be the most appropriate. Patients who report good or fair relief of symptoms without excessive morbidity or mortality may be said to have acceptable palliation. Those patients who report poor relief of symptoms or have excessive morbidity or mortality have not been properly palliated.

Alimentary Tract Intubation

Patients with incurable gastric cancer treated with feeding jejunostomy, with or without gastrostomy, usually have a poor

TABLE 29-1. *Symptoms in patients with gastric cancer*

	Percentage of patients			
Symptom	Adashek (N501)	Diehl (N164)	Meyers (N255)	Ekbom (N144)
Pain	38	90	51	47
Weight loss	24	88	72	38
Vomiting	24		40	22
Weakness	17			13
GI bleeding	16	3	31	13
Vague abdominal discomfort			22	
Dyspepsia	16			1
Dysphagia	13	48	22	10
Anorexia	4		35	18
Obstruction		7		6
Perforation			1	1
Asymptomatic		1		4

Adapted from Vezeridis MP, Wanebo HJ. Gastric cancer. In: McKenna RJ, Murphy GP, eds. Cancer Surgery. Philadelphia: JB Lippincott, 1994

outcome. ReMine in 1979 described 13 patients treated with palliative enterostomy. More than half of these patients survived less than 3 months, and most of the patients reported no relief of symptoms.[12] There is obviously a selection bias because patients treated with this modality alone invariably have very advanced cancers. However, it is clear that this treatment usually does not produce relief of symptoms, and further that these patients have a short survival time, making this an unacceptable form of palliation. However, there are a few situations in which this treatment may be justifiable. When preoperative symptoms include excessive vomiting leading to dehydration, placement of gastrostomy and jejunostomy tubes may obviate the need for continued intravenous hydration and nasogastric tube decompression. This may therefore allow sufficient administration of fluids so that the patient may leave the hospital for the remainder of his or her life. In situations in which the tumor is deemed unresectable, gastrojejunostomy can usually be performed for bypass, which has the added benefit of allowing the patient to receive oral intake. In such situations, distal jejunostomy allows early enteral feeding. This adjunctive use of alimentary tract intubation is reasonable if the goal is eventually to restore oral intake. Finally, if chemotherapy is planned, feeding jejunostomy allows for continued enteral feeding despite the nausea that is so frequently associated with this form of treatment.

Gastroenteric Anastomosis

Gastroenteric anastomosis has been the treatment chosen in up to 70% of patients with unresectable gastric cancer in some

TABLE 29-2. *Qualities of acceptable palliation*

1. Low associated morbidity and mortality
2. Effective relief of symptoms
3. Reasonable quality of life
4. Possible increased survival time.

TABLE 29-3. *Determinants of incurability*

1. Malignant Ascites
2. Distant Metastases
3. Unresectability
4. Carcinomatosis.

series.[12] The principal indication for this therapy was preoperative symptoms of obstruction or findings of near-obstruction or unresectability at exploration. Operative mortality tends to be relatively high after gastroenteric anastomosis and is most likely related to the extent of disease and debility in these patients. Table 29-4 compares operative mortality, 1-year survival, and effectiveness of palliation in a number of large series of patients with gastric cancer deemed incurable. The proportion of patients reporting fair or good palliation after gastroenteric anastomosis is inconsistent between series. Whereas Ekbom and Gleysteen achieved this in 80% of 20 patients treated with gastroenteric anastomosis, ReMine reported acceptable palliation in only 32% of 98 patients.[12,13] The anastomotic leak rate tends to be less than after resection, but the overall perioperative mortality is approximately equivalent to that with resection. The low rate of good palliation combined with the uniformly low 1-year survival rate after gastroenteric anastomosis makes this therapy less than optimal in most situations.

Resectional Techniques

Partial, total, or extended gastric resection have often been used to treat incurable gastric cancer. Operative mortality with gastric resection tends to be no worse and perhaps even better than that with nonresectional surgical therapy. Relief of symptoms is good in most cases, with 85% to 95% of patients reporting good or fair palliation in most series.[13–15] The notable exception to this is the series reported by ReMine, where 64% reported acceptable palliation after subtotal resection (see Table 29-4). Also encouraging is the generally improved survival seen after resection. Again, it is often difficult to compare survival between patients undergoing resection and those undergoing nonresectional surgery because no randomized trial has been conducted and disease stage tends to vary between the different treatment groups. However, several authors have attempted to deal with this problem by stratifying patients according to various characteristics. Haugstvedt[16] first evaluated specific patient characteristics using a multivariate analysis to identify independent predictors of survival. He then used these factors to estimate survival within similar groups of patients undergoing resectional or nonresectional surgery. Using the Cox proportional hazards model, he estimated a 25% and 18% improvement in 1-year survival for stage III and IV gastric cancer, respectively, comparing resectional surgery with nonresectional surgery (Table 29-5). Hallissey and colleagues also showed that survival after resection was clearly improved over bypass or intubation even in the presence of distant metastases or tumor too advanced locally to be resected for cure.[5] Many other investigators since the mid-1950s have consistently shown improved survival in patients treated with palliative resection over those treated with bypass alone.[12–15,17]

Controversy still exists regarding the management of patients

TABLE 29-4. *Results after surgical palliation of gastric cancer*

	Gastroenteric anastamosis					Subtotal gastrectomy					Total gastrectomy				
Series	N	Mortality	1-year survival	Good result	Comp	N	Mortality	1-year survival	Good result	Comp	N	Mortality	1-year survival	Good result	Comp
Remine 1979[12]	98	3.1%	12%	32%	NR	44	6.5%	33%	64%	NR	6	0%	16%	NR	NR
Ekbom 1980[13]	20	25%	0%	80%	20%	40	15%	16%*	88%†	22%	15	27%	16%*	88%†	33%
Boddie 1983[14]	21‡	23.8%	5%	60%	NR						45	17.8%	40%	85.7%	NR
Bozzetti 1987[16]	80	10%	18%	NR	NR	61†	11.5%	39%†	NR	NR	61†	11.5%†	39%†	NR	NR
Haugstvedt 1989[37]	70	24%	9%	NR	NR	118	14%	36%	NR	NR	64	13%	43%	NR	NR
Butler 1989[18]											27	4%	55%	NR	48%
Monson 1991[15]											53	8%	70%	87%	NR
Lo 1991[38]	51	22%	NR§	60%	55%										

* 2-year survival reported instead of 1-year survival.
† Subtotal and total gastrectomy considered as a group.
‡ Includes exploration with gastroenteric anastamosis and exploration alone.
§ Median survival 14 weeks.

TABLE 29-5. *Survival (estimated by Cox proportional hazards model) by type of surgery given similar age (70 yr), preoperative weight loss (5 kg), and stage*

	Survival		
	Median (mo)	1-year (%)	2-year (%)
STAGE III			
Resectional surgery	9	38	20
Nonresectional surgery	4.5	13	3
STAGE IV			
Resectional surgery	6	23	2
Nonresectional surgery	3	5	0

Adapted from Haugstvedt T, Asgaut V, Eide GE, Soreide O. The survival benefit of resection in patients with advanced stomach cancer: the Norwegian multicenter experience. World J Surg 1989;13: 617.

with extensive metastatic disease. Many studies have shown the same improvement in survival with palliative resection over gastroenteric anastomosis in the presence of limited hepatic metastases as in patients without hepatic metastases. However, there is good evidence that when metastases are multiple and scattered throughout both lobes of the liver, survival is not improved, and in fact may be lessened, after palliative gastric resection.[17,18]

Significant disagreement exists regarding the use of total gastrectomy for palliation of incurable gastric cancer. Some authors believe that postoperative morbidity and mortality are too high to justify total gastrectomy for palliation,[12] whereas others have reported surprisingly good results. Monson and associates described extremely good outcome in 53 patients, achieving 87% acceptable palliation with only 8% mortality. Further, survival was excellent with median survival being 19 months, and 24% of patients living for more than 2 years.[15] Many believe that anastomotic leak rates are higher with the esophagoenteric anastomosis required after total gastrectomy. Although it is true that some series report a higher leak rate,[14] a number of others have reported rates as good as those reported after gastroenteric anastomosis.[15,19] Overall postoperative morbidity does appear to be somewhat higher after total gastrectomy than after partial gastrectomy. Ekbom and Gleysteen reported 33% incidence of postoperative complications after total gastrectomy, compared with 22% and 20% after partial gastrectomy and gastroenteric anastomosis, respectively.[13] Butler and coworkers reported a 48% overall complication rate after total gastrectomy, but a perioperative mortality rate of only 4%.[19] With these figures demonstrating excellent relief of symptoms with low mortality, total gastrectomy should be considered a viable option for palliation if necessary.

Finally, the surgeon is at times faced with a proximal cancer of the gastroesophageal junction that is incurable. Boddie and colleagues demonstrated good palliation with extended survival in those patients treated with limited esophagogastric resection.[14] In these situations, it appears that esophagogastrectomy with esophagogastric anastomosis is the treatment of choice.

NONOPERATIVE PALLIATION

There are a number of situations in which nonoperative techniques may be indicated in the palliation of gastric cancer. These include patient refusal of surgery, clear preoperative indicators of incurability, and associated comorbid risk factors making major gastric surgery unacceptable. These techniques are all directed toward relief of dysphagia, obstruction, or bleeding, and are therefore most applicable in tumors of the gastric cardia, where dysphagia is a common symptom. There have been reports of effectiveness as well in treatment of cancer recurrence at gastroenteric anastomoses.[20,21] The available endoscopic techniques include dilation, laser tumor ablation, placement of rigid endoprostheses, and ethanol-induced tumor necrosis.

Endoscopic Dilation

Dilation has been used effectively for strictures of the esophagus, particularly benign strictures such as those caused by caustic ingestion and those associated with Barrett's epithelium. The use of endoscopic dilation alone for carcinoma of the gastroesophageal junction may provide some relief of obstruction and dysphagia, but this relief usually is short lived. More promising is the use of dilation in conjunction with one of the other mentioned modes of palliation. Dilation is often helpful before stent placement or in conjunction with ethanol injection. As with esophageal dilation, the surgeon must bear in mind the possibility of perforation of the gastroesophageal junction with use of either pneumatic or rigid dilation.

Laser Tumor Ablation

Laser tumor ablation has been used extensively as a palliative technique in stenotic, obstructing, or bleeding malignant tumors of the gastroesophageal junction and cardia, and less commonly in distal gastric lesions.[22–24] Almost exclusively used has been the neodymium-yttrium-aluminum garnet laser. In general, laser therapy is carried out with intravenous sedation only, and requires several treatments to be effective in reestablishing a lumen (Fig. 29-1). One to six treatments may be required and can be undertaken with a 48-hour interval between treatments. Effectiveness of palliation has been good in all series, with acceptable relief of obstruction and dysphagia achieved in 90% to 95% of patients. The major complication of this technique is perforation, and most series report a perforation rate of 2% to 5%, with an associated mortality of 1% to 4%. This technique is attractive because it can be performed on an outpatient basis without general anesthesia, it has a high rate of success with low morbidity and mortality, and it can be repeated as necessary for progression and regrowth of tumor. One significant disadvantage, however, is the cost associated with the necessary equipment, making the availability of this form of therapy limited. As expected, survival does not seem to be enhanced, with median survival times averaging 4 to 6 months.[22,25–27]

Placement of Rigid Endoprostheses

Endoscopic placement of rigid prostheses has become an accepted form of treatment for incurable malignant strictures of the esophagus and gastric cardia.[22,25,28–35] A variety of stents have been used, including simple rigid tubes and, more recently, self-expanding, steel mesh prostheses (Figs. 29-2 and 29-3).[20]

As expected, the stents are not at all effective in treating bleeding, but have been highly effective in relieving dysphagia and allowing resumption of oral intake. Virtually all patients have improvement in swallowing immediately after tube placement. A criticism of this form of palliation historically has been that although after placement all patients can swallow liquids, many patients cannot eat a solid diet, and have to remain on semisolid or liquid diets for the remainder of their lives.[31] In fact, with standard stents only 10% to 15% of patients could resume a normal diet after placement.[26] However, with newer, nonstandard tubes, the proportion of patients able to eat a regular, solid diet has risen considerably.[20,22,26] The procedure itself most commonly requires general anesthesia to perform the dilation that is required before prosthesis placement. In some cases, multiple dilations—each requiring anesthesia—are needed before stent placement.[31] Complications related to this procedure include perforation, hemorrhage, aspiration, and migration of prosthesis. The combined incidence of these complications varies from 5% to 20% between series, with mortality rates ranging from 0% to 8% (Table 29-6). As with laser therapy, survival time tends to be poor, with average survival times of less than 6 months reported in the literature. Compared with laser ablation of tumors, stent placement has the advantage of a stable lumen that usually does not require further manipulation once it is in place. The disadvantages include the need for general anesthesia, a higher complication rate, and the possibility of gastroesophageal reflux and its inherent complications if the stent crosses the gastroesophageal junction.

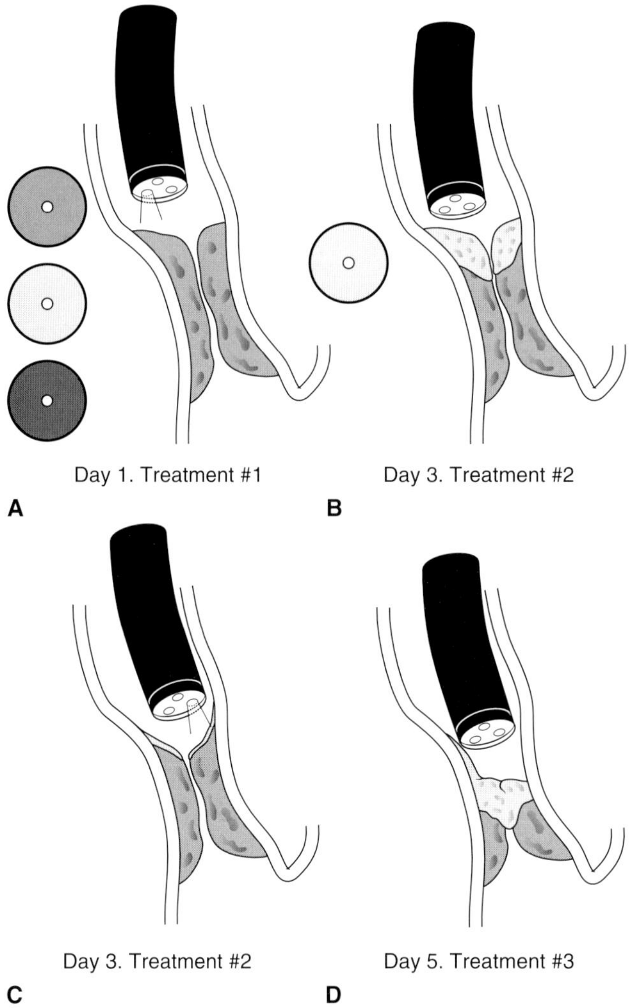

FIG. 29-1. Techniques of endoscopic laser therapy for obstructing neoplasm of the gastric cardia **(A)** Endoscope advanced to the superior margin of the tumor. Laser waveguide passed through biopsy channel aiming at the tumor. The circles at the left represent cross sections of the tumor at the superior margin. The *upper gray circle* represents the tumor surface before laser therapy. After initial laser treatment, the treated area will be coagulated and appear whitish-yellow (*middle*). With continued treatment, the vaporized tissue is blackened. **(B)** Appearance day 3, 48 hours after laser treatment. Previously treated tissue now necrotic. The cross section shows the whitish-yellow color. **(C)** Appearance day 3 after removal of necrotic laser-treated tissue. Second treatment can now begin. **(D)** Appearance day 5. Sequence performed on day 3 will be repeated at a more distal level. (From Flesicher D, Sivak MV. Endoscopic Nd:YAG laser therapy as palliative treatment for advanced adenocarcinoma of the gastric cardia. Gastroenterology 1984;87:815.)

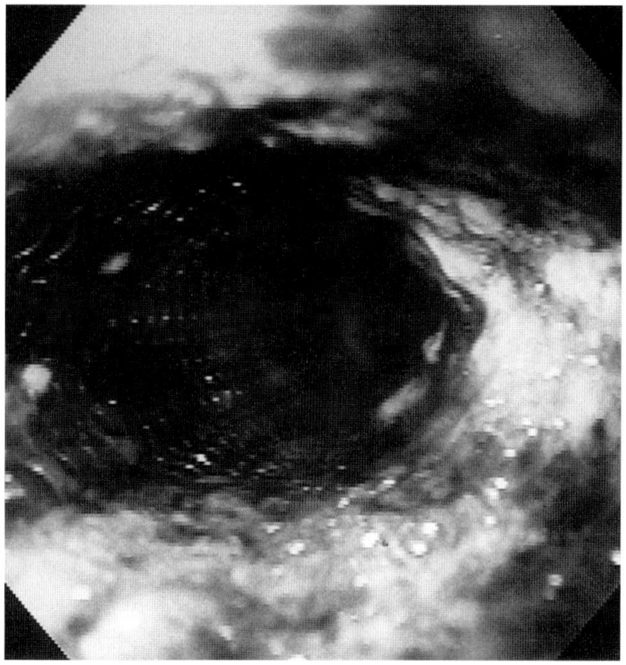

FIG. 29-2. Endoscopic view of an 18 mm nitinol self-expanding metal esophageal stent (Microvasives), immediately following placement. The stent maintains luminal patency of the gastroesophageal junction in a patient with unresectable adenocarcinoma.

Ethanol-Induced Tumor Necrosis

The use of ethanol injection to induce tumor necrosis and thereby relieve obstructive symptoms has been described for malignancies of both the esophagus and gastric cardia.[36,37] The technique itself can be performed under intravenous sedation only and is often used in conjunction with dilation. Absolute ethanol is injected directly into the tumor mass in an attempt

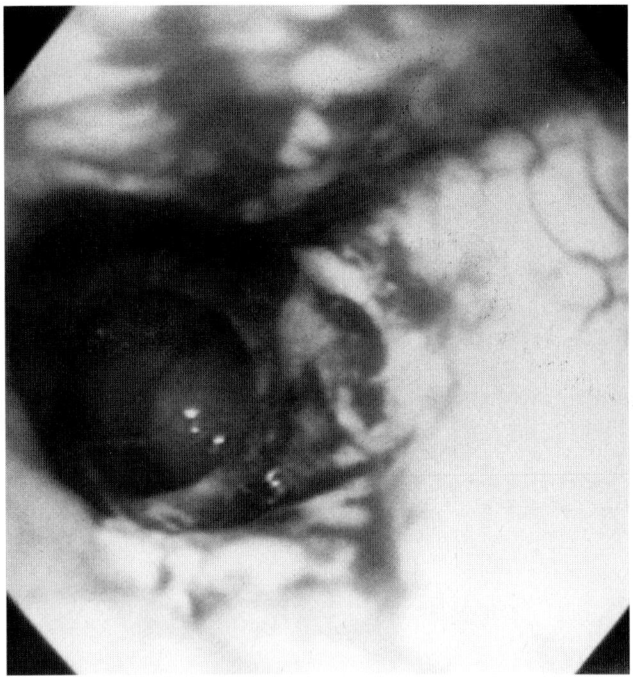

FIG. 29-3. Endoscopic view of a similar stent placed across a gastroesophageal junction tumor. This picture was taken 6 months after placement of the stent. Tumor ingrowth through the metal mesh is apparent, but luminal patency is maintained. Gastric rugae are visible at the distal aspect of the stent. (Photo by Paul Ackerman, MD.)

to inject all visible tumor. Multiple treatments are often required and a period of approximately 1 week is allowed between treatments. This time period allows for necrosis and sloughing of tumor. Virtually all patients experience improvement in dysphagia, but rarely are patients able to tolerate regular, solid diets after treatment.[36] Complications are rare with this technique, and, as expected, survival is poor after this therapy.

SUMMARY

Gastric cancer continues to be a disease for which cure is often not attainable and palliation must be the goal. In most cases, operative exploration is necessary clearly to establish incurability. When operative therapy is possible, it offers the best palliation, including in most cases some prolongation of survival. Of the available operative techniques, resection offers the most consistent relief of symptoms with improved survival. If total gastrectomy is required for palliative resection, it should be considered a viable option, in the understanding that each case needs to be evaluated individually and that severely debilitated patients may not do well with extensive resections. If extensive hepatic metastases are present, resection is not likely to extend life significantly, and gastroenteric anastomosis may be considered. Alimentary tract intubation for feeding purposes alone usually is not effective in palliation and should not be considered as treatment for incurable gastric cancer. In those situations in which incurability can be established with certainty before surgery, and the patient is severely debilitated or refuses surgery, consideration should be given to one of the available nonoperative forms of palliative treatment.

TABLE 29-6. *Morbidity and mortality related to endoscopic prosthesis placement*

	Morbidity		
Series	Perforation	Hemorrhage	Aspiration Mortality
Buset, 1987[21]	7.8	3.4	2.2
Gasparri, 1987[30]	2	NR	NR
Loizou, 1991[24]	13	0	0

All numbers reported as percentages.
NR, not reported.

REFERENCES

1. Silverberg E, Lubera J. Cancer statistics 1989. CA Cancer J Clin 1989; 1:3.
2. Bringaze W, Chappuis C, Cohn I, et al. Early gastric cancer. Ann Surg 1986;204:103.
3. Dalton R, Eisenberg B. Rationale for the current surgical management of gastric adenocarcinoma. Oncology 1994;8:99.
4. Wanebo HJ, Kennedy BJ, Chmeil J, et al. Cancer of the stomach: a patient care study by the American College of Surgeons. Ann Surg 1993;218:583.
5. Hallissey MT, Allum WH, Roginski C, Fielding JWL. Palliative surgery for gastric cancer. Cancer 1988;62:440.
6. Douglass HO, Nava HR. Gastric adenocarcinoma: management of the primary disease. Semin Oncol 1985;12:32.
7. Lawrence WT, Lawrence W Jr. Gastric cancer: the surgeon's viewpoint. Semin Oncol 1980;7:400.
8. Cady B, Rossi RL, Silverman ML, Piccione W, Heck TA. Gastric adenocarcinoma. Arch Surg 1989;124:303.
9. Meyers WC, Damiano RJ, Postlethwait RW, Rotolo FS. Adenocarcinoma of the stomach: changing patterns over the last 4 decades. Ann Surg 1987;205:1.
10. Diehl JT, Hermann RE, Cooperman AM, Hoerr SO. Gastric carcinoma: a ten year review. Ann Surg 1983;198:9.
11. Deziel DJ, Millikan K. Palliative operations for advanced gastric carcinoma. In: Economou SG, Witt TR, Deziel DJ, Saclarides TJ, Staren ED, Bines SD, eds. Adjuncts to cancer surgery. Malvern, PA: Lea & Febiger, 1992:312.
12. ReMine WH. Palliative operations for incurable gastric cancer. World J Surg 1979;3:721.
13. Ekbom GA, Gleysteen JJ. Gastric malignancy: resection for palliation. Surgery 1980;88:476.
14. Boddie AW, Mcmurtrey MJ, Giacco GG, Mcbride CM. Palliative total gastrectomy and esophagogastrectomy: a reevaluation. Cancer 1983; 51:1195.
15. Monson JRT, Donohue JH, Mcilrath DC, Farnell MB, Ilstrup DM. Total gastrectomy for advanced cancer: a worthwhile palliative procedure. Cancer 1991;68:1863.
16. Haugstvedt T, Asgaut V, Eide GE, Soreide O. The survival benefit of resection in patients with advanced stomach cancer: the Norwegian multicenter experience. World J Surg 1989;13:617.
17. Bozzetti F, Bonfanti G, Audisio RA, et al. Prognosis of patients after palliative surgical procedures for carcinoma of the stomach. Surg Gynecol Obstet 1987;164:151.
18. Koga S, Hiroki K, Hiroyuki K, et al. Therapeutic significance of noncurative gastrectomy for gastric cancer with liver metastasis. Am J Surg 1980;140:356.
19. Butler JA, Dubrow TJ, Trezona T, Klassen M, Nejdl RJ. Total gastrectomy in the treatment of advanced gastric cancer. Am J Surg 1989; 158:602.
20. Topazian M, Ernest R, Grendell J. Palliation of obstructing gastric cancer with steel mesh, self-expanding endoprostheses. Gastrointest Endosc 1992;38:58.

21. Brennan FN, McCarthy JH, Laurence BH. Endoscopic Nd-YAG laser therapy for palliation of upper gastrointestinal malignancy. Med J Aust 1990;153:27.
22. Buset M, des Marez B, Baize M, et al. Palliative endoscopic management of obstructive esophagogastric cancer: laser or prosthesis?. Gastrointest Endosc 1987;33:357.
23. Flesicher D, Sivak MV. Endoscopic Nd:YAG laser therapy as palliative treatment for advanced adenocarcinoma of the gastric cardia. Gastroenterology 1984;87:815.
24. Swain CP, Bown SG, Edwards DAW, Salmon PR. Neoplastic gastric outflow tract obstruction relieved at endoscopy by argon laser. Gastrointest Endosc 1984;30:31.
25. Loizou LA, Grigg D, Atkinson M, Robertson C, Bown SG. A prospective comparison of laser therapy and intubation in endoscopic palliation for malignant dysphagia. Gastroenterology 1991;100:1303.
26. Brown SG. Palliation of malignant dysphagia: surgery, radiotherapy, laser, intubation alone or in combination? Gut 1991;32:841.
27. Mason RC, Bright N, McColl I. Palliation of malignant dysphagia with laser therapy: predictability of results. Br J Surg 1991;78:1346.
28. Den Hartog Jager FCA, Bartelsman JFWM, Tytgat GNJ. Palliative treatment of obstructing esophagogastric malignancy by endoscopic positioning of a plastic prosthesis. Gastroenterology 1979;11:1008.
29. Atkinson M, Ferguson R. Fiberoptic endoscopic palliative intubation of inoperable esophagogastric neoplasms. Br Med J 1977;1:266.
30. Tytgat GNJ, Huibregtse K, Bartelsman JFWM, Den Hartog Jager FCA. Endoscopic palliative therapy of gastrointestinal and biliary tumours with prostheses. Clin Gastroenterol 1986;155:249.
31. Gaspari G, Casalengo PA, Camadona M, et al. Endoscopic insertion of 248 prostheses in inoperable carcinoma of the oesophagus and cardia: short-term and long-term results. Gastrointest Endosc 1987;33:354.
32. Bennett JR. Intubation of gastro-oesophageal malignancies: a survey of current practice in Britain 1980. Gut 1981;22:336.
33. Celestin LR, Etienne J, Raimbert P, Fallouh H, Sultan R. Traitement endoscopiques des stenoses oesophagiennes par prothese de Celestin. Nouvelle Presse Medicale 1980;31:2155.
34. Cusumano A, Ancona E, Simminni A, Pesavento G, Maccari T, Bardini R. Ruolo delle dilatazioni e dell'intubazione con protesi per via endoscopica nel trattamento delle stenosi dell'esofago. Giorn Gastroent End 1978;1:201.
35. Jones BD, Davies PS, Smith PM. Endoscopic insertion of palliative oesophageal tubes in oesophagogastric neoplasms. Br J Surg 1981;68:197.
36. Payne-James JJ, Spiller RC, Misiewicz JJ, Silk DBA. Use of ethanol-induced tumor necrosis to palliate dysphagia in patients with esophagogastric cancer. Gastrointest Endosc 1990;36:43.
37. Spiller RC, Misiewicz JJ. Ethanol-induced tumour necrosis for palliation of malignant dysphagia. Lancet 1987;2:792.
38. Lo NN, Kee SG, Nambiar R. Palliative gastrojejunostomy for advanced carcinoma of the stomach. Ann Acad Med 1991;20:356.
39. Adashek K, Sanger J, Longmire WP Jr. Cancer of the stomach: review of consecutive ten years intervals. Ann Surg 1979;189:6.
40. Vezeridis, MP, Wanebo HJ. Gastric cancer. In: McKenna RJ, Murphy GP, eds. Cancer surgery. Philadelphia: JB Lippincott, 1994:63.

Surgery for Gastrointestinal Cancer: A Multidisciplinary Approach, edited by Harold J. Wanebo.
Lippincott-Raven Publishers, Philadelphia, © 1997.

CHAPTER 30

Radiation and Combined Modality Therapy for Cancer of the Stomach

Stephen R. Smalley and Stephen K. Williamson

RADIATION THERAPY FOR CANCER OF THE STOMACH

Radiation therapy, judiciously administered, has a limited but well-established role in the care of those afflicted with gastric cancer. Most patients who have the potential for receiving benefit from radiation therapy are faced with an extremely poor prognosis overall and are quite compromised with respect to their overall general health. Because patients are facing such significant psychological difficulties and because their health and quality of life are so significantly compromised, both by their disease and by the substantial toxicity of therapy, it is imperative that management of gastric cancer be performed by experienced clinicians who work together to integrate and individualize therapy according to the unique needs of the individual patient and family. Furthermore, the efficacy of radiation therapy is maximized when it is administered in concert with concomitant chemotherapy and expert surgical and general medical care.

RADIATION THERAPY WITH OR WITHOUT CHEMOTHERAPY FOR LOCALLY UNRESECTABLE OR POSTOPERATIVE RESIDUAL DISEASE

Most nonmetastatic gastric cancer can be resected, often with curative intent. Occasionally, however, either the general medical condition of the patient or unusual anatomic aspects of the tumor do not allow a curative resection. Furthermore, it is not unusual for surgical margins to be either frankly positive or compromised on careful histopathologic review of those who are fortunate enough to receive a gross total excision. Table 30-1 summarizes several series that document a 7% to 32% incidence of microscopically positive margins among those undergoing resection.[1–6] Careful assessment of resection margins is an extremely important issue because most of those with positive margins are destined to suffer local failure. The radial or circumferential margins of the surgical specimens are the margins most likely to be microscopically positive and are not routinely evaluated in many pathology departments. This is especially problematic in view of the rising incidence of gastroesophageal carcinoma, which, in most T3,4 primary tumors, has either markedly compromised or microscopically involved radial margins. Therefore, consideration of the management of those with either nonmetastatic but locally unresectable or postoperative residual (positive resection margins) tumors is important because this is not an uncommon problem.

Radiation therapy has the capability of salvaging a small but consistently reproducible percentage of patients who present with locally advanced disease. The results of radiotherapeutic management of locally unresectable or postoperative residual gastric cancer are shown in Table 30-2.[1,7–18] The series tabulated in this table represent a wide variety of radiation therapy techniques and philosophies regarding concomitant chemotherapy, as well as a heterogeneous group of patient subsets. Undoubtedly, this is responsible, in part, for the wide range of 5-year survivals, which range from 0% to 20%. Realistically, with appropriately selected patients, not much more than 5% to 10% will be cured with currently available therapy. Although radiation therapy with or without chemotherapy has substantial toxicity (see discussion later) and only a limited ability to cure, the survivals and cures demonstrated in Table 30-2 establish it as a reasonable therapeutic option for those who are reasonably healthy and willing to accept the expected morbidity of therapy. Nevertheless, these results are far from acceptable, and thoughtfully designed clinical trials are necessary to attempt to improve them.

Several general treatment principles are evident from an evaluation of the radiation therapy literature for locally unresectable gastric cancer; these are discussed in the following sections.

Stephen R. Smalley, Clinical Professor of Radiation Oncology, University of Kansas Medical Center, Therapeutic Radiologists, Inc., 6400 Prospect, Suite 240, Kansas City, MO 64131.

Stephen K. Williamson, Associate Professor of Medicine, University of Kansas Medical Center, 39th and Rainbow Boulevard, Kansas City, KS 66160-7353.

TABLE 30-1. *Microscopic margin positivity in resected gastric specimens*

Authors	No. margin positive/no. resected (%)
Bleiberg, et al[1]	22/111 (20%)
Slot, et al[2]	16/58 (28%)
Gez, et al[3]	7/22 (32%)
Siewert, et al[4]	71/307 (23%)
Gill, et al[5]	1/14 (7%)
Allum, et al[6]	78/436 (18%)

Surgical Debulking

Surgical debulking is associated with consistently improved survival compared with those who receive irradiation for unresected disease.[7,11,19,20] Some of this apparent survival advantage for surgical debulking may simply be a result of selection bias. Certainly, those amenable to subtotal resection may have less tumor burden and more favorable medical conditions than those who are either medically inoperable or who have tumors that are not amenable to resection. However, surgical debulking has been reported to improve tolerance of gastric radiation therapy[21] and has the added advantage of providing palliation of tumor-related obstruction, bleeding, and other problems before the initiation of therapy. Therefore, surgical debulking is likely to both improve the patient's prospect of cure and diminish the toxicity of subsequent radiation therapy with or without chemotherapy. The value of the debulking operation is maximized when it is integrated into the patient's overall management. The multidisciplinary team approach potentially uses this procedure to ensure adequate nutrition during radiation therapy plus chemotherapy (through feeding tube placement), delineate tumor sites (through placement of surgical clips), and relieve pain (through celiac blocks when appropriate).

Concomitant Chemotherapy

The administration of 5-fluorouracil (5-FU) concomitantly with radiation consistently improves both survival and palliation.[1,8,16,22,23] Several prospectively randomized trials have systematically tested the role of concomitant 5-FU. The Mayo Clinic randomized 48 patients with histologically confirmed locally unresectable gastric adenocarcinoma in a phase III study.[23] Patients received 35 to 40 Gy to the tumor nodal area and were randomized in a double-blind fashion to receive either 5-FU (15 mg/kg intravenous bolus; days 1 to 3) or saline placebo on the same schedule. Survival was statistically significantly improved in the 5-FU group ($P < 0.01$). Mean survival was 6 months with saline injections plus radiation therapy versus 13 months with 5-FU plus radiation therapy. Twelve percent of the 5-FU plus radiation therapy group survived 5 years, versus none in the placebo plus radiation therapy group. Bleiberg and colleagues[1] randomized 115 patients with either curative or palliative gastric cancer resections to either radiation therapy alone (55.5 Gy; 1.85 Gy/fraction; 5 days/week; continuously), versus radiation therapy plus concomitant chemotherapy, versus radiation therapy plus postradiation therapy chemotherapy, versus radiation therapy plus concomitant and postradiation ther-

TABLE 30-2. *Radiation therapy with or without chemotherapy for locally unresectable or postoperative residual gastric cancer*

Series	No. of patients	Therapy	Survival 1-Year	Survival 2-Year	Survival 5-Year
Gastrointestinal Tumor Study Group[7]	45	(25 Gy + 5-FU) × 2—break—5-FU + meCCNU	(44%)	(25%)	(20%)
Nordman[8]	19	30–50 Gy (37% with concomitant 5-FU)	10/19 (53%)	5/19 (26%)	NS
Haas, et al[9,10]	11	(FAM + 15 Gy) × 3—break—FAM × 4	9/11 (82%)	1/11 (9%)	1/11 (9%)
Thirlwell, et al[11]	15	46 Gy + 5-FU 500 mg/m² IV q wk—5-FU + meCCNU	7/15 (50%)	5/15 (33%)	NS
Klaasen, et al[12]	26	40 Gy + 5-FU then 5-FU weekly	(37%)	0/26 (0%)	
Asakawa, et al[13]	96	≥50 Gy with concomitant 5-FU	55/96 (57%)	25/96 (26%)	11/96 (11%)
Schein, et al[14]	30	FAM–(22.5 Gy + 5-FU) × 2—FAM × 6	(70%)*	(15%)*	
Mayo Clinic[15,16]	25	35–40 Gy + 5-FU 15 mg/kg d 1–3	(36%)*		3/25 (12%)†
	23	35–40 Gy + saline	(18%)*	0/23	0/23 (0%)†
Abe, et al[17]	14	Intraoperative radiation therapy 20–40 Gy	11/14 (79%)	5/14 (36%)	3/14 (21%)
Wieland and Hymmen[18]	106	60 Gy			5/106 (5%)
Bleiberg, et al[1]	12	55.5 Gy + 5-FU 575 mg/m² IV d 1–4; then 5-FU 750 mg/m² q 2 wk × 18 mo			2/12 (16%)

5-FU, 5-fluorouracil; *meCCNU,* methyl CCNU (semustine); *FAM,* combination chemotherapy consisting of 5-FU, doxorubicin (Adriamycin), and mitomycin-C; *NS,* not stated.
* Estimated from actuarial curves.
† Randomized trial.

apy 5-FU. Among those patients with incompletely resected tumors, all long-term survivors received both concomitant and postradiation therapy chemotherapy. In addition, statistically significant overall survival advantage was observed in those who received 5-FU plus radiation therapy (log rank $P = 0.04$), and this advantage was strongest for those who received postradiation therapy 5-FU as a component of their management. Therefore, all patients who are to receive radiation therapy for locally unresectable or postoperative residual gastric cancer should be considered for concomitant and postoperative 5-FU chemotherapy.

Prognostic Variables

It is well established that a variety of patient and tumor variables are powerfully associated with outcome. Those who have suffered a substantial amount of pretherapy weight loss and those who have poor overall performance status have a much inferior outcome and tolerance of therapy.[12] Female gender may also confer a favorable outcome.[20] As would be anticipated, survival is superior in those with lower tumor stage.[13,17,24] Japanese investigators have called attention to the importance of the Borrmann classification with regard to tumor response, survival, and palliation.[13,19,24,25] Several investigators have noted that those with Borrmann type IV (linnita plastica) disease have an extraordinarily poor outcome with combined radiation therapy plus 5-FU. This clinicopathologic presentation is such a powerful adverse prognostic factor that these patients should be considered almost uniformly incurable. Cardia or gastroesophageal junction adenocarcinomas, which are increasing in incidence, may have different epidemiologic factors and a different tumor biology.[26–28] The overall prognosis of cardia or gastroesophageal lesions is inferior to that in other locations in the stomach.[29,30] The etiology for this inferior prognosis is probably multifactorial but may, in part, relate to the much greater incidence of aneuploidy compared with antral or body primary locations.[31] The next several years will almost certainly see the identification of a cornucopia of molecular biologic and immunohistochemically defined prognostic variables.[31,32] An evaluation of all of these prognostic variables in light of the patient's overall clinical situation will, it is hoped, lead to improvements in both our understanding and management of these patients.

POSTOPERATIVE ADJUVANT RADIATION THERAPY WITH OR WITHOUT CHEMOTHERAPY

There is no documented survival benefit to postoperative radiation therapy with or without chemotherapy, or chemotherapy alone, in margin-negative, completely resected gastric cancer. However, there is a significant amount of interest in exploring combined radiation therapy and chemotherapy in future gastric surgical adjuvant trials. Clearly, the cure rates associated with completely resected gastric cancer leave room for improvement. In patients fortunate enough to have no evidence of metastatic disease but with extension of the primary through the stomach wall, 5-year survival is only approximately 45%.[33,34] Those with lymph node metastasis have only a 15% to 20% cure rate,[33,35] and this already dismal cure rate is further diminished by the increasing number of metastically involved lymph nodes and increasing distance of the lymph nodes from the primary tumor through the bowel wall.[34,35] Furthermore, locoregional failure after complete resection of gastric carcinoma is not at all uncommon. A variety of reports have evaluated the incidence of tumor recurrence in the locoregional area and have consistently reported significant problems with local failure. Pattern-of-failure series are usually determined either by clinical (physical examination, radiographic, and laboratory-based failure determination), reoperation (failure sites determined by laparotomy), or autopsy methodologies. Both reoperative and autopsy series more reliably assess the locoregional area for tumor recurrence, and therefore more accurately delineate the presence of failure at this area. A summary of several pattern-of-failure analyses is shown in Table 30-3 These pattern-of-failure series consistently establish that locoregional failure occurs in 50% or more of patients who have either extension of the primary tumor through the full thickness of the stomach wall or have metastatically involved lymph nodes.[35–40] Furthermore, as depicted in Table 30-3, the tumor bed, regional undissected lymph nodes, and the anastomosis or stump are the most common sites of locoregional failure. Some have concluded that this unsatisfactorily high rate of local failure is a result of inadequate surgical technique, which could be corrected by implementation of more extensive lymph node dissection. A complete discussion of this topic is addressed elsewhere in this textbook. However, it is worth noting insofar as failure patterns are concerned, that the University of Minnesota reoperative series did not demonstrate significant alterations in either failure rates or subsites of failure when aggressive lymph node dissections were performed.[36] Furthermore, a randomized comparison of R1 versus R2 resections in patients with T1–3, N1–2 gastric cancer has been performed. This showed no change in relapse probability at 3 years.[41] Furthermore, evaluation of another randomized trial between R1 and R2 dissection has demonstrated extremely high rates of noncompliance in both Japanese and Western surgeons participating in separate randomized trials.[42] Therefore, there is grounds for considerable skepticism that more extensive lymph node dissection will substantially alter patterns of failure or that definitive evidence of the efficacy of more extensive

TABLE 30-3. *Pattern-of-failure series in resected gastric cancer*

	Failure sites (%)			
Study methodology	Gastric bed	Anastomosis/stump	Node(s)	Abdominal wound
Clinical series[36]	21%	25%	8%	—
Reoperation[35]	54%	26%	42%	5%
Autopsy[37–40]	52–68%	54–60%	52%	—

lymph node dissection will be at hand within the next several years.

Furthermore, surgical series have documented that approximately 20% of all local recurrences are completely resectable at the time of original recurrence, and that perhaps as many as 20% of these patients may be cured with salvage surgery.[43] The demonstration that a significant portion of those who fail only in the locoregional area can be cured with surgical resection, lends credence to the pattern-of-failure analyses, which suggest that 20% to 40% of those who fail will fail only in the locoregional area.[35,36]

In summary, available evidence indicates that locoregional failure is common after resection of high-risk gastric cancer. Indeed, most cases with either extension through the full thickness of the gastric wall or with positive lymph nodes have postoperative subclinical residual disease in the locoregional area. Furthermore, 20% to 40% of these fail only in the locoregional area, and a small but definable proportion of these can be salvaged with surgical reresection. The fact that combined modality therapy can cure some with postoperative residual disease or unresectable tumor makes postoperative adjuvant combined modality therapy a reasonable strategy to use in these high-risk patients. Indeed, the demonstration that combined modality therapy works most effectively when there is minimal residual disease makes this adjuvant strategy even more attractive.

SUMMARY AND CRITIQUE OF ADJUVANT RADIATION THERAPY TRIALS

Several pilot studies have used combined radiation therapy and chemotherapy in high-risk, completely resected gastric cancer. For example, Gunderson and colleagues[21] used postoperative radiation therapy (45 to 52 Gy; 1.8 Gy/d) usually in combination with 5-FU-containing chemotherapy. In this cohort, which was largely composed of modified Astler-Coller B2 to C1–3 stage tumors, there was a 43% overall disease-free survival. Therapy was tolerable and the disease-free survival was somewhat encouraging. Robinson and Cohen used radiation therapy (30 to 40 Gy; 2 Gy/d) and 5-FU in 94 consecutive stage B and C patients.[44] This cohort had a significantly improved survival compared with historical control patients of similar stage who underwent only a surgical resection. Obviously, the lack of a concurrent control group makes interpretation of any of these pilot studies inconclusive. Nevertheless, these and other trials have demonstrated that moderate-dose radiation therapy and concomitant chemotherapy is both tolerable and sufficiently encouraging to warrant a formal phase III evaluation.

There are three flawed, but prospectively randomized, phase III comparisons of radiation therapy with or without chemotherapy. Takahashi and Abe[45] randomized patients to receive either resection alone or resection plus intraoperative radiation therapy (IORT). A single fraction of 28 to 35 Gy was used in those randomized to IORT. The radiation was delivered with a pentagonal treatment cone positioned at the tumor bed and high-risk lymphatic regions, which the authors defined as the left gastric, common hepatic, celiac, and splenic nodal areas. Of note, the residual stomach, intestinal anastomosis, and colon were displaced from the IORT field. The results are shown in Table 30-4. There was no apparent advantage for patients with early (node-negative, nonmuscle-invasive) tumors, of whom most were cured with surgery alone. However, patients with more advanced primary tumors or with involved nodes had an improved survival of approximately 15% to 20% in stages II, III, and IV. This improvement of approximately 20% reflects about the same proportion of patients defined in the pattern-of-failure series who are destined to fail only in the locoregional bed.[35,36] Although the IORT Gastric Surgical Adjuvant Trial is intriguing, patients were randomized on the basis of the day of their hospital admission to receive either surgery alone or IORT. Therefore, this randomization was susceptible to clinical bias affecting treatment selection, and failed to stratify for important prognostic factors between the groups.

TABLE 30-4. *Intraoperative radiation therapy gastric surgical adjuvant trial*

Stage	Treatment	No. of patients	5-Year survival
I	Surgery + IORT	24	87%
	Surgery	43	93%
II	Surgery + IORT	20	84%
	Surgery	11	62%
III	Surgery + IORT	30	62%
	Surgery	38	37%
IV	Surgery + IORT	27	15%
	Surgery	18	0%

IORT, intraoperative radiation therapy.

Modified from Takahashi M, Abe M. Intra-operative radiotherapy for carcinoma of the stomach. Eur J Surg Oncol 1986;12:247.

Moertel and others at the Mayo Clinic also performed a prospectively randomized trial among 62 patients with poor-prognosis, completely resected gastric tumors.[15] Patients were randomized to receive either surgery alone or surgery followed by radiation (37.5 Gy in 4 to 5 weeks) with concomitant 5-FU (15 mg/kg/d for 3 days by intravenous bolus). Sixty-two were entered on study, of whom 39 were randomized to treatment and 23 to observation alone. When analyzed by initial randomization assignment, the 39 randomized to radiation therapy plus 5-FU—regardless of treatment actually received (see discussion later)—had a statistically improved relapse-free and overall survival. However, a prerandomization scheme was used in which only those patients randomized to treatment were asked to provide informed consent. Unfortunately, 10 of the 39 randomized to adjuvant therapy refused randomization and were therefore simply observed. Unexpectedly, the 10 randomized to therapy but refusing to participate in the trial had a 5-year recurrence-free survival of 20%, versus 17% for the 29 randomized to and receiving therapy and 4% for those randomized to observation. Locoregional recurrence was decreased in those who received adjuvant therapy. Locoregional failure occurred in 39% of the 29 randomized to and agreeing to adjuvant therapy, in contrast to 54% of the 33 patients who were untreated either because they were randomized to observation or because they refused therapy. The 15% decrease in locoregional failure is encouraging. Nevertheless, although the survival of those randomized and treated with adjuvant radiation therapy plus 5-FU was clearly superior to those randomized to no additional therapy, the surprisingly good outcome of those randomized but refusing adjuvant therapy complicates interpretation of this trial.

Last, Allum and others have reported a prospective, randomized trial of observation alone versus radiation therapy alone versus chemotherapy in high-risk, completely resected gastric cancer.[6] Patients were stratified by age, duration of symptoms, and stage. A total of 436 were randomized and stratified by treating institution, age, length of symptoms, and stage of disease. Patients were eligible if they had either extension of the tumor through the full thickness of the gastric wall, positive regional lymph nodes, or incompletely resected locoregional disease. Patients with either metastatic or completely unresectable, locally advanced gastric cancer were not eligible. Therefore, 29% had known residual disease, 18% had involvement of the surgical margin, and 14% had only palliative surgical procedures. In this sense, a substantial proportion of these patients were treated for known residual tumors and would not be included in surgical adjuvant trials as usually defined in the United States. Chemotherapy consisted of 5-FU, doxorubicin, and mitomycin-C. Radiation therapy was to consist of 45 Gy in 25 fractions, with or without 5-Gy boost volumes. Minimum follow-up was 1 year. Only 117 of 153 (76%) of those randomized to receive radiation therapy actually received treatment. In addition, only 102 (66% of those randomized) received at least 90% of the protocol-defined dose. Finally, no evaluation of the protocol-defined radiation therapy fields was reported. No survival differences were seen between any of the three groups. Those randomized to radiation therapy manifested only a 15% locoregional failure at the time of first recurrence, as opposed to 39% in those who received surgery alone. The fact that the British study did not deliver concomitant chemotherapy with radiation, included a large proportion of patients with residual gastric cancer who would not ordinarily be eligible for gastric surgical adjuvant as designed in the United States, and had such a large number of radiation therapy protocol violations, makes any interpretation of this trial less than definitive.

In summary, several pilot studies and three methodologically flawed but intriguing phase III trials appear to confirm that adjuvant therapy decreases locoregional failure and can be administered with acceptable, although significant, toxicity. A large, U.S.–Canadian intergroup trial is being conducted that will, it is hoped, definitively establish the role of postoperative combined modality therapy.

ROLE OF RADIATION THERAPY IN THE NEOADJUVANT SETTING

The fact that less than half of those with newly detected gastric cancer are candidates for a potentially curative surgical resection has prompted a number of investigators to explore therapies delivered before resection. This neoadjuvant or protoadjuvant therapy is delivered in an effort to convert surgically unresectable to resectable tumors and to provide some impact on distant, subclinical, micrometastatic disease. Table 30-5 summarizes the resection and locoregional failure rates when neoadjuvant chemotherapy is used for locally unresectable gastric cancer. A review of these trials indicates the importance of patient selection factors, because the resectability rate ranges widely (29% to 38%), as does the curative resection rate (8% to 76%). However, a review of these trials indicates that, overall, neoadjuvant chemotherapy allows potentially curative resection only in approximately half of patients who are deemed healthy and otherwise suitable candidates for such an aggressive and potentially toxic approach. Furthermore, the two series that have reported locoregional failure rates for curative resections after neoadjuvant chemotherapy have observed a consistently high (approximately 74%) rate of failure in the locoregional area (personal communication, R. J. C. Verschueren, MD, University Hospital Groningen, Oostersingel, The Netherlands, 1988).[48,51]

These data indicate that neoadjuvant chemotherapy by itself is a far from entirely satisfactory therapy. The addition of radiation therapy within the context of carefully controlled and monitored clinical trials could be used both to improve resectability rates and to diminish the extremely high rate of locoregional failure after curative resections.

RADIATION THERAPY TOXICITY

Anorexia, nausea, and fatigue are almost ubiquitous problems during gastric radiation therapy. We have a very poor understanding of the pathophysiologic processes by which gastric radiation produces either fatigue or anorexia and nausea and vomiting. Animal models are quite limited and imperfect. Wang and associates[52] performed experiments testing the impact of

TABLE 30-5. *Resection and locoregional failure rates in neoadjuvant trials for locally unresectable gastric cancer*

Authors	No. of patients	No. resected (%)	No. of "curative" resections (%)	No. of LRF after resection (%)
Wilke, et al[46]	27		7/27 (26%)	
Leichman, et al[47]	38	33/38 (87%)	29/38 (76%)	
Wilke, et al[48]	34	10/34 (29%)		9/12 (75%)
Lerner, et al[49]	13	5/13* (38%)	1/13 (8%)	
Ajani, et al[50]†	26	23/26 (88%)	15/26 (58%)	
Verschueren, et al[51]‡	19	7/19 (37%)		5/7 (71%)
Total		78/130 (60%)	52/104 (52%)	14/19 (74%)

* Four of five resections were incomplete.

† Gastroesophageal or esophageal adenocarcinomas.

‡ Additional data according to R.J.C. Verschueren, MD, University Hospital Groningen, Oostersingel, The Netherlands (personal communication, 1988).

LRF, locoregional failure.

chemoreceptor trigger zone ablation, abdominal vagotomy, and abdominal sympathectomy on radiation therapy-induced emesis. Chemoreceptor trigger zone ablation eliminated emesis, whereas visceral deafferentation delayed but did not prevent it. Therefore, although it is possible that visceral afferents may play some role in the acute emetogenic effects of radiation therapy, other factors, potentially chemical in nature and mediated by the chemoreceptor trigger zone, may be more important. In addition, radiation therapy can alter gastric motility and prolong gastric emptying, which could certainly accentuate the anorexia, early satiety, and nausea associated with radiation therapy.[53]

The nutritional and gastrointestinal complications of gastric radiation therapy require careful support and multidisciplinary management. The importance of nutritional complications is emphasized by the Gastrointestinal Tumor Study Group experience,[7] in which a minimum 13% treatment-related mortality accrued from either nutritional or septic (usually neutropenic) events. Caudry and colleagues[20] observed that nutritional complications prevented almost 20% of patients from completing planned radiation therapy for gastric cancer. Others have reported no severe or life-threatening nutritional compromise.[11,14,21]

Clearly, it is imperative that gastrointestinal complications be managed aggressively and proactively. Patients who are treated after gastrectomy may have an improved tolerance of gastric irradiation. If patients are being treated postoperatively for residual tumor, it is helpful if the surgeon can place clips during surgery to allow the postoperative radiation therapy to be more precisely focused. Careful treatment planning and judicious use of beam blocking also minimize the integral volume of normal tissue irradiated. If surgeons discover factors during surgery that may warrant postoperative therapy, placement of feeding jejunostomy tubes markedly facilitates nutritional care of patients during radiation therapy. Finally, it is the authors' clinical practice prophylactically to administer antiemetic therapy before radiation therapy in all patients receiving upper abdominal treatment. 5-Hydroxytryptamine receptor (5-HT_3) blockers are more likely to be effective than are other, more traditional antiemetics such as prochlorperazine or metoclopramide. 5-HT_3 blockers are much more expensive than other antiemetics and there is no clear demonstration of the efficacy of antiemetic therapy in this context. Myelosuppression resulting in serious and, rarely, lethal toxicity is also reported in many of the combined modality trials.[9,11,12,14,21] Radiation therapy alone would produce some myelosuppression, but only rarely of a clinically significant nature. When standard doses of 5-FU are used with radiation for gastric cancer, serious problems with sepsis or bleeding should be uncommon if blood counts are monitored twice weekly.[9,11,21]

Late effects consist of either gastritis, uncomplicated gastric ulcers, or ulcers complicated by perforation or obstruction.[53] Using modern radiation therapy machines and techniques and daily dose fractions of 1.8 to 2.0 Gy/d, severe late effects should be uncommon in doses of 40 to 45 Gy or less. Chiefly, doses in this range may produce gastritis, which usually responds to medical therapy. However, doses of 45 to 50 Gy may produce a 5% to 10% incidence of late gastric effects, whereas doses of 55 to 60 Gy or more carry a 10% to 15% risk of chronic toxicity.[20,54] It is the authors' practice prophylactically to administer histamine receptor (H_2) blockers to all patients prophylactically when 40 Gy or more will be administered to any significant volume of stomach or proximal duodenum. The impact of either H_2 blockers or sucralfate therapy prophylactically on late gastric complications is unknown.

PALLIATIVE ROLE OF RADIATION THERAPY

Radiation therapy can provide considerable relief of local gastric cancer symptoms. Problems such as obstruction, bleeding, and pain all can respond to palliative radiation therapy. Approximately 50% to 75% of patients have had symptomatic improvement of these problems in a variety of trials.[8,22,55–57] Palliation may be improved by concomitant 5-FU administration,[8,22,53,57] and when patients have satisfactory overall general health and performance scores as well as a relatively small tumor bulk.[53] The duration of palliation is variable but ranges from 4 to 18 months.[8,22,55,57] Given the rising incidence of gastroesophageal junction tumors and the use of laser palliation, it is important to note that most who are palliated by laser therapy will suffer recurrence of symptoms within a few weeks of treatment.[58] Pilot data[58] and a randomized trial[59] clearly document the value of radiation therapy in significantly prolonging the duration of palliation after laser therapy.

REFERENCES

1. Bleiberg H, Goffin JC, Dalesio O, et al. Adjuvant radiotherapy and chemotherapy in resectable gastric cancer. Eur J Surg Oncol 1989;15:535.
2. Slot A, Meerwaldt JH, van Putten WLJ, Treurniet-Donker AD. Adjuvant postoperative radiotherapy for gastric carcinoma with poor prognostic signs. Radiother Oncol 1989;16:269.
3. Gez E, Sulkes A, Yablonsky-Peretz T, Weshler Z. Combined 5-fluorouracil (5-FU) and radiation therapy following resection of locally advanced gastric carcinoma. J Surg Oncol 1986;31:139.
4. Siewert JR, Lange J, Bottcher K, Holscher M, Weiser HF, Gossner W. Stomach cancer: the current situation from the surgical viewpoint. Dtsch Med Wochenschr 1987;112:622.
5. Gill PG, Jamieson GG, Denham J, et al. Treatment of adenocarcinoma of the cardia with synchronous chemotherapy and radiotherapy. Br J Surg 1990;77:1020.
6. Allum WH, Hallissey MT, Ward LC, Hockey MS. A controlled, prospective, randomised trial of adjuvant chemotherapy or radiotherapy in resectable gastric cancer: interim report. Br J Cancer 1989;60:739.
7. Gastrointestinal Tumor Study Group (GITSG). A comparison of combination chemotherapy and combined modality therapy for locally advanced gastric carcinoma. Cancer 1982;49:1771.
8. Nordman E. Value of megavolt therapy in gastric carcinoma. Bull Cancer 1976;63:217.
9. Haas CD, Mansfield CM, Leichman LP, et al. Combined nonsimultaneous radiation therapy and chemotherapy with 5-FU, doxorubicin, and mitomycin for residual localized gastric adenocarcinoma: a Southwest Oncology Group Pilot Study. Cancer Treat Rep 1983;67:421.
10. Haas L, Vaitkevicius V, Bukowski R, et al. Southwest Oncology Group (SWOG) pilot study of radiotherapy (R) + 5-fluorouracil (F) + Adriamycin (A) + mitomycin C (M) in patients with minimal residual gastric cancer. Proceedings of the American Society of Clinical Oncologists 1980;21:342.
11. Thirlwell MP, Keable HE, Kost K, et al. Combination of 5-fluorouracil (5-FU) plus semustine (MECCNU) with and without radiotherapy (RT) in advanced gastric and pancreatic carcinoma. Proceedings of the American Society of Clinical Oncologists 1981;22:449.
12. Klaassen DJ, MacIntyre JM, Catton GE, et al. Treatment of locally unresectable cancer of the stomach and pancreas: a randomized comparison of 5-fluorouracil alone with radiation plus concurrent and maintenance 5-fluorouracil. An Eastern Cooperative Oncology Group Study. J Clin Oncol 1985;3:373.
13. Asakawa H, Otawa H, Yamada S, Matsumoto K. Combination therapy

of gastric carcinoma with radiation and chemotherapy. Tohoku J Exp Med 1982;137:445.
14. Schein PS, Smith FP, Dritschillo A, et al. Phase I–II trial of combined modality FAM plus split-course radiation (FAM-RT-FAM) for locally advanced gastric and pancreatic cancer: a Mid-Atlantic Oncology Program study [abstract]. Proceedings of the American Society of Clinical Oncologists 1983;2:126.
15. Moertel CG, Childs DS, O'Fallon JR, et al. Combined 5-fluorouracil and radiation therapy as a surgical adjuvant for poor prognosis gastric carcinoma. J Clin Oncol 1984;2:1249.
16. Holbrook MA. Radiation therapy. Current concepts in cancer. Gastric cancer: treatment principles. JAMA 1974;228:1289.
17. Abe M, Takahashi M, Yabumoto E, et al. Clinical experiences with intraoperative radiotherapy of locally cancers. Cancer 1980;45:40.
18. Wieland C, Hymmen U. Megavoltage therapy for malignant gastric tumors. Strahlentherapie 1972;40:20.
19. Asakawa H, Takeda T. High energy x-ray therapy of gastric carcinoma. Journal of the Japanese Society of Cancer Therapy 1973;8:362.
20. Caudry M, Escarmant P, Maire JP, et al. Radiotherapy of gastric cancer with a three field combination: feasibility, tolerance and survival. Int J Radiat Oncol Biol Phys 1987;13:1821.
21. Gunderson LL, Hoskins B, Cohen AM, et al. Combined modality treatment of gastric cancer. Int J Radiat Oncol Biol Phys 1983;9:965.
22. Falkson G. Halogenated pyrimidines as radiopotentiators in the treatment of stomach cancer. Prog Biochem Pharmacol 1965;1:695.
23. Moertel CG, Childs DS Jr, Reitemeier RJ, et al. Combined 5-fluorouracil and supervoltage radiation therapy of locally unresectable gastrointestinal cancer. Lancet 1969;2:865.
24. Dent DM, Werner ID, Novis B, et al. Prospective randomized trial of combined oncological therapy for gastric carcinoma. Cancer 1979;44:385.
25. Tsukiyama I, Akine Y, Kajiura Y, Ogino T, Yamashita K, Egawa S. Radiation therapy for advanced gastric cancer. Int J Radiat Oncol Biol Phys 1988;15:123.
26. MacDonald WC, MacDonald JB. Adenocarcinoma of the esophagus and/or gastric cardia. Cancer 1987;60:1094.
27. Meyers WC, Damiano RJ, Postlethwait RW, Rotolo FS. Adenocarcinoma of the stomach: changing patterns over the last 4 decades. Ann Surg 1987;205:1.
28. Yamada Y, Kato Y. Greater tendency for submucosal invasion in fundic area gastric carcinomas than those arising in the pyloric area. Cancer 1989;63:1757.
29. Fein R, Kelsen DP, Geller N, et al. Adenocarcinoma of the esophagus and gastroesophageal junction: prognostic factors and results of therapy. Cancer 1985;56:2512.
30. Hartley LC, Evans E, Windsor CJ. Factors influencing prognosis in gastric cancer. Aust N Z J Surg 1987;57:5.
31. Nanus DM, Kelsen DP, Niedzwiecki D, et al. Flow cytometry as a predictive indicator in patients with operable gastric cancer. J Clin Oncol 1989;7:1105.
32. Sugiyama K, Yonemura Y, Miyazaki I. Immunohistochemical study of epidermal growth factor and epidermal growth factor receptor in gastric carcinoma. Cancer 1989;63:1557.
33. Dockerty MB. Pathologic aspects of primary malignant neoplasms of the stomach. In: ReMine WH, Priestley JT, Berkson J, eds. Cancer of the stomach. Philadelphia: WB Saunders, 1964:173.
34. Kennedy BJ. TNM classification for stomach cancer. Cancer 1970;26:971.
35. Gunderson LL, Sosin H. Adenocarcinoma of the stomach: areas of failure in a reoperation series (second or symptomatic looks): clinicopathologic correlation and implications for adjuvant therapy. Int J Radiat Oncol Biol Phys 1982;8:1.
36. Landry J, Tepper JE, Wood WC, Moulton EO, Koerner F, Sullinger J. Patterns of failure following curative resection of gastric carcinoma. Int J Radiat Oncol Biol Phys 1990;19:1357.
37. Horn RC. Carcinoma of the stomach: autopsy findings in untreated cases. Gastroenterology 1955;29:515.
38. McNeer G, Vandenberg H, Donn FY, et al. A critical evaluation of subtotal gastrectomy for the cure of cancer of the stomach. Ann Surg 1957;134:2.
39. Stout AP. Pathology of carcinoma of the stomach. Arch Surg 1943;46:807.
40. Thomson FB, Robins RE. Local recurrence following subtotal resection for gastric carcinoma. Surg Gynecol Obstet 1952;95:341.
41. Dent DM, Madden MV, Price SK. Randomized comparison of R1 and R2 gastrectomy for gastric carcinoma. Br J Surg 1988;75:110.
42. Bunt AMG, Hermans J, Boon MC, et al. Evaluation of the extent of lymphadenectomy in a randomized trial of Western- versus Japanese-type surgery in gastric cancer. J Clin Oncol 1994;12:417.
43. Douglass HO Jr. Potentially curable cancer of the stomach. Cancer 1982;50:2582.
44. Robinson E, Cohen Y. The combination of surgery, radiotherapy and chemotherapy in the treatment of gastric cancer. Recent Results Cancer Res 1977;32:177.
45. Takahashi M, Abe M. Intra-operative radiotherapy for carcinoma of the stomach. Eur J Surg Oncol 1986;12:247.
46. Wilke H, Preusser P, Fink U, et al. Neoadjuvant chemotherapy with etoposide/adriamycin/cisplatin (EAP) in locally advanced gastric cancer [abstract]. Proceedings of the American Society of Clinical Oncologists 1988;7:100.
47. Leichman L, Silberman H, Leichman CG, et al. Preoperative systemic chemotherapy followed by adjuvant postoperative intraperitoneal therapy for gastric cancer: a University of Southern California pilot program. J Clin Oncol 1992;10:1933.
48. Wilke H, Preusser P, Fink U, et al. Preoperative chemotherapy in locally advanced and nonresectable gastric cancer: a phase II study with etoposide, doxorubicin, and cisplatin. J Clin Oncol 1989;7:1318.
49. Lerner A, Gonin R, Steele GD Jr, Mayer RJ. Etoposide, doxorubicin, and cisplatin chemotherapy for advanced gastric adenocarcinoma: results of a phase II trial. J Clin Oncol 1992;10:536.
50. Ajani JA, Roth JA, Ryan B, et al. Intensive preoperative chemotherapy with colony-stimulating factor for resectable adenocarcinoma of the esophagus or gastroesophageal junction. J Clin Oncol 1993;11:22.
51. Verschueren RJC, Willemse PHB, Sleijfer DT, de Vries EGE, Mulder NH. Combined chemotherapeutic–surgical approach of locally advanced gastric cancer [abstract]. Proceedings of the American Society of Clinical Oncologists 1988;7:93.
52. Wang S, Renzi A, Chinn H. Mechanism of emesis following x-irradiation. Am J Physiol 1958;193:335.
53. Smalley SR, Evans RG. Radiation morbidity to the gastrointestinal tract and liver. In: Plowman P, McElwain TJ, Meadows AT, eds. The complications of cancer management. London: Butterworth, 1989.
54. Nelson J, Boyce J, Macasaet M, et al. Incidence, significance, and follow-up of para-aortic lymph node metastases in late invasive carcinoma of the cervix. Am J Obstet Gynecol 1977;128:336.
55. Mantell BS. Radiotherapy for dysphagia due to gastric carcinoma. Br J Surg 1982;69:69.
56. Henderson IWD, Lipowska B, Lougheed MN. Clinical evaluation of combined radiation and chemotherapy in gastrointestinal malignancies. AJR 1968;102:545.
57. Falkson G, Van Eden EB, Sandison AG. A controlled clinical trial of fluorouracil plus imidazole carboxamide dimethyl triazeno plus vincristine plus bis-chloroethyl nitrosourea plus radiotherapy in stomach cancer. Med Pediatr Oncol 1976;2:111.
58. Sargeant IR, Loizou LA, Tobias JS, Blackman G, Thorpe S, Brown WG. Radiation enhancement of laser palliation for malignant dysphagia: a pilot study. Gut 1992;33:1597.
59. Sander R, Hagenmueller F, Sander C, Riess G, Classen M. Laser versus laser plus afterloading with iridium-192 in the palliative treatment of malignant stenosis of the esophagus: a prospective, randomized, and controlled study. Gastrointest Endosc 1991;37:433.

Surgery for Gastrointestinal Cancer: A Multidisciplinary Approach, edited by Harold J. Wanebo.
Lippincott-Raven Publishers, Philadelphia, © 1997.

CHAPTER 31

Gastric Lymphoma

Isha A. Mustafa, Jeffrey Clark, Jila Khorsand, and Harold J. Wanebo

The gastrointestinal tract is the most common site of extranodal non-Hodgkin's lymphomas, accounting for approximately 40% of all extranodal lymphoma.[1] Although most malignant lymphomas of the gastrointestinal tract involve the stomach, this is usually associated with disease either elsewhere in the gastrointestinal tract or secondary to primary nodal lymphoma. The stomach is the most common site of primary gastrointestinal lymphomas, yet these account for less than 5% of all gastric neoplasms.[2] A near doubling in the incidence of primary gastric lymphoma since the early 1980s has been reported; however, this may simply represent improvement in diagnosis and changes in the definition of primary gastric lymphoma. In addition, there does appear to be an increasing number of patients with acquired immunodeficiency syndrome (AIDS)-associated gastrointestinal lymphomas, but this represents only a small percentage of the overall increase in the incidence of gastrointestinal lymphoma.[4]

The rare nature of this tumor is represented by continuing controversy over its optimal treatment. The treatment of early-stage gastric lymphoma, preoperative workup, intraoperative diagnosis, and the extent of resection, as well as postoperative adjuvant therapy, are still subjects of debate. We explore these issues in this chapter.

POSSIBLE ETIOLOGIC FACTORS

The risk for development of a gastric lymphoma does not appear to be related to the limited amount of lymphoid tissue normally present in the stomach. A possible association of atrophic gastritis, especially that associated with *Helicobacter pylori* infection and autoimmune or immune deficiency states (including human immunodeficiency virus-seropositive individuals with AIDS), with gastric lymphomas has been reported, but no causal relationship has been established.[5–10] The possible relationship between infection with *H pylori* and gastric lymphoma is addressed in more detail latter in the chapter. Although gastric lymphomas are occasionally seen in patients with other diseases or malignancies, there is no clear etiologic association with these other disease states. Familial occurrences of gastric lymphoma have been rarely reported, so that genetic factors that enhance the risk for development of gastric lymphoma may be involved in rare instances.[11]

CLINICAL FEATURES

In 1961, Dawson and colleagues defined primary gastric lymphoma as a gastric lesion without palpable superficial lymphadenopathy on initial presentation, no mediastinal lymph node involvement on chest radiography, white blood cell count and differential counts within normal limits, a predominant gastric lesion with only adjacent lymph nodes obviously affected on laparotomy, and no tumor in the spleen or the liver.[12]

The median age at diagnosis is between 54 and 60 years, with a slight male predominance (male-to-female ratio of approximately 1.5 overall, although this varies from less than 1 to approximately 3 in various studies). Patients with low-grade lymphomas tend to be younger than those with high-grade lesions.

Presenting symptoms are usually vague. There are no distinguishing clinical features that differentiate gastric lymphoma from other gastric neoplasms or even benign peptic ulcer disease. Symptoms are insidious and include anorexia, early satiety, weight loss and fatigue. B symptoms such as fever and night sweats occur in less than 10% of patients. Most present with pain mimicking peptic ulcer disease. The pain is epigastric and often relieved with the administration of H_2 antagonists, thus often precluding further workup and resulting in delay of diagnosis. Approximately half of patients who present for evaluation have an epigastric mass. Obstruction and perforation are uncommon but have been reported to occur, though certainly less frequently than in patients with gastric carcinoma. Gross hemorrhage is uncommon in primary gastric lymphomas, however 50% of patients experience occult blood loss, with resultant anemia in about half of these patients.

Isha A. Mustafa, Fellow, Division of Surgical Oncology, Brown University, Providence, RI.

Jeffrey Clark, Division of Medical Oncology, Department of Medicine, Harvard Medical School, M6 Hospital, Boston, MA.

Jila Khorsand, Department of Pathology, Brown University and Roger Williams Medical Center, Providence, RI.

Harold J. Wanebo, Director, Division of Surgical Oncology, Brown University, Surgeon in Chief, Roger Williams Medical Center, Providence, RI.

RADIOLOGIC IMAGING

Barium study of the upper gastrointestinal tract is useful although not diagnostic. Most patients with primary gastric lymphoma show some abnormality when studied after a barium meal. Some have changes resembling peptic ulceration, whereas others may have a mass effect suggestive of carcinoma. Still others may have nonspecific finding such as thickened rugal folds.

Computed tomography (CT) scan may be used to assess the extent of disease and can be helpful in preoperative staging of those patients who have no obvious adenopathy on physical examination. Because of the difficulty in analyzing regional gastric nodes by CT scan, some authors have found a significant rate of false-negative studies when patients were staged with preoperative CT scan, resulting in pathologic upstaging of the disease after resection.[13]

Endoscopic ultrasound has been used to evaluate the extent of invasion of the gastric wall and involvement of regional lymph nodes,[14] and has been shown to be more accurate than endoscopy, radiologic evaluation by CT scan, or barium studies in both detecting and staging gastric lymphoma. Endoscopic ultrasonography has a sensitivity between 83% and 87% with a specificity of 97%, and a positive predictive value between 83% and 87%.[15,16] Bolondi and colleagues described three distinct endosonographic patterns of gastric lymphoma.[17] The first is a polypoid pattern with protrusions into the gastric lumen; second, localized hypoechoic infiltration; and third, diffuse, extended, or longitudinal hypoechoic infiltration of the gastric wall. Pathognomonic for the diagnosis of gastric lymphoma was localized mucosal ulceration with extended infiltration of the second and third layers. A later study by Suekane and coworkers described four distinct patterns that correlated with histologic types.[18] These were categorized as follows: mass-forming, superficially spreading, diffusely infiltrating, and mixed. In addition to diagnosing and staging disease, endoscopic ultrasound has also been used to follow patients treated with radiation or chemotherapy.

Transabdominal ultrasound has not proved to be practical in either diagnosing gastric lymphoma or determining the extent of intraabdominal disease after the diagnosis has been made by other means.

ENDOSCOPIC EVALUATION

The endoscopic appearance of gastric lymphoma is greatly variable and includes tumorous and polypoid changes, polypoid mucosal folds either with or without ulceration, ulcers, and gastritis. Non-Hodgkin's lymphoma involving the gastrointestinal tract may be more common than is usually diagnosed,[19] but studies have not shown any benefit to performing routine endoscopy simply to rule out gastrointestinal involvement when the diagnosis can be made based on disease either in the lymph nodes themselves, or in other extranodal sites such as the bone marrow. There has been no evidence to demonstrate a change in therapy in a significant number of patients to warrant endoscopy as a routine method for either diagnosing or staging secondary gastrointestinal lymphoma.

With regard to primary gastric lymphoma, biopsy provides a positive tissue diagnosis in 60% to 80% of cases when endoscopy has been performed for gastrointestinal symptoms. Because of the tendency for submucosal infiltration, the biopsy should include the submucosa of the gastric wall. Cytologic analysis is not useful, with an overall sensitivity of less than 50%.[20]

The effectiveness of endoscopy in staging is limited in gastric lymphoma because the size of the tumor is often underestimated due to the submucosal nature of this disease. In addition, endoscopy cannot be used to determine the depth of invasion or obtain information regarding nodal status or the extent of distant disease. Hence, endoscopy should be used as part of the workup of gastrointestinal symptoms but should not be used to stage the disease.

PATHOLOGY

On gross inspection, lesions may resemble diffuse gastritis, localized ulcers, or polypoid tumors. The gastric antrum and prepyloric region are the mostly commonly involved sites (20% to 60%) for primary gastric lymphoma. The body is involved 15% to 40% of the time, whereas the fundus is involved in only 1% to 15% of cases.[21,22,23–25] Twenty-five to 50% are ulcerative, 25% to 40% polypoid–exophytic, and 25% to 40% linitis-like. The median size of these lymphomas is approximately 6 to 7 cm in diameter at the time of diagnosis.[21,22,25]

The quality of local gastrointestinal immune response is believed to be determined by the selective migration through post-capillary high endothelium of lymphocytes into precise areas such as Peyer's patches. In the murine model, cell adhesion molecules present on endothelial cells of the venules within these specific sites have been shown to play a role in the lymphocyte homing process.[26] How these mechanisms function in the stomach and what initiates the accumulation of lymphoid tissue within the stomach that leads to the development of primary gastric lymphoma is unclear.

Gastric lymphomas are characterized by various histologic features such as cytologic type, grade, and immunophenotype (B cell vs. T cell). These characterizations have been modified over the years to reflect the increased understanding of gastrointestinal immunology and associated lymphoid tissue, as well as improved diagnostic techniques differentiating one type of lymphoma and cell line from others. Most (>90%) primary gastric lymphomas are non-Hodgkin's B-cell lymphomas that include low-grade B-cell lymphoma of mucosa associated lymphoid tissue (MALT) and high-grade B-cell lymphoma.[22,27–29]

The term "pseudolymphoma" was used in the past to describe lesions with a prolonged clinical course and histomorphologic features suggesting a reactive process. Brooks and Enterline described them as mass lesions of the stomach composed of small lymphocytes with a low mitotic index, lacking atypia of the germinal centers, and usually without associated nodal involvement.[30,31] These may represent slow-growing or very low-grade lymphomas that progress to aggressive disease over time. With the remarkable advances in immunology and molecular biology, and applicability of newly developed techniques in routine surgical pathology, lymphoid infiltrates in-

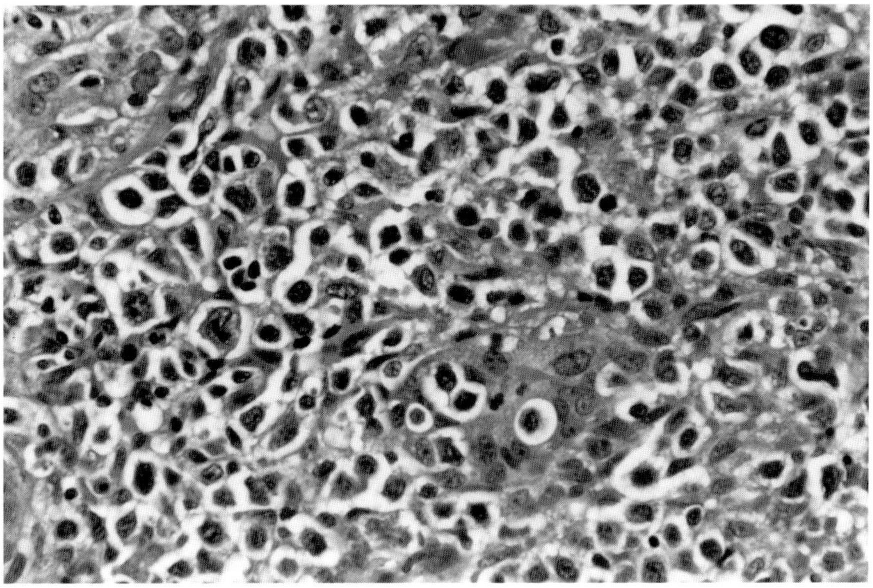

FIG. 31-1. Mucosa-associated lymphoid tissue lymphoma with monocytoid B-cell areas. Neoplastic lymphocytes display monocytoid features with abundant clear cytoplasm. (Original magnification ×400)

volving the stomach are diagnosed with greater accuracy today, making the term "pseudolymphoma" nearly archaic.

In the early to middle 1980s, Isaacson and colleagues introduced the concept of MALT,[32,33] and suggested that gastrointestinal lymphomas are unlike their nodal counterparts in origin and mode of dissemination, with a tendency to remain localized for long periods of time. Because of the unique clinical and pathologic characteristics that separate MALT lymphomas from other extranodal lymphomas, they are difficult to classify using the Working Formulation (see Table 31-2) and therefore are usually described using the updated Kiel classification (see Table 31-3).

Morphologically, low-grade MALT lymphoma is characterized by the presence of large, nonneoplastic lymphoid follicles and a dense neoplastic lymphoid infiltrate in a perifollicular location. These lymphocytes are of small to medium size, with abundant cytoplasm and irregular nuclei that Isaacson named centrocyte-like (CCL) cells. The CCL cells at times reveal abundant clear cytoplasm resembling monocytoid B lymphocytes (Fig. 31-1). A significant morphologic feature of low-grade MALT lymphoma is the lymphoepithelial lesion, characterized by clusters of atypical CCL cells infiltrating the mucosal structures (Fig. 31-2). Presence of lymphoepithelial lesion in gastric biopsies with dense, atypical lymphoid infiltrate is highly suggestive of low-grade MALT lymphoma.

Zukerberg and colleagues were able to establish histologic criteria associated only with lymphomas and not present in benign inflammatory lesions. This is important because it is often difficult to discern between benign inflammatory infiltrates and early lymphoma, especially with endoscopic biopsy specimens.[34] The histologic features Zukerberg and colleagues found to be associated only with lymphoma were prominent lymphoepithelial lesions, Dutcher bodies (prominent intranuclear pseudoinclusions that are periodic acid–Schiff positive or immunoglobulin positive with immunostaining),[35] and moderate cytologic atypia. Features present in both lymphomas and benign inflammatory infiltrates are dense lymphoid infiltrates, rare or questionable lymphoepithelial lesions, ulceration, muscularis mucosa invasion, and mild cytologic atypia. Immunohis-

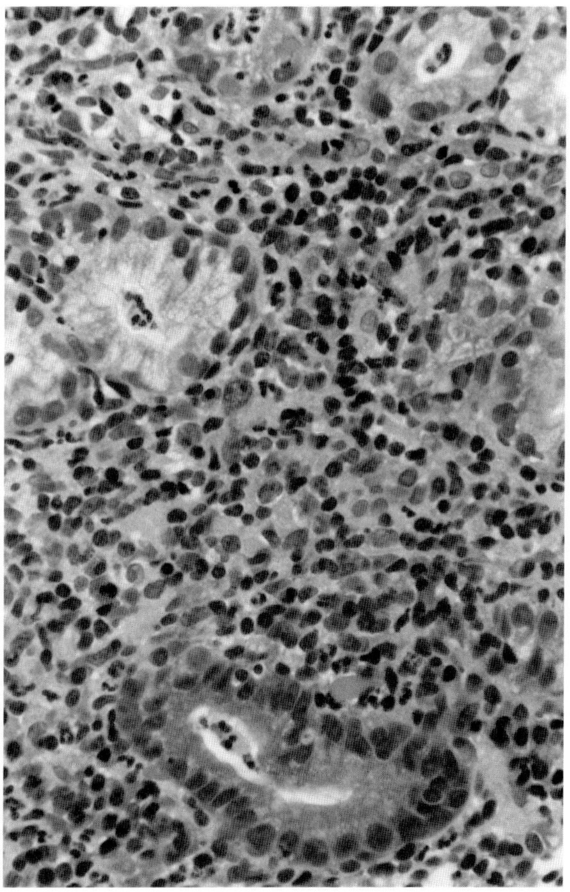

FIG. 31-2. Low-grade mucosa-associated lymphoid tissue lymphoma. Dense lymphoid infiltrate composed of small lymphocytes with irregular nuclei. (Original magnification ×400.)

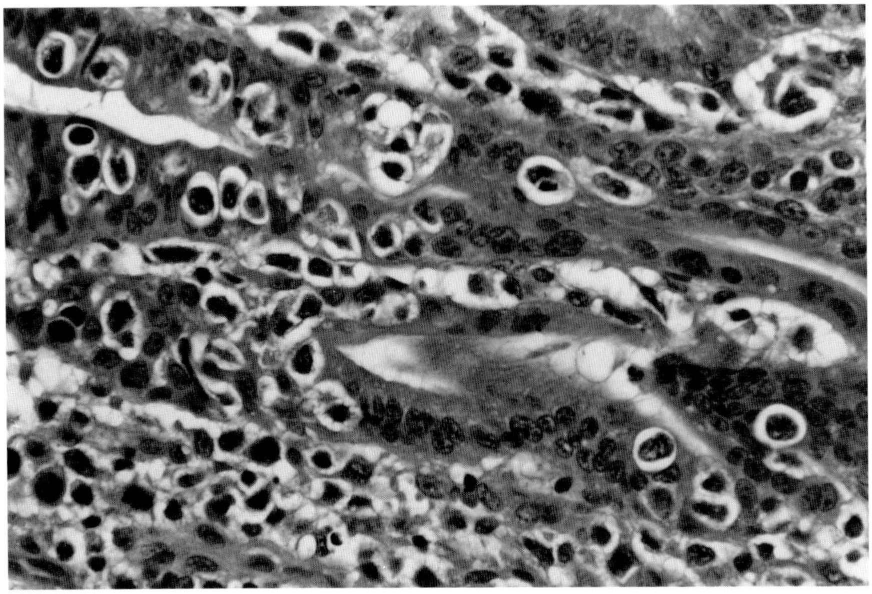

FIG. 31-3. Lymphoepithelial lesion. Neoplastic lymphocytes infiltrating gastric glands. (Original magnification ×400.)

tologic features include monotypic immunoglobulin staining (either IgMλ or IgMκ) but polytypic germinal centers. In addition, most express the pan-B-cell marker CD20.

The lymphoepithelial lesion described as part of MALT show great variability in the extent of epithelial destruction. In some, the lumen of the gastric glands is intact (Fig. 31-3). In others, there are many intraepithelial CCL cells with marked destruction of the normal glandular architecture. The cytoplasm of these epithelial cells also changes and becomes eosinophilic in appearance and larger, with a more central nucleus. In others there are no identifiable glandular structures. Eosinophilic epithelial cells are present within the diffuse lymphoma (Fig. 31-4). This may represent the end stage of the lymphoepithelial lesion, demonstrating total destruction of the gastric glands by neoplastic cells.[36] Papadaki and Isaacson postulated that the close association of the neoplastic CCL cells and epithelial cells suggests the presence of either an antigen or receptor on the plasma membrane of the epithelial cell through which the effects are mediated. This is yet to be proven. The same authors state that MALT lymphomas represent the neoplastic equivalent of the normal lymphocyte–epithelial cell interaction and that progression occurs along one of two lines: 1) cytoplasmic organelles remain intact although the epithelial cells become distorted and separate from surrounding cells because of the CCL cells; these cells then lose orientation and cease to have controlled function; 2) swelling of the cellular compartments and disintegration of plasma membranes results in loss of organelles, leaving only partially membrane-bound cytoplasmic ground substance. This may account for the observation of eosinophilic cytoplasm.

Genomic studies, as well as histologic studies of MALT lymphoma, point to these tumors being distinct from their nodal

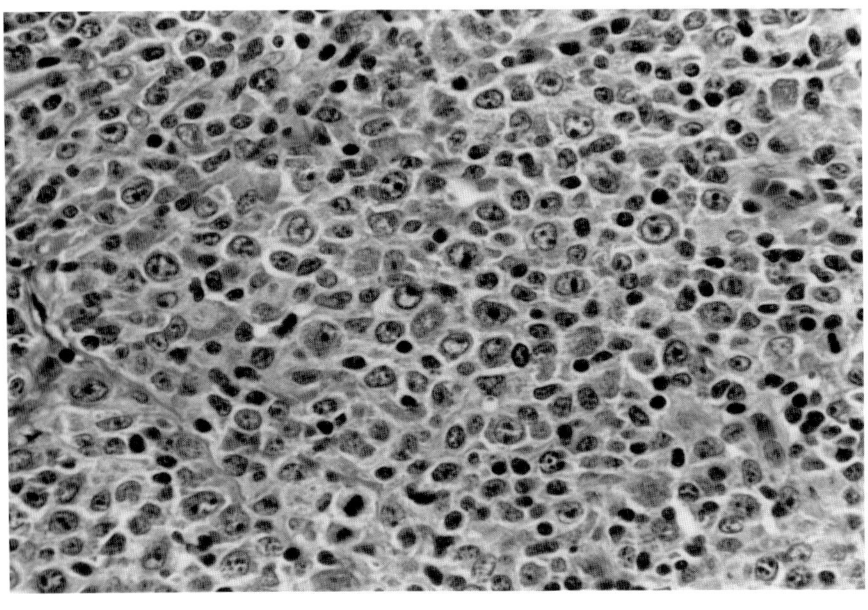

FIG. 31-4. High-grade mucosa-asociated lymphoid tissue lymphoma. Large neoplastic lymphoid cells with vesicular nuclei and prominent nucleoli. (Original magnification ×400.)

counterparts. *myc* rearrangements, associated with Burkitt's lymphoma, have not been demonstrated in MALT lymphomas. Similarly *BCL2* gene rearrangement, which is frequent in centroblastic/centrocytic lymphoma, and *BCL1* rearrangement associated with several types of node-based lymphomas, have not been detected in MALT lymphomas.[37]

HELICOBACTER PYLORI AND GASTRIC LYMPHOMA

Half of the world's population is infected with *H pylori,* yet it was not until 1983 when Warren and Marshall discovered this spiral urease-producing organism in the human stomach.[38] There have been causal relationships drawn between the presence of *H pylori* and the subsequent development of peptic ulcer disease and gastric carcinoma. The EUROGAST study found a sixfold increased risk of gastric cancer in populations infected with *H pylori* compared to those not infected.[39] An attempt has been made to establish a relation between *H pylori*-induced chronic gastritis and the subsequent development of gastric lymphoma.

As stated earlier, the normal stomach does not contain lymphoid tissue. Organized mucosa-associated lymphoid follicles are acquired in the stomach in association with infection by *H pylori.*[40,41] *H pylori* infection has been demonstrated in 92% of patients with gastric MALT lymphoma, compared with a 50% to 60% infection rate in the population at large.[42] This is comparable to percentages of *H pylori* infection in peptic ulcer disease and gastric carcinoma, where the organism has been implicated as a causative factor. The mechanism of this is postulated to be similar to the acquisition of MALT in other sites such as the thyroid and salivary glands due to the inflammatory autoimmune disorders, Hashimoto's thyroiditis and Sjögren's syndrome.[43,44] Based on this theory, the development of lymphoma begins with infection by *H pylori,* which leads to chronic antral gastritis. This results in intestinal metaplasia and accumulation of organized lymphoid follicles, followed by dysplasia and finally the development of carcinoma or lymphoma. Hussel and coworkers showed that gastric MALT lymphoma could be stimulated in vitro to proliferate in the presence of a specific strain of *H pylori.*[45] This is a T-cell–dependent and IL-2 effect of the B lymphocytes. Despite these arguments, no proven clonal progression has been demonstrated from *H pylori*-induced chronic gastritis and the formation of primary gastric non-Hodgkin's lymphoma. It has been proposed that *H pylori* infection is merely a promoter and that other factors must exist for MALT lymphoma to develop. This suggests that *H pylori* may be a necessary factor but not sufficient to be a singular cause of gastric lymphoma. Data from Africa and India, where *H pylori* infection is nearly 100% but the incidence of peptic ulcer disease and gastric cancer is low, seem to support this hypothesis.[46,47]

Whether *H pylori* is a causative factor or a promoter of the growth of primary gastric lymphoma is not clear. There are many reports of cases in which eradication of infection leads to either cure or regression of MALT lymphoma. This may prove to have significant implications for the treatment of low-grade primary gastric lymphoma, because therapy with bismuth, omeprazole, amoxicillin, and metronidazole is certainly better tolerated than either chemotherapy or surgery. However, because there is an incidence of recurrence after such therapy, some authors have suggested follow-up surveillance endoscopy and biopsy, reserving conventional surgery and/or chemotherapy, with or without radiation, as second-line treatment for patients who fail antibiotic therapy.[48–53]

STAGING AND PROGNOSTIC FACTORS

Once a diagnosis of lymphoma has been established, appropriate staging studies include thorough physical examination (including palpating for an enlarged spleen and examination of all lymph node-bearing areas), evaluation of the cells on the peripheral blood smear to look for lymphomatous involvement, chest radiography (and chest CT scan if indicated by any abnormalities on the chest radiograph or symptoms), abdominopelvic CT, bilateral bone marrow aspirations, and biopsies and gallium scan. In addition, these patients should have indirect laryngoscopy to rule out involvement of Waldeyer's ring.[54]

Several classification schemes describe gastrointestinal lymphoma. These are based on systems originally designed for nodal lymphomas. The most widely used systems attempt to organize histologic subtype and are summarized in Tables 31-1 through 31-3.

Staging systems have traditionally been based on the Musshoff modification of the Ann Arbor staging system for nodal Hodgkin's lymphomas. Stage I is disease confined to the stomach. Stage II comprises tumors of the stomach with regional lymph node involvement. Stage III includes nodal involvement on both sides of the diaphragm. Stage IV is diffuse (i.e., bone marrow) involvement. This system has been criticized with respect to its use in gastrointestinal lymphoma because these are non-Hodgkin's lymphomas that have behavior characteristics distinct from nodal lymphomas. Because of the inadequacies of this system in correlating stage with survival, Lim and colleagues defined a type of TNM system in 1977.[55] The letter E is used to denote the fact that these are extranodal lymphomas. This system has the advantage of addressing the issue of tumor depth of invasion, and is summarized in Table 31-4. Similarly, Shimodaira and colleagues[56] have proposed a staging system

TABLE 31-1. *Rappaport classification of gastrointestinal lymphomas*

Histiocytic lymphoma-diffuse
Lymphocytic lymphoma
poorly differentiated:
nodular
diffuse
mixed nodular and diffuse
well differentiated:
diffuse
Mixed histiocytic and lymphocytic
nodular
diffuse
Composite lymphoma
"Mediterranean type" lymphoma
Burkitt's lymphoma
Undifferentiated non-Burkitt's
Hodgkin's disease
Unclassified lymphoma

TABLE 31-2. *Working formulation*

LOW GRADE	
Small lymphocytic, consistent with CLL, plasmacytoid	A
Follicular, predominantly small cleaved cell, diffuse areas, sclerosis	B
Follicular, mixed, small cleaved and large cell, diffuse areas, sclerosis	C
INTERMEDIATE GRADE	
Follicular, predominantly large cell, diffuse areas, sclerosis	D
Diffuse, small cleaved cell, sclerosis	E
Diffuse, mixed, small and large-cell sclerosis, epithelioid cell component	F
Diffuse, large cell, cleaved cell, noncleaved cell, sclerosis	G
HIGH GRADE	
Large cell, immunoblastic, plasmacytoid, clear-cell, polymorphous epithelioid cell component	H
Lymphoblastic convoluted cell, non-convoluted cell	I
Small noncleaved cell, Burkitt's follicular areas	J

which appears to correlate quite well with survival statistics. This system is summarized in Table 31-5.

In addition to depth of invasion, other tumor characteristics have been associated with a poorer prognosis, and include size greater than 5 cm, regional lymph node involvement, distant metastases, high grade, and diffuse versus nodular histologic type. Low-grade lymphomas have the best survival, followed by lymphomas in transformation and then high-grade lymphomas, which have the worst survival, with 5-year survival rates being approximately 90%, 70% and 50% respectively. Tumor penetration beyond the serosa lowers the 5-year survival from 75% to 90% to 50% to 60%. One study suggests that, as is true of non-Hodgkin's lymphomas in general, age greater than 65 years and elevated lactic dehydrogenase are negative prognostic factors.[25]

TABLE 31-3. *Kiel classification*

LOW-GRADE MALIGNANCY	
Lymphocytic, chronic lymphocytic leukemia	A
Lymphocytic, other	B
Lymphoplasmacytoid	C
Centrocytic	D
Centroblastic-centrocytic	
Follicular, without sclerosis	E
Follicular, with sclerosis	F
Follicular and diffuse, without sclerosis	G
Follicular and diffuse, with sclerosis	H
Diffuse	I
Low grade malignant lymphoma, unclassified	J
HIGH-GRADE MALIGNANCY	
Centroblastic	K
Lymphoblastic	
Burkitt's type	L
Convoluted cell type	M
Other (unclassified)	N
Immunoblastic	O
High grade malignant lymphoma, unclassified	P
Malignant lymphoma, unclassified	Q
Composite lymphoma	R

TABLE 31-4. *Modified TNM staging of gastric lymphoma*

Stage	Extent of involvement
IA	Mucosa only
IB	Submucosal penetration
IC	Serosal penetration
II	Any degree of gastric wall involvement with positive perigastric nodes in the immediate vicinity of the primary tumor
III	Any degree of gastric wall involvement with positive lymph nodes distant from the primary tumor or on both curvatures of the stomach; no distant metastases
IV	Distant metastases including spleen and liver

TREATMENT

Optimal treatment approaches for patients with different stages and histologic types remain undefined. Most have undergone either subtotal or total gastrectomies. The classic therapy for gastric lymphoma has been resection. In recent years, attempts have been made to improve survival with the addition of chemotherapy or radiation therapy. In addition, some suggest

TABLE 31-5. *TNM staging*

TNM staging system definitions

T1	Tumor invades the lamina propria or submucosa
T2	Tumor invades the muscularis propria
T3	Tumor invades the subserosa
T4	Tumor invades serosa without invasion of adjacent structures
T5	Adjacent structures invaded
N0	No regional lymph node metastases
N1	Perigastric lymph nodes within 3 cm of the edge of the primary tumor
N2	Perigastric lymph nodes more than 3 cm from the edge of the primary tumor or in lymph nodes along the left gastric common hepatic, splenic, or celiac arteries
N3	Paraaortic and hepatoduodenal lymph nodes and/or other intraabdominal lymph nodes
M0	No distant metastases
M1	Distant metastases present

TNM stage and percent 5 year survival

Stage	T	N	M	Five-year survival rate (%)
I	T1	N0, N1	M0	100
II	T1	N2	M0	88.9
	T2, T3	N0, N1, N2	M0	
III	T4, T5	any N	M0	52.1
	any T	N3, N4	M0	
IV	any T	any M	M1	25.0

Shimodaira M, Tsukamoto Y, Niwa Y, et al. A proposed staging system for primary gastric lymphoma. Cancer 1994;73(1):2709.

this disease be treated completely without surgical intervention. The debate regarding optimal therapy for primary gastric lymphoma is by no means settled. Because of the rate nature of this disease, and thus the small size of the studies available, there are data to both support and refute almost all sides of the issue.

The application of surgical exploration in primary gastric lymphoma is multifold. In some instances, this is the only method of securing a histologic diagnosis. On the occasion that the patient presents with bleeding, obstruction, or perforation, surgery remains the only therapy. Surgical pathologic staging may be the only accurate way to assess the extent of disease because all forms of radiologic, ultrasonographic, and combined endoscopic evaluation have only an 80% to 90% accuracy.

Stage of disease and resectability are the only two consistent factors that have significant influence on survival.[57–59] Whether margins are positive or negative has not proven to have a statistical significance in predicting outcome in several studies. Most studies show resection to be beneficial in stages IE and IIE disease only. Talamonti and associates, however, reported that even in the fact of disseminated disease, the 5-year survival rate with resection in combination with chemotherapy is 81%, compared with 6% treated without resection.[60] With regard to the extent of resection, studies show that radical resection is not necessary and that subtotal gastrectomy is usually sufficient treatment and better tolerated than more extensive excision.[61,62]

There have been reports of long-term survival and even cure in patients treated without surgery.[25,63,64] Several series show 5-year survival rates of 58% to 83% in unresected patients, with up to 10% death in the induction chemotherapy group in one study.[65,68] Chemotherapy alone for treatment of early-stage primary gastric lymphoma is debatable because survival data in most studies show either reduced survival or at best survival equal to that with surgical resection. In addition, there are morbidities associated with chemotherapy, including bone marrow suppression and peripheral neuropathies. As stated earlier, there is also some mortality with chemotherapy.

Radiation therapy has most often been given in the adjuvant setting after subtotal gastrectomy. Radiation therapy doses have ranged from 10 to 40 Gy. Most commonly, either 20 to 25 Gy is given to the whole abdomen with a 15-Gy boost to the epigastric region, or, alternatively, 40 Gy is administered to the epigastric area only.[25] Good long-term disease control rates have been reported in a few series using this approach, especially for patients with small volumes of residual disease after surgery. However, because most relapses are not local, it is difficult to know what the role of radiation therapy is in this disease in the absence of controlled, randomized studies. Consistent with this are a number of studies that suggest that, in general, for patients with high-grade lymphomas, postoperative adjuvant radiation therapy does not appear to add significantly to their survival.[24,67,69,71] Radiation therapy has also been used as primary therapy for patients with stage IE disease, with 5-year survival results comparable to those seen in patients who underwent both surgery and radiation therapy. Because of the varied treatment regimens used and the small numbers of patients in each study, prospective, randomized trials are still needed to define fully what role either primary or postoperative adjuvant radiation therapy may play in treating specific subsets of patients with gastric lymphoma.

Several studies have explored the issue of adjuvant chemotherapy either to prevent recurrence of disease or to treat recurrence of disease after resection. Favorable results with adjuvant chemotherapy have been documented by several groups.[55,58] Pasini and colleagues[72] looked at 53 patients with stages IE and IIE primary gastric lymphoma; 34 had poor prognostic features including high or intermediate grade, positive margins, serosal invasion, and tumor mass larger than 5 cm. Patients with poor prognostic features were given postoperative polychemotherapy (mostly the CHOP [cyclophosphamide, hydroxydaunomycin, Oncovin, and prednisone] regimen). In this study, the 10-year overall survival rate in low-risk patients was 89% when treated with resection alone (68% disease-free survival, with another two thirds of patients rescued with chemotherapy after recurrence). This compares with 87% 10-year overall survival in patients with poor prognostic features treated with resection followed by postoperative chemotherapy. These data suggest that adjuvant chemotherapy may improve survival in patients with poor prognostic features and those who have recurrence after resection. This study and others[73] also demonstrate that primary gastric lymphoma with good prognostic features can be cured in a significant percentage of patients with resection alone (Table 31-6).

Shiu and coworkers published a study in 1986 comparing resection (92% were subtotal gastrectomies) with resection plus total abdominal radiation therapy or resection with adjuvant

TABLE 31-6. *Percent 5 year survival for alternative primary treatment modalities of stage IE and IIE gastric lymphoma*

Author	Year	Number of patients	Treatment modality: number of patients in each group given Surgery	Radiation	Chemotherapy	Combined
Rackner	1991	36	15 (80)	10 (65)	11 (45)	
Thirlby	1993	22	15 (75)	7 (45)		
Ben-Yosef	1994	24	2 (66)			22 (70)*
Shimodaira	1994	75	40 (90)			35 (94)**
Shui	1986	29	5 (100)			24 (95)*
Pasini	1993	53	19 (90)			34 (100)**
Pytel	1994	31	6 (100)			25 (80)*

Similar results for stages IIIE and IVE are not given due to difficulty in distinguishing primary and secondary gastric lymphomas. Treatment modalities and methods of reporting survival statistics vary immensely among the studies listed.

* Denotes varying combinations of surgery, chemotherapy and radiation therapy.

** Denotes surgical resection in combination with chemotherapy.

chemotherapy) mostly CHOP and variations of CHOP).[74] Five-year survival is 95% for stage IE and 100% for resectable stage IIE lesions based on these data. Patients treated with total abdominal radiation received 3700 cGy including a boost to the stomach bed and paraortic nodes. Tumors of favorable histologic type achieved dose-related local control, whereas tumors of unfavorable histologic type, such as diffuse histiocytic lymphoma, which is the most common histologic subtype, did not show a dose–response relationship. The local relapse rate after radiation for stages IE and IIE disease ranged from 14% to 22%. There were no operative or perioperative deaths in this study. Combined modality therapy did result in morbidity, including bone marrow depression, malabsorbtion, and nutritional complications. From these data, they proposed optimizing treatment of primary gastric lymphoma based on extent and stage of disease. The choice of which adjuvant therapy to use is debatable, with chemotherapy being equal to or superior to total abdominal radiation in terms of survival advantage and fewer associated morbidities. Studies by Dworkin and colleagues and Hockey and associates found no benefit to postoperative radiation.[75,76] Similarly, there does not appear to be an advantage to using both adjuvant modalities as opposed to one.[50]

The wide variety of treatments used has precluded any firm conclusions about optimal therapy of patients with primary gastric lymphoma. In the absence of definitive data from randomized trials, a reasonable approach is surgically to resect patients with apparently resectable disease, approximately 60% to 70% of patients. The potential roles for adjuvant chemotherapy or radiation therapy for patients with high-grade lesions need to be addressed in large, multicenter, prospective, randomized, controlled studies.

Based on data from the previously mentioned studies as well as many other published accounts, several guidelines have been set forth. For tumors limited to the gastric mucosa and submucosa, recurrence is infrequent, and therefore resection alone is sufficient. Tumors with deep penetration but not involving the serosa should be considered for adjuvant therapy (either radiation therapy or chemotherapy) because relapse is more likely to occur. Adjuvant therapy is indicated when the serosa is invaded, the tumor is greater than 7 cm in diameter, or there is regional nodal disease (stage IIE). In more locally advanced unresectable disease, gross residual disease, or when there are metastases, chemotherapy is the treatment of choice and radiation should be added to control local bulky disease. Liver and nodal biopsies should also be done as part of staging at laparotomy. Consideration should also be given to splenic biopsy with possible removal of the spleen if it is involved with lymphoma.

As discussed earlier, the treatment of MALT lymphomas with antibiotic therapy and H_2 antagonists is still under investigation. This may prove to be the treatment of choice for these early-stage lesions, with other conventional therapies reserved only for those patients who either do not respond or who have recurrence. Certainly, reliable follow-up is essential regardlesss of the treatment option.

Gastric lymphoma remains a disease for which large, multicenter, prospective, randomized clinical trials are needed to address the questions concerning the roles of surgery, radiation therapy, and chemotherapy in treating patients with different histologic types and stages.

SUMMARY

The etiology, diagnosis, and treatment of primary gastric lymphoma are by no means clear. As more is learned about the immunology of the gastrointestinal tract and the natural history of extranodal lymphomas, especially the early-stage and MALT tumors, perhaps optimal and less invasive treatment regimens will become solidified. At present, it appears that surgery still plays an important role in the diagnosis, staging, and treatment of primary gastric lymphoma and is an integral part of multidisciplinary approach to this disease.

REFERENCES

1. Herrmann R, Panahon AM, Barcos MP, Walsh D, Statzman L. Gastrointestinal involvement in non-Hodgkin's lymphoma. Cancer 1980;46:215.
2. Burgess HN, Dockerty MB, ReMine WH. Sarcomatous lesions of the stomach. Ann Surg 1971;173:758.
3. Severson RK, Davis S. Increasing incidence of primary gastric lymphoma. Cancer 1990;66:1283.
4. Cappell MS, Botros N. Predominantly gastrointestinal symptoms and signs in 11 consecutive AIDS patients with gastrointestinal lymphoma: a multicenter, multiyear study including 763 HIV-seropositive patients. Am J Gastroenterol 1994;89:545.
5. Louie S, Schwartz R. Immunodeficiency and the pathogenesis of lymphoma and leukemia. Semin Hematol 1980;15:117.
6. Louie S, Daoust P, Schwartz R. Immunodeficiency and the pathogenesis of non-Hodgkin's lymphoma. Semin Oncol 1980;7:267.
7. Abe T, Yachi A, Yabana T, et al. Gastric non-Hodgkin's lymphoma associated with Behcet's disease. Intern Med 1993;32:663.
8. Isaacson PG. Extranodal lymphomas: the MALT concept. Verh Dtsch Ges Pathol 1992;76:14.
9. Greiner A, Marx A, Heesemann J, et al. Idiotype identity in MALT-type lymphoma and B cells in *Helicobacter pylori* associated chronic gastritis. Lab Invest 1994;70:572.
10. Parsonnet J, Hansen S, Rodriguez L, et al. *Helicobacter pylori* infection and gastric lymphoma. N Engl J Med 1994;330:1267.
11. Isaacson PG. Gastric lymphoma and *Helicobacter pylori.* N Engl J Med 1994;330:1310.
12. Dawson IMP, Cornes JS, Morson BC. Primary malignant lymphoid tumors of the intestinal tract: report of 37 cases with a study of factors influencing prognosis. Br J Surg 1961;49:80.
13. Mentzer SS, Osteen RT, Rosenthal DS, et al. Surgical therapy of localized abdominal non-Hodgkin's lymphomas. Surgery 1988;103:609.
14. Taal BG, der Hartig J, Tytgat G. The endoscopic spectrum of non-Hodgkin's lymphoma of the stomach. Endoscopy 1987;19:190.
15. Caletti GC, Brocchi E, Gibilaro M, et al. Sensitivity specificity and predictive value of endoscopic ultrasonography (EUS) in the diagnosis and assessment of gastric lymphoma. Gastrointest Endosc 1990;36:195A.
16. Caletti GC, Ferrari A, Brocchi E, Barbara L. Accuracy of endoscopic ultrasonography in the diagnosis and staging of gastric cancer and lymphoma. Surgery 1993;113:1.
17. Bolondi L, Casanova P, Caletti GC, et al. Primary gastric lymphoma versus gastric carcinoma: endoscopic US evaluation. Radiology 1987;165:821.
18. Suekane H, Lida MM, Yao T, et al. Endoscopic ultrasonography in primary gastric lymphoma: correlation with endoscopic and histologic findings. Gastrointest Endosc 1993;39:139.
19. Fischbach W, Kestel W, Kirchner T, Mossner J, Wilms K. Malignant lymphomas of the upper gastrointestinal tract: results of a prospective study in 103 patients. Cancer 1992;70:1075.
20. Sherman ME, Anderson C, Herman L, Ludwig ME, Erozan YS. Utility of gastric brushings in the diagnosis of malignant lymphoma. Acta Cytol 1994;38:169.
21. Radaszkiewicz T, Drgosics B, Bauer P. Gastrointestinal malignant lymphomas of the mucosa-associated lymphoid tissue: factors relevant to prognosis. Gastroenterology 1992;102:1628.
22. Cogliatti SB, Schmid U, Schumacher U, et al. Primary B-cell gastric lymphoma: a clinicopathological study of 145 patients. Gastroenterology 1991;101:1159.
23. Isaacson PG, Wright DH. Malignant lymphoma of mucosa-associated

lymphoid tissue: a distinctive type of B-cell lymphoma. Cancer 1982; 52:1410.
23. Ruskone-Fourmestraux A, Aegerter P, Delmer A, et al. Primary digestive tract lymphoma: a prospective multicentric study of 91 patients. Gastroenterology 1993;105:1662.
24. Amer MH, El-Akkad S, Gastrointestinal lymphoma in adults: clinical features and management of 300 cases. Gastroenterology 1994;106: 846.
25. Schwartz RJ, Conners JM, Schmidt N. Diagnosis and management of stage IE and stage IIE gastric lymphomas. Am J Surg 1993;165:561.
26. Streeter PR, Rouse BTRN, Butcher EC. Immunohistologic and functional characterisation of vascular addressin involved in lymphocyte homing into peripheral lymph nodes. Cell Biol 1988;107:1853.
27. Radaszkiewicz T, Drgosics B, Bauer P. Gastrointestinal malignant lymphomas of the mucosa-associated lymphoid tissue: factors relevant to prognosis. Gastroenterology 1992;102:1628.
28. Franssila KO, Jaser N, Sivula A. Gastrointestinal non-Hodgkin's lymphoma: a population based clinicopathological study of 111 adult cases with a follow-up of 10–15 years. APMIS 1993;10:631.
29. Grody WW, Magidson JG, Weiss LM, et al. Gastrointestinal lymphomas: immunohistochemical studies on the cell of origin. Am J Surg Pathol 1985;9:328.
30. Brooks JJ, Enterline HT. Primary gastric lymphoma: clinicopathological study of 58 cases with long-term follow-up and literature review. Cancer 1983;51:701.
31. Brooks J, Enterline H. Gastric pseudolymphoma: its three subtypes and relation to lymphoma. Cancer 1983;51:476.
32. Isaacson PG, Wright DH. Malignant lymphoma of mucosa-associated lymphoid tissue: a distinctive type of B-cell lymphoma. Cancer 1983; 52:1410.
33. Isaacson PG, Spencer J. Malignant lymphoma of mucosa associated lymphoid tissue. Histopathology 1989;11:445.
34. Zukerberg LR, Ferry JA, Southern JF, Harris NL. Lymphoid infiltrates of the stomach: evaluation of histologic criteria for the diagnosis of low-grade gastric lymphoma on endoscopic biopsy specimens. Am J Surg Pathol 1990;14:1087.
35. Dutcher TF, Fahey JL. The histopathology of the macroglobulinemia of Waldenstrom. J Nat Cancer Inst 1959;22:887.
36. Papadaki L, Wotherspoon AC, Isaacson PG. The lymphoepithelial lesion of gastric low-grade B0-cell lymphoma of mucosa-associated lymphoid tissue (MALT): an ultrastructural study. Histopathology 1992;21:415.
37. Wotherspoon AC, Pan L, Diss TC, Isaacson PG. A genomic study of low grade B-cell lymphomas, including lymphomas of mucosa associated lymphoid tissue (MALT). J Pathol 1990;162:135.
38. Warren JR, Marshall BJ. Unidentified curved bacilli on gastric epithelium in active chronic gastritis. Lancet 1983;1:1273.
39. The EUROGAST Study Group. An international association between *Helicobacter pylori* infection and gastric cancer. Lancet 1993;341: 1359.
40. Wyatt JI, Tathbone BJ. Immune response of the gastric mucosa to *Campylobacter pylori.* Scand J Gastroenterol 1988;23(Suppl 142):44.
41. Stolte M, Eidt S. Lymphoid follicles in the antral mucosa: immune response to *Campylobacter pylori.* J Clin Pathol 1989;42:1269.
42. Wotherspoon AC, Ortiz-Hidalgo C, Falzon MR, Isaacson PG. *Helicobacter pylori*-associated gastritis and primary B-cell gastric lymphoma. Lancet 1991;338:1175.
43. Hyjek E, Smith WJ, Isaacson PG. Primary B-cell lymphoma of salivary glands and its relationship to myoepithelial sialadenitis. Hum Pathol 1988;19:766.
44. Hyjek E, Isaacson PG. Primary B-cell lymphoma of the thyroid and its relationship to Hashimoto's thyroiditis. Hum Pathol 1988;19:1315.
45. Hussell T, Isaacson PG, Crabtree JE, Spencer J. The response of cells from low-grade B-cell gastric lymphoma of mucosa-associated lymphoid tissue to *Helicobacter pylori.* Lancet 1993;342:571.
46. Holcombe C. *Helicobacter pylori:* the African enigma. Gut 1992;33: 429.
47. Grahan DY, Adam E, Reddy GT, et al. Seroepidemiology of *Helicobacter pylori* infection in India: comparison of developing and developed countries. Dig Dis Sci 1991;36:108.
48. Wotherspoon AC, Doglioni C, Diss Rc, Pan L, Moschini A, de Boni M, Isaacson PG. Regression of primary low-grade B-cell gastric lymphoma of mucosa-associated lymphoid tissue type after eradication of *Helicobacter pylori.* Lancet 1993;342:575.
49. Roggero E, et al. Eradication of *Helicobacter pylori* infection in primary low-grade gastric lymphoma of mucosa-associated lymphoid tissue. Ann Intern Med 1995;122:767.
50. Weber DM, Dimopoulos MA, Anadu DP, Pugh WC, Steinbach G. Regression of gastric lymphoma of mucosa-associated lymphoid tissue with antibiotic therapy for *Helicobacter pylori.* Gastroenterology 1994; 107:1835.
51. Okazaki K, Morita M, Yamamoto Y. Gene rearrangements, *Helicobacter pylori* and gastric MALT lymphoma. Lancet 1994;343:1636.
52. Montalban C, Monzanal A, Boixeda D, Redondo C, Bellas C. Treatment of low-grade gastric MALT lymphoma with *Helicobacter pylori* eradication. Lancet 1995;345:798.
53. Harris AW, Misiewicz JJ. Antibiotic treatment for low-grade gastric MALT lymphoma. Lancet 1994;343:1503.
54. Paulsen J, Lennert K. Low grade B-cell lymphoma of mucosa-associated lymphoid tissue type in Waldeyer's ring. Histopathology 1994; 24:1.
55. Lim FE, Hartman AS, Tan E, et al. Factors in the prognosis of gastric lymphoma. Cancer 1977;39:1715.
56. Shimodaira M, Tsukamoto Y, Niwa Y, Goto H, Hase S, Hayakawa T. A proposed staging system for primary gastric lymphoma. Cancer 1994; 73(1):2709.
56. Pytel J, Sigon R, Bidoli EK, et al. Primary gastric non-Hodgkin's lymphoma: does surgery still play any role? Eur J Surg Oncol 1994;20: 525.
57. Rackner VL, Thirlby RC, Ryan JA. Role of surgery in multimodality therapy for gastrointestinal lymphoma Am J Surg 1991;161:570.
58. Thirlby RC. Gastrointestinal lymphoma: a surgical perspective. Oncology 1993;7:29.
59. Talamonti MS, Sawes LG, Joehl RJ, et al. Gastrointestinal lymphoma: a case for primary surgical resecion. Arch Surg 1990;125:972.
60. Weingrad DN, DeCosse JJ, Sherlock P, Straus D, Liegerman PH, Filippa DA. Primary gastrointestinal lymphoma: a 30 year review. Cancer 1982;49:1258.
61. Shiu MH, Karas M, Nisce BJ, et al. Management of primary gastric lymphoma. Ann Surg 1982;195:196.
62. Maor MH, Maddux B, Osborne M, et al. Stages IE and IIE non-Hodgkin's lymphomas of the stomach: comparison of treatment modalities. Cancer 1984;54:2330.
63. Econommopoulos T, Alexopoulos C, Stathakis N, et al. Primary gastric lymphoma: the experience of a general hospital. Bri J Cancer 1985; 52:391.
64. Salles G, Raoul H, Tilly H, et al. Aggressive primary gastrointestinal lymphomas: review of 91 patients treated with the LNH-84 regimen. A study of the Groupe d'Etude des Lymphomes Agressifs. Am J Med 1991;90:77.
65. Burgers JMV, Taal BG, Van Heerde P, et al. Treatment results of primary stage I and II non-Hodgkin's lymphoma of the stomach. Radiother Oncol 1988;11:319.
66. Maor MH, Velasquez WS, Fuller LM, Silvermintz KB. Stomach conservation in stages IE and IIE gastric non-Hodgkin's lymphomas. J Clin Oncol 11988;1990;8:266.
67. Aviles A, Diaz-Maqueo JC, de la Torre A, et al. Is surgery necessary in the treatment of primary gastric non-Hodgkin's lymphoma? Leuk Lymphoma 1991;5:365.
68. Romaguera JE, Velasquez WS, Silvermintz KB, et al. Surgical debulking is associated with improved survival in stage I–II diffuse large cell lymphoma. Cancer 1990;66:267.
69. Jones RE, Willis S, Innes DJ, et al. Primary gastric lymphoma: problems in staging and management. Am J Surg 1988;155:118.
70. Bozzetti F, Audisio RA, Giardini R, et al. Role of surgery in patients with primary non-Hodgkin's lymphoma of the stomach: an old problem revisited. Br J Surg 1993;80:1101.
71. Pasini F, Abrosetti A, Sabbioni R, et al. Postoperative chemotherapy increases the disease-free survival in primary gastric lymphomas stage IE and IIE. Eur J Cancer 1994;30A:33.
72. Mentzer SJ, Osteen RT, Pappas TN, et al. Surgical therapy of localized abdominal non-Hodgkin's lymphomas. Surgery 1988;103:609.
73. Shiu MH, Nisce LZ, Pinna A, et al. Recent results of multimodal therapy of gastric lymphoma. Cancer 1986;58:1389.
74. Dworkin B, Lightdale CJ, Weingrad DN, et al. Primary gastric lymphoma: a review of 50 cases. Dig Dis Sci 1982;27:986.
75. Hockey MS, Powell J, Crocker J, et al. Primary gastric lymphoma. Br J Surg 1987;74:483.

PART IV

Pancreatic Cancer

Surgery for Gastrointestinal Cancer: A Multidisciplinary Approach, edited by Harold J. Wanebo.
Lippincott-Raven Publishers, Philadelphia, © 1997.

CHAPTER 32

Management of the Apparent Periampullary Malignancy: Preoperative Evaluation and Operative Treatment

David R. Farley and Michael G. Sarr

The identification of a mass in the head of the pancreas in any patient is an ominous sign. Because most of these periampullary masses prove to be a pancreatic ductal adenocarcinoma, such a lesion usually foreshadows the eventual demise of most patients. Most such neoplasms are unresectable, and the onus is on the physician and surgeon alike to characterize the tumor in a timely, cost-effective manner and to resect those malignancies that remain regionally confined. Palliation of the remaining majority of patients is often necessary and difficult. The objective of this chapter is to present a strategy for a timely and cost-effective preoperative evaluation of the patient with extrahepatic biliary obstruction or a mass in the head of the pancreas; appropriate considerations in preoperative and intraoperative decision making; and a realistic rationale for tumor resection or operative palliation.

ETIOLOGY

To know best how to diagnose and subsequently treat patients with extrahepatic biliary obstruction or a mass in the head of the pancreas, it is imperative that physicians have an understanding of the relative frequencies of the possible neoplasms—benign and malignant—that cause such a radiographic finding. Although each patient obviously cannot reflect the broader incidence of neoplasm in the region of the pancreatic head, knowledge of such frequencies streamlines an otherwise expensive diagnostic process.

Unfortunately, the most common neoplasm of the periampullary region is pancreatic ductal adenocarcinoma (Table 32-1). The incidence of pancreatic cancer appears to have increased in the first six decades of the 1900s, but now has stabilized for reasons unknown. Nevertheless, it represents the most common cause of extrahepatic biliary obstruction in patients older than 50 years of age. Epidemiologic studies have consistently shown an association with increasing age, smoking, male gender, and chronic calcific pancreatitis, with a less consistent association with diabetes mellitus, gastrectomy, and alcohol intake. There is the rare family with an apparent hereditary trait. Despite more aggressive surgical resections and improved postoperative survival times, this disease remains fatal in greater than 99% of patients.[1] Endoscopic, radiologic, and surgical reports classify malignant periampullary neoplasms into pancreatic (60% to 80%), ampullary (5% to 20%), biliary (5% to 10%), and duodenal (5% to 10%).[2–4] However, the relative frequency of each of these specific neoplasms varies with the authors' primary specialty. For instance, surgical series addressing curative resections have a larger percentage of ampullary cancers because they are more often resectable. Although infrequent, metastatic disease, including renal cell carcinoma, melanoma,[5] and lung cancer or lymphoma,[6] may cause a mass in the head of the pancreas along with benign diseases, the most common being pancreatitis. Because a pancreatic malignancy is the most common mass in this region, this chapter is appropriately weighted to address the management of tumors thought to be pancreatic ductal adenocarcinoma.

PREOPERATIVE EVALUATION

Because the list of differential diagnoses is not long, the preoperative evaluation of the patient with a periampullary mass should be simple: define if the mass is malignant or benign, and, if malignant, determine if it is resectable. Unfortunately, the "standard evaluation" for such a disease process is too frequently redundant and inappropriately expensive.

Before the advent of the current techniques of flexible endoscopy, angiography, transcutaneous ultrasonography, and computed tomography (CT), the initial work-up for vague epigastric

David R. Farley, Division of G.I. and General Surgery, Mayo Clinic, Rochester, MN 55905
Michael G. Sarr, Division of G.I. and General Surgery, Mayo Clinic, Rochester, MN 55905

TABLE 32-1. *Relative frequencies of conditions associated with extrahepatic biliary obstruction or periampullary mass*

Condition	Frequency
Ductal adenocarcinoma of pancreas	85%
Ampullary carcinoma	5%
Pancreatitis*	5%
Other neoplasms	5%
Duodenal carcinoma	
Distal bile duct carcinoma	
Islet cell tumors	
Periampullary villous adenomas	
Cystadenoma/carcinoma	
Metastatic neoplasms (melanoma, renal cell, lung)	

* Without the usual past medical history of pancreatitis

pain, jaundice, or weight loss included routine blood studies and a barium upper gastrointestinal radiographic examination. Even today, some abnormality on upper gastrointestinal film is identified in about a third of patients with pancreatic cancer.[7] However, this outdated diagnostic work-up lacks specificity and sensitivity; more important, it offers no useful data on staging, and surgeons historically were forced to take nearly all patients to the operating room. Celiotomy all too often led to the discovery of an advanced malignancy and a nontherapeutic or palliative operation. Resection for cure was rare. With modern imaging modalities, fine-needle aspiration, and advanced serologic and molecular testing, a few notable changes have occurred. Although resection for cure remains rare (<15%) when all patients presenting with pancreatic cancer are considered, the significant change since the early 1970s has been the elimination of surgical exploration in patients with advanced disease at the price of expensive diagnostic tests for everyone. Careful scrutiny of each test in our armamentarium to diagnose and stage tumors of the periampullary region is worthwhile to help devise a concise, efficient, safe, and cost-effective evaluation of the patient with a presumed periampullary malignancy.

History and Physical Examination

An accurate history and physical examination of patients with vague abdominal or back discomfort, jaundice, or weight loss is imperative. Although such a statement seems obvious, it is worth remembering that the shorter the delay in diagnosis, the smaller the tumor with more favorable staging and a greater chance of resection for cure.[8] Although advances in imaging techniques may not subsequently improve survival,[9] early clinical signs can help to direct eventual treatment. Abdominal pain and especially central mid-back pain about the level of T12–L1 associated with a peripancreatic mass usually denotes a more advanced stage of disease,[8] whereas the new onset of diabetes mellitus in patients older than age 50 years, especially with other abdominal complaints, should raise the question of pancreatic cancer.[10,11] A meticulous physical examination looking specifically for signs of distant disease (ascites, periumbilical mass, left supraclavicular Virchow's node), coupled with a careful history, including details of abdominal pain, gallstones, alcohol consumption, and so forth, remains vital to streamlining the diagnostic evaluation.

Serologic Screening

A complete blood cell count, chemistry panel, and serum amylase are routine studies suggested before general anesthesia and operative exploration in the patient with extrahepatic biliary obstruction. An array of serologic tests has been developed to screen for the diagnosis of malignancy, especially pancreatic malignancy. None, however, is sufficiently specific or sensitive enough to diagnose or exclude pancreatic cancer (Table 32-2). Tumor markers with the greatest sensitivity and specificity include carcinoembryonic antigen, CA 19-9, CA 242, and DU-PAN-2.[12–14] Because none of these markers is sensitive or specific, they remain of unproven efficacy as screening tools for early detection of cancer. Although CA 19-9 levels are frequently normal early in the course of pancreatic cancer, increased levels have been reported to be helpful in attempting to differentiate malignancy versus pancreatitis[15]; however, this marker alone is not specific enough to determine treatment. These tumor markers may actually be of more benefit postoperatively as markers of recurrence; a prolonged or sustained decrease in CA 19-9 after curative resection suggests a better prognosis and may be useful in follow-up.[10]

Serum activities of various pancreatic enzymes have been used to screen for pancreatic cancer. Serum galactosyltransferase II, ribonuclease, and elastase levels may be increased with pancreatic malignancy, but, as with the tumor markers, none of these three enzymes is sufficiently sensitive and specific to be the basis for treatment options.[10] Similarly, although greater than 70% of men with pancreatic cancer have plasma testosterone : dihydrotestosterone ratios of less than 5 (normal$\geq$10),[16] such information is of no use clinically in individual patients as either a screening test or a diagnostic marker. In summary,

TABLE 32-2. *Tumor "markers" proposed for use in screening or postoperative follow-up in patients with pancreatic cancer*

ONCOFETAL ANTIGENS
Pancreatic oncofetal antigen
Oncofetal pancreatic antigen
Fetal acinar pancreatic protein
PA 8-15
Carcinoembryonic antigen*
MUCIN ANTIGENS
CA 19-9*
CA 50*
CA 242*
BW 494
DU-PAN-2
Y PAN-1
ONCOGENES
ERB B2
*KRAS**

* Best candidate markers with greatest sensitivity and specificity.

current serologic testing for accurate diagnosis or as a means of directing therapy is of no proven clinical efficacy.

The introduction of powerful, innovative techniques of molecular biology may, in the future, prove to be of use both in diagnostic and screening evaluations. As with other malignancies, a host of genetic abnormalities have been described in the malignant tissue of patients with pancreatic cancer, including point mutations in the *KRAS* or *ERBB2* oncogenes, deletion of other genes, or loss of regions of specific chromosomes encoding the tumor suppressor genes *P53*, *DCC*, *MTS1*, and *P16*.[17] To be detected, these abnormalities currently require tissue specimens from biopsies of the resected tumors. However, the ability to screen duodenal or pancreatic ductal aspirates or even stool specimens in the near future for objective genetic abnormalities specific for pancreatic cancer is not unrealistic.

Imaging

In an algorithm designed to evaluate the patient with presumed extrahepatic biliary obstruction (Fig. 32-1), radiologic imaging is crucial. The goals of imaging are twofold: to obtain a near-certain diagnosis, and to stage the disease. Transabdominal ultrasonography or thin-slice or "spiral" CT, in conjunction with endoscopic retrograde cholangiopancreatography (ERCP), provide the standard from which to obtain the necessary information about the periampullary region. Proponents exist for each technique, but the bottom line remains that none is precise in predicting tumor resectability. Often the best technique is that in which the radiologist is most experienced reading, because ultimately each test is only as good as the person performing and reading it. Bakkevold and colleagues[8] demonstrated prospectively in 472 patients that the preoperative assessment of a "resectable" mass in the head of the pancreas was accurate in only 42%. The positive predictive value of ultrasonography was 29%, CT 35%, and ERCP 43%. Conversely, the imaging of unresectable tumors was more accurate with CT and ultrasonography, with positive predictive values of 97% and 95%, respectively. ERCP (75%) was less accurate.

Freeny and associates[18] similarly have shown that state-of-the-art abdominal CT is quite accurate in diagnosing pancreatic cancer (97%) and, more important, in identifying unresectable pancreatic cancer (95%). However, only 13 of 18 (72%) "radiographically resectable" patients were able to undergo a curative resection. Because no single test has proven to be the gold standard in identifying resectability, physicians in the past have erred on the side of obtaining multiple studies (angiography, endoscopic ultrasonography, magnetic resonance imaging) in the attempt to avoid an unnecessary operation. Our own bias has been (and continues to be) to use abdominal CT as the primary diagnostic study. If the patient has a good performance status and the tumor appears "resectable" on CT, we proceed directly with operative exploration. Even if the neoplasm proves unresectable, we believe that operative biliary decompression provides superior palliation in these good-risk patients with a good performance status (see section on Palliation). In contrast, if evidence of unresectability is present, we use fine-needle aspiration as a means of obtaining an objective tissue diagnosis to justify use of radiation therapy for palliation in conjunction with an endobiliary stent. If fine-needle aspiration will not alter the management plan, it is not used, especially preoperatively in patients in whom exploration is planned.[19] Thin-section CT in fact may be the best study, including operative exploration, to delineate resectability around the superior mesenteric vein.[20]

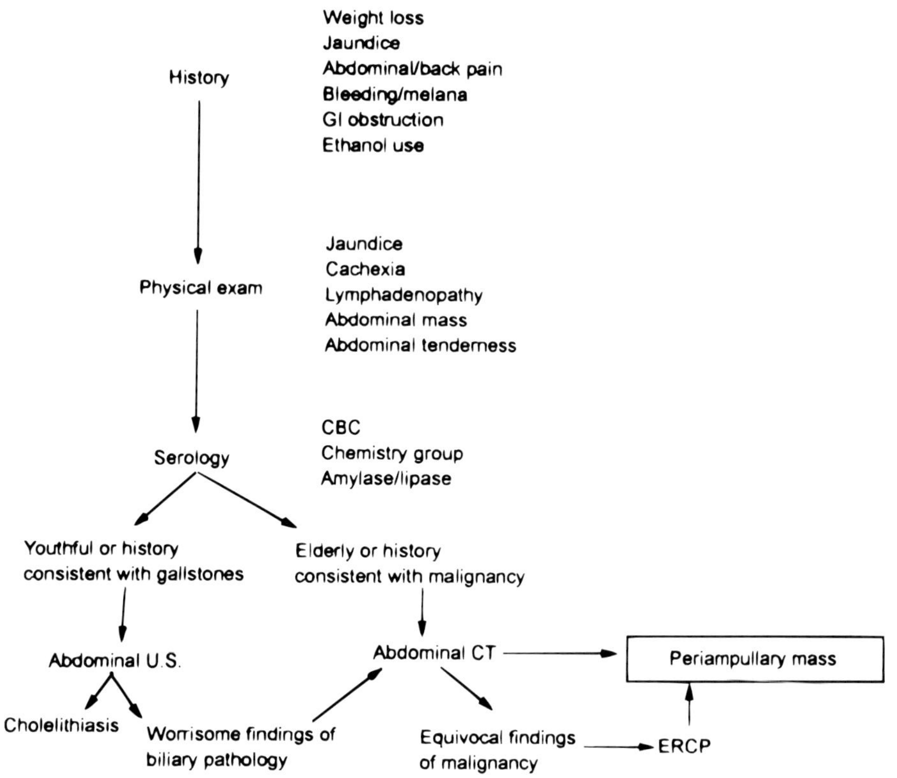

FIG. 32-1. Algorithm for diagnosis of a periampullary mass. *CBC,* complete blood count; *CT,* computed tomography; *ERCP,* endoscopic retrograde cholangiopancreatography; *GI,* gastrointestinal; *US,* ultrasound.

Although magnetic resonance imaging has proven of superior sensitivity in recognizing hepatic metastases in islet cell tumors, it has no significant advantage over CT in patients with periampullary neoplasms.

Angiography remains for us an expensive and invasive study that affords little or no additional information. Others, however, have used it routinely,[21,22] touting its ability both to stage pancreatic cancer and identify anatomic vascular anomalies of the pancreatohepatic axis; others use it selectively in reoperative settings.[20] Although angiography delineates the vascular anatomy and shows an abnormality in 34% of patients,[23] the assessment of tumor invasion of vascular structures lacks specificity, and the delineation of vascular anomalies rarely alters the surgical approach for the experienced pancreatic surgeon.[24] For instance, a replaced left hepatic artery should be immediately evident, but in (and of) itself does not affect the operation. A replaced right hepatic artery arising from the superior mesenteric artery should be evident by the presence of an arterial pulse posteriorly in the hepatoduodenal ligament and can be easily preserved during a conventional pancreatoduodenectomy. Angiography is not useful in evaluating tumor size, location, or lymph node involvement.[25]

Endoscopic retrograde cholangiopancreatography also has a controversial role in evaluating periampullary tumors and the proximal (hepatic) extent of the biliary obstruction imaged successfully by CT (or ultrasonography). Internists tout its diagnostic and palliative capabilities because pancreatograms are normal in only 3% of all patients with pancreatic cancer, whereas surgeons note the potential morbidity and mortality of this procedure, especially if it fails to add information that would alter management.[19] We agree with the *Policy and Procedure Manual* of the American Society for Gastrointestinal Endoscopy, which states, ''Endoscopic retrograde cholangiopancreatography is generally not indicated as further evaluation of pancreatic malignancy which has been demonstrated by ultrasonography or CT *unless* management will be altered.''[26] Use of an endoscopic approach for palliative endobiliary stenting in inoperable situations or for securing the diagnosis in patients with atypical findings on CT is warranted, but the over-liberal use of ERCP for the purpose of preoperative biliary stenting is of no benefit, as has been confirmed repeatedly[27–29]; moreover, colonization of the biliary tree occurs, leading to bacterobilia and a greater risk of postoperative sepsis. We have found ERCP of the most benefit in the patient with a periampullary mass and a history of pancreatitis. Interestingly, pancreatic duct aspiration for cytologic sampling of ductal epithelium for malignancy has proven sensitive in 76%, with a specificity approaching 100%.[30] Use of molecular biology techniques to look for genetic abnormalities may also be of potential diagnostic benefit in recognizing early lesions (see discussion earlier). Used selectively, ERCP is beneficial in managing selected patients with periampullary masses, but its routine use with occasional sphincterotomy and endobiliary stenting and its associated risks of pancreatitis (1% to 7%), hemorrhage (1% to 2%), and duodenal perforation (1% to 4%) is unacceptable and unjustified.[31]

Newer imaging modalities of scintigraphy with positron emission tomography scanning, radiolabeled antibodies, and pancreatic duct endoscopy may prove useful, but experience is limited, and the tests remain expensive.[10] Endoscopic ultrasonography appears to offer potentially important information in preoperative staging. *Invasion* of the retropancreatic superior mesenteric vein/portal vein junction by pancreatic cancer, as opposed to just displacement or compression, appears to be better visualized by endoscopic ultrasonography. Possibly endoscopic ultrasonography should be reserved for the patient in whom CT suggests vascular compression or invasion, or close proximity by the mass.

Fine-Needle Aspiration

Fine-needle aspiration is an excellent study to obtain with relative safely an objective tissue diagnosis. It is the diagnostic study of choice if radiologic imaging shows the periampullary lesion to be unresectable, and palliative operative intervention is not needed or contraindicated because of medical comorbidity precluding exploration for resection. Although some use fine-needle aspiration reluctantly because of the concern of tumor dissemination,[32,33] we agree that CT-guided fine-needle aspiration of the pancreas is a safe, accurate, and minimally invasive way to obtain a definitive diagnosis in unresectable patients who will not need palliative operative bypass and who are candidates for palliative radiation therapy or chemotherapy. To prevent possible tumor dissemination, Warshaw and Fernandez-del Castillo[10] have advised low-dose radiation (10 Gy) before fine-needle aspiration, but such a strategy is unfounded. With experience, cytopathologists are expert in obtaining the histologic diagnosis if the tumor has been accurately sampled. There appears to be *no justification* for its use in patients who are going to undergo exploration for potential resection.[19]

Preoperative Laparoscopy

Laparoscopy before aggressive exploration is currently fashionable. Warshaw, Cuschieri, and others[21,33–35] have used laparoscopy with peritoneal washings in patients with resectable-appearing tumors by CT and angiography. They have shown that 40% to 70% of patients with no findings of unresectable metastatic disease on radiologic examination will have small distant metastases seen on laparoscopy.[34] Similarly, 12 of 40 patients (30%) with tumors deemed resectable by CT will have positive cytologic findings on peritoneal washings,[21] which confers a dismal prognosis. Only one such patient had a ''resectable'' tumor. Unlike CT (45%) and angiography (54%), laparoscopy appears to be a reasonable study to identify resectable pancreatic tumors (90% resectable if laparoscopy findings favorable). Laparoscopic accuracy at defining unresectability was 89%, compared with 92% for CT and 95% for angiography.

Laparoscopic ultrasonography has been used to help identify favorable tumors to resect. In a small study of 12 patients, Murugiah and associates[36] were able to resect six pancreatic neoplasms found to be free of distant disease. Routine laparoscopic evaluation identified four patients with distant metastatic disease, including four with hepatic metastases, two with peritoneal metastases, and one with malignant ascites. Two other patients proved to be unresectable by the findings of laparoscopic ultrasonography. Overall, laparoscopic ultrasonography identified four patients with additional findings: hepatic metastases (four), worrisome peripancreatic lymph nodes (four), local invasion beyond the pancreas (two), and portal vein involvement (four). One patient was identified correctly with an anomalous origin of the superior mesenteric artery.

Our own approach has been to refrain from routine laparoscopic exploration because, except in select patients, findings of small distant metastases in the patient with an excellent performance status will not necessarily change our suggested treatment; that is, we do not believe that endoscopic endobiliary stenting provides as effective and long-lasting palliation and superior quality of life as does operative biliary bypass in patients with a good performance status who are expected to live longer than 6 months. With this management bias, the findings at laparoscopy are not used to determine management and thus the test is redundant. In the future, the use of preoperative ''neoadjuvant'' protocols of chemotherapy plus radiation therapy[37,38] may prove of benefit—if so, then diagnostic laparoscopy will be able to select appropriate candidates for this treatment approach before exploration for resection.

OPERATIVE MANAGEMENT

With a clinically resectable neoplasm in an otherwise healthy patient, the decision for exploratory celiotomy should be straightforward. In contrast, borderline radiographic findings, poor patient performance status, unusual patient history, or absent signs of malignant disease make the decision for formal celiotomy more difficult. Despite health care reform in this country, which often advises us that less is better than more, we remain committed to celiotomy with resection or bypass as indicated to provide the patient with the greatest chance of cure or palliation of symptoms to provide the best quality of remaining life. In our hands, such an approach translates to Whipple resection if possible, palliative biliary or enteric bypass if indicated, and celiac axis block. The reasoning for such a scheme is logical (Fig. 32-2).

Whipple Resection

The Whipple resection (pancreatoduodenectomy) for periampullary malignancies remains the gold standard of therapy no matter the etiology—bile duct, ampulla, duodenal, or pancreatic. It remains a good operation even for worrisome masses that turn out to be associated with chronic pancreatitis.[39] We concur with Carter, who states, ''When in doubt, regard the Whipple operation as the most effective and reliable method of providing the pathologist with a biopsy of the head of the pancreas.''[40] We advocate this ''radical'' approach because the only chance for ''cure'' or for prolonged palliation is resection. Moreover, although most periampullary neoplasms are pancreatic ductal cancers, a ''resectable'' periampullary neoplasm increases the likelihood of this being a nonpancreatic primary and thus confers a much greater chance of cure. After a full abdominal exploration reveals no evidence of distant peritoneal or hepatic metastasis, a wide-extended Kocher maneuver with takedown of the ligament of Treitz is performed, and biopsy

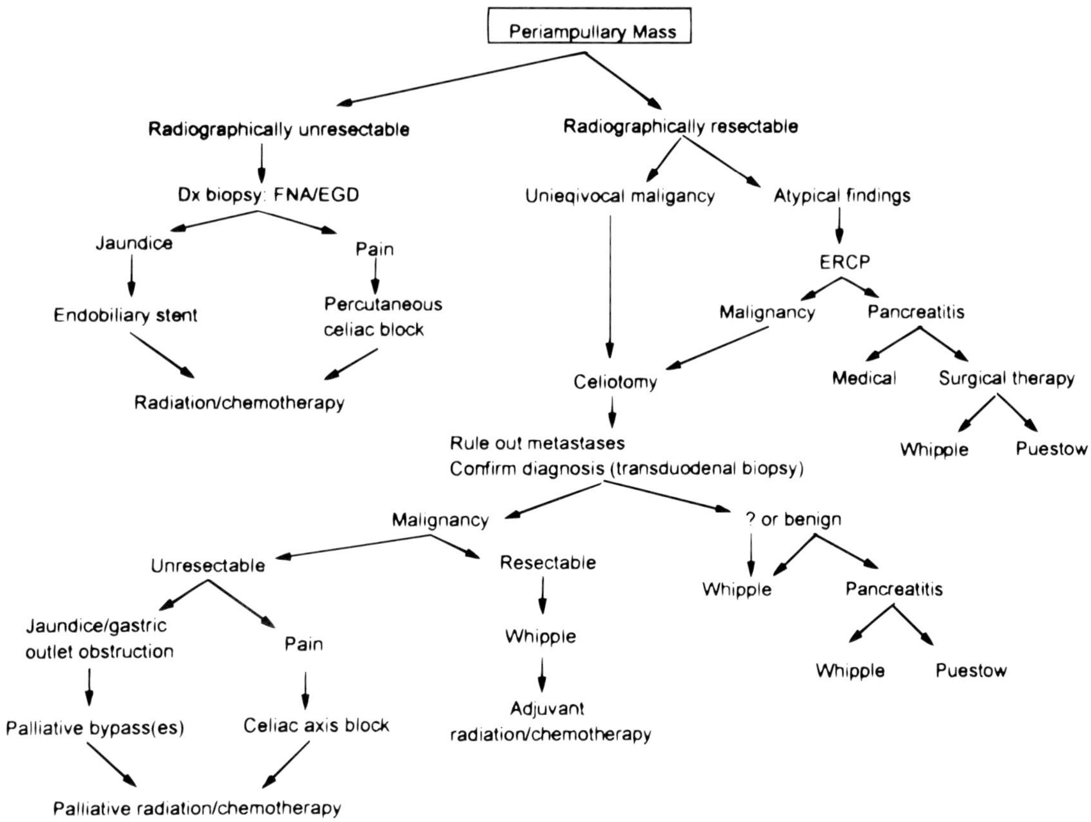

FIG. 32-2. Therapeutic algorithm for a periampullary mass. *FNA,* fine-needle aspiration; *EGD,* esophagogastroduodenoscopy; *ERCP,* endoscopic retrograde cholangiopancreatography.

specimens of palpable adenopathy outside the confines of planned resection (hepatoduodenal ligament, superior pancreatic and celiac axis, base of small bowel mesentery) are taken and sent for frozen-section analysis. Mobilizing the backside of the neck of the pancreas off the superior mesenteric vessels is the final step before confirming "resectability." At this point, with no evidence of advanced disease, the neoplasm, whether benign or malignant, can be safely resected.

The operative mortality for the Whipple procedure is less than 4% in experienced hands.[4,41,42] Significant morbidity, however, still occurs in up to 50% of patients.[43] Survival for all periampullary masses is contingent on several factors: the primary origin of tumor, vascular or lymphatic invasion (macrometastasis and micrometastasis), and tumor grade.[42,44] Despite evidence of negative factors of survival and the overall poor outlook for this group of patients as a whole, we have no data that support the idea that resecting fewer tumors affords greater survival. Therefore, we advise resection if possible because it remains the only true chance for cure. If the neoplasm is resectable, the Whipple procedure affords 5-year survivals of 90% or more for masses associated with pancreatitis, 30% to 50% for duodenal or periampullary cancers, 10% to 20% for cholangiocarcinoma, and 5% to 20% for pancreatic cancer. Glucose control is retained in approximately 90% and exocrine function is preserved in nearly 75% with this procedure.[45]

Alternatives to Whipple Resection

Reasonable alternatives to Whipple resection exist in selected patients. Total pancreatectomy, pylorus-preserving pancreaticoduodenectomy (PPPD), and extensive nodal dissection with pancreaticoduodenectomy (R2 or R3) have been adopted as standard therapy by other groups. Total pancreatectomy has been advocated by Moosa and Davies,[46] among others,[47] as a better cancer operation affording wider soft tissue margins and nodal clearance (and avoiding a pancreatic anastomosis). Brooks and others[48] have claimed that cancers of the head of the pancreas are associated with multicentric disease distant to the primary mass in up to 34% of patients. More recent work by Kloppel and colleagues[49] has challenged this concept of multicentricity, suggesting that the "multicentricity" does not involve invasive ductal carcinoma or even carcinoma in situ, but rather a ductal hyperplasia, the significance of which is unknown. Despite the proposed benefits of total pancreatectomy, it has not been proven to provide any better long-term survival than a Whipple resection.[45] The loss of pancreatic endocrine and exocrine function coupled with the morbidity of splenectomy and higher incidence of marginal ulceration makes total pancreatectomy less acceptable for most patients.[50] Total pancreatectomy is warranted, however, in several selective situations, including when the pancreatic anastomosis is unsafe; the pathologic pancreatic margin is involved with tumor or carcinoma in situ; mucinous ductal ectasia of the entire ducts exists[51]; and when patients have a strongly defined family history of pancreatic cancer.[52] Preoperative pancreatic insufficiency is a relative indication for total pancreatectomy, but the lack of intraportal glucagon and other islet cell regulatory peptides after total pancreatectomy may be as important physiologically as the loss of insulin in causing serious and potentially fatal metabolic sequelae,[45] including steatohepatitis and even cirrhosis.

Pylorus-preserving pancreaticoduodenectomy was first described in 1944. Devised to help preserve more normal gastrointestinal function, at least 52% of all patients have delayed gastric emptying requiring nasogastric decompression for more than 1 week after PPPD.[53] More important, Moosa and Davies[46] and others[53] maintain that PPPD may not allow adequate resection of periampullary tumors. Roder and coworkers[54] noted significantly better survival ($P < 0.05$) in patients having Whipple resection than in those undergoing PPPD for pancreatic cancer, but Grace and colleagues[55] found no statistical difference in survival in a large review of the literature. Some data suggest a better long-term nutritional status after PPPD. We continue to prefer Whipple resection to PPPD for the advantage of wider resection margins along the duodenum and a lesser incidence of marginal ulceration.[50]

Fortner[56] has been an advocate of aggressive resections in the face of advanced periampullary cancer (Fortner I involves resection of the pancreatic head along with a segment of portal vein; Fortner II similarly involves resection of tumor-encased arteries with the specimen). Such aggressive resections, however, do not appear to improve survival. Similarly, although much has been published about extended en bloc lymph node dissections (so-called R1, R2, and R3 resections), Satake and colleagues[57] found no overall survival benefit for 57 patients undergoing R2 resection compared with 72 patients undergoing Whipple resection. Although the ability to resect for curative intent was markedly better with R2 resection in stage III and IV disease, clinically there proved to be no long-term survival advantage. Obviously, small tumors confined to the pancreas or periampullary region (stage I) remain the most curable tumors. Although tumors less than 3.0 cm in size frequently remain clinically curable, microscopic extension to neural, lymphatic, and vascular structures is often prominent. Kayahara and associates[58] note that "curative resections" have only 1- to 2-mm margins, and small pancreatic tumors are not necessarily early lesions. Because retropancreatic spread occurs early, they advise extensive nodal dissection in all patients. We agree that the ability to diagnose periampullary malignancy usually occurs after the presence of nodal extension. Cubilla and colleagues[59] reported that 19 of 22 patients undergoing Whipple resection for pancreatic cancer had positive lymph nodes. Indeed, multiple studies have shown that aggressive resection is indicated for early pancreatic cancer (small tumors *confined* to the pancreas, free of nodal, neural, or vascular involvement).[60] However, as Trede, Cameron and colleagues[4,61] have shown, the standard pancreaticoduodenectomy in properly selected patients can be done safely (<2% mortality) with long-term success (5-year survival rate of 20% to 25%). Disease beyond the confines of a standard Whipple resection foreshadows short survival, and resection for metastatic tumor has always been contraindicated.

Palliation

Most patients with a mass in the head of the pancreas are beyond the possibility of resection for cure. Therefore, surgeons and physicians alike should acknowledge their predominant role of providing optimal palliation (as opposed to resection) in most patients with pancreatic cancer. Operative palliation must be considered carefully, because celiotomy with palliative bypass(es) carries a 30-day operative mortality of up to 10%. Operative palliation of jaundice and gastric outlet obstruction is effective, but should be undertaken only for patients with a good performance status who are able to tolerate general anesthesia and with some expectation of living more than several months.

Biliary decompression can be obtained percutaneously, endoscopically, or surgically. Decompression before planned surgical intervention is of no benefit,[27–29] and its routine use should be terminated.[19] Percutaneous transhepatic drainage is an effective means of acute symptomatic palliation for elderly, ill patients unable to tolerate operative bypass. Although complications of bleeding, sepsis, or biliary leak are uncommon, the external drain is inconvenient and nutritionally depleting. Therefore, conversion to either a percutaneous internal drainage or to an endoprosthesis should be undertaken. A primary endoscopic approach to placement of a biliary stent is usually recommended over a transhepatic approach. Endoscopic placement is less uncomfortable, avoids an external drainage tube (even if only transiently), and avoids the potential morbidity of a transhepatic puncture approach. In contrast, endoscopic biliary stents require a sphincterotomy and may not be technically possible in patients with advanced disease. In this situation, a combined percutaneous transhepatic and endoscopic tandem technique may prove the best means for nonoperative placement of an endoprosthesis.

Several randomized, prospective trials found no difference in survival between endobiliary or external biliary stent placement and surgical bypass for patients with malignancy causing obstructive jaundice.[62–65] Patients with endoscopic stents required more frequent readmission for stent occlusion with recurring jaundice and cholangitis. Our preference for operative palliation of jaundice in the good-risk patient stems from four benefits it provides: establishment or confirmation of the unresectable disease process; a more durable long-term palliation of jaundice without requiring multiple stent changes; the ability to palliate established or impending duodenal obstruction; and palliation of back pain associated with malignancy.

Therefore, otherwise healthy (Eastern Cooperative Oncology Group performance status 0 or 1) but *symptomatic* patients with unresectable tumors of the periampullary region should undergo surgical biliary bypass. Operative bypass appears to be a better means of palliation.[66] The best method, but also the most involved procedure, involves a side-to-side Roux-en-Y hepaticojejunostomy. This procedure is performed far distant from the site of future tumor progression within the biliary tree, and long-term palliation of biliary obstruction is therefore conferred.[67] Younger patients or patients with longer expected survival tolerate the procedure well and avoid the complications of "lesser" biliary bypasses.[66] Bringing up a loop of jejunum (as opposed to a Roux-en-Y limb) to create a simple side-to-side hepaticojejunostomy is quick and often successful,[67] but it may be technically more difficult, and anastomotic leaks subsequently involve both biliary and gastrointestinal tracts.

Cholecystojejunostomy is a quick and easy method for biliary diversion and may be favored for selected patients. The incidence of cholangitis and recurrent jaundice, however, approaches 10% to 15% after this procedure related to cystic duct occlusion from local tumor progression. Such complications after choledochoenteric bypass are rare. The 30-day operative mortality for both procedures is approximately 5% to 10%. Although cholecystojejunostomy is performed more frequently,[7] knowledge that the cystic duct enters the common bile duct quite distally in 10% of humans[68] should mandate confirmatory intraoperative cholangiography with this procedure. Several authors have found that in a significant percentage of patients after cholecystoenteric bypass, recurrent obstructive jaundice developed secondary to malignant cystic duct obstruction.[69–71] Choledochoduodenostomy has been advocated by several groups, but concerns about local tumor progression with subsequent anastomotic occlusion (estimated 20% to 40%) have been used to argue against this form of operative bypass in patients with periampullary malignancies. Therefore, in the good-risk patient, hepaticojejunostomy to a Roux-en-Y limb is the procedure of choice.

Up to 34% of patients undergoing palliative biliary bypass alone eventually have duodenal obstruction.[66] For this reason, some surgeons advocate routine duodenal bypass by means of a gastroenterostomy. Palliative gastrojejunostomy does not increase operative mortality, but delays hospital discharge in up to 20% of patients because of transient functional problems with gastric emptying in the early postoperative period.[72] Meinke and coworkers[73] defined the risk of subsequent gastric outlet obstruction to be greater than 25% if patients met two or more of the following criteria: age younger than 60 years, hemoglobin less than 11.5 g/dL, absence of liver metastases, presence of jaundice, and projected survival greater than 3 months. Not everyone believes enteric bypass is justified. Van der Schelling and colleagues[74] studied 142 patients with advanced cancer of the pancreatic head and noted that palliative or prophylactic gastrojejunostomy was associated with greater hospital morbidity; functional gastric outlet obstruction developed in 32 patients (23%), and 10 later had recurrent obstructive symptoms after palliative gastrojejunostomy. Our preference remains for the liberal use of prophylactic palliative gastrojejunostomy in younger patients with smaller tumors in whom a prolonged postoperative survival is expected (>6 months), or for palliative bypass either for impending obstruction or in the rare patient with symptoms or radiographic evidence of duodenal obstruction. The realization that in a sizable percentage of patients (20% to 30%) nausea and vomiting may be unrelated to frank obstruction is understood. A collective review of 1865 unresectable patients revealed that 13% required reoperation because of gastric outlet obstruction, and an additional 10% to 20% of patients were presumed to have died with duodenal obstruction that might have been prevented.[7]

Technical considerations for creating the palliative gastrojejunostomy in our opinion favor the antecolic isoperistaltic loop gastrojejunostomy, but good results have been reported by others with use of retrocolic approaches.[67] Although Roux-en-Y drainage minimizes intestinal reflux, the added time necessary, the extra anastomosis, the risk of anastomotic ulcer, and the brief expected survival negate any benefit of the Roux-en-Y configuration. One group has advocated antrectomy with gastrojejunostomy as a means of minimizing the postoperative gastric stasis that often complicates palliative or prophylactic duodenal bypass.[75]

Abdominal or back pain from malignancy can be devastating and debilitating. As early as 1908, Chauffard[76] pointed out that 50% to 90% of patients with pancreatic cancer experienced severe, incapacitating pain. Some 20% to 60% of patients experience relief of their pain solely with biliary or intestinal bypass. Intraoperative chemical splanchnicectomy (celiac plexus block) is expeditious and easy (Fig. 32-3). Injections of 20 to 30 mL of 50% ethanol or 6% phenol along both sides of the celiac

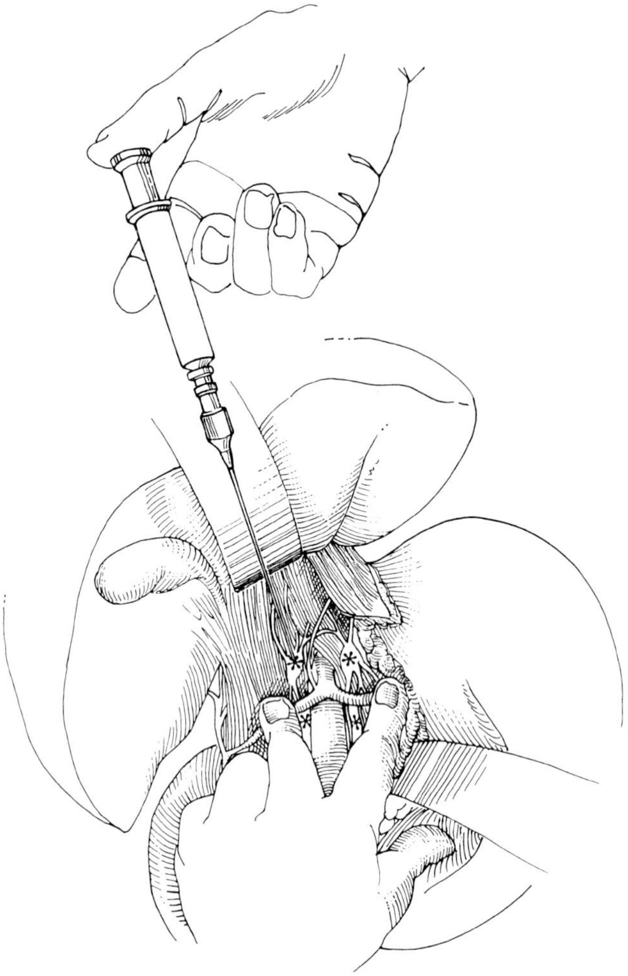

FIG. 32-3. Technique of celiac axis block. The retroperitoneal peritoneum is left intact over the celiac axis. The middle finger feels the pulse of the common hepatic artery and the index finger feels the splenic artery. Injections are made 10 mm above and below these fingers (stars on Figure). It is easiest to use a 20-gauge spinal needle.

axis afford significant relief in most patients. Flanigan and Kraft[77] found that greater than 80% of patients with chemical splanchnicectomy obtained immediate relief, and greater than 50% had permanent relief of pain. Recurrent discomfort can be managed with subsequent percutaneous chemical neurolysis of the celiac ganglion and possible radiation therapy[7,78] Lillemoe and colleagues[79] performed a prospective, randomized study of the use of chemical splanchnicectomy in patients with unresectable pancreatic cancer. Although their study confirmed the benefit in treating established pain and in preventing the development of future back pain, they also found surprisingly (and inexplicably) a greater survival as well. Because of its ease, safety, efficacy, and possible survival benefit, intraoperative celiac plexus block should be at least entertained in all patients with unresectable periampullary and pancreatic cancers.

ADDITIONAL THERAPY

Because the overall outlook for patients with periampullary cancers is dismal, preoperative, intraoperative, and postoperative adjuvant therapy should be considered. Studies have clearly shown survival benefit for the use of postoperative radiation and chemotherapy.[80,81] Intraoperative radiation therapy allows increased radiation dosage while minimizing tissue damage. Although considerable enthusiasm exists today in Europe and Japan for intraoperative radiation therapy, its superiority over external beam irradiation has not been established.[82,83] Preoperative neoadjuvant chemotherapy plus radiation therapy to improve curative resections has been recommended by some,[37,38] but confirmatory data remain elusive.

REFERENCES

1. Gudjonsson B, Levistone E, Spiro U. Pancreatic diagnostic accuracy and survival statistics. Cancer 1978;1:2494.
2. Michelassi F, Erroi F, Dawson PJ, et al. Experience with 647 consecutive tumors of the duodenum, ampulla, head of the pancreas, and distal common bile duct. Ann Surg 1989;210:544.
3. Geer RJ, Brennan MF. Prognostic indicators for survival after resection of pancreatic adenocarcinoma. Am J Surg 1993;165;68.
4. Crist DW, Sitzmann JV, Cameron JL. Improved hospital morbidity, mortality and survival after the Whipple procedure. Ann Surg 1987; 206:3:358.
5. England MD, Sarr MG. Metastatic melanoma: an unusual cause of obstructive jaundice. Surgery 1990;107:595.
6. Behrns KE, Sarr MG, Strickler JG. Pancreatic lymphoma: is it a surgical disease. Pancreas 1994;9:662.
7. Sarr MG, Cameron JL. Surgical management of unresectable carcinoma of the pancreas. Surgery 1982;91:123.
8. Bakkevold KE, Arnesjo B, Kambestad B. Carcinoma of the pancreas and papilla of Vater: assessment of resectability and factors influencing resectability in stage I carcinomas. A prospective multicentre trial in 472 patients. Eur J Surg Oncol 1992;18:494.
9. Gillen P, Peu ALG. Failure to improve survival by improved diagnostic techniques in patients with malignant jaundice. Br J Surg 1986;73:631.
10. Warshaw AL, Fernandez-del Castillo C. Pancreatic carcinoma. N Engl J Med 1992;326:455.
11. Gullo L, Pezzilli R, Morselli-Labate AM, and the Italian Pancreatic Cancer Study Group. Diabetes and the risk of pancreatic cancer. N Engl J Med 1994;331:81.
12. Parker N, Makin CA, Ching CK, et al. A new enzyme-linked lectin-mucin antibody sandwich assay (CAM17.1/WGA) assessed in combination with CA19-9 and peanut lectin binding assay for the diagnosis of pancreatic cancer. Cancer 1992;70:1062.
13. Pasanen PA, Eskelinen M, Partanen K, Pikkarainen P, Penttila I, Alhava E. Receiver operating characteristic (ROC) curve analysis of the tumor markers CEA, CA50, and CA242 in pancreatic cancer: results from a prospective study. Br J Cancer 1993;67:852.
14. Toshkov I, Mogaki M, Kazakoff K, Pour PM. The patterns of coexpression of tumor-associated antigens CA 19-9, TAG-72, and DU-PAN-2 in human pancreatic cancer. Int J Pancreatol 1994;15:97.
15. Frebourg T, Bercoff E, Manchon N, et al. The evaluation of CA 19-9 antigen level in the early detection of pancreatic cancer. Cancer 1988; 62:2287.
16. Robles-Diaz G, Diaz-Sanchez V, Mendez JP, Altamirano A, Wolpert E. Low serum testosterone/dihydrotestosterone ratio in patients with pancreatic carcinoma. Pancreas 1987;2:684.
17. Simon B, Weinel R, Hohne M, et al. Frequent alterations of the tumor suppressor genes p53 and DCC in human pancreatic carcinoma. Gastroenterology 1994;106:1645.
18. Freeny PC, Traverso LW, Ryan JA. Diagnosis and staging of pancreatic adenocarcinoma with dynamic computed tomography. Am J Surg 1993; 165:600.
19. Temudom T, Sarr MG, Douglas MG, Farnell MB. An argument against routine percutaneous biopsy, ERCP, or biliary stent in patients with clinically resectable periampullary masses: a surgical perspective. Pancreas 1995;11:283.
20. Tyler DS, Evans DB. Reoperative pancreaticoduodenectomy. Ann Surg 1994;219;2:211.
21. Warshaw AL, Gu Z-Y, Wittenberg J, Waltman AC. Preoperative stag-

ing and assessment of resectability of pancreatic cancer. Arch Surg 1990;125:230.
22. Dooley WC, Cameron JL, Pitt HA, Lillemoe KD, Yue NC, Venbrux AC. Is preoperative angiography useful in patients with periampullary tumors? Ann Surg 1990;211:649.
23. Rong GH, Sindelar WF. Aberrant peripancreatic arterial anatomy: considerations in performing pancreatectomy for malignant neoplasms. Ann Surg 1987;53:726.
24. Murugiah M, Windsor JA, Redhead DN, et al. The role of selective visceral angiography in the management of pancreatic and periampullary cancer. World J Surg 1993;17:796.
25. Mackie CR, Noble UG, Cooper MJ, Collins P, Block GE, Moosa AR. Prospective evaluation of angiography in the diagnosis and management of patients suspected of having pancreatic cancer. Ann Surg 1979; 189:11.
26. American Society for Gastrointestinal Endoscopy. Policy and procedure manual for gastrointestinal endoscopy: guidelines for training and practice, 1990. Manchester, MA: American Society for Gastrointestinal Endoscopy, 1990.
27. Pitt HA, Gomes AS, Lois JF, Mann LL, Deutsch LS, Longmire WP Jr. Does preoperative percutaneous biliary drainage reduce operative risk or increase hospital cost. Ann Surg 1985;201:545.
28. Hatfield ARW, Tobas R, Terblanche J, et al. Preoperative external biliary drainage in obstructive jaundice: a prospective controlled clinical trial. Lancet 1982;2:896.
29. McPherson GAD, Benjamin IS, Hodgson HJF, Bowley NB, Allison DJ, Blumgart LH. Preoperative percutaneous transhepatic biliary drainage: the results of a controlled trial. Br J Surg 1984;71:371.
30. Nakaizumi A, Tatsuta M, Vehara H, et al. Cytologic examination of pure pancreatic juice in the diagnosis of pancreatic carcinoma: the endoscopic retrograde introduction catheter aspiration cytologic technique. Cancer 1992;70:2610-2614.
31. Sarr MG, Fishman EK, Milligan FD, Siegelman SS, Cameron JL. Pancreatitis or duodenal perforation after peri-Vaterian therapeutic endoscopic procedures: diagnosis, differentiation, and management. Surgery 1986;100:461.
32. Willett CG, Lewandowski K, Warshaw AL, Efird J, Compton CC. Resection margins in carcinoma of the head of the pancreas: implications for radiation therapy. Ann Surg 1993;217:144.
33. Warshaw AL. Implications of peritoneal cytology for staging of early pancreatic cancer. Am J Surg 1991;161:26.
34. Warshaw AL, Tepper JE, Shipley WV. Laparoscopy in the staging and planning of therapy for pancreatic cancer. Am J Surg 1986;151:76.
35. Cuschieri A. Laparoscopy for pancreatic cancer: does it benefit the patient. Eur J Surg Oncol 1988;14:41.
36. Murugiah M, Paterson-Brown S, Windsor J, Miles W, Garden OM. Early experience of laparoscopic ultrasonography in the management of pancreatic carcinoma. Surg Endosc 1993;7:177.
37. Yeung RS, Weese JL, Hoffman JP, et al. Neoadjuvant chemoradiation in pancreatic and duodenal carcinoma: a phase II study. Cancer 1993; 72:2124.
38. Evans DB, Rich TA, Byrd DR, et al. Preoperative chemoradiation and pancreticoduodenectomy for adenocarcinoma of the pancreas. Arch Surg 1992;127:1335.
39. Stone WM, Sarr MG, Nagorney DM, McIlrath DC. Chronic pancreatitis: results of Whipple resection and total pancreatectomy. Arch Surg 1988;123:815.
40. Carter DC. Cancer of the head of pancreas or chronic pancreatitis?: a diagnostic dilemma. Surgery 1992;111:602.
41. Trede M, Schwall G, Saeger HD. Survival after pancreatoduodenectomy. Ann Surg 1990;211:447.
42. Nitecki SS, Sarr MG, Colby TV, van Heerden JA. Long-term survival after resection for ductal adenocarcinoma of the pancreas: is it really improving? Ann Surg 1995;221:59.
43. Miedema BW, Sarr MG, van Heerden JA, Nagorney DM, McIlrath DC, Ilstrup D. Complications following pancreaticoduodenectomy: current management. Arch Surg 1992;127:945.
44. Monson JRT, Donohue JH, McEntee GP, et al. Radical resection for carcinoma of the ampulla of Vater. Arch Surg 1991;126:353.
45. Sarr MG, Behrns KE, van Heerden JA. Total pancreatectomy: an objective analysis of its use in pancreatic cancer. Hepatogastroenterology 1993;40:418.
46. Moosa AR, Davies R. Pancreatic cancer. In: Moody FG, ed. Surgical treatment of digestive disease. 2nd ed. Chicago: Year Book Medical Publishers, 1990:528.
47. Ihse I, Lilja P, Arnesjo B, Bengmark S. Total pancreatectomy for cancer: an appraisal of 65 cases. Ann Surg 1977;186:675.
48. Collins JJ, Craighead JE, Brooks JR. Rationale for total pancreatectomy for carcinoma of the pancreatic head. N Engl J Med 1966;274:599.
49. Kloppel G, Lohse T, Bosslet K, Ruckert K. Ductal adenocarcinoma of the head of the pancreas: incidence of tumor involvement beyond the Whipple resection line: histologic and immunocytochemical analysis of 37 total pancreatectomy specimens. Pancreas 1987;2:170.
50. Grant CS, van Heerden JA. Anastomotic ulceration following subtotal and total pancreatectomy. Ann Surg 1979;190:1.
51. Rickaert F, Cremer M, Deviere J, et al. Intraductal mucin-hypersecreting neoplasms of the pancreas: a clinicopathologic study of eight patients. Gastroenterology 1991;101:512.
52. Lynch HT, Fusaro L, Lynch JF. Familial pancreatic cancer: a family study. Pancreas 1992;7:511.
52a. Braasch JW, Rossi RL, Watkins E, Deziel DJ, Winter PF. Pyloric and gastric preserving pancreatic resection: experience with 87 patients. Ann Surg 1986;204:411.
53. Sharp KW, Ross CB, Walter SA, et al. Pancreatoduodenectomy with pyloric preservation for carcinoma of the pancreas: a cautionary note. Surgery 1989;105:645.
54. Roder JD, Stein HJ, Huttl W, Siewert JR. Pylorus-preserving versus standard pancreaticoduodenectomy: an analysis of 110 pancreatic and periampullary carcinomas. Br J Surg 1992;79:152.
55. Grace PA, Pitt HA, Longmire WP. Pylorus-preserving pancreatoduodenectomy: an overview. Br J Surg 1990;77:968.
56. Fortner JG. Pancreatectomy for cancer of the pancreas, ampulla and other related sites. Ann Surg 1984;199:418.
57. Satake K, Nishiwaki H, Yokomatsu U, et al. Surgical curability and prognosis for standard versus extended resection for T_1 carcinoma of the pancreas. Surg Gynecol Obstet 1992;175;259.
58. Kayahara M, Nagakawa T, Ueno K, Ohta T, Takeda T, Miyazaki I. An evaluation of radical resection for pancreatic cancer based on the mode of recurrence as determined by autopsy and diagnostic imaging. Cancer 1993;72:2118.
59. Cubilla AL, Fitzgerald PJ, Fortner JG. Pancreas cancer–duct cell adenocarcinoma: survival in relation to site, size, stage, and type of therapy. J Surg Oncol 1978;10:465.
60. Nagakawa T, Kobayashi H, Ueno K, et al. The pattern of lymph node involvement in carcinoma of the head of the pancreas. Int J Pancreatol 1993;13:15.
61. Trede M, Schwall G, Saeger H-D. Survival after pancreatoduodenectomy: 118 consecutive resections without an operative mortality. Ann Surg 1990;211:447.
62. Andersen JR, Sorensen SM, Kruse A, Rokkjaer M, Matzen P. Randomised trial of endoscopic endoprosthesis versus operative bypass in malignant obstructive jaundice. Gut 1989;30:1132.
63. Shepherd HA, Royle G, Ross APR, Arthur M, Colin-Jones D. Endoscopic biliary endoprosthesis in the palliation of malignant obstruction of the distal common bile duct: a randomized trial. Br J Surg 1988; 75:1166.
64. Bornman PC, Harries-Jones R, VanStiegman G, Terblanche J. Prospective controlled trial of transhepatic biliary endoprosthesis versus bypass surgery for incurable carcinoma of the head of the pancreas. Lancet 1986;1:69.
65. Hatfield ARW. Palliation of malignant obstructive jaundice: surgery or stent. Gut 1990;31:1339.
66. Sarr MG, Cameron JL. Surgical palliation of unresectable carcinoma of the pancreas. World J Surg 1984;8:906.
67. Watanapa P, Williamson RCN. Single-loop biliary and gastric bypass for irresectable pancreatic carcinoma. Br J Surg 1993;80:237.
68. Howard JM, Jordan GL Jr. Surgical diseases of the pancreas. Philadelphia: JB Lippincott, 1960.
69. Blievernicht SW, Neifeld JP, Terz JJ, Lawrence KW Jr. The role of prophylactic gastrojejunostomy for unresectable periampullary carcinoma. Surg Gynecol Obstet 1980;151:794.
70. Elmslie RG, Slavotinek AH. Surgical objectives in unresected cancer of the head of the pancreas. Br J Surg 1972;59:508.
71. Richards AB, Chir M, Sosin H. Cancer of the pancreas: the value of radical and palliative surgery. Ann Surg 1973;177:325.
72. Sarr MG, Gladen HE, Beart RW Jr, and van Heerden JA. Role of

gastroenterostomy in patients with unresectable carcinoma of the pancreas. Surg Gynecol Obstet 1981;152:597.
73. Meinke WB, Twomey PL, Guernsey JM, Frey CF, Higgins G, Keehn R. Gastric outlet obstruction after palliative surgery for cancer of the head of the pancreas. Arch Surg 1983;118:550.
74. van der Schelling GP, van den Bosch RP, Klinkenoij JHG, Mulder P, Jeckel J. Is there a place for gastroenterostomy in patients with advanced cancer of the head of the pancreas. World J Surg 1993;17:128.
75. Lucas CE, Ledgerwood AM, Bender JS. Antrectomy with gastrojejunostomy for unresectable pancreatic cancer-causing duodenal obstruction. Surgery 1991;110:583.
76. Chauffard MA. Le cancer du corps du pancreas. Bulletin de l'Academe Medicine 1908;60:242.
77. Flanigan DP, Kraft RO. Continuing experience with palliative chemical splanchnicectomy. Arch Surg 1978;113:509.
78. Singh SM, Longmire WP Jr, Reber HA. Surgical palliation for pancreatic cancer: the UCLA experience. Ann Surg 1990;212:132.
79. Lillemoe KD, Cameron JL, Kaufman HS, Yeo CJ, Pitt HA, Sauter PK. Chemical splanchnicectomy in patients with unresectable pancreatic cancer: a prospective randomized trial. Ann Surg 1993;217:447.
80. Gastrointestinal Tumor Study Group. Further evidence of effective adjuvant combined radiation and chemotherapy following curative resection of pancreatic cancer. Cancer 1987;59:2006.
81. Foo ML, Gunderson LL, Nagorney DM, et al. Patterns of failure in grossly resected pancreatic ductal adenocarcinoma treated with adjuvant irradiation ± 5 fluorouracil. Int J Radiat Oncol Biol Phys 1993; 26:483.
82. Dobelbower R Jr, Konski AA, Merrick UW III, Brown DG, Schifteling D, Kamen C. Intraoperative electron beam radiation therapy (IOEBRT) for carcinoma of the exocrine pancreas. Int J Radiat Oncol Biol Phys 1991;20:113.
83. Zerbi A, Fossati V, Parolini D, et al. Intraoperative radiation therapy adjuvant to resection in the treatment of pancreatic cancer. Cancer 1994;73:2930.

Surgery for Gastrointestinal Cancer: A Multidisciplinary Approach, edited by Harold J. Wanebo.
Lippincott-Raven Publishers, Philadelphia, © 1997.

CHAPTER 33

Diagnosis and Treatment of Cancers of the Ampulla, Terminal Bile Duct, and Duodenum: Indications for Pylorus-Preserving Pancreaticoduodenectomy

Edward H. Livingston and Ronald K. Tompkins

BACKGROUND

Carcinoma of the ampulla and terminal bile duct are infrequent tumors. Because of their early involvement of the bile duct, they present early in the course of the disease with jaundice. In contrast to pancreatic carcinoma, these tumors present as smaller lesions and are associated with a better long-term survival after resection. Duodenal tumors differ in that they characteristically do not present until they are much larger. Unless they originate close to the bile duct or ampulla, they may grow unnoticed for many months because the liquid content of the duodenum may pass by the tumor until it is nearly obstructing. These lesions have a poorer prognosis than ampulla and terminal bile duct cancers, but a better prognosis than pancreatic cancer.

HISTORY OF PYLORUS-PRESERVING RESECTION

Pylorus preservation for periampullary tumors dates back to Whipple's initial description of a pancreatic resection. In this initial report, a two-stage operation was described with a gastrojejunostomy, distal bile duct ligation, and cholecystogastrostomy being performed in the first stage (Fig. 33-1). The pancreatic resection was performed in a second stage with oversewing of the pylorus, leaving the antrum and pylorus as a blind stump.[1] Later reports of a one-stage procedure describe what has evolved into the "classic" Whipple resection that includes distal gastrectomy.[2,3] Complications of dumping, early satiety, and stomal ulceration at the gastrojejunostomy led Watson to perform the first pylorus-preserving pancreaticoduodenectomy (PPPD), in which the duodenum was anastomosed to the alimentary canal[4] (Fig. 33-2). Watson's patient, who had a carcinoma involving the papilla of Vater, underwent a two-stage procedure, the first stage being an antecolic cholecystojejunostomy. In the second stage, performed 35 days later, the head of the pancreas, most of the duodenum, and the distal bile duct were resected. Watson divided the duodenum 1 inch beyond the pylorus and divided the right gastric artery as well. The cut end of the pancreas was oversewn with four mattress sutures after the main and accessory pancreatic ducts were ligated. The loop of jejunum afferent to the previously constructed cholecystojejunostomy was divided 4 inches proximal to that anastomosis and this short segment was anastomosed end to end to the duodenum.

The patient's postoperative course was complicated by early bile fistula, and oral fluids that had been started in the first 12 hours were discontinued because of repeated vomiting. The second and third 12-hour periods were complicated by wound hemorrhage requiring two pints of blood transfusion. Oral fluids were again tried in the third 12-hour period, but vomiting resulted and oral fluids were stopped until the fourth 12-hour period, and the patient did not vomit until the next day (postoperative day 3). By postoperative day 5, the patient was vomiting less and peptonized milk alternating with water was given by mouth. By postoperative day 6 the patient was taking egg and milk. Daily morning stomach washouts had shown residual fluids of 4 to 12 ounces. However, by the 9th postoperative day the patient began vomiting again and this increased to the 15th

Edward H. Livingston, Assistant Professor of Surgery and Assistant Dean, UCLA School of Medicine, Assistant Chief of Surgery, VA Medical Center, West Los Angeles, 10833 Le Conte Avenue, Los Angeles, CA 90095-6904

Ronald K. Tompkins, Professor and Chief, Gastrointestinal Surgery, UCLA School of Medicine, 10833 Le Conte Avenue, CA 90095-6904

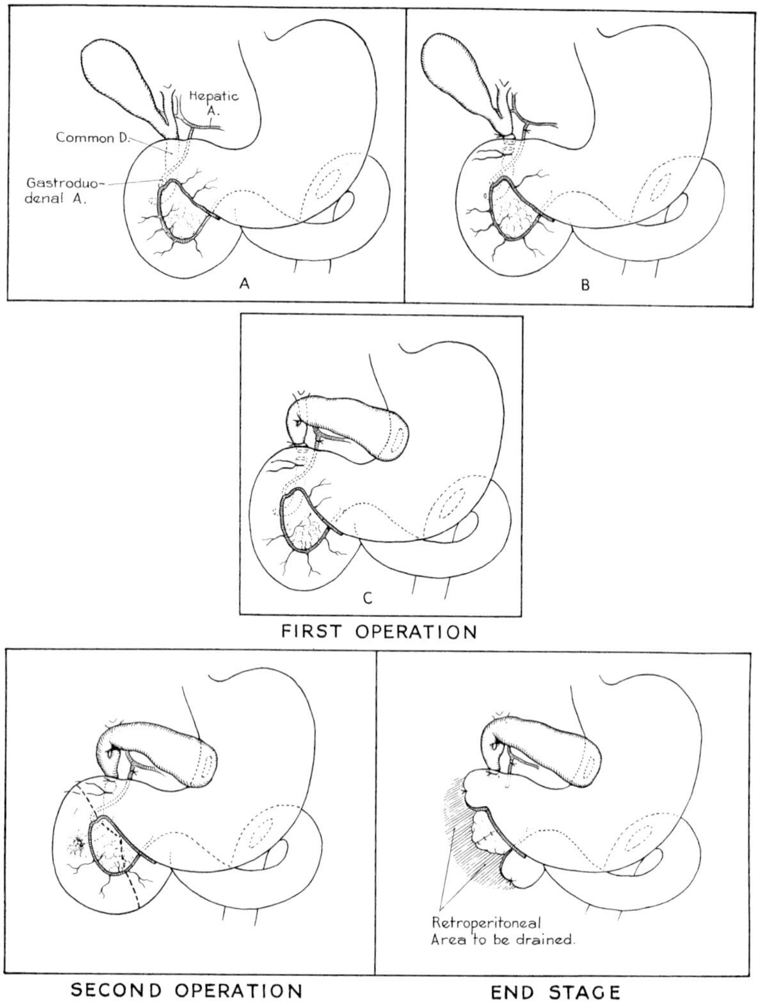

FIG. 33-1. Pancreaticoduodenectomy as first described by Whipple. (Whipple AO, Parsons WB, Mullens CT. Treatment of carcinoma of the ampulla of Vater. Ann Surg 1935;102:763.)

postoperative day, when a Witzel jejunostomy was surgically placed. On the 18th postoperative day, a barium upper gastrointestinal study showed considerable gastric retention after 24 hours, and by the 22nd postoperative day reoperation was done to drain a subhepatic abscess. By the 26th postoperative day the jejunostomy tube was removed and the patient was taking semisolids by mouth. Six months after the second-stage procedure, the patient was doing housework and shopping and had gained 11 pounds.

Watson claimed ''distinct advantages'' for his two-stage pylorus-preserving technique: the first-stage procedure is limited and relieves biliary obstruction efficiently; and the second stage preserves the stomach intact, does not leave a long loop of jejunum exposed to acid, and should protect against anastomotic ulcer. In his discussion, he pointed out that the ''ideal operative treatment of ampullary carcinoma would be a one-stage block resection'' but that this was precluded by biliary obstruction, which was present in almost all patients.

However, Watson's report received little attention and the Whipple resection with distal gastrectomy became the standard operation. This was thought more adequately to ensure clear margins of resection as well as avoid stomal ulceration by performing a distal gastrectomy.[5–7] PPPD was reintroduced by Longmire and Traverso in 1978 in their report of two patients (one with chronic pancreatitis and the other with duodenal carcinoma) undergoing pancreatic resection (Fig. 33-3).[8,9] The rationale was to improve gastric function and reduce stomal ulceration by preserving the pylorus in those patients who did not appear to need a wide gastric margin.

DIAGNOSIS

The evaluation of these lesions is relatively straightforward. Patients with bile duct or ampullary lesions typically present with jaundice. Initial evaluation of jaundiced patients at this institution begins with *ultrasound*, which often does not demonstrate the lesion but invariably shows dilated bile ducts. Ultrasound has the advantages of being portable, requiring minimal, if any, patient preparation in the urgent setting, and not involving ionizing radiation. The ability to image bile duct tumors is limited, but the presence of a ''common channel'' sign on ultrasound is suggestive of malignant obstruction. The common channel is characterized by a thin-walled, dilated gallbladder continuous with a dilated common bile duct--an ultrasonic Courvoisier's sign (Fig. 33-4). One series found the sign present in 11 of 24 patients with surgical jaundice, all of whom proved to have malignant etiologies (6 with pancreatic and 5 with peri-

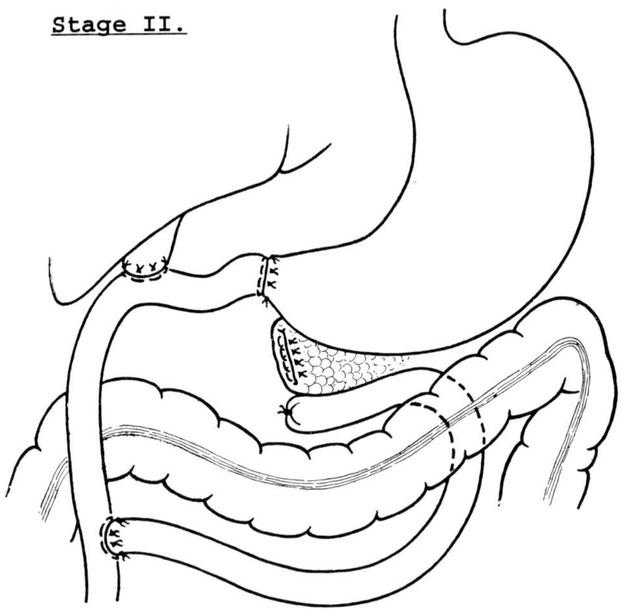

FIG. 33-2. Pylorus-preserving pancreaticoduodenectomy as described by Watson. (Watson K. Carcinoma of the ampulla of Vater: a successful radical resection. Br J Surg 1944;3331:368.)

ampullary carcinoma). Of the 13 jaundiced patients without the sign, only 2 had malignant disease.[10]

The next step in the evaluation of the jaundiced patient in this institution is to obtain a *cholangiogram*. If the ductal dilatation on ultrasound extends into the extrahepatic system and suggests a lower bile duct obstruction, an endoscopic retrograde cholangiogram is selected. In addition to the cholangiogram, this examination provides the best opportunity to observe the ampulla and duodenum as well as a mechanism to obtain biopsy specimens or cytologic brushings of the areas. In some poor-risk patients who are not deemed surgical candidates, endoscopic stenting may be carried out at the same procedure. In cases in which ultrasound shows only intrahepatic ductal dilatation, or the status of the extrahepatic bile duct cannot be determined, a cholangiogram by way of the percutaneous transhepatic route is selected. Lesions in the upper bile duct are discussed in other chapters.

Some authors have proposed that the jaundiced patient with malignant obstruction is better studied with an abdominal *computed tomography (CT) scan* with oral contrast.[11] If a mass in the pancreatic head is encountered without evidence of metastasis, further workup adds little and the patient should proceed to surgical exploration.[12] CT has an 85% to 90% sensitivity in the diagnosis of pancreatic carcinoma, and has the added advantage of evaluating the rest of the abdomen for metastatic disease. Although the diagnostic accuracy of CT for tumors of the bile duct, ampulla, and duodenum is less than that for pancreatic carcinoma, these tumors occasionally are seen on CT scan.

The future utility of CT scanning may be greatly enhanced by the advent of *helical (''spiral'') CT*, which has greater resolution capabilities not only for tumors but for vessels in the area (Fig. 33-5). Ongoing studies to evaluate this technology in diagnosis and staging should be completed in the near future.

Patients with duodenal carcinoma usually present with gastric obstruction or pain; however, those with disease involving the duodenum around the ampulla present with jaundice as well. Approximately 20% of these patients present with anemia, but acute gastrointestinal hemorrhage is unusual in our experience.[13] These symptoms typically were evaluated with a contrast upper gastrointestinal radiograph, but initial endoscopy

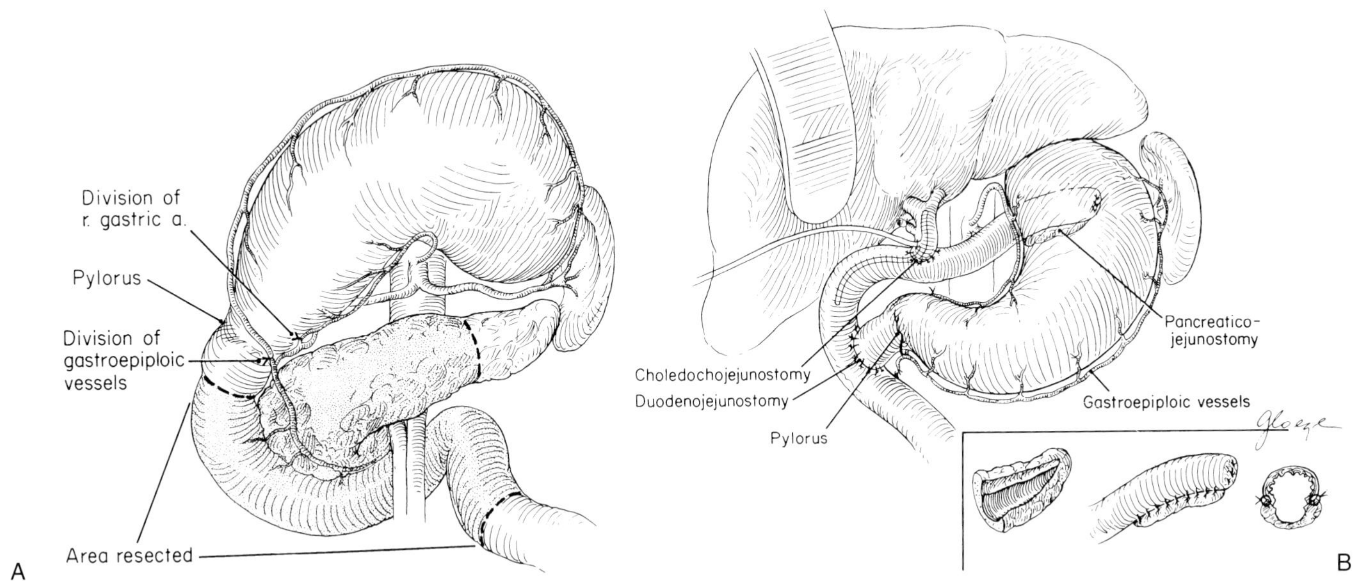

FIG. 33-3. (A) Pylorus-preserving pancreaticoduodenectomy as described by Traverso and Longmire. Dashed lines denote areas of the pancreas and duodenum to be resected. **(B)** Ligation of the right gastric and gastropyloric vessels preserves the vascular arcade on lesser and greater curvatures of the stomach, with an intact blood supply to pylorus and first portion of duodenum. (Traverso LW, Longmire WP Jr. Preservation of the pylorus in pancreaticoduodenectomy. Surg Gynecol Obstet 1978;146:959.)

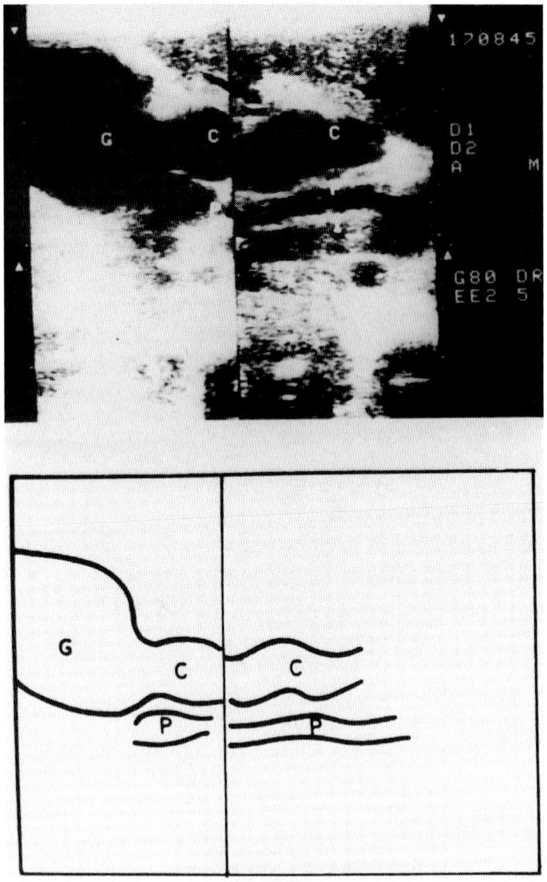

FIG. 33-4. Common channel sign suggestive of malignant bile duct obstruction. (Dwivedi M, Acharya SK, Tandon BN. The ultrasonographic "common channel" sign: a characteristic feature of malignant obstruction of the lower end of common bile duct. J Clin Gastroenterol 1989;11:233.)

with biopsy is now more frequently applied. It is important that the endoscopist examine the duodenum beyond the ampulla so as not to miss distal duodenal lesions. Preoperative CT scanning of the abdomen in these patients may be done to assess vessel invasion and metastatic disease. However, because these patients are often obstructed, surgery is most frequently required to palliate this symptom, even when metastatic disease is found.

The utility of *endoscopy* is increasing in the diagnosis of lesions of the ampulla, distal bile, duct and duodenum. Endoscopy is the most reliable method for diagnosing ampullary and duodenal tumors. In addition, *endoscopic retrograde cholangiopancreatography* may be performed to delineate the biliary and pancreatic ductal anatomy. Cytologic analysis of brushings from these ducts averages 40% in providing the correct diagnosis of biliary carcinomas. More recent studies of *endoscopic ultrasound* have been encouraging in the diagnosis of small lesions in the distal bile ducts. Accuracy rates of 84% to 88% in staging ampullary carcinoma have been reported.[14] In addition, some observers are able to detect metastases in lymph nodes around the periampullary region with this technology. Its proper use in the preoperative evaluation of patients with periampullary lesions remains to be shown by careful clinical trials.

Although some authors have proposed that any patient considered for a Whipple procedure should have preoperative *angiography*, this has not been the policy at the University of California, Los Angeles (UCLA) School of Medicine. It is an exceptional patient in our institution who requires preoperative evaluation by this technique. The use of *Doppler ultrasound* to evaluate the superior mesenteric and portal veins has been proposed as a less invasive technique than angiography.[15] However, we have not depended on this modality to rule out operation in any of our patients.

Magnetic resonance imaging scans, intravenous cholangiograms, or *radionuclide imaging* have not been helpful in the evaluation of these patients, and have the added disadvantage of being very expensive.

TREATMENT

On the basis of prospective, randomized trials at our institution as well as others, preoperative percutaneous biliary drainage has not been used.[16,17] Studies of preoperative drainage have shown no benefit in reducing operative mortality risk, but have demonstrated a higher morbidity risk, including serious postoperative infectious complications.[15] In addition, reports of seeding of the tube tract by malignant cells have raised additional concerns regarding preoperative intubation.[18]

There has been no conclusive physiologic advantage demonstrated for either of the two major procedures, PPPD or standard Whipple resection. Both appear to have similar outcomes in terms of nutrition and survival rate. Technical details for the Whipple resection are presented in other chapters. Many surgeons claim that PPPD is technically less demanding than the standard Whipple procedure, and this may be the main reason

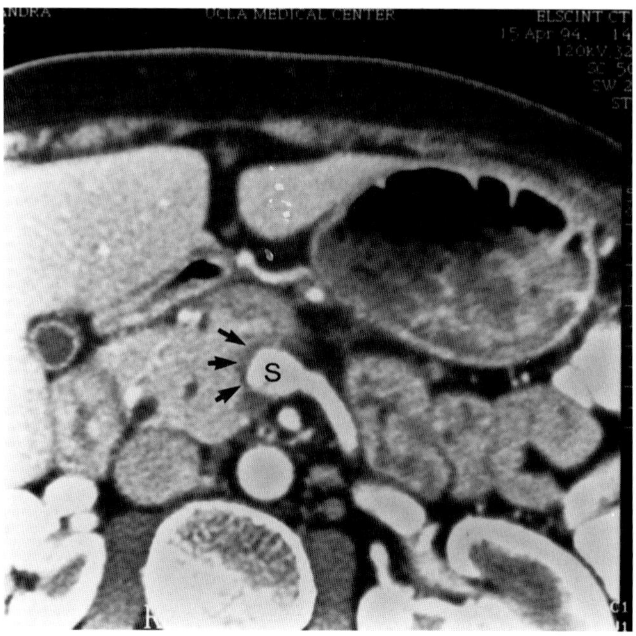

FIG. 33-5. Spiral (helical) computed tomography image of pancreatic tumor *(arrows)* surrounding superior mesenteric vein (S). This detail was not seen on conventional computed tomography scan in this patient. Tumor was unresectable at operation.

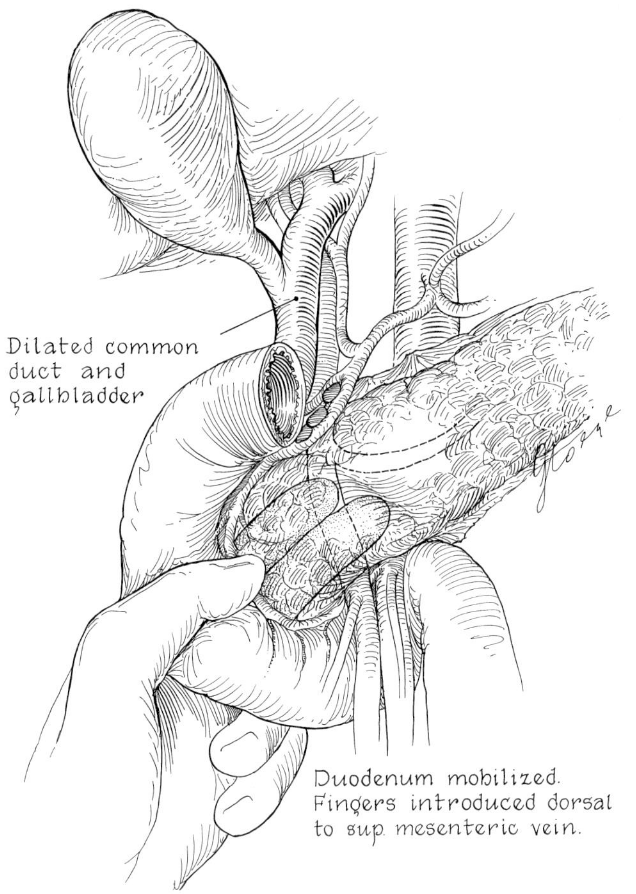

FIG. 33-6. Extended Kocher maneuver. The hepatic flexure of the colon, the duodenum, and the head of the pancreas are completely mobilized. This enables palpation of the periampullary area to assess resectability, but, more important, enables compression and control of the portal vein between the thumb and fingers in the event it is injured. (Longmire WP Jr. The technique of pancreaticoduodenal resection. Surgery 1966;59:344.)

for selecting it over the standard procedure in patients in whom either procedure would be applicable.

Pylorus-Preserving Pancreaticoduodenectomy: Technical Considerations

The best exposure is obtained by means of bilateral subcostal incisions, except in the case of patients with an acute costal angle in whom an upper midline incision is preferable. The abdomen should be thoroughly explored for the presence of carcinomatosis or liver metastasis. The lesser sac is opened, exposing the entire anterior pancreatic surface. An extended Kocher maneuver is made so that the mesenteric vessels can be palpated from behind the pancreas. This key maneuver also allows for compression of the portal vein to control bleeding if it should be injured later in the dissection. Careful palpation of the hepatoduodenal ligament is performed to assess for high nodal metastasis (Fig. 33-6).[19]

For patients with bile duct carcinoma, it is imperative to perform an early bile duct exploration, including choledochoscopy. Examination of the upper bile ducts reveals diffuse tumors beyond the extent of resection in 7% to 12% of cases.[20,21]

The decision to proceed with PPPD may now be made. If the tumor is small, at least 5 cm from the pylorus, and with no metastases apart from paraduodenal lymph nodes, the operation may be performed. The line of resection across the duodenum is at least 2 cm distal to the pylorus. This area is cleared of investing tissues, but care is taken to preserve the right gastric artery as well as the vagal innervation of the pylorus and antrum. The gastroduodenal artery is divided at its junction with the hepatic artery, preserving the right gastric artery. The gastroepiploic artery along the greater curvature of the stomach is preserved and divided at its junction with the anterior pancreaticoduodenal artery on the head of the pancreas.[22]

Once the duodenum is divided, the superior mesenteric vein is identified either by following the middle colic vein to the inferior surface of the pancreas, or by its location at the most medial extent of the extended Kocher incision. The portal vein is identified after performing a cholecystectomy and dividing the common bile duct above the junction of the cystic and common bile ducts. The superior mesenteric and portal veins are bluntly dissected from the posterior surface of the neck of the pancreas. The neck of the pancreas is then divided with electrocautery.

After carefully ligating the branches to the pancreas from the superior mesenteric vein, the uncinate process is now exposed. The inferior pancreaticoduodenal artery is divided and ligated. The uncinate process is then divided between clamps close to the superior mesenteric artery. The dissection is carried inferiorly, taking the short mesenteric vessels of the third portion of the duodenum between clamps and ligatures up to the point where the mesentery passes behind the superior mesenteric vessels. The ligament of Treitz is identified and the jejunum is divided just beyond it. After ligation of jejunal mesenteric vessels, the cut end of the jejunum is passed beneath the superior mesenteric vessels. The dissection of the duodenal mesentery is completed from above the colon to the right of the mesenteric vessels. The specimen can now be removed.

Reconstruction is performed by first creating the pancreaticojejunostomy. Although it may be possible to perform an end-to-end pancreaticojejunostomy in some cases, it is often easier technically to oversew the cut end of the jejunum and perform an end-to-side anastomosis, dunking the end of pancreas into the jejunum. This technique also avoids undue tension on the end of the jejunum, which might produce ischemia or leak at the anastomosis. A mucosa-to-mucosa anastomosis between the pancreatic duct and jejunum is made. A polyethylene or Silastic tube is placed in the duct and exited downstream through a jejunostomy to aid in splinting the duct for 3 to 6 weeks while healing takes place. Intestinal continuity is restored by next performing an end-to-side duodenojejunostomy approximately 12 inches beyond the pancreatic anastomosis. The bile duct is anastomosed end to side to the jejunum about 12 inches distal to the duodenal anastomosis (Fig. 33-7).

For those patients having metastatic disease or carcinomatosis, or locally advanced disease that precludes curative resection, palliative biliary bypass should be performed. Because gastric outlet obstruction also develops in 36% of these patients, gastrojejunostomy should be performed as well.[23]

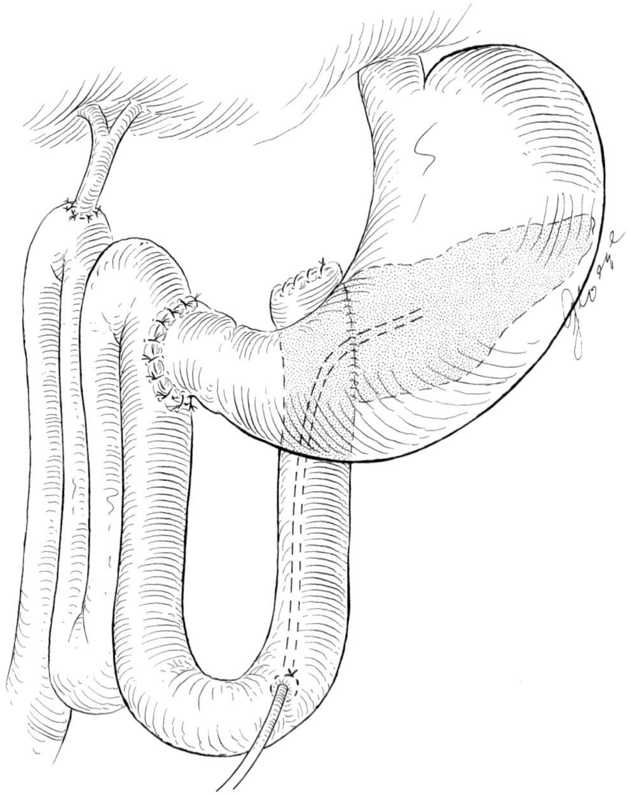

FIG. 33-7. Reconstruction after pylorus-preserving pancreaticoduodenectomy as practiced by the authors.

Pylorus-Preserving Pancreaticoduodenectomy: Outcomes

The short- and long-term results of PPPD compared with those in the standard Whipple resection has been extensively reviewed.[20,24]

Morbidity and Mortality

One major advantage of PPPD is that it is technically easier than the standard Whipple resection. The operative times and blood loss are less with PPPD, and patients have shorter hospital stays.[25] The overall morbidity and mortality for the procedure are no different than those for Whipple resection.[26,27] The major morbidity associated with PPPD is leakage of the pancreatic anastomosis, which has been reported to be reduced by functionally excluding the pancreaticojejunal anastomosis by Roux-en-Y anastomosis.[28,29]

Survival

The most controversial issue related to the PPPD is the adequacy of resection and whether leaving the antrum and duodenum compromises survival. There have not been any randomized, controlled trials comparing the two operations with regard to survival differences. Although one series has suggested decreased survival with PPPD compared with Whipple resection, it is impossible to exclude selection bias as leading to this result.[27] Conceivably, patients with greater likelihood for cure preferentially received the more radical Whipple operation if that was the bias of the operating surgeon.

Most studies report similar survivals for the two operations.[25,30] In an analysis of 69 patients undergoing pancreaticoduodenectomy for malignancy at UCLA between 1975 and 1984, 18 had ampullary carcinomas, 5 had duodenal carcinomas, and 5 had distal bile duct carcinomas.[26] Survival for all 28 patients was 58% for 5 years; for ampullary carcinoma it was 62%, and for bile duct cancer it was 52%. Five patients with duodenal carcinoma treated by PPPD had a 5-year survival of 60%.

The UCLA experience for carcinoma of the duodenum treated between 1954 and 1986 has been reported.[13] Of the 24 patients treated, pancreaticoduodenectomy with intent to cure was performed in 15 (62.5%). Median survival for patients with negative nodes was 42 months. Patients with positive paraduodenal nodes or regional nodal metastases had median survivals of 16.5 and 6 months, respectively. Two patients had survived over 5 years at the time of report (8.3%), reflecting the poorer prognosis in the older series of patients treated before 1975, compared with the more recent series referred to earlier.

Gastric Emptying

The greatest criticism of PPPD relates to concern for prolonged delays in gastric emptying after the procedure. Compared with the standard Whipple resections, several reports have documented prolonged gastric stasis in the immediate postoperative period.[30–33] A transient delay in emptying might be caused by gastric dysrhythmias immediately after PPPD.[34] However, other studies have found durations of gastric ileus equivalent to those that occur after standard Whipple resection,[26,35,36] and have attributed the ileus to other abdominal complications.[34] Objective assessments of gastric emptying within 2 months or longer by fluoroscopy or isotopic studies[30,37–40] have demonstrated relatively normal gastric emptying patterns. Small bowel transit has been observed to be increased, which may explain the dumping syndrome occasionally observed in patients after PPPD.[39] Isotopic emptying studies demonstrated abnormalities of emptying as well as biliary reflux in patients undergoing both operations, but symptoms were less frequent than the isotopic studies would predict.[41] An extensive review of the literature by Grace and colleagues found only 5% of reported PPPD patients experienced delayed gastric emptying, suggesting that this potential complication is overrated.[24]

Nutrition

Whipple patients almost never regain their preoperative weight.[42] Although most studies demonstrating this can be criticized because patients undergoing Whipple resection tend to have more extensive disease, postoperative early satiety and dumping may play a role in this process. Detailed nutritional studies of PPPD and Whipple patients showed that their objective nutritional parameters such as vitamins A and B_{12}, carotene, iron, and iron-binding capacity were about the same.[43]

However, PPPD patients usually regain their preoperative weight,[25,30,42] suggesting the potential for restoration of normal nutritional function after PPPD.

Marginal Ulceration

Another reason PPPD has been advocated is to attempt to reduce the rate of marginal ulceration that might occur by performing a gastrojejunostomy. Basal and stimulated gastric acid secretion is reduced after PPPD[40] and no hypergastrinemia is observed.[44] However, the incidence of marginal ulceration after PPPD is about 5%,[30,43] similar to that after standard Whipple operation.[5,26,35] Thus, incidence of marginal ulceration cannot be a criterion for the choice of either of these operations.

Therefore, the theoretic advantages of PPPD over the Whipple procedure of less marginal ulceration and better long-term nutritional status have not been proven to be of clinical significance. The operation is regarded as technically easier than the standard Whipple procedure. Because survival statistics for PPPD with periampullary and distal bile duct tumors are similar to those for standard Whipple resection, PPPD can be advocated for these lesions. Duodenal carcinomas present a special problem in selection of PPPD over Whipple. In cases of tumors localized to the third or fourth portion of the duodenum, PPPD may be a safe choice. However, we have observed patients with tumors in the second portion of the duodenum in whom complete duodenal resection is necessary to ensure adequate margins. A special problem arises in patients with villous adenomas of the duodenum, which have a 60% or greater likelihood of malignancy. Many of these patients have associated field defects in the duodenal mucosa or villous tumor changes over large areas of the mucosa (Fig. 33-8). In these patients, PPPD might leave behind neoplasm-prone mucosa and hence is best avoided.

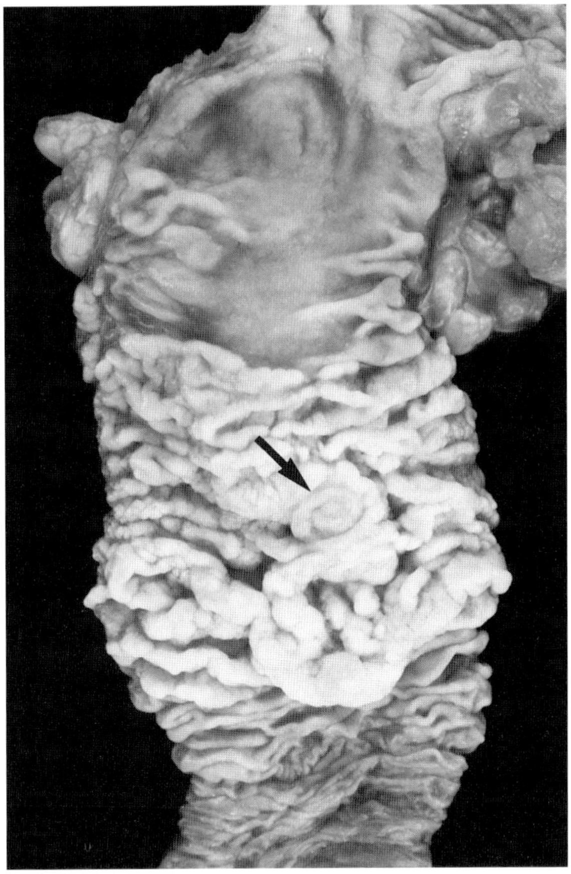

FIG. 33-8. Gross specimen removed by standard Whipple procedure from a patient with a villous adenoma of papilla of Vater *(arrow)*. The mucosal field defect extends proximally and distally from the papilla, and the margins would not be adequate if the pylorus preservation technique had been used. (Pylorus is at top of figure.) See color Figure 33-8.

Chemotherapy

In 1988, a new protocol was begun at UCLA for chemotherapeutic treatment of patients with advanced cancer of the pancreas, bile duct, and periampullary region, including duodenum.[45] The treatment consists of constant intravenous (IV) infusion, by pump, of 5-fluorouracil 200 mg/m^2/d. Calcium leucovorin 30 mg/m^2 is given by IV bolus on day 1 and at weekly intervals. Mitomycin-C 10 mg/m^2 IV is given on day 1 and at intervals of 6 weeks, not to exceed 15 mg per dose. Dipyridamole 75 mg four times daily is also given by mouth.

Although this regimen has been used primarily in patients with unresectable, poorly resected, or recurrent cancers, the results have been unusually good. For example, in 38 stage II and III pancreatic cancer patients treated at UCLA to date, 17 (45%) are responders (4 complete and 13 partial). The complete responses range from 13 to 45 months. Median survival for this group of patients has not yet been attained, but will exceed 15 months. One patient with bile duct cancer who was simply intubated because of peritoneal metastases at operation is alive with controlled disease on this chemotherapy regimen more than 6 years after operation. In a group of seven bile duct cancer patients with stage III or IV disease, the median survival was 17 months.

SUMMARY

The PPPD has been demonstrated to be technically easier than the standard Whipple procedure with antrectomy. There is no convincing evidence that it conveys any superior long-term physiologic or nutritional benefits, however. Studies of survival data show no differences between PPPD and standard Whipple procedures for lesions of the ampulla, distal bile duct, or duodenum. The decision as to whether to perform this procedure or the older Whipple procedure with antrectomy remains with the operating surgeon and should be based on his or her assessment of the tumor at the time of operation.

REFERENCES

1. Whipple AO, Parsons WB, Mullens CT. Treatment of carcinoma of the ampulla of Vater. Ann Surg 1935;102:763.
2. Trimble IR, Parsons JW, Sherman CP. A one-stage operation for the cure of carcinoma of the ampulla of Vater and the head of the pancreas. Surg Gynecol Obstet 1941;73:711.
3. Whipple AO. The rationale for cancer of the pancreas and ampullary region. Ann Surg 1941;114:612.

4. Watson K. Carcinoma of the ampulla of Vater: a successful radical resection. Br J Surg 1944;31:368.
5. Grant CS, van Heerden JA. Anastomotic ulceration following subtotal and total pancreatectomy. Ann Surg 1979;190:1.
6. Scott JW, Dean RH, Parker T, Avant G. The role of vagotomy in pancreaticoduodenectomy. Ann Surg 1980;191:688.
7. Warren KW, Veidenheimer MC, Pratt HS. Pancreaticoduodenectomy for periampullary cancer. Surg Clin North Am 1967;47:639.
8. Longmire WP Jr, Traverso LW. The Whipple procedure and other standard operative approaches to pancreatic cancer. Cancer 1981;47: 1706.
9. Traverso LW, Longmire WP Jr. Preservation of the pylorus in pancreaticoduodenectomy. Surg Gynecol Obstet 1978;146:959.
10. Dwivedi M, Acharya SK, Tandon BN. The ultrasonographic "common channel" sign: a characteristic feature of malignant obstruction of the lower end of common bile duct. J Clin Gastroenterol 1989;11:233.
11. D'Agostino HB, van Sonnenberg E, Sanchez RB, O'Laoide R, Ogilvie S. Imaging and radiologic intervention of the biliary tree. In: Braasch JW, Tompkins RK, eds. Surgical disease of the biliary tract and pancreas. St. Louis: Mosby-Year Book, 1994:73.
12. Alvarez C, Livingston EH, Ashley SW, Schwarz, Reber HA. Cost-benefit analysis of the workup for pancreatic cancer. Am J Surg 1993; 165:53.
13. Lai ECS, Doty JE, Irving C, Tompkins RK. Primary adenocarcinoma of the duodenum: analysis of survival. World J Surg 1988;12:695.
14. Binmoeller KF, Soehendra N. Diagnostic and therapeutic endoscopic advances in pancreatic and ampullary neoplasms. In: Braasch JW, Tompkins RK, eds. Surgical disease of the biliary tract and pancreas. St. Louis: Mosby-Year Book, 1994:530.
15. Beazley RM, Hadjis N, Benjamin IS, Blumgart LH. Clinicopathologic aspects of high bile duct cancer. Ann Surg 1984;199:623.
16. McPherson GAD. Preoperative percutaneous transhepatic biliary drainage: the results of a controlled trial. Br J Surg 1984;71:1.
17. Pitt HA, Gomes AS, Lois JF, Mann LL, Deutsch LS, Longmire WP Jr. Does preoperative percutaneous biliary drainage reduce operative risk or increase hospital cost? Ann Surg 1985;201:545.
18. Chapman WC, Sharp KW, Weaver F, Sawyers JL. Tumor seeding from percutaneous biliary catheters. Ann Surg 1989;209:708.
19. Longmire WP Jr. The technique of pancreaticoduodenal resection. Surgery 1966;59:344.
20. Reding R, Buard J-L, Lebeau G, Launois B. Surgical management of 552 carcinomas of the extrahepatic bile ducts (gallbladder and periampullary tumors excluded). Ann Surg 1991;213:236.
21. Saunders KD, Longmire WP Jr, Tompkins RK. Diffuse bile duct tumors: guidelines for management. Am Surg 1991;57:816.
22. Grace PA, Pitt HA, Longmire WP Jr. Pancreatoduodenectomy with pylorus preservation for adenocarcinoma of the head of the pancreas. Br J Surg 1986;73:647.
23. Aston SJ, Longmire WP Jr. Pancreaticoduodenal resection: twenty years' experience. Arch Surg 1973;106:813.
24. Grace PA, Pitt HA, Longmire WP Jr. Pylorus preserving pancreatoduodenectomy: an overview. Br J Surg 1990;77:968.
25. Klinkenbijl JH, van der Schelling GP, Hop WC, van Pel R, Bruining HA, Jeekel J. The advantages of pylorus-preserving pancreatoduodenectomy in malignant disease of the pancreas and periampullary region. Ann Surg 1992;216:142.
26. Grace PA, Pitt HA, Tompkins RK, DenBesten L, Longmire WP Jr. Decreased morbidity and mortality after pancreatoduodenectomy. Am J Surg 1986;151:141.
27. Roder JD, Stein HJ, Huttl W, Siewert JR. Pylorus-preserving versus standard pancreaticoduodenectomy: an analysis of 110 pancreatic and periampullary carcinomas. Br J Surg 1992;79:152.
28. De Bernardinis G, Agnifili A, Gola P, et al. An original reconstructive method after pylorus-preserving pancreatoduodenectomy. Surg Today 1993;23:481.
29. Kingsnorth AN, Berg JD, Gray MR. A novel reconstructive technique for pylorus-preserving pancreaticoduodenectomy: avoidance of early postoperative gastric stasis. Ann R Coll Surg Engl 1993;75:38.
30. Braasch JW, Rossi RL, Watkins E, Deziel DJ, Winter PF. Pyloric and gastric preserving pancreatic resection. Ann Surg 1986;204:411.
31. Mosca F, Guilianotti PC, Arganini M, Brandi LS, Selli M. Pancreaticoduodenectomy with pylorus preservation. Italian Journal of Surgical Science 1984;14:313.
32. Warshaw AL, Torchina DL. Delayed gastric emptying after pylorus preserving pancreaticoduodenectomy. Surg Gynecol Obstet 1985;160: 1.
33. Williamson RCN, Cooper MJ. Resection in chronic pancreatitis. Br J Surg 1987;74:807.
34. Hocking MP, Harrison WD, Sninsky CA. Gastric dysrhythmias following pylorus-preserving pancreaticoduodenectomy: possible mechanism for early delayed gastric emptying. Dig Dis Sci 1990;35:1226.
35. Crist DW, Sitzmann JV, Cameron JL. Improved hospital morbidity, mortality and survival after the Whipple procedure. Ann Surg 1987; 206:358.
36. McAfee MK, van Heerden JA, Adson MA. Is proximal pancreatoduodenectomy with pyloric preservation superior to total pancreatectomy? Surgery 1989;105:347.
37. Williamson RC, Bliouras N, Cooper MJ, Davies ER. Gastric emptying and enterogastric reflux after conservative and conventional pancreatoduodenectomy. Surg 1993;114(1):82.
38. Hunt DR, McLean R. Pylorus-preserving pancreatectomy: functional results. Br J Surg 1989;76:173.
39. Patti MG, Pellegrini CA, Way LW. Gastric emptying and small bowel transit of solid food after pylorus-preserving pancreaticoduodenectomy. Arch Surg 1987;122:528.
40. Traverso LW, Longmire WP Jr. Preservation of the pylorus in pancreaticoduodenectomy: a followup. Ann Surg 1980;192:306.
41. Williamson RC, Bliouras N, Cooper MJ, Davies ER. Gastric emptying and enterogastric reflux after conservative and conventional pancreatoduodenectomy. Surgery 1993;114:82.
42. Braasch JW. Pancreaticoduodenal resection. Curr Probl Surg 1988;25: 321.
43. Fink AS, DeSouza LR, Mayer EA, Hawkins R, Longmire WP Jr. Long-term evaluation of pylorus preservation during pancreaticoduodenectomy. World J Surg 1988;12:663.
44. Pearlman NW, Stiegmann GV, Ahnen DJ, Schultz AL, Fink LM. Acid and gastrin levels following pyloric-preserving pancreaticoduodenectomy. Arch Surg 1986;121:661.
45. Isacoff WH, Botnick L, Tompkins RK. Treatment of patients with advanced tumors of the bile ducts with continuous infusion of 5-fluorouracil in conjunction with calcium leucovorin, mitomycin-c and dipyridamole [abstract]. Proceedings of the American Society of Clinical Oncologists 1993;12:225.

Surgery for Gastrointestinal Cancer: A Multidisciplinary Approach, edited by Harold J. Wanebo.
Lippincott-Raven Publishers, Philadelphia, © 1997.

CHAPTER 34

Laparoscopic Staging With Selected Resection in Pancreatic Cancer

Carlos Fernández-del Castillo and Andrew L. Warshaw

RATIONALE

Of all gastrointestinal malignancies, pancreatic cancer is the one with the worst prognosis: less than 20% of patients are alive 1 year after diagnosis, and the overall 5-year survival rate is only 3%.[1] As dismal as this may look, these numbers represent significant improvement in relation to the prognosis of pancreatic cancer patients in the early 1970s. Although earlier diagnosis or even a change in the biology of pancreatic cancer may account for part of this improvement, there is no question that it is also related to major advancements in surgical treatment as well as in our ability to stage the disease adequately. The once formidable morbidity and mortality associated with pancreatectomy have been abated, with several centers throughout the world now reporting operative mortality rates for pancreatoduodenectomy in the range of 0% to 3%, and commensurate declines in postoperative complications.[2–7] These same series and others also show very encouraging survival rates for *resected* patients, which go from 17% to 24% in unselected patients,[3,8,9] to as to high as 27% when only small (<2 cm) tumors are considered,[10] or even 57% in the absence of nodal metastases.[8] This contrasts markedly with data from a comprehensive review published in 1987 that shows that of 47,000 patients reported in 145 series, there were 3000 pancreatoduodenectomies and only 150 5-year survivors (0.1% of the total group; 3.5% of resected patients), with a mean operative mortality of 18%.[11] Since the late 1980s, the importance of preoperative staging has been more widely recognized and the tools to implement it have improved, with a concomitant tendency of surgeons to abandon the traditional approach of operating on all patients with pancreatic cancer. For all practical purposes, only those patients with pancreatic cancer who are surgically resected have an expectation for cure. This by itself justifies all efforts at precise preoperative staging, because the low operative morbidity and mortality of pancreatic resection, which are the results of accumulated experience, may not be available everywhere. Furthermore, even if staging shows that the patient is not resectable, there is a real benefit in knowing this beforehand, for the following reasons: a prognosis is established; in many instances surgery can be avoided altogether because jaundice, which is present in over 50% of patients, can be effectively relieved by endoscopic or transhepatic placement of stents, particularly now that expandable metal stents are available; and there are treatment alternatives, such as external beam or intraoperative radiation therapy, that may significantly prolong survival, but that obviously are applicable only to patients without distant metastases.

In our experience, only 15% of patients with pancreatic cancer are resectable, about 40% have a localized tumor that is no longer resectable, and the remaining 45% have distant metastases at the time the diagnosis is established. The reasons for unresectability in tumors that are still localized are usually invasion of the portal or superior mesenteric vein, or extensive retroperitoneal invasion. Distant metastases may be present anywhere in the body; however, at the time of diagnosis the usual sites are liver and peritoneum. Thus, a scheme for preoperative staging in pancreatic cancer should be able to allocate patients into these three categories (resectable, localized but unresectable, disseminated) by identifying these elements.

Computed tomography (CT) of the upper abdomen and angiography of the celiac and superior mesenteric vessels have traditionally been used for the purpose of staging in this disease. In many patients, CT scan may be all that is needed, because it readily detects intraparenchymal liver metastases or large tumors with obliteration of vascular structures and retroperitoneal tissues. If this is not the case, angiography follows to document the presence or absence of vascular compromise. However, although CT and angiography are accurate in identifying unresectability (their false-positive rates are 5% and 3%, respectively[12]), they are not good enough for prediction of

Carlos Fernández-del Castillo, Assistant Professor of Surgery, Massachusetts General Hospital and Harvard Medical School, 15 Parkman Street, Boston, MA 02114

Andrew L. Warshaw, Chief of General Surgery and Associate Chief of Surgical Services, Massachusetts General Hospital, Harold and Ellen Danser Professor of Surgery Harvard Medical School, 15 Parkman Street, Boston MA 02114

TABLE 34-1. *Frequency (%) of extranodal metastases of pancreatic cancer in autopsy studies*

Study	Site				
	Liver	Peritoneum	Lung	Adrenal	Ovary
Lee and Tatter[13] (N = 126)	78	41	40	24	11
Cubilla and Fitzgerald[14] (N = 119)	76	55	50	26	7
Halpert et al[15] (N = 120)	80	52	43	19	—
Bell[16] (N = 609)	68	40	27	12	2
Mean	76	47	40	20	7

resectability, misclassifying as many as 60% of patients, who then undergo an operation that will not benefit them.

Autopsy studies show that the peritoneum is the second most common site for extranodal involvement in pancreatic cancer, after the liver[13–16] (Table 34-1), with peritoneal metastases present in about 50% of patients at the time of death. This is considerably more than the 10% incidence found in periampullary tumors[13] or the 32% in colon cancer,[17] but is less than that in tumors well known for their propensity for peritoneal spread, such as ovarian cancer, in which the incidence can reach over 90%.[18]

Typically, peritoneal metastases are 1- to 2-mm nodules, although larger deposits found within the omentum are not uncommon. They may be present in the parietal peritoneum (Fig. 34-1), or in the serosal surfaces of the stomach, intestine, or liver (Fig. 34-2). The latter should be distinguished from parenchymal hepatic metastases, which are much larger and presumably are disseminated by way of the portal venous system. Unfortunately, this consideration is not made in the autopsy studies describing metastatic spread, and thus the true extent of peritoneal spread in pancreatic carcinoma is probably underestimated. The size of these lesions precludes their detection by CT or ultrasound, and at present they can be identified only by direct visualization. It is for this reason we believe that laparoscopy should form an integral part of the evaluation of patients with pancreatic cancer, complementing the information provided by CT and angiography.

TECHNICAL CONSIDERATIONS

The procedure can be performed in an outpatient setting, either under local anesthesia with intravenous sedation, or under general anesthesia. Previous intraabdominal surgery, particularly cholecystectomy or gastrectomy, may preclude adequate exploration of the liver surfaces and thus be a limiting factor. After an adequate pneumoperitoneum is obtained, a large trocar and subsequently the camera are inserted, usually through an infraumbilical incision. Visual examination of the lower abdomen and pelvis is completed first. Peritoneal and omental metastases can be found in this location, even in the absence of implants elsewhere. The laparoscope is then rotated to inspect the upper abdomen. Examination of the liver surfaces is particularly important, and to do this adequately it is necessary to insert a rod through a second, smaller trocar (5 mm) in the right upper quadrant of the abdomen. The rod is used to lift areas of the liver so that the undersurface can be inspected, or to push other viscera away from the area the surgeon wishes to see.

Specimens of peritoneal or omental nodules can be taken for

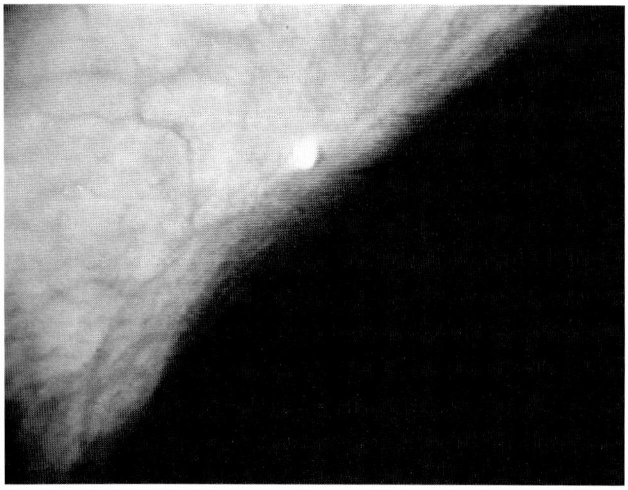

FIG. 34-1. Laparoscopic view of a peritoneal implant in pancreatic cancer.

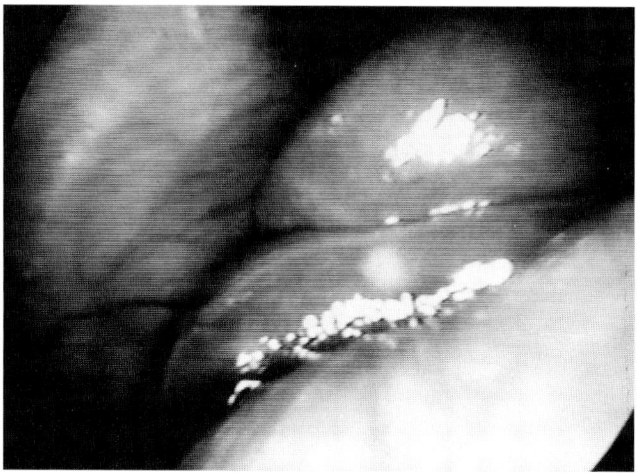

FIG. 34-2. Liver metastases in pancreatic cancer.

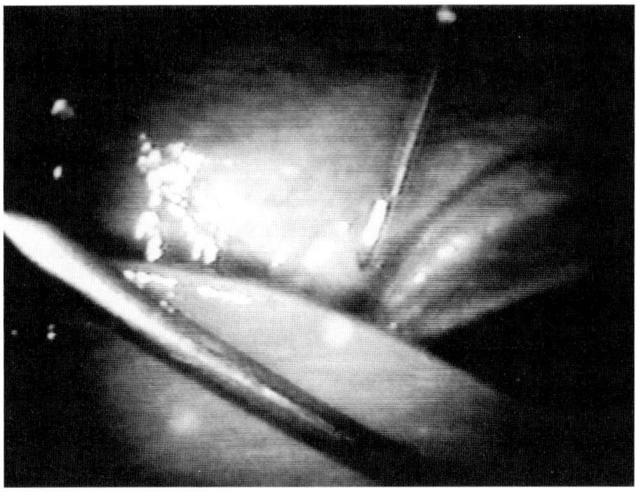

FIG. 34-3. Biopsy of small liver metastases is possible under direct visualization at the time of laparoscopy.

biopsy with forceps inserted through the second trocar. Nodules in the liver are most easily sampled with a cutting needle (eg, Tru-Cut) inserted directly through the abdominal wall (Fig. 34-3). Nodules smaller than 1 mm can be accurately sampled under direct vision. Samples of metastases on the pelvic peritoneum also can be taken with a cutting needle; however, because of their location, it is sometimes necessary to insert another trocar in the lower midline for the biopsy forceps. Enlarged lymph nodes can be successfully sampled with the cutting needle or by fine-needle aspiration.

In some cases, tumors of the head of the pancreas or uncinate process can be seen bulging through the mesocolon and can be sampled for biopsy directly. Laparoscopy also permits visualization of the body and tail of the pancreas by using either a supragastric approach (through the lesser omentum) or entering below the stomach (through the gastrocolic omentum or the mesocolon). This procedure, which has also been called pancreatoscopy, was first proposed by Meyer-Burg,[19] and was further developed by Ishida[20] and Cuschieri and colleagues.[21] For the supragastric approach, the operating table is raised to about 30°, and the lesser omentum under the left lobe of the liver is exposed by elevating the latter with the tip of the laparoscope. Next a forceps is inserted into the peritoneal cavity from the right upper part of the abdomen, and a lesser omentotomy is performed. The laparoscope is then inserted through this opening, the pancreatic body is visualized, and a sample taken for biopsy.

Cholangiography can also be performed at the time of laparoscopy, with transhepatic injection of contrast either to the gallbladder or to a dilated bile duct.[21] Laparoscopic cholecystojejunostomy has been described in patients with pancreatic cancer who at the time of laparoscopic staging are found to be unresectable.[22]

It has been our practice to use laparoscopy to help stage pancreatic cancer because of its unique capacity to detect small peritoneal metastatic disease. We do not think that direct visualization of the pancreatic tumor is necessary because a CT scan or ultrasonogram has already been obtained in most cases. Furthermore, the tumor can be sampled for biopsy percutaneously in most cases, and sampling perhaps should not be attempted in patients with potentially resectable tumors, as is discussed later. The only exception in which direct visualization of the tumor and biopsy is justified is in the patient with pancreatic cancer whom we know is unresectable by angiography, has no metastatic disease, and needs tissue diagnosis to receive radiation therapy. Diagnostic cholangiography is rarely needed by the time the patient is being staged; if there is any question about the diagnosis of pancreatic cancer, or if relief of jaundice is required before surgery, endoscopic retrograde cholangiopancreatography and stenting are done before staging.

RESULTS FROM CLINICAL STUDIES

The use of laparoscopy for staging in pancreatic cancer predates by many years the current surge of laparoscopic surgical procedures. Before the widespread availability of CT, laparoscopy was used extensively in Europe for the diagnosis and staging of various gastrointestinal cancers, including pancreatic.[23–26] Results of several published series describing the use of diagnostic laparoscopy in pancreatic cancer are given in Table 34-2.[12,20,21,27–29] The table also includes a more recent series of 74 patients staged by us over a 3-year period (January, 1991 through December, 1993).

The series published by Ivanov and Keranov[29] and the second one from Cuschieri[28] both show prevalences of peritoneal and liver metastases identified by laparoscopy of 70% or more. This is much higher than the range of 35% to 43% previously described by us and also reported by Ishida.[20] This discrepancy is accounted for by the exclusion in our studies of patients with liver or other distant metastases identified by CT or ultrasound. These patients clearly have now benefitted from laparoscopy because they are no longer candidates for resection or radiation and tissue for diagnosis can be obtained percutaneously with little morbidity.

Our experience from 1991 to 1993 shows that the prevalence of liver and peritoneal involvement identified by laparoscopy is significantly less than that found in the period from 1982 to 1989. There is no obvious explanation for this, although several possibilities exist. One is that refinements in CT now allow

TABLE 34-2. *Detection by laparoscopy of peritoneal and liver metastases in pancreatic cancer*

Study	Liver and peritoneal involvement (%)
Cuschieri, et al[21] 1978 (N = 23)	39
Ishida[20] 1983 (N = 71)	43
Warshaw, et al[27] 1986 (N = 40)	35*
Cuschieri[28] 1988 (N = 73)	70
Ivanov and Keranov[29] 1989 (N = 78)	73
Warshaw, et al[12] 1990 (N = 47)	36*
Current series 1994 (N = 74)	20*

* $P < 0.05$.

for identification of smaller liver and peritoneal metastases; however, if this were the case, we would expect to be doing less staging laparoscopies, which is not the case. Another possibility is that we are seeing patients at an earlier stage of the disease, which may well be a trend. A third possibility is that the biology of pancreatic cancer is changing, which is also suggested by the increased 5-year survival seen throughout the world.

Despite this relatively lower diagnostic yield, we still believe laparoscopy should form an integral part of the staging of patients with pancreatic cancer as a way to optimize resources and avoid unnecessary surgery. The current trend for more aggressive multimodality treatments in which radiation and chemotherapy precede resection underscores even more the necessity to exclude metastatic disease, because the morbidity, costs, and time commitment associated with this approach are not negligible. Other institutions share this belief and include laparoscopy in their protocols before selecting patients for this form of treatment.[30]

In our overall experience, the incidence of metastases identified by laparoscopy (and not detected by CT) is much higher in tumors of the pancreatic body and tail (26 of 45, 57%) than in tumors of the pancreatic head (25 of 116, 21%). This is probably the result of a more delayed diagnosis in tumors of the distal pancreas. In the habitual staging scheme for patients with presumptive pancreatic cancer, it is more cost effective to perform laparoscopy before angiography, because the latter is obviously not needed if the patient has distant metastases, whereas laparoscopy will still be required even if the patient has vascular involvement to determine if he or she is a candidate for external and intraoperative radiation treatment.

Peritoneal Cytology

Peritoneal carcinomatosis and ascites containing malignant cells are not uncommon in patients with advanced pancreatic cancer, but little is known about the prevalence of malignant cells within the peritoneal cavity in patients with small, apparently contained tumors. We investigated this issue by performing peritoneal washings in 40 patients with ''early'' pancreatic cancer (ie, localized by CT and angiography).[31] Washings were performed during laparoscopy or laparotomy by instilling 100 mL of normal saline into the subhepatic space, allowing it to disperse in the peritoneal cavity by tilting the operating table and agitating the abdominal wall, and then aspirating under direct vision. Cytologic smears and cell blocks prepared from centrifuged specimens were used and examined for the presence of malignant cells, using strict criteria for malignancy to avoid potential confusion with reactive mesothelial or inflammatory cells.

Malignant cells were found in 12 of the 40 patients (30%). Eight patients had small amounts of ascites, but malignant cells were encountered only in half of them. Six of the 40 patients had small liver metastases that were identified by laparoscopy, but none of them had positive peritoneal cytologic results (ie, malignant cells). A disturbing finding of the study was that positive cytologic results were significantly increased in patients who had undergone percutaneous needle biopsy earlier compared with those who had not (75% vs. 19%). This is consistent with observations made by other investigators of rapid intraabdominal spread and implantation after tumor manipulation and biopsy,[32,33] and should caution against the use of preoperative biopsy in potentially resectable patients. The likelihood of resectability was higher in patients with negative cytologic findings (13 of 25) compared with those positive for malignant cells (1 of 10), a fact that was also reflected in a significantly better survival. In another report of a small series of patients, preoperative peritoneal cytologic findings were positive in two of seven patients who had undergone a previous percutaneous biopsy with fine-needle aspiration, and negative in all eight patients without prior biopsy.[34]

In our more recent experience, peritoneal cytologic findings have been positive in only 9 of 57 patients (16%). This lower prevalence may be in agreement with the lower incidence of positive laparoscopic findings, or may be the result of a more limited use of preoperative biopsy of pancreatic tumors. Whenever histologic diagnosis is mandatory (eg, if the patient is to enter a protocol of intensive preoperative radiation and chemotherapy), our policy is to precede the biopsy by low-dose radiation (1000 cGy) to decrease the likelihood of peritoneal dissemination.

We are aware of only one other study evaluating peritoneal washings in pancreatic cancer. In it, Martin and Goellner[33] describe the presence of malignant peritoneal cells in 22% of 20 pancreatic cancer patients. They also describe a better prognosis for patients with negative washings.

REFERENCES

1. National Cancer Institute. Annual cancer statistics review 1973–1989. National Institutes of Health Publication No. 92-2789. Bethesda, MD: U.S. Department of Health and Human Services, 1992.
2. Grace PA, Pitt HA, Tompkins RK, DenBesten L, Longmire WP. Decreased morbidity and mortality after pancreatoduodenectomy. Am J Surg 1986;151:141.
3. Trede M, Schwall G, Saeger HD. Survival after pancreatoduodenectomy. Ann Surg 1990;211:447.
4. Singh SM, Longmire WP, Reber HA. Surgical palliation for pancreatic cancer: the UCLA experience. Ann Surg 1990;212:132.
5. Pellegrini CA, Heck CF, Raper S, Way LW. An analysis of the reduced morbidity and mortality rates after pancreaticoduodenectomy. Arch Surg 1989;124:778.
6. Geer RJ, Brennan MF. Prognostic indicators for survival after resection of pancreatic adenocarcinoma. Am J Surg 1993;165:68.
7. Cameron JL, Pitt HA, Yeo CJ, Lillemoe KD, Kaufman HS, Coleman J. One hundred and forty-five consecutive pancreaticoduodenectomies without mortality. Ann Surg 1993;217:430.
8. Cameron JL, Crist DW, Sitzmann JV, et al. Factors influencing survival after pancreaticoduodenectomy for pancreatic cancer. Am J Surg 1991; 161:120.
9. Warshaw AL, Fern ndez-del Castillo C. Medical progress: pancreatic carcinoma. N Engl J Med 1992;326:455.
10. Tsuchiya R, Noda T, Harada M, et al. Collective review of small carcinomas of the pancreas. Ann Surg 1986;203:77.
11. Gudjonsson B. Cancer of the pancreas: 50 years of surgery. Cancer 1987;60:2284.
12. Warshaw AL, Gu Z-y, Wittenberg J, Waltman AC. Preoperative staging and assessment of resectability of pancreatic cancer. Arch Surg 1990; 125:230.
13. Lee YN, Tatter D. Carcinoma of the pancreas and periampullary structures: pattern of metastasis at autopsy. Arch Pathol Lab Med 1984; 108:584.
14. Cubilla AL, Fitzgerald PJ. Tumors of the exocrine pancreas. In: Atlas of tumor pathology, 2nd series, fascicle 19. Washington, DC: Armed Forces Institute of Pathology, 1984;134.
15. Halpert B, Makk L, Jordan GL. A retrospective study of 120 patients with carcinoma of the pancreas. Surg Gynecol Obstet 1965;121:91.

16. Bell ET. Carcinoma of the pancreas: II. the relation of cancer of the pancreas to diabetes mellitus. Am J Pathol 1957;33:511.
17. Welch JP, Donaldson GA. The clinical correlation of an autopsy study of recurrent colorectal cancer. Ann Surg 1979;189:496.
18. Dvoretsky PM, Richards KA, Angel C, et al. Distribution of disease at autopsy in 100 women with ovarian cancer. Hum Pathol 1988;19:57.
19. Meyer-Burg J. The inspection, palpation and biopsy for the pancreas. Endoscopy 1972;4:99.
20. Ishida H. Peritoneoscopy and pancreas biopsy in the diagnosis of pancreatic diseases. Gastrointest Endosc 1983;29:211.
21. Cuschieri A, Hall AW, Clark J. Value of laparoscopy in the diagnosis and management of pancreatic carcinoma. Gut 1978;19:672.
22. Shimi S, Banting S, Cuschieri A. Laparoscopy in the management of pancreatic cancer: endoscopic cholecystojejunostomy for advanced disease. Br J Surg 1992;79:317.
23. Watt I, Stewart I, Anderson D, Bell G, Anderson JR. Laparoscopy, ultrasound and computed tomography in cancer of the oesophagus and gastric cardia: a prospective comparison for detecting intra-abdominal metastases. Br J Surg 1989;76:1036.
24. Kriplani AK, Kapur BM. Laparoscopy for preoperative staging and assessment of operability in gastric carcinoma. Gastrointest Endosc 1991;37:441.
25. Dagnini G, Caldironi MW, Marin G, Buzzaccarini O, Tremolada C, Ruol A. Laparoscopy in abdominal staging of esophageal carcinoma: report of 369 cases. Gastrointest Endosc 1986;32:400.
26. Chissov VI, Maksimov IA, Vinogradov AL. Laparoscopy in the diagnosis of gastric carcinoma spread. Khirurgiia (Mosk) 1981;11:13.
27. Warshaw AL, Tepper JE, Shipley WU. Laparoscopy in the staging and planning of therapy for pancreatic cancer. Am J Surg 1986;151:76.
28. Cuschieri A. Laparoscopy for pancreatic cancer: does it benefit the patient? Eur J Surg Oncol 1988;14:41.
29. Ivanov S, Keranov S. Laparoscopic assessment of the operability of pancreatic cancer. Khirurgiia (Sofiia) 1989;42:12.
30. Fuhrman GM, Charnsangavej C, Abbruzzese JL, et al. Thin-section contrast-enhanced computed tomography accurately predicts the resectability of malignant pancreatic neoplasms. Am J Surg 1994;167:104.
31. Warshaw AL. Implications of peritoneal cytology for staging of early pancreatic cancer. Am J Surg 1991;161:26.
32. Weiss SM, Skibber JM, Mohiuddin M, Rosato FE. Rapid intra-abdominal spread of pancreatic cancer. Arch Surg 1985;120:415.
33. Martin JK Jr, Goellner JR. Abdominal fluid cytology in patients with gastrointestinal malignancies. Mayo Clin Proc 1986;61:467.
34. Zerbi A, Balzano G, Bottura R, DiCarlo V. Reliability of pancreatic cancer staging classifications. Int J Pancreatol 1994;15:13.

Surgery for Gastrointestinal Cancer: A Multidisciplinary Approach, edited by Harold J. Wanebo.
Lippincott-Raven Publishers, Philadelphia, © 1997.

CHAPTER 35

Pylorus-Preserving Pancreaticoduodenectomy

Ricardo L. Rossi and Ronald F. Martin

GENERAL CONSIDERATIONS

The treatment of patients with carcinoma of the pancreas continues to be associated with poor results. However, surgical resection represents the only possibility of cure and may represent the best form of palliation in patients with resectable disease. In addition, it enables resection of other periampullary tumors associated with a better prognosis that clinically cannot be differentiated from pancreatic ductal carcinoma. In some series,[1] these tumors represent as many as 20% of the neoplasms thought clinically to be pancreatic carcinoma. In several multifactorial analyses, the presence of positive margins of resection is the most important prognostic factor related to recurrence and poor survival, followed by positive nodal involvement.[1,2] Therefore, the initial resection should be extensive enough to avoid the possibility of positive margins. Whether extensive lymphadenectomy improves survival or whether it provides better staging of the disease and is a prognostic indicator only is unproved.

Because the extent of local resection and the extent of lymphadenectomy are controversial issues, it is important to understand the local growth characteristics of pancreatic carcinoma and the patterns of progression of lymph node involvement. The relation of a tumor of the head of the pancreas to its surrounding structures is shown in Figure 35-1. The margin most frequently involved by tumor represents invasion of the peripancreatic fat around the head of the pancreas,[2] particularly in its posterior aspect, where the pancreas lies over the vena cava and aorta. This margin is only a few millimeters. Other margins of interest include the margin of the head of the pancreas and uncinate process as they relate to the superior mesenteric vessels, the neck of the pancreas where the gland is transected, and the distal common duct margin. Most resectable ductal carcinomas of the head of the pancreas are several centimeters away from the pyloric area. In a review of operative specimens of patients who underwent resection of the head of the pancreas, Cubilla and colleagues[3] noted that, in the presence of pancreatic ductal carcinoma, none of the nodes of the lesser curvature and greater curvature of the stomach and in only 1 of the 11 patients were the pyloric lymph nodes involved with metastatic disease. Pancreatic ductal carcinoma tended to metastasize to multiple lymph node groups, primarily the superior pancreatic head and body groups, the posterior pancreaticoduodenal group, and the inferior pancreatic head group. Similarly, Cooperman[4] found no extension of tumor proximal to the pylorus and no involvement of perigastric lymph nodes. Nagai and coworkers[5] reported that the location and extent of infiltration or interstitial carcinoma (ie, within lymphatic vessels, nerves, or connective tissue) paralleled lymph node metastasis, and added that even small pancreatic tumors are often metastatic to periaortic lymph node groups.

Kayahara and associates[6] studied the lymphatic pathways of the head of the pancreas to the periaortic lymph nodes on the basis of lymph node involvement after extended radical operations. The lymph nodes around the common hepatic artery, lymph nodes of the hepatoduodenal ligament, the posterior pancreaticoduodenal lymph nodes, lymph nodes around the superior mesenteric artery, paraaortic lymph nodes, and anterior pancreaticoduodenal lymph nodes were associated with a high rate of metastasis. Based on these results, it would appear that the main lymphatic pathway from the head of the pancreas to the periaortic lymph nodes is through lymph nodes around the superior mesenteric artery, and that pyloric and perigastric nodes would be involved predominantly in later stages of disease. Kayahara and associates[6] also noted that no relation existed between the size of the tumor and involvement of lymph nodes.

The operation described by Whipple and colleagues[7] in 1935 has undergone many modifications. In 1944, Watson[8] reported on the preservation of the pylorus after pancreaticoduodenectomy for ampullary carcinoma. In his operation, the cut end of the pancreas was oversewn and not anastomosed to the jejunum. In 1978, Traverso and Longmire[9] reported a pylorus-preserving procedure in two patients with chronic pancreatitis who required resection of the head of the gland for control of pain. They performed this modification in an attempt to decrease the sequelae of gastrectomy, such as the loss of gastric capacity and postgastrectomy syndromes (ie, dumping, diarrhea), and to improve the nutritional condition of these patients. They advised that the procedure not be carried out in patients with malignant disease.

Ricardo L. Rossi: Hospitale Admissions, Pontifica Universidad Catolica de Chile, Hospitole Clinico Escuela Medicina, Nord Marcleta 347, Casilla 114D, Santiago, Chile

Ronald F. Martin: 72 West Street, Portland, ME 04102

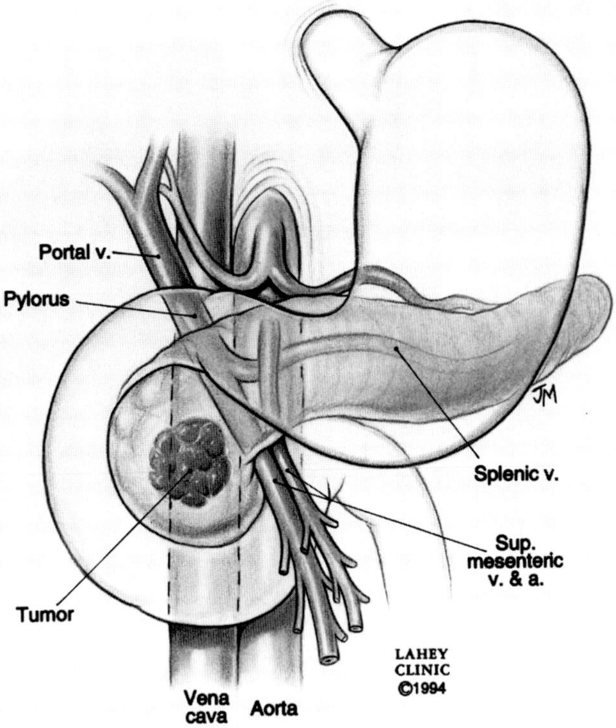

A

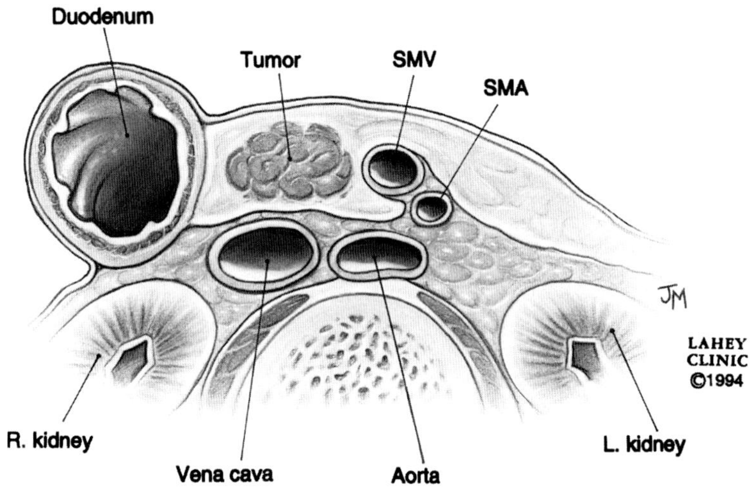

B

FIG. 35-1. Anatomic relationships of a pancreatic tumor. **(A)** Anteroposterior view shows proximity to superior mesenteric vessels. **(B)** Lateral view demonstrates the limited posterior margin over the aorta and vena cava. (Reprinted with permission of Lahey Clinic.)

However, since 1979, we have routinely been performing pylorus-preserving pancreaticoduodenectomy for the management of pancreatic and periampullary tumors as long as a negative duodenal margin of resection can be obtained and the antropyloric area appears viable. The premise for selecting this approach was that the margin most at risk of containing a malignancy was the posterior pancreatic margin and not the proximal duodenal margin. In addition, the few additional lymph node groups that could be removed with the standard Whipple operation (ie, lesser curvature and greater curvature nodes) are rarely involved. When they are involved, most patients have extensive nodal metastases of the peripancreatic nodes and periaortic nodes, and, therefore, operation is unlikely to affect survival. Our bias in the management of patients with pancreatic ductal adenocarcinoma is that the issue is not the proximal margin of resection of the duodenum but, rather, that our efforts should be directed to early diagnosis, further evaluation of preoperative, intraoperative, and postoperative adjuvant therapies, a better understanding of tumor biology, and the use of prospective, randomized trials for the evaluation of the role of more aggressive lymphatic clearance. It was believed that the pylorus-preserving operation probably represented a cancer operation that was similar to the standard Whipple operation with regard to survival and recurrence rates, was a lesser procedure, maintained gastric capacity and a functioning antropyloric duodenal complex, minimized gastrointestinal symptoms and sequelae of

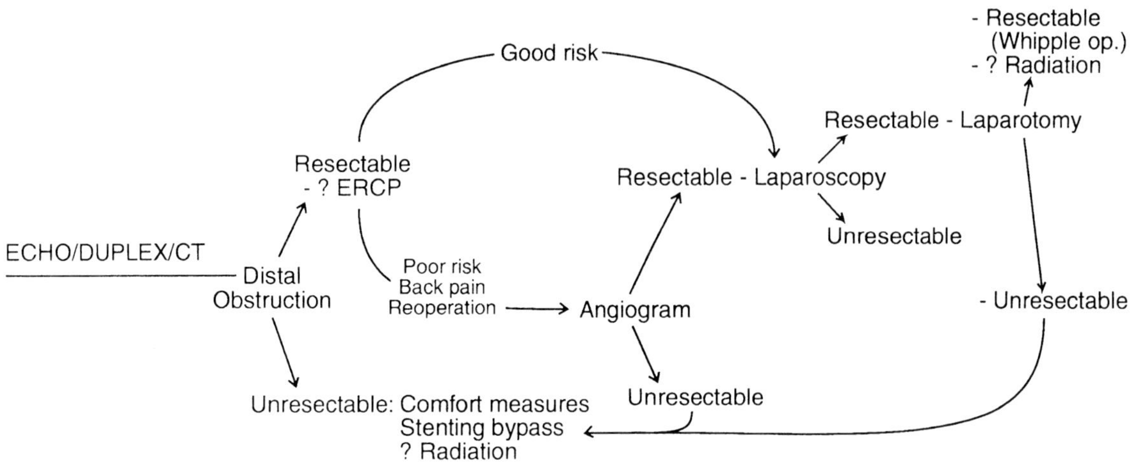

FIG. 35-2. Algorithm for the study of patients with distal obstructive jaundice.

gastric resection, and perhaps improved nutrition and quality of life.

Most patients have painless jaundice on presentation. Many diagnostic studies are available for the evaluation of these patients, but often they add little additional information while adding significantly to the cost of care. An algorithm of how we currently study these patients is shown in Figure 35-2. We favor a selective approach based on the clinical characteristics of the patient, the associated diseases and operative risks, and the information gained by initial ultrasonography and by dynamic computed tomography (CT) with images of good quality, including evaluation of the portal vein. Often, endoscopic retrograde cholangiopancreatography (ERCP) or angiography is not needed. We reserve ERCP for patients in whom CT does not reveal a mass, patients in whom we suspect a benign condition (ie, common duct stone, pancreatitis), patients who are thought to require stenting before surgery (ie, sepsis, malnutrition), or patients with unresectable disease. We do not obtain routine angiography in good-risk patients who appear to have patent superior mesenteric vessels on ultrasonography and CT because this study adds little to their management. We consider angiography for high-risk patients or for patients with back pain.

Pancreatic surgeons should be able to identify variations in vascular anatomy at the time of operation without the need for angiography.

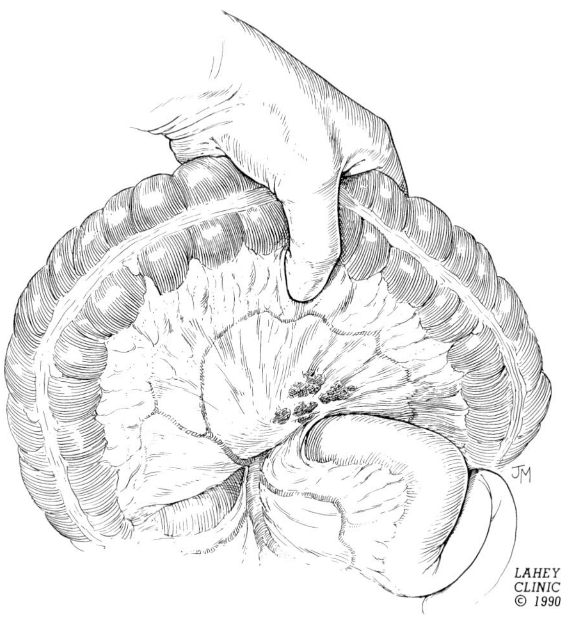

FIG. 35-3. The root of the mesentery and the angle of Treitz are assessed for invasion by tumor. (Reprinted with permission of Lahey Clinic.)

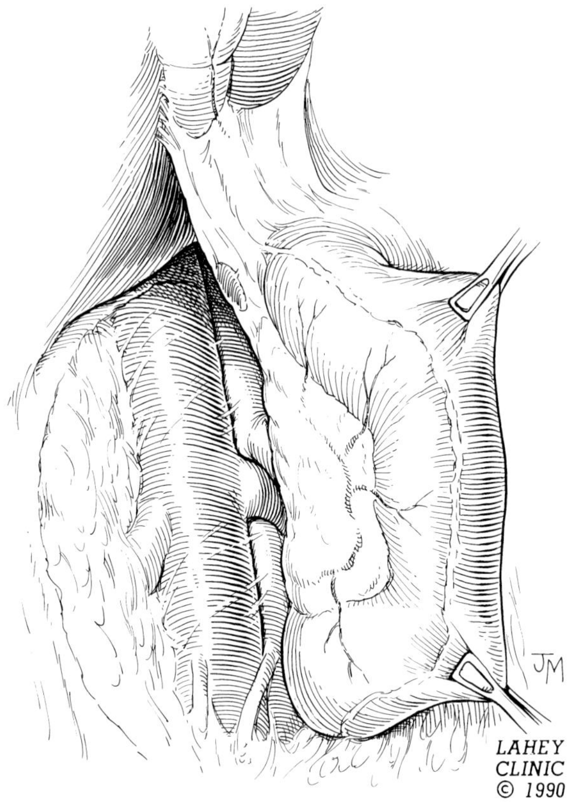

FIG. 35-4. Extensive Kocher maneuver is shown. (Reprinted with permission of Lahey Clinic.)

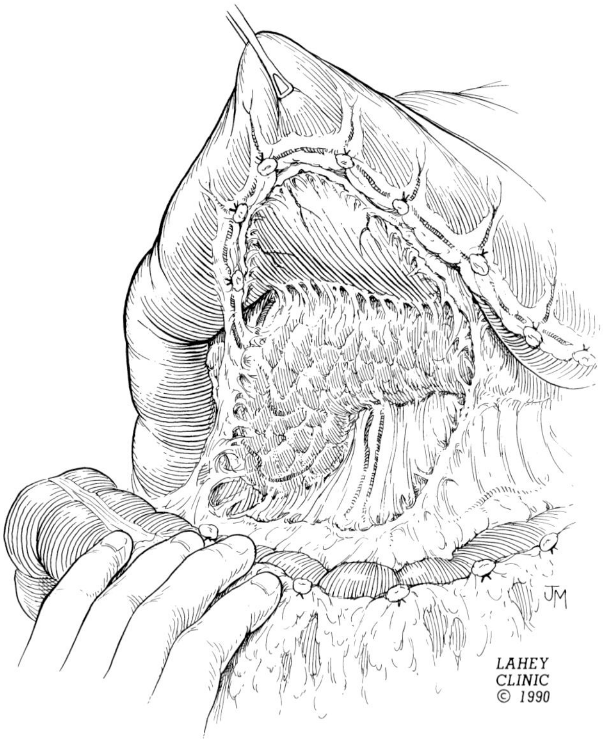

FIG. 35-5. The gastrocolic ligament is opened outside the gastroepiploic arcade, and the pancreas is exposed. (Reprinted with permission of Lahey Clinic.)

Gulliver and colleagues[10] reported that angiography would not have altered the outcome of patients studied previously with dynamic CT. Similarly, Freeny and associates[11] found that no tumors classified as resectable by CT were found to be unresectable by subsequent angiography. Dooley and coworkers[12] found that surgical resection was possible in 35% of patients with vessel encasement noted on angiography and in 77% of patients with normal results on angiography. Resection was not possible in any patient with total occlusion. The latter can currently be defined by ultrasonography. In our institution, the patient charges for ERCP with stenting is $4000. For superior mesenteric arteriography, the charge is $3500, with an added $896 fee for each additional vessel. The charge for percutaneous biopsy is $1800. Percutaneous biopsy is performed only in patients whose disease is thought to be unresectable or in patients whose condition is not suitable for surgery.

Patients whose disease is considered resectable undergo laparoscopy for staging, followed by laparotomy in the same procedure when the laparoscopic findings are negative. Patients with unresectable disease discovered during any stage of the evaluation are treated with comfort measures alone, decompression by either stenting or bypass, and radiation and chemotherapy on an individualized basis. Before operation, coagulopathy should be corrected as well as fluid and electrolyte imbalances, and prophylactic antibiotics are given.

TECHNIQUE

A bilateral subcostal incision is used, and the abdomen is explored to rule out metastatic disease. The root of the mesentery and the angle of Treitz are assessed for invasion by tumor (Fig. 35-3). An extensive Kocher maneuver is performed that permits examination and sampling of the common bile duct node, the hepatoduodenal ligament, and the periaortic area (Fig. 35-4). Gerota's fascia can be removed to optimize the margin in larger tumors.

The gastrocolic ligament is divided outside the gastroepiploic arcade to permit exposure of the pancreas while optimizing the blood supply to the antropyloric area (Fig. 35-5). The pancreas is exposed anteriorly. After the pancreas has been mobilized, additional peripancreatic, superior mesenteric, and celiac nodes can be sampled for staging. The local extent of disease can be appreciated better by palpation of the head of the gland (Fig. 35-6). At this time, palpation identifies any vascular anomalies, such as a replaced right hepatic artery arising in the superior mesenteric artery. This artery can be displaced and preserved during dissection and removal of the head of the pancreas (Fig. 35-7).

The inferior border of the pancreas is dissected, and the supe-

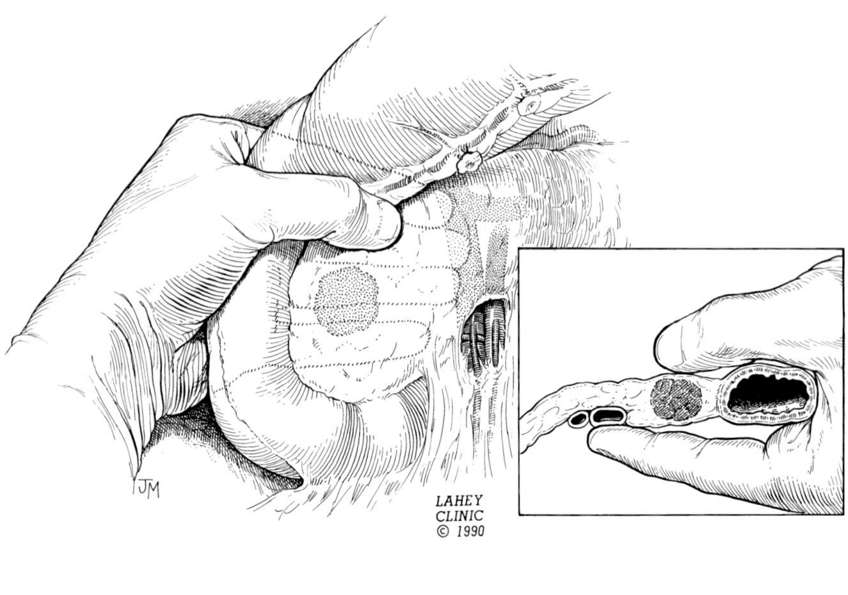

FIG. 35-6. The local extent of the tumor is assessed by palpation. The hepatoduodenal ligament is examined for a replaced right hepatic artery. (Reprinted with permission of Lahey Clinic.)

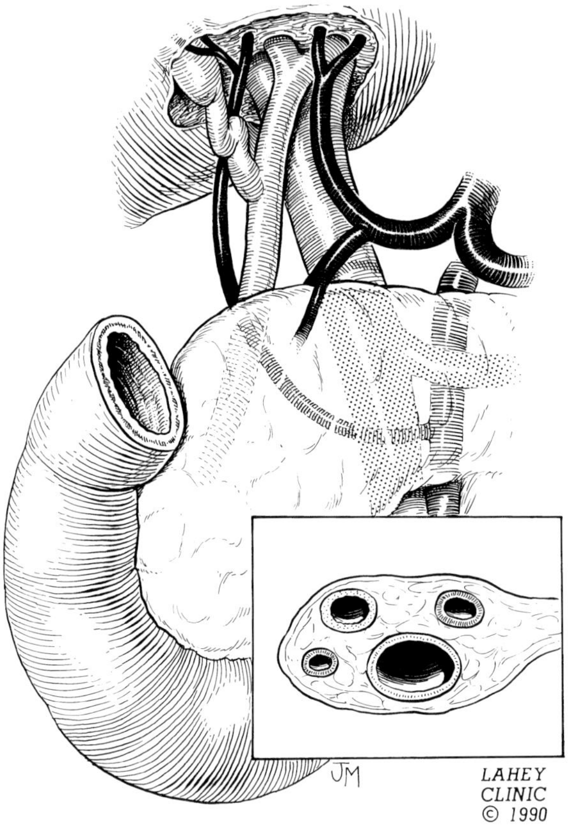

FIG. 35-7. The replaced right hepatic artery arises from the superior mesenteric artery. (Reprinted with permission of Lahey Clinic.)

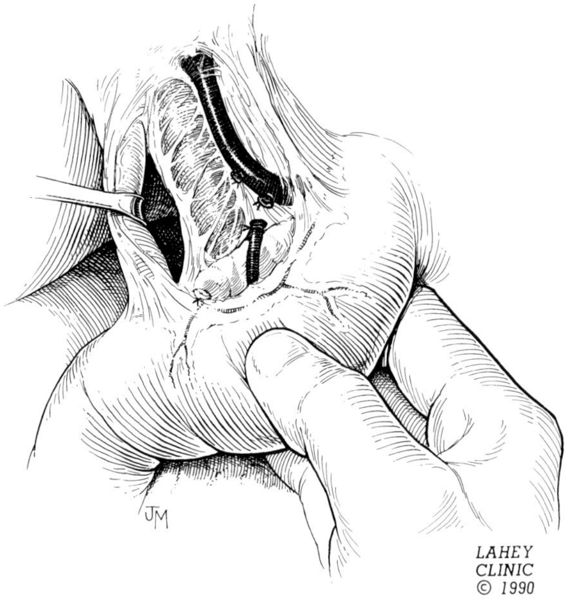

FIG. 35-9. The gastroduodenal artery is suture ligated and divided. (Reprinted with permission of Lahey Clinic.)

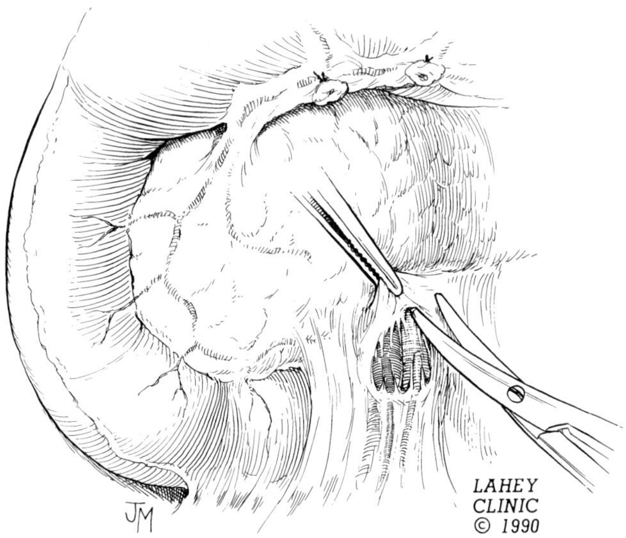

FIG. 35-8. The superior mesenteric vein is identified at the inferior border of the pancreas. (Reprinted with permission of Lahey Clinic.)

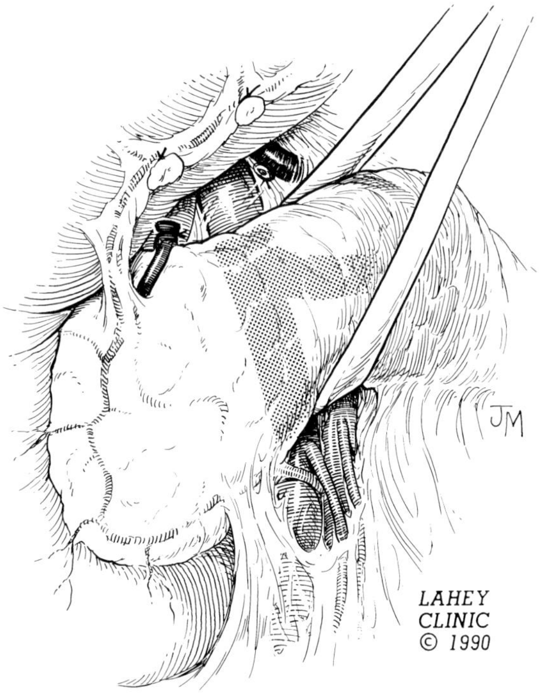

FIG. 35-10. The neck of the pancreas is elevated from the superior mesenteric vessels. (Reprinted with permission of Lahey Clinic.)

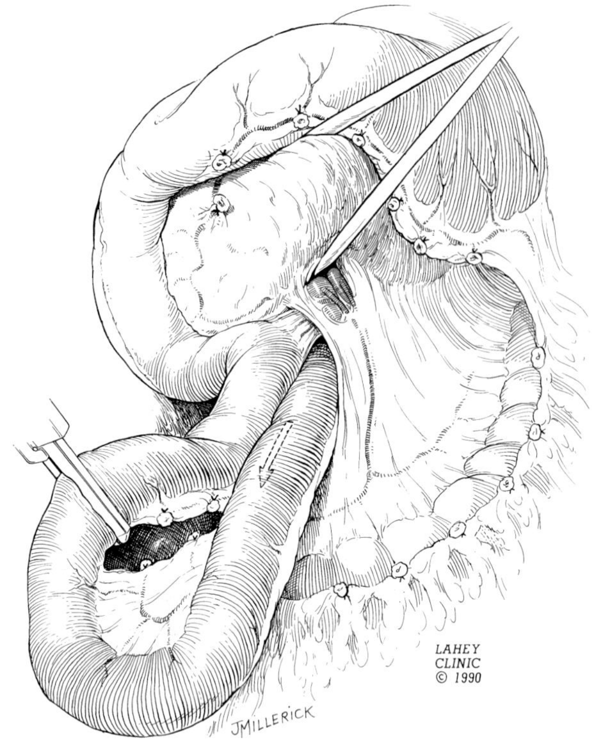

FIG. 35-11. The proximal jeujunum is mobilized, and the angle of Treitz is divided. The jejunum is brought under the superior mesenteric vessels and divided with a GIA stapler. (Reprinted with permission of Lahey Clinic.)

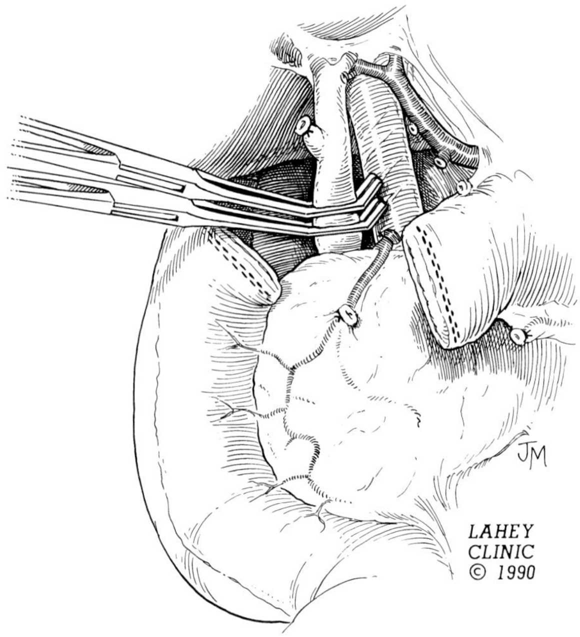

FIG. 35-13. The common duct is divided. (Reprinted with permission of Lahey Clinic.)

rior mesenteric vein is identified (Fig. 35-8). The common duct is displaced to the right, and the hepatic artery is palpated, identified, and dissected. The gastroduodenal artery is identified and dissected. A vascular clamp is applied to the gastroduodenal artery. The pulse of the hepatic artery is assessed, and when it decreases or disappears, the need for a vein graft from the aorta to the hepatic artery or celiac axis should be considered. When the pulse persists, the gastroduodenal artery is suture ligated and divided (Fig. 35-9). Division of the gastroduodenal artery facilitates identification of the portal vein in the superior border of the pancreas.

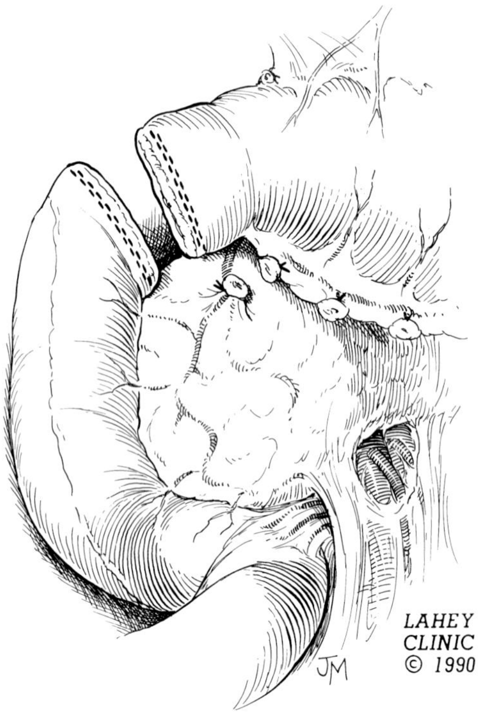

FIG. 35-12. The duodenum is divided, preserving the nerves of Latarjet. (Reprinted with permission of Lahey Clinic.)

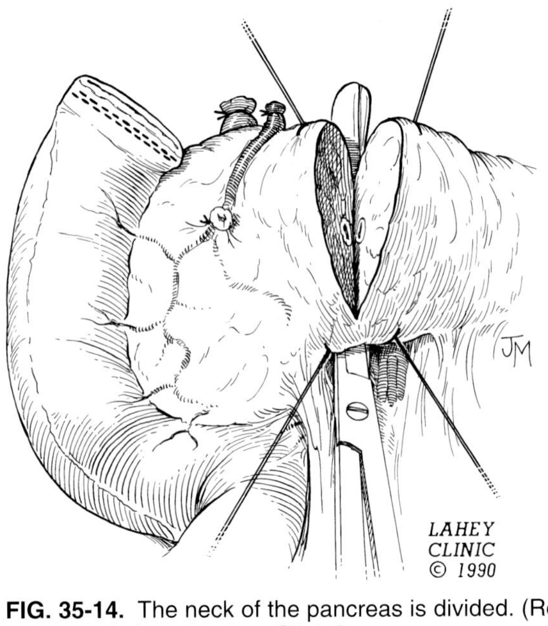

FIG. 35-14. The neck of the pancreas is divided. (Reprinted with permission of Lahey Clinic.)

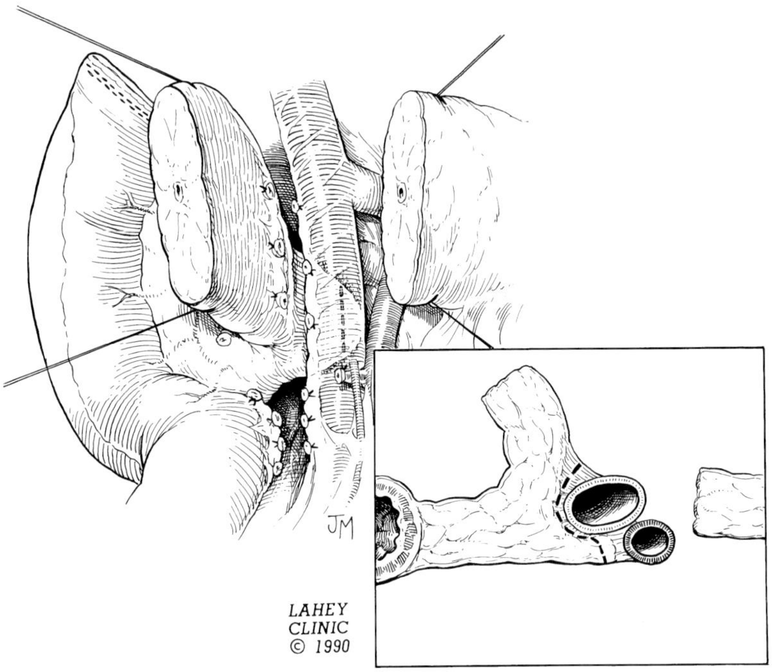

FIG. 35-15. Dissection of the head of the pancreas and uncinate process from the superior mesenteric vessels and portal vein is shown. (Reprinted with permission of Lahey Clinic.)

The pancreas is elevated from the superior mesenteric vessels by careful blunt dissection (Fig. 35-10). Additional information concerning local extent of disease to the superior mesenteric vessels and portal vein can be achieved at this time. When the lesion is thought to be resectable, mobilization of the angle of Treitz is completed, bringing the proximal jejunum to the right and under the superior mesenteric vessels. The proximal jejunum is divided with a gastrointestinal anastomosis stapler (United States Surgical Corp., Norwalk, CT; Fig. 35-11). Care is taken to ligate the short mesenteric branches between the proximal jejunum and the superior mesenteric artery to avoid bleeding.

The duodenum is dissected. The left gastroepiploic artery is suture ligated and divided over the pancreas, and the proximal duodenum is divided with the gastrointestinal anastomosis stapler about 4 cm from the pylorus. Care is taken not to injure the nerves of Latarjet and the blood supply of the antropyloric area (Fig. 35-12). Cholecystectomy is performed, and the middle third of the common duct is divided (Fig. 35-13).

The neck of the pancreas is divided between stay sutures of silk, and all bleeding points are suture ligated with silk (Fig. 35-14). The head of the pancreas is dissected from the superior mesenteric vein, and lateral branches of the portal vein are ligated. The uncinate process is exposed and dissected from the superior mesenteric artery (Fig. 35-15). The uncinate process is carefully dissected from the superior mesenteric artery, visualizing small branches and suture ligating them, or palpating the artery and clamping the uncinate process just to the right of the superior mesenteric artery. The anatomy after removal of the specimen is shown in Figure 35-16.

Gastrointestinal reconstruction is performed next, bringing the proximal jejunum in a retrocolic manner through the mesocolon. The pancreaticojejunostomy can be performed as a dunking technique in one (Fig. 35-17) or two layers (Fig. 35-18), or, as is my (RLR) preference, end-to-side two-layer mucosa-to-mucosa anastomosis (Fig. 35-19). End-to-side hepaticojejunostomy is performed with a single layer of absorbable monofilament sutures. Occasionally, the biliary anastomosis is stented. The T-tube is brought out through the hepatic duct primarily for decompression of the proximal jejunum and the pancreaticojejunostomy (Fig. 35-20).

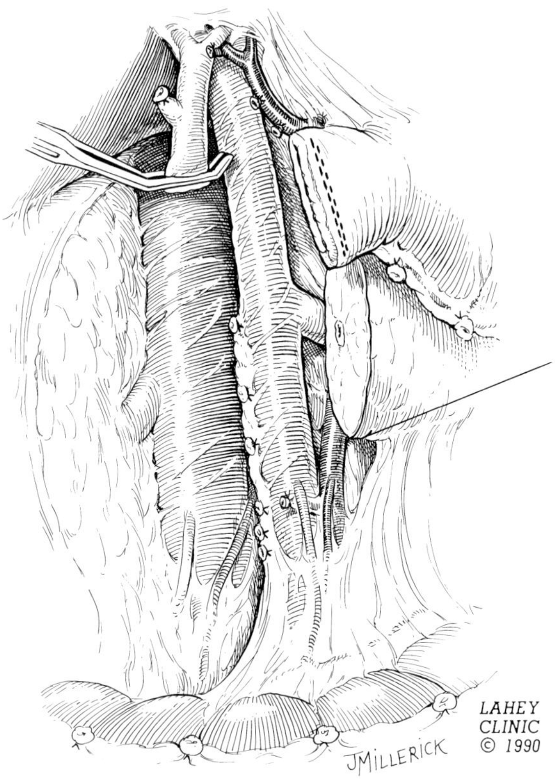

FIG. 35-16. Anatomy is shown after the specimen has been removed. (Reprinted with permission of Lahey Clinic.)

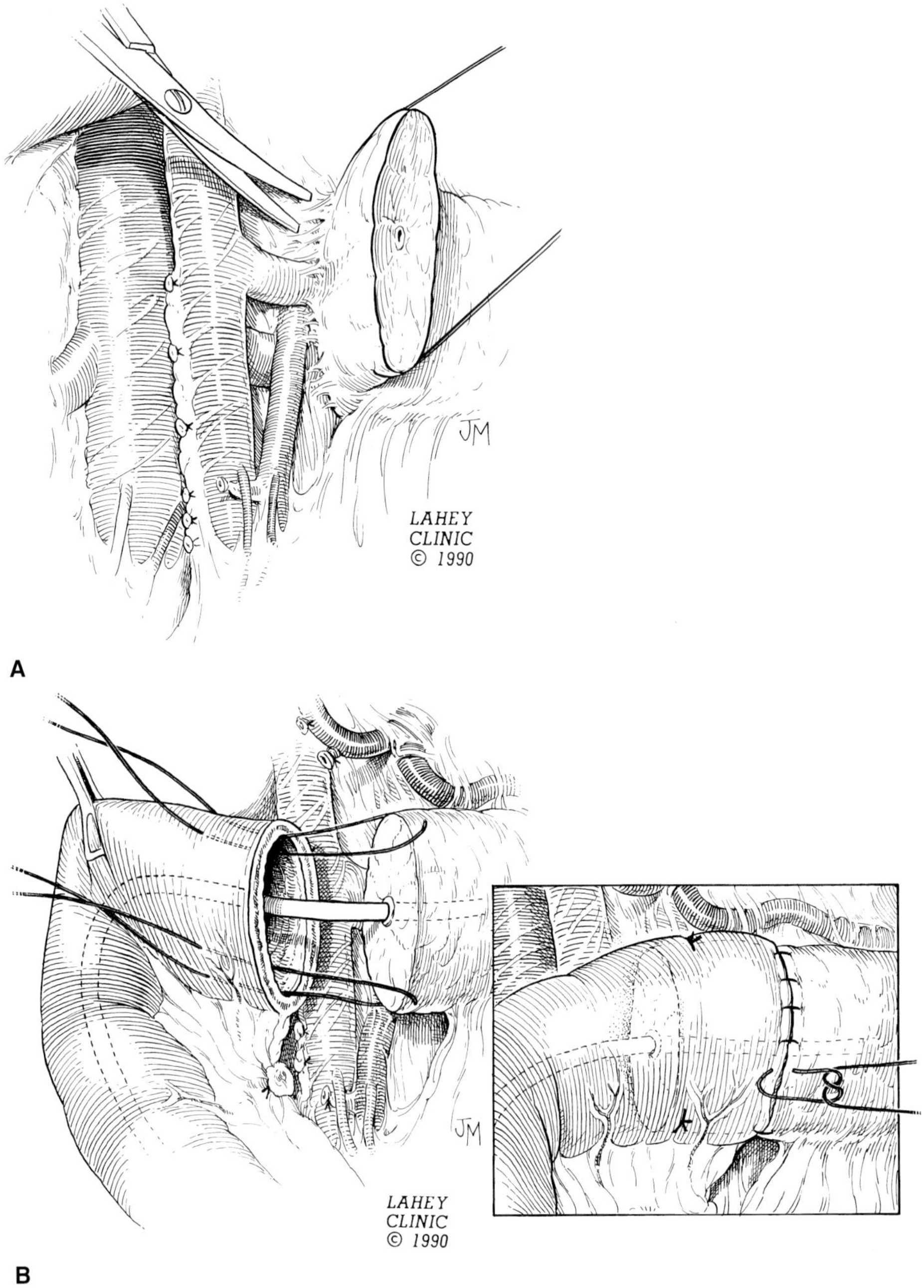

FIG. 35-17. (A) and **(B)** One-layer dunking pancreaticojejunostomy is shown. (Reprinted with permission of Lahey Clinic.)

Duodenojejunostomy is performed in an end-to-side manner, using an inner layer of interrupted absorbable sutures and an outer layer of interrupted silk. This is done in the infracolic position (Fig. 35-21). The completed procedure is shown in Figure 35-22. Attention to detail can minimize the frequency and severity of pancreatic fistula, and preserve the blood supply of the duodenum and the function of the nerves of Latarjet—factors that may be important in minimizing delay of gastric emptying early after the procedure.

RESULTS

Between November 1979 and June 1992, we performed 106 pylorus-preserving pancreaticoduodenectomies for primary neoplasm in the periampullary area and 48 for pancreatitis. Of the patients with carcinoma, proximal pancreatectomy was performed in 95 patients, and total pancreatectomy was performed in 11 patients. Resection of the portal vein was carried out in 10 patients. The 30-day operative mortality rate was 1.9%. The pathologic diagnoses were reviewed critically to define more accurately the site of origin of the tumor. The site of tumor and the procedure performed were correlated (Table 35-1).

Although 20% of patients had a positive histologic margin of resection, in no patient was carcinoma detected at the duodenal margin of resection. The incidence of carcinoma at the margin of resection was higher in patients with carcinoma of the pancreas (37%) compared with ampullary adenocarcinoma (11%), bile duct carcinoma (19%), and duodenal carcinoma (18%). A positive pancreatic margin was defined as tumor present in the

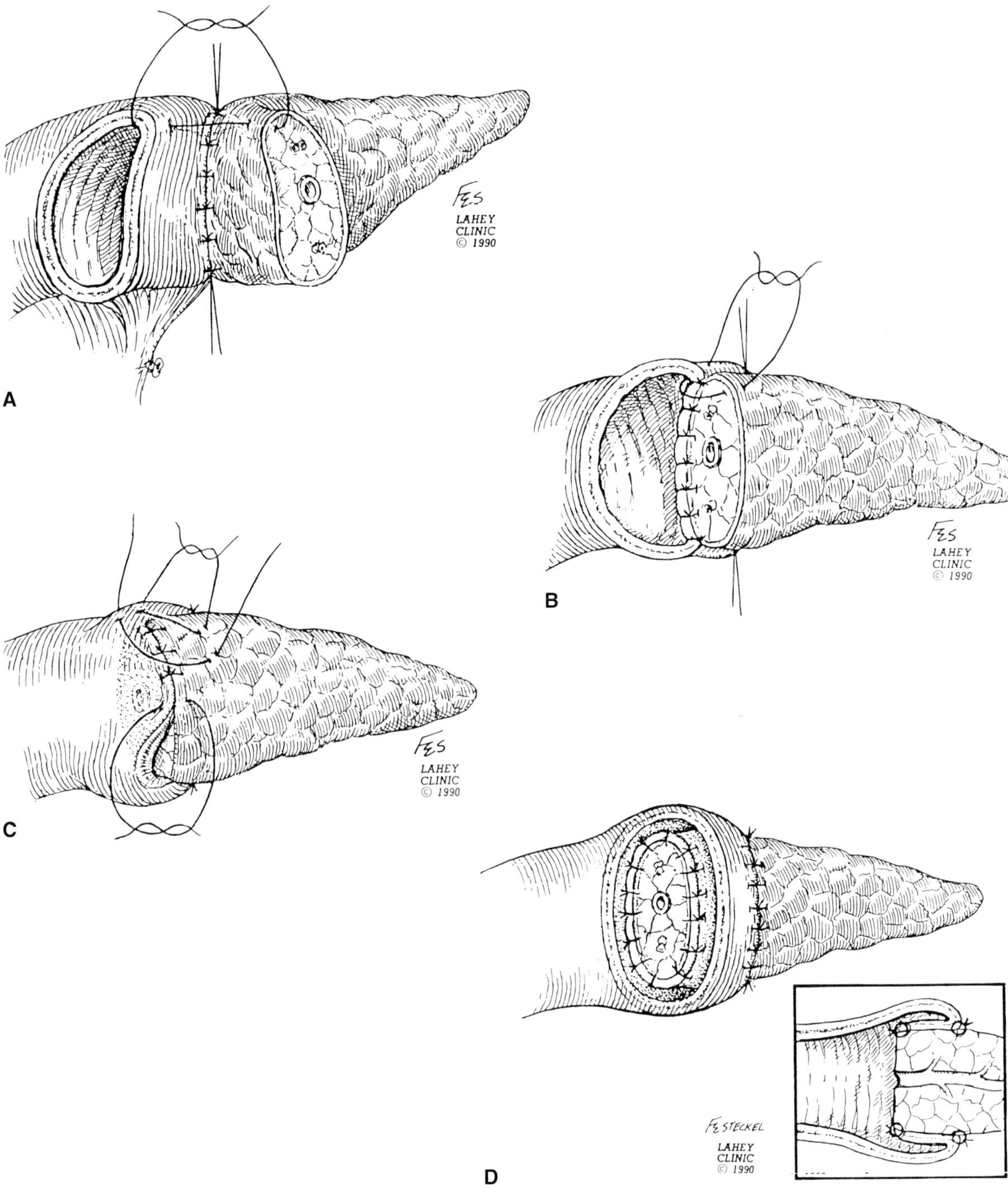

FIG. 35-18. (A–D) Two-layer dunking pancreaticojejunostomy is shown. (Reprinted with permission of Lahey Clinic.)

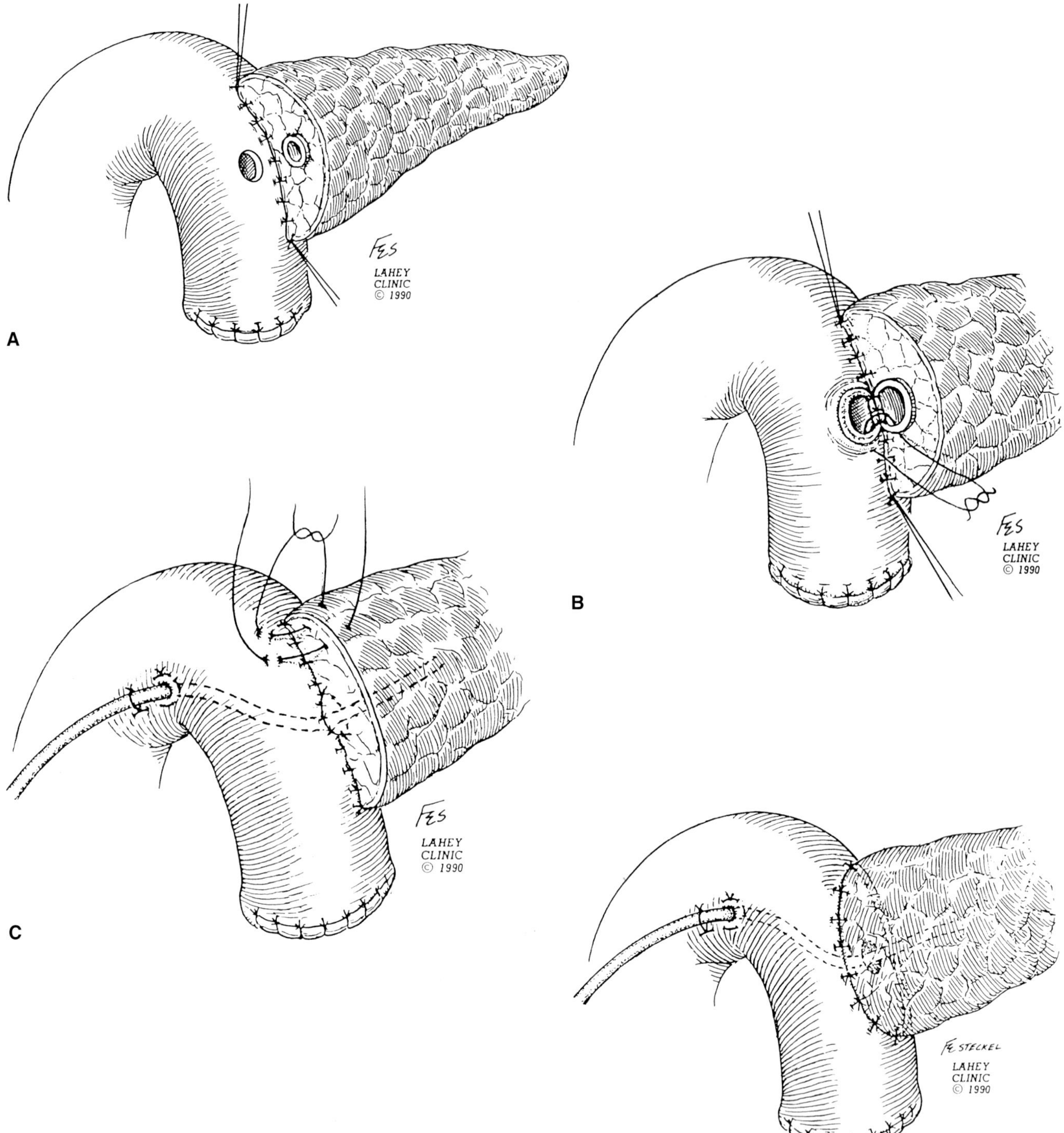

FIG. 35-19. (A–D) End-to-side mucosa-to-mucosa pancreaticojejunostomy is shown. (Reprinted with permission of Lahey Clinic.)

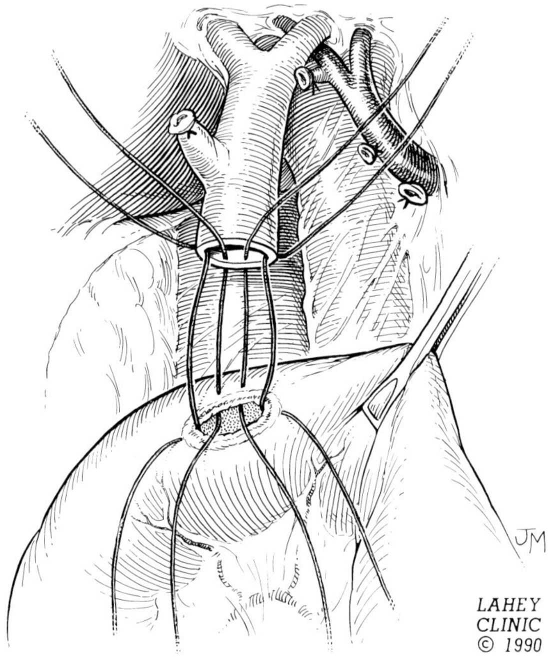

FIG. 35-20. Single-layer interrupted end-to-side hepaticojejunostomy is shown. (Reprinted with permission of Lahey Clinic.)

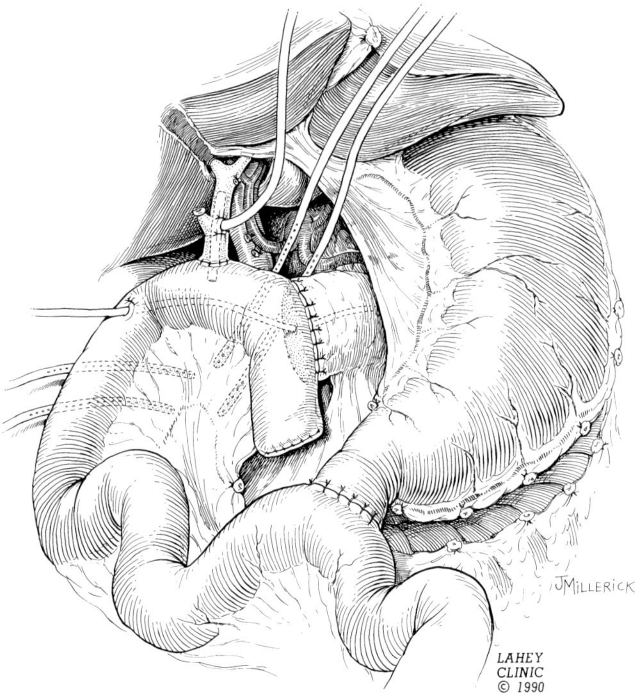

FIG. 35-22. Completed pylorus-preserving pancreatoduodenectomy is shown. (Reprinted with permission of Lahey Clinic.)

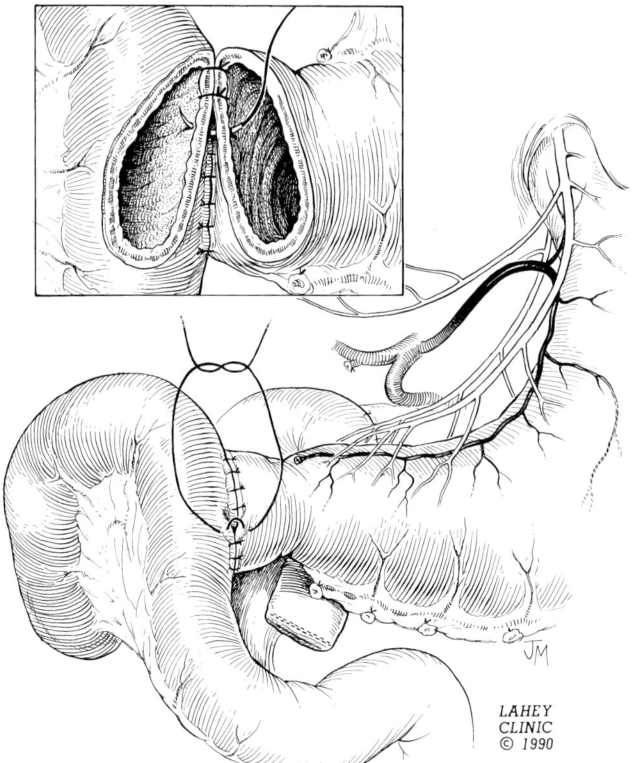

FIG. 35-21. Duodenojejunostomy is shown. (Reprinted with permission of Lahey Clinic.)

resected peripancreatic soft tissue or lymphatic channels. The presence of tumor at the pancreatic margin of resection occurred most commonly in the posterior pancreas or uncinate process. None of the patients had malignant involvement of the transection margin at the neck of the pancreas. We recommend routine frozen-section analysis of the transected margin of the neck of the pancreas at the time of operation.

The median size of the pancreatic ductal carcinoma was 2.5 cm (range, 1 to 6.5 cm). Of patients with pancreatic ductal carcinoma, 33% had stage I disease, 22% had stage II disease, and 44% had stage III disease. The location of positive margins at the site of origin of the primary tumor is seen in Table 35-2.

The median follow-up time was of 30 months (range, 6 to 156 months). Of the patients, 57% were using pancreatic enzyme supplementation. Diarrhea was present in 9% of patients, marginal ulceration was suspected in 7% of patients, and late gastric outlet obstruction occurred in 2% of the patients. None of the patients had the dumping syndrome.

Postoperative weight measurement available in 80 patients without clinical evidence of recurrence at the 6-month follow-up visit showed that 24 patients (30%) regained a median of 105% of their preoperative weight, 44% had a postoperative weight that was the same as or was within 10% of their preoperative weight, and the remaining 26% of patients had lost more than 10% of their preoperative weight.

The median survival for patients with ampullary adenocarcinoma was 52 months; for patients with pancreatic ductal adenocarcinoma, it was 18 months; for patients with carcinoma of the distal bile duct, it was 24 months; and for patients with duodenal carcinoma, it was 65 months. The 5-year survival rates were 45% ± 9% for patients with ampullary adenocarcinoma, 6.6% ± 6.1% for patients with pancreatic ductal carci-

TABLE 35-1. *Types of operations performed in 106 patients undergoing pylorus-preserving resection for carcinoma*

Type of cancer	No. of patients	No. patients undergoing proximal pancreatectomy (n = 95)		No. patients undergoing total pancreatectomy (n = 11)	
		Alone	With PVR*	Alone	With PVR*
Ampullary	34	31	0	3	0
Pancreatic ductal	27	15	7	4	1
Distal bile duct	24	23	0	0	1
Duodenal	11	11	0	0	0
Pancreatic islet cell	6	5	0	0	1
Cystadenocarcinoma	4	3	0	1	3
Total	106	88	7	8	3

* PVR, portal vein resection.

From Tsao JI, Rossi RL, Lowell JA. Pylorus-preserving pancreatoduodenectomy: is it an adequate cancer operation? Arch Surg 1994;129:407.

noma, 33.3% ± 10.7% for patients with distal bile duct carcinoma, 60.6% ± 15.7% for patients with duodenal carcinoma, and 75% ± 21.7% for patients with pancreatic islet cell carcinoma.

For patients with pancreatic ductal adenocarcinoma, tumor size of 2 cm or less was associated with a more favorable survival (16.7%; $P = 0.03$). Total pancreatectomy and portal vein resection were not associated with improved survival compared with results of pylorus-preserving pancreatectomy and results in patients without vein resection.

No prospective, randomized trial has compared the survival and metabolic advantages associated with pylorus-preserving pancreaticoduodenectomy with the standard Whipple operation. Pylorus-preserving pancreaticoduodenectomy has been reported[13] to be associated with shorter operative time and blood requirement than standard pancreaticoduodenectomy. Several reports[13–16] have failed to show a significant difference in survival at 3 and 5 years regardless of the type of resection performed (standard Whipple operation vs. pylorus-preserving pancreaticoduodenectomy) for pancreatic and other periampullary malignancies. As in our study, Cameron and associates[14] noted that no patients with pancreatic adenocarcinoma had positive duodenal margins. Klinkenbijl and colleagues[13] compared results of 47 pylorus-preserving pancreaticoduodenectomies with 44 standard Whipple operations for carcinoma and found no difference in involvement of margins between the two operations. Some reports[2,14–21] on survival of patients who had pancreatic resection for ductal pancreatic carcinoma are listed in Table 35-3. Possible improvement in median and 5-year survival rates for patients with pancreatic carcinoma that has been suggested by some authors[14] is explained by them as a possible change in biologic behavior of this tumor. Now that pancreatic and periampullary carcinomas are being treated more aggressively with resection, it must be kept in mind that other periampullary tumors are associated with a lower incidence of lymph node metastasis and local peripancreatic infiltration than pancreatic carcinoma[3,5]; therefore, they are proportionately more resectable, and long-term survival is superior to that associated with pancreatic carcinoma. The clinical ability to distinguish pancreatic from periampullary tumors is limited, as is the ability of the pathologist to distinguish the site of origin on every occasion.[1] Therefore, we strongly suggest that when reporting survival rates for patients with periampullary tumors and pancreatic carcinoma, a separate group of patients with indeterminate site of origin should be created. This categorization permits more accurate reporting of the sites of origin and better comparison of survival rates in the different series, and minimizes the possibility of including, as pancreatic carcinoma, other periampullary tumors more likely to be resectable and associated with a better prognosis.

TABLE 35-2. *Tumor involvement at resection margins in 106 patients undergoing pylorus-preserving pancreatoduodenectomy for periampullary carcinoma*

Type of cancer	No. of patients	Location of positive margin, no. patients				
		Duodenum	Bile duct	Pancreas*	Retroperitoneum	Vascular
Ampullary	34	0	0	1	3	0
Pancreatic duct	27	0	0	9	1	2
Distal bile duct	24	0	1	2	1	0
Duodenal	11	0	0	0	2	0
Pancreatic islet cell	6	0	0	0	0	0
Cystadenocarcinoma	4	0	0	0	0	1
Total	106	0	1	12	7	3

* Peripancreatic fat and uncinate; margin neck of pancreas negative in all patients.

From Tsao JI, Rossi RL, Lowell JA. Pylorus-preserving pancreatoduodenectomy: is it an adequate cancer operation? Arch Surg 1994;129:408.

TABLE 35-3. *Five-year survival associated with pancreatoduodenectomy for pancreatic carcinoma*

Study	Study period	No. of patients	Procedure	5-year survival, %
Jones et al,[17] 1985	1962–1983	34	Whipple	7
Tsuchiya et al,[18] 1986	1966–1983	91	Whipple	30*
Tarazi et al,[19] 1986	1980–1984	26	Whipple	4
Grace et al,[16] 1986	1975–1984	35	Whipple/PPPD	5
Trede et al,[20] 1990	1985–1989	44	Whipple	14†
Cameron et al,[14] 1991	1969–1990	89	Whipple/PPPD	19
Kozuschek et al,[15] 1994	1985–1992	68	Whipple/PPPD	15
Nitecki et al,[21] 1994	1981–1991	174	Whipple/PPPD	7
Tsao et al,[2]	1979–1992	27	PPPD	7‡

* Small carcinoma (<2 cm) stages 1 and 2.

† Resection only: Negative margins; 25% survival. Resection for pancreatic cancer: Positive margins; 0% survival.

‡ Survival for patients with tumors <2 cm was 17% ($P = 0.03$). PPPD, Pylorus-preserving pancreatoduodenectomy.

Adapted from Tsao JI, Rossi RL, Lowell JA: Pylorus-preserving pancreatoduodenectomy: is it an adequate cancer operation? Arch Surg 1994;129:410.

The incidence of marginal ulceration and bleeding gastritis after pylorus-preserving pancreaticoduodenectomy is lower or similar to that reported for standard pancreaticoduodenectomy with hemigastrectomy or antrectomy and vagotomy (4% to 7%).[22,23] Child and Frey[24] suggested that extended hemigastrectomy be performed rather than limited antrectomy—not because of the presence of carcinoma but to minimize marginal ulceration. Pearlman and coworkers[25] demonstrated that pylorus-preserving pancreaticoduodenectomy was not associated with hypergastrinemia or hyperacidemia.

Maintaining gastric capacity, normal gastric emptying, mixing, and a mechanism of trituration have been suggested as potential advantages of pylorus-preserving pancreaticoduodenectomy. If this were true, benefits should be noted in weight gain, decrease in the incidence of postgastrectomy syndromes, better absorption, and perhaps easier management of patients who are diabetic. A study[26] of gastric emptying performed late in the postoperative period at our institution using radioisotopic techniques confirmed that the gastric emptying for solids and liquids after pylorus-preserving pancreaticoduodenectomy was similar to that for normal control subjects. In addition, enterogastric reflux is significantly decreased with pylorus-preserving pancreaticoduodenectomy compared with patients undergoing gastric resection. Using digital subtraction radiologic techniques to study gastric and pyloric motility, Kozuschek and associates[15] demonstrated that gastric motility was normal in all five patients studied. The transit time to the cecum was also preserved, whereas it was considerably faster in patients who underwent the standard Whipple operation. Doty and Meyer[27] suggested that vagotomy and antrectomy impaired absorption of fat from solids but not from liquid dietary sources because of the failure of mixing and trituration of the stomach. The study of Kozuschek and associates[15] compared results of pylorus-preserving pancreaticoduodenectomy in 28 patients with results of the standard Whipple operation in 14 patients who were operated on in the same period of time, although the study was not a prospective, randomized one. After pylorus-preserving pancreaticoduodenectomy, 75% of patients had achieved their preoperative weight by 6 months, and 86% by 12 months. The respective figures for the standard Whipple operation were 35% and 43% (Fig. 35-23), a difference that was statistically significant. Our data[28] comparing both operations for chronic pancre-

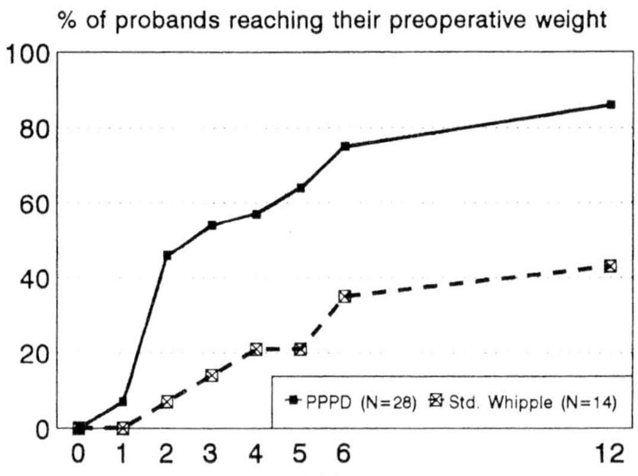

	0	1	2	3	4	5	6						12
PPPD (N=28)	0	7	46	54	57	64	75						86
Std. Whipple (N=14)	0	0	7	14	21	21	35						43

Time in months

FIG. 35-23. Weight gain after pylorus-preserving pancreatoduodenectomy (PPPD) and standard Whipple operation is shown ($P < 0.05$). (Reproduced from Kozuschek W, Reith HB, Waleczek H, Haarmann W, Edelmann M, Sonntag D. A comparison of long term results of the standard Whipple procedure and the pylorus preserving pancreatoduodenectomy. J Am Coll Surg 1994;178:446, with permission.)

atitis showed that 65% of patients gain weight after pylorus-preserving pancreaticoduodenectomy and 42% gain weight after the Whipple operation. In a similar group of patients, Morel and colleagues[29] noted that 95% of patients gained weight after pylorus-preserving pancreaticoduodenectomy for pancreatitis, compared with 50% after the standard Whipple operation.

The report of Hongo and coworkers[30] suggested that the insulin requirement was affected by gastric emptying in patients who were diabetic. The insulin demand was affected by the fast gastric emptying of patients who underwent gastric resection compared with patients who had a normal antropyloric complex and emptying mechanism, another potential advantage of the pylorus-preserving pancreaticoduodenectomy.

CONCLUSIONS

Pylorus-preserving pancreaticoduodenectomy can achieve results as a cancer operation that are similar to those associated with the standard Whipple operation, while eliminating the side effects related to gastric resection. The resulting improved nutritional status of these patients represents a better quality of life and could result in improved tolerance of adjuvant cancer treatments. That the standard Whipple operation offers survival advantages in a subgroup of patients has not yet been proved. A prospective, randomized trial is needed to define the role of extensive nodal dissection.

REFERENCES

1. Martin FM, Rossi RL, Dorrucci V, Silverman ML, Braasch JW. Clinical and pathologic correlations in patients with periampullary tumors. Arch Surg 1990;125:723.
2. Tsao JI, Rossi RL, Lowell JA. Pylorus-preserving pancreatoduodenectomy: is it an adequate cancer operation? Arch Surg 1994;129:405.
3. Cubilla AL, Fortner J, Fitzgerald PJ. Lymph node involvement in carcinoma of the head of the pancreas area. Cancer 1978;41:880.
4. Cooperman AM. Cancer of the pancreas: a dilemma in treatment. Surg Clin North Am 1981;61:107.
5. Nagai H, Kuroda A, Morioka Y. Lymphatic and local spread of T1 and T2 pancreatic cancer: a study of autopsy material. Ann Surg 1986; 204:65.
6. Kayahara M, Nagakawa T, Kobayashi H, et al. Lymphatic flow in carcinoma of the head of the pancreas. Cancer 1992;70:2061.
7. Whipple AO, Parsons WB, Mullins CR. Treatment of carcinoma of ampulla of Vater. Ann Surg 1935;102:763.
8. Watson K. Carcinoma of ampulla of Vater: successful radical resection. Br J Surg 1944;31:368.
9. Traverso LW, Longmire WP Jr. Preservation of the pylorus in pancreaticoduodenectomy. Surg Gynecol Obstet 1978;146:959.
10. Gulliver DJ, Baker ME, Cheng CA, Meyers WC, Pappas TN. Malignant biliary obstruction: efficacy of thin-section dynamic CT in determining resectability. AJR Am J Roentgenol 1992;159:503.
11. Freeny PC, Marks WM, Ryan JA, Traverso LW. Pancreatic ductal adenocarcinoma: diagnosis and staging with dynamic CT. Radiology 1988;166(1 Pt 1):125.
12. Dooley WC, Cameron JL, Pitt HA, Lillemoe KD, Yue NC, Venbrux AC. Is preoperative angiography useful in patients with periampullary tumors? Ann Surg 1990;211:649.
13. Klinkenbijl JH, van der Schelling GP, Hop WC, van Pel R, Bruining HA, Jeekel J. The advantages of pylorus-preserving pancreatoduodenectomy in malignant disease of the pancreas and periampullary region. Ann Surg 1992;216:142.
14. Cameron JL, Crist DW, Sitzmann JV, et al. Factors influencing survival after pancreaticoduodenectomy for pancreatic cancer. Am J Surg 1991; 161:120.
15. Kozuschek W, Reith HB, Waleczek H, Haarmann W, Edelmann M, Sonntag D. A comparison of long term results of the standard Whipple procedure and the pylorus preserving pancreatoduodenectomy. J Am Coll Surg 1994;178:443.
16. Grace PA, Pitt HA, Tompkins RK, DenBesten L, Longmire WP Jr. Decreased morbidity and mortality after pancreatoduodenectomy. Am J Surg 1986;151:141.
17. Jones BA, Langer B, Taylor BR, Girotti M. Periampullary tumors: which ones should be resected? Am J Surg 1985;149:46.
18. Tsuchiya R, Noda T, Harada N, et al. Collective review of small carcinomas of the pancreas. Ann Surg 1986;203:77.
19. Tarazi RY, Hermann RE, Vogt DP, et al. Results of surgical treatment of periampullary tumors: a thirty-five-year experience. Surgery 1986; 100:716.
20. Trede M, Schwall G, Saeger H-D. Survival after pancreatoduodenectomy: 118 consecutive resections without an operative mortality. Ann Surg 1990;211:447.
21. Nitecki S, Sarr MG, Colby TV, van Heerden JA. Long term survival after resection for ductal carcinoma of the pancreas: is it really improving? (Abstract). In: Program, Meeting of the Society for Surgery of the Alimentary Tract, New Orleans, May 1994:114.
22. Itani KM, Coleman RE, Meyers WC, Akwari OA. Pylorus-preserving pancreatoduodenectomy: a clinical and physiologic appraisal. Ann Surg 1986;204:655.
23. Traverso LW. The superlative results of pylorus-preserving pancreaticoduodenectomy for severe complications of chronic pancreatitis. Japanese Journal of Gastroenterological Surgery 1992;25:2269.
24. Child CG III, Frey CF. Pancreaticoduodenectomy: surgical grand rounds—University of Michigan. Surg Clin North Am 1966;46:1201.
25. Pearlman NW, Stiegmann GV, Ahnen DJ, Schultz AL, Fink LM. Acid and gastrin levels following pyloric-preserving pancreaticoduodenectomy. Arch Surg 1986;121:661.
26. Braasch JW, Deziel DJ, Rossi RL, Watkins E Jr, Winter PF. Pyloric and gastric preserving pancreatic resection: experience with 87 patients. Ann Surg 1986;204:411.
27. Doty JE, Meyer JH. Vagotomy and antrectomy impairs absorption of fat from solid, but not liquid dietary sources. (Abstract) Gastroenterology 1987;92(5 Pt 2):1374.
28. Braasch JW. Pylorus-preserving pancreatoduodenectomy. In: Braasch JW, Tompkins RK, eds. Surgical diseases of the biliary tract and pancreas: multidisciplinary management. St Louis: Mosby-Year Book, 1994:565.
29. Morel P, Mathey P, Corboud H, Huber O, Egeli RA, Rohner A. Pylorus-preserving duodenopancreatectomy: long-term complications and comparison with the Whipple procedure. World J Surg 1990;14:642.
30. Hongo M, Satake K, Sanoyama K, et al. Regulation of insulin demand by gastric emptying in diabetics. (Abstract) Gastroenterology 1987; 92(5 Pt 2):1440.

Surgery for Gastrointestinal Cancer: A Multidisciplinary Approach, edited by Harold J. Wanebo.
Lippincott-Raven Publishers, Philadelphia, © 1997.

CHAPTER 36

Total Pancreatectomy for Cancer of the Head of the Pancreas

A. Rahim Moossa and Marquis Hart

The most appropriate operation for cancer of the head of the pancreas is a debatable topic that centers around two technical points: the extent of the pancreatic resection; and the extent of the peripancreatic excision. We believe that these two issues are intimately related because one facilitates the other.[1]

Total pancreaticoduodenectomy remains a controversial operation for the treatment of ductal adenocarcinoma of the head of the pancreas. In the 1950s, 1960s, and early 1970s, there was growing dissatisfaction with the poor survival results and the high operative mortality and morbidity associated with the conventional prototype pancreaticoduodenectomy for carcinoma of the pancreatic head. During that era, mortality rates of 20% to 40% were commonly reported and accepted. Complications that were usually fatal included intraoperative and postoperative hemorrhage, leakage from the pancreatojejunal anastomosis, intraabdominal sepsis, and multiorgan system failure. The 5-year survival rate of patients who survived the Whipple resection was dismally low, in the range of 0% to 5%. This state of affairs led several authorities to question whether any type of pancreaticoduodenectomy was ethically justifiable. Others approached the problem by searching for more effective operations to treat this dismal disease. As early as 1944, Priestley and colleagues from the Mayo Clinic had reported that long-term survival was possible after total pancreaticoduodenectomy.[2] Ten years later, Ross emphasized the multicentricity of pancreatic cancer and made a strong plea for total pancreatic extirpation in these cases.[3] By 1958, Milton Porter, working at Whipple's institution, had become a major advocate of the operation.[4]

The major setback in the popularity of total pancreatectomy came in 1960, when Howard and Jordan reported a collected series of total pancreatectomies performed by numerous surgeons at multiple institutions with an average mortality of 37%.[5] This review had a major impact on surgical practice, and total pancreatectomy was abandoned as an option for well over a decade, even though, in 1966, Collins and associates had made a strong case for total pancreatectomy as the ideal treatment for cancer of the head of the pancreas.[6]

In the early 1970s, there was a revival of interest in total pancreatectomy as the treatment for ductal adenocarcinoma in the head of the gland, and this coincided with several advances in surgical techniques, anesthesia, blood banking, intensive care monitoring, and patient selection and preparation, as well as in the treatment of metabolic disorders. The advantages of total pancreatectomy over a Whipple operation are largely theoretic and probably cannot be subjected to proper statistical validation. Failure to demonstrate a difference between two retrospective groups of noncomparable patients, however, does not necessarily imply that no such difference exists. We believe that comparison of noncomparable data should not be used to support any preconceived thesis.

In the past, total pancreatectomy was indiscriminately applied to patients with far-advanced pancreatic cancer. In addition, the operative mortality and morbidity were prohibitive. It must, however, be admitted at the outset that total pancreatectomy is not the ideal operation for *all patients* with cancer in the head of the pancreas.

In the late 1970s, support for total pancreatic extirpation came from various quarters. Remine, Brooks, Ishe, Moreno-Gonzales, Manabe, and Moossa all advocate total pancreatic extirpation in *selected* patients with stage I or II cancer of the head of the gland, for several reasons[7]:

1. *Experimental, clinical, and pathologic evidence strongly suggest that all ducts within the gland are exposed to the same carcinogenic stimuli and that cancer of the head of the gland, like cancer in many other organs, is potentially multifocal in origin.* Such multicentricity has been demonstrated in anything from 16% to 37% of cases. In addition, ductal epithelial hyperplasia, papillary hyperplasia, and carcinoma in situ have been found in as many as 41% of pancreatic cancer specimens. This compares with the results of routine autopsy specimens from patients dying

A. Rahim Moossa, Professor and Chair, Department of Surgery, University of Southern California, San Diego, UCSD Medical Center, 200 West Arbor Drive, San Diego, CA 92103-8400

Marquis Hart, Assistant Professor, Department of Surgery, University of Southern California, San Diego, UCSD Medical Center, 200 West Arbor Drive, San Diego, CA 92103-8401 without pancreatic cancer, whereby these changes are seen in only 9% of the normal gland. Admittedly, the rate of progression and the natural history of these histologic dysplastic changes are unknown. It is thus impossible to speculate how long these microscopic changes will take to evolve into a frankly invasive neoplasm.

2. *Direct extension, intraductal seeding, and regional lymphatic permeation have all been demonstrated in pancreatic cancer.* Extension of the malignancy into the line of pancreatic transection during a Whipple pancreaticoduodenectomy has been demonstrated histologically in many cases. Viable malignant cells are often exfoliated into an obstructed pancreatic ductal system and, if the gland is transected, this creates a potential seeding hazard for local recurrence. Every surgeon will admit that subtle forms of multicentricity or direct extension cannot be readily appreciated at operation because they are often outwardly invisible or impalpable. Associated obstructive pancreatitis often creates additional confusion. Even an experienced pathologist may have difficulty in providing a frozen-section histologic report on the surgical margins intraoperatively. This type of situation often leads to operative indecision and confusion over the exact site of pancreatic transection, which in turn leads to other time-consuming diagnostic maneuvers in the operating room. These dilemmas and difficulties are often eliminated by total pancreatectomy.
3. *Total pancreatectomy abolishes the need for pancreatojejunal anastomosis, which, even in expert hands, has a small risk of postoperative pancreatitis and anastomotic dehiscence.* Although the mortality and morbidity from this complication have been reduced appreciably since the early 1980s, it remains a serious complication. It is estimated that about 40% of all deaths after the Whipple operation in the 1970s were related to the pancreatojejunal anastomosis.
4. *There are appreciable data, emanating largely from Japan, that en bloc tissue dissection of all peripancreatic connective tissue and regional lymph nodes, as well as skeletonization of major vessels, substantially improve survival after pancreaticoduodenectomy of the Whipple type.*[8–10] There is no doubt that this potentially beneficial peripancreatic dissection can be performed more adequately if the entire gland is removed.
5. *The authors admit to a personal prejudice against partially resecting any gland that harbors a lethal cancer.* The fear of replacing one disease (ie, cancer) by another (ie, diabetes mellitus) is largely irrational in most instances. At least one third of all patients with pancreatic cancer are already diabetic at the time of diagnosis, and another 40% to 50% have abnormal glucose tolerance test results as defined by the American Diabetic Association age-adjusted criteria.[11] In addition, there is a high incidence of exocrine insufficiency after any type of pancreatojejunal anastomosis. Thus, the exocrine benefit of any remaining pancreatic tissue after a Whipple operation is often transient, variable, and doubtful, because many pancreatojejunostomies stenose after a variable period of time.

THE PLACE OF THE WHIPPLE OPERATION

Pancreaticoduodenectomy of the Whipple type is still considered to be the ideal operation for carcinoma of the ampulla of Vater, the duodenum or the distal common bile duct, for islet cell tumors that cannot be safely enucleated, and for chronic pancreatitis with dominant disease involving the head and the uncinate process. The debatable issue is whether it is the optimum procedure for all cases of exocrine cancer arising in the head of the gland. The Mayo Clinic group have reviewed their experience of several years with the Whipple operation versus total pancreatectomy for cancer of the head of the pancreas and have demonstrated no difference in survival between the two operations. No attempt was made to standardize the stages of the disease and the performance status of the patients in either group. In addition, the operations were performed over two to three decades by numerous surgeons without any type of randomization. Yet, based on this review, their recommendation is that the Whipple operation should be performed in the first instance for cancer of the head of the pancreas and should be converted into a total pancreatectomy only under three circumstances: if a safe pancreatojejunal anastomosis cannot be constructed; if there is tumor extension at the transection line on frozen-section histologic examination of the pancreas; or if the patient is already an insulin-requiring diabetic.[12]

The impact of this publication and its interpretation has had a profound influence on surgical practice. In addition, many surgeons in the 1980s had already abandoned total pancreatectomy based on a few anecdotal unpleasant experiences. By and large, total pancreatectomy was relegated to the operation for patients with far-advanced tumors. Brooks and Culebras and others have rightly pointed out that the results of total pancreatectomy are best when the operation is performed for stage I or II tumors.[13,14]

THE EXTENT OF PERIPANCREATIC DISSECTION

In 1973, Joseph Fortner developed the ''regional'' approach to pancreatic cancer and emphasized the resection of one or all the major vessels near the neck of the pancreas, namely the portal vein–superior mesenteric vein (PV-SMV) axis, the superior mesenteric artery, and the celiac axis.[15,16] These vessels were then reconstructed by end-to-end anastomosis or by an interposition graft. Unfortunately, whereas the operation satisfies the Halstedian concept of cancer surgery, it was wrongly performed for patients with far-advanced disease. As a result, the mortality and morbidity were high and the salvage rate was minimal. It is now generally accepted that resection of the major *arteries* does not improve survival. However, resection of the major vein (PV-SMV) is clearly desirable *if it will allow adequate soft tissue and lymphatic clearance.* Ishikawa and colleagues compared two consecutive groups of patients: group R-1 (receiving standard pancreaticoduodenectomy), and group R-2 (receiving a wider range of lymphatic and soft tissue excision, including the paraaortic region) as well as a more extensive pancreatic resection, leaving only a small stump of the gland in situ.[8] Mortality was similar in both groups, but the 3-year cumulative survival was 13% in the R-1 group compared with 38% in the R-2 group. Virtually all the deaths from cancer recurrence occurred within 3 years of operation. The cumulative rate of death from local recurrence decreased from 67% in the R-1 group to 16% in the R-2 group at 3 years ($P < 0.05$). Even among patients with nodal involvement, there was no 3-year survivor in the R-1 group, but there was 27% survival in the R-2 group ($P < 0.05$). The authors emphasized that extended clearance of the regional lymph nodes and soft tissue in the peripancreatic region benefits the patient with ductal adenocarcinoma of the head of the pancreas, provided that the tumor is not greater than 4 cm in diameter and provided that there is no obvious retroperitoneal extension at the time of operation. The same authors developed criteria for excision of the major veins in cases of pancreatic cancer.[10] The extent of the venous invasion determines whether the operation is worthwhile. If the PV-SMV axis is involved for a distance greater than 1.2 cm, or to an extent of half the circumference of major vein, than major venous resection does not improve survival. On the other hand, with a lesser extent of venous invasion, 59% 5-year survival can be achieved by segmental resection of the PV-SMV, with end-to-end anastomosis and meticulous dissection of the surrounding connective lymphatic tissues and skeletonization of the remaining vessels.

Manabe and coworkers also emphasize the radical nature of the lymphatic and peripancreatic soft tissue excision and report the best 5-year survival rate in the literature for both stage I to II and stage III to IV cancer in the head of the pancreas.[9] In their hands, total pancreaticoduodenectomy gave the best results. Their 5-year survival for stage I and II cancer is 41%, and for stage III to IV, 17.4%.

Nagakawa (personal communication)[7] also espouses the concept of a regional dissection and emphasizes the importance of a microscopically curative procedure to obtain the best chance of cure. His 3- and 5-year survival rates for cancer of the head of the pancreas are 31.7% and 27.8%, respectively.

THE PLACE OF THE PYLORUS-PRESERVING PROCEDURE

Considering the data discussed previously, the pylorus-preserving pancreaticoduodenectomy clearly does not satisfy the requirements of an adequate cancer operation. The operation was originally designed by Longmire and Traverso for benign disease of the pancreas.[17] In theory, the patient can eat normal-sized meals and does not contract dumping syndrome, but long-term follow-up and evaluation of symptoms, as well as studies of gastric emptying, have not demonstrated any significant difference between patients undergoing this operation and those undergoing the standard pancreaticoduodenectomy. This senior author believes that the pylorus-preserving operation should not be applied to cancer in the periampullary region because it further reduces the small surgical margins and may well short-change the individual patient by compromising an already small chance of cure. In spite of these dangers, it must be admitted that the pylorus-preserving operation is enjoying an ever-increasing popularity for all types of periampullary cancers in several centers across the world.

PREOPERATIVE CONSIDERATIONS

Selection of the patient and good preoperative preparation are essential. The general clinical assessment of the patient should be thorough and specific investigative procedures should be kept to a minimum. Computed tomography is the single most valuable preoperative study. Endoscopic retrograde cholangiopancreatography is performed only if indicated, largely to exclude benign disease such as choledocholithiasis, and should be performed just before operation to eliminate the development of biliary sepsis. Percutaneous transhepatic biliary decompression or endoscopic biliary decompression are *not* routinely advised preoperatively. Celiac and superior mesenteric arteriography is reserved for situations when the surgeon anticipates specific difficulties such as before reoperations, for obese patients, for patients who have had previous radiation therapy, for giant tumors that are likely to distort the normal vascular anatomy, or when the surgeon anticipates that he or she may have to do a major vascular resection with reconstruction.

The patient should be kept well hydrated, with intravenous fluids as necessary, and a diuresis should be maintained to prevent the risk of renal failure in the jaundiced patient. Vitamin K should be administered routinely. Anemia is occasionally corrected by blood transfusion if it is severe and is affecting the patient's general condition. Although packed red blood cells, fresh frozen plasma, and platelets are made routinely available, most cases of total pancreaticoduodenectomy can be performed without any blood transfusion. Cardiopulmonary function and renal function should be assessed routinely and intensive pulmonary physiotherapy started before surgery. Chronologic age of the patient is no longer a contraindication for major pancreatic resection. Physiologic age as assessed by the patient's functional status provides a much better criterion for selection or exclusion.

THE NEED FOR TISSUE DIAGNOSIS BEFORE A MAJOR RESECTIVE PROCEDURE

As recently as the early 1970s, the feeling of most surgeons was that an operation of the magnitude of a pancreaticoduodenectomy or total pancreaticoduodenectomy should not be performed without a definite tissue diagnosis of malignant disease. Times have changed. Because the mortality and morbidity of all forms of pancreaticoduodenectomies resections have decreased drastically since the 1970s, every surgeon should be prepared to accept an occasional benign pathology report.[18,19] The earlier the tumor, the more difficult it is to achieve a more positive diagnosis by any needle biopsy technique, preoperatively or intraoperatively. The only hope of averting the tragedy of not resecting a potentially curable lesion is by performing the resection as an "excisional biopsy," provided that it can be done safely. Thus, pancreatic biopsy should not be performed in a "knee-jerk" fashion without any planning whenever a pancreatic abnormality is encountered during an imaging technique or at laparotomy. Before proceeding with a pancreatic biopsy, the surgeon must plan how to proceed if the biopsy shows cancer and how to proceed if the biopsy does not. We believe that a pancreatic biopsy is justified only if the result is likely to influence the patient's future management. On the other hand, unresectable or metastatic tumors must always be sampled until a definite diagnosis is made, no matter how tedious or time consuming the job may be. This removes any element of doubt about the diagnosis and obviates the need for a second laparotomy if the patient survives longer than anticipated.[20,21]

RESULTS AND POSTOPERATIVE MANAGEMENT

The operative mortality of total pancreatectomy in expert hands is of the order of 1% to 2%. The immediate postoperative morbidity is less than 20%, if one includes relatively trivial complications such as atelectasis, superficial wound infections, thrombophlebitis at intravenous sites, inability to control blood sugar adequately during the early postoperative phase, and the like. This is in contradistinction to the standard Whipple operation, whereby the complication rate is of the order of 40% to 50%, largely related to the pancreatojejunal anastomosis and to the delay in gastric emptying.

The long-term survival of extirpative pancreatic surgery is directly dependent on the pathologic stage of the tumor. The main issue relating to the staging of pancreatic cancer is that it can only be done by the pathologist *after* the lesion has been resected. In 1981, we defined an "early" pancreatic cancer as one that satisfied the following criteria[22]:

1. Small lesion, namely, 2 cm or less in diameter.
2. No microscopic lymph node involvement. Here, the pathologist must examine at least 40 to 50 nodes of the submitted specimen before he or she can be sure that there is no lymph node disease.
3. No peripancreatic involvement. The retroperitoneum and the pseudocapsule of the pancreas must not be invaded by tumor either at operation or by histologic examination of the margins of resection.
4. No invasion of major vessels. These include the PV-SMV axis and superior mesenteric artery and the celiac axis.
5. No distant metastases at careful abdominal exploration.

This definition corresponds to stage I of the classification recommended by the Japanese Pancreatic Association. The first 64 cancers that we resected in our experience yielded 17 "early" tumors. They were all located in the head of the pancreas, but only 11 of the 17 were diagnosed before surgery. Four of the 17 were "incidental" cancers found after a total pancreatectomy for alleged pancreatitis. It must also be emphasized that 5 of the 17 patients eventually died from pancreatic cancer metastases between 3 to 6 years after surgery, implying that our classification is not perfect. However, 8 of the 17 patients survived over 5 years. There were two 10-year and two 15-year survivors.

The Japanese Pancreatic Association undertook a collective review of "small" carcinomas of the pancreas and collected 106 such cases.[23] By definition, these are tumors that are 2 cm in diameter or less. The resectability rate was 99% and the perioperative mortality rate was 3.9%. Of the 106 small carcinomas studied, only 44% belonged to stage I, and therefore are "early" by our previous definition. However, the cumulative survival data are impressive: 89.5% of patients with stage I disease survived at 1 year, 52% at 3 years, 37% at 5 years, and 37% at 10 years. Even for patients with stage II disease there was a 74% 1-year survival, 44% 3-year survival, and 26% 5-year survival. Thus, these data support our previous clinical impression that resection, even if does not confer immortality on every patient, provides the best palliation in terms of duration of survival, time away from hospital, and freedom from symptoms.

Patients with cancer in the head of the pancreas are usually elderly and are in a high-risk category because they often have other common disorders as comorbid factors. Thus, there is a high attrition rate with time because of metastatic disease as well as other unrelated conditions. Cardiovascular disease, cerebrovascular disease, primary lung cancer, colorectal cancer, and prostatic cancer are not uncommon. One patient in our series died of insulin overdose.

Total pancreatectomy should be seriously considered for *selected* patients with *relatively early* cancer in the head of the pancreas, especially if they are already diabetic, provided that these patients can be appropriately rehabilitated and educated to manage the metabolic sequelae.[24] It is essential to help the totally pancreatectomized patient manage his or her lifestyle in as easy a way as possible. This is performed by appropriately educating the patient, the close relatives, and the referring primary care physicians. The totally pancreatectomized patient is exquisitely sensitive to insulin because of the absence of pancreatic glucagon as a counterregulatory hormone. The patient must be instructed to eat small, frequent meals regularly. The diet must have a low fat content, and the patient must take regular enzyme supplements with each meal. The patient must check his or her blood glucose or urine fractionals at least twice daily. An occasional glycosuria or hyperglycemia, per se, is of no consequence. The patient should use a combination of long-acting and regular insulin given as one injection in the morning, and supplemented in the evening as deemed necessary by a further injection. The patient must be instructed never to miss meals and to carry sugar with him or her at all times. The patient must take sugar immediately if any untoward symptom such as dizziness, confusion, drowsiness, sweatiness, tachycardia, headache, or weakness develops. It is sometimes useful to allow the individual patient to experience one or two hypoglycemic attacks while in the hospital for him or her to see that these symptoms are rapidly alleviated by taking additional sugar.

In summary, total pancreatectomy with regional lymphadenectomy appears to be the best operation in a highly selected population with a relatively small cancer in the head of the pancreas. Twenty-five to 30% 5-year survival is not an unreasonable goal or expectation at the present time. Postoperative adjuvant therapy with radiation therapy and 5-fluorouracil as a radiosensitizer has emerged as an important adjunct to increased survival and to decrease local recurrence.[25] Whether this additional treatment should be given postoperatively to all patients or to selected patients with nodal metastases or extrapancreatic tumor extension is not yet settled.

REFERENCES

1. Moossa AR. Invited commentary on total pancreatectomy in ductal adenocarcinoma of the pancreas with special reference to resection of the portal vein in multicentric cancer. World J Surg 1993;17:126.
2. Priestley JT, Comfort MW, Radcliffe J Jr. Total pancreatectomy for hyperinsulinism due to islet cell adenoma: survival and cure after 16 months after operation: presentation of metabolic studies. Ann Surg 1944;119:211.
3. Ross DE. Cancer of the pancreas: a plea for total pancreatectomy. Am J Surg 1954;87:20.
4. Porter M. Total pancreatectomy. In: Maingot R, ed. Abdominal operations. 6th ed. New York: Appleton-Century-Crofts, 1976:963.
5. Howard JM, Jordan GL. Cancer of the pancreas. Curr Probl Cancer 1977;62:36.
6. Collins JJ, Craighead JE, Brooks JR. Rationale for total pancreatectomy for carcinoma of the pancreatic head. N Engl J Med 1966;274:559.

7. Moossa AR. Tumors of the pancreas. In: Moossa AR, Robson M, Schimpff S, eds. Comprehensive textbook of oncology. 2nd ed. Baltimore: Williams & Wilkins, 1991:958.
8. Ishikawa O, Ohhigashi H, Sasaki Y, et al. Practical usefulness of lymphatic and connective tissue clearance for carcinoma of the pancreatic head. Ann Surg 1988;208:215.
9. Manabe T, Oshio G, Baba N, et al. Radical pancreatectomy for ductal cell adenocarcinoma of the head of the pancreas. Cancer 1984;64:113.
10. Ishikawa O, Ohhigashi H, Imaoko, et al. Preoperative indications for extended pancreatectomy for locally advanced pancreas cancer involving the portal vein. Ann Surg 1992;215:231.
11. Schwartz SS, Zeidler A, Moossa AR, et al. A prospective study of glucose tolerance, insulin, C-peptide and glucagon responses in patients with pancreatic carcinoma. Dig Dis Sci 1978;23:1107.
12. Van Heerden JA, McIlrath DC, Ilstrup M, et al. Total pancreatectomy for ductal adenocarcinoma of the pancreas: an update. World J Surg 1988;12:658.
13. Brooks JR, Culebras JM. Cancer of the pancreas: palliative operation, Whipple procedure, or total pancreatectomy? Am J Surg 1976;1:416.
14. Brooks JR, Brooks DC, Levine JD. Total pancreatectomy for ductal cell carcinoma of the pancreas: an update. Ann Surg 1989;209:405.
15. Fortner JG. Regional resection of cancer of the pancreas: a new surgical approach. Surgery 1973;73:307.
16. Fortner JG. Surgical principles for pancreatic cancer: regional, total, and subtotal pancreatectomy. Cancer 1981;47:1712.
17. Traverso LW, Longmire WP Jr. Preservation of the pylorus in pancreatoduodenectomy. Surg Gynecol Obstet 1978;146:959.
18. Trede M, Schwall G, Saeger HD. Survival after pancreatoduodenectomy: 118 consecutive resections without an operative mortality. Ann Surg 1990;211:447.
19. Crist DW, Cameron JL. Current status of pancreatoduodenectomy or periampullary carcinoma. Hepatogastroenterology 1989;36:478.
20. Moossa AR. Biopsy of pancreatic masses. In: Burns JP, Bank S, eds. Disorders of the pancreas: current issues in diagnosis and management. New York: McGraw-Hill, 1992:345.
21. Moossa AR. Re-operation for pancreatic cancer. Arch Surg 1979;114:502.
22. Moossa AR, Levin B. The diagnosis of early pancreatic cancer: the University of Chicago experience. Cancer 1981;47:1688.
23. Tsuchiya R, Takatoshi N, Harada N, et al. Collective review of small carcinomas of the pancreas. Ann Surg 1986;203:77.
24. Ishe I, Andren-Sandberg A, Andersson R, et al. The role of total pancreatectomy in pancreatic cancer. Journal of Hepatobiliary and Pancreatic Surgery 1994;1:546.
25. Kalser MH, Allenberg S. Pancreatic cancer: adjuvant combined radiation and chemotherapy following curative resection: GITSG randomized study. Arch Surg 1985;120:899.

Surgery for Gastrointestinal Cancer: A Multidisciplinary Approach, edited by Harold J. Wanebo.
Lippincott-Raven Publishers, Philadelphia, © 1997.

CHAPTER 37

Regional Pancreatectomy: Translateral Retroperitoneal Approach

Takukazu Nagakawa

Surgical outcomes for pancreatic cancer are not as good as those for cancer of other organs. Some surgeons are of the opinion that resection of pancreatic cancer is ineffective. On the other hand, a number of reports recommend total pancreatectomy and the excision of lymph nodes and lymphatic vessels for the radical cure of pancreatic carcinoma.[1,2] En bloc resection of the invaded portion of the portal vein and superior mesenteric vein is performed to remove the regional extension of pancreatic cancer affecting the adjacent major blood vessels. In 1973, Fortner[3] succeeded in performing an end-to-end anastomosis after resection of the portal vein. In our clinic at Kanazawa University we developed a translateral retroperitoneal approach that facilitated combined portal resection,[4,5] and have performed this procedure for pancreatic carcinoma since 1973.

This chapter discusses the indications for extensive radical surgery for pancreatic carcinoma, the morbidity of the procedure, and its effect on prognosis.

MATERIALS AND METHODS

The elements of extended radical pancreatectomy by the translateral retroperitoneal approach include complete excision of the lymph nodes and nerve plexuses of the trunks of both celiac axes and the superior mesenteric artery. Adequate lymphadenectomy requires wide retroperitoneal dissection of the retroperitoneal nodes from the peripancreatic and adrenal glands above to the iliac bifurcation below. The extent of the pancreatectomy depends on the site of the cancer: for localized cancer of the head of the pancreas, the pancreas is transected from the left of the aorta and celiac artery, combined with resection of the portal vein. For nonlocalized cancer of the head, a total pancreatectomy with resection of the portal vein is performed. In all cases the translateral retroperitoneal approach facilitates an adequate lymphadenectomy.

Since 1973, 216 patients with pancreatic cancer underwent surgical exploration, 147 of whom had cancer of the head of the pancreas. Cystoadenocarcinoma, islet carcinoma, and carcinoma of the inferior bile duct and papilla of Vater were not included in this study. These 216 patients comprised 148 men and 68 women, and at the time of operation their ages ranged between 31 and 82 years, the mean being 62.9 years. One hundred forty-seven patients had cancer of the head of the pancreas, 53 had cancer in the body and tail, and 16 had cancer extending throughout the entire pancreas. Resection was performed in 104 patients (48.1%), including 58 patients who underwent curative resection based on macroscopic criteria (Table 37-1). The long-term results of cancer of the body and tail of the pancreas were poor in all instances. This chapter describes the results of surgery for cancer of the head of the pancreas only, and evaluates histopathologically the local extent of the tumor, the staging of the cancer, and the presence of cancer at the surgical margin in specimens from 51 patients with carcinoma of the head of the pancreas who survived the operation and underwent macroscopic curative resection.

Tumor size was classified into t1 (<2.0 cm in diameter), t2a (2.1 to 3.0 cm in diameter), t2b (3.1 to 4.0 cm in diameter), t3 (4.1 to 6.0 cm in diameter), and t4 (>6.1 cm in diameter). The local extent of disease was evaluated as s0 (anterior capsule of the pancreas not invaded), s1 (slightly invaded), or s2 (invasion of the capsule), and rp0, rp1, or rp2, depending on whether the retroperitoneal tissue had been invaded. Invasion of the portal vein was evaluated as pv0 (negative invasion), pv1 (positive invasion to the adventitia or media of the portal vein), or pv2 (positive invasion to the intima or the internal lumen of the portal vein accompanied by retroperitoneal invasion). Invasion into the surgical margin of resection was classified as ew0 (negative invasion), ew1 (positive invasion within 5 mm of the surgical margin), and ew2 (positive invasion). Invasion of the extrapancreatic nerve plexus was classified from plx0 to plx2 according to the grade of invasion, but this assessment was included in the evaluation of invasion of the surgical margin.

Lymph node metastasis (n factor) was evaluated and the stages were classified according to the General Rules published by the Japan Pancreas Society.[6,7]

The generalized Wilcoxon test was used for statistical analysis and differences were considered significant if the probability of the observed results was less than 0.05. The survival rate was shown by the Kaplan-Meier method.

Second Department of Surgery, School of Medicine, Kanazawa University, Takaramachi, 13-1, Kanasawa, 920 Japan.

TABLE 37-1. *Surgical cases of pancreatic carcinoma**

Carcinoma types	Surgical cases No.	Resected cases No.	Resected cases %	Macroscop. curative cases No.	Macroscop. curative cases %	Microscop. curative cases No.	Microscop. curative cases %
Head of the pancreas	147	72	49.0	58	39.5	39	26.5
Body and tail of the pancreas	53	30	56.6	3	5.7	2	3.8
Entire pancreas	16	2	12.5	1	6.3	1	6.3
TOTAL	216	104	48.1	62	28.7	42	19.4

* Results from Kanazawa University School of Medicine, November 1973 through December 1993.

TECHNIQUE OF RETROPERITONEAL DISSECTION BY THE TRANSLATERAL RETROPERITONEAL APPROACH

The abdomen is opened through a chevron incision in the epigastric region.

Retroperitoneal Dissection

Using an electric scalpel, the retroperitoneum is entered by incising the peritoneum at the lower margin of the liver, carrying the incision inferiorly about 3 cm laterally along the right side of the duodenum (Fig. 37-1). The incision is extended further along the right margin of the ascending colon to the cecum, and the duodenocolic ligament is divided. The duodenum is mobilized and elevated along with the pancreas, the ascending colon, and the transverse colon, thus allowing full access to the retroperitoneum.

The right kidney is first exposed at the lateral aspect of the duodenum, and the fatty tissue attached to it is removed. The right renal artery and vein are now visible. The dissection then proceeds leftward, exposing the inferior vena cava. Care should be taken not to damage the suprarenal vein. Once the inferior vena cava is fully exposed, the dissection is directed inferiorly to remove the soft tissue and lymph nodes along the vena cava. During this maneuver, the testicular or ovarian vein is ligated and dissected.

Care should be taken not to injure the right ureter. Dissection of the retroperitoneum is carried as far as the bifurcation of the common iliac artery. At this point, dissection proceeds superiorly, exposing the abdominal aorta. Small-caliber vessels to the inferior vena cava and from the abdominal aorta are ligated and divided. The lymph nodes around both renal arteries, particularly the right renal artery, are dissected carefully, and the vessels are retracted with vascular tape (Fig. 37-2). Particular attention should be paid to the dissection around the root of the inferior mesenteric artery and the left ureter. Exposure of the abdominal aorta is carried as far as the root of the superior mesenteric artery. The field of dissection is shifted to the retroperitoneum in the vicinity of the foramen of Winslow, exposing the inferior vena cava and left renal vein. Next, as much fatty tissue and as many lymphatics around the left side of the abdominal aorta as possible are ligated to prevent excessive postoperative lymphorrhea.

Treatment of the Transverse Mesocolon, Dissection of the Hepatoduodenal Ligament, Cholecystectomy, and Gastrectomy

The greater omentum is divided at its attachment to the transverse colon, and the transverse mesocolon is divided by an

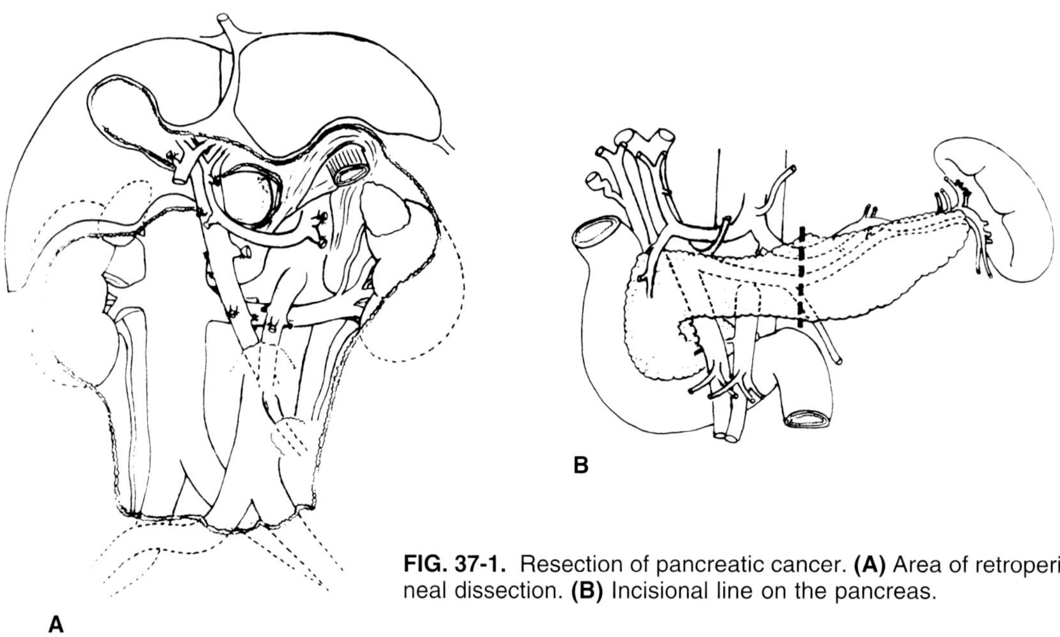

FIG. 37-1. Resection of pancreatic cancer. **(A)** Area of retroperitoneal dissection. **(B)** Incisional line on the pancreas.

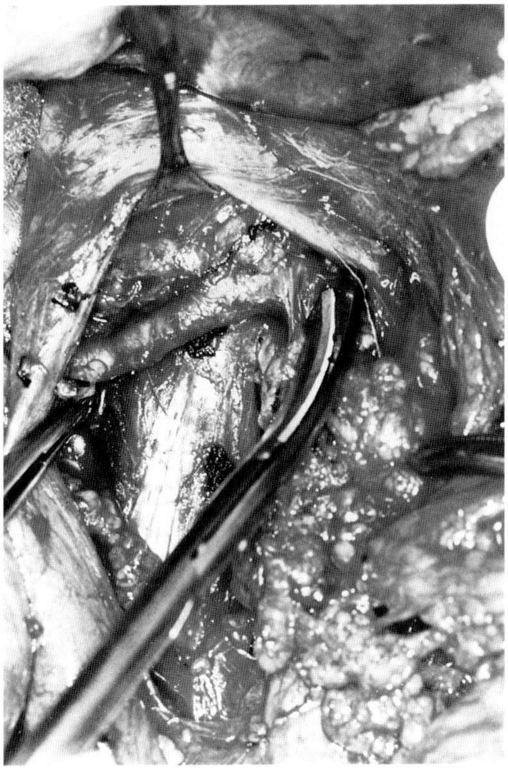

FIG. 37-2. Dissection around the right renal artery. The left renal vein is hung up and the right renal artery is exposed.

electric scalpel 3 cm distal to its attachment to the pancreas. The middle colic artery and vein are ligated and divided. It is advisable in the subsequent procedure to keep several centimeters of the superior mesenteric vein free distally (Fig. 37-3).

Attention now shifts to the hepatoduodenal ligament. The gastroduodenal artery is ligated and divided at its root, the lesser omentum is divided along the lower margin of the liver, and the stomach is resected. Total gastrectomy is performed in conjunction with total pancreatectomy, and subtotal gastrectomy is done when a proximal pancreatoduodenectomy is performed.

Dissection Around the Celiac Artery and Left Upper Quadrant of the Retroperitoneum, and Division of the Pancreas

Keeping the stomach elevated toward the right, the lymph nodes around the root of celiac artery are removed en bloc with the ganglion and nerve plexus. The pancreas is divided along the line of the celiac axis, and the splenic vein is ligated and divided as in a standard pancreatoduodenectomy. The dissection is directed toward the left border of the abdominal aorta. Lymph nodes around the left renal artery are dissected at this time (Fig. 37-4). This establishes a connection with the site of the initial dissection, inferiorly. The splenic artery is ligated and divided in a total pancreatectomy. This maneuver exposes the common hepatic artery.

Dissection Around the Superior Mesenteric Artery

The jejunum is transected 10 to 20 cm from the ligament of Treitz. The jejunal crus, which had been divided, is lifted upward from the opening of the previously mentioned incision. The jejunal crus and pancreas are pulled downward and to the right, and the superior mesenteric vein is pulled to the left with a hook. This maneuver exposes the superior mesenteric artery along with its nerve plexus. The nerve plexus can be separated from the vessels easily using Kelly hemostats (Fig. 37-5). However, the surgeon must take care not to avulse any small vessels arising from the superior mesenteric artery. The dissection is continued to the root of the superior mesenteric artery (Fig. 37-6). The nerve plexus is dissected using scissors, and the superior mesenteric artery is divided between ligatures. At this point all retroperitoneal soft tissue and ganglia can be removed en bloc together with the pancreas (Fig. 37-7). In patients with early stage (I and II) cancers, a thin layer of nerve plexus around the superior mesenteric artery and the left ganglion at the root of the celiac artery are preserved.

Combined Resection of the Portal Vein

When a combined resection of the portal vein is required, the procedures for handling the portal vein described previously

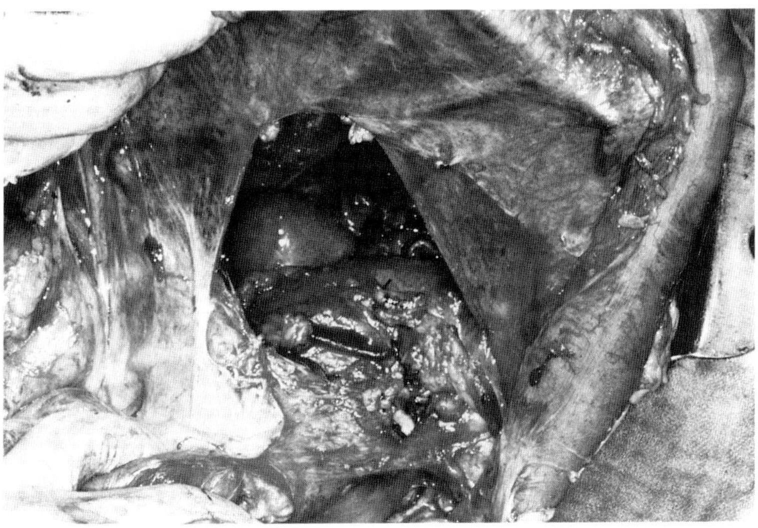

FIG. 37-3. Division of the transverse mesocolon. The mesocolon is divided by an electric scalpel 3 cm from the attachment of the pancreas. The middle colic artery and vein are ligated and divided.

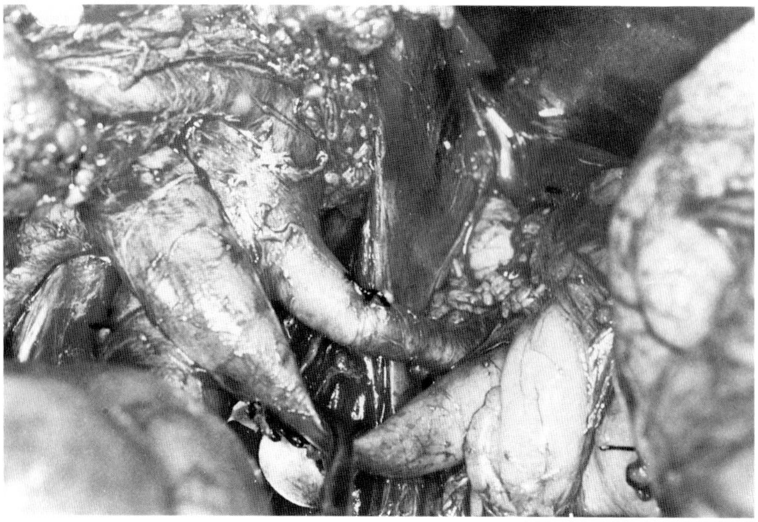

FIG. 37-4. Dissection at the left border of the abdominal aorta. The left renal vein is pulled down and the left renal artery is exposed from the root. The root of the celiac axis and the diaphragmatic crus are visible.

can be dispensed with. Once the retroperitoneum has been dissected, the portal vein can be divided at the upper and lower margins of the pancreas and removed with the pancreas. An end-to-end anastomosis of the portal vein can be performed easily using 5-0 Prolene sutures (Fig. 37-8).

A reconstruction technique is illustrated in Figure 37-9. A common reconstruction includes a single jejunal limb that is anastomosed to the stomach (end to side), pancreas (end to side), and common duct (end to side). Silastic stents are placed in the pancreatic duct and in the common hepatic duct and exited through the abdominal wall. These are removed at selected times once drainage has subsided to a minimum level, as described in the following section.

Abdominal Drainage

In an attempt to prevent the fatal complications of pancreatic leakage, we developed a new method of intraabdominal drainage that involves continuous suction.

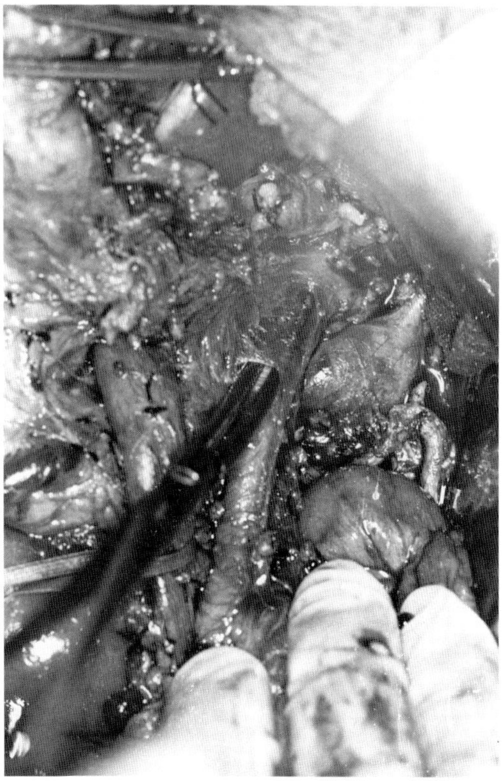

FIG. 37-5. Dissection around the superior mesenteric artery, showing the technique for approaching the artery. Kelly hemostats are used to resect the nerve tissue around the artery.

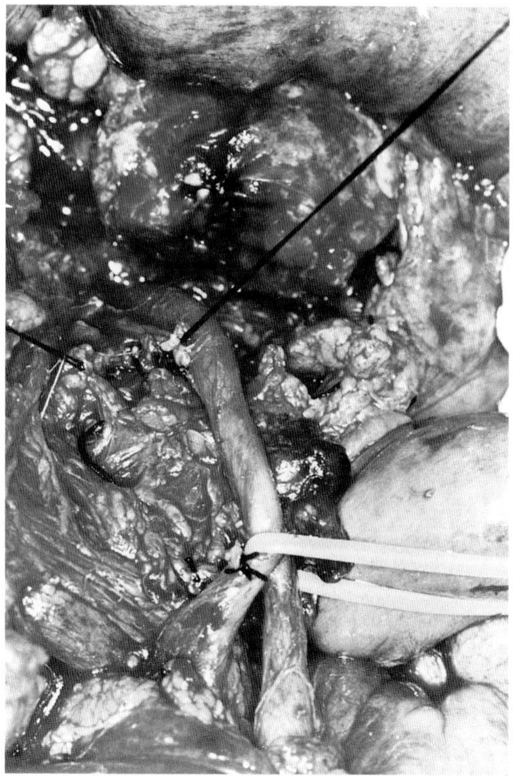

FIG. 37-6. Dissection around the superior mesenteric artery. The inferior pancreatoduodenal artery is ligated and divided, and the artery is exposed.

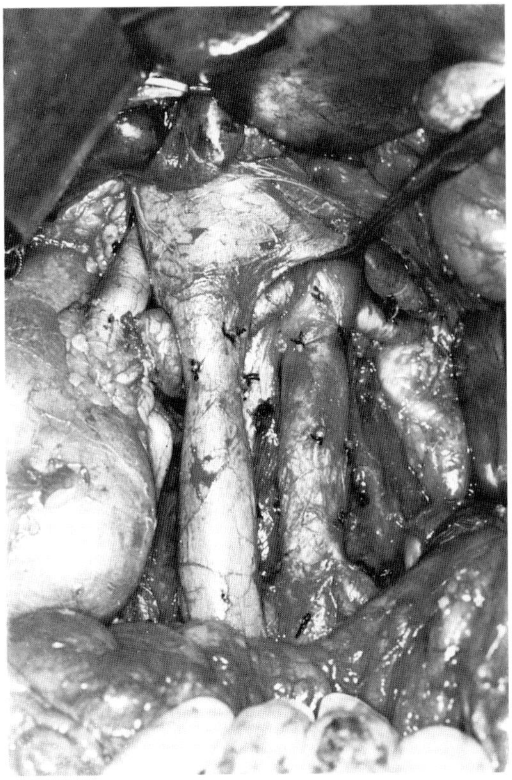

FIG. 37-7. Appearance of the retroperitoneum after completion of the dissection. The abdominal aorta and inferior vena cava have been completely skeletonized. Both renal arteries and veins are exposed.

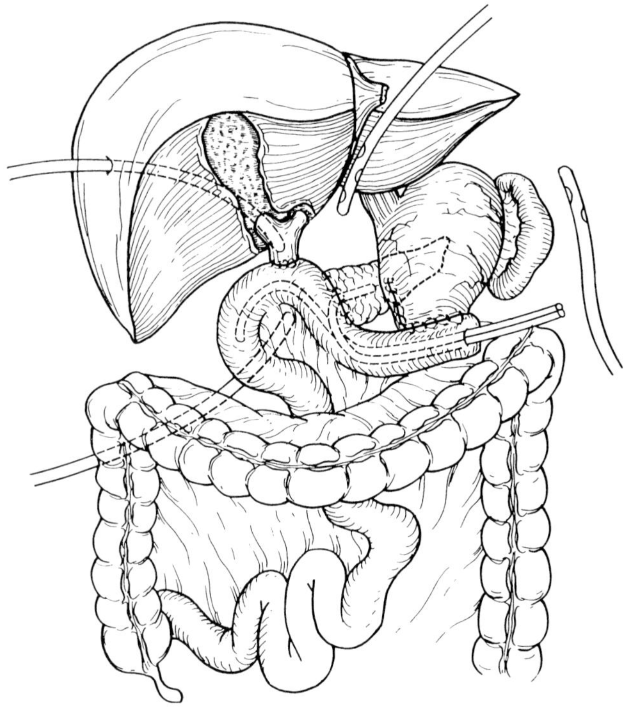

FIG. 37-9. Abdominal drainage. Imanaga's reconstruction is shown.

First, an 18-Fr, double-lumen sump tube is positioned beside the pancreaticoenterostomy with Penrose drains and a duple drain, ensuring that the sump drain tube is not kinked (see Fig. 37-9).

Immediately after the operation, continuous suction drainage is begun at a pressure of about -20 cm H_2O. We usually use the common thoracic pump as the suction machine. When the sump tube does not work effectively, it should be changed in the ward and the position immediately checked by a plain abdominal roentgenogram.

The amylase level and bacterial cultures of the sump tube fluid should be examined regularly to monitor for early detection of dehiscence of the pancreaticoenterostomy. The sump tube should be removed when it is draining less than 50 mL and the amylase level has normalized.

Two Penrose and one duple or ϕ con tubes are inserted toward the pancreaticoenterostomy, after which fluid from the abdominal cavity is allowed to exclude passively. The other abdominal drainage techniques are the same as those used for the continuous intraabdominal drainage (CISD) method.

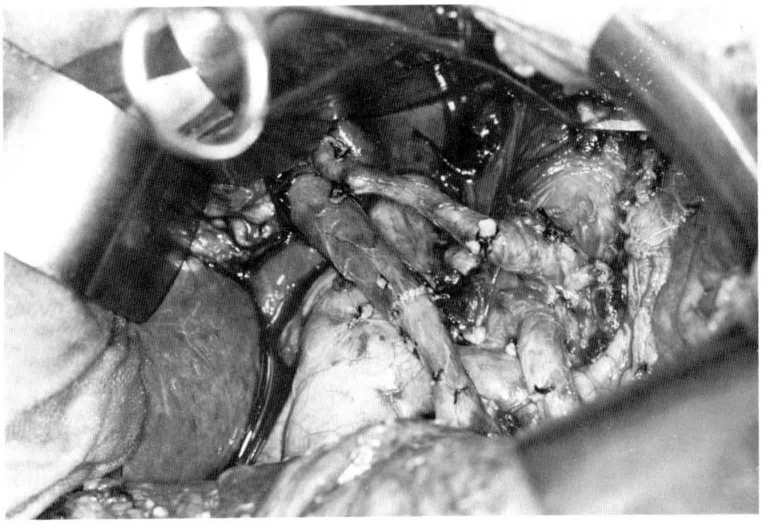

FIG. 37-8. Anastomosis after combined resection of the portal vein. The roots of the dissected celiac axis and superior mesenteric artery are visible.

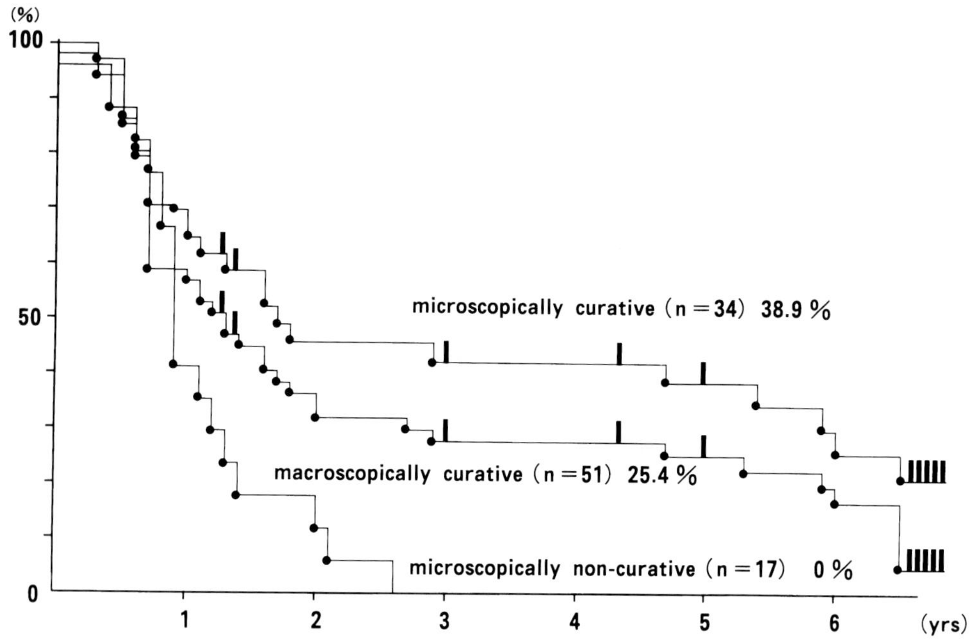

FIG. 37-10. Cumulative survival rates according to the type of curative resection for carcinoma of the head of the pancreas (Kaplan-Meier method). Percentages are given for 5-year survival rates.

RESULTS

Postoperative Surgical Results

Of the 58 patients who underwent macroscopically curative resection, 4 (6.9%) died within 30 days from peritonitis or intraperitoneal hemorrhage, and another 3 died within 60 days from sepsis or hepatorenal failure. Major postoperative complications included wound infection, postoperative hemorrhage, pneumonia, and hepatic and renal insufficiency. Including minor complications, the incidence of complications was 32.8%.

The postoperative survival rates of the 51 patients who tolerated the operation among the 58 macroscopically curatively resected patients are shown in Figure 37-10; 14 patients survived for 3 or more years (27.8%), 10 of whom have survived for 5 years (25.4%). Among these 51 patients, 34 underwent curative resection by microscopic criteria, and 17 had microscopically noncurative resections. Respective 5-year survival rates were 38.9% and 0%.

Diarrhea and nutritional disturbance were observed in most of the patients as late postoperative complications.

Prognosis According to Stage of Disease

1. Tumor size (Fig. 37-11): There was no correlation between tumor size and prognosis.

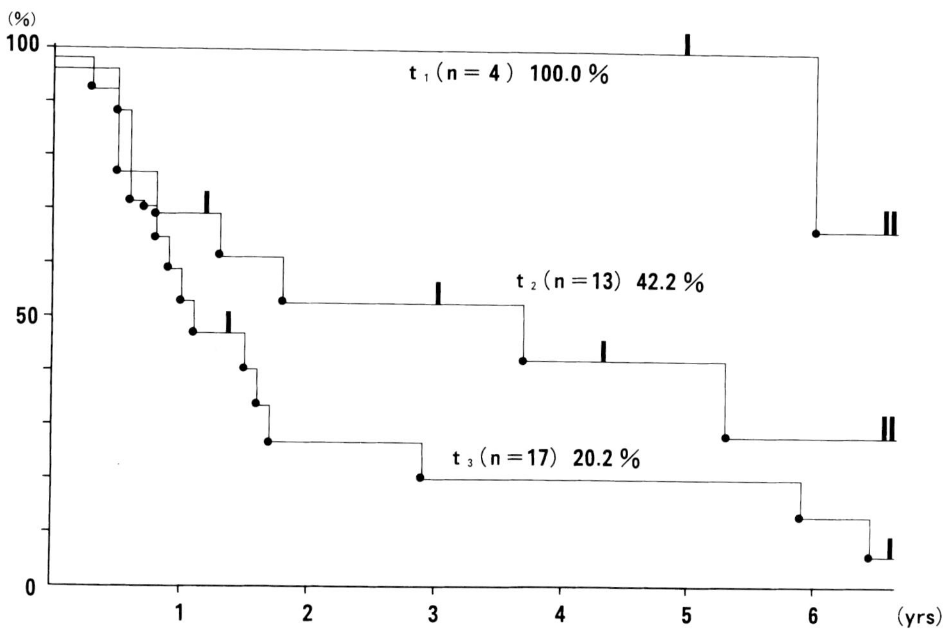

FIG. 37-11. Survival rates according to tumor size (t).

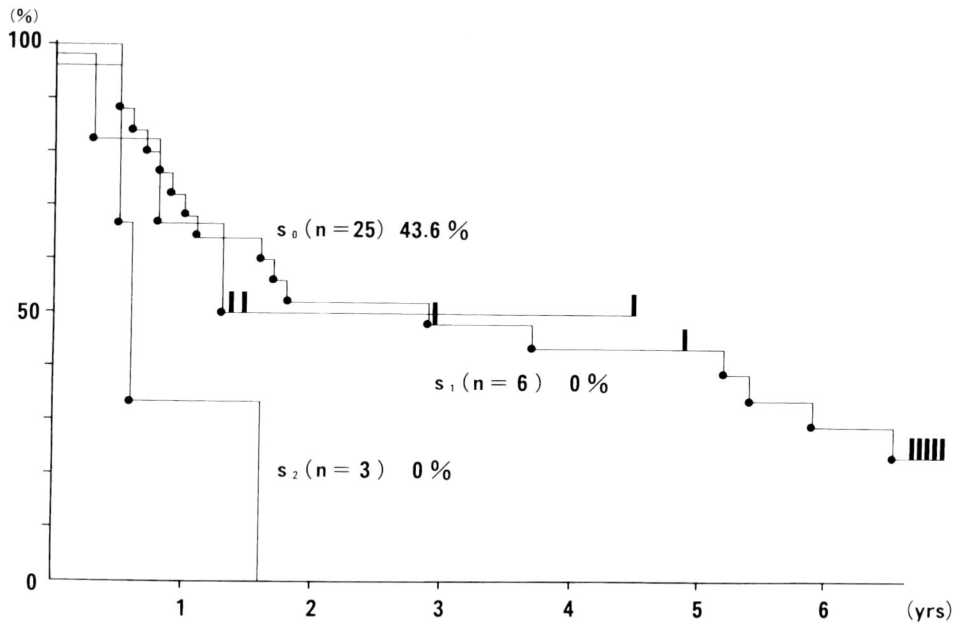

FIG. 37-12. Survival rates according to invasion of the anterior pancreatic capsule (s).

2. Invasion of the capsule of the pancreas (s0, s1, and s2; Fig. 37-12): Three patients with s2 disease died early, whereas the s0 patients (n = 25) had a 5-year survival rate of 43.6%. The difference between the s0 and s2 survival curves was significant at the 0.05 level.
3. Retroperitoneal invasion (rp0, rp1, and rp2; Fig. 37-13): There were 5-year survivors in all three groups, but the survival curve for rp0 was significantly higher than that for rp2 ($P < 0.05$). Five of the patients with rp1 or rp2 disease survived more than 3 years. There were 5-year survivors in the pv1 group, but there was no statistical difference in survival rates between pv0 and pv1. In evaluating the correlation of retroperitoneal invasion and invasion of the portal vein, cancer cells were found within 3.0 mm of the vein in 16 of the 21 cases in which an evaluation was possible.
4. Invasion at the surgical margin of resection (Fig. 37-14): All patients with microscopic evidence of cancer at the resection margin were dead within 3 years. In those patients with a negative margin, a 5-year survival rate of 49.2% was seen. Cancer at the resection margin was a statistically significant factor at the $P < 0.05$ level.
5. Lymph node metastasis (Fig. 37-15): Lymph nodes were positive in 39 patients. All patients with n2 disease were dead within 3 years, whereas three patients with n1 nodes survived more than 3 years, and patients with n0 disease had a 5-year survival rate of 76.9%. There was a significant difference between n0 and n1 survival curves ($P < 0.05$).

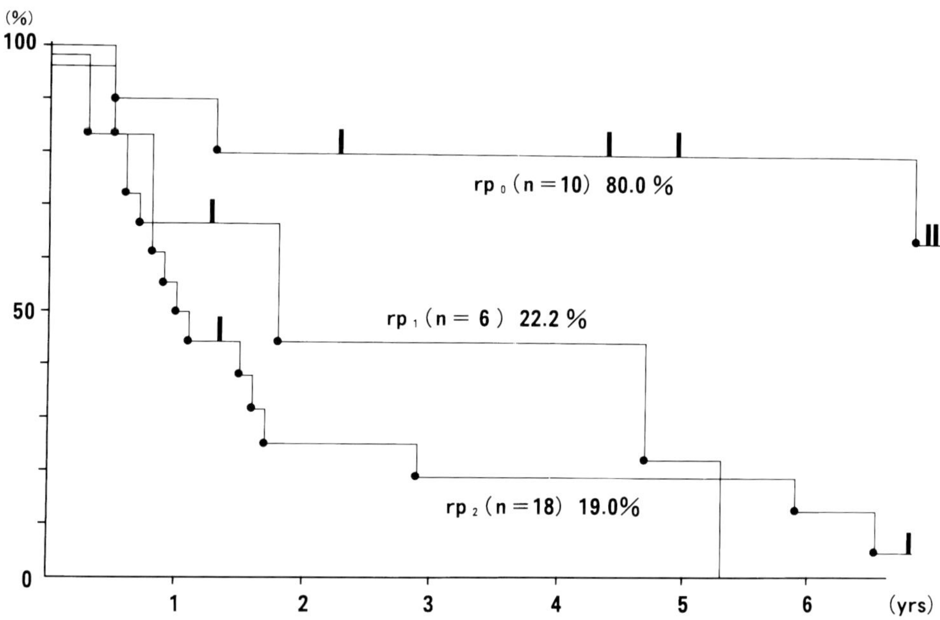

FIG. 37-13. Survival rates according to invasion of the retroperitoneal tissue behind the pancreas (rp).

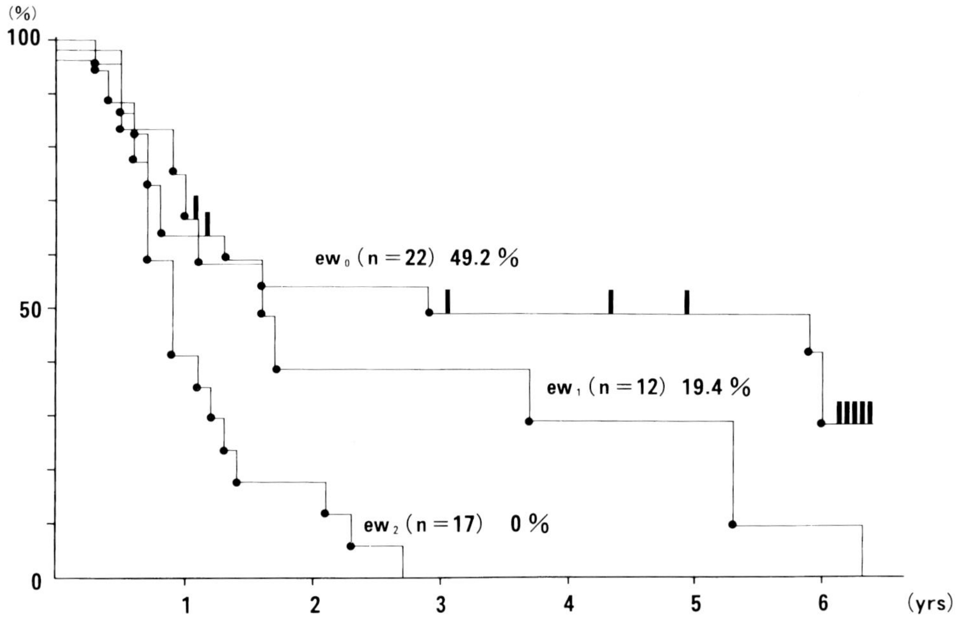

FIG. 37-14. Survival rates according to invasion of the excisional margin (ew). Survival was significantly better in patients with ew0 compared to ew2 ($P < 0.05$). Percentages are given for 5-year survival rates. *ew0,* negative invasion; *ew1,* invasion within 5 mm of surgical margin; *ew2,* positive invasion.

In all of our patients with metastases to the paraaortic lymph nodes, the nodes around the superior mesenteric artery were also affected. There were three patients with a single metastasis to the paraaortic lymph nodes who lived for more than 1 year.

6. Anatomic stage of disease (Fig. 37-16): All patients with stage IVb disease were dead within 2 years, and there was no statistical difference in survival between stages I, II, and III.

Survivals Longer Than 3 Years

Fourteen patients survived for 3 years or more. Among these 14 patients, there were 4 with n1 or n2, 6 with rp1 or rp2, 3 with plx1, and 2 with ew1 disease. Macroscopically resected cancer by our extended technique carries a 5-year survival rate of 25%; this is in contrast to the 16.6% survival reported by the Japanese Pancreas Society (Fig. 37-17).

DISCUSSION

The resection rate for pancreatic carcinoma is increased when advanced techniques such as en bloc resection of the portal vein are used. At the same time, the mortality of extensive operations for pancreatic cancer can be reduced by using ancillary techniques such as percutaneous transhepatic biliary drainage and perioperative nutritional support. Despite these approaches,

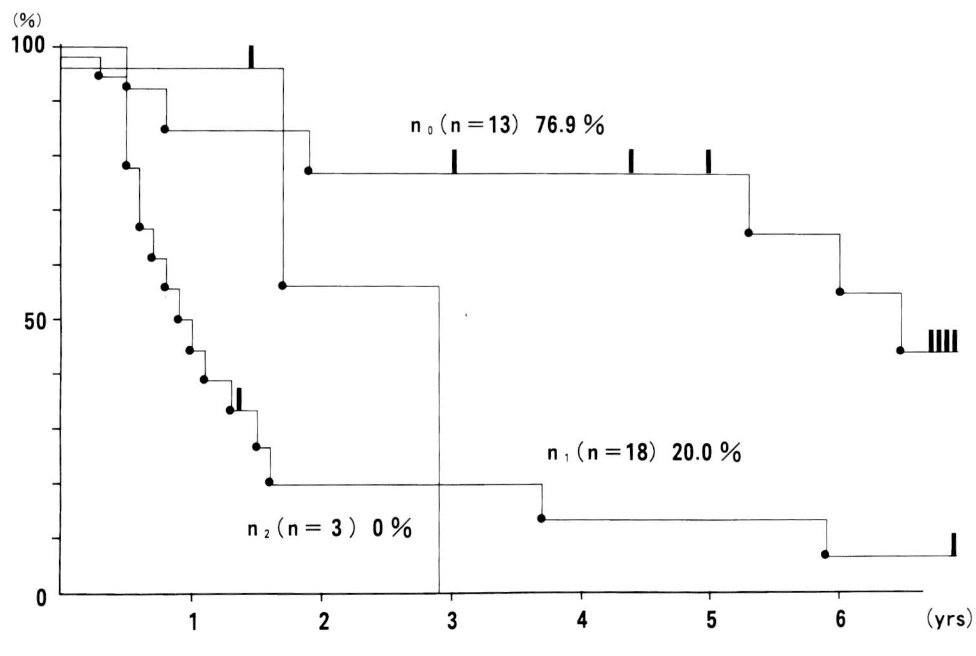

FIG. 37-15. Survival rates according to lymph node metastasis (n).

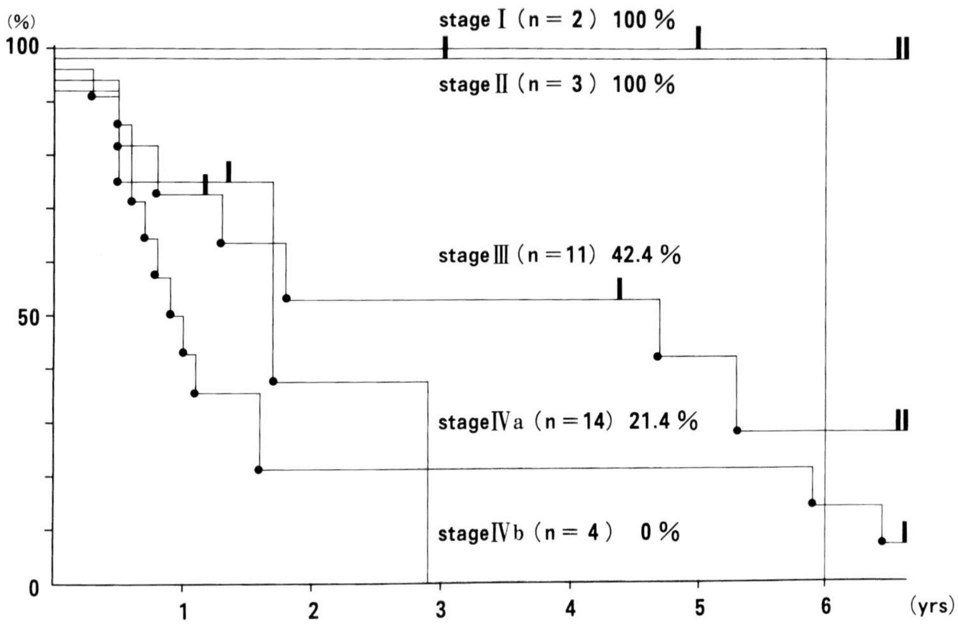

FIG. 37-16. Survival rates according to cancer stage. Survival was significantly better in patients with stage Tá and Uá disease compared with those with stage Wáb disease ($P < 0.005$). Percentages are given for 5-year survival rates. Stage I: t1, s0, rp0, pv0, and n0; stage II: s0, rp0, pv0, and n1; stage III: s1, rp1, pv1, or n2; stage IVa: n2 and s2, rp2, or pv2; stage IVb: others.

however, the 5-year survival rate is still disappointing, ranging from 2.3% to 14.3% for cancer of the head of the pancreas.[5,8–17] Because of the dissatisfaction with long-term survival rates after radical surgery, some authors suggest that a bypass should be used as the procedure of choice.[18,19]

In Japan, extensive surgery has been debated and discussed since the early 1980s. Figure 37-17 shows the cumulative survival rates of 7235 patients with pancreatic cancer in Japan between 1981 and 1989.[20] These results show that the survival rate with resection is better than that with palliative surgery or other operations. Based on the results in our clinic, we believe that there is rational support for the approach of extended radical pancreatectomy, given the long-term survival rates in patients with rp2, ew1, and n1 disease. These results would not have been achieved if a standard radical pancreatectomy had been performed.

The safety of en bloc resection of the portal vein is reasonably well established,[21] although the necessity for routine removal of the portal vein is not clear. The results of invasion of the portal vein in our patients suggested that a resection that did not include the periportal tissues would have left cancer cells in the operative field.

Invasion of the extrapancreatic nerve plexus was correlated with invasion of the surgical margin of resection in our patients, which shows that an extensive dissection of the extrapancreatic nerve plexus and the superior mesenteric nerve plexus is necessary for curative resection of cancer of the head of the pancreas.

The most serious nutritional disturbances were related mainly to the diarrhea that occurred after the operation. This problem is related to the excision of sympathetic nerves to the small intestine, and can be affected by the method of reconstruction. We investigated this problem clinically and experimentally, and

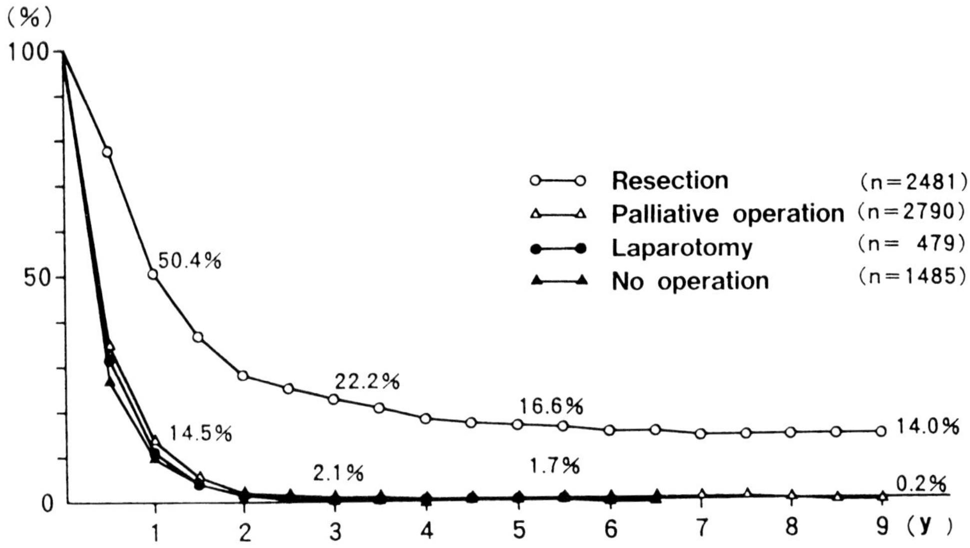

FIG. 37-17. Cumulative survival rates of pancreatic cancer in Japan.

found that the degree of disturbance correlates with the extent of nerve dissection. Furthermore, reconstruction by the Imanaga method,[22] in which the stomach, pancreas, and bile duct are reconstructed in that order, led to more favorable results than other methods, such as the Child reconstruction.[23] Because this disorder is caused by the complete excision of lymph vessels and resection of nerve plexuses, excision leaving a thin layer of the superior mesenteric nerve plexus[24,25] is recommended in patients with stage I and II disease.

According to the results reported here, our extensive surgery seems to resolve the problems of local extension of pancreatic cancer, particularly retropancreatic invasion, but does not resolve the problems of lymphatic metastases, particularly around the superior mesenteric artery and the abdominal aorta. However, some patients with lymphatic metastases around the superior mesenteric artery or the abdominal aorta survived for 2 years. We think that combined resection of the superior mesenteric artery or the abdominal aorta may be necessary to improve the surgical results of cases of positive lymphatic metastases around these arteries.

Postoperative complications and mortality are significant problems in such extensive surgery. The operative bleeding volume was 5 to 10 L during the beginning of this series, but has been decreased to 1 to 2.5 L. The postoperative complications also have been decreased, and an operative death within 60 postoperative days has not been experienced since 1992. These results suggest that extensive surgery for pancreatic cancer should not be abandoned, and that we should continue to explore the value of extended surgery with properly selected patients.

CONCLUSIONS

We have compared our extended resection with conventional resection of pancreatic cancer according to the General Rules published by the Japan Pancreas Society. There was no statistical difference in survival based on tumor size or stage; however, there was a significant difference in the survival curves according to presence of invasion of the anterior capsule of the pancreas (S0, S1, S2), presence of invasion of the retroperitoneal tissue (rp0, rp1, rp2), invasion at the surgical margin of resection (ew0, ew2) or extent of lymph node metastases (n0, n1). This comparison suggests that extended radical pancreatectomy could be considered the procedure of choice for pancreatic cancer that has spread to the retroperitoneum and extrapancreatic nerve plexus. Use of this procedure in patients with early stage disease may also merit consideration, as indicated by the favorable survival results in patients with t1 or t2 and n0 tumors.

REFERENCES

1. Pliam MB, ReMine WH. Further evaluation of total pancreatectomy. Arch Surg 1975;110:506.
2. Brooks JR, Culebras JM. Carcinoma of the pancreas: palliative operation, Whipple procedure, or total pancreatectomy? Am J Surg 1979; 131:516.
3. Fortner JG. Regional resection of cancer of the pancreas. Surgery 1979; 73:307.
4. Nagakawa T, Konishi K, Kurachi M, Miyazaki I. Retroperitoneal dissection for pancreatic carcinoma: translateral retroperitoneal approach. Igaku no Ayumi 1979;111:339 (in Japanese).
5. Nagakawa T, Kurachi M, Konishi K, Miyazaki I. Translateral retroperitoneal approach in radical surgery for pancreatic carcinoma. Japanese Journal of Surgery 1982;12:229.
6. The Japan Pancreas Society. The general rules for surgical and pathological studies on cancer of the pancreas. Tokyo: Kanehara Shuppan, 1993 (in Japanese).
7. Pour PM, Konishi Y, Kloeppel, Longnecker DS. Staging for carcinoma of the pancreas: Japanese stage classification compared to UICC stage classification. In: Japan Pancreas Society. Atlas of exocrine pancreatic tumors. New York: Springer-Verlag, 1994:247.
8. Sato T, Saito Y, Noto T, Matsuno S. Follow-up studies of radical resection for pancreaticoduodenal cancer. Ann Surg 1977;186:581.
9. Tsuchiya R, Tomioka T, Izawa K, et al. Collective review of small carcinomas of the pancreas. Ann Surg 1986;283:77.
10. Nakase A, Matsumoto Y, Uchida K, Honjo I. Surgical treatment of cancer of the pancreas and the periampullary region: cumulative results in 57 institutions in Japan. Ann Surg 1977;185:52.
11. Fortner JG. Surgical principles for pancreatic cancer: regional total and subtotal pancreatectomy. Cancer 1981;47:1712.
12. Nix GA, Schmitz PIM, Wilson JHP, van Blankenstein M, Groeneveld CFM, Hofuijk R. Carcinoma of the head of the pancreas. Gastroenterology 1984;87:37.
13. Bjorck S, Svensson JO, Macpherson S, Edlund Y. Cancer of the head of the pancreas and choledochoduodenal junction: a clinical study of 88 Whipple resections. Acta Chir Scand 1981;148:353.
14. van Heerden JA. Pancreatic resection for carcinoma of the pancreas: Whipple versus total pancreatectomy—an institutional perspective. World J Surg 1984;8:880.
15. Kummerle F, Ruckert K. Surgical treatment of pancreatic cancer. World J Surg 1984;8:889.
16. Longmire WP Jr. Cancer of the pancreas: palliative operation, Whipple procedure, or total pancreatectomy. World J Surg 1984;8:872.
17. Grace PA, Pitt HA, Longmire WP. Pancreatoduodenectomy with pylorus preservation for adenocarcinoma of the head of the pancreas. Br J Surg 1986;73:647.
18. Crile G Jr. The advantages of by-pass operation over radical pancreatoduodenectomy in the treatment of pancreatic carcinoma. Surg Gynecol Obstet 1970;130:1049.
19. The Japan Pancreas Society. Report on registration of cases of pancreatic cancer in 1989 (in Japanese). Yohichi Saito: Tokyo, 1990.
20. Nakao A, Horisawa M, Kondo T, et al. Total pancreatectomy combined with resection of the portal vein employing portal perfusion method. Shujutsu 1983;37:1 (in Japanese).
21. The Japan Pancreas Society. The statistical results of pancreatic cancer in Japan for 10 years. Yohichi Saito: Tokyo, 1991.
22. Imanaga H. A new method of pancreaticoduodenectomy designed to preserve life and pancreatic function. Surgery 1960;47:577.
23. Child CG III. Pancreaticojejunostomy and other problems associated with the surgical management of carcinoma involving the head of the pancreas. Ann Surg 1944;119:845.
24. Nagakawa T. Extended radical operation for carcinoma of the pancreatic head region. Surgical Therapy 1985;52:186 (in Japanese).
25. Nagakawa T, Mori K, Kayahara M, et al. Three-dimensional studies on the structure of the tissue surrounding the superior mesenteric artery. Int J Pancreatol 1994;15:129.

Surgery for Gastrointestinal Cancer: A Multidisciplinary Approach, edited by Harold J. Wanebo.
Lippincott-Raven Publishers, Philadelphia, © 1997.

CHAPTER 38

Intraoperative Radiation Therapy in Resected Carcinoma of the Pancreas

William F. Sindelar

BACKGROUND

Carcinoma of the pancreas has a relatively low incidence of 9 per 100,000 in the United States but is the fourth leading cause of overall cancer mortality.[1] Gudjonsson found that of 22,319 patients collected from 85 published series from 1949 to 1986, only 0.4% underwent resection and lived at least 5 years after diagnosis.[2] The current relative 5-year survival rate for the disease is less than 5%.[2]

The dismal overall survival in patients with pancreatic cancer results from three major factors. First, the natural history of pancreatic cancer often involves the early dissemination of malignant cells, frequently during the preclinical phase of the disease. The second factor relates to the lack of sufficiently sensitive screening and diagnostic techniques to identify truly localized disease at early stages, which is the most likely to be cured. The third factor related to poor survival is the paucity of effective therapeutic agents for advanced pancreatic cancer, which accounts for the extent of malignancy in at least 70% to 80% of patients at the time of presentation.[1,3]

TREATMENT METHODS AND RESULTS

Surgical resection is the only therapeutic modality capable of curing pancreatic cancer, although long-term survival is observed in only a few patients. In a literature review of 2398 resected patients, Gudjonsson found only 92 individuals (3.8%) who survived 5 years or longer.[2] In certain series of highly selected patients undergoing pancreatic resection, 5-year survival rates as high as 18% to 25% have been reported.[4–6] In part, the increments in long-term survival have been attributed to declining morbidity and mortality after pancreatic resection in the last decade.[7–9]

When potentially complete resections are performed in patients with carcinoma of the pancreas, local recurrences are common and are observed in at least 50% of cases.[10] The observation of local recurrence as the initial site of disease relapse in many resected patients suggests that improvements in the treatment of local disease could provide therapeutic benefit. Extended resections have been described and are used at some centers,[11,12] but local failures still occur after the most aggressive surgical extirpations.[13] Radiation therapy is used widely to promote the local control of a variety of malignancies and is used frequently in the treatment of advanced cancers of the pancreas.[14] Radiation therapy has been used as an adjunct to surgical resection and, combined with 5-fluorouracil chemotherapy, has been demonstrated to improve survival after resection compared with surgery alone.[15] However, the toxicity of external-beam radiation therapy (EBRT) to the upper abdomen is considerable, and the high doses of radiation necessary to control residual disease after resection often are tolerated poorly.

INTRAOPERATIVE RADIATION THERAPY

Intraoperative radiation therapy (IORT) involves the administration of large single doses of radiation during operative procedures directly to surgically exposed tissues. IORT offers the opportunity to deliver high doses of radiation to areas of neoplastic involvement while simultaneously minimizing the risk of radiation toxicity by limiting the dose to surrounding radiosensitive normal tissues, which may be physically shielded or displaced from the radiation treatment volume. IORT was explored in various malignancies during the 1970s in Japan, with reports of benefit in both disease control and survival in selected patients with various types of malignancies.[14,16,17]

Several early clinical trials investigated IORT as a potential treatment modality in pancreatic cancer. An early pilot series was reported by Goldson in which 19 patients demonstrated the feasibility of defining IORT in pancreatic cancer.[18] A larger Japanese experience of 108 patients with pancreatic cancer demonstrated a median survival of 6 months in patients with advanced disease.[19] The Massachusetts General Hospital accu-

William F. Sindelar: Surgery Branch, National Cancer Institute, National Institutes of Health, Building 10, Room 2B42, Bethesda, MD 20892.

mulated a series of 16 patients with unresectable pancreatic cancer who were treated with IORT in combination with EBRT. These patients had an encouraging median survival of 18 months.[20] Further experience in treating selected patients with IORT at the Massachusetts General Hospital suggested a median survival of 17 months, considerably longer than that expected from conventional therapies for pancreatic carcinoma.[21] Large early experiences with IORT in unresectable pancreatic carcinoma also were accumulated at the Mayo Clinic, where the median survival was 11 months for 44 patients who had unresectable pancreatic cancer without distant metastasis.[22] Disease progression was clinically documented in 71% of treated patients, although only 7% were considered to have progressed within the IORT field. The Radiation Therapy Oncology Group conducted a multi-institutional phase I-II trial of IORT in locally advanced pancreatic carcinoma.[23] Patients received IORT at the time of palliative biliary and gastric surgical bypass. Postoperative EBRT therapy was delivered concomitantly with 5-fluorouracil chemotherapy. The median survival of 51 patients who received IORT according to protocol was 9 months. The Radiation Therapy Oncology Group study suggested little effect of IORT on survival, although local tumor progression appeared to be controllable with little overall radiation-related toxicity.

INTRAOPERATIVE RADIATION THERAPY COMBINED WITH PANCREATIC RESECTION

The feasibility of using IORT in combination with pancreatic resection for cancer was demonstrated by 1983 at the National Cancer Institute,[24] where a patient with advanced cancer was described to be disease-free for more than 19 months after extended pancreatectomy with portal vein resection and IORT delivered to the resection bed and regional nodal basins. Because of the technical complexity of delivering IORT in combination with extensive pancreatic surgery, relatively few institutions accumulated a significant experience with IORT as an adjunct to pancreatectomy.

The use of IORT with pancreatic resection was explored early at Kyoto University.[25,26] Twenty-three patients underwent potentially curative resection of pancreatic cancer and had IORT (25 to 30 Gy) delivered to the resection bed. In addition, conventional EBRT was given before or after surgery to most patients (total EBRT dose, 60 to 70 Gy). The 5-year survival rate was 19% for patients receiving IORT. Eighteen patients had resections that were considered to be noncurative because of disease extension or nodal involvement. These patients received IORT and EBRT. The noncuratively resected patients receiving IORT had a median survival of 14 months, significantly longer than the 4-month median survival of a comparative series of noncuratively resected patients who received no radiation therapy.

Hiraoka and colleagues at Kumamoto University resected 12 patients with pancreatic cancer and administered adjunctive IORT (30 Gy), comparing the clinical results with those of 12 patients undergoing similar resections without radiation therapy.[27] Although there were 4 treatment-related deaths in the series, no deaths occurred among patients receiving IORT. At 12 months, 50% of adjunctive IORT patients and 25% of surgery alone patients were still alive. In a subsequent report, Hiraoka treated 16 patients with extended pancreatectomy, including wide nodal dissection and portal vein resection, and delivered IORT (30 Gy) to the resection bed.[28] Nine patients underwent extended pancreatectomy alone. At 5 years, 29% of the IORT patients were alive, compared with none of the non-IORT patients. Prospective comparative studies evaluating IORT in resectable pancreatic cancer are summarized in Table 38-1.

A comparative study of IORT in patients with resectable pancreatic cancer was reported from the University of Milan by Zerbi and associates.[29] Ninety patients underwent pancreaticoduodenectomy between 1985 and 1993. IORT (13 to 20 Gy) was delivered to the tumor bed in 43 patients. No IORT was given to 47 patients. No postoperative adjunctive radiation therapy or chemotherapy was administered. Tumor size, adequacy of resection, morbidity, and mortality were similar between IORT and non-IORT patients. IORT significantly improved the median time to relapse (13 months for IORT patients, 8 months for surgery alone patients) and the local control rate (27% local recurrence for IORT patients, 57% for surgery alone patients). At 1 year, the overall survival rate was higher in IORT patients (71%) compared with surgery alone patients (49%). Similarly, a higher survival rate at 2 years was observed in IORT patients (24%) compared with non-IORT patients (16%). The observed survival differences were not statistically significant because of small patient numbers.

A prospectively randomized controlled clinical trial of IORT in resectable pancreatic cancer was performed at the National Cancer Institute. Twenty-four patients with completely resected adenocarcinoma of the pancreatic head were randomly assigned to receive IORT (20 Gy) to the resection bed or standard treatment (standard control therapy was defined as 45 to 55 Gy of postoperative EBRT for patients with extrapancreatic extension or nodal disease; control patients with disease confined within the pancreatic capsule received surgery alone, without postoper-

TABLE 38-1. *Prospective comparative studies of intraoperative radiotherapy in resected carcinoma of pancreas*

Institution	Type study	Treatment groups	No. patients	Survival		
				1-year	2-year	5-year
Kumamoto University	Nonrandomized	Extended resection	9	—	—	0%
		Extended resection + IORT	16	—	—	29%
University of Milan	Nonrandomized	Resection	47	49%	16%	—
		Resection + IORT	43	71%	24%	—
National Cancer Institute	Randomized	Extended resection + EBRT	12	42%	17%	0%
		Extended resection + IORT	12	50%	33%	17%

IORT, intraoperative radiotherapy; EBRT, external beam radiotherapy.

ative EBRT). Nineteen patients had locally advanced disease that would be considered unresectable by conventional criteria and underwent extensive extirpating surgery. The overall perioperative mortality rate was 27%, and the morbidity rate was 71%. Mortality and morbidity rates did not differ statistically between IORT and control groups. The median survival of IORT patients was 18 months, compared with 12 months for control patients. Local recurrences occurred in all of 12 control patients (100%) but in only 4 of 12 IORT patients (33%). One IORT patient remains alive without evidence of disease more than 10 years after therapy at the National Cancer Institute. Because of small patient numbers, statistically significant survival differences were not reached between IORT and control groups.

CONCLUSIONS

Available studies indicate that the combination of IORT and pancreatic resection is feasible and does not lead to substantially increased morbidity and mortality compared with surgical resection alone. However, IORT must be considered an experimental treatment. IORT permits higher doses of radiation to be delivered to intraabdominal sites than conventional fractionated radiotherapeutic techniques, with acceptable toxicity to most normal tissues. The higher total doses seem to enhance local control rates in pancreatic carcinoma after resection with IORT, as compared with conventional surgical treatment alone. Although major improvements in survival have not been seen in most reports of IORT used as an adjunct to pancreatic resection, it seems reasonable to speculate that the enhanced local control provided by IORT may have some ultimate survival benefit. It is probable that any enhancement of survival provided by improved local control will become more apparent if effective systemic therapeutic adjuncts become available that reduce the incidence of widespread metastases, the usual late clinical finding in patients who die of pancreatic cancer.

In institutions with the capability to deliver IORT, this technique should be considered routinely in patients with locally advanced pancreatic carcinoma in whom resection appears technically possible, even if an extended operation may be necessary to extirpate the disease. Alternatively, in centers without the capability to deliver IORT, referral of patients to facilities with IORT should be contemplated. The application of IORT in such patients should be performed within the context of approved trials designed to evaluate the efficacy and toxicity of IORT in specific clinical situations. The referral and inclusion of patients with pancreatic malignancies will be important in the final assessment of the role of IORT in the armamentarium of cancer treatment.

REFERENCES

1. Warshaw AL, Fernandez-Del Castellio C. Pancreatic carcinoma. N Engl J Med 1992;326:455.
2. Gudjonsson B. Cancer of the pancreas: 50 years of surgery. Cancer 1987;60:2284.
3. Warshaw AL, Swanson RS. Pancreatic cancer in 1988: possibilities and probabilities. Ann Surg 1988;208:541.
4. Crist DW, Sitzmann JV, Cameron JL. Improved hospital morbidity, mortality, and survival after the Whipple procedure. Ann Surg 1987; 206:358.
5. Trede M, Schwall G, Saefer H-D. Survival after pancreatoduodenectomy. Ann Surg 1990;211:447.
6. Cameron JL, Crist DW, Sitzmann JV, et al. Factors influencing survival after pancreaticoduodenectomy for pancreatic cancer. Am J Surg 1991; 161:120.
7. Grace PA, Pitt HA, Tompkins RK. Decreased morbidity and mortality after pancreatoduodenectomy. Am J Surg 1986;151:141.
8. Pellegrini CA, Heck CF, Raper S, et al. An analysis of the reduced morbidity and mortality rates for pancreaticoduodenectomy. Arch Surg 1989;124:778.
9. Cameron JL, Pitt HA, Yeo CJ, et al. One hundred and forty-five consecutive pancreaticoduodenectomies without mortality. Ann Surg 1993; 217:430.
10. Tepper J, Nardi G, Suit HD. Carcinoma of the pancreas: review of the MGH experience from 1963 to 1973. Analysis of surgical failure and implications for radiation therapy. Cancer 1978;37:1519.
11. Fortner JG. Regional resection of the pancreas: a new surgical approach. Surgery 1973;73:307.
12. Fortner JG. Regional pancreatectomy for cancer of the pancreas, ampulla, and other related sites. Tumor staging and results. Ann Surg 1984;199:418.
13. Sindelar WF. Clinical experience with regional pancreatectomy for adenocarcinoma of the pancreas. Arch Surg 1989;124:127.
14. Johnstone PAS, Sindelar WF, Kinsella TJ. Experimental and clinical studies of intraoperative radiation therapy. Curr Probl Cancer 1994; 18:249.
15. Kalser MH, Ellenberg SS. Pancreatic cancer: adjuvant combined radiation and chemotherapy following curative resection. Arch Surg 1985; 120:899.
16. Abe M, Yabumoto E, Takahashi M, et al. Intraoperative radiotherapy of gastric cancer. Cancer 1974;34:2034.
17. Abe M, Takahashi M, Yabumoto E, et al. Clinical experiences with intraoperative radiotherapy of locally advanced cancers. Cancer 1980; 45:40.
18. Goldson AL. Preliminary clinical experience with intraoperative radiotherapy. J Natl Med Assoc 1978;70:493.
19. Abe M, Takahashi M, Yabumoto E, et al. Techniques, indications and results of intraoperative radiotherapy of advanced cancers. Radiology 1975;116:693.
20. Wood W, Shipley WU, Gunderson LL, et al. Intraoperative irradiation for unresectable pancreatic carcinoma. Cancer 1982;49:1272.
21. Shipley WU, Wood WC, Tepper JC, et al. Intraoperative electron beam irradiation for patients with unresectable pancreatic carcinoma. Ann Surg 1984;200:289.
22. Gunderson LL, Martin JK, Kvols LK, et al. Intraoperative and external beam irradiation ± 5-FU for locally advanced pancreatic cancer. Int J Radiat Oncol Biol Phys 1987;13:319.
23. Tepper JE, Noyes D, Krall JM, et al. Intraoperative radiation therapy of pancreatic carcinoma. A report of RTOG-8505. In: Abe M, Takahashi M, eds. Intraoperative radiation therapy. Proceedings of the Third International Symposium on Intraoperative Radiation Therapy. New York: Pergamon Press, 1991:231.
24. Sindelar WF, Kinsella T, Tepper J, et al. Experimental and clinical studies with intraoperative radiotherapy. Surg Gynecol Obstet 1983; 157:205.
25. Manabe T, Shibamoto Y, Ono K, et al. Combined modality treatment for cancer of the pancreas: Intraoperative and external radiotherapies. In: Abe M, Takahashi M, eds. Intraoperative radiation therapy. Proceedings of the Third International Symposium on Intraoperative Radiation Therapy. New York: Pergamon Press, 1991:246.
26. Manabe T, Baba N, Ono K, et al. Radical pancreatectomy with intraoperative radiation therapy for pancreatic head cancer. In: Abe M, Takahashi M, eds. Intraoperative radiation therapy. Proceedings of the Third International Symposium on Intraoperative Radiation Therapy. New York: Pergamon Press, 1991:249.
27. Hiraoka T, Watanabe E, Mochinaga M, et al. Intraoperative irradiation combined with radical resection for cancer of the head of the pancreas. World J Surg 1984;8:766.
28. Hiraoka T. Extended radical resection of cancer of the pancreas with intraoperative radiotherapy. Ballieres Clin Gastroenterol 1990;4:985.
29. Zerbi A, Fossati V, Parolini D. Intraoperative radiation therapy adjuvant to resection in the treatment of pancreatic cancer. Cancer 1994; 73:2930.

Surgery for Gastrointestinal Cancer: A Multidisciplinary Approach, edited by Harold J. Wanebo.
Lippincott-Raven Publishers, Philadelphia, © 1997.

CHAPTER 39

Radiation Therapy for Unresectable Cancer of the Pancreas

Mohammed Mohiuddin

Although the incidence of cancer of the pancreas has increased since the 1940s, cure of this disease remains elusive. Gudjonsson in a review of 590 studies of 22,319 patients observed a 5-year survival of only 0.4%.[1] Surgery is considered the only curative modality, but the retroperitoneal location of the pancreas and its relative inaccessibility continue to hamper early diagnosis, and less than 10% of patients are candidates for surgical resection. In a series of 410 patients seen at Thomas Jefferson University Hospital (TJUH), only 23 were resectable and of these only 7 (2%) had disease totally confined to the pancreas (stage I).[2] Approximately half of all patients who are surgically unresectable, however, have localized disease without evidence of distant metastases. Modern imaging techniques such as computed tomography, ultrasound, endoscopic retrograde cholangiopancreatography, and magnetic resonance imaging have enabled us to define better the extent of these locally extensive tumors and to offer expanded options for their nonsurgical treatment. High-dose external radiation, interstitial implantation, intraoperative radiation therapy (IORT), and chemotherapy have been used either alone or in a variety of combinations. These modalities have enabled us effectively to palliate the symptoms of this disease and have also extended short-term survival of patients.

EXTERNAL BEAM RADIATION

In the orthovoltage era, cancer of the pancreas was considered a radioresistant tumor, and for many decades radiation therapy for this disease was thought of as only of palliative value. Effective radiation doses could not be delivered to the pancreas because of the inherent limitations of the low-energy x-rays and the potential for damage to the surrounding critical organs such as the kidneys, stomach, bowel, and liver. With the advent of megavoltage (>1 MV) irradiation, there has been a realization that with good treatment techniques, adequate radiation doses can be safely delivered to control pancreatic cancer.

University of Kentucky, 800 Rose Street, Lexington, KY 40536

Miller and Fuller,[3] in a review of 91 patients with pancreatic cancer, found that 3 of 12 patients treated with teleradium had long periods of palliation (12, 28, and 40 months), whereas only 2 patients treated with orthovoltage beams had long survival (14 and 18 months). The authors noted that upper abdominal radiation therapy was surprisingly well tolerated, and there was a general improvement in patients with relief of pain and jaundice after doses of 5000 cGy or higher. Other authors have found no palliative benefit at lower radiation doses (3.5 Gy) in patients with unresectable tumors.[4]

In an effort to improve patient tolerance of higher doses of radiation (6.0 Gy), Haslam and colleagues[5] used a double-split course technique (20 Gy/2 weeks, followed by 2 weeks of rest, then 20 Gy/2 weeks rest and a further 2.0 Gy). The split course approach was used to allow patient recovery from debilitating effects of large-field upper abdominal radiation. In patients treated with curative intent, a median survival of 7.5 months (range, 2 to 76 months) was obtained, with one patient alive for longer than 8 years. They also found that in patients receiving concurrent chemotherapy, the median survival was 11 months compared with 8 months for those treated with radiation therapy alone. Good palliation was obtained in 45% of the patients and moderate to fair palliation in 24%.

With the advent of whole-body computed tomography scans, greater accuracy in tumor localization has been obtained. Dobelbower and associates[6] used a technique of small-volume, multiple-field irradiation—so-called "precision high-dose" radiation therapy"—to escalate further the radiation doses to the pancreatic tumors. The tumor extent was delineated surgically by using radiopaque clips in addition to computed tomography scan localization. Cerrobend custom blocking techniques were used to limit dose to surrounding organs, and a combination of high-energy photons (45 MV) and electrons (15 to 40 MV) was used to deliver tumor doses of 60 to 70 Gy in 7 to 9 weeks at 1.8 Gy per fraction. This approach to precision high-dose radiation therapy was well tolerated, with only 2 of 40 reported patients showing delayed normal tissue toxicity (gastritis or bleeding). Care in treatment planning is essential if such high radiation doses are to be delivered without exceeding the tolerance of

TABLE 39-1. *Minimal and maximal tolerance dose levels*

Organ	Total dose 5/5 (cGy)	Total dose 50/5 (cGy)
Liver	3500	4500
Stomach	4500	5000
Small bowel	4500	6500
Colon	4500	6500
Kidney	2500	4000

the surrounding critical normal organs (Table 39-1). Three-dimensional tumor and normal tissue localization is best achieved using all possible imaging techniques available. The placement of radiopaque clips to delineate the margin of the neoplasm at the time of surgical exploration is helpful. Normal tissue localization can be further improved by obtaining anterior, posterior, and cross-table lateral simulation films using intravenous pyelograms to localize the kidneys. The locations of the spinal cord, stomach, and liver also need to be delineated to minimize the whole-organ dose to these structures. Good patient immobilization should be maintained throughout treatment for accurate reproduction of the daily treatment set-up. Tumor volume should include generous right and left lateral borders, especially in the region of the extrahepatic bile duct and in the region of the porta hepatis, because pancreatic tumors have a tendency to spread along this route. A 3-cm margin in the lateral direction and a 2-cm medial margin is often adequate. On the lateral fields, the anterior field margin can be less generous (approximately 1 cm) because this border is usually well defined by the placement of surgical clips; however, the posterior margin needs to include the retroperitoneal spread of disease and should encompass at least 1 cm of the anterior extent of the vertebral bodies (Fig. 39-1). At least 50% of the renal parenchyma should be outside the high-dose treatment volume, and the dose to this volume should be kept below 25 Gy. The dose to the spinal cord should be limited to 45 Gy. After a dose of 45 to 50 Gy, the treatment volume should be reduced to treat the tumor with limited margins (1 cm) and radiation continued to doses of 60 to 65 Gy (Fig. 39-2).

A clear benefit of external beam radiation is the alleviation of pain due to retroperitoneal extension of disease. In the TJUH experience, pain was relieved in 22 of 32 patients treated with external radiation alone.[6] Median survival also appeared to be improved. However, in spite of high doses delivered with precision external beam radiation techniques, local persistence/recurrence of disease still remains significant (50%),[7] and additional approaches to dose escalation need to be used for improved results.

RADIOACTIVE IMPLANTATION

In the early years of radiation therapy, the inability effectively to deliver adequate doses of external radiation with orthovoltage equipment led to experimentation with interstitial implantation techniques to treat unresectable pancreatic cancer. Handley[8] was the first actually to implant radioactive sources into the pancreas. Between 1925 and 1933, he treated 7 patients with radium needles using 1 to 9 tubes and a dose range of 675 to 1800 mg/h. Two patients died within 25 days of surgery, but one patient had relief of pain and gained weight; another patient was treated on two occasions, 1 year apart, and on each occasion his tumor responded with relief of symptoms and he lived 26 months after the initial diagnosis. Another patient was well 14 years after treatment, although histologic confirmation of cancer was lacking in this long-term survivor. These early results suggested the potential benefit of radioactive implantation techniques in palliating unresectable cancers.

Pack and McNeer[9] performed the first permanent implants of radioactive sources (gold-filtered radon seeds) in biopsy-proven human pancreatic cancer. One patient was treated with

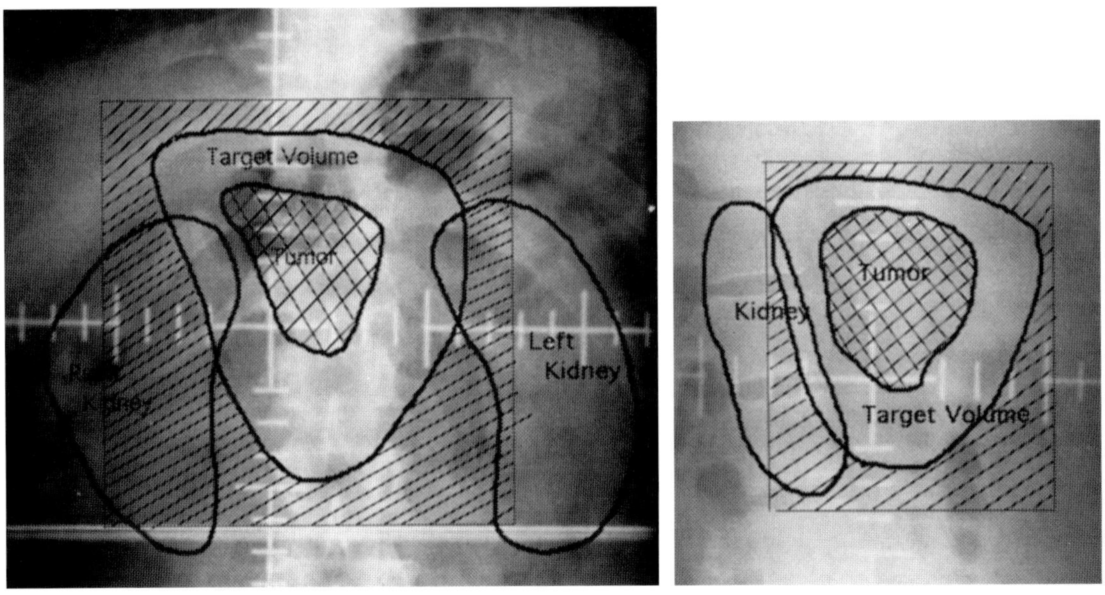

A B

FIG. 39-1. (A) Anteroposterior and **(B)** lateral field arrangements for external beam radiation for unresectable cancer of the pancreas.

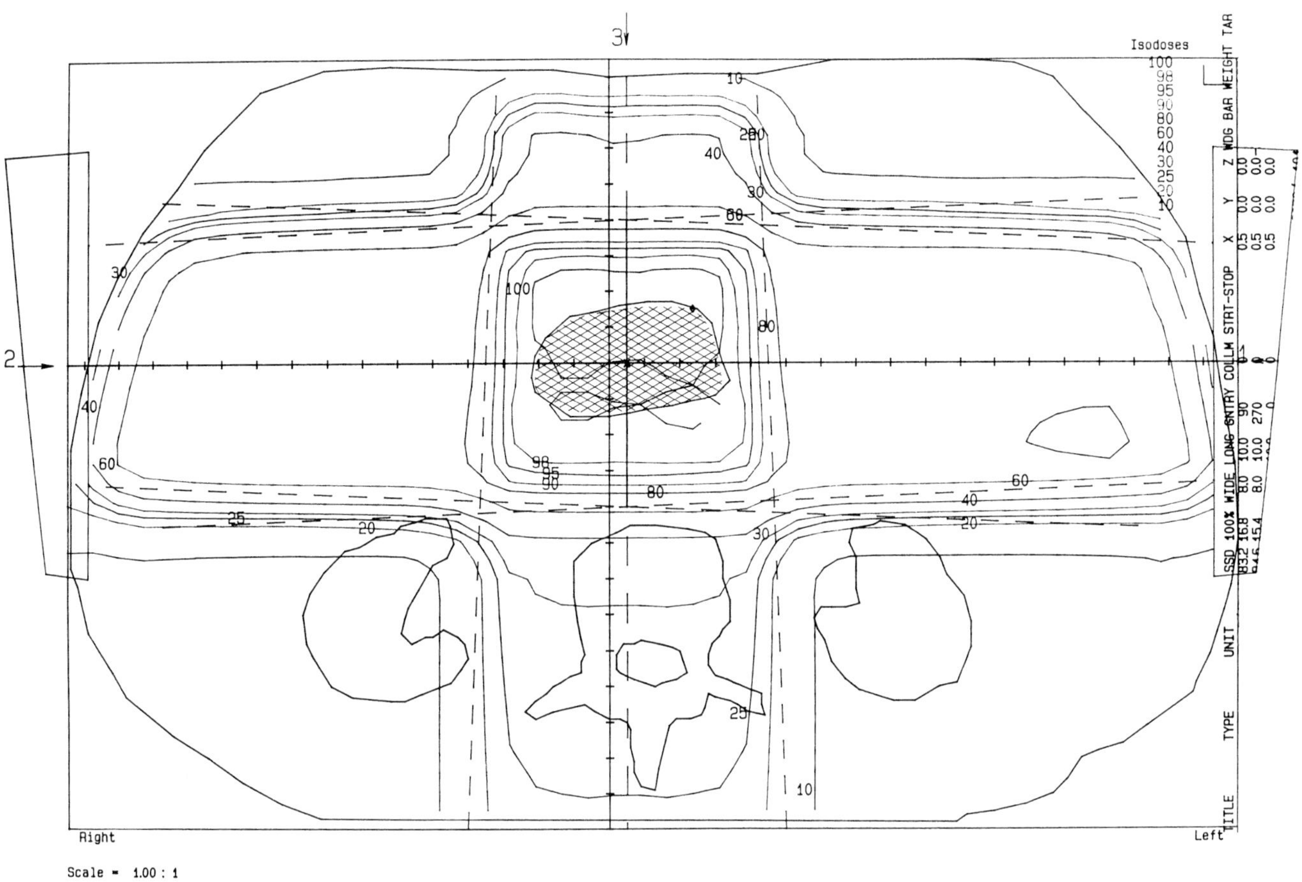

FIG. 39-2. Dose distribution for external beam radiation for unresectable cancer of the pancreas.

implant alone, one with implant plus 200 kVp external beam therapy, and one with implant plus fractionated teleradium therapy. The first two patients died after 3 and 6 months, respectively, but both experienced some improvement of symptoms. The patient treated with implant plus teleradium therapy survived 16 months. Twenty additional patients were subsequently treated. Of these, none had biopsy confirmation of cancer, and two patients survived over 1 year (17 and 28 months). Ten of the 23 patients received significant palliation. Also noted was that all but one patient had definite tumor regression and improved appetite and weight gain. These results were encouraging and have led to investigations of a potential role for permanent radioactive implantation techniques for this disease.

In the modern era, Fortner and coworkers[10] treated patients with interstitial implantation of iodine 125 or iridium 192 to deliver localized tumor doses of 160 Gy and compared their experience with patients treated with bypass surgery alone. They reported that the median survival of patients was improved from 3 to 6 months. Ten of the treated patients were alive longer than 1 year. More important, they observed that pancreatic pain was relieved in 80% of the patients treated by interstitial implantation, compared with 62% treated by external beam radiation and 50% of those treated with bypass alone. The use of implantation directly into the pancreatic tumor allowed for significant escalation of radiation dose yet spared radiation to the surrounding normal tissues. In an update of this experience, Peretz and colleagues[11] confirmed the improved palliation of pancreatic cancer pain in patients undergoing iodine 125 implantation. A median survival of 7 months was disappointing, but in patients with small tumors (T1N0) a survival of 18.5 months (median) was observed.

Shipley and colleagues[12] reported that the survival of 12 patients with small tumors treated with permanent iodine 125 implantation was similar to that of patients treated by a pancreaticoduodenectomy (Whipple procedure).

A series of studies using combined iodine 125 implantation, external beam radiation, and chemotherapy were undertaken at TJUH.[13] The early experience indicated a high incidence of perioperative mortality (34%) and morbidity (30%). With the development of a unified team approach and experience with these procedures, the morbidity and mortality of the procedures were substantially reduced.[13] The major cause of perioperative morbidity and mortality seems to be related to the inadvertent implantation of areas of normal pancreas or acute pancreatitis rather than the tumors. Pancreatic leaks, autodigestion of tissues, fistulization, pseudocysts, and abscess formation have been the major perioperative problems. A more conservative approach to implanting clearly defined areas of tumor and not the junctional areas of normal pancreas has resulted in substantially reduced morbidity and mortality from the procedure.

Iodine 125 implantation requires thorough exploration of the abdominal cavity to be certain that there are no metastatic foci in the liver or peritoneal surfaces. Adequate surgical exposure of the anterior surface of the pancreas is essential. The tumor is measured in a three-dimensional format, anteroposterior and lateral dimensions obtained, and an equivalent volume estimation made. Assessment of the number of seeds to be implanted is based on the activity of the seeds and the prescribed radiation dose ascertained by using established nomograms.[14] A dose of 120 to 160 Gy over the period of complete isotope decay is generally used with permanent iodine 125 implants. With other isotopes these doses need to be modified. Based on the number of seeds required for the implant, the number of needles to be placed in the tumor is mapped out and the tumor is implanted, avoiding areas of pancreatitis or normal pancreas. The prescribed number of seeds is implanted through the needles with the use of applicators to obtain an even distribution of seeds through the tumor volume, and the needles are withdrawn after placement of the seeds. Occasionally, bleeding can occur after withdrawal of the needles, and it is important to make sure that absolute hemostasis is achieved after the implant procedure to avoid displacement of the radioactive seeds. Hemostasis can be achieved using local pressure with a peanut or by applying small sutures. Biliary and gastrointestinal bypass procedures can be accomplished after radioactive implantation. The energy of the gamma rays emitted from the iodine 125 is low (70 kV), and the dose to the operator undertaking these bypasses is insignificant but should be monitored.

The surface of the pancreas is then covered with an omental fat pad to prevent attachment of the adjacent stomach and colon to the surface of the pancreas because this can result in delivery of an unnecessary radiation dose to these organs. Excessive radiation dose has been associated with an increased risk of late gastrointestinal bleeding, especially when implants have been combined with high-dose external beam radiation. Postoperative stereoshift or orthogonal radiographs can be obtained for dosimetric recalculation of tumor volume and the delivered radiation dose.

The most recent experience at TJUH[13] in patients treated with a combination of iodine 125 implantation followed by external beam radiation therapy and chemotherapy indicates a significant reduction in perioperative mortality (<5%). High rates of clinical local control of primary tumor (71%) have also been achieved. Patients were treated with a planned total dose of 160 Gy from the iodine 125 implant, followed by perioperative chemotherapy on day 10 postsurgery (5-fluorouracil [5-FU], semustine). This was followed by combined external radiation (55 to 60 Gy) at week 4 and further 5-FU chemotherapy. A median survival of 12 months was obtained, with 2- and 5- year survivals of 27% and 14%, respectively.

Although these survival results appear promising, early and late morbidity remains a significant factor. The most serious complication was late gastrointestinal bleeding. Patients often manifested a diffuse pattern of gastritis 12 to 18 months after treatment. The cause of the gastritis appears to be multifactorial. The high doses of radiation, the chemotherapy, and biliary reflux all result in dissolution of the mucous barrier that protects the gastric epithelium. This can lead to punctate ulceration of the mucous membrane or to a pattern of diffuse gastritis and chronic bleeding. Although these toxicities remain a concern, the 14% 5-year survival in this study is encouraging and suggests that some patients with unresectable pancreatic cancer may potentially be curable with aggressive combined local and systemic treatment.

INTRAOPERATIVE RADIATION THERAPY

Intraoperative radiation therapy is an area of increasing clinical interest, especially for tumors of the abdomen. The concept of IORT is similar to that of interstitial or intracavitary radiation, in which large doses of radiation can be delivered to specified small tumor volumes with relative sparing of the adjacent normal tissues, thereby increasing the ratio of tumor control to normal tissue toxicity. The extent of the tumor can be more precisely defined at surgery, and radiation can be applied directly to it. Normal structures can be mobilized away from the tumor to avoid any direct or scattered radiation to these areas. Application of IORT itself is not new, having first been described in 1915 with the use of orthovoltage radiation. More recently, however, the availability of electron beam accelerators stirred interest in the use of this technique as an adjunct to the conventional use of external radiation for pancreatic cancers. The well defined characteristics of high-energy electrons, as well as the minimal shielding requirements and the relatively easy access to the anterior surface of the pancreas, make this approach well suited to this disease.

Although the early Japanese experience used IORT as a single modality, the most effective use of IORT appears to be as a boost in conjunction with high-dose external radiation and chemotherapy. The biologic effect of a large single dose of radiation is two to three times that of similar doses of fractionated treatment, and a large single dose is likely to be more biologically effective than radiation delivered with permanent implants, especially radioactive sources with a long half-life such as iodine 125 (60 days). The higher dose of radiation is also likely to have a marked cell-killing effect on hypoxic foci that are often the limiting factor in the radiocurability of large tumors.

The Japanese[15] undertook the first extensive studies in the use of electron beam IORT for pancreatic cancer. Their initial experience demonstrated that using single doses of IORT alone could palliate pain in approximately 70% of patients with unresectable cancers. This modality was introduced into the United States in 1976 at Howard University, and subsequently has undergone trials at several institutions[16–19] and within the Radiation Therapy Oncology Group. The chief advantage of IORT for the treatment of localized pancreatic cancer is the ability to deliver high radiation doses directly to the area of the tumor without violating the tumor itself, as occurs with the insertion of needles for radioactive implantation. This is likely to reduce the perioperative morbidity and mortality associated with instrumentation of the pancreas. In addition, radiation exposure to the surrounding dose-limiting normal structures can also be reduced by retracting the dose-limiting structures away from the field of radiation and by placement of the rigid treatment cone, which helps keep normal viscera from encroaching into the radiation field. The choice of electron energy can be tailored to varying thicknesses of the tumor.

Intraoperative radiation therapy in combination with external beam radiation can be delivered either at the time of initial exploration or after a course of preoperative external beam radiation. Combined with systemic chemotherapy, studies have reported a median survival ranging from 12 to 14 months for unresectable carcinoma of the pancreas.[17–19] Survival of patients after IORT does not appear to be better than with the use of radioactive implantation for these tumors, but perioperative

TABLE 39-2. *Intraoperative external beam radiationtherapy for unresectable pancreatic cancer*

Institution	Schedule	No. of patients	Local control	Median survival (mo)
Massachusetts General Hospital[20]	20 Gy IORT + 50 Gy ext + 5-FU	76	69%	13
Mayo Clinic[21]	20 Gy IORT + 45–50 Gy ext + 5-FU	37	66%	13
Kyoto[19]	10–25 Gy IORT + 45 Gy ext	20	—	12
Thomas Jefferson University Hospital[18]	20 Gy IORT + 59–60 Gy ext + 5-FU	39	60%	12

IORT, intraoperative radiation therapy; *ext,* external beam radiation therapy; *5-FU,* 5-fluorouracil.

morbidity and mortality appear to be reduced significantly (Table 39-2).

Carefully delivered IORT, avoiding inner portions of the duodenal mucosa, has resulted in reduced overall long-term complications in the TJUH study. Early morbidity has been reduced from 32% after iodine 125 implantation to 15%, and late morbidity has been reduced from 34% to 8%. One of the unanticipated benefits of IORT has been rapid palliation of pancreatic cancer pain after treatment. Pain relief can occur within 24 hours of IORT, and 50% to 75% of patients have remained pain free for the rest of their lives.[18,19]

Local control of disease is often difficult to monitor in pancreatic, but ranges from 60% to 65% with IORT, slightly lower than that reported with interstitial implantation, which may be related to the lower dose of external beam radiation often used with IORT in current treatment programs.

A few studies have investigated the use of misonidazole as a radiation sensitizer in conjunction with IORT, and although early results appeared promising, more recent data indicate that there appears to be no benefit from the addition of the sensitizer to IORT.[20]

COMBINED MODALITIES: RADIATION THERAPY AND CHEMOTHERAPY

A variety of systemic chemotherapeutic agents have been explored in the treatment of pancreatic cancer to overcome the aggressive natural history of this disease, which is associated with early dissemination of tumor, especially to the liver and peritoneal cavity. 5-FU remains the most effective cytotoxic agent and is also known to be an effective radiation sensitizer.[21] This has led to the development of combined modality approaches with 5-FU and radiation to treat this and other gastrointestinal tumors.[22,23] A combined approach of adjunctive radiation and chemotherapy has been shown to improve local control and survival for resected pancreatic cancers.[24]

In unresectable pancreatic cancer, Moertel and colleagues[21] delivered modest doses of radiation to the upper abdomen with large 20 × 20 cm fields in combination with 5-FU, 15 mg/kg by rapid intravenous infusion on the first 3 days of radiation. Patients treated with this combined modality approach had a median survival of 10.4 months, compared with 6.3 months for patients treated with radiation alone ($P < 0.05$). The Gastrointestinal Tumor Study Group[22] undertook the first randomized trial for patients with unresectable carcinomas. Three treatment arms were used, 4000 cGy plus 5-FU, 6000 cGy plus 5-FU, and 6000 cGy alone. The radiation was delivered in a split-course fashion at 2000 cGy in 10 fractions over 2 weeks, followed by a 2-week rest period. The 5-FU was administered intravenously in doses of 500 mg/m^2 on the first 3 days of each cycle of radiation therapy and weekly thereafter. Median survival in the radiation-alone arm was 17 weeks, compared with 32 weeks for the 4000 cGy plus 5-FU arm, and 44 weeks for the 6000 cGy plus 5-FU arm. This study strongly suggests that the therapeutic benefit was a result of both the radiation dose and the use of 5-FU in conjunction with it. Several other combinations of drugs and radiation have been used, but none has shown any further advantage over 5-FU and radiation alone (Table 39-3).

In spite of these aggressive approaches, patients continue to fail with distant metastases, and more recent approaches have focused on the search for biologic response modifiers to enhance the efficacy of 5-FU together with radiation.

SUMMARY

For unresectable pancreatic carcinoma, the use of carefully delivered IORT and postoperative external beam radiation in combination with systemic chemotherapy appears to offer the

TABLE 39-3. *Combined external beam radiation and chemotherapy for unresectable pancreatic cancer*

Institution	Schedule	No. of patients	Local control	Median survival (mo)
GITSG[22]	60 Gy/10 wk	25	77%	5.2
	40 Gy/6 wk + 5-FU	83	74%	9.6
	60 Gy/10 wk + 5-FU	86	73%	9.2
GITSG[25]	60 Gy/10 wks + 5-FU	73	42%	8.4
	60 Gy/10 wks + doxorubicin	70	49%	7.5
Mayo Clinic[21]	40–60 Gy/6 wk + chemotherapy	122	20%	12.6
Thomas Jefferson University Hospital[2]	63–70 Gy/7–9 wk + 5-FU	46	28%	7.3

GITSG, Gastrointestinal tumor study group; *5-FU,* 5-fluorouracil.

best palliation and a median survival approaching 1 year. There is long-term salvage of a small number of patients. However, patients continue to fail with both local, regional, and distant disease. The development of new options for systemic therapy is essential for further improvements in the survival of these patients.

REFERENCES

1. Gudjonsson B. Cancer of the pancreas: 50 years of surgery. Cancer 1987;60:2284.
2. Mohiuddin M, Rosato F, Schuricht A, Barbot D, Biermann W, Cantor R. Carcinoma of the pancreas: the Jefferson experience 1975–1988. Eur J Surg Oncol 1994;20:13.
3. Miller TR, Fuller LM. Radiation therapy of carcinoma of the pancreas. AJR Am J Roentgenol 1958;80:787.
4. Moertel CG, Frytak S, Hahn RG, and the Gastrointestinal Tumor Study Group. Therapy of locally unresectable pancreatic carcinoma: a randomized comparison of high dose (6000 rads) radiation alone, moderate dose radiation (4000 rads + 5-fluorouracil), and high dose radiation + 5-fluorouracil. Cancer 1981;48:1705.
5. Haslam JB, Cavanaugh PJ, Stroup SL. Radiation therapy in the treatment of irresectable adenocarcinoma of the pancreas. Cancer 1973;32: 1341.
6. Dobelbower RR, Borgelt BB, Strubler KA, Kutcher GJ, Suntharalingam N. Precision radiotherapy for cancer of the pancreas: technique and results. Int J Radiat Oncol Biol Phys 1980;6:1127.
7. Whittington R, Dobelbower RR, Mohiuddin M, Rosato FE, Weiss SM. Radiotherapy of unresectable pancreatic carcinoma: a six year experience with 104 patients. Int J Radiat Oncol Biol Phys 1981;7:1639.
8. Handley WS. Pancreatic cancer and its treatment by implanted radium. Ann Surg 1934;100:215.
9. Pack GT, McNeer G. Radiation treatment of pancreatic cancer. AJR Am J Roentgenol 1938;40:708.
10. Fortner JG, D'Angio GJ, Hilaris BS, et al. Iodine-125 implantation for unresectable cancer of the pancreas. Postgrad Med 1970;47:226.
11. Peretz T, Nori D, Hilaris B, et al. Treatment of primary unresectable carcinoma of the pancreas with I-125 implantation. Int J Radiat Oncol Biol Phys 1989;17:931.
12. Shipley WU, Nardi GG, Cohen AM, Ling CC. Iodine-125 implant and external beam irradiation in patients with localized pancreatic carcinoma: a comparative study to surgical resection. Cancer 1980;45:709.
13. Mohiuddin M, Cantor RJ, Biermann W, Weiss SM, Barbot D, Rosato FE. Combined modality treatment of localized unresectable adenocarcinoma of the pancreas. Int J Radiat Oncol Biol Phys 1988;148:79.
14. Waterman FM, Strubler KA. Absorbed dose determinations for interstitial I-125 boost therapy. Med Phys 1980;7:437.
15. Abe M, Yamano K, Imura T, et al. Intraoperative radiotherapy of abdominal tumors: part 1. intraoperative irradiation to carcinoma of the pancreas head and biliary system. Nippon Acta Radiologica 1969;29: 75.
16. Tepper JE, Nardi GL, Suit HD. Carcinoma of the pancreas: review of MGH experience from 1963 to 1973: analysis of surgical failure and implications for radiation therapy. Cancer 1976;37:1519.
17. Roldan G, Gunderson L, Nagorney D, et al. External beam vs. intraoperative and external beam irradiation for locally advanced pancreatic cancer. Cancer 1988;61:1110.
18. Mohiuddin M, Regine W, Rosato F, et al. A comparison of intraoperative radiation therapy (IORT) and I-125 implantation for cancer of the pancreas. In: Intraoperative Radiation Therapy, Proceedings of the 4th International Symposium, 1994:315.
19. Abe M, Shibamoto T, Takahashi M, Manabe T, Tobe T, Inamoto T. Intraoperative radiotherapy in carcinoma of the stomach and pancreas. World J Surg 1987;11:459.
20. Tepper JE, Shipley WU, Warshaw AL, et al. The role of misonidazole combined with intraoperative radiation therapy in the treatment of pancreatic carcinoma. J Clin Oncol 1987;5:579.
21. Childs DS, Moertel DG, Holbrook MA, Reitemeir RJ, Colby MY. Treatment of malignant neoplasms of the gastrointestinal tract with a combination of 5-fluorouracil and radiation. Radiology 1965;84:143.
22. Gastrointestinal Tumor Study Group. A comparison of combination chemotherapy and combined modality therapy for locally advanced gastric carcinoma. Cancer 1982;49:1771.
23. Krook JE, Moertel CG, Gunderson LL, et al. Effective surgical adjuvant therapy for high risk rectal carcinoma. N Engl J Med 1991;324:709.
24. Gastrointestinal Tumor Study Group. Further evidence of effective adjuvant combined radiation and chemotherapy following curative resection of pancreatic cancer. Cancer 1987;59:2006.
25. Gastrointestinal Tumor Study Group. Treatment of locally unresectable carcinoma of the pancreas: comparison of combined-modality therapy (chemotherapy plus radiotherapy) to chemotherapy alone. J Natl Cancer Inst 1988;80:751.
26. Gastrointestinal Tumor Study Group. Radiation therapy combined with Adriamycin or 5-fluorouracil for the treatment of locally unresectable pancreatic carcinoma. Cancer 1985;56:2563.

Surgery for Gastrointestinal Cancer: A Multidisciplinary Approach, edited by Harold J. Wanebo.
Lippincott-Raven Publishers, Philadelphia, © 1997.

CHAPTER 40

Preoperative Adjuvant Therapy for Cancer of the Pancreas

John P. Hoffman

Preoperative radiation therapy (RT) was suggested in print by Tepper and colleagues in 1975.[1] The concept was introduced in the discussion of a study that reported a 50% rate of local or regional recurrence in patients with pancreatic exocrine cancer treated by pancreatoduodenectomy. A small cohort of patients already were being treated in this fashion by surgeons and radiotherapists in another Boston institution as early as 1972.[2,3] The results of this trial apparently were not as interesting to workers in the field as was the addition of chemotherapy (CTX) to RT and its use as an adjunct to surgery (regardless of its timing), because no more studies of preoperative RT were reported until 1989.[4] The next decade brought reports from four institutions where trials of preoperative irradiation with CTX were conducted between 1986 and 1991.[5–9] In addition, the Eastern Cooperative Oncology Group (ECOG) performed a phase II trial of preoperative RT and CTX (EST PD289).

This chapter discusses what has been learned from these experiences.

THEORETIC ADVANTAGES OF PREOPERATIVE CHEMOTHERAPY AND RADIATION THERAPY

The only justifications for the preoperative sequencing of RT in the two early papers from Tufts-New England Medical Center were to increase resectability and perhaps reduce the number of viable cells being shed into the circulation at the time of surgery.[2] Otherwise, the goals of local or regional control could be achieved as well by postoperative RT, which had the added virtue of sparing the time, expense, and complications of RT for patients with distant metastases discovered at surgery.

Other potential advantages of preoperative RT were enumerated later:

1. A decrease in the ability of tumor cells to implant on the surgical incisions at the time of operation.[4]
2. Improved tolerance to RT (with or without CTX), because patients do not have to recover from a recent operation[6] and do not have fixed small bowel in the RT portal.[10]
3. Improved ability to deliver the planned RT dose, especially to patients in whom prolonged operative complications would have severely delayed or prevented the delivery of postoperative RT.[6]
4. Improved effectiveness of RT because cancer cells in the target area are relatively less hypoxic (better vascularity) than after pancreatoduodenectomy.[6]
5. The ability to screen out many patients who initially possess distant micrometastases that become detectable during the 10- to 12-week delay before pancreatectomy, sparing them a celiotomy or futile pancreatectomy.[6,11]
6. A potential reduction in the number of pancreatojejunostomy leaks because of the increased fibrous tissue in the pancreatic remnant.[10,12]

The results of the various trials are examined for evidence of these putative advantages.

PREOPERATIVE RADIATION THERAPY WITHOUT CHEMOTHERAPY

Two papers were published within 3 years from Tufts-New England Medical Center describing patients treated with RT followed by surgery.[2,3] Seventeen patients were treated with 40 to 50 Gy (75% received between 44 and 46 Gy) and were described in 1980.[2] Four patients were treated with 40 to 46 Gy and were described in 1983.[3] The authors do not believe that any patient was described twice. The 17 patients in the first report had large cancers (13 were more than 5 cm in diameter, but the method of determining size was not reported). These lesions involved the body of the pancreas in 3 patients and the body and head of the pancreas in 4 patients. Sixteen of the patients underwent exploratory celiotomy to determine resectability, and 11 were considered to have unresectable cancers because of the "involvement" of portal or superior mesenteric vessels. Three other patients had cancers of "borderline" re-

Department of Surgery, Fox Chase Cancer Center, 7701 Burholme Avenue, Philadelphia, PA 19111-2497 sectability, and 2 had unresectable cancers as defined by the surgeon. Bypasses were done in 15 patients. Five patients required a second celiotomy for tissue diagnosis because the first surgeon judged pancreatic biopsy to be "too risky."[2] The interval between initial celiotomy and the initiation of RT was not reported.

All the patients received at least 4000 cGy through parallel opposed portals. One patient had a myocardial infarction, 1 had distant metastases, 1 had both distant and local progression, and 3 had local progression obviating reexploration. Eleven underwent another celiotomy with the intention of pancreatic resection between 3 and 8 weeks after RT. Four were found to harbor distant abdominal metastases and 1 was found to be locally unresectable. The other 6, all of whom had tumors confined to the head of the pancreas, underwent Whipple procedures. One patient died after surgery of renal shutdown, 1 died later of unknown causes, 2 who had positive pancreatic margins died of local and distant recurrences, and 2 lived free of disease for more than 5 years.

Four patients with pancreatic cancers treated by a similar technique were described 3 years later.[3] Patients with unresectable tumors and those with positive pancreatic margins were excluded from the report. One patient survived 7 years until a paraaortic recurrence developed. Another was described without recurrence at 15 months after surgery. Two others died 8 and 14 months after surgery of peritoneal and liver metastases, respectively.

The authors of the early paper reported marked tumor shrinkage in 5 of the 17 patients. Because all the patients underwent resection, the authors speculated that future patients could be monitored for shrinkage and resection performed only if it occurred. They did not comment on the histologic reactions to the RT, but did observe that the most dramatic shrinkage occurred in a patient with only "microscopic residual disease."[2] The later paper reported tumor shrinkage in 3 of the 4 patients, but only 1 had histologic evidence of a response. This patient, who had not undergone a previous exploration, initially was believed to have an ampullary cancer, but the tumor was determined to have arisen in the pancreas at final pathology. This conclusion is not entirely convincing, because the histologic findings were reported to reveal no residual tumor.[3] No other patients with pancreatic cancer have had complete pathologic responses to RT, with or without CTX. However, several complete pathologic responses have been reported in patients with ampullary and duodenal carcinomas.[11]

Ishikawa and associates also were interested in the histologic effects of preoperative RT.[4] They treated 12 patients with pancreatic cancers and observed tumor shrinkage in all cases. However, 3 patients displayed little evidence of a histologic effect. This was attributed to surrounding pancreatitis, which lowered the oxygen tension in the tumors. Their system for measuring histologic effects to RT is the first reported in pancreatic cancer.

PREOPERATIVE RADIATION THERAPY WITH CHEMOTHERAPY

Radiation Therapy, Two 96-Hour 5-Fluorouracil Infusions, and Bolus Mitomycin C

The first trial that added CTX to preoperative RT was developed at the Fox Chase Cancer Center (FCCC) in 1986 and first reported in 1990.[5] Work from a phase III Gastrointestinal Tumor Study Group (GITSG) trial and phase II experiences from several centers had established the superiority of combination CTX and RT over RT alone.[13–17] However, none of these experiences were in the adjuvant setting. The type of CTX used most commonly was 5-fluorouracil alone, although CTX concurrent with RT had evolved to include mitomycin C with bolus 5-fluorouracil at Thomas Jefferson University Hospital.[14] RT concurrent with a different regimen of 5-fluorouracil and mitomycin C had been tested at FCCC in many patients with esophageal cancer. This regimen, consisting of two 96-hour infusions of 5-fluorouracil (1000 mg/m^2) during days 2 through 5 and 29 through 32, and a single injection of mitomycin C (10 mg/m^2) on day 2 of the RT, was used to treat a total of 66 patients (with 61 pancreatic and 5 duodenal cancers) from 1986 to 1994. RT was given by a three- or four-field technique at 180-cGy fractions (five per week), with a cone down after 3960 cGy to a field 1 to 2 cm from the margins of the lesion to a total of 5040 cGy.[5,10,11] The pilot study had accrued 23 patients before the opening of the ECOG protocol PD289, which consisted of exactly the same regimen, with stricter eligibility requirements. The ECOG trial began in late 1990 and closed 3 years later, with 64 patients accrued. Because the data have not been published, the findings are not discussed here, except to say that the evolution of the accrual to this study mirrored that of the FCCC pilot. That is, patients with extremely advanced local or regional cancer initially were chosen to participate in the trial, such that the eligibility criteria had to be rendered more exclusive as the trial progressed. During the 3-year period of the ECOG trial, the FCCC pilot continued to accrue patients with periampullary cancers not known to be pancreatic in origin, those with lesions larger than 5 cm in greatest diameter, those with tumors of adenosquamous histology, and those treated with the RT and CTX regimen outside FCCC or its network hospitals. This added 12 patients with pancreatic cancer and 3 with duodenal or bile duct cancer to the FCCC study. Thirty-five patients with pancreatic cancer from the FCCC pilot and 26 patients accrued to the ECOG study from FCCC are discussed as 61 patients with pancreatic cancer treated at FCCC.

Radiation Therapy and Continuous Infusion of 5-Fluorouracil Plus Intraoperative Radiation Therapy

A regimen of RT and a continuous infusion (5 d/wk) of 5-fluorouracil (300 mg/m^2) plus intraoperative RT was used at the M.D. Anderson Cancer Center (MDACC) beginning in 1988.[6,7,18,19] A new protocol with a different schedule of external-beam RT (300 cGy in 10 fractions) was begun in 1993. The original trial enrolled 51 patients.

External-Beam Radiation Therapy and Continuous Infusion of 5-Fluorouracil

A regimen of external-beam RT and a continuous infusion (7 d/wk) of 5-fluorouracil at a lower dosage (225 mg/m^2, because there was no weekend break) was administered to 16 patients with unresectable pancreatic cancer between 1990 and 1991.[8] Another 7 patients were added from another institution the next year[20] (JM Jessup, personal communication, July

TABLE 40-1. *Trials of preoperative radiation therapy with or without chemotherapy*

Institution (ref.)	Years of trial	Number of patients	Radiation therapy	Chemotherapy
Tufts[2,3]	1972–1981	17 + 4	40–50 Gy, 2 Gy/fraction, AP-PA ports	None
Osaka[4,12]	Before 1987	12 + 10	50 Gy, 2 Gy/fraction, AP-PA ports	None
Fox Chase[5,10,11]	1986–1994	Pilot study 36, ECOG Trial 26	50.4 Gy, 1.8 Gy/fraction, 3 or 4 fields	5-FU (96 h, days 2–5, 29–32), mitomycin C (Day 2)
M.D. Anderson[6,7,18,19]	1988–1993	28?	45–50.4 Gy, 1.8 Gy/fraction; IORT (10–20 Gy)	5-FU (continuous infusion 5 d/wk, 300 mg/m^2)
New England Deaconness, Dartmouth[8,20]	1990–1992	23	At least 45 Gy 45 Gy	5-FU (continuous infusion 7 d/wk, 225 mg/m^2)
Roger Williams[9]	1990	14		5-FU, cisplatin

AP-PA, anteroposterior-posteroanterior; *IORT,* intraoperative radiation therapy.

1994). The RT given is not reported in detail, but it is stated that all patients received at least 45 Gy.

External-Beam Radiation Therapy, 5-Fluorouracil, and Cisplatin

Wanebo and colleagues conducted a pilot protocol including external-beam RT, 5-fluorouracil, and cisplatin in which patients underwent full operative staging for resectability and preliminary biliary and gastric bypass before the CTX and RT.[9]

All the trials described are summarized in Table 40-1.

INDICATIONS FOR PREOPERATIVE ADJUVANT THERAPY

Metastases are found on presentation in 45% to 50% of patients with pancreatic cancer.[21,22] The classification of patients without metastases varies according to the criteria used to determine resectability, but can include those with easily resectable stage T1a lesions, larger but resectable lesions (T1b to stage III), unresectable lesions because of local or regional factors, and unresectable lesions because of occult distant metastases discovered at celiotomy. Ten percent of resected cancers are smaller than 2 cm in diameter, and less than half these tumors are confined to the pancreas (ie, they have not invaded through the capsule or spread to regional nodes).[23–25] Between 1% and 78% of patients undergo resection, depending on which patients are placed in the denominator (ie, all of those who have pancreatic masses without further nonoperative analyses of resectability, or all of those who undergo angiography, laparoscopy, computed tomography (CT), or magnetic resonance imaging to determine resectability).[26–29] However, these percentages describe the fraction of patients who actually undergo resection among those who are operated on with the intention of resection. The fewer the tests for resectability, the more operations are done for unresectable tumors and the lower is the resectability rate.

Sener and associates studied 2401 patients with pancreatic cancer in the state of Illinois from 1978 to 1984.[30] Clinical stage I to III cancer was present in 744 patients, clinical stage IV cancer in 945 patients, and cancer of unknown stage in 712 patients. Pancreatic resection was performed in 204 patients (27%).

Tepper and colleagues described 114 patients who underwent laparotomy without resection.[1] Thirty-five (31%) had no evidence of distant disease but did not undergo resection because of medial or posterior extension to large blood vessels. The only reason for unresectability was vascular encasement in 20 of 39 unresectable cases reported by Warshaw and associates.[29] Thirty percent to 50% of potentially resectable cases are found to be unresectable because of direct extension and 50% to 70% because of occult distant metastases. Of those with direct extension, no data are available regarding the percentage with tumor approximation or narrowing of the superior mesenteric vein (SMV) or portal vein without encasement of the neighboring superior mesenteric artery (SMA) or hepatic artery. The Fox Chase Cancer Center experience indicates that about one fifth have arterial involvement, but this may be a high estimate because of the tertiary referral nature of our institution, where we see more patients who are declared hopeless at their primary treatment centers.

Preoperative therapy is of no use in the 60% to 70% of patients who have obvious or occult metastatic pancreatic cancer. Of the three remaining groups, preoperative RT and CTX might benefit all except those with true SMA or hepatic artery encasement. End results information, however, will include mostly those patients in the third group (ie, locally unresectable because of SMV encroachment), a few in the group that would make up most contemporary series of resections, and probably none in the tiny group with cancers smaller than 2 cm in diameter. An exact algorithm of indications awaits phase III testing in each of the categories (surgery alone versus preoperative versus postoperative RT in stage T1a cancers, preoperative versus postoperative RT in the two more advanced tumor groups). Meanwhile, in view of the demonstrated safety of preoperative RT or RT plus CTX, it seems reasonable to use this approach for all but the smallest of pancreatic cancers.[7,10]

LIMITATIONS OF PREOPERATIVE ADJUVANT THERAPY

Several problems face the physician who wishes to deliver preoperative adjuvant RT with or without CTX. First, a diagnosis must be established. The simplicity of obtaining a biopsy at resectional surgery is much less frustrating than the difficult, sometimes impossible, task of obtaining samples of the tumor adequate for cytologic interpretation. Of 21 patients referred to this author's institution after exploratory celiotomy, only 15 had adequate material for diagnosis, necessitating further attempts at percutaneous biopsy and, in 1 patient, a second celiotomy after three separate CT-directed fine-needle aspirations (FNAs) had failed in obtaining diagnostic material. Of 29 patients in whom celiotomy had not been done and tissue was required for diagnosis, a single procedure was successful in 22 cases (76%; 18 under CT direction, 2 by ultrasound, and 2 under fluoroscopic direction). Five patients required two procedures, and 2 needed three FNAs under CT guidance. In 3 patients with negative CT-directed FNAs, diagnoses were made from tissue obtained at endoscopic retrograde cholangiopancreatography (ERCP). Diagnoses were made by ERCP (2 patients) or percutaneous transhepatic cholangiography (1 patient) brushings in only 3 of 56 patients.

There appears to be a learning curve for radiologists performing these biopsies, and it is helpful to have a cytopathologist with a scanning microscope present at the aspirations so that another needle pass can be taken at the first sitting if adequate tissue is not obtained. If a stent is in place, this author prefers to use FNA directed to the area of the original stricture under fluoroscopic guidance (Fig. 40-1). This is particularly valuable in patients with lesions that are too small to appreciate by CT. It is extremely frustrating to have a patient with a small cancer found at a previous exploratory celiotomy in whom "shave" biopsies or no biopsies were taken and no stent is available to guide the radiologist because a biliary bypass was done and the stent was removed.

In the hands of an experienced radiologist, it usually is as easy to obtain diagnostic material from a small cancer as a larger one, provided the mass can be seen on a CT image. Diagnostic tissue can be obtained by the method illustrated in Figure 40-1. However, Graham and associates have reported that the number of false-negative biopsy results increases with decreasing cancer size, such that a patient with a 3-cm cancer has only a 50% chance of having a positive result from a biopsy obtained by FNA.[31] The method clearly depends on the skill of the interventional radiologist. Nevertheless, even with the most talented radiologist, the added waiting, pain, and possible tumor cell contamination that a single FNA entails are enough to discourage some clinicians and patients from using preoperative adjuvant therapy until there is solid evidence that the method is superior to postoperative treatment.

In regard to the possibility that cells may be shed into the peritoneal cavity by percutaneous FNA, Warshaw and colleagues have suggested that the technique produces inoperability and poorer prognoses.[32] However, their study was retrospective and did not include details such as tumor size and reason for unresectability, so the conclusions are not convincing.[32] Nevertheless, it would be ideal if the diagnosis could be made at initial ERCP. This awaits the development of transduodenal biopsy techniques using endoscopic ultrasound. This author has found no difference in resectability, survival, or recurrence patterns in patients whose diagnoses have been established by FNA compared with those who diagnoses have been established by open or other biopsy techniques. For added protection, fine needles are available that are surrounded by coaxial sheaths that may prevent cancer cells from being drawn out into the peritoneal cavity by the biopsy needle.

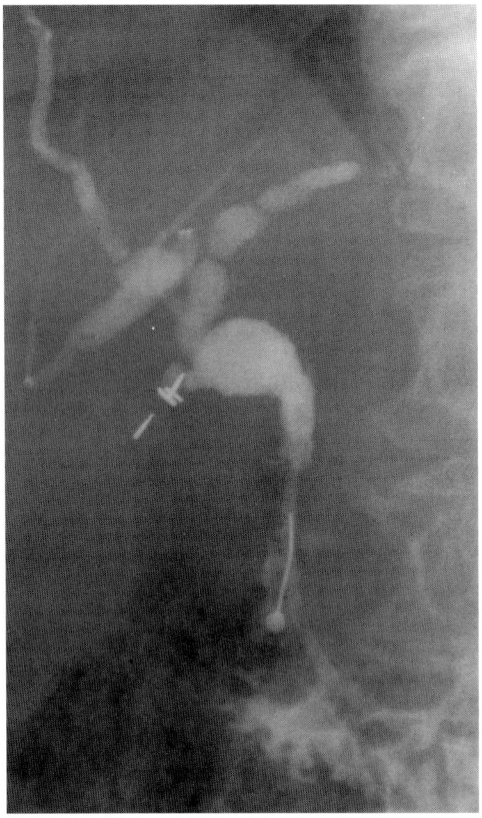

FIG. 40-1. Radiograph taken after radiopaque dye was injected transhepatically into an intrahepatic duct. Some of the dye has traversed stent placed into the duodenum at endoscopic retrograde cholangiopancreatography. The needle overlying the stent has been positioned just below the stricture noted by the cholangiogram. The fine-needle aspirate was done from this area and was successful in obtaining material for a diagnosis of pancreatic cancer.

Another limitation of preoperative RT and CTX is that a patient with an obstructing tumor of the pancreatic head without an operative bypass requires a functioning internal stent. This author's experience with internalized stents in these patients is disconcerting. Of seven ERCP-placed stents, four have required replacement by transhepatic stents, and of three internal transhepatic stents, one has required conversion to an external transhepatic stent. Perhaps the RT and CTX produce an excess of necrotic material that obstructs the internal stents, or perhaps the patients are hypovolemic from their treatments and side effects, causing biliary secretions to sludge. All 19 patients who had transhepatic stents also required tube changes within the 11 or 12 weeks before surgery. This is accomplished more readily and easily than with the endoscope. This author usually changes the stents every 4 to 6 weeks (sooner if dilated ducts or alkaline phosphatase elevations are observed), and replaces the 8.5F tubes with 10F tubes at the first exchange.

Other, less vexing limitations of preoperative RT and CTX are the obligatory delays to the beginning of therapy resulting from the use of multiple treatment modalities (eg, visits to the radiation and medical oncologist, set-up and simulation times) and the increased difficulty at some operations in dissecting irradiated, fibrotic tumor margins from the central vessels (SMV and SMA). The latter is a problem only in those cancers that probably could not have been resected with clear margins without the preoperative therapy.

Finally, even the best imaging and laparoscopic techniques are not as good as thorough, open surgical staging and resectability determinations. Inevitably, more patients are given RT and CTX when staging is done without surgery than when resection is performed first, followed by adjuvant therapy. This number also is increased by those patients without demonstrable metastases at the initiation of RT who display distant metastases at restaging 3 to 4 weeks after the completion of RT or at celiotomy with the intention of tumor resection. This increase supports the use of preoperative therapy, because of its potential for reducing the number of futile resections.

The lack of surgical and pathologic staging in these patients at the time of initial treatment is the major limitation of any comparison of preoperative and postoperative adjuvant therapies. Unless newer imaging and laparoscopic techniques that rival pathologic staging are discovered, the only way to determine the actual differences among preoperative and postoperative adjuvant therapies is through a prospective, randomized trial of patients who have had an initial tissue diagnosis before trial entry.

COMPLICATIONS OF PREOPERATIVE ADJUVANT THERAPY

The complications that occurred in 33 patients who underwent pancreatectomy after the FCCC RT and CTX program are listed in Table 40-2. Four of the patients had duodenal carcinomas and 4 underwent palliative pancreatectomies (3 with excision of liver metastases, 1 with replacement of the hepatic artery and SMV). Complications unique to these postirradiation procedures were ascites after total pancreatectomy in 7 of the 11 patients so treated and an electrocautery injury to the right ureter requiring ureteroureterostomy over a stent. The right ureter often is pulled far medially by the RT to a position overlying the inferior vena cava. It must be identified clearly before the Kocher maneuver is begun. Ascites was uncommon after Whipple resection but is almost the rule after total pancreatectomy. Peritoneovenous shunting was required in 1 patient and several had severe abdominal distention and fluid and electrolyte problems for several weeks after surgery. The ascites always resolved within 2 to 3 months. The fluid was chylous in only 1 patient. Because care was taken to ligate paraaortic and mesenteric lymphatics, the ascites in these patients was not as marked. It is possible that the RT narrowed lymphatic pathways in the mesentery, mesocolon, and retroperitoneal areas, so that injury to remaining lymph vessels produced more than the usual disruption in fluid dynamics.

Other series report complication rates similar to those of patients treated without preoperative RT. Three different series have shown a reduction in the incidence of pancreaticojejunal leaks after RT.[7,10,12] Presumably, this is because of fibrosis in the remaining pancreatic tail, which therefore holds sutures more securely. It is doubtful that decreased pancreatic juice production is responsible, because some patients are able to eat normally without pancreatic enzyme replacement. Among 20 cases of Whipple resection performed after RT and CTX at FCCC, there have been 4 chemical amylase leaks (amylase in the drain fluid greater than serum amylase for at least one determination) and 1 clinical leak that required percutaneous drainage. Of 15 duct-to-mucosa anastomoses, 3 had chemical leaks and 1 of these was in a patient with a splenic artery ligation within the substance of the pancreas for a splenic artery aneurysm. The 1 clinical leak and another chemical leak were noted in 5 patients with intussuscepted anastomoses. This author prefers the former technique of anastomosis.

The mortality rate at FCCC was 3.4% (1 of 29) for standard resections after CTX and RT, and rose to 6% (2 of 33) when palliative resections were counted (including 1 death 3 days after hepatic artery and SMV resection and replacement). Two patients had prolonged hospitalizations (79 and 144 days) from efferent loop obstruction and respiratory failure, respectively. One left the hospital, but returned with a hepatic abscess from a retracted biliary stent and died 5 months after Whipple resection. The other remains free of disease 68 months after her tissue diagnosis. Mortality rates from other series are similarly low. Two patients from the Tufts series had renal failure, 1 in the postoperative period associated with multisystem organ failure.[2,3] The other case occurred many years after treatment,

TABLE 40-2. *Complications after pancreatic resection and preoperative chemotherapy or radiation therapy (Fox Chase Cancer Center)*

Type of complication	Total pancreatectomy (n = 9)	Whipple procedure (n = 20)	Distal pancreatectomy (n = 2)	Total pancreatectomy with vessel replacement (n = 2)
Ascites	5 (56%)	2 (10%)	0	2 (100%)
ARDS	1	1	0	1
Efferent loop obstruction	0	1	0	0
Cholangitis	3	2	0	0
Upper gastrointestinal hemorrhage	1	0	0	0
Pancreatojejunostomy leak (clinical)	0	1	0	0
Psychosis	1	2	0	0
Gastric atony	0	1	0	0
Injured right ureter	0	1	0	0
Number of patients with complications	5 (56%)	7 (35%)	0	2 (100%)

ARDS, adult respiratory distress syndrome.

consistent with renal damage from the RT given through opposed anteroposterior-posteroanterior portals.

RESULTS OF PREOPERATIVE ADJUVANT THERAPY

Three of 10 patients survived more than 5 years after preoperative RT (without CTX) followed by resection.[2,3] However, 1 of the patients could have had an ampullary rather than a pancreatic primary lesion. This cannot be evaluated because the patient had a complete pathologic response to the therapy. Ishikawa and associates reported only one recurrence during a short follow-up period (2 to 39 months) after preoperative RT and resection.[4] A more recent analysis of 23 patients treated with preoperative RT recorded a 74% resectability rate and a significantly lower local recurrence rate than that of patients undergoing surgery alone (O Ishikawa, personal communication, July 1994). However, 3- and 5-year survival rates were the same as those associated with surgery alone (28% versus 32% and 22% versus 26%, respectively). Resectability, local recurrence, operative mortality, and survival rates from all the trials are provided in Table 40-3.

There is no evidence that the addition of CTX to RT improves local tumor control or survival. The FCCC results show a 3- and 5-year projected survival rate of 40% with follow-up of 9 to 69 months for the 25 patients who underwent resection. Median survival is 22 months (Fig. 40-2). Only 3 of the 14 patients with recurrence had any local component of recurrence, and this was found after extensive distant recurrence had been detected.

Thirty patients who underwent resection after preoperative RT and continuous (Monday through Friday) infusion of 5-fluorouracil at MDACC had an 18-month median survival. Only 3 of 18 patients with recurrence had local recurrence as the first recurrence site (DB Evans, personal communication, July 1994). The local recurrence data from these two series are the strongest indicators that preoperative RT and CTX may be more effective than postoperative RT and CTX; the local recurrence rate was 43% in the GITSG trial and 25% in a report from Whittington and colleagues in which the FCCC regimen of RT and CTX was used in the postoperative setting.[33,34] However, the median survival is no better than the 18 to 21 months of the registry and treatment group in the GITSG trial and only slightly better than the 16 months of the patients described by Whittington.[33,34] Only the GITSG series is mature enough to have established these median survival times. Enough patients are still alive with or without recurrence in the FCCC, MDACC, and University of Pennsylvania series that their median survival rates may be significantly longer in the future.

The effects of RT and CTX have included modest reductions in tumor size as measured by CT, but significant histologic responses. The FCCC CT results showed 5 patients with an increase in the size of the tumor within the RT field, 34 with a stable measurement, and 17 with a minimal (less than 50% reduction in the product of the greatest perpendicular diameters—15 patients) or partial (greater than 50% reduction in the product of the diameters—2 patients) decrease. Four of 27 patients had greater than 90% histologic reduction of cancer cells, 9 had 75% to 89% reduction, and 9 had 50% to 74% reduction, but none had a complete pathologic response. The experience is similar at MDACC, where 4 of 17 specimens had greater than 90% local cancer cell destruction.[7]

Because the results from studies of preoperative RT and CTX are not clearly better than those from contemporary series of patients treated by surgery alone or surgery followed by RT and CTX, it is important to compare as many prognostic parameters as possible to assess the distribution of patient and tumor characteristics, and thus the relative value of these approaches. This is made more difficult by the presumed alteration of most histopathologic features (eg, diminution of nodal involvement, decrease in tumor size and cellularity) in the groups treated by preoperative RT.[10] Thus the only measures for comparing prognostic features are those obtained by pretreatment imaging and blood tests.

It is impossible to define all the prognostic features that affect outcome in any group of patients, which is why a phase III randomized trial is the most reliable means of determining differences in treatment programs. However, until such a trial is performed and completed, it is important that authors presenting treatment results closely define the prognostic parameters of the cohorts treated.

Imaging tests are the main means of comparison. Tumor size and invasion of neighboring structures are the major prognostic variables for patients who are presumed to have localized cancers. Pancreatic cancer size has been shown by many to be one of the most important prognostic determinants.[35–40] However, few have shown that size determined by imaging studies approximates that measured in the pathology laboratory.[4] This

TABLE 40-3. *End results for 248 patients having preoperative radiation therapy with or without chemotherapy*

Institution (ref.)	Respectability	Operative mortality	Local recurrence	Survival
Tufts[2,3]	3/17 (18%)	9%	33% (2/6)	2/6 5-Year
Osaka[4,12]	17/23 (74%)	NS	Less than those treated with surgery alone	1-Year 75%, 3-year 28%, 5-year 22%
Fox Chase[5,10,11]	25/61 (41%)	1/25	3/25 (All with distant metastases first)	Median survival 22 months; 3- and 5-year survival 40%
M.D. Anderson[6,7,18,19]	30/51 (59%)	1/30	NS	Median survival 18 months in 30 patients with resection
New England Deaconness, Dartmouth[8,20]	3/23 (13%)	0/3	0/3	15, 42 Months NED, 39 months AWR

NS, not stated; *NED,* no evidence of disease; *AWR,* alive with recurrence.

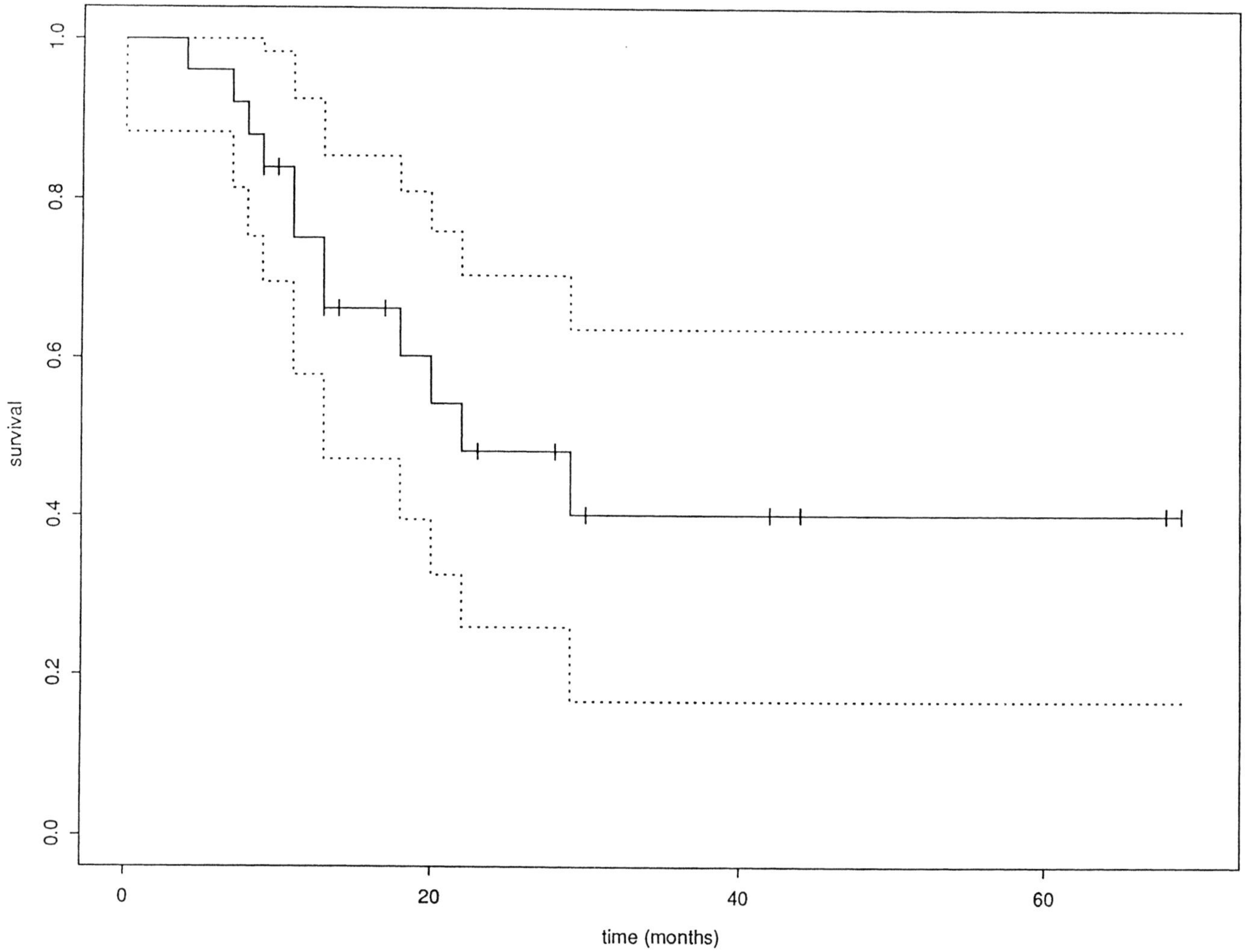

FIG. 40-2. Kaplan-Meier survival curve depicting the fates of 25 patients undergoing resection of pancreatic cancer at Fox Chase Cancer Center after preoperative chemotherapy and radiation therapy. Dotted lines indicate the 95% confidence intervals. Data as of March 31, 1994.

author has examined tumor size as measured by CT and CT portography within a week or two of measurement in the pathology laboratory. The correlation between CT measurements and actual tissue measurements was excellent with tumors larger than 2 cm or smaller than 5 cm in diameter, but four specimens measured in the pathology laboratory as less than 2 cm were judged to be at least 1.5 cm larger by radiology. Of the 29 cancers evaluated by two radiologists, only 20 of the measurements (69%) were within 1 cm of the actual diameter. The nine specimens that caused the most difficulty for the radiologists were two with diffuse mucinous tumors throughout the gland (underestimated by 2.5 cm); one 7-cm mass with a cystic center composed of necrotic cells (overestimated by 2.5 cm, perhaps because of deformity or release of fluid in the pathology laboratory); four small masses (1 to 1.5 cm in diameter), smaller than the normal diameter of the pancreatic head; and two tumors with inexplicably inaccurate size estimates. The last two specimens were from patients with previous biliary-enteric bypasses and RT and CTX. One was a 2.5-cm tumor overestimated by 2.5 cm, and the other was a 4.5-cm tumor underestimated by 1.75 cm. Of the nine cases in which errors of at least 2 cm were made by at least one radiologist, six tumors were measured as larger than they actually were. Spiral and thin-section CT with bolus enhancement probably would improve the ability of radiologists to estimate pancreatic tumor size.[41] However, current techniques are reasonably accurate for tumors larger than 2 cm in diameter.

Gross duodenal invasion can be observed by the endoscopist, but capsular and perineural invasion go unnoticed by even the most sophisticated imaging techniques. Invasion, encasement, and encroachment of neighboring portal, superior mesenteric, and splenic veins, and hepatic, superior mesenteric, and splenic arteries are other important tumor attributes that can be measured, but often are not described in reports of end results. Ishikawa and associates have observed a correlation between survival and the level of SMV involvement.[42] Evans and colleagues have used the fat around the SMA as a boundary for unresectability, although they have not published the fates of those patients with positive SMA margins who underwent resection.[41]

This author has used both systems and finds that neither is invariably accurate in determining resectability, except in pa-

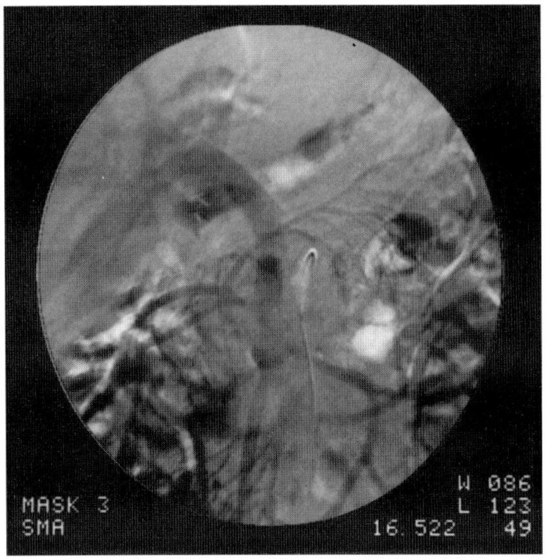

FIG. 40-3. Normal superior mesenteric vein as seen in a late view after superior mesenteric arteriography.

tients with total tumor encasement of the SMA. Although only 1 of 7 patients with SMV occlusion underwent resection, 15 of 31 with lesser SMV encroachment did so. In addition, 1 patient with a cancer of the pancreatic body and tail had an occluded splenic vein and artery in addition to SMA tumor encroachment, but has survived without recurrence 69 months after her tissue diagnosis, CTX, and RT, and 65 months after her subtotal distal pancreatectomy with lateral superior mesenteric venorrhaphy.[10] The number of patients who have undergone resection in this series is too small to produce a reliable correlation between SMV, portal vein, or SMA encroachment and survival after resection. Ishikawa and colleagues showed that no patients who had tumors with SMV or portal vein occlusion or with bilateral impingement had long survival after extended pancreatectomy alone.[42] This author had only 5 such patients, but 1 with SMV occlusion survived 29 months after tissue diagnosis and 1 with bilateral impingement is alive without recurrence 42 months after diagnosis. An example of a normal SMV is shown in Figure 40-3, and venograms of a patient with bilateral SMV impingement at the time of diagnosis and improvement to unilateral impingement after CTX and RT are shown in Figure 40-4. Figure 40-5 demonstrates a disadvantage of this system. The venogram must be interpreted alongside a CT scan with contrast medium in the SMV. This patient originally had been judged to have bilateral SMV impingement. This finding was revised to no impingement after the CT portogram was examined. Of 6 patients who underwent SMV (5 patients) or splenic artery (2 patients, one with both) resection because of tumor adherence or occlusion (2 patients) demonstrated by angiography, none had histologic evidence of blood vessel invasion, even into the adventitia. Preoperative CTX and RT may change the angiographic indications for tumor resectability and vessel resection.

We at Fox Chase Cancer Center have developed a grading system for scoring tumors as they approach the SMA, as seen by CT. It includes four categories: normal fat plane surrounding the SMA, involved ("dirty") fat around the SMA, tumor touching the SMA, and tumor surrounding the SMA (Figs. 40-6 through 40-8). Only 32 of 53 scans were judged by two radiologists to fall clearly into one category. However, only 2 patients had scans that produced variance by more than one category. These were 2 patients with scans judged to be normal by one radiologist and to have no intervening tumor or SMA fat by the other. Again, the numbers of patients are insufficient to produce sound correlations, but the rate of resectability was 33% (6 of 18) for patients with any component of SMA and tumor continuity, and 53% (17 of 32) for those with a tissue plane between the tumor and the SMA, either free or "dirty." As expected, there appear to be more long-term survivors in the first two groups, but statistical significance has not been reached.

FUTURE DIRECTIONS FOR PREOPERATIVE ADJUVANT THERAPY

The four major questions to be answered by further work are as follows:

1. Is preoperative RT with CTX any better than the same regimens applied after resection? (Corollaries: How many

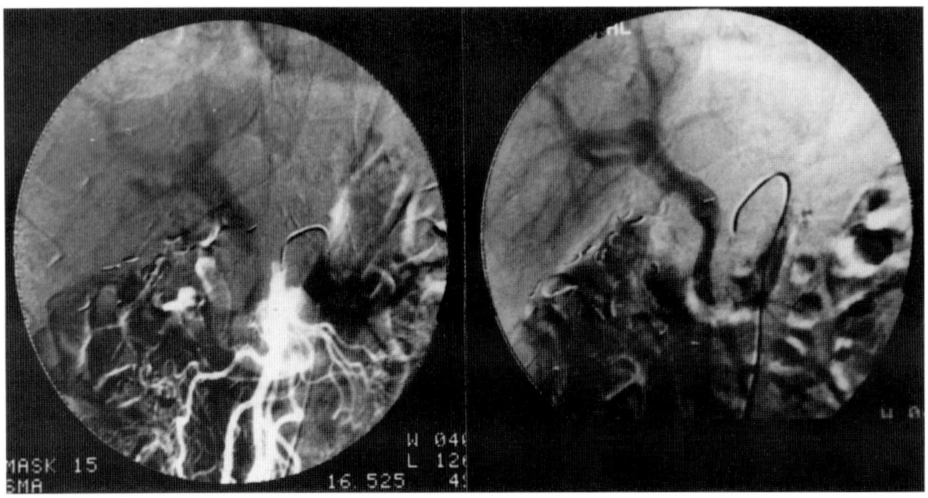

FIG. 40-4. *Left,* bilateral superior mesenteric vein impingement found before chemotherapy and radiation therapy for a 4 cm pancreatic adenocarcinoma. *Right,* the same patient 4 weeks after the completion of chemotherapy and radiation therapy. The superior mesenteric vein narrowing has decreased and appears as a unilateral narrowing. The left venogram is a grade IV impingement as defined by Ishikawa and colleagues, whereas the right panel is grade III.[42]

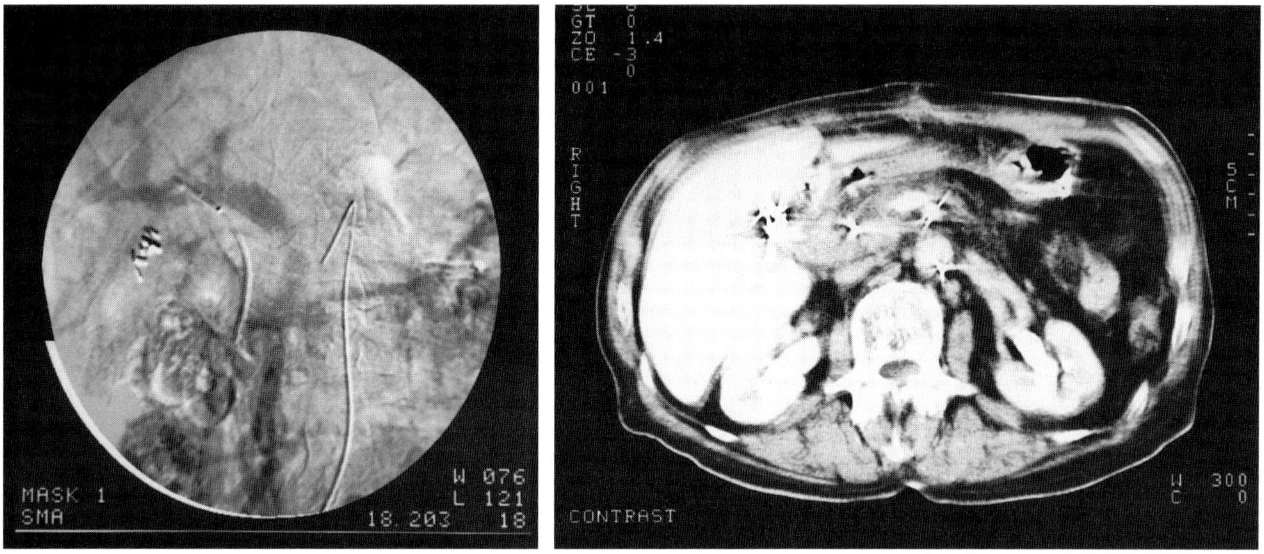

FIG. 40-5. (A) Superior mesenteric vein appearing to show bilateral tumor impingement. **(B)** Computed tomographic portogram showing no tumor impingement on the superior mesenteric vein. The three bright, stellate images represent the catheters in the aorta and superior mesenteric artery *(center)* and in the intrapancreatic bile duct *(left)*.

tumors are converted from unresectable to resectable by the adjuvant therapy? Are any of them cured? Are there patients with complications after resection that would prohibit postoperative RT? Is their survival reduced?)

2. What is the optimal RT dosage or technique for these patients and what is the optimal radiopotentiator?
3. Is there a systemic therapy that will be effective against these cancers, and is it the same as the radiopotentiating agent?
4. What are the limits of resectability for patients treated with preoperative CTX and RT?

All but the last of these questions require phase III trials for reliable answers. Regarding the relative values of preoperative and postoperative RT and CTX, surgeons have too many different selection criteria for resection and too few nonoperative staging parameters to allow the comparison of individual series of patients treated by these methods. Individual surgeons probably have enough different selection criteria to mandate a phase III comparison of two different postoperative RT and CTX regimens, in which at least the histologic prognostic variables are available. Furthermore, not enough information is available regarding the relative prognostic importance of central vascular proximity, perineural invasion, capsular invasion, differentiation, mitotic and proliferation indices, and size to be sure of the prognosis for any given tumor.

The series of patients receiving postoperative RT and CTX may contain patients more rigidly selected for small cancers and those distant from the SMV, because larger, more central lesions are less likely to be deemed resectable by surgeons treat-

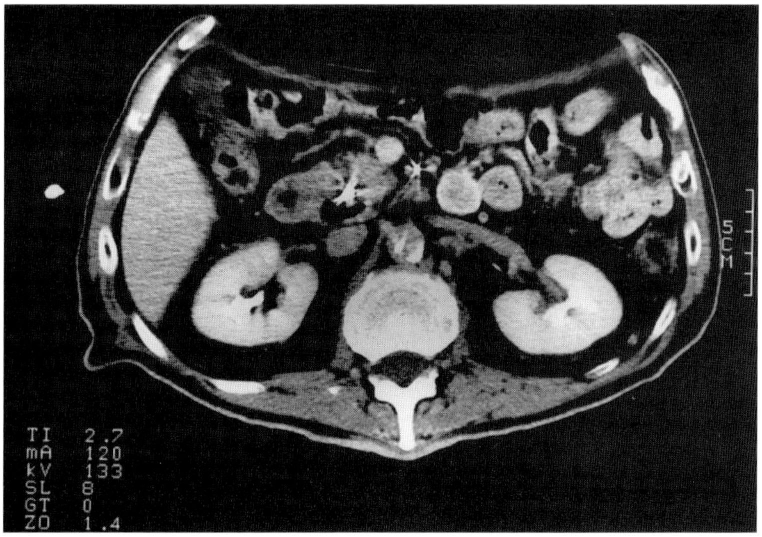

FIG. 40-6. Normal fat plane around the superior mesenteric artery. The bright, stellate image is the arterial catheter within the superior mesenteric artery.

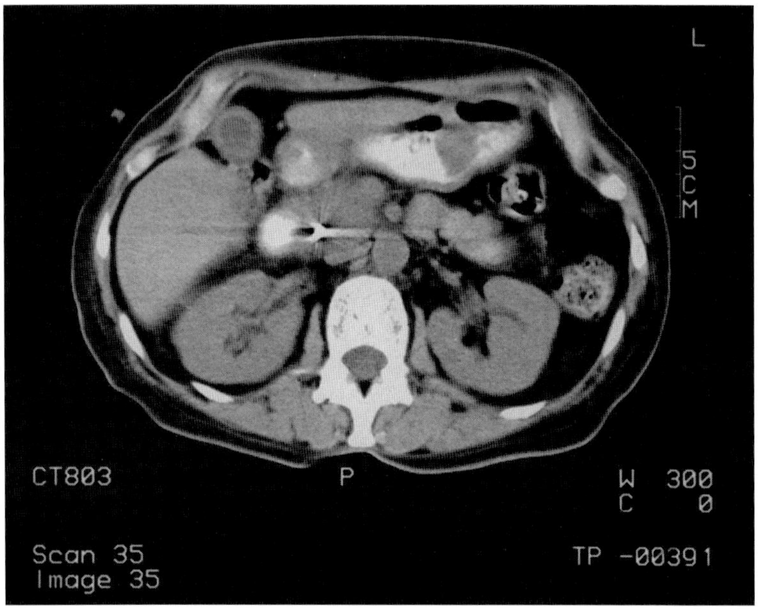

FIG. 40-7. Computed tomographic scan showing fat denser than normal ("dirty fat") surrounding the superior mesenteric artery (center of picture, directly above aorta).

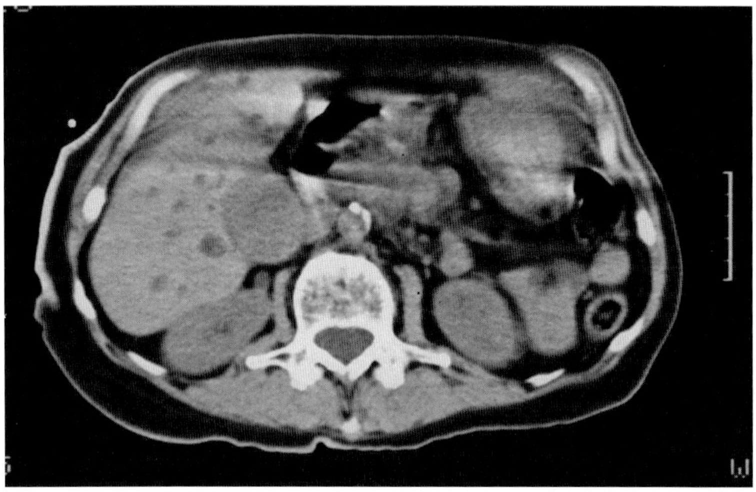

FIG. 40-8. Large adenocarcinoma of the pancreas within the uncinate process and pancreatic body. The superior mesenteric artery has been pushed far to the left of its normal position. The cancer is touching the right side of the artery, obliterating the fat plane.

ing patients without previous irradiation. Experience with preoperative irradiation has led many to proceed with resection in any case in which there are no distant metastases and in which the tumor appears to be separate from the SMA, regardless of its proximity to the SMV. However, resection criteria vary with individual surgeons and individual patients, and CT estimates of tumor size usually are equal to or exceed actual size, particularly in the smaller tumors, biasing analyses against postoperative RT sequencing.

It may be that the outcome differences for the two techniques are so small that they cannot be detected by anything but a study with unattainably large numbers of patients. It is probable that even modest benefits of one method over another will be overshadowed by the majority of patients with distant metastases. Nevertheless, if there are benefits of one method over another, it is important to try to obtain that knowledge, because even after superior drugs are discovered, optimal local or regional tumor eradication techniques probably still will be desirable.

REFERENCES

1. Tepper J, Nardi G, Suit H. Carcinoma of the pancreas: review of MGH experience from 1963 to 1973: analysis of surgical failure and implications for radiation therapy. Cancer 1976;37:1519.
2. Pilepich MV, Miller HH. Preoperative irradiation in carcinoma of the pancreas. Cancer 1980;46:1945.
3. Kopelson G. Curative surgery for adenocarcinoma of the pancreas/ampulla of Vater: the role of adjuvant pre or postoperative radiation therapy. Int J Radiat Oncol Biol Phys 1983;9:911.
4. Ishikawa O, Ohigashi H, Teshima T, et al. Clinical and histopathological appraisal of preoperative irradiation for adenocarcinoma of the pancreatoduodenal region. J Surg Oncol 1989;40:143.
5. Weese JL, Nussbaum ML, Paul AR, et al. Increased resectability of locally advanced pancreatic and periampullary carcinoma with neoadjuvant chemoradiotherapy. Int J Pancreatol 1990;7:177.
6. Evans DB, Byrd DR, Mansfield PF. Preoperative chemoradiotherapy for adenocarcinoma of the pancreas: rationale and techniques. Am J Clin Oncol 1991;14:359.
7. Evans DB, Rich TA, Byrd DR, et al. Preoperative chemoradiation and pancreaticoduodenectomy for adenocarcinoma of the pancreas. Arch Surg 1992;127:1335.

8. Jessup JM, Steele G Jr, Mayer RJ, et al. Neoadjuvant therapy for unresectable pancreatic adenocarcinoma. Arch Surg 1993;128:559.
9. Wanebo HJ, Posner M, Glicksman A, et al. Integrated modality protocol for carcinoma of the pancreas: pilot program. (Abstract) Proc Am Soc Clin Oncol 1991;10:A499.
10. Hoffman JP, Weese JL, Solin LJ, et al. A single institutional experience with preoperative chemoradiotherapy for stage I-III pancreatic adenocarcinoma. Am Surg 1993;59:772.
11. Yeung RS, Weese JL, Hoffman JP, et al. Neoadjuvant chemoradiation in pancreatic and duodenal carcinoma: a phase II study. Cancer 1993; 72:2124.
12. Ishikawa O, Ohigashi H, Imaoka S, et al. Concomitant benefit of preoperative irradiation in preventing pancreas fistula formation after pancreatoduodenectomy. Arch Surg 1991;126:885.
13. Moertel CG, Frytak S, Hahn RG, et al. Therapy of locally unresectable pancreatic carcinoma: a randomized comparison of high dose (6000 rads) radiation alone, moderate dose radiation (4000 rads) + 5-fluorouracil, and high dose radiation + 5-fluorouracil. The Gastrointestinal Tumor Study Group. Cancer 1981;48:1705.
14. The Gastrointestinal Tumor Study Group. A multi-institutional comparative trial of radiation therapy alone and in combination with 5-fluorouracil for locally unresectable pancreatic carcinoma. Ann Surg 1979;189:205.
15. Shipley WU, Wood WC, Tepper JE, et al. Intraoperative electron beam irradiation for patients with unresectable pancreatic carcinoma. Ann Surg 1984;200:289.
16. Mohiuddin M, Cantor RJ, Biermann W, et al. Combined modality treatment of localized unresectable adenocarcinoma of the pancreas. Int J Radiat Oncol Biol Phys 1988;14:79.
17. Roldan GE, Gunderson LL, Nagorney DM, et al. External beam versus intraoperative and external beam irradiation for locally advanced pancreatic cancer. Cancer 1988;61:1110.
18. Evans DB, Termuhlen PM, Byrd DR, Ames FC, Ochran TG, Rich TA. Intraoperative radiation therapy following pancreaticoduodenectomy. Ann Surg 1993;218:54.
19. Tyler DS, Evans DB. Reoperative pancreaticoduodenectomy. Ann Surg 1994;219:211.
20. Jessup JM, Colacchio T, Valone F, et al. Phase I/II neoadjuvant trial for locally advanced pancreas adenocarcinoma. (Abstract) Proc Am Soc Clin Oncol 1993;12:201.
21. Carter SK, Comis RL. The integration of chemotherapy into a combined modality approach for cancer treatment. VI. Pancreatic adenocarcinoma. Cancer Treat Rev 1975;2:193.
22. Fernandez-Del Castillo C, Warshaw AL. Laparoscopy for staging in pancreatic carcinoma. J Surg Oncol 1993;2(Suppl 1):25.
23. Hermanek P. Staging of exocrine pancreatic carcinoma. Eur J Surg Oncol 1991;17:167.
24. Manabe T, Miyashita T, Ohshio G, et al. Small carcinoma of the pancreas: clinical and pathologic evaluation of 17 patients. Cancer 1988; 62:135.
25. Tsuchiya R, Tomioka T, Izawa K, et al. Collective review of small carcinomas of the pancreas. Ann Surg 1986;203:77.
26. Connolly MM, Dawson PJ, Michelassi F, Moossa AR, Lowenstein F. Survival in 1001 patients with carcinoma of the pancreas. Ann Surg 1987;206:366.
27. Michelassi F, Erroi F, Dawson PJ, et al. Experience with 647 consecutive tumors of the duodenum, ampulla, head of the pancreas, and distal common bile duct. Ann Surg 1989;210:544.
28. Dooley WC, Cameron JL, Pitt HA, Lillimoe KD, Yue NC, Venbrux AC. Is preoperative angiography useful in patients with periampullar tumors? Ann Surg 1990;211:649.
29. Warshaw AL, Gu Z, Wittenberg J, Waltman AC. Preoperative staging and assessment of resectability of pancreatic cancer. Arch Surg 1990; 125:230.
30. Sener SF, Fremgen A, Imperato JP, Sylvester J, Chmiel JS. Pancreatic cancer in Illinois: a report by 88 hospitals on 2,401 patients diagnosed 1978-84. Am Surg 1991;57:490.
31. Graham RA, Bankoff M, Hediger R, Shaker HZ, Reinhold RB. Fine-needle aspiration biopsy of pancreatic ductal adenocarcinoma: loss of diagnostic accuracy with small tumors. J Surg Oncol 1994;55:92.
32. Warshaw AL. Implications of peritoneal cytology for staging of early pancreatic cancer. Am J Surg 1991;161:26.
33. Gastrointestinal Tumor Study Group. Further evidence of effective adjuvant combined radiation and chemotherapy following curative resection of pancreatic cancer. Cancer 1987;59:2006.
34. Whittington R, Bryer MP, Haller DG, Solin LJ, Rosato EF. Adjuvant therapy of resected adenocarcinoma of the pancreas. Int J Radiat Oncol Biol Phys 1991;21:1137.
35. Nix GAJJ, Bubbleman C, Wilson JHP, Schütte HE, Jeekel J, Postema RR. Prognostic implications of tumor diameter in carcinoma of the head of the pancreas. Cancer 1991;67:529.
36. Bakkevold KE, Arnesjø B, Kambestad B. Carcinoma of the pancreas papilla of Vater—assessment of resectability and factors influencing resectability in stage I carcinomas. A prospective multicentre trial in 472 patients. Eur J Surg Oncol 1992;18:494.
37. Bøttger T, Zech J, Weber W, Sorger K, Junginger T. Relevant factors in the prognosis of ductal pancreatic carcinoma. Acta Chir Scand 1990; 156:781.
38. Cubilla AL, Fitzgerald PJ, Fortner JG. Pancreas cancer-duct cell adenocarcinoma: survival in relation to site, size, stage and type of therapy. J Surg Oncol 1978;10:465.
39. Geer RJ, Brennan MJ. Prognostic indicators for survival after resection of pancreatic adenocarcinoma. Am J Surg 1993;165:68.
40. Cameron JL, Crist DW, Sitzmann JV, et al. Factors influencing survival after pancreaticoduodenectomy for pancreatic cancer. Am J Surg 1991; 161:120.
41. Fuhrman GM, Charnsangavej C, Abbruzzese JL, et al. Thin-section contrast-enhanced computed tomography accurately predicts the resectability of malignant pancreatic neoplasms. Am J Surg 1994;167: 104.
42. Ishikawa O, Ohigashi H, Imaoka S, et al. Preoperative indications for extended pancreatectomy for locally advanced pancreas cancer involving the portal vein. Ann Surg 1992;215:231.

Surgery for Gastrointestinal Cancer: A Multidisciplinary Approach, edited by Harold J. Wanebo.
Lippincott-Raven Publishers, Philadelphia, © 1997.

CHAPTER 41

Surgical Management of Endocrine Tumors of the Gastrointestinal Tract

Norman W. Thompson

Gastrointestinal tract neuroendocrine tumors include those found in the stomach and intestine as well as those occurring in the pancreas. They arise in more than 20 different types of endocrine cells that, in aggregate, comprise the largest endocrine gland in the body.[1–3] They are often functionally active, causing pathophysiologic findings that may be the first clue to their presence. A number of distinctive syndromes have been elucidated that can be related to specific hormone hypersecretion.[4] In some patients, the tumors may be physiologically silent until their local mass effect or distant metastases cause pain, jaundice, bleeding, or obstruction.[5–7] Other tumors, such as those occurring in the appendix or rectum, are most often found incidental to an operative procedure for which the endocrine tumor was unsuspected.[8] In general, all gastroenteropancreatic tumors should be considered potentially malignant, although this expression depends on the site of origin and tumor size more often than histopathologic status per se. Based on their cell type and peptide or amine production, neuroendocrine tumors of the diffuse gastrointestinal endocrine system are conveniently divided into those involving the foregut, midgut, and hindgut. The foregut tumors include those occurring in the stomach, duodenum, and proximal jejunum, and those in the midgut from the proximal to mid-jejunum through the right colon.[3] Hindgut tumors rarely are seen in the colon and occur primarily in the rectum. Neuroendocrine tumors arising in the pancreas may be grouped with those in the foregut, although because they usually arise from islet cells, they may be considered separately from those of the diffuse neuroendocrine system. For purposes of discussion, the surgical management of these tumors is related to the organs in which they occur, beginning with the foregut.

STOMACH

At one time, it was estimated that gastric endocrine tumors accounted only about 3% of all neuroendocrine gut neoplasms.[8,9] More recently, studies suggest the incidence of gastric carcinoids accounts for at least 10% or more of all such tumors.[1–3,6,10–13] This probably represents increased recognition rather than a true increase in incidence because it has occurred since endoscopic examination of the stomach became widespread.[14,15] The interest in gastric carcinoids has increased considerably since the mid-1970s, during which time their occurrence with certain disease states has led to a better understanding of their pathogenesis and prognosis.[10,11,13,16] Gastric neuroendocrine tumors are now classified based on their association with several hypergastrinemic conditions, and as those that occur sporadically as single tumors, usually arising in normal mucosa. The most common are those occurring with chronic atrophic gastritis with or without pernicious anemia and arising in a background of enterochromaffin cell-like (ECL) hyperplasia, induced by hypergastrinemia, which is a promoting growth factor for these cells. Most of these tumors are less than 1 cm in diameter, well differentiated, and confined to the mucosa and submucosa of the upper two thirds of the stomach. They are frequently multiple and grossly present as polyploid tumors. Lymph node metastases do occur, but in fewer than 10% of these patients and primarily when the tumors are 2 cm in diameter or larger. ECL tumors also arise in patients with hypergastrinemia associated with the Zollinger-Ellison syndrome (ZES), but only in those with an underlying multiple endocrine neoplasia type I syndrome (MEN I).[12,17–20] It would appear that a genetic predisposition to the development of these tumors occurs in patients with gastrinomas, and that hypergastrinemia alone is not sufficient to induce these tumors without atrophic gastritis. ECL tumors occur in only about 10% of patients with this combination of diseases and have been recognized only since the early 1980s. Tumors are usually small, but larger ones have been reported that may be associated with lymph node metastases.

Well differentiated neuroendocrine tumors arising sporadically in the gastric mucosa are frequently 2 cm or larger at the time of discovery and often show angioinvasion or invasion within the stomach wall. These tumors comprise approximately 20% of all gastric neuroendocrine tumors, but represent an im-

T. Nagakara: Chief, Division of Endocrine Surgery, University of Michigan, 465 Hillspur, Ann Arbor, MI 48105.

portant group because more than 60% of these solitary lesions have been associated with lymph node metastases and at least half of these with liver metastases.[3,21] These tumors are also usually composed of ECL cells and rarely are associated with an atypical carcinoid syndrome of the histamine type. As a rule, tumors less than 1 cm in diameter usually follow a benign course, whereas tumors larger than 2 cm must be considered malignant and frequently associated with metastases. Tumor size of gastric carcinoids appears to be a fundamental risk factor for metastatic dissemination, and surgical management is commonly based on the size of these lesions.

The surgical management of gastric carcinoids is also predicated on the degree of differentiation and pathogenesis. Tumors associated with chronic atrophic gastritis up to 1.5 cm in diameter are usually benign and can be removed endoscopically.[10,11,14,15,21–24] Those larger than 1.5 cm in diameter have low-grade malignant behavior but also may be removed endoscopically, providing there is no evidence of deep gastric wall invasion. Some have recommended that lesions measuring 1 cm or larger should be surgically removed because this offers the possibility of clearing any regional lymph node metastases, which may be present in a small percentage of cases.[22,25,26] All tumors larger than 2 cm should be removed surgically. Antrectomy has been proposed for those patients with multiple small tumors, ECL hyperplasia, atrophic gastritis, and hypergastrinemia.[26–31] A theoretic basis for this procedure is that hypergastrinemia is the promoting growth factor for tumor development. In our experience with four patients undergoing this procedure, the larger carcinoids were excised and regional lymph nodes along the left gastric artery were cleared. In one case, a single, 1-cm liver metastasis was locally excised. In each of these cases, subsequent endoscopic follow-up revealed regression of remaining small carcinoids and ECL hyperplasia. Although our experience with antrectomy has been excellent, other reports suggest regression may not occur in all patients.[26] Antrectomy should be limited to patients with low-grade carcinoidosis, with no expectation that large, locally invasive or metastatic tumors will respond consistently. In some patients with multiple large tumors, total gastrectomy may be indicated.[21]

In patients with MEN I ZES, the malignancy rate of gastric carcinoids may lie somewhere between that associated with chronic atrophic gastritis and that seen with solitary carcinoids. The presence of lymph node metastases has been reported, but liver metastases have not been described. Although reports are limited, it seems likely that carcinoids in these patients may be treated similarly to the carcinoids seen in chronic atrophic gastritis, with management of smaller tumors primarily by endoscopic removal and surgical excision for tumors larger than 1 cm in diameter.[12,17–20] The antrum is not the source of the hypergastrinemia and its excision is not indicated in this syndrome. There have been no cases reported of ECL tumors in which a MEN I patient has been rendered eugastrinemic after an attempt to cure the ZES component. We are following a patient in which this was achieved after removing three duodenal gastrinomas and performing a distal pancreatectomy for other neuroendocrine tumors. At the time of exploration, two ECL tumors (1.5 and 2.0 cm) were surgically excised. Subsequently, the patient has remained eugastrinemic and has had regression of her diffuse carcinoidosis.

Sporadic singular gastric carcinoids are generally more aggressive and usually have been disseminated at the time of diagnosis. These tumors may arise in the antrum as well as the body or fundus of the stomach. The sporadic gastric carcinoid occurs as a solitary tumor in nonatrophic gastric mucosa without associated endocrine cell proliferation. This feature distinguishes the sporadic gastrinoma from the other types previously discussed.[11,13,32] Regional lymph node metastases have been described in 20% to 50% of patients at diagnosis, and liver metastases have ultimately developed in as many as two thirds of these patients. The carcinoid syndrome has been reported to occur in 5% to 30% of patients and is usually the atypical type characterized by a bright red, severe flush, cutaneous edema, lacrimation, and bronchoconstriction related to histamine secretion. Patients with tumors 5 cm in diameter or larger and showing atypical morphology have a 5-year survival rate that has been reported to be only 20%. Smaller tumors showing more differentiation are associated with a comparably more favorable outcome. Moderate cellular atypia, an increased rate of mitoses, angioinvasion, deep gastric wall invasion, and a size greater than 2 cm are features related to distant metastases and eventual tumor-related death. Because the available evidence indicates that sporadic gastric carcinoids usually are malignant in behavior, surgical ablation should always be undertaken. Those with typical histologic features and measuring less than 1 cm may be removed endoscopically, but all larger tumors require operative excision and regional lymph node clearance. Tumors larger than 2 cm with atypical histologic features or gastric wall invasion are appropriately treated by gastrectomy and lymph node dissection.[21]

DUODENAL CARCINOIDS

According to the World Health Organization classification, all endocrine tumors of the duodenum are referred to as carcinoids, although a number of investigators have proposed the term "neuroendocrine tumor" as more appropriate.[1,3] In the neuroendocrine tumor classification, all tumors are distinguished according to the site of origin. They are then further subdivided into neoplasms that have benign behavior, those that have uncertain behavior (benign or low-grade malignancies), tumors with definite low-grade malignant behavior, and high-grade malignant tumors. The main criteria for this biologic categorization are histologic differentiation, angioinvasion, direct invasion of neighboring organs, and the presence of metastases. An additional criterion is size. The third principle is the incorporation of the hormonal function, which can often be related to clinical behavior. Those tumors without a hormonal syndrome are considered as nonfunctioning. This new classification does not include neoplasms that have been termed mixed exocrine–endocrine or amphicrin tumors. For practical clinical purposes, we continue to refer to functioning neuroendocrine tumors of the duodenum by the hormonal syndrome they produce (eg, gastrin hypersecretion as gastrinomas). Neuroendocrine tumors of the duodenum account for approximately 2% of gastroenteropancreatic tumors.[6,9] There are five major types of neuroendocrine tumors that can be distinguished in the duodenum. The most common is gastrin producing and accounts for 60% of tumors. About one third of these have been functional and associated with ZES,[3,21] but about two thirds of those tumors staining positive for gastrin have not been associated with hypergastrinemia or ZES. Most of these latter behave in a benign fashion. Most current studies suggest that approximately 40% of patients with sporadic ZES have a duodenal gastrinoma.[33–41] Since the mid-1980s, in our experience, the incidence has been 60%.[40,41] In ZES occurring in the MEN I syndrome, approximately 90% of patients harbor at least one duodenal gastrinoma with or without other gastrinomas arising in the pancreas.[25,34,36,37,40–49] In both sporadic and familial patients with ZES, these tumors arise in the first or second portion but occasionally may be found in the distal or duodenum proximal jejunum. Most commonly, they are less than 1 cm in diameter, but are associated with lymph node metastases in a high percentage of cases (50% to 60%). Nevertheless, liver metastases are rare and occur late in the course of the disease (<10%). In general, these tumors are classified as low-grade malignancies.

The second type of tumor secretes somatostatin. Fifteen to 20% of all duodenal neuroendocrine tumors are in this category.[3,50–52] These tumors usually occur in the ampullary region and are characterized by local invasion into the muscular layer and lymph node metastases. They are considered nonfunctional clinically. Histologically they are further characterized by the presence of psammoma bodies.[52] These tumors are not associated with the MEN I syndrome, but approximately one third are found in patients with neurofibromatosis type I. In this group of patients, they may also be associated with pheochromocytomas.[53] They are considered nonfunctioning, low-grade malignant tumors.

The third type comprises gangliocytic paragangliomas, and these occur in the periampullary region or ampulla.[3,54,55] The gangliocytic component is characteristic and the endocrine tumor cells usually stain positive for pancreatic polypeptide (PP) and S-100 as well as somatostatin. They are often larger than 2 cm in diameter and are usually benign; even though larger tumors may show local invasion, metastases are extremely rare.

The fourth type is derived from cells producing serotonin, calcitonin, or PP, or all three. These are rare duodenal carcinoids not associated with functional syndromes, and are characteristically benign.

The fifth type is a poorly differentiated neuroendocrine tumor that is invariably aggressive with a relatively poor prognosis. These high-grade malignant tumors are composed of poorly differentiated intermediate or small cells, usually arising in the ampullary region.

Duodenal gastrinomas are a particularly important group of neuroendocrine tumors that have been recognized with increasing frequency as the cause of ZES since the late 1980s.[36,37,41,43] Because of their small size and frequent association with lymph node metastases, they were often unrecognized in the past. They were the most likely cause of failed operations for ZES in more than 40% of patients explored in the past when no tumor was detected.[41] Because of their small size and submucosal location, they are rarely detected by preoperative endoscopic examination, even when performed with ultrasonography.[56,57] In evaluating patients with sporadic ZES proven biochemically by hypergastrinemia, hyperchlorhydria, and a positive secretin stimulation test, a computed tomography or magnetic resonance imaging scan is performed to screen for hepatic metastases. If none is present, we then perform endoscopic ultrasonography (EUS) of the entire pancreas through the stomach and duodenum. Because nearly all pancreatic gastrinomas are at least 1 cm in diameter, a negative EUS examination implies an extrapancreatic gastrinoma that is found, with rare exceptions such as the liver or ovary, in the duodenum. Despite careful mobilization of the entire duodenum and bimanual examination, only about half are palpable. Even with the aid of transillumination of the duodenum, one third of these tumors remain undetected unless a duodenotomy is performed.[38] Palpable tumors are usually locally invasive into the submucosa. In sporadic cases these tumors are invariably singular. Surgical treatment includes excision of a full-thickness ellipse of duodenal wall around a palpable tumor to ensure its complete excision.[40] Rarely, a large duodenal gastrinoma in the inner curvature of the duodenum may require a Whipple procedure for its excision.[42,58] After a duodenotomy closure in two layers, a peripancreatic and periduodenal lymph node dissection should be performed routinely because at least 50% of even the smallest duodenal gastrinomas have been associated with lymph node metastases.[21,33,34,36,39–41,43,45–47,58–60] We include all lymph nodes on both surfaces of the pancreatic head, those along the common bile duct and in the porta hepatis, and those along the hepatic artery to the celiac axis. Duodenal gastrinomas less than 0.5 cm in diameter are usually not invasive and can be enucleated with the mucosa overlying them. In patients without a palpable tumor, a 6- to 8-cm duodenotomy is performed and both the proximal and distal duodenum is inverted so that the mucosa can be palpated and tumors as small as 1 to 2 mm identified.[41]

In MEN I ZES, a duodenotomy should be routinely performed regardless of the presence of other neuroendocrine tumors in the pancreas. Most pancreatic neuroendocrine tumors in MEN I patients are not gastrinomas but are potentially malignant.[25,36,37,46–49] We routinely perform a distal pancreatectomy and enucleate any tumors in the head or uncinate process, in addition to a long duodenotomy to allow complete exposure of the duodenal mucosa. In contrast to sporadic ZES, MEN I duodenal neuroendocrine tumors are frequently multiple.[36,37,47] Most commonly they are in the first and second portion of the duodenum, but not infrequently they may occur in the third portion as well. In most cases, enucleation can be performed without the necessity of multiple duodenotomies. Nevertheless, whenever a tumor is larger than 0.5 cm and adherent to the underlying submucosa, a full-thickness excision should be performed. A lymph node dissection is likewise indicated because the incidence of metastatic disease is similar to that occurring in sporadic cases.

Somatostatin-rich carcinoids occur almost exclusively in the ampulla of Vater and may cause obstructive jaundice or bleeding. Metastases to regional lymph nodes or the liver are present in 45% of patients.[3,21,52] Depending on the size of the tumors and presence or absence of liver metastases, they may be locally excised or treated by pancreaticoduodenectomy.[21,61–63] In patients with neurofibromatosis, the adrenal glands should always be evaluated before surgery, and if a pheochromocytoma is detected, the patient should be adequately prepared with α blockade before operation.[53] The pheochromocytoma should be removed before proceeding with treatment of the duodenal somatostatinoma. We have encountered one patient with a locally invasive ampullary tumor causing both jaundice and necrotizing pancreatitis. Because of the necrotizing pancreatitis involving the distal portion of the pancreas, a Whipple procedure was contraindicated. Through a duodenotomy, a wedge excision of the ampulla was accomplished with total removal of the tumor, allowing free drainage of pancreatic juice into the duodenum. The bile duct was reconstructed with a hepatodochoduodenostomy. This patient had an uneventful postoperative recovery and has had no recurrence of tumor.

Ganglioparagangliomas are rare and occur almost exclusively in the second portion of the duodenum.[3,54,55] Because they are generally benign, they can be locally excised, usually through a duodenotomy, with an excellent postexcision prognosis.

Poorly differentiated neuroendocrine tumors arising in the duodenum are fortunately very rare. They occur in the ampulla of Vater and present with jaundice. A Whipple procedure is indicated in those without liver metastases, but the prognosis, regardless of the procedure, is poor and a rapidly fatal course usually ensues.

MIDGUT CARCINOIDS

This group of tumors includes those arising in the small bowel, appendix, cecum, and ascending colon, and characteristically they secrete serotonin and kinins. When metastatic to the liver, they are the most common cause of the classic carcinoid syndrome. Carcinoid tumors distal to the proximal jejunum account for about 90% of all carcinoids of the gastrointestinal tract. At autopsy, the prevalence of carcinoid tumors has been found to be 0.14% to 0.34%.[2,3,6,8,9,64] The appendix is the most common location and is the site for 45% of all gastroenteropancreatic carcinoids.[60,65–72] These tumors are found in about 0.17% of surgical appendectomy specimens. Those occurring in the distal jejunum and ileum account for approximately 28% of all carcinoid tumors.[60,64,70,73–76] The overall incidence of gastrointestinal carcinoid tumors is estimated to be 1.5 per 100,000 individuals.[70] In contrast to foregut carcinoids, midgut carcinoids arising from enterochromaffin cells are rich in serotonin content and, when metastatic to the liver, are the most common cause of the classic carcinoid syndrome with flushing and diarrhea. Over 80% of small bowel carcinoids occur within the ileum and 40% occur within 2 feet of the ileocecal valve. Primary tumors often elicit a significant local fibrotic reaction that can cause small bowel obstruction or mesenteric infarction. In most cases the signs and symptoms of small bowel carcinoid tumors lead to a diagnosis of small bowel obstruction. Obstruction usually is not caused by the primary tumor per se but by the plastic reaction, which leads to shrinking of the mesentery and kinking of the bowel. In one large series of 145 patients with carcinoid tumors, only 12 had a correct preoperative diagnosis and all 12 had definite signs of the carcinoid syndrome.[8] Small bowel infarction resulting from metastatic carcinoid tumor in the mesentery was traditionally considered to be caused by compression of the mesenteric vessels. However, it is more likely to be the result of a unique pathophysiologic vascular process designated "subadventitial elastosis." This occurs in vessels that are contiguous to metastatic lymph nodes and probably is induced by secretory products from the tumor that result in the development of a thick layer of elastic tissue beneath the adventitia that, in its extreme, may completely collapse the vessel, causing its obstruction. As a result, areas of infarction may develop that are either proximal or distal to the primary tumor.[76] There is an almost linear relationship between tumor size and the risk for metastases, reaching 85% for tumors larger than 2 cm. The extent of the disease, considering lymph node and liver involvement, is a definitive predictor for outcome. The overall 5-year survival rates range from 50% to 60%. They decrease from 75% or higher for local disease to 60% for those with positive nodes confined to the mesentery, and to 20% to 35% if liver metastases are present.[6,64,70,73–80]

All small bowel carcinoids should be considered malignant. There is no indication for limited resection, and resections including the lymph node drainage should always be performed. This allows histopathologic staging, resection of occult lymph node metastases, and prevention of local complications due to desmoplastic reaction. Furthermore, a meticulous intraoperative examination of the remaining small bowel is mandatory because multicentric carcinoid tumors are present in 20% to 40%. In addition, adenocarcinomas in other parts of the gastrointestinal tract may occur simultaneously in 8% to 29%.[6,70,76] It is our policy to remove all involved lymph nodes whenever feasible, including those at the base of the mesentery, providing integrity of the superior mesenteric artery and vein can be maintained. In patients with the carcinoid syndrome confirmed before surgery by high levels of 5-hydroxyindoleacetic acid in the urine and the typical flush, wedge resection of liver lesions is accomplished when possible. In the unusual patient with a single liver metastasis confined to one lobe, a surgical lobectomy or segmentectomy is performed. In most patients, multiple metastases are found in both lobes of the liver. It is our feeling that patients who have the carcinoid syndrome should undergo resection of their primary tumor and as many lymph nodes as is feasible. Even though this is not a curative procedure, it may avoid symptomatic small bowel obstruction, alleviate diarrhea, and prevent small bowel infarction. In addition, a cholecystectomy should also be performed to prevent complications resulting from the use of long-acting somatostatin.[73,77–80]

Several principles should be emphasized in the preoperative evaluation of the patient with the carcinoid syndrome. Because of the high incidence of right-sided cardiac valvular disease, a careful evaluation of the cardiac status should be performed before considering operative intervention. Some of these patients may require either dilatation of the pulmonary or tricuspid valves or even valve replacement, particularly those who have been in heart failure. Second, all patients with the carcinoid syndrome should be prepared with long-acting somatostatin (octreotide) before their operation to prevent intraoperative carcinoid crisis due to massive release of serotonin and vasoactive kinins. Without this precaution, severe hypotension, hypertension, or a cardiac arrest can occur during surgery. Octreotide has proven to be nearly 100% effective in preventing this complications.[70,76]

CARCINOID TUMORS OF THE APPENDIX

As noted earlier, the appendix is by far the most common site of carcinoid tumors that are detected during life. These account for 35% to 48% of all carcinoid tumors. Fortunately, carcinoid tumors in this location have the best prognosis, and more than 99% survive 5 years or longer.[67] Whether this stems from an earlier diagnosis resulting from symptoms of appendicitis or from removal of the tumor at the time of an incidental appendectomy is not entirely clear.[60,68] However, 70% to 90% of all carcinoid tumors of the appendix are less then 1 cm in diameter, and 4% to 25% are 1 to 2 cm in diameter.[67,69,70] Very few are larger than 2 cm. Metastases from tumors less than 1 cm in diameter are nil, and between 0% and 1% for tumors between 1 and 2 cm. The only real risk occurs in patients with tumors that are 2 cm in diameter or larger, because metastases occur in from 20% to 75%. Those with carcinoids at the base of the appendix with local invasion not completely removed at the time of appendectomy are also at risk for recurrence unless treated by a more extensive resection.[65,67,71,72] Another explanation for the less aggressive clinical behavior of appendiceal carcinoids is that they arise in a different cell of origin, the subepithelial enterochromaffin cell, and not the mucosal enterochromaffin cell typical in small bowel carcinoids.[60,66] Surgical treatment consists of appendectomy, which is considered adequate for all lesions up to 1 cm. Appendectomy alone is probably still sufficient for most lesions in the range of 1 to 2 cm, although those with histologic evidence of invasion of the mesoappendix should be considered for a more extensive operation. In nearly all series, appendiceal carcinoids less than 2 cm in diameter have had a benign course.[67] For tumors 2 cm or larger, right hemicolectomy including the lymphatic drainage is the procedure of choice. For tumors between 1.5 and 2 cm, the extent of the resection must be determined by the surgeon with the help of the pathologist after evaluating whether the mesoappendix subserosal lymphatics or base of the appendix has been invaded.[65,70]

Carcinoid tumors involving the colon, distal to the appendix, account for only about 5% of all carcinoid tumors. These are found predominantly in the right colon, and these patients usually present with abdominal pain and weight loss.[81–83] These tumors have a less pronounced tendency to produce regional node metastases but are associated with a significantly higher incidence of liver metastases.[70] Even though lymph node metastases occur in a third or less, a standard colon cancer resection, including lymphatic drainage, is the procedure of choice. This is indicated for all carcinoid tumors of the colon that are 2 cm or larger, which most are at the time of diagnosis. The overall 5-year survival rates reported for colon carcinoids averages only 37%.[70,81,83]

CARCINOID TUMORS OF THE RECTUM

Rectal carcinoids represent the third most common carcinoid lesion in the gastrointestinal tract. These tumors account for about 16% of all such carcinoids.[84,85] Approximately 1 in 2500 proctoscopic examinations discloses a rectal carcinoid tumor, usually presenting as a yellowish submucosal nodule on the anterior or lateral walls of the rectum.[86] Fewer than 50% cause any symptoms, and these consist of transanal bleeding (18%) constipation (17%), rectal pain (7%), and pruritus ani (3%). Aside from bleeding, which can be related to mucosal erosion over the tumor, all of the other symptoms attributed to these tumors are probably coincidental but were helpful in leading to the diagnosis. Characteristically, rectal carcinoids are hormonally inactive, and even with extensive liver metastases, the carcinoid syndrome is absent. Nevertheless, immunohistochemical staining typically shows neuron-specific enolase, chromogranin, and other peptides.[87,88] In addition, many rectal carcinoids have been associated with an elevated prostatic acid phosphatase (80%) and an elevated carcinoembryonic antigen in 25%.[70,89] Because simultaneous adenocarcinomas of the gastrointestinal tract or internal female genitalia are found in conjunction with rectal carcinoid tumors in 7% to 9%, careful evaluation of the entire colon is always indicated as well as a careful pelvic examination in female patients.

There is general agreement that lesions smaller than 2 cm can be treated by local excision. Lesions less than 1 cm in diameter may be removed by endoscopic excision, and a local surgical excision may be adequate for most tumors 1 to 2 cm in diameter, although there is a small risk of metastatic disease being present. Larger carcinoids, with invasion to the muscle layers, should be treated by a standard cancer resection. When transmural invasion has been found by histopathologic study of lesions between 1 and 2 cm initially treated by local resection. A second operative procedure should be performed. Muscular invasion should be considered as an additional criterion for combined abdominal perineal resection. When distant metastases have been detected before or at the time of operation, only local measures should be applied to palliate local symptoms such as bleeding or obstruction.[70,84–86]

ISLET CELL TUMORS OF THE PANCREAS

Islet cell tumors of the pancreas are relatively rare, occurring in about 1 in 100,000 of the general population per year.[35,90] Their recognition is important because they can cause significant morbidity and mortality from either their functional activity or malignant behavior. Early diagnosis can lead to surgical cure in many patients and appropriate operative management can result in excellent long-term palliation in other patients when the extent of malignant disease precludes total excision.[7,79,90]

There are three basic questions that should be answered before treatment when a patient with islet cell tumor is encountered. First, is the tumor functional? Is it secreting a peptide hormone that can be measured, and if so, what systemic effects is the hormone having on the health of the patient? The most common functional tumors are gastrinomas and insulinomas causing ZES and hypoglycemic syndrome, respectively. At one time, insulinomas were considered the most frequent functional tumor, but with better recognition, gastrinomas are diagnosed equally as often. The other functional pancreatic tumors in decreasing order of frequency are VIPomas (tumors secreting vasoactive intestinal polypeptide), glucagonomas, somatostatinomas, GRFomas (tumors secreting growth hormone-releasing factor), and adrenocorticotropic hormone-secreting tumors. All of these tumors are rare in comparison to insulinomas and gastrinomas. Approximately 50% of tumors may secrete two or more functional hormones, although concurrent clinical syndromes are rare.[25] PPomas are more common than some of the other tumors noted previously. Because they cause no specific symptoms, they are considered with other nonfunctional tumors.[5] This group comprises approximately 15% to 30% of all islet cell tumors. Because of the life-threatening effects of hormone hypersecretion, the initial treatment of some functional tumors may be drug therapy such as the use of octreotide (Sandostatin) to control diarrhea in VIPoma patients or omeprazole to decrease acid secretion in gastrinoma patients.[79]

Second, is the tumor benign or malignant? This question may not always be answerable until a surgical exploration has been performed or years of follow-up have transpired. Of the functional tumors, the insulinoma is least likely to be malignant (10%), whereas most glucagonomas are malignant when diagnosed because of hormonal symptoms.[35,91] As a general rule, more than 50% of functional tumors are malignant, and an even higher incidence has been noted in nonfunctional tumors that caused symptoms and were not just detected incidentally. For many islet cell tumors, histopathologic features may not be determinate in differentiating benign from malignant tumors. More often malignancy is established based on lymph node or liver metastases. Whether there are liver metastases or local infiltration into the superior mesenteric vessels by the primary tumor is important from the surgeon's viewpoint. Islet cell tumors metastatic only to lymph nodes are potentially curable by surgical resection when the primary tumor can be resected. Invasion of the superior mesenteric vein is not a contraindication to performing a Whipple procedure if otherwise indicated for an islet cell tumor.[7] Grafting the superior mesenteric vein with a jugular vein should be considered when venous involvement is the only limitation to total excision of an islet cell tumor. Because the liver is such a common site for metastatic disease, either a computed tomography or magnetic resonance imaging scan should be obtained routinely in the preoperative assessment of patients with islet cell tumors.

We also perform EUS in all patients with islet cell tumors. In addition to localizing most small pancreatic tumors, EUS can also assess whether the tumor is locally infiltrating into pancreatic parenchyma (malignant).[56,57]

Third, is the tumor sporadic (nonfamilial) or a component of MEN I syndrome? The answer to this question is essential in ZES patients because more than 25% are determined to be MEN I and have multifocal disease in the pancreas and duodenum. It is also important in all other patients with islet cell disease in determining the appropriate operation to perform. The answer can be obtained by a carefully obtained family history (50%) or by minimal biochemical screening for hyperparathyroidism (calcium and parathyroid hormone levels), and pituitary adenoma (prolactin), adrenocorticotropic hormone, or growth hormone if clinically indicated.

The surgical treatment of the two most common functional islet cell tumors is outlined in more detail.

The management of gastrinomas can be divided into those that are sporadic and those associated with MEN I. As a general rule, all patients in either group who present without liver metastases are candidates for a potentially curative operation once the diagnosis has been confirmed by finding a combination of acid hypersecretion, hypergastrinemia, and a positive secretin stimulation test. A computed tomography or magnetic resonance imaging scan is done to screen for hepatic metastases and, if negative, a EUS is performed to evaluate the entire pancreas. Sporadic gastrinomas arising in the pancreas are solitary and nearly always larger than 1 cm in diameter.[36] Such tumors should be detectable (localized) by EUS in nearly all patients in which the entire pancreas can be studied.[57] If EUS is negative, it implies that the gastrinoma is extrapancreatic and most likely in the duodenum. Further localization may be unnecessary but can be confirmed by the Imamura intraarterial secretin stimulation test, which regionalizes the hypersecretion of gastrin to the distribution of the gastroduodenal artery.[44] The procedure we perform for pancreatic gastrinomas in the head or uncinate is enucleation unless the tumor is locally infiltrating. In those rare cases without liver metastases, a Whipple procedure may be indicated. In most patients with a sporadic duodenal gastrinoma, a duodenotomy is performed, designed to excise the palpable tumor with a margin. A vertical duodenotomy is performed, centered in the second portion of the duodenum, when no tumor is palpable. Most small tumors (0.5 cm or less) are not palpable and require a careful mucosal search for detection. These can be enucleated. In either case, a peripancreatic lymph node dissection must be performed, including nodes on both surfaces of the pancreas, along the common bile duct, porta hepatis, and hepatic artery to the celiac because more than 50% have micrometastases.[40,41] Although controversial, we believe that most MEN I patients with ZES can be made eugastrinemic by a multifaceted operation consisting of distal pancreatectomy (other islet cell tumors), enucleation of any palpable or ultrasonically detected tumors in the head or uncinate, duodenotomy and excision of one or more duodenal gastrinomas, and peripancreatic lymph node dissection.[47,48]

There is little controversy in the management of insulinoma. More than 80% are sporadic and benign. Only about 5% are associated with MEN I, and although 10% to 15% may be malignant by strict criteria, only 5% are malignant as defined by liver metastases. The diagnosis must be confirmed by biochemical testing (insulin : glucose ratio >0.3, elevated proinsulin or C-peptide). The only controversy pertains to the extent of preoperative localization because of the small size of many insulinomas and the possibility of no tumor being found (hyperplasia or nesidioblastosis). Although many expensive noninvasive and invasive localization studies are available, we use only EUS when an islet-cell tumor has been identified (90%).[57,91] If no tumor is detected, we prefer the Doppman-Imamura intraarterial calcium stimulation test, which measures insulin from the right hepatic vein.[35,92] Elevated insulin levels from multiple arterial regions strongly suggest islet cell hyperplasia, whereas a single region implies an occult adenoma, which should be found at exploration with or without intraoperative ultrasound. Enucleation is the procedure of choice for nearly all insulinomas of the head or uncinate as well as body or tail when feasible without duct injury. Rarely, a Whipple procedure may be necessary for a large, infiltrating, locally malignant insulinoma of the head.[7,90] In MEN I patients, multiple tumors are frequent, although not all are insulinomas.[25,46,93] We perform a distal pancreatectomy and enucleate any tumors in the head and uncinate.[47] A duodenectomy is not indicated unless the basal serum gastrin has been proven to be elevated and a subsequent secretin test shown to be positive. Extrapancreatic insulinomas have not been encountered in MEN I patients and are extremely rare in sporadic cases.

REFERENCES

1. Capella C, Heitz PHU, Höfler H, Solcia E, Klöppel G. Revised classification of neuroendocrine tumors of the lung, pancreas and gut. Digestion 1994;55(Suppl 3):11.
2. Capella C, Riva C, Rindi G, et al. Histopathology, hormone products and clinicopathological profile of endocrine tumors of the upper small intestine: a study of 44 cases. Endocrine Pathology 1991;2:92.
3. Klöppel G, Heitz PU, Capella C, Solcia E. Pathology and nomenclature of human gastrointestinal neuroendocrine tumors and related lesions. World J Surg 1996;20:132.
4. Debas HT, Mullvihill SJ. Neuroendocrine gut neoplasms: important lessons from uncommon tumors. Arch Surg 1994;129:965.
5. Eckhauser FE, Cheung PS, Vinik AI, et al. Non-functioning malignant neuroendocrine tumor of the pancreas. Surgery 1986;100:978.
6. Thompson GB, van Heerden JA, Martin JK, Schutt AJ, Ilstrup DM,

Carney JA. Carcinoid tumors of the gastrointestinal tract: presentation, management and prognosis. Surgery 1985;98:1054.
7. Thompson NW, Eckhauser FE. Malignant islet cell tumors of the pancreas. World J Surg 1984;8:1.
8. Godwin JD. Carcinoid tumors: an analysis of 2837 cases. Cancer 1975; 36:560.
9. Williams ED, Sandler M. The classification of carcinoid tumors. Lancet 1963;1:238.
10. Gough DB, Thompson GB, Crotty TB, et al. Diverse clinical and pathologic features of gastric carcinoid and the relevance of hypergastrinemia. World J Surg 1994;18:473.
11. Rindi G, Luinetti O, Cornaggia M, et al. Three subtypes of gastric argyrophil carcinoid and the gastric neuroendocrine carcinoma: a clinicopathologic study. Gastroenterology 1993;104:994.
12. Solcia E, Capella C, Fiocca R, Rindi G, Rosai J. Gastric argyrophil carcinoidosis in patients with Zollinger-Ellison syndrome due to type I multiple endocrine neoplasia: a newly recognized association. Am J Surg Pathol 1990;14:503.
13. Thomas RM, Baybick JH, Elsayed AM, Sobin LH. Gastric carcinoids: an immunohistochemical and clinicopathologic study of 104 patients. Cancer 1994;73:2053.
14. Sjoblom SM, Sipponen P, Jarvinen H. Gastroscopic follow-up of pernicious anemia patients. Gut 1993;34:28.
15. Sjoblom SM, Sipponen P, Miettenen M, et al. Gastroscopic screening for gastric carcinoids and carcinoma in pernicious anemia. Endoscopy 1988;20:52.
16. Solcia E, Bordi C, Creutzfeldt W, et al. Histologic classification of non antral gastric endocrine growths in man. Digestion 1988;41:185.
17. Cadiot G, Lehy T, Mignon M. Gastric endocrine cell proliferation and fundic argyrophil carcinoid tumors in patients with the Zollinger-Ellison syndrome. Acta Oncol 1993;32:135.
18. Goldfain D, Le Bodic MF, Lavergne A, Galian A, Modigliani R. Gastric carcinoid tumors in patients with Zollinger-Ellison syndrome on long-term omeprazole. Lancet 1989;1:776.
19. Lehy T, Cadiot G, Mignon M, Ruszniewski P, Bonfils S. Influence of multiple endocrine neoplasia type 1 on gastric endocrine cells in patients with the Zollinger-Ellison syndrome. Gut 1992;33:1275.
20. Mignon M, Lehy T, Bonnefond A, Ruszniewski P, Labeille D, Bonfils S. Development of gastric argyrophil carcinoid tumors in a case of Zollinger-Ellison syndrome with primary hyperparathyroidism during long-term antisecretory treatment. Cancer 1987;59:1959.
21. Åkerström G. Management of carcinoid tumors of the stomach, duodenum and pancreas. World J Surg 1996;20:173.
22. Ahlman H, Dahlstrom A, Enerbach L, et al. Two cases of gastric carcinoids: diagnostic and therapeutic aspects. World J Surg 1988;12:356.
23. Borch K, Renvall H, Liedberg G. Gastric endocrine cell hyperplasia and carcinoid tumors in pernicious anemia. Gastroenterology 1985;88: 638.
24. Hodges JR, Isaacson P, Wright R. Diffuse enterochromaffin-like (ECL) cell hyperplasia and multiple gastric carcinoids: a complication of pernicious anemia. Gut 1981;22:237.
25. Åkerström G, Johansson H, Grama D. Surgical treatment of endocrine pancreatic lesions in MEN I. Acta Oncol 1991;30:542.
26. Wangberg B, Grimelius L, Granerus G, Conradi N, Jansson S, Ahlman H. The role of gastric resection in the management of multicentric argyrophil gastric carcinoids. Surgery 1990;108:851.
27. Eckhauser FE, Lloyd RV, Thompson NW, Raper SE, Vinik AI. Antrectomy for multicentric, argyrophil gastric carcinoids: a preliminary report. Surgery 1988;104:1046.
28. Hirschowitz BI, Griffin J, Pellegrin D, Cummings OW. Rapid regression of enterochromaffin-like cell gastric carcinoids in pernicious anemia after antrectomy. Gastroenterology 1992;102:1409.
29. Kern SE, Yardly JH, Lazenby AJ, et al. Reversal by antrectomy of endocrine cell hyperplasia in the gastric body in pernicious anemia: a morphometric study. Mod Pathol 1990;3:561.
30. Olbe L, Lundell L, Sundler F. Antrectomy in a patient with ECL-cell gastric carcinoids and pernicious anemia. Gastroenterology International 1988;1:340.
31. Richards AT, Hinder RA, Harrison AC. Gastric carcinoid tumor associated with hypergastrinemia and pernicious anemia: regression of tumors by antrectomy. S Afr Med J 1987;75:51.
32. Lasson A, Alwmark A, Nobin A, Sundler F. Endocrine tumors of the duodenum: clinical characteristics and hormone content. Ann Surg 1983;197:393.
33. Bornman PC, Marks IN, Mee AS, Price S. Favorable response to conservative surgery for extra-pancreatic gastrinomas with lymph node metastases. Br J Surg 1987;74:198.
34. Imamura M, Kanda M, Takahashi K, et al. Clinicopathological characteristics of duodenal microgastrinomas. World J Surg 1992;16:703.
35. Norton JA. Neuroendocrine tumors of the pancreas and duodenum. Curr Probl Surg 1994;31:77.
36. Pipeleers-Marichal M, Donow C, Heitz PU, Kloppel G. Pathologic aspects of gastrinomas in patients with Zollinger-Ellison syndrome with and without multiple endocrine neoplasia type I. World J Surg 1993; 17:481.
37. Pipeleers-Marichal M, Somers G, Willems C, et al. Gastrinomas in the duodenums of patients with multiple endocrine neoplasia type I and the Zollinger-Ellison syndrome. N Engl J Med 1990;322:723.
38. Sugg SL, Norton JA, Fraker DL, et al. A prospective study of intraoperative methods to diagnose and resect duodenal gastrinomas. Ann Surg 1963;218:138.
39. Thom AK, Norton JA, Axiotis CA, Jensen RT. Location, incidence and malignant potential of duodenal gastrinomas. Surgery 1991;110: 1086.
40. Thompson NW, Pasieka J, Fukuuchi A. Duodenal gastrinoma duodenotomy and duodenal exploration in the surgical management of the Zollinger Ellison syndrome. World J Surg 1993;17:455.
41. Thompson NW, Vinik AI, Eckhauser FE. Microgastrinomas of the duodenum: a cause of failed operations for the Zollinger-Ellison syndrome. Ann Surg 1989;209:396.
42. Delcore R, Friesen SR. The role of pancreaticoduodenectomy for primary duodenal wall gastrinomas in patients with the Zollinger-Ellison syndrome. Surgery 1992;112:1.
43. Donow C, Pipeleers-Marichal M, Schroder S. Surgical pathology of gastrinoma: site, size multicentricity, association with multiple neoplasia type I and malignancy. Cancer 1991;68:1329.
44. Imamura M, Minematsu S, Suzuki T, et al. Usefulness of selective arterial secretin injection test for localization of gastrinoma in the Zollinger-Ellison syndrome. Ann Surg 1987;205:230.
45. Modlin IM, Lawton GP. Duodenal gastrinoma: the solution to the pancreatic paradox. (Editorial) J Clin Gastroenterol 1994;19:184.
46. Shepherd JJ, Challis DR, Davies PF, et al. Multiple endocrine neoplasia, type I: gastrinomas, pancreatic neoplasms, microcarcinoids, the Zollinger-Ellison syndrome, lymph nodes and hepatic metastases. Arch Surg 1993;128:1133.
47. Thompson NW. Surgical management of hyperparathyroidism and endocrine disease of the pancreas in the multiple endocrine neoplasia type I patient. J Intern Med 1995;238:269.
48. Thompson NW. Surgical treatment of the endocrine pancreas and pancreas and Zollinger-Ellison syndrome in the MENI syndrome. Henry Ford Hospital Medical Journal 1992;40:195.
49. Thompson NW, Bondeson AG, Bondeson L, Vinik AI. The surgical management of gastrinoma in MEN I syndrome patients. Surgery 1989; 106:1081.
50. Attanoos R, Williams GT. Epithelial and neuroendocrine tumors of the duodenum. Semin Diagn Pathol 1991;8:149.
51. Burke AP, Federspiel BH, Sobin LH, Shekitka KM, Helwig EB. Carcinoids of the duodenum: A histologic and immunohistochemical study of 65 tumors. Am J Surg Pathol 1989;13:828.
52. Dayal Y, Doos WG, O'Brien MJ, Nunnemacher G, DeLellis RA, Wolfe HJ. Psammomatous somatostatinomas of the duodenum. Am J Surg Pathology 1983;7:653.
53. Wheeler MH, Curley IR, Williams ED. The association of neurofibromatosis pheochromocytoma, and somatostatin rich duodenal carcinoid tumor. Surgery 1986;100:1163.
54. Hamid QA, Bishop AE, Rode J, et al. Duodenal gangliocytic paragangliomas: a study of 10 cases with immunocytochemical neuroendocrine markers. Hum Pathol 1986;17:1151.
55. Perrone T, Sibley RK, Rosai J. Duodenal gangliocytic paraganglioma: an immunohistochemical and ultrastructural study and a hypothesis concerning its origin. Am J Surg Pathol 1985;9:31.
56. Rosch T, Lightdale CH, Botet JF, et al. Localization of pancreatic endocrine tumors by endoscopic ultrasonography. N Engl J Med 1992; 326:1721.
57. Thompson NW, Czako PF, Fritts LL, et al. Role of endoscopic ultrasonography in the localization of insulinomas and gastrinomas. Surgery 1995;116:1131.

58. Declore R Jr, Cheung LS, Friesen SR. Characteristics of duodenal wall gastrinomas. Ann J Surg 1990;160:621.
59. Friesen SR. Are "aberrant nodule gastrinomas" pathogenetically similar to "lateral aberrant thyroid" nodules? Surgery 1990;107:236.
60. Lundqvist M, Wilander E. A study of the histopathogenesis of carcinoid tumors of the small intestine and appendix. Cancer 1987;60:201.
61. Hatzitheoklitos E, Büchler MW, Friess H, et al. Carcinoid of the ampulla of Vater: clinical characteristics and morphologic features. Cancer 1994;73:1580.
62. Ricci JL. Carcinoid of the ampulla of Vater: local resection or pancreaticoduodenectomy. Cancer 1993;71:686.
63. Rottner DW, Fernandez-del Castillo C, Brugge WR, Washaw AL. Defining the criteria for local resection of ampullary neoplasms. Arch Surg 1996;131:366.
64. Moertel CG, Sauer G, Dockerty MB, Baggenstoss AH. Life history of the carcinoid tumor of the small intestine. Cancer 1961;14:901.
65. Gouzi JL, Laigneau P, Delalande JP, et al. Indication for right hemicolectomy in carcinoid tumors of the appendix. Surg Gynecol Obstet 1993;176:543.
66. Iwafuchi M, Watanabe H, Ajioka Y, Shunoda T, Iwashida A, Ito S. Immunohistochemical and ultrastructural studies of twelve argentaffin and six argyrophil carcinoids of the appendix vermiformis. Hum Pathol 1990;21:773.
67. Moertel CG, Weiland LH, Nagorney DM, Dockerty MB. Carcinoid tumors of the appendix: treatment and prognosis. N Engl J Med 1987; 317:1699.
68. Parkes SE, Muir KR, Al-Sheyyab M, et al. Carcinoid tumors of the appendix in children 1957–1986: incidence, treatment and outcome. Br J Surg 1993;80:502.
69. Roggo A, Wood W, Ottinger LW. Carcinoid tumors of the appendix. Ann Surg 1993;217:385.
70. Stinner B, Kisker O, Zielke A, Rothmund M. Surgical management of carcinoid tumors of small bowel, appendix, colon and rectum. World J Surg 1996;20:183.
71. Syracuse DC, Perzin KH, Price JB, Weidel PD, Mesa-Tejada R. Carcinoid tumors of the appendix: mesoappendiceal extension and nodal metastases. Ann Surg 1979;190:58.
72. Thirlby RC, Kasper CS, Jones RC. Metastatic carcinoid tumor of the appendix: report of a case and review of the literature. Dis Colon Rectum 1984;27:42.
73. Deguchi H, Dequchi K, Tsukada T, et al. Long-term survival in patients with malignant carcinoid treated with high dose octreotide. Intern Med 1994;31:100.
74. Jaffe BM. Surgery for gut hormone producing tumors. Am J Med 1987; 82:68.
75. Makridis C, Öberg K, Juhlin C, et al. Surgical treatment of mid-gut carcinoid tumors. World J Surg 1990;14:377.
76. Strodel WE, Talpos G, Eckhauser FE, Thomson NW. Surgical therapy for small bowel carcinoid tumors. Arch Surg 1983;118:391.
77. Arnold R, Trautmann ME, Creuttzfeldt W, et al. Somatostatin analogue octreotide and inhibition of tumor growth in metastatic endocrine gastroenteropancreatic tumors. Gut 1996;38:430.
78. Lamberts SWJ, Krenning EP, Reubi JC. The role of somatostatin and its analogs in the diagnosis and treatment of tumors. Endocr Rev 1991; 12:400.
79. Maton PN. Use of octreotide acetate for control of symptoms in patients with islet cell tumors. World J Surg 1993;17:504.
80. Saltz L, Trochonowsky, G, Buckley M, et al. Octreotide as an antineoplastic agent in the treatment of functional and non-functional neuroendocrine tumors. Cancer 1993;72:244.
81. Ballantyne GH, Savoca PE, Flannery JT, Ahllman MH, Modlin IM. Incidence and mortality of carcinoids of the colon: data from the Connecticut tumor registry. Cancer 1992;69:2400.
82. Berardi RS. Carcinoid tumors of the colon (exclusive of the rectum). Dis Colon Rectum 1972;15:383.
83. Rosenberg JM, Welch JP. Carcinoid tumors of the colon: a study of 72 patients. Am J Surg 1985;149:775.
84. Burke M, Shepherd N, Mann CV. Carcinoid tumors of the rectum and anus. Br J Surg 1987;74:358.
85. Federspiel BH, Burke AP, Sobin LH, Shekitka KM. Rectal and colonic carcinoids: a clinicopathologic study of 84 cases. Cancer 1990;65:135.
86. Jetmore AB, Ray JE, Gathright JB Jr, McMullen K, Hicks T, Timmcke AE. Rectal carcinoids: the most frequent carcinoid tumor. Dis Colon Rectum 1992;35:717.
87. Alumets J, Alm P, Falkmer S, et al. Immunohistochemical evidence of peptide hormones in endocrine tumors of the rectum. Cancer 1981; 48:2409.
88. Fiocca R, Rindi G, Capella C, et al. Glucagon, glicentin, proglucagon, PYY, PP and pro-PP-icosapeptide immunoreactivities of rectal carcinoid tumors and related nontumor cells. Regul Pept 1987;29:9.
89. Fukayama M, Hayashi Y, Shiozawa Y, Okabe S, Kolke M. Human chorionic gonadotropin alpha-subunit in rectal carcinoids. Am J Pathol 1989;135:1065.
90. Grant CS. Surgical management of malignant islet cell tumors. World J Surg 1993;17:498.
91. Pasieka JL, McLeod MK, Thompson NW, Burney RE. Surgical approach to insulinomas: assessing the need for preoperative localization. Arch Surg 1992;127:442.
92. Doppman JL, Miller DL, Chang R, et al. Intraarterial calcium stimulation test for detection of insulinoma. World J Surg 1993;17:439.
93. O'Riordain DS, O'Brien T, van Heerden JA, et al. Surgical management of insulinoma associated with multiple endocrine neoplasia type I. World J Surg 1994;18:488.

Surgery for Gastrointestinal Cancer: A Multidisciplinary Approach, edited by Harold J. Wanebo.
Lippincott-Raven Publishers, Philadelphia, © 1997.

CHAPTER 42

Chemotherapy for Advanced Upper Gastrointestinal Malignancy (Esophagus, Stomach, Pancreas)

James D. Ahlgren

ROLE OF CHEMOTHERAPY IN ADVANCED GASTROINTESTINAL CANCER

The role of chemotherapy in advanced gastrointestinal cancer is palliative, that is, to ameliorate symptoms, or to delay their onset. There is usually no curative potential, but patients who respond to chemotherapy may still achieve significant benefit. Those who have an objective response to chemotherapy may obtain marked (although often brief) improvement in the quality of their lives. Patients who achieve major responses may live longer, although a survival benefit at the median level among all patients is difficult to demonstrate. In addition, subjective responses, particularly reduction in pain, may occur more frequently than objective response rates indicate. However, given the limited potential of chemotherapy, quality of life must be the primary goal of treatment planning in advanced disease.

Among upper gastrointestinal malignancies, the probability of achieving an objective response varies widely with the site. Carcinomas of the esophagus and stomach tend to be more chemosensitive, with objective response rates as high as 50% or higher. Carcinoma of the pancreas is much more chemoresistant, with response rates usually below 20%.

The potential for toxicity is important in the choice of a chemotherapy regimen. This is particularly so when the potential for response is low. Any potential benefit in quality of life must be balanced against quality reduction due to side effects. These issues should be discussed openly with the patient, along with the limited objectives of therapy, so that the patient can make an informed decision whether to undertake treatment.

Particularly important is the continued need for rational clinical trials in the chemotherapy of upper gastrointestinal cancer. These are common malignancies and many patients are candidates for chemotherapy. If improved regimens are to to be found, it will be through appropriate clinical trials. However, in patients with advanced disease, it is difficult to justify highly aggressive regimens when the intent is palliative. Trials of chemotherapy in upper gastrointestinal cancer should incorporate quality of life evaluation as a major endpoint.

James D. Ahlgren: Division of Hematology/Oncology, George Washington University Medical Center, 2150 Pennsylvania Avenue, NW, Washington, DC 20037-2396

SOME SPECIAL PROBLEMS IN INTERPRETING THE RESULTS OF CHEMOTHERAPY IN GASTROINTESTINAL CANCER

An inconsistency in interpreting older trials in chemotherapy for gastrointestinal cancer arises from changes over the years in response criteria. In colorectal cancer, for example, Moertel and Reitemeyer documented reports of response rates to 5-fluorouracil (5-FU) chemotherapy ranging all the way from 8% to 85%.[1] This variability was largely the result of differing response criteria; before the introduction of standardized response criteria[2] by the cooperative groups, various criteria were applied in different trials, and with varying degrees of rigor. Some early trials scored subjective responses, and others interpreted objective response criteria very liberally.

Even with current uniform response criteria, a significant problem remains. Most trials have allowed the use of hepatomegaly, as measured by physical examination, as a criterion for measurable disease. A 30% reduction in palpable hepatomegaly is commonly accepted as evidence for a partial response. This measurement is subjective, highly variable, and is influenced by factors other than tumor size.

Uren and colleagues[3] compared liver dimensions on radionuclide scan (with rib marker) with those determined by the referring physician by palpation. Only 56% of livers extending 10 cm or more below the costal margin, and only 66% of those 15 cm or more below, were detected by palpation. In only 12 of 21 patients with hepatic metastases was the liver palpated and thought to be enlarged, although all livers extended below the costal margin on scan (median 9 cm, range 3 to 26 cm). In 19 of 38 patients free of metastases by scan, livers were palpated and thought to be enlarged.

To evaluate the subjectivity of liver measurement by palpation, Warr and associates arranged for patients to be examined blindly by different oncologists. Comparing all observations for each patient, they showed that without any treatment at all, there would have been an 18% false-positive determination of partial response based on the standard criteria for assessment of hepatomegaly.[4]

In metastatic gastrointestinal cancer, the liver is the site of measurable disease in a significant fraction of patients. True objective response rates are low in many gastrointestinal cancers; this is especially true for those of the pancreas. The overestimation of response rate by physical determination of hepatomegaly is probably a major reason for unrealistically high response rates reported in early trials, rates that are not confirmed in trials in which computed tomography (CT) or other imaging is required to substantiate response. This is particularly a problem in evaluating the activity of single agents (eg, 5-FU), because most single-agent trials cited in the literature are from periods when flexible response criteria were the rule. Thus, many historic data pertaining to single-agent response rates in gastrointestinal cancer are significantly overstated.

Another problem, giving an opposite bias, is unique to pancreatic cancer.[5] Unfortunately, CT imaging of pancreatic cancer may not immediately reflect the effect of chemotherapy. Ductal carcinomas of the pancreas (and biliary system, as well) tend to provoke a rather vigorous desmoplastic reaction (Fig. 42-1). Even when chemotherapy is successful, this reactive fibrous tissue may not immediately shrink, so that the appearance of the tumor on CT scan may not reflect the true proportion of tumor kill. This effect may underestimate the response to chemotherapy. Metastatic deposits also often contain a major desmoplastic component. This desmoplastic reaction is intimately associated with the tumor cells and may reduce penetration of chemotherapy drugs to the tumor cells; it may be a factor contributing to the low response rate of these tumors.

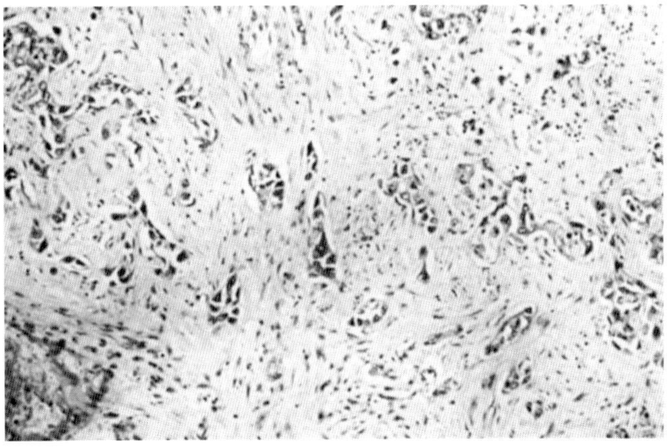

FIG. 42-1. Ductal carcinoma of the pancreas. A vigorous proliferation of fibroblasts is seen. This fairly typical desmoplastic reaction is characteristic of pancreatic and biliary cancers. (Courtesy Arnold M. Schwartz, MD, PhD, Department of Pathology, The George Washington University Medical Center, Washington, DC. Reproduced with permission from Ahlgren JD, Hill MC, Roberts IM. Pancreatic cancer: patterns, diagnosis and approaches to treatment. In: Ahlgren JD, Macdonald JS, eds. Gastrointestinal Oncology. Philadelphia: JB Lippincott, 1992:197.)

In summary, several factors can confuse the interpretation of available data on the chemotherapy of gastrointestinal cancer. Individually, these factors can tend either to overstate or understate the actual effectiveness of the therapy; however, the major bias in historic trials is one of overstatement.

DRUG RESISTANCE IN GASTROINTESTINAL CANCER

The fundamental reason for the wide difference in chemosensitivity of cancers from different gastrointestinal organs is drug resistance. A number of important mechanisms of drug resistance exist. One of the most important is the P-glycoprotein, coded by the *PGY1* (multidrug resistance 1, mdr-1) gene.[6] An explanation for this phenomenon has emerged since the identification by Ling and coworkers[7] of a 170-kd membrane protein (P-glycoprotein) associated with this class of resistance. It was already known from drug uptake and release kinetics that the reduced drug accumulation in resistant cells could involve active efflux of drug, rather than defective transport inward. Further studies suggested that P-glycoprotein was implicated in active outpumping of drug. Identification and cloning of the gene (*PGY1*) coding for P-glycoprotein[8,9] led to identification of hydrophobic membrane-spanning domains of the protein, as well as adenosine triphosphate-binding sites, consistent with its role as an energy-dependent transmembrane pump.

The initial study of P-glycoprotein–mediated multidrug resistance was stimulated by the investigation of acquired resistance and by the observation that acquired resistance to agents with differing modes of action often developed simultaneously. However, de novo resistance is more important than acquired resistance in gastrointestinal cancer. Although almost any cancer can develop increased expression of *PGY1* in response to chemotherapy, only a few tissues possess high P-glycoprotein levels before the selection pressure of chemotherapy. These tissues include the normal kidney, liver, lower gut, and adrenal.[6,10]

Sequence and structure of P-glycoprotein are highly conserved through evolution. Similar transmembrane transport proteins have been demonstrated in diverse species, from bacteria[11] onward. Such a highly conserved protein must have an important normal role. It functions as an active efflux pump for a wide variety of xenobiotics, and its localization in normal kidney and liver suggest that P-glycoprotein serves as the pump by which these organs clear the blood of toxic natural products. Toxins cleared by the liver must pass through the small intestine and colon before elimination. Because these organs are permeable to a variety of substances, a similar efflux pump mechanism would be required in the mucosal lining of these organs to prevent reabsorption of excreted toxins, as well as to protect the body from absorption of toxic ingested xenobiotics. P-glycoprotein is also expressed in most pancreatic carcinomas.[10] Probably for similar reasons, glutathione-S-transferase,[12] another detoxification mechanism, is also overexpressed in the same anatomic distribution. Above the papilla of Vater, where the gastrointestinal tract does not act as a conduit for toxins excreted in the bile, the expression of drug resistance mechanisms is significantly lower.[13] The net result is significantly reduced effectiveness of most drugs in several gastrointestinal cancers, including those of the pancreas, hepatobiliary system, and large and small bowel. The major drug class *not* influenced by *PGY1* and glutathione-S-transferase is the fluorinated pyrimidines.

CHEMOTHERAPY FOR SPECIFIC UPPER GASTROINTESTINAL CANCERS

Chemotherapy for Advanced Esophageal Cancer

Esophageal cancer probably represents the most chemosensitive malignancy among those of the upper gastrointestinal organs. Drug resistance mechanisms are not usually expressed de novo in the esophagus, presumably because of its limited absorptive capacity and its location well above the entry of the bile stream. The chemosensitivity of esophageal cancers is beginning to be exploited in combined regimens for initial therapy of limited disease. Indeed, many of the response data in esophageal cancer are derived from studies of neoadjuvant therapy of regional disease, before surgery or radiation therapy, and may somewhat overstate the response expectation in more advanced disease. Palliative responses are common in advanced disease, however, even though long-term results in advanced disease remain quite poor.

The relative chemosensitivity of squamous carcinoma versus adenocarcinoma of the esophagus has been debated. Some early studies suggested that prognosis with adenocarcinoma was poorer than with squamous carcinoma. However, one study in which cisplatin/5-FU/vinblastine chemotherapy was combined before surgery with radiation therapy showed comparable chemosensitivity and actually superior initial survival with adenocarcinoma than with squamous carcinoma.[14] Cisplatin/5-FU–based regimens probably have comparable efficacy with either histologic type. In addition, regimens active in gastric cancer appear to have activity in esophageal adenocarcinoma, but have not been adequately tested in squamous carcinoma of the esophagus.

Activity of Individual Drugs in Esophageal Cancer

Many drugs have activity in esophageal cancer[15] (Table 42-1). The most important are cisplatin and 5-FU, and these two drugs form the basis for most combination regimens in use today.

Data on the use of of cisplatin as a single agent in esophageal cancer come largely from series that included a large percentage of previously treated patients. An overall response rate of 23% is obtained by summing the results from four published series[16–19] involving 86 patients (see Table 42-1). These trials used dose intensities ranging from 17 to 35 mg/m²/wk. The largest single series, reported by the Southwest Oncology Group (SWOG), produced a 26% response rate among 35 patients, all of whom received cisplatin as second-line chemotherapy[16]; there were three complete responses in that series (9%).

With the demonstrated superiority of infusional schedules, bolus 5-FU is no longer used in the treatment of esophageal cancer. One early study of bolus 5-FU by the the Eastern Cooperative Oncology Group yielded a response rate of 17% among 23 previously treated patients.[20] Infusional schedules have made 5-FU an important drug for esophageal carcinoma. The schedule most commonly used today in combination chemotherapy regimens is a 4- to 5-day infusion of the order of 800 to 1000 mg/m²/d, given every 3 to 4 weeks. This is largely based on extrapolation of results with this same schedule in squamous cancers of the head and neck, because good single-agent response data do not exist for this schedule in esophageal cancer. However, Lokich and colleagues evaluated the effect of a protracted 5-FU infusion (PIF), given for 6 weeks at 300 mg/m²/d.[21] Among 13 patients with previously untreated, locally advanced esophageal cancer, the response rate was 77% (11/13, 1 complete response [CR]) at 6 weeks. Data are lacking on 5-FU with leucovorin, *N*-(phosphonacetyl)-L-aspartic acid (PALA), and other modifiers, except for a small trial of bolus 5-FU with interferon-α, which produced a 27% response rate among 11 patients.[22]

More data on infusional 5-FU monotherapy in esophageal cancer are needed, both with the widely used 5-day schedule, and to confirm Lokich and colleagues' results with PIF. Trials with leucovorin and other modulators are also needed. However, given the high response rates repeatedly shown with combination therapy, it will now be difficult to justify trials of monotherapy on untreated patients.

Paclitaxel (Taxol) showed a 32% response rate in one trial,[23] and appears to have considerable promise. It is being evaluated in combination regimens. Other agents with useful response in esophageal carcinoma include mitomycin-C,[20] paclitaxel,[23] bleomycin,[24–26] doxorubicin,[27] methotrexate,[28] vindesine,[29–31] and mitoguazone (MGBG).[32]

Combination Chemotherapy for Esophageal Cancer

Many chemotherapy trials in esophageal cancer have been in the setting of initial therapy for localized disease, before surgery or radiation therapy. These patients in general have been of better performance status, and with less tumor burden, than those with advanced disease. It may be expected, therefore, that results in advanced disease will not be as good. Response evaluation has usually been by CT and endoscopy; however, a higher level of response evaluation is available in those trials where surgery followed the chemotherapy. In these trials, a few pathologically documented CRs were seen, offering the hope that, with improvements, chemotherapy may eventually offer a long-term survival benefit for at least some patients. The most widely used combination therapy is cisplatin/5-FU; taxol-based combinations are being actively investigated.

Cisplatin/Infusional 5-FU

Cisplatin and 5-FU are synergistic, both in laboratory models[33] and in the clinic. Cisplatin increases the intracellular level of methylenetetrahydrofolate,[34] which may in part explain the synergy. An early study of cisplatin combined with equitoxic doses of bolus 5-FU versus 5-FU as a 5-day infusion showed significant superiority for the infusional schedule in squamous carcinoma of the head and neck.[35] This short term

TABLE 42-1. *Drugs with single-agent activity in esophageal cancer*

Drug	No. patients	Percent responses	Reference(s)
Cisplatin	86 (4 trials)	23 (6 CR)	16–19
5-FU (bolus)	23 (1 trial)	17	20
5-FU (5-d infus.)	inadequate data		
5-FU (PIF)	13 (1 trial)	77 (1 CR)	21
5-FU/leucovorin	inadequate data		
Mitomycin C	24 (1 trial)	42	19
Paclitaxel	50 (1 trial)	32 (1 CR)	23
Bleomycin	25 (2 trials)	24 (2 CR)	24–26
Doxorubicin	34 (2 trials)	18	20,27
Methotrexate	70 (2 trials)	34 (1 CR)	20,28
Vindesine	120 (3 trials)	20 (3 CR)	29–31
Mitoguazone	23 (1 trial)	17	32

Adapted with permission from Ahlgren JD. Esophageal cancer: chemotherapy and combined modalities. In: Ahlgren JD, Macdonald JS, eds. Gastrointestinal oncology. Philadelphia: JB Lippincott, 1992:135.

(4- to 5-day) infusion schedule has been generally adopted for the combination of 5-FU and cisplatin, in esophageal cancer as well as in head and neck cancer.

Results with cisplatin/5-FU in esophageal cancer have been impressive in previously untreated patients with localized disease (Table 42-2). Customary schedules have been cisplatin, 60 to 100 mg/m^2 either on day 1 or divided over 4 to 5 days, plus 5-FU as a continuous 4- to 5-day infusion at a dose rate of 800 to 1000 mg/m^2/d. The largest preoperative series is that of of Hilgenberg and coworkers at Massachusetts General Hospital.[36,37] They treated 59 patients with squamous cancer of the esophagus with two cycles of 5-FU (1 gm^2/d as a 4-day infusion) plus cisplatin (100 gm/m^2 on day 4). Patients were restaged by CT, endoscopy, and barium swallow before surgery. Overall objective response rate was 66% (38/59), with 39% (23/59) CRs. After restaging, 47 (80%) patients underwent resection, with 3 (5% of the original cohort) showing pathologic CR. Two other trials[38,39] have reported similar response rates with this combination.

Lester and associates[40] added methotrexate (120 mg/m^2 with leucovorin rescue) to the cisplatin/5-FU combination. Of 34 evaluable patients, 24 (71%, 3 pathologic CRs at esophagectomy) responded.

Other Combination Regimens

The combination of paclitaxel with cisplatin appears to be highly active in esophageal carcinoma. However, results at present are only preliminary. The combination of paclitaxel, cisplatin, and 5-FU was reported to produce 44% objective responses (17/39, 1 CR).[41]

The other regimen that has seen significant investigation in esophageal carcinoma is the combination of cisplatin and bleomycin, usually with a third drug (Table 42-3). Bleomycin also exhibits synergy with cisplatin in some models. It has been suggested that synergy is maximized by infusional schedules of bleomycin, possibly because of prolonged inhibition of DNA repair enzymes.[42]

Three trials of the combination of cisplatin and bleomycin alone have yielded objective response rates of 14% to 24%.[43–45] Kelsen and associates added vindesine to the cisplatin/bleomycin combination and observed an increased response rate of 55% in each of two trials, 91 patients in all.[46,47] A SWOG trial in previously treated patients yielded a 29% response rate.[48] Other drugs that have been used with the cisplatin/bleomycin combination include methotrexate[49,50] and mitomycin-C,[51] both with response rates in the 50% range.

Kelsen and associates studied the cisplatin/MGBG/vindesine combination, substituting MGBG for bleomycin to avoid the pulmonary toxicity of the latter agent. In their initial report, 8 of 20 patients (40%) achieved a response.[52] Forastiere and coworkers substituted vinblastine for vindesine, and reported a 44% response rate among 29 patients treated with cisplatin/MGBG/vinblastine.[53] A small series with cisplatin/MGBG/vindesine/methotrexate appeared active, with five of eight patients responding.[54] The FAP combination (bolus 5-FU, doxorubicin, and cisplatin), which has been more widely used in gastric can-

TABLE 42-2. *Clinical trials using cisplatin/infusional 5-FU with subsequent pathologic evaluation in esophageal carcinoma*

Drug dose cisplatin	mg/m^2 FUra	Freq	Pts	Clinical response rate	Path responses/ pts resected	Reference(s)
100	1000/d × 4	q3w × 2	59	38 (66%), 39% CR	3/47 (5%)*	Hilgenberg et al[36,37]
100	1000/d × 5	q3w × 2	26	11 (42%), 12% CR	0/14	Kies et al[38]
20 × 5	1000/d × 5	q3w × 2–6	25	18 (72%), 44% CR	2/NS (8%)*	Ajani et al[39]

* Pathologic CR rate as a percentage of initial cohort of patients.

Reproduced with permission from Ahlgren JD. Esophageal cancer: chemotherapy and combined modalities. In: Ahlgren JD, Macdonald JS, eds. Gastrointestinal oncology. Philadelphia: JB Lippincott, 1992:135.

TABLE 42-3. *Some clinical trials of regimens based on cisplatin and bleomycin in esophageal carcinoma*

Drug doses (mg/m²)					
Cisplat	Bleomycin	Other drug	Freq	Response rate	Reference
120	10/d infus × 8	—	q4w	4/17 (24%)	Bosset[44]
120	10 + 10/d infus × 4		q4w	6/43 (14%)	Coonley[45]
120	10 + 10/d infus × 4	VDS 3qw	q4w	29/53 (55%)	Kelsen[46]
120	10 + 10/d infus × 4	VDS 3qw	q4w	21/38 (55%)	Kelsen[47]
50	15 (dl)	VDS 3qw	q3w	7/27 (29%)	Dinwoodie[48]
50 (d4)	10 IM qw	MTX 40 d1, 14	q3w	5/10 (50%)	Vogl[49]
50 (d3)	10 IM qw	MTX 40 d1, 15	q3w	8/31 (26%)	DeBasi[50]

Reproduced with permission from Ahlgren JD. Esophageal cancer: chemotherapy and combined modalities. In: Ahlgren JD, Macdonald JS, eds. Gastrointestinal oncology. Philadelphia: JB Lippincott, 1992:135.

cer, has also been tested in esophageal cancer. Among 21 patients, 7 (33%) responded, with 5 CRs.[55] However, no responses were seen among 19 untreated patients receiving carboplatin/vinblastine.[56]

Clearly, combination chemotherapy is active in esophageal cancer. However, there are few large studies of palliative chemotherapy in advanced esophageal cancer, so it is difficult to evaluate the effect on survival. Most of the more recent studies have been in patients with locoregional disease and good performance status. A prospective trial in patients with advanced disease is needed to prove a survival benefit.

Chemotherapy for Advanced Gastric Cancer

Gastric cancer has moderate chemosensitivity, and was the first gastrointestinal cancer for which an effective combination chemotherapy regimen (bolus 5-FU, doxorubicin, and mitomycin-C [FAM]) was devised.[57] There have been reports of long-term survival in patients with advanced disease treated with chemotherapy, but such survival must be considered a rare event. However, useful palliation is often achieved.

Activity of Individual Drugs in Gastric Cancer

De novo expression of multidrug resistance mechanisms is variable in gastric cancer, but is considerably less frequent than in cancers of the lower gut, where it is almost universal.[13,58,59] Thus, a fairly wide spectrum of antitumor drugs (Table 42-4) have activity in gastric cancer, although 5-FU remains the most important single agent. Historically, 5-FU was administered in bolus schedules. Reviews of the early experience suggest a response rate for bolus 5-FU of the order of 20%,[60] although this may be optimistic, considering the flexibility of response criteria in many early trials. Both PIF schedules[61] and the use of leucovorin as a modulator[62–64] appear to increase the response rate of 5-FU to the 30% range. Still unapproved in the United States but widely used elsewhere are the 5-FU–related

TABLE 42-4. *Drugs with single-agent activity in gastric cancer*

Drug	No. patients	Percent responses	Reference(s)
5-FU (bolus)	392*,†	21	60
5-FU (5-d infus.)	inadequate data		
5-FU (PIF)	13 (1 trial)	31	61
5-FU/leucovorin	127 (3 trials)†	17 (1 CR)	62–64
Tegafur	31 (2 trials)	29	65,66
UFT	18 (1 trial)	6	67
Doxorubicin	68*,†	25	60
Epirubicin	48 (2 trials)†	25	69,70
Cisplatin	50 (3 trials)†	24 (2 CR)	71–73
Mitomycin C	211*,†	30	60
Etoposide	inadequate data		
Methotrexate	28 (1 trial)	11	74
Triazinate	26 (1 trial)	15	74
Trimetrexate	26 (1 trial)	19	75
methyl-CCNU	37	8	60
BCNU	23 (1 trial)	17	76
Chlorambucil	18 (1 trial)	17	77
Nitrogen mustard	23 (1 trial)	13	78

* Response may be overstated due to nonstandardized response criteria.
† Combined results of 2 or more trials using different schedules.

TABLE 42-5. *FAM and SMF regimens*

Week	1	2	3	4	5	6	7	8	9
FAM REGIMEN (Macdonald et al[57])									*
5-FU 600 mg/m^2	X	X			X	X			R
Doxorubicin 30 mg/m^2	X				X				E
Mitomycin-C 10 mg/m^2	X								P
									E
SMF REGIMEN (Wiggans et al[142])									A
5-FU 600 mg/m^2	X	X			X	X			T
Streptozotocin 1 gm/m^2	X	X			X	X			
Mitomycin-C 10 mg/m^2	X								*

oral prodrug tegafur (Ftorafur)[65,66] and its mixture with uracil (UFT).[67,68] These appear comparable in efficacy to PIF.

Probably the next most important class of drugs in gastric cancer are the anthracyclines. Both doxorubicin[60] and epirubicin[69,70] appear to have response rates of the order of 25%. Cisplatin has a response rate of the order of 20%,[71–73] whereas early data for mitomycin-C suggest a response rate as high as 30%.[60] Other drugs with lesser activity include antifols[74,75] and the nitrosoureas.[76] Earlier literature also suggests some activity for conventional alkylating agents[77,78] and hydroxyurea.[60] The topoisomerase II inhibitor etoposide appears to have strong activity in combination regimens,[79,80] although single-agent data are not available. Adequate data are not yet available on the newer topoisomerase I inhibitors irinotecan and topotecan.

Combination Chemotherapy in Gastric Cancer

Combination chemotherapy is more effective than therapy with single agents in gastric cancer, at least in terms of response rate. The FAM regimen[57] (Table 42-5) was the first combination regimen to show efficacy in any gastrointestinal malignancy. Since its initial publication in 1980, numerous confirmatory trials[81–84] have substantiated a response rate of the order of 40% in metastatic gastric cancer (Table 42-6). FAM can be considered the prototype first-generation regimen for gastric cancer, and has usually performed equally well as or better than similar regimens in which other agents, chiefly nitrosoureas, were added or substituted. Nevertheless, in spite of a useful rate of palliation, no survival advantage is seen with FAM[83] or with any of the other first-generation combinations. Median survival in patients with measurable metastatic disease treated with first-generation combinations is approximately 9 to 12 months. Complete tumor responses are rare with these regimens, usually less than 5%.

TABLE 42-6. *Results with FAM chemotherapy in advanced gastric cancer*

Study	Response rate	98% Confidence interval
Macdonald et al[57] (1980)	27/62 (44)	.31–.56
Douglass et al[81] (1984)	18/46 (39%)	.24–.54
Beretta et al[82] (1982)	20/45 (44%)	.29–.60
Cullinan et al[83] (1985)	5/13* (39%)	.14–.68
Bitran et al[84] (1979)	6/11† (55%)	.24–.87
(Total)	76/177 (43%)	

* Measurable gastric cancer patients only.
† Previously untreated patients only.

An optimum chemotherapy regimen for gastric cancer is yet to be devised, but newer-generation regimens have been introduced in the hope of influencing survival in patients with advanced disease (Table 42-7). The potential improvements of these newer regimens over FAM include the use of more optimal scheduling or modulators with the 5-FU and the introduction of newer agents, particularly etoposide and cisplatin. The newer-generation regimens appear to result in a higher percentage of complete remissions (Table 42-8), and it is hoped that a survival benefit will be confirmed.

One of the earliest second-generation regimens was the FAMTX combination of Klein and colleagues[85] (see Table 42-7). In this regimen, a high dose of methotrexate, 1.5 g/m^2, is administered 1 hour before a single dose of 1.5 g/m^2 of 5-FU. Leucovorin rescue, 15 mg orally every 6 hours, is administered for 2 days, beginning 24 hours after the methotrexate. Doxorubicin, 30 mg/m^2, is administered on day 14, and the cycle repeated every 4 weeks. This is a toxic regimen, with life-threatening neutropenia and thrombocytopenia in over 10% of patients. However, in the original 100 patients treated by Klein and colleagues, the overall response rate was 59%, with 12% CRs. A confirmatory trial by the European Organization for Research in the Treatment of Cancer (EORTC) yielded a lower overall response rate of 33%, but again 13% CRs,[86] and then a randomized phase III trial by the same group yielded a 41% overall response rate (6% CR), versus 9% for FAM.[87] Kelsen and colleagues performed a randomized trial between FAMTX and EAP (see next paragraph), with a 33% response rate (10/30, 10% CR).[88] Another phase II trial of FAMTX with the methotrexate dose reduced to 1.0 g/m^2 resulted in a 50% response rate (15/30) with 10% CR.[89]

Preusser and colleagues introduced the EAP regimen, an aggressive schedule of etoposide, doxorubicin, and cisplatin (see Table 42-7). In their original report, a 64% response rate, with 21% CR, was reported among 64 patients.[79] Using minor scheduling rearrangements and a slightly lower dose of etoposide ("VAP"), Katz and associates also reported a high response rate, 72% overall, 12% CR, among 25 patients.[90] A confirmatory trial in the United States could not reproduce these response

TABLE 42-7. *Some newer generation regimens for gastric cancer*

Day	1	2	3	4	5	6	7	8	14
FAMTX REGIMEN (Klein et al[85])									
Methotrexate 1.5 gm/m^2	X								
5-FU 1.5 gm/m^2*	X								
Leucovorin 15 mg po q6h		X	X						
Doxorubicin 30 mg/m^2									X
EAP REGIMEN (Preusser et al[79])									
Doxorubicin 20 mg/m^2	X						X		
Cisplatin 40 mg/m^2		X						X	
Etoposide 120 mg/m^2				X	X	X			
VAP REGIMEN (Katz et al[90])									
Etoposide 100 mg/m^2	X	X	X						
Doxorubicin 20 mg/ms^2	X							X	
Cisplatin 40 mg/m^2		X						X	
ELF REGIMEN (Wilke et al[80])									
Etoposide 120 mg/m^2	X	X	X						
Leucovorin 300 mg/m^2	X	X	X						
5-FU 500 mg/m^2	X	X	X						

* 5-FU administered 1 hour after methotrexate; leucovorin begins 24 hours after methotrexate for a total of 8 doses.

rates, however, reporting 33% overall responders (8% CR) among 36 patients,[91] and Kelsen and colleagues' randomized trial against FAMTX produced a response rate of only 20% without any CRs.[88] This is also a toxic regimen, with toxic deaths in each of these studies.

The same German group that developed EAP also has described a less intense regimen, ELF, in which etoposide is combined with 5-FU/leucovorin (see Table 42-7). This was intended for patients considered too debilitated to tolerate EAP, but proved to have impressive performance as well. In the initial publication, response was 48% among 34 patients, with 12% CR (one pathologically documented).[80] An update when the series had reached 51 patients reported responses holding at 53% (12% CR), with 11-month median survival.[92]

Several other regimens have shown promising response rates in preliminary reports. The combination of 5-FU, leucovorin, doxorubicin, and cisplatin yielded a 41% response rate (13/32, 1 CR) in adenocarcinoma of the stomach and gastroesophageal junction.[93] The combination of 5-FU (5-day infusion) with cisplatin has been studied in two trials[94,95] both of which reported 43% response rate (36/83, 5% CR, and 17/40, respectively). The combination of cisplatin, epirubicin, and 5-FU was reported to yield a 47% response rate (28/62, 7 CR).[96] A similar regimen with leucovorin resulted in a 43% response rate (37/85, 4 CR) in a randomized trial against FAM[97]; a more intensive weekly regimen combining 5-FU, cisplatin, epirubicin, and leucovorin, with glutathione and granulocyte colony stimulating factor protection, had a response rate of 68% among 40 patients in the preliminary report.[98]

Summary and Outlook

Truly effective chemotherapy for gastric cancer continues to fascinate oncologists. Slow but steady progress is being made. Useful palliation of advanced disease is achieved in roughly 50% of cases, with CRs in over 10%. However, survival benefit remains elusive. It is hoped that this will be achieved with further improvements.

TABLE 42-8. *Results with newer generation combination regimens for gastric cancer*

Regimen	No. patients	Percent response	Survival	Reference
FAMTX	100	59% (12% CR)	9 mos	Klein et al[85]
	67	33% (13% CR)	6 mos	Wils et al[86]
	81	41% (6% CR)	10 mos	Wils et al[87]
	30	33% (10% CR)	7 mos	Kelsen et al[88]
(1 gm/m^2 mtx)	30	50% (10% CR)	10 mos	Murad et al[89]
EAP	67	64% (21% CR)	9 mos	Preusser et al[79]
	33	33% (8% CR)	6 mos	Lerner et al[91]
	30	20% (0 CR)	6 mos	Kelsen et al[88]
VAP	25	72% (12% CR)	6 mos	Katz et al[90]
ELF	51	53% (12% CR)	11 mos	Wilke et al[92]

Chemotherapy for Advanced Pancreatic Cancer

Activity of Individual Drugs in Pancreatic Cancer

The fundamental problem with chemotherapy in pancreatic cancer is the lack of any individual drug with strong activity.[5] Drug resistance mechanisms may contribute, as may problems of drug penetration due to the vigorous desmoplastic reaction that usually surrounds pancreatic cancer deposits. The major drug *not* influenced by the multidrug resistance mechanisms is 5-FU. However, even 5-FU is less effective in pancreatic cancer than in most other gastrointestinal sites.

5-Fluorouracil and 5-Fluorouracil With Modulators

5-Fluorouracil, with and without modulators, is currently the most important drug in pancreatic cancer (Table 42-9). It was the first drug reported to be active in pancreatic cancer.[99,100] Those reports used bolus schedules. Carter and Comis reviewed 15 small trials of bolus 5-FU[101] in pancreatic cancer. These individual trials reported response rates ranging from 0% to 67%, comparable to the wide range of early results in colorectal cancer noted earlier.[1] An overall response rate for bolus 5-FU of 26% in 251 patients has been cited by O'Connell[102] and Moertel.[103] However, these reports draw heavily on early studies using poorly defined or undocumented response criteria. Even eliminating from these compilations four series from the early 1960s that cited response rates of 46% to 67%, the remaining overall response rate of 15% in 169 patients is still probably an overstatement.[104] The situation probably parallels that in colorectal cancer, where response rates of 20% to 25% are cited in the older literature, but cannot be supported by data from several more recent phase III trials in which stringently applied response criteria were used. Five such trials reported response rates for bolus 5-FU of 7% to 12%[99–109]; four of these trials had response rates below 10%. Because virtually all broad trials of 5-FU in gastrointestinal malignancies have yielded lower response rates in patients with pancreatic cancer than in those with colorectal cancer, the true objective response rate of bolus 5-FU in pancreatic cancer is likely to be no greater than 10%.

Improved scheduling or the use of modulators such as leucovorin can substantially improve the response of bolus 5-FU. Most of the comparative studies have been carried out in colorectal cancer, where the addition of appropriate schedules of leucovorin to bolus 5-FU,[105,107–109] or the use of PIF schedules,[106,110–112] increase the response rate of 5-FU to the 30% to 35% range. Bolus 5-FU with leucovorin has been evaluated in pancreatic cancer in two phase II trials. The high-dose weekly Gastrointestinal Tumor Study Group (GITSG) schedule of 5-FU/leucovorin (which had a 30% response rate in colorectal cancer[107]) was evaluated in a joint trial by Dana-Farber and Roswell Park. In pancreatic cancer, this regimen yielded only 3 partial responses (7%) among 42 patients.[113] Another phase II trial at Memorial Sloan-Kettering used a schedule similar to the high-dose Mayo/North Central Cancer Treatment Group (NCCTG) regimen (26% response in colorectal cancer[108]); this study produced no objective responses and only one minor response among 20 patients.[114] These results do not indicate that bolus 5-FU alone (with historical higher response rates) is a better regimen than 5-FU with leucovorin, but should be interpreted as being more plausible than the older results with bolus 5-FU alone, being based on more stringently applied objective response criteria. They also confirm the lower overall responsiveness of pancreatic cancer than colorectal cancer. We are inclined to believe the more recent results with 5-FU plus modulators, and to conclude that the true response rate of bolus 5-FU is lower still.

Surprisingly, there is still no published trial of PIF alone in pancreatic cancer. Nevertheless, it is reasonable to extrapolate the same pharmacologic advantage that has been clinically demonstrated in colorectal cancer.[106] Our own limited clinical experience suggests a response rate of PIF in pancreatic cancer of about 15%.

Another 5-FU modulator that has been studied extensively in colorectal cancer is interferon-α, with response rates of 26% to 76% reported in that disease.[115–117] This combination was evaluated in 46 patients with pancreatic cancer by Pazdur and associates; only 2 (4%) achieved partial responses.[118] Two phase II trials combining 5-FU with both leucovorin and interferon-α in pancreatic cancer resulted in response rates of 12% (4/32)[119] and 14% (8/57),[120] but a third trial of the same combination among 20 patients yielded no objective responses and high toxicity.[121]

TABLE 42-9. *Published activity of 5-FU with or without modulators in pancreatic cancer*

Schedule	No. patients	Percent response	Reference
5-FU (bolus)	169 (11 trials)*	15*	Ahlgren[104]
Protracted infusional 5-FU (PIF)		inadequate data	
5-FU + leucovorin			
(GITSG schedule)	42	7	DeCaprio et al[113]
(5-day schedule)	20	0	Crown et al[114]
5-FU + α-interferon	46	4	Pazdur et al[118]
5-FU + leucovorin	32	12	Scheithauer et al[119]
+ α-interferon	57	14	Bernhard et al[120]
	21	0	Schneider et al[121]
5-FU (24-h infusion)			
± PALA (phase I)	17	18	Ardalan et al[122]
+ PALA (phase II)	35	14 (1 CR)	Rosvold et al[123]

* Compilation of 11 published trials, some early, which probably overestimates true response rate substantially (see text). True response rate of bolus 5-FU is probably less than 10%.

Another 5-FU modulator, PALA, was evaluated by Ardalan and coworkers in a phase I and II trial of weekly 24-hour infusions of 5-FU with and without PALA in a mixed population that included both colorectal and pancreatic cancer.[122] Among the 17 patients with pancreatic cancer, the response rate was 3/17 (18%), with two of the three responders receiving PALA along with the 5-FU. The same combination was tested at full dose (2.6 g/m^2 5-FU, 250 mg/m^2 PALA, both as a weekly 24-hour infusion) in pancreatic cancer by Rosvold and colleagues, with a response rate of 14% (5/35, 1 CR).[123]

Other Drugs

Other than 5-FU, drugs with documented activity (marginal to modest) in pancreatic cancer include antimetabolites, alkylating agents, and antibiotics (Table 42-10). Mitomycin-C is probably the most active drug after 5-FU. Early trials showed fairly similar response rates between 5-FU and mitomycin-C. Carter and Comis[101] combined the results of four very small published series (44 patients in all) and obtained a response rate of 27%. This probably significantly overestimates the true response rate, for the same reasons as noted earlier for 5-FU. However, mitomycin-C has useful activity in pancreatic cancer, and has been used in a number combination regimens.

The anthracyclines also have some activity in pancreatic cancer. Doxorubicin was studied by GITSG in a randomized trial in which methotrexate and actinomycin-D formed the other two arms.[124] The response rate was 13% (2/15) in previously untreated patients and 8% (2/25) overall, including patients who had failed previous chemotherapy. Epirubicin was studied by EORTC,[135] and yielded a response rate of 20% (8/40, 2 CRs). This is an impressive response rate, in that all responses were documented by CT or sonograms. Some responses developed as late as the fourth course, perhaps suggesting delayed resolution of the fibrosis normally associated with pancreatic ductal carcinoma.

The nitrosoureas, another class of agents active in gastrointestinal malignancies, have been studied in pancreatic cancer. The chloroethylnitrosoureas, carmustine (BCNU), lomustine (CCNU), and semustine (methyl-CCNU), are probably roughly equivalent in their efficacy in pancreatic cancer. Although they have activity,[101,133,134] they are probably inferior to mitomycin-C and the anthracyclines (see Table 42-10). Streptozotocin differs from the chloroethylnitrosoureas in that it is a monofunctional alkylator and does not cross-link DNA. It was initially explored because of its unique activity in islet cell tumors of the pancreas. Because of this, and its relatively lower myelotoxicity than the chloroethylnitrosoureas, it was also tried in combina-

TABLE 42-10. *Other drugs with reported single-agent activity in pancreatic cancer*

Drug	No. patients	Percent response	Reference(s)
ANTIMETABOLITES			
Methotrexate	25	4	Schein et al[124]
Gemcitabine	63	NS*	Rothenberg et al[125]
	63	NS*	Moore et al[126]
ALKYLATORS			
Melphalan	58 (2 trials)	5	Horton et al[127] Smith et al[128]
Ifosfamide	116 (4 trials)†	10	Loehrer et al[129] Bernard et al[130] Ajani et al[131] GITSG[132]
BCNU	22	0	Moertel et al[133]
CCNU	19 (CTEP-IS data)	16‡	Comis & Carter[101]
Methyl-CCNU	83 (2 trials)	7	Moertel et al[133] Moertel et al[134]
Streptozotocin	27 (CTEP-IS data)	11‡	Comis & Carter[101]
Cisplatin, Carboplatin		inadequate data	
ANTIBIOTICS			
Mitomycin C	44 (4 trials)	27‡	Comis & Carter[101]
Doxorubicin	25	13§	Schein et al[124]
Epirubicin	40	20	Wils et al[135]
Actinomycin D	28	7	Schein et al[124]
OTHER AGENTS			
Hexamethylmelamine	55	8§	GITSG[136]
Vindesine	15	7	Smith et al[137]

NS: not stated.
* 17/36 patients had clinical response (≥50% reduction in pain of narcotic use or ≥20% rise in KPS.
† Some early trials excluded; see text.
‡ Response may be overstated due to nonstandardized response criteria.
§ Excluding previously treated patients.

Adapted with permission from Ahlgren JD. Pancreatic cancer: Chemotherapy for advanced disease. In: Ahlgren JD, Macdonald JS, eds. Gastrointestinal oncology. Philadelphia: JB Lippincott, 1992:227.

tion regimens in pancreatic cancer. The only published data on single-agent activity of streptozotocin in pancreatic adenocarcinoma come from National Cancer Institute records on 27 patients, and suggest a relatively low response rate of 8%.[101]

There have been anecdotal reports of occasional responses to the classic alkylating agents, including mechlorethamine, cyclophosphamide, and chlorambucil, but only melphalan and ifosfamide have been evaluated in prospective trials. The two small trials of melphalan[127,128] reported minimal activity. Loehrer and colleagues[129] reported 6 responses (22%) among 27 evaluable patients treated with ifosfamide, after early reports from Egypt[138,139] suggested much greater activity. However, three other U.S. trials reported only marginal activity.[130–132] Combining all U.S. trials, the overall response rate is 10% among 116 patients (see Table 42-10).

Cisplatin has been reported anecdotally to have useful activity in pancreatic cancer, although essentially no prospective single-agent trials have been reported for either cisplatin or carboplatin. However, cisplatin continues to be explored in combination regimens. Actinomycin-D, amsacrine, aziridinylbenzoquinone (AZO), etoposide, methotrexate, and mitoxantrone have all been studied adequately to rule out more than minimal activity, whereas hexamethylmelamine and vindesine appeared to have marginal activity in small trials. Among the current experimental agents, gemcitabine and irinotecan are currently in trials in pancreatic cancer, and appear to have promise. Gemcitabine has been evaluated using clinical benefit ($\geq$ 50% reduction in pain or narcotic use, or increase in Karnofsky performance score by $\geq$ 20%, maintained for at least 4 weeks) rather than objective response as the primary endpoint. In this context it resulted in a clinical benefit in 27% of patients who had failed 5-FU,[125] and showed a greater rate of clinical benefit than 5-FU (P = 0.0025) in previously untreated patients.[126]

Combination Chemotherapy in Pancreatic Cancer

There has been hope that improved therapeutic results might be obtained with combination chemotherapy in pancreatic cancer, because several classes of drugs have at least some activity. However, this hope is yet to be realized. No combination regimen has yet been able to demonstrate any survival advantage, and objective response rates have been below 20% in the larger trials. Two regimens have shown high response rates in small single-institution trials. In both cases, however, larger trials of the same regimens have had disappointing outcomes.

The most widely used combination regimens in pancreatic cancer have been based on 5-FU and mitomycin-C, plus a third drug. The first two regimens to be introduced, FAM and SMF (streptozotocin, mitomycin-C, and 5-FU; see Table 42-5), are still widely used in the community. FAM was initially studied in gastric cancer, where it reliably produces a response rate of 35% to 40%,[57] Early single-institution trials in pancreatic cancer produced encouraging response rates around 40%.[140,141] The SMF regimen was conceived as an alternative to FAM, intended specifically for pancreatic cancer. It also produced promising results in early single-institution trials,[142,143] as well as a 34% response rate among 56 patients in a SWOG trial.[144] Unfortunately, these early results have never been repeated. A larger trial of FAM by GITSG produced only a 9% response rate.[145] Next, two randomized trials comparing FAM and SMF were organized (Table 42-11). A prospective three-arm GITSG trial produced response rates of 14% for both FAM and SMF.[146] In an even larger two-arm trial organized by Cancer and Acute Leukemia Group B, FAM again produced a 14% response (9/63), versus only 4% (3/66) for SMF.[147]

TABLE 42-11. *Randomized prospective trials comparing FAM and SMF in pancreatic cancer*

Group	Response		Reference
	FAM	SMF	
GITSG	14%	14%	GITSG[146]
CALGB	14%	4%	Oster et al[147]

Other variations of the FAM regimen have also been tested in pancreatic cancer. A combination (FAM-S) incorporating both mitomycin-C and streptozotocin, produced promising results in a small initial study.[148] Addition of chlorozotocin[149] or methyl-CCNU[150] to FAM have both produced disappointing results. Other combinations based on 5-FU with chloroethylnitrosoureas, although less extensively studied than FAM and SMF, have also been uniformly discouraging. A prospectively randomized study comparing 5-FU/methyl-CCNU (FMe) with 5-FU/mitomycin-C (FM) was reported by SWOG, and resulted in a 5% response rate (2/43) for FMe versus 22% (10/45) for FM.[151] The FAP combination was explored by Moertel and colleagues in two studies with response rates of 21% and 15%.[152,153]

The results of all of these trials suggest that the response rates of FAM, SMF, and their variants in pancreatic cancer are substantially less than those which were seen in the early single-institution studies. Even more disappointing is the fact that neither of these regimens nor any other has had any impact on survival. Even in the single-institution trials that produced high response rates, median survival has remained less than 6 months, with only 10% or so surviving for as long as 1 year. A large trial by the Veterans Administration Surgical Oncology Group randomized 152 patients with advanced pancreatic cancer between a regimen of 5-FU + CCNU and supportive care only.[154] Survival of the chemotherapy group was actually poorer than the control group (3.0 vs. 3.9 months), but the difference was not significant. In another trial with survival as the primary outcome, NCCTG randomized 144 patients with advanced pancreatic carcinoma among three arms: FAM, FA (without mitomycin-C), and bolus 5-FU monotherapy.[83] All three treatments showed identical median survival of 5 months.

Only a single trial has suggested that chemotherapy could prolong survival in pancreatic cancer, compared with supportive care.[155] That small trial of the Mallinson regimen (an induction cycle of 5-FU, cyclophosphamide, methotrexate, and vincristine, followed by maintenance with 5-FU and mitomycin-C) could not be confirmed in a much larger phase III trial by the NCCTG.[153] In the latter study, median survival with the Mallinson regimen was only 19.5 weeks, not significantly different from the 15.2 weeks of the 5-FU monotherapy control arm. There is still no good evidence for a survival benefit from any chemotherapy in pancreatic cancer (Table 42-12).

It would appear that new agents will be required before there are any breakthroughs in the development of truly effective chemotherapy for pancreatic cancer. One avenue for exploration

TABLE 42-12. *Advanced pancreatic cancer: comparison of survival in large chemotherapy trials with the natural history of the disease*

Center or group	Treatment	Median survival (weeks)
GITSG[146]	FAM	12
	SMF	18
CALGB[147]	FAM	26
	SMF	18
SWOG[144]	SMF	21
	MF	18
NCCTG[83]	FAM	18
	FA	21
	F	21
NCCTG[153]	Mallinson regimen	19
	FAP	15
MSKCC[156]	(Natural history of unresectable disease)	17–22

Abbreviations: GITSG, Gastrointestinal Tumor Study Group; CALGE, Cancer and Acute Leukemia Group B; SWOG, Southwest Oncology Group; NCCTG, North Central Cancer Treatment Group; MSKCC, Memorial Sloan-Kettering Cancer Center; F, fluorouracil; A, doxorubicin; M, mitomycin C; P, cisplatin; S, streptozotocin.

Reproduced with permission form Ahlgren JD. Chemotherapy for pancreatic cancer. Cancer 1996; 78(3 suppl.).

with current agents would be the integration of 5-FU with modulators, or of PIF, into combination regimens. PIF has some promise in this regard because it has almost no myelotoxicity. Thus, full therapeutic doses of other drugs should be possible. This approach has been explored by the Mid-Atlantic Oncology Program in phase II trials of PIF with weekly low-dose cisplatin and carboplatin. With approximately 55 patients in each trial, the PIF/cisplatin trial showed a response rate of only 16%, but an encouraging 1-year survival of 25%,[157] The PIF/carboplatin trial (as yet unpublished) showed a response rate of 19% in preliminary analysis, with very low toxicity. Another phase II trial based on PIF, in which weekly leucovorin and dipyridamole were added to modulate the 5-FU and mitomycin-C was the second cytotoxic drug, was reported to produce a very high response rate in locally advanced patients. That trial yielded objective responses in 17 of 46 patients (37%, 4 CRs), with median survival greater than 15 months, and 4 patients converted to resectability after chemotherapy.[158] If confirmed, this result would be substantially better than other combinations evaluated thus far.

Summary and Outlook

The promise of combination chemotherapy in pancreatic cancer is yet to be realized. No regimen has demonstrated repeatable response rates greater than 20%, and no regimen can be considered standard therapy. Participation in rational clinical trials is to be encouraged, but the palliative nature of chemotherapy and quality-of-life issues must always be borne in mind. Regimens based on low-toxicity infusional schedules of 5-FU, or on 5-FU with modulators, continue to be explored. The potential appears limited, but should probably be better than the status quo.

REFERENCES

1. Moertel CG, Reitemeyer RJ. Advanced gastrointestinal cancer: clinical management and chemotherapy. New York: Harper and Row, 1969.
2. Oken MM, Davis TE, Creech RH, et al. Toxicity and response criteria of the Eastern Cooperative Oncology Group. Am J Clin Oncol 1982; 5:549.
3. Uren RF, Hutcherson RJ, Stephen MS, Wong J. Liver scanning in patients with suspected metastatic malignant disease. Med J Aust 1976;ii:477.
4. Warr D, McKinney S, Tannock I. Influence of measurement error on assessment of response to anticancer chemotherapy: proposal for new criteria of tumor response. J Clin Oncol 1984;2:1040.
5. Ahlgren JD. Chemotherapy for pancreatic cancer. Carcinoma 1996; 78(suppl).
6. Fojo AT, Ueda K, Slamon DJ, et al. Expression of a multidrug-resistance gene in human tumors and tissues. Proc Natl Acad Sci U S A 1987;84:265.
7. Kartner N, Riorden JR, Ling V. Cell surface P-glycoprotein associated with multidrug resistance in mammalian cell lines. Science 1983;221: 1285.
8. Roninson IB, Chin JE, Choi K, et al. Isolation of human *mdr* DNA sequences amplified in multidrug-resistant KB carcinoma cells. Proc Natl Acad Sci U S A 1986;83:4538.
9. Gros P, Croop J, Roninson I, et al. Isolation and characterization of DNA sequences amplified in multidrug-resistant hamster cells. Proc Natl Acad Sci U S A 1986;83:337.
10. Gottesman MM, Pasten I. Biochemistry of multidrug resistance mediated by the multidrug transporter. Annu Rev Biochem 1993;62:385.
11. Gros P, Croop J, Housman D. Mammalian multidrug resistance gene: complete cDNA sequence indicates strong homology to bacterial transport proteins. Cell 1986;47:371.
12. Morrow CS, Cowan KH. Glutathione S-transferases and drug resistance. Cancer Cells 1990;2:15.
13. Park J-G, Kramer BS, Lai S-L, et al. Chemosensitivity patterns and expression of human multidrug resistance-associated MDR1 gene by human gastric and colorectal carcinoma cell lines. J Natl Cancer Inst 1990;82:193.
14. Forastiere AA, Orringer MB, Perez-Tamayo C, et al. Concurrent chemotherapy and radiation therapy followed by transhiatal esophagectomy for local-regional cancer of the esophagus. J Clin Oncol 1990;8:119.
15. Kelsen D. Chemotherapy of esophageal cancer. Semin Oncol 1984; 11:159.
16. Panettiere FJ, Leichman LP, Tilchen EJ, Chen TT. Chemotherapy for advanced epidermoid carcinoma of the esophagus with single-agent cisplatin: final report on Southwest Oncology Group study. Cancer Treat Rep 1984;68:1023.
17. Ravry M, Moore M. Phase II pilot study of cisplatinum (II) in advanced squamous cell esophageal cancer. (Abstract) Proceedings of the American Association of Cancer Research/American Society of Clinical Oncology 1980;21:353.
18. Davis S, Shanmugathasa M, Kessler W. *cis*-Dichlorodiammine platinum(II) in the treatment of esophageal carcinoma. Cancer Treat Rep 1980;64:709.
19. Engstrom PF, Lavin PT, Klaassen DJ. Phase II evaluation of mitomycin and cisplatin in advanced esophageal carcinoma. Cancer Treat Rep 1983;67:713.
20. Ezdinli EZ, Gelber R, Desai DV, et al. Chemotherapy of advanced esophageal carcinoma: Eastern Cooperative Oncology Group experience. Cancer 1980;46:2149.
21. Lokich JJ, Shea M, Chaffey J. Sequential infusion of 5-fluorouracil followed by concomitant radiation for tumors of the esophagus and gastroesophageal junction. Cancer 1987;60:275.
22. Strack M, Wadler S, Lyver A, Wiernik P. Phase II trial of fluorouracil (5FU) and recombinant alpha-2a-interferon (rIFNα2a) in patients (pts) with advanced carcinoma of the esophagus. (Abstract) Proceedings of the American Society of Clinical Oncology 1990;9:119.
23. Ajani JA, Ilson DH, Daugherty K, et al. Activity of Taxol in patients with squamous cell carcinoma and adenocarcinoma of the esophagus. J Natl Cancer Inst 1994;86:1086.
24. Ravry M, Moertel CG, Schutt AJ, et al. Treatment of advanced squa-

mous cell carcinoma of the gastrointestinal tract with bleomycin (NSC 125066). Cancer Chemother Rep 1973;57:493.
25. Kolaric K, Maričic Z, Dujnovic I, et al. Therapy of advanced esophageal cancer with bleomycin, irradiation and combination bleomycin and irradiation. Tumori 1976;62:255.
26. Bonnadonna G, de Lena M, Monfardini S, et al. Clinical trial of bleomycin in lymphomas and solid tumors. Eur J Cancer Clin Oncol 1972; 8:205.
27. Roth A. Combination of chemotherapy and irradiation: a new approach to the treatment of locally advanced esophageal cancer. Recent Results Cancer Res 1988;110:30.
28. Advani SH, Saikia TK, Swaroop S. Anterior chemotherapy in esophageal cancer. Cancer 1985;56:1502.
29. Kelsen DP, Bains MF, Cvitkovic E, Golbey R. Vindesine in the treatment of esophageal carcinoma: a phase II study. Cancer Treat Rep 1979;63:2019.
30. Bezwoda WR, Derman DP, Weaving A, Nisselbaum M. Treatment of esophageal cancer with vindesine: an open trial. Cancer Treat Rep 1984;68:783.
31. Japanese Esophageal Oncology Group (Iizuka T, Kakegawa T, Ide H, et al). A phase II study of vindesine in the treatment of esophageal carcinoma: Japanese Esophageal Oncology Group. Jpn J Clin Oncol 1989;19:380.
32. Faldson G. Methyl-GAG (NSC 32946) in the treatment of esophagus cancer. Cancer Chemother Rep 1971;55:209.
33. Schabel FM Jr, Trader MW, Laster WR Jr, et al. *cis*-dichlorodiammineplatinum(II): combination chemotherapy and cross-resistance studies with tumors of mice. Cancer Treat Rep 1979;63:1459.
34. Scanlon KJ, Newman EM, Lu Y, Priest DG. Biochemical basis for cisplatin and 5-fluorouracil synergism in human ovarian carcinoma cells. Proc Natl Acad Sci U S A 1986;83:8923.
35. Kish JA, Ensley JF, Jacobs J, et al. A randomized trial of cisplatin (CACP) + 5-fluorouracil (5-FU) infusion and CACP + 5-FU bolus in recurrent and advanced squamous cell carcinoma of the head and neck. Cancer 1985;56:2740.
36. Hilgenberg AD, Carey RW, Wilkins EW Jr, et al. Preoperative chemotherapy, surgical resection, and selective postoperative therapy for squamous cell carcinoma of the esophagus. Ann Thorac Surg 1988; 45:357.
37. Carey RW, Hilgenberg AD, Grillo HC, et al. Esophageal carcinoma: long term follow-up of patients treated by neo-adjuvant chemotherapy, surgery and possible postoperative radiation and/or chemotherapy. (Abstract) Proceedings of the American Society of Clinical Oncology 1990;9:105.
38. Kies MS, Rosen ST, Tsang T-K, et al. Cisplatin and 5-fluorouracil in the primary management of squamous esophageal cancer. Cancer 1987;60:2156.
39. Ajani J, McMurtrey M, Rich T, et al. Combined modality therapy with effective prolonged systemic component for the locally advanced squamous cell carcinoma of the esophagus (SCCE). (Abstract) Proceedings of the American Society of Clinical Oncology 1987;6:82.
40. Lester EP, Pate JW, Memula NG, et al. Esophageal carcinoma: results of initial chemotherapy with methotrexate (MTX), leucovorin (L), cisplatinum (CDDP), and 5-fluorouracil (5-FU). (Abstract) Proceedings of the American Society of Clinical Oncology 1990;9:115.
41. Ajani JA, Ilson D, Bhalla A, et al. Taxol®, cisplatin, and 5-FU (TCF): a multi-institutional phase II study in patients with carcinoma of the esophagus. (Abstract) Proceedings of the American Society of Clinical Oncology 1995;14:203.
42. Okayuma S, Mishina H. Consecutive therapy of cancer aimed at perpetuation of repairable damage: a hypothesis unifying radiotherapy and chemotherapy. J Clin Hematol Oncol 1980;10:83.
43. Kelsen DP, Cvitkovic E, Bains M, et al. *Cis*-dichlorodiammineplatinum(II) and bleomycin in the treatment of esophageal carcinoma. Cancer Treat Rep 1978;62:1041.
44. Bosset JF, Hurteloup P, Bontemps P, et al. A phase II trial of bleomycin and cisplatin (CDDP) in advanced oesophagus carcinoma. (Abstract) International Cancer Congress, (abstract) 1982:41.
45. Coonley DJ, Bains M, Hilaris B, et al. Cisplatin and bleomycin in the treatment of esophageal carcinoma: a final report. Cancer 1984; 54:2351.
46. Kelsen DP, Bains M, Hilaris B, et al. Combination chemotherapy of esophageal carcinoma using cisplatin, vindesine, and bleomycin. Cancer 1982;49:1174.
47. Kelsen DP, Minsky B, Smith M, et al. Preoperative therapy for esophageal cancer: a randomized comparison of chemotherapy versus radiation therapy. J Clin Oncol 1990;8:1352.
48. Dinwoodie WR, Bartolucci AA, Lyman GH, et al. Phase II evaluation of cisplatin, bleomycin and vindesine in advanced squamous cell carcinoma of the esophagus: a Southeastern Cancer Study Group trial. Cancer Treat Rep 1986;70:267.
49. Vogl SE, Greenwald E, Kaplan BH. Effective chemotherapy of esophageal cancer with methotrexate, bleomycin, and cis-diamminedichloroplatinum II. Cancer 1981;48:2555.
50. DeBasi P, Salvagno L, Endrizzi L, et al. Cisplatin, bleomycin and methotrexate in the treatment of advanced oesophageal cancer. Eur J Cancer Clin Oncol 1984;20:743.
51. Kukla L, Lad T, McGuire WP, Thomas P. Multimodality therapy of squamous carcinoma of the esophagus. (Abstract) Proceedings of the American Association of Cancer Researchers/American Society of Clinical Oncology 1981;22:449.
52. Kelsen DP, Fein R, Coonley C, et al. Cisplatin, vindesine, and mitoguazone in the treatment of esophageal cancer. Cancer Treat Rep 1986; 70:255.
53. Forastiere AA, Gennis M, Orringer MB, Agha FP. Cisplatin, vinblastine, and mitoguazone chemotherapy for epidermoid and adenocarcinoma of the esophagus. J Clin Oncol 1987;5:1143.
54. Vogl SE, Camacho F, Berenzweig M, Ruckdeschel J. Chemotherapy for esophageal cancer with mitoguazone, methotrexate, bleomycin, and cisplatin. Cancer Treat Rep 1985;69:21.
55. Gisselbrecht C, Calvo F, Mignot L, et al. Fluorouracil (F), Adriamycin (A) and cisplatin (P) (FAP): combination chemotherapy of advanced esophageal carcinoma. Cancer 1983;52:974.
56. Lovett D, Kelsen D, Eisenberger M, Houston C. A phase II trial of carboplatin and vinblastine in the treatment of advanced squamous cell carcinoma of the esophagus. Cancer 1991;67:354.
57. Macdonald JS, Schein PS, Woolley PV, et al. 5-Fluorouracil, doxorubicin and mitomycin (FAM) combination chemotherapy for advanced gastric cancer. Ann Intern Med 1980;93:533.
58. Goldstein LJ, Galski H, Fojo A, et al. Expression of a multidrug resistance gene in human cancers. J Natl Cancer Inst 1989;81:116.
59. Mizoguchi T, Yamada K, Furukawa T, et al. Expression of MDR1 gene in human gastric and colorectal carcinomas. J Natl Cancer Inst 1990;82:1679.
60. Comis R. Integration of chemotherapy into combined modality treatment of solid tumors. Cancer Treat Rev 1974;221.
61. Miyuihan T, Hansen R, Anderson T, et al. Continuous 5-fluorouracil infusion in advanced gastric carcinoma. Am J Clin Oncol 1988;11: 461.
62. Machover D, Goldschmidt E, Chollet P, et al. Treatment of advanced colorectal and gastric adenocarcinomas with 5-fluorouracil and high dose folinic acid. J Clin Oncol 1986;4:685.
63. Arbuck SG, Douglass HO Jr, Trave F, et al. A phase II study of 5-fluorouracil and high dose folinic acid in gastric carcinoma. J Clin Oncol 1987;5:115.
64. Berenberg JL, Goodman PJ, Oishi N, et al. 5-Fluorouracil (5FU) and folinic acid (FA) for the treatment of metastatic gastric cancer. (Abstract) Proceedings of the American Society of Clinical Oncology 1989;8:101.
65. Bjerkeset T, Fjosne H. comparison of oral Ftorafur and intravenous 5-fluorouracil in patients with advanced cancer of the stomach, colon, or rectum. Oncology 1986;43:212.
66. Palmeri S, Gebbia V, Russo A, et al. Oral tegafur in the treatment of gastrointestinal tract cancer: a phase II study. Br J Cancer 1990;61: 475.
67. Malik STA, Talbot D, Clarke PI, et al. Phase II trial of UFT in advanced colorectal and gastric cancer. Br J Cancer 1990;62:1023.
68. Saltz LB, Leichman CG, Young CW. A fixed-ratio combination of uracil and ftorafur (UFT) with low dose leucovorin: an active oral regimen for advanced colorectal cancer. Cancer 1995;75:782.
69. Cazap E, Bruno M, Levy D, et al. Phase II trial of 4′-epidoxorubicin (4′epi-dx) in advanced gastric cancer. (Abstract) Proceedings of the American Society of Clinical Oncology 1986;5:91.
70. DeVries E, Nanninga AG, Greidanus J, et al. A phase II study of a 21 day continuous infusion schedule with epirubicin in advanced gastric cancer. Eur J Cancer Clin Oncol 1989;25:1509.
71. Lacave A, Izarzugaza I, Aparicio L, et al. Phase II clinical trial of

cis-dichlorodiammineplatinum in gastric cancer. Am J Clin Oncol 1983;6:35.

72. Beer M, Cocconi G, Ceci G, et al. A phase II study of cisplatin in advanced gastric cancer. Eur J Cancer Clin Oncol 1983;19:717.
73. Leichman L, McDonald B, Dindogru A, et al. Cisplatin: an active drug in the treatment of disseminated gastric cancer. Cancer 1984; 53:18.
74. Bruckner H, Lokich J, Stablein D. Studies of Baker's antifol, methotrexate and razoxane in advanced gastric cancer: a Gastrointestinal Tumor Study Group report. Cancer Treat Rep 1982;66:1713.
75. Asbury RF, Cuaan A, Haller D, Eastern Cooperative Oncology Group (ECOG). Phase II study of trimmetrexate (TMTX) in metastatic gastric cancer. (Abstract) Proceedings of the American Society of Clinical Oncology 1990;9:126.
76. Schnitzler G, Queisser W, Heim M, et al. Phase III study of 5-FU and carmustine versus 5-FU, carmustine and doxorubicin in advanced gastric cancer. Cancer Treat Rep 1986;70:477.
77. Moore G, Bross I, Aussman R, et al. Effects of chlorambucil (NSC-3088) in 374 patients with advanced cancer. Cancer Chemother Rep 1968;52:661.
78. Hurley J, Ellison E, Carey L. Treatment of advanced cancer of the gastrointestinal tract with antitumor agents. Gastroenterology 1961; 41:557.
79. Preusser P, Wilke H, Achterrath W, et al. Phase II study of the combination of etoposide, doxorubicin and cisplatin in advanced measurable gastric cancer. J Clin Oncol 1989;7:1310.
80. Wilke H, Preusser P, Fink U, et al. High dose folinic acid/etoposide/5-fluorouracil in advanced gastric cancer: a phase II study in elderly patients or patients with cardiac risk. Invest New Drugs 1990;8:65.
81. Douglass HO, Lavin PT, Goudsmit A, et al. An Eastern Cooperative Oncology Group evaluation of combinations of methyl-CCNU, mitomycin-C, Adriamycin, and 5-fluorouracil in advanced measurable gastric cancer (EST 2277). J Clin Oncol 1984;2:1372.
82. Beretta G, Fraschini P, Labianca R, Luporini G. The value of FAM poly-chemotherapy in advanced gastric carcinoma. (Abstract) Proceedings of the American Society of Clinical Oncology 1982;1:103.
83. Cullinan S, Moertel CG, Fleming T, et al. A comparison of three chemotherapeutic regimens in the treatment of advanced pancreatic and gastric carcinoma: fluorouracil *vs* fluorouracil and doxorubicin *vs* fluorouracil, doxorubicin, and mitomycin. JAMA 1985;253:2061.
84. Bitran JD, Desser RK, Kozloff MF, et al. Treatment of metastatic pancreatic and gastric adenocarcinomas with 5-fluorouracil, Adriamycin and mitomycin-C (FAM). Cancer Treat Rep 1979;63:2049.
85. Klein H, Wickramanayake P, Farrokh G. 5FU, Adriamycin and methotrexate: a combination protocol (FAMTX) for treatment of metastatic stomach cancer. (Abstract) Proceedings of the American Society of Clinical Oncology 1986;5:84.
86. Wils J, Bleiberg H, Dalesio O, et al. An EORTC Gastrointestinal Group evaluation of the combination of sequential methotrexate and 5-fluorouracil, combined with Adriamycin in advanced measurable gastric cancer. J Clin Oncol 1986;4:1799.
87. Wils JA, Klein HO, Wagener DJTh, et al. Sequential high-dose methotrexate and fluorouracil combined with doxorubicin—a step ahead in the treatment of advanced gastric cancer: a trial of the European Organization for Research and Treatment of Cancer Gastrointestinal Tract Cooperative Group. J Clin Oncol 1991;9:827.
88. Kelsen D, Atiq OT, Saltz L, et al. FAMTX versus etoposide, doxorubicin, and cisplatin: a random assignment trial in gastric cancer. J Clin Oncol 1992;10:541.
89. Murad AM, Santiago FF, Petroianu A, et al. Modified therapy with 5-fluorouracil, doxorubicin, and methotrexate in advanced gastric cancer. Cancer 1993;72:37.
90. Katz A, Gansl R, Simon S, et al. Phase II trial of VP16, Adriamycin, and cisplatinum in patients with advanced gastric cancer. (Abstract) Proceedings of the American Society of Clinical Oncology 1989;8: 98.
91. Lerner A, Steele GD, Mayer RJ. Etoposide, doxorubicin, cisplatin chemotherapy for advanced gastric adenocarcinoma: results of a phase II trial. J Clin Oncol 1992;10:536.
92. Wilke H, Preusser P, Fink U, et al. New developments in the treatment of gastric carcinoma. Semin Oncol 1990;17(Suppl 2):61.
93. Vaughn DJ, Holroyde C, Meropol NJ, et al. A phase II trial of 5-fluorouracil, leucovorin, Adriamycin, and cisplatin (FLAP) in patients with advanced gastric and gastroesophageal junction adenocarcinoma: a Penn Cancer Center Clinical Trials Group (PCCTG) and Roswell Park Cancer Institute (RPCI) trial. (Abstract) Proceedings of the American Society of Clinical Oncology 1995;14:197.
94. Rougier Ph, Ducreux M, Mahjoubi M, et al. Efficacy of combined 5-fluorouracil and cisplatinum in advanced gastric carcinomas: a phase II trial with prognostic factor analysis. Eur J Cancer 1994;30A: 1263.
95. Ohtsu A, Shimada Y, Yoshida S, et al. Phase II study of protracted infusional 5-fluorouracil combined with cisplatinum for advanced gastric cancer: report from the Japan Clinical Oncology Group (JCOG). Eur J Cancer 1994;30A:2091.
96. Di Lauro L, Capomolla E, Vici P, et al. Cislatin, epirubicin and fluorouracil (PEF) for advanced measurable gastric carcinoma. (Abstract) Proceedings of the American Society of Clinical Oncology 1995;14: 206.
97. Cocconi G, Bella M, Zironi S, et al. Fluorouracil, doxorubicin, and mitomycin combination versus PELF chemotherapy in advanced gastric cancer: a randomized trial of the Italian Oncology Group for Clinical Research. J Clin Oncol 1994;12:2687.
98. Cascinu S, Labianca R, Fedeli A, et al. Phase II trial of intensive weekly chemotherapy for advanced gastric cancer using 5-fluorouracil (5FU); cisplatin (CDDP); epi-doxorubicin (epi-ADR); glutathione (GSH) and granulocyte colony stimulating factor (G-CSF): an Italian Gastrointestinal Tumors Group (GISCAD) study. (Abstract) Proceedings of the American Society of Clinical Oncology 1995;14:190.
99. Cornell GN, Cahow CE, Frey C, et al. Clinical experience with 5-fluorouracil (NSC-19893) in the treatment of malignant disease. Cancer Chemother Rep 1960;9:23.
100. Hurley JD, Ellison EH. Treatment of advanced cancer with 5-fluorouracil. Ann Surg 1960;152:568.
101. Carter SK, Comis L. The integration of chemotherapy into a combined modality approach for cancer treatment: VI. pancreatic adenocarcinoma. Cancer Treat Rev 1975;2:193.
102. O'Connell MJ. Current status of chemotherapy for advanced pancreatic and gastric cancer. J Clin Oncol 1985;3:1032.
103. Moertel CG. Chemotherapy of gastrointestinal cancer. Clin Gastroenterol 1976;5:777.
104. Ahlgren JD. Pancreatic cancer: chemotherapy of advanced disease. In: Ahlgren JD, Macdonald JS, eds. Gastrointestinal oncology. Philadelphia: JB Lippincott, 1992:227.
105. Erlichman C, Fine S, Wong A, Elhakim T. A randomized trial of fluorouracil with folinic acid in patients with metastatic colorectal carcinoma. J Clin Oncol 1988;6:469.
106. Lokich JJ, Ahlgren JD, Gullo JJ, et al. A prospective randomized comparison of continuous infusion fluorouracil with a conventional bolus schedule in metastatic colorectal carcinoma: a Mid-Atlantic Oncology Program study. J Clin Oncol 1989;7:425.
107. Petrelli N, Douglass HO, Herrera L, et al. The modulation of fluorouracil with leucovorin in metastatic colorectal carcinoma: a prospective randomized phase III trial. J Clin Oncol 1989;7:1419.
108. Poon MA, O'Connell MJ, Moertel CG, et al. Biochemical modulation of fluorouracil: evidence of significant improvement in survival and quality of life in patients with advanced colorectal carcinoma. J Clin Oncol 1989;7:1407.
109. Petrelli N, Herrera L, Rustum Y, et al. A prospective randomized trial of 5-fluorouracil versus 5-fluorouracil and high-dose leucovorin versus 5-fluorouracil and methotrexate in previously untreated patients with advanced colorectal carcinoma. J Clin Oncol 1987;5:1559.
110. Lokich JJ, Ahlgren JD, Cantrell J, et al. A prospective randomized comparison of protracted infusional 5-fluorouracil with or without weekly bolus cisplatin in metastatic colorectal carcinoma: a Mid-Atlantic Oncology Program study. Cancer 1991;67:14.
111. Caudry M, Bonnel C, Floquet A, et al. A randomized study of bolus fluorouracil plus folinic acid versus 21-day fluorouracil infusion alone or in association with cyclophosphamide and mitomycin C in advanced colorectal carcinoma. Am J Clin Oncol 1995;18:118.
112. Leichman CG, Fleming TR, Muggia FM, et al. Phase II study of fluorouracil and its modulation in advanced colorectal cancer: a Southwest Oncology Group study. J Clin Oncol 1995;13:1303.
113. DeCaprio JA, Mayer RJ, Gonin R, Arbuck SG. Fluorouracil and high-dose leucovorin in previously untreated patients with advanced adenocarcinomas of the pancreas: results of a phase II trial. J Clin Oncol 1991;9:2128.
114. Crown J, Casper ES, Botet J, et al. Lack of efficacy of high-dose

leucovorin and fluorouracil in patients with advanced pancreatic adenocarcinoma. J Clin Oncol 1991;9:1682.
115. Wadler S, Schwartz EL, Goldman M, et al. Fluorouracil and recombinant alfa-2a-interferon: an active regimen against advanced colorectal carcinoma. J Clin Oncol 1989;7:1769.
116. Kemeny N, Younes A, Seiter K, et al. Interferon alpha-2a and 5-fluorouracil for advanced colorectal carcinoma: assessment of activity and toxicity. Cancer 1990;66:2470.
117. Pazdur R, Ajani JA, Patt YZ, et al. A phase II study of fluorouracil and recombinant interferon alfa-2a in previously untreated advanced colorectal carcinoma. J Clin Oncol 1990;8:2027.
118. Pazdur R, Ajani JJ, Abbruzzese JL, et al. Phase II evaluation of fluorouracil and recombinant α-2a-interferon in previously untreated patients with pancreatic adenocarcinoma. Cancer 1992;70:2073.
119. Scheithauer W, Pfeffel F, Kernek G, et al. A phase II trial of fluorouracil, leucovorin, and recombinant alpha-2b-interferon in advanced adenocarcinoma of the pancreas. Cancer 1992;70:1864.
120. Bernhard H, Jäger-Arand E, Bernhard G, et al. Treatment of advanced pancreatic cancer with 5-fluorouracil, folinic acid and interferon alpha-2A: results of a phase II trial. Br J Cancer 1995;71:102.
121. Schneider CJ, Vaughn DJ, Holroyde B, et al. Phase II trial of 5-FU, leucovorin, and interferon alpha 2A in metastatic pancreatic carcinoma: a Penn Cancer Clinical Trials Group (PCCTG) trial. (Abstract) Proceedings of the American Society of Clinical Oncology 1995;14: 189.
122. Ardalan B, Singh G, Silberman H. A randomized phase I and II study of short-term infusion of high-dose fluorouracil with or without N-(phosphonacetyl)-L-aspartic acid in patients with advanced pancreatic and colorectal cancers. J Clin Oncol 1988;6:1053.
123. Rosvold E, Schilder R, Walczak J, et al. Phase II trial of PALA in combination with 5-fluorouracil in advanced pancreatic cancer. Cancer Chemother Pharmacol 1992;29:305.
124. Schein PS, Lavin PT, Moertel CG, et al. Randomized phase II clinical trial of Adriamycin, methotrexate, and actinomycin-D in advanced measurable pancreatic carcinoma: a Gastrointestinal Tumor Study Group report. Cancer 1978;42:19.
125. Rothenberg ML, Burris HA III, Andersen JS, et al. Gemcitabine: effective palliative therapy for pancreas cancer patients failing 5-FU. (Abstract) Proceedings of the American Society of Clinical Oncology 1995;14:198.
126. Moore M, Andersen J, Burris H, et al. A randomized trial of gemcitabine (GEM) versus 5FU as first-line therapy in advanced pancreatic cancer. (Abstract) Proceedings of the American Society of Clinical Oncology 1995;14:199.
127. Horton J, Gelber R, Engstrom P, et al. Trials of single agent and combination chemotherapy for advanced cancer of the pancreas. Cancer Treat Rep 1981;65:65.
128. Smith DB, Kenny JB, Scarffe JH, et al. Phase II evaluation of melphalan in adenocarcinoma of the pancreas. Cancer Treat Rep 1985;69: 917.
129. Loehrer PJ, Williams SD, Einhorn LH, Ansari R. Ifosfamide: an active drug in the treatment of adenocarcinoma of the pancreas. J Clin Oncol 1985;3:367.
130. Bernard S, Noble S, Wilcosky T, et al. A phase II trial of ifosfamide (IFOS) plus N-acetyl cysteine (NAC) in metastatic measureable pancreatic carcinoma (PC). (Abstract) Proceedings of the American Society of Clinical Oncology 1986;5:328.
131. Ajani JA, Abbruzzese JL, Goudeau P, et al. Ifosfamide and mesna: marginally active in patients with advanced carcinoma of the pancreas. J Clin Oncol 1988;6:1703.
132. Gastrointestinal Tumor Study Group. Ifosfamide is an inactive substance in the treatment of pancreatic carcinoma. Cancer 1989;64:2010.
133. Moertel CG, Schutt AJ, Reitemeier RJ, Hahn RG. Therapy of gastrointestinal cancer with the nitrosoureas alone and in drug combination. Cancer Treat Rep 1976;60:729.
134. Moertel CG, Douglass HO, Hanley J, Carbone PP. Phase II study of methyl-CCNU in the treatment of advanced pancreatic carcinoma. Cancer Treat Rep 1976;60:1659.
135. Wils J, Bleiberg H, Blijham G, et al. Phase-II study of epirubicin in advanced adenocarcinoma of the pancreas. Eur J Cancer Clin Oncol 1985;21:191.
136. Gastrointestinal Tumor Study Group. Phase II trials of hexamethylmelamine, dianhydrogalactitol, razoxane, and beta-2′-deoxythioguanosine as single agents against advanced measurable tumors of the pancreas. Cancer Treat Rep 1985;69:713.
137. Smith FP, Stablein DM, Schein PS. Phase II combination chemotherapy trials in advanced measureable pancreatic cancer. (Abstract) Proceedings of the American Society of Clinical Oncology 1984;3:150.
138. Gad-El-Mawla N, Ziegler JL. Ifosfamide treatment of pancreatic cancer. Cancer Treat Rep 1981;65:357.
139. Gad-El-Mawla N. Ifosfamide in advanced pancreatic cancer: a 5-year experience. Cancer Chemother Pharmacol 1986;18(Suppl):55.
140. Smith FP, Hoth DF, Levin B, et al. 5-Fluorouracil, Adriamycin, and mitomycin-C (FAM) chemotherapy for advanced adenocarcinoma of the pancreas. Cancer 1980;46:2014.
141. Bitran JD, Desser RK, Kazloff MF, et al. Treatment of metastatic pancreatic and gastric adenocarcinomas with 5-fluorouracil, Adriamycin, and mitomycin C (FAM). Cancer Treat Rep 1979;63:2049.
142. Wiggans RG, Woolley PV, Macdonald JS, et al. Phase II trial of streptozotocin, mitomycin-C and 5-fluorouracil (SMF) in the treatment of advanced pancreatic cancer. Cancer 1978;41:387.
143. Bukowski RM, Aberhalden RT, Hewlett JS, et al. Phase II trial of streptozotocin, mitomycin-C and 5-fluorouracil in adenocarcinoma of the pancreas. Cancer Clinical Trials 1980;3:321.
144. Bukowski RM, Balcerzak SP, O'Bryan RM, et al. Randomized trial of 5-fluorouracil and mitomycin C with or without streptozotocin for advanced pancreatic cancer. Cancer 1983;52:1577.
145. Theologides A, Cooper MR, Rafla S, et al. Fluorouracil + Adriamycin + mitomycin C in advanced pancreatic cancer. (Abstract) Proceedings of the American Society of Clinical Oncology 1982;1:90.
146. Gastrointestinal Tumor Study Group. Phase II studies of drug combinations in advanced pancreatic carcinoma: fluorouracil plus doxorubicin plus mitomycin C and two regimens of streptozotocin plus mitomycin C plus fluorouracil. J Clin Oncol 1986;4:1794.
147. Oster MW, Gray R, Panasci L, Perry MC. Chemotherapy for advanced pancreatic cancer: a comparison of 5-fluorouracil, Adriamycin, and mitomycin (FAM) with 5-fluorouracil, streptozotocin, and mitomycin (FSM). Cancer 1986;57:29.
148. Bukowski RM, Schacter LP, Groppe CW, et al. Phase II trial of 5-fluorouracil, Adriamycin, mitomycin C, and streptozotocin (FAM-S) in pancreatic cancer. Cancer 1982;50:197.
149. Smith FP, Rustgi VK, Schertz G, et al. Phase II study of 5-FU, doxorubicin, and mitomycin (FAM) and chlorozotocin in advanced measurable pancreatic cancer. Cancer Treat Rep 1982;66:2095.
150. Karlin DA, Stroehlein JR, Bennetts RW, et al. Phase I–II study of the combination of 5-FU, doxorubicin, mitomycin, and semustine (FAMMe) in the treatment of adenocarcinoma of the stomach, gastroesophageal junction, and pancreas. Cancer Treat Rep 1982;66:1613.
151. Buroker T, Kim PN, Groppe C, et al. 5-fluorouracil infusion with mitomycin-C *vs* 5-FU infusion with methyl-CCNU in the treatment of advanced upper gastrointestinal cancer. Cancer 1979;44:1215.
152. Moertel CG, Rubin J, O'Connell MJ, et al. A phase II study of combined 5-fluorouracil, doxorubicin, and cisplatin in the treatment of advanced upper gastrointestinal adenocarcinomas. J Clin Oncol 1986; 7:1053.
153. Cullinan S, Moertel CG, Wieand HS, et al. A phase III trial on the therapy of advanced pancreatic carcinoma: evaluations of the Mallinson regimen and combined 5-fluorouracil, doxorubicin and cisplatin. Cancer 1990;65:2207.
154. Frey C, Twomey P, Keehn R, et al. Randomized study of 5-FU and CCNU in pancreatic cancer: report of the Veterans Administration Surgical Adjuvant Cancer Chemotherapy Group. Cancer 1981;47:27.
155. Mallinson CN, Rake MO, Cocking JB. Chemotherapy in pancreatic cancer: results of a controlled, prospective, randomised, multicentre trial. Br Med J 1980;281:1589.
156. Brennan MF, Kinsella TJ, Casper ES. Cancer of the pancreas. In: DeVita VT Jr, Hellmans, Rosenberg SA, eds. Cancer: principles and practice of oncology, 4th ed. Philadelphia: JB Lippincott, 1993:849.
157. Rothman H, Cantrell JE Jr, Lokich J, et al. Continuous infusion 5-fluorouracil plus weekly cisplatin for pancreatic carcinoma: a Mid-Atlantic Oncology Program study. Cancer 1991;68:264.
158. Isacoff WH, Reber H, Tompkins R, et al. Continuous infusion (CI) 5-fluorouracil (5-FU), calcium leucovorin (LV), mitomycin-C (Mito C) and dipyridamole (D): treatment for patients with locally advanced pancreatic cancer. (Abstract) Proceedings of the American Society of Clinical Oncology 1995;14:198.

PART V

Liver, Bile Duct, and Gallbladder

Surgery for Gastrointestinal Cancer: A Multidisciplinary Approach, edited by Harold J. Wanebo.
Lippincott-Raven Publishers, Philadelphia, © 1997.

CHAPTER 43

Hepatocarcinoma: Results With Resection (Western Experience)

Bernard Nordlinger and Emmanuel Tarla

Hepatocellular carcinoma (HCC) is common worldwide and causes more than 1 million deaths each year, primarily in Asia and sub-Saharan Africa.[1] In these high-risk regions, where the incidence is 30 per 100,000 inhabitants per year, it is a major public health problem. In North America and Northern Europe, HCC is less common, with fewer than 2 new cases diagnosed per 100,000 inhabitants per year.[2] In certain Latin European areas, however, the rate is higher than in other Western European countries, with an annual incidence of up to 10 per 100,000 for men.[3] These geographic differences in incidence between high-risk areas and Western countries seem to be attributable mainly to causative factors such as viral hepatitis B or C and alimentary hepatotoxins.[1] In North America and France, alcoholism is an important cause of the cirrhosis that leads to HCC.[4–8] In other Latin European countries, viral hepatitis is the principal cause of cirrhosis.[2,9] Liver cirrhosis is present in up to 90% of all patients with HCC and appears to be a major prognostic factor, increasing mortality and morbidity. The clinical presentation, treatment, and long-term results of HCC associated with liver cirrhosis or occurring in a previously normal liver are different.[10]

Twenty years ago, HCC usually was discovered at an advanced and inoperable stage. The prognosis remains poor today in symptomatic forms of the disease, which are unresectable in 90% of cases because of tumor size or severe underlying cirrhosis.[11] Most patients with untreated HCC die of hepatic failure or hemorrhage,[9] with a 1-year survival rate of 3% and a mean survival time of 4 months from the onset of symptoms.[12] However, improvements in the early detection of HCC through careful follow-up of high-risk patients,[13] better selection of patients for surgery, and the use of new procedures in liver surgery have improved the results of surgical resection, which usually is considered the treatment of choice for this disease.[14] In addition, new treatment modalities for HCC have become available during the last decade, such as transplantation, hepatic arterial chemoembolization, and percutaneous ethanol injection.[15,16]

Bernard Nordlinger, Centre de chirurgie digestive, Hôpital Saint Antoine, 184, rue du Fg Saint Antoine, 75571, Paris, France Cédex 12

Emmanuel Tarla, Centre de chirurgie digestive, Hôpital Saint Antoine, 184, rue du Fg Saint Antoine, 75571, Paris, France Cédex 12

PREOPERATIVE EVALUATION

Before a patient with HCC and cirrhosis of the liver can undergo surgery, it must be determined whether the tumor is resectable, whether liver function is sufficient to allow partial liver resection, and whether the patient can tolerate major liver surgery.

TUMOR STAGING

In general, asymptomatic HCC grows slowly, with a tumor volume doubling time estimated at 1 to 19 months.[1,17] The lesion should be diagnosed early, when it is potentially resectable and before symptoms such as right upper quadrant pain or an abdominal mass have developed. Because of the good results reported by Asian groups, systematic screening for tumor markers in high-risk patients and noninvasive imaging techniques are being used more often in Western countries, increasing the rate of discovery of small, asymptomatic tumors.[1,18,19]

Many modes of presentation can lead to the diagnosis of HCC, but regular follow-up of patients with chronic liver disease should be the most common one. Serum α-fetoprotein (AFP) assessment is the principal biochemical screening test for HCC. A sharp or progressive rise in the serum AFP level is uncommon in uncomplicated cirrhosis and requires further investigation, which may lead to the early detection of small tumors.[20] In most cases of symptomatic HCC, the serum AFP level is higher than 1000 ng/mL, but in two thirds of cases of small, asymptomatic HCC, the level is lower than 200 ng/mL.[1] The serum level of AFP is roughly proportional to the size of the tumor,[21] but only 60% to 95% of tumors secrete AFP. In fibrolamellar carcinoma, the serum AFP level often is within normal limits.[22,23] An increased serum AFP concentration is not specific for HCC and also can be seen in other conditions, such as chronic hepatitis.[1] However, the association of an elevated AFP level (particularly above 500 ng/mL) and a focal intrahepatic lesion on ultrasonography establishes the diagnosis in most cases.[7] HCC also can be discovered after spontaneous rupture, which is a common circumstance of diagnosis in Asia[24] and Africa. In a French multicenter study, 5.6% of 196 HCCs associated with cirrhosis were discovered after the tumors ruptured.[5]

The preoperative staging of HCC, particularly in cirrhotic livers, should address three questions:

1. Is there a liver tumor?
2. Is it an HCC?
3. Is it resectable according to the site, number, and vascular relations of liver deposits?

Regardless of the imaging technique used, the radiologist's report should provide the surgeon with a precise liver map analyzing the following factors:

1. The site of the tumor based on segmental anatomy[25]
2. The number and size of the tumor or tumors
3. The relations between the tumor, the portal branches, and the major hepatic veins
4. The volume and percentage of remnant liver parenchyma after the planned resection
5. The extrahepatic contiguous dissemination (eg, diaphragm, right adrenal)
6. The distant metastases to lung, bone, or peritoneum

Ultrasonography

Small HCCs usually appear as hypoechoic lesions, but in encapsulated tumors, the fibrous capsule may cast acoustic shadows. Any focal lesion discovered by sonography in a patient with chronic liver disease should be considered a possible HCC, particularly if it was not present on previous examinations. However, differentiation of HCC from regeneration nodules or benign hepatic tumors can be difficult and may require other imaging techniques.[26] Sonography may help to guide percutaneous biopsy if doubt persists in spite of the use of different imaging methods. In Europe, as in Asia, ultrasonography is the first imaging modality used when HCC is suspected, because it is the most sensitive procedure for small lesions[27] and can detect asymptomatic tumors measuring 1 cm.[28]

Computed Tomography

HCCs usually appear as low-density areas when compared with surrounding liver parenchyma. They also may be isodense, in which case differentiation is not possible without contrast enhancement. Computed tomography (CT) is a noninvasive method that can detect most tumors larger than 3 cm.[29]

Angiography

Mesenteric arteriography may be required before surgery for precise localization of the tumor and evaluation of the vascular anatomy or any aberrant arterial supply. In addition, CT performed 1 to 3 weeks after superior mesenteric artery injection of ultrafluid Lipiodol has a high sensitivity for the detection of small HCC and the discovery of daughter nodules within the liver.[30]

When the diagnosis remains uncertain in spite of the use of several imaging techniques,[26] a percutaneous needle biopsy can be performed. This procedure is associated with a risk of bleeding because of the high vascularity of HCC, particularly in superficial tumors.[6] In addition, iatrogenic tumor dissemination along the needle track has been reported after percutaneous or laparoscopic biopsy.[31–34] Laparoscopic vision-directed biopsy could be helpful in identifying superficial lesions that may be missed by imaging techniques.[35] However, in many cases the diagnosis is probable, preoperative biopsy can be avoided, and the lesion is identified during surgery with ultrasound-directed biopsy of the suspect area.

ASSESSMENT OF LIVER FUNCTION

Abdominal surgery in patients with cirrhosis carries an increased risk of mortality and morbidity.[5] In a series of 100 consecutive patients with liver cirrhosis operated on mainly for biliary tract disease, the operative mortality and morbidity rates were 30% each. Sepsis with multiple organ failure was responsible for 90% of deaths.[36] Postoperative complications are a major problem after abdominal surgery in patients with cirrhosis. Although liver surgery in general has become safer, the treatment of HCC with underlying cirrhosis remains a challenge. The main problems after liver resection in patients with cirrhosis are related to insufficient hepatic reserve, poor regeneration of cirrhotic parenchyma, and hemorrhage resulting from portal hypertension.[37,38] The liver is less able to regenerate in patients with cirrhosis, although complete restoration of the residual liver is possible[38] and major hepatectomy has proven successful in selected patients.[39–41]

Liver resection for HCC and cirrhosis has two opposing objectives:

1. To satisfy the principles of cancer surgery and remove the primary tumor with a sufficient margin of normal liver parenchyma (at least 1 cm)[42]
2. To preserve enough liver parenchyma to reduce the risk of postoperative liver failure

The ideal would be to evaluate the risk of postoperative liver failure before surgery. A history of upper gastrointestinal bleeding, delirium tremens, or hepatic encephalopathy must be investigated. Patients with jaundice, encephalopathy, and ascites refractory to medical management because of advanced hepatocellular insufficiency are not candidates for major liver surgery.[43] Repeated liver biopsy in nontumorous tissue may be necessary before surgery if acute alcoholic hepatitis is suspected.[5] In cases of acute alcoholic hepatitis and active chronic hepatitis, elective hepatic resection should be delayed until the hepatitis has resolved.[5,44]

Some liver function tests have been proposed to assess liver function before resection. Most authors consider liver resection to be contraindicated if the bilirubin level is higher than 20 mg/L, the serum albumin level is lower than 30 g/L, and the prothrombin time is less than 50%.[43,45] Although the evaluation is not perfect, the Child-Pugh's classification remains useful for estimating the risk of postoperative liver failure.[46,47] Hepatic functional capacity also can be estimated by indocyanine green clearance.[48,49] Morbidity and mortality would be expected to be higher after liver resection in patients with slow indocyanine green clearance. The risk of postoperative liver failure could be appreciated by measuring the nontumorous volume of liver parenchyma with three-dimensional CT. This imaging procedure could predict the percentage of functional parenchyma that would remain after resection.[50,51]

In patients with good liver function (ie, Child's grade A), the postoperative risk of major liver resection is similar to that of patients with normal, noncirrhotic remnant liver. In patients with Child's grade B liver function, major hepatectomy should not be performed; in these cases, segmentectomy or subsegmentectomy should be undertaken. Patients with Child's grade C liver function usually are considered incapable of undergoing resection of liver tumors.

PATIENT EVALUATION

The general status of the patient must be evaluated carefully because associated illness, such as chronic renal failure, ischemic heart disease, or chronic lung disease, increases operative risk. The age of the patient also must be considered before major liver surgery because liver regeneration capacity is reduced in elderly individuals.[52]

TECHNICAL CONSIDERATIONS

Surgical Anatomy of the Liver

The principles of liver surgery are based on the segmental anatomy described by Couinaud.[25] The liver is divided into eight segments based on the division of the portal and hepatic veins. The right lobe includes four segments (V, VI, VII, and VIII) and the left lobe contains three segments (II, III, and IV). Segment I lies posteriorly between the porta hepatis and inferior vena cava.

Routes of Access

The most commonly used incision is a bilateral subcostal incision running two or three fingerbreadths below each costal margin, with a possible upward extension to the xiphoid process. This gives a wide exposure and can be enlarged into the chest through the sixth or seventh interspace if necessary.

Vascular Clamping

Intraoperative hemorrhage is a main determinant of short-term prognosis after hepatic resection.[53,54] Vascular occlusion is used to reduce perioperative blood loss. A Pringle maneuver can be performed,[55] or a complete hepatic vascular exclusion can be used if the tumor is large or located close to the vena cava or hepatic veins.[56]

Portal Triad Clamping

Temporary portal triad clamping (Pringle maneuver) can be used in all liver resections and usually is sufficient, except in bulky or posterior tumors. Normal liver parenchyma can tolerate 60 to 90 minutes of normothermic ischemia.[57–59] Normothermic liver ischemia of up to 1 hour also is well tolerated in cirrhotic livers.[56] Intermittent clamping with periods of reperfusion has been proposed to reduce the duration of ischemia.[60] However, it may increase blood loss and have undesirable effects because of repeated reperfusion injuries.

Hepatic Vascular Exclusion

The risk of massive hemorrhage and air embolism resulting from injury to the vena cava or hepatic veins is especially high during the excision of large and posterior tumors. To prevent this possibility, hepatic vascular exclusion is used to isolate the liver and retrohepatic inferior vena cava completely by occluding the portal triad and the inferior vena cava above and below the liver. Hepatic vascular exclusion usually is well tolerated, even in patients with liver cirrhosis, provided continuous hemodynamic monitoring is performed.[57] In case of poor hemodynamic tolerance, venovenous bypass can be used, as in liver transplantation.

Liver refrigeration associated with "in situ" or "ex situ" liver surgery has been proposed in bulky tumors requiring vascular reconstruction.[61–63] These surgical procedures rarely have been applied in cirrhotic livers.

Surgical Procedures

The surgical procedures used for liver resection of HCC are anatomic resections following anatomic plans or nonanatomic resections such as wedge resections. All types of resections, from tumorectomies to major resections, can be applied to the surgery of HCC.[64–67] Technically, the type of liver excision performed depends on the size, number, and location of the tumors, the relation of the tumors to the hepatic veins and vascular pedicles, and the need to remove with the tumors a margin of healthy parenchyma (at least 1 cm).[39,66] A sufficient amount of functional liver parenchyma should be preserved, particularly in cases of cirrhosis, because of the risk of postoperative liver failure.

Tumorectomy and wedge resection usually are adequate for small lesions that are superficial and easily accessible. Small HCCs that are located deep in the liver or close to major pedicles may require major resection. Segmentectomy resects with the tumor a complete liver segment and the whole area at risk for the development of daughter nodules from portal vein dissemination. A free margin of at least 1 cm is considered adequate for resection of HCCs.[4,39,66] When the tumors are located in one or two liver segments, resection of each segment can be performed. Because it preserves most nontumorous liver parenchyma, segmentectomy is the procedure of choice in well-compensated cirrhosis of Child's grade A or B.[35,65]

Major liver resections resect at least three contiguous liver segments in their entirety. Right lobectomy resects segments

V, VI, VII, and VIII. Left lobectomy resects segments II, III, and IV. Right trisegmentectomy concerns segments IV to VIII, and left lateral segmentectomy concerns segments II and III, but most authorities do not consider this a major resection. In the French multicenter study, the mortality rate was no higher after major hepatectomy than after bisegmentectomy.[5] Resection of involved contiguous structures, such as the diaphragm or right adrenal, can be carried out at the same time as removal of the tumor.

Intraoperative Ultrasonography

The use of intraoperative ultrasonography has been a major advance in the surgery of HCC in patients with liver cirrhosis. It has improved the adequacy of conventional resections and led to the development of new surgical procedures over the last 10 years.[68,69] Tumors detected before surgery and those that may have been missed on preoperative imaging tests can be identified with ultrasonography, although they cannot be palpated because of the cirrhosis of the liver. Operative ultrasound should be performed again after complete mobilization of the liver to detect nodules smaller than 1 cm.[70] If neoplastic thrombi in the portal vein or other unsuspected intrahepatic lesions are detected by ultrasound, resection may be contraindicated.[71] In addition to the detection of tumors, Makuuchi and associates have described the use of ultrasound to guide subsegmentectomy.[72] Under perioperative ultrasound guidance, a balloon catheter can be inserted into the portal branch supplying the segment to be resected. By simultaneously clamping the appropriate hepatic artery branch and inflating the balloon, total vascular exclusion of one liver segment is obtained and guides elective resection.[70] Thrombosis of the portal vein has been observed after the use of this technique.[4] Ultrasound also can be used during anatomic resections to locate the anatomic planes of division and identify major portal and hepatic veins.[70]

Parenchymal Transection

Transection of the parenchyma in long anatomic planes prevents major vessel injuries and reduces blood loss and tissue devitalization. Liver transection can be performed by finger fracture[35] or by crushing the hepatic tissue with Kelly forceps. It also can be performed by new techniques using the ultrasonic dissector,[73] contact yttrium-aluminum-garnet laser,[74] or water jet dissector.[75] Once vessels and bile ducts have been isolated, hemostasis can be obtained with sutures or vascular clips. Absorbable vascular clips reduce the artifacts induced by metal clips on follow-up CT scans.

Treatment of the Section Area

The section area can be left untreated if good hemostasis has been obtained. It also can be covered with dehydrated fibrin (biologic glue), microcrystalline collagen powder, or an omental patch to decrease the risk of postoperative bleeding and biliary leakage.[35,58,76] Argon beam coagulation also can be used.[77] No randomized study has been performed to compare these methods.

Postoperative Drainage

Drainage after elective hepatic resection remains controversial. The space left empty by the removal of liver parenchyma can be filled by fluid accumulation, blood, or bile, leading to intraperitoneal sepsis. Although most liver surgeons continue to drain the abdominal cavity after liver resection, some have suggested avoiding drainage in cirrhotic patients.[78,79] A randomized study has compared the influence of closed-suction drainage with no drainage on the incidence of postoperative complications after elective hepatic resection.[80] This series included 81 patients, 19 of whom were undergoing resection for HCC associated with liver cirrhosis. After major liver resection, the rate of intraabdominal postoperative complications (eg, subphrenic fluid collection, hematoma) was similar in the drainage group and the nondrainage group. After minor liver resection, the patients without drainage had fewer complications. However, because of the small number of patients with cirrhosis in the study, no firm conclusions could be drawn about this interesting group in whom avoidance of drainage can prevent leakage of ascitic fluid.

COMPLICATIONS OF SURGERY

In patients undergoing liver resection for HCC, operative mortality depends on the extent of resection and the presence of associated cirrhosis. In patients with cirrhosis, mortality rates higher than 50% have been reported after major liver resection.[40] However, with better adaptation of the extent of liver resection to the status of liver function, operative mortality rates in patients with cirrhosis now range from 7% to 25%.[4,5,35,71,81] Some series report no postoperative deaths.[65] But death can occur, even when less than 5% of the functional liver parenchyma has been resected.[4] In patients with normal parenchyma, the operative mortality rate ranges from 3% to 7.3%[10,81] and is similar to that associated with the resection of other types of liver tumors, including fibrolamellar carcinoma.[82] Intraoperative deaths usually are caused by uncontrollable bleeding from hepatic veins or injury to the inferior vena cava.[83] Postoperative deaths usually result from hepatic failure, hemorrhage, sepsis, or ascites.[84] The morbidity rate in patients with cirrhosis who undergo hepatic resection is high (17% to 50%), and hepatic failure is the most common postoperative complication.[35,71,81]

Hepatic Failure

Hepatic failure can complicate any surgical procedure in a patient with cirrhosis, regardless of whether it involves the liver.[5] After liver resection, this risk is linked to preoperative hepatic function, to the importance of parenchymal removal, and to perioperative hemorrhage.[53,57] Hepatic functional capacity should be assessed before surgery as precisely as possible to avoid postoperative liver failure. Poor liver function increases the risk of bleeding during surgery, which in turn can precipitate postoperative liver failure. Death resulting from progressive and isolated liver failure caused by excessive resection of functional parenchyma is rare. In general, liver failure is precipitated by the addition of a complication of liver resection, such as sepsis, bile fistula, renal dysfunction, gastrointestinal bleeding, ascites, or portal thrombosis.

Postoperative Hemorrhage

Postoperative bleeding is another common complication that carries significant morbidity and mortality. It is the second most important mortality factor after the resection of HCC complicating cirrhosis. In patients with cirrhosis, hemorrhage during and after surgery can result from multiple factors, including liver dysfunction, thrombocytopenia, coagulopathy, and portal hypertension. Postoperative variceal bleeding may be induced by acute portal hypertension after major liver resection.[85] Some authors have suggested concomitant treatment of esophageal varices or the construction of a portosystemic shunt in these cases to prevent variceal hemorrhage.[86,87] Paquet and colleagues recommend that patients with histories of variceal bleeding or with large varices be treated with prophylactic sclerotherapy.[35]

Postoperative Ascites

Postoperative ascites is common after any surgical procedure in patients with cirrhosis.[88] In a French multicenter survey, postoperative ascites was observed in 36% of patients, and in 50% of those who had preoperative ascites.[5] Ascites is a major factor contributing to postoperative morbidity and mortality. The accumulation of ascites increases the risk of wound dehiscence, fluid leakage, and secondary sepsis, with the subsequent risk of multiple organ failure. In liver cirrhosis, immune defenses are impaired and patients are susceptible to bacterial infections of ascitic fluid. Ascitic fluid infection may lead to septicemia and peritonitis, with a mortality rate of 60%.[5]

As with resection for other liver tumors, local postoperative complications also can occur. Cirrhosis does not seem to increase the risk of postoperative bile fistula or subphrenic abscess.[66]

The postoperative course after resection of HCC associated with cirrhosis depends mainly on preoperative liver function. In patients with good hepatic function, mortality and morbidity rates are similar to those associated with surgery for other liver tumors, such as colorectal metastases.[89]

LONG-TERM RESULTS

After curative surgery of HCC, survival depends on evolution of the underlying cirrhosis and recurrence of the cancer. The overall long-term prognosis after curative resection of HCC in patients with cirrhosis remains poor, with a 5-year survival rate of 17% to 25%.[8,39,81,90]

Cancer Recurrence

Recurrence of carcinoma is the main cause of death after surgical resection of HCC. The cumulative intrahepatic recurrence rate 5 years after surgical resection of asymptomatic HCC in patients with cirrhosis is as high as 100% in some series.[39] In half the cases, recurrence occurs during the first year after surgical resection, and in two thirds of the cases, it occurs in the first 2 years.[39,91] After surgical resection of HCC, recurrence occurs in the liver in 80% to 93% of cases.[39,91,92] Less than 20% of recurrences are extrahepatic, located in lung, bone, or brain. In most cases, extrahepatic and intrahepatic recurrences are associated. The high rate of recurrence after resection of HCC suggests the possible benefit of postoperative adjuvant chemotherapy. However, the efficacy of this approach needs to be proven in prospective randomized trials.

FACTORS ASSOCIATED WITH AN INCREASED RISK OF RECURRENCE

Knowledge of the factors associated with an increased risk of cancer recurrence is important for more accurate selection of good surgical candidates and avoidance of unnecessary surgery in poor candidates. Unfortunately, prognostic factors are difficult to evaluate in HCC because of the heterogeneity of the criteria analyzed in different series. In addition, most of the factors can be determined only after resection and histologic examination of the resected specimen.

Margin of Resection

The amount of healthy parenchyma that is removed with the tumor is an important prognostic factor. In general, a margin of 1 cm is thought to be adequate.[39,42,85] If the margin is smaller, early recurrence can occur in up to 62.5% of patients.[93] If the margin is adequate, 80% of recurrences should appear at a distance from the cut surface of the liver because they are more likely to be related to synchronous or metachronous multifocal HCC than to insufficient excision.[39] There is no proof that recurrences occur less often after major compared with minor resections, provided the tumor is resected completely, with a margin of more than 1 cm.

Portal Invasion

One of the characteristics of HCC is invasion and dissemination through portal veins. While the tumor increases in size, the walls of small portal veins may be invaded and tumor thrombi may develop within the portal vein lumina. Friable fragments may break off and be carried distally by portal venous flow. Tumor fragments then can grow and form daughter nodules. Surgical resection should remove the primary tumor with a sufficient margin of normal liver parenchyma and the entire liver segment that is susceptible to house the development of daughter nodules resulting from portal vein thrombi.[72] To prevent recurrence, it has been suggested that segmentectomy be performed under perioperative ultrasonographic guidance with selective occlusion of the branch of the portal vein,[72] because most recurrences appear in the same liver segment as the primary tumor.

Tumor Size

The influence of tumor size is an important prognostic factor.[39,94,95] In most studies, the recurrence rate increases with tumor size and the survival rate is higher in patients with small tumors. The cumulative intrahepatic recurrence rate is higher in patients with tumors larger than 5 cm.[39,94,95] Tumor size also affects the rate of resectability, and is higher in patients with tumors smaller than 5 cm.

Pathologic Factors

The most definitive pathologic feature is the presence or absence of a capsule around the tumor. Several studies have shown fewer recurrences after resection of encapsulated tumors.[18,71,93] In patients with nonencapsulated tumors, the recurrence rate is high regardless of tumor size.[93] The fibrous capsule surrounding the tumor could act as a barrier against tumor spread into adjacent parenchyma and small portal veins.[96]

The best candidates for resection, according to the characteristics of the tumor, probably are patients with tumors that are smaller than 5 cm, encapsulated, solitary, and without portal vein invasion.

Fibrolamellar carcinoma of the liver has a better prognosis after surgical resection, and its detection is important. The resectability rate exceeds 50% and major resection should be considered whenever technically feasible.[23,97] The recurrence rate of 20% to 50% at 5 years is lower than for other forms of HCC, and long-term survival of more than 5 years has been reported.[98] If tumor removal is not possible with a partial liver resection, total hepatectomy and transplantation should be considered.[98]

Treatment of Intrahepatic Recurrence After Resection of Hepatocellular Carcinoma

No medical treatment has been proven to cure recurrent intrahepatic HCC, and repeated resection should be considered every time it is technically feasible.[23,97] Serial serum AFP determinations and hepatic imaging with ultrasound and CT are indicated after resection of HCC to detect recurrence at a preclinical stage.[1,99] The resectability rate for recurrent HCC confined to the liver and without evidence of distant metastatic disease has been estimated at 20% to 25%.[91] Even for a small recurrent tumor, resection may be impossible because of poor liver function or inaccessible tumor location. Whenever feasible, the procedure of choice is an anatomic resection segmentectomy or subsegmentectomy, with resection of the tumor and a margin at least 1 cm of normal liver parenchyma.[100,101] In patients with Child's grade A cirrhosis, morbidity and mortality rates are low. Although liver regeneration is poor after resection in cirrhotic livers, a second hepatic resection may be possible in some patients who already have undergone a major excision, as long as liver function is good.[100,101] Survival rates of 26% to 38% at 5 years have been reported after surgical resection of recurrent HCC.[91,102]

CONCLUSION

In Western countries, surgical resection is considered the treatment of choice for selected patients with HCC and normal liver parenchyma or mild to moderate liver dysfunction. The best results are obtained with solitary tumors smaller than 5 cm. Total hepatectomy and orthotopic liver transplantation, which had been considered an option for patients with larger tumors, is associated with a high rate of recurrence and limited by the shortage of donors. It seems better indicated in patients with small tumors. Future studies must compare the results of partial liver resection and orthotopic liver transplantation for small tumors. For large tumors, no effective treatment is available.

REFERENCES

1. Di Bisceglie AM, Rustgi VK, Hoofnagle JH, Dusheiko GM, Lotze MT. NIH conference: hepatocellular carcinoma. Ann Intern Med 1988;108:390.
2. Colombo M, De Franchis R, Del Ninno E, et al. Hepatocellular carcinoma in Italian patients with cirrhosis. N Engl J Med 1991;325:675.
3. Boutron MC, Faivre J, Milan C, Bedenne L, Hillon P, Klepping C. Primary liver cancer in Côte d'Or (France). Int J Epidemiol 1988;17:21.
4. Bismuth H, Houssin D, Ornowski J, Meriggi F. Liver resections in cirrhotic patients: a Western experience. World J Surg 1986;10:311.
5. Belghiti J, Gillet M. Chirurgie digestive chez le cirrhotique. Paris: Springer-Verlag, 1993:15.
6. Chlebowski RT, Tong M, Weissman J, et al. Hepatocellular carcinoma: diagnostic and pronostic features in North American patients. Cancer 1984;54:1461.
7. Durand F, Buffet C, Pelletier G, Hagege H, Ink O, Etienne JP. Hepatocellular carcinoma. N Engl J Med 1993;328:64.
8. Nagorney DM, Van Heerden JA, Ilstrup DM, Adson MA. Primary hepatic malignancy: surgical management and determinants of survival. Surgery 1989;106:740.
9. Cottone M, Virdone R, Fusco G, et al. Asymptomatic hepatocellular carcinoma in Child's A cirrhosis. Gastroenterology 1989;96:1566.
10. Smalley SR, Moertel CG, Hilton JF, et al. Hepatoma in the non cirrhotic liver. Cancer 1988;62:1414.
11. Sitzmann JV, Abrams R. Improved survival for hepatocellular cancer with combination surgery and multimodal treatment. Ann Surg 1993;217:149.
12. Nagasue N, Hirofumui H, Hamada T, et al. The natural history of hepatocellular carcinoma. Cancer 1984;54:1461.
13. Kobayashi K, Sugimoto T, Makino H, et al. Screening methods for early detection of hepatocellular carcinoma. Hepatology 1985;5:1100.
14. Heyward WL, Lanier AP, McMahon BJ. Early detection of primary hepatocellular carcinoma. JAMA 1985;254:3052.
15. Okuda K. Hepatocellular carcinoma: recent progress. Hepatology 1992;15:948.
16. Farmer DG, Rosove MH, Shaked A, Busuttil RW. Current treatment modalities for hepatocellular carcinoma. Ann Surg 1994;219:236.
17. Colombo M. Hepatocellular carcinoma. J Hepatol 1992;15:225.
18. Okuda K, Ohtsuky T, Obata H, et al. Natural history of hepatocellular carcinoma and prognosis in relation to treatment. Cancer 1985;56:918.
19. Dusheiko GM, Hobbs KD, Burroughs AK. Treatment of small hepatocellular carcinomas. Lancet 1992;340:285.
20. Okuda K. Diagnosis of hepatocellular carcinoma. In: Okuda K, ed. The International Association for the Study of the Liver/The Asian Pacific Association for the Study of the Liver. Postgraduate course, Hong Kong, 1982.
21. Tang YZ, ed. Subclinical hepatocellular carcinoma. New York: Springer-Verlag, 1985.
22. Craig JR, Peters RL, Edmonson HA, Omata M. Fibrolamellar carcinoma of the liver. A tumor of young adolescents and young adults with distinctive clinico-pathologic features. Cancer 1980;46:372.
23. Soreide O, Czemiak A, Bradpiece H, Bloom S, Blumgart L. Characteristics of fibrolamellar hepatocellular carcinoma. A study of nine cases and a review of the literature. Am J Surg 1986;151:518.
24. Lai ECS, Wu KM, Choi TK, Fan ST, Wong J. Spontaneous ruptured hepatocellular carcinoma. An appraisal of surgical treatment. Ann Surg 1989;210:24.
25. Couinaud C. Le foie: etudes anatomiques et chirurgicales. Paris: Masson, 1957.

26. Nagasue N, Yukaya H, Chang YC, et al. Hepatocellular pseudotumor (regenerating nodule) in the cirrhotic liver mimicking hepatocellular carcinoma. Br J Surg 1988;75:1124.
27. Takashima T, Matsui O, Suzuki M, et al. Diagnosis and screening of small hepatocellular carcinomas: comparison of radionuclide imaging, ultrasound, computed tomography, hepatic angiography and alpha-1-fetoprotein assay. Radiology 1982;145:635.
28. Igidbashin V, Jibin L, Goldberg B. Hepatic ultrasound. Semin Liver Dis 1989;9:16.
29. Kunstlinger F, Federle MP, Moss AA, Marks W. Computed tomography of hepatocellular carcinoma. AJR Am J Roentgenol 1980;134:431.
30. Yumoto Y, Jinno K, Tokuyama K, et al. Hepatocellular carcinoma detected by iodized oil. Radiology 1985;154:19.
31. Haskell CM, Selch MT, Ramming KP. Primary neoplasms of the liver. In: Haskell CM, ed. Cancer treatment. 3rd ed. Philadelphia: WB Saunders, 1990:276.
32. Ferruci JT Jr, Wittenberg J, Margolies MN, Carey RW. Malignant seeding of the tract after thin-needle aspiration biopsy. Radiology 1979;30:345.
33. Nduka CC, Monson JRT, Menzies-Gow N, Darzi A. Abdominal wall metastases following laparoscopy. Br J Surg 1994;81:648.
34. Russi EG, Pergolizzi S, Mesiti M, et al. Unusual relapse of hepatocellular carcinoma. Cancer 1992;70:1483.
35. Paquet KJ, Koussouris P, Mercado MA, Kalk JF, Müting D, Rambach W. Limited hepatic resection for selected cirrhotic patients with hepatocellular or cholangiocellular carcinoma: a prospective study. Br J Surg 1991;78:459.
36. Garrison RN, Cryer HM, Howard DA, Polk HC. Clarification of risk factors for abdominal operations in patients with hepatic cirrhosis. Ann Surg 1984;199:648.
37. Lee CS, Chao CC, Lin TY. Partial hepatectomy on cirrhotic patients with a right lateral tumor. Surgery 1985;98:942.
38. Nagasue N, Yukaya H, Ogawa Y, et al. Human liver regeneration after major hepatic resection. A study of normal liver and livers with chronic hepatitis and cirrhosis. Ann Surg 1987;206:30.
39. Belghiti J, Panis Y, Farges O, Benhamou JP, Fekete F. Intrahepatic recurrence after resection of hepatocellular carcinoma complicating cirrhosis. Ann Surg 1991;214:114.
40. Huguet C, Nordlinger B, Vacher B, et al. Résection chirurgicale des hépatocarcinomes. Etude rétrospective de 42 cas. Gastroenterol Clin Biol 1985;9:244.
41. Bismuth H, Houssin D, Castaing D. Major and minor segmentectomies "règlées" in liver surgery. World J Surg 1982;6:10.
42. Lee CS, Sung JL, Hwang LY, et al. Surgical treatment of 109 patients with symptomatic and asymptomatic hepatocellular carcinoma. Surgery 1986;99:481.
43. Elias D. Chirurgie du carcinome hépatocellulaire sur cirrhose. Actualisation des éléments décisionnels et perspectives nouvelles. Gastroenterol Clin Biol 1987;11:795.
44. Powell-Jackson P, Greenway B, Williams R. Adverse effects of exploratory laparotomy in patients with unsuspected liver disease. Br J Surg 1982;69:449.
45. Belghiti J, Menu Y, Cherqui D, Nahum H, Fekete F. Traitement chirurgical des carcinomes hépatocellulaires sur cirrhose. Intérêt de l'échotomographie per-opératoire. Gastroenterol Clin Biol 1986;10:244.
46. Child CG. The liver and portal hypertension. Philadelphia: WB Saunders, 1954.
47. Pugh RNH, Murray-Lyon IM, Dawson JL, et al. Transection of the esophagus for bleeding esophageal varices. Br J Surg 1973;60:646.
48. Matsumata T, Kanematsu T, Yoshida Y, Toshiya F, Yanaga K, Sugimachi K. The indocyanine green test enables prediction of postoperative complications after hepatic resection. World J Surg 1987;11:678.
49. Bismuth H, Chiche L, Adam R, Castaing D, Diamond T, Dennison A. Liver resection versus transplantation for hepatocellular carcinoma in cirrhotic patients. Ann Surg 1993;218:145.
50. Hashimoto D, Dohi T, Tsuzuki M, et al. Development of a computed-aided surgery system: three dimensional graphic reconstruction for treatment of liver cancer. Surgery 1991;109:589.
51. Okamoto E, Kyo A, Yamanaka N, Tanaka N, Kuwata K. Prediction of the safe limits of hepatectomy by combined volumetric and functional measurements in patients with impaired hepatic function. Surgery 1984;95:586.
52. Bucher NLK, Swaffield MN, DiTroia JF. Influence of age upon incorporation of thymidine 2-C14 into DNA of regenerating rat liver. Cancer Res 1964;24:509.
53. Ekberg H, Tranberg KG, Andersson R, et al. Major liver resection: perioperative course and management. Surgery 1986;100:1.
54. Delva E, Barberousse JP, Nordlinger B, et al. Hemodynamic and biochemical monitoring during major liver resection with use of hepatic vascular exclusion. Surgery 1984;95:309.
55. Pringle JH. Notes on the arrest of hepatic hemorrhage due to trauma. Ann Surg 1908;48:541.
56. Huguet C, Nordlinger B, Bloch P, Conard J. Tolerance of the human liver to prolonged normothermic ischemia. Arch Surg 1978;113:1448.
57. Delva E, Camus E, Nordlinger B, et al. Vascular occlusions for liver resections. Operative management and tolerance to hepatic ischemia: 142 cases. Ann Surg 1989;209:211.
58. Hannoun L, Borie D, Delva E, et al. Liver resection with normothermic ischaemia exceeding 1 h. Br J Surg 1993;80:1161.
59. Huguet C, Gavelli A, Chieco PA, et al. Liver ischaemia for hepatic resection: where is the limit? Surgery 1992;11:251.
60. Elias D, Desruennes E, Lasser P. Prolonged intermittent clamping of the portal triad during hepatectomy. Br J Surg 1991;78:42.
61. Fortner JG, Shiu MH, Kinne DW, et al. Major hepatic resection using vascular isolation and hypothermic perfusion. Ann Surg 1974;180:644.
62. Pichlmayr R, Grosse H, Hauss J, Gubernatis G, Lamesch P, Bretschneider HJ. Technique and preliminary results of extracorporeal liver surgery (bench procedure) and of surgery on the in situ perfused liver. Br J Surg 1990;77:21.
63. Hannoun L, Panis Y, Balladur P, et al. Ex-situ in-vivo liver surgery. Lancet 1991;337:1616.
64. MacIntosh L, Minuk GY. Hepatic resection in patients with cirrhosis and hepatocellular carcinoma. Surg Gynecol Obstet 1992;174:245.
65. Franco D, Smadja C, Kahwaji F, Grange D, Kemeni F, Traynor O. Segmentectomies in the management of liver tumors. Arch Surg 1988;123:519.
66. Franco D, Smadja C, Meakins JL, et al. Improved early results of elective hepatic resection for liver tumors: one hundred consecutive hepatectomies in cirrhotic and non cirrhotic patients. Arch Surg 1989;124:1033.
67. Schwartz SI. Hepatic resection. Ann Surg 1990;211:1.
68. Makuuchi M, Hasegawa H, Yamazaki S. Intraoperative ultrasonic examination for hepatectomy. Jpn J Clin Oncol 1981;11:367.
69. Sheu JC, Lee CS, Sung JL, et al. Intraoperative hepatic ultrasonography: an indispensable procedure in resection of small hepatocellular carcinomas. Surgery 1985;97:97.
70. Castaing D, Garden OJ, Bismuth H. Segmental liver resection using ultra-sound guided selective portal venous occlusion. Ann Surg 1989;201:20.
71. Gozzetti G, Mazziotti A, Cavallari A, et al. Clinical experience with hepatic resections for hepatocellular carcinoma in patients with cirrhosis. Surg Gynecol Obstet 1988;166:503.
72. Makuuchi M, Hasegawa H, Yamazaki S. Ultrasonically guided segmentectomy. Surg Gynecol Obstet 1985;162:346.
73. Putnam CW. Techniques of ultrasonic dissection in resection of liver. Surg Gynecol Obstet 1983;157:474.
74. Schröder T, Hasselgren PO, Brackett K, Joffe SN. Techniques of liver resection. Comparison of suction knife, ultrasonic dissector, and contact neodymium-YAG laser. Arch Surg 1987;122:116.
75. Persson BG, Jeppsson B, Tranberg KG, et al. Transection of the liver with a water-jet. Surg Gynecol Obstet 1989;168:267.
76. Sakon M, Monden M, Gotoh M, et al. Use of microcrystalline collagen powder and fibrinogen tissue adhesive for hemostasis and prevention of rebleeding in patients with hepatocellular carcinoma associated with cirrhosis of the liver. Surg Gynecol Obstet 1989;168:453.
77. Postema RR, Ten Kate FJW, Terpstra OT. Less hepatic tissue necrosis after argon beam coagulation than after conventional electrocoagulation. Surg Gynecol Obstet 1993;176:177.
78. Franco D, Karaa A, Meakins JL, Borgonovo G, Smadja C, Grange G. Hepatectomy without abdominal drainage: results of a prospective study in 61 patients. Ann Surg 1989;6:748.
79. Smadja C, Berthoux L, Meakins JL, Franco D. Patterns of improvement in resection of hepatocellular carcinoma in cirrhotic patients: results of a non drainage policy. HPB Surg 1989;1:141.
80. Belghiti J, Kabbej M, Sauvanet A, Vilgrain V, Panis Y, Fekete F.

Drainage after elective hepatic resection. A randomized trial. Ann Surg 1993;218:748.
81. Ringe B, Pichlmayr R, Wittekind C, Tusch G. Surgical treatment of hepatocellular carcinoma: experience with liver resection and transplantation in 198 patients. World J Surg 1991;15:270.
82. Starzl TE, Iwatsuki S, Shaw B, Nalesnik MA, Farhi DC, Van Thiel DH. Treatment of fibrolamellar hepatoma with partial or total hepatectomy and transplantation of the liver. Surg Gynecol Obstet 1986;162:145.
83. Iwatsuki S, Gei WP. Specific complications in surgery of the liver. Surg Clin North Am 1977;57:409.
84. Iwatsuki S, Starzl TE. Personal experience with 400 hepatic resections. Ann Surg 1988;208:421.
85. Nagasue N, Yukaya H, Ogawa Y, Higashi T. Portal pressure following partial to extensive hepatic resections in patients with and without cirrhosis of the liver. Ann Chir Gynaecol 1983;72:18.
86. Nagasue N, Yukaya H, Ogawa U, et al. Morbidity and mortality after major hepatic resection in cirrhotic patients with hepatocellular carcinoma. HPB Surg 1988;1:45.
87. Kanematsu T, Takenaka K, Furuta T, Ezaki T, Sugimachi K, Inokuchi K. Acute portal hypertension associated with liver resection. Analysis of early postoperative death. Arch Surg 1985;120:1303.
88. Aranha GV, Greenlee HB. Intra-abdominal surgery in patients with advanced cirrhosis. Arch Surg 1986;121:275.
89. Nordlinger B, Jaeck D. Treatment of hepatic metastases of colorectal cancer. Paris: Springer-Verlag, 1992:141.
90. Iwatsuki S, Starzl TE, Sheahan DG, et al. Hepatic resection versus transplantation for hepatocellular carcinoma. Ann Surg 1991;214:221.
91. Nagao T, Inoue S, Yoshimi F, et al. Postoperative recurrence of hepatocellular carcinoma. Ann Surg 1990;211:28.
92. Kanematsu T, Matsumata T, Takenaka K, et al. Clinical management of recurrent hepatocellular carcinoma after primary resection. Br J Surg 1988;75:203.
93. Franco D, Capussotti L, Smadja C, et al. Resection of hepatocellular carcinoma: results in 72 European patients with cirrhosis. Gastroenterology 1990;98:733.
94. The Liver Cancer Study Group of Japan. Primary liver cancer in Japan. Clinicopathologic features and results of surgical treatment. Ann Surg 1990;211:277.
95. Ohnishi K, Tanabe Y, Ryu M, et al. Prognosis of hepatocellular carcinoma smaller than 5 cm in relation to treatment: study of 100 patients. Hepatology 1987;7:1285.
96. Kemeny F, Vadrot J, Wu A, et al. Morphological and histological features of resected hepatocellular carcinoma in cirrhotic patients in the West. Hepatology 1989;9:457.
97. Nagorney DM, Adson MA, Weiland LH, et al. Fibrolamellar hepatoma. Am J Surg 1985;149:113.
98. Starzl TE, Iwatsuki S, Shaw B, Nalesnik MA, Farhi DC, Van Thiel DH. Treatment of fibrolamellar hepatoma with partial or total hepatectomy and transplantation of the liver. Surg Gynecol Obstet 1986;162:145.
99. Nagasue N, Yukaya H, Chang Y, et al. Assessment of pattern and treatment of intra hepatic recurrence after resection of hepatocellular carcinoma. Surg Gynecol Obstet 1990;171:217.
100. Huguet C, Bona S, Nordlinger B, et al. Repeat hepatic resection for primary and metastatic carcinoma of the liver. Surg Gynecol Obstet 1990;171:398.
101. Lange JF, Leese T, Castaing D, Bismuth H. Repeat hepatectomy for recurrent malignant tumors of the liver. Surg Gynecol Obstet 1989;169:119.
102. Nagasue N, Yukaya H, Ogawa Y, et al. Second hepatic resection for recurrent hepatocellular carcinoma. Br J Surg 1986;73:434.

Surgery for Gastrointestinal Cancer: A Multidisciplinary Approach, edited by Harold J. Wanebo.
Lippincott-Raven Publishers, Philadelphia, © 1997.

CHAPTER 44

Resectional Approaches to Hepatocellular Carcinoma: Japanese Experience

Shigeki Arii and Takayoshi Tobe

The number of patients with hepatocellular carcinoma (HCC), a common malignancy in Japan and Southeast Asia, has been increasing over the last 10 years. The development of noninvasive diagnostic modalities such as computed tomography and ultrasonography, in addition to the policy of providing medical follow-up to patients with chronic liver disease, has contributed to the early detection of HCC. Surgical treatment, perioperative management, and the evaluation of hepatic functional reserve have improved considerably. Consequently, the number of resectable cases has been increasing steadily, and both the operative death rate (Fig. 44-1) and the long-term survival rate have improved markedly.[1–4]

In this chapter, the status of resection as an approach to the treatment of HCC in Japan is described.

SURGICAL INDICATIONS

The crucial surgical indications are thought to be hepatic functional reserve and the extent of tumor formation. In this regard, much effort has been made to clarify the indications for surgery, to achieve a more radical excision, and to evaluate liver function more precisely. In this section, recent developments and the general consensus in regard to these problems are discussed.

Evaluation of Hepatic Functional Reserve

About 90% of HCCs in Japan are associated with chronic liver disease (Table 44-1). As a result, hepatic functional reserve varies considerably among individuals. In general, the most useful indicators of hepatic functional reserve are considered to include total protein, albumin, and bilirubin levels, cholinesterase activity, prothrombin time, and indocyanine green clearance rate. However, accurate assessment of functional reserve necessitates a combination of indicators, because hepatic integrity is reflected by a variety of functions.

The Liver Cancer Study Group of Japan has established a simple system for the evaluation of liver function, as summarized in Table 44-2.[5] Furthermore, using clinical and basic studies, a variety of sophisticated liver function tests have been devised as follows. Ozawa and colleagues clarified the control of hepatic functional reserve by mitochondrial adenosine triphosphate synthetic ability, which can be correlated with the oral glucose tolerance test.[6] There are two discernible oral glucose tolerance test patterns. One is a parabolic pattern in which the hepatic energy charge is within the normal range; the other is a linear pattern in which the energy charge is below normal. Other studies have revealed that acetoacetate/β-hydroxybutyrate levels in arterial blood can be correlated with the redox potential of mitochondria, facilitating perioperative management.[7] Noguchi and Mizumoto established the measurement of the ICGRmax of the putative remnant liver by multiplying the ICGRmax value for the whole liver by the remaining liver volume as calculated using computed tomography.[8] The ICGRmax scores obtained for the remnant liver can be classified as follows. Most of the patients in whom the preoperative ICGRmax of the remnant liver was above 0.4 mg/kg/min had a good postoperative prognosis, irrespective of the type of hepatectomy performed. Of those patients who had an ICGRmax between 0.4 and 0.2 mg/kg/min, severe postoperative liver dysfunction occurred in about 50%. All patients with a value below 0.2 mg/kg/min had an extremely poor prognosis. Hepatectomy should not be considered in such cases. Yamanaka and Okamoto proposed the equation, $Y = -110 + 0.942 \times$ resection rate (%) $+ 1.36 \times$ indocyanine green retention rate (%) $+ 1.17 \times$ patient's age $+ 5.94 \times$ indocyanine green maximal removal rate (mg/kg/min), for the prediction of postoperative liver failure, by multivariate analysis of their results.[9] As shown in this formula, they stressed the indocyanine green value and patient age in their evaluation of liver functional reserve, and concluded

Shigeki Arii, First Department of Surgery, Faculty of Medicine, Kyoto University, 54-Shogoin Kawara-cho, Sakyo-ku, Kyoko 606, Japan
Takayoshi Tobe, First Department of Surgery, Faculty of Medicine, Kyoto University, 54-Shogoin Kawara-cho, Sakyo-ku, Kyoko 606, Japan

TABLE 44-1. *Changes in liver parenchyma accompanying hepatocellular carcinoma (n= 1976)*

Fibrosis	157 (7.9%)
Cirrhosis*	1458 (73.8%)
B-type	1131 (57.2%)
B′-type	218 (11.0%)
A-type	48 (2.4%)
A′-type	44 (2.2%)
F-type	17 (0.9%)
Others	162 (8.2%)
None	199 (10.1%)

* According to Miyake's classification of cirrhosis, A-, B-, and F-types almost correspond to postnecrotic, posthepatitic, and nutritional cirrhosis, respectively.

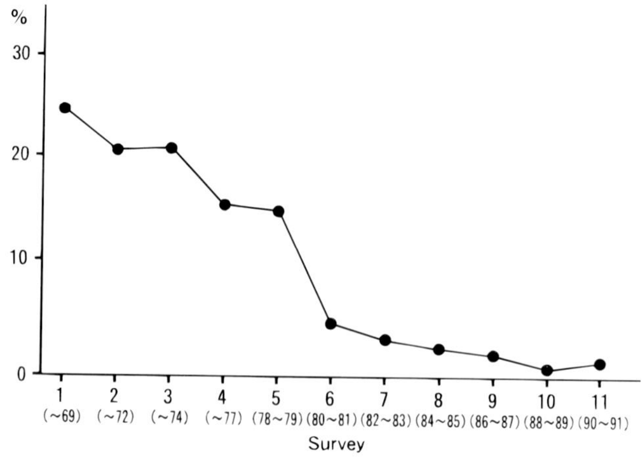

FIG. 44-1. Change in operative death rates.

that a Y value of greater than 50 points indicated a high risk of posthepatectomy liver failure.

Extension of the Surgical Indications

The amount of hepatic parenchyma that can be removed safely is limited severely by the hepatic functional reserve. Therefore, resectability is dependent on both the extent of the cancer and the functional capacity of the remnant liver. A dilemma arises between the need for radical excision and the need to maintain adequate postoperative liver function. To avoid life-threatening liver failure after extensive hepatectomy, percutaneous transhepatic portal branch embolization (PTPE) was devised (Fig. 44-2). In 1920, Rous and Larimore found that the hepatic lobe serviced by the portal branch that was ligated shrank, whereas the nonligated lobe hypertrophied.[10] Honjo and associates attempted portal branch ligation as a therapy for unresectable liver cancer, and also performed a two-stage surgery involving portal branch ligation with hepatic resection of the ligated lobe about 1 month later.[11] Based on this surgical protocol, embolization of the portal branch by ultrasonically guided percutaneous transhepatic portal catheterization subsequently was devised to expand the surgical indications and to attain the radial surgical excision desired.[12]

After PTPE, the embolized lobe tends to become smaller and the nonembolized lobe tends to become larger. The increase in the volume of the nonembolized lobe depends on the area embolized. Serum levels of aspartate aminotransferase and alanine aminotransferase usually are increased after PTPE, but are lower than those after transarterial embolization (TAE), and typically return to baseline levels within 2 weeks. Most patients experience mild abdominal pain and a low-grade fever, which subside within 3 to 4 days after PTPE. Hepatic resection is performed about 3 to 4 weeks later.

TECHNICAL CONSIDERATIONS

The follow-up study by the Liver Cancer Study Group of Japan documented a gradual but definite increase in the use of limited resection (Table 44-3). In the 1970s, Japanese liver surgeons tried to resect widely to attain radical excision or to circumvent technical problems. During this period, severe complications and postoperative deaths were encountered with high frequency because of the limited functional reserve in cirrhotic livers. Limited but anatomically precise hepatectomies in cirrhotic livers now have become prevalent, as described elsewhere in this chapter.

Standard Procedures: Right Hepatectomy, Left Hepatectomy, Right Trisegmentectomy, Left Trisegmentectomy, and Lateral Segmentectomy

In principle, the operative procedures comprise selection of the appropriate skin incision (eg, bilateral subcostal, oblique costoabdominal); detachment of the liver; cholecystectomy and dissection of the portal veins, hepatic arteries, and bile ducts at the porta hepatis; parenchymal resection along the intersegmental line; and dissection and ligation of the hepatic vein,

TABLE 44-2. *The liver cancer study group of Japan system for evaluation of liver function*

Fingings	Clinical Stage I	II	III
Ascities	None	Treatment effective	Treatment ineffective
Seru bilirubin (mg/dL)	Below 2	2–3	Over 3.0
Serum albumin (g/dL)	Over 3.5	3–3.5	Below 3.0
Indocyanine green R_{15} (%)	Below 15	15–40	Over 40
Prothrombin activity value (%)	Over 80	50–80	Below 50

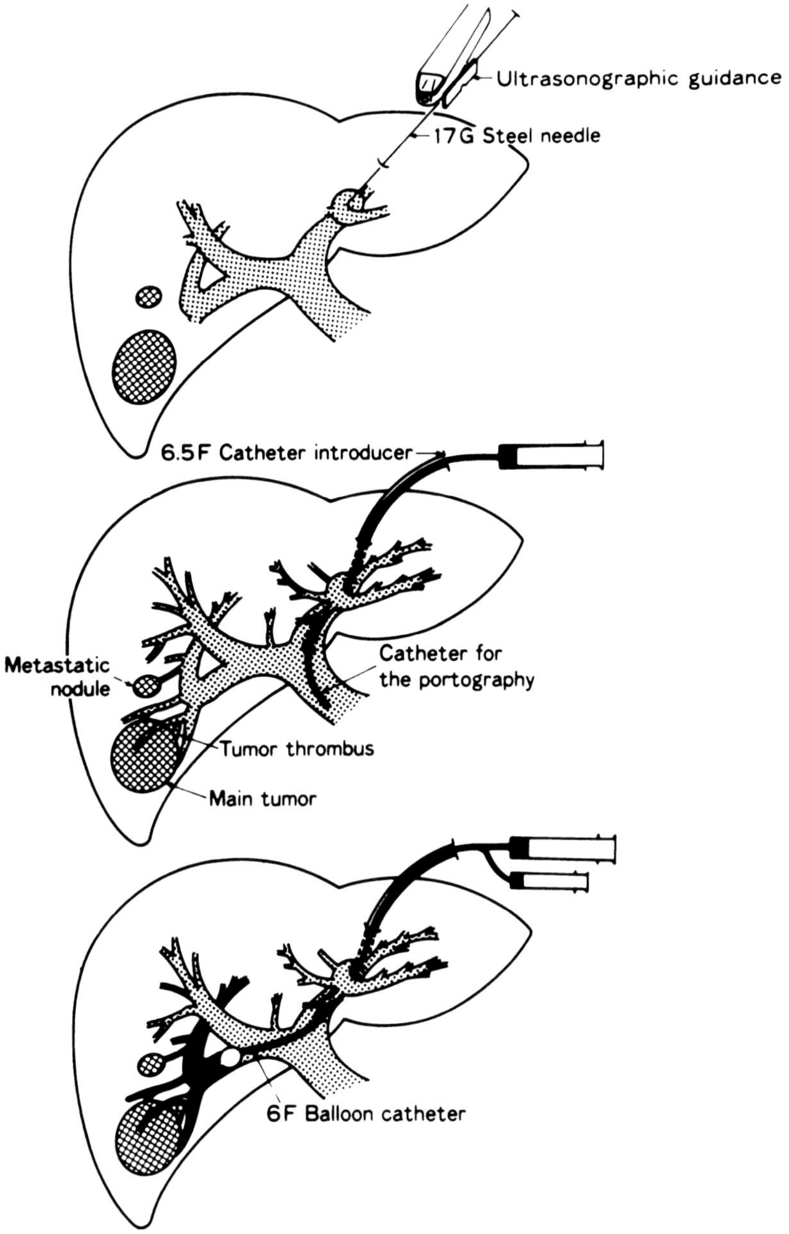

FIG. 44-2. Procedure for percutaneous portal branch embolization. (Kinoshita H, Sakai K, Ozawa K, et al. Preoperative portal vein embolization for hepatocellular carcinoma. World J Surg 1986;10:803.)

TABLE 44-3. *Changes in the mode of hepatectomy*

Procedure	4th (1968–1977)	5th (1978–1979)	6th (1980–1981)	7th (1982–1983)	8th (1984–1985)	9th (1986–1987)	10th (1988–1989)	11th (1990–1991)
Extended right/left hepatectomy	40 (13.9%)	43 (15.4%)	64 (10.5%)	48 (5.5%)	61 (4.9%)	79 (4.4%)	123 (4.7%)	124 (3.7%)
Right/left hepatectomy	123 (42.7%)	111 (39.8%)	202 (33.1%)	227 (26.2%)	257 (20.6%)	298 (16.7%)	440 (17.0%)	542 (16.2%)
Segmentectomy*	91 (31.6%)	58 (20.8%)	106 (17.3%)	201 (23.2%)	263 (21.1%)	404 (22.6%)	517 (20.0%)	743 (22.2%)
Subsegmentectomy†	—	—	—	—	—	463 (25.9%)	623 (24.0%)	755 (22.6%)
Partial resection	34 (11.8%)	67 (24.0%)	239 (39.1%)	389 (45.0%)	668 (53.5%)	542 (30.3%)	888 (34.3%)	1179 (35.3%)
Total	288	279	611	865	1249	1786	2591	3343

* Segmentectomy means resection of the anterior segment, posterior segment, medial segment, lateral segment, and caudate lobe.

† Subsegmentectomy means resection of one Couinaud's segment.

depending on the type of hepatectomy. Some of these steps sometimes are reversed, especially the last four. Posterior segmentectomy (Couinaud's 6 and 7),[13] anterior segmentectomy (Couinaud's 5 and 8), and medial segmentectomy (Couinaud's 4) are based on these procedures.

Procedure for Suprahilar Ligation of the Portal Pedicles

Suprahilar ligation of the portal pedicles, a sophisticated technique that is useful for the resection of subsegments of the right lobe (Couinaud's 5, 6, 7, and 8), first was reported by Takasaki, Yamanaka, and Okamoto.[14] The technique does not require the dissection of each branch of the portal vein, hepatic artery, and bile duct, all of which are encased in Glisson's sheath. This procedure is comprised of the following steps: detachment and dislocation of the right portal pedicle; dissection and isolation of segmental and subsegmental pedicles by encircling each with tape (bifurcation points of these pedicles in each segment or subsegment are so close to the porta hepatis that their roots can be accessed without dissecting much of the liver parenchyma)(Fig. 44-3); identification of the segmental or subsegmental areas by temporary occlusion of the pedicles; and resection of the target area.

Ultrasonically Guided Subsegmentectomy)

Ultrasonically guided subsegmentectomy first was reported by Makuuchi and associates.[15] The procedure is performed as follows. The liver is mobilized and the probe for the ultrasonographic apparatus is placed on its surface (Fig. 44-4). The relation between the tumor and the adjacent blood vessels is examined (Fig. 44-5). The location of the tumor is ascertained again to identify the Glisson's vessels, which perfuse the tumor-bearing subsegment. Then, under the guidance of ultrasonography, a 22-gauge needle is inserted into the parenchyma and the tip of the needle is placed in the portal vein.

Figure 44-6 shows the needle inserted into the right anterosuperior branch of the portal vein, with the tip of the needle placed about 1 cm distal to the base of the right anterosuperior branch. After the location of the needle has been confirmed, indigo carmine is injected until the surface of the liver is clearly stained. On the ultrasonogram, the flow of the staining solution in the portal vein can be seen clearly as a current of echogenic tiny spots. The further injection of 1 to 2 mL of dye into the parenchyma (''tattooing'') adjacent to the vessels to be ligated is a useful procedure, because it renders the ligation point at the transection of the parenchyma readily visible. After the ultrasonically guided preparation, hemihepatic vascular occlusion at the hepatic hilum is carried out to reduce blood loss during the parenchymal transection.

Removal of Tumor Thrombi in the Portal Vein

Tumor thrombi in the portal vein are characteristic of HCC, and are related closely to the incidence of intrahepatic metastasis and to the overall prognosis.[14] Of particular concern is portal thrombosis in the main trunk or the first branches of

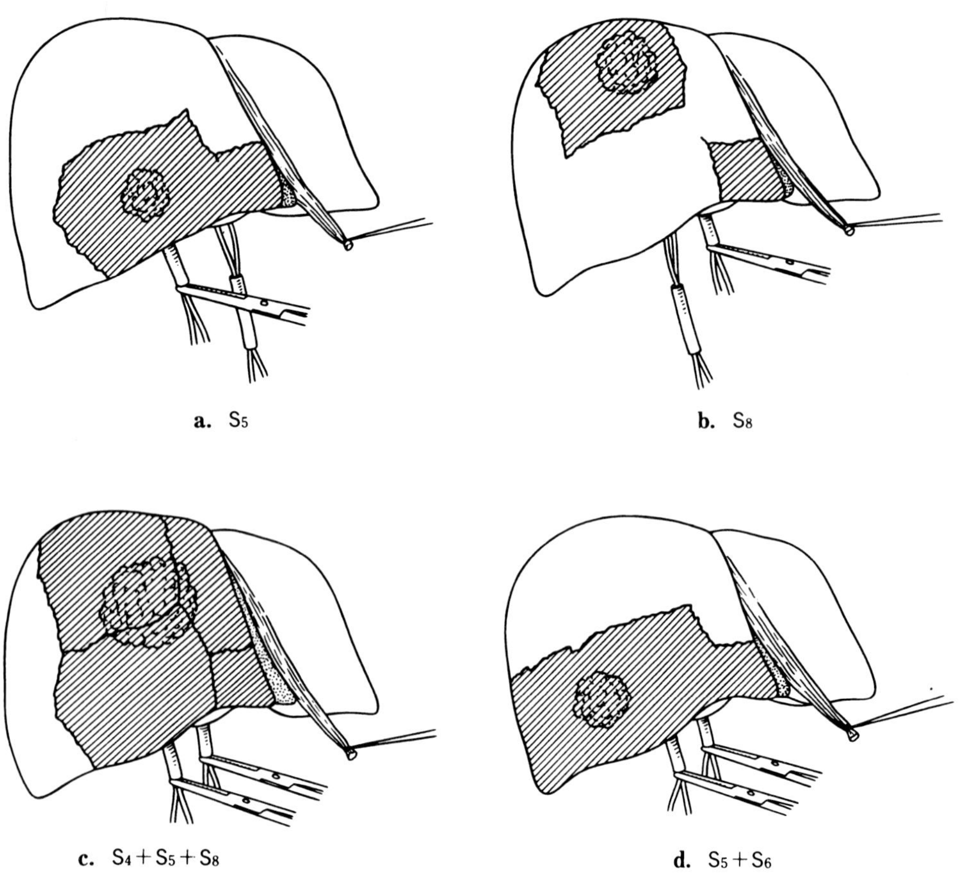

FIG. 44-3. Procedure for suprahilar ligation of the portal pedicles. (Okamoto E, Yamanaka N. Anatomical resection of the right hepatic subsegments preceded by suprahilar ligation of the portal pedicles. In: Tobe T, Kameda, H, Okudaira M, et al, eds. Primary liver cancer in Japan. Springer-Verlag, 1992:229.)

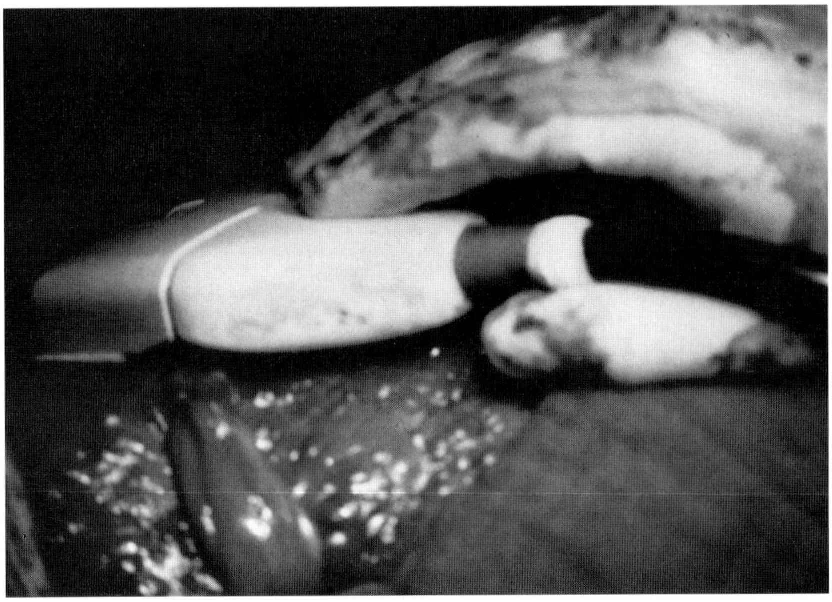

FIG. 44-4. Intraoperative ultrasonography.

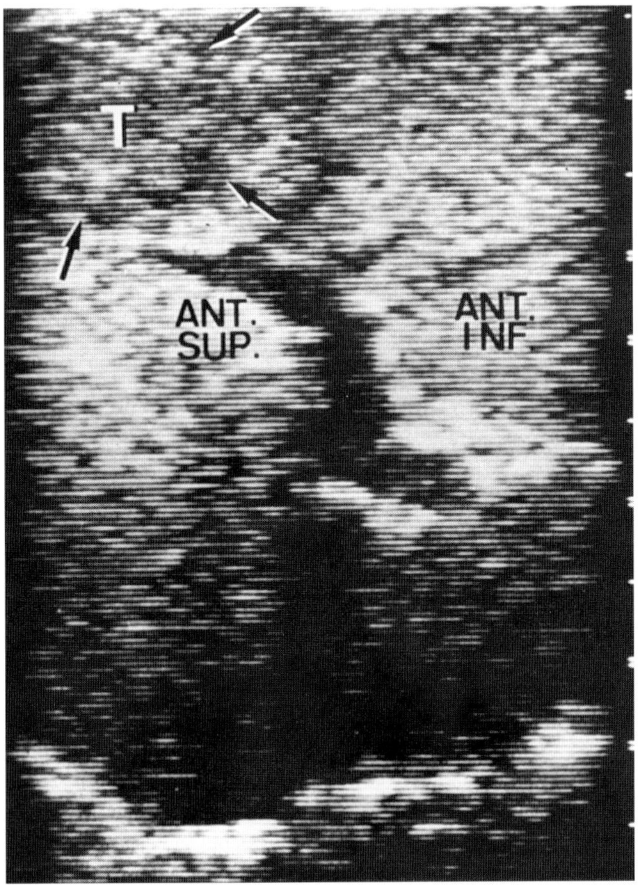

FIG. 44-5. Intraoperative ultrasonography. *T*, tumor *(arrows)*; *ANT. SUP.*, portal branch of the anterosuperior segment; *ANT. INF.* portal branch of the anteroinferior segment.

the portal vein, which can cause portal hypertension, inducing esophageal variceal bleeding. Kumada and Ozawa reported that the removal of tumor thrombi in the remnant portal vein contributes to portal decompression, the feasibility of arterial embolization, and increased resectability of the main tumor.[16] They demonstrated three different techniques: the balloon catheter method, the bypass method, and the open method (Fig. 44-7). It is important that the resection be carried out to the division of Glisson's vessels, which perfuse the tumor-bearing area. This procedure is followed by portal reconstruction and the open method. Kumada and Ozawa recommended the catheter method as the first choice for the management of tumor thrombi in the portal confluence, and the open method for tumor thrombi that develop in secondary branches. They also indicated that elevated serum bilirubin levels in patients with cirrhosis are a contraindication to this procedure, but slight ascites is not. Seven of 13 patients treated by this approach are still alive (mean survival time, 16 months), but the technique is regarded as an emergency procedure primarily for the avoidance of lethal impendence.

COMPLICATIONS OF SURGERY

Posthepatectomy Liver Failure

Postoperative liver failure is the most serious complication of hepatectomy, and is associated with an extremely high mortality rate. The causes of hepatic failure are thought to include excessive removal of liver tissue, hypoxia, hypotension, massive bleeding, and severe infection. The major signs of liver failure are increased jaundice, uncontrollable ascites, encephalopathy, and hemorrhagic diathesis. Effective therapy for these conditions remains to be established, and the development of improved liver support systems is urgently needed.

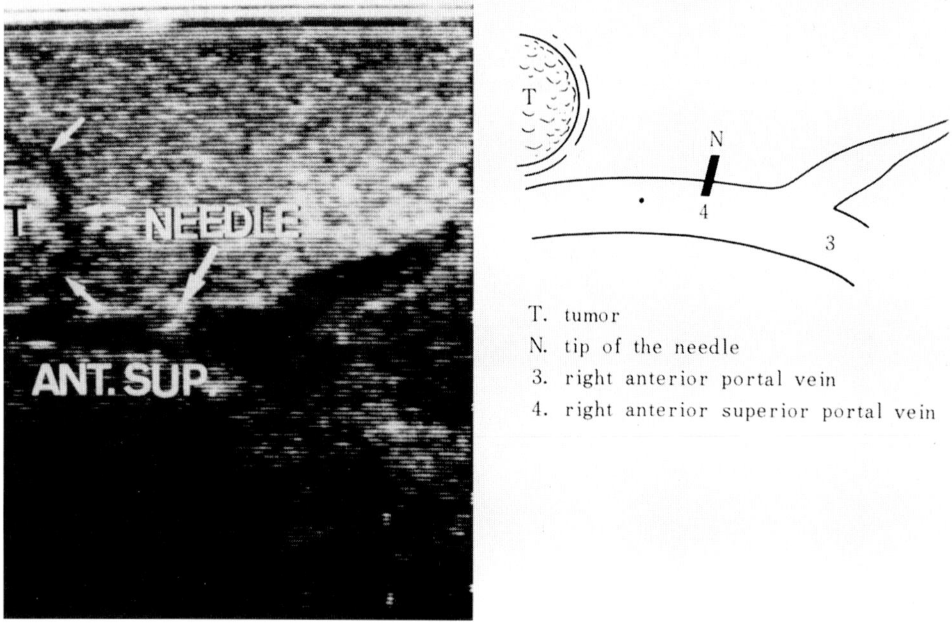

FIG. 44-6. Intraoperative ultrasonography. The needle was inserted into the right anterosuperior portal vein for the injection of dye.

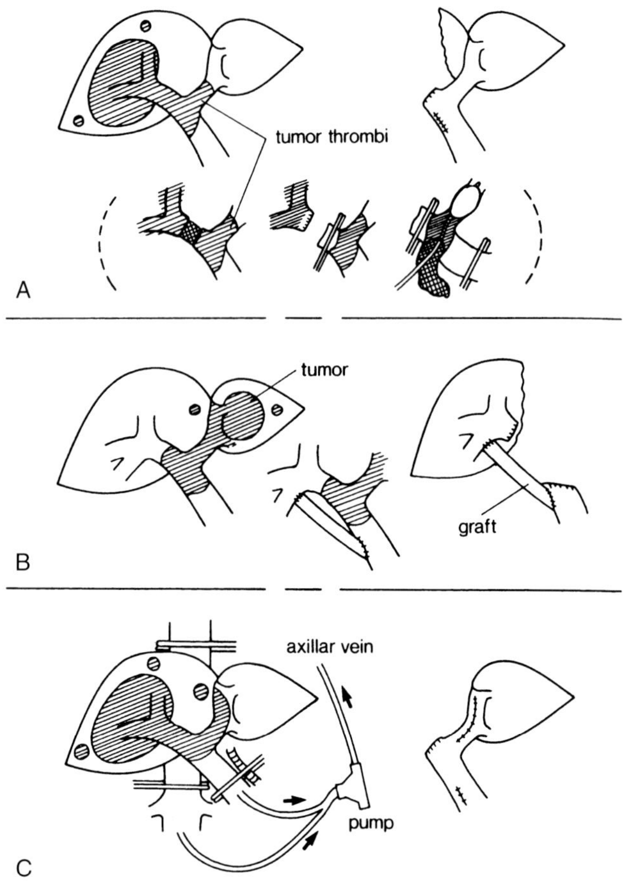

FIG. 44-7. Operative procedures for removal of tumor thrombi of the portal confluence. **(a)** Balloon catheter method. **(b)** Bypass method. **(c)** Open method. (Kumada K, Ozawa K, Okamoto R, et al. Hepatic resection for advanced hepatocellular carcinoma with removal of portal vein tumor thrombi. Surgery 1990;108.

Jaundice

Temporary jaundice with serum bilirubin levels of about 2 to 5 mg/dL is common after hepatectomy and subsides within 7 to 10 days in most cases. However, if there is a background of hepatic cirrhosis, jaundice may persist for more than 10 days. In the experience of these authors, the serum bilirubin level is the most reliable predictor of posthepatectomy liver failure, and more than 10 mg/dL of bilirubin in the serum at 1 week after surgery signifies progressive liver failure. When massive blood transfusions are administered during surgery, indirect bilirubin predominates in the early postoperative period. Thereafter, the ratio of direct bilirubin to indirect bilirubin increases progressively with the development of hepatic failure. Postoperative hepatitis, bile duct stenosis, and recurrent liver cancer should be differentiated from posthepatectomy liver failure. Although plasmapheresis helps reduce bilirubin levels, its effect usually is transient. Ursodeoxycholic acid and steroid hormones also have been used, but their effect is limited in most cases.

Ascites

Along with jaundice and hepatic encephalopathy, ascites is one of the most important pathophysiologic signals of impaired hepatic function. In patients with liver cirrhosis, fluid tends to accumulate as a result of sodium retention. After surgery, it is common to see ascitic fluid being discharged through the abdominal drain. When this discharge is massive (more than 500 mL/d), a low-sodium diet, restricted fluid intake, and diuretic therapy are required in postoperative management. Urine output should be maintained at about 2000 mL/d. When hyponatremia is not present, chlorothiazide and furosemide are the first-choice diuretics. However, when the ascites appears to be intractable, aldosterone antagonists combined with other kinds of diuretics often are effective. Spironolactone (50 mg) and chlorothiazide (50 mg) or furosemide (40 mg) can be administered two times a day. When diuretics are used, serum electrolyte levels should be monitored carefully to prevent hypokalemia and hyponatremia. If hypokalemia occurs, a potassium chloride solution should be administered. Hyponatremia usually is caused by excess water. In such cases, water intake should be restricted. Sodium intake should be restricted because the urinary excretion of sodium is impaired in hepatic cirrhosis. A shunt from the peritoneal cavity to the subclavian vein is indicated for massive and intractable ascites.

Postoperative Bleeding

Postoperative bleeding can be fatal in cirrhotic patients. The most common sites of bleeding are the cut surface of the hepatic parenchyma, the dissected area of the diaphragm, and the right adrenal gland. After hepatectomy, the production of clotting factors in the liver is likely to depend mainly on the hepatic functional reserve. The most significant factor that contributes to postoperative bleeding is the degree of liver cirrhosis. Fresh blood, which is rich in clotting factors, is preferable for blood transfusions to cirrhotic patients during surgery. In addition, hemostasis is facilitated if the anticipated area of bleeding is coated with fibrin gel. When postoperative bleeding occurs, the induction of an irreversible state of shock should be prevented. Hypotension of long duration frequently induces irreversible hepatic failure, especially in cirrhotic patients. Therefore, when no hemodynamic improvement is apparent using conservative methods, repeated laparotomy should be carried out promptly.

Bile Leakage

Leakage of bile from the cut surface of the hepatic parenchyma sometimes is intractable, even when there is no stricture downstream from the bile duct. To prevent bile leakage, these authors routinely perform a ''leak test,'' in which the extravasation of dye infused with a catheter inserted from the stump of the cystic duct to the common bile duct is examined. In addition, a drainage tube should be placed close to the cut surface of the liver. When the drainage is insufficient and retained bile is contaminated with bacteria, subphrenic abscesses may occur. If the bile leakage continues for 2 to 3 months, surgical treatment should be considered.

Adult Respiratory Distress Syndrome

Although the causative mechanism of the adult respiratory distress syndrome (ARDS) after hepatectomy is not well understood, the condition is encountered frequently. The initial sign, which precedes chest radiographic findings, is a decrease in PaO_2 levels with blood gas analysis. Pardy and Dudley suggested that the occurrence of ARDS after hepatectomy is related closely to impaired hepatic function, because the liver is working with the reticuloendothelial system as a prepulmonary filter.[17] Because the liver accounts for about 85% of the reticuloendothelial system in the whole body,[18] extensive reduction in the volume of the reticuloendothelial system may be an important factor in the development of ARDS. When the Pao_2 does not increase above 65 mm Hg, even with oxygen administration using a face mask, endotracheal intubation and assisted ventilation with positive end-expiratory pressure should be performed. The administration of diuretics contributes to the improvement of ARDS, and a steroid hormone (Solu-Medrol) sometimes is indicated in compromised patients.

Acute Renal Failure

When oliguria or anuria occurs despite adequate fluid infusion, acute renal failure should be suspected, and serum blood urea nitrogen and creatinine levels should be determined. In particular, persistent jaundice frequently induces renal failure (the hepatorenal syndrome). The ratio of serum creatinine to urinary creatinine usually is less than 5, and the ratio of blood urea nitrogen to serum creatinine is between 20 and 30 in acute renal failure. Hemodialysis is indicated when the blood urea nitrogen level is more than 60 mg/dL, the serum creatinine level is more than 4 to 5 mg/dL, and the serum potassium level is more than 6.5 mEq/L. In many cases, acute renal failure occurs in association with multiple organ failure.

Disseminated Intravascular Coagulation

Bacterial infection and endotoxemia induce the development of disseminated intravascular coagulation (DIC) with high frequency in cirrhotic patients, because liver cirrhosis is thought to predispose to DIC. DIC should be suspected if the following findings are observed: a thrombocyte count less than 15,000/mm, a fibrinogen level less than 160 mg/dL, and a prothrombin time longer than 15 seconds. Further, if the value of fibrinogen degradation products is abnormally high, DIC should be diagnosed and treated with heparin. Heparin, 150 to 500 U/kg/d, usually is administered by continuous intravenous infusion. The drug acts indirectly by enhancing the function of antithrombin III. Therefore, antithrombin III should be added externally when serum antithrombin III levels are decreased. Therapy for DIC should be initiated as soon as the condition is strongly suspected or its occurrence is predicted.

Multiple Organ Failure

The most life-threatening state after hepatectomy is multiple organ failure. Eiseman and colleagues first reported that advances in the field of surgery that permit survival despite the failure of several vital organs have created a new clinical syndrome, which they termed *multiple organ failure*.[19] Multiple organ failure consists of the failure of several or all of the following systems: liver, lung, kidney, and clotting system. In general, multiple organ failure is an end-stage condition. No established therapy is available, although aggressive treatment of each organ system may contribute to survival.

SURVIVAL RATES AFTER HEPATECTOMY

The Liver Cancer Study Group of Japan has been conducting a nationwide survey of Japanese patients with HCC since 1965. Up to December 31, 1991, more than 40,000 patients from more

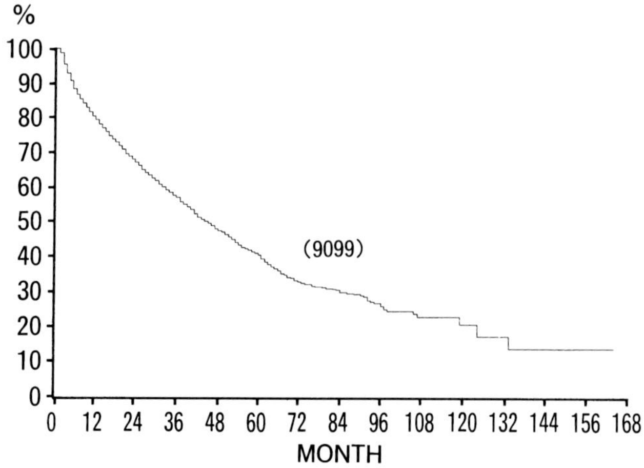

FIG. 44-8. Survival rates of patients with hepatocellular carcinoma who undergo hepatic resection.

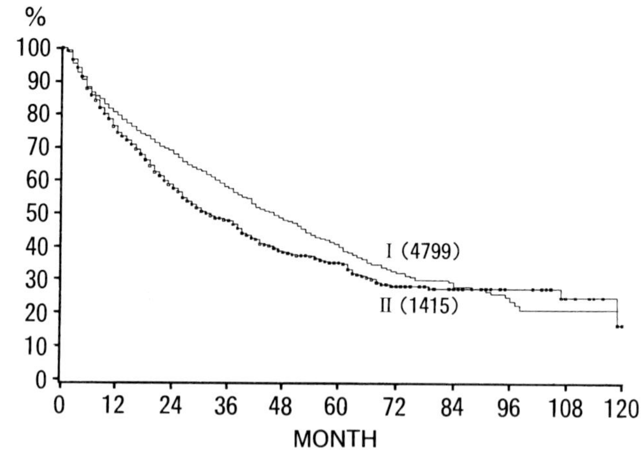

FIG. 44-10. Survival rates in relation to positivity for hepatitis B surface antigen (HBsAg). *I,* HBsAg-negative; *II,* HBsAg-positive.

than 600 hospitals had been registered in a computer at Kyoto University.

Cumulative survival rates calculated by the method of Cutler-Ederer are described for this follow-up study. The overall 1-, 2-, 3-, 5-, and 8-year survival rates were 80.3%, 68%, 57.5%, 40.8%, and 26.4%, respectively (Fig. 44-8). The survival rates in relation to clinical and histopathologic factors are listed below.

Age

When the patients were divided into three age groups (younger than 40 years, 40 to 59 years, and older than 60 years), a significant difference was observed between the survival rates of the two older groups. Patients younger than 40 years seemed to survive longer than older patients. The survival rate of the younger group during the relatively early postoperative period was lower than that of the older groups (Fig. 44-9).

Gender

No significant difference was observed between males and females, although the latter tended to survive longer than the former.

Hepatitis B Surface Antigen

The survival rate was significantly higher among HBsAg-negative patients than among HBsAg-positive patients (Fig. 44-10).

α-Fetoprotein

When the patients were divided into five groups according to their serum α-fetoprotein levels (0 to 20, 21 to 200, 201 to 1000, 1001 to 10,000, and more than 10,000 ng/mL), their survival rates correlated with their α-fetoprotein values. As the α-fetoprotein values increased, the survival rates decreased (Fig. 44-11).

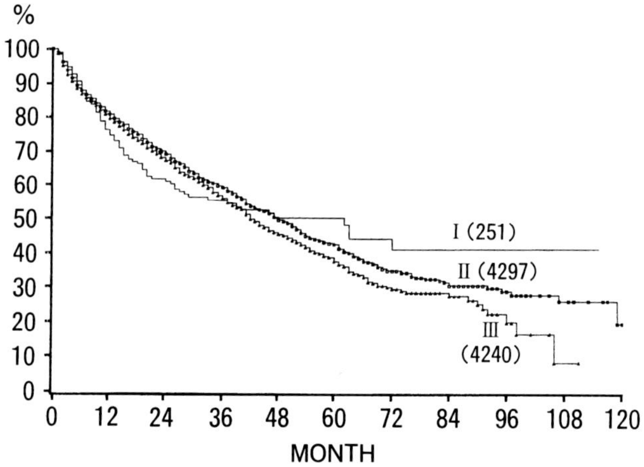

FIG. 44-9. Survival rates in relation to age. *I,* younger than 40 years; *II,* 41 to 60 years; *III,* Older than 60 years.

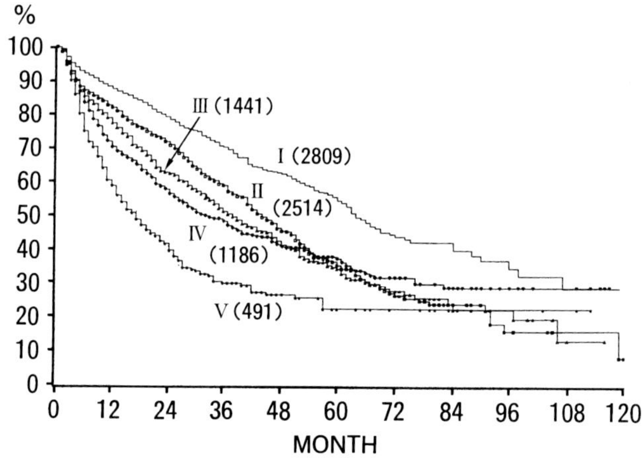

FIG. 44-11. Survival rates in relation to serum level of α-fetoprotein. *I,* 0–20 ng/mL; *II,* 21–200 ng/mL; *III,* 201–1000 ng/mL; *IV,* 1001–10,000 ng/mL; *V,* ≥10,001 ng/mL.

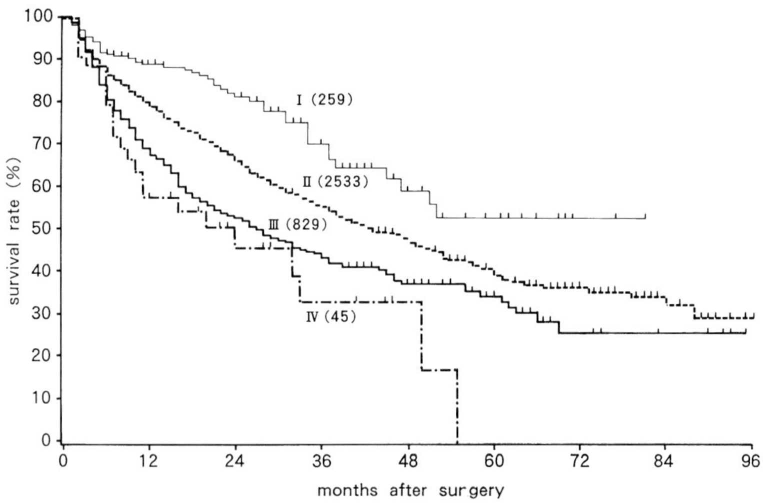

FIG. 44-12. Survival rates in relation to Edmondson-Steiner classification.

Grade of Anaplasia of Cancer Cells (Edmondson-Steiner Classification)

There was a significant correlation between survival rate and Edmondson-Steiner classification (Fig. 44-12).

Tumor Size

In patients with tumors smaller than 2 cm in diameter, the 1-, 2-, 3-, and 5-year survival rates were 89.8%, 82.6%, 73.1%, and 54.9%, respectively. Patients with tumors larger than 2 cm in diameter had a poorer prognosis (2.1 to 5 cm: 1 year, 85.1%; 2 years, 74.4%; 3 years, 64.1%; 5 years, 44.6%). The differences among these three groups (0–2 cm, 2.1 ~ 5.0 cm, 5.1 ~ 10 cm) were significant (Fig. 44-13).

Tumor Number

The survival rates of the patients with solitary tumors were 84.1% at 1 year, 73.6% at 2 years, 63.9% at 3 years, and 46.8% at 5 years, whereas those of the patients with two tumors were 79.1% at 1 year, 65.2% at 2 years, 52.7% at 3 years, and 36.2% at 5 years. There was a significant difference in survival between the patients with single tumors and those with two or more tumors, but no significant difference between those with two tumors and those with three tumors (Fig. 44-14).

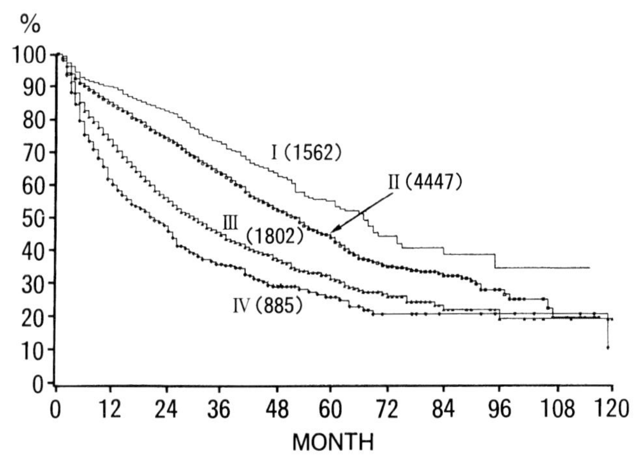

FIG. 44-13. Survival rates in relation to tumor size in maximal diameter. *I,* 0–2 cm; *II,* 2.1–5 cm; *III,* 5.1–10 cm; *IV,* greater than 10.1 cm.

Infiltration of Cancer Cells Into the Tumor Capsule

The infiltration of cancer cells into the fibrous capsule of the tumor was related to a low survival rate. In the patients without capsular infiltration, 1-, 2-, 3-, and 5-year survival rates were 85.5%, 75.5%, 65.6%, and 47.5%, respectively, whereas in the patients with infiltration, they were 77.6%, 62.2%, 51.1%, and 35.4%, respectively (Fig. 44-15).

Invasion of the Portal Vein by Tumor

There was a significant difference in survival associated with the presence or absence of portal vein invasion by tumor. In the absence of portal vein invasion, survival rates were 85.6% at 1 year, 74.9% at 2 years, 64.6% at 3 years, and 45.7% at 5 years, whereas in the presence of portal vein invasion, they were 61.8% at 1 year, 45% at 2 years, 33.9% at 3 years, and 27.5% at 5 years (Fig. 44-16).

Accompanying Liver Cirrhosis

The patients with chronic hepatitis had a significantly higher survival rate than the patients with liver cirrhosis. However, there was no significant difference between the patients without chronic liver disease and the other two groups. This result was attributable to the low survival rate in the early postoperative period of the patients without pathologic livers, although these patients had apparently survived longer (Fig. 44-17).

Surgical Curability

Surgical curability was defined by the general rules for the clinical and pathologic study of primary liver cancer established

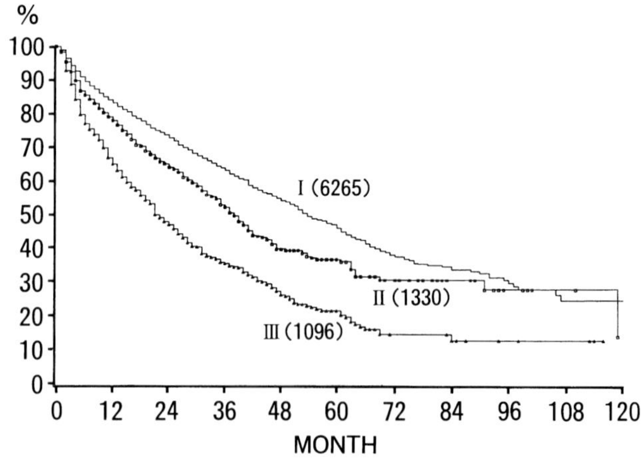

FIG. 44-14. Survival rates in relation to number of tumors. *I,* solitary tumor; *II,* two tumors; *III,* three or more tumors.

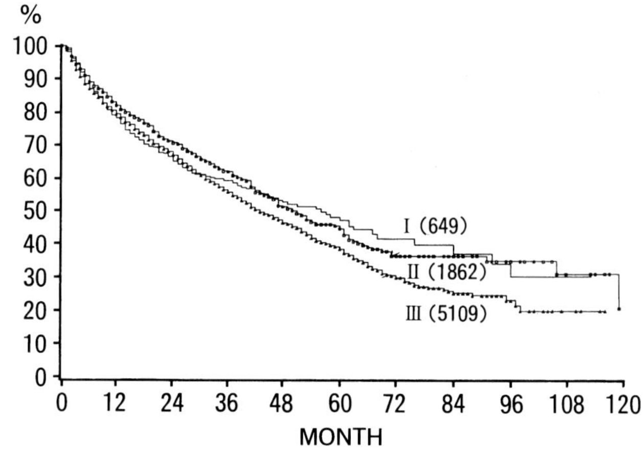

FIG. 44-17. Survival rates in relation to accompanying liver cirrhosis. *I,* no chronic liver disease; *II,* fibrosis or chronic hepatitis; *III,* liver cirrhosis.

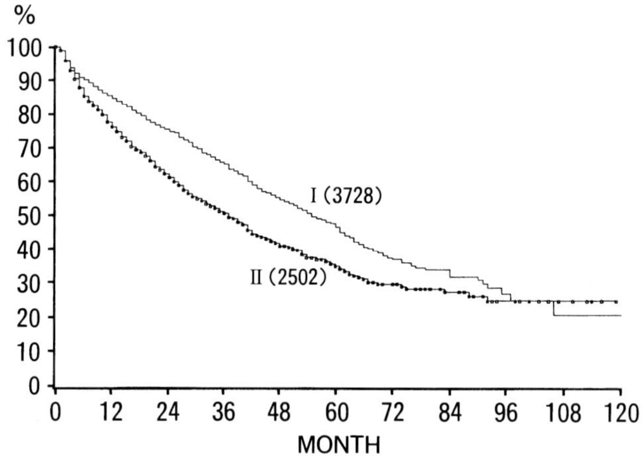

FIG. 44-15. Survival rates in relation to capsular infiltration of cancer cells. *I,* absence of capsular infiltration; *II,* presence of capsular infiltration.

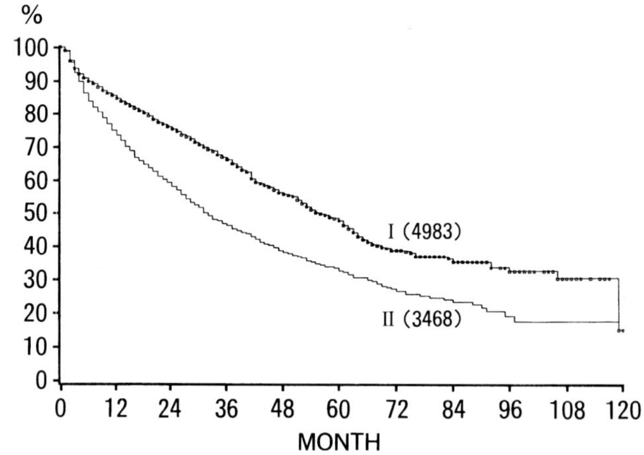

FIG. 44-18. Survival rates in relation to surgical curability. *I,* curative operation; *II,* noncurative operation.

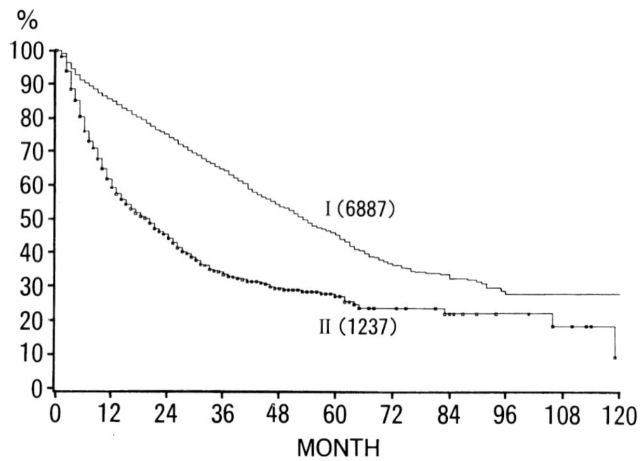

FIG. 44-16. Survival rates in relation to portal involvement. *I,* absence of portal involvement; *II,* presence of portal involvement.

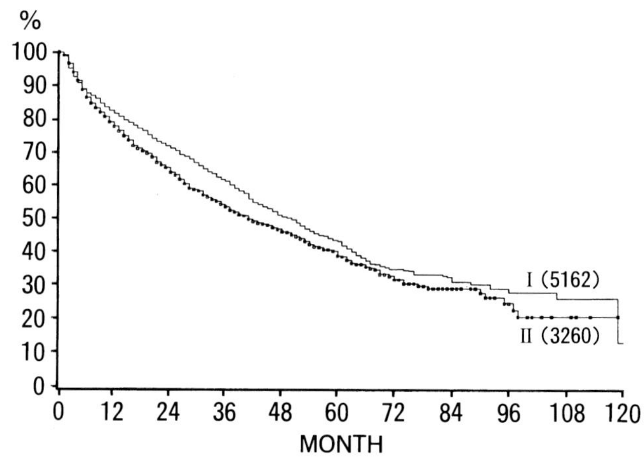

FIG. 44-19. Survival rates in relation to 1-cm cancer-free margin. *I,* presence of 1-cm cancer-free margin; *II,* absence of 1-cm cancer-free margin.

by the Liver Cancer Study Group of Japan. The patients who underwent curative resection had a higher survival rate than those who underwent noncurative resection (Fig. 44-18).

One-Centimeter Cancer-Free Margin

Controversy has existed regarding the critical distance between the edge of the tumor and the cut surface necessary to attain maximum curability. In this survey, the survival rates were calculated in relation to a 1-cm cancer-free margin. The patients who underwent hepatic resection with a 1-cm cancer-free margin survived longer than those without such a margin (Fig. 44-19).

REFERENCES

1. Okuda K. The Liver Cancer Study Group of Japan. Primary liver cancers in Japan. Cancer 1980;45:2663.
2. The Liver Cancer Study Group of Japan. Primary liver cancer in Japan—sixth report. Cancer 1987;60:1400.
3. The Liver Cancer Study Group of Japan. Primary liver cancer in Japan. Clinicopathologic features and results of surgical treatment. Ann Surg 1990;211:277.
4. The Liver Cancer Study Group of Japan. Predictive factors for long term prognosis after partial hepatectomy for patients with hepatocellular carcinoma in Japan. 1994;74:2772.
5. The Liver Cancer Study Group of Japan. The general rules for the clinical and pathological study of primary liver cancer. Jpn J Surg 1989; 19:98.
6. Ozawa K, Ida T, Yamada T, et al. Significance of glucose tolerance as prognostic sign in hepatectomized patients. Am J Surg 1976;131: 541.
7. Ozawa K, Aoyama K, Yasuda Y, et al. Metabolic abnormalities associated with postoperative organ failure—a redox theory. Arch Surg 1983; 118:1245.
8. Noguchi T, Imai T, Mizumoto R. Preoperative estimation of surgical risk of hepatectomy in cirrhotic patients. Hepatogastroenterology 1990; 37:165.
9. Yamanaka N, Okamoto E, Kuwata K, et al. A multiple regression equation for prediction of posthepatectomy liver failure. Ann Surg 1984;200:658.
10. Rous P, Larimore LD. Relation of the portal blood to liver maintenance. J Exp Med 1920;31:609.
11. Honjo I, Suzuki T, Ozawa K, et al. Ligation of a branch of the portal vein for carcinoma of the liver. Am J Surg 1975;130:296.
12. Kinoshita H, Sakai K, Hirohashi K, et al. Preoperative portal vein embolization for hepatocellular carcinoma. World J Surg 1986;10:803.
13. Couinaud C: Bases anatomiques des hépatectomies gauche et droite réglées. Techniques qui en découlent. J Chir (Paris) 1954;70:933.
14. Okamoto E, Yamanaka N. Anatomical resection of the right hepatic subsegments preceded by suprahilar ligation of the portal pedicles. In: Tobe T, et al, eds. Primary liver cancer in Japan. Springer-Verlag, 1992:229.
15. Makuuchi M, Hasegawa H, Yamazaki S. Ultrasonically guided subsegmentectomy. Surg Gynecol Obstet 1985;161:346.
16. Kumada K, Ozawa K, Okamoto R, et al. Hepatic resection for advanced hepatocellular carcinoma with removal of portal vein tumor thrombi. Surgery 1990;108:821.
17. Pardy BJ, Dudley HAF. Post-traumatic pulmonary insufficiency. Surg Gynecol Obstet 1977;144:259.
18. Arii S, Shibagaki S, Tobe T, et al. Changes in the reticuloendothelial phagocytic function following partial hepatectomy of rats. J Lab Clin Med 1985;105:668.
19. Eiseman B, Beart R, Norton L. Multiple organ failure. Surg Gynecol Obstet 1977;144:323.

Surgery for Gastrointestinal Cancer: A Multidisciplinary Approach, edited by Harold J. Wanebo.
Lippincott-Raven Publishers, Philadelphia, © 1997.

CHAPTER 45

Surgical Resection of Small Hepatocellular Carcinoma

Zhao-You Tang, Ye-Qin Yu, and Xin-Da Zhou

Hepatocellular carcinoma (HCC), a fatal malignancy prevalent in Southeast Asia and Africa, is responsible for 250,000 deaths every year worldwide. About 45% (110,000) of these deaths occur in China.[1] The prognosis of HCC was dismal for decades, but has begun to improve steadily. In the United States, 5-year relative survival rates were 2% between 1960 and 1963, 3% between 1970 and 1973, 4% between 1974 and 1976, and 6% between 1983 and 1988.[2] At the authors' institution, 5-year survival rates also have improved during the past 3 decades.[3] It is widely accepted that surgery plays a major role in prolonging the survival of patients with HCC. Unfortunately, only 5% to 10% of patients with HCC are candidates for resection, and the 5-year survival rate after the resection of large tumors is less than 20%. However, the use of α-fetoprotein (AFP) serologic surveys and ultrasonographic monitoring in high-risk populations is expanding the role of HCC surgery.

BRIEF HISTORICAL AND LITERATURE REVIEW

The discovery of AFP in 1956, particularly AFP detectable in the sera of patients with HCC, provided a new clue to the diagnosis of asymptomatic small HCC.[4] Unfortunately, the value of AFP serologic surveys in early detection was not widely acknowledged because of the dismal results of AFP screening in Africa.[5] However, the discovery of small tumors (5 cm or less) was reported early in 1975 by Okuda and colleagues during follow-up monitoring of AFP levels.[6] In China, AFP serologic surveys with agar gel diffusion assays were conducted between 1971 and 1973. Of the 343,999 individuals screened, 147 asymptomatic patients were found to have elevated AFP levels, and 88.4% of them were proven to have HCC during 2 to 10 months of follow-up.[7] More impressive results were obtained after passive reverse hemagglutination assays and radiorocket electrophoresis autography came into use in 1974.[8] The first report of resection of small HCC was published by Yu and Sang in 1975.[9] In 1977, Tang and Qian reported 33 cases of resection for subclinical HCC, with a 2-year survival rate of 77%.[10] In Shanghai, nearly 2 million individuals were screened between 1971 and 1976. Of the 300 patients found to have HCC, 134 (44.7%) had subclinical disease, and the 3-year survival rate after resection was 57.1%.[11] In 1979, the authors reported a 3-year survival rate of 70.5% after resection of small HCC in 30 patients.[12] The 2-year survival rate after resection of subclinical HCC was 69% in a report from a high-risk area of China (Qidong County) in 1981.[13] Papers concerning resection of small or subclinical HCC have been published since the 1970s.[14–21]

Five- and 10-year survival rates have become available from long-term follow-up studies. As listed in Table 45-1, 5-year survival rates after resection of small HCC varied from 11% to 72.5%, but most were around 40% to 60%.[20,22–29] Ten-year survival rates were higher after limited resection than after lobectomy (50.6% versus 38.5%).[20] Five-year survival rates after resection of small HCC (less than 2 cm) were even better (60.5% in a series of 347 patients, 61% in a series of 23 patients, and 100% in a series of 14 patients).[30–32] In the authors' series, the increasing use of limited resection and growing experience with resection of tumors in segment VIII led to an increase in resectability rates for small HCC, from 75% in the 1970s to 93.3% in the 1980s[20,33] (see Table 45-1).

IMPLICATIONS OF RESECTION OF SMALL HEPATOCELLULAR CARCINOMA

Based on 2 decades of long-term follow-up studies, the implications of resection of small HCC are summarized.

Long-term Survival Data

When Curutchet and colleagues summarized the worldwide data from 1905 through 1970, only 45 patients with 5-year

Z-Y Tang, Liver Cancer Institute, Shanghai Medical University, Shanghai 200032, China.
Y-Q Yu, Liver Cancer Institute, Shanghai Medical University, Shanghai 200032, China.
X-D Zhou, Liver Cancer Institute, Shanghai Medical University, Shanghai 200032, China.

TABLE 45-1. *Selected series of patients undergoing resection of small hepatocellular carcinoma with 5-year survival rates*

Author	Number of patients	Five-year survival (%)
1985 Nakanishi et al[22]	25	72.5
1985 Kanematsu et al[23]	32	22.2
1986 Wu et al[24]	70	64.0
1987 Okamoto et al[25]	79	46.0
1988 Huang[26]	50	48.7
1990 Yamanaka et al[27]	124	47.0
1991 Lai et al[28]	39	11.0
1993 Makuuchi et al[29]	349	43.7
1994 Tang et al (This series)	407	64.3 (10–year, 49.5)

survival were found.[34] By December 1991, 135 5-year survivors had been treated at the authors' institution, 69 (51.1%) of whom underwent resection of small HCC.[3]

Five-Year Survival Data

In the authors' institution, the 5-year survival rate was 3% in the 1960s and 12.2% in the 1970s. The rate increased to 40.2% in the 1980s in association with a rise in the percentages of small tumors in the series (2.2%, 11.8%, and 30.6%).[3]

Effectiveness in Comparison With Resection of Large Hepatocellular Carcinoma

In the authors' institution, 381 patients with small HCC were compared with 1261 patients with large HCC. Patients with small HCC had a higher resectability rate (90.6% versus 43.9%) and a lower operative mortality rate (2% versus 5.8%). The number of long-term survivors was similar (69 versus 66) in both groups, but the number of patients with small HCC was only one third the number of patients with large HCC.[3]

Research and Changing Concepts

Studies on the resection of small HCC have stimulated research on HCC markers, imaging, and related basic aspects (eg, precancerous lesions and adenomatous hyperplasia, unicentric or multicentric origin of HCC, ploidy pattern, kinetic change of biologic characteristics during HCC evolution, expression of hepatitis B virus X gene, and p53 mutation).[35–39] Interest in the early diagnosis, extent of resection, management of recurrence, and natural history of HCC has been renewed.[40–42]

GENERAL DATA FROM THE AUTHORS' SERIES

From January 1967 to December 1992, 445 patients with pathologically and surgically proven small HCC (5 cm or less) were treated at the Liver Cancer Institute of Shanghai Medical University. The median age of the patients was 50 years (range, 21 to 76 years), and the male : female ratio was 11.7 : 1 (410 males and 35 females). Two hundred seventy patients (60.8%) had histories of hepatitis, with a median duration of disease of 13 years (range, 1 to 33 years). Serum HBsAg was detected in 312 (75.4%) of 414 patients, and the rate of anti-HBcAg positivity was 78.6%. Associated liver cirrhosis was found in 92.3% of patients, with micronodular cirrhosis in 27.8% and macronodular cirrhosis in 64.5%.

Of the 445 patients treated, 238 (53.5%) were detected through general population screening or regular health check-ups using AFP, ultrasonography, or both, and 80 (18%) were discovered through high-risk population screening. Only 127 (28.5%) of the patients had clinical symptoms and signs.

Laboratory evaluation revealed elevated AFP levels in 344 (78.4%) of 439 patients (21 to 500 μg/L in 29.2%, greater than 500 μg/L in 49.2%). Here, the entire series includes large HCC. γ-Glutamyl transpeptidase levels were abnormal in 150 (35.1%) of 427 patients.

Ultrasonography was positive in 386 (96.5%) of 400 patients, computed tomography (CT) in 267 (95.7%) of 279 patients, angiography in 40 (85.1%) of 47 patients, and ^{99m}Tc-pyridoxyl-5-methyl trytophan (PMT) scanning in 21 (43.8%) of 48 patients.

Operative findings in the 445 patients revealed a single HCC nodule in 345 patients (77.5%), HCC of the right lobe in 277 patients (62.3%), HCC of the left lobe in 92 patients (20.7%), HCC of the hilar area or caudal lobe in 39 patients (8.8%), and bilateral HCC in 37 patients (8.3%).

The treatment modalities used in the series were as follows: resection in 407 patients (91.5%), cryosurgery or laser vaporization in 17 patients (3.8%), hepatic artery ligation or cannulation in 16 patients (3.6%), intralesional ethanol injection in 2 patients (0.5%), and exploration laparotomy in 3 patients (0.7%). The operative mortality rate within 30 days after resection was 1.7% (7 of 407 patients).

Pathologic examination of the surgical specimens revealed HCC differentiation of grade I in 7.1% of patients, grade II in 85.6%, grade III in 7.4%, and grade IV in 0%. Well-encapsulated tumors were found in 76.2% of patients, no tumor embolus was found in 66.5%, gross tumor embolus was found in 3.4%, and microscopic tumor embolus was found in 30.1%.

Reoperation was done for recurrence or lung metastasis in 60 patients. The median interval between the first and second operations was 18 months (range, 2 to 195 months). Repeated resection was performed in 47 patients (78.3%), cryosurgery or laser vaporization in 6 patients (10%), hepatic artery ligation or cannulation in 2 patients (3.3%), intralesional ethanol injection in 2 patients (3.3%), and lung resection in 2 patients (5%).

Survival rates were calculated by the life-table method using a microcomputer. The 1-, 2-, 3-, 4-, 5-, and 10-year survival rates for the entire series of 445 patients were 87.4%, 76.5%, 71%, 64.7%, 60.3%, and 44.8%, respectively, and those for the 407 patients who underwent resection were 88.7%, 79.6%, 74.9%, 68.4%, 64.3%, and 49.5%, respectively.

The 5- and 10-year survival rates for the 69 patients treated between January 1967 and December 1982 were 46.4% and 30.4%, and those for the 376 patients treated between January 1983 and December 1992 were 65.7% and 54.8%.

The 1-, 3-, 5-, and 10-year survival rates for the 60 patients who underwent reoperation were 98.3%, 75.4%, 60.8%, and 37.9%, respectively, when calculated from the first operation, and 79.3%, 51.8%, 46.0%, and 30.7%, respectively, when calculated from the second operation.

SURGICAL INDICATIONS FOR SMALL HEPATOCELLULAR CARCINOMA

Accurate Diagnosis

In the authors' institution, the rate of AFP positivity was 72.2% in 1464 inpatients, similar to the rate of 72.4% reported by the Ninth National Liver Cancer Survey in Japan.[43] From 1981 to 1991, AFP levels were greater than 20 μg/L in 75.4% of patients with small HCC (5 cm or less).[20] Therefore, AFP levels were useful in the diagnosis of small HCC, particularly in Asian patients. The diagnostic criteria for AFP were levels consistently greater than 500 μg/L for 1 month, or greater than 200 μg/L for 2 months without coexisting active liver disease (ie, abnormal serum alanine aminotransferase levels, bilirubin levels, or prothrombin times) and with the exclusion of pregnancy or teratoma of the gonads. Abnormal prothrombin (des-γ-carboxy prothrombin) was helpful in detecting non–AFP-producing HCC, but was less sensitive for small HCC. Imaging modalities were useful for the diagnosis and localization of small HCC. The rate of positivity for ultrasonography was as high as 96.5% in this series, which was similar to the 92.2% reported by Shinagawa and colleagues.[44] Small HCC (3 cm or less) usually showed a hypoechoic area with a halo image (capsule), whereas most small hemangiomas were hyperechoic and without a halo.[45] On CT, the injection of contrast medium usually demonstrated rapid filling of the hypodense area and revealed a totally hyperdense area in small hemangiomas, which was helpful in differentiating these lesions from small HCC.[46] Tumor vessels and tumor staining usually were found in small HCC using angiography. The rate of positivity of angiography for small HCC was 77.8% for lesions measuring 1 to 2 cm, 88.5% for lesions measuring 2 to 3 cm, 71.4% for lesions measuring 3 to 4 cm, and 88.9% for lesions measuring 4 to 5 cm,[47] and was 85.1% in the authors' series. CT with Lipiodol revealed many small HCC lesions that were not found by other techniques.[48] The detection rate of magnetic resonance imaging was 97.5% in lesions measuring more than 2 cm, but only 33.3% in lesions measuring less than 2 cm.[49] ^{99m}Tc-PMT delayed hepatobiliary scintigraphy also was useful in the diagnosis of small HCC, detecting 33.3% of lesions measuring less than 2 cm, 41.2% of lesions measuring 2 to 3 cm, 60% of lesions measuring 3 to 4 cm, and 54.2% of lesions measuring 4 to 5 cm. The smallest lesion detected measured 1.2 cm. Only HCC and hepatic adenomas could be detected on PMT scanning.[50] The detection rates for the 89 lesions measuring less than 2 cm were 97.8% for ultrasonography, 75.4% for angiography, 61.6% for magnetic resonance imaging, and 54% for CT.[51] In general, 1-cm lesions were not difficult to detect using serum markers and imaging techniques. Using a sensitive kit for the detection of hepatitis B virus markers in Chinese patients with HCC, one or more markers for hepatitis B virus were found in as many as 97.4% of 114 patients.[52] Therefore, a complete absence of serum hepatitis B virus markers can help to exclude HCC in China.

Hepatic Functional Reserve

To estimate surgical risk and guide the selection of surgical procedures, parameters for evaluating hepatic functional reserve have been reviewed thoroughly by Mizumoto and Noguchi. Serum bilirubin; albumin; prothrombin time; indocyanine green retention rate at 15 minutes, indocyanine green disappearance rate, or indocyanine green maximal removal rate; and Child's classification are the parameters used most commonly in Japan.[53]

In the authors' institution, a reversed serum albumin-to-globulin ratio, impaired prothrombin time (less than 50% of the normal value), or high bilirubin level (greater than 2 mg/dL) is a contraindication to surgery. A serum γ-glutamyl transpeptidase level is of value for assessing resectability and predicting prognosis.[54]

Tumor Status

Surgery is not recommended when there are more than three tumor nodules. Tumors located in the hepatic hilar area are not unresectable, but a second-stage resection after cytoreductive therapy is suggested when the tumor measures around 5 cm and is close to major vessels, and curative resection is difficult.

Contraindications

Besides obvious disorders in important organs (eg, heart, lung, kidney) and severe systemic diseases (eg, diabetes), jaundice, ascites, distant metastasis, and tumor emboli in the main trunk of the portal vein are contraindications to surgery. Ultrasonography is of great value in detecting emboli in the main trunk of the portal vein.

PREOPERATIVE PREPARATION

Ultrasonography

In the authors' institution, the chief surgeon must perform preoperative ultrasonography to guide the operative position and incision, to estimate the distance between the tumor nodule and major vessels, to determine satellites, to plan the extent of resection, and to evaluate the severity of cirrhosis.

Preoperative Routine

Meticulous preoperative management is necessary because of the close association of HCC with liver cirrhosis (92.3% in this series, primarily macronodular cirrhosis) and the fact that the risk of right lobectomy with cirrhosis rises as tumor size decreases. The routine should include intravenous administration of glucose, vitamin C, and vitamin K; plasma or albumin, if needed; an oral antibiotic immediately before surgery; and Chinese herbs to strengthen host defenses or improve liver function.

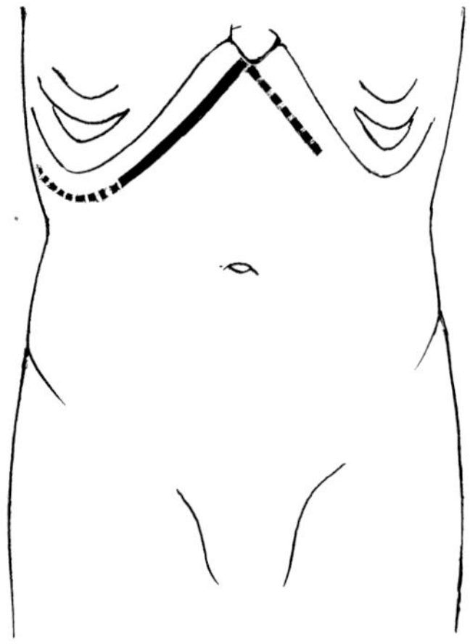

FIG. 45-1. Incision for resection of small hepatocellular carcinoma.

SURGICAL PROCEDURE FOR SMALL HEPATOCELLULAR CARCINOMA

Anesthesia and Blood Transfusion

General anesthesia with a sufficient oxygen supply is suggested. Transfusion with fresh blood through an upper extremity is superior to banked blood given through a lower extremity.

Position and Incision

Preoperative ultrasonography is helpful to guide the patient's position according to the tumor site. As shown in Figure 45-1, a right subcostal incision is used routinely. An extension in the left subcostal direction usually is needed for left lobe resection. An extension toward the 12th rib is helpful for right posterior resection. When a strong retractor is used, a transthoracic abdominal incision seldom is needed.

Selection of Surgical Treatment

Resection remains the treatment of choice for small HCC; 91.5% of the patients with small HCC who were candidates for surgery in the authors' series underwent resection. However, in patients with severe cirrhosis or with tumors close to major vessels, cryosurgery using −196°C liquid nitrogen with repeated freezing and thawing cycles, or high-power yttrium-aluminum-garnet laser vaporization are alternatives to resection, particularly when the tumor is on the surface of the liver.[55] Hepatic artery ligation or cannulation or both on the affected side is indicated for multiple or deep-seated unresectable small tumors. Intralesional ethanol injection is another alternative for unresectable small HCC.

TABLE 45-2. *Types of resection in small hepatocellular carcinoma*

Types of resection	Number of patients	Percentage
Local resection	278	68.3
Left lateral segmentectomy	35	8.6
Left himihepatectomy	29	7.1
Left trisegmentectomy	1	0.3
Right posterior labectomy	34	8.3
Right hemihepatectomy	4	1.0
Middle lobectomy	7	1.7
Two-site resection	19	4.7
Total	407	100.0

Types and Extent of Resection

The types of resection used in the authors' series are listed in Table 45-2. Because of the significant association of liver cirrhosis with HCC in this series, and because right lobe small HCC accounted for 62.3% of cases, limited resection was used, particularly in those patients with small HCC located in the right lobe of a cirrhotic liver. As shown in Figure 45-2, the types of limited resection include wedge-shaped resection or partial hepatectomy for a tumor in the peripheral part of the liver, spindle-shaped resection for a tumor in the central part of the liver, and enucleation for a tumor located close to the hepatic hilum. However, left lateral segmentectomy usually is used for small HCC at that segment. Left lobectomy also was used for small HCC located at the medial segment of the left lobe when cirrhosis was not severe or hepatic functional reserve was adequate. However, quadrate lobe resection is effective for small HCC at that location. Based on the results of a long-term follow-up study, resection with a margin of about 2 cm (depending on tumor size) from the tumor capsule was accepted as curative therapy for small HCC. In this series, the 10-year survival rate was 51.5% in the 313 patients who underwent limited resection or left lateral segmentectomy, compared with

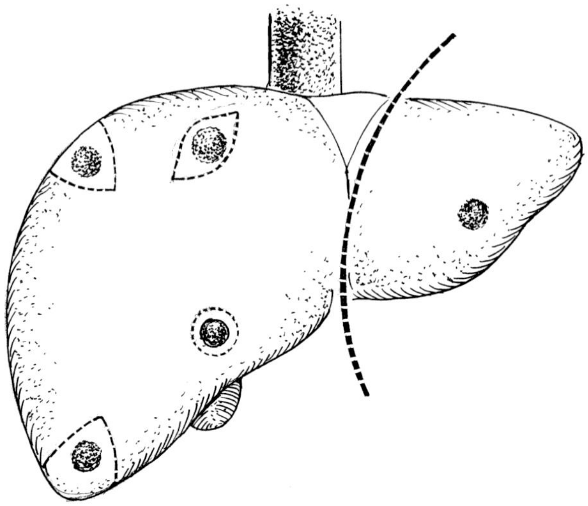

FIG. 45-2. Types of resection for small hepatocellular carcinoma.

TABLE 45-3. *Long-term results of limited resection versus lobectomy for small hepatocellular carcinoma*

Survival	Limited resection and Left lateral segmentectomy (n = 313)	Lobectomy (n = 94)
1-Year	91.7%	79.6%
3-Year	77.7%	66.3%
5-Year	66.7%	56.7%
10-Year	51.5%	39.6%

39.6% in the 94 patients who underwent lobectomy (Table 45-3). The increased use of limited resection (from 64% in the 1970s to 81.6% in the 1980s) has resulted in a rise in the resectability rate (from 75% to 93.3%, respectively).[20] Similar findings also have been reported by Kanematsu and associates.[56] Ultrasonographically guided subsegmentectomy or anatomic resection of the right hepatic subsegments preceded by suprahilar ligation of the portal pedicle also has been advocated.[57,58] In patients without coexisting cirrhosis, the use of standard lobectomy remains advisable. However, livers removed at transplantation have shown strong evidence of a multicentric origin of HCC.[59] This suggests that the background of multicentricity may not be eliminated by limited or massive resection. Careful assessment of the extent of resection in a cirrhotic liver is one of the key factors of successful resection (see Tables 45-2 and 45-3).[60]

Techniques for Minimizing Blood Loss

Approaches to minimizing blood loss during resection include the following:

Good exposure and fresh blood transfusion
Step-by-step resection and ligation of intrahepatic vessels without hilar occlusion
Use of a hepatic clamp or interrupted mattress suture
Temporal occlusion of the hepatic hilum using a rubber tube
Complete vascular occlusion, including the inferior vena cava
Hemihepatic occlusion
Suprahilar ligation of the portal pedicle

In noncirrhotic livers, hilar occlusion and quick resection is a good choice if occlusion is needed. Repeated episodes of occlusion lasting less than 20 minutes each are better than one prolonged episode.

In cirrhotic livers, interrupted mattress suture was used for peripheral tumors, followed by step-by-step resection with ligation of the intrahepatic ducts (Figs. 45-3 and 45-4). Temporal occlusion of the first hepatic hilum was used for tumors seated deep in the liver or near the hepatic hilum. The occlusion time should not exceed 15 minutes for cirrhosis and 10 minutes for severe cirrhosis. Repeated occlusion is necessary for complicated resections. For resection of tumors in segment VIII (Fig. 45-5) at the authors' institution, occlusion of the hepatic hilum was adequate in most patients (25 of 32) and the average occlusion time was 14 minutes. The longest occlusion time was 45 minutes (three 15-minute episodes). However, a tape placed at the suprahepatic and infrahepatic inferior vena cava without occlusion helps to control massive bleeding. Complete vascular occlusion with hypothermic perfusion no longer is used at the authors' institution. The 5-year survival rate was 28.6% for 32 patients (mean tumor diameter, 5 cm).[33] The authors agree with Taniguchi and colleagues that occlusion of the hepatic hilum results in a higher postoperative elevation of the alanine aminotransferase level as compared with unilateral occlusion or no occlusion, and vascular inflow exclusion may not be essential for successful hepatic resection.[61] Intraoperative ultrasonography is a good guide for resection.

Management of the Cut End and Drainage

The cut end should be approximated by suture without tension, or covered by a piece of falciform ligament or omentum

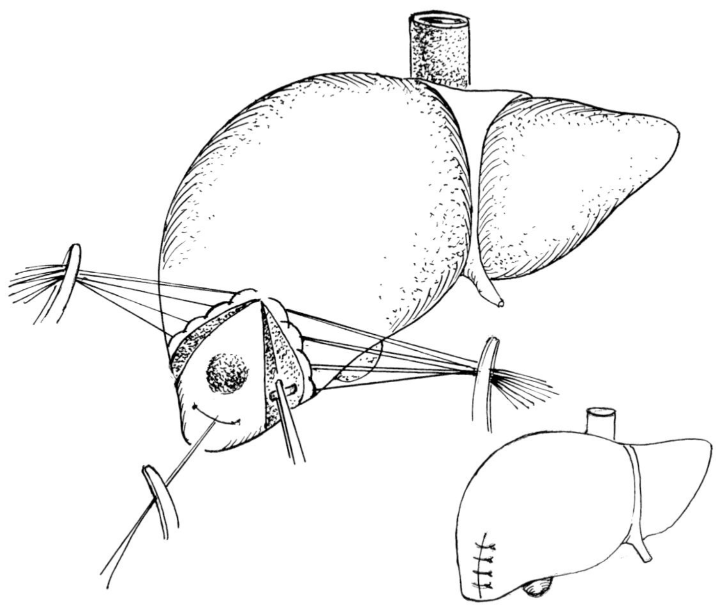

FIG. 45-3. Wedge-shaped resection. Cut end approximated by suture.

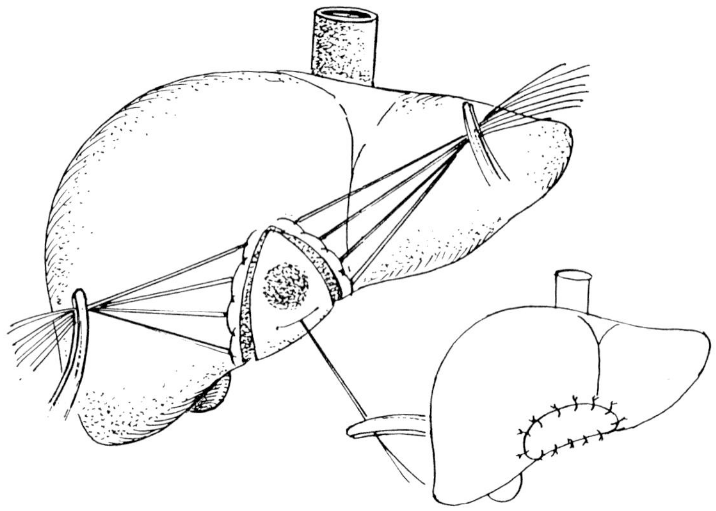

FIG. 45-4. Limited resection of quadrate lobe. Cut end covered by falciform ligament.

with pedicle. A deep mattress suture crossing the cut end is helpful to eliminate dead space. Adequate drainage using both a rubber tube and a cigarette drain is important.

OPERATIVE MORTALITY AND POSTOPERATIVE COMPLICATIONS

The operative mortality rate (death within 30 days) after resection of small HCC was 1.7% in 362 patients in a report by Makuuchi and associates,[29] and also was 1.7% in the authors' series of 407 patients. These rates are much lower than those associated with resection of large HCC.

The causes of the 7 operative deaths in the authors' series included hepatic failure in 5 patients, 4 of whom died between days 20 and 30, and 1 of whom had gastrointestinal bleeding and died on day 7. All 5 of the patients had coexisting severe macronodular cirrhosis. Limited resection was performed in all cases. Resection was done after transcatheter arterial embolization in 1 patient, and hepatic artery cannulation was added in 1 patient. One elderly patient died of multiple organ failure. One died of septicemia 5 days after bloodless resection with hypothermic perfusion.

The key factors to a low operative mortality rate after resection of small HCC are careful patient selection, adequate preoperative care, careful determination of the extent of resection in cirrhotic livers, good exposure, limited blood loss, short duration of occlusion of the hepatic hilum, transfusion with fresh blood, and avoidance of unnecessary surgical procedures in severely cirrhotic livers (eg, hepatic artery cannulation, cholecystectomy).

Postoperative complications after resection of small HCC were less common than after resection of large HCC. Hepatic dysfunction remained the primary problem with resection of small HCC in cirrhotic livers. An unexplained high pulse rate, marked increase in the serum bilirubin level (greater than 5 mg/dL), marked prolongation of the prothrombin time (less than 20% of the normal value), and early appearance of ascites were poor prognostic findings. Early and aggressive treatment with albumin, fresh plasma, glucose, vitamin K, antibiotics, and oxygen were needed. Chest fluid often was found with resection of small HCC in the right lobes of cirrhotic livers. Aspiration of chest fluid and injection of *Corynebacterium parvum* or mitomycin C helped to control protein loss, and albumin also was required. Subdiaphragmatic abscess was less common when drainage was adequate. Ultrasonically guided aspiration with injection of antibiotics was the treatment of choice. The bile leakage that plagues massive hepatic resection of large HCC occurred less frequently in resection of small HCC, except in small tumors located at the hepatic hilum. Adequate drainage with a tube was necessary. Temporal ascites was a common complication of resection of small HCC in cirrhotic livers. Al-

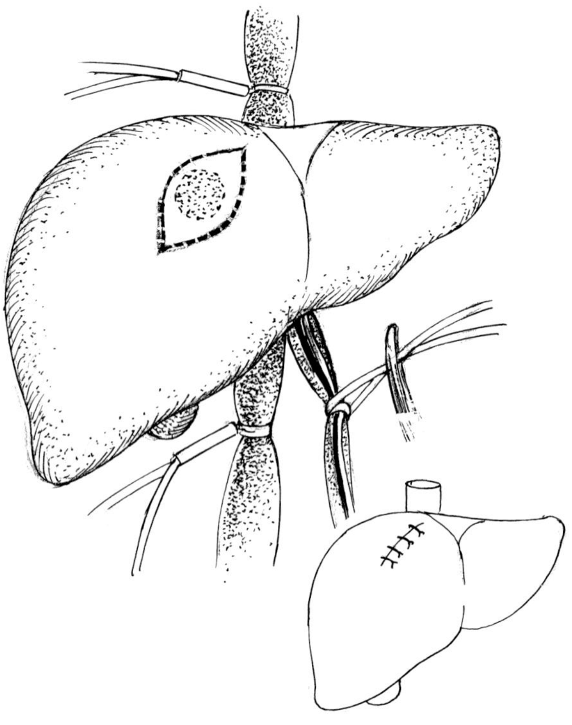

FIG. 45-5. Resection of small hepatocellular carcinoma segment VIII under complete occlusion.

bumin and diuretics were used routinely. Aspiration of ascites seldom was helpful. Secondary bleeding was encountered infrequently, except in patients with prolonged prothrombin times. Conservative treatment was used unless an active bleeding site was found. Routine postoperative studies included hepatic and renal function tests, AFP levels, and ultrasonography.

PATHOLOGY OF SMALL HEPATOCELLULAR CARCINOMA

In the authors' series of small HCC, the pathologic findings revealed a single HCC nodule in 77.5% of cases, an Edmondson grade I to II tumor in 92.7%, a well-encapsulated tumor in 76.2%, and a tumor embolus in 66.5%. These findings coincided with reports in the literature indicating that most small HCC were well differentiated, more diploid, single, encapsulated tumors that became progressively less differentiated, more aneuploid, multiple nodules with poor encapsulation as they progressed to large HCC.[41,62–64] In a comparison of small HCC (less than 3 cm) and large HCC, Cong and Wu found that 66.7% of small tumors were diploid, 16% were associated with invasion of the capsule, 20% were associated with tumor emboli, and 75% were associated with 5-year survival after resection. In contrast, 92.3% of large tumors were aneuploid, 84% were associated with invasion of the capsule, 80% were associated with tumor emboli, and 46.2% were associated with 5-year survival after resection.[38] Therefore, 3 cm may be the size at which changes in DNA stem lines and biologic characteristics occur. All these findings strongly support the use of early resection.

MANAGEMENT OF SUBCLINICAL RECURRENCE

The 1-, 3-, and 5-year recurrence rates after resection of small HCC in the authors' series were 6.5%, 25.7%, and 43.5%, respectively.[65] In the literature, the recurrence rate after resection of small HCC was 54.2% at 14.9 months, and 5-year survival rates varied markedly between the 49 patients without recurrence (48.9%) and the 58 patients with recurrence (11%).[66] The following factors favored recurrence: tumor size greater than 2.2 cm, infiltration of the capsule, deep seating of the tumor in the liver, invasion of the portal vein, and metastasis within the liver.[67] For early detection of subclinical recurrence, AFP levels and ultrasonography should be performed every 2 to 3 months and chest radiography every 6 months for 5 to 10 years after resection of small HCC.

At the authors' institution, early detection of subclinical (without symptoms and signs) recurrence and repeated resection were important in managing recurrence after resection of small HCC. In a series of 407 patients, 60 patients underwent reoperation. Repeated resection of liver recurrence was performed in 47 patients, lung resection in 3 patients, and cryosurgery, laser vaporization, hepatic artery ligation or cannulation, or ethanol injection in the remainder. The 5-year survival rate was 60.8% after the first resection and 46% after the second operation. Limited resection was the choice for repeated resection.

Transcatheter arterial embolization and ultrasonically guided percutaneous ethanol injection are alternatives when reoperation is contraindicated. In the literature, 5-year survival rates after recurrence treated with or without transcatheter arterial embolization were 14.9% in 32 patients and 0% in 23 patients.[66] Nakajima and associates reported 5-year survival rates after recurrence of 92% in 14 patients who underwent resection, 22% in 22 patients who underwent transcatheter arterial embolization, and 0% in 21 patients who received no treatment.[68]

Reoperation may prolong survival after resection of small HCC, and also may provide curable outcome. The 10-year survival rate after reoperation was as high as 30.7% in the authors' series. However, reoperation for subclinical recurrence was limited by the multicentric origin of the tumors.[37,69,70]

TABLE 45-4. *Factors influencing prognosis in patients with small hepatocellular carcinoma (HCC)*

Prognostic factors	Number of patients	3-Year survival (%)	5-Year survival (%)
Entire series	445	71.0	60.3
Cirrhosis			
None	34	92.0	75.8
Micronodular	123	71.3	65.9
Macronodular	284	68.2	56.2
Number of HCC nodules			
One	345	75.5	64.6
More than one	100	55.5	44.8
Encapsulation			
Good	329	77.5	66.2
Poor	103	51.5	42.2
Treatment			
Resection	407	74.9	64.3
No resection	38	33.5	20.9

PROGNOSIS

As shown in Table 45-4, analysis of the factors influencing the prognosis of small HCC revealed that patients with single tumor nodules, well-encapsulated tumors, no cirrhosis or micronodular cirrhosis, and resectional therapy had better outcomes than did patients with more than one tumor nodule, poorly encapsulated tumors, macronodular cirrhosis, and nonresectional treatment.

The encouraging overall 5-year survival rate of 60.3% in this series was mainly a result of resection. As shown in Table 45-5, the 5-year survival rate was 64.3% with resection, compared with only 28.3% with cryosurgery or laser vaporization. Hepatic

TABLE 45-5. *Survival of patients with small hapatocellular carcinoma according to treatment group*

Treatment	Number of patients	1-Year survival (%)	3-Year survival (%)	5-Year survival (%)
Resection	407	88.7	74.9	64.3
Cryosurgery/laser	17	87.9	37.7	28.3
Hepatic artery	16	73.3	34.7	—
ligation/	2	33.3	—	—
cannulation	3	20.0	—	—
Ethanol injection				
Exploration only				

TABLE 45-6. *Comparison of survival of patients with small hepatocellular carcinoma in the periods 1967–1982 and 1983–1992*

Survival rate (%)	1967–1982 (n = 69)	1983–1992 (n = 376)
1-Year	82.6	88.5
3-Year	59.4	74.4
5-Year	46.4	65.7

artery ligation or cannulation was even less effective (see Table 45-5).

The 5-year survival rates after resection of small HCC (less than 2 cm) were even better: 61% in 23 patients and 100% in 14 patients with T1N0M0 lesions.[31,32] Unfortunately, vascular invasion was found in some of the minute tumors.

The overall 5-year survival rate after resection of small HCC in this series increased by about 20% from the period 1967 to 1982 to the period 1993 to 1992 (Table 45-6). This may be attributable to the increase in resectability and the rising number of repeated resections performed for subclinical recurrence between 1983 and 1992.[20]

CONCLUSION

The resection of small tumors has altered dramatically the clinical outlook in HCC. It has been more effective than the resection of large tumors. The primary objective is to make every effort to eradicate small HCC by resection or alternative procedures as long as hepatic functional reserve is acceptable. Repeated resection for subclinical recurrence may prolong survival further. Problems such as multicentricity, biologic characteristics (particularly early vascular invasion), and coexisting Child's grade C cirrhosis remain to be studied.

ACKNOWLEDGMENT

The authors wish to express their appreciation to Drs. HW Wang and HC Sun for their help in preparing this manuscript.

REFERENCES

1. Parkin DM, Stjernsward J, Muir CS. Estimates of the worldwide frequency of twelve major cancers. Bull World Health Organ 1984;62:163.
2. Boring CC, Squires TS, Tong T. Cancer statistics, 1993. CA Cancer J Clin 1993;43:7.
3. Tang ZY, Yu YQ, Zhou XD. Evolution of surgery in the treatment of hepatocellular carcinoma from the 1950s to the 1990s. Semin Surg Oncol 1993;9:293.
4. Tatarinov Y. Detection of embryo-specific globulin in the blood sera of patients with primary liver tumors. Vopr Med Khim 1964;10:90.
5. Masseyeff RF. Factors influencing alpha fetoprotein biosynthesis in patients with primary liver cancer and other diseases. Gann Monograph of Cancer Research 1973;14:3.
6. Okuda K, Kotoda K, Obata H, et al. Clinical observation during a relatively early stage of hepatocellular carcinoma, with special reference to serum alpha fetoprotein levels. Gastroenterology 1975;69:226.
7. Xu KL. Large-scale AFP screening for hepatocellular carcinoma in China. In: Fishman WH, ed. Oncodevelopment markers: biologic, diagnostic, and monitoring aspects. New York: Academic Press, 1983:395.
8. Sun TT, Wan LC, Chang YL, et al. Radiorocket electrophoresis autography (RREA) through labelled antigen for AFP assay and its application in sero-epidemiological investigation on primary hepatocellular carcinoma. Chin Med J (Engl) 1979;92:17.
9. Yu YQ, Sang LA. Early diagnosis and resection of primary liver cancer. Tumor Prevention, Treatment and Study 1975;3:1 (in Chinese).
10. Tang ZY, Qian SQ. Surgical treatment of primary liver cancer. Jiangsu Medicine 1977;3:501 (in Chinese).
11. Shanghai Coordinating Group for Research in Liver Cancer, China. Diagnosis and treatment of primary hepatocellular carcinoma in early stage—report of 134 cases. Chin Med J (Engl) 1979;92:801.
12. Tang ZY, Yu YQ, Lin ZY, et al. Small hepatocellular carcinoma—clinical analysis of 30 cases. Chin Med J (Engl) 1979;92:455.
13. Zhu YR. AFP serosurvey and early diagnosis of liver cell cancer in Qidong area. Chinese Journal of Oncology 1981;3:35 (in Chinese).
14. Tang ZY, Yu YQ, Zhou XD, Zhou NQ. Surgical treatment of subclinical hepatocellular carcinoma (HCC) and its ultimate outcome. A comparative study of 74 cases of subclinical HCC and 229 cases of clinical HCC undergone surgery. Journal of Experimental and Clinical Cancer Research 1983;2:261.
15. Tang ZY. Surgical treatment of subclinical hepatocellular carcinoma. In: Tang ZY, ed. Subclinical hepatocellular carcinoma. Berlin: Springer, 1985:63.
16. Tang ZY, Yu YQ, Yang BH. Subclinical hepatocellular carcinoma. In: Wagner G, Zhang YH, eds. Cancer of the liver, esophagus, and nasopharynx. Berlin: Springer, 1987:64.
17. Tang ZY. Surgical treatment of subclinical cases of hepatocellular carcinoma. In: Okuda K, Ishak KG, eds. Neoplasms of the liver. Tokyo: Springer, 1987:367.
18. Tang ZY, Yu YQ, Zhou XD, et al. Surgery of small hepatocellular carcinoma--analysis of 144 cases. Cancer 1989;64:536.
19. Tang ZY. Small hepatocellular carcinoma. In: Tang ZY, Wu MC, Xia SS, eds. Primary liver cancer. Berlin: Springer, 1989:191.
20. Tang ZY, Yu YQ, Zhou XD, Yang BH, Lin ZY. Small hepatocellular carcinoma—three decades' experience. In: Jiang SJ, Xiao SD, eds. Proceedings of 1992 Shanghai International Symposium on Gastroenterology. Shanghai: Shanghai Scientific and Technical Literature Publishers, 1992:52.
21. Tang ZY, Yu YQ, Zhou XD, Yang BH, Ma ZC, Lin ZY. Subclinical hepatocellular carcinoma: an analysis of 391 patients. J Surg Oncol 1993;3:55.
22. Nakanishi Y, Sano H, Watanabe S, Kenno T. Concept and problems of early stage of primary liver cancer. Journal of Japanese Surgical Society 1985;86:1082.
23. Kanematsu T, Sonoda T, Takenaka K, et al. The value of ultrasound in the diagnosis and treatment of small hepatocellular carcinoma. Br J Surg 1985;72:23.
24. Wu MC, Zhang XH, Chen H, et al. Hepatic resection for primary liver cancer. Chin Med J (Engl) 1986;99:175.
25. Okamoto E, Yamanaka N, Toyosaka A, Tanaka N, Yabuki K. Current status of hepatic resection in the treatment of hepatocellular carcinoma. In: Okuda K, Ishak KG, eds. Neoplasms of the liver. Tokyo: Springer, 1987:353.
26. Huang XY. The role of small hepatocellular carcinoma (HCC) surgery in the improvement of overall HCC prognosis. Journal of Practical Oncology 1988;3:8 (in Chinese).
27. Yamanaka N, Okamoto E, Toyosaka A, et al. Prognosis factors after hepatectomy for hepatocellular carcinoma. Cancer 1990;65:1104.
28. Lai ECS, Ng IOL, You KT, et al. Hepatic resection for small hepatocellular carcinoma: the Queen Mary Hospital experience. World J Surg 1991;15:654.
29. Makuuchi M, Kosuge T, Takayama T, et al. Surgery of small liver cancers. Semin Surg Oncol 1993;9:298.
30. Arii S, Tobe T. Results of surgical treatment: follow up study by Liver Cancer Study Group of Japan. In: Tobe T, Kameda H, Okudaira M, et al, eds. Primary liver cancer in Japan. Tokyo: Springer, 1992:243.
31. Nagao T, Nagashima I, Inoue S, Omori Y, Kawano N, Morioka Y. Hepatic resection for minute hepatocellular carcinoma. Japanese Journal of Surgery 1992;22:110.
32. Zhou XD, Tang ZY, Yu YQ, et al. Solitary minute hepatocellular carcinoma—a study of 14 patients. Cancer 1991;67:2855.
33. Yu YQ, Zhou XD, Tang ZY, Xu DB, Feng XS. Experience with resection of segment VIII of liver for hepatocellular carcinoma. Semin Surg Oncol 1993;9:305.

34. Curutchet HP, Terz JJ, Kay S, Lawrence W Jr. Primary liver cancer. Surgery 1971;70:467.
35. Chen Y, Tang ZY, Liu KD, et al. Accumulation of mutant p53 protein correlates with elevation of serum AFP in human hepatocellular carcinoma. Hapatology 1992;15:843.
36. Eguchi A, Nakashima O, Okudaira S, Sugihara S, Kojiro M. Adenomatous hyperplasia in the vicinity of small hepatocellular carcinoma. Hepatology 1992;15:843.
37. Liang XH, Loncarevic IF, Tang ZY, Yu YQ, Zentgraf HZ, Schroder CH. Resection of hepatocellular carcinoma: oligocentric origin of recurrent and multinodular tumors. J Gastroenterol Hepatol 1991;6:77.
38. Cong WM, Wu MC. Small hepatocellular carcinoma—DNA content and biological characteristics. Chin Med J (Engl) 1989;102:783.
39. Aoki K, Sakamoto M, Hirohashi S. Nucleola organizer regions in small nodular lesions representing early stage of human hepatocarcinogenesis. Cancer 1994;73:289.
40. Tang ZY. A new concept on the natural course of hepatocellular carcinoma. Chin Med J (Engl) 1981;94:585.
41. Tang ZY, Ying YY, Guo TJ. Hepatocellular carcinoma: changing concepts in recent years. In: Popper H, Schaffner F, eds. Progress in liver diseases. New York: Grune & Stratton, 1982:637.
42. Ebara M, Ohto M, Shinagawa T, et al. Natural history of minute hepatocellular carcinoma smaller than three centimeters complicating cirrhosis. A study in 22 patients. Gastroenterology 1986;90:289.
43. Liver Cancer Study Group of Japan. Summary of the data from a follow-up study by the Liver Cancer Study Group of Japan. In: Tobe T, Kameda H, Okudaira M, et al, eds. Primary liver cancer in Japan. Tokyo: Springer, 1992:445.
44. Shinagawa T, Ohto M, Kimura K, et al. Diagnosis and clinical features of small hepatocellular carcinoma with emphasis on the utility of real time ultrasonography—a study on 51 patients. Gastroenterology 1984; 86:495.
45. Xu ZZ. Ultrasonography of primary liver cancer. In: Tang ZY, Wu MC, Xia SS, eds. Primary liver cancer. Berlin: Springer, 1989:305.
46. Su XZ. Computed tomography of hepatoma. In: Tang ZY, Wu MC, Xia SS, eds. Primary liver cancer. Berlin: Springer, 1989:318.
47. Sumida M, Ohto M, Ebara M, Kimura K, Okuda K, Hirooka N. Accuracy of angiography in the diagnosis of small hepatocellular carcinoma. Am J Roentgenol 1986;147:531.
48. Yumoto Y, Jinno K, Tokuyama K, et al. Hepatocellular carcinoma detected by iodized oil. Radiology 1985;154:15.
49. Ebara M, Ohto M, Watanabe Y, et al. Diagnosis of small hepatocellular carcinoma: correlation of MR imaging and tumor histologic studies. Radiology 1986;159:371.
50. Chen SL, Zhao HY, Yuan AN, Tang ZY, Ma ZC. Diagnosis value of ^{99m}Tc-PMT delayed hepatobiliary imaging in small hepatocellular carcinoma—an analysis of 62 cases. Chinese Journal of Oncology 1991;13:30 (in Chinese).
51. Ebara M, Ohto M, Kondo F. Strategy of early diagnosis of hepatocellular carcinoma. Ann Acad Med Singapore 1989;18:83.
52. Cao YZ, Tang ZY. Presence of HBV DNA, HBV antigens, and HBV antibodies in hepatocellular carcinoma. In: Tang ZY, Wu MC, Xia SS, eds. Primary liver cancer. Berlin: Springer, 1989:9.
53. Mizumoto R, Noguchi T. Hepatic functional reserve and surgical indication in primary liver cancer. In: Tobe T, Kameda H, Okudaira M, et al, eds. Primary liver cancer in Japan. Tokyo: Springer, 1992:185.
54. Lu JZ, Yu YQ. Clinical value of gamma-glutamyl transpeptidase in primary liver cancer. In: Tang ZY, Wu MC, Xia SS, eds. Primary liver cancer. Berlin: Springer, 1989:284.
55. Zhou XD, Tang ZY, Yu YQ, et al. The role of cryosurgery in the treatment of hepatic cancer: a report of 113 cases. J Cancer Res Clin Oncol 1993;120:100.
56. Kanematsu T, Takenaka K, Matsumata T, Furuta T, Sugimachi K, Inokuchi K. Limited hepatic resection effective for selected cirrhotic patients with primary liver cancer. Ann Surg 1984;199:51.
57. Makuuchi M, Hasegawa H, Yamazaki S. Ultrasonically guided subsegmentectomy. Surg Gynecol Obstet 1985;161:346.
58. Okamoto E, Yamanaka N. Anatomical resection of the right hepatic subsegments preceded by suprahilar ligation of the portal pedicles. In: Tobe T, Kameda H, Okudaira M, et al, eds. Primary liver cancer in Japan. Tokyo: Springer, 1992:229.
59. Cameron RG, Greig PD, Farber E, et al. Small encapsulated hepatocellular carcinoma of the liver: provisional analysis of pathogenetic mechanisms. Cancer 1993;72:2550.
60. Makuuchi M, Mori T, Gunven P, et al. Safety of hemihepatic occlusion during resection of the liver. Surg Gynecol Obstet 1987;164:155.
61. Taniguchi H, Takahashi T, Shioaki Y, Itoh A, Oguro A. Vascular inflow exclusion and hepatic resection. Br J Surg 1992;79:672.
62. Okuda K. Early recognition of hepatocellular carcinoma. Hepatology 1986;6:729.
63. Kenmochi K, Sugihara S, Kojiro M. Relationship of histologic grade of hepatocellular carcinoma (HCC) to tumor size, and demonstration of tumor cells of multiple different grades in single small HCC. Liver 1987;7:18.
64. Kondo F, Kondo Y. Hepatocellular carcinoma of the early stage: morphology and developmental process. J Surg Oncol 1993;3:1665.
65. Tang ZY. Efforts in the past decades to improve ultimate outcome of primary liver cancer. In: Tang ZY, Wu MC, Xia SS, eds. Primary liver cancer. Berlin: Springer, 1989:469.
66. Takayasu K, Muramatsu Y, Moriyama N, et al. Clinical and radiologic assessments of the results of hepatectomy for small hepatocellular carcinoma and therapeutic arterial embolization of postoperative recurrence. Cancer 1989;64:1848.
67. Shirabe K, Kanematsu T, Matsumata T, Adachi R, Akazawa K, Sugimachi K. Factors linked to early recurrence of small hepatocellular carcinoma after hepatectomy. Hepatology 1991;14:802.
68. Nakajima Y, Ohmura T, Kimura J, et al. Role of surgical treatment for recurrent hepatocellular carcinoma after hepatic resection. World J Surg 1992;17:792.
69. Esumi M, Aritaka T, Arii M, et al. Clonal origin of human hepatoma determined by integration of hepatitis B virus DNA. Cancer Res 1986; 46:5767.
70. Chen PJ, Chen DS, Lai MY, et al. Clonal origin of recurrent hepatocellular carcinoma. Gastroenterology 1989;96:527.

Surgery for Gastrointestinal Cancer: A Multidisciplinary Approach, edited by Harold J. Wanebo.
Lippincott-Raven Publishers, Philadelphia, © 1997.

CHAPTER 46

Resection Versus Transplantation for Malignancy of Liver and Bile Duct

Burckhardt Ringe, Arved Weimann, Günther Tusch, and Rudolf Pichlmayr

Liver and bile duct malignancies play a significant role worldwide, with considerable differences in geographic distribution and incidence, causes and risk factors, tumor types, and growth patterns. Most of these neoplasms have a similar, and overall fatal, prognosis. Spontaneous survival usually is limited to a few months, and most untreated patients die of systemic, rather than local, malignant disease.

Systematic screening of well-known risk groups and the introduction of high-quality noninvasive imaging techniques has led to earlier diagnosis. Improved understanding of the epidemiology and biology of these tumors, and especially the assessment of clinicopathologic factors influencing their prognosis, has laid the foundation for a more reliable judgment, including the indications for treatment.[1–3]

The wide therapeutic spectrum available ranges from conservative to surgical measures. With few exceptions, however, the mainstay is still an operation with the goal of radical tumor removal. This approach offers the best chance for long-term symptom-free survival and potential cure. Because of this, and because the liver no longer is the surgeon's "no man's land," the treatment of hepatobiliary malignancies falls clearly into the surgical domain.

Based on growing experience with the anatomy and functional capacity of the liver and advances in operative and anesthetic management, significant effort has been put forth to perfect the technique of partial hepatectomy. Various modifications of inflow and outflow occlusion and in vivo or ex vivo protection (including liver autotransplantation) have resulted in an increase in resectability and ischemic tolerance, adding to the safety of traditional hepatobiliary surgery.[4,5]

Nevertheless, most liver and bile duct malignancies are unresectable because of local anatomic restriction, advanced tumor stage, or functional impairment resulting from underlying cirrhosis. Total hepatectomy followed by liver allotransplantation and multivisceral ("cluster") resection have been suggested to extend the limits of conventional resectability. The former approach has been used in several centers for many years, generating a wealth of fundamental data.[6–14]

It remains unclear whether partial or total hepatectomy is the superior procedure. The advantages of resection include lower morbidity and mortality, more widespread applicability, and limited cost. Its disadvantages include unresectability in most cases, multicentric tumor origin, and persistence of the oncogenic risk in cirrhosis. The advantages of transplantation include extended resectability, significant palliation in many cases, and potential long-term cure in some cases. Its disadvantages include doubtful cure of tumor, limited donor resources, and the adverse effects of lifelong immunosuppression.

In trying to identify the optimal therapeutic modality for patients with liver and bile duct malignancies, these considerations must be taken into account, along with the relevant clinical experience. In this chapter, the overall role of liver transplantation for liver and bile duct malignancies in the authors' center is analyzed, following earlier retrospective studies, then the use of resection versus transplantation in selected tumor types is examined more specifically. In the discussion of these updated and comparative results, the present status is summarized, including the authors' personal views, focusing on the practical consequences for clinical decision-making and the performance of adequate surgical therapy.

ROLE OF TRANSPLANTATION

The liver transplant program at the Medizinische Hochschule Hannover has been in existence since 1972. Up to December

Burckhardt Ringe, Georg-August-Universität Göttingen, Klinik für Transplantationschirurgie, Robert-Koch-Str. 40, 37075 Göttingen, Germany

Arved Weimann, Medizinische Hochschule Hannover, Klinik für Abdominal- und Transplantationschirurgie, Konstanty-Gutschow-Str. 8, 30625 Hannover, Germany

Günther Tusch, Medizinische Hochschule Hannover, Klinik für Abdominal- und Transplantationschirurgie, Konstanty-Gutschow-Str. 8, 30625 Hannover, Germany

Rudolf Pichlmayr, Medizinische Hochschule Hannover, Klinik für Abdominal- und Transplantationschirurgie, Konstanty-Gutschow-Str. 8, 30625 Hannover, Germany

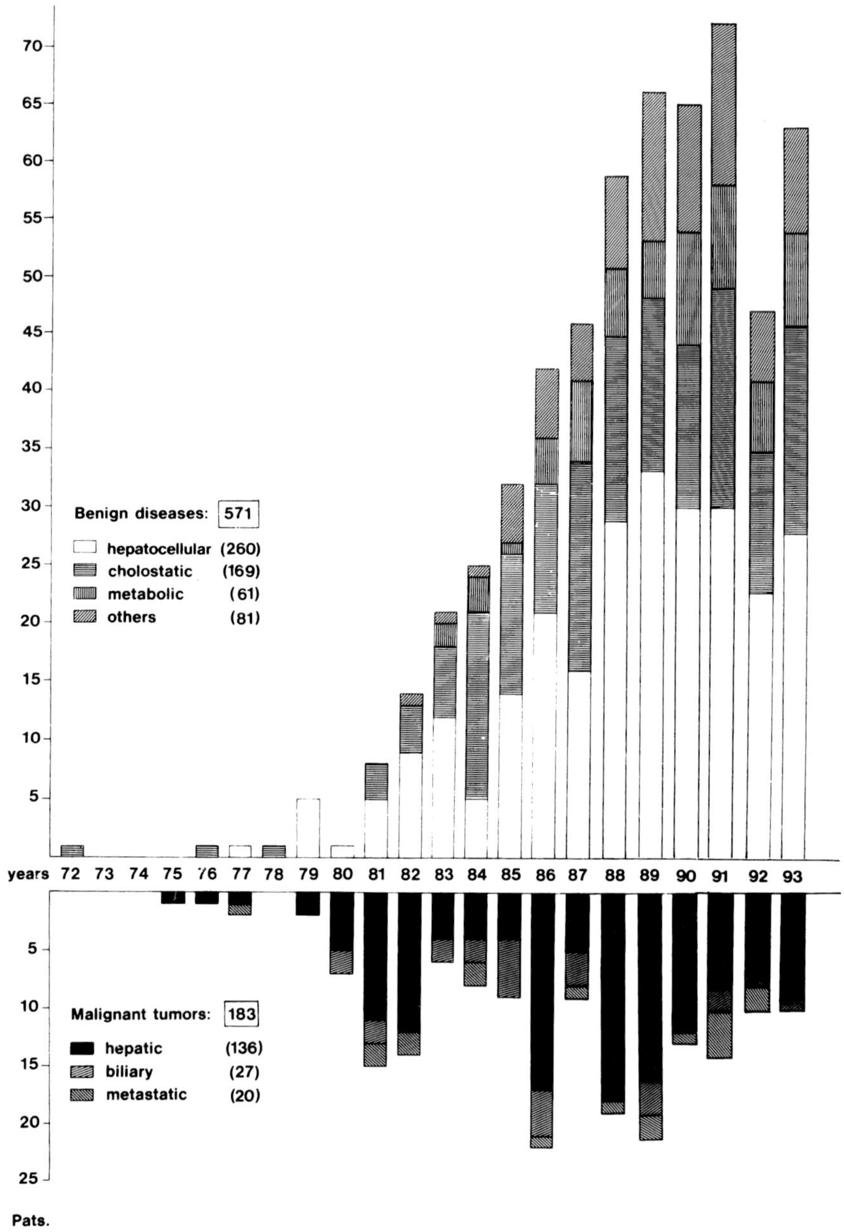

FIG. 46-1. Development of indication categories for liver transplantation in 754 patients. *MHH,* Medizinische Hochschule Hannover, 1972–1993.

31, 1993, 754 adult and pediatric patients had received a total of 897 allografts. In 183 recipients (24%), total hepatectomy was performed for different types of hepatic, biliary, and metastatic malignancies (Fig. 46-1). Leading indications in this category were as follows: hepatocellular carcinoma with (HCC^+) or without (HCC^-) cirrhosis in 68 and 28 cases, respectively; proximal bile duct carcinoma (BDC) in 25 cases; intrahepatic cholangiocellular carcinoma (CCC) in 21 cases; liver metastases from various endocrine tumors in 11 cases; and the fibrolamellar variant of primary liver cancer (FLC) in 7 cases. The other, less common, histopathologic types are listed in Table 46-1.

Resection or partial hepatectomy has always been the principal therapeutic strategy for patients with hepatobiliary malignancies in this center, and is carried out whenever feasible. The use of total hepatectomy and transplantation is considered only in patients with technically and functionally unresectable lesions or recurrent tumors after previous resection. Systematic regional lymphadenectomy, preoperative chemoembolization, and adjuvant therapy have been added to radical tumor excision, as suggested by newly established protocols.

All patients and liver specimens undergo a standard workup, including a complete pathologic evaluation and tumor classification in accordance with the TNM system. The immunosuppressant regimens used have varied over time, and are based mainly on azathioprine, cyclosporine, and FK506 as one of three or four different components. No recipient has been lost to follow-up, and information regarding survival and recurrence is available until the patient's death or the end of 1993. In analyzing the results of this series, it must be kept in mind that it is a retrospective, almost historical series including a long-lasting learning phase that still is not complete.

TABLE 46-1. *Histopathologic diagnosis and patient survival after liver transplantation for malignancy (Medizinische Hochschule Hannover, 1972–1993)*

Type of tumor	Patients (n)	Median (mo)	1 mo % (n)	1 y % (n)	3 y % (n)	5 y % (n)
Primary liver cancer	136	10.7	83.7 (113)	46.6 (59)	26.3 (27)	22.8 (15)
Hepatocellular carcinoma (HCC^-)	28	14.0	85.7 (24)	55.9 (15)	29.8 (8)	25.6 (4)
Hepatocellular carcinoma in cirrhosis (HCC^+)	68	10.2	80.7 (54)	47.4 (30)	24.7 (12)	19.8 (6)
Fibrolamellar carcinoma (FLC)	7	—	100.0 (7)	71.4 (5)	57.1 (3)	57.1 (3)
Cholangiocellular carcinoma* (CCC)	21	5.2	76.2 (16)	13.2 (2)	0	—
Others (OPT)	12	—	100.0 (12)	58.3 (7)	50.0 (4)	50.0 (2)
Hepatoblastoma	4		(4)	(2)	(2)	(1)
Epithelioid hemangioendothelioma	5		(5)	(4)	(2)	(1)
Hemangiosarcoma	2		(2)	(0)	—	—
Cystadenocarcinoma	1		(1)	(1)	—	—
Biliary cancer	27	12.7	81.5 (22)	55.6 (15)	20.8 (5)	16.7 (4)
Proximal bile duct carcinoma (BDC)	25	15.5	88.0 (22)	60.0 (15)	22.5 (5)	18.0 (4)
Gallbladder carcinoma	2	—	0	—	—	—
Secondary liver cancer	20	10.9	70.0 (14)	48.8 (9)	48.8 (4)	48.8 (1)
Endocrine tumor	11	—	90.9 (10)	81.8 (9)	81.8 (4)	81.8 (1)
Others	9	0.98	44.4 (4)	0	—	—
Colorectal carcinoma	4		(2)	(0)	—	—
Melanoma	2		(1)	(0)	—	—
Choriocarcinoma	2		(1)	(0)	—	—
Pancreatic carcinoma	1		(0)	—	—	—

* Including 3 patients with mixed hepatocholangiocellular carcinoma.

Overall, the actuarial survival rate after liver transplantation for malignancy was only 25% at 5 years. Although hospital morbidity and mortality decreased over time and with more experience, most patients died of tumor recurrence within 3 years of operation. Seventeen liver recipients are alive and disease-free with follow-up periods ranging from 5 to 18 years. Their original tumors were HCC in 8 cases, FLC in 3 cases, BDC in 3 cases, and hepatoblastoma, epithelioid hemangioendothelioma, and endocrine metastasis in 1 case each. Late tumor recurrence beyond 5 years has been an exception, occurring in only 4 patients, 3 of whom died soon after diagnosis. The fourth patient, who originally underwent transplantation for stage IV HCC in hepatitis B virus cirrhosis, received a second liver 6 years later for concomitant recurrence of both diseases—complete cirrhosis and the original cancer within the liver only—and is now alive and tumor-free 2 years after repeated transplantation.

A rough comparison of the three major indication categories revealed a significantly better prognosis for metastatic compared with primary hepatic and biliary tumors (Fig. 46-2). More specific analysis of primary liver cancers alone showed fairly similar 5-year survival rates for HCC^+ and HCC^- (19.8% and 25.6%, respectively), whereas the rates for FLC and other tumor types were almost twice as high (57.1% and 50%, respectively; Fig. 46-3).

The term *cholangiocarcinoma* should be defined precisely, distinguishing between two forms: the intrahepatic, peripheral type, or CCC, and the extrahepatic BDC. The pathologic anatomic location, clinical presentation, and prognosis of the two forms are different. Compared with a maximum survival of only 25 months in 1 patient with stage II CCC, 4 transplant recipients are alive 5 years after transplantation for BDC (Fig. 46-4).

The difference in outcome is even more pronounced in patients with various types of liver metastases. The longest survivor with a primary colorectal tumor died after 10 months. In contrast, 9 of 11 patients with secondary tumors from endocrine lesions are still alive, including 5 with well-controlled recurrences (Fig. 46-5). Except for those disease-free long-term survivors who may be definitively cured, most patients with hepatobiliary malignancies have experienced significant palliation and prolonged symptom-free survival.

In summarizing the overall results of transplantation for malignancy in this series according to tumor type, the following prognostic groups could be identified (see Table 46-1):

1. Fatal prognosis
   Patients with CCC or liver metastases from other than endocrine tumors seemed to be incurable. They had a high operative mortality rate, partly because of lack of surgical experience and poor patient selection, and partly because of the extremely high risk of early tumor recurrence with no long-term survival at all. A comparable fatal outcome was seen in the few patients with hemangiosarcoma, and gallbladder cancer as an incidental finding.
2. Intermediate or undetermined prognosis
   Median, early, and late survival rates were similar in patients with HCC^+, HCC^-, and BDC. Most of the tumors recurred within 3 years after transplantation, but several patients survived beyond 5 or even 10 years without any recurrence, obviously cured of their malignancies.
3. Favorable prognosis
   By far the best chance for disease-free long-term survival was seen in patients with FLC, hepatoblastoma, and epithelioid hemangioendothelioma. Although transplantation for endocrine metastases was followed by recurrent tumor out-

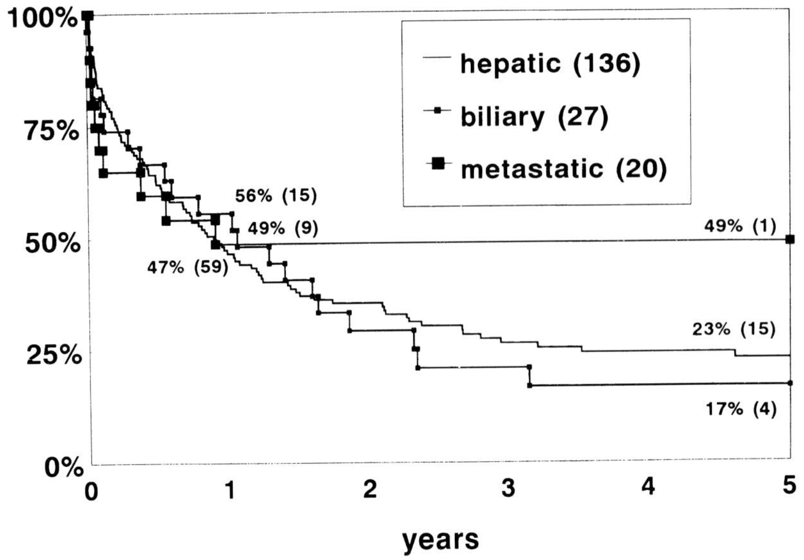

FIG. 46-2. Actuarial patient survival after liver transplantation for malignancy: hepatic versus biliary versus metastatic cancer (Medizinische Hochschule Hannover, 1972–1993).

side the liver in about 50% of cases (usually with good palliation), prolonged survival seemed to be the rule.

RESECTION VERSUS TRANSPLANTATION

To elucidate more clearly the role and prognosis of different surgical treatment options, patients with the most common primary tumors of the liver and bile duct were incorporated in a retrospective analysis, comparing resection with transplantation. It must be emphasized again, however, that this was not a randomized or prospective study, which means that the selection criteria for each group were different: resection always had the first priority, whereas transplantation was chosen only in unresectable cases. This bias must be considered when evaluating the results.

Corresponding data for partial and total hepatectomy followed by transplantation were available for the same institution and period (Table 46-2). In addition to the 183 transplant recipients already described, a total of 360 patients underwent resection for HCC^{-} (135 patients), HCC^{+} (38 patients), FLC (16 patients), CCC (46 patients), or BDC (125 patients). The date of follow-up was December 31, 1993.

Similar to transplantation, conventional liver resection was performed using a standardized operative technique according to the following major principles: dissection along the vascular anatomy and intrahepatic segmentation, hemostasis usually facilitated by inflow occlusion of the hepatoduodenal ligament, and the objective of radical tumor excision without residual deposits. Ten patients underwent various modifications of in vivo (2 patients), ante vivo (1 patient), or ex vivo (7 patients) resection, including hepatic protection with Bretschneider solution. Combined liver and bile duct resection (including segment I in 43 cases) was performed in 95 of 125 cases with cancer at the biliary bifurcation, and hilar resection alone was performed in 30 cases. Preoperative and postoperative adjuvant chemo-

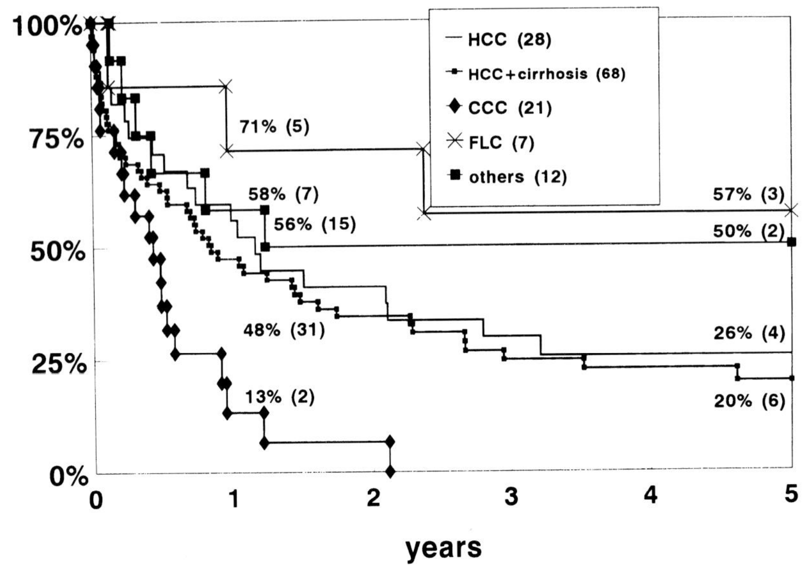

FIG. 46-3. Actuarial patient survival after liver transplantation for primary hepatic cancer: hepatocellular carcinoma (HCC) versus HCC + cirrhosis versus cholangiocellular carcinoma (CCC) versus the fibrolamella variant of primary liver cancer (FLC) versus others (Medizinische Hochschule Hannover 1972–1993).

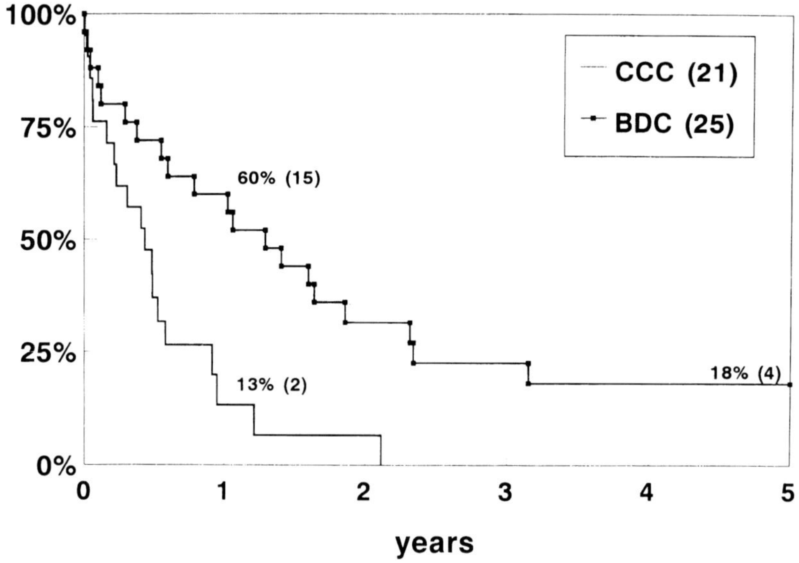

FIG. 46-4. Actuarial patient survival after liver transplantation for cholangiocellular (CCC): CCC versus bile duct cancer (BDC) (Medizinische Hochschule Hannover, 1972–1993).

therapy and radiation therapy were not used routinely. Pathologic evaluation and staging following the TNM guidelines was obligatory, and formed the basis for assessment of the relevant prognostic determinants within the different tumor type and treatment groups.

Hepatocellular Carcinoma Without Cirrhosis

As expected, there was an uneven distribution of HCC^- and HCC^+, and of tumor stage. More patients who underwent resection had noncirrhotic livers (135 of 173, or 78%) and early stage I or II tumors (54 of 173, or 31%), as compared with transplant recipients, who had significantly more cirrhosis (68 of 96, or 71%) and advanced malignancies (82 of 96, or 85%), emphasizing again the selection criteria of anatomic and functional unresectability used in the latter population.

The overall survival data for HCC^- were superior in patients who underwent resection as compared with transplantation (median survival, 31.8 versus 14 months). Thirty-day mortality rates were 9.7% and 14.3% in the two groups, respectively. Long-term actuarial survival rates at 1, 3, 5, and 10 years were 68.3%, 44.8%, 38.2%, and 32% for resection, and 55.9%, 29.8%, 25.6%, and 19.2% for transplantation, respectively.

The advantage of resection over transplantation was particularly evident when tumor stage was evaluated (Fig. 46-6). Resection for stage II HCC^- in 42 patients produced the best 5- and 10-year survival rates in the entire series (62.5% and 58.1%, respectively). There were only 2 comparable transplant recipients. One had a centrally located solitary tumor, which might have been resectable today, but she underwent transplantation in 1975 and is still alive. The other had undergone a previous liver resection deemed to be nonradical. However, at transplantation, no residual tumor was found (explaining stage 0) and

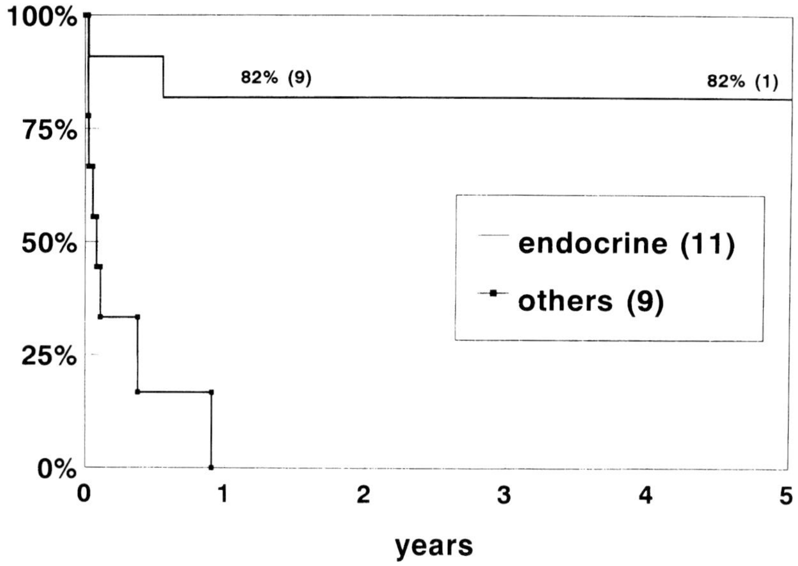

FIG. 46-5. Actuarial patient survival after liver transplantation for metastases: endocrine versus others (Medizinische Hochschule Hannover, 1972–1993).

TABLE 46-2. *Comparative patient survival after resection versus transplantation for malignancy*

Tumor type	TNM Stage	Resection						
		Patients (n)	Median (mo)	1 mo % (n)	1 y % (n)	3 y % (n)	5 y % (n)	10 y % (n)
HCC^-		135	31.8	90.3 (120)	68.3 (80)	44.8 (43)	38.2 (31)	32.0 (6)
	0/II	—/42	121.4	92.6 (37)	82.2 (29)	73.3 (22)	62.5 (15)	58.1 (3)
	III	41	61.9	92.7 (38)	80.2 (30)	54.6 (15)	50.7 (13)	40.1 (2)
	IVA/B	45/7	10.6	86.5 (45)	47.4 (21)	14.5 (6)	9.1 (3)	6.1 (1)
HCC^+		38	12.0	78.4 (26)	47.3 (14)	16.8 (3)	16.8 (2)	—
	I/II	1/11	22.8	90.9 (10)	72.7 (7)	26.0 (2)	26.0 (1)	—
	III	9	10.2	66.7 (6)	44.4 (4)	14.8 (1)	14.8 (1)	—
	IVA/B	15/2	4.8	76.5 (10)	27.5 (3)	—	—	—
FLC		16	44.6	100.0 (16)	86.7 (13)	53.8 (8)	40.0 (6)	—
	I/II	0/5	77.4	100.0 (5)	100.0 (5)	80.0 (4)	60.0 (3)	—
	III	6	24.9	100.0 (6)	66.7 (4)	33.3 (2)	16.7 (1)	—
	IVA/B	5/0	—	100.0 (5)	100.0 (4)	50.0 (2)	50.0 (2)	—
CCC		46*	12.8	95.7 (37)	65.1 (20)	25.5 (6)	16.0 (3)	—
	I/II	0/12	31.5	91.7 (9)	81.5 (7)	34.9 (3)	34.9 (3)	—
	III	16	12.8	100.0 (12)	73.3 (7)	31.4 (2)	—	—
	IVA/B	17/1	8.6	94.4 (16)	47.7 (6)	13.1 (1)	—	—
BDC		125	19.9	89.5 (108)	64.8 (66)	33.2 (29)	26.9 (18)	7.4 (1)
	I/II	11/37	48.3	93.8 (43)	72.2 (29)	52.0 (19)	42.3 (11)	—
	III	14	11.8	92.9 (13)	46.3 (4)	23.1 (2)	—	—
	IVA/B	60/3	16.6	85.7 (52)	62.6 (33)	20.3 (8)	20.3 (7)	6.5 (1)

* Including mixed hepatocholangiocellular carcinoma: 8 resected, 3 transplanted.

HCC$^-$, hepatocellular carcinoma, *HDD*$^+$· hepatocellular carcinoma in cirrhosis; *FLC,* fibrolamellar carcinoma; *CCC,* cholangiocellular carcinoma; *BDC,* proximal bile duct carcinoma.

the patient has survived 5 years. Few patients with advanced HCC^- were long-term survivors in either group.

Hepatocellular Carcinoma in Cirrhosis

Of 106 patients with HCC^+, 24 (23%) had stage I and II tumors, 51 had stage IVA tumors, and 10 had stage IVB tumors. There were no significant differences between the treatment groups, except for 6 small tumors discovered incidentally after total hepatectomy.

The 30-day mortality rates were similar after resection and transplantation (21.6% and 19.3%, respectively), as were the gross actuarial survival rates at 5 years (16.8% and 19.8%, respectively). After resection, 7 of 38 patients survived beyond 2 years. Five of these patients are still alive after 29 to 99 months, including 2 with recurrences, which were treated effectively by chemoembolization and subsequent transplantation in 1 case each. Eleven of the 20 liver recipients who reached the 2-year follow-up point are still alive after 25 to 87 months, and only 2 have had tumor recurrence.

Again, the most striking difference between resection and transplantation for HCC^+ became obvious when tumor stages were compared (Fig. 46-7). Twelve patients in each treatment

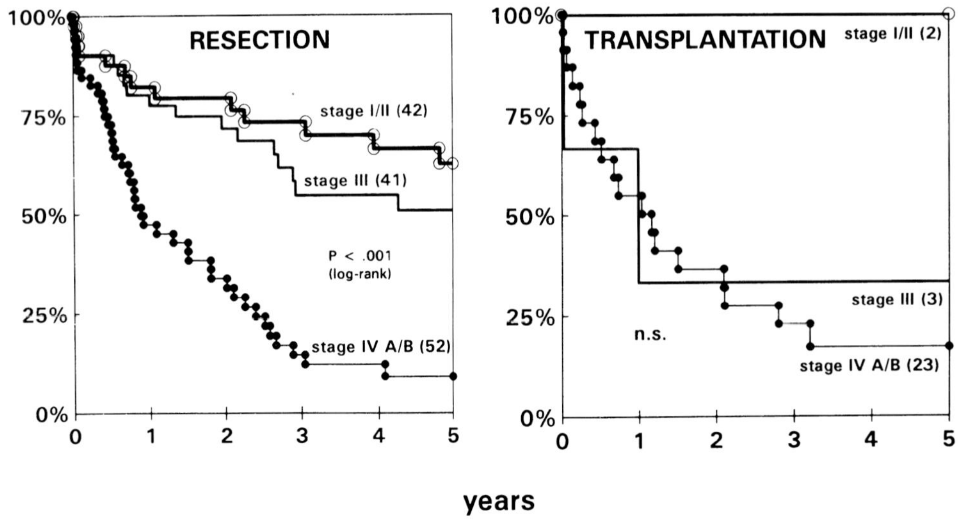

FIG. 46-6. Comparative actuarial patient survival after liver resection and transplantation for hepatocellular carcinoma without cirrhosis (HCC^-) according to tumor stage (Medizinische Hochschule Hannover, 1972–1993).

of the liver and bile duct (Medizinische Hochschule Hannover, 1972–1993)

Transplantation						
Patients (n)	Median (mo)	1 mo % (n)	1 y (%) (n)	3 y % (n)	5 y % (n)	10 y % (n)
28	14.0	85.7 (24)	55.9 (15)	29.8 (8)	25.6 (4)	19.2 (2)
1/1	—	100.0 (2)	100.0 (2)	100.0 (2)	100.0 (2)	50.0 (1)
3	11.9	66.7 (2)	33.3 (1)	33.3 (1)	33.3 (1)	—
17/6	14.0	87.0 (20)	54.9 (12)	22.9 (5)	17.2 (1)	17.2 (1)
68	10.2	80.7 (54)	47.4 (30)	24.7 (12)	19.8 (6)	—
5/7	—	91.7 (11)	83.3 (8)	69.4 (4)	69.4 (1)	—
12	8.4	90.0 (10)	36.4 (4)	18.2 (1)	18.2 (1)	—
36/8	8.8	75.0 (33)	40.9 (18)	17.5 (7)	12.0 (4)	—
7	—	100.0 (7)	71.4 (5)	57.1 (3)	57.1 (3)	—
0/2	—	100.0 (2)	100.0 (2)	50.0 (1)	50.0 (1)	—
1	—	100.0 (1)	100.0 (1)	100.0 (1)	100.0 (1)	—
4/0	—	100.0 (4)	50.0 (2)	50.0 (1)	50.0 (1)	—
21*	5.2	76.2 (16)	13.2 (2)	—	—	—
0/4	25.4	75.0 (3)	75.0 (1)	—	—	—
2	8.6	100.0 (2)	0	—	—	—
13/2	3.6	73.3 (11)	6.7 (1)	0	—	—
25	15.5	88.0 (22)	60.0 (15)	22.5 (5)	18.0 (4)	—
1/8	37.8	88.9 (8)	88.9 (8)	55.6 (5)	44.4 (4)	—
4	23.9	100.0 (4)	75.0 (3)	—	—	—
10/2	5.8	83.3 (10)	33.3 (4)	0	—	—

group had early stage tumors. The 5-year survival rates were 26% after resection and 69.4% after transplantation. Even taking into account that the tumors were incidental in 6 of the 12 transplant recipients (ie, the indication for liver replacement was cirrhosis and not tumor), the results were still better in patients with stage I and II tumors. The incidental finding alone could not explain the better survival; this was determined by early tumor stage. In patients with stage IVA and IVB tumors, the longest survival after resection has been 30 months, compared with 5 years for at least 12% of transplant recipients, 4 of whom are still alive (3 free of disease and 1 with an intrahepatic recurrence who underwent repeated transplantation).

Partial hepatectomy for HCC$^+$ was not incompatible with prolonged survival in selected patients, but total hepatectomy and transplantation demonstrated a remarkable prognostic benefit over resection, particularly in patients with early stage tumors and those few who had unresectable advanced malignancies. This may be an indication of extended surgical resectability and improved oncologic cure.

Fibrolamellar Carcinoma

The more favorable prognosis of FLC has been recognized for a long time by several authors. A previous analysis by these authors did not confirm this optimistic view in general, but pointed out the positive influence of early tumor stage on survival as one possible explanation. An updated analysis of the

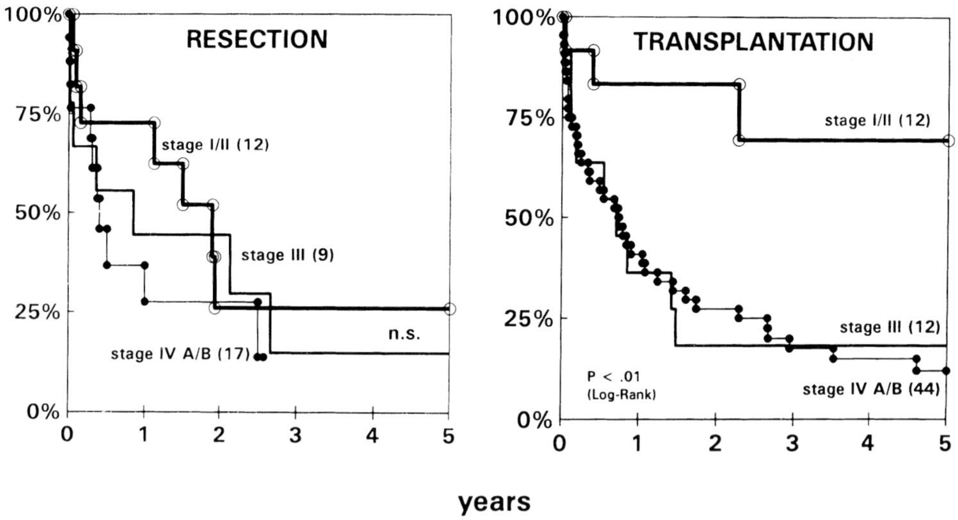

FIG. 46-7. Comparative actuarial patient survival after liver resection and transplantation for hepatocellular carcinoma in cirrhosis (HCC$^+$) according to tumor stage (Medizinische Hochschule Hannover, 1972–1993).

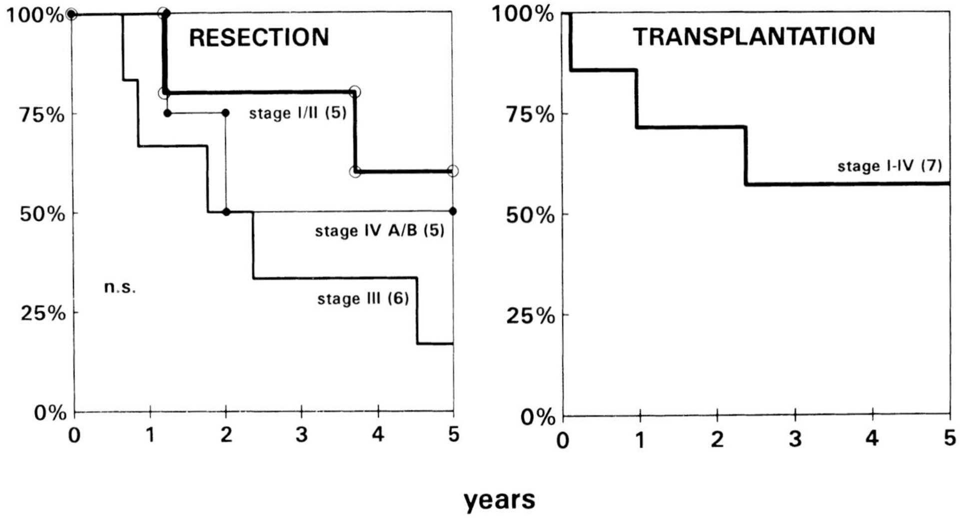

FIG. 46-8. Comparative actuarial patient survival after liver re-section and transplantation for fibrolamellar carcinoma (FLC) according to tumor stage (Medizinische Hochschule Hannover 1972–1993).

series, which now includes 16 resected and 7 transplanted patients, confirmed this impression.

Overall, there was no operative mortality and there was a long-term advantage of transplantation over resection, with 5-year survival rates of 57.1% and 40%, respectively, again related to tumor stage (Fig. 46-8). The rate of recurrent disease was high in both treatment groups (13 of 16 resected patients and 4 of 7 transplanted patients). After partial hepatectomy, 5 patients are still alive, including 2 without recurrence, as compared with 4 liver recipients, 2 of whom also are free of disease. The most beneficial effect of surgery in patients with FLC has been prolonged palliation rather than cure.

Cholangiocellular Carcinoma

As with HCC$^-$, the distribution and incidence of early and late tumor stages in CCC were different in the two groups of patients, with more advanced cases undergoing transplantation. Thirty-day mortality rates were 4.3% after partial hepatectomy and 23.8% after total hepatectomy. The difference reflected the learning curve and the selection of patients in poor clinical condition. A direct comparison of both approaches revealed a highly significant overall survival advantage at 1 year for patients who underwent resection (65.1%) compared with transplantation (13.2%).

Whereas the prognosis in the resected group basically was determined by tumor stage, with 1- and 5-year survival rates of 81.5% and 34.9%, respectively, among patients with stage II tumors, and no long-term survivors among patients with stage III, IVA, or IVB tumors, the situation was completely different after transplantation (Fig. 46-9). Regardless of tumor stage, the median survival of all patients was only 5.2 months, and there were no tumor-free long-term survivors in this series. Based on these results, transplantation does not appear to have any place in the treatment of CCC, whereas resection is indicated in early cases.

Proximal Bile Duct Carcinoma

In both the resection and the transplantation groups, tumors of stages I to III and stages IVA to IVB each accounted for about half the cases of BDC. According to Bismuth's classification, more than 90% of the tumors were stage III to IV. The 30-day mortality rates for both types of surgery were comparable (10.5% and 12%, respectively).

In regard to long-term outcome, the survival rates were slightly better at 1 and 5 years after resection (64.8% and 26.9%, respectively) as compared with transplantation (60% and 18%, respectively). When resection alone was examined more closely, the results after hilar resection were similar to those after combined hilar and liver resection. Multivariate analysis showed a significant influence of residual cancer, vascular invasion, regional lymph node infiltration, and TNM stage. The 5-year survival rate was 42.3% in patients with stage I to II tumors, compared with 0% in those with stage III tumors, and 20.3% in those with stage IVA or IVB tumors (Fig. 46-10).

The prognosis of liver transplantation for BDC was determined by local tumor extent, parenchymal invasion, lymph node status, and tumor stage. No patients with positive regional lymph nodes survived beyond 16 months. Tumor staging showed a clear benefit for patients with stage I to II tumors, with a 5-year actuarial survival rate of 44.4%. Maximum survival in patients with stage III or IV tumors was only 28 months. Four patients who had early stage tumors at the time of transplantation are alive and free of disease, 3 after 8 to almost 10 years. Compared with transplantation, resection for biliary cancer produced a slight advantage in overall survival and favorable results for stage I to II tumors.

Transplantation for Intrahepatic Tumor Recurrence After Resection

A subgroup of 15 patients was identified who underwent secondary liver transplantation for intrahepatic tumor recurrence or nonradical surgery for microscopic residual cancer, after a total of 18 previous resections (Table 46-3). Included were 2 patients in whom the prolonged anhepatic phase between extended procedures—finally leading to complete hepatectomy—was bridged with a temporary portacaval shunt until an allograft became available, an approach previously described by the authors' group. The remaining patients had intervals of

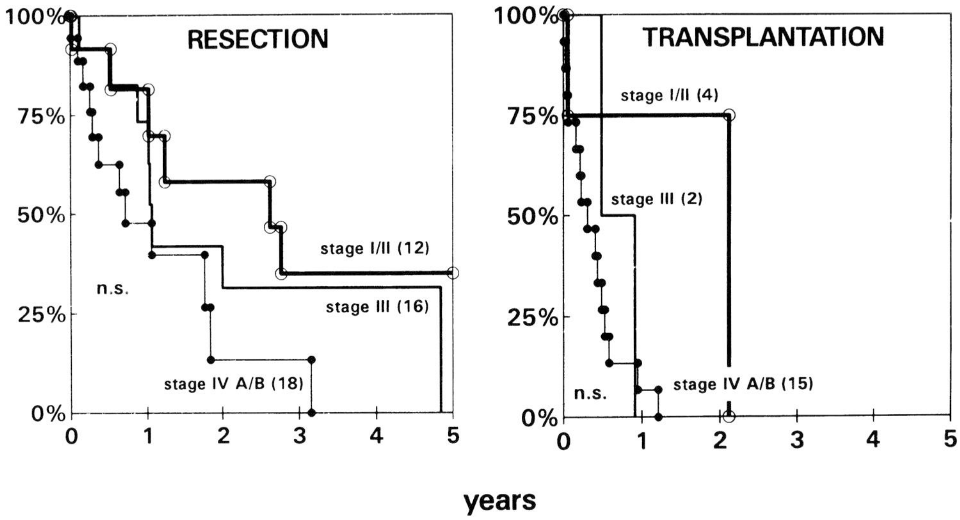

FIG. 46-9. Comparative actuarial patient survival after liver resection and transplantation for cholangiocellular carcinoma (CCC) according to tumor stage (Medizinische Hochschule Hannover 1972–1993).

2 to 72 months between partial and total hepatectomy. Tumor stage at the time of liver replacement was advanced in most cases (stage IVA or IVB in 9 patients). In 1 patient, no cancer cells could be found in the hepatectomy specimen, in accordance with stage 0.

Four of the 15 patients (27%) died early (within 7 to 44 days) of non–tumor-related causes. Three other liver recipients died of diffuse recurrence of their original cancer at 9 to 27 months, and 1 additional patient died of a de novo tumor in the brain at 67 months. Seven patients remain alive, including 4 who are free of disease after 10, 85, 91, and 103 months of follow-up, respectively. The individual risk and success rates in this small series of patients were remarkable, emphasizing the long-term outcome of transplantation—also when performed subsequently to resection.

DISCUSSION

The principal role of radical surgery for malignancy of the liver and bile duct is undisputed worldwide because it offers the greatest chance for disease-free long-term survival or complete cure. For several medical and nonmedical reasons, partial hepatectomy or resection is considered the operation of choice, and the experience with this approach is vast and international in scope.[15–20]

The limitations of resectional surgery in daily practice, deriving mainly from anatomic and functional contraindications, have stimulated scientific research and clinical interest, leading to many significant innovations in technical expertise and safety, and to the extension of indications for surgery and the improvement of patient survival. The surgical choices available today can be daunting, especially when trying to select the right therapy for the right patient at the right time.

Total hepatectomy and subsequent transplantation has become an attractive approach for many hepatobiliary conditions, and is the standard therapy for many benign end-stage diseases when other treatments fail.[21] The particular attractiveness and role of transplantation as a valuable therapy for liver and bile duct malignancies is founded on the assumption that it nearly fulfills the ultimate goal and traditional oncologic principles, surgery of gastrointestinal cancer. Unfortunately, the clinical

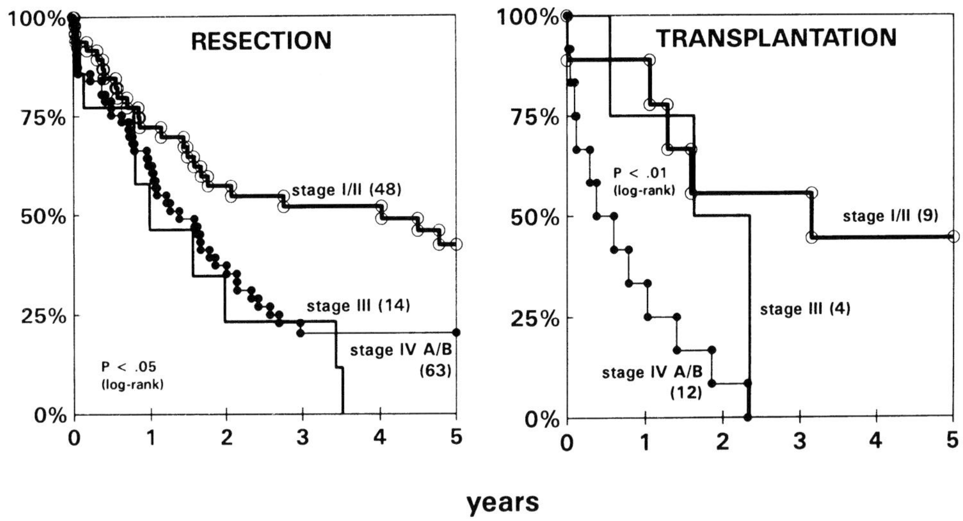

FIG. 46-10. Comparative actuarial patient survival after liver resection and transplantation for proximal bile duct carcinoma (BDC) according to tumor stage (Medizinische Hochschule Hannover, 1972–1993).

TABLE 46-3. *Results of transplantation for intrahepatic recurrence after previous resection (Medizinische Hochschule Hannover, 12/31/93)*

Type of tumor	Patient (liver transplant)	Type of resection	Interval	Tumor stage at transplantation	Outcome
HCC⁻	225	L segmentectomy	11 mo		
		L lobectomy	9 mo	III	AFD 91 mo
	245	L extended lobectomy (R1)	2 mo	0	DFD 67 mo
	344	R lobectomy	16 mo	III	DFD 9 d
	507	R atypical resection	50 mo		
		L atypical resection	39 mo	IVA	AWD 51 mo
	532	R extended lobectomy (R1)	4 mo	IVB	DWD 7 d
HCC⁺	266	Atypical resection (R1)	4 mo	IVA	AFD 85 mo
	397	R atypical segmentectomy	29 mo	IVA	DWD 27 mo
FLC	402	L lobectomy	26 mo	III	AWD 63 mo
	671	R lobectomy	72 mo	IVA	AWD 30 mo
CCC	815	Ex situ resection*	1 d	II	AFD 10 mo
BDC	16	Hilar resection	19 mo	IVA	DWD 9 mo
	23	Hilar resection (R1)	32 mo	IVA	DFD 36 d
	45	Local extirpation (papilloma)	9 mo		
		Local extirpation	13 mo	IVA	DWD 44 d
	160	Hilar resection (R1)	7 mo	IVA	AFD 103 mo
	268	Hilar resection and L extended lobectomy*	1 d	II	DWD 22 mo

* Subsequent total hepatectomy and temporary portocaval shunt

L, left; *R*, right; *R1*, microscopic residual tumor; *AFD*, alive, free of disease; *AFD*, alive, with disease; *DFD*, died, free of disease; *DWD*, died, with disease; *HCC⁻*, hepatocellular carcinoma; *HCC⁺*, hepatocellular carcinoma in cirrhosis; *FLC*, fibrolamellar carcinoma; *CCC*, cholangiocellular carcinoma; *BDC*, proximal bile duct carcinoma.

experience does not support these high expectations, and death resulting from tumor recurrence is still a reality.

Despite considerable advances and improved assessment of general and individual prognostic factors, optimal patient selection remains a dilemma. The need to develop innovative multimodality treatment concepts that include resection and transplantation as complementary approaches, together with adjuvant chemotherapy or radiation therapy, has been expressed often, but has not been attempted in randomized prospective trials.[6,22,23]

Basic criteria for assessing the efficacy of therapy center around resectability, operative morbidity and mortality, radical tumor removal, tumor-free survival, and long-term cure. For accurate comparison of the results of different forms of therapy and studies by different authors, it is essential that the same nomenclature be used for pathologic tumor classification and staging, such as the TNM system. This issue has been addressed many times.[24–27] In reviewing the role of resection versus transplantation for hepatobiliary malignancy, two crucial questions need to be answered.

Can Transplantation Be Considered as an Alternative Option in Conventionally Unresectable Lesions—Is There a Gain in Surgical Resectability of the Tumor?

The answer to this almost classic question, in spite of the short history of modern hepatobiliary surgery, is undoubtedly affirmative. It has been shown repeatedly in several series from various centers, and has been confirmed by the experience of these authors, that the limits of conventional resectability can be overcome by total hepatectomy.[28–32] Intrahepatic anatomic restrictions, such as large or diffuse tumor mass, multiple bilobar location, vascular invasion, and extensive biliary infiltration, and severe functional limitations, such as Child's class B or C cirrhosis, have become amenable to surgery with acceptable risk. Even in patients with more advanced, extrahepatic malignancies, such as regional lymph node infiltration or invasion of adjacent structures and organs, complex multivisceral "cluster" resection and en bloc upper abdominal exenteration has been performed with at least technical success.

Despite the fact that transplantation has increased surgical resectability, the prognoses of primary and secondary hepatobiliary malignancies (ie, specific characteristics of disease recurrence and individual patient survival) still are determined largely by histopathologic tumor type and stage. In principle, and in common with other malignancies, tumors in limited and early stages have significantly better outcomes than those in late and advanced stages. This holds true for HCC, in which the influence of underlying cirrhosis plays an additional role (see below) because it has a direct bearing on the choice of resection versus transplantation.

Whether FLC really has a better prognosis remains to be proved. Overall long-term survival seems to be improved, but this also is influenced strongly by early TNM stage. However, most patients who undergo resection or transplantation eventually experience tumor recurrence, so good palliation over a prolonged period is the major benefit from either radical operation.[33–35]

The use of transplantation does not seem advisable in patients with unresectable CCC, and may be contraindicated, because no tumor-free long-term survivors have been observed. Resection is the only treatment option with an acceptable prognosis in patients with early CCC.[36–41] Patients with other, rare primary liver tumors, such as hepatoblastoma and epithelioid hemangioendothelioma, benefit from transplantation, often experiencing disease-free survival for many years, if they are not eligible for conventional resection.[42,43]

The role of transplantation in BDC has been disputed for many years, with recommendations ranging widely. Curative tumor removal has been shown to provide the best results in terms of survival and palliation. This goal can be achieved by hilar and liver resection in about half of all patients, but selected patients with unresectable tumors or local recurrence may be good candidates for transplantation.[44–46]

Hepatic metastases from various primary tumors usually are not accepted as an indication for total hepatectomy and liver replacement, with one exception: the prognosis of neoplasms of endocrine origin is significantly better in terms of long-term patient survival and good palliation, despite frequent tumor recurrence.[47]

Between conventional resection and transplantation, various modifications of in situ, ante situ, or ex vivo "bench" surgery, including autotransplantation, have found a place. These techniques have proven feasible in primary and, especially, secondary liver tumors, but are unsuitable in cases of BDC with severe cholestasis. Although resectability could be extended, further experience and follow-up is needed to determine whether radical removal also can be improved.[5,48,49]

Should Transplantation Be Performed as the Superior Approach in Potentially Resectable Tumors—Is There a Gain in Oncologic Radical Resection for the Patient?

The most important question regards the prognostic relevance of different treatment modalities, and cannot be answered simply. However, reevaluation of the appropriate data suggests that some traditional points of view and attitudes may need to be altered. A careful evaluation of the comparative results of the authors' analysis suggests the following conclusions.

In patients with HCC$^-$, there is no advantage of total hepatectomy. Resection is the treatment of choice and results in good long-term survival, especially in early stage tumors. In contrast, transplantation seems to be superior in cases of HCC$^+$. This benefit is obvious in unresectable lesions, particularly those in stages I and II, including incidental cancers. Cirrhotic patients with suspected or confirmed small HCC may be ideal candidates for transplantation, because both the cirrhosis and the underlying oncogenic potential are controlled better and longer by total rather than partial hepatectomy.[50–52]

The answer to the second question can be a straightforward "yes." In selected cases (eg, patients with potentially resectable stage I to II HCC$^+$), transplantation may be justified, and even the best choice. Before this practice is adopted widely, however, the following considerations warrant attention: public health and financial concerns; limited donor resources, which could be ameliorated by the more frequent or principal use of split grafts; and the influence of immunosuppression on tumor progression, which must be explored more intensively, and could explain the extremely poor outcome of CCC.[53,54]

Going one step further, it may be possible to achieve extensive extrahepatic tumor removal in both early and advanced tumors through various types of combined or multivisceral procedures that do not directly address the tumor itself. Examples of such logical oncologic approaches in principle include obligatory regional lymphadenectomy, caudate lobectomy, ligamentectomy, and even the standard performance of partial or total pancreatectomy in cases of BDC, with the goal of eradicating all tumor growing along the duct and perineural tissue.[55–57] Only the practical application of such aggressive procedures in a systematic fashion will show whether the prognosis can be significantly improved.

TABLE 46-4. *Prognostic role of resection (LRx) versus transplantation (LTx) for hepatobiliary malignancy*

	Long-term survival					
	Early tumor stage			Advanced tumor stage		
Histological tumor type	LRx		LTx	LRx		LTx
HCC$^-$	+ + + +	>	(+ + + +)	+	<	+ +
HCC$^+$	+	>	+ + + +	0	<	+ +
FLC	+ + + +	>	(+ + + +)	+ +	<	(+ + +)
CCC	+ + +	>	+ + +	0	=	0
BDC	+ + +	>	0	+	>	0

( ), Few patients eligible; *0,* none; +, fairly low (<10%); + +, low (10%–25%); + + +, medium (25%–40%); + + + +, high (>40%); *HCC$^-$*, hepatocellular carcinoma; *HCC$^+$*, hepatocellular carcinoma in cirrhosis; *FLC,* fibrolamellar carcinoma; *CCC,* cholangiocellular carcinoma; *BDC,* proximal bile duct carcinoma.

Based on the clinical experience thus far, some final conclusions regarding the prognostic role of surgery are necessary (Table 46-4). Resection is still a valid first-line therapy for most patients with malignancies of the liver and bile duct. It is the best or only treatment option for patients with resectable primary tumors, such as HCC$^-$, FLC, CCC, and BDC. Transplantation is useful in exceptional unresectable lesions without extrahepatic spread and in cases of intrahepatic recurrence after previous partial hepatectomy. Total hepatectomy as the therapy of choice has been shown to be superior in a few well-selected types and stages of cancer, such as early HCC$^+$. Its use instead of resection, however, must be weighed against all other options, and always should be part of prospective therapeutic concepts.

We should not hesitate to consider new possibilities, because the overall prognosis of liver and bile duct malignancy is far from satisfactory. Every effort must be made to improve the palliation of symptomatic tumors and prolong survival. In evaluating innovative therapies and setting new standards, we must be courageous but also critical enough to balance the risks and benefits for individual patients.

REFERENCES

1. Okuda K, Ishak KG, eds. Neoplasms of the liver. Tokyo: Springer, 1987.
2. Hermanek P, Sobin LH, eds. TNM classification of malignant tumors. 4th ed. Berlin: Springer, 1987.
3. Wanebo HJ, Vezeridis MJ. Hepatoma. J Surg Oncol 1993;3(Suppl):40.
4. Huguet C, Gavelli A, Chieco A, et al. Liver ischemia for hepatic resection: where is the limit? Surgery 1992;111:251.

5. Pichlmayr R, Grosse H, Hauss J, Gubernatis G, Lamesch P, Bretschneider HJ. Technique and preliminary results of extracorporeal liver surgery (bench procedure) and of surgery on the in situ perfused liver. Br J Surg 1990;77:21.
6. Starzl TE, Koep LJ. Surgical approaches for primary and metastatic liver neoplasms, including total hepatectomy with orthotopic liver transplantation. Prog Clin Cancer 1978;7:181.
7. O'Grady JG, Polson RJ, Rolles K, Calne R, Williams R. Liver transplantation for malignant disease. Ann Surg 1988;207:373.
8. Ringe B, Wittekind C, Bechstein WO, Bunzendahl H, Pichlmayr R. The role of liver transplantation in hepatobiliary malignancy. Ann Surg 1989;209:88.
9. Ismail T, Angrisani L, Gunson BK, et al. Primary hepatic malignancy: the role of liver transplantation. Br J Surg 1990;77:983.
10. Olthoff K, Millis M, Rosove MH, Goldstein LI, Ramming KP, Busuttil RW. Is liver transplantation justified for the treatment of hepatic malignancies? Arch Surg 1990;125:1261.
11. Penn I. Hepatic transplantation for primary and metastatic cancers of the liver. Surgery 1991;110:726.
12. Haug CE, Jenkins RL, Rohrer RJ, et al. Liver transplantation for primary hepatic cancer. Transplantation 1992;53:376.
13. Starzl TE, Todo S, Tzakis A, et al. Abdominal organ cluster transplantation for the treatment of upper abdominal malignancies. Ann Surg 1989; 210:374.
14. Moreno-Gonzales EM, Gomez R, Garcia I, et al. Liver transplantation in malignant hepatic neoplasms. Am J Surg 1992;163:395.
15. Iwatsuki S, Starzl TE. Personal experience with 411 hepatic resections. Ann Surg 1988;208:421.
16. Franco D, Capussotti L, Smadja C, et al. Resection of hepatocellular carcinomas. Results in 72 European patients with cirrhosis. Gastroenterology 1990;98:733.
17. Belghiti J, Panis Y, Farges O, Benhamou JP, Fekete F. Intrahepatic recurrence after resection of hepatocellular carcinoma complicating cirrhosis. Ann Surg 1991;214:114.
18. Tang ZY, Yu YQ, Zhou XD, Yang BH, Ma ZC, Lin ZY. Subclinical hepatocellular carcinoma: an analysis of 391 patients. J Surg Oncol 1993;3(Suppl):55.
19. Nagasue N, Kohno H, Chang YC, et al. Liver resection for hepatocellular carcinoma—results of 229 consecutive patients during 11 years. Ann Surg 1993;217:375.
20. Gozzetti G, Mazziotti A, Grazi GL, et al. Surgical experience with 168 primary liver cell carcinomas treated with hepatic resection. J Surg Oncol 1993;3(Suppl):59.
21. Gordon RD, Bismuth H. Liver transplant registry report. Transplant Proc 1991;23:58.
22. Bronowicki JP, Nisand G, Alticri M, et al. Compared results of resection (RX), orthotopic liver transplantation (OLT), and transcatheter oily chemoembolization (TOCE) in the treatment of Okuda's stage I hepatocellular carcinoma (HCC). Gastroenterology 1993;104(Suppl): A881.
23. Farmer DG, Rosove MH, Shaked A, Busuttil RW. Current treatment modalities for hepatocellular carcinoma. Ann Surg 1994;219:236.
24. Ringe B, Pichlmayr R, Wittekind C, Tusch G. Surgical treatment of hepatocellular carcinoma: experience with liver resection and transplantation in 198 patients. World J Surg 1991;15:270.
25. Iwatsuki S, Starzl TE, Sheahan DG, et al. Hepatic resection versus transplantation for hepatocellular carcinoma. Ann Surg 1991;214:221.
26. Tanikawa K. Indication of liver transplantation for hepatocellular carcinoma in Japan. Japanese Journal of Surgery 1992;22:395.
27. McPeake JR, O'Grady JG, Zaman S, et al. Liver transplantation for primary hepatocellular carcinoma: tumor size and number determine outcome. J Hepatol 1993;18:226.
28. Söreide O, Czerniak A, Blumgart LH. Large hepatocellular cancers: hepatic resection or transplantation? BMJ 1985;291:853.
29. Pichlmayr R, Weimann A, Steinhoff G, Ringe B. Liver transplantation for hepatocellular carcinoma: clinical results and future aspects. Cancer Chemother Pharmacol 1992;31(Suppl 1):S157.
30. Calne RY. Resection of large liver tumours: lessons from transplantation surgery. Lancet 1993;342:386.
31. Pichlmayr R, Weimann A, Ringe B. Indications for liver transplantation in hepatobiliary malignancy. Hepatology 1994;20:33S.
32. Pichlmayr R, Weimann A, Lamesch P, Ringe B. Liver transplantation for hepatocellular carcinoma, with additional reference to bench surgery. Journal of Hepato-Biliary-Pancreatic Surgery 1994;2:133.
33. Starzl TE, Iwatsuki S, Shaw BW Jr, et al. Treatment of fibrolamellar hepatoma with partial or total hepatectomy and transplantation of the liver. Surg Gynecol Obstet 1986;162:145.
34. Berman MA, Burnham JA, Sheahan DG. Fibrolamellar carcinoma of the liver: an immunohistochemical study of nineteen cases and a review of the literature. Hum Pathol 1988;19:784.
35. Ringe B, Wittekind C, Weimann A, Tusch G, Pichlmayr R. Results of hepatic resection and transplantation for fibrolamellar carcinoma. Surg Gynecol Obstet 1992;175:299.
36. Chen MF, Jan YY, Wang CS, Jeng LB, Hwang TL. Clinical experience in 20 hepatic resections for peripheral cholangiocarcinoma. Cancer 1989;64:2226.
37. Yeo CJ, Pitt HA, Cameron JL. Cholangiocarcinoma. Surg Clin North Am 1990;70:1429.
38. Yamamoto J, Kosuge T, Takayama T, et al. Surgical treatment of intrahepatic cholangiocarcinoma: four patients surviving more than five years. Surgery 1992;111:617.
39. Schlinkert RT, Nagorney DM, van Heerden JA, Adson MA. Intrahepatic cholangiocarcinoma: clinical aspects, pathology and treatment. HPB Surg 1992;5:95.
40. Ringe B, Weimann A, Lamesch P, Nashan B, Pichlmayr R. Liver transplantation as an option in patients with cholangiocellular and bile duct carcinoma. In: Sugarbaker P, ed. Hepatobiliary cancer. Boston: Kluwer, 1994:259.
41. Pichlmayr R, Lamesch P, Weimann A, Tusch G, Ringe B. Surgical treatment of cholangiocellular carcinoma. World Journal of Surgery 1995;19:83.
42. Kelleher MB, Iwatsuki S, Sheahan DG. Epithelioid hemangioendothelioma of liver. Clinicopathological correlation of 10 cases treated by orthotopic liver transplantation. Am J Surg Pathol 1989;13:999.
43. Koneru B, Flye MW, Busuttil RW, et al. Liver transplantation for hepatoblastoma. Ann Surg 1991;213:118.
44. Pichlmayr R, Ringe B, Lauchart W, Bechstein WO, Gubernatis G, Wagner E. Radical resection and liver grafting as the two main components of surgical strategy in the treatment of proximal bile duct cancer. World J Surg 1988;12:68.
45. Pichlmayr R, Weimann A, Steinhoff G, Ringe B. Chirurgische Eingriffe bei proximalen Gallenwegstumoren. Chirurg 1992;63:539.
46. Bismuth H, Nakache R, Diamond T. Management strategies in resection for hilar cholangiocarcinoma. Ann Surg 1992;215:31.
47. Makowka L, Tzakis AG, Mazzaferro V, et al. Transplantation of the liver for metastatic endocrine tumors of the intestine and pancreas. Surg Gynecol Obstet 1989;168:107.
48. Kumada K, Yamaoka Y, Morimoto T, et al. Partial autotransplantation of the liver in hepatocellular carcinoma complicating cirrhosis. Br J Surg 1992;79:566.
49. Yanaga K, Kishikawa K, Shimada M, et al. Extracorporeal hepatic resection for previously unresectable neoplasms. Surgery 1993;113: 637.
50. Belli L, Romani F, Belli LS, et al. Reappraisal of surgical treatment of small hepatocellular carcinomas in cirrhosis: clinicopathological study of resection or transplantation. Dig Dis Sci 1989;34:1571.
51. Romani F, Sansalone CV, Rimoldi P, et al. Liver transplantation for small HCC in cirrhosis. Transpl Int 1992;5(Suppl 1):S215.
52. Bismuth H, Chiche L, Adam R, Castaing D, Diamond T, Dennison A. Liver resection versus transplantation for hepatocellular carcinoma in cirrhotic patients. Ann Surg 1993;218:145.
53. Yokoyama I, Carr B, Saitsu H, Iwatsuki S, Starzl TE. Accelerated growth rates of recurrent hepatocellular carcinoma after liver transplantation. Cancer 1991;68:2095.
54. O'Grady JG, Johnson PJ, Zaman S, Calne RY, Williams R. Decreased rate of growth of hepatocellular carcinoma recurrence after liver transplantation in patients maintained on cyclosporine immunosuppression. Transplant Proc 1988;20(Suppl 3):394.
55. Mimura H, Kim H, Ochiai Y. Radical block resection of hepatoduodenal ligament for carcinoma of the bile duct with double catheter bypass for portal circulation. Surg Gynecol Obstet 1988;167:527.
56. Sugiura Y, Nakamura S, Iida S, et al. Extensive resection of the bile ducts combined with liver resection for cancer of the main hepatic duct junction: a cooperative study of the Keio Bile Duct Cancer Study Group. Surgery 1994;115:445.
57. Neuhaus P, Blumhardt G. Extended bile duct resection—a new oncological approach to the treatment of central bile duct carcinomas? Langenbecks Arch Chir 1994;379:123.

Surgery for Gastrointestinal Cancer: A Multidisciplinary Approach, edited by Harold J. Wanebo.
Lippincott-Raven Publishers, Philadelphia, © 1997.

CHAPTER 47

Surgical Management of Metastatic Colorectal Cancer of the Liver

M. Margaret Kemeny

Colorectal cancer is one of the leading health problems in the industrialized world. No progress has been made in preventing this disease. The only method of ensuring a successful outcome is early detection of primary and metastatic lesions.

Unlike some other malignancies, colorectal cancer follows a predictable pattern in its spread. Disease that is small and contained in the mucosa virtually never spreads beyond the colon. When disease does get beyond the wall of the colon or rectum, it usually goes to the lymph nodes first, although bloodstream seeding can occur before lymph node spread. If the cancer seeds the blood, the first area of metastasis is the liver in more than half the cases. From the liver, the disease spreads to other organs, most commonly the lung.

Reducing metastatic spread is of major concern, and many large trials have been conducted in an attempt to refine adjuvant chemotherapy into a more effective means of preventing dissemination. This involves improving the available chemotherapeutic agents, establishing better criteria for the use of chemotherapy, and defining the optimal schedule for the delivery of adjuvant treatment (ie, before, during, or after surgery).

When disease does metastasize to the liver, early discovery is important to allow for the implementation of treatment options that produce a cure in almost one third of patients. After curative surgery for colorectal cancer, patients are followed up closely with carcinoembryonic antigen levels and imaging studies. More and more patients with potentially resectable hepatic metastases are being identified, resulting in a more extensive knowledge base regarding treatment options.

Isolated liver metastases are the first sign of metastatic disease in about 23% of patients with colorectal cancer. A large study from Germany established this statistic by observing more than 5000 patients from the time of operation to the development of recurrence. Of these patients, 23% had isolated liver metastases synchronously (ie, at the time of resection of the primary colorectal tumor) or metachronously (ie, at any time after the colorectal resection).[1] In the United States, more than 150,000 new cases of colorectal cancer are detected each year. If 23% of these patients have isolated liver metastases, 37,500 patients will be eligible for some sort of regional hepatic therapy. Multiple studies have shown that 9% (3300) of recurrences are solitary, another 20% (7500) are potentially resectable, and the rest consist of multiple unresectable lesions (Fig. 47-1). The optimal therapy for all three of these categories remains the subject of investigation, but enough information has been amassed over the last 2 decades that the treatment of resectable disease can be discussed with some degree of scientific certainty.

Resection of liver metastases has been the mainstay of treatment for more than 3 decades in patients with solitary metastases from primary colorectal tumors. Many large studies from single institutions and a large multi-institutional hepatic registry have confirmed that resection of a solitary lesion results in permanent eradication of disease in 25% to 30% of patients.[1–11] No form of systematic chemotherapy can produce equal results. In two matched control studies of 120 patients with solitary lesions who did not undergo resection because of patient or physician preference, no patients survived for 5 years.[1,2]

Morbidity and mortality rates associated with hepatic resection have been declining over the last 20 years. Centers at which liver surgery is common report mortality rates of 5% or less for hepatic resection. Centers at which liver metastases are resected should be able to produce similar mortality rates.

Several factors influence patient prognosis after hepatic resection: number of metastases, margin of resection, and length of time to recurrence. The degree of significance of each of these factors varies between different studies. This variation is difficult to explain. One possibility is that most of these trials are not randomized studies directly examining these prognostic variables. Another is that many of the individual studies are too small to produce a definitive statement about most of these variables.

Chief of the Division of Surgical Oncology, North Shore University Hospital, New York University School of Medicine, 300 Community Drive, Manhasset, NY 11030

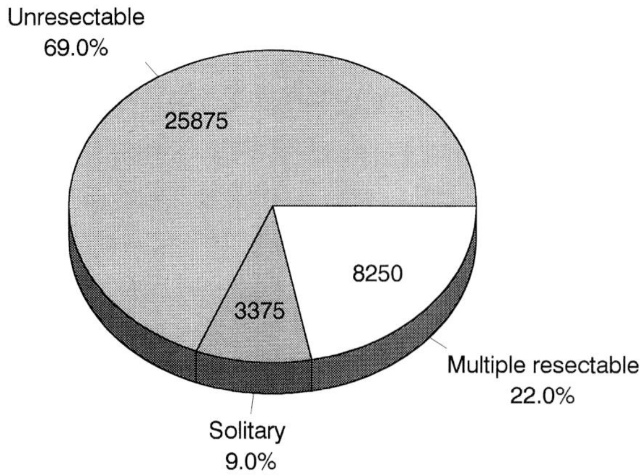

FIG. 47-1. Isolated liver metastases from colorectal cancer (37,500 cases per year).

POTENTIALLY RESECTABLE METASTASES: NUMBER OF LESIONS RESECTABLE

The consensus among groups treating liver metastases is that solitary metastases should be resected and that 5-year survival rates for these patients should be at least 25% to 30%. For patients with multiple hepatic metastases, work done during the past 2 decades has produced certain guidelines. There is widespread agreement that when two or three hepatic metastases are resected, the 5-year survival rate is equal to that after resection of a solitary lesion. This is true regardless of the location of the metastases (ie, unilobar or bilobar). Most groups believe that three hepatic metastases are the maximum for resection.[1–11]

Table 47-1 outlines 5-year survival data after resection of multiple metastases from various groups around the world, reflecting the effect of number of metastases on survival.[1–3,9,10] Conflicting evidence has made it difficult to ascertain the precise number of metastases that should be treated by resection. In a large series from Paris of 97 patients who underwent resection of hepatic metastases from primary colorectal tumors, there was no difference in survival between the 19 patients who had 4 or more metastases and the 78 patients who had 1 to 3 metastases.[4] The 4-year survival rate was 90% among patients with 4 or more metastases and 50% among patients with 1 to 3 metastases; the difference was not statistically significant. In an even larger retrospective study of 266 patients from Erlangen, Germany, there was no difference in survival between patients who underwent resection of 1 metastasis compared with those who underwent resection of more than 2 metastases.[1] The same study also showed similar survival among the 20 patients who underwent resection of more than 4 metastases and the 187 patients who underwent resection of 1 to 3 metastases. In contrast, in a report from the New England Deaconess Hospital, the presence of more than 3 hepatic metastases was found to be a poor prognostic factor, despite resection.[12] In a multi-institutional study from Holland of more than 100 patients who underwent resection for liver metastases, there were no 5-year survivors among patients with 3 or more metastases.[9] In a large study from Milan, only 7 patients had more than 3 metastases; 40% of these patients survived for 5 years.[10] It is difficult to draw a definitive conclusion regarding the exact number of metastases for which resection is beneficial. The discrepancies between the results of these studies cannot be explained except by postulating the existence of a selection bias at various institutions that contributed to the outcomes. A clear answer awaits the performance of a large randomized study specifically evaluating the number of hepatic metastases that should be treated by resection.

A small randomized, prospective study done at the City of Hope Medical Center compared the treatment of multiple metastases (2 to 15 lesions) with resection versus continuous hepatic artery infusion of floxuridine (FUDR).[13,14] There were no significant differences in survival between the 10 patients in the resection group and the 15 patients in the hepatic infusion group. Further prospective work with larger groups of patients needs to be carried out to establish whether resection of 4 or more metastases results in increased survival compared with other forms of treatment.

MARGIN OF RESECTION

Several factors other than the number of metastatic lesions also are important prognostic indicators for patients undergoing resection of liver metastases. As with the number of metastases, there is no uniform agreement about which of these factors are the most significant. The margin of resection necessary to prevent recurrence has been a matter of debate for many years. Precise measurement of this margin often is difficult, especially in cases where the ultrasonic dissector (Cavitron) has been used. Normal hepatic parenchyma may be dispersed with the dissector, leaving no obvious margin of normal liver parenchyma on the specimen when there actually may have been at least a 1-cm margin between the tumor and the edge of the liver parenchyma that is left behind.

Most studies of resection of various liver tumors use a 1-cm margin as the minimal acceptable distance. In the analysis of more than 200 hepatic resections from Erlangen, Germany, the extent of clear margins had no significance for disease-free survival.[6] In the studies from Holland and Paris, the size of

TABLE 47-1. *Survival after hepatic resection*

Group	Number of patients	Solitary metastasis (%)	Two to three metastases (%)	More than three metastases (%)
Milan[10]	95	38	—	40
Paris[4]	97	45	50	88
Rotterdam[9]	117	26	10	0
Registry[3]	789	37	37	18
Erlangen[1]	207	30	31	48

the margin also was not a significant prognostic indicator of survival.[4,9] In contrast, the data from the hepatic registry compiled by Hughes showed the extent of the margin to be significant, with 5-year survival rates of 44% for patients with margins of more than 1 cm compared with 26% for those with margins of 1 cm or less.[3] The discrepancies in these findings may be related to the small number of patients in most of the studies and to the fact that precise measurement of margins of resection often is difficult to accomplish.

SYNCHRONOUS AND METACHRONOUS METASTASES

For many years, numerous centers performing resection of liver metastases observed no differences in survival between patients in whom the metastases were discovered at the time of primary colorectal resection and those in whom they appeared after treatment of the colorectal disease.[3,9,10,15,16] These findings were surprising, because the synchronous appearance of metastases with the primary lesion is associated with a worse prognosis in most tumors. The contradiction was elucidated through the hepatic registry compiled by Hughes (Table 47-2). Information was amassed regarding hepatic resection for more than 750 patients and the survival data were divided according to the interval between diagnosis of the primary tumor and appearance of the liver metastases. Three groups were studied: 223 patients with synchronous metastases, 199 patients with metastases that appeared within 12 months of the primary surgery, and 360 patients with metastases that appeared more than 12 months after the primary surgery. No survival difference was observed between the first two groups, which had 5-year survival rates of 24% and 28%, respectively. The third group had a significantly better 5-year survival rate of 40%.[3] This study demonstrated that many prognostic questions dealing with subgroups and survival can be answered definitively only when there are large numbers of patients in each group. The registry data show that patients with relatively slow-growing hepatic metastases isolated to the liver (over the course of 1 year after colon resection) appear to survive longer when they are treated by hepatic resection. In addition, the interval between resection of the primary tumor and appearance of the metastases is a prognostic factor and not an exclusionary condition for hepatic resection. Even patients with the poorer prognosis associated with synchronous lesions had a 5-year survival rate of 24% after hepatic resection.

EXTRAHEPATIC DISEASE

Disease outside the liver in a patient with liver metastases usually is incurable. The most common intraabdominal site of extrahepatic disease is the portal lymph nodes. In a study at the City of Hope Medical Center, 125 patients with colorectal cancer underwent laparotomy with metastatic disease confined to the liver on preoperative computed tomography; 43 (34%) were found to have extrahepatic intraabdominal metastases. Fifteen of the 43 patients had portal node involvement, 12 had celiac node involvement, 11 had peritoneal seeding, 4 had retroperitoneal node involvement, and 1 had an omental nodule.[13]

Whether the frequent portal node involvement represents disease spread from the liver metastases or the primary tumor is unknown. It is reasonable to believe that it might be from the liver metastases, because it is a sign of advancing disease that is incurable by resection. Because even microscopic involvement of a portal lymph node is a contraindication to hepatic resection, the portal lymph nodes must be sampled before major resection is undertaken. Hughes' hepatic registry included no 5-year disease-free survivors among patients with extrahepatic intraabdominal disease, despite resection of both the hepatic and extrahepatic disease.[3]

Extraabdominal metastatic disease outside the liver is found most commonly in the lungs. Liver resection in the presence of lung metastases usually is unwarranted. Occasional patients with solitary hepatic or pulmonary metastases have benefited from resection of both sites. In these individual cases, the prognostic factors and the patients' conditions must be assessed carefully to determine whether the potential morbidity of hepatic and pulmonary resection is greater than the potential benefit.

STAGE OF PRIMARY COLORECTAL CANCER

Most studies over the past 2 decades have shown that patients whose primary colorectal cancers are confined to the colon or

TABLE 47-2. *Survival after hepatic resection: synchronous versus metachronous*

Study Group	Number of patients	Synchronous	Number of patients	5-Year survival (%)	*P* value
Milan[10]	95	Yes	28	31	NS
		No	67	28	
Rotterdam[9]	117	Yes	38	15	NS
		No	79	22	
Erlangen[6]	173	Yes	85	32	0.05
		No	88	45	
Hepatic Registry[3]	789	Yes	223	24	0.02
		1–12 mo	199	28	
		<12 mo	360	40	
Paris[4]	97	Yes	35	52	NS
		No	62	52	
Italy[16]	212	Yes	99	18	NS
		No	113	22	

NS, not significant.

TABLE 47-3. *Survival after hepatic resection: stage of primary*

Group	Dukes[1] stage	Number of patients	5-Year survival	*P* value
Milan[10]	B	29	47	0.02
	C	50	24	
Hepatic Registry[3]	B	250	35	0.001
	C	338	28	
Paris[4]	B	39	52	NS
	C	58	53	
Rotterdam[9]	B	53	26	NS
	C	54	11	
Erlangen[1]	B	49	53	0.01
	C	119	32	
Italy[16]	B	69	32	0.001
	C	116	11	

NS, not significant.

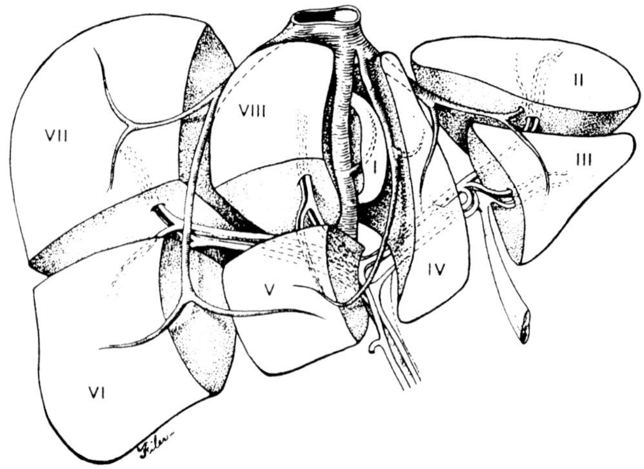

FIG. 47-2. Couinaud's eight hepatic segments (subsegments).

rectum have a better survival rate after liver resection than do patients whose primary cancers have spread to the regional lymph nodes (Table 47-3). Patients with lymph node involvement may be more prone to systemic metastases. Again, the initial involvement of regional lymph nodes is not an exclusionary criterion for hepatic resection, but simply a prognostic tool.

In the hepatic registry, the 5-year survival rates were 35% for the 250 patients with negative lymph nodes and 28% for the 338 patients with involved mesenteric nodes.[3] This included data from Germany, where patients with Duke's A and B cancers who did not have liver metastases were compared with patients with Duke's A and B cancers who had resected liver metastases. No significant difference in long-term survival was observed between these two groups. These data support the concept that the liver may be the only site of disease in patients with isolated liver metastases, and that this possibility is more probable if the mesenteric lymph nodes were not involved with the primary cancer.

OPERATIVE MORBIDITY AND MORTALITY

As the worldwide experience with hepatic resection has expanded, the morbidity and mortality accompanying these procedures has declined. In the larger studies, the operative mortality rate has ranged from 2.7% to 13% (Table 47-4). Mortality data include intraoperative deaths and deaths occurring during the first 30 days after operation. The worldwide average seems to be about 5%.

The morbidity rate in these series ranges from 5% to 34% (see Table 47-4). Increased familiarity with hepatic anatomy, especially the segmental information supplied by Couinaud (Fig. 47-2), which divides the liver into eight segments, has made it possible to perform resection along anatomic lines not previously appreciated.

New intraoperative equipment also has facilitated large hepatic resections. The ultrasonic dissector (Cavitron) is used widely and has expedited hepatic parenchymal dissection for many surgeons. This instrument delivers pulsed jets of water that can disperse the loosely connected cells of the hepatic parenchyma while leaving the more cohesive bile duct and vascular wall intact. In this manner, the vessels can be recognized more easily and bleeding can be controlled better.

Most centers report a mean blood loss of 3 U accompanying major hepatic resection (see Table 47-4). Because of the current medical environment and concerns about AIDS and hepatitis, blood transfusions often are limited. Measures to avoid transfusion have included using the intraoperative cell saver during resection. In a matched control study from Japan, hepatic resection was performed for primary liver cancer using the cell saver in 54 patients and no autologous blood in 50 patients.[17] No differences were observed in disease-free or overall survival rates. A retrospective study from California reported similar findings.[18] These studies demonstrated that the cell saver can be used safely in patients with malignancies without fear of disseminating the disease.

Other techniques for reducing blood loss include hepatic vas-

TABLE 47-4. *Morbidity and mortality associated with hepatic resections*

Institution	Number of patients	Morbidity (%)	Mortality (%)	Mean Transfusions (U)
Roswell Park[5]	62	30	8	3.8
New England Deaconess[12]	66	18	2.7	3
Erlangen[6]	266	22	5.6	NA
Rotterdam[9]	118	34	7.6	3.2
Milan[10]	100	5	13	NA

NA, not available.

cular occlusion maneuvers, which were developed for hepatic transplantation.[19–27] If the hepatic vasculature is totally isolated, resection can be carried out in a bloodless field. To accomplish this total vascular exclusion of the liver, clamps must be placed on the vena cava proximal to the entrance of the hepatic veins and on the vena cava below the liver but above the adrenal vein entrance. The portal triad, including the portal vein and the hepatic artery, also must be occluded. The average avascular time for the liver during vascular exclusion reported by Bismuth and colleagues from Paris was 46 minutes, with a range of 20 to 70 minutes.[19] In the same series, among 51 patients treated by the total vascular occlusion technique, there was 1 postoperative death of hepatic failure, 3 biliary fistulas, 3 subhepatic collections, and 7 cases of right basilar atelectasis. Almost all patients had a transient rise in the transaminase level 2 days after surgery, which returned to normal after 2 weeks. Numerous other centers have reported on this technique of vascular occlusion, which is becoming accepted as the procedure of choice for large central tumors and for tumors at the hepatic veins and near the vena cava. However, exposing patients to the hemodynamic changes accompanying total vascular occlusion probably is not necessary for the more standard hepatic procedures involving wedge resections or lobectomies.

As the trend has shifted from resecting only solitary lesions to resecting multiple metastases, the type of operation has changed from lobectomy to segmentectomy to subsegmental metastasectomies. Despite the fact that subsegmental metastasectomies require the resection of multiple areas of the liver, complication rates have declined as lobectomies have been replaced by lesser procedures. Sometimes, trisegmentectomies or extended lobectomies are still necessary to remove all the tumor. In general, even after extensive liver resection, the remaining liver function is not as much of a problem with this group of patients as it is with patients undergoing resection for hepatocellular carcinoma. Patients with colorectal cancer usually have normal liver parenchyma outside the carcinoma, whereas patients with hepatocellular cancer almost always have concomitant cirrhosis induced by alcohol or virus. For this reason, the preoperative work-up for patients with metastatic disease does not need to include an analysis of liver function other than the standard liver function tests and the prothrombin time.

Another new device is intraoperative ultrasound. Using this form of ultrasound increases the operating surgeon's ability to identify all the metastatic disease present in the liver. This should allow for more curative resections, because small outlying metastases can be appreciated; eventually, this should result in fewer hepatic recurrences after resection. No definitive studies have provided this information.

RECURRENCE AFTER RESECTION

Patterns of recurrence after hepatic resection were not well studied for many years. However, institutions with large series of hepatic resections of colorectal metastases have been recording sites of relapse after resection (Table 47-5). In a report from Heidelberg on recurrence after hepatic resection, 59 patients (78%) had recurrence, 28 confined to the liver.[28] In a more selected series of 77 patients described by Fortner over the last 20 years, only 45 had recurrence after liver resection.[29] Most of the hepatic resections done in this series were lobectomies, probably all were for solitary lesions, and the intervals between diagnosis of the primary tumors and development of the recurrences were not specified. In this study, only 17% of patients had recurrent disease in the liver. In three other studies from Europe, recurrence rates ranged from 49% to 60%. The liver was the only site of recurrence in 29% to 66% of patients who had relapses.[4,9,10]

A large study from Tokyo reported a 60% recurrence rate, with 29% restricted to the liver.[30] Evaluating the data as a whole, it appears that resection of multiple metastases from the liver has been followed by recurrent disease in more than half the patients, and that recurrence has been confined to the liver in about one third. There is no evidence that particular surgical techniques decrease the likelihood of regional recurrence. Information from Fortner suggests that in selected patients with solitary lesions, lobectomy with wide margins may decrease the local recurrence rate. However, this study has biases.

RESECTION OF RECURRENCE IN THE LIVER AFTER HEPATIC RESECTION

At least 50% to 75% of patients have a recurrence after liver resection. Of these recurrences, about one third are confined to the liver or appear initially in the liver. Several centers have reported on their experience with repeated resection of these hepatic recurrences.[32–39]

In a study from Memorial Sloan-Kettering Cancer Center, 44 (9%) of 499 patients who underwent hepatic resection had a hepatic recurrence that was reexplored for a possible second resection.[36] Of these 44 patients, 19 had unresectable disease and 25 went on to have a second hepatic resection. There was no 30-day operative mortality in these 25 patients and the morbidity rate was 28%. The median disease-free survival was 9 months, with a median survival of 30 months.

In a report from Paris of 181 patients who underwent curative liver resection, 60 had isolated liver recurrences.[34] Ten of these patients underwent a second liver resection. There were no operative deaths. The mean intraoperative blood loss was almost 6 U. Six patients had a major complication and 1 died of liver failure 16 days after surgery. The 5-year overall and disease-free survival rates were 30% and 18%, respectively.

Eleven cases of repeated hepatic resection were reported from Milan.[33] There was 1 operative death and 5 postoperative complications. The median blood loss was 2 U. In the short median follow-up time of 17 months, 4 patients remained disease-free.

The Registry of Repeat Resections of Hepatic Metastases is a compilation of data from 20 institutions around the world.[32] Information has been gathered on 170 patients who have undergone repeated liver resection for colorectal metastases. The mortality and morbidity rates are not significantly different from those associated with initial resection. The survival rate is essentially the same at 5 years (25%).

Sufficient evidence is available to reinforce the concept that for a few patients (around 10%) who have isolated hepatic recurrence after hepatic resection, the treatment that offers the best results is repeated hepatic resection. The operative morbidity and mortality may be slightly higher for this group, but are not statistically significant. The overall survival for patients having successful eradication of recurrent disease should be the same as for patients undergoing initial hepatic resection. There

TABLE 47-5. *Patterns of recurrence after hepatic resection*

Group	Number of patients	Number of recurrences (%)	Liver only (%)	Liver plus other (%)	Extrahepatic only (%)
Heidelberg[28]	75	59 (78)	28 (47.5)	8 (13.5)	23 (39)
Memorial (Fortner)[29]	77	45 (58)	8 (17)	NA	37 (83)
Milan[10]	100	69 (69)	28 (40.5)	13 (19)	28 (40.5)
Paris[4]	97	48 (49)	32 (66)	NA	13 (27)
Tokyo[30]	107	64 (60)	34 (53)	6 (9)	32 (50)
Netherlands[9]	108	69 (69.5)	21 (29)	14 (21)	34 (69)
Hepatic Registry[31]	607	344 (56)	149 (40)	42 (11)	106 (25)

NA, not available.

does not seem to be any contraindication to repeated resection, as long as patients are free of disease in all extrahepatic sites.

ADJUVANT THERAPY AFTER RESECTION

Despite the surgical advances that have widened the indications for hepatic resection and reduced the morbidity and mortality, most patients still die of metastatic disease, even after resection. Further, most patients have liver metastases as part of their relapse.

Adjuvant chemotherapy is the standard therapy for patients with stage III colorectal cancer, using systemic agents that are based on 5-fluorouracil (5-FU) therapy. Many patients with liver metastases already have received some adjuvant therapy for their primary cancers.

The efficacy of systemic therapy for liver metastases has been limited. The best available approach is a combination of 5-FU and leucovorin. However, when all the data regarding this drug regimen were evaluated by metanalysis, the overall response rate was only 23%, with a median survival of 11.5 months.[40] No randomized studies have been completed that demonstrate a survival benefit when 5-FU and leucovorin are given after liver resection.

Continuous hepatic artery infusion of FUDR, a 5-FU analogue, has yielded a higher response rate in liver metastases than any other form of chemotherapy. Overall objective response rates of 50% or higher have been reported in numerous studies of patients with disease confined to the liver, with an average of 40% replacement of the hepatic parenchyma with tumor.[41–43] In some reports of selected patients, objective responses have been seen in more than 80% of patients treated with continuous hepatic artery infusion.[13]

Because of the apparent increased response rates seen with this new treatment modality, the use of continuous hepatic artery infusion of FUDR after liver resection was investigated in a randomized study at the City of Hope Medical Center.[13,14] Among a small group of 11 patients with solitary hepatic metastases, 6 underwent hepatic resection followed by continuous hepatic artery infusion of FUDR. None of these patients had recurrent hepatic disease. Of the 5 patients who underwent resection only, 4 had hepatic recurrence. Despite the small size of this group, the difference in disease-free survival between the patients who underwent resection alone (8 months) and those who underwent resection followed by continuous hepatic artery infusion of FUDR (30 months) was statistically significant.

Another group of 15 patients had multiple hepatic metastases and were treated with resection followed by continuous hepatic artery infusion of FUDR. Again, none had initial recurrence in the liver. All but 1 had recurrence in extrahepatic sites, primarily the lung.

This regional therapy given after hepatic resection was accompanied by numerous side effects, some of them serious. The most significant was the biliary sclerosis or sclerosing cholangitis that affected one fourth of the patients. The patients who had undergone resection seemed to be more vulnerable to this complication than the patients with unresected liver metastases. When the interval between resection and the initiation of chemotherapy was lengthened to at least 6 to 8 weeks, the chemotherapy was tolerated better and there was a marked reduction in the incidence of biliary sclerosis. In addition, the dosage of the infusion was decreased after it was discovered that the biliary sclerosis was dose-dependent. The usual starting dosage was reduced from 0.3 mg/kg/d to 0.1 mg/kg/d. In a study from California, decreasing the starting dosage reduced the incidence of biliary sclerosis by more than 50%.[43] In patients who had lobectomies, the dosage was decreased even further to 0.05 mg/kg/d.

In the City of Hope Medical Center study, there was no additional morbidity accompanying hepatic resection when the pump was placed at the same setting. The operative time was lengthened minimally. There were no operative deaths in this series.[13]

Although placement of the hepatic pump has been shown to be safe, the actual benefit of intrahepatic therapy after liver resection has not been established. An intergroup study is being conducted in the United States and Australia to answer this question.

CONCLUSION

Many advances have been made in the surgical treatment of hepatic metastases from colorectal cancer, including technical surgical innovations and refinement of the selection criteria for hepatic resection. Prognostic variables have been delineated over the last decade that aid in treatment decisions. Additional therapy after surgery is under investigation. All these advances have resulted in significantly improved patient outcomes. The results of ongoing trials and the initiation of more randomized controlled studies with large numbers of patients may provide clues to the questions that remain unanswered.

REFERENCES

1. Scheele J, Stangl R, Altendorf-Hofmann A. Hepatic metastases from colorectal carcinoma: impact of surgical resection on the natural history. Br J Surg 1990;77:1241.
2. Wilson SW, Adson MA. Surgical treatment of hepatic metastases from colorectal cancers. Arch Surg 1976;111:330.
3. Hughes K, Scheele J, Sugarbaker PH. Surgery for colorectal cancer metastatic to liver. Surg Clin North Am 1989;69:339.
4. Elias D, Lasser P, Rougier P, Debaene B. Another failure in the attempt of definition of the indications to the resection of liver metastases of colorectal origin. J Chir (Paris) 1992;129:59.
5. Petrelli N, Gupta B, Piedmonte M, Herrera L. Morbidity and survival of liver resection for colorectal adenocarcinoma. Dis Colon Rectum 1991;34:899.
6. Scheele J, Stangl R, Altendorf-Hofmann A, Gall FP. Indicators of prognosis after hepatic resection for colorectal secondaries. Surg 1991;110:13.
7. Adson MA, van Heerden JA, Adson MH, Wagner JS, Ilstrup DM. Resection of hepatic metastases from colorectal cancer. Arch Surg 1984;119:647.
8. Gennari L, Doci R, Bignami P, Bozzetti F. Surgical treatment of hepatic metastases from colorectal cancer. Ann Surg 1986;203:49.
9. van Ooijen B, Wiggers T, Meijer S, et al. Hepatic resections for colorectal metastases in the Netherlands. A multi-institutional 10-year study. Cancer 1992;70:28.
10. Doci R, Gennari L, Bignami P, Montalto F, Morabito A, Bozzetti F. One hundred patients with hepatic metastases from colorectal cancer treated by resection: analysis of prognostic determinants. Br J Surg 1991;78:797.
11. Adson M, Beart RW. Elective hepatic resections. Surg Clin North Am 1977;57:339.
12. Cady B, Stone MD, McDermott WV, et al. Technical and biological factors in disease-free survival after hepatic resection for colorectal cancer metastases. Arch Surg 1992;127:561.
13. Kemeny MM, Goldberg D, Beatty D, et al. Results of a prospective randomized trial of continuous regional chemotherapy and hepatic resection as treatment of hepatic metastases from colorectal primaries. Cancer 1986;57:492.
14. Wagman LD, Kemeny MM, Leong L, et al. A prospective, randomized evaluation of the treatment of colorectal cancer metastatic to the liver. J Clin Oncol 1990;8:1885.
15. Schlag P, Hohenberger P, Herfarth C. Resection of liver metastases in colorectal cancer—competitive analysis of treatment results in synchronous versus metachronous metastases. Eur J Surg Oncol 1990;16:360.
16. Fegiz G, Ramacciato G, Gennari L, et al. Hepatic resections for colorectal metastases: the Italian multicenter experience. J Surg Oncol Suppl 1991;2:144.
17. Fujimoto F, Okamota E, Yamanaka N, et al. Efficacy of autotransfusion in hepatectomy for hepatocellular carcinoma. Arch Surg 1993;128:1065.
18. Zulim RA, Rocco M, Goodnight JE, Smith JG, Krag DN, Schneider PD. Intraoperative autotransfusion in hepatic resection for malignancy. It is safe? Arch Surg 1993;128:206.
19. Bismuth H, Castaing D, Garden J. Major hepatic resection under total vascular exclusion. Ann Surg 1989;210:13.
20. Emre S, Schwartz ME, Katz E, Miller CM. Liver resection under total vascular isolation. Variations on a theme. Ann Surg 1993;217:15.
21. Hannoun L, Borie D, Delva E, et al. Liver resection with normothermic ischaemia exceeding 1 h. Br J Surg 1993;80:1161.
22. Elias D, Desrruennes, Lasser P. Prolonged intermittent clamping of the portal triad during hepatectomy. Br J Surg 1991;78:42.
23. Huguet C, Gavelli A, Addario Chieco P, et al. Liver ischemia for hepatic resection: where is the limit? Surgery 1992;111:251.
24. Yanaga K, Matsumata T, Nishizaki T, Shimada M, Sugimachi K. Alternate hemihepatic vascular control technique for hepatic resection. Am J Surg 1993;165:365.
25. Huguet C, Addario-Chieco P, Gavelli A, Arrigo E, Harb J, Clement RR. Technique of hepatic vascular exclusion for extensive liver resection. Am J Surg 1992;163:602.
26. Stephen MS, Sheil-Ross AG, Thompson JF, Wilson T, Boland SL. Aortic occlusion and vascular isolation allowing avascular hepatic resection. Arch Surg 1990;125:1482.
27. Delva E, Camus Y, Nordlinger B, et al. Vascular occlusions for liver resections. Operative management and tolerance to hepatic ischemia: 142 cases. Ann Surg 1989;209:211.
28. Hohenberger P, Schlag P, Schwarz V, Heergarth C. Tumor recurrence and options for further treatment after resection of liver metastases in patient with colorectal cancer. J Surg Oncol 1990;44:245.
29. Fortner JG. Recurrence of colorectal cancer after hepatic resection. Am J Surg 1988;155:378.
30. Sugihara K, Hojo K, Moriya Y, Yamasaki S, Kosuge T, Takayama T. Pattern of recurrence after hepatic resection for colorectal metastases. Br J Surg 1993;80:1032.
31. Hughes K, Simon R, Songhorabodi S, et al. Resection of the liver for colorectal carcinoma metastases: a multi-institutional study of patterns of recurrence. Surgery 1986;100:278.
32. Fernandez-Trigo V, Shamsa F, Aldrete J, et al. Repeat liver resections from colorectal metastases. In: Sugarbaker P, ed. Hepatobiliary cancer. Kluwer Academic Publishers, 1994.
33. Bozzetti F, Bignami P, Montalto F, Doci R, Gennari L. Repeated hepatic resection for recurrent metastases from colorectal cancer. Br J Surg 1992;79:146.
34. Vaillant JC, Balladur P, Nordlinger B, et al. Repeat liver resection for recurrent colorectal metastases. Br J Surg 1993;80:340.
35. Griffith KD, Sugarbaker PH, Chang AE. Repeat hepatic resections for colorectal metastases. Surgery 1990;107:101.
36. Yuman F, Blumgart LH, Cohen A, Fortner J, Brennan MF. Repeat hepatic resections for metastatic colorectal cancer. Ann Surg 1994;220:657.
37. Que FG, Nagorney DM. Resection of "recurrent" colorectal metastases to the liver. Br J Surg 1994;81:255.
38. Nordlinger B, Vaillant JC, Guiguet M, et al. Liver resections for recurrent colorectal metastases: 143 cases. J Clin Oncol 1994;12:1491.
39. Lange JF, Leese T, Castaing D, Bismuth H. Repeat hepatectomy for recurrent malignant tumor of the liver. Surg Gynecol Obstet 1989;169:119.
40. Advanced Colorectal Cancer Meta-Analysis Project. Modulation of fluorouracil by leucovorin in patients with advanced colorectal cancer: evidence in terms of response rate. J Clin Oncol 1992;10:896.
41. Rougier P, Laplanche A, Huguier M, et al. Hepatic arterial infusion of floxuridine in patients with liver metastases from colorectal carcinoma: long-term results of a prospective randomized trial. J Clin Oncol 1992;10:1112.
42. Hohn DC, Stagg RJ, Friedman MA, et al. A randomized trial of continuous intravenous versus hepatic intraarterial floxuridine in patients with colorectal cancer metastatic to the liver: the Northern California Oncology Group trial. J Clin Oncol 1989;7:1646.
43. Kemeny N, Daly J, Reichman B, et al. Intrahepatic or systemic infusion of flurodeoxyuridine in patients with liver metastases from colorectal carcinoma. A randomized trial. Ann Intern Med 1987;107:459.

Surgery for Gastrointestinal Cancer: A Multidisciplinary Approach, edited by Harold J. Wanebo.
Lippincott-Raven Publishers, Philadelphia, © 1997.

CHAPTER 48

Operative Approaches to Hepatocellular Carcinoma in the Cirrhotic Patient

Wing-Yiu Lui and Gar-Yang Chau

Hepatocellular carcinoma (HCC) is one of the most common malignancies, and has been difficult to treat successfully. Nearly 1 million patients around the world die of this disease each year.[1] Among the various therapeutic approaches to HCC, surgery remains the only method that offers a chance of cure. In Eastern and Western countries, 60% to 75% of HCC occurs in cirrhotic livers.[2–5] The high incidence of cirrhosis associated with HCC makes surgical management even more difficult. To achieve good clinical results, the operative approach to HCC in cirrhotic patients should include careful patient selection, meticulous surgical technique, intensive postoperative care, and close follow-up.

PATIENT SELECTION AND PREOPERATIVE EVALUATION

The resectability rate of HCC occurring in cirrhotic patients is increasing. Resection rates vary between 15% and 60%.[6–9] When HCC is diagnosed, two key factors determine whether surgical resection is feasible: the extent of liver involvement and the hepatic functional reserve. Tumors in cirrhotic livers tend to be smaller than those in noncirrhotic livers. However, the incidence of multifocal tumors, which may result from intrahepatic metastasis through the portal blood flow or from multicentric origins, is higher in cirrhotic patients. Up to 54.9% of resected lesions occurring in cirrhotic livers are multifocal.[10] In general, the extent of hepatic involvement by the tumor, rather than its size or number, indicates whether exploration and resection is warranted. Useful studies for preoperative evaluation of intrahepatic tumor involvement are abdominal ultrasonography, computed tomography (CT), and hepatic arteriography (including indirect arterial portography). To avoid seeding along the needle tract or into the peritoneal cavity, these authors usually do not perform preoperative histologic diagnosis of the tumor by ultrasound- or CT-guided needle biopsy. This procedure is used only when the diagnosis of malignancy is in doubt.

Patients with tumor involving more than two anatomic segments, or two nonadjacent segments, are not candidates for surgical resection. Patients with tumor involving the portal vein up to the first branch can undergo resection safely, but the possibility of intrahepatic metastasis is high under these conditions. Although resection of tumor involving the main portal vein, main hepatic vein, or inferior vena cava has been reported, the procedure should be regarded as merely palliative.[11] Tumor invading adjacent structures, such as the diaphragm, adrenal glands, or colon, may be resected for cure en bloc.

When the tumor is considered to be anatomically resectable, the functional reserve of the liver should be evaluated carefully. These authors assess hepatic function using Pugh's grades of severity of liver disease and the indocyanine green retention rate. Pugh's grading system is based on five clinical and laboratory parameters: encephalopathy, ascites, serum bilirubin level, serum albumin level, and prothrombin time. On the basis of this classification system, cirrhotic patients can be separated into three groups with different operative risk, ranging from good in grade A to poor in grade C[12] (Table 48-1). These authors use the indocyanine green retention test routinely in cirrhotic patients and find it to have substantial prognostic value. The test is a reflection of hepatic blood flow. Briefly, 0.5 mg/kg of indocyanine green is injected intravenously and the venous blood is sampled at 5, 10, and 15 minutes. From these readings, the indocyanine green retention rate is calculated. Patients with a high retention rate have significant hepatic dysfunction and would be expected to have higher morbidity and mortality after hepatic resection. Indocyanine green studies are especially useful in identifying patients with significantly impaired hepatic function who otherwise seem to have compensated cirrhosis[13] (ie, their routine serum chemical liver profiles and coagulation studies are near normal limits).

W-Y Lui, Department of Surgery, Veterans General Hospital–Taipei, National Yang-Ming Medical University, Taipei, Taiwan, ROC

Gar-Yang Chau, Department of Surgery, Veterans General Hospital–Taipei, National Yang-Ming Medical University, Taipei, Taiwan, ROC

TABLE 48-1. *Pugh's grading of severity of liver disease*

Clinical and biochemical measurement	Points scored for increasing abnormality		
	1	2	3
Encephalopathy	None	1 and 2	3 and 4
Ascites	Absent	Slight	Moderate
Bilirubin (mg/dL)	12	23	>3
Albumin (gm/dL)	>3.5	2.8–3.5	<2.8
Prothrombin time (seconds prolonged)	1–4	4–6	>6

Scoring: grade 1 (5–6), grade B (7–9), grade C (10–15). (Adapted from Pugh RN, Murray-Lyon IM, Dawson JL, Pietroni MC, Williams R. Transection of the esophagus for bleeding esophageal varices. Br J Surg 1973;60:646.)

A variety of other studies using complex techniques have been proposed to predict postsurgical outcome. These include ^{198}Au-colloid uptake studies[14] and hepatic mitochondrial redox tolerance tests.[15] All these measurements can be regarded as tools for excluding high-risk patients from consideration for resection. Table 48-2 provides a flow chart for surgical decision-making based on the assessment of hepatic function.

In patients with evidence of portal hypertension, such as marked splenomegaly or leukopenia and thrombocytopenia, preoperative esophagogastroscopy should be performed to detect varices. Because there is a risk of increased portal pressure after hepatectomy,[16,17] a concomitant surgical procedure (eg, esophageal devascularization and splenectomy) or endoscopic sclerotherapy is necessary for patients with previous bleeding or risky varices. These authors have performed concomitant operations with satisfactory results.[18]

OPERATIVE CONSIDERATIONS

Hepatic resection can be divided into anatomic resection (lobectomy, segmentectomy, subsegmentectomy) and nonanatomic resection (wedge resection). Higher local tumor recurrence rates have been reported with nonanatomic wedge resection than with anatomic resection.[19] In the experience of these authors, intrahepatic invasion (portal venous invasion with microemboli or tumor capsular infiltration) is the most important adverse prognostic factor for tumor recurrence after hepatic resection. The results of our prospective study in 68 consecutive cases of small HCC (Table 48-3, unpublished data) and the results of other studies indicate that there is a high incidence of intrahepatic invasion, macroscopic or microscopic, even in small tumors.[20] Therefore, anatomic resection (lobectomy, segmentectomy) or systematic subsegmentectomy as described by Makuuchi[21] (removal of the entire portal unit) is the operative procedure of choice for the treatment of small HCC in cirrhotic patients with adequate hepatic functional reserve. Local tumor wedge resection is indicated only in patients with poor hepatic functional reserve.

OPERATIVE TECHNIQUES

Incision

Good exposure is the key to successful hepatic resection. For resection over the right lobe of the liver, an inverted T-shaped abdominal wall incision usually is used. An upper midline incision is made from the junction of the xiphoid process and the left costal arch to 2 cm above the umbilicus, then is curved and extended laterally to the right midaxillary line (Fig. 48-1*A*). For procedures such as left lobectomy or lateral segmentectomy, an upper abdominal bilateral subcostal incision is used, with an extension up to the xiphoid process (see Fig. 48-1*B*). Both costal arches are retracted cranially with a Kent abdominal retractor. Good exposure is obtained with this method, and these authors have found that thoracotomy is not necessary for hepatic resection in cirrhotic patients. The liver should be mobilized fully by dividing the round, falciform, bilateral coronary, and triangular ligaments. After extensive mobilization, the liver can be rotated out of the abdominal cavity with complete exposure of the whole organ. At this time, the liver should be inspected and palpated carefully to evaluate its condition, including its consistency, and to detect any additional tumor nodules missed during preoperative assessment and any invasion of the surrounding tissue by the tumor.

Intraoperative Ultrasound

Intraoperative ultrasound can help the surgeon to define accurately the location and nature of the lesions and to perform safe hepatic resection. It is an indispensable tool and is used routinely by these authors for liver resection. It adds about 15 to 20 minutes to the operative procedure. In a series of 110 cases of hepatic resection for HCC, the sensitivity of intraoperative ultrasound in detecting small HCC nodules was 92%, better than that of preoperative ultrasound (75%), CT (70%), or angiography (83%). Some important ultrasonographic features of HCC have been described[22]: the tumor margin typically is round and smooth; the lesion may have a thin ''halo'' sign; the internal echo has a mosaic pattern; there is a small, star-shaped and scattered anechoic area; and there are enhanced posterior echoes with lateral shadows. Several pitfalls also have been encountered in the use of intraoperative ultrasound. First, mistaken

TABLE 48-2. *Flow chart for surgical decision-making based on assessment of hepatic function*

Pugh's grade		A	B	C
ICG 15′	<10%	10%–20%	20%–30%	30%–40%
Right lobectomy		Left lobectomy	Subsegmentectomy	Enucleation
Segmentectomy		Segmentectomy	Wedge resection	
		Subsegmentectomy		

ICG 15′, indocyanine green 15 minutes retention rate.

TABLE 48-3. *Incidence of daughter nodule formation and microscopic invasion of surrounding liver tissue in 68 resected small hepatocellular carcinomas*

		Invasion to		
Tumor size (cm)	Daughter nodule	Microvessels	Capsule	Outside capsule
1–2 (n = 18)	8 (44.4%)	7 (38.8%)	1/8 (12.5%)	5/8 (62.5%)
2.1–3 (n = 24)	12 (50%)	11 (45.8%)	2/17 (11.7%)	7/17 (41.2%)
3.1–5 (n = 26)	14 (53.8%)	14 (53.9%)	2/15 (13.3%)	10/15 (66.6%)

characterization of the important intrahepatic structures, such as portal vein branches, bile ducts, and hepatic vein branches, may result in excessive or inadequate resection of the liver parenchyma. This can be avoided only by identifying the structures meticulously with the guidance of an experienced surgeon. Second, undetected malignant tumor may be left in the liver remnant because nodules smaller than 0.5 cm in diameter can be overlooked, even with careful scanning. Third, undiagnosed malignant lesions may be deemed benign and left in the liver remnant. Intraoperative ultrasonography still is unable to reveal definitely whether a lesion is malignant or benign. When HCC is well differentiated or present in an extremely cirrhotic liver with prominent regenerative nodules, the lesions may be obscured by the surrounding liver tissue and definite characterization of all the suspected nodules may be difficult. When any lesion is questionable, histologic confirmation by frozen section should be undertaken using ultrasound-guided fine-needle biopsy. It is the policy of these authors to abandon liver resection if histologically positive nodules are detected in more than two segments or in two nonadjacent segments.

Inflow Occlusion and Dissection of the Liver Parenchyma

An operative strategy for the tumor should be established as the intraoperative ultrasonography is completed. Anatomic resection is performed after isolation and division of the portal pedicles supplying the areas to be resected. Total or partial vascular inflow occlusion at the hilus is useful in reducing operative blood loss, especially during a nonanatomic resection.[23] Total inflow occlusion (the Pringle maneuver) can be accomplished by clamping the hepatoduodenal ligament with an intestinal clamp.[24] Partial inflow disruption is achieved by occluding only the vessels at the operative site (unilateral exclusion of the right or left side) using a tape to encircle the vessels and a rubber tube for the snare (Fig. 48-2). Normal liver can tolerate normothermic ischemia for up to 60 minutes.[25,26] Cirrhotic liver, because of its increased vulnerability to ischemia, should be occluded for only 15 minutes, followed by 5 minutes of reperfusion. This procedure can be repeated intermittently until hepatic resection is complete. Selective inflow occlusion can reduce the ischemic insult to the remnant liver by maintaining blood flow to the nonoperative site, and also is helpful in demarcating the resectional line based on a color change on the liver's surface (Fig. 48-3). When the tumor is located in the left lateral segment of the left lobe (segments II and III by Couinaud's nomenclature[27]) or in the posterior segment of the right lobe (segments VI and VII), selective inflow occlusion may be accomplished by clamping the left or right branch of the inflow pedicles. When resection involves tumor located in the anterior segment (segments V and VIII) of the right lobe or in the medial segment (segment IV) of the left lobe, or when central bisegmentectomy is planned, vascular occlusion of the right and left sides may be carried out alternatively.[28,29] On some occasions, total occlusion of hepatic inflow is necessary when the operative

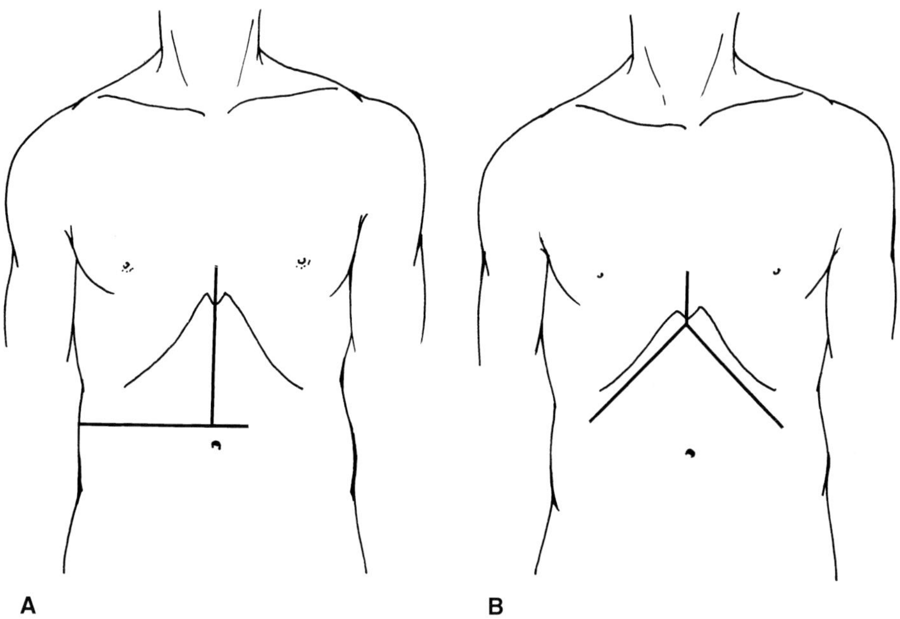

FIG. 48-1. Incisions for hepatic resection. (**a**) Inverted T-shaped incision. (**b**) Bilateral subcostal incision.

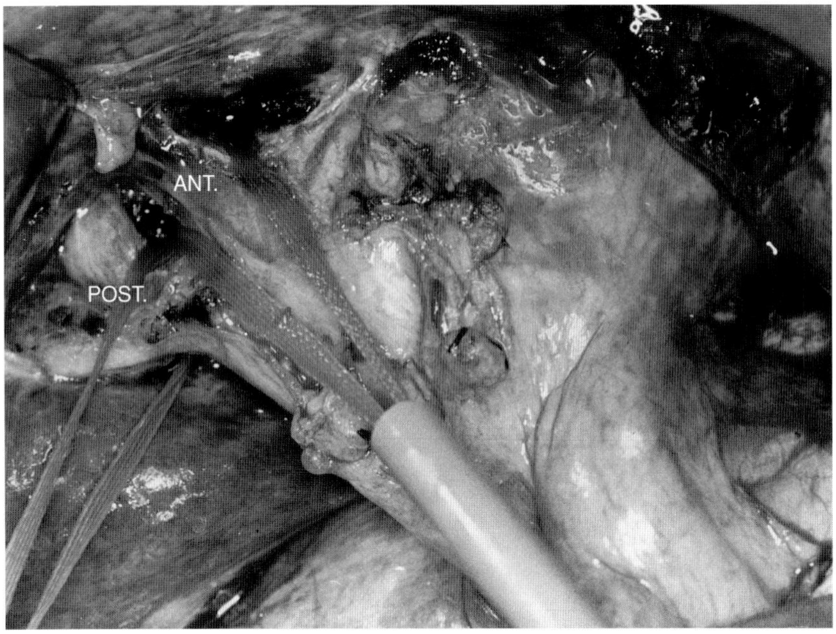

FIG. 48-2. Operative photograph at the liver hilus. The right anterior and posterior branches of the portal pedicles have been dissected out. Vessel loops encircle the branches preparing for partial inflow occlusion. *Ant*, anterior segment portal branch; *post*, posterior segment portal branch.

site receives significant blood supply from the opposite lobe, leading to unexpected blood loss. Another important bleeding source during parenchymal dissection is the hepatic vein and its branches. Inflow occlusion does not prevent bleeding from the hepatic veins resulting from retrograde flow from the vena cava, and some authors have advocated performing total vascular exclusion (clamping the vena cava below and above the liver) to reduce such blood loss.[30,31] Because the walls of the hepatic veins are much weaker than those of the hepatic arteries or portal veins, the hepatic veins should be handled carefully and their branches ligated diligently during parenchymal dissection. This decreases hepatic venous hemorrhage and obviates the need for total vascular exclusion by caval clamping. Transection of the liver parenchyma can be performed slowly and carefully by crushing the parenchyma with a small Kelly clamp (tissue-fracture technique). Use of the ultrasonic surgical aspirator for hepatic resection has proved to be efficient and safe in both hilar dissection and parenchymal transection. Small intraparenchymal vascular structures can be cauterized and divided. To minimize the chance of postoperative bleeding or bile leakage, vessels larger than 1 mm in diameter and all biliary structures should be ligated meticulously with 3/0 silk before resection. Vascular and biliary structures must be identified and ligated in a bloodless field to prevent iatrogenic injury to the vital structures, so a clean intraparenchymal operative area should be maintained diligently. Retraction of bleeding vessels

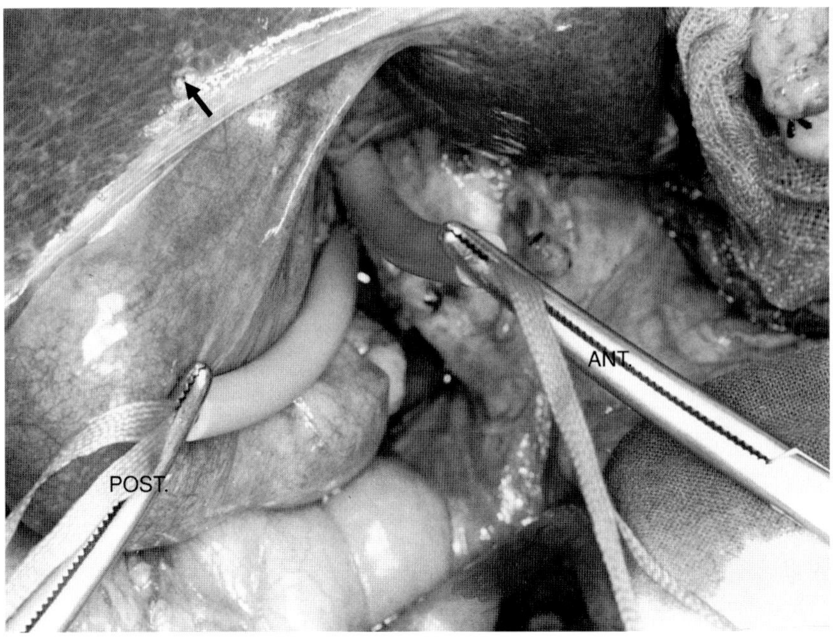

FIG. 48-3. Vessel loops occlude the portal inflow using the tourniquet during liver parenchymal dissection. Note the demarcation between segments S4 and S5 (*arrow*). *Ant*, anterior segment portal branch; *post*, posterior segment portal branch.

TABLE 48-4. *Complications in 110 cirrhotic patients undergoing hepatic resection for hepatocellular carcinoma**

Complication	Number of patients
Hepatic insufficiency	3
Subphrenic fluid collection	7
Gastric ulcer bleeding	1
Hemoperitoneum	1
Renal insufficiency	1
Bile leakage	6
Massive ascites	8
Massive pleural effusion	4
Drain-site infection	4
Ileus	1
Urinary tract infection	3
Wound infection	3
Acute psychosis	1

* Two patients eventually died.

into the liver substance should be avoided. If this occurs, the bleeding should be occluded immediately by oversewing with 3/0 nonabsorbable suture on atraumatic needles. Hemostasis of minor bleeding in the raw surface can be achieved by covering the area with Surgicel divided in tiny pieces and applying pressure for a few minutes. Biliary leakage can be detected by injecting saline through the cystic duct, and the leakage sites can be repaired carefully with absorbable suture. Before the abdomen is closed, drainage of the subphrenic region and the space left empty by removal of the liver parenchyma usually is required, using two or three silicone rubber closed-suction drains inserted through a separate stab incision.

POSTOPERATIVE CARE

Ascites accumulation after hepatic resection is common in cirrhotic patients. It should be controlled before and after surgery, because a high proportion of postoperative complications after resection of HCC result from ascites formation and leakage.[32] Restriction of fluid (40 mL/kg/d) and sodium (40 to 50 mEq/d) should be instituted immediately after operation. Salt-poor albumin (0.2 g/kg/d) and fresh-frozen plasma must be given to maintain effective plasma oncotic pressure, and diuretics (spironolactone alone or in combination with furosemide) usually are necessary to provide adequate natriuresis. Use of these regimens in the first several postoperative days usually reduces the development of ascites. Most patients can begin a low-sodium (1 to 2 g) liquid diet by the third postoperative day. Prophylactic antibiotics consisting of second-generation cephalosporins in combination with aminoglycosides are given for 3 days, or longer if there are signs of septic complications. The drainage tubes can be removed when the drainage fluid becomes serous and less than 100 mL/d. As soon as patients have recovered from anesthesia, respiratory care involving hourly coughing and deep breathing exercises using an incentive spirometer should be initiated to reduce the possibility of atelectasis and pulmonary infection.

PERIOPERATIVE MORBIDITY AND MORTALITY

In most reported series, the operative mortality rate after hepatic resection for malignancy is 2% to 5%.[33] This low rate is related to refined operative techniques and increased understanding of liver anatomy and physiology. However, liver resection in cirrhotic patients remains a potentially risky procedure, for several reasons. Patients with liver cirrhosis have an increased susceptibility to bacterial infection because of vascular shunting (intrahepatic and extrahepatic) and reticuloendothelial system dysfunction.[34–36] Hepatic resection may facilitate bacterial translocation from the gut into the portal circulation. Cirrhosis is characterized by secondary aldosteronism, which is heightened by the traumatic response to injury.[37] As a result, fluid may collect easily in the abdominal and pleural cavities after operation, resulting in infection and sepsis. There is an increased risk of perioperative hemorrhage as a result of portal hypertension, hypersplenism, and coagulopathy. The regenerative ability of the cirrhotic liver is impaired after resection. The reported operative mortality rate for liver resection in cirrhotic patients ranges from 6.9% to 18%, and the morbidity rate ranges from 20% to 50%.[38–40] In the authors' series of 110 consecutive resections, the overall operative mortality rate was 1.8% (Table 48-4).

SURVIVAL AFTER RESECTION OF HEPATOCELLULAR CARCINOMA IN THE CIRRHOTIC PATIENT

The long-term prognosis of cirrhotic patients with HCC is better after hepatic resection than after treatment by nonresectional methods.[41,42] However, as a whole, the results of treat-

TABLE 48-5. *Series reports of factors associated with intrahepatic tumor recurrence after surgical resection of hepatocellular carcinoma*

Authors	Number of patients	Significant risk factors for tumor recurrence
Bismuth et al. (1993)[42]	120	Tumor size >3 cm, more than 2 modules, diffuse form, presence of portal thrombus
Nagasue et al. (1993)[43]	201	Satellite nodules, venous invasion, presence of cirrhosis, absence of capsule formation, cut margin 0.5 cm
Arii (1992)[44]	112	Tumor size >2 cm, 3 tumor nodules, capsule infiltration, portal involvement, tumor stage II
Chiu (1992)[45,46]	238	Tumor size >5 cm, multiple/daughter nodule types, aneuploid tumors with more than one G0/G1 peak
Chiu (1993)[47]	55	Increased proliferative capacity (18%) of the nontumor part

ment are unsatisfactory. Five-year survival rates range from 22% to 44%.[43–45] In the authors' series of 186 cirrhotic patients with HCC who underwent hepatic resection, the 1-, 3-, and 5-year overall survival rates were 82.2%, 55.2%, and 39.2%, respectively, and the disease-free survival rates were 67.9%, 42.9%, and 36.3%, respectively. Intrahepatic cancer recurrence is the major cause of death after partial hepatectomy, followed by cirrhosis-associated hepatic failure and variceal bleeding.[46,47] By analyzing the disease-free survival rates in relation to clinical and histopathologic factors, several important prognostic indicators of tumor recurrence have been delineated in different centers (Table 48-5). Patients with these high-risk factors for tumor recurrence must be observed closely after hepatic resection. Survival after tumor recurrence can be improved by repeated resection of the tumor.[48,49] When repeated resection is not feasible, treatment by transcatheter arterial chemoembolization, targeted chemotherapy, or percutaneous alcohol injection also is effective in prolonging survival.[50–52] In addition, mutidisciplinary adjuvant therapy is necessary to improve long-term survival in this subgroup of high-risk patients.

SUMMARY

Successful hepatic resection for HCC in cirrhotic patients depends on well-directed preoperative evaluation, careful patient selection, meticulous operative technique, and intensive perioperative care. This procedure can be performed with acceptably low mortality and morbidity rates. Surgical treatment of HCC in cirrhotic patients may prolong survival and offer a chance of cure.

REFERENCES

1. Rustgi VK. Epidemiology of hepatocellular carcinoma. Ann Intern Med 1988;108:309.
2. The Liver Cancer Study Group of Japan. Primary liver cancer in Japan. Cancer 1984;54:1747.
3. Tang Z, Yu Y, Zhou X. Factors influencing primary liver cancer resection survival rate. Chin Med J (Engl) 1981;94:749.
4. Lee NW, Ong GB. The surgical management of primary carcinoma of the liver. World J Surg 1982;6:66.
5. Johnson PJ, Portman KB, Eddleston ALWF, Williams R. Hepatocellular carcinoma in Great Britain: influence of age, sex, HBsAg status, and etiology of underlying cirrhosis. Gut 1978;19:1022.
6. MacIntosh EL, Minuk GY. Hepatic resection in patients with cirrhosis and hepatocellular carcinoma. Surg Gynecol Obstet 1992;174:245.
7. Nagasue N, Yukay H, Ogawa Y, et al. Clinical experience with 118 hepatic resections for hepatocellular carcinoma. Surgery 1986;99:694.
8. Bismuth H, Houssin D, Ornowski J, Merrigi F. Liver resections in cirrhotic patients: a western experience. World J Surg 1986;10:311.
9. Kinami Y, Takashima S, Miyazaki I. Hepatic resection for hepatocellular carcinoma associated with liver cirrhosis. World J Surg 1986;10:294.
10. Toshiyuki H. A study on the relation between the intrahepatic extensive mode of hepatocellular carcinoma and the degree of the fibrosis of the adjacent noncancerous liver. The Japanese Journal of Gastroenterological Surgery 1992;25:36.
11. Yamaoka Y, Kumada K, Ino K, et al. Liver resection for hepatocellular carcinoma with direct removal of tumor thrombi in the main portal vein. World J Surg 1992;16:1172.
12. Pugh RN, Murray-Lyon IM, Dawson JL, Pietroni MC, Williams R. Transection of the esophagus for bleeding esophageal varices. Br J Surg 1973;60:646.
13. Mimura H, Takakura N, Ohno Y, et al. Determination of the extent of feasible hepatic resection from hepatic blood flow. World J Surg 1986;10:302.
14. Mimura H, Takakura N, Ohno Y, et al. Determination of the extent of fissible hepatic resection from hepatic blood flow. Worl J Surg 1986;10:320.
15. Mori K, Ozawa K, Yamamoto Y, et al. Response of hepatic mitochondrial redox tolerance test as a new prediction of surgical risk in hepatectomy. Ann Surg 1990;211:438.
16. Kanematsu T, Takenaka K, Furata T, Ezaki T, Sugimachi K, Inokuchi K. Acute portal hypertension associated with liver resection. Analysis of early postoperative death. Arch Surg 1985;120:1303.
17. Nagasue N, Yukaya H, Ogawa Y, Higashi T. Portal pressure following partial to extensive hepatic resection in patients with and without cirrhosis. Ann Chir Gynaecol 1983;72:18.
18. Chau GY, Yui TC, Loong CC, King KL, Chiu JH, Lui WY. Concomitant surgical treatment of hepatocellular carcinoma and esophageal varices. (Abstract) Hepatogastroenterology 1993;3(Suppl 1):83.
19. MacIntosh EL, Minuk GY. Hepatic resection in patients with cirrhosis and hepatocellular carcinoma. Surg Gynecol Obstet 1992;174:245.
20. Ohto M, Kondo F, Ebara M. Pathology diagnosis and treatment for small liver cancer. In: Tobe T, Kameda H, Okudaira M, et al, eds. Primary liver cancer in Japan. Tokyo: Springer-Verlag, 1992:365.
21. Makuuchi M, Hasegawa H, Yamasaki S. Ultrasonically guided subsegmentectomy. Surg Gynecol Obstet 1985;161:356.
22. Makuuchi M. Intraoperative ultrasonography for hepatic surgery. In: Makuuchi M, ed. Abdominal intraoperative ultrasonography. Tokyo-New York: Igaku-Shoin, 1987:1.
23. Bismuth H. Surgical anatomy and anatomical surgery of the liver. World J Surg 1982;6:3.
24. Pringle JH. Notes on the arrest of hepatic hemorrhage due to trauma. Ann Surg 1908;48:541.
25. Huguet C, Nordlinger B, Bloch P, et al. Tolerance of the human liver to prolonged normothermic ischemia. Arch Surg 1978;113:1448.
26. Delva E, Barberousse JP, Nordlinger B, et al. Hemodynamic and biochemical monitoring during major liver resection with use of hepatic vascular exclusion. Surgery 1984;95:309.
27. Couinaud C. Le foie. Etudes anatomiques et chirurgicales. Paris: Masson, 1957:1.
28. Hasegawa H, Makuuchi M, Yamazaki S, et al. Central bisegmentectomy of the liver: experience in 16 patients. World J Surg 1989;13:786.
29. Taniguchi H, Takahashi T, Shioaki Y, Itoh A, Oguro A. Vascular inflow exclusion and hepatic resection. Br J Surg 1992;79:672.
30. Bismuth H, Castaining D, Garden J. Major hepatic resection under total vascular exclusion. Ann Surg 1989;210:13.
31. Smadja C, Elias D. Resection of hepatocellular carcinoma in cirrhosis: operative technique. Eur Clin Digest Dis Suppl Series Vol 1. Hepatogastroenterology 1992;39:103.
32. Kanematsu T, Takenaka K, Matsumata T, Furuta T, Sugimachi K, Inokuchi K. Limited hepatic resection effective for selective cirrhotic patients with primary liver cancer. Ann Surg 1984;199:51.
33. James V, Sitzmann JV, Greene PS. Perioperative predictors of morbidity following hepatic resection for neoplasm. Ann Surg 1994;219:13.
34. Rimola A, Soto R, Bory F, et al. Reticuloendothelial system phagocytic activity in cirrhosis and its relation to bacterial infections and prognosis. Hepatology 1984;4:53.
35. Hiroshi Y. Bacterial infection in cirrhosis, with and without hepatocellular carcinoma. Am J Gastroenterol 1993;12:2067.
36. Warren WD, Millikan WJ. The liver and portal vein. In: Dudrick SJ, Baue AE, Eiseman B, MacLean LD, Rowe MI, Sheldon GF, eds. Manual of perioperative and postoperative care. Philadelphia: WB Saunders, 1983:422.
37. Hemming AW, Scudamore CH, Shackleton CR, Pudek M, Erb SR. Indocyanine green clearance as a predictor of successful hepatic resection in cirrhotic patients. Am J Surg 1992;163:515.
38. Franco D, Capussotti L, Smadja C, et al. Resection of hepatocellular carcinomas. Results in 72 European patients with cirrhosis. Gastroenterology 1990;98:733.
39. Shijo H, Okazaki M, Higashihara H, Koganemaru F, Okumura M. Hepatocellular carcinoma: a multivariate analysis of prognostic features in patients treated with hepatic arterial embolization. Am J Gastroenterol 1992;87:1154.
40. Okuda K, Ohtsuki T, Obata H, et al. Natural history of hepatocellular carcinoma and prognosis in relation to treatment. Cancer 1985;56:918.

41. Sasaki Y, Imaoka S, Masutani S, et al. Influence of coexisting cirrhosis on long-term prognosis after surgery in patients with hepatocellular carcinoma. Surgery 1992;112:515.
42. Bismuth H, Chiche L, Adam R, Castaing D, Diamond T, Dennison A. Liver resection versus transplantation for hepatocellular carcinoma in cirrhotic patients. Ann Surg 1993;218:145.
43. Nagasue N, Uchida M, Makino Y, et al. Incidence and factors associated with intrahepatic recurrence following resection of hepatocellular carcinoma. Gastroenterology 1993;105:488.
44. Arii S, Tanaka J, Yamazoe Y, et al. Predictive factors for intrahepatic recurrence of hepatocellular carcinoma after partial hepatectomy. Cancer 1992;69:913.
45. Chiu JH, Kao HL, Wu LH, Chang HM, Lui WY. Prediction of relapse or survival after resection in human hepatomas by DNA flow cytometry. J Clin Invest 1992;89:539.
46. Jwo SC, Chiu JH, Chau GY, Loong CC, Lui WY. Risk factors linked to tumor recurrence of human hepatocellular carcinoma after hepatic resection. Hepatology 1992;16:1367.
47. Chiu JH, Wu LH, Kao HL, et al. Can determination of the proliferative capacity of the nontumor portion predict the risk of tumor recurrence in the liver remnant after resection of human hepatocellular carcinoma? Hepatology 1993;18:96.
48. Kanematsu T, Matsumata T, Takenaka K, Yoshida Y, Higashi H, Sugimachi K. Clinical management of recurrent hepatocellular carcinoma after primary resection. Br J Surg 1988;75:203.
49. Matsuda Y, Ito T, Oguchi Y, Nakajima K, Izukura T. Rationale of surgical management for recurrent hepatocellular carcinoma. Ann Surg 1993;217:28.
50. Takayasu K, Muramatsu Y, Moriyama N, et al. Clinical and radiologic assessments of the results of hepatectomy for small hepatocellular carcinoma and therapeutic arterial embolization for postoperative recurrence. Cancer 1989;64:1848.
51. Kanematsu T, Furuta T, Takenaka K, et al. A 5-year experience of lipiodolization: selective regional chemotherapy for 200 patients with hepatocellular carcinoma. Hepatology 1989;10:98.
52. Shiina S, Yasude H, Muto H, et al. Percutaneous ethanol injection in the treatment of liver neoplasms. AJR Am J Roentgenol 1987;149:949.

Surgery for Gastrointestinal Cancer: A Multidisciplinary Approach, edited by Harold J. Wanebo.
Lippincott-Raven Publishers, Philadelphia, © 1997.

CHAPTER 49

Regional Chemotherapy for Hepatic Neoplasms

Alan P. Venook and Robert S. Warren

Hepatic neoplasms are unique targets for regional chemotherapeutic approaches. The dual blood supply of the liver (portal venous and hepatic arterial) allows for the delivery of drugs or interruption of blood flow to tumors without the induction of significant damage in the nontumorous liver. The clinical course in many patients with hepatic neoplasms, particularly colorectal liver metastases or hepatocellular carcinoma (HCC), also argues for a regional approach, because the progression of intrahepatic cancer nearly always determines patient survival. Although selected chemotherapeutic agents may achieve markedly increased local concentrations when administered intraarterially, the observed increased response rate has not translated clearly into a survival advantage. This is attributable at least in part to the toxicities and complications that confounded early investigation in this field. Clear delineation of the technical and pharmacologic principles of the approach, and concomitant changes in therapy, have led to apparent improvement in results. However, the regional strategy remains limited by the lack of available and active chemotherapeutic agents, and may lend itself even more to the delivery of nonclassic anticancer agents, such as genes or biologicals.

RATIONALE FOR REGIONAL CHEMOTHERAPY

The regional administration of chemotherapy to patients with liver tumors is designed to increase efficacy and decrease systemic toxicity. Malignant cells in the liver derive more than 80% of their blood supply from the hepatic arterial circulation, whereas normal hepatocytes are supplied primarily by the portal circulation.[1] The administration of chemotherapy into the hepatic artery allows for the selective delivery of drug to the tumor with relative sparing of normal hepatocytes.

Theoretically, hepatic intraarterial (HIA) chemotherapy should result in an increase in the regional peak concentration as long as the dose administered is equal to or greater than the standard systemic dose. The regional area under the curve (AUC), however, is a function of the total body clearance of the specific drug being administered and the hepatic arterial flow rate, as demonstrated in this equation:

$$\text{Regional AUC} \propto 1 + \frac{\text{total body clearance (mL/min)}}{\text{hepatic artery flow (mL/min)}} \times \frac{\text{regional dose}}{\text{systemic dose}}$$

Therefore, a drug such as floxuridine (FUDR), with a high total body clearance, theoretically offers the greatest advantage when administered regionally. Hepatic arterial flow rate (normally about 400 mL/min) is not easily altered, but is inversely related to regional AUC.

To the extent that the hepatic extraction of a drug enables the regional drug dose to exceed the standard systemic dose, the regional AUC also will be greater. However, for the drugs most commonly used in this way (FUDR, 5-fluorouracil [5-FU], and mitomycin C), the regional-to-systemic dose ratio is not significantly greater than 1. This applies even for FUDR because of the dosage limitations imposed by its hepatobiliary toxicity. Other factors, such as tumor vascularity and the dose-response relation of the chemotherapeutic agent and the tumor, are crucial determinants of outcome.

The other potential advantage of regional chemotherapy is the minimization of systemic toxicity. A decrease in the systemic AUC should lead to such a result, but whether this occurs is related to the specifics of the hepatic extraction of the drugs used.[2] This is illustrated in the following equation:

$$\text{Fraction systemic AUC} = 100\% - \%\ \text{hepatic extraction}$$

So, for example, only 5% of a dose of FUDR, with a first-pass hepatic extraction of 95%, will reach the systemic circulation. 5-FU exhibits dose-dependent pharmacokinetics, such that rapid-bolus HIA injection leads to a bypassing of the liver and significant systemic levels compared with long-term HIA infusion, in which 80% of the drug is extracted by the liver. However, the

A. P. Venook, Department of Medicine, Division of Hematology/Oncology, University of California, San Francisco, CA 94143.
R. S. Warren, Department of Surgery, University of California, San Francisco, CA 94143.

TABLE 49-1. *Regional advantage for selected chemotherapies*

Drug AUC†	Clearance*	Hepatic extraction	Increase
FUDR	25,000	95%	65
5-FU‡	4,000	80%	10
Mitomycin C	500	10%	2

* Total body clearance of drug milliliters per minute.
† Estimated increase in AUC for intrahepatic administration assuming hepatic artery flow rate of 400 mL/min.
‡ By infusion; bolus pharmacokinetcs are different.
AUC, area under curve; *FUDR,* floxuridine; *5-FU,* 5-fluorouracil.

minimization of toxicity also reflects the decreased systemic dosing achieved and predicts for little antitumor activity in nonhepatic sites. Table 49-1 lists a variety of chemotherapeutic agents and their corresponding parameters when administered by hepatic arterial infusion.

CANDIDATE DISEASES FOR REGIONAL CHEMOTHERAPY

Although HCC is one of the most common cancers worldwide,[3] metastatic tumors account for most malignancies of the liver in the United States. Virtually every cancer can spread to the liver, but gastrointestinal primary cancers, whose drainage typically is through the portal circulation, and breast cancer are the most common sources of metastatic tumors of the liver.

Few of these patients are reasonable candidates for regional therapy, because even patients with tumors confined to the liver are likely to have micrometastases elsewhere. For example, only 2 of 22 patients with breast cancer apparently confined to the liver had long-term disease-free survival after resection of isolated liver metastases.[4] The data are no better for patients who undergo resection of liver metastases from a variety of other primary sites.[5] Although the failure to affect survival by resection does not exclude the potential value of regional therapy in some of these cases, it emphasizes the systemic nature of most of these metastatic tumors.

The biology of colorectal cancer metastatic to the liver sometimes is compatible with a regional chemotherapeutic approach. About one third of patients with fewer than four liver metastases are cured by surgical extirpation of the tumors,[6] and nearly 90% of patients with liver metastases from colorectal cancer succumb to hepatic failure.[7] Among patients treated with an HIA chemotherapy regimen, the initial site of failure is within the liver about two thirds of the time and treatment is terminated for intrahepatic progression in about the same fraction.[8] Because extrahepatic metastases develop in most of these patients, effective systemic therapy would be preferable, but a metanalysis of more than 1300 patients, about one third of whom had liver-only metastases, demonstrated a median survival of about 11 months whether 5-FU was used as a single agent or in combination with leucovorin in the standard systemic chemotherapeutic approach.[9]

HCC also is a logical candidate for regional approaches, and many different strategies, both surgical and chemotherapeutic, have been used.[10] As with colorectal cancer, hematogenous or local metastases develop in more than 60% of patients with HCC,[11] but most die of progressive intrahepatic tumor or liver disease. Unfortunately, these patients often have compromised organ function and may not tolerate regional therapeutic approaches. Primary biliary cancers, although localized, usually defy treatment by regional therapies.

Neuroendocrine tumors, both islet cell tumors of the pancreas and carcinoid tumors of the bowel metastatic to the liver, are additional candidates for regional therapy. These relatively indolent cancers, which cause symptoms through the release of hormones into the hepatic vein and from which most patients die of progressive liver metastases, may be palliated by liver-directed therapies. The same holds true for extremely rare tumors such as hemangioendothelioma metastatic to the liver.[12] Patients with uveal melanoma may be targeted for liver-directed therapy[13] because of the preponderance of liver metastases during their course and because of the relative inactivity of systemic chemotherapy in that disease.[14]

Although anecdotal reports may suggest some tumor responses in patients with other metastatic lesions within the liver (ie, sarcoma),[15] these patients almost always have systemic and hepatic metastases and it is unusual for liver-directed treatment to offer significant palliation.

EXPERIENCE WITH HEPATIC INTRAARTERIAL CHEMOTHERAPY

Based on the pharmacologic principles outlined earlier, there was much enthusiasm for HIA chemotherapy during the 1980s. Numerous pilot studies, most of which used FUDR as the basis for the treatment of patients with colorectal liver metastases, were conducted using percutaneously placed catheters.[16] The results, often based on liberal response criteria not acceptable in the current era, revealed response rates ranging from 34%[17] to 88%.[18] At the same time, this treatment became manifestly easier with the introduction of the completely implantable infusion device. Because of this technologic advance, treatment could be administered over long periods in the ambulatory setting. Such encouraging developments led to a rush to complete randomized trials testing the newer therapies against the conventional 5-FU–based systemic treatments. Unfortunately, in the haste to design and carry out these randomized trials, scant attention was paid to refinement of the surgical technique necessary for truly selective and safe HIA chemotherapy delivery, or to the appropriate dosage and duration of FUDR.

Surgical Considerations

Once it has been decided that an individual patient is a candidate for regional chemotherapy through a hepatic artery infusion pump, three steps in the surgical strategy must be undertaken. These are designed to accomplish bilobar hepatic perfusion and to prevent administration of chemotherapy to the stomach or duodenum (misperfusion). Despite the apparent simplicity of this procedure, the rate of complications has been unusually high in the past, and has correlated directly with the experience of the operating surgeon.[19]

The first step consists of preoperative angiographic evalua-

TABLE 49-2. *Factors influencing the successful and safe use of intra-arterial therapy*

Factor	Rationale
Radiographic documentation of absence of extrahepatic tumor	Avoidance of unnecessary surgery
Angiographic before operation definition of arterial anatomy and confirmation of portal vein patency	Identification of arterial anomalies Portal vein occlusion is an absolute contraindication to manipulation of the hepatic artery
Ligation of arterial feeders to stomach and duodenum (monitored with intraoperative fluorescein injection and Wood's lamp)	Prevention of gastrointestinal ulceration and hemorrhage
Cholecystectomy	Avoidance of drug-induced acalculous cholecystitis
Postoperative radionuclide angiography by pump catheter to exclude misdirection of flow	Prevention of gastrointestinal ulceration and hemorrhage
Careful monitoring of liver function tests with appropriate withholding, or even termination, of floxuridine	Prevention of biliary sclerosis

tion of the arterial supply of the liver. A celiac injection is performed initially, followed by selective angiography of the hepatic, left gastric, and superior mesenteric arteries. Variations from the conventional hepatic arterial anatomy occur in up to 50% of patients.[20] A thorough angiographic evaluation is necessary to identify replaced or accessory hepatic arteries before surgery. Armed with this anatomic information, the next step, exploratory laparotomy, can be undertaken.

The abdomen may be entered through a midline or right subcostal incision. Abdominal exploration is undertaken to exclude unresectable extrahepatic tumor. Particular attention is paid to the lymph nodes in the porta hepatis, along the common hepatic artery, and at the celiac axis. If no contraindication to pump placement is found, a cholecystectomy is performed. The common hepatic artery is identified as it approaches the hepatoduodenal ligament. Dissection of this vessel begins here and progresses to the gastroduodenal artery, which is dissected free for a distance of 2 to 3 cm and is ligated distally. Dissection along the proper hepatic artery also is carried out for a few millimeters. The right gastric artery is identified, ligated, and divided to prevent misperfusion to the stomach. Next, a careful dissection and ligation of the small vessels along the superior border of the distal stomach and proximal duodenum is carried out. This devascularization is important to minimize further the risk of misperfusion.[21]

Attention then is directed at identifying any variations in the hepatic lobar arterial supply. A replaced or accessory left hepatic artery usually can be found within the gastrohepatic ligament along the inferior edge of the liver. A replaced or accessory right hepatic artery most commonly is identified by palpation as it exits from behind the duodenum and courses posteriorly within the hepatoduodenal ligament. Accessory right or left hepatic arteries may be ligated and divided without untoward effects. Usually, the gastroduodenal artery is the vessel of choice for cannulation. In the past, it has been customary to perform a dual cannulation in the face of a replaced right or left hepatic artery. It is now clear that this is an unnecessary procedure in most individuals.[22] The replaced hepatic artery is clamped temporarily and if no obvious ischemia to the liver ensues, the vessel may be ligated. As long as at least one hepatic artery to either lobe of the liver originates at the take-off of the gastroduodenal artery, hepatic perfusion of the contralateral lobe develops, often within seconds of ligation of the variant lobar artery. On the rare occasion in which clamping of a replaced hepatic artery produces prolonged ischemia to one lobe, that vessel must be side-cannulated using a tapered catheter and a dual catheter pump or a second device.

When the gastroduodenal artery arises distal to the left hepatic artery, the left hepatic artery is ligated and cross-hepatic perfusion from the right lobe to the left is relied on for complete hepatic chemotherapy delivery. Methods to achieve complete hepatic perfusion through cannulation of the gastroduodenal artery in the face of several variations in the hepatic arterial anatomy are given in Figure 49-1. Occasionally, stenosis of the celiac axis leads to a reversal of flow through the gastroduodenal artery such that this vessel becomes the predominant arterial supply to the liver. In this case, the common hepatic artery may be ligated 2 or 3 cm from the take-off of the gastroduodenal artery. The hepatic artery then is cannulated such that the tip of the catheter lies just proximal to the take-off of the gastroduodenal artery without disrupting arterial flow to the liver.

Pump placement then is undertaken. A transverse incision is made on each side of the lower anterior abdominal wall and a pocket is created inferiorly, overlying the anterior rectus sheath, to accommodate the pump. Care is taken to avoid positioning the pump too close to the symphysis pubis or the anterosuperior iliac spine. Once the pump has been loaded with heparinized water and secured into its pocket, the catheter is passed through the abdominal wall, trimmed to an appropriate length, and inserted through an arteriotomy into the gastroduodenal artery. The catheter is advanced so that its tip is just at the take-off of the gastroduodenal artery, and is secured with silk ties on each side of the intraluminal lead. As a final step in the procedure, 5 mL of fluorescein is injected into the side port of the pump and the liver, stomach, and duodenum are examined with a Wood's lamp. This is done to ensure bilobar liver perfusion and to exclude misperfusion to the stomach or duodenum.

Complications of hepatic arterial infusion pump placement may occur early or late.[23,24] Early complications consist of arterial injury, including creation of an intimal flap leading to hepatic artery thrombosis, incomplete perfusion of the entire liver as a result of lack of recognition of an accessory hepatic artery, misperfusion to the stomach or duodenum, and pump pocket hematoma. These complications occur in fewer than 5% of patients. Operative mortality should approach that of open cholecystectomy. Late complications tend to be more common and consist of inflammation or ulceration of the stomach or duodenum, pump pocket infection, and thrombosis of the catheter.

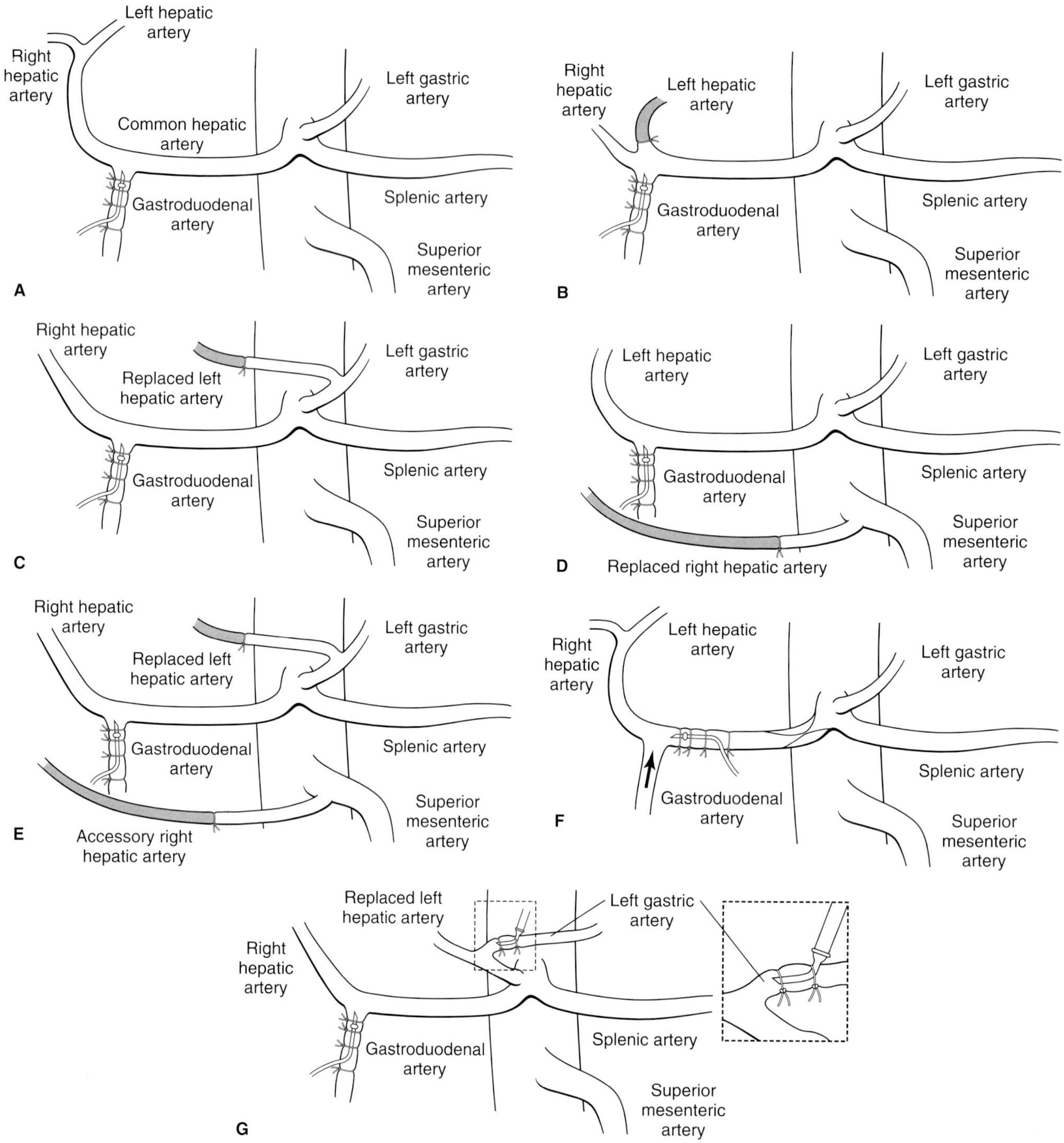

FIG. 49-1. **(A)** Standard hepatic arterial anatomy with distal ligation of gastroduodenal artery and cannulation of gastroduodenal artery. **(B)** Trifurcation variant of standard hepatic arterial anatomy with ligation of left hepatic artery and perfusion of entire liver through right hepatic artery through intrahepatic collaterals. **(C)** Replaced left hepatic artery arising from left gastric artery. Variant left hepatic artery is ligated with hepatic arterial perfusion through right hepatic artery. **(D)** Replaced right hepatic artery originating from superior mesenteric artery. Variant right hepatic artery is ligated with hepatic arterial perfusion through left hepatic artery. **(E)** Replaced left hepatic artery arising from left gastric artery and accessory right hepatic artery arising from superior mesenteric artery. Both variant vessels are ligated with perfusion of entire liver through normal right hepatic artery. **(F)** Proximal celiac or common hepatic artery stenosis, with reversal of flow through gastroduodenal artery. Proximal ligation of common hepatic artery is performed, with cannulation distal to ligature. Catheter tip is placed at junction of common hepatic and gastroduodenal arteries, with standard placement of bidirectional ligatures around catheter bead. **(G)** Dual cannulation of hepatic arteries with standard gastroduodenal artery cannulation combined with use of taper-tip catheter placed into replaced left gastric artery. Tip of taper catheter lies at junction of replaced left hepatic artery and common celiac trunk. Bead on taper-tip catheter is external to vessel and requires bidirectional fixation with suture ligatures to surrounding structures.

TABLE 49-3. *Randomized studies of intrahepatic versus systemic chemotherapy of colorectal liver metastases*

		Hepatic intraarterial		Intravenous		Response (%)	
Group/year	Number of randomized	Drug	Dose*	Drug	Dose	Hepatic intraarterial	Intravenous
MSKCC/1987	99	FUDR	0.3 mg/kg/d × 14 d	FUDR	0.15 mg/kg/d × 14 d	50	20
NCOG/1989	143	FUDR	0.3 mg/kg/d × 14 d	FUDR	0.075 mg/kg/d × 14 d†	42	10
NCI/1987	64	FUDR	0.3 mg/kg/d × 14 d	FUDR	0.125 mg/kg/d × 14 d	62	17
Mayo/1990	69	FUDR	0.3 mg/kg/d × 14 d	5-FU	500 mg/m^2 days 1–5	48	21
Rougier/1992	166	FUDR	0.3 mg/kg/d × 14 d	Physician choice		43	9
Mersh/1994	100	FUDR	0.2 mg/kg/d × 14 d	Physician choice		—	—

* Dosing convention is to report the actual dose delivered by the pump. MSKCC reports the total dose placed into the pump; because, on average, the pump delivers 60% to 65% of its volume in 14 days, the actual dose delivered is less than reported.

† Dose escalation if no toxicity.

MSKCC, Memorial Sloan-Kettering Cancer Center; *NCOG,* Northern California Oncology Group; *NCI,* National Cancer Institute; *FUDR,* Floxuridine; *5-FU,* 5-fluorouracil.

When antral or duodenal ulceration occurs during liver-directed chemotherapy, the possibility that chemotherapy misperfusion may be responsible can be evaluated by endoscopic examination of the stomach and duodenum with concomitant injection of methylene blue through the pump side port.[25] Immediate deep blue staining of the inflamed site warrants an angiographic search for a vessel responsible for the misperfusion. Once identified, the offending vessel often can be occluded using interventional radiologic techniques.

The general strategy used to maximize the safety and efficacy of this therapy is outlined in Table 49-2. Key technical points to consider in reducing the incidence of complications associated with this procedure include interruption of those vessels that might deliver chemotherapy retrograde from the liver to the stomach and duodenum, secure placement of the pump catheter to avoid advancement into the hepatic artery with subsequent thrombosis, and careful preoperative and intraoperative assessment of variant hepatic arterial anatomy.

Results of Clinical Trials

Six major prospective trials comparing systemic fluoropyrimidine chemotherapy (or no treatment) with HIA FUDR chemotherapy delivered by the implanted pump have been completed (Table 49-3). In all, nearly 600 patients were enrolled in these randomized studies, each of which clearly demonstrated superior response activity in the HIA arm compared with the systemic treatment group. Despite the apparent superiority of response, only two trials, those of Rougier and colleagues in France[26] and Allen-Mersh and associates in England,[27] demonstrated a survival benefit to the HIA group (Table 49-4). The control arm in both these studies, however, offered a no-treatment option, and only half the non–HIA-treated patients received any chemotherapy at all.

There are numerous possible explanations for the failure of trials with this active HIA therapy to demonstrate a survival benefit in these patients (Table 49-5). Although the response rates in these studies exceeded 50% in the HIA groups, few were complete responses. Furthermore, although the patients had, by definition, liver-only metastases from colorectal cancer at the initiation of therapy, extrahepatic metastases developed in many cases over time. Although few such patients died of extrahepatic tumor, the HIA therapy typically was discontinued as soon as other metastatic sites became apparent. To maintain equality in arms randomizing patients to laparotomy or no laparotomy, patients in these studies received HIA chemotherapy

TABLE 49-4. *Randomized studies of intrahepatic versus systemic chemotherapy for colorectal liver metastases*

	Median survival		
Group/year	Control	Hepatic intraarterial	Comment
MCKCC/1987	12	17	Crossover allowed
NCOG/1989	16	16.6	Crossover allowed
NCI/1987	11	16	Extrahepatic disease included
Mayo/1990	10.5	12.6	Time to liver progression: 6 versus 15.7 mo
Rougier/1992	11	15	50% of controls received chemotherapy
Mersh/1994	6.6	13.5	50% of controls received chemotherapy; quality of life analysis included

MSKCC, Memorial Sloan-Kettering Cancer Center; *NCOG,* Northern California Oncology Group; *NCI,* National Cancer Institute.

TABLE 49-5. *Flaws in randomized studies of hepatic intraarterial versus control therapy*

Crossover design may confound survival analysis.
Biliary toxicity excessive because of high-dose floxuridine.
Surgical complications restrict hepatic intraarterial chemotherapy.
Control arm 5-fluorouracil not modulated.

even if radiographically inapparent extrahepatic tumor was found in the abdomen; excluding such patients in the analysis would have given superior survival to HIA-treated patients in one of these studies.[28] Finally, the two largest studies, those of Kemeny and colleagues[29] and Hohn and associates,[30] each included the option of patient crossover to HIA therapy after failure of the systemic treatment. Given data documenting clinical responses to HIA therapy in patients who already have been treated with 5-FU–based chemotherapy,[8,31] a confounding of survival analysis is probable.

Another part of the explanation undoubtedly rests in the compromised HIA therapy that was delivered because of toxicity and complications. Without question, the delivered dosage of FUDR (0.3 mg/kg/d for 14 days) was too high, leading to hepatobiliary toxicity in nearly every patient and biliary sclerosis that required cessation of therapy in many.[32] Complications, including gastrointestinal misperfusion[21] and hepatic artery thrombosis, also crippled these randomized studies; for example, nearly one third of the 36 patients randomized to HIA therapy in the Mayo Clinic series never received any meaningful treatment.[33] Finally, the relative inability of fluoropyrimidines to generate durable responses in this chemotherapy-resistant disease may not be overcome even with the achievement of high local concentrations of drug.

Whatever the reason, the failure of these studies to demonstrate a survival advantage in the face of often-prohibitive hepatobiliary toxicity led to disenchantment with the therapy. However, a few centers continue to pursue the modality, and a series of phase II or randomized phase II studies suggests that modification of the original FUDR dosage and schedule may improve survival while diminishing toxicity (Table 49-6).

One strategy uses one sixth the original FUDR dosage (0.1 mg/kg/d for 7 days) alternating with HIA bolus 5-FU administered through the pump side port on days 15, 22, and 29 of each 5-week cycle.[8] None of 64 patients, 30 of whom previously had undergone unsuccessful systemic chemotherapy, had treatment limited by hepatobiliary toxicity, and the median survival of the untreated patients exceeded 2 years. The relative lack of anticancer activity was the dominant problem, in that progressive liver tumor was the initial site of failure (and cause of death) in most patients.

Modulation of FUDR with dexamethasone in an attempt to ameliorate an inflammatory aspect of the hepatobiliary toxicity[34] or to amplify biochemically the cytotoxicity with leucovorin[35] also has resulted in median survival of 2 years or more in patients with liver-only colorectal metastases, although still with a rare complication of biliary sclerosis. The advertised dosage of FUDR in both these studies was the conventional 0.3 mg/kg/d for 14 days, but it is critical to observe that these investigators erroneously report the total dose of drug in the entire pump; because the average pump delivers 2 cc/d of its 50-cc reservoir, about 56% of the 0.3 mg/kg/d (or 0.168 mg/kg/d) actually is delivered during the 14 days of treatment in these studies. Chronomodulation, or the infusion of FUDR with circadian time modification, also appears to ameliorate the hepatobiliary toxicity of HIA chemotherapy,[36] but it is not clear that significant clinical benefits are the result.

A definitive assessment of the role of HIA therapy awaits a non-crossover, randomized study between an HIA treatment and a systemic treatment in untreated patients with liver-only colorectal metastases. Such a protocol would need to include standard end points (ie, disease-free and overall survival) and cost and quality of life analyses. Such a phase III trial is being conducted by the Cancer and Leukemia Group B.

There is another large cohort of patients with liver-only colorectal metastases who already have received systemic 5-FU–based chemotherapy. Patients with metachronous liver metastases usually have advanced local colorectal cancers and have received a "standard" adjuvant chemotherapy, 5-FU with levamisole[37] or leucovorin.[38] Other patients have received front-line systemic chemotherapy with similar agents. In such patients, in whom further conventional chemotherapy offers little likelihood of significant clinical benefit,[39] HIA FUDR-based chemo-

TABLE 49-6. *Phase II results with alternative intrahepatic regimens*

Group/year	Number of patients	Hepatic intraarterial regimen	Response rate (%)	Toxicity*	Median survival (mo)
UCSF/1991	64†	FUDR 0.1 mg/kg/d × 7 d 5-FU 15 mg/kg on days 15, 22, 29	50	+	22.4
MSKCC/1992	25	FUDR 0.3 mg/kg/d × 14 d‡ Dexamethasone 20 mg	71	+ +	23
MSKCC/1994	42	FUDR 0.25–0.3 mg/kg/d × 14 d‡ Leucovorin 15–30 mg/m^2/d × 14 d	56	+ + +	24.2
MSKCC/1994		FUDR 0.3 mg/kg/d × 14 d‡ Leucovorin 15 mg/m^2/d × 14 d Dexamethasone 20 mg	78	+ +	24.8

* Toxicity: + = minimal; + + + + = severe.
† Includes 30 patients who previously had been treated with systemic chemotherapy.
‡ Dosing convention.
UCSF, University of California, San Francisco; *MSKCC,* Memorial Sloan-Kettering Cancer Center; *FUDR,* floxuridine; *5-FU,* fluorouracil.

therapy can be expected to produce responses in more than 30% of cases and a survival approaching 18 months.[31,40]

HIA infusional chemotherapy for HCC with agents such as FUDR, mitomycin C, and α-interferon[41,42] appears to be partially successful, with response rates as high as 50%. However, these responses usually are not durable and the patients treated in such trials tend to have a better performance status than the average patient with HCC. Further, long-term percutaneous catheterization of the hepatic artery or laparotomy for the placement of an infusion device may be ill-advised in patients with HCC, who may tolerate such invasive procedures poorly.[43] Given such realities and the lack of data generated on intraarterial therapy for HCC in randomized trials, any benefit is hard to measure, and it cannot be recommended as a standard practice. The same conclusion must be drawn for tumors other than colorectal cancer that have metastasized to the liver, because these are not likely to remain confined to the liver and, therefore, the morbidity of therapy is likely to outweigh the benefit.

HIA chemotherapy also can be viewed as a mode of augmenting the activity of radiation. Fluoropyrimidines have been used for their ''radiosensitizing'' properties in the conformal radiation therapy of patients with hepatobiliary tumors, with encouraging preliminary results.[44]

OTHER REGIONAL MODALITIES

Embolization and Chemoembolization

Given the preponderance of hepatic tumor blood flow from the hepatic artery compared with the portal vein,[1] occlusion of the hepatic artery can accomplish relatively selective tumor ischemia. Hepatic artery ligation can be done surgically, but requires a laparotomy and is only transiently effective[45] because of the rapid development of collateral vessels.[46] The interventional radiologist may interrupt arterial flow by the introduction of vaso-occlusive material into the vessel. Such a decrease in arterial flow increases the AUC achieved in the liver tumor bed compared with the systemic circulation when chemotherapy is infused into the hepatic artery.[47,48] The combination of these two strategies, called chemoembolization, theoretically could offer synergistic antitumor activity.

There is significant experience with chemoembolization for primary and metastatic liver tumors. Vaso-occlusive materials, including gelatin sponge, starch,[47] polyvinyl alcohol,[15,49] cross-linked bovine collagen,[50] and even autologous blood clot,[51] have been tried. The different sizes and degradability of these particles predict for different levels and duration of arterial blockage; the optimal material has not been determined.

HCC has been the tumor most often treated with chemoembolization. There are many series, each with different patient demographics, underlying types and stages of liver disease, chemotherapeutic dosages and combinations used, inclusion criteria (although most investigators exclude patients with thrombosed portal veins), vascular techniques, and sequencing and intervals of therapy.[52–58] Recognizing that these limitations make an overview statement about the activity of this modality simplistic, the efficacy in terms of conventional partial responses for chemoembolization of HCC is about 50%. Tumor liquefaction is seen on computed tomography in about two thirds of patients after this treatment and may be a persistent finding over many months. Histologically, this has been shown to correspond to tumor necrosis, although the significance of this finding in regard to overall outcome is uncertain.[59] Chemoembolization also has been used in the preoperative setting in an attempt to ''down-stage'' HCC. No prospective studies have been undertaken to assess this strategy, and the results of retrospective series fail to demonstrate any advantage.[60,61]

Although patients with small HCCs may achieve long-term survival after chemoembolization, and the results may be as good as those of resection,[62] the lack of randomized studies with this modality makes any conclusions about a survival advantage for some patients premature. Palliation of symptoms by chemoembolization cannot truly be assessed because no adequate measurements of quality of life have been reported in the myriad of studies. However, although the response rates are not superior to those of the intraarterial infusional strategies, they can be achieved, in some cases,[52] with a single treatment requiring only a few days in the hospital. Nonetheless, no definitive study has demonstrated the superiority of chemoembolization over infusional intraarterial therapy, other palliative therapies, or best supportive care for HCC.

Lipiodol

Lipiodol, lymphangiogram dye, is an ethyl ester of the fatty acid of poppy seed oil containing 38% iodine by weight. This agent concentrates in neoplastic tissue within the liver after administration into the hepatic artery.[63] The precise mechanism for this long-term deposition is unclear, although it is thought to relate to the abnormal vascularity and the lack of lymphatics in tumors. This attribute has led to the use of Lipiodol-enhanced computed tomography aorto-portography in the preoperative staging of patients with limited-stage HCC because of its sensitivity in identifying small satellite lesions that may be missed by other imaging modalities.[64]

The therapeutic use of Lipiodol has been explored in combination with lipophilic chemotherapeutic agents, with or without occlusive material,[65–67] administered into the hepatic artery. Studies demonstrate a 30% to 40% objective response rate and deposition of contrast medium within stable tumors for, in some cases, years. Analysis of this modality compared with others is necessary to verify a clinically relevant antitumor effect and to assess toxicity, because it is possible that Lipiodol might hasten the deterioration of liver dysfunction in patients with underlying cirrhosis.

Styrene-Maleic Acid-Neocarzinostatin

The conjugation of neocarzinostatin, a proteinaceous antibiotic, to copolystyrene-maleic acid enhances its in vitro cytotoxicity and offers numerous other pharmacologic improvements, including increased half-life, increased hydrophobia, and enhanced tropism to solid tumors.[68] Styrene-maleic acid-neocarzinostatin (SMANCS) has been used intraarterially with Lipiodol[69] or embolization material[70] in patients with a variety of hepatic neoplasms. Few data directly address the efficacy of SMANCS treatment alone in such patients and, as with the other modified intraarterial therapies, SMANCS has not been prospectively compared with untreated control patients or patients treated with other modalities.

Isolated Hepatic Perfusion

Taking advantage of classic pharmacologic principles, hepatic blood flow may be isolated and dosage-intensive chemotherapy delivered to the liver. This can be done with percutaneous catheters for blood diversion through an extracorporeal charcoal filtration chamber, with a reduction of chemotherapy "leak" into the systemic circulation.[71] Phase I studies with 5-FU and doxorubicin have identified the dosages to be used in phase II trials (T. Ravikumar, personal communication, 1993). It remains to be seen whether dosage-intensification of these drugs is adequate to overcome tumor resistance and improve the response rate for hepatic tumors enough to make such a technically difficult and invasive procedure worthwhile.

NEW STRATEGIES

For the future, it can only be hoped that a better understanding of the mechanisms of drug resistance or the development of new drugs will enable the formulation of better treatment strategies. More simplified drug delivery systems, such as liposomes,[72] might allow for significant pharmacologic manipulation without the need for major interventional procedures. New agents, including biologicals, may have improved therapeutic indices when administered regionally. Finally, the hepatic artery will be used as a vehicle for introducing wild-type genes, such as p53, which are mutant or absent in many patients with HCC and most patients with colorectal cancer.[73] Successful infection of such genetic material into tumors, perhaps through the regional infusion of liposomes[74] or virus particles, may be tumoricidal[75] or render the cancer cells chemosensitive.

CONCLUSIONS

The regional administration of chemotherapy for hepatic neoplasms is based on sound pharmacologic principles and appears to increase the activity of the anticancer agents. The toxicity and complications of the intraarterial approach have limited its utility, although newer treatment regimens and greater experience with the modality may make it more applicable. HIA infusional chemotherapy and variations such as chemoembolization, however, remain palliative therapies that should be used judiciously. Such a regional strategy may prove to be most useful with biologicals or gene-based therapies.

REFERENCES

1. Breedis C, Young G. The blood supply of neoplasms in the liver. Am J Pathol 1954;30:969.
2. Collins JM. Pharmacologic rationale for regional drug delivery. J Clin Oncol 1984;2:498.
3. Lotze M, Flickinger J, Carr B. Hepatobiliary neoplasms. In: Devita VT, Rosenberg SA, eds. Cancer: principles and practice of oncology. Philadelphia: JB Lippincott, 1993:883.
4. Elias D, Lasser P, Spielmann M, et al. Surgical and chemotherapeutic treatment of hepatic metastases from carcinoma of the breast. Surg Gynecol Obstet 1991;172:461.
5. Wolf RE, Goodnight JE, Krag DE, Schneider PD. Results of resection and proposed guidelines for patient selection in instances of noncolorectal hepatic metastases. Surg Gynecol Obstet 1991;173:454.
6. Steele GJ, Bleday R, Mayer RJ, Lindblad A, Petrelli N, Weaver D. A prospective evaluation of hepatic resection for colorectal carcinoma metastases to the liver: Gastrointestinal Tumor Study Group Protocol 6584. J Clin Oncol 1991;9:1105.
7. Goslin R, Steele Jr G, Zamcheck N, Mayer R, MacIntyre J. Factors influencing survival in patients with hepatic metastases from adenocarcinoma of the colon or rectum. Dis Colon Rectum 1982;25:749.
8. Stagg RJ, Venook AP, Chase JL, et al. Alternating hepatic intra-arterial floxuridine and fluorouracil: a less toxic regimen for treatment of liver metastases from colorectal cancer. J Natl Cancer Inst 1991;83:423.
9. Project Advanced Colorectal Cancer Metanalysis. Modulation of fluorouracil by leucovorin in patients with advanced colorectal cancer: evidence in terms of response rate. J Clin Oncol 1992;10:896.
10. Venook AP. Treatment of hepatocellular carcinoma: too many options? J Clin Oncol 1994;12:1323.
11. Yuki K, Hirohashi S, Sakamoto M, Kanai T, Shimosato Y. Growth and spread of hepatocellular carcinoma. Cancer 1990;66:2174.
12. Ishak KG, Sesterhenn IA, Goodman ZD, Rabin L, Stromeyer FW. Epithelioid hemangioendothelioma of the liver: a clinicopathologic and follow-up study of 32 cases. Hum Pathol 1984;15:839.
13. Carrasco CH, Wallace S, Charnsangavej C, Papadopoulos NEJ, Patt Y, Mavligit GM. Treatment of hepatic metastases in ocular melanoma. JAMA 1986;255:3152.
14. Nathan F, Sato T, Hart E, Berd D, Mastrangelo M. Response to combination chemotherapy of liver metastases from choroidal melanoma compared with cutaneous melanoma. Proceedings of the American Society of Clinical Oncology 1994;13:394.
15. Mavligit GM, Zukiwski AA, Salem PA, Lamki L, Wallace S. Regression of hepatic metastases from gastrointestinal leiomyosarcoma after hepatic arterial chemoembolization. Cancer 1991;68:321.
16. Stagg RJ, Lewis BJ, Friedman MA, Ignoffo RJ, Hohn DC. Hepatic arterial chemotherapy for colorectal cancer metastatic to the liver. Ann Intern Med 1984;100:736.
17. Grage TB, Vassilopoulos PP, Shingleton WW, et al. Results of a prospective randomized study of hepatic artery infusion with 5-fluorouracil versus intravenous 5-fluorouracil in patients with hepatic metastases from colorectal cancer: a Central Oncology Group study. Surgery 1979; 86:550.
18. Balch CM, Urist MM, Soong S-J, McGregor M. A prospective phase II clinical trial of continuous FUDR regional chemotherapy for colorectal metastases to the liver using a totally implantable drug infusion pump. Ann Surg 1983;198:567.
19. Campbell CA, Burns RC, Sitzmann JV, Lipsett PA, Grochow LB, Niderhuber JE. Regional chemotherapy devices: effect of experience and anatomy on complications. J Clin Oncol 1993;11:822.
20. Michels NA. Newer anatomy of the liver and its variant blood supply and collateral circulation. Am J Surg 1966;112:337.
21. Hohn DC, Stagg RJ, Price DC, Lewis B. Avoidance of gastroduodenal toxicity in patients receiving hepatic arterial 5-fluoro-2′-deoxyuridine. J Clin Oncol 1985;3:1257.
22. Rayner AA, Kerlan RK, Stagg RJ, Price DC, Hohn DC. Total hepatic arterial perfusion after occlusion of variant lobar vessels: implications for hepatic arterial chemotherapy. Surgery 1986;99:708.
23. Curley SA, Chase JL, Roh MS, Hohn DC. Technical considerations and complications associated with the placement of 180 implantable hepatic arterial infusion devices. Surgery 1993;114:928.
24. Shike M, Gillin JS, Kemeny N, Daly JM, Kurtz RC. Severe gastroduodenal ulcerations complicating hepatic artery infusion chemotherapy for metastatic colon cancer. Am J Gastroenterol 1986;81:176.
25. Frye J, Venook A, Ostroff J, et al. Hepatic intra-arterial methylene blue injection during endoscopy: a method of detecting gastroduodenal misperfusion in patients receiving hepatic intra-arterial chemotherapy via an implanted pump. Gastrointest Endosc 1992;38:52.
26. Rougier P, Laplanche A, Huguier M, et al. Hepatic arterial infusion of floxuridine in patients with liver metastases from colorectal carcinoma:

long-term results of a prospective randomized trial. J Clin Oncol 1992; 10:1112.
27. Allen-Mersh TG, Earlam S, Fordy C, Abrams K. Continuous hepatic artery floxuridine (FUDR) infusion prolongs overall and normal-quality survival in colorectal liver metastasis (CLM) patients. Proceedings of the American Society of Clinical Oncology 1994;13:202.
28. Chang AE, Schneider PD, Sugarbaker PH, Simpson C, Culnane M, Steinberg SM. A prospective randomized trial of regional versus systemic continuous 5-fluorodeoxyuridine chemotherapy in the treatment of colorectal liver metastases. Ann Surg 1987;206:685.
29. Kemeny N, Daly J, Reichman B, Geller N, Botet J, Oderman P. Intrahepatic or systemic infusion of fluorodeoxyuridine in patients with liver metastases from colorectal carcinoma. Ann Intern Med 1987;107:459.
30. Hohn DC, Stagg RJ, Friedman MA, et al. A randomized trial of continuous intravenous versus hepatic intraarterial floxuridine in patients with colorectal cancer metastatic to the liver: the Northern Oncology Group Trial. J Clin Oncol 1989;7:1646.
31. Kemeny N, Cohen A, Seiter K, et al. Randomized trial of hepatic arterial floxuridine, mitomycin, and carmustine versus floxuridine alone in previously treated patients with liver metastases from colorectal cancer. J Clin Oncol 1993;11:330.
32. Hohn D, Melnick J, Stagg R, et al. Biliary sclerosis in patients receiving hepatic arterial infusions of floxuridine. J Clin Oncol 1985;3:98.
33. Martin JK Jr, O'Connell MJ, Wieand HS, et al. Intra-arterial floxuridine vs systemic fluorouracil for hepatic metastases from colorectal cancer. Arch Surg 1990;125:1022.
34. Kemeny N, Seiter K, Niedzwiecki D, et al. A randomized trial of intrahepatic infusion of fluorodeoxyuridine with dexamethasone versus fluorodeoxyuridine alone in the treatment of metastatic cancer. Cancer 1992;69:327.
35. Kemeny N, Seiter K, Conti JA, et al. Hepatic arterial floxuridine and leucovorin for unresectable liver metastases from colorectal carcinoma. Cancer 1994;73:1134.
36. Hrushesky WJM, Von Roemeling R, Fraley EE, Rabatin JT. Circadian-based infusional chrono-chemotherapy controls progressive metastatic renal cell carcinoma. Semin Surg Oncol 1988;4:110.
37. Moertel CG, Fleming TR, MacDonald JS, et al. Levamisole and fluorouracil for adjuvant therapy of resected colon carcinoma. N Engl J Med 1990;322:352.
38. Wolmark N, Rockette H, Fisher B, et al. The benefit of leucovorin-modulated fluorouracil as postoperative adjuvant therapy for primary colon cancer: results from National Surgical Adjuvant Breast and Bowel Protocol C-03. J Clin Oncol 1993;11:1879.
39. Bruckner HW, Motwani BT. Chemotherapy of advanced cancer of the colon and rectum. Semin Oncol 1991;18:443.
40. Stagg R, Venook A, Frye J, et al. Hepatic intra-arterial FUDR/5-FU therapy for patients with metastatic colorectal cancer (CRC) to the liver who have failed systemic fluoropyrimidine therapy. Proceedings of the American Society of Clinical Oncology 1994;13:217.
41. Atiq OT, Kemeny N, Niedzwiecki D, Botet J. Treatment of unresectable primary liver cancer with intrahepatic fluorodeoxyuridine and mitomycin C through an implantable pump. Cancer 1992;69:920.
42. Patt YZ, Yoffe B, Charnsangavej C, et al. Low serum alpha-fetoprotein level in patients with hepatocellular carcinoma as a predictor of response to 5-FU and interferon-alpha-2b. Cancer 1993;72:2574.
43. Doci R, Bignami P, Bozzetti F, et al. Intrahepatic chemotherapy for unresectable hepatocellular carcinoma. Cancer 1988;61:1983.
44. Robertson JM, Lawrence TS, Dworzanin LM, et al. Treatment of primary hepatobiliary cancers with conformal radiation therapy and regional chemotherapy. J Clin Oncol 1993;11:1286.
45. Sparks FC, Mosher MB, Hallauer WC, et al. Hepatic artery ligation and postoperative chemotherapy for hepatic metastasis: clinical and pathophysiological results. Cancer 1975;35:1074.
46. Charnsangavej C, Chuang V, Wallace S, Soo C-S, Bowers T. Angiographic classification of hepatic arterial collaterals. Lancet 1982;144: 485.
47. Civalleri D, Esposito M, Fulco RA, et al. Liver and tumor uptake and plasma pharmacokinetic of arterial cisplatin administered with and without starch microspheres in patients with liver metastases. Cancer 1991;68:988.
48. Andersson M, Aronsen F, Balch C, et al. Pharmacokinetics of intra-arterial mitomycin-c with or without degradable starch microspheres (DSM) in the treatment of non-resectable liver cancer. Acta Oncol 1989;28:219.
49. Ajani JA, Carrasco H, Charnsangavej C, Samaan NA, Levin B, Wallace S. Islet cell tumors metastatic to the liver: effective palliation by sequential hepatic artery embolization. Ann Intern Med 1988;108:340.
50. Sternlicht M, Daniels JR, Sales SF, Daniels A. Effect of antimicrobial protection on tolerance to hepatic chemoembolization with a fibrous collagen carrier. Radiology 1989;170:1067.
51. Gunji T, Kawauchi N, Ohnishi S, et al. Treatment of hepatocellular carcinoma associated with advanced cirrhosis by transcatheter arterial chemoembolization using autologous blood clot: a preliminary report. Hepatology 1992;15:252.
52. Venook AP, Stagg RJ, Lewis BJ, et al. Chemoembolization for hepatocellular carcinoma. J Clin Oncol 1990;8:1108.
53. Ikeda K, Kumada H, Saitoh S, Arase Y, Chayama K. Effect of repeated transcatheter arterial embolization on the survival time in patients with hepatocellular carcinoma. Cancer 1991;68:2150.
54. Audisio RA, Doci R, Mazzaferro V, et al. Hepatic arterial embolization with microencapsulated mitomycin C for unresectable hepatocellular carcinoma in cirrhosis. Cancer 1990;66:228.
55. Yamada R, Sato M, Kawabata M, Nakatsuka H, Nakamura K, Takashima S. Hepatic artery embolization in 120 patients with unresectable hepatoma. Radiology 1983;148:397.
56. Lin D-Y, Liaw Y-F, Lee T-Y, Lai C-M. Hepatic arterial embolization in patients with unresectable hepatocellular carcinoma—a randomized controlled trial. Gastroenterology 1988;94:435.
57. Soga K, Nomoto M, Ichida T, Aoyagi Y, Ozaki T, Ichida F. Clinical evaluation of transcatheter arterial embolization and one-shot chemotherapy in hepatocellular carcinoma. Hepatogastroenterology 1988;35: 116.
58. Sakurai M, Okamura J, Kuroda C. Transcatheter chemo-embolization effective for treating hepatocellular carcinoma. Cancer 1984;54:387.
59. Takayasu K, Moriyama N, Muramtasu Y, et al. Hepatic arterial embolization for hepatocellular carcinoma. Radiology 1984;150:661.
60. Nagasue N, Galizia G, Kohno H, et al. Adverse effects of preoperative hepatic artery chemoembolization for resectable hepatocellular carcinoma: a retrospective comparison of 138 liver resections. Surgery 1989; 106:81.
61. Adachi E, Matsumata T, Nishizaki T, Hashimoto H, Tsuneyoshi M, Sugimachi K. Effects of preoperative transcatheter hepatic arterial chemoembolization for hepatocellular carcinoma. Cancer 1993;72: 3593.
62. Kanematsu T, Matsumata T, Shirabe K, et al. A comparative study of hepatic resection and transcatheter arterial embolization for the treatment of primary hepatocellular carcinoma. Cancer 1993;71:2181.
63. Nakakuma K, Tashiro S, Hiraoka T, et al. Studies on anticancer treatment with an oily anticancer drug injected into the ligated feeding hepatic artery for liver cancer. Cancer 1983;52:2193.
64. Ngan H. Lipiodol computerized tomography: how sensitive and specific is the technique in the diagnosis of hepatocellular carcinoma? Br J Radiol 1990;63:771.
65. Uchida H, Ohishi H, Matsuo N, et al. Transcatheter hepatic segmental arterial embolization using lipiodol mixed with an anticancer drug and gelfoam particles for hepatocellular carcinoma. Cardiovasc Intervent Radiol 1990;13:140.
66. Stuart K, Stokes K, Jenkins R, Trey C, Clouse M. Treatment of hepatocellular carcinoma using doxorubicin/ethiodized oil/gelatin powder chemoembolization. Cancer 1993;72:3202.
67. Vetter D, Wenger J-J, Bergeir J-M, Doffoel M, Bockel R. Transcatheter oily chemoembolization in the management of advanced hepatocellular carcinoma in cirrhosis: results of a western comparative study in 60 patients. Hepatology 1991;13:427.
68. Oda T, Maeda H. Binding to and internalization by cultured cells Of Neocarzinostatin and enhancement of its action by conjugation with lipophilic styrene-maleic acid copolymer. Cancer Res 1987;47:3206.
69. Ohtsuka N, Konno T, Miyauchi Y, Maeda H. Anticancer effects of arterial administration of the anticancer agent SMANCS with lipiodol on metastatic lymph nodes. Cancer 1987;59:1560.

70. Yumoto Y, Jinno K, Tokuyama K, et al. Trans-catheter hepatic arterial injection of lipiodol soluble anti-cancer agent SMANCS and ADR suspension in lipiodol combined with arterial embolization and local hyperthermia for treatment of hepatocellular carcinoma. Int J Hyperthermia 1991;7:7.
71. Beheshti M, Denny D, Glickman M, et al. Percutaneous isolated liver perfusion for treatment of hepatic malignancy: preliminary report. J Vasc Interv Radiol 1992;3:453.
72. Gabizon A, Shiota R, Papahadjopoulos D. Pharmacokinetics and tissue distribution of doxorubicin encapsulated in stable liposomes with long circulation times. J Natl Cancer Inst 1989;81:1484.
73. Harris CC, Hollstein M. Clinical implications of the p53 tumor-suppressor gene. N Engl J Med 1993;329:1318.
74. Zhu N, Liggitt D, Liu Y, Debs R. Systemic gene expression after intravenous DNA delivery into adult mice. Science 1993;261:209.
75. Baker S, Markowitz S, Fearon E, Willson J, Vogelstein B. Suppression of human colorectal carcinoma cell growth by wild-type p53. Science 1990;249:912.

Surgery for Gastrointestinal Cancer: A Multidisciplinary Approach, edited by Harold J. Wanebo.
Lippincott-Raven Publishers, Philadelphia, © 1997.

CHAPTER 50

Therapeutic Heat and Cold in Gastrointestinal Malignancies

F. Kristian Storm and David M. Mahvi

Extremes in temperature are lethal to cells, particularly temperatures that change abruptly (ie, within minutes), as a consequence of membrane disruption and protein denaturation. If differentially applied (or absorbed), these phenomena can be exploited to kill solid cancers while preserving normal adjacent tissues. For each modality—hyperthermia and cryotherapy—potentially therapeutic dose and time responses have been elucidated and clinically verified. As with most other forms of cancer treatment, multimodality therapy using neoadjuvant or adjuvant radiation therapy or chemotherapy in concert often enhances response and improves patient outcome. Most treatments using extremes in temperature are considered experimental in that efficacy and safety in any single individual remain largely unpredictable and the exact role, timing, extent, and frequency of treatment remain under intense evaluation. This chapter focuses on temperature therapy, with particular attention to its scientific rationale, background investigations, and early clinical trials that may lead to improved care for patients with gastrointestinal malignancies.

HYPERTHERMIA

Definitions

Ambient temperatures vary markedly throughout the body. For example, at a core temperature of 37°C, the skin and lungs are 33°C, the subcutaneous tissue is 35°C, and the liver and brain are 38°C. By consensus, hyperthermia occurs at 40°C (104°F) or above and may be whole-body, regional, or local, depending on the extent of the treatment field. Superficial hyperthermia is confined to the body wall, whereas deep hyperthermia is below the body wall. Visceral hyperthermia is heating of internal organs.

F. K. Storm, Comprehensive Cancer Center, University of Wisconsin School of Medicine, Madison, Wisconsin.
D. M. Mahvi, Comprehensive Cancer Center, University of Wisconsin School of Medicine, Madison, Wisconsin 53792.

Dose-Time Responses

Heat alone is capable of producing tumor death. Based on in vivo studies and clinical trials, thermal death time is nonlinear and approximates 100 hours at 40°C (104°F), 20 hours at 42°C (108°F), 3 hours at 45°C (113°F), and 5 to 6 minutes at 50°C (122°F). Because most tumors are heterogeneous in nature, with varying blood flow and heat dissipation characteristics, sustained uniform high-temperature heating above 43°C is achieved only rarely. Most trials using hyperthermia as a single agent have been abandoned in favor of combination thermal therapy, such as thermoradiotherapy or thermochemotherapy, in which enhanced or synergistic cytotoxicity occurs at low and more readily achieved temperatures (40° to 43°C).

Whole-Body Hyperthermia

Whole-body hyperthermia from 40° to 42°C has been produced by a variety of novel methods, including immersion in molten paraffin, enshroudment in hot water–circulating suits, and confinement in heated-air chambers. These physiologically stressful and labor-intensive techniques usually require substantial sedation or anesthesia, and may be associated with significant morbidity. Whole-body hyperthermia is administered in conjunction with chemotherapy; however, therapeutic drug doses have been possible only rarely with a few agents because of enhanced systemic drug toxicity. Evidence also suggests that whole-body hyperthermia has an adverse effect on lymphocytes, producing a transient state of immune paralysis. Although a multitude of anecdotal responses have appeared sporadically in the literature over the past 2 decades, overall clinical outcomes have remained disappointing, which has led to the abandonment of this technique at most centers.

Regional Hyperthermia

Regional hyperthermia, both superficial and deep visceral, most often uses some form of an electromagnetic field (ie, radiofrequency waves or microwaves) to produce heat within a portion of the body. Electromagnetic fields cause excitation of atoms, whose energy is dissipated as heat. The depth of penetration depends on the water content of the tissues under treatment and the wavelength (frequency, in megahertz) of the electromagnetic field. In general, simple microwave devices operating at 434 MHz, 915 MHz, and 2450 MHz have most of their energy absorbed by tissues with high water content (ie, muscle), which limits the depth of penetration to several centimeters. Similarly, simple radio wave devices operating at 13.5 MHz and 27 MHz have most of their incident power absorbed by tissues with low water content (ie, subcutaneous adipose), again limiting penetration in all but the leanest of patients. Superficial hyperthermia has been applied effectively, however, to a variety of surface and subsurface malignancies, most often in combination with radiation therapy. Locally advanced or recurrent perineal tumors are amenable to such therapy.

Internal visceral heating is made possible by a combination (array) of sophisticated microwave devices, or alternately, by radio wave magnetic-induction devices. These complex devices impart a substantial amount of energy below the surface, often at a depth of 10 to 20 cm, with surface tissue sparing. Steering or aiming such devices at specific tumor targets has proved largely impossible with current technology. However, these methods have been surprisingly useful in providing independent deep visceral tumor heating. Large electromagnetic fields are directed at a region of the body containing a tumor, the premise being that ''selective tumor heating'' occurs as a consequence of the relatively poor ambient blood flow present in most solid cancers and the inability of such cancers to substantially augment blood flow and dissipate incident heat as do normal adjacent tissues and organs. These techniques have allowed significant hyperthermia of 43°C or higher in regionally advanced, recurrent, and metastatic gastrointestinal lesions within the abdomen and pelvis, with an extremely low incidence of normal tissue toxicity (less than 0.5%).

Local Hyperthermia

Local hyperthermia involves the placement of small radiofrequency wave or microwave applicators or ultrasound transducers directly on or near tumor targets in an attempt to focus energy directly within the neoplasm. Such techniques have had limited success in visceral tumors because of body wall absorption and tissue-interface reflection of electromagnetic energy, and the inability of ultrasound acoustic energy to effectively traverse air-filled spaces (eg, bowel). However, tumors on or near the surface may be heated effectively in this manner, although clinical applications have been limited in gastrointestinal cancers.

Interstitial Hyperthermia

Interstitial hyperthermia is akin to and most often used in conjunction with radiation brachytherapy. In this method, an array of electrically conducting electrodes is placed directly within the tumor target. Heat is produced by passing radiofrequency wave currents through the tumor. The size and shape of the temperature field can be regulated precisely by the number and location of the electrodes. Moreover, the tube guides used for radium seed application also accept microelectrodes, allowing sequential radiation brachytherapy and interstitial hyperthermia. This invasive technique is limited to accessible and usually superficial tumors, such as anorectal or perineal lesions, or wound recurrences of gastrointestinal malignancies.

Immune Correlates

Although it appears that whole-body hyperthermia causes immune paralysis, many in vitro and in vivo studies and several anecdotal clinical experiences have suggested that local or regional hyperthermia may stimulate the immune system. It is speculated that moderate-dose hyperthermia may dissociate masking antibodies, and also, in the process of disrupting tumor cell membranes, may unmask tumor-associated antigens, improving immune recognition. However, these provocative theories remain unproven.

Thermotolerance

A substantial body of evidence in vitro, in animals, and in patients with cancer suggests that prolonged hyperthermia at 42° to 45°C is tumoricidal. The fact that many tumors do not respond to heat therapy in this temperature range (particularly when used as a single agent) has been attributed to thermotolerance induced in the cells during fractionated treatments. Thermotolerance is defined as an acquired, noninheritable, transient state of resistance to heat that can last for 48 to 72 hours. It is well known that sublethal heat exposure may protect cells against subsequent heating. Thermotolerance may be induced by brief heating (minutes) during fractionated exposure or by prolonged exposure (3 to 5 hours) at temperatures less than 42°C. Moreover, several tissue-cultured cell lines and solid tumors of different histologic types have displayed varying degrees of heat sensitivity to potentially therapeutic hyperthermia.

Originally, investigators attributed this phenomenon to the selection of phenotypically resistant cells, possibly the residents of a relatively heat-resistant part of the cell cycle. However, subsequent studies showed that thermotolerance could not be explained by cellular recovery from sublethal heat damage or from progression of cells into a resistant stage of the cell cycle. Although the definitive mechanism of thermotolerance has remained elusive, current hypotheses involve enhanced membrane stabilization as the cause of the acquired thermotolerance and apparent native thermoresistance observed in some tumors. Membrane stabilization may occur as a consequence of the release of one or more of the heat-shock proteins, which is a universally conserved response to cell stress (including heat stress), or to the release of prostaglandin E_2, both of which appear to confer thermoprotection to temperatures as high as 45°C.

Thermoradiotherapy Rationale

Solid tumors are comprised of a heterogeneous population of cells in various phases of the cell cycle, often under hypoxic conditions and at low pH. Combination hyperthermia exploits the fact that relatively radiation-resistant S-phase cells are relatively heat-sensitive. The presence of hypoxic foci within tumors also inhibits the efficacy of radiation therapy, whereas under similar conditions, hypoxic cells are at least as sensitive to hyperthermia as are oxygenated cells. Moreover, mild hyperthermia may introduce a significant increase in blood flow, improving oxygenation and, with it, the overall response to radiation therapy. In addition, although pH apparently has little or no relation to radiation sensitivity, when pH drops to 7.0 and below, as occurs centrally in most highly proliferative tumors, there is significant enhancement of hyperthermia sensitization. These thermal factors, alone and in combination, probably prevent repair of sublethal radiation damage and enhance lethal radiation injury, forming the scientific basis for combination thermoradiotherapy in which an additive or synergistic response is anticipated. Optimum enhancement with the highest therapeutic gain ratio occurs when hyperthermia and radiation therapy are administered within 1 to 2 hours of one another.

Thermochemotherapy Rationale

Heat acts synergistically with a spectrum of antineoplastic drugs. Heat also may overcome some forms of drug resistance by several potential mechanisms, including increased cell membrane permeability (improved drug uptake), inhibition of repair mechanisms, and temperature-dependent increases in drug action. Enhanced cytotoxicity may occur at temperatures as low as 39° to 41°C, although each class of drugs appears to have its own mode of action.

Several drugs show increased reaction rates with increased temperature. For example, the nitrosoureas (CCNU, methyl-CCNU) and cisplatin have rates of cell inactivation that are nearly linear at temperatures ranging from 39° to 43°C. Alternately, some drug interactions with heat do not follow simple Arrhenius kinetics and require threshold temperatures of 42° to 43°C before significant synergism occurs (eg, doxorubicin). Localized hyperthermia combined with nearly all the standard types and dosages of single and combination agents has produced objective responses in about one third of patients treated for advanced disease, without evidence of increased systemic drug toxicity by the intravenous or intraarterial route. Moreover, responses appear to be related to thermal dose. Maximum enhancement occurs within a narrow temperature range of 40° to 43°C, and prior drug resistance does not appear to confer heat resistance. Optimum enhancement occurs when heat and drug are administered simultaneously.

Clinical Trials

Several standard strategies exist using devices approved by the Food and Drug Administration for combination superficial hyperthermia (local and interstitial) and radiation therapy for locally advanced and recurrent accessible tumors of the head and neck, body wall, perineum, and anorectum. These protocols are based in large part on retrospective, nonrandomized, cumulative studies comparing radiation therapy with thermoradiotherapy that have shown an approximate doubling of response (30% to 35% versus 70% to 80%) with the addition of heat. The largest prospective, randomized trial was Radiation Therapy Oncology Group (RTOG) 81-04, which closed in 1987. Although the overall complete response rate was the same among patients without and with heat (28% versus 32%), probably because of the inability to heat effectively and uniformly the large tumors that comprised 78% of the study population, in tumors less than 3 cm in diameter that could be heated effectively (greater than 42.5°C for 45 minutes), 80% of patients who received combined therapy had a response duration of at least 12 months compared with only 15% of those who received radiation alone.

Investigative trials with various forms of deep visceral hyperthermia have been performed over the past 2 decades. Because most trials have used combination thermoradiotherapy or thermochemotherapy, it has been more difficult to dissect out and state with certainty the additional contribution of this experimental modality.

In one novel prospective drug study, 34 patients with metastatic colon carcinoma in the liver, hepatoma, and melanoma or sarcoma in the lung, who had documented disease progression while receiving chemotherapy alone, were treated subsequently with the same ineffective agent using the same dosage and route, but combined with regional hyperthermia from 41° to 45°C. Over 1 to 9 months, 15% of the tumors regressed and 56% stabilized.

In another prospective study, 51 patients with metastatic colorectal carcinoma in the liver were randomized to receive either intravenous 5-fluorouracil or intraarterial hepatic 5-fluorouracil, plus regional hyperthermia at 40°C or higher. This was a selected population of patients in that all were potentially operable with excellent activity status. The median survival of the entire population was 22 months, with no statistical differences between groups by route of drug administration. This overall outcome compared favorably with historic groups treated at the same institution with intravenous 5-fluorouracil alone (8 to 9 months) or intraarterial 5-fluorouracil alone (12 to 14 months).

Summary

Local superficial hyperthermia may be considered in combination with radiation therapy or chemotherapy in locally advanced or recurrent lesions of the perineum and anorectum in which an additive or synergistic response is anticipated. Deep visceral hyperthermia remains experimental, but may be applicable to gastrointestinal cancers in a protocol setting, particularly tumors that are refractory to conventional therapy or advanced disease within the pelvis and liver.

CRYOTHERAPY

Cryotherapy, like hyperthermia, is aimed at the local destruction of solid tumors. Unlike hyperthermia, there is no evidence that cryotherapy selectively targets malignant cells for destruction. Cryotherapy has been used effectively for many years in the treatment of cutaneous malignancies. The recent introduction of insulated probes capable of intraperitoneal solid organ treatment has sparked interest in the treatment of hepatic malignancies with cryotherapy.

Mechanism of Action and Dose-Time Response

The exact mechanism of cell destruction by cold is poorly understood. Possible mechanisms include the formation of ice crystals within the cell that rupture the cell membrane, coagulation necrosis of tissue microvasculature inducing cell death as a result of lack of blood supply, and osmotic effects of the freeze-thaw cycle. Effective hypothermic cell death requires a sustained temperature of −35°C. Experimental studies have demonstrated that two freeze-thaw cycles are superior to one, and that quick freezing (the maintenance of cold for 2 to 3 minutes) and slow thawing at body temperature are the most effective means of achieving cell death.

Immune Correlates

In addition to the local effects of cryotherapy, systemic antitumor immune responses have been observed in some animal studies. However, in nonimmunogenic tumors in vivo, and in clinical series, no tumor remissions have been observed in untreated lesions distant from the cryotherapy site.

Clinical Trials

The clinical application of cryotherapy has been driven by improvements in intraoperative ultrasonographic techniques. Intraoperative ultrasonography is the "gold standard" in the delineation of intrahepatic tumors, and many centers routinely perform intraoperative ultrasonography before resection or cryotherapy. However, ultrasonography is essential to localize hepatic tumors in their relation to the hepatic vasculature on the bile ducts, so that the cryoprobe can be inserted safely without disrupting any major blood vessels. Moreover, large adjacent vessels may act as a heat reservoir, making cryotherapy ineffective.

Unlike hyperthermia, precise identification of the therapeutic effectiveness of the freezing cycle is apparent and can be monitored by intraoperative ultrasound. The leading edge of the cryolesion can be identified as a hyperechoic area on the scan. The frozen portion of the liver is identified by acoustic shadowing posterior to the freeze site. The leading edge of the ultrasound transmission demonstrates cryolesions that correlate histologically with an area of coagulation necrosis. This leading edge of the cryolesion, however, is only 0° to −10°C, a temperature range that is inadequate to ensure tumor cell death. The cryolesion should be extended 0.5 to 1 cm beyond the visible margins of the hepatic lesion. The thermal gradient of the cryolesion is about 10°C/mm, and this safety margin should be sought to enhance the probability of local tumor control.

Clinical Results

Little in the way of long-term outcome data have been presented in the cryotherapy of hepatomas or liver metastases. There also have been no direct comparisons of cryosurgery with conventional hepatic resection for these tumors. Therefore, all clinical series must be considered anecdotal observations, and randomized comparisons of cryotherapy and hepatic resection are unlikely. Local failure at the cryotherapy site has been reported in 10% of patients with metastatic colorectal cancer in the liver. No 5-year survival statistics are available.

The morbidity of cryosurgery is related to the initial cryotherapeutic treatment, which occasionally causes a crack to occur in the liver parenchyma. This usually can be treated by packing and, occasionally, suture approximation of the liver capsule. In the series from the Deaconess Hospital in Boston, an occasional patient required packing of the liver, resulting in reexploration and removal of the packing material. Other postoperative complications have been similar to those observed with routine resective hepatic surgery (ie, infection at the site of resection or cryolesion and bilomas resulting from disruption of minor biliary ducts).

Limitations of Cryosurgery

The treatment of large intrahepatic lesions with the cryoprobe is technically difficult and requires the placement of multiple probes at various axes. Most such patients probably should undergo conventional hepatic resection. Lesions that are close to a major blood vessel also pose a particular problem with cryotherapy. A major vascular structure (in general, the vena cava) functions as a heat sink and does not allow adequate cooling at the periphery of the tumor adjacent to the blood vessel, making recurrence more probable.

Indications for Cryosurgery

The specific indications for cryosurgery continue to evolve. It is unlikely that cryosurgery will demonstrate greater local control rates or a decrease in the incidence of distal metastases, despite previous animal studies showing increased immunogenicity of tumors. Patients with hepatic tumors deemed unresectable by conventional surgery may be the population most affected by cryosurgery. Patients with significant comorbid disease who, in the opinion of the hepatic surgery team, would have unacceptable mortality related to liver resection may be ideal candidates for this form of therapy. Optimal candidates for cryotherapy are patients with insufficient hepatic reserve or comorbid diseases who cannot tolerate formal anatomic or extended nonanatomic liver resection, patients with lesions situated adjacent to vital anatomic sites not amenable to resection, and patients with bilateral disease in which one lesion is safely resectable but complete resection of an additional lesion would diminish hepatic reserve to a potentially dangerous level.

The ability of the cryoprobe to approach lesions deep in the liver without damaging significant amounts of surrounding liver tissue is a significant advantage for patients with compromised hepatic reserve, such as those with cirrhosis. The major indication for hepatic cryosurgery is bilateral disease in which resection would leave the patient with inadequate hepatic reserve. One example is a patient with a left lateral segment lesion requiring a left hepatic segmental lobectomy and a deep-seated right lesion that is not amenable to wedge resection. Such a patient would be served best by hepatic resection of the left lobe, followed by cryotherapy for the deep-seated right lesion.

Summary

The introduction of intraoperative ultrasonography has led to the investigation of hepatic cryosurgery for the treatment of primary and metastatic hepatic tumors. Animal studies and preliminary clinical trials have demonstrated that this procedure is potentially safe and has minimal mortality. The morbidity specifically related to the cryoprobe results from cracking of the liver capsule, which usually responds to local measures. Animal and human studies have demonstrated that the leading edge of the cryolesion is only 0° to −10°C, which is an inadequate temperature for the eradication of tumor. To ensure cell death, a tumor should be treated with two freeze-thaw cycles that include the tumor and a 1 cm-margin of normal adjacent liver.

The clinical application of this technique is evolving. The optimal candidates for cryotherapy include patients with insufficient hepatic reserve or comorbid disease who would not tolerate formal anatomic or nonanatomic liver resection, those with lesions situated in anatomic sites not amenable to resection, and those with bilateral disease in which one lesion is resectable but additional resection of a second lesion would diminish hepatic reserve to a dangerous level.

SUGGESTED READINGS

1. Steward JR, Bagshaw MA, Corry PM, et al. Hyperthermia as a treatment of cancer. Cancer Treatment Symposium 1984;1:135.
2. Hahn GM. Hyperthermia in cancer. New York: Plenum Press, 1982.
3. Storm FK, ed. Hyperthermia in cancer therapy. Boston: Hall, 1983; Chicago: Year Book, 1985.
4. Perez CA, Gillespie B, Pajak T, et al. Quality assurance problems in clinical hyperthermia and their impact on therapeutic outcome: a report by the Radiation Therapy Oncology Group. Int J Radiat Oncol Biol Phys 1989;16:551.
5. Storm FK, Baker HW, Scanlon EF, et al. Magnetic-induction hyperthermia: results of a 5-year multi-institutional national cooperative trial in advanced cancer patients. Cancer 1985;55:2677.
6. Storm FK, Scanlon EF, Baker HW, et al. Tumor stabilization after hyperthermia: an important criterion of response to thermal therapy. J Surg Oncol 1987;34:143.
7. Meyer JL, Kapp DS, Fessenden P, et al. Hyperthermic oncology: current biology, physics and clinical results. Pharmacol Ther 1989;42:251.
8. Storm FK. Clinical hyperthermia and chemotherapy. Radiol Clin North Am 1989;27(3):621.
9. Ravikumar TS, Kane R, Cady B, Jenkins R, Clouse M, Steele G Jr. A 5-year study of cryosurgery in the treatment of liver tumors. Arch Surg 1991;126:1520.
10. Ravikumar TS, Steele G Jr, Kane R, King V. Experimental and clinical observations on hepatic cryosurgery for colorectal metastases. Cancer Res 1991;51:6323.

Surgery for Gastrointestinal Cancer: A Multidisciplinary Approach, edited by Harold J. Wanebo.
Lippincott-Raven Publishers, Philadelphia, © 1997.

CHAPTER 51

Selection of Therapy for Bile Duct Cancer: A Rational Surgical Approach

Thomas H. Magnuson, John L. Cameron, and Henry A. Pitt

In 1957, Altemeier and colleagues described three patients with primary adenocarcinoma arising in the proximal biliary tree.[1] That report, along with a subsequent paper by Klatskin in 1969, stimulated interest in this relatively rare malignancy.[2] These authors observed the poor prognosis associated with cholangiocarcinoma and the fact that the diagnosis often was made only after the development of advanced unresectable disease. Over the last 3 decades, however, dramatic improvements in diagnostic imaging techniques and methods of preoperative preparation have resulted in the ability to identify which patients with cholangiocarcinoma may be amenable to resection. Similarly, advances in hepatobiliary surgery and perioperative care have decreased the morbidity of complex biliary resection and reconstruction. These advances now permit an aggressive surgical approach in many patients with cholangiocarcinoma with the possibility for long-term survival or improved palliation.

DIAGNOSIS AND STAGING

Most patients with cholangiocarcinoma initially have obstructive jaundice. Accurate diagnosis and clinical staging can be accomplished using a combination of imaging techniques, including computed tomography (CT), magnetic resonance imaging (MRI), sonography, cholangiography, and arteriography. Based on the radiologic appearance, cholangiocarcinoma can be classified by its anatomic distribution as involving primarily the intrahepatic, perihilar, or distal biliary tree. Findings at CT or MRI suggestive of an intrahepatic tumor are a mass without bile duct or gallbladder dilatation. In comparison, a hilar cholangiocarcinoma presents with a dilated intrahepatic biliary tree, a normal or collapsed gallbladder and extrahepatic biliary tree, and a normal pancreas. CT findings suggestive of a distal bile duct cholangiocarcinoma include a dilated intrahepatic and extrahepatic biliary tree, a distended gallbladder, and an enlarged pancreatic head or a normal pancreas. The primary tumor often is small and is visualized in only 20% of patients on CT. Newer spiral CT or MRI may prove to be more sensitive than traditional CT in detecting these small tumors (Fig. 51-1).

After documentation of bile duct dilatation by CT or ultrasound, biliary anatomy is defined further by percutaneous transhepatic cholangiography or endoscopic retrograde cholangiography. In tumors of the proximal biliary tree, percutaneous transhepatic cholangiography is favored because it allows better definition of the extent of proximal tumor involvement at the hepatic hilum and permits the preoperative placement of percutaneous transhepatic catheters. For neoplasms involving the bile duct bifurcation, both right and left hepatic ducts require visualization, and intubation with transhepatic catheters is the preferred initial step in management. For obstructing lesions in the distal common hepatic duct and below, a single right transhepatic stent is used. These transhepatic catheters are passed through the tumor and into the duodenum if possible. Although the preoperative placement of biliary drainage catheters does not decrease operative mortality, these transhepatic catheters are useful technical aids during surgery by allowing palpation of the catheter above the tumor during dissection and by serving as guides to facilitate the intraoperative placement of large-bore Silastic stents.

Visceral angiography also has proven useful in assessing the stage and resectability of proximal and distal bile duct tumors. Angiographic evidence of common hepatic artery or main portal vein encasement or occlusion usually precludes curative resection. In a series from The Johns Hopkins Hospital, of 97 patients with pathologically proven perihilar cholangiocarcinoma, 33% demonstrated arterial or venous encasement on preoperative arteriography.[3] Only 1 of these patients with left portal vein encasement was resected for cure. In this series, angiography alone predicted the clinical management in 71% of patients, whereas the combined predictive value of cholangiography and angiography was 79%.

T. H. Magnuson, Department of Surgery, The Johns Hopkins Medical Institutions, Baltimore, MD 21205.

J. L. Cameron, Department of Surgery, The Johns Hopkins Medical Institutions, Baltimore, MD 21205.

H. A. Pitt, Department of Surgery, The Johns Hopkins Medical Institutions, Baltimore, MD 21205.

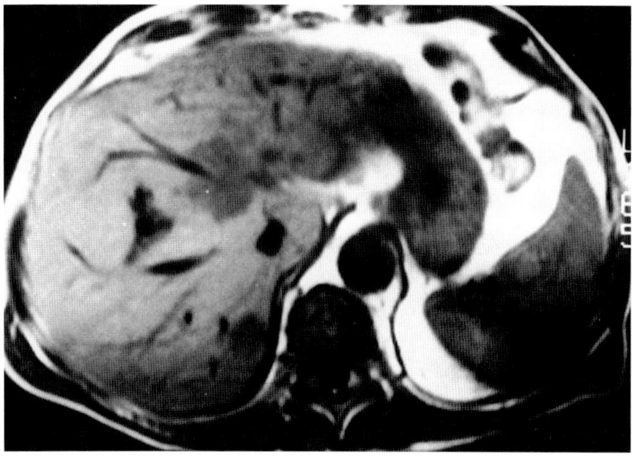

FIG. 51-1. Magnetic resonance scan, T1 image, demonstrating a cholangiocarcinoma *(dark)* surrounding the middle hepatic vein and also a second lesion posteriorly on the right. (Pitt HA, Dooley WC, Yeo CJ, Cameron JL. Malignancies of the biliary tree. Curr Probl Surg 1995;32:1.)

NONOPERATIVE MANAGEMENT

After preoperative staging, about 80% of patients are candidates for surgical exploration. The remaining 20% undergo nonoperative palliation. Radiographic evidence of bilobar hepatic involvement, extrahepatic disease, or main hepatic artery or portal vein encasement precludes curative resection. In addition, the overall medical condition of each patient warrants close inspection before surgical therapy is undertaken. Obstructive jaundice can have an adverse effect on a variety of metabolic processes, such as hepatic, renal, and immune function, and may increase operative morbidity.

Patients who are not candidates for surgery based on their overall medical condition or tumor extent may have their biliary tree decompressed by percutaneously or endoscopically placed drainage catheters. Proximal perihilar lesions are drained best through the percutaneous route. Bilateral catheters often are required for hilar lesions obstructing both the right and left ducts. Percutaneous transhepatic catheters are easy to reach and replace when they become occluded with sludge. These authors routinely flush the catheters with saline twice a day and exchange them over a guide wire every 2 to 3 months to maintain patency. The use of expandable metallic biliary stents has been advocated in patients with unresectable hilar and periampullary tumors.[4] Whether these indwelling metallic stents improve palliation and provide long-term patency is unclear.

OPERATIVE PALLIATION

The primary goal of surgical exploration is tumor resection. In good-risk patients without preoperative evidence of extrahepatic spread or locally unresectable disease, resection can be achieved in about 55% of cases. In the remaining patients, the finding at exploration of intraperitoneal tumor spread (15%) or extensive tumor involvement at the porta hepatis (30%) precludes resection.

Patients with widespread intraperitoneal tumors usually undergo minimal operative intervention. Transhepatic catheters placed preoperatively are left in place for postoperative biliary decompression. Cholecystectomy is performed to prevent the subsequent development of acute cholecystitis secondary to cystic duct obstruction by the indwelling biliary stents.[5] After operation, the transhepatic catheters can be exchanged under fluoroscopic guidance over guide wires for larger and softer catheters.

In patients with locally advanced unresectable tumors, several operative approaches to achieve palliative biliary decompression are available. Unresectable hilar tumors are palliated best with Roux-en-Y choledochojejunostomy. This approach begins with division of the common bile duct distal to the tumor and oversewing of the distal duct stump (Fig. 51-2*A*). Biopsies of the malignant stricture, using choledochoscopy if necessary, should be performed to establish a tissue diagnosis. Next, the proximal bile duct is dilated using progressively larger coudé catheters, replacing the preoperatively placed percutaneous transhepatic catheters with soft Silastic stents. This dilatation and catheter exchange is performed over guide wires inserted through the preoperatively placed catheters. Cholecystectomy is performed and a choledochojejunostomy is created using a 50-cm Roux-en-Y jejunal limb (see Fig. 51-2*B*). Compared with nonoperative palliation, this approach allows for removal of the gallbladder and avoidance of possible cholecystitis, placement of larger and softer stents, and positioning of the stents into a Roux-en-Y jejunal limb. Larger stents that drain into a defunctionalized limb of jejunum should reduce the incidence of subsequent cholangitis and help to minimize hepatic parenchymal dysfunction.

An alternative approach, used less frequently, in patients with locally advanced hilar cholangiocarcinoma is a biliary-enteric anastomosis proximal to the obstructing tumor. This technique is particularly useful when the tumor cannot be dilated from below and is predominantly right-sided. A Roux-en-Y hepaticojejunostomy can be fashioned to the left main hepatic duct at the base of segment IV or to the segment III bile duct exposed by tracing the falciform ligament into the umbilical fissure. For left-sided lesions, biliary-enteric bypass can be performed to the segment V duct after exposure through the gallbladder fossa.

In patients with unresectable distal bile duct tumors, palliative surgery is directed at relieving both biliary and duodenal obstruction and tumor-associated pain. Although unusual at initial diagnosis, symptomatic gastroduodenal obstruction occurs before death in up to 30% of patients with periampullary malignancies. For this reason, gastrojejunostomy should be performed during palliative surgery for unresectable distal bile duct tumors. In addition, many patients with unresectable tumors have severe epigastric and back pain. Chemical splanchnicectomy of the periaortic celiac plexus with 50% alcohol can be performed intraoperatively to help alleviate tumor-associated pain.[6] Biliary decompression is achieved with a choledochojejunostomy or hepaticojejunostomy. Cholecystojejunostomy should be reserved for patients with portal vein occlusion and multiple venous collaterals around the common bile duct. If a cholecystojejunostomy is performed, it is essential to document that the cystic duct enters the common bile duct several centimeters above the obstructing tumor so as to prevent recurrent jaundice.

The exact benefits, if any, that patients with cholangiocarcinoma derive from operative as opposed to nonoperative pallia-

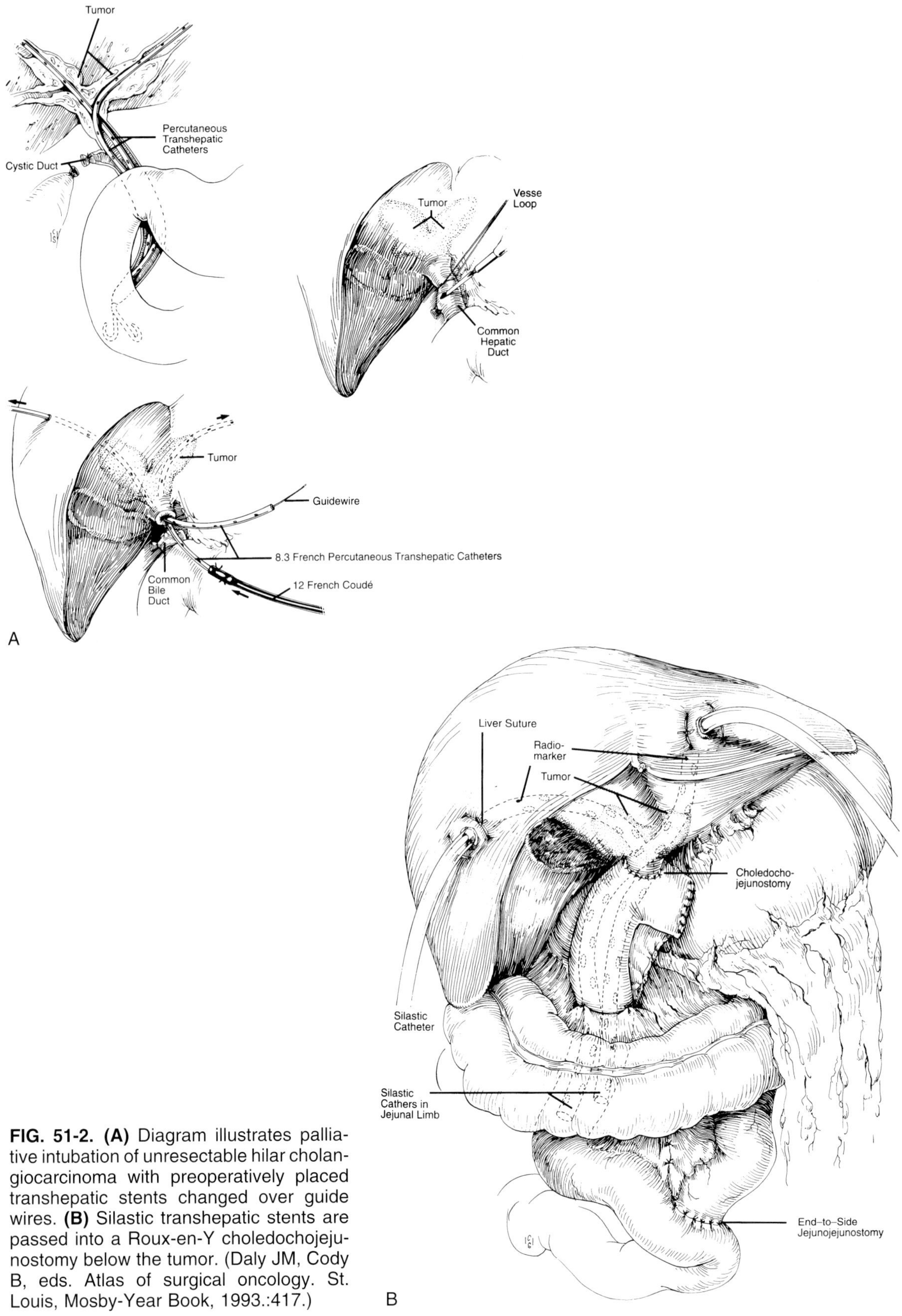

FIG. 51-2. (A) Diagram illustrates palliative intubation of unresectable hilar cholangiocarcinoma with preoperatively placed transhepatic stents changed over guide wires. **(B)** Silastic transhepatic stents are passed into a Roux-en-Y choledochojejunostomy below the tumor. (Daly JM, Cody B, eds. Atlas of surgical oncology. St. Louis, Mosby-Year Book, 1993.:417.)

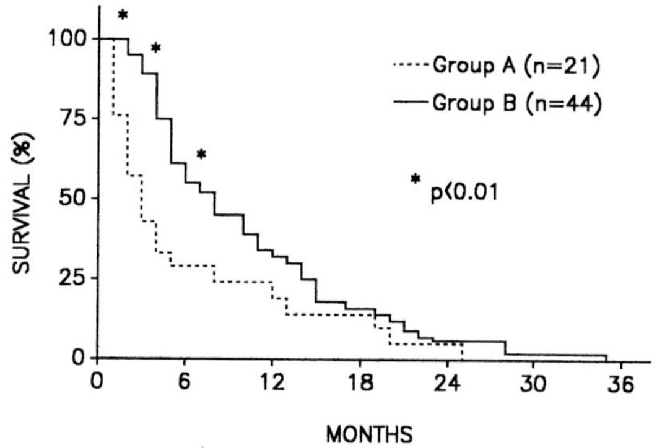

FIG. 51-3. Actuarial Kaplan-Meier survival for patients with unresectable perihilar cholangiocarcinoma treated with percutaneous stents (group A) or operatively placed large-bore Silastic stents (group B). Survival was improved ($P < .01$) in group B patients for the first 6 months. (Nordback IH, Pitt HA, Coleman JA, et al. Unresectable hilar cholangiocarcinoma: percutaneous versus operative palliation. Surgery 1994;115: 597.)

tion are difficult to determine. The differences in the morbidity and mortality of the two approaches may largely reflect selection bias. In a review of 65 patients with unresectable hilar cholangiocarcinoma treated at The Johns Hopkins Hospital, 21 patients were treated nonoperatively with percutaneous transhepatic stents and 44 patients underwent operative palliation.[7] The two groups were comparable with respect to multiple patient- and tumor-related parameters. The hospital mortality rate, however, was 14% in the nonoperative patients compared with 7% in the operatively palliated patients. The mean survival in the unoperated group was 5 months, significantly less than the 8-month mean survival observed in the operated group (Fig. 51-3). This retrospective study suggests that operative palliation with large-bore transhepatic stents and Roux-en-Y choledochojejunostomy may have some advantage over nonoperative palliation with transhepatic stents.

SURGICAL RESECTION

Operative resection of cholangiocarcinoma usually is approached through a midline vertical or right subcostal incision. A thorough exploration is performed initially to exclude tumor dissemination to the liver or peritoneal surfaces. The surgical procedure that is performed depends on the location of the tumor in the biliary tree.

Perihilar Cholangiocarcinoma

The perihilar area is the most common location for cholangiocarcinoma in patients with bile duct tumors requiring surgery. Dissection of the hepatic bifurcation is facilitated by two maneuvers. First, early mobilization of the gallbladder helps to expose the extrahepatic biliary tree. Palpation of the preoperatively placed transhepatic catheters also helps to identify the bile duct and hilar bifurcation (Fig. 51-4*A*). Second, early division of the distal extrahepatic biliary tree below the tumor aids in the technical aspects of proximal hepatic duct dissection. The distal bile duct stump is oversewn, and the proximal segment is reflected cephalad using the preoperatively placed transhepatic catheters as handles (see Fig. 51-4*B*). This maneuver facilitates exposure of the bile duct bifurcation and allows the underlying portal vein and hepatic artery to be dissected free under direct vision. The dissection proceeds circumferentially into the hepatic hilum beyond all gross tumor. The right and left hepatic ducts then are divided above the gross extent of the hilar cholangiocarcinoma, leaving the biliary stents exiting through the divided ducts.

After resection of the extrahepatic biliary tree and hepatic duct bifurcation, the previously placed transhepatic catheters are used to pull progressively larger coudé catheters and, eventually, large Silastic biliary stents through each of the lobar ducts (see Fig. 51-4*C*). The Silastic transhepatic stents are in proper position when all their side holes reside in the intrahepatic biliary tree and the upper portion of a 50-cm retrocolic Roux-en-Y jejunal limb that is used for the biliary-enteric anastomosis. Two separate end-to-side hepaticojejunostomies usually are performed over the Silastic stents exiting from the right and left hepatic ducts. The free ends of the stents exit the upper aspect of the liver capsule and are brought out through separate stab wounds in the upper abdomen. Mattress sutures are placed around the exit sites of the stents in the liver to prevent subsequent bile leakage in the early postoperative period.

In cases where hilar cholangiocarcinoma extends along the right or left hepatic duct into the hepatic parenchyma, appropriate hepatic lobectomy should be performed in addition to hilar resection. The need for hepatic lobectomy may be suspected at the time of preoperative cholangiography when peripheral neoplastic involvement of the right or left hepatic ducts is seen on radiography. Hepatic lobectomy is performed using standard techniques. Caudate lobe resection also may be required to achieve negative tumor margins. Biliary-enteric continuity is restored with a hepaticojejunostomy performed over a Silastic transhepatic stent. In selected cases in which tumor involves major vessels, segments of the hepatic artery or portal vein may be resected with subsequent vascular reconstruction. Both hepatic and vascular resection increase operative morbidity and mortality. However, improved 5-year survival has been reported in patients undergoing hepatic resection.[8,9]

Intrahepatic Cholangiocarcinoma

The operative management of intrahepatic or peripheral cholangiocarcinoma is similar to that of hepatocellular carcinoma. In most cases, hepatic lobectomy can be performed using standard resection techniques. Care must be taken, however, to achieve a negative bile duct margin if the tumor approaches the hepatic hilum. In general, the prognosis for resectable peripheral cholangiocarcinoma is better than that for hilar cholangiocarcinoma when negative margins can be obtained.

Selected patients with bilobar hepatic tumors and no evidence of extrahepatic spread may be considered candidates for total hepatectomy and orthotopic liver transplantation. However, the results of transplantation for cholangiocarcinoma have been disappointing, with the early recurrence of tumor being common.

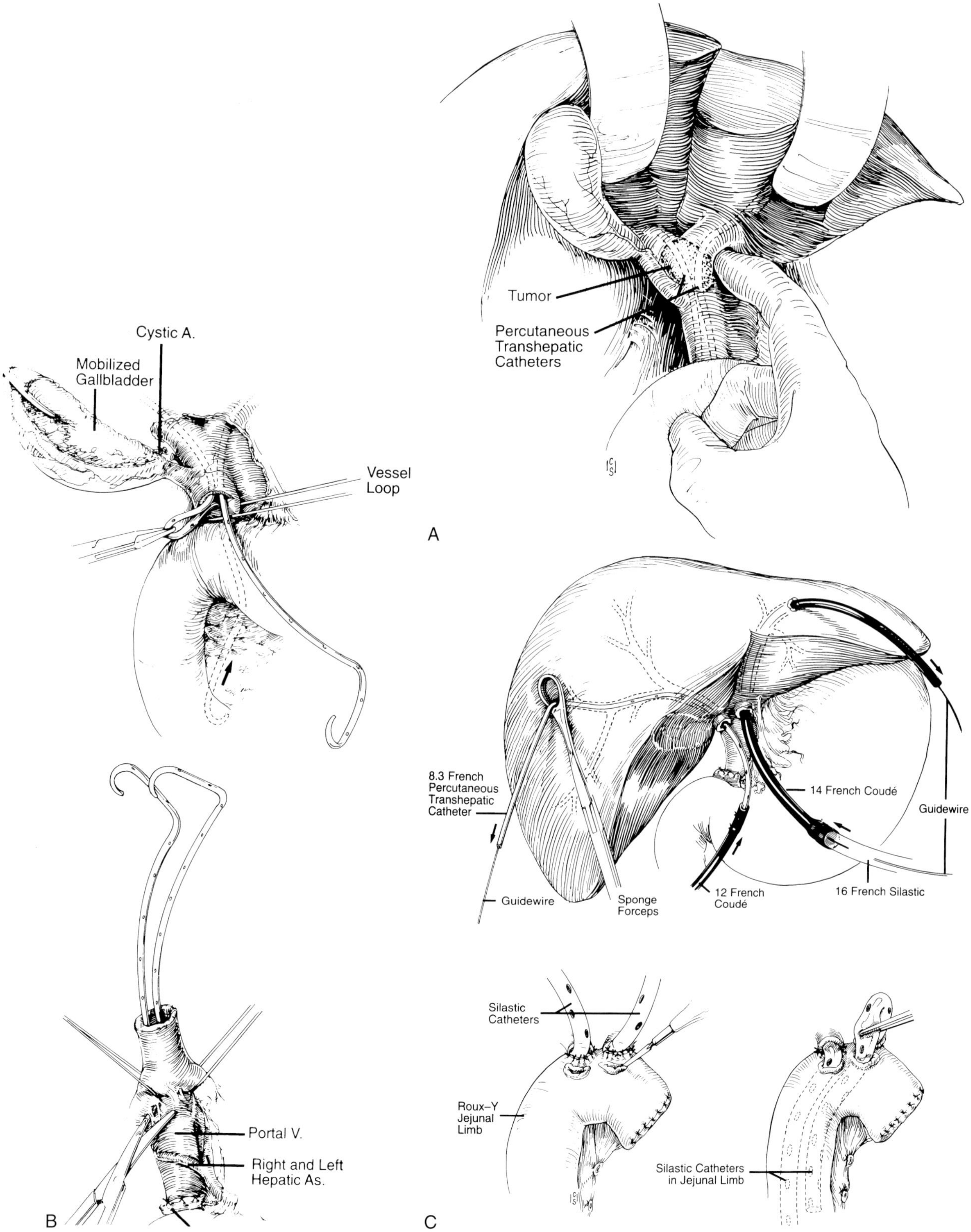

FIG. 51-4. (A) Diagram illustrates local resection of a perihilar cholangiocarcinoma with palpation of the percutaneous stent above the tumor. **(B)** Gallbladder mobilization and transection of common bile duct *(top),* and proximal resection *(bottom).* **(C)** Large coudé catheters and then Silastic stents are passed over guide wires *(top)* and bilateral hepaticojejunostomies are performed *(right* and *left).* (Daly JM, Cody B, eds. Atlas of surgical oncology. St. Louis, Mosby-Year Book, 1993.)

The best results have been reported in patients with negative hilar lymph nodes.[10,11]

Distal Cholangiocarcinoma

Patients with localized distal cholangiocarcinoma usually are treated with pancreatoduodenectomy. At initial exploration, a thorough inspection of the liver, peritoneal surfaces, and mesenteric lymph nodes is required to detect any spread of tumor outside the limits of resection, which would preclude further attempts at curative surgery. Duodenal and proximal pancreatic resection is performed in a standard fashion similar to that used for cancer of the pancreatic head. The pylorus is preserved if possible, and gastrointestinal continuity is reestablished by performing a pancreaticojejunostomy or pancreaticogastrostomy, hepaticojejunostomy, and duodenojejunostomy. The jejunum is brought up through a defect in the transverse mesocolon and the pancreaticojejunostomy is performed in an end-to-end or end-to-side fashion. Alternatively, the pancreas can be anastomosed to the adjacent stomach. The hepaticojejunostomy is performed in an end-to-side fashion. If a transhepatic catheter was placed before operation, it is used to stent the anastomosis. Otherwise, a T-tube is placed through the common hepatic duct. The final anastomosis is an end-to-side duodenojejunostomy to the 2-cm cuff of duodenum. Closed-suction drains are placed adjacent to the biliary and pancreatic anastomoses to control potential anastomotic leakage.

SURVIVAL

Perihilar Cholangiocarcinoma

Survival in patients with perihilar cholangiocarcinoma is highly dependent on the stage of disease at presentation and the resectability of the tumor. Between 1973 and 1989, 96 patients at The Johns Hopkins Hospital with hilar cholangiocarcinoma underwent surgical exploration with curative intent.[12] At exploration, 53 patients (55%) had resectable tumors. After resection, 14 of these 53 patients had obvious gross tumor left in situ and the remaining 39 patients were believed to have undergone curative surgery. Eight of these 39 patients required hepatic lobectomy to achieve negative tumor margins. The operative mortality rate for the entire group of 96 patients was 4%, and the 1-, 2-, and 5-year actuarial survival rates were 49%, 20%, and 5%, respectively. The 39 patients whose disease was resected completely had better survival rates at 1, 2, and 5 years of 70%, 41%, and 11%, respectively. The 14 patients with partially resected disease followed a clinical course similar to that of the 43 patients who underwent palliative operative stenting.

The role of hepatic resection for cholangiocarcinoma has been controversial. In a collective review of 389 patients with hilar cholangiocarcinoma, 201 patients treated by resection of the hepatic duct bifurcation were compared with 188 patients treated by hilar resection combined with hepatic lobectomy.[8] The operative mortality rate was 8% and the mean survival was 21 months in the patients who underwent hilar resection, compared with 15% and 24 months, respectively, in those who underwent hepatic lobectomy. These results suggest that operative mortality is increased but mean survival is improved only minimally with the addition of major liver resection for hilar cholangiocarcinoma. Nimura and associates have reported improved results with hepatic resection in selected patients with hilar cholangiocarcinoma, achieving an operative mortality rate of less than 5% and a 5-year survival rate of 34%.[9] This group routinely places multiple transhepatic catheters preoperatively to relieve jaundice and performs percutaneous flexible choledochoscopy to define the full extent of the tumor before major resection.

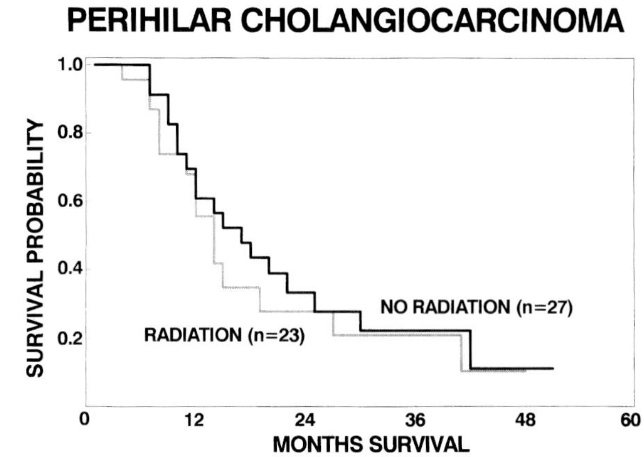

FIG. 51-5. Actuarial Kaplan-Meier survival for patients with perihilar cholangiocarcinoma who did (n = 23) or did not (n = 27) receive postoperative radiation. (Pitt HA, Nakeeb A, Abrams RA, et al. Perihilar cholangiocarcinoma: postoperative radiotherapy does not improve survival. Ann Surg 1995; 221(6):788.)

The benefit of adjuvant radiation therapy in the management of hilar cholangiocarcinoma remains controversial. Although several reports suggest improvement in survival with radiation therapy,[12,13] these have been retrospective reviews with inherent bias because of patient selection. A prospective study at The Johns Hopkins Hospital of operatively staged patients with perihilar cholangiocarcinoma compared 23 patients who received postoperative external-beam radiation therapy with 27 patients who received no adjuvant radiation therapy.[14] The two groups were comparable with respect to stage of disease, type of surgery, and multiple patient parameters. In this analysis, no survival advantage was achieved in the patients treated with radiation therapy (Fig. 51-5). Despite these results, further studies are needed to clarify the potential benefits of radiation therapy and its role in combination with other treatments or in the neoadjuvant setting.

Intrahepatic Cholangiocarcinoma

Intrahepatic bile duct tumors often become clinically evident only after the development of advanced disease. As a result, only 15% to 20% of these patients have resectable tumors at presentation. In resectable cases, standard hepatic lobectomy has been reported to result in median survival times of 18 to 30 months.[15,16] These results are somewhat more favorable than the prognosis of perihilar cholangiocarcinoma.

The results of complete hepatic resection and orthotopic liver transplantation for cholangiocarcinoma in general have been disappointing. Although 3-year disease-free survivors have been reported, operative mortality remains high and fewer than 10% of patients undergoing liver transplantation for cholangiocarcinoma have survived without tumor recurrence for 2 years. As a result, liver transplantation for cholangiocarcinoma remains experimental and should be reserved for selected, otherwise unresectable patients with bilateral intrahepatic lesions and no evidence of lymph node spread.

Distal Cholangiocarcinoma

The prognosis for patients with cholangiocarcinoma involving the distal common bile duct is more favorable than for patients with proximal lesions. These tumors often are difficult to differentiate from pancreatic cancer, which also has a worse prognosis. More than 50% of distal bile duct tumors are resectable for cure with standard pancreatoduodenectomy. The operative mortality rate usually is less than 5% and the 5-year survival rate is as high as 40%. Most patients with distal bile duct tumors should undergo surgical exploration and, if possible, tumor resection.

REFERENCES

1. Altemeier WA, Gall EA, Zinninger MM, et al. Sclerosing carcinoma of the major intrahepatic bile ducts. Arch Surg 1957;75:450.
2. Klatskin G. Adenocarcinoma of the hepatic duct at its bifurcation within the porta hepatis: an unusual tumor with distinctive clinical and pathologic features. Am J Med 1965;38:241.
3. Pitt HA, Dooley WC, Yeo CJ, Cameron JL. Malignancies of the biliary tree. Curr Probl Surg 1995;32:1.
4. Coons H. Metallic stents for the treatment of biliary obstruction: a report of 100 cases. Cardiovasc Intervent Radiol 1992;15:367.
5. Lillemoe KD, Pitt HA, Kaufman SL, Cameron JL. Acute cholecystitis occurring as a complication of percutaneous transhepatic drainage. Surg Gynecol Obstet 1989;168:348.
6. Lillemoe KD, Cameron JL, Kaufman HS, et al. Chemical splanchnicectomy in patients with unresectable pancreatic cancer: a prospective randomized trial. Ann Surg 1993;217:447.
7. Nordback IH, Pitt HA, Coleman JA, et al. Unresectable hilar cholangiocarcinoma: percutaneous versus operative palliation. Surgery 1994; 115:597.
8. Boerma EJ. Research into the results of resection of hilar bile duct cancer. Surgery 1990;108:572.
9. Nimura Y, Hayakawa N, Kamiya J, et al. Combined portal vein and liver resection for carcinoma of the biliary tract. Br J Surg 1991;78: 727.
10. Ringe B, Wittekind C, Bechstein WO, et al. The role of liver transplantation in hepatobiliary malignancy: a retrospective analysis of 95 patients with particular regard to tumor stage and recurrence. Ann Surg 1989;209:88.
11. Goldstein RM, Stone M, Tillery GW, et al. Is liver transplantation indicated for cholangiocarcinoma? Am J Surg 1993;166:768.
12. Cameron JL, Pitt HA, Zinner MJ, et al. Management of proximal cholangiocarcinoma by surgical resection and radiotherapy. Am J Surg 1990;159:91.
13. Verbeek PC, van Leeuwen DJ, van der Heyde MN, et al. Does additive radiotherapy after hilar resection improve survival of cholangiocarcinoma: an analysis in sixty-four patients. Ann Chir 1991;45:350.
14. Pitt HA, Nakeeb A, Abrams RA, et al. Perihilar cholangiocarcinoma: postoperative radiotherapy does not improve survival. Ann Surg 1995; 221:788.
15. Schlinkert RT, Nagorney DM, Van Heerden JA, et al. Intrahepatic cholangiocarcinoma: clinical aspects, pathology and treatment. HPB Surg 1992;5:95.
16. Yamamoto J, Kosuge T, Tukayama T, et al. Surgical treatment of intrahepatic cholangiocarcinoma: four patients surviving more than five years. Surgery 1992;111:617.

Surgery for Gastrointestinal Cancer: A Multidisciplinary Approach, edited by Harold J. Wanebo.
Lippincott-Raven Publishers, Philadelphia, © 1997.

CHAPTER 52

Resectional Approaches to Proximal Bile Duct Cancer

Peter W. T. Pisters and Leslie H. Blumgart

The selection of a therapeutic approach and palliative options for patients with proximal bile duct cancer has been addressed in detail in the preceding chapters. Although distant metastatic disease is uncommon at presentation, the locally advanced nature of the disease at the time of diagnosis often precludes curative resection. Nevertheless, many patients undergoing surgical exploration for hilar cholangiocarcinoma can undergo surgical resection. This subset of patients ranges from 20% to 40% of those explored and depends on the experience of the surgeon and the nature of the referral base. The proportion of patients who can undergo resection with curative intent probably is underappreciated by surgeons and gastroenterologists. Because surgical resection is the only curative therapy for proximal bile duct cancer, it is imperative that surgeons have a thorough understanding of the resectional approaches to these lesions.

PREOPERATIVE EVALUATION

Although the array of preoperative imaging techniques has been addressed elsewhere in this volume, several specific issues merit discussion. These include the assessment of vascular involvement (hepatic artery and portal vein), the presence of hepatic parenchymal invasion, and the presence of hepatic lobar atrophy.

Assessment of Vascular Involvement

It has been argued that preoperative assessment of vascular involvement is unnecessary for patients with localized hilar lesions because full operative exploration will reveal the extent of portal vein and hepatic artery involvement. In the authors' experience, however, accurate operative assessment of vascular involvement requires transection of the suprapancreatic common bile duct and elevation of the extrahepatic and hilar biliary ductal system with hilar vascular dissection. The dissection is sufficiently extensive that it should be undertaken only in cases in which preoperative imaging studies have indicated at least a potential for resectability.

Angiography remains the gold standard for the assessment of vascular involvement (Fig. 52-1). However, it is an invasive and relatively expensive approach. Data from the University of Bern suggest that duplex sonography may provide comparable assessment of vascular involvement, with accurate prediction of portal vein and hepatic arterial involvement in 19 of 22 patients.[1,2] Duplex ultrasound combined with helical computed tomography (CT) provides highly accurate vascular assessment (Fig. 52-2). Preliminary experience with this modality at the Memorial Sloan-Kettering Cancer Center confirms this impression, and duplex ultrasound has supplanted angiography for the assessment of localized hilar lesions at the authors' institution. This technique is comparably inexpensive, rapid, and considerably more convenient for the patient than selective mesenteric angiography.

Hepatic Parenchymal Invasion

Hepatic parenchymal involvement may be of a contiguous or discontiguous nature. Occasionally, surgical exploration reveals small, occult hepatic metastases distant from the hilus. These lesions may be associated with omental or peritoneal tumor implants and are essentially distant metastases. The presence of discontiguous hepatic involvement precludes curative resection.

Contiguous hepatic parenchymal involvement is common. This occurs because of the proximal location of these tumors and their intensely desmoplastic and locally invasive nature. Predominantly right ductal lesions commonly involve segments IV or V, whereas lesions originating in the left duct frequently extend to segments I or IV. This has two important implications for the biliary surgeon. First, the surgeon must be prepared to

Peter W. T. Pisters, Assistant Professor Surgical Oncology, The University of Texas M.D. Anderson Cancer Center, Houston, TX 77030

Leslie H. Blumgart, Enid A. Haupt Chair in Surgery, Diseases of the Liver and Biliary System, Memorial Sloan-Kettering Cancer Center, New York, NY 10021-6098

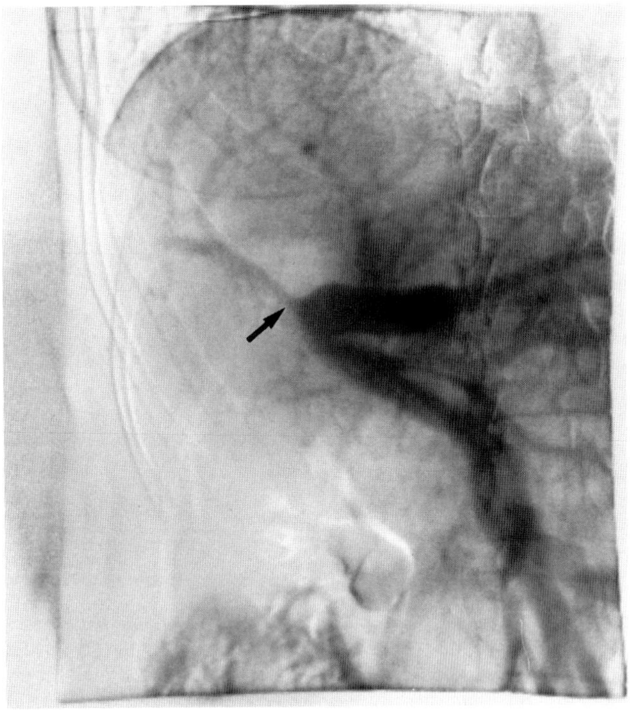

FIG. 52-1. Late-phase portography demonstrating severely compromised and almost occluded right portal vein *(arrow)* in a patient with locally advanced hilar cholangiocarcinoma.

perform en bloc hepatic resection to obtain negative histologic margins for most lesions originating at the hilus or in either ductal system. Second, the proximal origins of the caudate lobe biliary ducts are underappreciated by many surgeons. Extension into these ducts is common and en bloc caudate lobe resection is required for curative (negative microscopic surgical margins) resection of many lesions. The possibility of en bloc hepatic resection must be discussed with the patient and the anesthesiologist before operation.

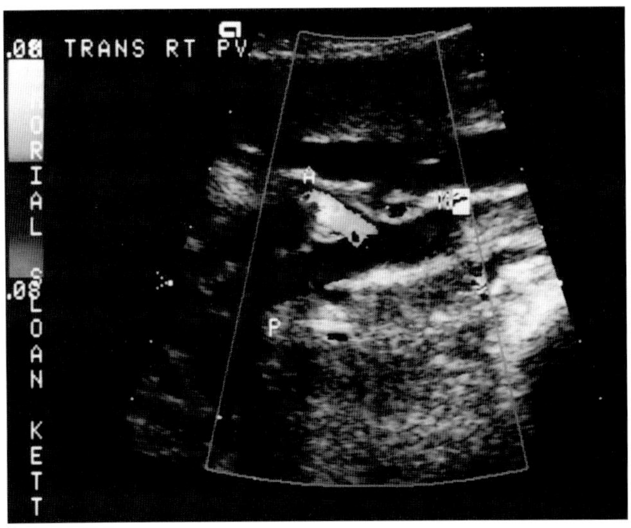

FIG. 52-2. Transverse sonographic view through the hepatic hilus demonstrating dilated bile ducts anteriorly with right anterior and posterior branches of the right portal vein. The significant anatomic detail that can be imaged using this technique is apparent.

Hepatic Lobar Atrophy

Hepatic lobar atrophy may be caused by obstruction of the portal vein, the hepatic artery, or, rarely, the hepatic vein.[3] In the setting of a hilar mass, lobar atrophy most commonly is associated with portal vein involvement. With the advent of routine CT scanning, atrophy is being identified with increasing frequency and may be present in as many as 50% of patients with localized hilar cholangiocarcinoma. Lobar atrophy (Fig. 52-3) at first may be a relatively subtle CT finding, but is of clinical significance in that it commonly is associated with vascular involvement and should alert the surgeon to the fact that, in the absence of contralateral vascular involvement, hepatic resection probably will be required to achieve negative microscopic margins.

Appreciation of gross atrophy is important because it may have a significant effect on the therapeutic strategy. The presence of significant right lobar atrophy is critical in planning an operative approach to right ductal lesions. With significant right lobar atrophy, the hypertrophied left lobe and the hilus of the liver usually are rotated posterolaterally toward the inferior vena cava and the spinal column, making the extended subcostal approach to the hilar dissection exceedingly difficult. When preoperative imaging studies demonstrate significant right lobar atrophy, a thoracoabdominal approach facilitates the hilar dissection before an en bloc right or extended right hepatic resection.

All clinicians including the biliary surgeon, interventional radiologist, and endoscopist should be cognizant of the implications of hepatic atrophy in formulating a therapeutic approach to these patients. For example, percutaneous or operative drainage of a grossly dilated duct within an atrophic segment may not be effective in relieving obstructive jaundice. Moreover, resection of hepatic parenchyma that leaves an atrophic remnant is dangerous and may be accompanied by postoperative liver failure.

ASSESSMENT OF RESECTABILITY

The Bismuth cholangiographic classification of hilar lesions incorporates only one component of the available preoperative data that affects the assessment of resectability (ie, the extent and distribution of intraductal tumor).[4] In clinical practice, however, the cholangiogram is integrated with other preoperative imaging studies, including CT and duplex ultrasound or selective mesenteric angiography. The triad of cholangiography, CT, and duplex ultrasound provides detailed preoperative assessment of numerous factors influencing resectability, including the site and extent of hepatic ductal involvement; the presence of ipsilateral, contralateral, or bilateral portal vein or hepatic artery involvement; the presence of hepatic lobar atrophy; the extent of contiguous or discontiguous hepatic parenchymal involvement; the presence of suspicious portal or periportal adenopathy; and the presence of gross extrahepatic disease. Preoperative staging of hilar cholangiocarcinoma should include

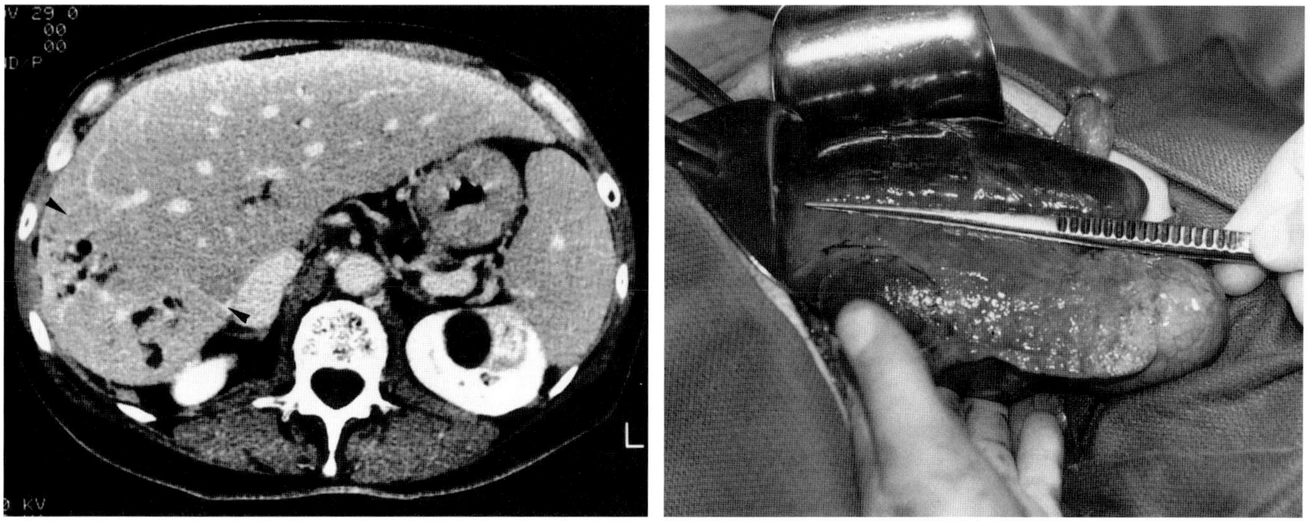

A B

FIG. 52-3. **(A)** Computed tomographic scan demonstrating severe right lobe atrophy (extent of right lobe indicated by *arrows*) with compensatory left lobe hypertrophy in a patient with hilar cholangiocarcinoma involving primarily the right hepatic ductal system. **(B)** Accompanying intraoperative photograph illustrating extensive right lobe atrophy. Forceps delineate the anatomic line between the right and left hepatic lobes, (atrophied right lobe is below forceps).

assessment of all these factors whenever possible. Ductal extension, portal vein involvement, and lobar atrophy should be evaluated assiduously. A preoperative staging system using these criteria is outlined in Figure 52-4. Uniform application of such a staging system would facilitate rational treatment planning and allow more direct comparison of different therapeutic strategies for this disease.

Based on the results of preoperative cholangiography, CT, and duplex ultrasound, unresectability is suggested by the following criteria:

1. Bilateral intrahepatic ductal spread of the disease so extensive as to preclude resection (or multifocal disease) on cholangiography
2. Involvement of the main trunk of the portal vein (except in unusual circumstances)
3. Bilateral involvement of hepatic arterial or portal venous branches
4. Vascular involvement contralateral to the cholangiographic origin of the tumor within the right or left biliary tree (except in unusual cases)
5. Discontiguous hepatic spread or extrahepatic disease

The presence of ipsilateral vascular invasion (portal vein or hepatic artery) does not contraindicate potentially curative resection with negative histologic margins. In such cases, hepatic resection with en bloc resection of the ipsilateral hilar vascular structures can be performed to effect complete tumor clearance. Such approaches sometimes are possible in patients with involvement of the contralateral portal vein or involvement at the confluence of the right and left portal veins.

The surgical assessment of resectability requires careful evaluation of the relation of the tumor mass to the hilar vascular structures and perihilar hepatic parenchyma. This may be difficult because preoperative percutaneous or endoscopic transtumoral biliary drainage generates an extensive periductal inflam-

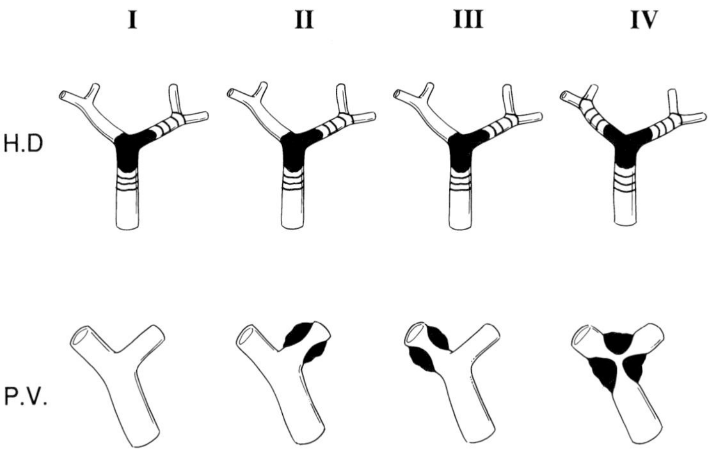

FIG. 52-4. Proposed preoperative staging system for localized hilar cholangiocarcinoma. This system evaluates the critical factors of bile duct extension, vascular involvement, and consequent hepatic lobar atrophy using the preoperative cholangiogram, computed tomogram and duplex sonogram or angiogram. The shaded areas and lines indicate the possible extent of ductal disease. Extrahepatic disease, if identified, is taken into account. Note that disease can extend into second-order bile ducts in each instance. Management strategies based on this preoperative staging system are as follows: stages I and II—surgical exploration with resection; stage III—surgical exploration with resection or bypass; stage IV—percutaneous drainage or intubation, or supportive care only. *HD,* hepatic ductal involvement; *PV,* portal vein involvement.

TABLE 52-1. *Internal drainage procedures in 28 patients undergoing palliative bypass surgery for unresectable hilar cholangiocarcinoma at the Memorial Sloan-Kettering Cancer Center (1991-1993)*

Procedure	Site	Number of patients
Rouxen-en-Y hepaticojejunostomy	Hilus	9
	Segment III	8
	Segment IV	1
	Right hepatic duct	3
	Left hepatic duct	1
	Right posterior duct	2
Roux-en-Y choledochojejunostomy*		1
Choledochoduodenostomy†		1
No internal drainage		2

* To provide access for trantumoral intubation and subsequent radiation therapy.
† After incomplete resection of papillary tumor at the hilus to allow subsequent endoscopy.

matory response that complicates assessment of resectability and the hilar dissection.[5] In fact, when the lesion is relatively locally advanced, the sclerotic nature of these tumors combined with the vascular inflammatory response elicited by the biliary stent may render an otherwise resectable lesion unresectable. Moreover, nearly one third of patients with malignant obstructive jaundice have bacterobilia.[6] When such covertly infected biliary trees are instrumented, cholangitis often is precipitated. Therefore, in the absence of preoperative biliary sepsis or organ failure, no patient with a hilar mass should have a biliary stent placed for "relief of jaundice" until the imaging studies have been reviewed by an experienced hepatobiliary surgeon. If absolute evidence of unresectability is evident on the imaging studies, nonoperative palliative approaches may be appropriate. The remaining patients should undergo surgical exploration for possible resection. Those who are found to be unresectable at exploration should undergo internal biliary-enteric drainage, which almost always can be accomplished in experienced hands. This point is emphasized in Table 52-1, which outlines 28 patients with pathologically confirmed hilar cholangiocarcinoma who were treated with palliative intent for unresectable disease at the Memorial Sloan-Kettering Cancer Center. Internal biliary-enteric drainage was accomplished in 26 of the patients. In the two patients in whom biopsy alone was performed, no internal drainage was attempted because of widespread carcinomatosis present at exploration.

A second clinical issue relative to assessment of resectability is the operative exposure. When tumor is present at the hilus of the liver, anterior dissection of the common bile duct and hilus does not permit adequate assessment of resectability. Complete assessment of resectability requires transection of the supraduodenal common bile duct with retrograde dissection in the plane between the common bile duct and the portal vein. This allows for anterior reflection of the extrahepatic biliary system and nodal clearance, and facilitates direct assessment of vascular involvement. If vascular involvement is found to preclude curative resection, a segment III biliary bypass can be performed for internal drainage with a choledochojejunostomy to reestablish continuity of the distal common bile duct and small bowel.

TECHNIQUES OF RESECTION

Resectional approaches to hilar cholangiocarcinoma can be divided into local resection and resection with en bloc hepatectomy. In a few patients in whom the lesions arise in the common hepatic duct, local resection can be performed. This involves resection of the entire supraduodenal bile duct, cystic duct, gallbladder, tumor, proximal hepatic ducts, and supraduodenal lymphatic tissues of the hepatoduodenal ligament. For more extensive tumors with unilateral hepatic parenchymal invasion, en bloc hepatic resection is required to effect extirpation with negative microscopic margins. Details of the exposure, dissection, and operation when hepatic resection is required are beyond the scope of this review. The chapters on hepatic resection address the salient technical points of hepatectomy. This description addresses the exposure and dissection of the hilar structures, and the biliary-enteric reconstruction when local resection is possible.

To assess the relation of the confluence of the bile ducts and

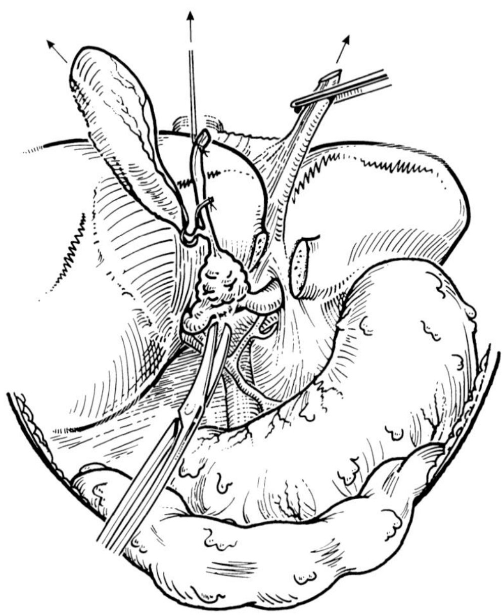

FIG. 52-5. The transected common bile duct, extrahepatic biliary apparatus, and related connective tissue and lymph nodes are reflected anterosuperiorly to facilitate dissection in the plane between the bile ducts and the nearby vessels. The tumor is elevated, and the portal vein and hepatic artery are dissected free.

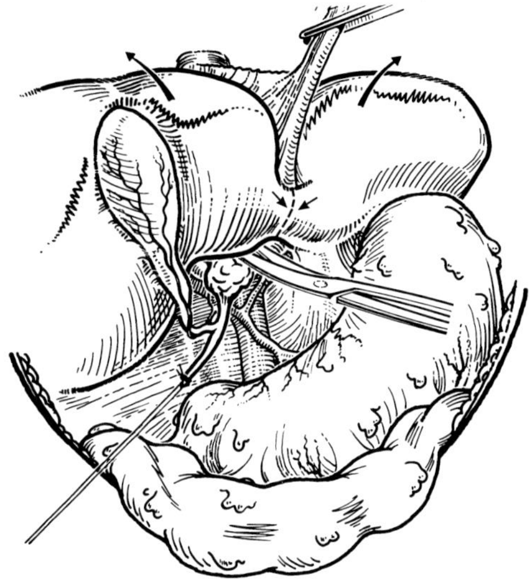

FIG. 52-6. Dissection at the base of segment IV to lower the hilar plate. Anterosuperior traction on the ligamentum teres facilitates the exposure. The bridge of hepatic parenchyma *(small arrows)* at the base of the umbilical fissure is still intact. The supraduodenal common bile duct has been divided and the plane between the duct and the portal vein and hepatic artery has been dissected to allow for accurate assessment of vascular involvement.

the related vessels, the common bile duct first must be transected in the immediate supraduodenal location and reflected anterosuperiorly (Fig. 52-5) to allow for the posterior dissection. The anterior dissection is facilitated by lowering the hilar plate at the base of segment IV[7,8] (Fig. 52-6). This allows for exposure of the anterior aspect of the confluence of the bile ducts and the proximal left hepatic duct. The extent of exposure usually is enhanced by dividing the bridge of hepatic tissue between the base of segment IV and the left lobe of the liver. With a combination of these techniques, segment IV can be mobilized and retracted anterosuperiorly to permit resection and reconstruction at the hilus.

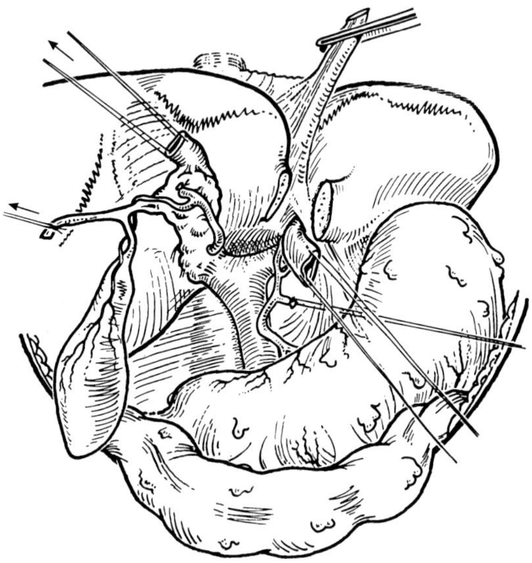

FIG. 52-7. The transected left hepatic duct, common bile duct, and gallbladder are reflected to the right to permit dissection of the right hepatic duct.

Elevation of the common bile duct and mobilized gallbladder, together with the related connective and lymphatic tissues of the hepatoduodenal ligament, exposes the vessels. This allows for dissection in the plane posterior to the tumor and anterior to the portal vein and hepatic artery (see Fig. 52-5). For local resection, it often is easiest to pursue dissection of the left hepatic duct first. This duct usually is longer and more extrahepatic in its course than the right duct. Once the proximal left hepatic duct is dissected, it is identified with stay sutures and transected, and a segment is sent for frozen section margin evaluation. The transected distal left hepatic duct, mobilized common bile duct, gallbladder, and related soft tissues then are reflected to the right (Fig. 52-7). This permits dissection of the right hepatic duct, which is mobilized, marked with stay sutures, and transected to complete the resection. A segment of the right duct also is sent for frozen section evaluation.

Several technical points merit further discussion. First, the surgeon must be aware of the frequent variations in the junction of the right hepatic sectoral ducts and the segment I (caudate lobe) ducts at the confluence of the liver.[9] These anomalies may not be apparent on the preoperative cholangiogram. After

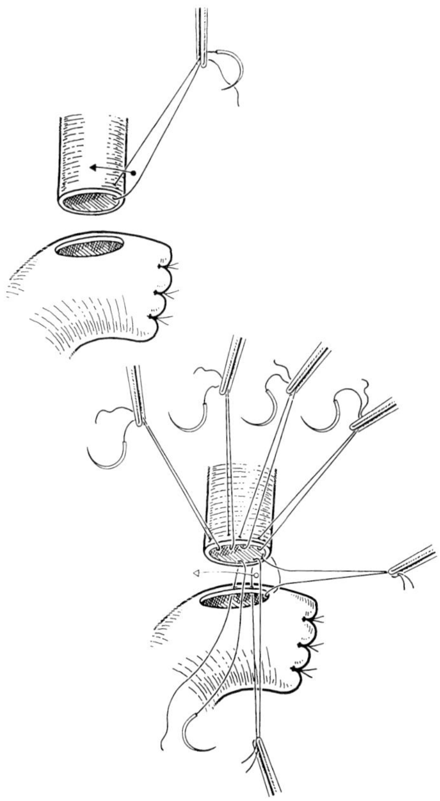

FIG. 52-8. (A) The hepaticojejunostomy is started by placing the anterior row of interrupted absorbable sutures into the bile duct. This allows for secure placement into the bile duct and permits gentle upward traction to facilitate exposure for the posterior row. **(B)** The posterior row of sutures is placed in an interrupted fashion with gentle traction on the anterior row for exposure.

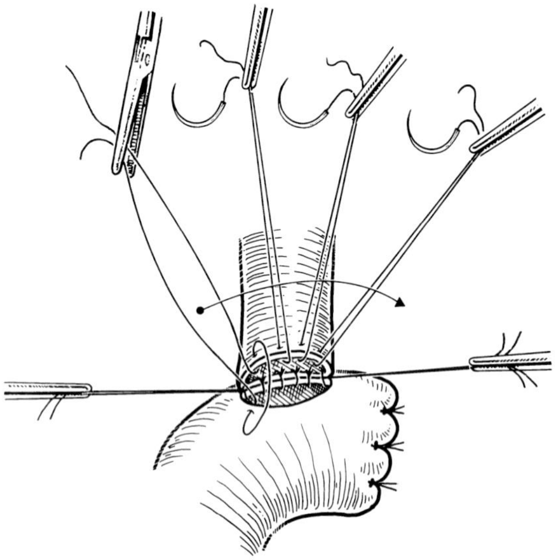

FIG. 52-9. Once the posterior row of the hepaticojejunostomy is tied, the anterior layer is completed. Silastic or other stents are not used.

local resection of the tumor, between two and five ducts may be exposed. Adjacent ducts then are sutured together so that there are no more than three separate ductal orifices for anastomosis. A 70-cm Roux-en-Y loop of jejunum is prepared and brought up, usually in a retrocolic fashion. The end-to-side hepaticojejunal anastomoses are performed using a single layer of interrupted 4-0 absorbable sutures[10,11] (Figs. 52-8 through 52-10). Sequential hepaticojejunostomies to multiple ducts at the hilus of the liver are exceedingly difficult to perform safely. Rather than work with one duct at a time, it is preferable to place the entire anterior layer of sutures to all exposed ducts first and then to place separately the entire posterior row of sutures. The jejunum then is parachuted down onto the hepatic ducts. The posterior sutures of all the ductal anastomoses are tied first. The individual anterior layers then are completed sequentially. Silastic or other stents are not used routinely.

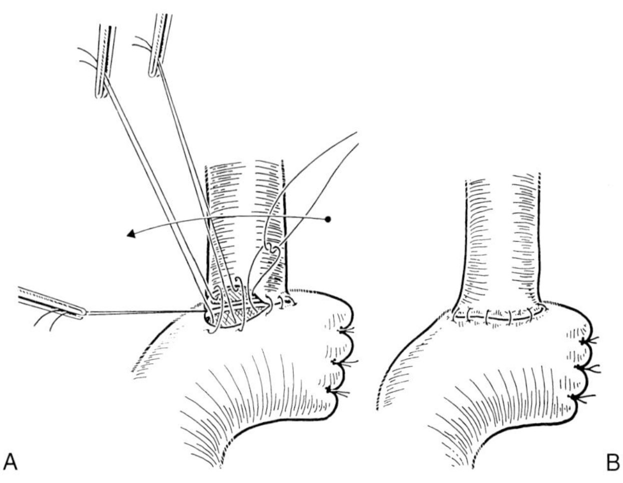

FIG. 52-10. **(A)** The anterior row of interrupted sutures is tied sequentially with the knots on the intraluminal surface. **(B)** Completed Roux-en-Y hepaticojejunostomy.

RESULTS OF SURGICAL RESECTION

Experience with resection of hilar cholangiocarcinoma remains modest, even in reports from major hepatobiliary centers. Interpretation of the literature often is difficult because patients with proximal and middle bile duct lesions are grouped together with patients with distal common bile duct lesions, incomplete resections frequently are combined with complete resections, and histologic margin status often is not included in the report, making it impossible to estimate the proportion of patients with true hilar cholangiocarcinoma resected with curative intent. Table 52-2 summarizes the experience of several investigators over the past decade.

Although it is difficult to compare these series directly, several issues merit comment. First, no institution has extensive experience with surgical resection for this disease. However, as specialized hepatobiliary centers become more common, some investigators are reporting a modest experience. Nagorney and colleagues report a 9-year experience with 171 patients with cholangiocarcinoma, 79 of whom had hilar lesions.[12] Blumgart has experience with 196 cases of hilar cholangiocarcinoma treated at the Hammersmith Hospital in London. Second, among the series that report both resected and unresected patients,[12–18] the resection rate ranges from 15% to 33%. When analyzed by preoperative intent, however, Baer and colleagues have demonstrated that the resectability rate is 70% among patients in whom preoperative imaging studies suggest resectability.[19] Therefore, state-of-the-art imaging studies permit reasonable preoperative assessment of the probability of a potentially curative resection.

The resection rate at a given hepatobiliary center is a function of the regional referral pattern. At the Royal Postgraduate Medical School at the Hammersmith Hospital, a resectability rate of 24% was observed in a series of 54 patients undergoing surgical exploration for hilar cholangiocarcinoma.[13] In a subsequent report from the University of Bern, the same senior investigator, using identical preoperative imaging protocols and indications for exploration and resection, recorded an overall resectability rate of 57% in 48 patients with hilar cholangiocarcinoma.[19]

These operations are complex and frequently involve an en bloc hepatic resection that is performed with a large tumor mass located at the hilus and usually in the presence of jaundice. However, operative morbidity and mortality rates have been acceptable. Several series from established hepatobiliary centers have reported no operative deaths in patients undergoing resectional procedures with curative intent, even among those undergoing en bloc hepatectomy.[14,17,20,21] This is in contrast to the more general multicenter experience of 97 patients reported by the French Surgical Association, in which the operative mortality rate was 16% for patients undergoing resection and 14% for patients requiring hepatic lobectomy in conjunction with bile duct resection.[22] With careful patient selection, the operative mortality rate for these resectional procedures should be around 5% in experienced hands. The incidence of reported postoperative morbidity depends on whether the data were collected prospectively or obtained retrospectively by review of hospital records. Prospective collection of complication data for patients undergoing major hepatobiliary procedures allows for accurate documentation of morbidity. Results of such data collection have demonstrated that complication rates for patients undergoing major hepatic resection and biliary reconstruction approach 50% (L.H. Blumgart, unpublished data).

TABLE 52-2. *Recent clinical series of hilar cholangiocarcinoma*

Institution/reference	Year	Total number of patients	Number with proximal or middle duct	Number operated	Number resected	Resection rate
Hammersmith/Glasgow[24]	1984	94	94	84	18	0.21
Lahey Clinic[14]	1984	109	95	109	16	0.15
Toronto[13]	1985	90	69	90	30	0.33*
MSKCC[17]	1989	52	52	52	14	0.27
Hammersmith[23]	1990	131	27	27	27	1.00†
Paris[16]	1992	122	122	122	23	0.19
Bern[19]	1993	48	48	37	21	0.57‡
Mayo Clinic[12]	1993	171	82	171	50	0.29§
UCSF[13]	1994	129	90	129	27	0.21
Keio BDCSG[25]	1994	158	158	158	83	0.53

* 0.22 for upper third lesions, 0.40 for middle third lesions.
† Includes resected patients only.
‡ 0.70 in those explored with curative intent.
§ Includes distal common bile duct lesions.
MSKCC, Memorial Sloan-Kettering Cancer Center; *USCF,* University of California at San Francisco; *Keio BDCSG,* Keio Bile Duct Cancer Study Group (Japan).

Most of these complications are minor; persistent major complications or reoperation are uncommon (less than 5%).

Several comments are warranted with regard to survival after resection of hilar cholangiocarcinoma. Among the authors who report median survival or the series in which it can be interpreted from published data (excluding series that include distal common bile duct lesions), the median survival after resection of hilar cholangiocarcinoma is consistent and ranges from 22 to 38 months. Five-year survival rates range from 16% to 22%.[12,18,23] Histologic margin status is of prognostic importance because at least three groups have observed significant survival differences when comparing patients with positive and negative microscopic surgical margins. Two groups have reported a 3-year survival rate of 50% in patients with negative histologic margins on final pathology as compared with 10% in patients with positive margins.[16,23] Similarly, Schoenthaler and colleagues have observed median survival times of 19 and 39 months for patients with positive and negative microscopic margins, respectively.[18] The apparent survival advantage of patients with negative histologic margins emphasizes the importance of achieving complete tumor clearance at the time of surgery.

SUMMARY

Hilar cholangiocarcinoma continues to pose significant challenges for surgeons and the array of medical specialists who participate in the care of these patients. Preoperative diagnosis is now possible in most cases. The diagnostic triad of cholangiography (usually percutaneous transhepatic cholangiography), duplex ultrasound, and high-resolution CT scanning permits accurate preoperative assessment of resectability in most cases. Angiography may be required in a few cases, primarily to exclude equivocal patients from exploration. After resection, residual disease, even if only microscopic, is a harbinger of poor outcome; most studies report a 3-year survival rate of 10% in such patients. This fact makes complete surgical resection with negative histologic margins the therapeutic goal of the hepatobiliary team. Given the propensity of these lesions to spread retrogradely along the bile duct and to invade adjacent hepatic parenchyma, the surgeon must be prepared to perform a difficult en bloc hepatic resection (frequently involving caudate resection for left-sided lesions) to effect complete tumor clearance. The results of such treatment demonstrate that complete resection is the best available therapy for patients with these difficult lesions.

REFERENCES

1. Looser CH, Stain SC, Baer HU, Triller J, Blumgart LH. Staging of hilar cholangiocarcinoma by duplex sonography: a comparison with operative findings. Br J Radiol 1992;65:871.
2. Triller J, Looser C, Baer HU, Blumgart LH. Hilar cholangiocarcinoma: radiological assessment of resectability. Eur J Radiol 1994;4:9.
3. Hadjis NS, Blumgart LH. Liver hyperplasia, hypertrophy and atrophy: clinical relevance. In: Blumgart LH, ed. Surgery of the liver and biliary tract. London: Churchill Livingstone, 1988:61.
4. Bismuth H, Corlette MB. Intrahepatic cholangioenteric anastomosis in carcinoma of the hilus of the liver. Surg Gynecol Obstet 1975;140:170.
5. Karsten TM, Davids PHP, van Gulik TM, et al. Effect of biliary endoprostheses on the extrahepatic bile ducts in relation to subsequent operation of the biliary tract. Journal of the American College of Surgeons 1994;178:343.
6. McPherson GAD, Blenkharm JI, Nathanson B, Bowley NB, Benjamin IS, Blumgart LH. Significance of bacteria in external biliary drainage systems: a possible role for antisepsis. Journal of Clinical Surgery 1982;1:22.
7. Hepp J, Couinaud C. L'abord et l'utilisation du canal hepatique gauche dans les reparations de la voie biliaire principale. Presse Med 1956;64:947.
8. Blumgart LH. Liver resection—liver and biliary tumours. In: Blumgart LH, ed. Surgery of the liver and biliary tract. London: Churchill Livingstone, 1988:1251.
9. Smadja C, Blumgart LH. The biliary tract and the anatomy of biliary exposure. In: Blumgart LH, ed. Surgery of the liver and biliary tract. London: Churchill Livingstone, 1988:11.
10. Blumgart LH, Kelley CJ. Hepaticojejunostomy in benign and malignant high bile duct stricture: approaches to the left hepatic ducts. Br J Surg 1984;71:257.
11. Blumgart LH. Hilar and intrahepatic biliary-enteric anastomosis. In:

Anonymous, ed. Surgery of the liver and biliary tract. London: Churchill Livingstone, 1988:899.
12. Nagorney DM, Donohue JH, Farnell MB, Schleck CD, Ilstrup DM. Outcomes after curative resections of cholangiocarcinoma. Arch Surg 1993;128:871.
13. Beazley RM, Hadjis N, Benjamin IS, Blumgart LH. Clinicopathological aspects of high bile duct cancer. Experience with resection and bypass surgical treatments. Ann Surg 1984;199:623.
14. Alexander F, Rossi RL, O'Bryan M, Khettry U, Braasch JW, Watkins E Jr. Biliary carcinoma. A review of 109 cases. Am J Surg 1984;147: 503.
15. Langer JC, Langer B, Taylor BR, Zeldin R, Cummings B. Carcinoma of the extrahepatic bile ducts: results of an aggressive surgical approach. Surgery 1985;98:752.
16. Bismuth H, Nakache R, Diamond T. Management strategies in resection for hilar cholangiocarcinoma. Ann Surg 1992;215:31.
17. Fortner JG, Vitelli CE, Maclean BJ. Proximal extrahepatic bile duct tumors. Analysis of a series of 52 consecutive patients treated over a period of 13 years. Arch Surg 1989;124:1275.
18. Schoenthaler R, Phillips TL, Castro J, Efird JT, Better A, Way LW. Carcinoma of the extrahepatic bile ducts. The University of California at San Francisco experience. Ann Surg 1994;219:267.
19. Baer HU, Stain SC, Dennison AR, Eggers B, Blumgart LH. Improvements in survival by aggressive resections of hilar cholangiocarcinoma. Ann Surg 1993;217:20.
20. Tompkins RK, Saunders K, Roslyn JJ, Longmire WP Jr. Changing patterns in diagnosis and management of bile duct cancer. Ann Surg 1990;211:614.
21. Bismuth H, Castaing D, Traynor O. Resection or palliation: priority of surgery in the treatment of hilar cancer. World J Surg 1988;12:39.
22. Reding R, Buard JL, Lebeau G, Launois B. Surgical management of 552 carcinomas of the extrahepatic bile ducts (gallbladder and periampullary tumors excluded). Results of the French Surgical Association Survey. Ann Surg 1991;213:236.
23. Hadjis NS, Blenkharn JI, Alexander N, Benjamin IS, Blumgart LH. Outcome of radical surgery in hilar cholangiocarcinoma. Surgery 1990; 107:597.
24. Blumgart LH, Hadjis NS, Benjamin IS, Beazley R. Surgical approaches to cholangiocarcinoma at confluence of hepatic ducts. Lancet 1984;1: 66.
25. Sugiura Y, Nakamura S, Iida S, et al. Extensive resection of the bile ducts combined with liver resection for cancer of the main hepatic duct junction: a cooperative study of the Keio Bile Duct Study Group. Surgery 1994;115:445.

Surgery for Gastrointestinal Cancer: A Multidisciplinary Approach, edited by Harold J. Wanebo.
Lippincott-Raven Publishers, Philadelphia, © 1997.

CHAPTER 53

Radiation Therapy for Bile Duct Cancer

Joel E. Tepper

The treatment of bile duct cancers has been poorly studied for a variety of reasons. First, the incidence of these tumors is low, making it difficult for any individual center to obtain a large experience with therapy. Second, the management of tumors originating in different portions of the biliary system can vary significantly. Tumors originating in the distal common bile duct are much more amenable to surgical resection and have a better prognosis. More proximal tumors are less likely to be technically resectable. It is difficult to develop a series with a consistent therapeutic approach. These tumors almost always are diagnosed after the patients have complete or nearly complete biliary obstruction, because they usually present with only obstructive symptoms.

Most would agree that surgical resection is the appropriate first-line therapy for patients who can withstand the surgical procedures and who have tumors that are potentially resectable for cure. However, the results of surgery are less than optimal, and even in patients with resectable lesions, it is appropriate to consider adjuvant therapy. In addition, a large percentage of patients have tumors that are not amenable to surgical resection, and consideration must be given to other approaches to palliate symptoms, to attempt to increase survival, and, sometimes, to produce a cure.

The experience with radiation therapy for tumors of the biliary tract is not extensive. However, a few reports have suggested a benefit to its use in a variety of clinical situations. Although radiation therapy has been used for primary treatment and as part of a program of adjuvant therapy, most of the data address its use for palliation.

ADJUVANT THERAPY

To justify the use of radiation therapy as an adjuvant to surgical resection, the rationale for the approach must be defined. The risk of local or regional failure after surgery alone is substantial. Radiation therapy is a localized treatment modality and may improve the outcome when used before or after surgery.

Professor and Chair, Department of Radiation Oncology, University of North Carolina School of Medicine, Chapel Hill, NC 27599-7512

Only limited information is available regarding failure patterns after surgical resection of biliary tract cancers. Kopelson and colleagues described a small series of 28 patients with extrahepatic bile duct, periampullary, and gallbladder cancers who underwent potentially curative surgical resection.[1] Thirteen of the 25 patients who survived operation had local or regional failure, representing 13 of the 16 patients who developed recurrent disease. Although these investigators analyzed a variety of sites within the portal region, the incidence of local failure was high. Other small series suggest a similarly significant risk of local relapse.

All published series evaluating the use of radiation therapy as an adjuvant to surgical resection are hampered by small patient numbers, lack of randomization, and substantial heterogeneity in the patient cohorts. Perhaps the largest adjuvant radiation therapy series is that of Cameron and associates.[2] Ninety-six patients were treated surgically. Fifty-three patients underwent resection; 38 of those patients received adjuvant external-beam radiation therapy and 27 also received an iridium-192 implant into a biliary stent. The use of postoperative radiation therapy produced no advantage in median survival, but the 3 patients who survived for 5 years received postoperative external-beam radiation therapy, and 2 of them received additional brachytherapy with iridium-192.

Mahe and colleagues from Lyon described patients treated for biliary tract cancer, some of whom received adjuvant radiation therapy.[3] Fourteen patients underwent complete gross resection, although 10 of these had positive margins. The patients were treated with external-beam radiation therapy or iridium implantation into the bile duct. The median survival was 27.5 months after complete gross resection and 13 months after incomplete gross resection.

RADIATION THERAPY ALONE

More information is available on the use of primary radiation therapy in patients with locally unresectable disease, but the series still are small and nonrandomized, and have relatively heterogeneous patient populations. Minsky and associates described 10 patients who underwent only biopsy or subtotal resection, and then were treated with 5000 cGy of external-beam irradiation and a 1500-cGy boost (in 8 patients) in addition to chemotherapy with 5-fluorouracil (5-FU) and mitomycin.[4] The 3-year actuarial survival rate was 50%, with a median survival of 16 months. Five patients were alive at the time of the analysis, having survived for 16 to 52 months. All patients who experienced treatment failure had local or regional failure as a component of their failure pattern.

Fields and Emami described 17 patients with extrahepatic bile duct cancers who were treated with external-beam radiation therapy with or without an iridium-192 implant.[5] The median survival was only 10.5 months, but survival was longer with an implant (15 months) than with external-beam radiation alone (7 months). However, there is potential bias in the analysis because patients with more extensive tumors would have been less likely to receive implants than patients with more limited disease. Local failure was the predominant cause of recurrent disease in these patients. Buskirk and colleagues described 16 patients with bile duct cancers who were treated with external-beam radiation (50 to 65 Gy) with or without a boost with iridium or intraoperative electron-beam radiation therapy (IORT).[6] Five of the patients were alive at a median follow-up of 18 months. Similar results have been reported by other investigators.[7] Veeze-Kuijpers and associates treated 42 patients with unresectable or residual disease using external-beam radiation therapy (3000 to 4000 cGy) plus an iridium-192 implant (2500 to 3000 cGy at 1 cm given in one or two sessions).[8] Median survival was 10 months, with 14% of patients surviving for more than 2 years. Patients who underwent resection with positive margins did better than those who did not undergo resection (median survival 15 months versus 8 months), and patients with nodal or hepatic involvement did worse than those without such involvement.

Alden and Mohiuddin reported the outcomes of 24 patients with unresected disease who received external-beam radiation therapy (46 Gy), an iridium-192 implant (25 Gy at 1 cm), and chemotherapy with 5-FU alone or in combination with doxorubicin (Adriamycin) or mitomycin C.[9] The 2-year survival rate was 30%, with a median survival of 12 months. These results were superior to those of a cohort of nonirradiated patients, in whom the 2-year survival rate was 17% and the median survival was 5.5 months. There appeared to be a survival benefit to higher radiation doses; patients who received more than 5500 cGy had a 2-year survival rate of 48% and a median survival of 24 months, compared with 0% and 6 months, respectively, in patients treated with lower radiation doses. The potential for bias in this study is substantial, but it does suggest that increased radiation doses provide a survival benefit.

The data from Grove and associates also suggest a benefit to the use of radiation therapy in patients with unresected disease.[10] The median survival was 12.2 months in a cohort of patients who received external-beam radiation therapy compared with 2.2 months in patients who received no external-beam radiation therapy. Hayes and colleagues reported similar findings, with median survival times of 12.2 and 2.2 months, respectively, in patients who received aggressive radiation therapy compared with patients who received only palliative treatment.[11] Other institutions have reported similar results (Table 53-1).

Todoroki and associates reported the results of an aggressive management strategy of surgical resection with IORT.[12] Patients with unresected biliary tract disease were given a single dose of IORT (2500 to 3000 cGy). The mean survival of patients with unresected tumors was 10.9 months. Recanalization of the duct was confirmed histologically in 8 autopsied patients. These investigators concluded that IORT increased the length and effectiveness of palliation in these patients.

TECHNIQUE

Two technical approaches have been used most commonly for the irradiation of bile duct cancers. The first is conventional external-beam radiation therapy, which has the advantage of delivering a moderately high dose of radiation to a relatively large volume of tissue. It is most effective in the treatment of bulky tumor masses, such as nodal disease or residual tumor after surgery, that are not limited to the bile duct. Typical radiation doses have been in the range of 4500 to 5000 cGy given daily for about 5 weeks, but higher doses have been used. External-beam radiation often is given in conjunction with 5-FU–based chemotherapy because this combination has proven more effective than radiation therapy alone in most sites in the gastrointestinal tract. The reason for this is unclear, although it is possible that 5-FU potentiates the effect of the radiation therapy by one of a variety of mechanisms, or that radiation modulates the efficacy of 5-FU, perhaps by altering the retention of 5-FU in the tumor.[13]

TABLE 53-1. *Radiation therapy for unresected biliary tract cancer*

Institution	Number of patients	Treatment technique	Median survival (mo)	2-Year survival (%)
USCF	30	54 Gy median	12	18
Washington University	9	external beam	7	0
	8	external beam implant	15	~26
MSKCC	10	50–65 Gy + 5-FU + mitomycin	16	50
MSKCC	8	Implantation and/or external-beam radiation	4.5	
Rotterdam	42	40 Gy + implantation	10	14
Cleveland Clinic	19	External-beam radiation	12.2	12 (est)
University of Utah	14	External-beam radiation and/or implantation	12.8	15 (est)
Jefferson Medical College	24	46 Gy + chemotherapy + implantation	12	30

UCSF, University of California–San Francisco; *MSKCC,* Memorial Sloan-Kettering Cancer Center; *5-FU,* 5-fluorouracil; *est,* estimated.

The second technical approach is intracavitary implantation of a radioactive isotope, such as iridium-192, into the bile duct. With this modality, the radioactive source is placed through a biliary stent either transhepatically or endoscopically into the bile duct so that it spans the portion of the duct that contains the tumor. Typically, a margin of 1 cm is implanted on each side of the lesion to ensure that the full length of the tumor is treated. The resulting radiation dose is localized, with the effective range of the radiation contained within a radius of about 1 cm from the stent. Because the treatment is so localized, high doses can be delivered to treat small tumors that remain in the bile duct after resection, or to provide palliation when the bile duct is obstructed by tumor. Typical doses used with this approach have been in the range of 2000 to 2500 cGy at a distance of 1 cm from the source. Implantation is limited by the fact that high radiation doses cannot be given to bulky tumor masses. These large tumors are not treated appropriately with implants alone.

Another technique that has been explored at a few centers is IORT. IORT can be used in addition to external-beam radiation therapy or resection.[15] This approach has the advantage of delivering a high radiation dose in a single fraction during surgery, with wider coverage than can be accomplished with an implant and a dose that is not limited to the bile duct itself. However, it still is not possible to treat large unresected tumor masses with IORT because the depth of penetration of the electron beam is limited to about 4 or 5 cm. Because the IORT field can be designed to avoid the stomach and small bowel, acute tolerance of the therapy usually is good.

IORT requires significant alterations in the infrastructure of the department of radiation oncology or the operating room. To provide the treatment in the operating room itself, it is necessary to install a radiation machine and the appropriate radiation shields. Alternatively, the patient can be transported from the operating room into a radiation therapy room that has been modified to allow part or all of the surgical procedure to be performed there. Both approaches require a significant institutional commitment.

Maximizing the palliative benefit of the therapy is important in patients with bile duct cancer. The most significant problem in these patients is biliary obstruction and infection. All stents are associated with a high incidence of infection, with recurring bouts of ascending cholangitis. Stents also become obstructed periodically, requiring replacement. This is accomplished easily if there is external access to the stent, but can be difficult if the stent is internalized. Surgical bypass, if possible, usually is the most lasting palliative procedure.

CONCLUSIONS

Local control and survival remain poor despite the use of radiation therapy as an adjuvant to surgical resection. It is unclear whether adjuvant radiation therapy improves survival rates or palliation. However, there is enough suggestion of benefit from radiation therapy to warrant continued study of its use as an adjuvant therapy. Unfortunately, it is unlikely that a randomized trial can be performed to formally test the benefit of adjuvant radiation therapy. It will be necessary to base therapeutic decisions on individual institutional trials.

In patients with unresected or incompletely resected tumors, the data consistently show an advantage to the use of adjuvant radiation therapy. However, it is probable that the patients who are most likely to receive radiation therapy are those with less advanced disease, making interpretation of the data difficult. It also seems unlikely that randomized trials can be performed for this clinical situation. It is difficult to determine how effective radiation therapy has been in any individual case, because there often is not a defined mass on radiographic studies by which to evaluate response. In addition, it is difficult to determine whether recurrent biliary obstruction is the result of tumor or secondary to the effects of therapy.

REFERENCES

1. Kopelson G, Galdabini J, Warshaw A, Gunderson L. Patterns of failure after curative surgery for extra-hepatic biliary tract carcinoma: implications for adjuvant therapy. Int J Radiat Oncol Biol Phys 1981;7:413.
2. Cameron J, Pitt H, Zinner M, Kaufman S, Coleman J. Management of proximal cholangiocarcinomas by surgical resection and radiotherapy. Am J Surg 1990;159:91.
3. Mahe M, Romestaing P, Talon B, et al. Radiation therapy in extrahepatic bile duct carcinoma. Radiother Oncol 1991;21:121.
4. Minsky B, Wesson M, Armstrong J, et al. Combined modality therapy of extrahepatic biliary system cancer. Int J Radiat Oncol Biol Phys 1990;18:1157.
5. Fields J, Emami B. Carcinoma of the extrahepatic biliary system: results of primary and adjuvant radiotherapy. Int J Radiat Oncol Biol Phys 1987;13:331.
6. Buskirk S, Gunderson L, Adson M, et al. Analysis of failure following curative irradiation of gallbladder and extrahepatic bile duct carcinoma. Int J Radiat Oncol Biol Phys 1984;10:2013.
7. Mittal B, Deutsch M, Iwatsuki S. Primary cancers of the extrahepatic biliary passages. Int J Radiat Oncol Biol Phys 1985;11:849.
8. Veeze-Kuijpers B, Meerwaldt J, Lameris J, van Blankenstein M, van Putten W, Terpstra O. The role of radiotherapy in the treatment of bile duct carcinoma. Int J Radiat Oncol Biol Phys 1990;18:63.
9. Alden M, Mohiuddin M. The impact of radiation dose in combined external beam and intraluminal IR-192 brachytherapy for bile duct cancer. Int J Radiat Oncol Biol Phys 1994;28:945.
10. Grove M, Hermann R, Vogt D, Broughan T. Am J Surg 1991;161:454.
11. Hayes J, Sapozink M, Miller F. Definitive radiation therapy in bile duct carcinoma. Int J Radiat Oncol Biol Phys 1988;15:735.
12. Todoroki T, Iwasaki Y, Okamura T, et al. Intraoperative radiotherapy for advanced carcinoma of the biliary system. Cancer 1980;46:2179.
13. Herskovic A, Heaston D, Engler M, Fishburn R, Jones RS, Noell KT. Irradiation of biliary carcinoma. Radiology 1981;139:219.

Surgery for Gastrointestinal Cancer: A Multidisciplinary Approach, edited by Harold J. Wanebo.
Lippincott-Raven Publishers, Philadelphia, © 1997.

CHAPTER 54

Treatment of Gallbladder Cancer

Harold J. Wanebo

Although an uncommon malignancy, carcinoma of the gallbladder is the fifth most common cancer of the gastrointestinal tract and the most common cancer of the biliary tract.[1] The diagnosis of gallbladder carcinoma is made incidentally at the time of exploration in 1% of patients undergoing surgical treatment for cholelithiasis.[1,2] Carcinoma of the gallbladder is more common in women; three fourths of the patients are women with a median age in the seventh decade. In most patients, the disease is advanced and unresectable. The overall prognosis, therefore, is rather dismal, with 5-year survival rates of less than 5% reported in most large published series.[1–27] However, in a small group of early lesions, surgery provides a reasonable probability of long-term survival. Radiation and chemotherapy have mostly a palliative role in the treatment of gallbladder carcinoma, and the experience with these treatment modalities is derived from their use in a limited number of patients.

SURGERY

In most reported series, the surgical management of gallbladder carcinoma has been quite variable. Of 100 patients reported in the University of Virginia series,[15] 92 were explored, and of these, only biopsy with or without a biliary–intestinal bypass procedure was performed in 44 patients. Of the remaining 48 in whom resection was feasible, 40 underwent cholecystectomy with or without common bile duct drainage and 8 had cholecystectomy with partial liver resection. The median survival after cholecystectomy alone was 6 months, with one long-term survivor living for 11 years; after cholecystectomy with common bile duct exploration or drainage with a T-tube, median survival was 4.5 months, with one long-term survivor living for 24 years; and after cholecystectomy with partial liver resection or wedge resection of the gallbladder bed, median survival was 14 months, again with one long-term survivor living for 6 years. The median survival among the 44 patients having miscellaneous nonresective procedures was 2 months, with no long-term survivors. Of the 46 patients in this series who could be staged according to the Nevin staging system,[11] only 6 had tumor confined to the mucosa or the muscularis, specifically, two stage I and four stage II lesions, with a 5-year survival of 40% in this small group.

There was only 1 5-year survivor and 3 2-year survivors among 21 patients with stage III disease. The overall 5-year survival rate was 5% after cholecystectomy with or without bypass and 13% after cholecystectomy with partial liver resection. These findings were similar to those reported in the University of Minnesota series.[17] There was a 46% survival rate in 11 patients with carcinoma confined to the gallbladder wall. There was one long-term survivor after cholecystectomy alone, whereas four of six patients who had more radical resections (i.e., cholecystectomy with lymphadenectomy or hepatic wedge resections) were long-term survivors. A 64% survival rate was observed in 11 patients with mucosal or submucosal lesions in a Scandinavian series reported by Bergdahl.[27] In the same series, the longest survival among 21 patients with cancer involving all layers of the gallbladder wall was 2.5 years. The overall survival rates in American series of patients staged according to American Joint Committee on Cancer criteria were 88% for in situ cancer, 60% for stage I, 24% for stage II, 9% for stage III, and 1% for stage IV (Fig. 54-1). The role of radical surgery in the treatment of gallbladder carcinoma has been reevaluated in the surgical literature. In a series of 113 patients with gallbladder carcinoma from Germany, 67% underwent resections, 30% for cure and 37% for palliation. The median survival was 14 months after curative resection, 5.8 months after palliative resection, and 3.6 months after exploration laparotomy only, palliative operation or no operation.[28]

In another series of 2567 patients with carcinoma of the gallbladder from Japan,[22] 20.6% were treated by radical resection. The 5-year survival was 97% for stage I, 58% for stage II, 25% for stage III, and 20% for stage IV. Even patients with stage V cancers had an 11% survival rate. These results are markedly superior to any of the European and American series and cannot be explained only on the basis of extent of the surgery.

In the Mayo Clinic series,[29] 36% of 111 patients with carcinoma of the gallbladder underwent resection. Cholecystectomy was performed in 20% and radical cholecystectomy in 16%. Radical cholecystectomy included resection of adjacent liver and regional node dissection. The median survival after radical

H. J. Wanebo: Director, Division of Surgical Oncology, Brown University, Chief of Surgery, Roger Williams Medical Center, 825 Chalkstone Avenue, Providence, RI 02908.

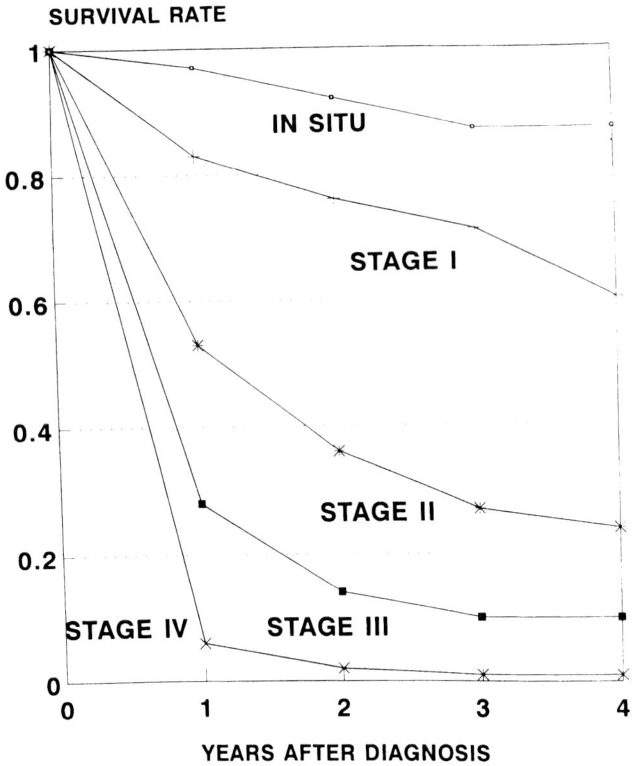

FIG. 54-1. Relative survival rates for 877 patients with gallbladder cancer according to the current American Joint Committee on Cancer staging classification. Data taken from the Surveillance, Epidemiology, and End Results Program of the National Cancer Institute for the years 1983 to 1987. Stage 0, 40 patients; stage I, 105 patients; stage II, 101 patients; stage III, 132 patients; stage IV, 499 patients. (From Beahrs OH, Henson DE, Hutter RVP, Kennedy BJ, eds. *Manual for staging of cancer.* Philadelphia: JB Lippincott, 1993:114.)

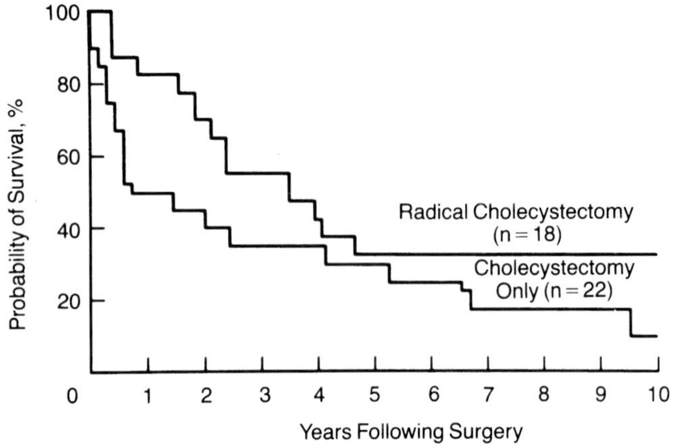

FIG. 54-2. Survival of patients with gallbladder carcinoma after curative surgery. Differences between radical resection and cholecystectomy only were not statistically significant ($P = 0.08$). (From Donohue JH, Nagorney DM, Grant CS, et al. Carcinoma of the gallbladder: does radical resection improve outcome? Arch Surg 1990;125:237, with permission.)

cholecystectomy was 3.6 years, whereas survival after simple cholecystectomy was 0.8 years. Although there was no overall difference in long-term survival, with 5-year survival rates of 33% for radical resection and 32% for cholecystectomy (Fig. 54-2), there was a significant difference in survival of patients with transmural tumor infiltration or nodal metastasis, with 29% of the patients surviving 5 years after radical cholecystectomy and no patients surviving 5 years after cholecystectomy alone (Fig. 54-3). Thus, in this study, radical cholecystectomy appeared to benefit some selected patients with carcinoma of the gallbladder.

In a study from Japan, Ogura and colleagues[30] reviewed 1686 cases of gallbladder carcinoma collected from 172 major hospitals. They found that the 3- and 5-year survival rates of 984 patients after radical resection were 66.2% and 50.7%, respectively, compared with 14.1% and 6.2%, respectively, in 702 patients after nonradical resection (Fig. 54-4). The authors recommended cholecystectomy alone in patients with tumors confined to the mucosa and more radical operations in patients with invasion beyond the mucosa. They suggested that the choice of the procedure should be defined by the extent of the tumor invasion and metastasis, with pancreaticoduodenectomy being indicated for tumors with metastases to the lymph nodes posterior to the head of the pancreas or with invasion of the duodenum, and major hepatic resection for tumors directly invading the liver.

However, Gagner and Rossi,[31] reviewing the experience with radical operations for carcinoma of the gallbladder in the United States, could not draw conclusions regarding the value of operations more extensive than simple cholecystectomy from the retrospective studies available in the literature, and suggested a randomized study comparing simple cholecystectomy to radical cholecystectomy.

Early asymptomatic carcinoma of the gallbladder found incidentally during cholecystectomy for benign disease has a substantial long-term survival rate. A Japanese study by Shirai and colleagues[32] reported a 5-year survival rate of 100% for patients with tumors confined to the mucosa or muscularis layers. Patients with tumors invading the perimuscular connective tissue,

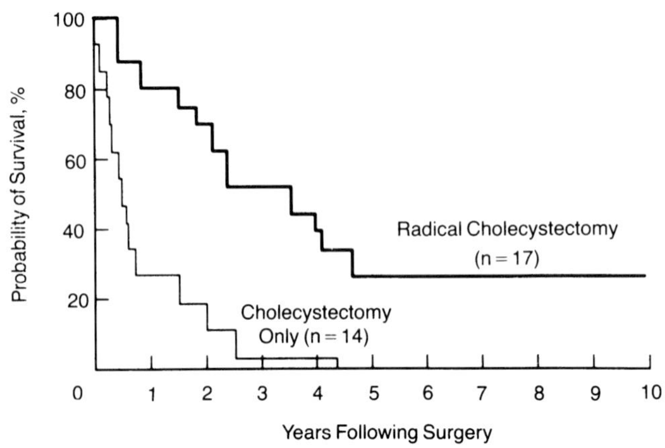

FIG. 54-3. Survival after curative resection for gallbladder carcinomas with transmural invasion or lymph node metastases. Survival after radical cholecystectomy was significantly better than after cholecystectomy only ($P < 0.001$). (From Donahue JH, Nagorney DM, Grant CS, et al. Carcinoma of the gallbladder: does radical resection improve outcome? Arch Surg 1990;125:237, with permission.)

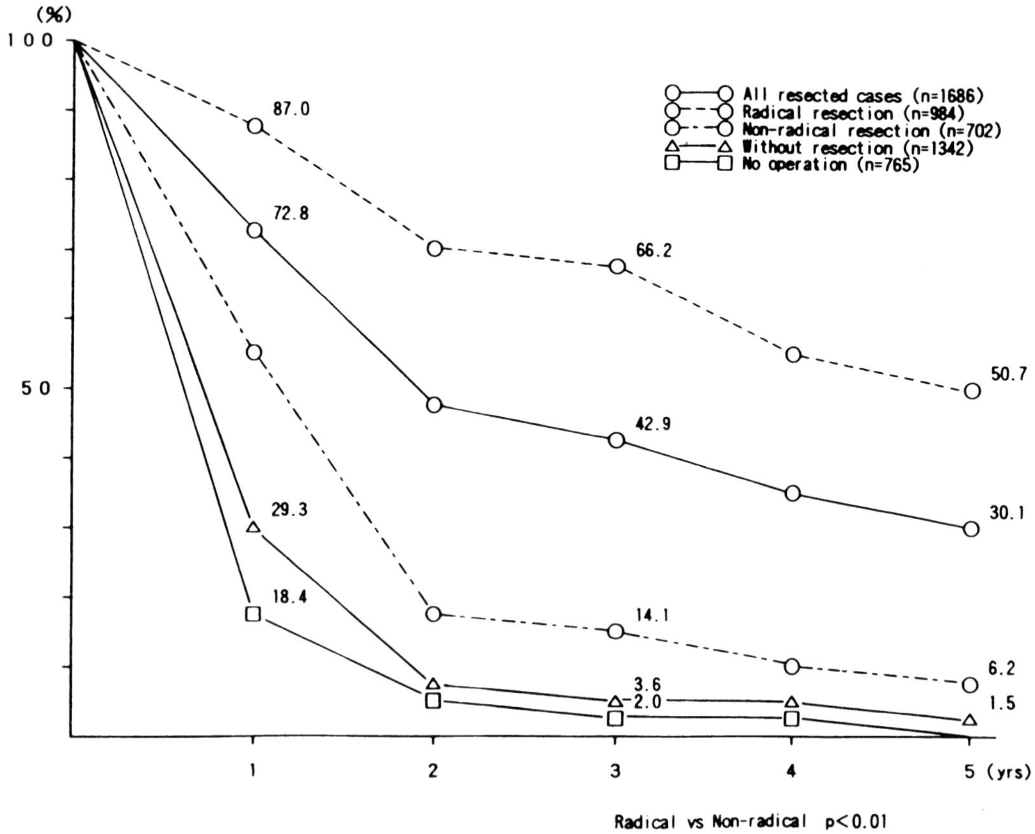

FIG. 54-4. Cumulative survival rates of gallbladder carcinoma according to treatment. Differences between radical and nonradical resections were statistically significant ($P < 0.01$). (From Ogura Y, Matsumoto V, Isaji S, et al. Radical operations for carcinoma of the gallbladder: present status in Japan. World J Surg 1991;15:337, with permission.)

without extension beyond the serosa or into the liver, had a 5-year survival rate of 40% after cholecystectomy alone and 90% after a radical second operation following the cholecystectomy, during which the inapparent carcinoma was diagnosed (Fig. 54-5).

Unfortunately, asymptomatic gallbladder carcinoma found incidentally during cholecystectomy for benign disease is a rather uncommon entity, accounting only for 5% to 10% of cases. At least 75% of patients have disease involvement beyond the scope of curative resection. However, surgery often offers the best palliation for these patients. Biliary obstruction is common and can be palliated with the use of various techniques. If the disease causes gastric or duodenal obstruction, surgical diversion is indicated. Diagnosis should be established in all patients with carcinoma of the gallbladder with proper biopsies during surgical exploration. The margins of unresectable tumors should be marked with radiopaque clips if external beam radiation therapy is being considered. Although the value of debulking by a simple cholecystectomy has not been definitely proved, this approach is recommended by some.

A large French Surgical Association study has shown survival of 20 to 22 months for T1–2 cancers, but poor survival (<7 months) for T3–4 cancers even with extended resection (Table 54-1). They did not show benefit with extended resection. Selected Japanese studies, notably Matsumoto and coworkers', have adopted an aggressive approach consisting of

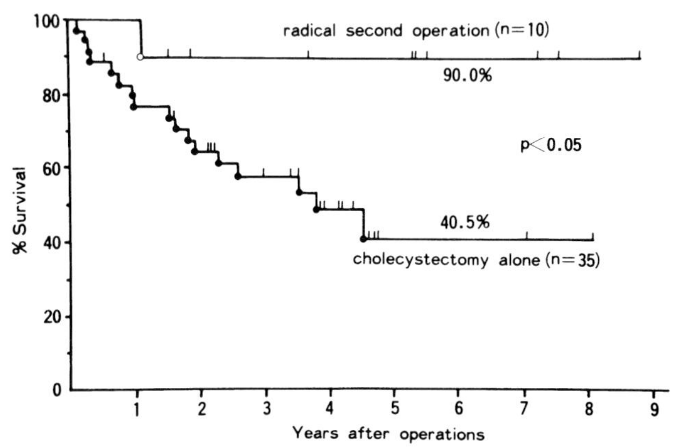

FIG. 54-5. Survival of patients with pT2 inapparent carcinoma of the gallbladder after cholecystectomy alone and cholecystectomy followed by a second radical operation. Patients after radical operations had a significantly better survival. (From Shirai Y, Yoshida K, Tsukada K, et al. Inapparent carcinoma of the gallbladder: an appraisal of a radical second operation after simple cholecystectomy. Ann Surg 1992;215:326, with permission.)

TABLE 54-1. *Recent series of resections*

Author	Pts.	Stage	Cholecystectomy	+ Hepatic resection	Billiary drainage	Exploratory laporotomy	Op mort	Survival: Med	Survival: 5 yrs
Cubertaford 1994[58]	724	T1S - 23 (4%)	23 (100%)	0	0	0	1 (4%)	>70 mos	0.93
		T1 - 20 (3%)	20 (100%)	0	9	0	1 (5%)	24 mos	0.2
		T2 - 58 (8%)	52 (88%)	0	4 (8%)	1 (2%)	1 (2%)	24 mos	0.28
		T3 - 58 (8%)	94 (41%)	13 (6%)	103 (45%)	18 (8%)	31 (13%)	24 mos	
		T4 - 390 (53%)	78 20%)	39 (10%)	102 (27%)	167 (43%)	94 (27%)	6 mos	
								3 mos	

MAJOR PROCEDURES FOR CURE
Cholecystectomy − 101
Cholecystectomy + Resection of Hepatic Bed — 35
Cholecystectomy + Resection Seg IV, V - 12
Cholecystectomy + R Hepatectomy - 5

Author	Pts.	Stage*	N	N0	N1	N2	N3	M1	Resection (%)	Survival: 2 yr DSF	Survival: Alive at
Bartlet et al, - 1994		T2	13	7	2	3	1	0	10 (77%)	60%	>3 yrs — 6
Memorial Sloan		T3	13	4	0	5	2	2	6 (46%)	83%	pts
Kettering		T4	30	3	1	12	8	18	6 (20%)	33%	>4 yrs — 5
	89	Total	58**	14	3	21	11	26	23 (40%)	61%	pts

23 pts.-Resection - Minimal liver bed
+ In dissectiontions
Trisegmentectomy - 43%
Hepatic Lobectomy - 13%
C Bile Duct Resection - 43%

35 pts.-Unresectable
Local Extha - 7
Distant Mets - 26

21 pts.-Previous Cholecystectomy
76% had residual disease/peritoneal/wound implant

Author	Pts.	Stage	Resection/ cholescystectomy: Simple	Resection/ cholescystectomy: Radical	Paliative RX	OP Mort	Survival: 1–2 yrs	Survival: 5 yrs
Oertli - 1993[59]	55	I/II - 23 (42%)	39 (62%)	2 (4%)	14 (25%)	9%	40%	7%
		III, IV - 32 (58%)						

Author	Stage	Curative Resection: T1/2	Curative Resection: T2	Op Mort	5 Yr. Survival: 1–2 yrs	5 Yr. Survival: 5 yrs
Ouchi 1993, 1994 [54,55]	(1960–78) 26	I/II 2 (8%) <30 mm 13 (50%)	8%	27%	12%	30%
	(1979–91) 25	I/II 9 (36%) <30 mm 20 (80%)	36%	76% (p < 001)	0%	60 (8%) p< 01

Author	Pts.	Stage	5 yr survivors: Yes	5 yr survivors: No	Operation	5 yr Survival vs. invasive: Mucosa	Muscularis	Subserosa	Invasive
Ouchi - BJ Surg - 8/94[55]	45	I - Mucosa	7	1	Extended Cholec - 24	100%	100%	78%	0%
		IIa - Muscularis	4	3	Simple Cholec - 19	71%	42%	0%	24%
		IIb - Submucosa	4	0	RHL - 2				
		III - Inv. serosa	0	9					
		IV - Serosa	2	10					

		Stage	Resection for cure	Survival 1–2 yrs	Survival 5 yrs
Chijiwa & Tanaka-1994[60]	48	I/II - 9 pts III - 23 Nla IV N1B/M1	63% had extended resection (cholecystectomy + hepatic bed) & LN dissection	0% >3 years	5 (56%) NED 50%

		Stage	Resection for cure	5 yr survival	Procedures		Curative	Op mort	Survival Overall	Survival Curative	Survival Non-Cure
Matsumoto - 1992[33]	48	I - 4	4	100%	Ext. cholectectomy	5	(4)		41 ± 28 mos	49 ± 25 mos	5 (0)
		II - 9	9	90%	Ext. cholec + duct ex.	25	(14)	1	22 ± 18 mos	33 ± 16 mos	8±
		III - 8	6	40%	Ext. cholec + PDR	4	(2)		19 ± 9 mos	26 ± 6 mos	
		IV - 27	9	20%	Hepatic resect + PDR	8	(4)	1	3–7 mos	1–7 mos	
					Hepatic resect + duct resect	6	(4)	(2–4%)	28 ± 20 mos	30 ± 21 mos	

		Stage	Resectable	Unresectable	Radical Resection	Survival 2 yrs	Survival 5 yrs
Nakamkura - 1994	60	IV	21	34	7 (hepato-pancreatic duodectomies - no Op depth)	29%	5.8%

		Stage		N−	N+	L+	L−	Operation (2nd)	Survival 1 yr	Survival 2 yr	Survival 3 yr
DeAretxababa - 1992[56]	54 44F/10M (Resectable) of 205 Pts	I - mucosa	7	—	—	—	—	Liver wedge IV, V + LN - 20	66%	5%	25%
		II - muscularis	9	8	—	1	7				
		II - subserosa	15	6	3	2	6	Hepatic resection - 3	19 pts died w/local recurrence/distant mets - 2–3 mos		
		III - serosa	13	2	4	5	1	+BD + LN + POR - 1			
		IV - serosa	10	0	2	2	0	LN + BD - 1			

* Invasive CA > T1 - into/through muscularis
** Two with no T
Median Survival = 8.6 mos.
Earlier Diagnosis = Better survival
N.B. - Favorable Prognostic Factors - Papillary, well differentiated tumors on mucosa, muscularis without vascular/neural invasion
Ultrasound dx - 3 of 34
Poor prognostic factor: Poorly differentiated/Age <40

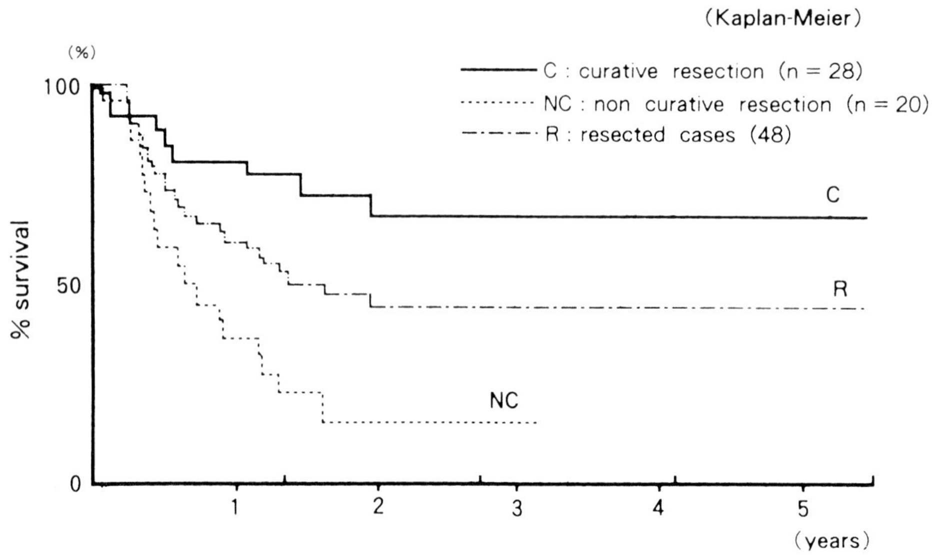

FIG. 54-6. Survival rates after resection of carcinoma of the gallbladder in 48 patients by curative and noncurative resections. (From Matsumoto Y, Fujii H, Hoyama H, et al. Surgical treatment of primary carcinoma of the gallbladder based on the histologic analysis of 48 surgical specimens. Am J Surg 1992;163:239, with permission.)

extended cholecystectomy and bile duct resection, pancreaticoduodenectomy, or hepatic resection.[33] They have achieved a survival of approximately 22 to 33 months overall with curative resection using this aggressive approach (see Table 54-1; Fig. 54-6). Their estimated 5-year survival for stage II disease was 80%, and for stage III it was about 40% (see Table 54-1; Fig. 54-7). It is not clear how many patients are actually surviving in this report. In a report presented by Bartlett[33a] from the Memorial Sloan-Kettering Cancer Center, radical resection was done in 23 of 58 patients explored without mortality. Five of these patients are alive at 4 years (see Table 54-1).

The aforementioned studies suggest that up to 20% of patients may survive with radical resection of stage II to III carcinoma of the gallbladder in the Western series, and in excess of this in the Japanese series. These data also suggest the need for additional therapy to supplement this aggressive approach.

An update of selected series (1992 to 1995) is given in Table 54-1.

Gallbladder Polyps

Polyps or small polypoid lesions in the gallbladder may be recognized by ultrasound. In the study by Edelman, 12 polyps were found in 461 cholecystectomy specimens (2% to 6%) removed laparoscopically. These lesions were shown to be adenomas, papillomas, cholesterolosis, or carcinomas. A carcinoma was identified in a 1.1-cm polyp, and two other polypoid lesions contained invasive cancer. The authors recommended an aggressive surgical approach, especially for polyps greater than 1.0 cm.[34]

A Japanese group has treated gallbladder polyps with percutaneous endoscopic polypectomy in patients who refused cholecystectomy. They inserted a cholecystoscope percutaneously into the gallbladder and removed cholesterol polyps in four patients and an adenoma in one patient. All retained a functional gallbladder postpolypectomy.[35]

In most cases, a laparoscopic cholecystectomy would seem

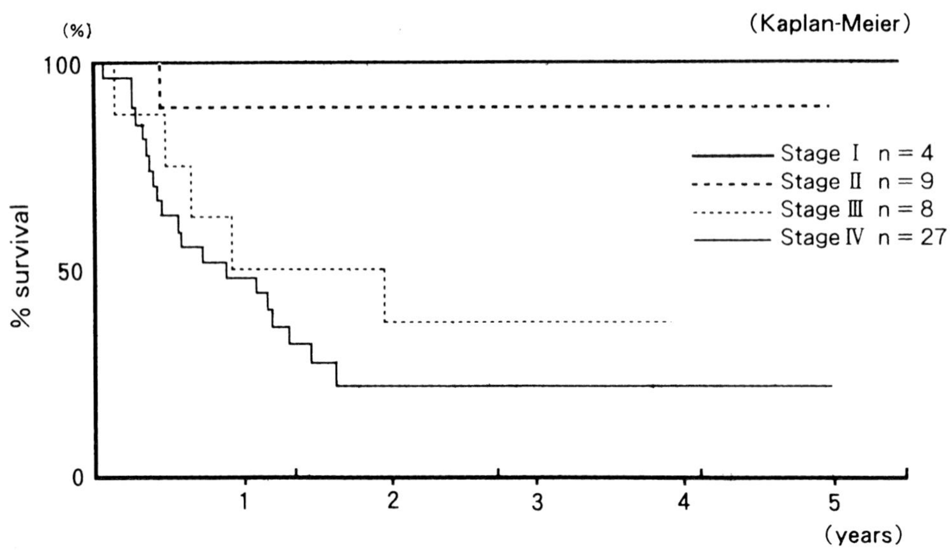

FIG. 54-7. Survival rates after resection of carcinoma of the gallbladder in 48 patients, by their stages. (From Matsumoto Y, Fujii H, Hoyama H, et al. Surgical treatment of primary carcinoma of the gallbladder based on the histologic analysis of 48 surgical specimens. Am J Surg 1992;163:239, with permission.)

to be the safest and most expeditious procedure, eliminating a target organ that is at risk for malignant transformation.

Gallbladder Cancer Discovered at Laparoscopic Cholecystectomy

The widespread use of laparoscopic cholecystectomy has uncovered a group of gallbladder cancers that hitherto usually went unrecognized and untreated by laparoscopic cholecystectomy.

The largest series thus far reported is by Fong and colleagues[36] (Table 54-2). Of their 10 cases, all had symptoms of cholelithiasis. Gallbladder surgery was suggested by imaging studies in three patients. In eight patients, cancer was suspected, and four had open laparotomy. A simple cholecystectomy was done in seven patients, the gallbladder was biopsied only in two patients, and one patient had a liver biopsy. Three patients had a radical resection within a median of 30 days (14 to 49 days), two had no evidence of disease at 5 and 13 months, and one was dead of disease at 7.1 months. The remaining seven were unresectable (two had bilobar metastases, four had intraperitoneal cancer, and one with retroperitoneal metastases had growth in the laparoscopic tract). Of another five patients reported in the literature, four had tumor implant at the port site. Our suggested management for this group of patients is "forewarned is forearmed." If the surgeon suspects gallbladder cancer, or is faced with questionable locally extensive benign disease, an open procedure should be planned. Laparoscopy with biopsy should be avoided (if the lesion is encountered laparoscopically, it is best not to sample it for biopsy it to reduce the hazard of seeding). A definitive resection as a possible gallbladder cancer should be planned. In such a case, en bloc resection of the gallbladder cancer (which can then be subjected to a careful confirmation biopsy), plus removal of nodes in the hepatoduodenal ligament and resection of segments IV and V of the liver is recommended. If the patient has locally extensive cancer or nodal metastases, postoperative radiation and chemotherapy should be given.

Technique of Radical Cholecystectomy

A better understanding of the rationale and technique of radical cholecystectomy requires knowledge of the venous and lymphatic drainage of the gallbladder as well as of the patterns of spread of gallbladder carcinoma. The venous net in the adventitia of the gallbladder wall drains either directly into the liver bed parenchyma by a number of small veins, or through a single vein into the ascending portal branch of hepatic segments V through VIII.[28,37] The gallbladder lymphatics drain first to the cystic node and the common duct nodes and then into the pancreaticoduodenal, celiac axis, and paraaortic nodes. Gallbladder carcinomas spread most commonly by direct extension and through the lymphatics. Direct extension involves adjacent structures such as liver, stomach, duodenum, pancreas, colon, omentum, and abdominal wall. Approximately 25% of 151 patients studied by Fahim and colleagues[37] had direct extension into the liver, primarily into the gallbladder bed, whereas 25% had metastases to the lymph nodes at the time of the initial surgery. At autopsy, metastases to the lymph nodes were found in 70% of the cases, whereas extension into the liver was present in 90% and involvement of the stomach, duodenum, or pancreas in 33% of the cases. Although direct extension to contiguous structures is frequent, peritoneal carcinomatosis is not common. This predominantly locoregional pattern of spread supports the assumption that radical cholecystectomy will provide long-term cure for some patients with carcinoma of the gallbladder.

For a radical cholecystectomy, we prefer an extended right or bilateral subcostal incision. After entering and exploring the abdomen, the liver is mobilized by dividing the round and falciform ligaments, and explored by careful palpation for presence of metastases. A Kocher maneuver is then performed with sharp dissection to include the peripancreatic nodes in the resection. The dissection is carried along the peripancreatic tissue to include the nodes along the celiac artery (no. 9), the hepatic artery (no. 8), the proper hepatic artery (no. 12) nodes, and the peripancreatic and retroperitoneal nodes (no. 13) (Fig. 54-8). Dissection is then carried along the entire length of the extrahepatic bile duct; the cystic duct is identified, dissected free at its junction

TABLE 54-2. *Gall bladder cancer, removed laparoscopically*

	Laparoscopic finding		
Pts.	Type	Stage	Surgical findings/Therapy
1	G.B.	polypoid	Intrahepatic Mets - → Radical Resection IV, V, Hepatic duodenal lig.[61]
2	G.B.	Benign Disease	Recur. Umbilical Port Site (21 d) (Peritoneal Tumor Implaint) Resected Port Site[62]
1	G.B.	Colecystitis	Tumor Implant Port Site and Liver Bed Resected G.B. Bed, laparoscopic scar - radiotherapy[63]
1	G.B.	Benign Disease	Umbilical Port Implant Recommend removal via nonporous bag[64]
10	G.B. cancers	Discovered laparoscopically	3 CA suspected by preop xray 8 had suspected CA and 4 had open procedure 7 pts. - simple cholecystectomy; 2 had biopsy, 1 had liver biopsy 3 pts. had radical resection; 2 NED - 5, 13 mos. - 1 DOD - 7 mos. 1 pt. Unresected; 2 liver mets, 5 intraretroperitoneal mets (2 port site)[36]

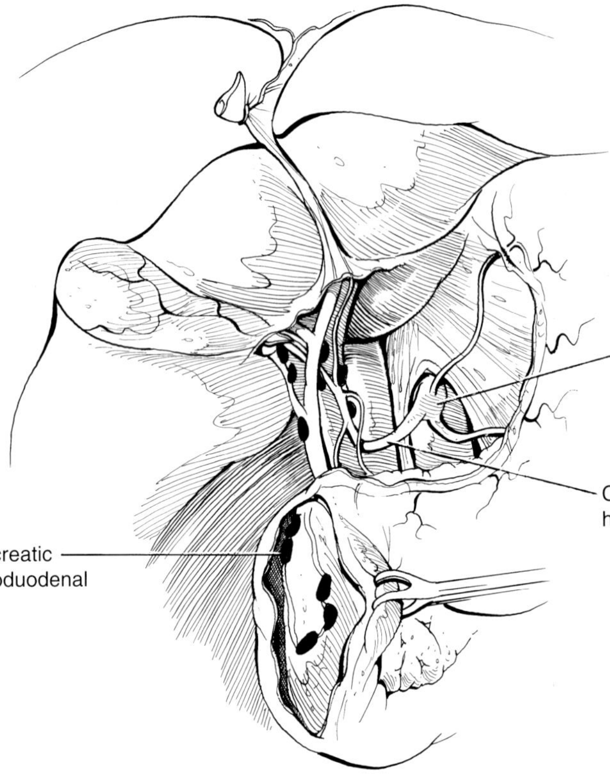

FIG. 54-8. Radical cholecystectomy. Lymphatic drainage of the gallbladder is shown. Lymph node dissection should include the celiac artery (no. 9), common hepatic artery (no. 8), gastroduodenal left proper hepatic artery (no. 12), and peripancreatic and retroduodenal nodes (no. 13).

to the common bile duct, and doubly ligated and divided. Dissection continues toward the porta hepatis and the cystic artery is identified, dissected free, and doubly ligated and divided. The areolar tissue and lymphatics of the triangle of Calot are dissected free of the bile duct to be included in the resection. Dissection is carried along the portal vein and the dissected tissue is left attached to the gallbladder to be removed in continuity with the final resection specimen (Fig. 54-9). The cystic duct node is included in the resection. If this node is grossly positive, the bile duct should be resected up to the bifurcation of the common bile duct or higher; reconstruction can be done with a Roux-en-Y choledochojejunostomy. The surgeon can access this area by elevating the ''hilar plate of Couinaud''. The fascial tissue separating the liver from the hepatic ducts and vessels can be incised allowing access to the hilar structures, in particular the right hepatic duct and right hepatic artery. Dissection continues along the porta structure into the base of the liver (about 4 cm), which will be the deep margin. Resection of the liver surrounding the gallbladder bed is started. The capsule of the anterior surface of the liver is divided using electrocoagulation, and dissection is then carried through the hepatic parenchyma. Blood vessels and intrahepatic biliary structures are controlled with clips or ligatures. A margin of normal hepatic parenchyma, preferably 3 to 4 cm, should be included in the specimen. Intraoperative ultrasonography is helpful in defining the extent of the tumor and its relation to major intrahepatic vessels. The dissection of the parenchyma is carried down to the level of the hepatic hilum, as described (Fig. 54-10). The right hepatic artery, right branch of the portal vein, and right hepatic duct are identified and preserved unless involved. If these structures are involved, a formal right hepatic lobectomy is warranted pending the medical status of the patient. The specimen containing the gallbladder with the surrounding liver parenchyma and the regional lymphatic tissue is removed. The hepatoduodenal nodes are dissected beginning at the celiac axis (no. 9), and then removing nodes at the common hepatic artery (no. 8) and the retroduodenal peripancreatic nodes (no. 13), to

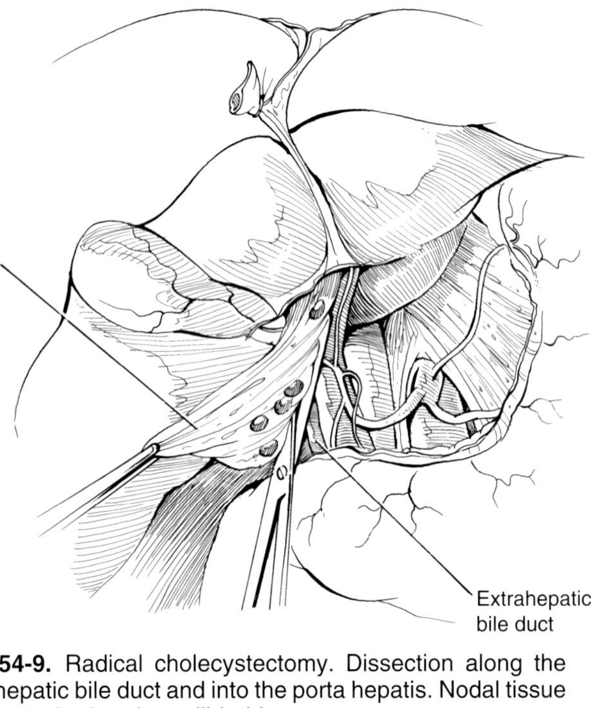

FIG. 54-9. Radical cholecystectomy. Dissection along the extrahepatic bile duct and into the porta hepatis. Nodal tissue is left attached to the gallbladder.

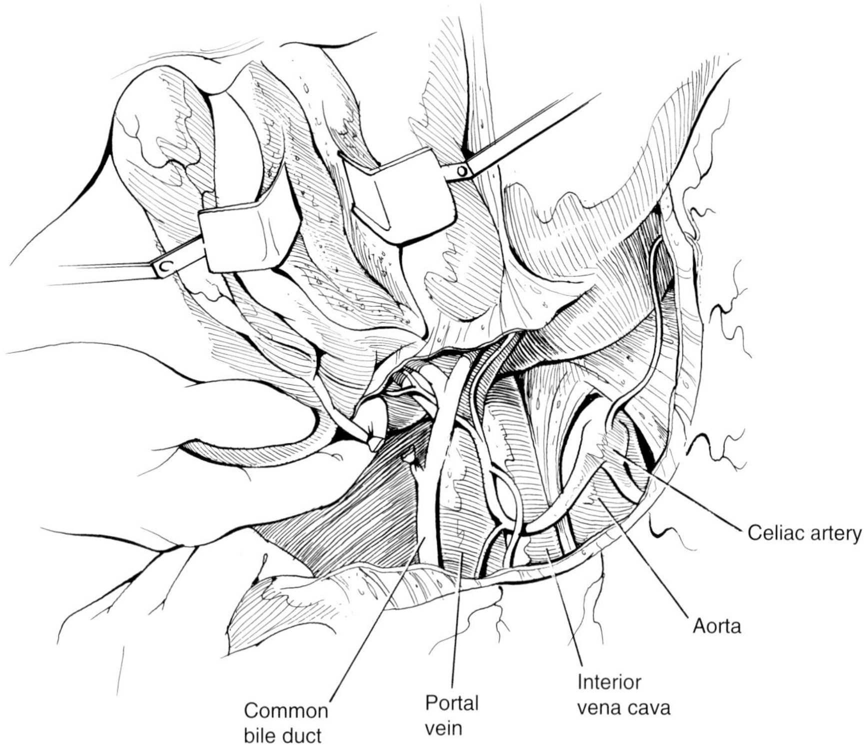

A

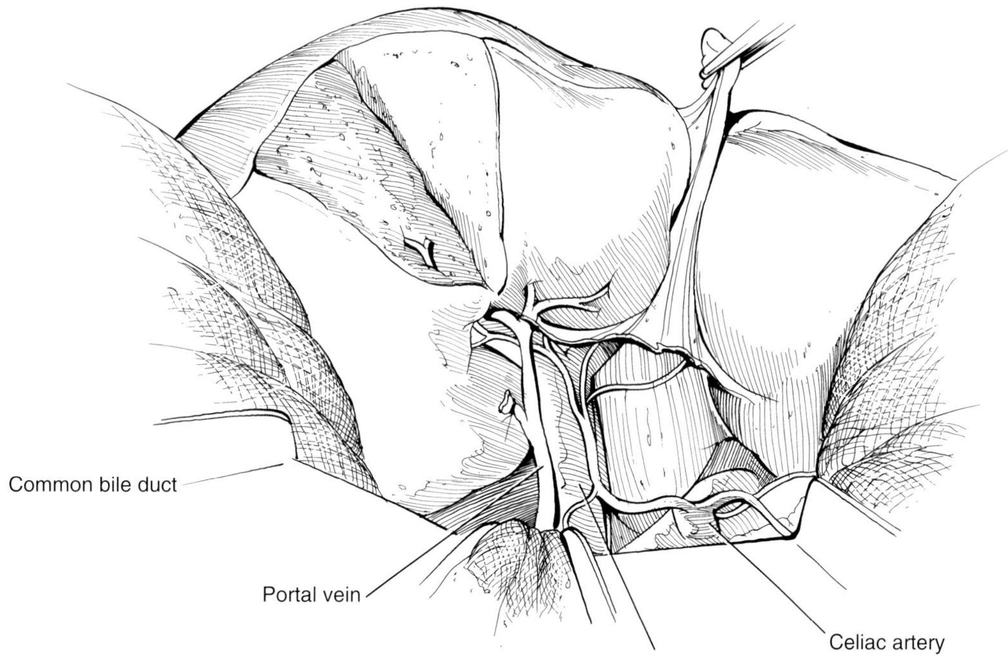

B

FIG. 54-10. Radical cholecystectomy. Resection of the liver parenchyma surrounding the gallbladder bed. This is accessed by resecting the liver tissue overlying the right hepatic duct and right hepatic artery **(A)** and extending the resection to include the full width of the gallbladder bed (segment IVB and V) **(B)**. Depth of liver tissue is approximately 4 cm.

the nodes along the hepatic artery proper (no. 12). The postero-superior pancreaticoduodenal and distal common duct nodes are then dissected from the posterior aspect of the head of the pancreas and the portal vein. Dissection continues along the portal vein and the hepatic artery to the level of the common hepatic artery origin. A closed suction drain is placed in the area of the liver transection after meticulous homeostasis and complete control of transected small biliary oradicles, and brought out through a separate small incision on the abdominal wall. The main incision is closed in layers. Although radical cholecystectomy is a straightforward procedure, it requires an in-depth knowledge of the anatomic variations of the vascular and biliary structures, which are quite common. Clear identification and preservation of the main vascular and biliary structures is of paramount importance in the performance of a safe, uncomplicated procedure.

RADIATION THERAPY

The limitations of surgery in adequately encompassing all resectable tumor in most patients become apparent from the pattern of failure after resection for carcinoma of the gallbladder.[38,39] Local recurrence is a common cause of death in patients who relapse after cholecystectomy.[38] In Kopelson and associates' review, local recurrence was present or was the cause of death of 86% of 110 patients who died within 5 years after simple cholecystectomy for gallbladder cancer.[38]

Radiation treatment data for gallbladder cancer are sparse. In a series of 51 patients treated at the Princess Margaret Hospital in Toronto with doses ranging from an average of 2600 cGy for palliation to 4000 cGy for curative intent, survival was stated to be significantly longer in patients receiving postoperative radiation therapy compared with those who had surgery alone.[40] Similar impressions of survival benefit with radiation were reported by other investigators, but the numbers are small.[38,41,42] In a retrospective review, the median survival of patients receiving postoperative radiation was 63 months, compared with 29 months in patients having surgery only. Prospective trials of adjuvant radiation therapy for gallbladder carcinoma have not been reported, and it is obvious that such trials are clearly needed.

The limited tolerance of the normal tissues surrounding the gallbladder to external beam radiation led to the introduction of intraoperative radiation. This technique enables the delivery of a large dose of radiation to the exact area of the tumor, while adjacent radiosensitive structures are retracted from the field. Intraoperative radiation can also be used as a boost to external beam radiation therapy. Preliminary reports indicate that the use of intraoperative radiation therapy may play a role in the curative and palliative management of gallbladder carcinoma.[43,44] In a series from Japan, 27 of 86 patients with stage IV carcinoma of the gallbladder underwent tumor resection. Of these, 17 received intraoperative radiation therapy with or without postoperative external beam radiation, 1 received postoperative external beam radiation, and 9 had resection only. The 3-year cumulative survival rate was 10.1% after resection plus intraoperative radiation, compared with 0% after resection alone[43] (Fig. 54-11). Although these results appear quite promising, further trials are necessary to establish firmly the efficacy of this treatment modality.

CHEMOTHERAPY

The infrequent occurrence of biliary cancer has limited the evaluation of its response to chemotherapy agents. Several drugs beneficial in other upper gastrointestinal malignancies have apparent single-agent activity in biliary cancer. Durations of response, however, have been very short, in the order of weeks.

The most commonly reported drug has been 5-fluorouracil. Bolus 5-fluorouracil has been reported to produce response rates ranging from 10% to 24%.[45,46] Other drugs with reported single-agent activity are mitomycin-C, doxorubicin, and the nitrosoureas, but the patient numbers are too small to draw reliable conclusions.[47–51] The available data on combination regimens are not sufficient to support reliable therapeutic decisions, and further trials in this direction are necessary.

Although regional chemotherapy has a reasonable rationale, based on anatomic considerations, it has not been adequately studied.[52,53] Adequate trials of adjuvant chemotherapy in gallbladder cancer have not been performed. In a small study of patients with gallbladder carcinoma, Oswalt and Cruz[53] re-

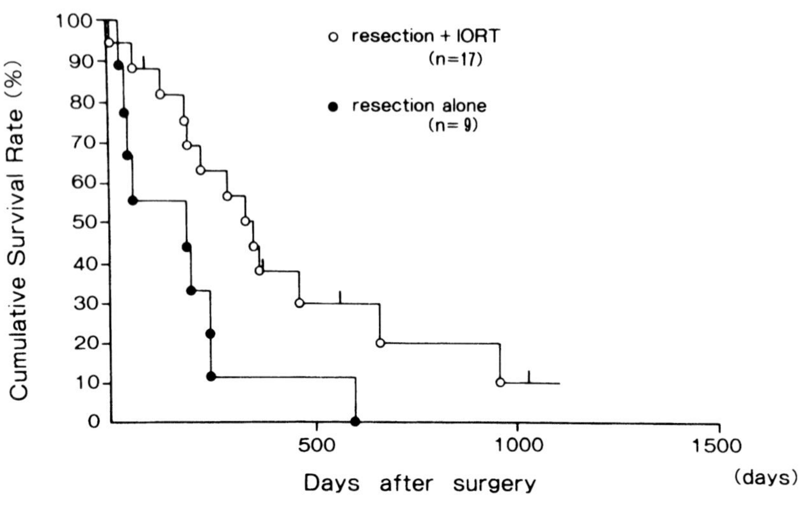

FIG. 54-11. Cumulative survival curves (Kaplan-Meier) for stage IV (TNM) carcinoma of the gallbladder. Comparison between resection alone and resection plus intraoperative radiation. Difference between the two curves was significant by the generalized Wicoxon test ($P < 0.05$). (From Todoroki T, Iwasaki Y, Orii K, et al. Resection combined with intraoperative radiation therapy [IORT] for stage IV [TNM] gallbladder carcinoma. World J Surg 1991;15:357, with permission.)

TABLE 54-3. *Other therapies*

Author	Pts.	Treatment	Median survival			Median survival		Chemo discontinued		
			Response	Responders	Non-responders	MMC	Historic controls	Progression	Toxicity	Other
Makela, NT & Kairaluoma - 1993	27	Superselective infusion of Mitomycin (MMC) Compared to 22 historic Controls	48%	14 mos	8 mos	14 mos	4 mos	8	7	1
			Pts. with tumor invasion > serosa—dead within 4 years							
			Chemo treatment with MMD—of value if CA restricted to gallbladder wall							

		Treatment	Eligible	Complete Protocol	Median F/U	Survival
Wolkov 1992 RTOG-8506	23	Intraoperative Radiation of Extra Hepatic Billiary Carcinoma Locally advanced billiary duct cancer - entered Phase I/II protocol Bulk of disease - important determinant of outcome	16	8	10.5 mos	2/8 >10 mos 6 dead - persistent/ recurrent tumor

ported a median survival of 20 weeks in 13 patients treated adjuvantly, compared to 8 weeks in nontreated patients. In the University of Minnesota series, 38 patients treated with chemotherapy or radiation had a median survival of 4.5 months, compared with a median survival of 3 months in a group of 14 patients treated with surgery alone ($P < 0.001$).[17] Clearly, well designed, randomized trails of adjuvant therapy for gallbladder carcinoma are urgently needed. Regional infusion with mitomycin-C has been studied by Makela and Kairaluoma[51]; the median survival was 14 months in the resected group versus 4 months in the histologic control group. There were no survivors who had serosal invasion. The chemotherapy protocol was not deemed successful and was discontinued (Table 54-3).

AN OPTIMAL APPROACH TO MANAGEMENT

The optimal surgical approach for carcinoma of the gallbladder has not been determined from any published clinical trial data, and, considering the infrequency of this cancer, it is unlikely that such data will be forthcoming in the near future.[54,55] Recommendations can be made on the basis of results of some of the larger clinical series. An important element in cancer management is knowledge of its pattern of spread. The major route of spread of gallbladder cancer appears to be locoregional rather than distant. Direct extension to the liver is common, with frequent spread to cystic, common duct, and retroduodenal and peripancreatic nodes.

A logical surgical approach would consist of total removal of the gallbladder, the underlying liver, and a dissection of the draining lymphatics as previously described. In the series reported by deAretxabalb and coworkers, these nodes were involved by cancer in about one third of the cases.[56] A right hepatic lobectomy is probably unnecessary in most cases, although it may make sense in selected patients because of clinical or anatomic considerations.

The surgeon should have a high index of suspicion for gallbladder cancer in selected cases, that is, the older patient with stones or a very thick-walled or calcified gallbladder.[57] If cancer is suspected, a small biopsy should be obtained before dissection of the gallbladder. This would prevent the unnecessary spillage of tumor cells that invariably occurs if a cholecystectomy is done and the carcinomatous communication between gallbladder and liver is disrupted. Tumor spillage may account for the frequent rapid dissemination of this disease in many patients after cholecystectomy.

In the event that a cholecystectomy was done for a clinically occult lesion, a reexploration with resection of the gallbladder bed and lymph node dissection should be considered for lesions invading beyond the mucosa. In the medically high-risk patient, the clinician could consider observation only for cancer limited to the mucosa or submucosa and radiation plus chemotherapy for lesions invading all layers, if the patient can tolerate this treatment. If a major resection is planned, a reasonable approach would be to resect a wedge of 3 to 4 cm of liver underlying the gallbladder bed along the gallbladder, if not previously resected, and a node dissection. Biopsy specimens of strategic areas in the resection site should be taken to ensure that the margins are clear. If all margins are clear, the nodes are negative, and the lesion seems confined to the gallbladder only, the clinician might observe the patient, obtaining frequent computed tomography scans. If the nodes are positive, the margins are positive, or the disease truly extends into the liver, postoperative radiation and chemotherapy would be indicated. The placement of radiopaque clips would facilitate radiation planning.

REFERENCES

1. Piehler JM, Crichlow RW. Primary carcinoma of the gallbladder. Surg Gynecol Obstet 1978;147:929.
2. Hamrick RE, Liner J, Hastings PR, et al. Primary carcinoma of the gallbladder. Ann Surg 1982;195:270.
3. Adson MA. Carcinoma of the gallbladder. Surg Clin North Am 1973; 53:1203.
4. Beltz WR, Condon RE. Primary carcinoma of the gallbladder. Ann Surg 1974;180:180.

5. Bossart PA, Patterson AH, Zintel HA. Carcinoma of the gallbladder: a report of seventy-six cases. Am J Surg 1962;103:366.
6. Chandler JJ, Fletcher WS. A clinical study of primary carcinoma of the gallbladder. Surg Gynecol Obstet 1963;117:297.
7. Donaldson LA, Busuttil A. A clinicopathological review of 68 carcinomas of the gallbladder. Br J Surg 1975;62:26.
8. Keill RH, DeWeese MS. Primary carcinoma of the gallbladder. Am J Surg 1973;125:726.
9. Litwin MS. Primary carcinoma of the gallbladder: a review of 78 patients. Arch Surg 1967;95:236.
10. Moossa AR, Anagnost M, Hall AW, et al. The continuing challenge of gallbladder cancer: survey of thirty years' experience at the University of Chicago. Am J Surg 1975;130:57.
11. Nevin JE, Moran TJ, Kay S, et al. Carcinoma of the gallbladder. Cancer 1976;37:141.
12. Robertson WA, Carlisle BB. Primary carcinoma of the gallbladder: review of fifty-two cases. Am J Surg 1967;113:738.
13. Thorbjarnarson B, Glenn F. Carcinoma of the gallbladder. Cancer 1959; 12:1009.
14. Vaittinen E. Carcinoma of the gallbladder: a study of 390 cases diagnosed in Finland 1953-1967. Ann Chir Gynaecol (Suppl) 1970;168:7.
15. Wanebo HJ, Castle WN, Fechner RE. Is carcinoma of the gallbladder a curable lesion? Ann Surg 1982;195:624.
16. Barr LH, Wright FH. Carcinoma of the gallbladder. Am Surg 1984; 50:275.
17. Morrow CE, Sutherland DE, Florack G, et al. Primary gallbladder carcinoma: significance of subserosal lesions and results of aggressive surgical treatment and adjuvant chemotherapy. Surgery 1983;94:709.
18. Friedman RB, Anderson RE, Gilchrist KW, et al. Prognostic factors in invasive gallbladder carcinoma. J Surg Oncol 1983;23:189.
19. Klamer TW, Max MH. Carcinoma of the gallbladder. Surg Gynecol Obstet 1983;156:641.
20. Dunbar LL, Adkins RB, Farringer J, et al. Carcinoma of the gallbladder and bile ducts: a retrospective review. Am Surg 1983;49:94.
21. Nagashima H, Watanabe A, Hayashi S, et al. Primary carcinoma of the gallbladder and the extrahepatic bile duct. Gastroenterology 1982; 17:246.
22. Tashiro S, Konno T, Mochinaga M, et al. Treatment of carcinoma of the gallbladder in Japan. Jpn J Surg 1982;12:98.
23. Albores-Saavedra J, Cruz-Ortiz H, Alcantra-Vazquez A, et al. Unusual types of gallbladder carcinoma: a report of 16 cases. Arch Pathol Lab Med 1981;105:287.
24. Koo J, Wong J, Cheng FC, et al. Carcinoma of the gallbladder. Br J Surg 1981;68:161.
25. Evander A, Ihse I. Evaluation of intended radical surgery in carcinoma of the gallbladder. Br J Surg 1981;68:158.
26. Gupta S, Udupa KN, Gupta S. Primary carcinoma of the gallbladder: a review of 328 cases. J Surg Oncol 1980;14:35.
27. Bergdahl L. Gallbladder carcinoma first diagnosed at microscopic examination of gallbladder removed for presumed benign disease. Ann Surg 1980;191:19.
28. Gall FP, Kockerling F, Scheele J, et al. Radical operations for carcinoma of the gallbladder: present status in Germany. World J Surg 1991; 15:328.
29. Donohue JH, Nagorney DM, Grant CS, et al. Carcinoma of the gallbladder: does radical resection improve outcome? Arch Surg 1990;125: 237.
30. Ogura Y, Matsumoto Y, Isaji S, et al. Radical operations for carcinoma of the gallbladder: present status in Japan. World J Surg 1991;15:337.
31. Gagner M, Rossi R. Radical operations for carcinoma of the gallbladder: present study in North America. World J Surg 1991;15:344.
32. Shirai Y, Yoshida K, Tsukada K, et al. Inapparent carcinoma of the gallbladder: an appraisal of a radical second operation after simple cholecystectomy. Ann Surg 1992;215:326.
33. Matsumoto Y, Fujii H, Hoyama H, et al. Surgical treatment of primary carcinoma of gallbladder based on histologic examination of 48 surgical specimens. Am J Surg 1992;163:239.
33a. Bartlett A, et al. Surgical resection of gall bladder cancer (abstract). Presentation to Society of Surgical Oncology, March 1996.
34. Edelman DS. Carcinoma of a gallbladder polyp: treated by laparoscopic laser cholecystectomy. Surg Laparosc Endosc 1993;3:142.
35. Ji ZL, Chen HR, Wang EH, et al. Percutaneous endoscopic polypectomy of gallbladder polyps. Endoscopy 1994;26:609.
36. Fong Y, Brennan MF, Turnbull A, Colt DG, Blumgart LH. Gallbladder cancer discovered during laparoscopic surgery. Arch Surg 1993;128: 1054.
37. Fahim RB, McDonald JR, Richard JC, et al. Carcinoma of the gallbladder: a study of its modes of spread. Ann Surg 1962;156:114.
38. Kopelson G, Harisiadis L, Tretter P, et al. The role of radiation therapy in cancer of the extra-hepatic biliary system: an analysis of thirteen patients and a review of the literature of the effectiveness of surgery, chemotherapy and radiotherapy. Int J Radiat Oncol Biol Phys 1977;2: 883.
39. Nagashima H, Watanabe A, Hayashi S, et al. Primary carcinoma of the gallbladder and the extrahepatic bile duct. Gastroenterology 1982; 17:246.
40. Hanna SS, Ride WD. Carcinoma of the gallbladder or extrahepatic bile ducts: the role of radiotherapy. Can Med Assoc J 1978;118:59.
41. Pilepich MV. Radiotherapy in carcinoma of the gallbladder. In: Wanebo HJ, ed. Hepatic and biliary cancer. New York: Marcel Dekker, 1978:447.
42. Treadwell TA, Harding WJ. Primary carcinoma of the gallbladder: the role of adjunctive therapy in its treatment. Am J Surg 1976;132:703.
43. Todoroki T, Iwasaki Y, Orii K, et al. Resection combined with intraoperative radiation therapy (IORT) for stage IV (TNM) gallbladder carcinoma. World J Surg 1991;15:356.
44. Busse PM, Cady B, Bothe A Jr, et al. Intraoperative radiation therapy for carcinoma of the gallbladder. World J Surg 1991;15:352.
45. Haskell CM. Cancer of the liver. In: Haskell CM, ed. Cancer treatment. Philadelphia: WB Saunders, 1980:319.
46. Falkson G, MacIntyre JM, Moertel CG. Eastern Cooperative Oncology Group experience with chemotherapy for inoperable gallbladder and bile duct cancer. Cancer 1984;54:965.
47. Crooke ST, Bradner WT. Mitomycin-C: a review. Cancer Treat Rev 1976;3:121.
48. vonEyben F, Hellekant C, Mattson M, et al. Mitomycin-C in advanced gallbladder carcinoma. Acta Radiol (Oncol) 1980;19:81.
49. Adolphson CC, Carpenter JT Jr. Response to doxorubicin and mitomycin in cholangiocarcinoma: a case report. Cancer Treat Rep 1982;66: 209.
50. Misra NC, Jaiswal MSD, Singh RV, et al. Intrahepatic arterial infusion of combination mitomycin-C and 5-fluorouracil in treatment of primary and metastatic liver carcinoma. Cancer 1977;39:1425.
51. Makela JT, Kairaluoma MI. Superselective intrahepatic chemotherapy with mitomycin C for gallbladder cancer. Br J Surg 1993;80:912.
52. Schmeck HJ, Bartels E, Viets, Arnold W. Intraduktale Chemotherapie eines Gallengangskarzinoms mit 5-Fluorouracil. Klin Wochenschr 1986;64:713.
53. Oswalt CE, Cruz AB. Effectiveness of chemotherapy in addition to surgery in treating carcinoma of the gallbladder. Rev Surg 1977;34: 436.
54. Ouchi K, Suzuki N, Saijo S. Do recent advances in diagnosis and operative management improve the outcome of gallbladder cancer? Surgery 1993;113:324.
55. Ouchi K, Suzuki S, Konno H, et al. Survival after surgery for carcinoma of the gallbladder. Br J Surg 1994;81:1655.
56. deAretxabalb X, Roa I, Burgos L. Gallbladder cancer in Chile: report on 54 potentially resectable tumors. Cancer 1992;69:60.
57. Polk HC. Carcinoma of the calcified gallbladder. Gastroenterology 1966;50:582.
58. Cubertaford P, Gainart A, Cucchiaró G. Surgical treatment of 724 carcinomas of the gallbladder. Results of the French Surgical Association Survey. Ann Surg 1994;219(3):275.
59. Oertli D, Herzog U, Tondell P. Primary carcinoma of the gallbladder: operative experience during a 16-year period. Eur J Surg 1993;159: 415.
60. Chijiwa K, Tanaka M. Carcinoma of the gallbladder: an appraisal of surgical resection. Surgery 1994;115:756.
61. Nishizaki T, Matsumata T, Hashizwme M, Maeda T, Otsuka K, Sugimachi K. Hepatic metastasis after laparoscopic cholecystectomy for polypoid gallbladder cancer following radical surgery. Surg Endos 1994;8:1436.
62. Wade TP, Comitalo JB, Andrusch, Godwin MN, Kamionski DL. Laparoscopic cancer surgery. Lesser form gallbladder surgery. Surg Endos 1994;8:698.
63. Kim HJ, Roy T. Unexpected gallbladder cancer with cutaneous surgery after laparoscopic cholecystectomy. South Med J 1994;87:817.
64. Nally L, Preshaw RM. Tumor implantation at umbilicus after laparoscopic cholecystectomy for unsuspected gallbladder carcinoma. Can J Surg 1994;37:243.

Surgery for Gastrointestinal Cancer: A Multidisciplinary Approach, edited by Harold J. Wanebo.
Lippincott-Raven Publishers, Philadelphia, © 1997.

CHAPTER 55

Treatment of the Patient With Hepatocellular Carcinoma

Brian I. Carr

The treatment of the patient with hepatocellular carcinoma (HCC) is driven is large part by an understanding of the biology and pathobiology of the disease. Some of the more important biologic principles are discussed in this chapter and form the basis for the therapeutic approach.

BIOLOGY OF HUMAN HEPATOCELLULAR CARCINOMA

Hepatocellular carcinoma is often a multifocal disease. Chronic dietary exposure of rats to a variety of hepatic carcinogens induces multilobar, multiple HCCs. The human cirrhotic liver contains vast numbers of cirrhotic nodules, any or all of which are putatively precursors of neoplastic transformation. Multiple tumors in humans have been shown to be independent clones of transformation by such means as hepatitis B virus integration patterns, showing that each malignant nodule appears to be an independent clone.[1]

HCC initially spreads throughout the liver. These tumors, particularly the larger ones, commonly are associated with satellite lesions. Whether HCC spreads directly or through the vasculature is unclear. However, a pathognomonic hallmark of the disease is vascular invasion, particularly portal venous infiltration. This can be discerned histologically on biopsy samples or resected specimens as HCC tumor cells infiltrating the walls of portal venous radicals or causing microthrombi, or macroscopically as portal venous thrombi on computed tomographic (CT) scan of the liver. Vascular invasion, together with tumor multifocality, is the strongest adverse prognostic factor for recurrence after resection, and especially after liver transplantation. Portal venous invasion must occur at an early stage, because it has been detected in HCCs smaller than 2 cm in diameter.[2] Particularly in the presence of cirrhosis with portal systemic shunting, this provides an obvious channel for systemic tumor dissemination.

Department of Surgery/Liver Transplant, University of Pittsburgh, Biomedical Science Tower, E1552, 200 Lothrop Street, Pittsburgh, PA 15213.

HCC is a systemic, blood-borne disease. Liver transplantation held the promise of being able to cure patients with unresectable HCC. However, disappointingly high recurrence rates in the transplanted liver and other organs after liver transplantation for apparent cure,[3–6] in spite of apparently negative metastatic work-up, has led to reevaluation of the clinical staging approach for HCC. As is true for breast and other cancers, our current ability to clinically stage HCC provides an underestimate of the extent of microscopic tumor invasion and tumor metastases. The most common forms of tumor spread are into the residual liver after resection or the new liver after transplantation; into the lungs, peritoneum, and osseous skeleton; and, less frequently, into the adrenals, brain, spleen, and other organs. In addition, direct evidence of hematogenous metastases has been provided by the finding of circulating cells in the bloodstream that have albumin messenger RNA, which is characteristic of hepatocellular origin.[7] Clinical evidence of recurrence in distant organs after liver transplantation and direct evidence of circulating tumor cells indicate that advanced stage HCC spreads hematogenously, and possibly at early stages.

HCC is relatively resistant to toxic chemotherapy and ionizing radiation. Many studies in the United States and Asia show that neither single nor combinations of cancer chemotherapeutic agents given by the standard intravenous route yield reproducible response rates in excess of 20%.[8] These agents which are thus of little benefit, include doxorubicin (Adriamycin), 5-fluorouracil, cisplatin, mitomycin C, *Vinca* alkaloids, and VP16. However the same agents when given into the hepatic artery produce a wide range of reported response rates, varying from 20% to 60%.[8] This probably is a result of the much higher drug concentrations that can be achieved with administration into the hepatic artery, which feeds most HCCs. This approach also takes advantage of the fact that the liver has a dual blood supply, in which the portal vein supplies about 80% of the oxygenated blood to the normal liver, whereas the hepatic artery provides about the same percentage to the tumor. Considerable cytotoxic chemotherapy can be administered to the tumor without the same level of damage to the normal liver. The concomitant use of some form of hepatic artery occlusion or embolization, with polyvinyl alcohol, starch, blood clot, gelatin sponge, microcapsules, steel coils, or simple physical obstruction, has been thought to enhance these objective response rates, although few convincing randomized studies have compared hepatic intraarterial chemotherapy with or without arterial occlusion.

The disadvantages of chemotherapy for HCC include potential damage to the underlying liver. Unlike most other human cancers, in which the tumor arises in an otherwise healthy body, HCC usually develops in a fundamentally diseased major organ. About 80% to 90% of all human HCCs in Asia and sub-Saharan Africa, and at least 50% of those in the United States, arise in association with chronic hepatitis or cirrhosis caused by long-term damage from hepatitis B or C virus, alcohol abuse, or, in Asia and Africa, dietary exposure to carcinogens (eg, aflatoxin B_1, sterigmatocystin, *N*-nitroso compounds, pyrrolizidine alkaloids). This imposes certain constraints on the use of cytotoxic chemotherapy, because the underlying liver often is damaged, and xenobiotic metabolism may be impaired, resulting in longer half-lives of the chemotherapeutic agents with enhanced systemic toxicities. Alternatively, the chemotherapy may enhance the damage to an already damaged liver, causing hepatic decompensation. No tests have proven useful in predicting the safety of chemotherapy or hepatic resection, including the indocyanine green clearance test, liver function tests, or measurements of liver size. However, hepatic intraarterial chemotherapy usually is safe when the bilirubin level is less than 2 mg/dL and the prothrombin time is less than 15 seconds. A rise of bilirubin greater than 3 mg/dL after any cycle of chemotherapy is normally a warning sign to not increase the dose of chemotherapy on subsequent cycles and to proceed with great caution even with the same dose. Because of the unpredictability of hepatic decompensation, this author uses 50% of the calculated dosage for the first cycle of treatment and increases the dosage by 25% increments for subsequent cycles, allowing each patient to act as his or her own hepatic tolerance control. In the event of sudden changes in the results of liver function tests, the dosage can be decreased or the treatment discontinued, forestalling irreversible hepatic decompensation.

The most specific blood tumor marker for HCC is α-fetoprotein. In one series, α-fetoprotein levels were elevated (greater than 20 ng/mL) in 49% of 450 patients with HCC. Because half of all patients with HCC do not have elevated α-fetoprotein levels, a normal value does not exclude the diagnosis. There was no clear relation between α-fetoprotein level and tumor size, although some of the largest tumors (greater than 20 cm in diameter) were associated with some of the highest levels (above 100,000 ng/mL). Patients with α-fetoprotein levels of 1 million had short survival times. The α-fetoprotein level remains the most useful screening test, together with twice-yearly hepatic ultrasound, in patients at high risk for the development of HCC, such as those with chronic hepatitis B or C virus infection, or those with cirrhosis who have a sudden change in the results of their liver function tests. In the last 15 years, the measurement of blood des-gamma-carboxy prothrombin (DCP or PIVKA-2), using an assay kit produced by the Eisai Company of Tokyo, Japan, has gained acceptance as a major supplement to α-fetoprotein determinations.[9,10] DCP levels are elevated (greater than 200 ng/mL) in more than 80% of patients with HCC, but are less specific than α-fetoprotein levels because they also are elevated in patients with hepatic failure, vitamin K dietary deficiency, warfarin (Coumadin) therapy, and obstructive jaundice. DCP is an immature form of prothrombin that is undercarboxylated and is secreted by HCCs. The tumors have a defect in the activity of the vitamin K–dependent prothrombin carboxylase, an enzyme necessary for the addition of amino-terminal carboxyl groups to prothrombin protein, which is required for the calcium-binding and coagulant functions of prothrombin. Evidence from patients with progressive liver disease who are unresponsive to chemotherapy indicates that α-fetoprotein and DCP levels are under independent control.

Other blood markers also have been proposed, including isoferritin, γ-glutamyl transpeptidase isoenzymes, variant alkaline phosphatase, and some lectin-binding variants of α-fetoprotein. However, none has achieved general clinical acceptance as a simple and useful marker for HCC.

DIAGNOSTIC PROCEDURES

Pathology

Accurate pathologic diagnosis, particularly histologic type, is essential to the proper treatment of the patient with HCC. Tumor variants, such as the fibrolamellar form and the childhood hepatoblastoma, have different prognoses and management than the normal adult type of HCC. In addition, the presence of microscopic vascular invasion has important adverse prognostic significance. Although fine-needle aspiration biopsy is easy to perform and often produces a confident diagnosis of malignancy, it does not demonstrate the architecture and pattern formation that can be determined with core tissue biopsy and usually is necessary to confirm the diagnosis. A variety of supportive stains are important in helping to make the diagnosis in difficult cases, such as the loss of reticulin staining, the presence of α-fetoprotein staining, and positive staining with polyclonal, but not monoclonal, carcinoembryonic antigen antibody. Gland formation makes the diagnosis of HCC unlikely, except in cases of mixed HCC and cholangiocarcinoma.

Radiology

Ultrasound evaluation of populations at risk because of high endemic levels of hepatitis B and C virus infection is time-honored, inexpensive, and useful for population screening. However, many tumors, particularly small ones, are overlooked on ultrasound, or confused with cirrhotic nodules. CT scanning of the abdomen and chest, together with bone scanning, is the primary means of assessing intrahepatic tumor size and extent, and extrahepatic spread. Brain scanning rarely is productive in the absence of specific symptoms. The abdominal CT scan is used to determine tumor size, tumor number, tumor sites and relation to main blood vessels within the liver, evidence of macroscopic vascular invasion as judged by obstruction of the main portal vein or its radicals, lymph node involvement in the porta hepatis or other abdominal lymph nodes, and evidence of hepatic dysfunction, including cirrhosis as judged by liver size, presence of ascites, shunting, varicose veins, splenomegaly, and other indices of portal hypertension. The standard CT scan is being superseded by the much faster and more accurate helical (spiral) CT scan, which produces many more images in only a few seconds. Using a bolus of rapidly injected dye, it provides

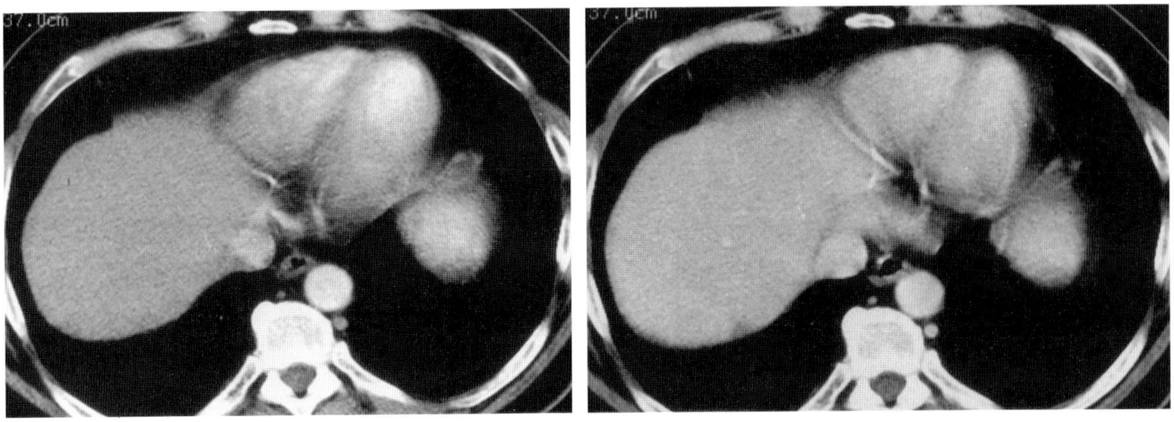

A B

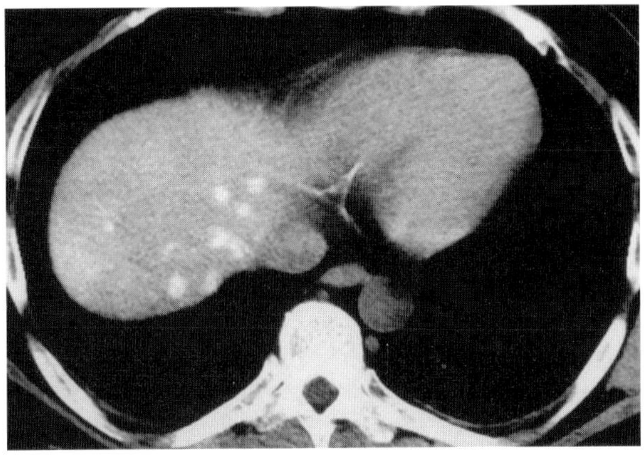

C

FIG. 55-1. Computed tomography (CT) of liver after intravenous contrast medium administration obtained on a helical CT scanner during the arterial phase (25 seconds) fails to identify a tumor. **(B)** Portal venous phase image obtained at the same level 30 seconds later also fails to visualize a tumor. **(C)** CT-arteriogram at the same level with contrast medium injected through a hepatic artery catheter shows numerous enhancing foci of hepatocellular carcinoma.

separate arterial- and venous-phase images. In addition, more numerous and smaller tumors can be diagnosed by CT-portography[11] or CT-arteriography (in the presence of portal hypertension) than by the current generation of CT or magnetic resonance imaging scanners (Fig. 55-1). This is important in planning resection, to ensure that residual disease is not left in the contralateral lobe, increasing the risk for postoperative recurrence. The uses and limitations of CT scanning, CT-portography, CT-arteriography, and ultrasonography have been reviewed elsewhere.[12] In addition, the importance of determining whether portal venous invasion is caused by malignant infiltration has led to the use of direct percutaneous biopsy of a thrombosed portal vein[13] under ultrasound guidance, to obtain direct evidence of portal venous and potential systemic spread. This is a routine practice in this author's institution when portal venous obstruction is seen on the CT scan.

DIAGNOSTIC EVALUATION

The initial patient evaluation includes an assessment of the tumor within the liver, metastases outside the liver, and hepatic function and hepatitis status.

Tumor Extent Within the Liver

The initial evaluation of the tumor within the liver is performed best by CT scanning. The objective is to determine the maximum diameter of the tumor, its location, the number of satellites, and the number of lobes involved. In addition, a reasonable assessment of lymph node enlargement can be made. Any involvement is proven through biopsy. Precise localization of the tumor is important in planning the extent of resection that is necessary or feasible. Portal venous invasion, as judged by obliteration or thrombus in a portal vein or radical, also is determined from the CT scan, with confirmatory biopsy.[13] In addition, the CT scan allows for determination of the size of the liver, the presence or absence of ascites, and other sequelae of portal hypertension, such as splenomegaly and the presence of varicose veins. For reasons that are unclear, some HCCs show up best on noncontrast CT images, some on contrast CT images, others on magnetic resonance but not CT images, and a few on ultrasound images but no other modalities. In patients being considered for resection, CT-portography or CT-arteriography also should be performed, because these techniques appear to be much more sensitive in revealing small lesions not otherwise detected on CT scanning (see Fig. 55-1*A*). Blood α-fetoprotein and DCP levels also should be drawn. At the time of CT-portography, it is common in many institutions to inject 5 to 15 mL of ethiodol (Lipiodol), which is taken up preferentially by many HCCs. This can be used for localization of the tumor for biopsy (Lipiodol on the pathology slides provides direct evidence of correct positioning of the tip of the biopsy needle in the tumor), and for the selective delivery of chemotherapy.

Evaluation of Extrahepatic Spread

HCC initially spreads throughout the liver and then predominantly to the regional lymph nodes and lungs. CT scanning of

TABLE 55-1. *Hepatocellular carcinoma*

Tumor size		Ascites		Albumin		Bilirubin	
>50 %	<50%			<3 g/dL	>3 g/dL	>3 mg/dL	3 mg/dL
(+)	(−)	(+)	(−)	(+)	(−)	(+)	(−)

Stage 1: All of the above indices are (−).
Stage II: 1 or 2 of the above indices are (+).
Stage III: 3 or 4 of the above indices are (+).

Okuda K, Ohtsuki T, Obata H, et al. Natural history of hepatocellular carcinoma and prognosis in relation to treatment: study of 850 patients. Cancer 1985;56:918.

the chest and abdomen usually is sufficient, together with bone scanning to exclude osseous metastases.

Liver Function and Hepatitis Status

Routine liver function tests usually are sufficient, although an indocyanine green clearance test may be included as part of the evaluation for resectability. Other widely used parameters of hepatic function include caffeine and antipyrine metabolism. Patients who are positive for hepatitis B E-antigen, and those who are positive for hepatitis B DNA are excluded from liver transplantation because of a high rate of recurrent hepatitis. All patients should undergo hepatitis B, C, and D serology determinations, and hepatitis B quantitative DNA or hepatitis C quantitative RNA testing should be performed in those with positive results. This information is likely to be useful for future refinements of hepatitis B and C virus exclusion criteria for liver transplantation, and for assessment of the hepatotoxicity of chemotherapy.

Staging of Hepatocellular Carcinoma

Two general types of staging systems have been used that have prognostic significance. The first is that of Okuda and colleagues, in which the size of the tumor and the degree of liver failure are used together as a scoring system[14] (Table 55-1). The second system is based on the TNM classification and was issued by the American Joint Committee on Cancer (Table 55-2).

The terms used in the TNM are defined as follows:

M1 = any metastases
N1 = any lymph node involvement by tumor

TABLE 55-2. *International (UICC) staging system for hepatocellular carcinoma*

Stage I:	T1 N0 M0
Stage II:	T2 N0 M0
Stage III:	T1 N1 M0
or	T2 N1 M0
or	T3 N0 M0
or	T3 N1 M0
Stage IVA:	T4 Any N M0
IVB:	Any distant metastases

T1 = a solitary HCC 2 cm or less in greatest diameter without vascular invasion
T2 = a solitary HCC 2 cm or less with vascular invasion, or a solitary tumor of any size greater than 2 cm without vascular invasion, or multiple tumors limited to one lobe but with no single lesion greater than 2 cm and all without vascular invasion
T3 = a solitary HCC greater than 2 cm in greatest diameter with vascular invasion, or multiple tumors limited to one lobe with none greater than 2 cm and with vascular invasion, or multiple tumors limited to one lobe with any lesion greater than 2 cm regardless of the presence or absence of vascular invasion
T4 = tumors in more than one lobe, or a tumor or tumors that also involve a major branch of the portal or hepatic vein

In general, this is a useful classification, except that stage III also includes nodal disease, which has a prognosis similar to that of metastatic disease. This is an important limitation of the staging classification, because stage III disease without nodal involvement has a relatively good prognosis after liver transplantation. The TNM staging system may require revision. This staging system also takes into account the fact that multiple small tumors may not be observed on radiology in the unresected specimen and that vascular invasion may not be clearly demonstrable in the unresected specimen. Therefore, this is essentially a pathologic classification, and when it is used clinically, it should be regarded as tentative until proven on the resected specimen.

THERAPY FOR HEPATOCELLULAR CARCINOMA

Partial and Complete Hepatectomy (Hepatic Resection and Transplantation)

Patients with noncirrhotic livers who have tumors smaller than 2 cm and no satellite lesions or vascular invasion are ideal candidates for long-term survival after therapy. Patients with chronic hepatitis who have similar types of HCC also do well.[15] These types of patients are rare in the United States but common in Asia, where the presence of endemic hepatitis makes it economically reasonable to perform routine screening, using hepatic ultrasonography and α-fetoprotein determinations every 6 to 12 months, to detect early HCCs in patients at risk. In this situation, percutaneous ethanol injections (PEI)[16] or segmental resection appear to produce long-term survival (greater than 5 years) and relatively long-term freedom from disease.[14,15] In addition, some recurrences can be treated by the same techniques. Many patients in the West, however, tend to present with symptoms, including abdominal pain, weight loss, or even on routine clinical evaluations in which the HCC was found as a surprise diagnosis. Most of these patients have TNM stage II, III, or IV tumors.

Stage II lesions, particularly those without vascular invasion, are treated best with resection. The standard of care usually includes resection for all stage II tumors, because they are limited to a single hepatic lobe and lack vascular invasion, even when there are multiple lesions.[17–21] It is not known whether the addition of preoperative neoadjuvant chemotherapy[25] or postoperative adjuvant chemotherapy by the intravenous or hepatic intraarterial route results in better survival, because few studies have compared directly resection with resection plus chemotherapy, particularly in the neoadjuvant setting. However, several studies have examined resection plus adjuvant or neoadjuvant chemotherapy with mixed, albeit somewhat disappointing, results.[21–24] Depending on the degree of cirrhosis, it may not be possible to resect a unilobar tumor, with or without vascular invasion, or multiple tumors extending throughout a lobe in patients with Child's class C or, often, Child's class B cirrhosis. Such patients may require liver transplantation for tumor extirpation. Given the high probability that new HCCs will develop in other cirrhotic nodules in patients with cirrhosis, limited stage I and II tumors in cirrhotic livers may have the best prognosis for long-term survival after liver transplantation. Even though such tumors may be technically resectable, liver transplantation probably has its maximum effect on this stage of HCC, because it removes the cirrhotic and preneoplastic nodules in the rest of the liver.

Stage III tumors present a problem. Recurrence rates after resection of solitary tumors with vascular invasion, and especially of multiple tumors with or without vascular invasion, are extremely high. The results of liver transplantation are not entirely clear. Some series show prolonged survival for patients with stage III lesions who undergo transplantation,[4] but other reports are less encouraging.[3] However, high recurrence rates for hepatitis B and C infections can limit survival in these patients, who may die of recurrent hepatitis and liver failure or recurrent tumor. The group of patients with hepatitis B and C that is least likely to have recurrent hepatitis in the transplanted liver is being defined in ongoing clinical studies. Studies also need to be performed comparing the treatment of stage III disease with resection versus transplantation, with and without neoadjuvant chemotherapy. In view of the increasing response rates to hepatic intraarterial chemotherapy (see below), randomized studies comparing resection or transplantation alone with resection or transplantation combined with hepatic intraarterial chemotherapy seem warranted.

Stage IVA Disease

Tumors involving both liver lobes and tumors infiltrating and causing obstruction of a major portal or hepatic vein branch are associated with extremely high recurrence rates within the liver after resection and both within and outside the liver after transplantation.[3,4,6] Pilot studies indicate that the addition of chemotherapy to liver transplantation may increase disease-free and absolute survival in this setting,[26–28] but no randomized study has been done, probably because of the small number of cases at any single institution.

Chemotherapy

Multiple studies have shown no increase in objective response rates or survival with the intravenous administration of single or multiple chemotherapeutic agents. However, there is growing evidence that several chemotherapeutic agents, alone or in combination, produce an objective response when given by the hepatic intraarterial route.[8,29] This response may be increased by the addition of some form of vascular occlusion or chemoembolization, although randomized studies comparing chemotherapy with and without concomitant occlusion or embolization have not demonstrated a convincing advantage of either approach.[30,31] This is attributable in part to the fact that the most extensive experience has been accumulated in Asia, where hepatic intraarterial chemotherapy is given in low dosages, and in part to the fact that different institutions use different drug combinations and dosages, and only some use additional arterial occlusive agents.[29,32–39] However, reproducible objective partial responses (a partial response is a 50% decrease of the product of two perpendicular diameters of the tumor as measured by CAT scan, such as a tumor that decreases from $5 \times 4 = 20$ cm to $3 \times 2 = 6$ cm) have been documented. An excess of 40% response rates (percentage of patients having a partial response) have now been achieved in several centers. Reported protocols include hepatic intraarterial cisplatin (100 mg/m^2), doxorubicin (Adriamycin, 20 mg/m^2) plus cisplatin (60 mg/m^2), and hepatic intraarterial infusion of 5-fluorodeoxyuridine, leucovorin, doxorubicin, and cisplatin. All these seem to be reasonable treatment regimens in terms of response rates, when given with or without ethiodol (Lipiodol), Gelfoam, or other vascular occlusive agents.

Several promising new approaches have been developed, including the use of conformal radiation therapy in addition to regional chemotherapy.[40] The advantage of conformal radiation is that significant portions of the normal liver can be protected from radiation toxicity, allowing higher doses of radiation to be applied to the tumor. The use of yttrium-90 microspheres has been reported to produce high response rates,[41] as has the use of styrene-maleic acid-neocarzinostatin mixtures (SMANCS), although the latter regimen has not been subjected to randomized study.[42] Multiple studies have used a range of chemotherapeutic agents, such as 5-fluorouracil, 5-fluorodeoxyuridine, doxorubicin, mitomycin C, or cisplatin, together with ethiodol (Lipiodol). Many institutions, particularly in Japan, use a combination of chemotherapy and Lipiodol and Gelfoam embolization. The reasoning behind this approach is that the Lipiodol opens small capillaries to chemotherapy access, whereas small amounts of Gelfoam cause hepatic artery slowing but not complete embolization of the arterial blood flow to the tumor. Large doses of Gelfoam often cause irreversible hepatic artery blockage. This has two adverse consequences. First, it can cause hepatic decompensation in a cirrhotic liver, especially in the presence of portal vein thrombus. Second, repeated chemotherapy cannot be given. Attempts have been made to deliver higher doses of chemotherapy using isolated hepatic perfusion. This has been accomplished by extracorporeal diversion of the blood through a charcoal filtration system, the idea being that the chemotherapy is infused into the liver and then removed from the blood before being returned to the general circulation.[43] It is too early to assess response rates in HCC for this logically attractive approach.

Future Directions

The use of more aggressive surgical therapy, including liver transplantation, and the production of higher response rates with high-dose hepatic intraarterial chemotherapy should lead to studies evaluating whether aggressive surgery combined with aggressive regional chemotherapy can produce higher response rates and longer survival than either modality alone. Surgery is capable of removing bulk tumor, whereas chemotherapy has the potential for removing micrometastatic disease. This is where current research is focused. However, neither approach takes into account the fact that advanced HCC tends to be a systemic disease.[7] Because no chemotherapeutic agent appears to work in a systemic fashion or against metastatic HCC, new forms of therapy are needed. Potential new therapeutic approaches involve inhibitors of known growth factors and growth factor receptors, such as suramin; antisense oligonucleotides or other inhibitors of known oncogenes, growth factor genes, and growth factor receptor genes; inhibitors of membrane and intracytoplasmic cell-signaling pathways, such as the protein tyrosine kinase inhibitors, including genistein, lavendustin A, erbstatin, herbimycin A, and their analogues, and the tyrphostins; inhibitors of angiogenesis and endothelial cell proliferation, such as the heparin analogues; modulators of chemotherapeutic agent drug resistance, including membrane-acting drugs such as phenothiazines, calcium-channel modulators, and cyclosporin A; and hormonal agents, especially antiandrogens, in view of the strong male predominance of HCC and the presence of androgen receptors in HCCs.

REFERENCES

1. Hsu H-C, Chiou T-J, Chen J-Y, Lee C-S, Lee P-H, Peng S-Y. Clonality and clonal evolution of hepatocellular carcinoma with multiple nodules. Hepatology 1991;13:923.
2. Ohto M, Kondo F, Ebara M. Pathology, diagnosis and treatment for small liver cancer. In: Tobe, et al, eds. Primary liver cancer in Japan. Toyko: Springer-Verlag, 1992:365.
3. Ringe B, Pichlmayr R, Wittekind C, Tusch G. Surgical treatment of hepatocellular carcinoma: experience with liver resection and transplantation in 198 patients. World J Surg 1991;15:270.
4. Iwatsuki S, Starzl TE, Sheahan D, et al. Hepatic resection versus transplantation for hepatocellular carcinoma. Ann Surg 1991;214:221.
5. Bismuth H, Chiche L, Adam R, Castaing D, Diamond T, Dennison A. Liver resection versus transplantation for hepatocellular carcinoma in cirrhotic patients. Ann Surg 1993;218:145.
6. Selby R, Kadry Z, Carr BI, Tzakis A, Madariaga J, Iwatsuki S. Liver transplantation for hepatocellular carcinoma. World J Surg 1995;19:33.
7. Kar S, Carr BI. Detection of liver cells in peripheral blood of patients with advanced stage hepatocellular carcinoma. Hepatology 1995;21:403.
8. Lotze MT, Flickinger JC, Carr BI. Hepatobiliary neoplasms in cancer. In: Devita VT, Hellman S, Rosenberg SA, eds. Principles and practice of oncology. 4th ed. Philadelphia: JB Lippincott, 1993:883.
9. Weitz IC, Liebman HA. Des-gamma-carboxy (abnormal) prothrombin and hepatocellular carcinoma: a critical review. Hepatology 1993;18:990.
10. Nakao A, Virji A, Iwaki Y, Carr BI, Iwatsuki S, Starzl TE. Abnormal prothrombin (des-carboxy prothrombin) in hepatocellular carcinoma. Hepatogastroenterology 1991;38:450.
11. Peterson MS, Baron RL, Dodd GD, et al. Hepatic parenchymal perfusion defects with CTAP: imaging-pathological correlation. Radiology 1992;185:149.
12. Baron RL. Understanding and optimizing use of contrast material for CT of the liver. AJR Am J Roentgenol 1994;163:323.
13. Dodd JD, Carr BI. Percutaneous biopsy of portal vein thrombus: a new staging technique for hepatocellular carcinoma. Am J Radiology 1993;161:229.
14. Okuda K, Ohtsuki T, Obata H, et al. Natural history of hepatocellular carcinoma and prognosis in relation to treatment: study of 850 patients. Cancer 1985;56:918.
15. Tang ZY. Subclinical hepatocellular carcinoma. Beijing: China Acad Publishers, 1985:1.
16. Ebara M, Ohto M, Sugiura N, et al. Percutaneous ethanol injection for the treatment of small hepatocellular carcinoma: study of 95 patients. J Gastroenterol Hepatol 1990;5:616.
17. Nagao T, Goto S, Kawano N, et al. Hepatic resection for hepatocellular carcinoma. Ann Surg 1987;205:33.
18. Tang ZY, Yu YQ, Zhou XD, et al. Surgery of small hepatocellular carcinoma. Cancer 1989;64:536.
19. Belli L, Romani F, Belli LS, et al. Reappraisal of surgical treatment of small hepatocellular carcinomas in cirrhosis. Dig Dis Sci 1989;34:1571.
20. Harada T, Shigemura T, Kodama S, Higuchi T, Ikeda S, Okazaki M. Hepatic resection is not enough for hepatocellular carcinoma. J Clin Gastroenterol 1992;14:245.
21. Franco D, Capussotti L, Smadja C, et al. Resectional hepatocellular carcinomas. Gastroenterology 1990;98:733.
22. Adachi E, Matsumata T, Nishizaki T, Hashimoto H, Tsuneyoshi M, Sugimagachi K. Effects of pre-operative trans catheter hepatic arterial chemoembolization for hepatocellular carcinoma. Cancer 1993;72:3593.
23. Izumi R, Shimizu K, Iyobe T, et al. Post-operative adjuvant hepatic-arterial infusion of lipiodol containing anti-cancer drugs in patients with hepatocellular carcinoma. Hepatology 1994;20:295.
24. Furuta T, Kanematsu T, Matsumata T, et al. Lipiodolization prolongs survival rates in post-operative patients with recurrent hepatocellular carcinoma. Hepatogastroenterology 1990;37:494.
25. Imaoka S, Sasaki Y, Shibata T, et al. A pre-operative chemoembolization therapy using lipiodol, cis-platin and gelatin sponge for hepatocellular carcinoma. Cancer Chemother Pharmacol 1989;23:S126.
26. Carr BI, Selby R, Madariaga J, Iwatsuki S, Starzl TE. Prolonged survival after liver transplantation and cancer chemotherapy for advanced stage hepatocellular carcinoma. Transplant Proc 1993;25:1128.
27. Cherqui D, Piedbois P, Pierga J-Y, et al. Multimodal adjuvant treatment and liver transplantation for advanced hepatocellular carcinoma. Cancer 1994;73:2721.
28. Stone MJ, Klintmalm GBG, Polter D, et al. Neoadjuvant chemotherapy and liver transplantation for hepatocellular carcinoma: a pilot study in 20 patients. Gastroenterology 1993;104:196.
29. Venook AP. Treatment of hepatocellular carcinoma: too many options? J Clin Oncol 1994;12:1323.
30. Chang J-M, Tzeng W-S, Pan H-B, Yang C-F, Lai K-H. Transcatheter emobolization with or without cis-platinum treatment of hepatocellular carcinoma. Cancer 1994;74:249.
31. Bruix J, Castells A, Montanya X, et al. Phase II study of trans-arterial embolization in European patients with hepatocellular carcinoma: need for controlled trials. Hepatology 1994;20:643.
32. Kardinal CG, Moertel CG, Wieand HS, et al. Combined doxorubicin and alpha interferon therapy of advanced hepatocellular carcinoma. Cancer 1993;71:2187.
33. Patt YZ, Charnsangavej C, Chuang LD, et al. Hepatic arterial infusion of FUDR, leucovorin, adriamycin and platinol (FLAP): effective palliation for nonresectable hepatocellular carcinoma. Proc ASCO 1992;11:474.
34. Carr BI, Iwatsuki S, Baron R, et al. Intra-hepatic arterial cis-platinum and doxorubicin with or without lipiodol for advanced hepatocellular carcinoma. Proc ASCO 1993;12:668.

35. Yoshikawa M, Saisho H, Ebara M, et al. A randomized trial of intrahepatic arterial infusion of 4-epidoxorubicin with lipiodol versus 4-epidoxorubicin alone in the treatment of hepatocellular carcinoma. Cancer Chemother Pharmacol 1994;33:S149.
36. Dazzi C, Fiorentini G, Graziani G, et al. Multi-agent chemoembolization in primary and metastatic hepatic tumors. Reg Cancer Treatment 1993;2:67.
37. Kato T, Saito Y, Niwa M, et al. Combination therapy of trans-catheter chemoembolization and percutaneous ethanol injection for unresectable hepatocellular carcinoma. Cancer Chemother Pharmacol 1994;33:S115.
38. Taniguchi K, Nakata K, Kato Y, et al. Treatment of hepatocellular carcinoma with trans-catheter arterial embolization. Cancer 1994;73:1341.
39. Carr BI. Spherex (degradable starch microspheres): a novel and safe emoblizing agent in the management of hepatocellular carcinoma. Proc ASCO 1994;13:605.
40. Robertson JM, Lawrence TS, Dworzanin LM, et al. Treatment of primary hepatobiliary cancers with conformal radiation therapy and regional chemotherapy. J Clin Oncol 1993;11:1286.
41. Lau W-Y, Leung W-T, Ho S, et al. Treatment of inoperable hepatocellular carcinoma with intra-hepatic arterial yttrium-90 microspheres: a phase I and II study. Br J Cancer 1994;70:994.
42. Konno T, Maeda H. Targeting chemotherapy of hepatocellular carcinoma: arterial administration of SMANCS/lipiodol. In: Okuda K, Ishak KG, eds. Neoplasms of the liver. New York: Springer-Verlag, 1987:343.
43. Kavikumar TS, Denny D, Bodden W, et al. Percutaneous isolated hepatic perfusion (PHIP) chemotherapy: phase I trial. Proc ASCO 1991;10:406.

Surgery for Gastrointestinal Cancer: A Multidisciplinary Approach, edited by Harold J. Wanebo.
Lippincott-Raven Publishers, Philadelphia, © 1997.

CHAPTER 56

Interventional Radiologic Techniques for the Diagnosis and Treatment of Hepatobiliary Malignancy

Chusilp Charnsangavej and Sidney Wallace

The role of the vascular and interventional radiologist in the diagnosis and treatment of hepatobiliary cancer has evolved since the late 1970s. During the late 1970s and early 1980s, angiography was commonly performed for the diagnosis of hepatic tumors, and embolization of unresectable tumors was used for palliative treatment and as an adjunct to intraarterial (IA) chemotherapy.[1–5] In the late 1980s, superselective catheterization for chemoembolization of various hepatic tumors with various agents underwent extensive investigation,[6–16] whereas the number of diagnostic angiographies performed continuously decreased. In the meantime, percutaneous aspiration biopsy became an important diagnostic procedure for patients with hepatobiliary cancer to confirm the diagnosis before treatment planning. In the late 1980s and early 1990s, applications of the percutaneous approach were extended to include tumor ablation by various chemical, physical, and mechanical agents.[17–33] The changing role of vascular and interventional radiology in the diagnosis and treatment of hepatobiliary cancer is the result of several factors, including: advances in imaging technology that make the diagnosis of many hepatic tumors more specific; the simplicity of the percutaneous approach, which is not only relatively cheap but accurate and effective; and the low morbidity of the percutaneous approach compared with embolization, chemoembolization, and surgery.

This chapter discusses the role of vascular and interventional radiology in hepatobiliary cancer and describes various techniques, their limitations, and their results. The chapter focuses on the treatment of hepatocellular carcinoma and hepatic metastases from colorectal carcinoma and neuroendocrine tumors, which are the most common hepatic tumors that are being treated.

Chusilp Charnsangavej: Department of Diagnostic Radiology, MD Anderson Cancer Center, 1515 Holcombe Boulevard, Houston, TX 77030

Sidney Wallace: Department of Radiology, MD Anderson Cancer Center, 1515 Holcombe Boulevard, Houston, TX 77030

DIAGNOSIS

Angiography and Computed Tomographic Angiography

Angiography is rarely performed solely for the diagnosis of hepatic tumors because various imaging techniques have shown high specificity in the diagnosis of lesions for which angiographic diagnosis was the previous gold standard. When the diagnosis remains in doubt, aspiration biopsy is usually performed regardless of whether angiography is available. Angiography is usually performed in conjunction with computed tomographic angiography (CTA) to provide vascular anatomic information before surgery.

Computed tomographic angiography is used for the staging of hepatic tumors when the patient is a surgical candidate. The technique is more sensitive in the detection of hepatic lesions than conventional CT scanning technique.[34–36] The technique includes CT arterial portography,[34–38] arterial contrast-enhanced CT,[39–41] and Lipiodol CT.[42–44] All of these techniques require an angiographic catheter placement, and therefore are invasive procedures, and are done in conjunction with an angiographic procedure.

Computed tomographic arterial portography is based on the fact that hepatic parenchyma enhances better if the contrast material can be delivered through the splanchnic circulation. The lesion in the liver receives no arterial enhancement during this phase of contrast enhancement; therefore, the lesion appears hypodense compared with the surrounding hepatic parenchyma. Studies have shown that the technique is highly sensitive in detecting hepatic lesions, 20% to 30% more sensitive than conventional dynamic bolus intravenous contrast enhancement.[34–36] However, the characteristics of the lesion cannot be defined by this technique; benign or malignant solid lesions appear the same. The study can also be subject to portal flow artefacts secondary to portal hypertension in cirrhosis, arterioportal venous shunts, or portal and hepatic vein occlusion.[37,38] The study must be interpreted in conjunction with a conventional contrast-enhanced scan. The examination requires a placement of a catheter in the superior mesenteric artery, avoiding and bypassing the replaced hepatic artery. CT is performed through the liver after delivery of contrast material (30% iodine concentration) at a rate of 2 mL/sec for 100 to 120 mL, with a scan delay of 20 to 30 seconds after the start of injection.

Contrast material can also be delivered directly into the hepatic artery by way of the catheter placed into the hepatic artery, and CT of the liver is performed during the arterial enhancement phase. The goal of this study is to identify small hepatic tumors that are hypervascular and become hyperdense compared with the hepatic parenchyma. The shortcomings of this study include the common variations in hepatic artery anatomy that limit enhancement only to portions of the liver that are supplied by the catheterized artery, and artefacts associated with nonspecific and nonuniform enhancement due to layering effects and previous regional chemotherapy.[41]

Iodized oil (Lipiodol; Laboratoires Andre Guerbet, Aulnay-sous-Bois, France) can also be used as an imaging agent delivered into the hepatic artery in conjunction with hepatic angiography and embolization. Lipiodol retained in small hepatic tumors can easily be recognized with high sensitivity when CT scans are done 7 to 14 days after injection, to allow absorption and clearing of Lipiodol from the normal parenchyma. The study is popular for the detection of small hepatocellular carcinomas after chemoembolization.[42–44]

Fine-Needle Aspiration Biopsy

Fine-needle aspiration (FNA) is a simple and relatively inexpensive technique for acquiring tissue for cytologic diagnosis. The keys to a successful FNA are the exact localization of the needle tip and the expertise of the cytopathologist. In the liver, we often use ultrasound or CT for imaging guidance to localize the needle, and we take extra care in making sure that the needle tip is in the proper location before obtaining the tissue. The sizes of the needle commonly used for FNA are 22 to 18 gauge; the tissue obtained from a 22-gauge needle is commonly processed for cytologic diagnosis, but when an 18- or 20-gauge needle is used, a tissue core for a histologic diagnosis is possible.

Fine-needle aspiration should not be performed in all lesions seen on imaging studies. FNA is commonly done when the diagnosis is uncertain and the result of the biopsy may influence the treatment. In most cases in which surgical resection is the treatment of choice, FNA is not necessary because of the risk of needle track seeding, even though it is very rare. A positive biopsy is highly accurate, but a negative biopsy does not rule out malignancy.

The risk with FNA is small; most contraindications are relative, but must be considered in patients who cannot be cooperative or have a severe bleeding tendency. These complications include bleeding and major vessel laceration, hemobilia, hepatic infarction, pneumothorax, and needle tract tumor seeding.[45] With experience, the accuracy of aspiration biopsy of lesions larger than 2 cm should be in the range of 95% to 100%.[46,47] Smaller and deeply located lesions may be more difficult to reach and can lower the yield of FNA.

NONSURGICAL THERAPEUTIC OPTIONS IN HEPATOBILIARY CANCER

Surgical resection is considered the gold standard for the treatment of hepatocellular carcinoma and hepatic metastasis from colorectal cancer because in selected patients, surgery may offer the chance for cure. However, only 10% to 20% of patients are operative candidates, and of these patients, the 5-year survival rates are only 20% to 30%, with an operative mortality of less than 5% and morbidity of 20% to 30%.[48–53] The low resectability rates result from the facts that hepatocellular carcinoma is often associated with liver cirrhosis, invasion through the capsules is common and results in intrahepatic spread, and hepatic metastases from colorectal cancer are infrequently solitary. For these reasons, researchers have continued to search for nonsurgical treatments to improve the survival rates in this disease.

Because the liver has a dual blood supply from the portal vein and the hepatic artery, and the tumor receives most of its blood supply from the hepatic artery, selective catheterization of the hepatic artery provides access for delivery of chemotherapeutic agents (IA chemotherapy), for injection of embolic materials to occlude the hepatic artery (embolization) so that the blood supply to the tumor can be cut off, or for delivery of both embolic materials and chemotherapeutic agents (chemoembolization) at the same time. Another approach is by a direct puncture of the tumor using ultrasound or CT guidance. Through the needle placed percutaneously directly into the tumor, absolute ethanol, a sclerosing agent, can be injected into the tumor to destroy the tumor cells. The techniques have been extended to use lasers for hyperthermia and photocoagulation, to apply high-intensity focused ultrasound to destroy the tissue, to apply radiofrequency electrocautery, and for cryotherapy application to freeze the tumor. This discussion focuses on treatments using the transarterial and percutaneous approaches.

Transarterial Approach

The goal of IA chemotherapy is to deliver high-dose chemotherapeutic agents into the hepatic artery, which supplies the tumors. Delivery of drugs in this manner provides a higher concentration of drugs to the tumor than can be achieved by systemic chemotherapy.[54–57] Several experimental and clinical studies have shown that a 20% to 30% higher response rate can be achieved.[58–64] However, the benefits of prolonged survival rates and improved quality of life are not well realized, and the patients are rarely cured.[58,60–64] The technique, therefore, did not gain enthusiastic support, particularly from interventional radiologists, and has not been used as a front-line therapy in many hepatic tumors, but rather has been used only after failure of other treatments and to test new regimens of drugs.

Chemoembolization is a technique that has been used for the treatment of nonresectable hepatic neoplasms since the early 1980s (Fig. 56-1). The technique combines embolization and chemotherapy in an attempt to "kill" the tumor; it is accomplished by delivery of chemotherapeutic agents and embolic agents into the blood vessels supplying the tumor. The rationale for combining embolization and chemotherapy is based on the theory that although embolic agents create ischemic effects on

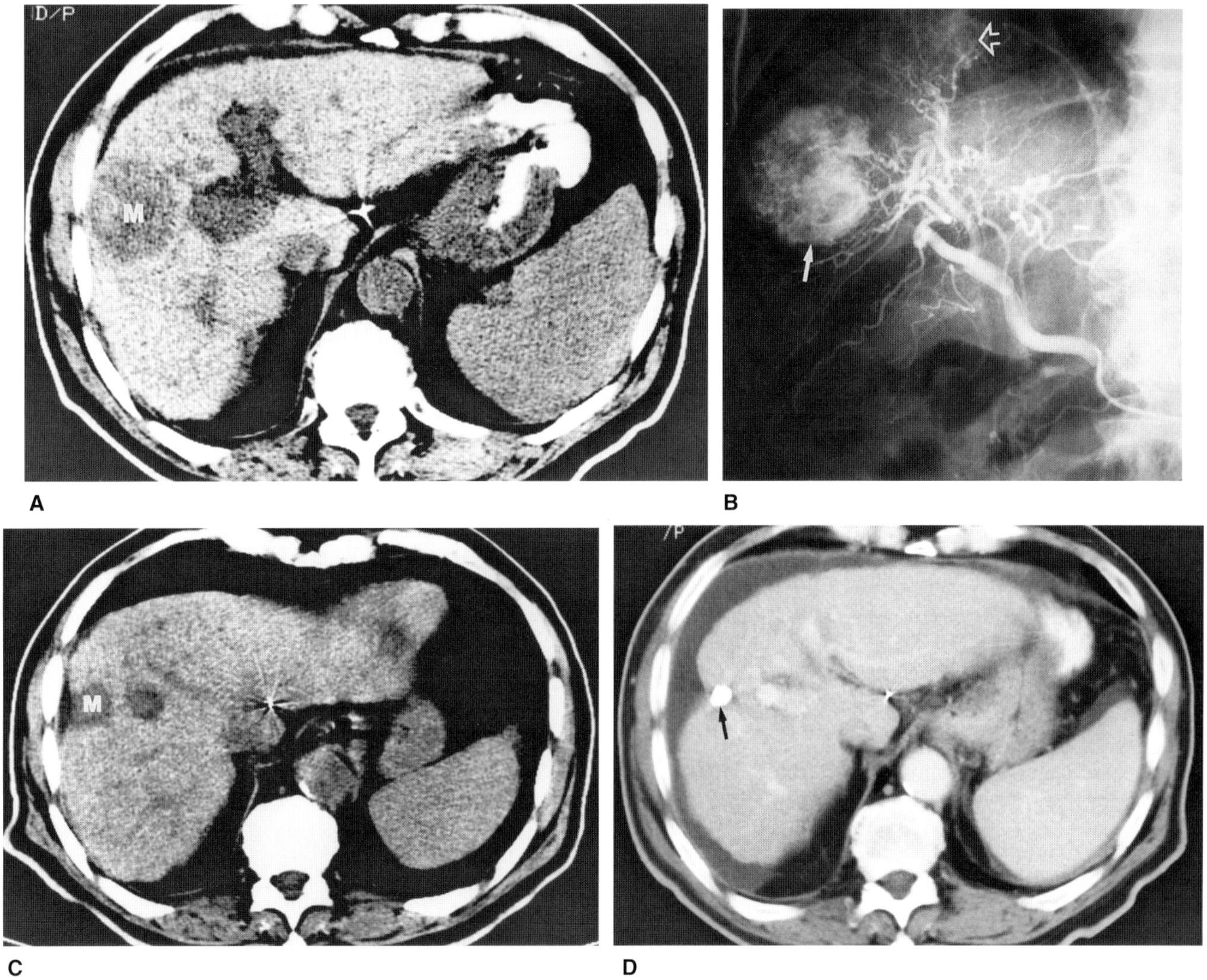

FIG. 56-1. A patient with multifocal hepatocellular carcinoma and liver cirrhosis treated with chemoembolization and absolute ethanol injection. **(A)** A 4-cm hypodense lesion (M) is shown in the right lobe of the liver on this computed tomography (CT) scan done without intravenous contrast enhancement. Note the irregular and nodular contour of the liver. **(B)** Hepatic angiogram showing two hypervascular lesions, one (*solid arrow*) corresponding to the lesion shown on CT, the other (*open arrow*) under the right hemidiaphragm. Chemoembolization was then performed with a mixture of polyvinyl alcohol foam and 50 mg of cisplatinum, 10 mg of doxorubicin, and 50 mg of floxuridine. **(C)** CT scan 3 months after chemoembolization shows the lesion (M) reduced in size to 1.5 cm. The hepatic artery was occluded and there was no access for the transarterial route. **(D)** Absolute ethanol and lipiodol were injected by direct puncture of the tumor nodule (*arrow*).

the tumor, they cannot completely kill all the tumor cells, particularly at the periphery of the tumor; adding chemotherapy helps destroy the tumor completely. In addition, embolization also decreases the speed of drug clearance by slowing down the blood flow through the tumor and increasing the contact time between the drugs and the tumor cells.

Chemoembolization is the method used to deliver sustained and slow-flow chemotherapeutic agents to the tumor. Several techniques have been used, including hepatic artery ligation and infusion with chemotherapeutic agents,[65,66] hepatic artery infusion after injection of biodegradable starch microspheres,[67,68] and embolization with ethylcellulose encapsulating mitomycin-C.[69] However, these techniques have not yielded significant clinical results. The techniques of chemoembolization that have gained wide clinical acceptance since the early 1980s are the use of embolic materials mixed with chemotherapeutic agents delivered into the arterial supply to the tumor, and the use of chemotherapeutic agents mixed with iodized oil injected into the artery, followed by Gelfoam embolization of the artery.[11–14]

Patient Selection and Pretreatment Evaluation

Not all patients with hepatic neoplasms benefit from a transarterial treatment approach. The benefits and the risk of complications from the procedure must be taken into consideration when selecting patients for treatment. Our experience in embolization of hepatic tumors in the early 1980s suggested that patients with extensive hepatic disease and impending hepatic failure would not benefit from embolization; rather, hepatic embolization in these patients could precipitate hepatorenal failure and result in death. Our unpublished data from a review of 400 patients who underwent hepatic embolization showed that in one third of the patients who had tumor replacement of more than 50% of the liver, serum lactic dehydrogenase levels above 425 mU/mL, serum glutamic oxaloacetic transaminase levels above 100 mU/mL, and serum bilirubin levels above 2 mg/dL, hepatic failure and death ensued within 1 month of embolization. Therefore, we adopt these criteria as contraindications to chemoembolization, and use other techniques as alternative treatment. In addition, in patients with extensive tumor involving the portal vein or in patients with cirrhosis of the liver, careful evaluation of the hemodynamics of the liver must be done and selective segmental embolization must be performed, particularly when hepatofugal flow of the portal vein is demonstrated. Such patients are at high risk for complications with IA chemotherapy, and if the treatment is absolutely necessary, the catheter must be placed superselectively into the hepatic artery that supplies only the tumor.

Technical Considerations

The goal of IA chemotherapy, hepatic embolization, or hepatic chemoembolization is to deliver the chemotherapeutic agents or embolic materials to the tumors in the liver without affecting the normal parenchyma or adjacent organs in the distribution of the hepatic artery.[70–73] To maximize this goal and minimize the complications of the treatment, which frequently are secondary to the unintentional or unavoidable infusion or embolization of normal organs in the distribution of the hepatic artery, it is necessary to understand the anatomy and hemodynamics of the hepatic artery and the blood supply to the tumor and adjacent organs.[74,75]

In pretreatment evaluation, CT with bolus intravenous contrast enhancement or magnetic resonance imaging are used to define the extent of the disease. We define not only the number and location of the tumors, but tumor extension into the portal or hepatic veins or evidence of bile duct obstruction. Knowledge of tumor extension helps define the plan for treatment by angiography. Tumor involvement of, or adjacent to, the diaphragm requires study of the inferior phrenic artery or the internal mammary artery. Involvement of the anterior medial segment of the left lobe requires study of not only the middle hepatic artery but the anterior segmental branch of the right hepatic artery and the left hepatic artery. A pedunculated mass from the right lobe and anterior medial segment of the left lobe may derive its blood supply from the gastroepiploic artery (the omentum), and a mass in the lateral segment may be supplied by the left gastric artery.

Diagnostic angiography must be carefully evaluated to obtain all information about the blood supply to the tumor, including variations in hepatic artery anatomy, and the potential collateral and parasitic arterial supply. This information is important for planning whether embolization or IA chemotherapy can be safely performed in one session, or must be done in a few consecutive sessions to achieve treatment goals and minimize complications.

Blood flow in the hepatic artery may vary depending on several factors, including vascularity of the tumor, the presence of arteriovenous shunting, and the presence of portal or hepatic vein obstruction. Increased blood flow in the hepatic artery may reverse the blood flow in the extrahepatic branches of the hepatic artery and facilitate catheter placement for embolization and infusion. However, in certain circumstances, it can also divert the blood flow away from the tumor into the normal parenchyma surrounding the tumor when the tumor is relatively hypovascular.[74] Understanding the anatomy and hemodynamics of the hepatic artery is necessary for proper catheter placement for embolization and infusion, and to improve the success of the treatment and minimize the complications.

Selective catheterization is required for most IA chemotherapy and chemoembolization procedures. Several factors must be taken into account for the position of catheter placement, including the vascularity of the tumor, the number and size of tumors, the experience of the angiographer, the type of catheter available, and the embolic material to be used. In general, the nodular type of hepatocellular carcinoma is hypervascular; tumor neovascularity draws the blood supply to the tumor. Selective catheterization may not be necessary, and the treatment can be performed from the proper hepatic artery after bypassing the gastroduodenal artery. In patients with multiple tumors involving both lobes of the liver, selective catheterization to each segment for embolization of each tumor nodule may not be practical. The treatment can be safely performed in the lobar artery unless there are other contraindications. On the other hand, a hypovascular tumor requires superselective catheterization to get as close to the tumor as possible.

Selecting a catheter for transarterial treatment depends largely on the experience of the angiographer performing the procedure. We prefer a 5-Fr or a 6.5-Fr tapered to 5-Fr polyethylene catheter (Cook, Inc., Bloomington, IN) with the tip formed to the anatomy of the hepatic artery. This catheter allows various embolic materials to be used, including polyvinyl alcohol foam (Ivalon; Unipoint, Inc., High Point, NC) and gelatin sponges (Gelfoam; Upjohn, Inc., Kalamazoo, MI) of various sizes. A newer coaxial catheter system using the Tracker microcatheter (Target Therapeutics, San Jose, CA) is easy to use, and selective catheterization to small and tortuous vessels can be accomplished in most cases. The disadvantages of this catheter system are its cost and limitations in the embolic materials that can be used; for IA chemotherapy, this catheter facilitates the treatment even in a tortuous and small hepatic artery. Embolization usually can be performed only with collagen (Angiostat; Regional Therapeutics, Pacific Palisades, CA), Gelfoam powder, or absolute ethanol as embolizing agents. We usually reserve this catheter for more difficult cases that requires complex superselective catheterization.

Embolization With Particulate Materials Mixed With Chemotherapeutic Agents

Some particulate materials are used for chemoembolization, including gelatin sponge, polyvinyl alcohol foam, and collagen. Gelatin sponge can be cut into pledgets of 1 mm^3, or it can be used in a powder form. When Gelfoam pledgets are used, they are soaked in chemotherapeutic agents that are dissolved in saline mixed with contrast material. Gelfoam powder and collagen are used by mixing them with a solution containing chemotherapeutic agents and contrast material through two syringes connected to each other by a connecting tube or a stopcock. The mixture of embolic particles and chemotherapeutic agents is flushed back and forth to form a slurry of materials that can be delivered through the catheter. At the M. D. Anderson Cancer Center, we mix a concentrated solution (10 to 15 mL) of chemotherapeutic agents with Ivalon suspension, which is prepared in our laboratory by the technique previously described. Ivalon suspension contains 10 mg Ivalon/mL. The mixture of Ivalon suspension and drugs is also flushed back and forth between two syringes before embolization.

Embolization With Iodized Oil and Chemotherapeutic Agents

This technique has been investigated extensively in Japan for chemoembolization of hepatic neoplasms subsequent to the earlier studies by Nakakuma and colleagues[6] and Konno and associates.[9] The technique uses an iodized oil (Lipiodol; or Ethiodol; Savage Laboratories, Melville, NY) mixed with a chemotherapeutic agent or a combination of agents to form an emulsion. The emulsion is then injected into the hepatic artery, followed by an injection of gelatin sponge particles of 1- to 3-mm diameter. The solution of chemotherapeutic agents should be mixed at a certain concentration so that the specific gravity of the solution is similar to that of the iodized oil, to make the emulsion more stable.[13] A usual dose of doxorubicin (60 mg) is dissolved in 3 to 5 mL of fluid and mixed with 5 to 20 mL of iodized oil at a 2 to 3 : 1 ratio (iodized oil : doxorubicin), depending on the size and vascularity of the tumor. The mixture is then shaken to homogenize the emulsion before it is used for embolization.

It has been demonstrated that iodized oil mixed in this manner carries the drug within the emulsion, and when the emulsion is injected into the hepatic artery it is trapped in the tumor vasculature,[6–8] in the sinusoid around the tumor,[76] and particularly in daughter nodules surrounding the main tumor.[6–8] Injection of the emulsion is usually limited to 20 mL of iodized oil because overflow into the portal vein,[77] the sinusoids, and then into the systemic circulation can occur. In fact, an experimental injection of iodized oil into the hepatic artery in rats showed that iodized oil was always shunted into the portal venules and the sinusoids immediately after the injection.[78] The gelatin sponge injected after the infusion of emulsion is designed to stop the flow in the hepatic artery so that the emulsion remains in the tumor vascular bed. Pharmacokinetic studies and examinations of surgical specimens have shown that by using this technique the concentration of doxorubicin remains high in the tumor compared with the normal parenchyma, and only a very small amount of the drug escapes into the systemic circulation during the treatment.[79] That the iodized oil emulsion remains in the main tumor, the daughter nodules, and satellite metastatic lesions while the emulsion in the normal parenchyma slowly disappears is believed to result from the absorption of the oil by the Kupffer cells in the liver, with reestablishment of flow in the normal parenchyma clearing the iodized oil into the systemic circulation. The oil droplets are then trapped in the lung and spleen, and phagocytosis of the oil by the reticuloendothelial cells occurs. Retention of oil in the tumor has been used in follow-up for recurrent disease, because iodized oil retained in the lesion can be easily seen on CT.[10,11]

Segmental Chemoembolization

More recently, a more aggressive technique of chemoembolization has been studied. Uchida and colleagues,[80] Nakamura and coworkers,[81] and Matsui and colleagues[82] performed chemoembolization through a superselective catheter placed in a segmental artery supplying tumors confined to that segment. Iodized oil mixed with chemotherapeutic agents was injected into the artery, but with an attempt to overflow the emulsion into the portal vein of that segment, followed by an injection of gelatin sponge similar to the technique described in the preceding section. This technique of ''overembolization'' created an infarction of the entire segment, including the tumor nodules and the parenchyma surrounding them, producing a result similar to that with segmental resection.

Selection of Chemotherapeutic Agents

The most common chemotherapeutic agents or combination of agents that have been used or investigated for chemoembolization are doxorubicin, cisplatinum, and mitomycin-C. Doxorubicin is commonly used as a bolus of 60 mg with a range of 40 to 100 mg for chemoembolization of hepatocellular carcinoma. The dose of doxorubicin should be reduced if the patients are jaundiced, or the drug is used in combination with other drugs. As a single agent, cisplatinum has been used at 2 mg/kg of body weight, to a total dose of 100 to 150 mg, for chemoembolization of hepatocellular carcinoma, metastatic colorectal carcinoma, metastatic ocular melanoma, and metastatic neuroendocrine tumors. Cisplatinum is not as easily resolved in fluid as is doxorubicin or mitomycin-C, but when mixed with embolic materials or iodized oil, cisplatinum can be delivered through the catheter without any difficulties. For mitomycin-C, the standard dose has been 10 to 20 mg, but it has been more commonly used in combination with other agents at 10 mg rather than as a single agent. When a combination of drugs is used, the dosage of each drug is usually reduced by one third or one half. For example, when a combination of doxorubicin, cisplatinum, and mitomycin-C is used for chemoembolization of hepatocellular carcinoma, doxorubicin is administered at 20 to 40 mg, cisplatinum at 50 to 75 mg, and mitomycin C at 10 mg. However, the dose of chemotherapeutic agents could vary if the agents are premixed and the dose is adjusted according the cessation of flow of the vessel.

At the M. D. Anderson Cancer Center, our practice with drug selection is usually arranged after discussion with our oncologists because many of our patients may have received prior treatment and may be resistant to or may not be able to tolerate certain drugs. The types of drugs that we use are similar to the regimen described previously, with a few exceptions: we may use vinblastine for IA infusion after embolization, or we may use floxuridine at 75 to 100 mg in addition to cisplatinum and doxorubicin in hepatocellular carcinoma. However, all of these

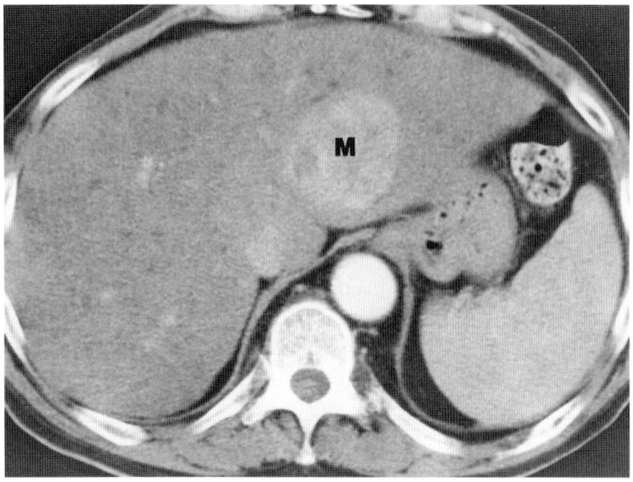

A

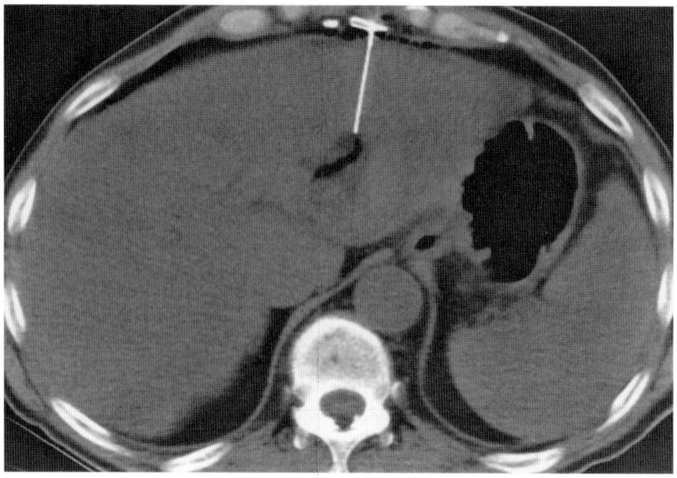

B

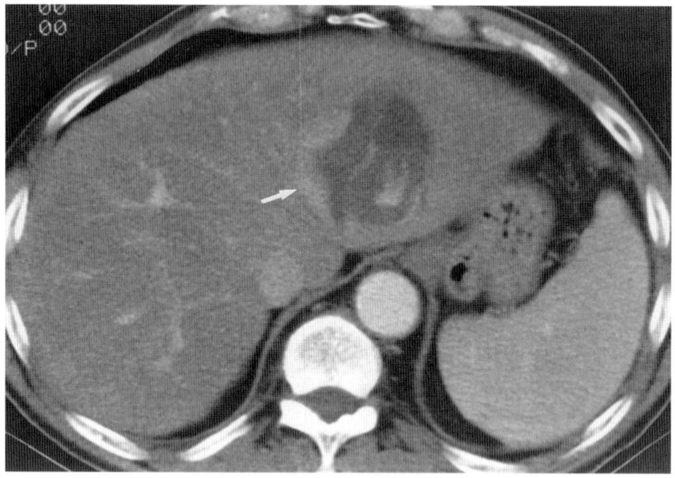

C

FIG. 56-2. A patient with hepatocellular carcinoma in cirrhotic liver. **(A)** Computed tomography (CT) of the liver during the bolus phase of intravenous contrast enhancement shows a 5-cm hypervascular mass (M) in segment 2. **(B)** The tip of the needle is in the lesion, the area of hypodense area is from absolute ethanol injection. **(C)** Incomplete necrosis of the tumor is shown on this CT scan, taken 1 month after absolute ethanol injection, with residual tumor nodule (*arrow*) seen at the periphery of the lesion.

combinations are adjusted according to the experience of each oncologist in treating different types of tumors.

Percutaneous Tumor Ablation Approach

Percutaneous tumor ablation using absolute ethanol has been a subject of extensive investigation and has gained popularity and enthusiastic support from many interventional radiologists and gastroenterologists for the treatment of small hepatocellular carcinoma in cirrhotic liver and selected hepatic metastases (Fig. 56-2). The technique is based on the concept that direct injection delivers absolute ethanol into the tumor. The toxic effects of ethanol on the tumor are the results of ethanol diffusion into the cells, producing cellular dehydration, protein denaturation, and immediate coagulation necrosis.[83–87] Ethanol diffusion into the surrounding tissue and vessels also produces vascular thrombosis and fibrosis, and therefore may prevent tumor seeding along the needle tract. Because the treatment uses a small volume of absolute ethanol and directs it to the tumor, systemic effects from absolute ethanol are minimal; but because only a small volume of absolute ethanol can be injected, this is also a limiting factor in the application of this technique to the treatment of large tumors.

The technique is well accepted by many interventional radiologists because it is much simpler and less expensive than catheterization techniques, and because of the increased detection of small hepatic tumors as a result of effective screening in Japan and certain regions of Europe. However, the results must still be viewed with caution because of the lack of sufficient histologic data to verify that 100% tumor necrosis is achieved in a large number of patients, and long-term survival and recurrent rates have yet to established.

Patient Selection and Pretreatment Evaluation

Most patients who undergo treatment by percutaneous injection with absolute ethanol have small hepatocellular carcinoma tumors and liver cirrhosis, and limited number of lesions. Several investigators have set guidelines for the treatment by limiting the size of the lesions to less than 5 cm and the number of lesions to not more than five.[21,23,24,86–89] Others have explored the safety and possibility of treating larger lesions.[87,90] In theory, the treatment is more likely to be effective against smaller lesions than larger lesions because it is not possible to diffuse absolute ethanol uniformly in a large lesion.

Unlike a transarterial approach, the percutaneous technique is not limited by poor liver function test results due to liver cirrhosis because the treatment is more localized and does not affect the surrounding parenchyma as much, if the proper technique is performed. Caution must be used in patients with coagulopathy and ascites, and in those who are uncooperative. Therefore, a patient with Child class C liver cirrhosis may not be a good candidate for this technique. Percutaneous seeding along the needle tract rarely occurred, but instances have been reported. Most patients experienced pain during injection, and fever can develop after the treatment.[86,87,90] Pain can be relieved by analgesics. Symptoms of alcohol intoxication are not infrequent and do not require any specific treatment.[86]

Technical Considerations

Percutaneous direct injection of absolute ethanol is commonly done under real-time ultrasound or CT guidance. A 22- to 18-gauge needle can be used. The needle tip is placed at the center of the lesion and absolute ethanol is injected into the lesion according to the calculated volume, $V = 4/3\pi(r + 0.5)^3$, where V is the total volume, and r is the radius of the lesion, as described by Shiina and associates.[86] The lesion is viewed by real-time ultrasound during injection, and should become hyperechoic when it is properly perfused by absolute ethanol.[87] When CT is used for guidance, the lesion should become hypodense immediately during injection.[91] The treatment is usually done under local anesthesia and can be divided into several sessions depending on the size of the lesion, the total volume of absolute ethanol required, and the patient's tolerance. In larger lesions, attempts have been made to deliver larger volumes by multiple injections in one session, but under general anesthesia. The technique is acceptable and practical without serious complications, according to Livraghi and colleagues,[87] but the margin of safety for a large-volume absolute ethanol injection has not been well established.

Results of Chemoembolization and Intraarterial Chemotherapy

The evidence that chemoembolization is effective in treating hepatocellular carcinoma was provided by histopathologic study of resected specimens after chemoembolization. Sakurai and colleagues,[7] Takayasu and associates,[8] and Yamada and coworkers[79] showed that almost 50% of the resected tumors became completely necrotic after embolization with gelatin sponge mixed with chemotherapeutic agents. The necrotic tumors also show on CT as areas of low density after embolization. Study of the resected specimens after chemoembolization with iodized oil mixed with chemotherapeutic agents and gelatin sponge showed improved results, with complete necrosis seen in 83% of the main tumors, 53% of the daughter nodules, and 17% of tumor thrombi in the portal venules.[11] The degree of tumor necrosis corresponded to the complete staining of the tumor by iodized oil as shown on CT after embolization. Most studies showed a significant decrease in the level of serum α-fetoprotein in 85% to 90% of cases.

Prolonged survival rates in patients who had chemoembolization for hepatocellular carcinoma have been reported. However, there is no randomized study comparing the patients who received no treatment and the patients who received treatment. Yamada and coworkers reported 1-, 2-, and 3-year survival rates of 51%, 28%, and 13%, respectively, among 793 patients who were treated with gelatin sponge mixed with doxorubicin and mitomycin-C.[79] The 1-, 2-, and 3-year survival rates increased to 72%, 55%, and 47% in 66 patients with tumors smaller than 6 cm. Nakamura and associates[13] demonstrated an improved result in patients who were treated with iodized oil, doxorubicin, and gelatin sponge embolization. The 1-, 2-, and 3-year survival rates of their 100 patients were 54%, 33%, and 18%, respectively, slightly but significantly better than the control group of patients who were embolized with Gelfoam and doxorubicin. The results of iodized oil chemoembolization reported by Ohishi and colleagues[14] also confirmed these findings, and in their 263 patients with tumors smaller than 5 cm the 1-, 2-, and 3-year survival rates improved to 79%, 52%, and 36%, respectively. It is not clear if there is a significant difference between the two techniques of chemoembolization, and there were no prospective, randomized studies to assess and compare them.

The results of segmental and subsegmental chemoembolization have been shown by Matsui and colleagues[82] and Uchida and coworkers[80] to be superior to those of chemoembolization alone. This is probably because of increased effectiveness of embolization of the daughter nodules and tumor invasion beyond the capsules. Recurrence rates, as reported by Matsui and colleagues,[82] were 18% at 1 year, 30% at 2 years, and 33% at 3 and 4 years after treatment. The 3-year survival rates were 55% to 78%, and the 4-year survival rate was 67%.

The results of chemoembolization for hepatocellular carcinoma in Europe and in the United States were not as good as the results from Japan. Venook and coworkers[92] reported a median survival period of 7 months in the 51 patients who were embolized with Gelfoam powder mixed with doxorubicin, cisplatinum, and mitomycin-C. Our experience at the M. D. Anderson Cancer Center was similar to that of Venook and coworkers, but we prefer Ivalon suspension as our embolic material. A 1-year survival rate of 59% was reported by Vetter and colleagues[15] in patients who received iodized oil chemoembolization. Van Beers and associates,[16] in a retrospective analysis of chemoembolization in 54 patients with hepatocellular carcinoma, found that the patients who had oil retention in the tumor of greater than 50% of the tumor size lived significantly longer than the patients who had oil retention of less than 50% (1- and 2-year survival rates of 82% and 65%, respectively, vs. 27% and 0%). They also observed that the tumors in those patients who had poor oil retention were infiltrative and hypovascular and more advanced, whereas the lesions that had oil retention greater than 50% were of nodular and hypervascular types. The findings in this study support our belief that the lesions that will benefit from chemoembolization are of the nodular type of hepatocellular carcinoma. This type of tumor is usually well capsulated and hypervascular and is seen more frequently and earlier in Japan, perhaps because of the screening program there. When the tumor is more advanced, associated with tumor thrombus and cirrhosis, or hypovascular, the treatment is less effective because of the inability to deliver the chemotherapeutic agents and embolic materials into the tumor.

The efficacy of different chemotherapeutic agents used for chemoembolization of hepatocellular carcinoma has not been well confirmed. Some studies suggest that cisplatinum may be more effective than the commonly used doxorubicin and mitomycin-C. However, the significance of these studies has yet to be evaluated.

The results of chemoembolization for hepatic metastases are less optimistic and more mixed. In the early 1980s, we used Ivalon mixed with cisplatinum for chemoembolization in a group of patients with metastatic colorectal carcinoma to the liver. The results of this treatment were not published because there was no evidence that the treatment produced a significant response or prolonged survival time in these patients, and the attempt to provide symptomatic relief from the tumor burden resulted in the adverse effects of pain and fever after chemoembolization. The study by Yamashita and colleagues,[93] who treated 68 patients with various hepatic metastases with iodized oil and chemotherapeutic agents, produced a response rate of 22% and a median survival of 10 months. A similar result was also observed by Inoue and associates,[94] showing a partial response rate of 16% and a median survival period of 11 months. We currently do not perform chemoembolization in patients with metastatic colorectal carcinoma because the results are not improved over a less aggressive approach using IA chemotherapy. However, our view differs from that of Lang and Brown[95] and Pentecost and coworkers,[96] who, encouraged by results of chemoembolization of hepatic metastases from colorectal cancer, believe that the technique can be recommended as palliative treatment.

Other types of hepatic metastases treated by chemoembolization at our institution are metastatic ocular melanoma, metastatic leiomyosarcoma, metastatic neuroendocrine tumors, and, on occasion, metastatic hypernephroma. For metastatic ocular melanoma, chemoembolization with cisplatinum and Ivalon produced a response rate of 46% and a median survival period of 11 months.[97] These are not common tumors, and most are treated on protocol study. The more common types of hepatic metastases from colorectal carcinoma and carcinoma of the breast are usually treated by systemic or IA chemotherapy. Our approach to chemoembolization of hepatic metastases is similar to that with hepatocellular carcinoma, that is, a hypervascular tumor is more likely to benefit from treatment than a hypovascular one. The goal of treatment, whether it is to provide symptomatic relief or to prolong survival, must be considered against the risk of complications.

Our experience in treating hepatocellular carcinoma at the M. D. Anderson Cancer Center led to our belief that the type of hepatocellular carcinoma seen at our institution and, perhaps, in the United States is different from the types of tumors commonly treated in Japan. The nodular type of hepatocellular carcinoma is seen in less than 25% of our patients. A more challenging problem is the treatment of an advanced hepatocellular carcinoma or recurrent disease after previous treatment. These types of tumors are more commonly seen in our practice. They are more difficult to treat because they are usually associated with arterioportovenous shunts, tumor thrombus in the portal and hepatic veins, and liver cirrhosis and portal hypertension. Direct injection of absolute ethanol and chemoembolization are not likely to be completed, and may be contraindicated. We treat these patients with arterial infusion of chemotherapeutic agents and take care to deliver most of the drugs into the tumor and avoid infusion of the normal adjacent structures. The current regimens use cisplatinum 50 to 75 mg/m^2 and doxorubicin 25 to 40 mg/m^2 infused over 2 hours each, followed by 3 to 4 days' continuous infusion of floxuridine 50 to 75 mg/m^2 and leucovorin 15 mg/m^2/d. This regimen yielded a response rate of 41% with a median time to disease progression of 13 months. The median survival duration was 15 months, and was better among patients with negative hepatitis B or hepatitis C serology.[98] Treatment using a slightly different regimen consisting of floxuridine, doxorubicin, and mitomycin-C yielded a response rate of 78% and a median survival of 11.5 months.[99]

Results of Percutaneous Direct Injection With Absolute Ethanol

The effectiveness of the treatment has been shown in histopathologic studies from specimens in patients who had surgical resection after absolute ethanol injection. Shiina and colleagues reported complete tumor necrosis in up to 70% of their selected cases, and the remaining cases showed 70% to 90% tumor necrosis.[83] Shiina and colleagues,[24] Ebara and coworkers,[89] and Tanikawa and associates[88] reported long-term survival rates ranging from 49% to 61% at 4 years and 39% to 48% at 5 years. Recurrence at the injected lesion is rare according to Shiina and colleagues, but more frequent at other regions of the liver; their series showed recurrence rates of up to 64% at 5 years.[24,86] The results reported by Shiina and colleagues combined treatments using direct injection of absolute ethanol and chemoembolization.[20,24] Long-term survival data for treatment of hepatic metastases by direct injection are not available, and the benefits of treating asymptomatic, small hepatic metastases by direct injection with absolute ethanol are not well established.

SUMMARY

The nonsurgical treatment of hepatic tumors must be put in perspective. The small, nodular type of hepatocellular carcinoma is the type that may benefit most from such treatment, but the choices of therapy are many. This type of tumor be recommended by the interventional radiologist to have a treatment either by a direct injection of alcohol or by segmental chemoembolization, but it is also the type that could be resected, and is less likely to be treated by an interventional radiologist if the patient is seen first by a surgeon. The results of the treatment are likely to be good, with a chance of 2-year survival approaching 75% or better, a 4-year survival rate of 50%, and a 5-year survival of 30% to 40%. However, there is no randomized study to date comparing the results of the various techniques, including surgery. The decision to choose one treatment modality above the others is based on the recurrence rate and the morbidity and mortality associated with the treatment. Percutaneous direct injection with absolute ethanol and segmental chemoembolization or the combination of both are low-morbidity and low-mortality procedures, whereas surgical resection has a 5% or lower mortality rate and 20% to 30% postoperative morbidity. The percutaneous direct injection technique is associated with a 60% recurrence rate at 4 to 5 years, whereas segmental chemoembolization is associated with a 33% recurrence rate at 4 years, and this number is similar to that with surgical resection. Currently, there is no effective treatment for a large, unresectable hepatocellular carcinoma, but the tumor can be palliated by IA chemotherapy, which yielded a median survival of 12 to 15 months. For hepatic metastasis from colorectal carcinoma, IA chemotherapy yielded response rates of 40% to 70% and a median duration of survival of 15 to 18 months. A justification for chemoembolization or percutaneous injection with absolute ethanol has not been well established. Future research should be designed to compare the results of treatment by surgical resection and nonsurgical techniques, to improve the techniques of chemoembolization and percutaneous direct injection to decrease recurrence rates, and to search for new techniques to treat large, unresectable lesions.

REFERENCES

1. Chuang VP, Wallace S. Hepatic artery embolization in the treatment of hepatic neoplasms. Radiology 1981;140:51.
2. Chuang VP, Wallace S. Hepatic arterial redistribution for intraarterial infusion of hepatic neoplasms. Radiology 1980;135:295.
3. Chuang VP, Wallace S, Soo CS, Charnsangavej C, Bowers T. AJR Am J Roentgenol 1982;138:289.
4. Yamada R, Sato M, Kawabata M, et al. Hepatic artery embolization in 120 patients with unresectable hepatoma. Radiology 1983;148:397.
5. Patt YZ, Chuang VP, Wallace S, Herch EM, Freireich EJ, Marligit GM. The palliative role of hepatic arterial infusion and arterial occlusion in colorectal carcinoma metastatic to the liver. Lancet 1981;1:349.
6. Nakakuma K, Tashiro S, Hiraoka T, et al. Studies on anticancer treatment with an oily anticancer drug injected into the ligated feeding hepatic artery for liver cancer. Cancer 1983;52:2193.
7. Sakurai M, Okamura J, Kuroda C. Transcatheter chemoembolization effective for treating hepatocellular carcinoma. Cancer 1984;54:387.
8. Takayasu K, Moriyama N, Muramatsu Y, et al. Hepatic arterial embolization for hepatocellular carcinoma. Radiology 1984;150:661.
9. Konno T, Maeda H, Iwai K, et al. Selective targeting of anticancer drug and simultaneous image enhancement in solid tumors by arterially administered lipid contrast medium. Cancer 1985;54:2367.
10. Ohishi H, Uchida H, Yoshimura H, et al. Hepatocellular carcinoma detected by iodized oil. Radiology 1985;154:25.
11. Takayasu K, Shima Y, Muramatsu Y, et al. Hepatocellular carcinoma: treatment with intraarterial iodized oil with and without chemotherapeutic agents. Radiology 1987;162:345.
12. Kasugai H, Kojima J, Tatsuta M, et al. Treatment of hepatocellular carcinoma by transcatheter arterial embolization combined with intraarterial infusion of a mixture of cisplatin and ethiodized oil. Gastroenterology 1989;97:965.
13. Nakamura H, Hashimoto T, Oi H, Sawada S. Transcatheter oily chemoembolization of hepatocellular carcinoma. Radiology 1989;170:783.
14. Ohishi H, Yoshimura H, Uchida H, et al. Transcatheter arterial embolization using iodized oil (Lipiodol) mixed with an anticancer drug for the treatment of hepatocellular carcinoma. Cancer Chemother Pharmacol 1989;23(Suppl):33.
15. Vetter D, Wenger JJ, Bergier JM, et al. Transcatheter oily chemoembolization in the management of advanced hepatocellular carcinoma in cirrhosis: results of a western comparative study in 60 patients. Hepatology 1990;13:427.
16. Van Beers B, Roche A, Cauquil P, et al. Transcatheter arterial chemotherapy using doxorubicin, iodized oil and Gelfoam embolization in hepatocellular carcinoma. Acta Radiol 1989;30:415.
17. Sheu J-C, Huang G-T, Chen, D-S, et al. Small hepatocellular carcinoma: intratumor ethanol treatment using new needle and guidance systems. Radiology 1987;163:43.
18. Shiina S, Yasuda H, Muto H, et al. Percutaneous ethanol injection in the treatment of liver neoplasms. AJR Am J Roentgenol 1987;149:949.
19. Livraghi T, Salmi A, Bolondi L, et al. Small hepatocellular carcinoma: percutaneous alcohol injection—results in 23 patients. Radiology 1988;168:313.
20. Shiina S, Tagawa K, Unuma T, et al. Percutaneous ethanol injection therapy of hepatocellular carcinoma: analysis of 77 patients. AJR Am J Roentgenol 1990;155:1221.
21. Tanaka K, Nakamura S, Numata K, et al. Hepatocellular carcinoma: treatment with percutaneous ethanol injection and transcatheter arterial embolization. Radiology 1992;185:457.
22. Livraghi T, Vettori C. Percutaneous ethanol injection therapy of hepatoma. Cardiovasc Intervent Radiol 1990;13:146.
23. Livraghi T, Bolondi L, Lazzaroni S, et al. Percutaneous ethanol injection in the treatment of hepatocellular carcinoma in cirrhosis: a study in 207 patients. Cancer 1992;69:925.
24. Shiina S, Tagawa K, Niwa Y, et al. Percutaneous ethanol injection therapy for hepatocellular carcinoma: results in 146 patients. AJR Am J Roentgenol 1993;160:1023.
25. Nolsoe CP, Torp-Pedersen S, Burcharth F, et al. Interstitial hyperthermia of colorectal liver metastases with a US-guided Nd-YAG laser with a diffuser tip: a pilot clinical study. Radiology 1993;187:333.
26. Amin Z, Donald JJ, Masters A, et al. Hepatic metastases: interstitial laser photocoagulation with real-time US monitoring and dynamic CT evaluation of treatment. Radiology 1993;187:339.
27. Dachman AH, McGehee JA, Beam TE, et al. US-guided percutaneous laser ablation of liver tissue in a chronic pig model. Radiology 1990;176:129.
28. Kopecky KK, Yang R, Sanghvi NT, et al. Liver tumor ablation with high-intensity focused ultrasound. Semin Intervent Radiol 1993;10:125.
29. McGahan JP, Brock JM, Tesluk H, et al. Hepatic ablation with use of radio-frequency electrocautery. Invest Radiol 1990;1992;3:291.
30. McGahan JP, Browning PD, Brock JM, et al. Hepatic ablation using radiofrequency electrocautery. Invest Radiol 1990;25:267.
31. Kane RA. Ultrasound-guided hepatic cryosurgery for tumor ablation. Semin Intervent Radiol 1993;10:132.
32. Onik G, Kane R, Steele G, et al. Monitoring hepatic cryosurgery with sonography. AJR Am J Roentgenol 1986;147:665.
33. Onik G, Rubinsky B, Zemel R, et al. Ultrasound-guided hepatic cryosurgery in the treatment of metastatic colon carcinoma: preliminary results. Cancer 1991;67:901.
34. Nelson RC, Chezmar JL, Sugarbaker PH, et al. Hepatic tumors: comparison of CT during arterial portography, delayed CT, and MR imaging for preoperative evaluation. Radiology 1989;172:27.
35. Heiken JP, Weyman PJ, Lee JKT, et al. Detection of focal hepatic masses: prospective evaluation with CT, delayed CT, CT during arterial portography, and MR imaging. Radiology 1989;171:47.
36. Soyer P, Levesque M, Elias D, et al. Detection of liver metastases from colorectal cancer: comparison of intraoperative US and CT during arterial portography. Radiology 1992;183:541.
37. Peterson MS, Baron RL, Dodd GD III, et al. Hepatic parenchymal perfusion defects detected with CTAP: imaging-pathologic correlation. Radiology 1992;185:149.
38. Fernandez MP, Bernardino ME. Hepatic pseudolesions: appearance of focal low attenuation in the medial segment of the left lobe at CT-arterial portography. Radiology 1991;181:809.
39. Prando A, Wallace S, Bernardino ME, et al. Computed tomographic arteriography of the liver. Radiology 1979;130:697.
40. Freeny PC, Marks WM. Computed tomographic arteriography of the liver. Radiology 1983;148:193.
41. Freeny PC, Marks WM. Hepatic perfusion abnormalities during CT angiography: detection and interpretation. Radiology 1986;159:685.
42. Ohishi H, Uchida H, Yoshimura H, et al. Hepatocellular carcinoma detected by iodized oil: use of anticancer agents. Radiology 1985;154:19.
43. Hayashi N, Yamamoto K, Tamaki N, et al. Metastatic nodules of hepatocellular carcinoma: detection with angiography, CT, and US. Radiology 1987;165:61.
44. Merine D, Takayasu K, Wakao F. Detection of hepatocellular carcinoma: comparison of CT during arterial portography with CT after intra-arterial injection of iodized oil. Radiology 1990;175:707.
45. Smith EH. Complications of percutaneous abdominal fine-needle biopsy. Radiology 1991;178:253.
46. Welch TJ, Sheedy PF, Johnson CD, et al. CT guided biopsy: prospective analysis of 1,000 procedures. Radiology 1989;172:493.
47. Charboneau JW, Reading CC, Welch TJ. CT and sonographically guided needle biopsy: current techniques and new innovations. AJR Am J Roentgenol 1990;154:1.
48. Hoover HC. Surgical resection of primary hepatomas and hepatic metastases. Semin Intervent Radiol 1993;10:169.
49. Nagao T, Inoue S, Goto S, et al. Hepatic resection for hepatocellular

carcinoma: clinical features and long-term prognosis. Ann Surg 1987; 205:33.
50. Malt RA. Current concepts: surgery for hepatic neoplasms. N Engl J Med 1985;313:1591.
51. Yamanaka N, Okamoto E, Toyosake A, et al. Prognostic factors after hepatectomy for hepatocellular carcinomas. Cancer 1990;1105.
52. Iwatsuki S, Starzl TE. Personal experience with 411 hepatic resections. Ann Surg 1988;204:421.
53. Steele G, Ravikumar TS. Resection of hepatic metastases from colorectal cancer. Ann Surg 1989;210:127.
54. Goodman LE, Seligman AM. Regional chemotherapy. In: Holland JF, Frei E III, eds. Cancer medicine. Philadelphia: Lea & Febiger, 1973: 730.
55. Creech O Jr, Krementz ET, Ryan RF, Winbald JN. Chemotherapy of cancer: regional perfusion utilizing an extracorporeal circuit. Ann Surg 1958;148:616.
56. Anderson JH, Gianturco C, Wallace S. Experimental transcatheter intraarterial infusion-occlusion chemotherapy. Invest Radiol 1981;16: 496.
57. Wright KC, Charnsangavej C, Wallace A, et al. Regional isolation-persfusion: an experimental percutaneous approach tested and compared with arterial occlusion-infusion. Cardiovasc Intervent Radiol 1984;7:294.
58. Kemeny N, Daly J, Reichman B, et al. Intrahepatic or systemic infusion of fluorodexoxyuridine in patients with liver metastases from colorectal carcinoma. Ann Intern Med 1987;107:459.
59. Mavligit GM, Patt YZ, Haynie TP, et al. Differential tumor regression in patients with bilobar hepatic metastases and dual arterial supply: evidence supporting the advantage of intraarterial over intravenous route of drug delivery. Selective Cancer Therapy 1989;5:37.
60. Chang AE, Schneider PD, Sugarbaker PH. A prospective randomized trial of regional vs systemic continuous 5 fluorodeoxyuridine chemotherapy in the treatment of colorectal liver metastases. Ann Surg 1987; 206:685.
61. Martin JK Jr, O'Connell MJ, Wieand HS, et al. Intraarterial floxuridine vs systemic fluorouracil for hepatic metastases of colorectal cancer: a randomized trial. Arch Surg 1990;125:1022.
62. Niederhuber JE, Ensminger W, Gyves J, et al. Regional chemotherapy of colorectal cancer metastatic to the liver. Cancer 1984;53:1336.
63. Kemeny N, Cohen A, Bertino JR, et al. Continuous intrahepatic infusion of floxuridine and leucovorin through an implantable pump for treatment of hepatic metastases from colorectal carcinoma. Cancer 1990;65:2446.
64. Patt YZ, Boddie AW Jr, Chaarnsangavej C, et al. Hepatic artery infusion with floxuridine and cisplatin: overriding importance of anti-tumor effect versus degree of tumor burdens as determinants of survival among patients with colorectal cancer. J Clin Oncol 1986;4:1356.
65. Fortner JG, Mulcare RJ, Solis A, et al. Treatment of primary and secondary liver cancer by hepatic artery ligation and infusion chemotherapy. Ann Surg 1973;178:162.
66. Guelessarian HP, Lawton LL, Condon RE. Hepatic artery ligation and cytotoxic infusion in treatment of liver metastases. Arch Surg 1972; 105:280.
67. Aronsen KF, Hellekant C, Holmberg J, et al. Controlled blocking of hepatic artery flow with enzymatically degradable microspheres combined with oncolytic drugs. Eur Surg Res 1979;11:99.
68. Dakhil S, Ensminger W, Cho KJ, et al. Improved regional selectivity of hepatic arterial BCNU with degradable microspheres. Cancer 1982; 50:631.
69. Kato L, Nemoto R, Mori H, et al. Arterial chemoembolization with microencapsulated anticancer drug. JAMA 1981;245:1123.
70. Carrasco CH, Freeny PC, Chuang VP, et al. Chemical cholecystitis associated with hepatic artery infusion chemotherapy. AJR Am J Roentgenol 1983;141:703.
71. Botet JF, Watson RC, Kemeny N, et al. Cholangitis complicating intraarterial chemotherapy in liver metastasis. Radiology 1985;156:335.
72. Hohn DC, Melnick J, Stagg RJ, et al. Biliary sclerosis in patients receiving hepatic arterial infusion of floxuridine. J Clin Oncol 1985;3:98.
73. Hohn DC, Stagg RJ, Price DC, et al. Avoidance of gastroduodenal toxicity in patients receiving hepatic artery 5-fluoro-2'-deoxyuridine. J Clin Oncol 1985;3:1257.
74. Charnsangavej C, Carrasco CH, Wallace S, et al. Hepatic arterial flow distribution in portal vein occlusion: its significance in hepatic artery infusion chemotherapy. Radiology 1987;165:71.
75. Cho KJ, Andrews JC, Williams DM, et al. Hepatic arterial chemotherapy: role of angiography. Radiology 1989;173:783.
76. Miller DL, O'Leary TJ, Girton M. Distribution of iodized oil within the liver after hepatic arterial injection. Radiology 1987;162:849.
77. Nakamura H, Hashimoto T, Oi H, Sawada S. Oil in the portal vein after arterial embolization. Radiology 1988;167:415.
78. Kan Z, Ivancev K, Hagerstrand I, et al. In vivo microscopy of the liver after injection of Lipiodol into the hepatic artery and portal vein in the rat. Acta Radiol 1989;30:419.
79. Yamada R, Kishi K, Sonomura T, et al. Transcatheter arterial embolization in unresectable hepatocellular carcinoma. Cardiovasc Intervent Radiol 1990;13:135.
80. Uchida H, Ohishi H, Matsuo N, et al. Transcatheter hepatic segmental arterial embolization using Lipiodol mixed with an anticancer drug and gelfoam particles for hepatocellular carcinoma. Cardiovasc Intervent Radiol 1990;13:140.
81. Nakamura H, Hashimoto T, Oi H, et al. Treatment of hepatocellular carcinoma by segmental hepatic artery injection of Adriamycin-in-oil emulsion with overflow to segmental portal veins. Acta Radiol 1990; 31:347.
82. Matsui O, Kadoya M, Yoshikawa J, et al. Small hepatocellular carcinoma: treatment with subsegmental transcatheter arterial embolization. Radiology 1993;188:79.
83. Shiina S, Tagawa K, Unuma T, et al. Percutaneous ethanol injection therapy for hepatocellular carcinoma: a histopathologic study. Cancer 1991;68:1524.
84. Burgener FA, Steinmetz SD. Treatment of experimental adenocarcinomas by percutaneous intratumoral injection of absolute ethanol. Invest Radiol 1986;22:472.
85. Festi D, Monti F, Casanova S, et al. Morphological and biochemical effects of intrahepatic alcohol injection in the rabbit. J Gastroenterol Hepatol 1990;5:402.
86. Shiina S, Niwa Y, Omata M. Percutaneous ethanol injection therapy for liver neoplasms. Semin Intervent Radiol 1993;10:57.
87. Livraghi T, Solbiati L. Percutaneous ethanol injection in liver cancer: method and results. Semin Intervent Radiol 1993;10:69.
88. Tanikawa K. Multidisciplinary treatment of hepatocellular carcinoma. In: Tobe T, Kameda H, Ohto M, et al, eds. Primary liver cancer in Japan. Tokyo: Springer-Verlag, 1992:327.
89. Ebara M, Ohto M, Suguira N, et al. Percutaneous ethanol injection for the treatment of small hepatocellular carcinoma: study of 95 patients. J Gastroenterol Hepatol 1990;5:616.
90. Redvanly RD, Chezmar JL, Strauss RM, et al. Malignant hepatic tumors: safety of high-dose percutaneous ethanol ablation therapy. Radiology 1993;188:283.
91. Redvanly RD, Chezmar JL. Percutaneous ethanol ablation therapy of malignant hepatic tumors using CT guidance. Semin Intervent Radiol 1993;10:82.
92. Venook AP, Stagg RJ, Lewis BJ, et al. Chemoembolization for hepatocellular carcinoma. J Clin Oncol 1990;8:1108.
93. Yamashita Y, Takahashi M, Koga Y, et al. Prognostic factors in liver metastases after transcatheter arterial embolization or arterial infusion. Acta Radiol 1990;31:269.
94. Inoue H, Kobayashi H, Itoh Y, et al. Treatment of liver metastases by arterial injection of Adriamycin/mitomycin C Lipiodol suspension. Acta Radiol 1989;30:603.
95. Lang EK, Brown CL Jr. Colorectal metastases to the liver: selective chemoembolization. Radiology 1993;189:417.
96. Pentecost MJ, Teitelbaum GP, Katz MD, et al. Chemoembolization in hepatic malignancy. Semin Intervent Radiol 1992;9:28.
97. Mavligit GM, Charnsangavej C, Carrasco CH, et al. Regression of ocular melanoma metastatic to the liver after hepatic arterial chemoembolization with cisplatin and polyvinyl sponge. JAMA 1988;260:974.
98. Patt YZ, Charnsangavej C, Yoffe B, et at. Hepatic arterial infusion of floxuridine, leucovorin, doxorubicin, and cisplatin for hepatocellular carcinoma: effects of hepatitis B and C viral infection on drug toxicity and patient survival. J Clin Oncol 1994;12:1204.
99. Patt YZ, Charnsangavej C, Boddie A, et al. Treatment of hepatocellular carcinoma with hepatic arterial floxuridine, doxorubicin, and mitomycin C (FUDRAM) with or without hepatic artery embolization: factors associated with longer survival. Regional Cancer Treatment 1989;2: 98.

PART VI

Lower Gastrointestinal Cancer

Surgery for Gastrointestinal Cancer: A Multidisciplinary Approach, edited by Harold J. Wanebo.
Lippincott-Raven Publishers, Philadelphia, © 1997.

CHAPTER 57

Surgical Endoscopy of the Large Bowel: "Tricks of the Trade"

Frederick L. Greene

Approximately 250,000 people in the United States are diagnosed as having cancer of the digestive organs each year.[1] Of this number, 150,000 new cases of colorectal cancer are diagnosed and approximately 60,000 deaths occur from this disease annually. Colorectal cancer is responsible for 20,000 deaths each year in Britain.[2] From these statistics alone, it is obvious that the introduction of endoscopic screening and therapeutic maneuvers has had a great importance in the lives of many of these people with neoplasia. In the gastrointestinal tract, more than 80% of these tumors arise from mucosal surfaces that are within the optical range of modern endoscopic equipment, and therefore both surveillance and therapeutic maneuvers become realistic options.

The approach endoscopically to large bowel neoplasia can be viewed from the aspects of surveillance, early diagnosis and biopsy, endoscopic ablation and excision, and follow-up techniques using the endoscope. The various "tricks" used in the foregoing are obviously developed through the surgical endoscopist's experience and depend also on using new and updated equipment that allows for facile passage of the endoscope and delivery of the therapeutic modality to a specified area of colon.

TECHNICAL CONSIDERATIONS

The technique of diagnostic and therapeutic colonoscopy depends on the creation of a mechanically clean colon. Without adequate patient preparation, attempts to visualize even a portion of the colon may not only be unrewarding but are dangerous. The experienced endoscopist recognizes early during the examination that the preparation is marginal and plans for a repeat attempt at examination on another day. Mechanical cleansing with polyethylene glycol/electrolyte solutions (PEG–electrolyte solutions) creates an appropriate environment whereby visualization and biopsy sampling can be safely performed. Although osmotic fluids are reported to remain within the colonic lumen and act by lavage, an increase in plasma volume does in fact occur to a small extent, and may lead to an increased intravascular volume in patients who are already compromised from congestive heart failure, renal disease, or other metabolic derangements.[3] For patients who are unable to drink 3 to 4 L of PEG–electrolyte solution, conventional bowel preparation with clear liquids over 2 to 3 days and cathartics such as magnesium citrate may be used.

If the patient has already had a barium study performed on the colon, it is useful to have this study available in the endoscopy suite to act potentially as a "road map" for the surgical endoscopist. In addition, information regarding the presence of benign diseases such as diverticulosis may be helpful to avoid pitfalls that may occur when large diverticula are intubated (Fig. 57-1). In addition, tortuosity of the colon may be visualized on a barium enema, and this study helps the endoscopist decide whether changing patient position may be helpful during insertion of the endoscope.

It is mandatory that the endoscope, whether it be a rigid proctoscope, flexible sigmoidoscope, or 180-cm colonoscope, be gently and effectively placed in the anal canal. Patients with increased anal tone may present difficult challenges; this barrier may be overcome by gentle digital introduction, using a slight traction technique as the endoscope is introduced (Fig. 57-2). The instrument should never be forced through the anal canal because tears of mucosa as well as irritation of hemorrhoidal venous plexuses may result. It is important to take time during this portion of the examination so that the patient remains comfortable, even though sedation has been used.

Once the endoscope has been positioned in the distal rectum, gentle insufflation of air is necessary to create the proper cavity for safe insertion. The beginning endoscopist usually creates a situation of overinsufflation, which makes the patient more uncomfortable during the endoscopic examination. The gentle application of insufflated air, as well as its removal, aid the migration of the scope proximally. Patients are always encouraged to pass flatus to avoid overdistention and the need for additional sedation.

The performance of safe colonoscopy is one of the most

Frederick L. Greene: Department of Surgery, University of South Carolina, Two Medical Park Road, Suite 402, Columbia, SC 29203

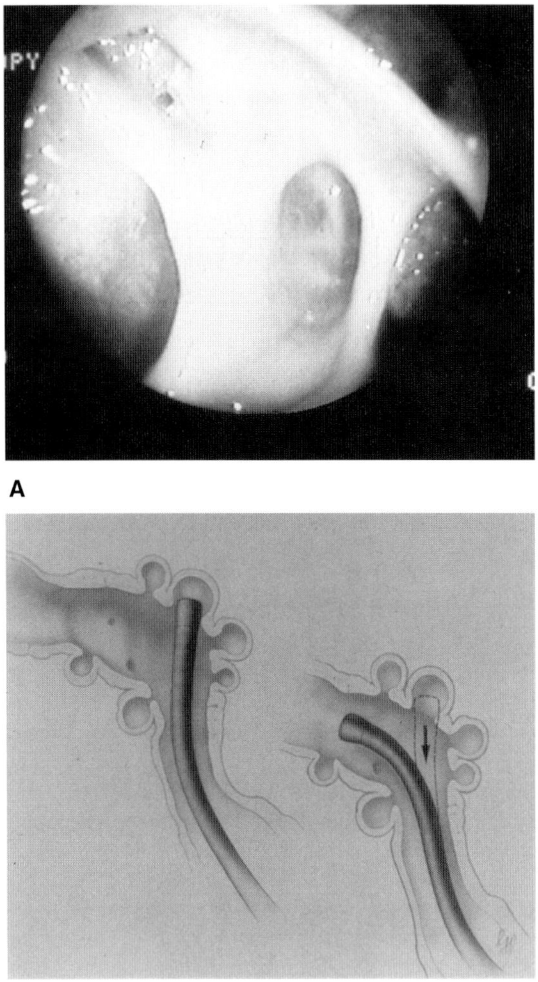

FIG. 57-1. (A) Intraluminal view showing extensive diverticulosis. **(B)** Inadvertent intubation of large diverticulum.

difficult and demanding endoscopic procedures performed in the gastrointestinal tract. Only through a long experience can the technique be mastered and a safe examination be accomplished. The goal of the colonoscopic examination is to intubate the entire colon to the cecum and then perform the complete examination on withdrawal of the instrument. The patient usually is placed in the left lateral decubitus position (Sims' position), but other positions may be necessary as demanded by the anatomy of the colon and the discomfort of the patient. In general, the distal rectum and sigmoid colon are the most difficult areas to intubate because of the tortuosity of these areas and the angulation of the rectosigmoid flexure, which occurs at 15 cm from the anal verge. The major ''trick'' to intubate this area effectively is to use torquing maneuvers by turning the instrument both clockwise and counterclockwise as insertion takes place under direct vision (Fig. 57-3). It is important always to have the lumen visible at all times to avoid inappropriate intubation of diverticula or perforation of the wall of the distal bowel. One of the frequent mistakes is to measure the position of abnormal findings using the centimeter guideline printed on the endoscope itself. It is important to note that stretching and an ''accordion'' phenomenon take place as the instrument is positioned and, therefore, it is unrealistic to rely too much on information based on the length of scope introduced during insertion. It is more appropriate to measure the position of an intraluminal lesion during withdrawal, when less of the colon is collapsed in a longitudinal fashion around the scope.

One of the common pitfalls and problems seen in colonoscopy is the inability to intubate the sigmoid colon effectively because of previous pelvic or abdominal surgical procedures. Taking a good history is important to determine whether adhesions may be present that may make the examination more difficult and may, in fact, require the use of a greater amount of intravenous sedation. Although the location of adhesions is important in the pelvic area, it is even more crucial to recognize that adhesions may form in the left upper quadrant and create a tethering effect around the spleen. If the area of the splenic flexure is forcibly straightened, a capsular tear may be created in the spleen that can manifest as significant hypotension several hours after the procedure. The message regarding adhesions is that gentle introduction of the colonoscope with careful insufflation of air should be the mainstay of the examination.

The introduction of the endoscope may be further hampered by diverticular disease, and the associated spasm may create a greater problem as the endoscope is introduced. A helpful adjunct for passage of the scope in this setting is the use of intravenous glucagon, 0.5 to 1 mg, which acts as an antispasmodic within 5 to 10 minutes after injection. Even patients who have no evidence of diverticula but who have a history of irritable

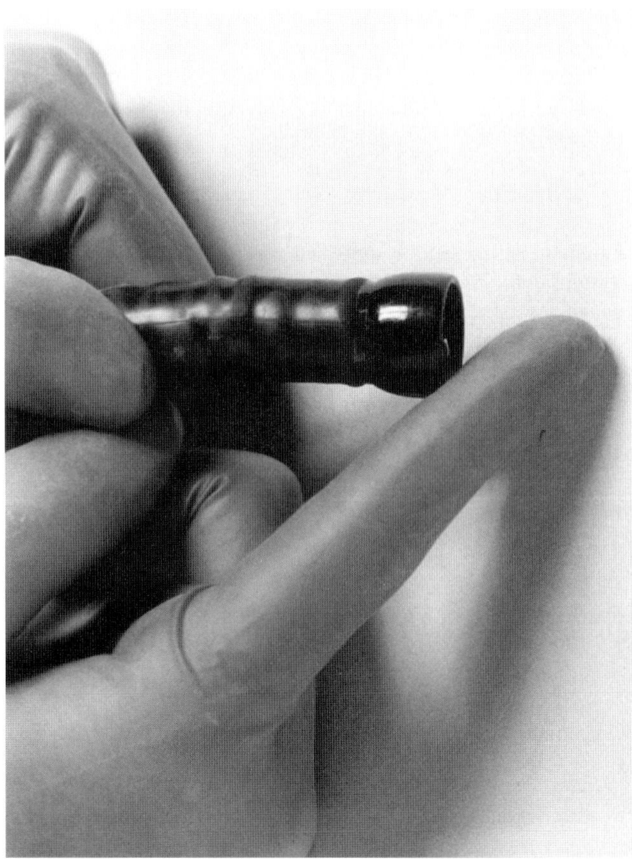

FIG. 57-2. Proper positioning of endoscopic tip during anal intubation.

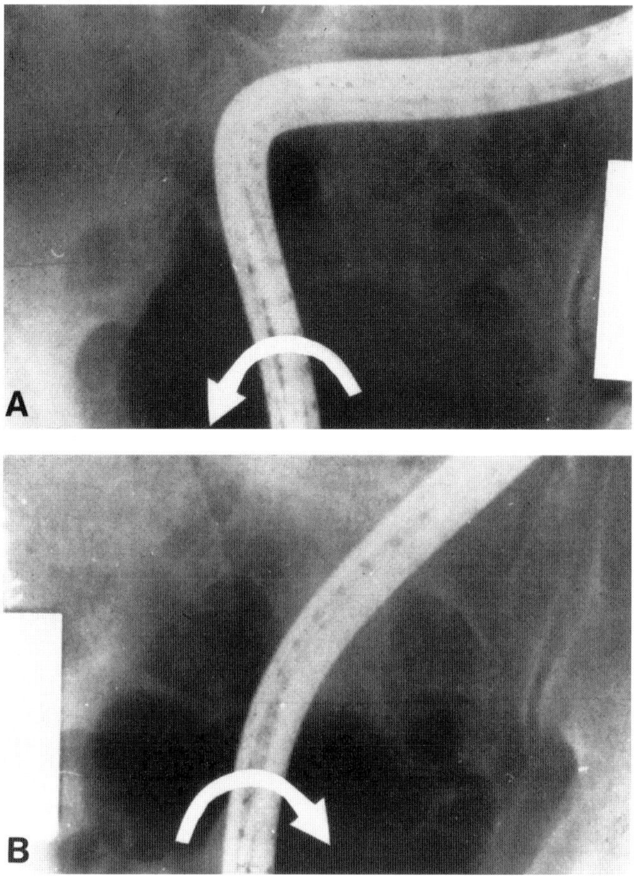

FIG. 57-3. Introduction of colonoscope using counterclockwise **(A)** and clockwise **(B)** torquing maneuvers.

bowel may benefit by intravenous glucagon early in the examination to avoid significant spasm enhanced by the procedure.

As mentioned previously, the goal of colonoscopy is to intubate completely the abdominal colon and to reach the cecum. The cecum is recognized by the "vaulted-church" appearance of its most proximal area (Fig. 57-4). Frequently, the ileocecal valve may be visualized, and may actually appear to be a "lesion" in the cecum to the unwary or inexperienced endoscopist (Fig. 57-5). The ileocecal valve may take many shapes, and can be quite polypoid in its appearance. If the ileocecal valve is easily seen, the distal ileum may also be intubated, which can be especially helpful when patients are examined who have diagnoses of inflammatory bowel disease and suspected neoplasia.

The major part of the diagnostic procedure is performed during withdrawal of the colonoscope, and here, attention to detail is especially important. If patients have been prepared using PEG–electrolyte solutions, a large amount of liquid may still reside in the colon, and if it is not effectively suctioned free, small lesions may remain undetected, especially in areas of dependency when the patient is in a lateral position. As mentioned previously, avoiding overinsufflation is very important, not only for patient comfort, but to avoid a compression effect on small lesions that may be significant in the diagnosis of colonic neoplasia. If a "napkin-ring" lesion is suspected from a prior barium enema or is visualized on the initial endoscopic

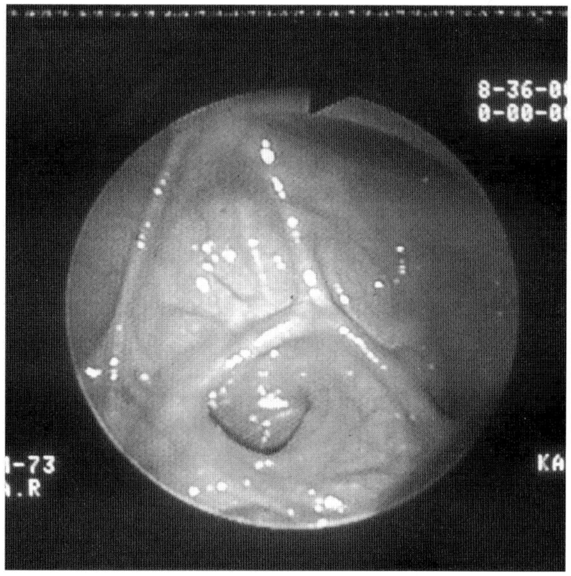

FIG. 57-4. Cecum, showing "vaulted-church" appearance.

examination, it is important to avoid overinsufflation with air because even a mildly obstructive lesion may produce a "valvular effect" and cause overdistention of the proximal colon, especially when the ileocecal valve is competent. If a large amount of air is placed in this setting, perforation of the cecum or right colon may occur even though the endoscope never reaches the proximal bowel. This scenario has been seen by the author even when flexible sigmoidoscopy is performed for a distal, moderately obstructing colonic lesion.

INSTRUMENT AND ACCESSORY ISSUES

The ability to perform adequate and safe endoscopy depends on the endoscopic physician being thoroughly familiar with the

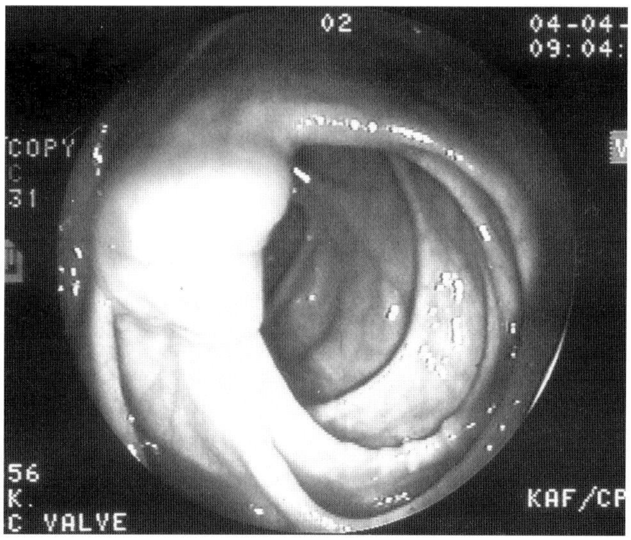

FIG. 57-5. Prominent ileocecal valve may mimic polypoid lesion.

instrumentation that he or she will be using in the examination. Since the early 1980s, significant improvements have been made in endoscopic equipment that necessitate continuous education on the part of the endoscopic physician to keep pace with changes in techniques and equipment. It is important to ensure that the light source, irrigating system, and insufflation mechanism are working appropriately before insertion of the endoscope.

In the modern era of endoscopy, the gastrointestinal assistant has become a valuable colleague of the medical and surgical endoscopist, but this phenomenon cannot replace the need for the physician to ensure that equipment is ready for use. In addition, ascertaining the availability of appropriate accessories such as biopsy forceps and cytology brushes is mandatory before the procedure. During the colonic examination for neoplasia, the likelihood of visualizing polypoid lesions in addition to a synchronous carcinoma is high, and therefore snare wire and cautery application always must be anticipated.

As is true with open surgical procedures, the need for prophylactic antibiotics may be indicated in patients with pacemakers, vascular grafts, or orthopedic hardware, or those with associated cardiac valvular disease. The antibiotic of choice must be appropriate to cover anaerobic organisms and should be given at least 10 to 15 minutes before the endoscopic procedure. An appropriate intravenous line is always necessary for patients undergoing full colonoscopy and should be in place for the administration of sedative drugs, which usually include midazolam and meperidine. One important consideration is to place the intravenous line in the right upper extremity because the patient is in a left lateral position for the examination; obstruction to venous inflow could develop by lying on the left side. An intravenous line on the left hand or arm may not function well because of this lateral decubitus position.

It is mandatory in the well equipped outpatient endoscopy suite to have proper monitoring devices, including pulse oximetry, sphygmomanometry, and electrocardiographic monitoring, if indicated. The gastrointestinal assistant plays an important role in helping to monitor the patient during the examination, and it is mandatory that proper monitoring devices be in place before beginning the endoscopic examination.

BIOPSY TECHNIQUES AND INTERPRETATION

Although technical ability to perform large bowel examination for neoplasia is important, it is equally, if not more, important to interpret findings correctly and to recognize when biopsy sampling should and should not be attempted. Because the outcome and long-term survival from carcinoma of the colon depend on finding lesions at an early time in their development, the casual endoscopist may overlook important small lesions if the examination is not done correctly and all areas of the colon are not inspected with care. Although it is not necessary to sample all hyperplastic (metaplastic) polyps, the experienced endoscopist recognizes these small lesions, which are approximately 3 to 4 mm in diameter, sessile, and relatively pale in appearance compared with adenomatous polyps (Fig. 57-6).

Although a concern regarding dissemination of tumor during endoscopic examination has been raised,[4] our studies have demonstrated that patients who have undergone preoperative endoscopic studies show no increase in tumor stage or worsened

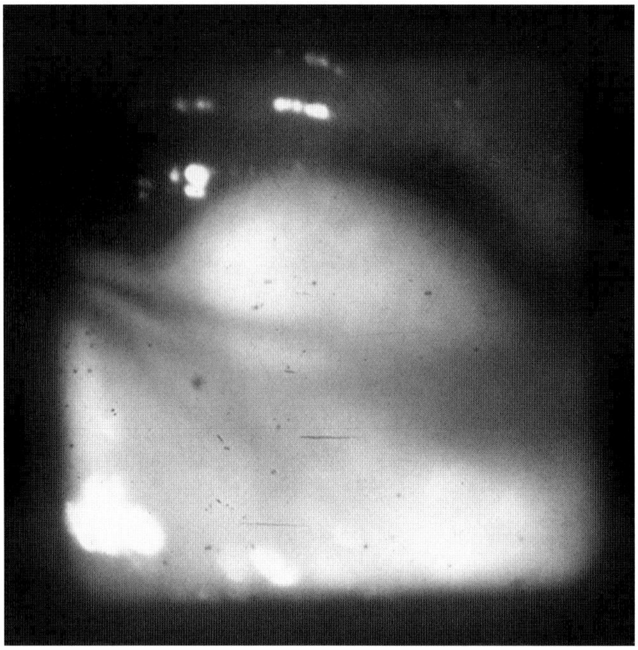

FIG. 57-6. Diminutive, hyperplastic polyp of colon.

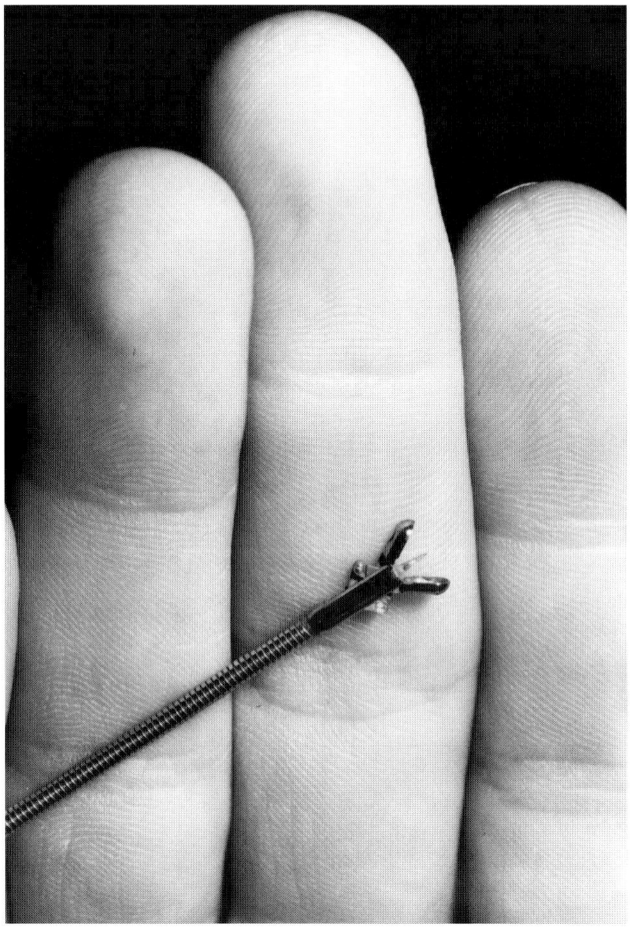

FIG. 57-7. Forceps used for colonoscopic biopsy.

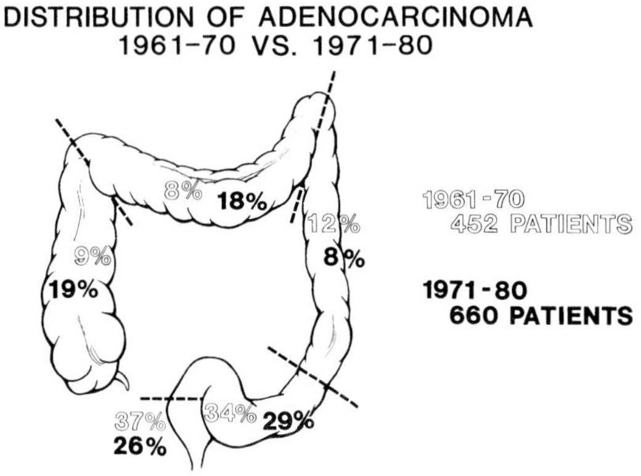

FIG. 57-8. Results of study showing distribution of colonic cancer over two decades.[7]

outcome compared with patients having no endoscopic study.[5] There are no data to suggest that contact between the endoscope and intraluminal colonic tumor causes significant shedding of cancer cells, either intraluminally or through vascular or lymphatic drainage.

Biopsy techniques for lesions interpreted as carcinoma are varied and should be carefully undertaken to avoid the "missed" lesion or the phenomenon of having a diagnosis returned as "inflammation only." Although the beginning endoscopist usually tries to sample in the central portion of an ulcerating tumor, the best and most productive area is the periphery of the crater of the ulceration. Because the biopsy forceps are small, measuring approximately 3 mm (Fig. 57-7), it is necessary mildly to force the biopsy forceps past the surface of the tumor to obtain a satisfactory histologic specimen, and to avoid the surface exudate, which only gives a picture of inflammation. The experienced endoscopist is able to interpret adequately if an adenocarcinoma is present and does not accept a diagnosis of "inflammation," but plans to reexamine endoscopically and resample to obtain adequate tissue. It is also mandatory to obtain three or four specimens from different areas of tumor to assess the lesion adequately.

During the diagnostic study of patients with colonic carcinoma, a major objective is to rule out additional lesions such as adenomatous polyps that occur in 40% to 50% of patients with colorectal cancer and may be seen in areas of the colon remote from the primary tumor.[6] It is important to examine all areas of the colon and to sample lesions that may change the operative technique and extent of a planned extirpative procedure. The endoscopist must remember that since approximately the 1940s, the traditional anatomic location for colorectal cancer and polyps has undergone a significant change in that a greater percentage of neoplastic lesions is located in the proximal colon. A number of studies, including our own,[7] have confirmed a "left-to-right shift" of cancer in the colon, and this has underlined the important concept that total colonoscopy must be accomplished in any patient with symptoms of colonic cancer (Fig. 57-8). Our studies have also confirmed that this proximal shift is seen more commonly in older patients (Fig. 57-9*A*), and especially in women older than 65 years of age[7] (see Fig. 57-9*B*). The finding of synchronous polyps in patients with proximal carcinoma of the colon remains an important concept, and these lesions should be searched for diligently during endoscopic studies for large bowel neoplasia.

ENDOSCOPY IN THE BLEEDING PATIENT

Since the development of colonoscopy in the early 1970s,[8] it has generally been recognized that application of this technique is not appropriate in patients who are acutely bleeding. Because of the inability adequately to clean the colon and to visualize the colonic lesion, the likelihood of perforation is increased during the examination. Because most carcinomas of the colon do not present with significant ongoing colonic bleeding, the opportunity for proper cleansing and nonemergent examination is usually the norm. On occasion, however, patients present with brisk bleeding that may be related to a colonic tumor, but because of the bleeding pattern, may mimic angiodysplasia or diverticulosis. It is important for the experienced endoscopist to attempt to cleanse the distal colon before any examination, and this is best accomplished using rigid proctoscopic techniques. Gentle lavage with saline is helpful to remove gross blood and clot and to ensure that rectal lesions are not missed. This scenario could lead to the inappropriate abdominal colectomy for a presumed diverticular bleed while a more distal lesion is overlooked because of the inability to palpate digitally or the inadequacy of the endoscopic view.

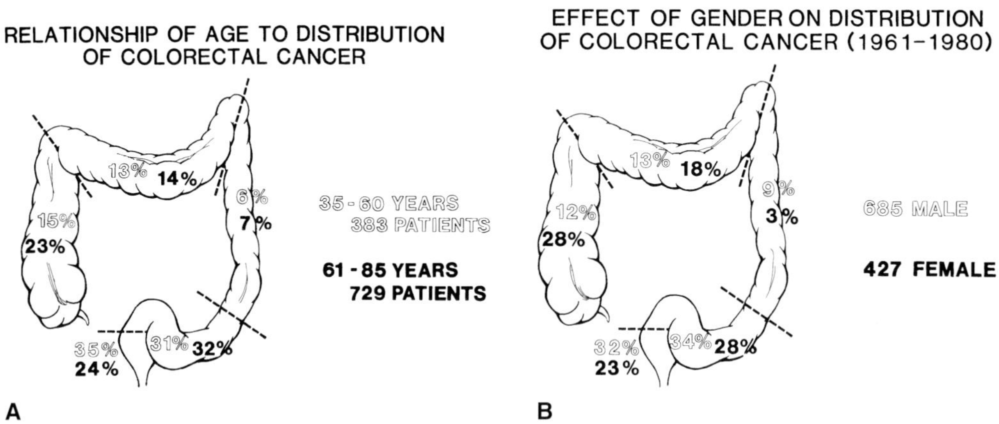

FIG. 57-9. (A) Changing distribution of colorectal cancer as a result of age.[7] **(B)** Changing distribution of colorectal cancer as a result of gender.[7]

COLONOSCOPIC POLYPECTOMY

The initial report of endoscopic polypectomy described the snaring and cauterization of an adenomatous polyp, performed in September, 1969. Since this original contribution by Wolff and Shinya,[9] the colonoscope has been the mainstay of polyp removal and has all but eliminated the necessity of transabdominal colotomy and polypectomy. Although most polyps removed through the colonoscope are pedunculated, the experienced endoscopist may also approach sessile lesions, especially villous tumors that are interpreted with reasonable assurance to be benign. Techniques using injection of the mucosa with saline to elevate the sessile lesion may facilitate endoscopic snare removal[10] (Fig. 57-10). Snare polypectomy of sessile lesions must be performed with caution because of the increased rate of perforation possible in this setting.

The preparation of the bowel is similar to that used in a traditional colectomy. Bowel preparation, both mechanical and antibiotic, reduces some potential septic hazards if perforation occurs. The initial report of colonoscopic polypectomy was delayed by the authors because of their concern that perforation might be a significant phenomenon; they therefore chose to complete more than 200 cases without complications before reporting the new procedure.[11] One of the important considerations during polypectomy is the cautery setting. As is true with open surgical procedures, a lower setting on the monopolar cautery of approximately 20 to 30 W and the use of a blended current for both cutting and coagulation are important considerations that minimize the probability of tissue destruction and late perforation.

Endoscopic polypectomy should be performed by personnel who have significant experience in diagnostic colonoscopy to minimize potential risks of the procedure. Although polyp removal is now within the purview of both the medical and surgical gastroenterologist, the surgeon is the best judge of the relation of the planned polypectomy to the overall treatment of the patient with additional neoplastic lesions in the colon. The finding of a significant number of polyps throughout the colon may indicate that total abdominal colectomy is warranted, rather than individual snare removal followed by a more limited resection.

One of the problems related to colonoscopic polypectomy is the difficulty of retrieving polyps once the stalk has been effectively divided using cautery. It is mandatory that polyps be recovered for histologic study, although every experienced colonoscopist realizes that occasionally a polyp cannot be retrieved during the procedure. The most efficacious method of polyp retrieval is to use the endoscopic suction to fix the excised polyp to the end of the instrument. In this way, the polyp may be retrieved, although occasionally the tissue is lost as the endoscope is withdrawn. Additional techniques have been developed using small baskets and atraumatic graspers that may hold the resected tissue better than the suction technique (Fig. 57-11). It is important to avoid crushing tissue during removal after polypectomy because any artefact maximizes the difficulty of pathologic interpretation. The effect of cautery on the base of

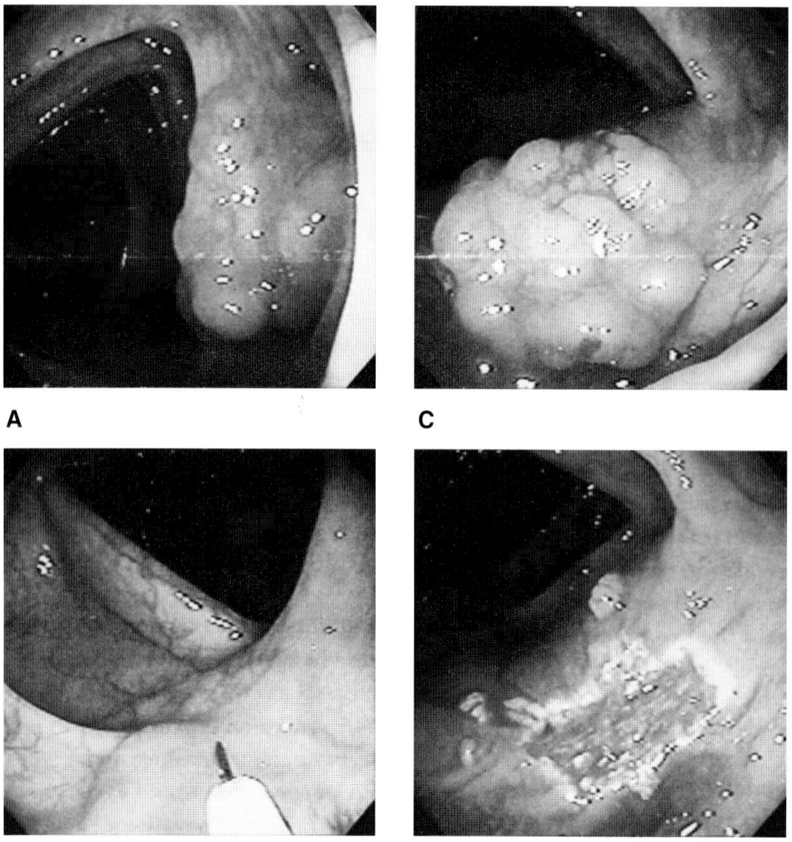

A C B D

FIG. 57-10. Technique of saline injection using sclerotherapy needle to elevate sessile polyp **(A–C).** After elevation, snare cautery of lesion may be safely undertaken, with resultant mucosal defect **(D).**

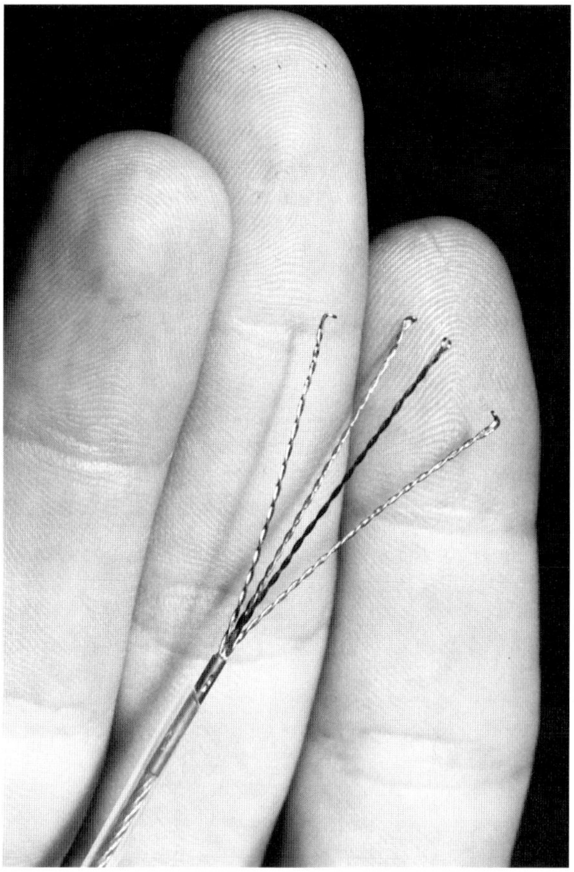

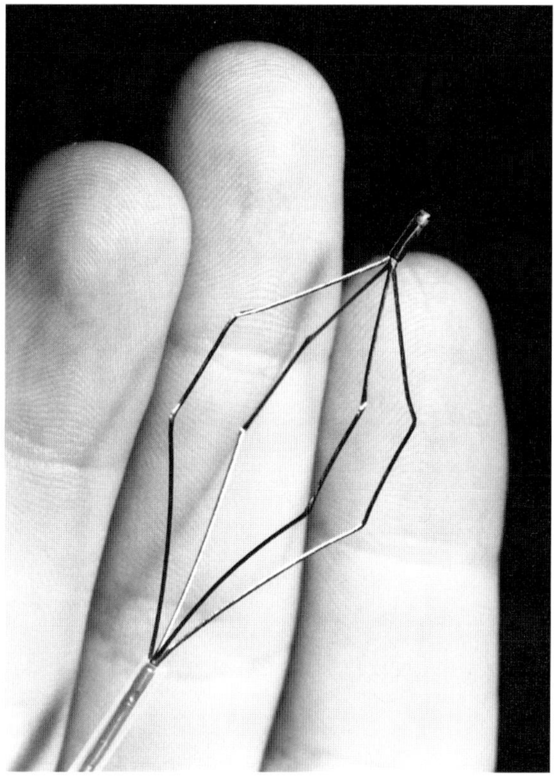

A B

FIG. 57-11. Atraumatic grasper **(A)** and basket **(B)** used for polyp removal after snare cauterization.

the polyp may create problems in deciding whether a polypoid carcinoma extends into the stalk. It is important for the surgical endoscopist to view the histologic investigation in the pathology laboratory to recognize some of the consequences of polypectomy and to help minimize problems of interpretation related to polypectomy technique.

One of the significant pitfalls leading to inappropriate interpretation and management is the performance of a "fractional" biopsy procedure that gives only a minimal amount of information relative to the true histologic type of the lesion. Not only does "fractional" biopsy give erroneous information regarding the benign or malignant nature of the polyp, but this maneuver underestimates the presence of tumor in making the diagnosis of tumor invasion (Fig. 57-12). To make a determination of invasion, entire removal of the polyp and complete sectioning is necessary. The proper orientation of the polyp by the pathologist is crucial to avoid misinterpretation and the findings previously seen in the entity termed "epithelial misplacement."[12] The astute endoscopist realizes all of the consequences of suboptimal biopsy and therefore uses techniques that remove the entire polyp. If this removal is not appropriate or is deemed unsafe, the endoscopist must realize that full-thickness excision should be achieved to make a proper histologic determination. This is accomplished with traditional open or newer laparoscopic extirpation.

COMPLICATIONS OF POLYPECTOMY

As mentioned previously, the skill of the endoscopist determines to a large degree whether the procedure can be accomplished safely. Even in the hands of the safe and experienced technician, however, untoward results occur, and these should at least be discussed when informed consent is obtained from the patient. Material risks include perforation and bleeding when polypectomy is anticipated. The overall complication rate in experienced hands should certainly not exceed 1%. Specific complications during polypectomy include bleeding, perforation, transmural burn, and snare entrapment.

Bleeding represents approximately 50% of the complications seen as a result of polypectomy.[13] The effective use of cautery and the avoidance of tearing during application of the snare wire reduce the likelihood of postpolypectomy bleeding. This bleeding may present as a slow ooze or brisk hemorrhage, and may be immediate or delayed. Many patients are on low-dose aspirin for a variety of reasons, and this fact should be elicited when history is taken to avoid the complication of bleeding secondary to platelet dysfunction. The use of aspirin-containing and nonsteroidal drugs should be curtailed at least 10 days before an attempted endoscopic procedure with planned polypectomy. In addition, patients on anticoagulation for cardiac or chronic venous disease should have their medication discontinued for at least 3 to 5 days before the procedure. In these pa-

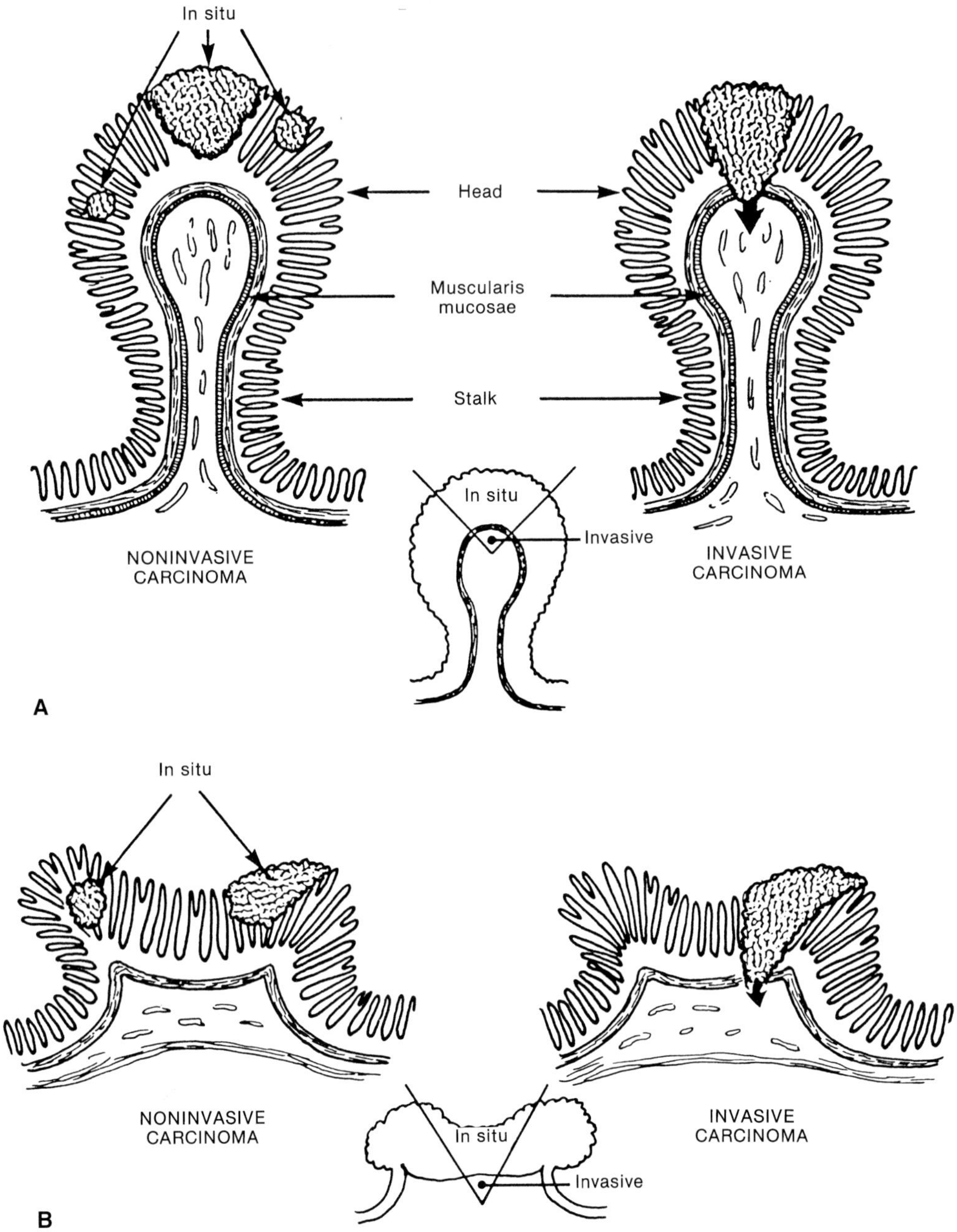

FIG. 57-12. Foci of superficial and invasive cancer in pedunculated **(A)** and sessile **(B)** polyp, showing the importance of avoiding "fractional biopsy."

tients, appropriate prothrombin times and partial thromboplastin times should be obtained.

Perforation may occur as a consequence of cautery effect during polypectomy. The application of increased cautery power may cause a transmural burn that classically manifests several hours to several days after the procedure. This potential complication is lessened by applying the snare wire in the midportion of a stalk, which avoids a tenting effect at the base of the stalk of the polyp (Fig. 57-13). Obviously, if sessile lesions are approached, the opportunity for perforation increases. By using a technique that elevates the sessile polyp from the surrounding mucosa through saline injection, the colonic wall may be protected when sessile lesions are removed. Perforation secondary to cautery effect may be diminished by using a lower-wattage setting and by carefully placing the snare wire before delivery of current.

On occasion, when a large polyp is approached, the snare wire may be closed prematurely, resulting in snare wire entrapment. This may occur during the removal of either a pedunculated or sessile polyp, and may lead to incomplete transection of the polyp and inability to remove the snare wire. On occasion, the wire should be left in place, and may only release as the polyp continues to slough. If the surgeon is concerned about the inability to remove the snare wire, a traditional celiotomy may be performed to avoid further complications of bleeding or perforation. In general, this problem should occur very infre-

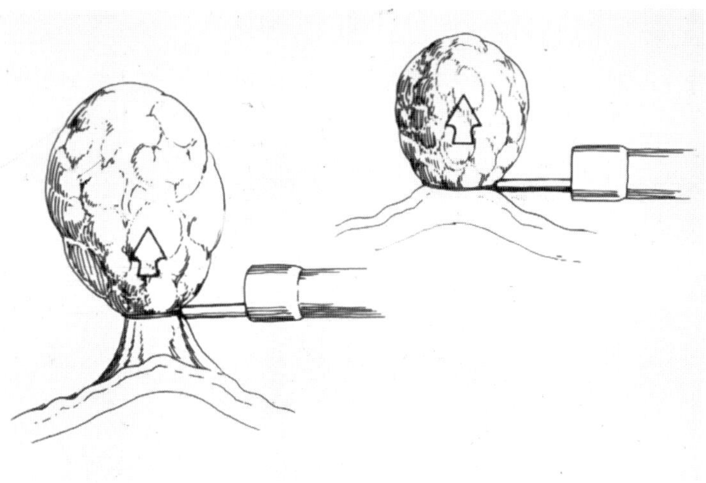

FIG. 57-13. Proper application of snare wire for removal of a pedunculated polyp.

quently because of the newer and more sophisticated accessories that are available for polypectomy. The problem of entrapment occurs when there is too much tissue in the snare or when the electrocautery is not effective, thus causing transection of tissue.

COMBINED USE OF INTRALUMINAL AND LAPAROSCOPIC TECHNIQUES

Although the traditional approach to intraluminal colonic cancer has limited the role of flexible endoscopy to one of diagnosis and excision or fulguration of small mucosal lesions, the advent of colonic extirpation, using newer laparoscopic techniques, has identified a potentially greater role for flexible instrumentation. The complete gastrointestinal surgeon should be facile in flexible endoscopy and laparoscopic techniques as well as traditional transabdominal operative maneuvers.

It becomes even more important in the age of "minimal access" colonic resection that an accurate determination of location be made before any attempt at laparoscopic removal. The inability to assess adequately the location of an intraluminal lesion through the laparoscope is a definite pitfall of this approach, and therefore preoperative localization, either with intramural dye or other markers,[14] is critical to ensure that laparoscopic resection is appropriately performed. Similarly, there may be a greater role for the synchronous application of colonoscopy and laparoscopy as a "rendezvous" procedure to help in the accurate identification of intraluminal neoplasia. Using concomitant intraluminal visualization of a colonic lesion, the laparoscopic surgeon may identify the transmural light, and therefore have an exact means of locating the tumor before beginning laparoscopic resection. This exciting use of our flexible equipment is only an extension of the intraoperative role for flexible endoscopy that has been the mainstay of many gastrointestinal surgeons since the early 1970s. Through the use of flexible endoscopic and rigid laparoscopic techniques, it is anticipated that carcinoma of the colon will be diagnosed at an earlier stage and potentially resected with less metabolic consequences than with previous transabdominal techniques. Only through the use of well designed clinical trials will this goal be realized.

REFERENCES

1. Boring CC, Squires BA, Tong T, Montgomery S. Cancer statistics, 1994. CA Cancer J Clin 1994;44:7.
2. Pollack A, Quirke P. Adenoma screening and colorectal cancer: the need for screening and polypectomy is unproved. Br Med J 1991;303:3.
3. Turnage RH, Guice KS, Gannon P, Gross M. The effect of polyethylene glycol gavage on plasma volume. J Surg Res 1994;57:284.
4. Sollenberger LL, Eisenstat TE, Rubin RJ. Is preoperative colonoscopy necessary in carcinoma of the colon and rectum? Am Surg 1988;54:113.
5. Howard ML, Greene FL. The effect of preoperative endoscopy on recurrence and survival following surgery for colorectal carcinoma. Am Surg 1990;56:124.
6. Schrock TR. Colonoscopy in the diagnosis and treatment of colorectal malignancy. In: Greene FL, Ponsky JL, eds. Endoscopic surgery. Philadelphia: WB Saunders, 1994:256.
7. Greene FL. Distribution of colorectal neoplasms: a left to right shift of polyps and cancer. Am Surg 1983;49:62.
8. Greene FL, Livstone EM, Troncale FJ. The role of fiberoptic colonoscopy in the diagnosis of colonic and rectal disease. Conn Med 1973;37:439.
9. Wolff WI. Colonoscopy: history and development. Am J Gastroenterol 1989;84:1017.
10. Williams CB. Colonoscopy: general aspects, polyps and cancer. In: Cotton PB, Tytgat GNJ, Williams CB, eds. Annual of gastrointestinal endoscopy. London: Current Science, Ltd., 1992:133.
11. Wolff WI, Shinya H. Polypectomy via the fiberoptic colonoscope. N Engl J Med 1973;288:329.
12. Greene FL. Epithelial misplacement in adenomatous polyps of the colon and rectum. Cancer 1974;33:206.
13. Wolff WI, Shinya. Therapeutic colonoscopy: polypectomy, management of bleeding and decompressive techniques. In: Greene FL, Ponsky JL, eds. Endoscopic surgery. Philadelphia: WB Saunders, 1994:235.
14. Hyman N, Waye JD. Endoscopic four quadrant tattoo for the identification of colonic lesions at surgery. Gastrointest Endosc 1991;37:56.

Surgery for Gastrointestinal Cancer: A Multidisciplinary Approach, edited by Harold J. Wanebo.
Lippincott-Raven Publishers, Philadelphia, © 1997.

CHAPTER 58

Surgery of the Polyposis Syndromes

James M. Church

The gastrointestinal polyposes are a group of rare conditions that present special challenges for the physician facing them. Included in this group are familial adenomatous polyposis (FAP), Peutz-Jeghers syndrome, juvenile polyposis, ganglioneuromatosis, and the Cronkhite-Canada syndrome. Of these, FAP is by far the most common.

FAMILIAL ADENOMATOUS POLYPOSIS

Familial adenomatous polyposis, the most common of the inherited polyposis syndromes, is still a rare disease. It occurs, on average, once in every 8000 births and accounts for less than 1% of all colorectal cancers. FAP is an autosomal dominant trait; this means that the mutation responsible for the disease is not on a sex chromosome but on one of the 22 other chromosomes (autosomes), and that only one mutated gene out of the 2 copies (alleles) needs to be inherited for the disease to be clinically manifest. The mutation causing FAP is primarily expressed as multiple colorectal adenomas, one or more of which, if untreated, ultimately becomes malignant (Fig. 58-1). FAP is both clinically fascinating and scientifically instructive. Its fascination is that it represents an amplified and accelerated version of colorectal carcinogenesis; its instruction comes from the opportunity it presents to study the adenoma–carcinoma sequence and the effects of potential modifiers, such as diet and nonsteroidal antiinflammatory drugs (NSAIDs), on it. For patients with FAP, however, it is neither fascinating nor instructive. They find it a frightening and sometimes lethal condition, for which at least one major abdominal surgery is certain.

Molecular Genetics

Familial adenomatous polyposis is caused by the mutation of a tumor suppressor gene (*APC*) on the long arm of chromosome 5.[1] Tumor suppressor genes hold the genetic code for proteins that suppress cell growth. Mutations of the *APC* gene that stop production of its growth-inhibiting protein predispose cells (colonocytes in particular) to neoplasia. When further genetic damage occurs, affecting other tumor suppressor genes, progressive loss of control of growth and differentiation occurs.[2] Activation of protooncogenes (genes coding for proteins that stimulate cell growth) is also part of the cascade of genetic changes that eventually produce the uncontrolled, undifferentiated cells of an invasive malignancy.

Genetic mutations can be inherited from a parent, acquired at conception, or happen during life (by exposure to carcinogens, or merely from aging). Mutations that are inherited or occur at conception affect every cell in the body, and this is the case with FAP. The *APC* gene mutations are inherited in 80% of FAP patients and occur during conception as germ cell mutations in 20%. Therefore, 80% of FAP patients are part of a family with the disease, and have the chance for screening and early diagnosis. Twenty percent have no family history and are usually diagnosed when symptoms occur.

Genetic Testing

In 1991, the gene, mutations of which are responsible for FAP, was identified and cloned.[1] Before this, genetic testing was based on linkage analysis, an often inconclusive method by which genetic markers close to the *APC* gene were linked to clinical evidence of the disease and used to identify those undiagnosed family members who were probably affected. Once the actual gene was identified, direct analysis of mutations was possible. Finding the mutation operating in a family is a labor-intensive exercise, because the gene is long and the mutations small. Once the mutation is found, however, it is easily analyzed in other family members. Over 200 mutations associated with FAP have been reported, with one or two "hot spots" on the gene. There is a correlation between the site of the mutation and severity of polyposis. Mutations in exons near the beginning of the gene[3,4] seem to produce mild or attenuated FAP, while those at the hot spots in exon 15 are usually associated with severe disease. This association may influence clinical management, encouraging early screening and total proctocolectomy in patients with exon 15G mutations.

James M. Church: Director, David G. Jagelman Center for Inherited Colorectal Cancer, Department for Colorectal Surgery, Cleveland Clinic Foundation, Cleveland Clinic Hospital, 9500 Euclid Avenue, Cleveland, OH 44195-5044

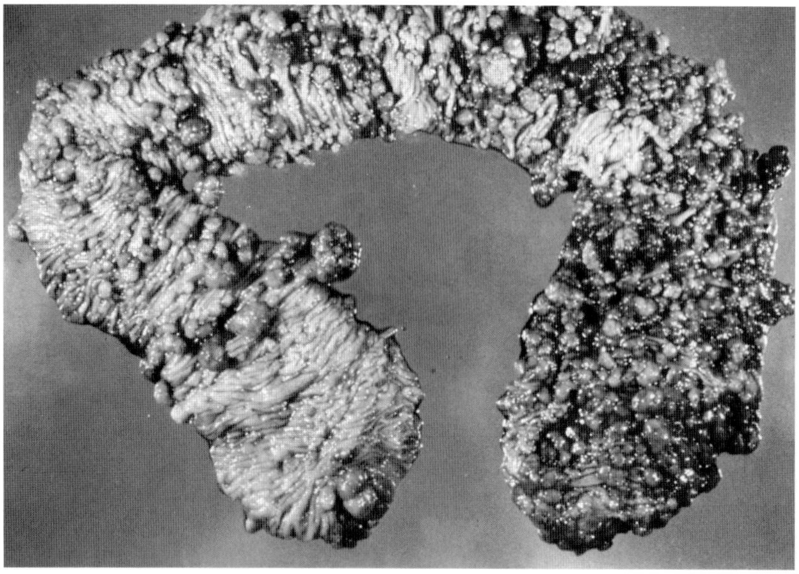

FIG. 58-1. Colectomy specimen of a patient with severe familial adenomatous polyposis. Note the large number of polyps; all are adenomas.

The normal *APC* gene codes for a protein whose loss of function predisposes to abnormal cell growth. Each mutation results in an abnormal (truncated) protein, or no protein at all. Technology has progressed to the point that this truncated protein can be identified and used as an absolute indication of inheritance of FAP.[3]

Diagnosis

Before genetic testing became available in 1988, members of an FAP family were screened with endoscopy. Based on the assumption that all those affected would have at least one rectosigmoid polyp, yearly proctoscopy or flexible sigmoidoscopy was sufficient to diagnose the disease. If genetic testing is unavailable in an institution, endoscopic screening is still satisfactory. Attempts to use extracolonic manifestations of FAP as markers of the disease (congenital hypertrophy of the retinal pigment epithelium, osteomas, epidermoid cysts) have not been successful because these are not universal features.

Patients with FAP can be diagnosed in one of three ways, summarized in Table 58-1:

1. By symptoms: Patients may be the first in their family with FAP (a ''spontaneous'' mutation), or they may not know their family history (adopted, or separated from affected relatives). Screening is not performed and diagnosis is made when symptoms prompt investigations. These are the patients who present late and may have a cancer.
2. By endoscopy: Patients may be part of a family and be diagnosed by screening endoscopy.
3. By genetics: Patients may be diagnosed by genetic analysis, without undergoing endoscopy.

Presentation

Familial adenomatous polyposis presents with a spectrum of severity, reflected in the age of presentation and the number of adenomas in the colon. At one end of the spectrum are patients who have thousands of polyps in their early teenage years and have cancer in their early third decade. At the other end are the patients with attenuated FAP, who reach their seventh decade with less than 100 small adenomas. The severity of the FAP is the major determinant of the timing of surgery and the selection of the operation to be used.

Extracolonic Manifestations

Because FAP is a generalized growth disorder, its effects can be seen in organs outside the colorectum. These are summarized

TABLE 58-1. *Diagnosis of familial adenomatous polyposis*

	By symptoms	By endoscopy	By genetics
Age	20–40 y	10–20 y	1–10 y
Family status	−ve or unknown	+ve	+ve
Symptoms	Yes	No	No
Endoscopy	Polyps/cancer	Polyps	Not done
Genetics	Not done	Not done	+ve
Timing of surgery	Now	When convenient	Teenage years

+ve, positive; −ve, negative.

TABLE 58-2. *Extracolonic manifestations of familial adenomatous polyposis*

Organ	Benign	Malignant
Endocrine	Adenoma	Thyroid, adrenal carcinoma
Bone	Osteoma	Osteogenic sarcoma
Stomach	Fundic gland polyp Adenoma	Carcinoma
Duodenum	Adenoma	Carcinoma
Bile duct	Papillary adenoma	Bile duct carcinoma
Small bowel	Adenoma	Carcinoma
Brain		Medulloblastoma* Glioblastoma*
Liver		Hepatoblastoma
Pancreas	Adenoma	Carcinoma
Fibrous tissue	Desmoid†	Desmoid†

* Turcot's syndrome.
† With epidermoid cysts and osteomas, Gardner's syndrome.

in Table 58-2. The tumors that most affect patients are duodenal adenomas and desmoid tumors.

The most common cause of death in patients with FAP is colorectal cancer. Next most common are desmoid tumors and periampullary carcinoma.[5]

Desmoid Tumors

Desmoid tumors are nonmetastasizing (therefore theoretically benign) tumors of fibroaponeurotic tissue that occur rarely in the general population but in 8% to 10% of polyposis patients. Desmoids tend to cluster in families and to occur after (perhaps stimulated by) surgery. They are usually intraabdominal (Fig. 58-2), where they infiltrate the small bowel mesentery and cause symptoms resulting from pressure effects on the bowel or adjacent organs. These intraabdominal desmoids are extremely difficult to excise completely because of their infiltrative nature, and recurrence is common.[6] Medical treatment with NSAIDs or estrogen blockers offers some hope of control, but sometimes cytotoxic chemotherapy is used in a last-ditch effort to control aggressive tumors. In general it is the natural history of the patient's desmoid, aggressive or benign, that determines the ultimate outcome. The influence of desmoid tumors on colorectal surgery in FAP is discussed later.

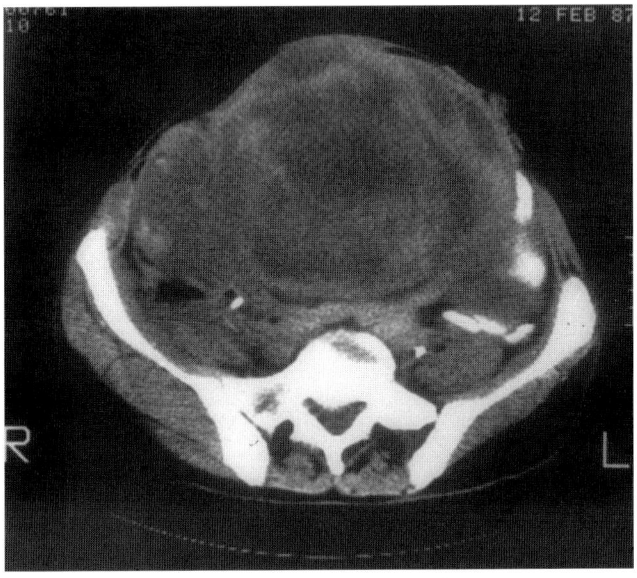

FIG. 58-2. Abdominal computed tomography scan of a patient with an intraabdominal desmoid, showing a large mass filling the abdomen. Surprisingly, such patients usually have few symptoms, other than the presence of the mass.

Duodenal and Ampullary Adenomas

The duodenal mucosa seems as vulnerable to the neoplasia-inducing effects of the *APC* gene mutation as the colorectum; perhaps the bile bathing the area is responsible for this. Prospective surveillance shows that 90% of FAP patients have adenomas here. Even when the ampulla of Vater looks normal, biopsies show dysplasia in 50% of cases.[7] Thankfully, periampullary carcinoma is rare. Surveillance is routine but prophylactic surgery is uncommon.

Nonsurgical Treatment of Familial Adenomatous Polyposis

Reports are accumulating that demonstrate antineoplastic effects of NSAIDs in FAP patients. Sulindac is the most often quoted agent, and it may both eradicate and suppress colorectal adenomas. The effect is not dependable, however; nor is it universal.[8] A note of caution has been sounded by recent reports of rectal cancer developing in patients whose rectal polyps were being suppressed by Sulindac.[9,10] NSAIDs should not be used as definitive treatment for FAP. They may be useful in temporizing treatment, when surgery needs to be delayed for some reason and there is concern about the adenomas.

SURGERY FOR FAMILIAL ADENOMATOUS POLYPOSIS

The aim of the surgical treatment of FAP is to intervene in the polyp–cancer sequence by removing the polyps before the transformation to malignancy occurs. This is done by prophylactic colectomy or proctocolectomy. Because FAP is a mucosal disease, it is analogous to ulcerative colitis. The surgical options are similar and are shown in Table 58-3, with their inherent advantages and disadvantages.

Choosing the Operation

The way in which an FAP patient presents has a strong effect on the choice of surgery. When the disease is discovered on screening, the patient is usually young and asymptomatic, just entering or about to enter adulthood. To take such a patient and make them incontinent, or slaves to an abnormal bowel habit, is to do them a disservice. Even total proctocolectomy (TPC) does not cure FAP, nor does it remove the need for regular

TABLE 58-3. *Options for the surgical treatment of familial adenomatous polyposis*

Option	Advantages	Disadvantages	Indications
TPC–ileostomy	Total removal of at-risk epithelium	Permanent ileostomy	Low rectal cancer
TPC, ileal pouch–anal anastomis	Total removal of at-risk epithelium (?) Restores normal defecation	Complex Many complications Worse bowel function Temporary stoma	High risk of rectal cancer Poor compliance with follow-up
Total colectomy–ileorectal anastomosis	Simpler Fewer complications Better function No stoma	Rectum at risk	Attenuated familial adenomatous polyposis Teenagers or younger Fewer than 20 rectal polyps Compliant patients
TPC–continent ileostomy	Total removal of at-risk epithelium Maintains continence	Permanent ileostomy High risk of complications and reoperation	Patients without an anus who do not like an end ileostomy

TPC, total proctocolectomy.

surveillance. In such patients, colectomy and ileorectal anastomosis (IRA) allows a good quality of life during the formative years, while substantially reducing the risk of large bowel cancer. Preoperative discussions focus on the need for regular postoperative surveillance of the rectum, and the possibility of further surgery.

A patient who is experiencing symptoms from a large number of colorectal adenomas needs TPC. Almost all these patients are suitable for an ileal pouch–anal anastomosis (IPAA). The critical decision is not which operation to perform, but which sort of IPAA to use. The two options, hand-sewn or stapled, are summarized in Table 58-4 and shown in Figure 58-3. Because the low rectum appears to be a "hot spot" for polyps after IRA, in most cases this area should be removed by mucosectomy with hand-sewn ileoanal anastomosis. In some patients (eg, the very young, those with relatively few rectal polyps, or those in whom an ultra-low stapled anastomosis is possible), a stapled anastomosis may be performed, with the residual anal mucosa kept under surveillance. Figure 58-4 shows a villous adenoma that developed in the residual rectal mucosa of a 16-year-old after a stapled IPAA. The adenoma and the residual rectum were excised transanally and a neo-IPAA constructed.

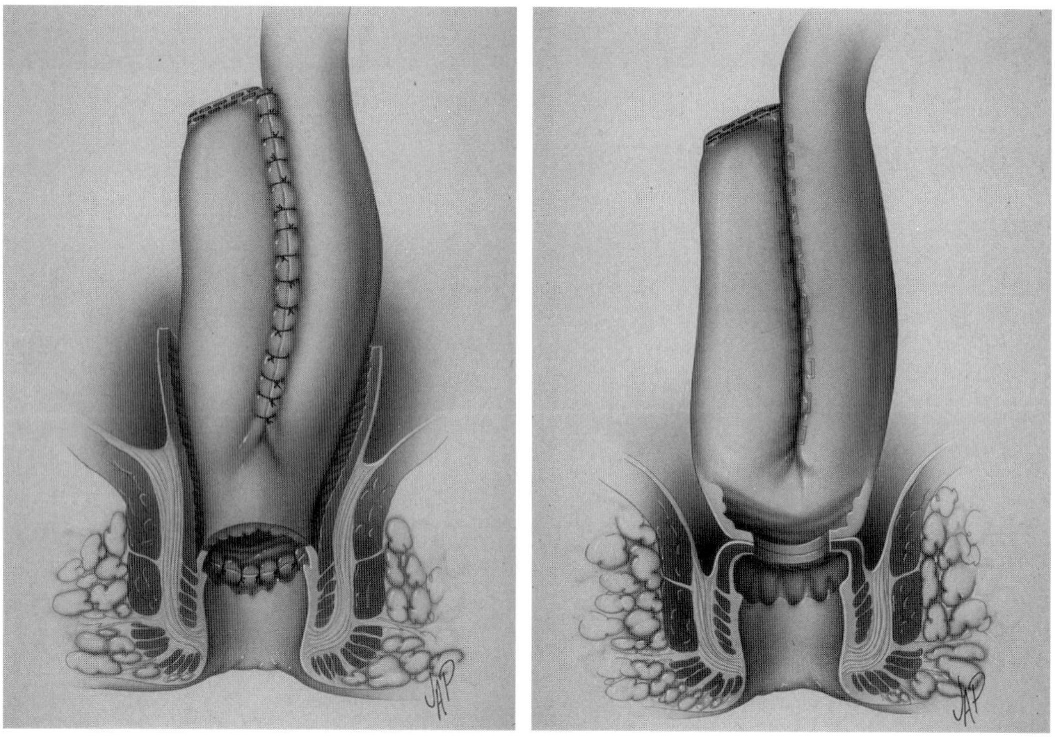

A **B**

FIG. 58-3. Diagrams of a hand-sewn **(A)** and a stapled ileal pouch–anal anastomosis **(B).** Note the small strip of residual rectum in the stapled procedure.

TABLE 58-4. *The ileal pouch–anal anastomosis: stapled or hand-sewn?*

	Advantages	Disadvantages
Stapled	Safer, quicker, better function allows omission of ileostomy	Leaves 1–2 cm of rectum
Hand-sewn	Removes all rectum (?)	More complications Longer, more leakage

If a patient presents with FAP and cancer, the top priority is to cure the cancer. Restorative proctocolectomy (with IPAA) is still possible as long as chances of cure are not compromised. If a colon cancer is incurable and surgery is to be palliative, IRA is a good choice.

Patients who present with a desmoid tumor or a strong family history of desmoid tumors deserve special consideration. Such patients are at risk for development of an intraabdominal desmoid after their colectomy, a desmoid that may make future abdominal surgery difficult or even impossible. Strong consideration should be given to TPC with or without IPAA as a first and (it is hoped) only operation. My practice is to premedicate these patients with sulindac (150 mg, twice daily) for 3 to 6 months, if circumstances permit.

A family history of desmoid tumors may make laparoscopic surgery more desirable, in that surgical trauma is minimized.

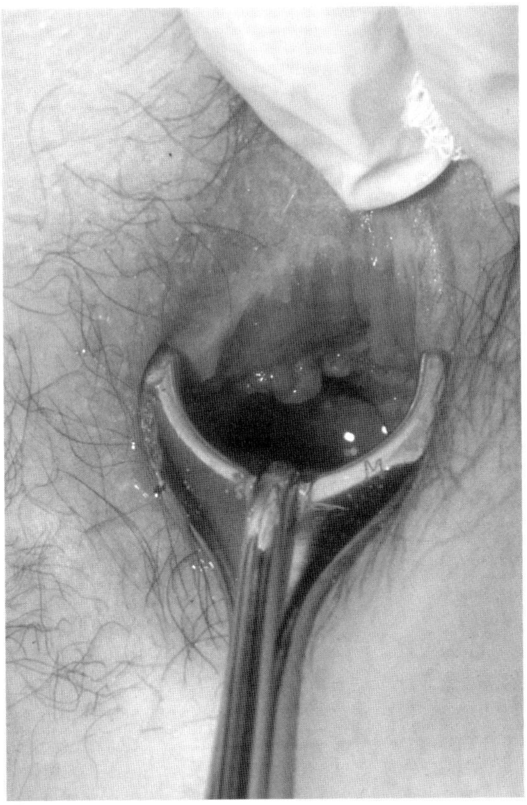

FIG. 58-4. A villous adenoma growing in the small strip of residual rectum after stapled ileal pouch–anal anastomosis.

TABLE 58-5. *Reasons for choice of total proctocolectomy and ileal pouch–anal anastomis in 33 patients treated at the Cleveland Clinic*

Reason	No. of patients
Carpeted rectum	14
Rectal cancer	6
Uncontrollable polyps	5
Large rectal polyp	2
Patient requests	2
Family history of desmoid	1
Surgeon preference	1
Status post total proctocolectomy, ileostomy	1
Unclear	1

The practicability of this theoretic advantage remains to be tested.

The choice of surgery is made by the patient with the advice of the surgeon. The surgeon should present a full range of options, with advantages and disadvantages of each. Only then can the patient make an informed choice. In a disease like FAP, the patient's choice is often influenced by the experience of other family members. If this experience has been bad, the Polyposis Registry Coordinator can have a role in counseling, and resolving fears and apprehensions. Factors retrospectively identified as being involved in the choice of TPC–IPAA at the Cleveland Clinic are listed in Table 58-5. Figure 58-5 is an algorithm summarizing some of the decision points in choosing an operation in a FAP patient. A rectum is "high risk" if there is a cancer in the colon or rectum, if the rectum has more than 20 polyps, or if the rectum has a large (>3 cm) polyp. A "low-risk" rectum contains only a few (<20) small adenomas.

The Continent Ileostomy

The continent ileostomy, or Kock pouch, is not described in detail here. It is an option for patients who are ineligible for a restorative resection, but can be offered only by surgeons with an ongoing experience in the procedure. Technical modifications have improved the results of the continent ileostomy,[11] but it remains a complex procedure with a marked "learning curve." The learning curve applies not only to performing the procedure but to caring for these patients in the postoperative period and beyond. Tertiary care centers are available to which potential candidates can be referred.

Laparoscopy in Familial Adenomatous Polyposis

Because most patients with FAP do not have a cancer at the time of prophylactic colectomy, they are good candidates for laparoscopic surgery. Teenagers who are diagnosed on screening stand to benefit most from such minimally invasive surgery. The lack of a large midline incision minimizes time away from school and from the sort of physical activities teenagers are wont to do. Figure 58-6 shows the incisions made for a laparoscopic colectomy and IRA in a 13-year-old girl. The colectomy part of a TPC–IPAA can be done in this way, although a larger

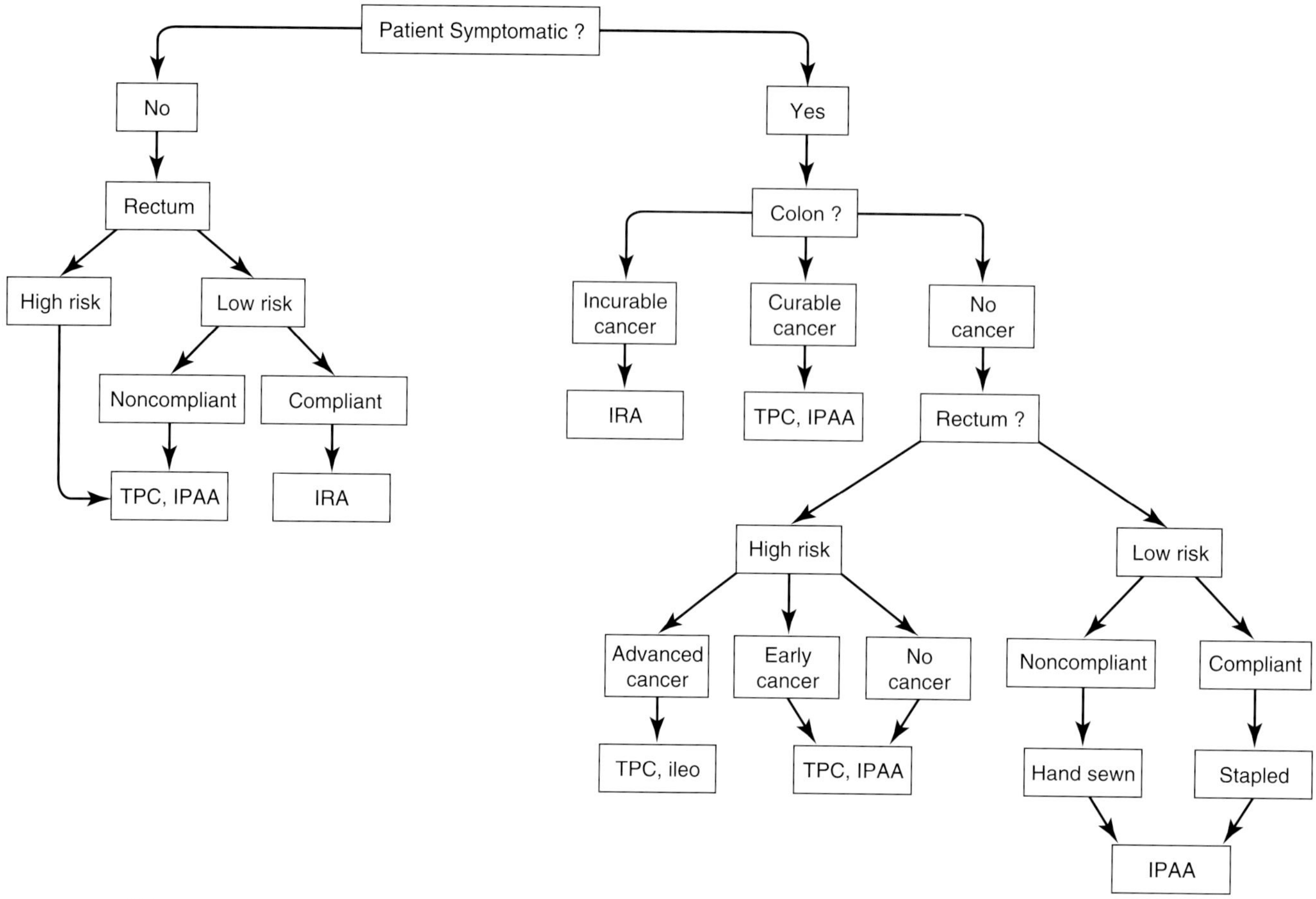

FIG. 58-5. An algorithm describing factors involved in choosing the surgical procedure for a patient with familial adenomatous polyposis. *IPAA*, ileal pouch–anal anastomosis; *IRA*, ileorectal anastomosis; *TPA*, total proctocolectomy.

incision is necessary to make the pouch. If this option can be offered, surgery is a less frightening prospect for the patient before the operation, and a more comfortable experience afterward.

Timing the Operation

Preoperative colonoscopy in FAP patients is important in helping determine the choice of operation, its timing, and even the techniques of resection. Large numbers of polyps in a symptomatic patient mean early surgery, as soon as it is convenient. Suspicion of a cancer means very early surgery, and a radical colectomy performed with oncologic technique (eg "No Touch"). An asymptomatic patient with modest numbers of small polyps may be able to wait 1 or 2 years for surgery, as long as endoscopic surveillance is performed yearly. In such patients the timing of surgery is a matter of convenience for the family, with school, vacations, sports, and insurance coverage all factors in the decision.

Preparation for Surgery

Almost all FAP patients are young and fit, and preoperative preparation can be limited to a comprehensive history and physical examination, with a minimum of testing. If a stoma is to be used, stoma marking should be done during the preoperative visit.

Patients can be cleared as outpatients and undergo gut lavage at home the evening before surgery. My patients arrive at the

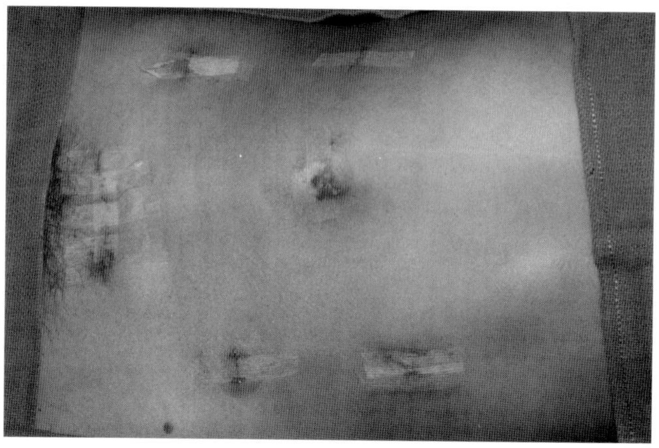

FIG. 58-6. The incisions made for laparoscopic colectomy and ileorectal anastomosis in a 13-year-old girl with mild, asymptomatic familial adenomatous polyposis.

hospital 2 hours before the scheduled operating time. They are taken to a precare facility for immediate preparation. Intravenous antibiotics (aerobic and anaerobic coverage) are given on call to the operating room, and calf compression stockings are routine. My preference is to use subcutaneous miniheparin as deep venous thrombosis prophylaxis. If epidural anesthesia is to be used, the catheter is inserted.

Operative Techniques

A modified lithotomy position is used to allow synchronous access to the anus and abdomen. Insert a urethral catheter and irrigate the rectum with saline and povidone–iodine.

Take the midline incision right down to the symphysis if a pouch is to be made, but leave it higher if an IRA is planned. In either case, the upper extent of the incision reaches at least to the mid-epigastrium, to allow take-down of the flexures. Abdominal exploration precedes the start of the dissection.

The Colectomy

If there is no suspicion of cancer, a conservative mesenteric resection is best. I preserve the omentum, take down the flexures, and then mobilize the right and left colons to the sacral promontory, and divide the bowel. Division of the mesentery is completed and the terminal ileum is sectioned flush with the cecum. If a cancer is suspected, divide the major vessels first, the rest of the mesentery next, and mobilize the bowel last.

After the Colectomy

I prefer to perform a stapled IRA, using a 29-mm circular stapling instrument. For a young child, a smaller stapler may be needed. Do not place the anastomosis in the sigmoid colon because this makes surveillance difficult.

If a proctectomy is planned, and no cancer is present, perform conservative surgery. Start the posterior dissection by entering the presacral space, keeping just behind superior rectal artery. Pull forward on the rectum to facilitate sharp dissection behind the mesorectum. Divide the rectosacral fascia sharply. Incise the peritoneum down each side of the rectum and across its front, in the cul-de-sac of the pelvis. Keep the lateral dissection close to the rectum, and divide lateral ligaments close in. Anteriorly, dissection proceeds close to the bowel, behind Denonvillier's fascia. Once the mesorectum is entirely mobilized, clear the lower rectum/upper anus circumferentially. At this point, the rectal irrigation tube should be palpable. I find bimanual palpation, with a finger in the rectum and a hand in the pelvis, valuable for assessing the extent of dissection. When the upper anus is reached a transverse stapler can be applied (if a stapled IPAA is intended) or the anal mucosectomy can be performed. First, remove the rectal tube and then apply a 30-mm transverse stapler. Check this staple line by insufflation of air. If there is a hole, it may be possible to pass the rod of the circular stapler through it.

If there is a rectal cancer, perform a standard cancer resection with wide margins. Do not do a stapled anastomosis.

The Pouch

Once the rectum has been removed, pack the pelvis and turn attention to the small bowel. I oversew the stapled end of the terminal ileum, using 3-0 Vicryl. Mark a point 20 cm upstream and tentatively pull down to see how well the pouch will fit. If the ileum reaches below the pubis, all will be well. If there is going to be some tension, make sure the terminal ileal mesentery is completely mobilized, make some horizontal slits in the peritoneum of the mesentery directly over the superior mesenteric artery (SMA), and consider making a window in the mesentery by dividing the terminal extension of the SMA. It is best to have preserved the ileocolic branch of the SMA if this window is to be made. If there is still a problem with length, an "S" pouch will reach 1 to 2 cm lower than a "J." Construct a "J" pouch with two 20-cm limbs of terminal ileum, using two applications of a 100-cm linear stapling instrument. An "S" pouch is made with three 15-cm limbs, and is sewn by hand. Test the pouch with air and saline. If a stapled IPAA is to be made, use a purse-string suture of 0 Prolene in the open end of the pouch.

The Ileal Pouch–Anal Anastomosis

This is the next step, after ensuring pelvic hemostasis.

Stapled

Stapled IPAA is quick and easy, but take care when inserting the stapler cartridge through the anus. When there is a very short rectal or anal stump and a relatively tight anus, it is easy for an assistant to thrust the stapler right through the transverse staple line, necessitating removal of the stump and transanal, hand-sewn anastomosis. I insert the stapler myself, bimanually, with one hand on the stapler and the other in the pelvis protecting the staple line. Protrude the stapler spike through the middle of the staple line. If possible, I use a 33-mm circular stapler because this should encompass all of a 30-mm transverse staple line. Once the stapler is fired and removed, check the "donuts" and test the anastomosis by air insufflation.

Hand-Sewn

Start anal mucosectomy by effacing the anus, either with sutures or a retractor. Using electrocautery set on pure coagulation, make a circumferential incision at the dentate line. The mucosa, normal except for the polyps, strips easily from the underlying muscle. Use epinephrine–saline and cautery to ensure a bloodless dissection. Stop the mucosectomy 3 cm above the dentate line and deepen the incision through the muscle to connect with the abdominal dissection. Pull the pouch through and anastomose it to the anus. I use interrupted sutures of 2/0 Vicryl, with deep and generous bites. If the pouch does not pull completely out of the anus, insert at least four sutures (one in each quadrant) through the dentate line before pulling the pouch down. Complete these sutures by inserting them through the pouch. Traction on the tied sutures facilitates completion of the anastomosis. Regardless of which type of anastomosis is used, make sure the pouch is not twisted when it is pulled down. Keep the cut edge of the mesentery straight.

The Ileostomy

If all has gone well and a stapled IPAA has been constructed, it is reasonable to omit an ileostomy. In this case, insert a soft rubber rectal tube transanally, to decompress the pouch. If an ileostomy is needed, pick the loop of terminal ileum closest to the pouch that will traverse the abdominal wall at the premarked site. In extremely obese patients, this is difficult and may be impossible.[12] Place an umbilical tape around the bowel at this site and mark afferent and efferent limbs with sutures. Make the trephine incision through the abdominal wall, check hemostasis, and pull the bowel through. Insert the stoma rod. Mature the stoma after the abdominal incision is closed by incising the bowel of the efferent loop transversely just above the skin and placing interrupted 3/0 catgut sutures between bowel and dermis.

Other Tubes

A nasogastric tube can usually be omitted, but always use a pelvic drain. If hemostasis is good a closed-suction drain is fine, but if there is some oozing, use a sump drain so that the pelvis can be irrigated.

Postoperative Care

Polyposis patients recover quickly because they are young and fit. As soon as there is evidence of resumption of gastrointestinal function, fluids should be started by mouth. Parenteral analgesia is maintained until oral fluids are tolerated, and the patient is mobilized early, into a chair on the first postoperative day. Compression stockings are kept on on while the patient is in bed. Pelvic drains are removed when they drain less than 50 mL/24 hours, and the urethral catheter when fluid balance is stable and the patient is sufficiently mobile to use the bathroom (3 or 4 days). Patients should be warned of early postoperative diarrhea. This usually settles when solid food is eaten. Patients with an ileostomy need to know how to care for it, and lessons begin as soon as the patient is able to comprehend and retain the instructions. Usually 3 days are needed to complete the "course" of lessons. The patient should have adequate supplies at discharge.

Follow-up for a wound check is scheduled in 6 weeks. I advise a bland diet during the first month, with little roughage. Ileostomy closure is scheduled for 3 months, after preclosure Gastrografin enema has ruled out any leak from the pouch or the anastomosis. Anal manometry allows a preoperative estimation of the quality of postoperative continence.

Patients who have undergone an IPAA without an ileostomy tend to have a longer postoperative recovery than those with diversion. Use of the newly created pouch causes more severe stool frequency and urgency than when the pouch has healed, and patients may need to spend more time in hospital. Antidiarrheals (I prefer loperamide, 2 to 4 mg up to four times daily) can be prescribed for all patients to control postoperative diarrhea.

Postoperative Surveillance

All Patients

All patients with FAP should undergo endoscopic surveillance of the duodenum. Periampullary carcinoma is second only to colorectal cancer in malignancies causing the death of FAP patients. Patients can be segregated according to the status of their duodenum. If there are no polyps, or only a few small adenomas, esophagogastroduodenoscopy every 5 years is adequate. For multiple small polyps, esophagogastroduodenoscopies every 2 to 3 years suffice. When there are large adenomas (>1 cm), or carpeting of the duodenum, yearly esophagogastroduodenoscopy is necessary. If biopsy shows severe dysplasia, polypectomy is necessary. This may mean duodenectomy using a pancreas-sparing technique[13] or a transduodenal mucosal resection. Polypectomy may be possible endoscopically, but recurrence is 100%. A pancreaticoduodenectomy should not be performed for benign disease.

After Ileorectal Anastomosis

Patients who have had an IRA need yearly proctoscopy to remove rectal adenomas. This is a commitment patients make before the surgery. A prime role for FAP registries is to monitor a patient's attendance and to ensure and facilitate follow-up. Financial concerns should not be allowed to limit attendance.

Technique

A clean rectum is important and sometimes hard to obtain. One Fleet enema is sufficient preparation as long as the examination is performed promptly. A rigid proctoscope enables more efficient removal of semisolid stool than a flexible endoscope, and polyp coagulation is easy with a suction-coagulator. Flexible endoscopy tends to be more comfortable for the patient and is necessary if there is still a rectosigmoid angle. It also gives a better overall view as the rectum can be distended with air. All polyps bigger than 2 mm should be treated.

The sensitivity of the rectum can be an issue. Some patients tolerate polyp coagulation well, whereas others need conscious sedation or even general anesthesia. The most important thing is to get a good examination and thorough treatment. If examination is suboptimal because of preparation, but no major lesion is seen, proctoscopy can be rescheduled in 6 to 9 months depending on the degree of physician concern. If the limiting factor is poor patient cooperation, an examination under anesthesia can be scheduled.

When a patient has had multiple examinations and polypectomies, the rectum becomes scarred and its sensitivity increases. Such rectums are difficult to examine and are the type in which a small ulcerated cancer can appear in between surveillance examinations. In these patients, the surgeon should have a low threshold for proctectomy.

There are two "hot spots" in the rectum where polyps tend to appear, and to which particular attention need be paid. These are up by the anastomosis, and down by the anus. Adenomas may not be obvious, and any unusual folds should be sampled for biopsy. Adenomas in the low rectum/upper anus may be difficult to remove without sedation or anesthesia, because this area is extra sensitive because of its proximity to the anal sphincters.

The surgeon should try to determine an impression of the pattern of rectal neoplasia evolving in each patient over the course of time. When the rectum is stable, surveillance can be more relaxed. If a rectum is unstable, with more polyps requiring more frequent examinations, proctectomy may be required.

Surveillance After Ileal Pouch–Anal Anastomosis

Patients post-IPAA need yearly examination, regardless of whether they have had a mucosectomy. If there is residual rectal mucosa, this is a "hot spot" for recurrent neoplasia and may need to be stripped out if persistent neoplasia occurs. Mucosectomy does not guarantee complete excision of rectal epithelium, and neoplasia can still occur in these patients. The pouch itself may develop adenomas. The natural history of ileal pouch neoplasia in FAP patients is unknown and deserves study. As time from pouch construction increases, and as pouches become more like colons, the significance of pouch adenomas may increase. It should be borne in mind that these are patients in whom the colorectal manifestation of FAP was severe enough to warrant TPC.

Technique

Ileal pouches are difficult to survey because of all the liquid and semisolid stool. Patients should take a liquid diet 1 day before their appointment and give enemas until the pouch is clear. Flexible endoscopy is best because small adenomas are easier to see. Large (>5 mm) adenomas should be treated.

Getting a look at the IPAA can be difficult, especially in patients who have had a hand-sewn anastomosis with some stricturing and tenderness in the area. A rigid anoscope is the best way of seeing this area; the pediatric-size scope with an integrated fiberoptic light source may need to be used.

The Effect of Desmoid Tumors on Surgery for Familial Adenomatous Polyposis

Desmoid tumors are specters that haunt surgeons operating on patients with FAP. Their presence, or the potential for their development, can have a profound influence on the type of operation that is, or can be, performed. There are three scenarios in which desmoid tumors influence surgery.

In the first scenario, a family history of desmoid tumors alerts the surgeon to a higher than usual (10%) risk of a desmoid developing in a patient. There are three ways to respond to this risk:

1. Perform TPC with IPAA regardless of the state of the rectum, based on the rationale that only one surgery will be needed and that this will minimize the risk of desmoid formation. The problem with this philosophy is that desmoids can occur in the mesentery of a pouch, and if they do, can cause severe problems leading to pouch excision (Fig. 58-7).
2. Perform laparoscopic IRA, with the rationale that surgical trauma is minimized and with it, the risk of a desmoid. The problem here is that there are no data to support this assumption, and that if a desmoid does develop and the rectum needs to come out, the desmoid may make an IPAA impossible.[11]
3. Avoid surgery as long as possible, treating polyps with sulindac. Counsel against pregnancy and the use of oral contraceptives. This is reasonable in patients with mild polyposis. When the colorectum is severely affected, it is dangerous to delay surgery.

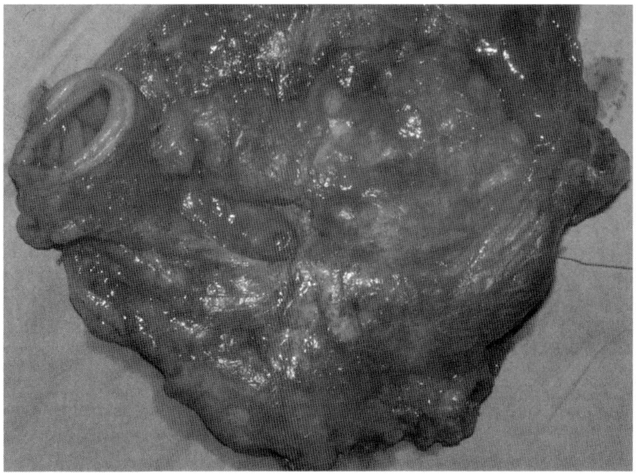

FIG. 58-7. An ileal pouch removed for recurrent bleeding from ulcers caused by a mesenteric desmoid tumor.

My recommendation is to delay surgery if the polyposis is mild. If it stays mild, choose a laparoscopic IRA when the patient is in his or her third decade; for severe polyposis, laparoscopic colectomy and IPAA at the time of presentation is reasonable. I premedicate such patients with sulindac for 3 months before surgery, hoping to inhibit any tendency to form desmoids (there are no data to support this suggestion).

In the second scenario, at laparotomy for colectomy or proctectomy, an unsuspected desmoid tumor is seen. Under these circumstances, it is unwise to proceed with an IPAA because of the risk of problems from progression of the desmoid and the possible desmoid-promoting effect of the mesenteric dissection and tension inherent in pouch procedures. If a desmoid-like reaction[6] is seen, where there is a whitish, plaque-like mesenteric reaction without a mesenteric mass or sclerosis, it is reasonable to proceed with an IPAA. The natural history of this desmoid-type reaction is unknown and the risk of a symptomatic desmoid developing after surgery is likely to be low, as long as the patient is not in a "desmoid family." If the patient has severe polyposis, proceed with proctectomy and ileostomy. Do not do a continent ileostomy. If the polyposis is mild and IRA was planned, it is reasonable to go ahead with this plan. After surgery, the desmoid must be closely monitored and treated if it enlarges. It is important to discuss the possibility of desmoid tumors and their effect on surgical strategy with the patient before the operation.

In the third scenario, a desmoid tumor develops in a patient

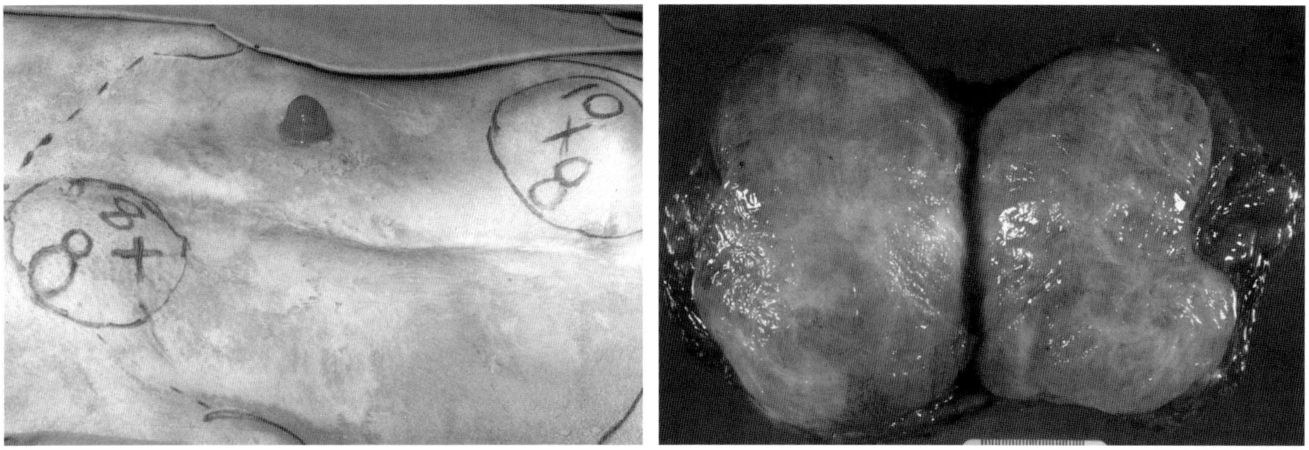

A B

FIG. 58-8. (A) Abdominal wall desmoid tumors ready for excision. After 4 years, there has been no recurrence. **(B)** Excised abdominal wall desmoid; the patient is different from the one shown in **(A).**

who has had his or her surgery for FAP. This is by far the most common scenario; symptomatic intraabdominal desmoid tumors present after abdominal surgery 80% of the time.

Intraabdominal desmoid tumors are difficult to treat. Complete excision is usually impossible because of their infiltrative growth pattern and their preferred site in the small bowel mesentery. If they are enlarging or symptomatic, treat with sulindac in combination with tamoxifen. If they continue to grow, chemotherapy, of the sort prescribed for sarcomas, is indicated. Surgery is reserved for treatable complications such as bowel obstruction. Attempts completely to excise intraabdominal desmoid tumors at the Cleveland Clinic were successful in only eight cases; even then, the tumor recurred in six.

Abdominal wall desmoids are more amenable to excision (Fig. 58-8). Request an abdominal computed tomography scan to assess their resectability because sometimes they are contiguous with intraabdominal tumors. Excise with at least 1-cm margins. The defect in the abdominal wall can be repaired with mesh.

Asymptomatic desmoids can be left alone and watched by clinical examination or computed tomography scan for signs of growth.

Results of Surgery for Familial Adenomatous Polyposis

The results of prophylactic proctocolectomy or colectomy in patients with FAP can be assessed in five areas:

1. The nature of the surgery
2. Morbidity and mortality
3. Bowel function
4. Neoplasia prevention
5. Quality of life and patient satisfaction

The two major choices in FAP surgery have been compared in each of these categories and the results for the first three areas can be seen in Table 58-6. There is no doubt that IRA is a quicker, less complex, and less bloody operation than IPAA, with fewer complications. It is not as good as IPAA in neoplasia prevention, but if patients are selected and followed correctly, this disadvantage is outweighed by the better bowel function and lower complication rate. A difference of 10% to 15% in complication rates is not very startling statistically, but its importance is magnified by the effects of the sometimes serious

TABLE 58-6. *Results of surgery for familial adenomatous polyposis: IRA versus IPAA (ileostomy closure excluded)*

	Mean duration time of operation* (h)	Mean blood loss (mL)*	Mean postoperative stay (d)		Complications			Bowel movements/day			Incontinence		
			CCF	St. Mark's	CCF[15]	St. Mark's[16]	Mayo clinic[17]	CCF[15]	St. Mark's[16]	Mayo clinic[17]	CCF[15]	St. Mark's[16]	Mayo clinic[17]
IRA	3.4 ± 0.3	423 ± 130	8.2	11	15%	24%	17%	3.8	3	5	18%	28%	17%
IPAA	4.8 ± 0.4†	913 ± 246†	9.4	24‡	28%	60%	26%	5.5	5.1	6	33%	40%	30%

* Results from CCF (±95% confidence limits).
†$P < 0.05$, Student's t Test.
‡ Includes ileostomy closure.
IRA, ileorectal anastomosis; *IPAA,* ileal pouch–anal anastomosis; *CCF,* Cleveland Clinic Foundation.
Ref (15) (16) (17).

TABLE 58-7. *Neoplasia after IPAA and IRA*

	No. of patients	Median follow-up (mo)	Mean no. of endoscopies per patient	Patients with polyps	Patients with coagulation
IRA	50	49	3.6	29	11
IPAA	40	46		3	3

IRA, ileorectal anastomosis; *IPAA*, ileal pouch–anal anastomosis.

complications on the lives of the patients. Similarly, a difference of two or three bowel motions per day may not look impressive on paper, but is more significant when translated into reality in the lives of these patients.

The effectiveness of each operation in neoplasia prevention is hard to assess because the follow-up of the earliest IPAA patients is now approaching 15 years. Most are much more recent than this. Rectal cancer after IRA is more thoroughly documented, but results from different centers differ considerably. Such results are probably irrelevant to surgery today, in that the high-risk patients are now routinely given an IPAA at their first surgery, and only those at low risk have an IRA. This selection should translate into a lower incidence of rectal cancer in the long run. Table 58-7 shows details of early endoscopic follow-up in patients operated at the Cleveland Clinic.

Patient satisfaction data are difficult to interpret in FAP. They are colored by the patient's presentation in that it is hard to satisfy asymptomatic patients and by the patient's expectations given his or her family's previous experience. The patient's appreciation of the risks of FAP and the value of prophylactic surgery also influences their satisfaction. If the right operation is chosen, if it is done well, and if the patient is kept informed and involved in preoperative and postoperative decision making, satisfaction will be high.

SURGERY OF OTHER POLYPOSIS SYNDROMES

Juvenile Polyposis

Juvenile polyposis is a rare condition in which multiple juvenile polyps occur throughout the colon and rectum. Juvenile polyps are hamartomas. They appear light red and multilobular on endoscopy (Fig. 58-9) and are found more commonly alone (70%) and in children. Juvenile polyposis presents as an inherited disorder with an autosomal dominant pattern. Rectal bleeding is the main symptom. There is a high incidence of colonic adenomas and an increased risk for carcinoma. Prophylactic surgery is indicated. The choice lies between colectomy and IRA, and proctocolectomy with IPAA, depending largely on the state of the rectum.[18]

Peutz-Jeghers Syndrome

Peutz-Jeghers syndrome defines a condition in which hamartomatous polyps of the large and small bowel are associated with patchy pigmentation around the mouth and in other parts of the body. This is also inherited in autosomal dominant fashion, although sporadic cases have been described. The polyps can grow to be quite large, at which point they cause symptoms by intussuscepting and obstructing the small bowel, or by bleeding. Patients with Peutz-Jeghers syndrome may undergo multiple abdominal operations because of repeated attacks of symptoms. There is an association with cancer, mainly of the colon and rectum, but also in extraintestinal sites.[19,20]

Troublesome colorectal and gastric polyps can be removed endoscopically, whereas symptomatic small bowel polyps require laparotomy and segmental resection, or enterotomy and polypectomy. During laparotomy, the site of polyps in the small bowel can be identified by the serosal umbilication produced by traction on the stalk (Fig. 58-10). All large polyps found at laparotomy should be removed. Surveillance for cancer of the gastrointestinal tract is a good idea, but detailed recommendations have not been made.

Intestinal Ganglioneuromatosis

Ganglioneuromatosis, a manifestation of neuromatosis, rarely affects the colon. In the handful of patients in whom it is described, it has been associated with slow-transit constipation. Because there is an association with multiple endocrine neoplasia, patients should be screened for tumors in the thyroid and adrenal glands. Treatment by subtotal colectomy and IRA is reasonable, if the constipation is bothersome. I have seen one case in which a patient with intestinal ganglioneuromatosis presented with a sigmoid colon carcinoma.

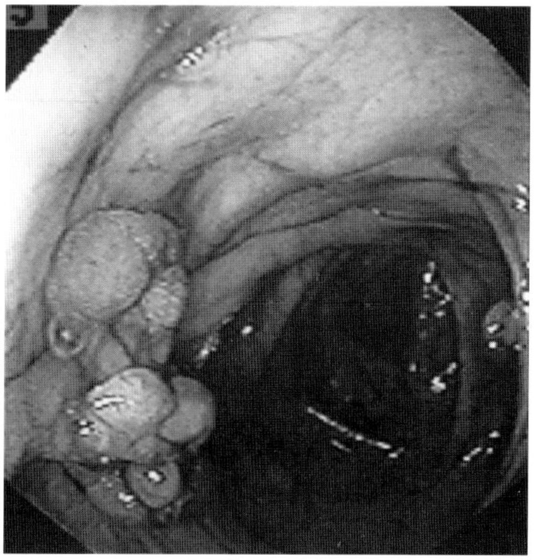

FIG. 58-9. Juvenile polyposis. Note the light red, multi-lobular appearance of the polyps. This patient presented with a colon cancer was initially diagnosed as having familial adenomatous polyposis. See also Color Figure 58-9.

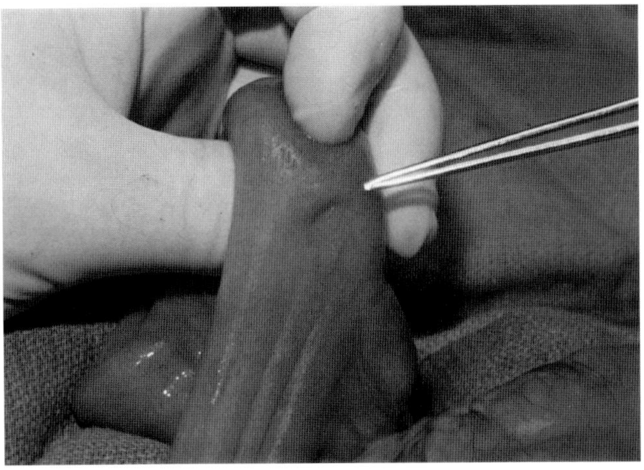

FIG. 58-10. The mid-small bowel in a patient with Peutz-Jeghers syndrome. Note the serosal dimpling caused by traction on a polyp stalk. See also Color Figure 58-10.

The world's reported experience with this condition is too small to calculate a risk of carcinoma, although I recommend colonoscopic surveillance if colectomy is not performed.

Cronkhite-Canada Syndrome

This association of generalized intestinal polyposis with alopecia, cutaneous pigmentation, and atrophy of the fingernails and toenails is extremely rare and not an inherited disorder. Diarrhea and malabsorption are common symptoms, and the condition is usually lethal. The polyps are hamartomas, but colon cancer has been described in association with Cronkhite-Canada syndrome.[21] Resection may be indicated if large numbers of polyps are in a confined area.[22]

REFERENCES

1. Groden J, et al. Identification and characterization of the familial adenomatosis polyposis coli gene. Cell 1991;66:601.
2. Vogelstein B, Fearon ER, Hamilton SR, et al. Genetic alterations during colorectal tumor development. N Engl J Med 1988;319:525.
3. Wu J, Paul P, McGannon EA, Church JM. Plyp density and surgical outcome correlate with location of APC mutations in familial adenomatous polyposis (in preparation).
4. Powell SM, Peterson GM, Krush AJ, et al. Molecular diagnosis of familial adenomatous polyposis. N Engl J Med 1993;329:1982.
5. Arvanitis ML, Jagelman DG, Fazio VW, et al. Mortality in patients with familial adenomatous polyposis. Dis Colon Rectum 1990;33:639.
6. Church JM. Desmoid tumors in familial adenomatous polyposis. Surgical Oncology Clinics of North America 1994;3:435.
7. Church JM, McGannon E, Hull-Boiner S, et al. Gastroduodenal polyps in patients with familial adenomatous polyposis. Dis Colon Rectum 1992;35:1170.
8. Giardello FM, Hamilton SR, Krush AJ, et al. Treatment of colonic and rectal adenomas with sulindac in familial adenomatous polyposis. N Engl J Med 1993;328:1313.
9. Thoron AG, Lynch HT, Smyrk TC. Rectal cancer in FAP patient after Sulindac. Lancet 1994;343:180.
10. Niv Y, Fraser GM. Adenocarcinoma in the rectal segment in familial polyposis coli is not prevented by Sulindac therapy. Gastroenterology 1994;107:854.
11. Fazio VW, Tjandra JJ. Technique for nipple valve fixation to prevent valve slippage in continent ileostomy. Dis Colon Rectum 1992; 35:1177.
12. Church JM. The ileal pouch-anal anastomosis in challenging patients: stretching the limits. Aust N Z J Surg 1995;65:104.
13. Chung RS, Church JM, Van Stolk R. Pancreas-sparing duodenectomy: indications, surgical technique and results. Surgery 1995;117:254.
14. Penna C, Tiret E, Parc R, et al. Operation and abdominal desmoid tumors in familial adenomatous polyposis. Surg Gynecol Obstet 1993; 177:263.
15. Church JM, Jagelman DG, Fazio VW, et al. The role of restorative proctocolectomy in the surgical treatment of familial adenomatous polyposis. Dis Colon Rectum (In press).
16. Madden MV, Neale KF, Nicholls RJ, et al. Comparison of the morbidity and function after colectomy and ileorectal anastomosis or restorative proctectomy for familial adenomatous polyposis. Br J Surg 1991; 78:789.
17. Ambroze WL, Dozois RR, Pemberton JH, et al. Familial adenomatous polyposis: results following ileal pouch-anal anastomosis and ileorectostomy. Dis Colon Rectum 1992;35:12.
18. Grosfield JL, West KW. Generalized juvenile polyposis coli. Arch Surg 1986;121:530.
19. Konishi F, Wyse NE, Muto T, et al. Peutz-Jeghers polyposis associated with carcinomas of the digestive organs: report of three cases and review of the literature. Dis Colon Rectum 1987;30:790.
20. Giardello FM, Welch SB, Hamilton SR, et al. Increased risk of cancer in the Peutz-Jegher's syndrome. N Engl J Med 1987;316:1511.
21. Rappaport LB, Sperling HV, Stravrides A. Colon cancer in Cronkhite-Canada syndrome. J Clin Gastroenterol 1986;8:199.
22. Cotterill JA, Day JL, Hughes JP, et al. The Cronkhite-Canada syndrome. Postgrad Med J 1973;49:268.

Surgery for Gastrointestinal Cancer: A Multidisciplinary Approach, edited by Harold J. Wanebo.
Lippincott-Raven Publishers, Philadelphia, © 1997.

CHAPTER 59

Surgical Resection for Colon Carcinoma

Philip H. Gordon

The first consideration in the operative management of colon carcinoma is access to the abdominal cavity. Incisions should be performed in a manner to provide maximum exposure for the planned resection. Most operations can be performed through a transverse incision. For a patient about to undergo a right hemicolectomy, an oblique right-sided abdominal incision is usually adequate and, if needed, can be extended. For transverse colon lesions, a supraumbilical transverse incision places access immediately in the area of the planned operation, and the incision can be extended in either direction should there be any difficulty encountered in taking down the flexures. For left-sided colonic lesions, a subumbilical transverse incision is usually employed. This permits adequate exposure for even a low anterior resection. Some surgeons prefer the use of a midline incision. For emergency operations, a midline incision is the access of choice.

The general principles advocated for all operations for carcinoma include removal of the primary lesion with adequate margins, including the areas of lymphatic drainage. Approximately half of the patients coming to operation already have metastatic disease to regional lymph nodes.[1] Controversy exists as to the appropriate extent of lymphatic dissection. The literature suggests that no survival advantage can be attributed to extended lymph node dissections for left colon and rectal carcinomas.[2–5] An exception is the isolated report by Enker and colleagues.[6] Without doubt, this operation does result in increased morbidity, with patients often suffering from impotence, bladder difficulties, and potential vascular problems. Surely, any marginal improvement is outweighed by the considerable morbidity.

For lesions located in the cecum or ascending colon, a right hemicolectomy to encompass the bowel served by the ileocolic, right colic, and right branch of the mid-colic vessels is recommended. For lesions involving the hepatic flexure, a more extended resection of the transverse colon is indicated. For lesions in the transverse colon, depending on the portion of the transverse colon, this segment of bowel is removed. Splenic flexure lesions require removal of the distal half of the transverse colon and the descending colon. Sigmoid lesions are appropriately treated by excision of the sigmoid colon. Some surgeons prefer more radical excisions, but there is no convincing evidence to suggest prolonged survival or decreased local recurrence.[2] Indeed, operative mortality and postoperative complications are reportedly higher.[2] For patients who have synchronous carcinomas in different portions of the colon, a subtotal colectomy is appropriate.

During the operation, certain intraoperative precautions have been proposed to eliminate or at least minimize dissemination of malignant cells. It has been postulated that handling of the primary lesion early in the operation promotes dissemination. This thesis was supported by the demonstration of malignant cells in the circulation,[7,8] a finding that led Turnbull and coworkers to popularize the early ligation "no-touch" technique, in which lymphovascular channels are ligated before any manipulation of the primary lesion. After using this maneuver, they reported improved survival rates for Dukes class C lesions.[9] However, this was not a controlled trial, and their results have not been duplicated. The technique has not been adopted by most surgeons as standard therapy.

In an effort to avoid implantation of malignant cells shed from the primary carcinoma, Cole and associates recommended encirclement of the bowel lumen proximal and distal to the primary lesion.[7] Wound edges can be covered to prevent implantation in the wound. In an effort to diminish the risk of implantation of malignant cells distal to the lesion, a host of cytotoxic agents (eg, Dakin's solution or bichloride of mercury), or simply distilled water, have been used to irrigate the distal bowel. None of these has been used in a clinical trial setting, and their value is in question. In an effort to diminish suture line implantation, iodized catgut enjoyed a brief burst of popularity.[10] The most recent effort is the intraluminal instillation of diluted formalin, in which case local recurrence was reportedly reduced to 2.6% from 14.3% for untreated patients.[11] None of the techniques, including irrigation of the peritoneal cavity, has been proven of value.

OPERATIVE TECHNIQUE

Right Hemicolectomy

The procedure is begun by incising the parietal peritoneum from just below the terminal ileum toward the hepatic flexure.

Philip H. Gordon: Director, Colon and Rectal Cancer, The Sir Mortimer B. Davis Jewish General Hospital, 3755 Chemin De La Cote-Sainte-Catherine, Montreal, Quebec H3T 1E2, Canada

This can be done with a Metzenbaum scissors or by use of diathermy. If feasible, the colon is encircled above and below the carcinoma with umbilical tapes. The right colon is elevated from the retroperitoneum, with care taken not to injure the ureter, gonadal vessels, duodenum, or inferior vena cava. Peritoneal division is continued around the hepatic flexure and horizontally along the upper border of the transverse colon. The lesser sac is opened by dividing the gastrocolic ligament. Mobilization is continued for as far as the resection is anticipated. Next, the greater omentum is transected vertically. The medial aspect of the peritoneum is then incised along the planned area of resection. The ileocolic, right colic, and right branch of the mid-colic vessels are divided in turn. The small vessels adjacent to the small bowel and transverse colon at the level of the proposed transection are divided between clamps, and hemostasis secured. The two ends of bowel are now ready for division, and whether the surgeon adopts a stapling technique or suture technique directs how the bowel is handled.

Surgeons who advocate the no-touch isolation technique ligate the lymphovascular structures as the initial maneuver of the operation. An incision is made in the root of the mesentery, and the trunks of the vessels are identified, divided, and ligated before any mobilization. The major concern with this method is the potential need to deal with the ureter, gonadal vessels, and duodenum without the benefit of adequate exposure, which may keep these structures out of harm's way. Its efficacy in terms of long-term survival advantage has not been supported in surgical trials against standard operative procedures. In a multicenter, prospective, randomized, controlled trial, Wiggers and colleagues compared the no-touch isolation technique with a conventional technique.[12] Both overall and corrected survival data did not differ between the two groups, although there was a tendency toward reduction in the number of and time to occurrences of liver metastases with the no-touch technique.

My preference for the reestablishment of intestinal continuity is to use staplers to create a functional end-to-end anastomosis.[13] Once the site of transection is selected, a small area is cleared and a linear anastomosing instrument is applied in the mesenteric–antimesenteric plane. If the bowel is not completely transected and stapled closed, the open area will be where an opening would have been made anyway to create the functional end-to-end anastomosis.

It is often easier to close the mesentery before the anastomosis is constructed, especially with a right hemicolectomy and in patients who are overweight. Completing this step before the anastomosis also diminishes the possibility of the error of rotation of the ileum.

The antimesenteric borders are aligned, and at each corner an amount of tissue is excised just adequate to insert the fork of the anastomosing instrument. The instrument is inserted its full length, and the halves of the instrument are mated. The anastomosis should be checked to see that it is being created through the antimesenteric border and that no fat, omentum, mesentery, sponge, or viscus is trapped. The "sleeping suture of Steichen" is placed at the end of the anastomosis on the antimesenteric border of the bowel to diminish any possible tension on the anastomosis. The halves of the instrument should be gently separated because excessive force may result in disruption of the anastomosis. Some bleeding at the suture line is not uncommon and may be controlled by sponge compression, light cautery, or suture ligature. Excessive cautery may result in a weakened anastomosis and may predispose to leakage. Heavy bleeding should be controlled by fine sutures.

The staple lines should be staggered when the linear stapler is applied. This modification was suggested by Chassin and coworkers to avoid too many intersecting staple lines, which may create an ischemic point with potential for a leak.[14] Allis clamps are applied to the tissues being approximated to prevent a portion of the bowel circumference from slipping back as the jaws of the instrument compress the tissue. The instrument is fired and the excess tissue cut away before release of the instrument to avoid injury to the anastomosis. The anastomosis is checked to ensure that it is complete and no leak is present.

When a hand-sutured anastomosis is elected, the bowel edges are transected obliquely to ensure adequate blood supply at the bowel edges to be anastomosed. Most modern surgeons prefer end-to-end anastomoses. Even in a situation in which there is a disparity in size of the bowel lumina, as occurs in anastomoses of the ileum to transverse colon, the discrepancy can be readily overcome by division of the antimesenteric border of the ileum. Considerable controversy has been engendered over whether to use a one-layer or two-layer anastomosis. The type of suture material has created further controversy. The two-layer technique that I have used successfully in the past consists of a posterior row of 4-0 silk placed on a fine atraumatic needle into the seromuscular layer. An inner layer of 4-0 chromic catgut is placed through the full thickness of the bowel wall, begun on one edge and continued on the posterior wall in a simple running over-and-over suture, but on the anterior half adopting the Connell suture. The anterior seromuscular layer is then completed with 4-0 silk sutures.

A growing number of surgeons have favored a single-layer inverting interrupted technique. A posterior interrupted single layer of an absorbable suture such as 3-0 or 4-0 Vicryl or Dexon has been used. This is then continued on the anterior wall. Care must be taken not to invert excessive amounts of tissue, thereby causing narrowing of the lumen. Some surgeons prefer to use a Gambee suture for the single-layered anastomosis.

Copious saline irrigation of the abdominal cavity is performed to remove blood, bacteria, and debris. Drains are not necessary. Wounds are closed with continuous absorbable sutures for the peritoneum and fascia, and subcuticular continuous absorbable material for the skin.

Resection of Transverse Colon

The appropriate operation for a carcinoma of the transverse colon has been somewhat controversial; the reason is that depending on the portion of the transverse colon involved, lymphatic drainage may occur through the middle colic or right colic and possibly left colic branches. For a lesion located in the mid-transverse colon, a transverse colectomy is in order.

The procedure might begin by division of the greater omentum from the greater curvature of the stomach, either above or below the gastroepiploic arterial arcade, with care taken not to injure the wall of the stomach. In the event of a very redundant transverse colon, the omentum may be divided vertically on either side at the proposed proximal and distal lines of resection of the colon. For a short transverse colon, the entire omentum may be included in the resected specimen. To avoid tension on the anastomosis, either one or both of the hepatic and splenic flexures requires mobilization. It is often technically easier to resect the right and transverse colon rather than attempt to mobilize both flexures.

Mobilization of the splenic flexure is facilitated by incising the lateral peritoneal attachment along the descending colon. As the splenic flexure is approached, great care must be exercised to avoid injury to the spleen. The lienocolic ligament can be accentuated by passage of a finger along the colonic wall from the descending colon side toward the splenic flexure. The ligament can then be clamped and divided, or divided with the use of a cautery. Great caution should be exercised in this maneuver because there are frequently numerous adhesions to the splenic capsule. The peritoneum is incised on the mesocolon, and in so doing, the splenic flexure is mobilized downward and to the right, exposing the retroperitoneum. If the greater omentum becomes a limiting factor, division of the omentum is begun. The trunk of the middle colic vessel and the smaller vessels are secured. The bowel is divided and an anastomosis created, as previously described. When reconstituting the mesenteric defect between the ileum and the descending colon, care must be exercised to avoid narrowing of the duodenojejunal junction.

For lesions at or near the hepatic flexure or the ascending colon, a right hemicolectomy is performed. For lesions near the splenic flexure, a partial left colectomy with anastomosis of the transverse colon to the proximal sigmoid is performed.

Resection of Descending Colon

For descending colon lesions, the left branch of the middle colic artery remains intact, but the left colic artery and, depending on the level of the lesion, the first sigmoid vessels are ligated. The anastomosis is performed between the distal transverse and proximal sigmoid colon. Some surgeons advocate a formal left hemicolectomy.

Sigmoid Resection

There is some controversy as to the most appropriate procedure for removal of a sigmoid carcinoma. One school of thought advocates the necessity for a radical left hemicolectomy with anastomosis of the transverse colon to the rectum. However, a growing number of surgeons realize that the extended resection has not resulted in increased survival rates. Patients with lymphatics involved to the root of the inferior mesenteric artery who have these resected have no increased survival over patients who have a less radical procedure.[4] It would therefore seem that the extra mobilization with its potential risks and prolonged operating time are not justified. The exact extent of the resection depends on the portion of the sigmoid colon involved. For lesions of the proximal sigmoid, an anastomosis is performed between the descending colon and distal sigmoid; for those of the distal sigmoid, an anastomosis is performed between the proximal sigmoid and upper rectum; and for those of the mid-portion of the sigmoid, depending on the redundancy of the colon, an anastomosis is performed between the sigmoid–descending junction and the rectosigmoid. The splenic flexure is not routinely mobilized, but depending on the location of the lesion and the redundancy of the colon, it may indeed require mobilization to avoid tension on the anastomosis.

The patient may be placed in the supine position, but for more distal lesions it is preferable to have the patient in the modified lithotomy position so simultaneous access can be obtained through the abdomen and rectum. This access is necessary to allow use of the circular stapling device or inspection of the anastomosis by proctosigmoidoscopy.

The procedure is initiated by incising the peritoneum along the white line of Toldt in the left paracolic gutter, freeing the distal descending colon and the sigmoid from their developmental attachments from the splenic flexure to the pelvic brim. In the mid-portion of the sigmoid mesocolon, there is the intersigmoid fossa, a small depression in the peritoneum that acts as a guide to the underlying ureter. Care is taken to protect the left ureter and gonadal vessels. The peritoneum over the medial aspect of the mesosigmoid is incised toward the root of the inferior mesenteric artery to the level of the proposed ligation, and then downward toward the pelvis. The inferior mesenteric artery distal to the left colic vessel is then divided and ligated. Smaller vessels leading toward the planned lines of resection are secured and the bowel transected proximally and distally. The anastomosis is then created according to the surgeon's method of choice, but if the anastomosis is low, my preference is to use the circular stapler. For surgeons who deem it necessary to perform the radical left hemicolectomy, the operation is conducted much along the same lines by combining the mobilization of the sigmoid, splenic flexure, and distal transverse colon. The notable difference is the level at which the vessels are secured. To accomplish this, the posterior parietal peritoneum is incised to expose the inferior mesenteric vessels. The artery is tied flush with the aorta, and the vein is ligated separately at the level of the duodenum.

MANAGEMENT OF ADVANCED DISEASE

Complicated Carcinomas

Obstruction

When complete obstruction of the colon arises because of a carcinoma, the recommended treatment depends on the level of the colon that is obstructed as well as the beliefs and experience of the treating surgeon.[15,16] If the patient can be stabilized and demonstrates evidence of resolution of the occlusion, bowel preparation and elective resection is the ideal solution. For the unresolved right-sided colonic obstruction, it is generally accepted that the treatment of choice is a resection and primary anastomosis removing the right and proximal transverse colon.[17] When the obstruction is located in the distal transverse colon, a growing number of surgeons have adopted the procedure of an extended right hemicolectomy followed by a primary ileodescending anastomosis.

For patients with an obstruction of the left side of the colon, a larger number of options are available. Traditionally, these patients underwent a three-stage operation, with the first stage being a transverse colostomy or possible cecostomy, followed by resection and anastomosis, and finally by closure of the colostomy as a third stage. More recently, some surgeons have recommended a subtotal colectomy with primary ileosigmoid or even ileorectal anastomosis. Advantages offered by this operation include no stoma problems, a one-stage procedure with single hospitalization, and shorter hospital stay with financial savings. Others have recommended resection with a proximal colostomy and mucous fistula or Hartmann's procedure, whereas still others have recommended resection of the primary disease combined with on-table lavage and a primary anastomosis.[18,19] Some authors have reported a higher 5-year survival rate when patients with an obstructing carcinoma were treated by primary resection as opposed to staged resection,[20,21] whereas others have not,[22] but this at the cost of a higher operative mortality.[20,23]

Still bolder surgeons have performed a resection with primary anastomosis in the absence of bowel preparation.[24] More recently, an intracolonic bypass has been suggested as treatment.[25] Still others have suggested a primary resection with anastomosis and proximal diversion. Kronborg conducted a randomized trial in which he compared the traditional staged procedures with an initial transverse colostomy, followed by curative resection, and subsequent colostomy closure with immediate resection, end colostomy, and mucous fistula with subsequent reanastomosis. He found no difference in mortality or carcinoma-specific survival between the two treatments.[26]

My preference is to extend the primary resection for lesions as far as the sigmoid colon. It appears well worthwhile to cleanse the bowel distal to the obstruction, and a primary anastomosis can then be effected between the terminal ileum and the sigmoid colon. By eliminating a second or third hospitalization, and a temporary colostomy, palliation is better for those patients who ultimately die of their recurrent disease. If the lesion is so distal that there would be little remaining reservoir after resecting all the obstructed colon proximal to the carcinoma, a reasonable alternative is to cleanse the bowel distal to the carcinoma and perform a primary resection, and on-table lavage, with a primary anastomosis. In the very debilitated patient, consideration should be given to a right transverse colostomy. In the exceptional case in which the obstructing lesion is deemed unresectable, a bypass should be performed.

There have been preliminary reports on the role of preresectional laser recanalization for obstructing carcinomas of the colon and rectum. Eckhauser and colleagues reported on the use of the neodymium : yttrium–aluminum garnet laser successfully to accomplish decompression and allow for a formal bowel preparation and a definitive one-stage operation.[27]

Perforation

For patients in whom a free perforation of the carcinoma itself develops, the aim of therapy should be to remove the diseased segment. Otherwise, contamination will continue. In a situation in which the patient already has a generalized peritonitis, it is inappropriate to perform a primary anastomosis, and in this event the proximal bowel is brought out as a stoma and the distal bowel as a mucous fistula, or closed as a Hartmann's pouch. For a right-sided perforation, a similar procedure can be performed. Another option is to resect the perforated diseased bowel and perform a primary anastomosis with a proximal diversionary stoma, either proximal colostomy or loop ileostomy.

Under circumstances in which there is a left-sided obstructing lesion and a perforation of the right colon, a viable option is a subtotal colectomy encompassing removal of the perforated colon and the malignancy in one operation. A subtotal colectomy might even be considered in the circumstance in which there is only left-sided perforation, because this operation fulfills the criterion of removing the diseased and unprepared bowel. Another option for management of the patient with a perforation remote from the diseased segment is to bring out the perforated segment as a stoma, either a colostomy or cecostomy.

Bleeding

Massive bleeding from a carcinoma is an unusual complication, but when it arises, it has the built-in advantage of being a colonic cathartic. Therefore, if bleeding is of the magnitude that urgent operation is required, mechanical cleansing is automatically present, and the affected portion of bowel is resected with a primary anastomosis.

Involvement of Adjacent Viscera

It is estimated that attachment to adjacent viscera occurs in 6% to 12% of all colon carcinomas without distant metastases.[28,29] To perform an adequate curative operation, it sometimes becomes necessary to excise en bloc a part or all of the attached viscus. Not infrequently, these adhesions are inflammatory in nature and not the result of malignant infiltration, so that the prognosis is often better than what might originally have been anticipated (Table 59-1).

Exceptions to these recommendations are when the duodenum or bladder base is extensively involved, in which case the primary lesion is removed and the structures at risk marked with metal clips. Under these circumstances, the morbidity and mortality of the radical operation involving an anterior exenteration or Whipple procedure probably outweigh any possible benefit to be derived from a superradical operation. In exceptionally good-risk patients, consideration may be given to a total pelvic exenteration.

Palliative Procedures

One of the most unsatisfying situations facing any surgeon who operates on patients with colon carcinoma is recommending a major abdominal procedure, with its potential complications, to a patient who has definite evidence of incurable disease. The decision regarding operative intervention is usually reached with some trepidation, because many of these patients are in poor physical condition and have a limited life expectancy. But even for patients with metastatic carcinoma of the large bowel, resection to eliminate the potential complications of obstruction, massive bleeding, and the effects of local invasion of the primary lesion may be worthwhile. In the unusual circumstance of a totally unresectable lesion, it can usually satisfactorily be bypassed.

In the presence of metastatic disease, survival depends on the nature and extent of the metastases. For example, Joffe and Gordon noted survival with unilobar liver metastases to be 16.9

TABLE 59-1. *Nature of adhesions between colon carcinoma and adjacent viscus*

Author*	No. of patients	Adhesions (%) Carcinomatous	Adhesions (%) Inflammatory	5-Year survival (%)	Operative mortality (%)
El-Domeiri, et al, 1970[237]	10	80	20	50	10
Jensen, et al, 1970[238]	60	70	30	47	22
McGlone, et al, 1982[239]	24	66	34	79	8
Pittam, et al, 1984[240]	44	33	67	46	14
Eldars, et al, 1985[241]	84	68	32	35	6
Glass, et al, 1986[242]	69	49	51	70	—
Gall, et al, 1987[235]	121	55	45	52	12
Hunter, et al, 1987[236]	28	39	61	61	0

* Reference numbers apply to references in Gordon.[1]

From Gordon PH. Malignant neoplasms of the colon. In: Gordon PH, Nivatvongs S, eds. Principles and practice of surgery for the colon, rectum and anus. St. Louis: Quality Medical Publishing, 1992:549.

months, whereas with bilobar metastases, survivorship was only 8.5 months.[30] Cady and coworkers noted a mean survivorship of 13 months,[31] Takaki and associates, 12 months,[32] and Goslin and colleagues, a similar survivorship.[33] Recommendation for resection under these circumstances should be tempered by the presence of extensive hepatic replacement or jaundice, marked ascites, or massive peritoneal seeding, in which case life expectancy is very short and no benefit could be accrued from a resection. Poor prognostic factors deduced were patients with extensive liver metastases, those older than 75 years of age, and a previous history of cardiovascular disease.[30]

OPERATIVE COMPLICATIONS

As with any operation, the potential for intraoperative or postoperative complications is ever-present. General complications such as wound infection, wound dehiscence, and early postoperative small bowel obstruction are not addressed. Problems such as bladder dysfunction and sexual dysfunction, which are more often encountered in rectal operations, also are not discussed. The surgeon must be aware of the possibility of a peroneal nerve palsy or compartment syndrome when the lower extremities are placed in stirrups. A number of potential complications specifically related to the resection are described.

Anastomotic Leak

One of the most devastating complications after bowel surgery is the development of an anastomotic leak. However, for the most part, a bowel anastomosis usually heals per primum. Anastomotic healing depends on the patient's general and local condition. Conditions such as malnutrition, particularly hypoalbuminemia, diabetes, irradiation, shock, severe blood loss, and unprepared or poorly prepared bowel determine the risk to healing. Technical factors such as adequate blood supply, freedom from tension, healthy bowel ends, and careful opposition of bowel wall are of great importance.

An anastomotic leak usually becomes apparent between 5 and 7 days after surgery. Early dehiscence (within 48 hours) is usually serious because fecal spillage gives rise to generalized peritonitis. The early signs of an anastomotic leak are signs of sepsis, including fever, leukocytosis, localized or generalized tenderness, generalized ileus with abdominal distention, and tachycardia. The evaluation for an anastomotic leak depends on the patient's condition. If generalized peritonitis is obvious, along with other signs of sepsis, an urgent or emergent exploratory celiotomy is indicated. Any investigation to confirm the diagnosis is unnecessary and only delays treatment. Antibiotics to cover both aerobes and anaerobes should be started immediately.

For an anastomotic leak that develops after 48 hours, plain abdominal films are useful. In stapled anastomoses, the line or the ring of staples is broken. If the anastomotic leak is not apparent but is suspected, a gentle Gastrografin enema is the most accurate method of identifying its presence. Proctoscopy or flexible sigmoidoscopy may or may not be able to identify the dehiscence. Computed tomography scan cannot diagnose an anastomotic leak, but the presence of accumulated fluid may suggest that a leak has occurred. The management of an anastomotic leak with generalized peritonitis should aim at dismantling the anastomosis, with the proximal end brought out as a colostomy or ileostomy and the distal end closed or brought out as a mucous fistula. For a left colon anastomosis, occasionally the inflammatory reaction is so dense that it becomes impossible to take down the anastomosis safely. In this situation, a diverting transverse colostomy or ileostomy and drain placement near the anastomosis should be performed. There is no place to repair the anastomotic dehiscence or reanastomose at this time.

Anastomotic Bleeding

Early postoperative bleeding is uncommon regardless of whether the technique used is a one-layer, a two-layer, or a stapled anastomosis. The diagnosis of anastomotic bleeding is difficult and usually is achieved by deduction. Proctoscopy or flexible sigmoidoscopy can be performed if the anastomosis is in the lower left colon. Colonoscopy should not be done in the early postoperative period because of the danger of disrupting the anastomosis. Selective arteriography is one option, with the possibility of stopping the bleeding with vasopressin.

The management of anastomotic hemorrhage is initially conservative. Any bleeding diathesis should be corrected. Bleeding from a low anastomosis in the anorectum can be controlled by an anal approach with suture or electrocoagulation of the bleeding point. Blood transfusion may be necessary. Very rarely, a laparotomy and reanastomosis are considered.

Splenic Injury

Operative injury to the spleen accounts for 20% to 40% of all splenectomies performed in hospitals in the United States. Neither the incidence of this mishap nor its complications have lessened appreciably in the last three decades.[34]

The injury is invariably an avulsion of the splenic capsule, caused either by tearing of the normal splenic attachments (ie, the gastrosplenic, splenocolic, phrenicosplenic, and phrenicocolic ligaments), or by traction on the greater omentum. A common site of capsular tear is in a small area on the anterior or medial aspect of the lower pole of the spleen. Very little traction is needed to pull it off the spleen and cause bleeding. Another area common for a splenic tear is at the hilum. To avoid capsular tear, these folds should be incised before any traction is placed on the greater omentum and stomach and before mobilization of the splenic flexure is begun. For a safe exploration of the left upper quadrant and mobilization of the splenic flexure, it is important to have adequate exposure and assistants. Every attempt should be made to save the spleen. Most capsular tears can be managed by compressing the bleeding points with collagen pledgets. A splenectomy is reserved only as a last resort.

Ureteral Injury

Because of its proximity to the colon, intraoperative injuries to the ureters can occur, particularly when there are severe adhesions in that region from multiple previous operations, a malignancy, an inflammatory process, or previous radiation. Intraoperative ureteral injuries are uncommon during colorectal operations. Only 20% to 30% of iatrogenic ureteral injuries are recognized or detected at the time of operation[35]; this is crucial, because an immediate repair of the injury results in good healing. When recognition is delayed, the outcome becomes unpredictable and the incidence of nephrectomy increases sevenfold.[36] There are four danger zones where the ureter is most frequently injured during colorectal procedures[37]: during ligation of the inferior mesenteric artery; near the cul-de-sac where the ureter crosses the vas deferens, and at the sacral promontory; during division of the lateral stalks of the rectum; and during reperitonealization, when the ureter may be included in ligatures. The left ureter is more commonly injured than the right in colonic operations.[38] Types of injuries include ligation, crush injury, transection (partial or complete), and ischemic injury.[39]

Visual inspection is the most reliable means of assessing ureteral integrity. If there is doubt, methylene blue can be injected intravenously. Extravasation of blue-tinged urine or dye confirms the diagnosis. For the delayed diagnosis, retrograde pyelography is the most sensitive radiographic tool for identifying ureteral extravasation or obstruction from ligation.[39]

Injuries detected during operation or within the first few days after operation in a stable patient should be repaired immediately. When the patient is unstable or the detection is delayed for several days or weeks, the patient should undergo immediate proximal urinary diversion followed by delayed repair. In most cases, proximal urinary diversion may be achieved by placement of a percutaneous nephrostomy catheter.[39]

When the ureter has been inadvertently ligated during operation, often all that is necessary is removal of the suture. If the ureter has been crushed and is nonviable, a repair should be performed. The general principles of ureteral repair include debridement of nonviable tissues, a tension-free anastomosis, and a mucosa-to-mucosa reapproximation. When a difficult operation is anticipated, such as may occur with a large malignant mass, risk of ureteral injuries can be minimized by preoperative placement of ureteral catheters.

SURVIVAL AFTER OPERATION FOR COLON CARCINOMA

There is tremendous variation in the way survival data are reported in the literature, and this makes comparison of various series difficult. Nevertheless, with full recognition of the limitations of the exercise, an effort has been made to extract a number

TABLE 59-2. *Results of curative operation for colon carcinoma*

Author*	No. of patients	Resectability rates (%)	Operative mortality (%)	5-Year	
				Crude	Corrected
Slaney, 1971[292]	3094	—	—	42	52
Welch, et al, 1974[148]	1193	—	3	54	—
Corman, et al, 1979[4]	1008	95	4	—	—
Pihl, et al, 1980[293]	434	—	7	—	76
Stefanini, et al, 1981[294]	436	81	3	—	—
Zhou, et al, 1983[295]	302	71	2	73	—
Umpleby, et al, 1984[296]	439	—	13	27	59
Isbister, et al, 1985[297]	1505	—	—	43	—
Wied, et al, 1985[298]	442	—	—	47	—
Glass, et al, 1986[242]	413	—	3	—	82
Davis, et al, 1987[299]	405	—	3	38	52
Moreaux, et al, 1987[300]	646	—	1	78	—
Brown, et al, 1988[301]	550	85	7	—	—
Enblad, et al, 1988[302]	38,166	—	3	—	46

* Reference numbers apply to references in Gordon.[1]

From Gordon PH. Malignant neoplasms of the colon. In: Gordon PH, Nivatvongs S, eds. Principles and practice of surgery for the colon, rectum and anus. St. Louis: Quality Medical Publishing, 1992:556.

TABLE 59-3. *5-Year survival according to stage after curative resection*

	Dukes class A			Dukes class B			Dukes class C		
Author*	N	Cr. (%)	Corr. (%)	N	Cr. (%)	Corr. (%)	N	Cr. (%)	Corr. (%)
Gilbertsen, 1971[303]	359	67	—	174	51	—	173	33	—
Murray, et al, 1975[304]	21	81	—	166	63	—	80	49	—
Corman, et al, 1979[4]	225	81	95	332	62	90	204	35	55
Pihl, et al, 1980[293]	109	—	88	208	—	78	90	—	60
Eisenberg, et al, 1982[305]	101	—	75–87†	274	—	64–85†	501	—	39–43†
Isbister, et al, 1985[297]	172	64	—	427	58	—	354	32	—
Davis, et al, 1987[299]	24	71	96	125	65	87	85	36	52

* Reference numbers apply to references in Gordon.[1]
† Range depending on portion of colon affected.
N, number of patients; *Cr.,* crude data; *Corr.,* corrected data.

From Gordon PH. Malignant neoplasms of the colon. In: Gordon PH, Nivatvongs S, eds. Principles and practice of surgery for the colon, rectum and anus. St. Louis: Quality Medical Publishing, 1992:556.

of representative series of reasonable size, and these have been tabulated in Tables 59-2 and 59-3. Devesa and associates, in a review of 22 series, determined that the corrected 5-year survival rates for patients with large bowel carcinoma operated on for cure varies from 44% to 68%.[40]

Survival rates for patients who present with obstructing and perforating carcinomas are considerably more dismal. Operative mortality for obstructing carcinoma ranges from 2% to 23%, with a reasonable expectation of about 15% and a crude 5-year survival ranging from 9% to 78%, with a reasonable expectation of about 25%.[1] For perforated carcinoma, operative mortality ranges from 14% to 38%, with a reasonable expectation in the 20% to 30% range, and a 5-year crude survival rate ranging from 7% to 43%, with a reasonable expectation of about 25%.[1]

REFERENCES

1. Gordon PH. Malignant neoplasms of the colon. In: Gordon PH, Nivatvongs S, eds. Principles and practice of surgery for the colon, rectum and anus. St. Louis: Quality Medical Publishing, 1992.
2. Busuttil RW, Foglia RP, Longmire WP. Treatment of carcinoma of the sigmoid colon and upper rectum: a comparison of local segmental resection and left hemicolectomy. Arch Surg 1977;112:920.
3. Dwight RW, Higgins GA, Keehn RJ. Factors influencing survival after resection in cancer of the colon and rectum. Am J Surg 1969;117:512.
4. Grinnell RS. Results of ligation of inferior mesenteric artery at the aorta in resections of carcinoma of the descending and sigmoid colon and rectum. Surg Gynecol Obstet 1965;170:1031.
5. Pezim ME, Nicholls RJ. Survival after high or low ligation of the inferior mesenteric artery during curative surgery for rectal cancer. Ann Surg 1984;200:729.
6. Enker WE, Laffer VT, Black GE. Enhanced survival of patients with colon and rectal cancer is based upon wide anatomic resection. Ann Surg 1979;190:350.
7. Cole WH, Packard D, Southwick HW. Carcinoma of the colon with special reference to the prevention of recurrence. JAMA 1954;155:1549.
8. Fisher ER, Turnbull RB Jr. The cytologic demonstration and significance of tumor cells in the mesenteric venous blood in patients with colorectal carcinoma. Surg Gynecol Obstet 1955;100:102.
9. Turnbull RB Jr, Kyle K, Watson FR, et al. Cancer of the colon: the influence of the no-touch technique on survival rates. Ann Surg 1967;166:420.
10. Cohn I Jr, Floyd CE, Atik M. Control of tumor implantation during operations of the colon. Ann Surg 1963;157:825.
11. Long RTL, Edwards RH. Implantation metastases as a cause of local recurrence of colorectal carcinoma. Am J Surg 1989:157:194.
12. Wiggers T, Jeekel J, Arends JW. No-touch isolation technique in colon cancer: a controlled prospective trial. Br J Surg 1988;75:409.
13. Gordon PH, Dalrymple S. The use of staples for reconstruction after colonic and rectal surgery. In: Ravitch MM, Steichen FM, eds. Principles and practice of surgical stapling. Chicago: Year Book Medical Publishers, 1987:402.
14. Chassin JL, Rifkind KM, Turner JW. Errors and pitfalls in stapling gastrointestinal anastomoses. Surg Clin North Am 1984;64:441.
15. Amsterdam E, Krispin M. Primary resection with colocolostomy for obstructive carcinoma of the left side of the colon. Am J Surg 1985;150:558.
16. White CM, Macfie J. Immediate colectomy and primary anastomoses for acute obstruction due to carcinoma of the left colon and rectum. Dis Colon Rectum 1985;28:155.
17. Smithers BM, Theile DE, Cohen JR, et al. Emergency right hemicolectomy in colon carcinoma: a prospective study. Aust N Z J Surg 1986;56:749.
18. Konishi F, Muto T, Kanazawa K, et al. Intraoperative irrigation and primary resection for obstructing lesions of the left colon. Int J Colorectal Dis 1988;3:204.
19. Meijer S, Hoitsma HFW, van Loenhout RM. Intraoperative antegrade irrigation in complicated left-sided colonic cancer. J Surg Oncol 1989;40:88.
20. Fielding LP, Wells BW. Survival after primary and staged resection for large bowel obstruction caused by cancer. Br J Surg 1974;61:16.
21. Umpleby HC, Williamson RCN. Survival in acute obstructing colorectal carcinoma. Dis Colon Rectum 1984;27:299.
22. Welch JP, Donaldson GA. Recent experience in the management of cancer of the colon and rectum. Am J Surg 1974;127:258.
23. Ohman U. Prognosis in patients with obstructing colorectal carcinoma. Am J Surg 1982;143:742.
24. Goodall RG, Park M. Primary resection and anastomosis of lesions obstructing the left colon. Can J Surg 1988;31:167.
25. Ravo B. Colorectal anastomotic healing and intracolonic bypass procedure. Surg Clin North Am 1988;68:1267.
26. Kronborg O. The missing randomized trial of two surgical treatments for acute obstruction due to carcinoma of the left colon and rectum. Int J Colorectal Dis 1986;1:162.
27. Eckhauser ML, Imbembo AL, Mansour EG. The role of pre-resectional laser recanalization for obstructing carcinomas of the colon and rectum. Surgery 1989;106:710.
28. Gall FP, Tonak J, Altendorf A. Multivisceral resections in colorectal cancer. Dis Colon Rectum 1987;30:337.
29. Hunter JA, Ryan JA, Schultz P. En bloc resection of colon cancer adherent to other organs. Am J Surg 1987;154:67.
30. Joffe J, Gordon PH. Palliative resection for colorectal carcinoma. Dis Colon Rectum 1981;24:355.
31. Cady B, Monson DO, Swinton NW Sr. Survival of patients after colonic

resection for carcinoma with simultaneous liver metastases. Surg Gynecol Obstet 1970;131:697.
32. Takaki HS, Ujiki GT, Shields TS. Palliative resection in the treatment of primary colorectal cancer. Am J Surg 1977;133:548.
33. Goslin R, Steele G, Zamcheck N, et al. Factors influencing survival in patients with hepatic metastases from adenocarcinoma of the colon or rectum. Dis Colon Rectum 1982;25:749.
34. Morgenstern L. The avoidable complications of splenectomy. Surg Gynecol Obstet 1977;145:525.
35. Zinman LM, Libertino JA, Roth RA. Management of operative ureteral injury. Urology 1978;12:290.
36. McGinty DM, Mendez R. Traumatic ureteral injuries with delayed recognition. Urology 1977;10:115.
37. Higgins CC. Ureteral injuries during surgery: a review of 87 cases. JAMA 1967;199:82.
38. Melick WF. Complications of colonic and rectal surgery: the causes and management of postoperative urologic complications. Dis Colon Rectum 1973;16:7.
39. Presti JC, Carroll PR. Intraoperative management of the injured ureter. Perspectives in Colon and Rectal Surgery 1988;1:98.
40. Devesa JM, Morales V, Enriquez, JM. Colorectal cancer: the basis for a comprehensive follow-up. Dis Colon Rectum 1988;31:636.

Surgery for Gastrointestinal Cancer: A Multidisciplinary Approach, edited by Harold J. Wanebo. Lippincott-Raven Publishers, Philadelphia, © 1997.

CHAPTER 60

Surgical Management for Rectal Cancer

Jeffrey W. Milsom and Kirk A. Ludwig

Despite expanding interest in chemotherapy and radiation therapy in the management of rectal cancer, nearly all curative treatment for this disease requires some type of surgical resection. Rectal cancer is a common malignancy in the United States, and by itself (apart from cancer of the colon) is the sixth most common internal malignancy, with 39,000 new cases predicted in 1996.[1] Although the diagnosis of rectal cancer carries with it the stigma of requiring a permanent colostomy, with current techniques and new instrumentation, few patients now require such an operation to effect permanent cure of their disease. Even when this becomes necessary, modern stomal appliances are so effective that most colostomates enjoy normal lives.

The purpose of this chapter is to define the role of major surgical resections in the treatment of rectal carcinoma. We hope to provide the reader with insights into the relevant anatomy, the appropriate preoperative and intraoperative evaluations, and some of the controversies surrounding rectal cancer surgery. Important concepts regarding sphincter and pelvic nerve preservation along with maintenance of sound oncologic principles also are highlighted.

HISTORY

Over the last 150 years, from a time when simple laparotomy was accompanied by a significant mortality rate to the present day, when radical, complex, sphincter-saving procedures are performed on a routine basis, the surgical management of rectal cancer has changed dramatically. It is still in a state of evolution. The history of rectal cancer surgery can be viewed as a progression through three primary phases: reducing perioperative morbidity and mortality, improving long-term survival with more radical surgery, and balancing long-term survival with acceptable long-term functional outcome.

Jeffrey W. Milsom: Staff Surgeon, Head, Section of Colorectal Research, The Cleveland Clinic Foundation, Department of Colorectal Surgery, Desk A111, 9500 Euclid Avenue, Cleveland, OH 44195-5044

Kirk A. Ludwig: The Cleveland Clinic Foundation, Department of Colorectal Surgery, 9500 Euclid Avenue, Cleveland, OH 44195

The high operative mortality after laparotomy in the early 19th century led to the use of the perineal approach for excision of rectal cancers. Using such an approach, in 1826, Jacques Lisfranc of Paris reported probably the first successful excision of the rectum for cancer.[2] Little is known about subsequent rectal cancer surgery until the latter half of the 1800s. Anesthesia and asepsis led to dramatic advances in this time period, and up until the 1930s the most popular operative treatment for rectal cancer was the perineal excision, championed by the London surgeon Lockhart-Mummery.[3] This was a two-stage undertaking with a preliminary laparotomy for staging, and creation of a sigmoid loop colostomy. After preparatory irrigation of the distal limb, 2 weeks after the laparotomy, a perineal excision of the rectum was performed. In a series of 370 patients, the operative mortality using this approach was 11.6% and the 5-year survival was 40%.[4]

As early as 1883, Vincenz Czerny proposed that removal of a tumor by the perineal approach was inadequate, at least in part because he was unable to complete a rectal excision from below. He thus became the earliest advocate of the combined abdominal and perineal approach for removing a rectal cancer and its pedicle.[5] After noting the modes of spread of rectal tumors in autopsies of patients who died of rectal cancer, Ernest Miles, in 1908, proposed that Czerny's operation failed to eradicate the *zone of upward spread*. Noting the need for a more proximal lymphadenectomy, he modified the procedure to excise the lymphovascular pedicle "along the parietal attachments of the pelvic mesocolon and in the adjacent parietal peritoneum . . . as far as the group of lymph nodes situated over the bifurcation of the common iliac artery." He advocated total rectal excision, including the anal canal and sphincters, wide excision of the pelvic floor, and ligation of the main sigmoid artery at its origin with preservation of the inferior mesenteric artery (IMA).[6] Although Miles' procedure contained most of the requisite elements of a radical oncologic resection, widespread acceptance was delayed[6] when in 1914 a 36% operative mortality was reported in his first 61 patients.[7] In 1923, Hartmann developed his operation for rectal cancers, whereby the sigmoid colon and intraperitoneal rectum are excised and the distal anorectum is turned-in and left in situ.[8]

By the 1930s, improvements in anesthetic management, surgical technique, and preoperative and postoperative care had reduced perioperative mortality of the "Miles procedure" to acceptably low levels, and this became the gold standard for the surgical treatment of rectal cancer. The operation was refined over time, with the most lasting modification being the change to a synchronous approach popularized by Lloyd-Davies of London.[9] The cumbersome turning of the patient between the abdominal and perineal phases of the procedure was replaced by the preferred two-team approach, with the patient placed in a modified lithotomy position for the entire operation. Improving survival with radical resections was the major focus of rectal cancer surgery at this time.

Exactly how radical a resection was needed for acceptable survival became the next issue. In 1916, William Mayo reported that sphincter-saving surgery for rectal cancer *at any height* above the sphincters decreased survival (20% 5-year survival compared with 40% to 50% with complete proctectomy).[10] Thirty-two years later, Claude Dixon, a member of Mayo's own department, proved this concept erroneous when he demonstrated in over 400 patients that low mortality (2% to 6%) and excellent 5-year survival (63.7%) could be achieved with radical rectal resection and anastomosis of descending colon to rectum.[11] Sphincter preservation was becoming an exciting new possibility for many rectal cancer patients.

In 1945, Bacon described his pull-through technique, whereby the descending colon is anastomosed to the everted anus.[12] He later reported that patients with mid-rectal tumors treated with his sphincter-saving pull-through operation had a survival equivalent to those undergoing abdominal perineal resection. In 1961, Turnbull and Cuthbertson, in Cleveland, and Cutait and Figlioni, of São Paulo, Brazil, independently described a two-staged pull-through procedure for effecting a very low coloanal anastomosis.[13,14] In 1966, Parks of St. Mark's Hospital in London first described the coloanal anastomotic technique still in vogue today.[15]

As sphincter-saving procedures gained acceptance, the goal of rectal cancer surgeons became the achievement of both good oncologic and functional results. Stated in other terms, surgeons asked how far the oncologic limits could be safely pushed without compromising survival.

An improved understanding of the adequacy of the distal margin was of prime importance in the adoption of sphincter-preserving protection. In 1951, Goligher and colleagues reviewed 1500 rectal cancer specimens and detected distal microscopic spread in 6.5%, with less than 2% greater than 2 cm; this led to the arbitrary 5-cm distal margin rule.[16]

The minimally accepted distal resection margin has been justifiably shortened since that time, with Williams and colleagues,[17] Pollett and Nicholls,[18] and others demonstrating no decrease in survival or local recurrence rates with even a 2-cm margin of distal resection. In these series, moreover, most patients demonstrating significant distal intramural spread did poorly as a result of extrapelvic metastatic disease, not local recurrence problems. The distal margin has been shown to be only one of the important concepts in oncologic rectal surgery. R. J. Heald, of Basingstoke, England, has reminded surgeons of the importance of total mesorectal excision in reducing the risk of local recurrence with sphincter-saving procedures.[19]

Further success in sphincter-saving resections came with the introduction of reliable, mass-produced, end-to-end circular staplers in 1977.[20] Patients who would otherwise have undergone abdominoperineal resection could now be offered very low anterior resection with a stapled anastomosis.

Advances in the understanding of rectal tumor biology, anorectal physiology and pelvic anatomy combined with advanced instrumentation mean that most rectal cancers can be completely and safely excised with restoration of intestinal continuity. In addition, improvements in ostomy surgery techniques and care have allowed maintenance of active lifestyles even when a stoma is necessary.

Many areas of controversy still exist, and the debate over optimal surgical treatment of rectal cancer still rages on many fronts. These points of controversy center mainly on the appropriate extent of resection; this is covered in more detail later in this chapter and elsewhere in this text.

RELEVANT ANATOMY OF THE RECTUM AND PERIRECTAL TISSUES

The rectum, enshrouded as it is by the rigid bony ring of the pelvis and the soft tissues of the neurovascular and genitourinary systems, presents formidable challenges to the surgeon wishing to extirpate some portion of it. By convention, the rectum is usually divided into thirds. Because of variations in body habitus and length of the anal canal, it is difficult to assign precise lengths to each third of the rectum, but in general the upper third extends from the sacral promontory proximally to the anterior peritoneal reflection (distally), making it lie approximately 10 to 15 cm above the anal verge on proctoscopic examination.

The middle rectal segment begins (proximally) at the anterior peritoneal reflection (10 to 11 cm from the anal verge) and extends to 5 or 6 cm above the verge.

The lower third of the rectum begins 5 or 6 cm from the verge and ends at the top of the anal sphincters (the top of the surgical anal canal).

The upper portion of the "surgical" anal canal begins at the top of the anal sphincters and extends to the anal verge (or anal margin), which is grossly denoted by the junction of hair- and nonhair-bearing skin seen at this location.

The literature of sphincter-sparing rectal cancer surgery is rife with confusion about precisely where tumors are located, primarily because most surgeons reporting on tumor location do so with reference to distance from the anal verge. The problem with this convention in tumors of the middle and lower rectum is that the surgical anal canal length is highly variable (Fig. 60-1), and may range from 2 to 7 cm depending on sex and body habitus. Thus, a tumor with its lower margin at 8 cm from the anal verge in a thin woman may lie well within the mid-rectum, with 5 or 6 cm of clearance above the anal sphincters. In a heavily-muscled man with a tumor at the same distance above the verge, this tumor may only lie 1 or 2 cm above the sphincters! The surgical implications of this type of difference are tremendous, and thus a profound understanding of these anatomic variations is crucial in providing expert care in rectal cancer management.

The plentiful blood supply of the rectum and pelvic tissues ensures, in nearly all instances, that major portions of the rectum and its blood supply may be removed, yet the remainder of the organ will survive. Superiorly, the IMA is the major source of vascular inflow to the upper rectum by way of the superior rectal

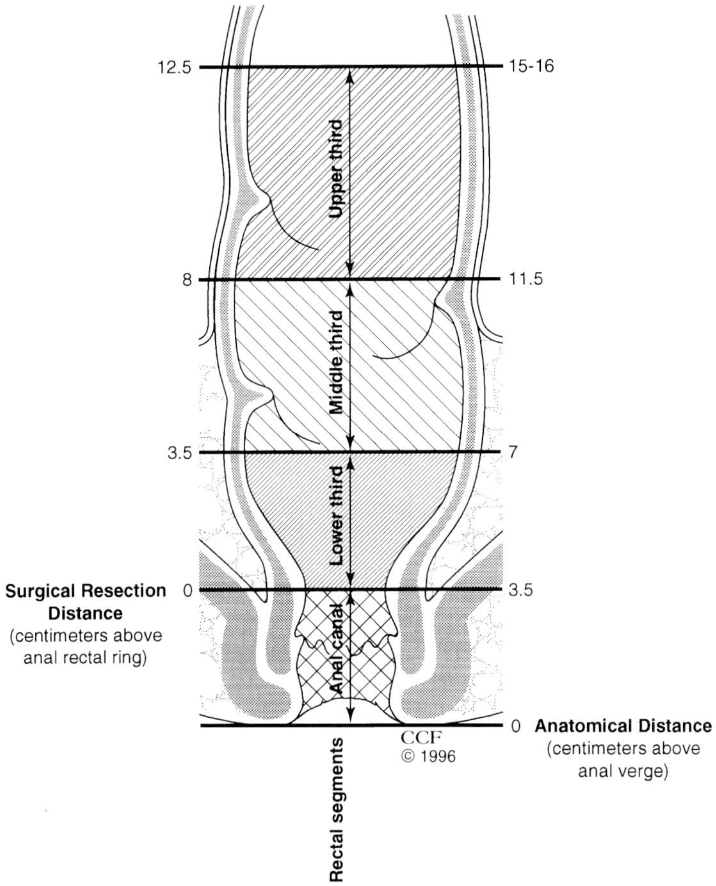

FIG. 60-1. Surgical and purely anatomical regions of the rectum as they relate to the anal sphincters and pelvic floor.

(hemorrhoidal) artery, which represents the terminal branch of the IMA. Anterolaterally, in the region of the mid-rectum, the middle rectal arteries are branches of the internal iliac vessels of the pelvis. These vessels are often diminutive, and may be absent in half or more of patients.[21] Inferiorly, branching from the internal pudendal vessels, are the inferior rectal arteries. These supply the anal sphincters and lower rectum up through the pelvic floor and along the wall of the rectum. They are the important vascular supply to the distal rectal segment in instances of sphincter-sparing surgery.

An understanding of the innervation of the rectum and adjacent pelvic structures is also crucial to the performance of safe and effective rectal cancer surgery. The rectum is surrounded by both the sympathetic and parasympathetic components of the autonomic nervous system. The sympathetic nerves cascade as a plexus from the preaortic region, just posterior to the IMA, bifurcating at the sacral promontory and then running laterally and inferiorly down the pelvic sidewalls. The parasympathetic nerves branch from sacral nerve roots two to four (S2–S4) and, intertwined with the sympathetic nerves, form the lateral stalks of the rectum, imparting to it the tough, fibrous consistency that leads this region of the pelvis also to be called the lateral "ligaments." As is discussed later, these nerves govern important motor and sensory functions to the pelvic organs, and their disruption at surgery leads to serious postoperative morbidities after proctectomy.

The lymphatic drainage of the rectum is especially complex because, unlike other portions of the intestinal tract, drainage is through the portal (mesenteric) as well as the systemic (internal iliac) circulations. Drainage follows the course of the vascular supply, as described earlier; thus, spread of rectal cancer may occur along the inferior mesenteric and superior rectal vessels as well as to the lateral pelvic wall (along the middle rectal vessels).

In performing proctectomy, several fascial planes surrounding the rectum are of surgical significance. The mesorectum, surrounding the posterior one half or more of the rectum, is enveloped by a thin, fibrous covering called the fascia propria. This forms an important oncologic barrier to primary and lymphatic spread to extrarectal pelvic tissues, and should be preserved intact in rectal dissection. It is immediately anterior to the fascia propria of the sacrum, and the potential space between these layers should represent the posterior extent of dissection for proctectomy. The surgical significance of this is discussed later. At the level of approximately S3, the rectosacral (Waldeyer's) fascia attaches itself to the presacral fascia, then travels interiorly to the region of the anorectal junction. This fascia must often be intentionally divided to mobilize the rectum safely and thoroughly to the pelvic floor.

Anteriorly, the plane between the rectum and the prostate and seminal vesicles contains another important fascial layer: Denonvillier's fascia. This also may represent an important boundary to tumor growth anteriorly, and must often be incised purposefully in the performance of complete rectal mobilization and safe separation of the rectum from the seminal vesicles and prostate (Fig. 60-2).

There are many other aspects of important surgical anatomy that the surgeon performing proctectomy for rectal cancer will

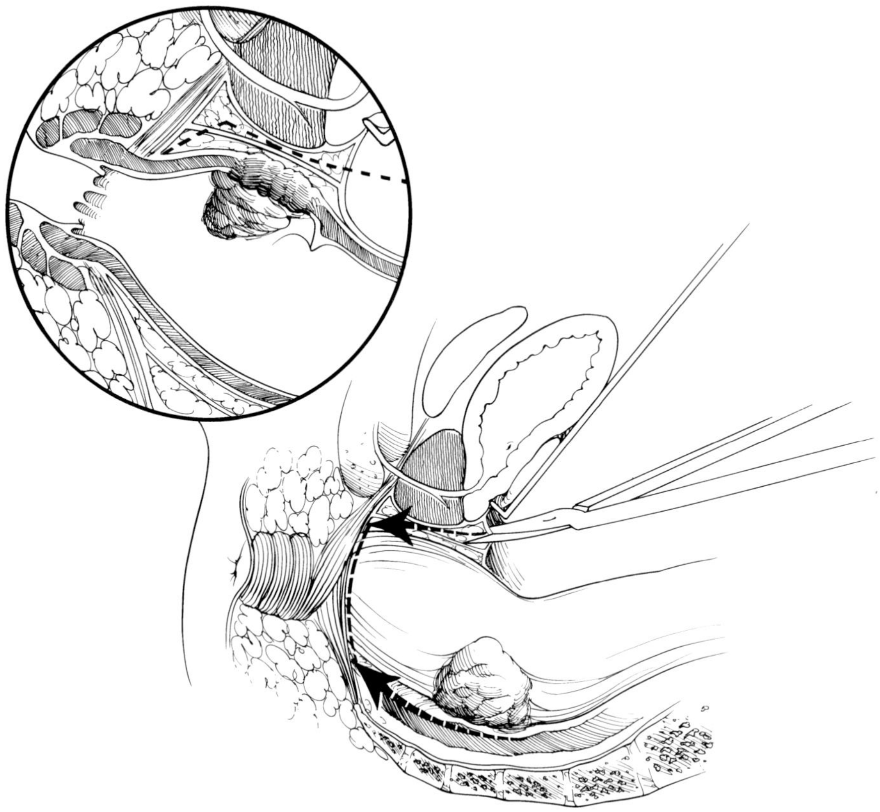

FIG. 60-2. Denonvillier's fascia may present an important boundary to tumor growth anteriorly, and must often be incised purposefully, superiorly, and inferiorly in anteriorly-situated tumors. (From Daly JM, Cady B, and Low DW, eds. *Atlas of Surgical Oncology.* St. Louis, Mosby Year Book 1992.)

encounter. These are highlighted in the section on Technical Details.

SURGICAL OPTIONS

Operations for middle and lower rectal cancers can be broadly divided into local procedures and radical extirpative operations. Local procedures are described elsewhere in the text. This chapter focuses on radical extirpative operations requiring a laparotomy. These can be divided into resectional procedures with permanent stoma (abdominoperineal resection and Hartmann's procedure) and sphincter-saving resectional procedures (low anterior resection, coloanal anastomotic procedures, and colonic J-pouch procedures). Each of these procedures is briefly defined in this section.

Resectional Procedures With Permanent Stoma

The *abdominoperineal resection*, according to Miles, ought to remove the following structures: the entire rectum, including the anal canal and sphincters, considerable parts of the levator ani muscles and ischiorectal fat, practically all the sigmoid colon and mesocolon, including the superior hemorrhoidal and inferior mesenteric vessels and glands lying in its base, and a portion of the pelvic peritoneum adjacent to the rectum. This operation is the most radical for mid- and low-rectal tumors and is considered the gold standard against which all other rectal cancer operations are judged. Although the abdominal and perineal portions of the operation originally required repositioning the patient, the operation today is usually performed with the patient in the modified lithotomy position using a two-team synchronous approach. The operation concludes with creation of an end-sigmoid colostomy, usually placed in the left lower abdomen.

Hartmann's procedure begins as the abdominal portion of the abdominoperineal resection. The rectal resection, however, ends at a point several centimeters distal to the tumor. The proctosigmoid specimen is resected and the distal rectal segment is either stapled or sutured over and a permanent left-sided colostomy is established.

Sphincter-Saving Resectional Procedures

The *low anterior resection* is distinguished from the anterior or high anterior resection in that the latter resections apply to lesions of the upper rectum (11 to 16 cm from the anal verge) typically located above the peritoneal reflection of the rectum. Mobilization of the rectum for low anterior resection is identical to that for abdominoperineal resection, and involves the following:

1. Complete circumferential opening of the pelvic peritoneum around the rectum
2. Division of the lateral ligaments (neurovascular pedicles) of the rectum
3. Elevation of the rectum posteriorly out of the presacral space, nearly always to the anorectal ring
4. Dissection of the anterior attachments of the rectum to the prostate or the vagina.

Because most of the blood supply to the sigmoid colon is also sacrificed in low anterior resection, the sigmoid colon, as well as the rectum, is resected (proctosigmoidectomy) before anastomosis of the descending colon to rectum. Complete mobilization of the splenic flexure is usually required to fashion a tension-free anastomosis deep within the pelvis.

In *coloanal anastomotic procedures*, the entire rectum, mobilized in a fashion identical to that for low anterior or abdominoperineal resection, is removed just above the level of the anorectal ring. In the method originally described by Parks in 1966,[15] the anal mucosa from the dentate line cephalad to the transection line is then excised transanally. By Parks' description, the well mobilized descending colon is then brought down through the anorectal remnant and anastomosed to the dentate line, usually by a hand-suturing technique "through the anal canal, which is held open by retractors or sutures." The anastomosis usually is protected temporarily with a diverting stoma.

The *colonic reservoir (or colonic J-pouch)* involves folding the distal 8- to 10-cm segment of the terminus of the descending colon on itself after proctosigmoidectomy and forming a J-shaped reservoir, the most dependent part of which is anastomosed to the anal sphincters in a circular stapled or hand-sewn side-to-end fashion. The addition of a pouch may improve the functional results of very low anterior or coloanal anastomotic procedures.

Other Procedures

Less commonly used over the last several decades are the so-called *pull-through techniques* for preservation of the anal sphincters and bowel continuity. These procedures involve rectal mobilization and transection similar to that in a coloanal procedure, but the descending colon is *pulled through* the anal orifice and sutured primarily to an everted anal canal (Bacon technique) or allowed to protrude through the anus for up to 10 to 12 days, at which time excess colon is trimmed away and a coloanal anastomosis is fashioned (as described by Turnbull and Cuthbertson,[13] Cutait and Figlioni,[14] and others). Functional outcome after these operations has been inferior to that with primary coloanal anastomosis, and they are rarely used in modern surgery. Their limited role, however, is described later in this chapter.

Use of *combined abdominal–transsacral procedures* has been described for removal of the rectum and more direct visualization of the lower rectum and anal sphincters for lower colorectal and coloanal anastomosis. Abdominosacral approaches require healing of an extra incision (the sacral one), they can injure the pelvic floor and sphincters, and they can be complicated by anastomotic leaks, leading to a troublesome fecal fistula. These procedures are rarely, if ever, required if adequate transabdominal and transperineal approaches are used. They are not discussed further in this chapter.

PREOPERATIVE EVALUATION

Surgical treatment for rectal cancer ranges from local, transanal procedures performed by a single surgeon on an outpatient basis to major extirpative operations requiring a complex multidisciplinary approach. Confronted with rectal cancer, the surgeon has many therapeutic options from which to choose. A thorough preoperative evaluation allows the surgeon to choose the proper course of action based on the condition of the patient and the extent of the tumor. The preoperative evaluation is designed to answer the following questions:

1. Is the patient fit for a major pelvic operation?
2. What is the exact location of the tumor? This location is best judged in relation to the top of the anorectal ring, not the anal verge.
3. How large is the tumor, what are its histologic features, what is its stage, and is there evidence of local or distant spread?
4. What is the status of the bowel proximal to the lesion?
5. What is the functional status of the sphincters?

The evaluation begins with a thorough history. Excision of a rectal cancer low in the pelvis is a major surgical endeavor and warrants a careful assessment of the overall medical condition of the patient. Cardiac, pulmonary, renal, and hematologic status must be suitable to allow for 2 to 4 hours of general anesthesia with a reasonable expectation for postoperative recovery and healing of the operative wounds. In the past, postoperative infectious complications were the primary cause of postoperative mortality. However, postoperative cardiopulmonary complications are now the principal cause of death.[22] A thorough preoperative evaluation allows the surgeon to identify risk factors and take appropriate steps to avoid postoperative complications. Although advanced age alone is not a contraindication to major surgery, the greater incidence of multiple comorbid diseases in the elderly patient must be recognized and taken into consideration. In general, the higher the operative risks, the more flexible the surgeon must be in choosing the appropriate therapy. A thorough history of bowel movement frequency and anal continence should be taken, especially if a sphincter-saving procedure is contemplated.

A standard abdominal examination is performed with special attention paid to the liver edge, the inguinal and supraclavicular lymph nodes, the presence of jaundice, the overall size of the patient, and the relative size of the pelvis. A careful digital examination of the rectum is most important. With the examining finger, the surgeon palpates the sphincters and assesses the resting and maximal squeeze pressures generated by the patient. Next, the *height of the tumor above the anorectal ring* (the top edge of the sphincters) is noted, as well as the tumor size and extent (Fig. 60-3). Approximate staging and fixation are determined as well as the relation to adjacent organs (vagina, cervix, and uterus in women and the prostate in men) and musculoskeletal components of the pelvis. In women, a bimanual pelvic examination must be performed to evaluate the pelvis thoroughly.

During rigid sigmoidoscopy, the distance of the tumor from the anal verge is noted, the gross morphologic features (eg, sessile, pedunculated, extent of circumferential involvement) are recorded, and the lesion is sampled for biopsy. At least one of the samples should be taken from the edge of the tumor so that characteristics of the advancing edge of the growth can be evaluated. "Palpation" with the sigmoidoscope also may aid in assessing fixation in tumors proximal to the examining finger. The height of the tumor with regard to the surgical procedure being contemplated should *not* be assessed with the flexible sigmoidoscope because this is unreliable.

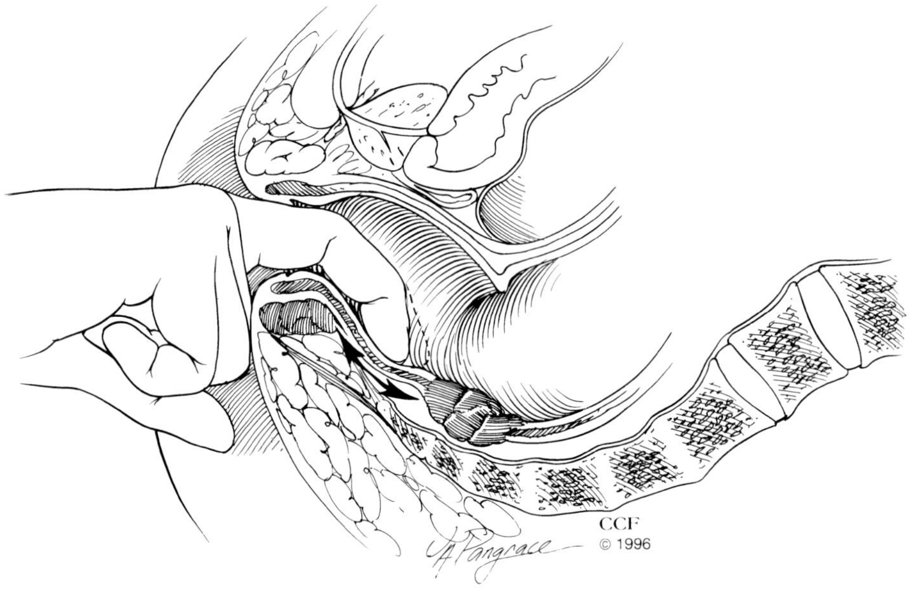

FIG. 60-3. The height of a rectal tumor *above* the anorectal ring (the top edge of the anal sphincters) is the most relevant factor in assessing a patient for a sphincter-saving operation.

Of patients with rectal cancer, *2% to 8%* harbor a more proximal synchronous carcinoma, and *30% to 40%* have a proximal polyp.[23–32] For this reason, all patients without significant obstruction should undergo an evaluation of the proximal bowel with either a barium enema or preferably a colonoscopy. Colonoscopy is preferred because of its sensitivity and accuracy in identifying lesions as well as its therapeutic potential. In the face of a nearly obstructing lesion, an intraoperative evaluation of the proximal bowel can be made by palpation and gentle colonoscopy after the anastomosis is completed.

Routine laboratory blood studies should include a complete blood count, electrolyte panel, clotting studies, liver function tests, and a preoperative carcinoembryonic antigen serum assay. Elevation of the serum carcinoembryonic antigen to greater than 20 ng/mL has been strongly associated with distant metastases,[33] and this information may assist in the decision to offer a less radical procedure. A type and cross-match for at least two units of packed red blood cells should be procured. Patients with normal preoperative hematocrit levels should be encouraged to autodonate 1 or 2 units of blood before surgery (a unit can be donated every week up to 72 hours before surgery) while the patient is simultaneously given an iron supplement. In nearly all patients, a starting hematocrit of 30% is quite acceptable at the time of rectal cancer surgery.

Imaging Studies

Computed tomography (CT) and magnetic resonance imaging (MRI) are frequently used before surgery to assess depth of tumor invasion into or through the rectal wall, status of the perirectal lymph nodes, involvement of adjacent organs, and presence of distal metastatic disease. Because neither study effectively visualizes the individual layers of the rectal wall, both are unreliable in assessing the depth of tumor penetration unless there is gross tumor penetration of the bowel wall (large T3 or T4 cancers).[34–40] CT and MRI can both visualize enlarged perirectal lymph nodes. However, neither is accurate in identifying normal lymph nodes or normal-size lymph nodes with metastases.[40–43] CT is valuable in assessing involvement of adjacent organs, as is MRI.

Detecting distant metastatic disease, hepatic metastases in particular, is the single best use for preoperative CT or MRI: CT has an accuracy of 90% to 95% in detecting liver metastases before surgery,[41,42,44,45] and MRI may prove to be even more accurate.

Computed tomography and MRI, because of their ineffectiveness in determining depth of tumor invasion and status of perirectal lymph nodes, are of limited use in determining which tumors are amenable to local therapy. However, in patients being considered for this type of therapy, a CT scan of the liver is warranted because no operative assessment of the liver is possible. If any preoperative adjuvant therapy is contemplated, CT scanning of the abdomen, pelvis, and chest is strongly suggested because it allows for detection of extrapelvic, specifically hepatic or pulmonary, metastases that would render such therapy, in patients who might otherwise be candidates, senseless.

If preoperative CT scanning reveals potential adjacent pelvic organ involvement, intravenous pyelography should be considered. This can often be performed in concert with (immediately after) the CT scan, with the intravenous dye from the CT scan sufficing to visualize the ureters, to rule out ureteral involvement by tumor. Routine chest radiographs should always be taken to assess for occult pulmonary metastases and to evaluate grossly cardiopulmonary status.

Anorectal Physiology Laboratory Studies

Endoluminal ultrasound (ELUS) is a minimally invasive, rapid, and well tolerated office procedure that appears to be the most accurate means of staging rectal cancers.[46] Although the procedure is quite operator dependent and a learning curve is involved,[47] ELUS is assuming a more important and extensive role in the preoperative evaluation of rectal cancer patients.[48]

ELUS plays a key role in determining which tumors can be treated by local measures. The preoperative ability to stage these tumors accurately also allows for more rational use of preoperative radiation therapy. ELUS is the most accurate modality available for assessing depth of invasion, with accuracy rates as high as 83% to 90%.[46,49–51] Studies have shown that ELUS assesses depth of wall penetration better than either CT or MRI.[52] It is also the most accurate study for determining the extent of mesorectal lymph node metastases, with an accuracy in predicting positive lymph nodes reported to be in the 70% to 80% range.[53] In an attempt to increase the accuracy of preoperative staging, ELUS has been used to sample suspect pararectal lymph nodes for biopsy. Preliminary experience provides evidence that ELUS-guided biopsy sampling of pararectal lymph nodes is safe and feasible and yields useful decision-making data.[54] Data also suggest that ELUS is accurate in predicting adjacent organ involvement.[48]

Anorectal manometry is used to evaluate and quantitate anorectal sphincter pressures at rest and with maximal squeeze efforts. When considering a sphincter-saving procedure in a patient complaining of minor incontinence, a normal manometric examination may reassure the surgeon that these complaints are secondary to secretions caused by the tumor or the pelvic pressure of a pelvic mass. Conversely, manometric studies indicating a very weak sphincter, substantiated by electromyelography studies showing denervation of the sphincters, would argue against a restorative procedure.

PATIENT SELECTION: MATCHING THE PATIENT AND THE OPERATION

Once the surgeon has ascertained that the patient is a suitable candidate for laparotomy and proctectomy, then certain preoperative and intraoperative maneuvers should be undertaken to maximize safety and operative results. Significant medical conditions, particularly related to cardiovascular, pulmonary, or diabetic problems, should be optimized, using appropriate consultation as necessary. Although greater than 90% of our elective surgical patients undergo outpatient mechanical bowel cleansing, any patient with significant underlying medical conditions or an obstructing tumor that might preclude a thorough bowel preparation, or any patient judged unreliable, is admitted the day before surgery. A 42- to 72-hour clear liquid diet combined with gentle laxative (citrate of magnesia 5 to 10 ounces orally every 4 to 6 hours) is used if significant obstruction is present. In the unobstructed patient, we use a mechanical preparation of clear liquids for 24 hours before surgery, then polyethylene glycol (4 L) or sodium phosphate (3 ounces plus added liquid) to purge the intestinal tract thoroughly of food. If there is concern about bowel preparation because of the obstruction, after hospital admission, some gentle tap water enemas (300 to 500 mL) can also be administered to cleanse the distal bowel.

Preoperative planning for a temporary or permanent stoma must also be considered. This means that potential sites on the right and left sides of the abdomen should be marked. An enterostomal therapy nurse may be of major assistance, both in choosing satisfactory sites and in counseling the patients before surgery. Bilateral stoma marks are important because temporary diversion *with* colorectal anastomosis may be preferable using a loop ileostomy. The rationale for this is as follows: If a locally advanced tumor is found that precludes anastomosis, a permanent (left-sided) colostomy may be preferable. Temporary diversion in concert with colorectal anastomosis using a left-sided colostomy is undesirable because the marginal artery of the colon (leading to the anastomosis) may be jeopardized. A right-sided loop colostomy for temporary diversion is often large and foul smelling, and the liquid stool is no easier for the patient to deal with than the smaller and relatively odorless loop ileostomy. The loop ileostomy also seems technically easier to close than the right-sided colostomy, mainly because of its smaller size.

ONCOLOGIC PRINCIPLES IN RECTAL SURGERY

Extent of Resection

General principles of oncologic colorectal surgery have been well established over the last century. These include proximal ligation of the vascular pedicle, thorough regional lymphadenectomy, and wide en bloc resection of tumor-bearing soft tissue and mesentery. However, the exact extent of resection necessary during a rectal cancer operation still generates considerable discussion.

High Versus Low Ligation of the Inferior Mesenteric Artery

A high versus low ligation of the IMA continues to stir controversy, yet the literature on the subject is quite clear; no good evidence exists to support the concept that a high ligation (ligation proximal to the left colic artery) improves survival. Miles,[6] in his initial description of the abdominoperineal resection, proposed ligating the IMA below the left colic artery. In that same year, 1908, Moynihan[56] championed a radical concept of ligating the IMA flush with the aorta, based on the concept that oncologic surgery is related directly to "anatomy of the lymphatic system."[56] Cuthbert Dukes and colleagues substantiated this concept by demonstrating that lymphatic extension of rectal cancer was remarkably constant, nearly always following the path of the IMA to the aorta.[55,57] Goligher, in a study examining the blood supply of the sigmoid colon and mesentery, reported that the distance between the IMA origin at the aorta and the take-off of the left colic artery averaged 4 cm, and that as many as 10 lymph nodes could be retrieved from this margin.[58] Subsequent studies reported an 11% to 22% incidence of positive nodes between the origin of the left colic artery and IMA.[59,60]

There would seem to be obvious value in resecting these involved lymph nodes, but a number of studies have shown this not to be the case. Bacon and associates reported a 5% increase in survival with high ligation in his series, but statistical significance was not reached.[59] Grinnell and Hint, early advocates of high ligation,[61] reversed their opinion on the value of high ligation in 1965 when they were unable to show increased survival after high ligation.[62] More recently, in a large study from St. Mark's Hospital involving over 1300 resections, no difference in crude or age-corrected 5-year survival rates for any Dukes' classification could be demonstrated after high ligation.[63] Further analysis of data from St. Mark's confirmed that the level of ligation has no effect on patient survival.[64]

Two pathologic features of rectal cancer probably explain the failure of high ligation to improve survival: the lymphatic and hematogenous drainage of the rectum is through multiple vessels coursing through the pelvis along the inferior mesenteric vessels and the internal iliac vessels, and even through inguinal routes; and involvement of nodes at the base of the IMA suggests that cancer cells have already spread elsewhere in the lymphatics outside the reach of surgery.

Despite the fact that it does not appear to influence survival, high ligation of the IMA does have some technical merit in that it allows for a more complete mobilization of the left colon, which facilitates a tension-free low pelvic or anal anastomosis. Ischemia of the left colon after high ligation is of some concern, especially in patients with known or suspected atherosclerotic disease. It may also lead to a higher morbidity rate. Our approach to proximal ligation is as follows: a high ligation of the IMA is attempted if safe and disease appears localized to the pelvis. If a high ligation could be hazardous or unduly prolong the operation (as with evidence or suspicion of mesenteric vascular disease, obesity, or major underlying medical problems), a ligation and division of the IMA distal to the left colic artery is logical because this is unlikely adversely to affect long-term survival. We prefer to ligate the inferior mesenteric vein at the inferior edge of the pancreas or adjacent to the IMA. A high ligation of the vein also frees the colon to move caudally to the pelvis for a low anastomosis.

Distal Margin of Resection

The historical shift from radical abdominoperineal resection for all rectal tumors to the use of sphincter-saving techniques in most cases has resulted primarily from a better understanding of what constitutes an adequate distal resection margin. Mayo recommended abdominoperineal resection for any rectal cancer.[10] Dixon showed, 32 years later, that a low morbidity and mortality as well as a high 5-year survival (63.7%) could be achieved after a sphincter-saving, low anterior resection.[11] In 1949, Best and Blair demonstrated that the use of a 3.5 cm distal margin was oncologically safe in treating nearly all rectal cancers.[65] In 1951, Goligher and colleagues reported on a pathologic review of 1500 rectal cancer specimens. They found distal intramural spread in only 6.5% and spread of more than 2 cm in less than 2%.[66] Based on these data, the somewhat arbitrary "5-cm distal margin" concept was developed. In the 1980s, Williams and colleagues[67] and Pollett and Nicholls[18] proposed that perhaps even a 2-cm distal resection margin was justifiable. In Williams and colleagues' report, in 50 patients with rectal cancer, 76% had no intramural spread, whereas 14% had distal spread less than 1 cm. Of the five patients with distal spread greater than 1 cm, all had poorly differentiated Dukes' C tumors and all had distant metastatic disease within 3 years of operation. A 5-cm distal margin did not favorably affect survival. Pollett and Nicholls, in their review of 334 patients treated for rectal cancer at St. Mark's Hospital, were also unable to show any survival advantage or reduction in local recurrence rates when distal resection margins greater than 5 cm were compared with those less than 2 cm.

The literature regarding the distal resection margin is somewhat problematic in that authors measure the margin in various ways. Weese and colleagues determined that a 5-cm margin in situ became a 2.4-cm margin in the "fixed, unpinned" state in 10 rectal cancer specimens.[68] We prefer to ascertain the distal resection margin in the following manner: the rectum is completely mobilized to the pelvic floor when proctectomy is undertaken. When a sphincter saving procedure is attempted, the 2-cm margin distal to the tumor is estimated using the distance of "two fingerbreadths" on the unstretched rectum in situ. Electrosurgery is used to mark the rectal wall at this point, and a complete mesorectal excision down to this level is undertaken. After resection, we routinely open the specimen on the back table of the operating room and measure the distal margin. If less than 2 cm in a given area, a frozen section of the area in question is taken to rule out the possibility of intramural extension, especially if unfavorable histology was documented on preoperative biopsy. Unfavorable histology and a margin of less than 2 cm would lead to an abdominoperineal resection in most cases.

If the tumor is exophytic or a villous lesion and seems well encompassed by the resection, even a 1-cm margin in the gross evaluation of the specimen is acceptable. Use of preoperative radiation in a low-lying lesion ($<$5 cm from the top of the anal sphincters) might justify acceptance of a margin of 1 to 2 cm because the periphery of an irradiated lesion would be less likely to contain malignant cells.

Based on a 2-cm distal margin, sphincter-saving operations can be justified in most cases, with recurrence rates identical to those after abdominoperineal resection.[66,68–71]

Radial Margin and Complete Mesorectal Resection

Obtaining an adequate distal margin of resection is of little value if the lateral margins are not clear. Clear margins must be obtained cicumferentially around the tumor. The wide variation in local recurrence rates (2% to 50%) may be explained on the basis of inadequate lateral or radial margins of resection.[72–75] Quirke and colleagues[76] and Heald and associates[77,78] are responsible for emphasizing this important concept. Quirke and colleagues studied the degree of lateral spread in rectal cancer in a group of 52 patients, 23 of whom underwent abdominoperineal resection and 29 of whom were treated by sphincter-saving operations. They noted spread of cancer to the lateral margin in 13 patients. Local recurrence developed in 11 of these patients and in only 1 patient who had negative lateral or radial margins. Exacting surgical technique (avoiding "coning in" on the rectum) is the critical technical component in achieving clear lateral margins. In nearly all cases of curative rectal cancer surgery, the lateral dissection should be flush with the endopelvic fascia of the pelvic sidewall.

Complete mesorectal excision also seems to be a valid concept in avoiding local recurrence. Heald maintains that local recurrence results from spread into the mesorectum. His pathologic studies have demonstrated microscopic foci of tumor cells in the mesorectum 2 cm distal to the tumor.[77] Reporting a local recurrence rate of 2% to 3% and an 85% survival at 9 years in one series, Heald and Ryall argue emphatically that complete mesorectal excision is a key in obtaining good results with sphincter-saving operations.[19] Our experience with 391 rectal cancer patients treated with wide pelvic clearance and complete mesorectal excision and colorectal anastomosis supports these concepts. At 5-year follow-up, we found a 5% incidence of isolated local pelvic recurrence and an overall 9% combined local and distant recurrence rate (unpublished data, Cleveland Clinic Department of Colorectal Surgery, 1995).

Several authors have suggested extending the lateral resection to the internal iliac nodes beneath the endopelvic fascia.[78,79] We have not routinely practiced this type of dissection and believe that there is little evidence to support its use.

En Bloc Resections

The presence of a locally advanced (stage T4) tumor with direct invasion into other organs or structures is seen in 5% to 20% of patients with rectal cancer. This fixation does not necessarily preclude a curative operation if the tumor is localized.[80–83] The major morbidity of wide, excisional surgical procedures in the pelvis (as high as 39% in some series)[82] must, however, be balanced against the long-term cure rate.

When history and physical examination suggest invasion of adjacent pelvic structures, careful preoperative staging is undertaken. CT scans of the pelvis and abdomen are typically used. We have also found ELUS to be accurate in detecting adjacent organ involvement. Adjacent structures most commonly involved include the pelvic sidewall (89%), the vagina (81%), the small intestine (20% to 30%), and the uterus (24%).[81]

If preoperative staging suggests a stage T4 lesion, we suggest preoperative external beam radiation therapy during a period of 4 to 6 weeks in a dose of 40 to 50 Gy. This may downstage a rectal cancer, and may convert a lesion from fixed to mobile. Often, 5-fluorouracil is given at the beginning and end of the radiation therapy to enhance effects of the radiation.

After a suitable recovery period (4 to 6 weeks), patients undergo operation. If involvement of the urinary tract is suspected, a urologist should be consulted and the patient advised about the possible need for urinary diversion. At operation, if thorough abdominal and pelvic exploration reveals localized disease, contiguous organ involvement is an indication for en bloc resection. Any adhesions between the tumor and adjacent organs should be assumed malignant, and excision with 1 to 2 cm of adjacent normal tissue is undertaken. The bladder and vagina are easily managed in this fashion. Involvement of the bladder trigone is usually an indication for cystectomy and urinary diversion. Five-year survival rates for node-negative disease under these circumstances may be as high as 50% to 90%. Positive nodes reduce the likelihood of survival to 20% to 29% at 5 years.[80–82]

Sacral resection is warranted when localized sacral involvement is present and the patient is a good operative risk. The sacrum may be safely excised up to the S2–S3 junction without fear of bony instability.[84] Sugarbaker has reported survival in excess of 3 years in four of six patients undergoing partial sacrectomy and en bloc resection.[85] Consideration of sacral resection should prompt consultation with an orthopedic surgeon skilled in pelvic bony surgery.

Final Preparations for Major Oncologic Pelvic Surgery

Certain preoperative and intraoperative strategies help to ensure smooth conduct of an operation and good results. Medical conditions such as cardiopulmonary disease or diabetes are evaluated before surgery with the help of appropriate medical consultation. Physiologic parameters are optimized before and during surgery, and it is helpful to plan for invasive intraoperative monitoring if it may be needed. Preoperative nutritional status should not be ignored, and patients with significant weight loss should be considered for nutritional supplementation. A thorough preoperative staging workup allows for appropriate preoperative administration of adjuvant therapy, it allows the surgeon to plan the operation with the patient, it minimizes intraoperative surprises, and it maximizes the chance for a good outcome.

The patient is placed on the operating table in the supine position. With induction of anesthesia, broad-spectrum prophylactic antibiotics are administered (we usually use a third-generation cephalosporin in combination with metronidazole). After suitable general anesthesia is achieved, pneumatic sequential compression stockings for deep venous thrombosis prophylaxis are applied and the legs are placed in specialized padded lithotomy stirrups (Dan-Allen Co., Lakewood, OH). These stirrups support the foot and lower calf but place no pressure on the peroneal nerve at the fibular head. Thus a neuropraxia, even after an extended operation, is highly unlikely. The foot of the table is dropped and the buttocks are pulled to the end of the table so that the anus is easily accessed. A towel role is occasionally used to elevate the sacrum. The lower extremities are abducted only enough to allow access to the perineum. With the knees flexed, the hips are flexed only slightly so that the legs do not encroach on the abdominal field. A bladder catheter is placed and taped in place over the right thigh at the inguinal crease.

A rectal washout is then gently performed using warm saline through a large mushroom catheter connected to a 3-L irrigation bag. When the rectal effluent is clear, a final digital examination and rigid proctoscopy are done to reassess the relation of the tumor to the anal sphincters. The rectal tube is then replaced and 60 to 100 mL of povidone–iodine is instilled into the rectum. A bag is secured to the tube and it is left in place to drain the rectum.

The entire abdomen, genitalia, and perineum are then prepared and draped into the field with a separate drape covering the perineum/pelvis. The abdomen is entered through a long midline incision and a thorough and systematic exploration is carried out *away* from the pelvis. Suspect areas are sampled and sent for frozen-section analysis. A careful bimanual examination of the liver is performed and intraoperative ultrasonography is used to investigate any suspect liver lesion. The distal sigmoid colon is then encircled with a woven tape and tied down to isolate the proximal colon from the lumen of the rectum. The colon is palpated and the pelvis is surveyed. For tumors above the peritoneal reflection, the operative course can usually be outlined at this time. For tumors below the peritoneal reflection, final operative decision making is deferred until the pelvic dissection is complete.

TECHNICAL DETAILS

Proctosigmoidectomy

General Concepts

If the rectal tumor appears to be resectable, the preliminary steps of any operation to remove the rectum are nearly identical, whether performing a low anterior resection with colorectal anastomosis, a coloanal anastomosis, or abdominoperineal resection. Thus, the early part of this section focuses on the mobilization and vascular ligation phases of rectal resection. Special aspects of the anastomotic preparation (low anterior resection, coloanal anastomosis, colonic J-pouch) or perineal resection (abdominoperineal resection with permanent stoma) are dealt with in individual subsequent sections.

Vascular Isolation and Ligation

After ligating the sigmoid colon with a heavy tape (as described earlier), the small bowel is reflected cephalad and to the right. The base of the sigmoid mesentery, specifically the inferior mesenteric pedicle, is grasped by the surgeon's nondominant hand, and the peritoneum encircling the IMA and inferior mesenteric vein is incised just to the right of the origin of the IMA to the sacral promontory. The surgeon's fingertips are swept posterior to these vessels, and the hypogastric (sympathetic) nerve plexus is bluntly dissected posteriorly away from the IMA and inferior mesenteric vein, leaving it in situ. Further sharp dissection at the base of the IMA should allow for preservation of most of the preaortic sympathetic nerve fibers travelling to the pelvis. By mobilizing the sigmoid colon from its retroperitoneal attachments, this may allow for identification of the left ureter and gonadal vessels. These structures must be unequivocally identified and swept clear of the IMA and inferior mesenteric vein to allow for safe ligation of the vessels.

Each vessel is isolated and doubly ligated with size 0 or 2-0 ligatures. If the IMA is calcified, it may be wise to suture-ligate it after initial tying. "High ligation," above the left colic artery, is performed in nearly all patients for oncologic reasons (see the section on High Versus Low Ligation of the IMA, previously), as well as to allow the left colon to extend completely into the pelvis without tethering of the mesentery by the connected left colic artery (Fig. 60-4). In a clinical situation in which vascular insufficiency from the middle colic artery is possible, preservation of the left colic artery is advisable.

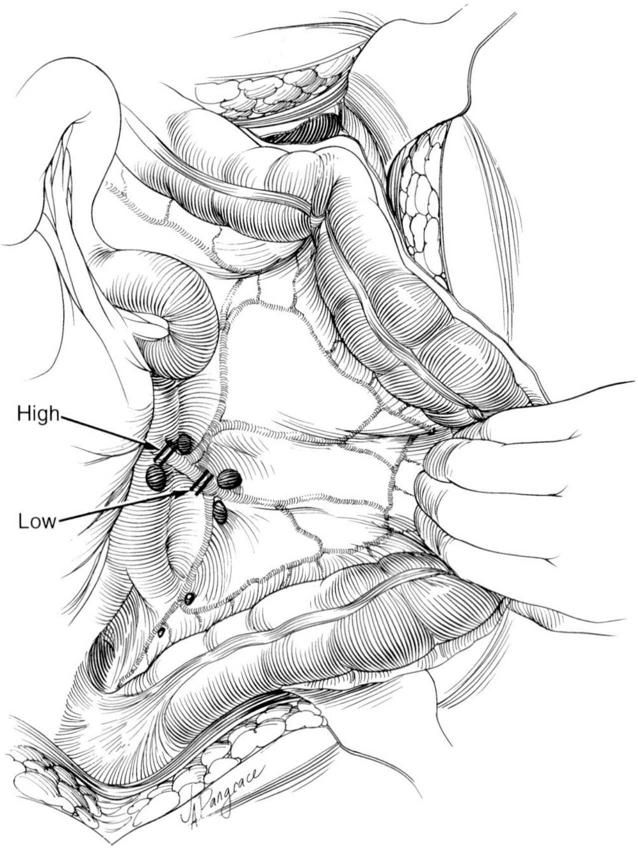

FIG. 60-4. The differentiation between a high versus low ligation of the inferior mesenteric artery relates to whether or not the ligation is above (high ligation) or below (low ligation) the left colic artery. (From Wanebo HJ. Colorectal Cancer, St. Louis: Mosby-Year Book, 1993.)

Mobilizing the Descending and Sigmoid Colon

After mobilizing the sigmoid colon from the sacral promontory to the lateral aspect of the left iliac fossa, the anterior aspect of Gerota's fascia is carefully separated from the posterior portion of the sigmoid and descending colon mesentery. This allows for easy elevation of the left colon away from its lateral peritoneal attachments up to the splenic flexure. If exposure of the splenic flexure becomes tedious, either the abdominal wall incision should be extended or the dissection should continue by detaching the omentum from the left portion of the transverse colon. After doing this, the transverse and descending colon may be grasped simultaneously (the omego maneuver) to enhance exposure and ultimate takedown of the splenic flexure. Extreme care must be taken in detaching the posterior mesenteric attachments of the splenic flexure region, because the marginal vessels of the left colon are at risk for injury during this dissection. These vessels are the lifeline of the mobilized bowel, bringing blood from the middle colic vasculature to the left colon (Fig. 60-5).

Mobilizing the Rectum Down to the Pelvic Floor

After vascular ligation/division and left colon mobilization, the pelvic dissection commences. Frequently, at this juncture, the inferior mesenteric vascular pedicle is divided on its left (lateral) edge all the way to the bowel at the junction between the sigmoid and descending colon, then the bowel is occluded with clamps and divided as well.

The rectum is mobilized and freed from surrounding structures by first incising the lateral, peritoneal reflections just below the sacral promontory, then by mobilizing it posteriorly from the sacral hollow. This is accomplished by sharp dissection in the plane between the fascia propria of the rectum and the presacral fascia (Fig. 60-6). Inadvertent dissection too posteriorly (usually when blunt dissection of the rectum is attempted) risks tearing of the presacral veins. These veins drain directly through the sacral periosteum and connect to the basivertebral venous system, and may bleed profusely (Fig. 60-7). Because of this, sharp dissection for the entire posterior mobilization is advised. Control of presacral bleeding, should it occur, is usually best accomplished with fingertip pressure, then by placement of a thumbtack-like device directly into the sacral bone over the bleeding vessel. This usually results in rapid control of the hemorrhage. It is possible that if there is no direct involve-

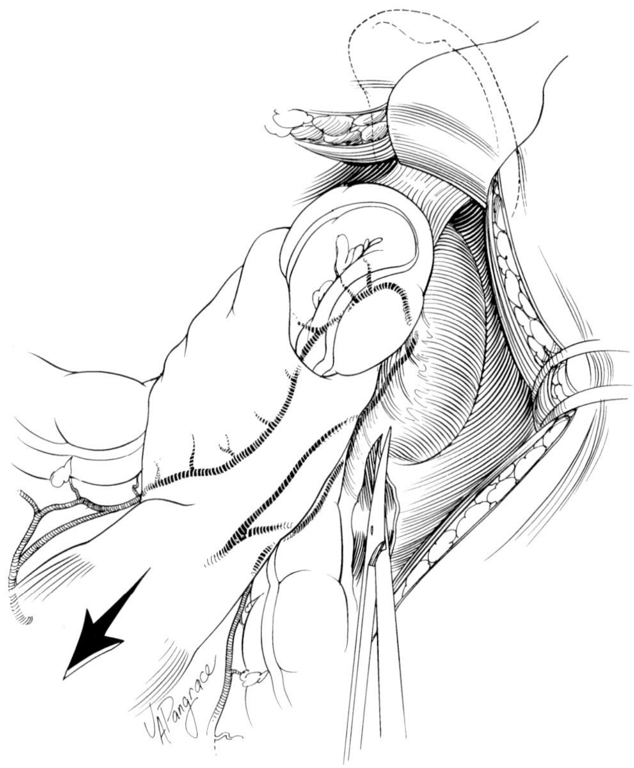

FIG. 60-5. The marginal artery, the lifeline of the left and descending colon, must be protected as the left colonic mesentery is separated from its retroperitoneal attachments.

ment of the tumor posteriorly, the presacral hypogastric nerves may be separated from the fascia propria of the rectum and preserved, because they lie just on top of the presacral fascia. Nerve preservation in the pelvis during rectal cancer surgery is being considered with increasing enthusiasm, and is a focus of interest in several institutions interested in rectal cancer, including ours.

The ligamentous lateral stalks of the rectum are approached after posterior dissection down to the pelvic floor. Lighted, long, narrow pelvic retractors (Brite Trac 10-inch by 1.5-inch blades; Codman, New Brunswick, NY) are of great assistance in supplying traction on the pelvic sidewalls. Electrosurgical dissection is used to divide these nerve-laden structures bilaterally because very few vessels are actually present within them. With a posterior-to-anterior approach, much of the nerve tissue supplying the pelvic organs other than the rectum may be preserved (unless the primary tumor is located at or just adjacent to the lateral stalks). Under direct vision, the lateral stalks must be dissected close to the pelvic sidewall if the tumor is in proximity to them. After adequate dissection bilaterally, the anterior plane is dissected using strong anterior retraction with a narrow retractor, and with equally forceful posterior and upward traction on the rectum (Fig. 60-8). This dissection may be assisted by having a perineal surgeon supply pressure between the ischial tuberosities using a fist or (in women) intravaginally using a sponge stick. The dissection is complete when the anorectal ring is reached (in women) or the caudal portion of the prostate is approached (in men).

Careful bimanual palpation of the pelvic structures by the surgeon may be warranted to define the anterior planes (Fig. 60-9). An anteriorly placed tumor may invade the vagina, the space between the rectum and Denonvillier's fascia, or bladder. These structures must then be considered for en bloc resection.

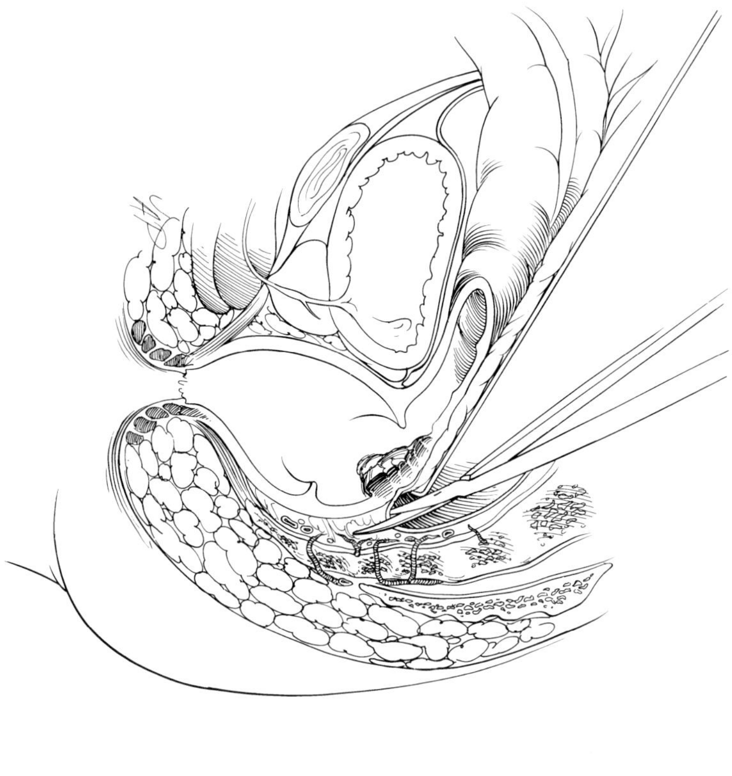

FIG. 60-6. Sharp dissection of the rectum posteriorly, between the fascia propria of the rectum and the presacral fascia, is the best technique to avoid inadvertent entry into the presacral plane with possible injury to presacral vessels. (From Daly JM, Cady B, and Low DW, eds. Atlas of Surgical Oncology, St. Louis: Mosby-Year Book, 1992.)

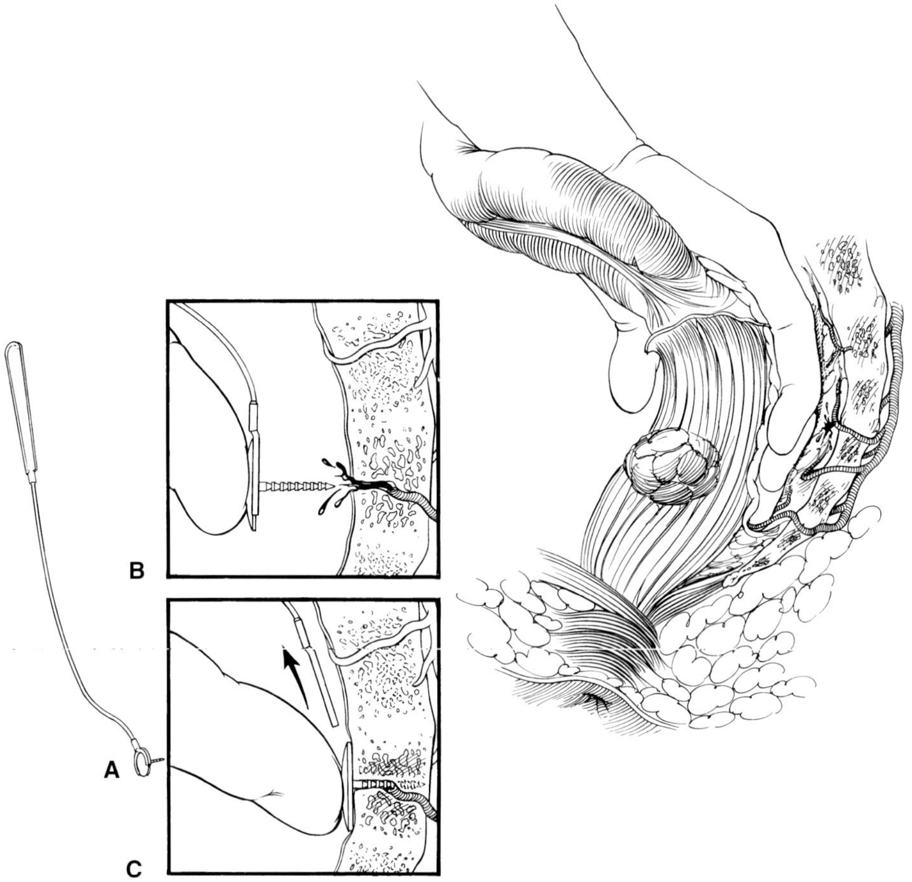

FIG. 60-7. Inadvertent tearing of presacral vessels may occur when blind, blunt dissection of the posterior rectum is performed. **(A)** Should presacral bleeding occur, a thumbtack device mounted on an applicator can be useful to stop the bleeding. **(B)** After locating the precise site of bleeding, the thumbtack device is placed directly over this spot; **(C)** then, the thumbtack is manually driven into the sacral bone. This usually results in immediate and effective hemostasis.

Once the complete, circumferential dissection to the pelvic floor has been attained, carefully avoiding "coning in" on the rectum during dissection (Fig. 60-10), a final decision regarding a sphincter-sparing operation (low anterior resection with circular stapled anastomosis, proctectomy with coloanal anastomosis) versus abdominoperineal excision must be made.

Any evidence for sphincter or pelvic floor involvement of the primary tumor mandates complete proctectomy with permanent

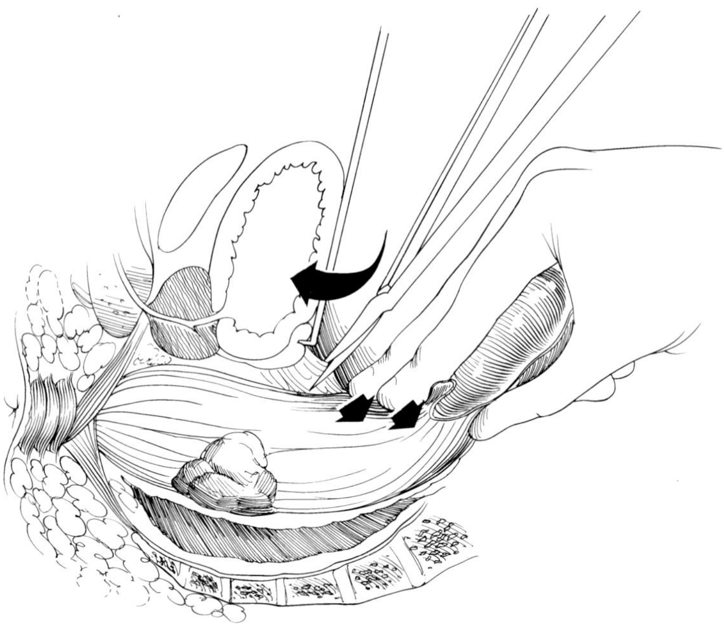

FIG. 60-8. Anterior dissection of the rectum entails adequate posterior retraction of the rectum by the surgeon's nondominant hand, with anterior retraction maintained by a deep pelvic retractor. (From Daly JM, Cady B, and Low DW, eds. Atlas of Surgical Oncology, St. Louis: Mosby-Year Book, 1992.)

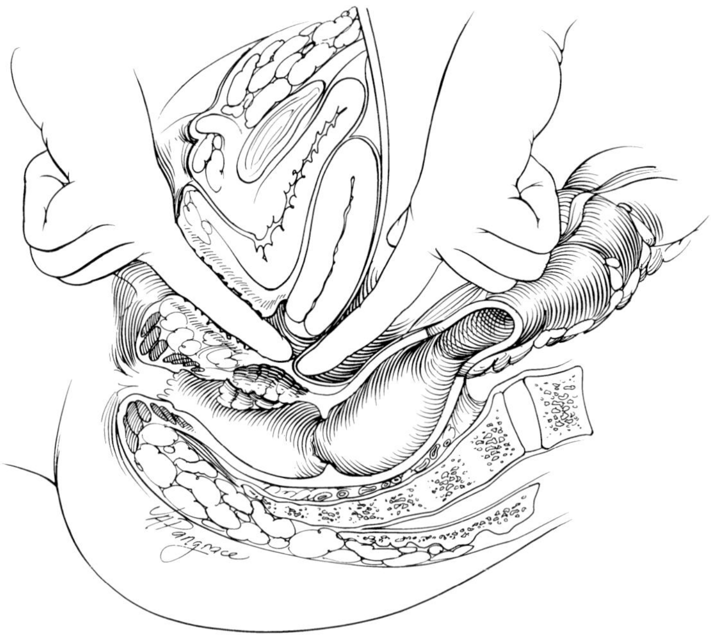

FIG. 60-9. Careful bimanual palpation of pelvic structures may be warranted. The surgeon should place an extra sterile glove or sleeve over the palpating hand, passed transvaginally or transrectally. Proper tissue planes for dissection can be more fully appreciated using this technique. (From Wanebo HJ. Colorectal Cancer, St. Louis: Mosby-Year Book, 1993.)

colostomy (Fig. 60-11). If mobilization has permitted greater than 2 cm of rectal wall clearance between the lower edge of the tumor and the top of the anal sphincters, then it may be reasonable to consider a sphincter-saving operation (Fig. 60-12).

Low Anterior Resection

The low anterior resection is the optimal procedure for tumors lying at or slightly below the peritoneal reflection (the mid-rectum) in a patient with good anal sphincter function and

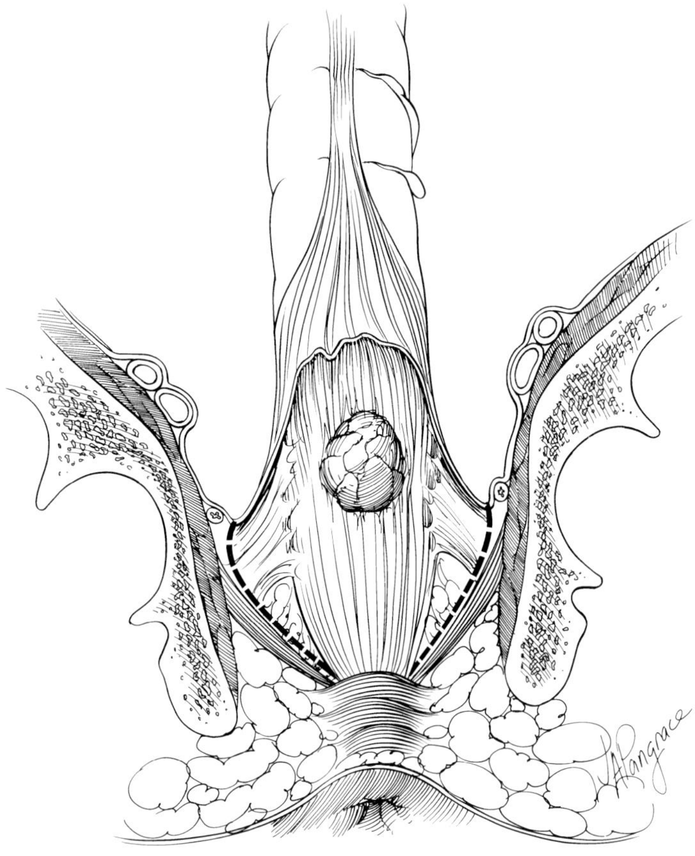

FIG. 60-10. Lateral dissection along the pelvic sidewall entails avoidance of "coning in" on the rectum during pelvic dissection. (From Wanebo HJ. Colorectal Cancer, St. Louis: Mosby-Year Book, 1993.)

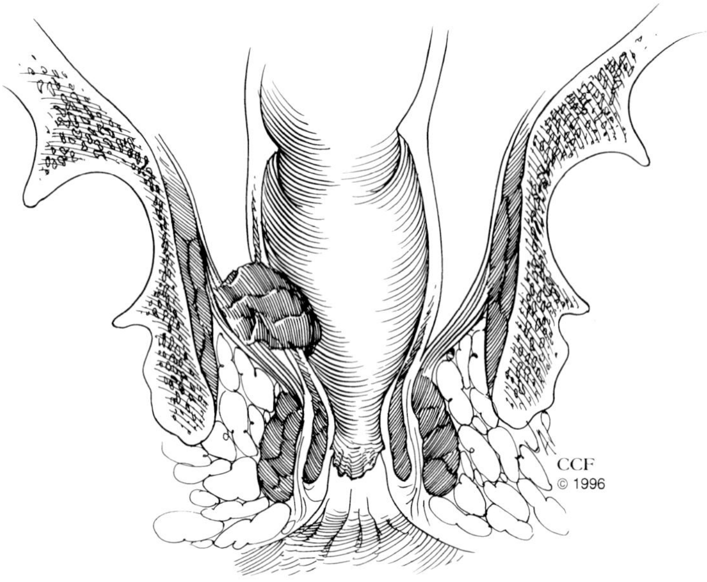

FIG. 60-11. Any contiguous pelvic floor involvement by a rectal cancer, even if it appears to be clear of the anal sphincters, also mandates consideration for complete proctectomy with permanent colostomy.

acceptable operative risk factors. Certain small tumors in the upper portion of the low rectum (3 to 4 cm above the anal sphincters) may also be amenable to this type of operation, but complete circumferential mobilization of the rectum must be achieved. This thorough freeing of the rectum may provide an additional 2 to 3 cm elevation of the tumor above the pelvic floor (Fig. 60-13).

The distal margin of the tumor may be estimated at the time of induction of anesthesia and placement of the patient in the modified lithotomy position, but the final judgment must rest

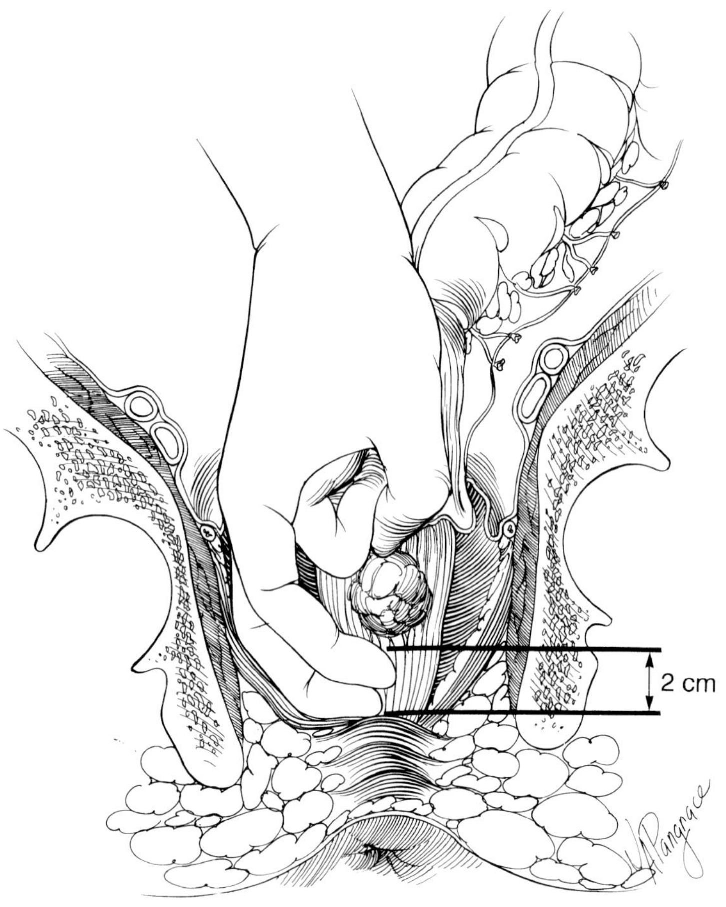

FIG. 60-12. Placing two fingertips below the tumor is a reasonable means to estimate a 2 cm margin of clearance between the lower edge of a rectal cancer and the pelvic floor. (From Wanebo HJ. Colorectal Cancer, St. Louis: Mosby-Year Book, 1993.)

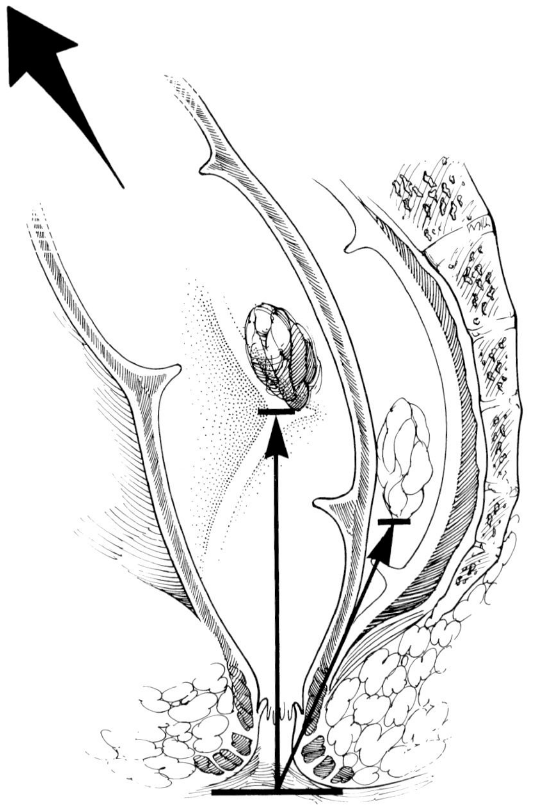

FIG. 60-13. Thorough moblization of the rectum all the way to the pelvic floor may elevate the tumor an additional 2 to 3 cms above the anal sphincters. (From Wanebo HJ. Colorectal Cancer, St. Louis: Mosby-Year Book, 1993.)

after full rectal mobilization, often with the surgeon using bimanual palpation of the tumor to estimate clearance above the pelvic floor. If a 2-cm distal resection margin can be achieved below the tumor, then low anterior resection may be a reasonable option.

Radial Margin

The distal margin of tumor clearance in a radial direction around the tumor is likely to be as important as the distal rectal clearance. Quirke and colleagues were intrigued by the wide variations in local recurrence rates seen after proctectomy for cancer (between 2% and 50%), and systematically analyzed lateral soft tissue spread in 52 rectal cancer patients.[76] There was local recurrence in 12 of 14 patients with histologically positive margins at the lateral resection margins, whereas only 1 of the other 38 patients with negative radial margins manifested any local recurrence. This concept is also likely to be responsible for the low local recurrence rates reported after the ''total mesorectal excision'' concept championed by R. J. Heald.[19,77]

Concept of Distal Rectal Washout

Although there is no definite proof that the rectum should be irrigated with a cytotoxic solution before formation of a distal rectal anastomosis, at our institution we prefer to do this because it is theoretically appealing, inexpensive, and takes relatively little time. To accomplish this, long, narrow pelvic retractors are placed deep in the pelvis anterior to the rectum and a right-angled bowel clamp is placed 2 cm below the cancer and closed. An assistant, working from between the legs, gently places an irrigating syringe transanally and irrigates the rectum thoroughly with a cytotoxic agent (Fig. 60-14). We use 40% ethanol, followed by a saline washout to avoid any risk of igniting the alcohol with electrosurgery. If it is feasible to pass a 30-mm linear stapler below the bowel-occluding clamp, this is done, and a double-stapled anastomosis is performed. If this is not feasible, then the rectum is divided with electrosurgery just below the bowel clamp and a size 0 polypropylene purse-string suture is placed. This is accomplished carefully, using strategically placed long, narrow pelvic retractors and perianal pressure (Fig. 60-15). As the rectum is divided gradually, the leading edge is grasped with a long Babcock clamp so the rectal wall, usually under considerable tension, does not recede from the surgeon's view as the purse-string suture is placed.

After distal rectal management and specimen removal, the proximal colon also is prepared for anastomosis with a similar purse-string suture placement, then the center rod and anvil of the largest possible circular stapler, nearly always a 31-mm one (Premium CEEA; United States Surgical Corp., Norwalk, CT), is placed into the bowel lumen and the purse-string securely tied. The stapler is thoroughly lubricated and gently passed transanally. If any anal stenosis is present, dilation using two fingertips is recommended before trying to pass the instrument. This lessens any risk of rectal injury by forceful dilation of the anal sphincters with the stapler, which can then rapidly ''pop'' through the sphincters and inadvertently tear the rectum. The stapler head is quickly recognized in the rectum by the operating surgeon. Once the top of the remaining rectum is reached by the stapler head, the instrument's wing nut is unscrewed counterclockwise, causing the center shaft to protrude up through the rectum. If the rectum has been closed with a linear stapler, then a sharp spike on the center shaft should protrude through the rectum just adjacent to the staple line (preferably posteriorly). Once the center shaft is fully extended, the plastic spike is removed from the shaft, and the center post protruding from the proximal bowel is securely placed into it (Fig. 60-16). If a purse-string has been placed, this is tied about the center rod, and the two ends of the stapler are joined and the instrument is fully tightened down over the bowel ends using clockwise screwing of the instrument's wing nut. The instrument is fired, and the wing nut is again used to loosen the anvil slightly from the stapler head. The instrument is gently rotated, and removed from the rectum.

Anastomotic integrity is assessed by directly palpating the anastomosis transanally; evaluating the ''completeness'' of each tissue ''donut'' on the stapler center shaft, removed from the rectum and colon anastomotic sites; and direct visualization with the rigid proctoscope, which is also used to insufflate air into the rectum after filling the pelvis with warm saline. The surgeon then looks for air bubbles emanating from the anastomosis. Absence of any air bubbles is reliable in predicting good anastomotic healing, but there is at least a 4% false-negative rate.[86]

If any questions remain about tissue integrity, including concern over irradiated tissue, steroid use, diabetes, excessive intra-

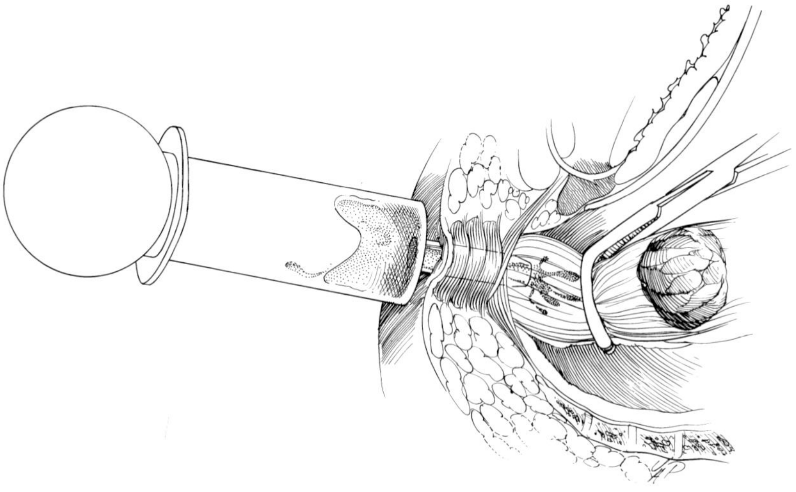

FIG. 60-14. Distal washout of the rectum after complete mobilization entails distal cross-clamping below the tumor with transanal irrigation using an irrigating syringe filled with a cytotoxic agent. This manuever should be done gently to avoid any trauma to the anal sphincters or lower rectum.

operative bleeding, instability of the patient, and so forth, it is wise to consider use of a diverting loop ileostomy placed through the rectus sheath in the right lower quadrant. This can usually be closed in 2 to 3 months after the patient has achieved medical stability and a healed anastomosis.

Coloanal Anastomosis

This technique uses a primary endoanal suturing technique, and has been appropriately termed a ''pull-to'' procedure.[15] When it becomes apparent, after complete rectal mobilization, that adequate distal rectal clearance if not possible without excision of the entire rectum above the pelvic floor, then this procedure is an option.

The perineal phase of this anastomotic technique begins by effacing the anus with six to eight heavy sutures placed at the lower edge of the anal sphincters. An abdominal surgery assistant tucks a laparotomy pad behind the rectum all the way down at the anorectal junction, then the anus and rectum are irrigated with a cytotoxic solution. To minimize bleeding during the transanal dissection, the anal submucosa is infiltrated with an epinephrine-containing solution (at a dilution of 1 : 200,000). Dissection of the mucosa begins at the dentate line and is continued cephalad for 5 to 10 mm (Fig. 60-17). This dissection is then deepened entirely through the muscularis propria into the surrounding perirectal tissues for 1 to 2 cm. This lower rectal segment is then sutured closed with a running absorbable stitch. A cytotoxic solution is again used to irrigate this area, and then dissection is carried further cephalad, circumferentially, until the rectum is entirely disconnected from the pelvic tissues.

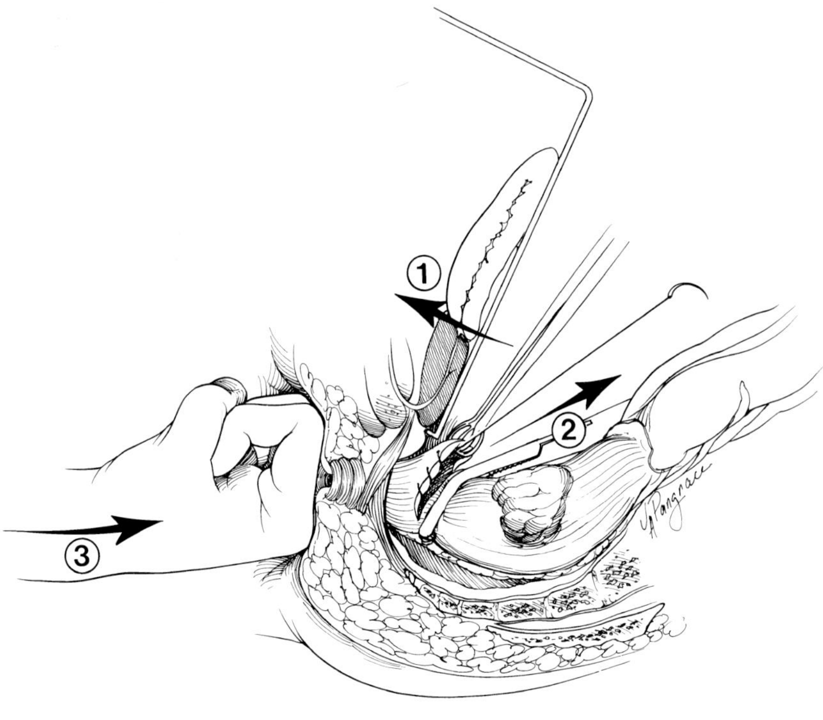

FIG. 60-15. Exposure of the distal rectum for placement of a circumferential purse-string entails: (*1*) anterior retraction with a long narrow instrument; (*2*) gentle cephalad traction on the rectum; and (*3*) perineal pressure with an assistant's fist or fingertips. (From Daly JM, Cady B, and Low DW, eds. Atlas of Surgical Oncology, St. Louis: Mosby-Year Book, 1992.)

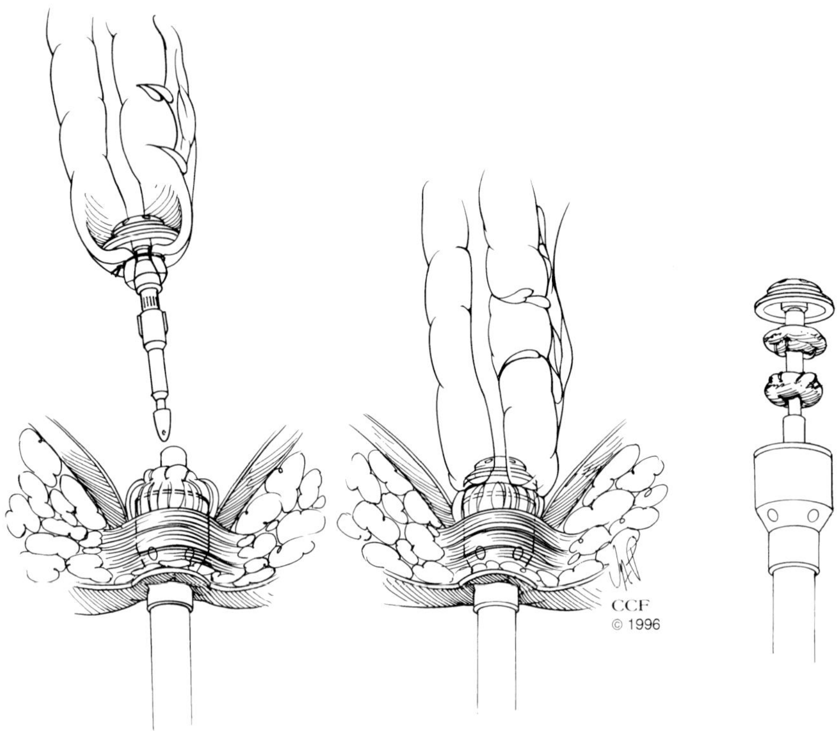

FIG. 60-16. Circular stapled low colorectal anastomosis, after placement of the distal rectal purse-string, entails passage of the protruding center rod from the proximal bowel into the receptacle center post of the transanally placed circular stapler, then careful apposition of the bowel ends by tightening of the wing nut on the circular stapling instrument. Finally, proximal and distal tissue donuts must be checked for completeness after extraction of the circular stapler.

The specimen is removed, the pelvis is irrigated, and a long Babcock clamp is passed transanally up into the pelvis to grasp the end of the mobilized left colon and carefully pull it down into the anal canal. This end of the colon has usually been closed with a linear stapling device; thus, when it presents at the anal orifice, it is opened and sequentially sutured anteriorly, laterally, and posteriorly (Fig. 60-18). Additional sutures are placed so that four or five per quadrant are in place at the completion of the anastomosis (Fig. 60-19). Palpation is used to verify anastomotic integrity, and then the anal retraction sutures are removed and a temporary loop ileostomy is created in the right lower quadrant.

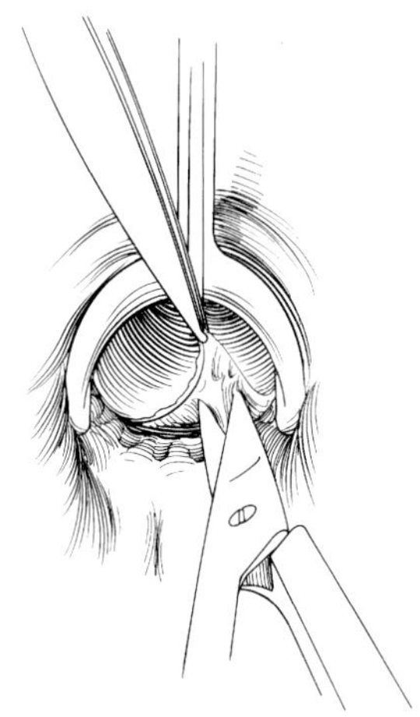

FIG. 60-17. In the performance of coloanal anastomosis, dissection of the distal rectal mucosa begins posteriorly at the dentate line, then continuing cephalad for at least 5 to 10 millimeters. (From Wanebo HJ. Colorectal Cancer, St. Louis: Mosby-Year Book, 1993.)

When is a classically described ''pull-through'' operation performed? These techniques[12–14] are performed in our practice only when there is an urgent need to complete the operation without taking time to create the coloanal anastomosis. The distal rectum is transected by everting the anorectum, then by pulling the specimen (rectum) through the anus. The proximal colon, still attached to the specimen is drawn through the anus so 2 to 3 cm of it protrudes beyond the everted anus. The specimen is transected at this point, the proximal bowel rapidly sutured to the everted anus, and this segment may be further secured with a gauze stent wrapped around the colon.[12,13] Ten or 12 days later, assuming the patient is in a good medical condition, he or she is returned to the operating room and the excess intestine is trimmed and a primary coloanal anastomosis created. The anus either retracts spontaneously, or it may be reduced by gentle massage at the second procedure.

Colonic Reservoir (J-Pouch)

One of the main drawbacks to the very low colorectal or coloanal anastomosis may be a poor functional outcome, with fecal urgency or soilage that may remain for many months or even permanently. These troubling sequelae of the low anastomosis may be caused by the operative anal manipulation, loss of the rectal reservoir capacity, and preoperative radiation therapy. In the late 1980s, a colonic J-shaped reservoir was proposed to ameliorate some of the functional deficiencies of the low anastomosis.[87]

This should be a rapid modification of the coloanal procedure, wherein the distal 6 to 10 cm of the preserved left colon

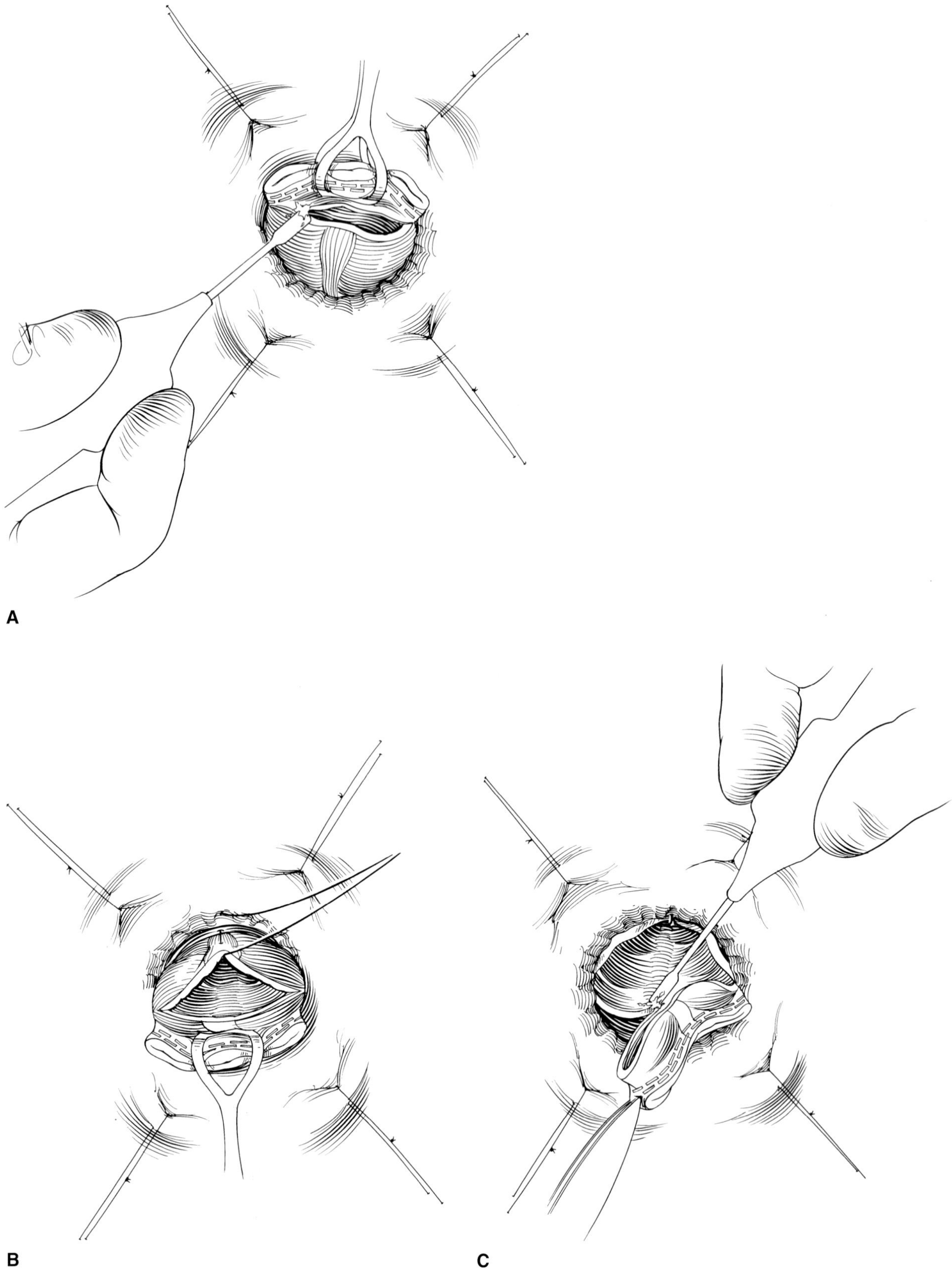

FIG. 60-18. (A) After delivering the closed end of the descending colon transanally using a Babcock clamp passed transanally, the anterior wall of the colon is opened using electrosurgery. **(B)** An anterior suture is placed first; and **(C)** lateral sutures are next placed after complete removal of the stapled end of the colon. (From Wanebo HJ. Colorectal Cancer, St. Louis: Mosby-Year Book, 1993.)

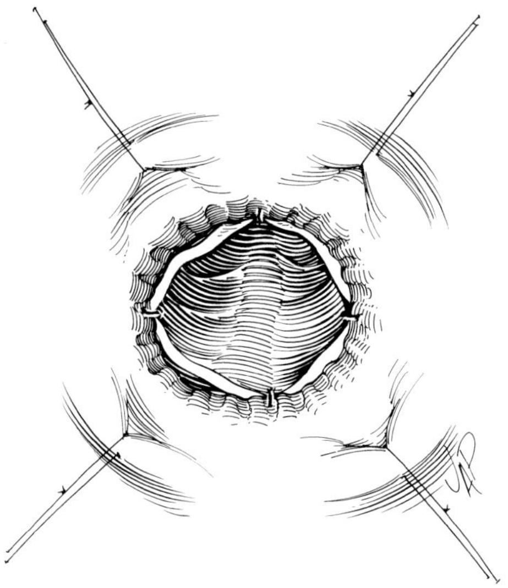

FIG. 60-19. After placement of four quadrant sutures, two or three additional sutures are placed between them to complete the anastomosis. (From Wanebo HJ, Colorectal Cancer, St. Louis, Mosby Year Book, 1993.)

is folded on itself; then a J-pouch is created using a linear cutting stapler (with a length of 6 cm or longer) (Fig. 60-20). The anastomosis is performed either by circular stapler or by hand-sewn technique. This anastomosis should be protected, in nearly all instances, with a diverting loop ileostomy. Anastomosis and pouch integrity are ensured at 2 to 3 months after surgery with a water soluble enema before stoma closure.

Abdominoperineal Resection With Permanent Stoma

When the rectal tumor lies within 2 or 3 cm of the top of the anal sphincters, or in certain circumstances when even a bit higher, abdominoperineal resection with complete circumferential excision of the anal sphincters and wide excision of the pelvic floor musculature should be carried out.

Rectal pedicle dissection, ligation, and mobilization should be identical to that performed for the low anterior resection. The only difference in proximal surgery may be that, because the proximally preserved colon need not be mobilized into the pelvis, complete left colonic mobilization is unnecessary unless the colon otherwise will not reach the anterior abdominal wall for stoma formation.

Thus, after complete circumferential rectal mobilization as in low anterior resection, the surgeon should perform bimanual palpation to ensure that complete mobilization has been performed, then move to the perineal phase. At our institution, we usually take a one-team approach, performing rectal mobilization first, then perineal excision second. In instances when this operation is performed on a high-risk patient and operative time is being kept to a minimum, a combined two-team approach (synchronous abdominal and perineal surgery) is used.

The perineal phase begins with careful positioning of the legs so that the hips are flexed at about 90° relative to the body, with the anus resting at or just below the bottom edge of the operating table.

The anus is sutured closed with a circumferential purse-string suture, and then the perineum is prepared and draped in sterile fashion.

A circumferential elliptical incision is created around the anus, encompassing skin and subcutaneous tissue for at least 2 to 3 cm outside of the anal margin (Fig. 60-21).

The focus of the early dissection should be posterior, then lateral to the anus. Subcutaneous tissue is excised until the pelvic floor is reached, and then the anococcygeal ligament and pelvic floor are incised. Once the pelvic floor is breached in the posterior midline (Fig. 60-22), the surgeon should proceed in a posterior-to-anterior direction through the pelvic floor, using the nondominant hand to retract the anorectum medially while an assistant retracts the perineal tissues laterally.

The anterior phases of the dissection are left until last. Tissue planes anteriorly may be confusing, and (in men) urethral injury especially must be avoided. Often the specimen may be delivered through the dissection onto the perineum while anterior structures remain attached. This usually allows for better visualization of the anterior perineum (Fig. 60-23).

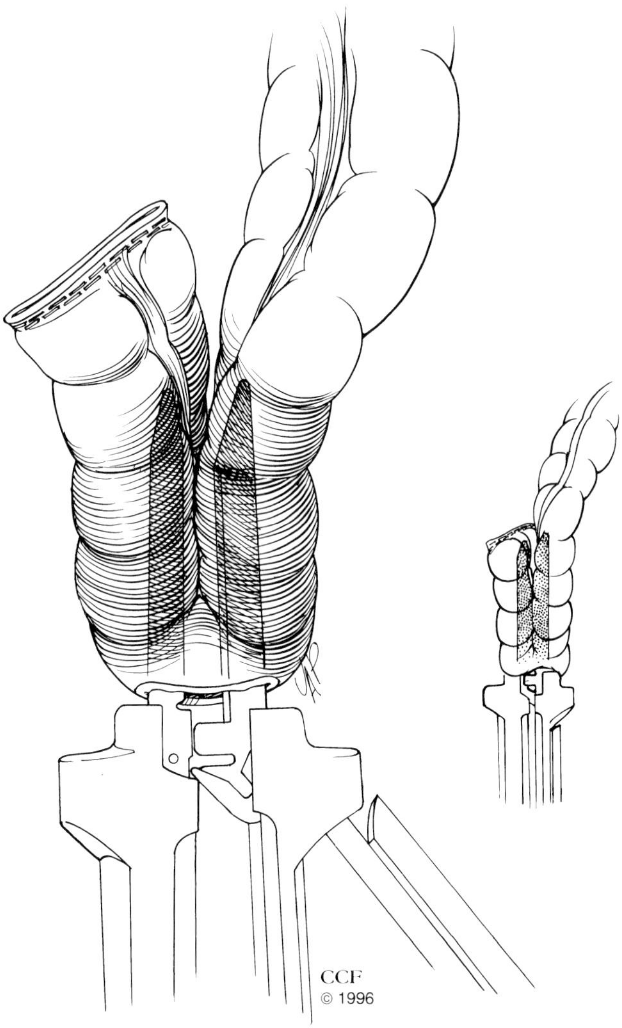

FIG. 60-20. A colonic J-pouch can be created using a GIA-type stapler 6 cm or longer in length, choosing the coloanal anastomotic site on the dependent, antimesenteric portion of the bowel.

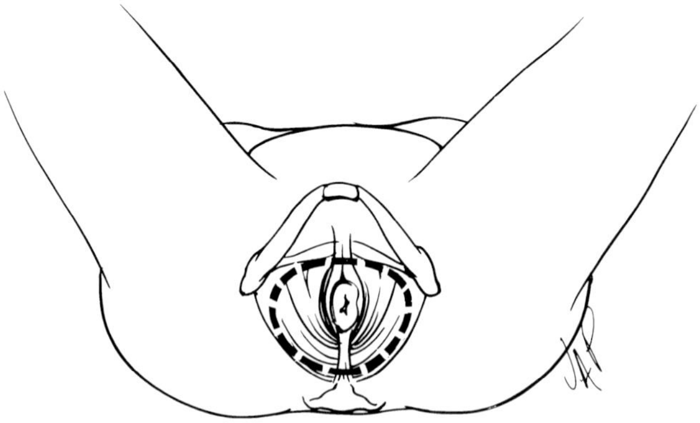

FIG. 60-21. Although incision of the skin and subcutaneous tissues around the anus may only be 2 to 3 cms around the anal orifice, pelvic floor dissection should pass out to nearly the pelvic side walls for most low rectal cancer excisions.

The superficial transverse perineal muscles and the perineal body are transected, then the stout muscular fibers of the pelvic floor (puborectalis) are encountered bilaterally and cut with electrosurgery. Anterior fibers of the pelvic floor muscles and the rectourethralis muscle are next incised, with care taken to observe that in men the prostate lies close underneath (superior to) this muscle. Careful dissection is necessary to avoid inadvertent prostatic/urethral injury or entry into the rectum. Once this plane has been opened, usually all that remains are some fibrous attachments of the rectum to the prostate. These may be incised by carefully palpating above, and by continuing to follow the plane between rectum and prostate (Fig. 60-24). In women, particularly with anteriorly placed tumors, it is reasonable to excise all or part of the posterior vaginal wall to ensure wide excision of the tumor (Fig. 60-25).

Once these steps have been accomplished, the rectum is removed, the pelvis copiously irrigated, and soft tissues of the pelvic floor opposed with interrupted absorbable sutures. If there is sufficient muscle to bring together, then this may be the only layer closed besides the skin. Otherwise, subcutaneous tissues are closed in one layer, then skin sutures are placed. We usually drain the pelvis using a right lower quadrant abdominal drain, allowing for complete perineal closure.

The colostomy is formed by the abdominal team in routine fashion, usually leaving the lateral peritoneal space open because it is quite large and, in our experience, not prone to any clinically important herniations.

OUTCOME AFTER LOW ANTERIOR RESECTION VERSUS ABDOMINOPERINEAL RESECTION

Although the abdominoperineal resection maintains an important place in the surgical management of rectal cancer, most patients with rectal cancer can be treated with sphincter-saving procedures, the low anterior resection being used most commonly. Numerous reports document the trend toward more sphincter-preserving resections.[19,68,88] In one study, the use rate of low anterior resection for treatment of rectal cancer rose from 46% from 1973 to 1978 to 62% from 1979 to 1983.[82]

The shift toward low anterior resection began with Claude Dixon's report from the Mayo Clinic documenting low operative morbidity and mortality with good outcomes after anterior resection for patients with carcinoma of the rectum.[11] However, the major increase in use of low anterior resection came with the introduction and widespread use of the circular stapler for fashioning a safe, reliable, straightforward colorectal anastomosis even in the depths of the pelvis. Technical refinements in pelvic surgery and a better appreciation of the anatomic requirements for a successful oncologic low anterior resection have also contributed. Finally, a better understanding of tumor biology and growth characteristics with regard to patterns of intramural and extramural spread also supported the shift toward the low anterior resection.

There has been reluctance among some surgeons to recommend the widespread use of low anterior resection based on the fear that in preserving the distal rectum, anal canal, and

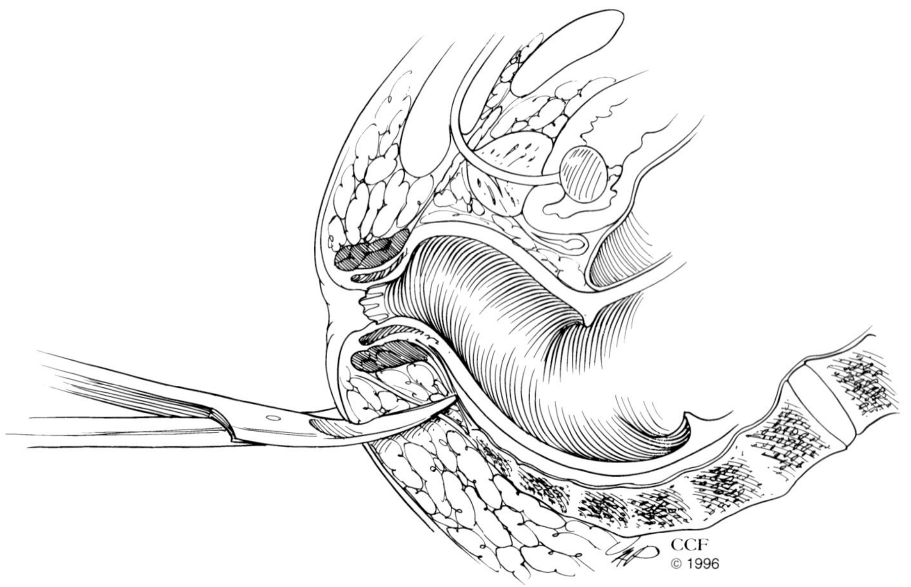

FIG. 60-22. The pelvic floor should initially be breached in the posterior midline, usually with scissor dissection.

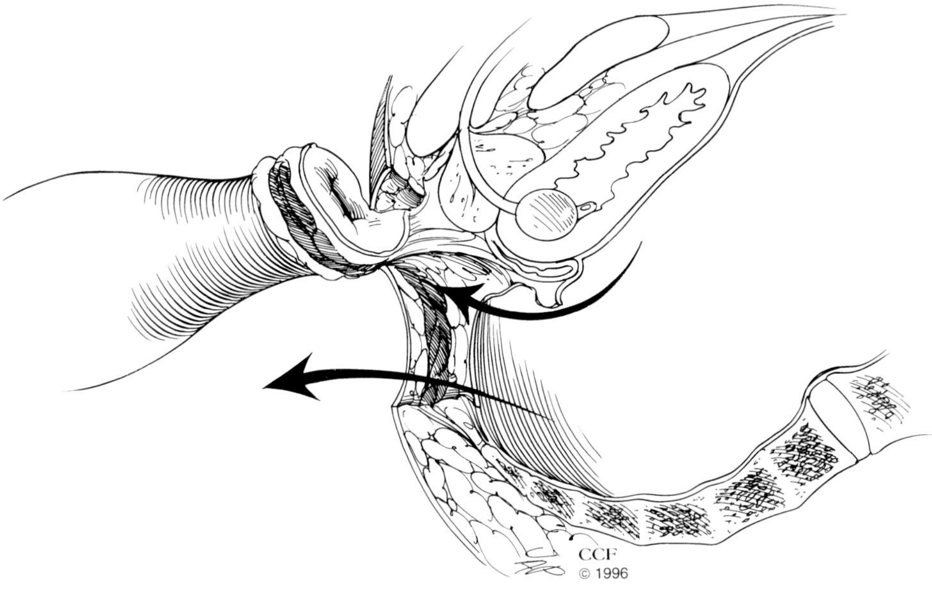

FIG. 60-23. Delivery of the specimen, after dividing the pelvic floor posteriorly and laterally, will usually allow for better visualization of the structures of the anterior perineum.

sphincters, a less-than-adequate oncologic operation is performed. Specifically, there has been a fear that distal and lateral resection margins could be compromised, resulting in high rates of local recurrence and reduced cure rates. In addition, there have been concerns over the functional outcome, especially in the elderly, after a low pelvic anastomosis.

Multiple studies document the fact that distal resection margins of less than 5 cm are adequate, and a 2-cm margin is perfectly reasonable in most situations. Histopathologic studies show that most rectal cancers do not demonstrate distal intramural spread, and retrograde (distal) lymphatic extension is equally rare. When these conditions do exist, the overall prognosis is poor despite the choice of operation. Therefore, in gaining a 5-cm distal margin on a routine basis, many patients lose their sphincters unnecessarily. Actually, the length of the distal resection margin (as long as it is clear of gross disease) does not seem to be a significant factor in predicting local recurrence. Pollett and Nicholls evaluated local recurrence and 5-year survival rates in 334 patients surviving radical restorative operations for rectal adenocarcinoma and found no difference in local recurrence rates or long-term survival based on distal resection margin (<2 cm, 2 to 5 cm, >5 cm).[18] Data from the Large Bowel Cancer Group Project from England showed that differences in local recurrence rates after low anterior resection and abdominoperineal resection were not a result of lesser distal resection margins because the margin of clearance was not different in those who did and did not have a local recurrence, and because for each centimeter of distal clearance there was

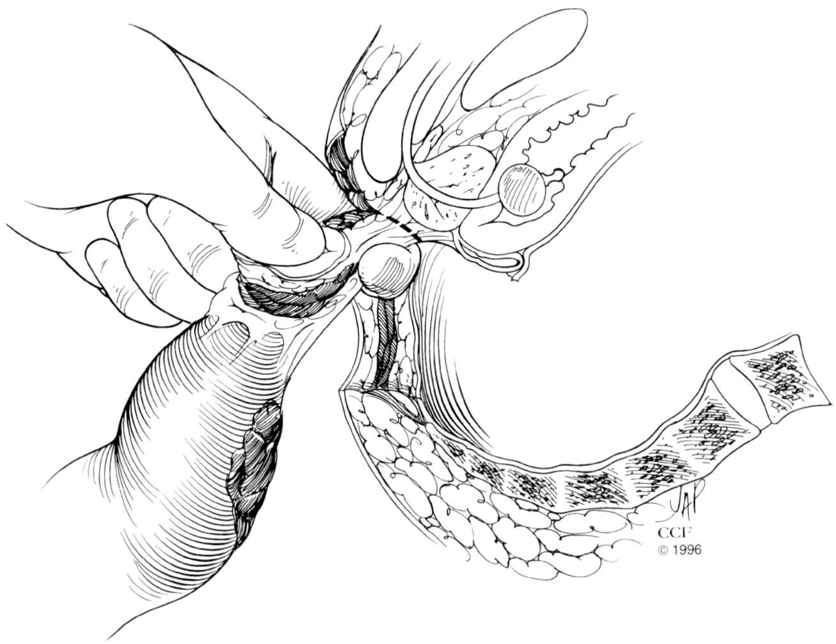

FIG. 60-24. Once the specimen has been delivered posteriorly, anterior structures can then be precisely dissected between the anorectum and the prostate using visualization and palpation.

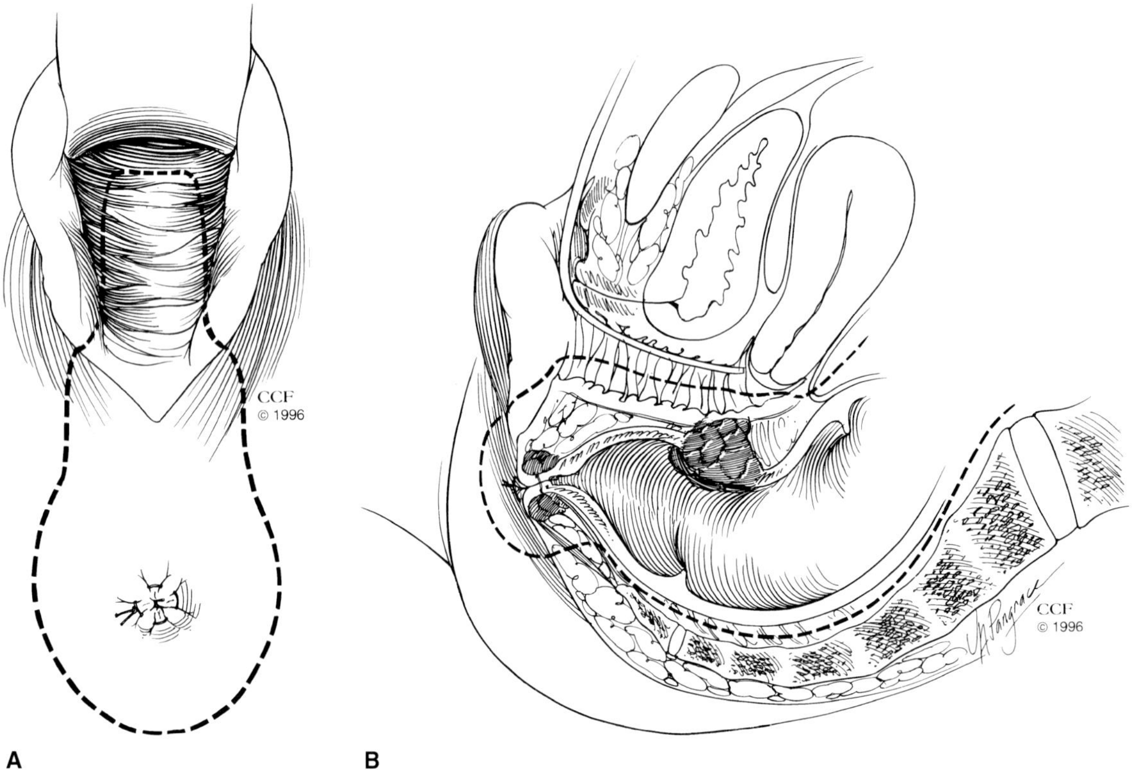

FIG. 60-25. In females with anteriorly placed tumors, it is reasonable to excise nearly all of the posterior vaginal wall in order to insure complete clearance around the tumor. **(A)** Perineal view. **(B)** Mid-saggittal view.

a consistently greater probability of recurrence for anterior resection.[72]

Lateral margins are as important, if not more important, than distal margins. A properly performed low anterior resection should not compromise the lateral margin of clearance. Keeping the dissection on the endopelvic fascia of the pelvis and performing complete mesorectal excision for low tumors should provide margins that are as good as those obtained with abdominoperineal resection. ''Coning down'' must be avoided during both types of procedures. The low anterior resection should not result in a lesser operation if there is meticulous adherence to the standard anatomic principles of oncologic surgery.

Whether a low anterior resection compromises long-term outcome compared with abdominoperineal resection will probably never be addressed in a prospective, randomized trial because of informed consent issues, but there are numerous retrospective and noncontrolled, prospective studies in the literature that address this issue. Williams and colleagues reported no significant difference in local recurrence rates (14% vs. 18%) or 5-year survival when comparing low anterior resection and abdominoperineal resection in 133 patients with rectal tumors located 3 to 12 cm from the anal verge.[67] Heimann and coworkers reported similar rates (16% vs. 17%) of local recurrence in their series of 320 patients undergoing either low anterior resection or abdominoperineal resection for middle and upper rectal tumors.[89] The University of Chicago also reported no difference in local recurrence.[90] Finally, Heald and colleagues reported extremely low rates of local recurrence (<5%) after low anterior resection.[91]

Two large series do, however, show significantly higher recurrence rates after low anterior resection. The National Surgeon's Adjuvant Breast and Bowel Project (NSABP) study[92] documented a local recurrence rate of 13% in 181 patients undergoing low anterior resection and 5% for 232 patients undergoing abdominoperineal resection. Despite this difference, there was no decrease in overall survival after the sphincter-preserving operation (71% vs. 66% 5-year survival for low anterior vs. abdominoperineal resection). Data from the Large Bowel Cancer Project[72] showed that the local recurrence rates after low anterior resection and abdominoperineal resection were 18% and 12%, respectively. No long-term survival data were reported. Operative mortality should not be different between the two operations.

On theoretic grounds, the results of low anterior resection should not be different from abdominoperineal resection if the operation is performed according to accepted principles of rectal cancer surgery: proximal pedicle ligation, wide resection of mesentery and soft tissue, and resection with adequate margins. As the literature is reviewed, it becomes clear that recurrence rates vary widely between surgeons. Heald, an ardent advocate of total mesorectal excision, reports recurrence rates of 5% or less,[91] whereas others report rates ranging from 11% to 56%.[93,94] Surgeon-to-surgeon variability can be explained only on technical grounds, highlighting the importance of surgical technique in achieving good local control.[95–98]

Functional results after low anterior resection are good and the contention that a permanent sigmoid colostomy provides superior functional results for most patients is incorrect in most cases. Several reports have detailed functional results after low anterior resection.[99–101] Almost all patients achieve continence for solid stool, although a few have difficulties with liquid feces or gas.[102–104] There is a period of adaptation that can last as long as 18 months. During this time, stool frequency decreases and control improves. In comparing quality of life after sphincter-preserving surgery and abdominoperineal resection, low anterior resection appeared to cause less social and psychologic trauma than a permanent colostomy.

OUTCOME AFTER COLOANAL ANASTOMOSIS

In the course of resection for low- and mid-level rectal tumors, there comes a point at which the only bowel left distally for anastomosis is that of the anal canal. Anastomosis at this level is referred to as a coloanal anastomosis. In the past, this type of anastomosis was completed by everting the distal rectal segment, or by using one of the pull-through techniques described by Bacon[12] or Turnbull and Cuthbertson.[13] These techniques were cumbersome and associated with poor functional outcomes because of the dissection required to evert the anal canal or the prolonged dilation of the sphincters required by the pull-through.

In 1972, Parks described his transanal technique for low rectal anastomosis, whereby the colon was anastomosed to the anal canal using an anal retractor that obviated the need for rectal eversion or resorting to a pull-through technique.[105] Although initially advocated for benign disease, the technique and its variations have now been adapted for use in malignant disease. This is a natural extension of current enthusiasm for sphincter-saving resections. The appreciation that margins less than 5 cm are acceptable combined with proper technique in completely mobilizing the rectum and its mesentery to the pelvic floor, down into the inlet of the anal sphincter mechanism, have opened the way for these techniques. Also, experience with ileal pouch–anal anastomosis has led to increased appreciation for the technique. There are a variety of methods for achieving a coloanal anastomosis: transanal, transsphincteric, hand-sewn or stapled, straight coloanal, or colonic J-pouch–anal. With all of the techniques, two major issues surround the operation: is the oncologic outcome acceptable in terms of local control and long-term survival, and are the functional results acceptable?

Enker and colleagues reported on 41 patients undergoing coloanal anastomosis with histologically proven invasive adenocarcinoma of the rectum (0 to 11 cm from the anal verge), 37 with curative intent.[106] With an almost equal distribution of Dukes' A, B, and C lesions in their series, they reported that with a median follow-up of 31 months, 30 patients were disease free, 5 were alive with disease, 3 died of disease, 2 died of other causes, and 1 patient underwent an abdominoperineal resection 7 months after the initial operation for a suture line recurrence, and was free of disease 3 years later. Sixty-four percent of the patients had full continence, and in Enker's personal series 86% were fully continent.

Using a synchronous abdominotranssphincteric resection and coloanal anastomosis in 65 patients with low rectal cancer (4 to 9 cm from anal verge), Lazorthes and colleagues[107] reported that in the 29 patients treated for potential cure, 82% were alive without recurrence after 3 years. Local recurrence occurred in four patients (6%). In the 51 patients without postoperative pelvic sepsis or anastomotic leak, 46 of 51 were continent for stool and the remaining 5 complained of only occasional minor soiling.

The Mayo Clinic reported that in 18 patients undergoing operation for rectal adenocarcinoma an average of 8 cm from the anal verge, at mean follow-up of 20 months,[108] 5 patients experienced recurrence of the tumor, 4 had distant recurrence only, and 1 had both local and distant disease. Two patients, both with Dukes' C lesions, had died of disease at the time of follow-up. Functional results were good. Cancer patients had a mean of 2.6 stools per day, and in the series overall, fecal continence was achieved by 84%, with 61% of patients having 3 stools or less per day.

A more recent study from France reported good results in 162 patients undergoing resection for rectal cancers (mean distance from anal margin was 7 cm) treated with proctectomy and colonic pouch–anal anastomosis.[109] The 5-year local recurrence rate was 10%, with an actuarial 5-year survival of 79%. Ninety-six percent had satisfactory continence. A German group reported on 63 patients undergoing coloanal anastomosis for rectal cancer, 57 with curative intent.[110] With a mean follow-up of 6.7 years, the local recurrence rate was 11%, distant recurrence with or without local failure occurred in 33%, and the 5-year survival was 62%. Eighty-five percent of patients had good continence.

The group from Memorial Sloan-Kettering has a large experience with these operations, and in 1994 reported that in 134 patients treated by low anterior resection and coloanal anastomosis, the actuarial 5-year survival was 73%.[111] Among 36 patients who relapsed, distant metastatic disease was present in 86% and pelvic recurrence was detected in only 13 patients, an actuarial rate of 11% at 5 years. Functional results reported elsewhere demonstrated overall function to be excellent in 28%, good in 28%, fair in 32%, and poor in 12%.[112] Median stool frequency was two per day, with 22% of patients reporting four or more stools per day. Fecal continence was complete in 51% of patients, with 21% reporting incontinence to gas only, minor leak in 23%, and significant leak in 5%. Complete evacuation of the neorectum was problematic in 32%.

Overall, a review of the literature shows that sphincter preservation for distal rectal tumors can be accomplished with low anterior resection and coloanal anastomosis with acceptable oncologic and functional outcomes. As in all oncologic resections, it seems that optimal results are obtained with careful patient selection and strict attention to operative detail.

LOCAL RECURRENCE AFTER USE OF THE CIRCULAR STAPLER

A logical concern in the 1980s, when an explosive growth in the use of circular staples for colorectal anastomoses occurred, was whether use of these instruments led to an increase in the local recurrence of rectal cancers. Part of this concern was fueled by the concomitant *decrease* in the frequency of abdominoperineal resections being performed.

Despite the paucity of and difficulty in conducting well constructed studies randomizing between low anterior and abdominoperineal resections for rectal cancer, there simply has been no convincing evidence that use of the circular stapling instrument contributes to an increase in local recurrence (Table 60-1).

There has been an additional concern that use of the circular

TABLE 60-1. *Incidence of local recurrence after abdominoperineal excision compared to low anterior resection (or restorative procedure), primary using a circular stapling instrument*

		No. of cases		Local recurrence (%)	
Authors	Year	APR	LAR	APR	LAR
Morson et al[113]	1963	1596	177	9.7	7.3
Slanetz et al[114]	1972				
Duke's B			25	23	
Duke's C			38	33	
McDermott et al[115]	1982	107	310	17	19
Rich et al[116]	1983	110	28	31	29
Phillips et al[72]	1984	478	370	12	18
Williams and Johnston[117]	1984	83	71	8	11
Williams et al[67]	1985	100	33	19	14
Heimann et al[89]	1986	118	202	17	16
Amato et al[118]	1991	69	78	10	12
Dixon et al[119]	1991	61	150	5	4

stapler to construct a colorectal anastomosis at low anterior resection may lead to an increased risk for local recurrence. Two early series on use of the circular stapler reported local recurrence rates of 28% and 32%.[120,121] It is likely that these high recurrence rates resulted from the very early experience in using the circular stapler, or from its use in very advanced lesions. There has been little or no repetition of such data in later studies. Several clinical studies have reported low recurrence rates after stapled anastomoses, even in those cases with anastomoses performed within several centimeters of the anus.[19,118] In addition, a prospective, multicenter, controlled trial of 294 patients randomized to undergo either a sutured or stapled anastomosis after colorectal cancer excision (with 109 patients undergoing colorectal anastomosis) revealed no difference in local recurrence between sutured versus stapled anastomosis, and an increased cancer-specific mortality rate in the sutured compared with the stapled group.[122]

Thus, as long as the oncologic principles enumerated in this chapter are adhered to, we believe there should be no increase in morbidity or mortality related to use of the circular stapler.

LONG-TERM OVERALL SURVIVAL DATA

The most critical evaluation of success in an operative procedure for cancer must lie in successful long-term survival. Drawing conclusions from the literature may be difficult, for a variety of reasons (different populations, age groups, and staging systems used), but most series have evaluated patients according to tumor stage (using Dukes' classification system), type of operation, and 5-year survival (Table 60-2). Overall survival has been most strongly correlated with tumor stage.[72,130,131]

A detailed discussion of the many other important factors involved in analyzing survival data is beyond the scope of this chapter. Patients undergoing ''curative'' rectal cancer surgery (defined as those patients with no definable residual disease after surgical and histopathologic evaluation) have in general a greater than 50% 5-year survival, with survival rates approaching 80% to 90% if the tumor is confined to the rectal wall.

Another important factor that may potentially have a heavy impact on outcome is the surgeon or institution performing the surgery. The issue of local recurrence according to consultant surgeon performing the operation was raised in 1984 by the British Large Bowel Cancer project[72] and submitted to a multifactorial analysis. After stratification for sex and Dukes' classification, there were persistent and significant differences between individual operators (ranging between 5% or less to 20%).

CONCLUSIONS

The modern development of rectal cancer surgery, barely more than a century old, was initially concerned with radical tumor extirpation combined with attempts to keep operative mortality to a minimum. Function was rationally sacrificed to survival in the earliest surgical endeavors.

Abdominoperineal excision was and is a valued procedure in the treatment of rectal cancer, yet the frequency of its use has diminished markedly with improvements in rectal mobilization, dissection, use of the circular stapler, and in the understanding of pelvic anatomy and pelvic floor function.

TABLE 60-2. *Crude five-year survival after curative rectal cancer surgery*

Authors	No. of cases	Dukes' A (%)	Dukes' B (%)	Dukes' C (%)
Whittaker and Goligher (1976)[123]	407	80	62	33
Patel, et al (1977)[124]	435	65	63	30
Localio, et al (1983)[125]	646	89	57	36
Hojo (1986)[126]	273	93	73	49
Davis, et al (1987)[127]	235	75	55	31
Michelassi, et al (1988)[128]	154	—	60	43
Milsom, et al (1995)[129]	609	85	74	59

Proctosigmoidectomy with sphincter preservation should not be considered a less radical approach to certain rectal cancers that lie 2 to 3 cm (or more) above the top of the anal sphincters. Distal intramural spread of rectal cancers beyond 2 cm occurs only in rare instances.[16]

The functional results after low colorectal anastomosis seem to be highly satisfactory, and there is evidence that new techniques in function preservation are emerging: the colonic J-pouch and pelvic nerve preservation. What role(s) laparoscopic techniques may play in the management of rectal cancer is still uncertain. Certain centers, including ours, are evaluating the use of laparoscopy versus conventional surgery in certain rectal cancers in a prospective, randomized fashion.[132]

The surgeon who chooses to treat rectal cancer patients must be the central coordinator of care for these patients because surgery remains the most potent therapy for nearly all cases of rectal cancers. A detailed understanding of pelvic anatomy, the biologic behavior of these tumors, and appropriate oncologic surgical technique allows for preservation of intestinal continuity in the vast majority of patients.

REFERENCES

1. Wingo PA, Tong T, Bolden S. Cancer statistics 1995. Ca Cancer J Clin 1995;45:8.
2. Lisfranc J. Mémoire sur l'excision de la partie inférieure du rectum devenue carcinomateuse. Mémoires de l'Académie Royale de Médecine, Paris 1833;3:810.
3. Lockhart-Mummery JP. Resection of the rectum for cancer. Lancet 1920;1:20.
4. Gabriel WB: Perineo-abdominal excision of the rectum in one stage. Lancet 1834;2:69.
5. Czerny V. Casuistische Mittheilugen aus der Chirurg Klin zer Heidelberg. Munich: Munch Med Wochenschr 1894;11.
6. Miles WE. A method of performing abdominoperineal excision for carcinoma of the rectum and of the terminal portion of the pelvic colon. Lancet 1908;1:1812.
7. Miles WE. Cancer of the rectum. London: Harrison, 1926.
8. Hartmann H. Chirurgie du rectum. Paris: Masson et cie, 1931.
9. Turner GG, Pounet CA, Lloyd-Davies OV. Discussion on radical excision of carcinoma of rectum with conservation of sphincters. Proc R Soc Med 1948;41:813.
10. Mayo WJ. The radical operation for cancer of the rectum and rectosigmoid. Transactions of the American Surgical Association 1916;34: 261.
11. Dixon CF. Anterior resection for malignant lesions of the upper part of the rectum and lower part of the sigmoid. Ann Surg 1948;128:425.
12. Bacon HE. Evolution of sphincter muscle preservation and reestablishment of continuity in the operative treatment of rectal and sigmoid cancer. Surg Gynecol Obstet 1945;181:113.
13. Turnbull RB, Cuthbertson AM. Abdominorectal pullthrough resection for cancer and for Hirschsprung's disease. Cleveland Clinic Quarterly 1961;28:109.
14. Cutait DE, Figlioni FJ. A new method of colorectal anastomosis is abdominoperineal resection. Dis Colon Rectum 1961;4:335.
15. Parks AG. Benign tumors of the rectum. In: Rob C, Smith R, Morgan CN, eds. Clinical surgery: abdomen and rectum and anus. 2nd ed. London: Butterworths, 1966:541.
16. Goligher JC, Dukes CE, Bussey HJR. Local recurrences after sphincter saving excisions for carcinoma of the rectum and rectosigmoid. Br J Surg 1951;39:119.
17. Williams NS, Dixon MF, Johnston O. Reappraisal of the 5-centimetre rule of distal excision for carcinoma of the rectum: a study of dietary intramural spread and of patients survival. Br J Surg 1983;70:150.
18. Pollett WG, Nicholls RJ. The relationship between the extent of distal clearance and survival and local recurrence rates after curative anterior resection for carcinoma of the rectum. Ann Surg 1983;198:159.
19. Heald RJ, Ryall RDH. Recurrence and survival after total mesorectal excision for rectal cancer. Lancet 1986;1:1479.
20. Beart RW Jr, Kelly KA. Randomized prospective evaluation of the EEA stapler for colorectal anastomosis. Am J Surg 1981;141:143.
21. VanDamme JP, Bonte J. Vascular anatomy in abdominal surgery. New York: Thieme Medical Publishers, 1990:76.
22. Neviloh J, Dordiks H, Dordik M, et al. Changing patterns in the morbidity and mortality of colorectal surgery. Am J Surg 1991;162:83.
23. Floyd CE, Stirling CT, Cohn I Jr. Cancer of the colon, rectum and anus: review of 1687 cases. Ann Surg 1966;163:829.
24. Travieso CR Jr, Knoepp LF Jr, Hanle PH. Multiple adenocarcinomas of the colon and rectum. Dis Colon Rectum 1972;15:1.
25. Brahme F, Ekelund GR, Morden JG, et al. Metachronous colorectal polyps: comparison of development of colorectal polyps and carcinoma in persons with and without histories of polyps. Dis Colon Rectum 1974;17:166.
26. Heald RJ, Bussey HJR. Clinical experiences at St. Mark's Hospital with multiple synchronous cancers of the colon and rectum. Dis Colon Rectum 1975;18:6.
27. Reilly JC, Rusin LC, Theuerkauf FJ Jr. Colonoscopy: its role in cancer of the colon and rectum. Dis Colon Rectum 1982;25:532.
28. Pagana TJ, Ledesmn EJ, Mittlman A, et al. The use of colonoscopy in the study of synchronous colorectal neoplasms. Cancer 1984;53: 356.
29. Langevin JM, Nivatvongs S. The true incidence of synchronous cancer of the large bowel: a prospective study. Am J Surg 1984;147:330.
30. Thorson AG, Christensen MA, Davis SJ. The role of colonoscopy in the assessment of patients with colorectal cancer. Dis Colon Rectum 1986;29:306.
31. Isler JT, Brown PC, Lewis FG, et al. The role of preoperative colonoscopy in colorectal cancer. Dis Colon Rectum 1987;30:435.
32. Barillari P, Ramacciato G, De Angelis R, et al. Effect of preoperative colonoscopy on the incidence of synchronous and metachronous neoplasms. Acta Chir Scand 1990;156:163.
33. Wanebo HJ, Rae B, Pinsky CM, et al. Preoperative carcinoembryonic antigen level as a prognostic indicator in colorectal cancer. N Engl J Med 1978;299:466.
34. Shank B, Dershaw DO, Caravelli J, et al. A prospective study of the accuracy of preoperative computed tomographic staging of patients with biopsy-proven rectal carcinoma. Dis Colon Rectum 1990;33: 285.
35. Adalsteinsson B, Glimelius B, Graffman S, et al. Computed tomography in staging of rectal carcinoma. Acta Radiol Diagn 1985;26:45.
36. Koehler, Fieldberg MAM, van Waes PFG. Preoperative staging of rectal cancer with computerized tomography. Cancer 1984;54:512.
37. Dixon AK, Fry IK, Morson BC, et al. Preoperative computed tomography of carcinoma of the rectum. Br J Radiol 1981;54:655.
38. Butch RJ, Stark DD, Wittenberg J, et al. Staging of rectal cancer by MR and CT. AJR Am J Roentgenol 1986;146:1155.
39. Guinet C, Buy J-N, Ghassain MA, et al. Comparison of magnetic resonance imaging and computed tomography in preoperative staging of rectal cancer. Arch Surg 1990;125:385.
40. Hodgman CG, Mac Carty RL, Wolf BG, et al. Preoperative staging of rectal carcinoma by computed tomography and 0.15T magnetic resonance imaging: preliminary report. Dis Colon Rectum 1986;29: 446.
41. Freemy PC, Marks WM, Ryan J, et al. Colorectal carcinoma evaluation with CT: preoperative staging and detection of postoperative recurrence. Radiology 1986;158:347.
42. Thompson WM, Halvoren RA, Foster WL Jr, et al. Preoperative and postoperative CT staging of rectosigmoid carcinoma. AJR Am J Roentgenol 1986;146:703.
43. Dooms GC, Hricats H, Crooks LE, et al. Magnetic resonance imaging of the lymph nodes: comparison with CT. Radiology 1984;153:719.
44. Zaunhauer W, Hoectel M, Fuchs WA. Computed tomography in carcinoma of the rectum. Gastrointest Radiol 1981;6:79.
45. Reing JW, Dwyer AJ, Miller DL, et al. Liver metastasis detection: comparative sensitivities of MR imaging and CT scanning. Radiology 1987;162:43.
46. Benyon J, Roe AM, Foy DMA, et al. Preoperative staging of local invasion in rectal cancer using endoluminal ultrasound. J R Soc Med 1987;80:23.
47. Orrom WJ, Wong WO, Rothenberger DA, et al. Endorectal ultrasound

in the preoperative staging of rectal tumors: a learning experience. Dis Colon Rectum 1990;33:654.
48. Milsom JW, Lavery IC, Stolfi VM, et al. The expanding utility of endoluminal ultrasonography in the management of rectal cancer. Surgery 1992;112:832.
49. Romano G, de Rora P, Vallone G, et al. Intrarectal ultrasound and computed tomography in the pre- and postoperative assessment of patients with rectal cancer. Br J Surg 1985;72(Suppl):5117.
50. Boscaini M, Masorri L, Moatori A. Transrectal ultra-sonography: three years experience. Int J Colorectal Dis 1986;1:203.
51. Hildebrandt V, Feifel G, Schwarz HP, et al. Endorectal ultrasound: instrumentation and clinical aspects. Int J Colorectal Dis 1986;1:203.
52. Rifkin MD, Wechsler RJ. A comparison of computed tomography and endorectal ultrasound in staging rectal cancer. Int J Colorectal Dis 1986;1:219.
53. Milsom JW, Graffner HO. Intrarectal ultrasonography in rectal cancer staging and in the evaluation of pelvic disease. Ann Surg 1990;212:602.
54. Milsom JW, Czyrko C, Hull TL, et al. Preoperative biopsy of pararectal lymph nodes in rectal cancer using endoluminal ultrasonography. Dis Colon Rectum 1994;37:364.
55. Gordon-Watson C, Dukes C. The treatment of carcinoma of the rectum with radium with an introduction in the spread of cancer of the rectum. Br J Surg 1930;17:643.
56. Moynihan BGA. The surgical treatment of cancer of the sigmoid flexure and rectum. Surg Gynecol Obstet 1908;6:463.
57. Gabriel WB, Dukes C, Bussey HJ. Lymphatic spread of cancer of the rectum. Br J Surg 1935;23:395.
58. Goligher JC. The blood supply of the sigmoid colon and rectum. Br J Surg 1949;37:157.
59. Bacon HF, Dirbas F, Myers TB, et al. Extensive lymphadenectomy and high ligation of the inferior mesenteric artery for carcinoma of the left colon and rectum. Dis Colon Rectum 1958;1:457.
60. Sugarbaker PH, Corlew S. Influence of surgical techniques on survival in patients with colorectal cancer: a review. Dis Colon Rectum 1982;25:545.
61. Grinnel RS, Hint RB. Ligation of the inferior mesenteric artery at the aorta in resection for carcinoma of the sigmoid and rectum. Surg Gynecol Obstet 1952;94:526.
62. Grinnel RS. Results of ligation of inferior mesenteric artery at the aorta in resections of carcinoma of the descending and sigmoid colon and rectum. Surg Gynecol Obstet 1965;120:1031.
63. Pezim ME, Nicholls RJ. Survival after high or low ligation of the inferior mesenteric artery during curative surgery for rectal cancer. Ann Surg 1984;200:729.
64. Surtees P, Ritchie JK, Philips RKS. High versus low ligation of the inferior mesenteric artery in rectal cancer. Br J Surg 1990;77:618.
65. Best RR, Blair JB. Sphincter preserving operations for rectal carcinoma as related to the anatomy of the lymphatics. Ann Surg 1949;128:425.
66. Goligher JC, Dukes CE, Bussey HJR. Local recurrence after sphincter saving excisions for carcinoma of the rectum and rectosigmoid. Br J Surg 1951;39:199.
67. Williams NS, Durdey P, Johnston D. The outcome following sphincter-saving resection and abdomino-perineal resection for low rectal cancer. Br J Surg 1985;72:595.
68. Weese JL, O'Grady MG, Ottery FD. How long is the five centimeter margin? Surg Gynecol Obstet 1986;163:101.
69. Anderberg B, Enhlad P, Sjodahl R, et al. Recurrent rectal carcinoma after anterior resection and rectal stapling. Br J Surg 1983;70:1.
70. Hurst PA, Proust WG, Kelly JM, et al. Local recurrence after low anterior resection using the staple gun. Br J Surg 1982;69:275.
71. Rosen CB, Beart RW, Alstrup DM. Local recurrence of rectal carcinoma after hand sewn and stapled anastomosis. Dis Colon Rectum 1985;28:305.
72. Phillips RKS, Hittinger R, Blesovsky L, Fry JS, Fielding LP. Local recurrence following "curative" surgery for large bowel cancer: II. the rectum and rectosigmoid. Br J Surg 1984;71:17.
73. Pilipshen SJ, Heiliveil M, Quan SHQ, Sternberg SS, Enker WE. Patterns of pelvic recurrence following definitive resections of rectal cancer. Cancer 1984;53:1354.
74. Rao AR, Kazan AR, Chan PM, Gilbert HA, Nusebaum H, Hintz BL. Patterns of recurrence following curative resection alone for adenocarcinoma of the rectum and sigmoid colon. Cancer 1981;48:1492.
75. Case AW, Millior RR, Pfaff WW. Patterns of recurrence following surgery alone for adenocarcinoma of the colon and rectum. Cancer 1976;37:2861.
76. Quirke P, Dundey P, Dixon MF, Williams NW. Local recurrence of rectal adenocarcinoma due to inadequate surgical resection. Lancet 1986;1:996.
77. Heald RJ, Husband EM, Ryall RDH. The mesorectum in rectal cancer surgery: the clue to pelvic recurrence? Br J Surg 1982;69:613.
78. Hojo K, Savada T, Moriya Y. An analysis of survival, voiding and sexual function after wide ileopelvic lymphadenectomy in patients with carcinoma of the rectum, compared with conventional lymphadenectomy. Dis Colon Rectum 1989;32:128.
79. Enker WE, Heiliveil ML, Hertz REL, et al. En bloc pelvic lymphadenectomy and sphincter preservation in the surgical management of rectal cancer. Ann Surg 1986;203:426.
80. Pittman MR, Thornton H, Ellis H. Survival after extended resection for locally advanced carcinomas of the colon and rectum. Ann R Coll Surg Engl 1984;66:81.
81. Orkin BA, Dozois RR, Beart RW, et al. Extended resection for locally advanced primary adenocarcinoma of the rectum. Dis Colon Rectum 1989;32:286.
82. Boey J, Wong J. Pelvic exenteration for locally advanced colorectal carcinoma. Ann Surg 1982;195:513.
83. Bonfanti G, Bozzetti F, Fori R, et al. Results of extended surgery for cancer of the rectum and sigmoid. Br J Surg 1982;69:305.
84. Wanebo HJ, Gaber DL, Whitehall R, Morgan RF, Constable WC. Pelvic recurrence of rectal cancer: options for curative resection. Ann Surg 1987;205:482.
85. Sugarbaker PH. Partial sacrectomy for en bloc excision of rectal cancer with posterior fixation. Dis Colon Rectum 1982;26:208.
86. Beard JD, Nicholson ML, Sayers RD, Lloyd D, Everson NW. The intraoperative air testing of colorectal anastomoses: a prospective randomized trial. Br J Surg 1990;77:1095.
87. Lazorthes F, Fages P, Chiotasso P, Lemozy J, Bloom E. Resection of the rectum with construction of a colonic reservoir and coloanal anastomosis for carcinoma of the rectum. Br J Surg 1976;73:136.
88. Lockhart-Mummery HE, Ritchie JK, Hawley PR. The results of surgical treatment for carcinoma of the rectum at St. Mark's Hospital from 1948 to 1972. Br J Surg 1976;63:673.
89. Heimann TM, Szporn A, Bolnick K, Aufses Jr AH. Local recurrence following surgical treatment of rectal cancer: comparison of anterior and abdominoperineal resection. Dis Colon Rectum 1986;29:862.
90. Michelassi F, Vannucci L, Ayala JJ, et al. Local recurrence after curative resection of colorectal adenocarcinoma. Surgery 1990;108:787.
91. Mac Farlane JK, Ryall RDH, Heald RJ. Mesorectal excision for rectal cancer. Lancet 1993;341:457.
92. Wolmark N, Fisher B. An analysis of survival and treatment failure following abdominoperineal and sphincter-saving resection in Dukes' B and C rectal carcinoma. Ann Surg 1986;204:480.
93. Williams NS, Johnston D. Survival and recurrence after sphincter saving resection and abdominoperineal resection for carcinoma of the middle third of the rectum. Br J Surg 1984;71:278.
94. Floyd CE, Corley RG, Cohn I. Local recurrence of carcinoma of the colon and rectum. Am J Surg 1965;109:153.
95. Phillips RKS, Hittinger R, Blesovsky L, et al. Local recurrence following "curative" surgery for large bowel cancer: I. the overall picture. Br J Surg 1984;71:12.
96. Fielding LP. Surgeon-related variability in the outcome of cancer surgery. J Clin Gastroenterol 1988;10:130.
97. Mc Ardle CS, Hole D, Hansell D, et al. Preoperative study of colorectal cancer in the West of Scotland: 10-year follow-up. Br J Surg 1990;77:280.
98. Mc Ardle CS, Hole D. Import of variability among surgeons on postoperative morbidity and mortality and ultimate survival. Br Med J 1991;302:1501.
99. Williams NS, Johnston D. The quality of life after rectal excision for low rectal cancer. Br J Surg 1983;70:460.
100. Prupe-Phillips W. Follow-up study of patients with colostomies. Am J Surg 1971;122:27.
101. Devlin HB, Plant JA, Griffith M. Aftermath of surgery for anorectal cancer. Br Med J 1971;3:413.
102. Cade D, Gallagher P, Schofield PF, Turner L. Complications of ante-

rior resection of the rectum using the EEA stapling device. Br J Surg 1981;68:339.
103. Heald RJ. Towards fewer colostomies: the import of circular stapling device on the surgery of rectal cancer in a district hospital. Br J Surg 1980;60:198.
104. Parks AG, Percy JP. Resection and sutured colo-anal anastomosis for rectal carcinoma. Br J Surg 1982;69:301.
105. Parks AG. Transanal technique in low rectal anastomosis. Proc R Soc Med 1972;65:47.
106. Enker WE, Stearns MW Jr, Janov AJ. Perianal coloanal anastomosis following low anterior resection for rectal carcinoma. Dis Colon Rectum 1985;8:576.
107. Lazorthes F, Fages P, Chicotasso P, Bugat R. Synchronous abdominotransphincteric resection of low rectal cancer: new techniques for direct colo-anal anastomosis. Br J Surg 1986;73:573.
108. Drake DB, Pemberton JH, Beart RW, et al. Coloanal anastomosis in the management of benign and malignant rectal disease. Ann Surg 1987;206:600.
109. Berger A, Tiret E, Parc R, et al. Excision of the rectum with colonic J-pouch anal anastomosis for adenocarcinoma of the low and mid rectum. World J Surg 1992;16:470.
110. Braun J, Treutner KH, Winkeltan G, et al. Results of intersphincteric resection of the rectum with direct coloanal anastomosis for rectal carcinoma. Am J Surg 1992;63:407.
111. Poty PB, Enker WE, Cohen AM, Lammers GY. Treatment of rectal cancer by low anterior resection with coloanal anastomosis. Ann Surg 1994;219: 365.
112. Poty PB, Enker WE, Cohen AM, et al. Long-term functional results of coloanal anastomosis for rectal cancer. Am J Surg 1994;167:90.
113. Morson BC, Vaughn EG, Bussey HJR. Pelvic recurrence after excision of rectum for carcinoma. Br Med J 1963;2:13.
114. Slanetz CA, Herter FP, Grinnell RS. Anterior resection versus abdominoperineal resection for cancer of the rectum and rectosigmoid: an analysis of 524 cases. Am J Surg 1972;123:110.
115. McDermott F, Hughes E, Pihl E, Milne J, Price A. Long term results of restorative resection and total excision for carcinoma of the middle third of the rectum. Surg Gynecol Obstet 1982;154:833.
116. Rich T, Gunderson L, Lew R, Galdibini JJ, Cohen AM, Donaldson G. Patterns of recurrence of rectal cancer after potentially curative surgery. Cancer 1983;52:1317.
117. Williams NS, Johnston D. Survival and recurrence after sphincter saving resection and abdominoperineal resection for carcinoma of the middle third of the rectum. Br J Surg 1984;71:278.
118. Amato A, Pescatori M, Butti A. Local recurrence following abdominal/perineal excision and anterior resection for rectal carcinoma. Dis Colon Rectum 1991;34:317.
119. Dixon AR, Maxwell WA, Thornton Holmes J. Carcinoma of the rectum: a 10-year experience. Br J Surg 1991;78:308.
120. Reid JD, Robins RE, Atkinson KG. Pelvic recurrence after anterior resection and EEA stapling anastomosis for potentially curable carcinoma of the rectum. Am J Surg 1984;147:629.
121. Hurst PA, Prout WG, Kelly JM, Bannister JJ, Walker RT. Local recurrence after low anterior resection using the staple gun. Br J Surg 1982; 69:275.
122. Akyol AM, McGregor JR, Galloway DJ, Murray G, George WD. Recurrence of colorectal cancer after sutured and stapled large bowel anastomosis. Br J Surg 991;78:1297.
123. Whitaker M, Goligher JC. The prognosis after surgical treatment for carcinoma of the rectum. Br J Surg 1976;63:673.
124. Patel SC, Towen EB, Langer B. Twenty-five years of experience with radical surgical treatment of carcinoma of the extra peritoneal rectum. Surgery 1977;82:460.
125. Localio SA, Eng K, Coopa GE. Abdominal resection for mid rectal cancer: a 15 year experience. Ann Surg 1983;198:320.
126. Hojo K. Anastomotic recurrence after sphincter saving resection for rectal cancer: length of distal clearance of the bowel. Dis Colon Rectum 1986;29:11.
127. Davis NE, Evans EB, Cohen JR, et al. Colorectal cancer: a large unselected Australian series. Aust N Z J Surg 1987;57:153.
128. Michelassi F, Block GE, Vanucci L, et al. A 5 to 21 year follow-up and analysis of 250 patients with rectal adenocarcinoma. Ann Surg 1988;208:379.
129. Milsom JW, Kitago K, Böhm B, Lavery IC, Church JM, Fazio VW. Recurrence and survival after curative colorectal cancer surgery: Cleveland Clinic experience. (Research study in progress).
130. Phillips RKS, Fry JS, Hittinger R. Prediction of outcome after curative resection for large bowel cancer. Lancet 1986;2:904.
131. Hermanek P. Colorectal carcinoma: histopathological diagnosis and staging. Baillieres Clin Gastroenterol 1989;3:511.
132. Milsom JW, Böhm B, Hammerhofer KA, et al. Laparoscopic versus conventional oncologic resection in colorectal cancers: a prospective randomized study. Research Procedures Committee #4237, Cleveland Clinic Foundation. (Trial in progress).

Surgery for Gastrointestinal Cancer: A Multidisciplinary Approach, edited by Harold J. Wanebo.
Lippincott-Raven Publishers, Philadelphia, © 1997.

CHAPTER 61

Abdominopelvic Lymphadenectomy With Autonomic Nerve Preservation for Carcinoma of the Rectum: Japanese Experience

Takayuki Akasu and Yoshihiro Moriya

In the 1950s, abdominopelvic lymph node dissection (APLD) for rectal cancer was first advocated by Deddish[1] and Sauer and Bacon[2] to reduce the local recurrence rate and improve the survival rate. They reported 5%[3] to 8%[4] improvement in 5-year survival rates for the patients with APLD compared with patients who underwent conventional resection. However, the improvement was not statistically significant; moreover, resulting urinary and sexual dysfunctions were severe.[4] Similar disappointing results were reported for following years.[5] Thus, APLD was abandoned except in a few institutions,[6,7] and instead of APLD, adjuvant radiation therapy and chemoradiation therapy have been investigated intensively.[8,9] In addition, new surgical approaches such as total mesorectal excision[10] and autonomic nerve-preserving pelvic sidewall dissection[11] have been practiced.

In Japan, in the 1970s, the authors began to use APLD and modify it (extended abdominopelvic lymphadenectomy [EAPL]).[12–14] The modification includes more complete pelvic lymphadenectomy[11,13] and combined resection of the internal iliac artery and vein (IIAV).[13–15] These operations resulted in significant improvement in survival.[13,15] In addition, to deal with urinary and sexual dysfunction, abdominopelvic lymphadenectomy with autonomic nerve preservation (APLANP) was created in the 1980s.[12,16]

In this chapter, the techniques of APLANP are presented and its results are reviewed.

PATIENTS AND METHODS

Between 1980 and 1992, 663 patients with invasive rectal adenocarcinoma located below the lower edge of the second sacral bone underwent surgical resection at the National Cancer Center Hospital in Japan. Of these, 276 patients (42%) underwent APLANP with curative intent, 272 (41%) underwent curative EAPL without nerve preservation, and 115 (17%) underwent palliative surgery due to distant metastasis, peritoneal dissemination, paraaortic lymph node metastasis, or positive surgical margins. In this study, medical records of 276 patients with APLANP were reviewed. There were 175 men (63%) and 101 women (37%), with a median age of 60 years (range, 34 to 92 years). Pathologic TNM stages[17] of these patients are shown in Table 61-1. The location of the tumor was at or below the peritoneal reflection (Rb) in 208 patients (75%) and above the peritoneal reflection (Ra) in 68 patients (25%). No patient underwent adjuvant radiation therapy.

All of the patients were closely followed in the outpatient clinic and were periodically examined for recurrence. Survival and disease-free survival distributions were estimated using the Kaplan-Meier product-limit method. Urinary function and sexual function were studied by interviewing the patients. Erectile function of male patients was evaluated by measuring nocturnal penile tumescence[18] with the Rigiscan device (Dacomed Corp., Minneapolis, MN).

Classification of Extent of Lymph Node Dissection

Figure 61-1 summarizes our classification of the extent of lymph node dissection. Abdominopelvic lymphadenectomy consists of upward dissection (UD) and lateral dissection (LD).

Upward dissection is classified into resection of the mesorectum (UD1), division of the inferior mesenteric artery just below the left colic artery and lymph node dissection below it (UD2), division of the root of the inferior mesenteric artery and lymph node dissection below it (UD3), and paraaortic lymph node dissection (extended upward dissection; UD4).

Lateral dissection is classified into mesorectal excision

Takayuki Akasu: Staff Surgeon, Department of Surgery, National Cancer Center Hospital, 1-1, Tsukiji 5-Chome, Chuo-Ku, Tokyo 104, Japan
Yoshihiro Moriya: Head, Department of Surgery, National Cancer Center Hospital, 1-1, Tsukiji 5-Chome, Chuo-Ku, Tokyo 104, Japan

TABLE 61-1. *Pathologic TNM stage and type of autonomic nerve preservation and lymph node dissection actually performed*

pTNM stage	No. of patients	Type of nerve preservation* NP1	NP2	NP3	With extended lateral dissection
Stage I	99	67	24	8	18 (18%)
Stage II	63	18	26	19	31 (49%)
Stage III	114	33	43	38	62 (54%)
Total	276	118	93	65	111 (40%)
With extended lateral dissection		13 (11%)	40 (43%)	58 (89%)	

* See text for explanation of nerve preservation procedures.

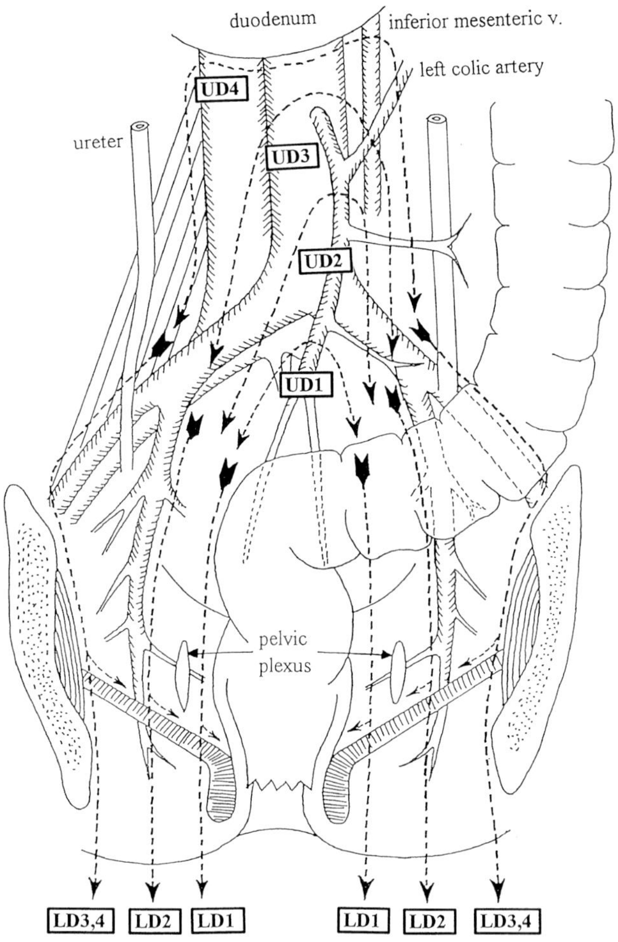

FIG. 61-1. Classification of the extent of abdominopelvic lymphadenectomy, which consists of upward dissection (UD) and lateral dissection (LD). *UD1*, resection of the mesorectum; *UD2*, division of the inferior mesenteric artery just below the left colic artery and lymph node dissection below it; *UD3*, division of the root of the inferior mesenteric artery and lymph node dissection below it; *UD4*, paraaortic lymph node dissection (extended upward dissection); *LD1*, mesorectal excision; *LD2*, dissection along the internal iliac artery and vein (IIAV); *LD3*, complete pelvic lymph node dissection, which includes complete clearance of the obturator space and skeletonization of the IIAV and its branches (extended lateral dissection); *LD4*, complete pelvic lymphatic clearance with combined resection of the IIAV.

(LD1), dissection along the IIAV (LD2), complete pelvic lymph node dissection including complete clearance of the obturator space and skeletonization of the IIAV and its branches (extended lateral dissection) (LD3), and complete pelvic lymphatic clearance with combined resection of the IIAV (LD4).

Classification of Autonomic Nerve Preservation

A schema of the pelvic autonomic nervous system is shown in Figure 61-2. Figure 61-3 summarizes our classification of pelvic autonomic nerve preservation. There are four major categories, including complete autonomic nerve preservation (NP1), preservation of the bilateral pelvic plexus (NP2), preservation of the unilateral pelvic plexus (NP3), and complete resection of the autonomic nerve (NP4). NP2 and NP3 are subdivided into NP2a and NP2b, and NP3a and NP3b, respectively, where "a" corresponds to complete preservation of each pelvic plexus, and "b" corresponds to preservation of the lower part of each pelvic plexus.

Preoperative and Intraoperative Staging and Choice of Surgery

Each patient was initially evaluated by digital examination. More recently, transrectal ultrasonography has been used for initial evaluation. When invasion through the muscularis propria or lymph node involvement was suspected, the patient was further examined with computed tomography or magnetic resonance imaging. T-stage and involvement of regional lymph nodes were accurately evaluated with transrectal ultrasonography. Other organ invasion and lateral pelvic lymph node involvement were more accurately diagnosed with computed tomography and magnetic resonance imaging.

Extent of dissection and nerve preservation were determined by both preoperative and intraoperative evaluation of tumor stage and location. Preoperative and intraoperative staging and type of surgery are summarized in Table 61-2. In the case of Rb tumors, the distal clearance margin was usually more than 2 cm from the anal edge of the tumor. In the case of Ra tumors, the distal clearance margin was usually more than 4 cm from the anal edge of the tumor.

When preoperative and intraoperative evaluation revealed TNM stage I[17] tumor, mesorectal excision with complete autonomic nerve preservation (LD1 + NP1) was performed. The

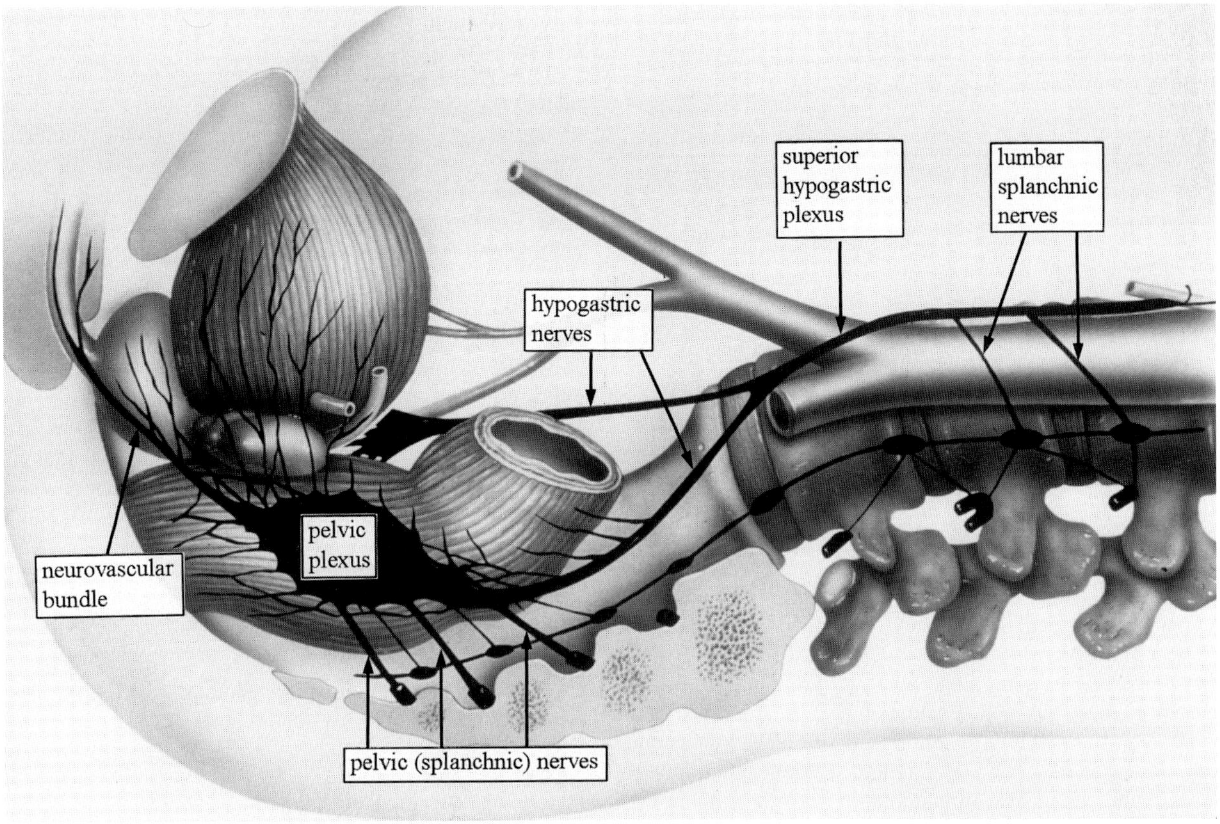

FIG. 61-2. Schema of the pelvic autonomic nervous system.

extent of upward dissection was determined by the location and T-stage of the tumor.

Stage II tumor was treated with extended lateral dissection (LD3) and bilateral or unilateral pelvic plexus preservation (NP2 to NP3). The level of upward dissection was determined according to the location and extent of the tumor (UD3 to UD4). In the case of Ra tumor, bilateral pelvic plexuses were preserved.

Stage III tumor was treated with extended lateral dissection (LD3) or combined resection of the IIAV (LD4) according to the extent of the involved lymph nodes. Nerve preservation and upward dissection were determined according to the location and extent of the tumor (NP2 to NP4, UD3 to UD4). In the case of Ra tumor, bilateral pelvic plexuses were preserved.

When computed tomography or magnetic resonance imaging examination or intraoperative palpation of the IIAV and obtura-

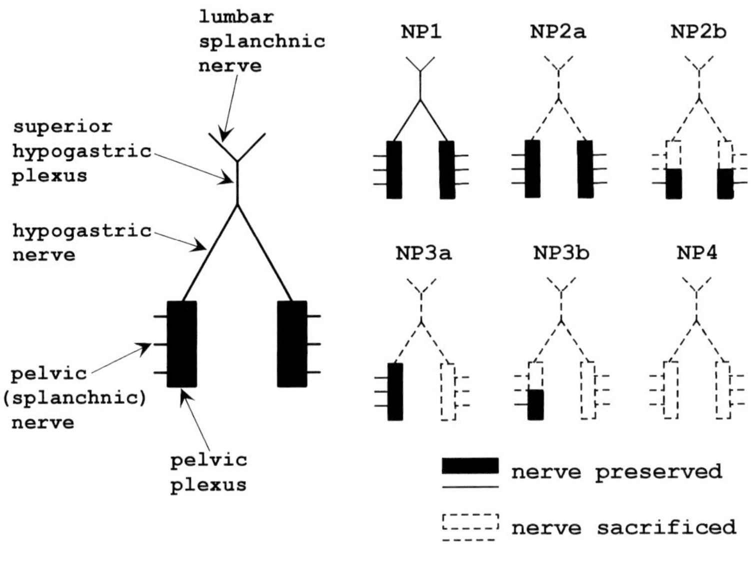

FIG. 61-3. Classification of pelvic autonomic nerve preservation. *NP1*, complete autonomic nerve preservation; *NP2*, preservation of the bilateral pelvic plexus; *NP3*, preservation of the unilateral pelvic plexus; *NP4*, complete resection of the autonomic nerve; *a*, complete preservation of each pelvic plexus; *b*, preservation of the lower part of each pelvic plexus.

TABLE 61-2. *Preoperative and intraoperative staging and type of surgery**

Preoperative and intraoperative TNM stage	Nerve preservation	Lateral dissection	Upward dissection
Stage I	NP1	LD1	UD1–3
Stage II	NP2–3	LD3	UD3–4
Stage III	NP2–4	LD3–4	UD3–4
Lateral node positive	NP3–4	LD4	UD4

* See text for explanation of types of surgery.

tor space revealed lymph node involvement along the IIAV or in the obturator space, the IIAV of the affected side were resected and complete en bloc lateral pelvic dissection was performed (LD4). In this case, the pelvic plexuses were preserved unilaterally or removed completely (NP3 or NP4).

In addition to the location and extent of the tumor, age, risk, gender, and histopathologic diagnosis of the tumor affected the type of surgery. In general, patients older than 80 years of age or poor-risk patients did not undergo EAPL. In female patients, preservation of the superior hypogastric plexus and hypogastric nerves was not considered because removal of those nerves did not influence subsequent sexual and urinary function. In cases of poorly differentiated adenocarcinoma, signet ring cell carcinoma, carcinoma with marked lymphatic infiltration, or scirrhous carcinoma, more radical dissection was performed.

Details of Operative Procedures

Paraaortic Lymph Node Dissection (Extended Upward Dissection, UD4)

The patient is placed in a moderate Trendelenburg position with flexed and abducted thighs and flexed knees. A long median incision is made to ensure wide visualization of both the abdominal and pelvic cavities. The entire abdomen is explored thoroughly to confirm the absence of peritoneal dissemination, liver metastasis, and involvement of paraaortic lymph nodes above the third portion of the duodenum.

The dissection starts with mobilization of the mesosigmoid. After the mesosigmoid is fully mobilized and retracted to the right, the left ureter and testicular (or ovarian) vessels are retracted laterally. There are several small arteries from the aorta to the ureter (ureteric arteries). They are tied and cut. Loose connective tissues between the aorta and the ureter is dissected until the left psoas muscle is exposed.

Retracting the mesosigmoid to the left, the peritoneum of the right side of the root of the mesosigmoid is cut. Again, the right ureter and testicular (or ovarian) vessels are retracted laterally, the ureteric arteries are cut, and the right psoas muscle is exposed. After the right wall of the vena cava is identified, dissection of the lymphatic and adipose tissues surrounding the vena cava is started from the right edge to the left. The lymphatics along the right common iliac vein and along the vena cava just below the duodenum are ligated and cut. There are several small veins branching directly from the vena cava that are also tied and cut.

After the paracaval lymphatic and adipose tissues are completely dissected, the right wall of the aorta can be identified under the right lumbar splanchnic nerves and the lymphatic and adipose tissues. They are also removed en bloc and the right and anterior wall of the aorta is exposed. There are several small arteries branching directly from the aorta, all of which are tied and cut. The root of the inferior mesenteric artery can then be seen, and is doubly ligated and cut. The lymphatics along the right common iliac artery and along the aorta just below the duodenum are ligated and cut.

The inferior mesenteric vein and left colic artery are tied and cut at the level of lower edge of the duodenum. Then the sigmoid arteries, mesosigmoid, marginal artery, and sigmoid colon are divided. Retracting the oral sigmoid colon cephalad and the anal colon caudad, the left lumbar splanchnic nerves and the lymphatic and adipose tissues are ligated and cut. All paraaortic lymphatics should be ligated. If these are left open, chylorrhea occasionally ensues.

Next, the lymphatic and adipose tissues around the left wall of the aorta are dissected down to the left common iliac artery. Finally, the lymphatics surrounding the left common iliac artery are tied and cut, and the en bloc paraaortic lymph node dissection is completed (Fig. 61-4).

Extended Lateral Node Dissection (LD3)

The dissection is started from the aortic bifurcation. The lymphatic and adipose tissues surrounding the aortic bifurcation and the common iliac arteries and veins are dissected en bloc with the paraaortic lymph node and mesorectum.

To facilitate further pelvic lymph node dissection, the retrorectal space and the rectoprostatic space (or rectovaginal space) are opened. Retracting the mesorectum caudad with the retractor, the retrorectal space is opened by sharp dissection using scissors or electrocautery under direct vision. Initially, the median part is opened to the Waldeyer's fascia, and then the lateral part is opened to expose the median aspects of the pelvic nerves. To prevent bleeding, blunt finger dissection should be avoided.

Next, retracting the bladder (or uterus) anteriorly with the deep pelvic retractor and retracting the rectum posteriorly with the surgeon's nondominant hand, the rectoprostatic space (or rectovaginal space) are opened. The dissection begins at the median part and ends at the rectovesical ligament (or rectouterine ligament). Denonvilliers' fascia is removed.

Retracting the rectum to the left, extended lymph node dissection of the right pelvic wall is started. First, medial surfaces of the right common iliac artery and vein are exposed, and then medial surfaces of the IIAV and all their branches, including the umbilical ligament, superior and inferior vesical vessels, and pudendal vessels, are dissected. The middle rectal artery, which is usually located between the roots of the superior and inferior vesical arteries, is cut at its root. Finally, the posterior wall of the bladder is exposed, and the rectum is suspended only by nerve fibers from the sacrum and genitourinary organs, which correspond to the pelvic nerves and genitourinary branches from the pelvic plexus, respectively. These nerves are ligated and cut as far from the rectum as possible. The lymphatic

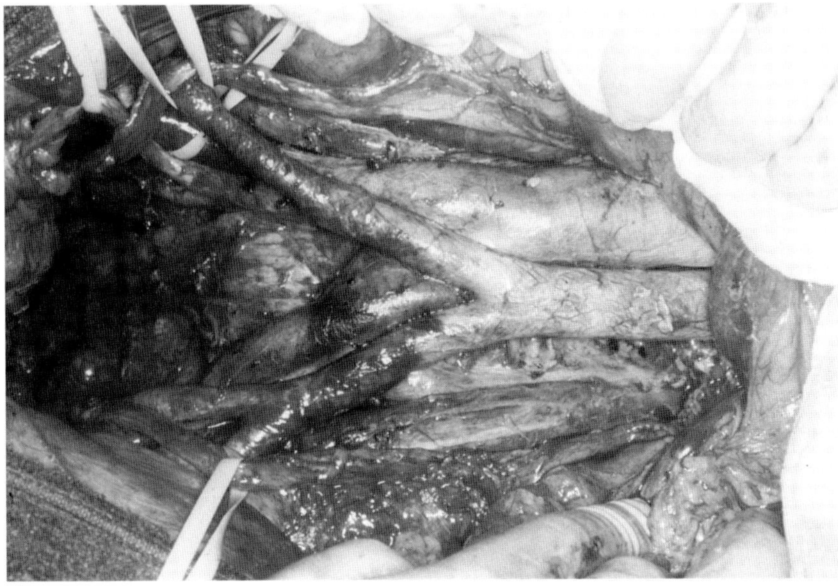

A

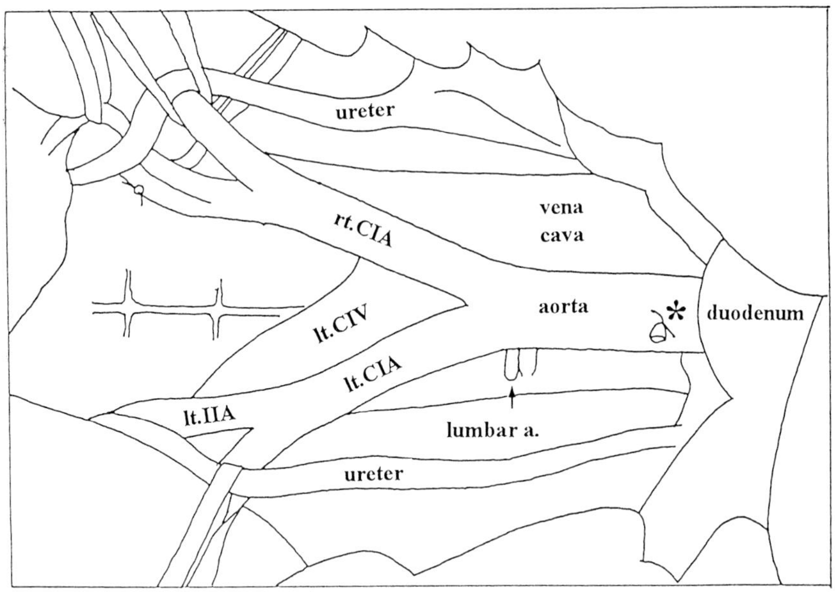

B

FIG. 61-4. Photograph **(A)** and schematic diagram **(B)** of the abdomen and pelvis after completion of paraaortic lymph node dissection (UD4). *CIA*, common iliac artery; *CIV*, common iliac vein; *IIA*, internal iliac artery; *, cut end of the inferior mesenteric artery.

and adipose tissues along these vessels are resected en bloc with the mesorectum.

After the same procedure is done on the left side, the rectum is supported only by the puborectalis muscle. According to the location and extent of the tumor, low anterior resection or Miles' operation is performed.

Next, lymph node dissection of the right obturator space is done. The lymphatic and adipose tissues around the right common iliac and external iliac arteries and veins are dissected. At the bifurcation of the external and internal iliac vessels, the obturator space is opened, and the root of the right obturator nerve is found. The lateral aspect of the obturator space is dissected, and the obturator internis muscle is fully exposed. Preserving the obturator nerve, dorsal and medial aspects of the obturator space are dissected, and lateral aspects of the IIAV and their branches, including the umbilical ligament, superior and inferior vesical vessels, and pudendal vessels, are exposed. The obturator artery, which is usually identified between the roots of the superior and inferior vesical arteries, is cut if needed. Finally, the posterolateral wall of the bladder is exposed, and the obturator space is cleared completely, and the IIAV and their branches are skeletonized (Fig. 61-5).

As described earlier, if the branches of the IIAV are preserved, en bloc resection of the obturator nodes is impossible. If the en bloc resection is needed in cases with involvement of the obturator nodes or internal iliac nodes, which is detected at preoperative examination or intraoperative inspection and palpation, resection of most of the branches of the IIAV or, preferably, combined resection of the IIAV is recommended.

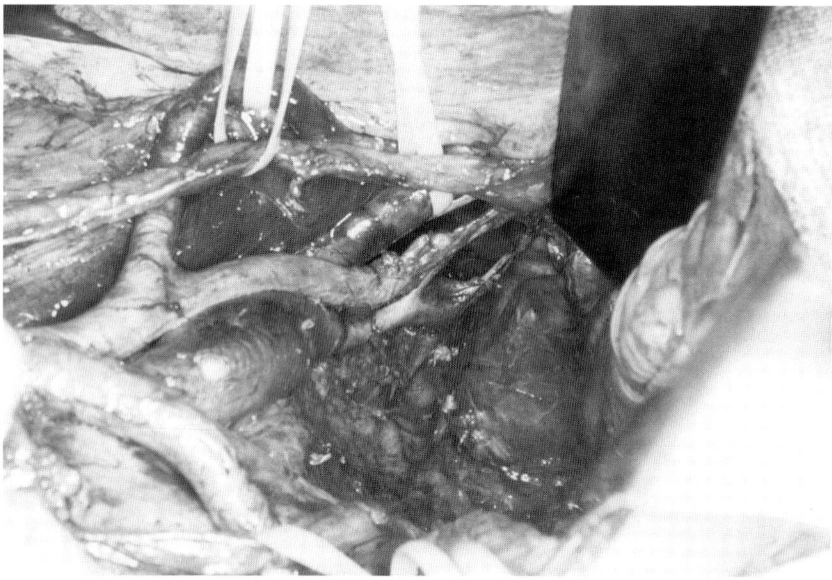

A

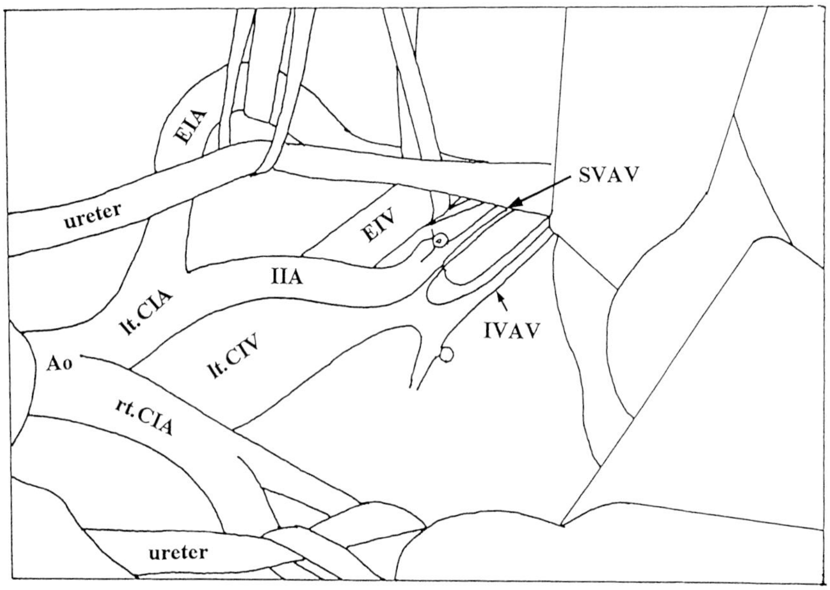

B

FIG. 61-5. Photograph **(A)** and schematic diagram **(B)** of the left pelvic wall after completion of extended lateral node dissection (LD3). *Ao*, aorta; *CIA*, common iliac artery; *CIV*, common iliac vein; *EIA*, external iliac artery; *EIV*, external iliac vein; *IIA*, internal iliac artery; *SVAV*, superior vesical artery and vein; *IVAV*, inferior vesical artery and vein.

Combined Resection of Internal Iliac Artery and Vein (LD4)

After dissection of the common iliac artery and vein, the roots of the IIAV are identified and dissection along these vessels is continued. The internal iliac artery is doubly suture-ligated and cut at its root or beyond the superior vesical artery, unless it compromises the dissection. To ensure blood supply to the bladder, at least the unilateral superior vesical artery should be preserved. The root of the internal iliac vein is also ligated and cut. All branches of the IIAV that penetrate the pelvic wall are carefully tied and cut. Finally, the internal pudendal artery and vein are tied and cut. Thus, the lymphatic and adipose tissues along the obturator space and IIAV are completely resected en bloc with the rectum, and the muscular pelvic sidewalls and the sacral nerve roots are exposed (Fig. 61-6).

Autonomic Nerve Preservation

As described previously, there are several variations in autonomic nerve preservation (see Fig. 61-3). Nerve preservation can be performed either bilaterally or unilaterally and can be combined with EAPL in accordance with the tumor extension (see Table 61-1). These procedures should be performed under direct vision to avoid nerve injury and bleeding, which makes identification of nerves difficult. We always use sharp dissection during these procedures and avoid mass ligation, which may accidentally injure the nerves.

Complete Autonomic Nerve Preservation (NP1)

After mobilization of the mesosigmoid, the superior hypogastric plexus can be easily identified between the mesorectum and

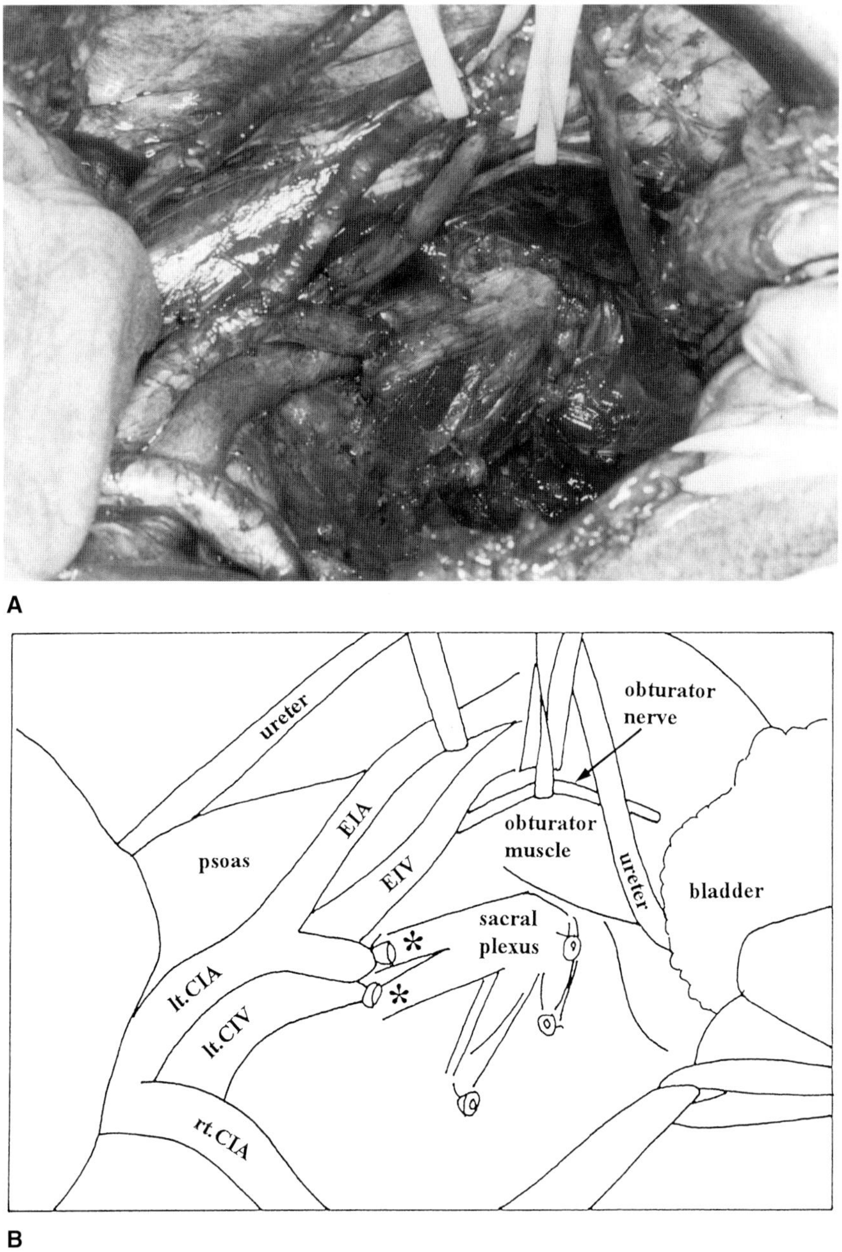

FIG. 61-6. Photograph **(A)** and schematic diagram **(B)** of the left pelvic wall after completion of extended lateral dissection with combined resection of the internal iliac artery and vein (LD4). *CIA*, common iliac artery; *CIV*, common iliac vein; *EIA*, external iliac artery; *EIV*, external iliac vein; *, cut ends of the internal iliac artery and vein.

the aortic bifurcation (see Fig. 61-2). Cutting several thin nerve branches, the plane between the superior hypogastric plexus and the mesorectum is dissected cephalad, and the root of the inferior mesenteric artery is reached. The inferior mesenteric artery is cut at its root or beyond the left colic artery according to the tumor extension, and the mesosigmoid and sigmoid colon are divided.

Retracting the rectum anteriorly, the plane between the superior hypogastric plexus and the mesorectum is dissected caudad. About 2 to 3 cm below the aortic bifurcation, the superior hypogastric plexus bifurcates into the right and left hypogastric nerves. Between these nerves, the retrorectal space is opened until the roots of the pelvic nerves can be seen as white, firm fibers.

After mobilization of the anterior wall of the rectum, the plane between the pelvic plexus and the rectum is dissected. Numerous thin nerve branches connect the pelvic plexus and the rectum. They all are cut. The peripheral branch of the middle rectal artery is identified among the nerve fibers and is cut. During this procedure, traction of the rectum and the countertraction of the plexus are important for good visualization of the correct plane. Thus, the rectum is freely mobilized and is sustained only by the puborectalis muscle (Figs. 61-7 and 61-8).

When abdominoperineal resection is needed, special care should be taken not to injure the neurovascular bundles (see Fig. 61-3), which lie in the posterolateral aspects of the prostate (Fig. 61-9).

Complete Preservation of the Pelvic Plexus (NP2a or NP3a)

After completion of lymph node dissection around the aorta and common iliac vessels, dissection is continued to expose the

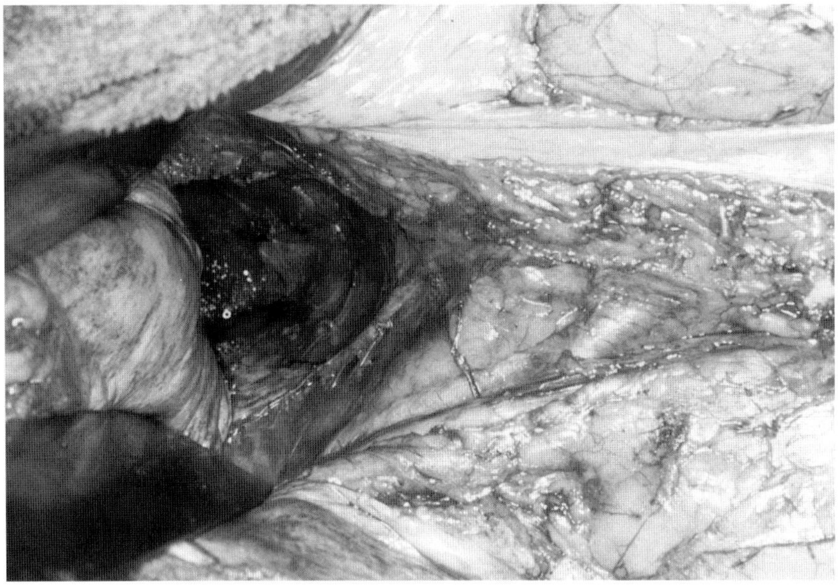

A

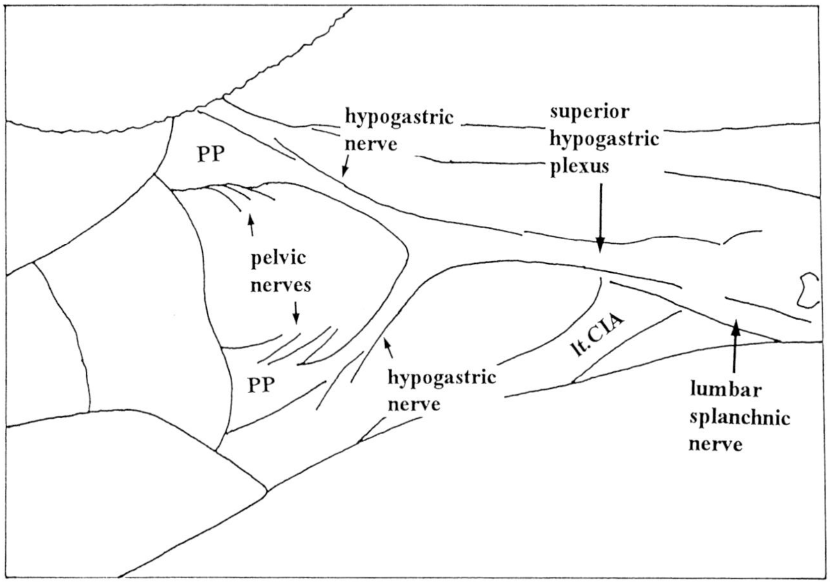

B

FIG. 61-7. Photograph **(A)** and schematic diagram **(B)** of the abdomen and pelvis after completion of complete autonomic nerve preservation (NP1). *CIA*, common iliac artery; *PP*, pelvic plexus.

IIAV until the cephalic edge of the pelvic plexus, which lies on the course of the pelvic nerves, is exposed. By incising the cephalic border of the pelvic plexus and cutting the hypogastric nerve, the plane of dissection is changed from the perivascular plane to the perirectal plane. Then the pelvic nerves and plexus are dissected from the rectum as described earlier. Thus, the pelvic plexus remains in situ.

Extended lateral dissection (LD3) can be performed with preservation of the plexus. However, the nerve preservation compromises lymph node dissection to some degree. After dissection of the obturator space, the lymphatic and adipose tissues between the IIAV and the plexus are removed. During this procedure, the root of the middle rectal artery is identified and the lymph node around this artery is dissected en bloc. At the end, the plexus remains as a thin plate of nerves measuring about 4 cm in diameter.

Preservation of the Lower Part of the Pelvic Plexus (NP2b or NP3b)

The lower part of the pelvic plexus can be preserved with resection of the upper part of the plexus. After lymph node dissection along the IIAV is continued down to the planned level, by incising the plexus, the plane of the dissection is changed from the perivascular plane to the perirectal plane. The fourth pelvic nerve is usually the thickest and can be easily identified and serve as a landmark (Fig. 61-10).

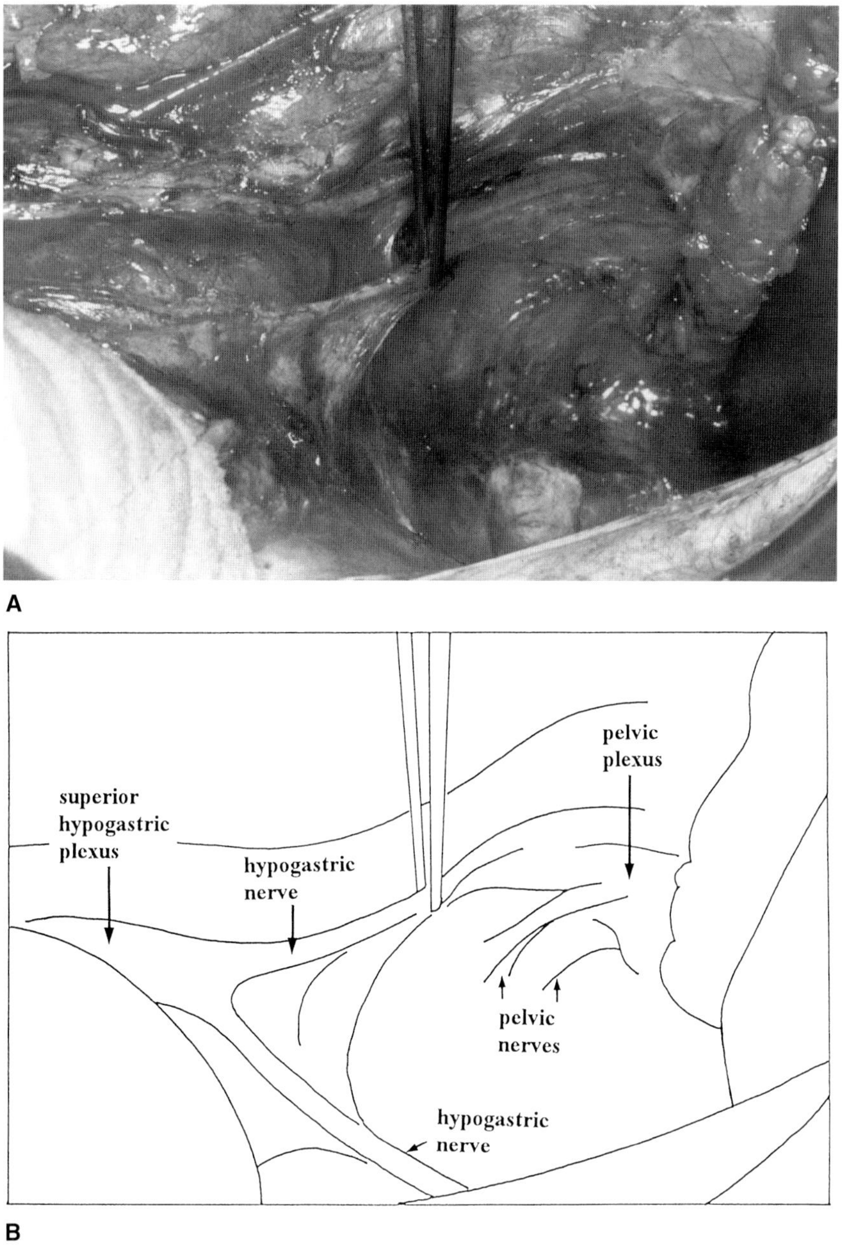

FIG. 61-8. Photograph **(A)** and schematic diagram **(B)** of the left pelvic wall after completion of complete autonomic nerve preservation (NP1).

RESULTS

Type of Surgery and Extent of Lymph Node Dissection and Nerve Preservation

Of 276 patients who underwent APLANP, 187 (68%) had a sphincter-saving procedure and 89 (32%) had abdominoperineal resection.

Pathologic TNM stage and type of nerve preservation and lymph node dissection actually performed are shown in Table 61-1.

Of 99 patients with stage I disease, 67 (70%) were staged correctly and underwent appropriate surgery (NP1), and 32 (30%) were overstaged and underwent excessive surgery (NP2 or NP3).

Of 177 patients with stage II and III disease, 126 (71%) underwent NP2 or NP3, 51 (29%) underwent NP1, and 93 (53%) underwent extended lateral dissection.

Morbidity and Mortality

Median operating time and blood loss according to the type of surgery are listed in Table 61-3. Both operating time and blood loss increased as the extent of the dissection expanded.

Of 276 patients with APLANP, 73 suffered postoperative complications (morbidity, 26%). Of these, 28 patients had anastomotic leakage, 31 had wound infection, 12 had bowel obstruction, and 20 had other complications. Only one patient died within 30 days after surgery, as a result of anastomotic leakage and diffuse peritonitis (mortality, 0.4%).

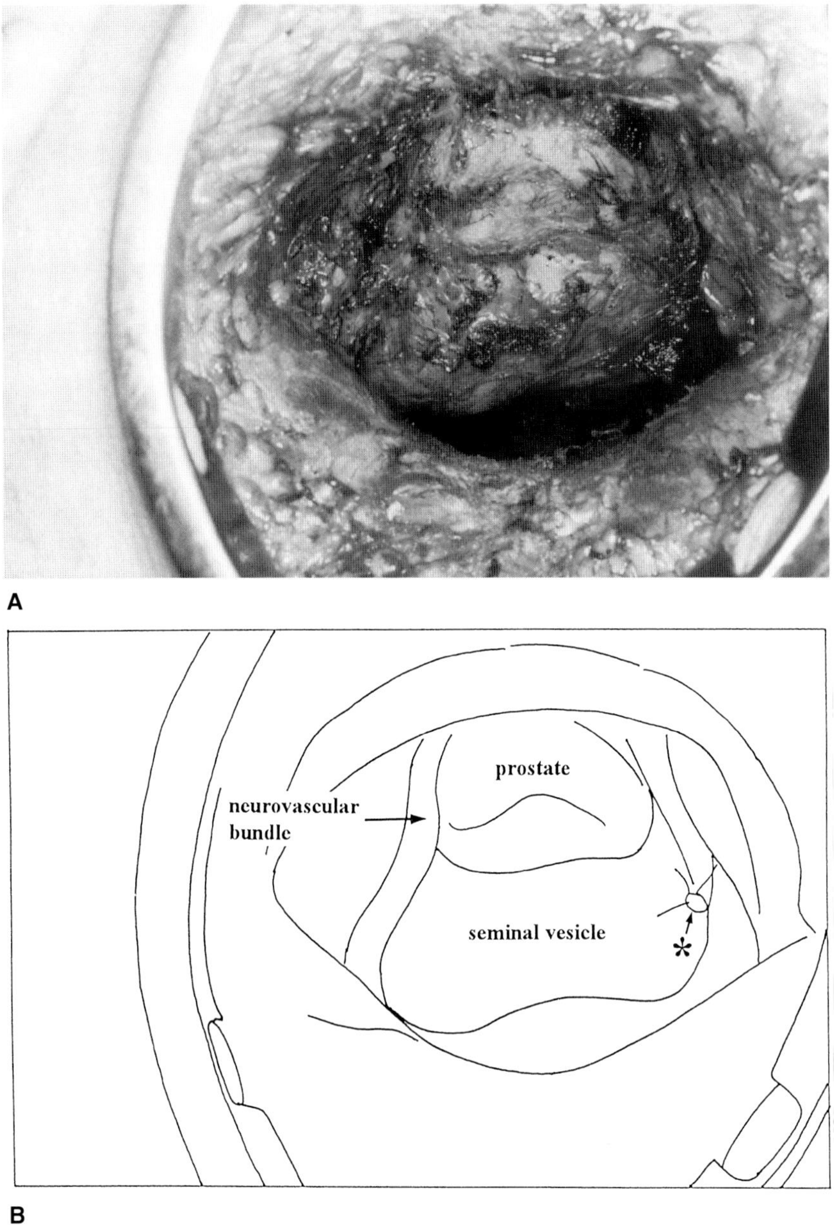

FIG. 61-9. Photograph **(A)** and schematic diagram **(B)** of the perineal phase of the abdominoperineal resection. In this case, the neurovascular bundle of the left side is resected, and that of the right side is preserved. *, Cut end of the neurovascular bundle.

TABLE 61-3. *Type of surgery, operating time, and blood loss*

Type of surgery*	No. of patients	Median operating time (min)	Median blood loss (g)
NP1	118	240	370
NP2	93	310	670
NP3	65	330	720
NP4†	272	350	1270

* See text for explanation of types of surgery.

† Extended abdominopelvic dissection without autonomic nerve preservation.

Urinary Function

Time to recovery of spontaneous urination according to type of autonomic nerve preservation is shown in Table 61-4. Of 143 patients who underwent APLANP and were interviewed, 120 (84%) could urinate spontaneously within 60 days after surgery. Time to recovery of spontaneous urination and incidence of prolonged urinary dysfunction necessitating self-catheterization were associated with the extent of nerve preservation. It was remarkable that 100% of the patients with complete nerve preservation (NP1) and 86% of the patients with bilateral pelvic plexus preservation (NP2) could urinate spontaneously, and even in cases with unilateral pelvic plexus preservation, 61% of the patients could urinate.

Preservation of urinary sensation was associated not only with the type of nerve preservation but with preservation of the

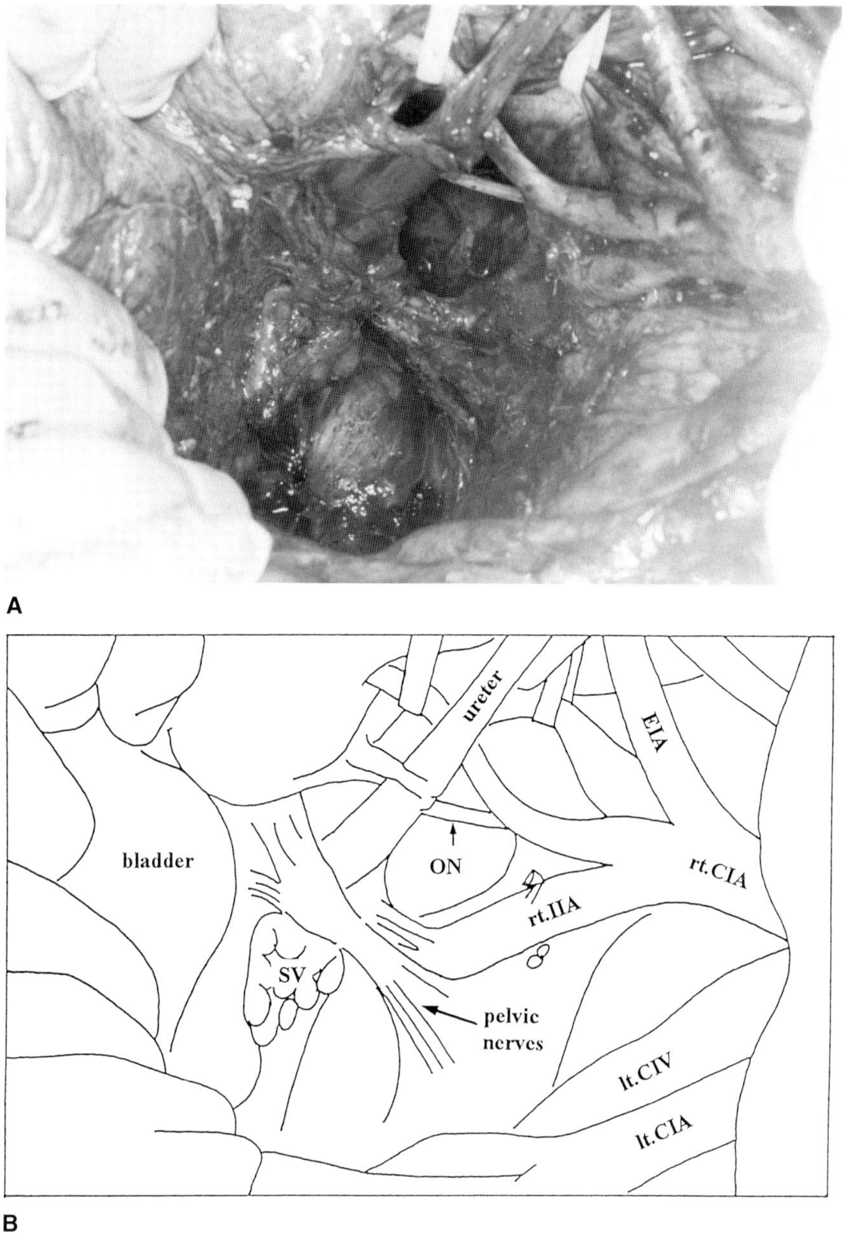

FIG. 61-10. Photograph **(A)** and schematic diagram **(B)** of the right pelvic wall after completion of preservation of the lower part of the pelvic plexus (NP2b or NP3b) with extended lateral dissection (LD3). *CIA*, common iliac artery; *CIV*, common iliac vein; *EIA*, external iliac artery; *IIA*, internal iliac artery; *ON*, obturator nerve; *SV*, seminal vesicle.

TABLE 61-4. *Type of nerve preservation and time to recovery of spontaneous urination*

Postoperative days	Type of nerve preservation (%)* NP1 (n = 56)	NP2 (n = 43)	NP3 (n = 44)	Overall (%) (n = 143)
<10	39 (70)	10 (23)	2 (5)	51 (36)
10–29	12 (21)	14 (33)	16 (36)	42 (29)
30–59	5 (9)	13 (30)	9 (20)	27 (19)
60<	0 (0)	6 (14)	17 (39)	23 (16)

* See text for explanation of nerve preservation procedures.

TABLE 61-5. *Type of autonomic nerve preservation and preservation of the sphincter and urinary sensation*

	Type of nerve preservation (%)*			
	NP2		NP3	
Urinary sensation	SSP (n = 30)	APR (n = 13)	SSP (n = 18)	APR (n = 26)
Normal	13 (43)	0 (0)	2 (11)	0 (0)
Mildly impaired	15 (50)	9 (69)	12 (67)	14 (53)
Severely impaired	2 (7)	4 (31)	4 (22)	12 (46)

*See text for explanation of nerve preservation procedures.
SSP, sphincter-saving procedure; *APR*, abdominoperineal resection.

anal sphincter (Table 61-5). The incidence of prolonged urinary dysfunction was also associated with preservation of the anal sphincter.

Sexual Function

Male sexual function according to type of nerve preservation is shown in Table 61-6. Of 73 patients who were interviewed, 47 (64%) answered that they were potent to a certain degree, and 30 (41%) could ejaculate. In general, preservation of sexual function was more difficult than that of urination. Preservation of male sexual function was also associated with the extent of nerve preservation. In particular, the incidence of impotence was high in patients with unilateral pelvic plexus preservation (NP3). Like urinary dysfunction, the incidence of impotence was also associated with preservation of the anal sphincter. The incidence of impotence was higher with abdominoperineal resection than in the sphincter-saving procedure. The incidence of impotence also depends on the experience of the surgeon; that is, it decreases as the surgeon gains experience in nerve preservation.

TABLE 61-6. *Male sexual function after autonomic nerve preservation**

	Type of nerve preservation (%)†		
Sexual function	NP1 (n = 38)	NP2 (n = 10)	NP3 (n = 25)
ERECTION			
Normal	17 (45)	0 (0)	0 (0)
Impaired	20 (53)	4 (40)	6 (24)
Absent	1 (2)	6 (60)	19 (76)
EJACULATION			
Normal	13 (34)	0 (0)	0 (0)
Impaired	16 (42)	1 (10)	0 (0)
Absent	9 (24)	9 (90)	25 (100)

* Male patients younger than 65 years of age were interviewed 1 or more years after surgery.
† See text for explanation of nerve preservation procedures.

TABLE 61-7. *Pattern of nocturnal penile tumescence and other sexual function after autonomic nerve preservation**

	Type of nerve preservation†			
	NP1		NP3	
Sexual function	SSP (n = 6)	APR (n = 2)	SSP (n = 1)	APR (n = 1)
PATTERN OF NOCTURNAL PENILE TUMESCENCE				
Normal	5	2	0	0
Shortened episode	0	0	1	0
Flat	1	0	0	1
ERECTION (INTERVIEW)				
Normal	5	2	0	0
Impaired	0	0	1	0
Absent	1	0	0	1
EJACULATION (INTERVIEW)				
Normal	5	2	0	0
Impaired	0	0	0	0
Absent	1	0	1	1

* Male patients younger than 65 years of age were interviewed and examined by Rigiscan 1 or more years after surgery.
† See text for explanation of nerve preservation procedures.
SSP, sphincter-saving procedure; *APR*, abdominoperineal resection.

To evaluate erectile function objectively, nocturnal penile tumescence in 10 patients was measured with the Rigiscan device (Table 61-7). Of eight patients with complete nerve preservation (NP1), seven showed a normal nocturnal penile tumescence pattern, and one showed a flat pattern; this patient had undergone abdominosacral coloanal anastomosis and suffered

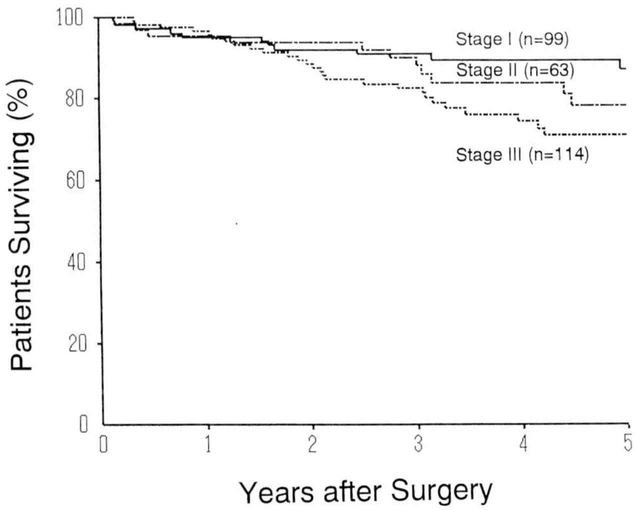

FIG. 61-11. Survival curves according to pathologic TNM stage. Five-year survival rates of stage I, II, and III patients who underwent abdominopelvic lymphadenectomy with autonomic nerve preservation were 87%, 78%, and 71%, respectively.

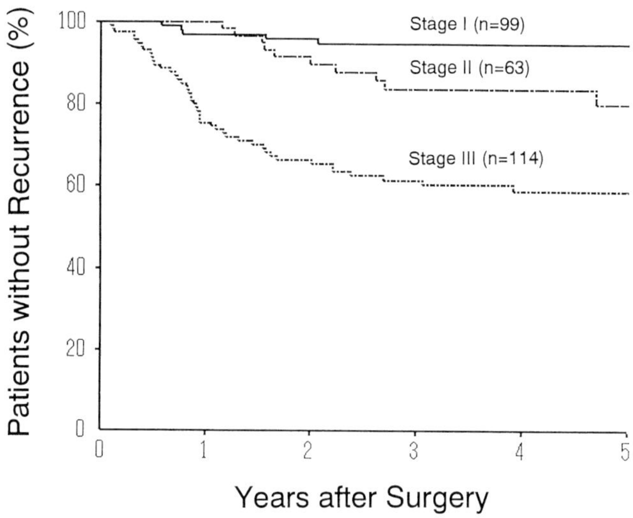

FIG. 61-12. Disease-free survival curves according to pathologic TNM stage. Five-year disease-free survival rates of stage I, II, and III patients who underwent abdominopelvic lymphadenectomy with autonomic nerve preservation were 95%, 80%, and 59%, respectively.

from injury of bilateral neurovascular bundles. Of two patients with unilateral pelvic plexus preservation (NP3), one showed a shortened episode of nocturnal penile tumescence, and one showed a flat pattern who had undergone extended lateral dissection with combined resection of the left IIAV and preservation of the right pelvic plexus (LD4 + NP3). Those results were similar to the results of the interview.

Survival

Survival and disease-free survival curves for the pathologic TNM stages are shown in Figures 61-11 and 61-12, respectively. The overall 5-year survival rate of the patients with APLANP was 78%, and the overall 5-year disease-free survival rate was 76%. Five-year survival rates of pathologic TNM stage I, II, and III patients with APLANP were 87%, 78%, and 71%, respectively (see Fig. 61-11). Five-year disease-free survival rates of stage I, II, and III patients were 95%, 80%, and 59%, respectively (see Fig. 61-12).

Of 276 patients with curative APLANP, 66 (24%) had recurrence, including intrapelvic recurrence in 19 patients (7%), liver metastasis in 22 (8%), lung metastasis in 19 (7%), and other sites in 6 (2%). The rates of intrapelvic recurrence in pathologic stage I, II, and III patients were 2%, 3%, and 15%, respectively.

DISCUSSION

More than 40 years have passed since the origination of APLD for rectal cancer. During this period, in Western countries, skepticism about the efficacy of APLD overcame enthusiasm for it because of statistically insignificant improvements in survival rates[3–5] and inevitable urinary and sexual dysfunction.[4] Thus, instead of APLD, adjuvant radiation therapy and chemoradiation therapy have been investigated intensively.[8,9] In addition, new surgical approaches such as total mesorectal excision[10] and autonomic nerve-preserving pelvic sidewall dissection[11] have been practiced. These contributed to improved survival and disease-free survival rates.

On the other hand, in Japan, some modifications of the original APLD have been made (EAPL). The first modification was a more accurate dissection of the pelvic lymphatic tissues, which completely skeletonized the intrapelvic vessels and exposed the muscular pelvic walls.[13] The second modification was the combined resection of the IIAV,[13–15] which enabled complete en bloc resection of the pelvic lymph nodes and the perivascular lymphatic tissues. We described the details of these procedures because there are varying degrees of possible dissections, and such variations can possibly influence survival.

In retrospective studies, APLD had a significant advantage over conventional dissection,[13,15] reducing the death rate by 14% (88% vs. 74%) in pathologic TNM stage II disease, and reducing the death rate by 18% (61% vs. 43%) in stage III disease.[13] The survival rate of patients with stage III disease treated by EAPL alone is even higher than the reported survival rate of patients with stage II to III disease treated by conventional resection and chemoradiation therapy.[9]

Even in the presence of lymph node involvement along the IIAV or in the obturator space, 49% of patients were disease free for 5 years after EAPL.[14] Results of total mesorectal excision[10] and autonomic nerve-preserving pelvic sidewall dissection[11] are quite satisfactory, and local recurrence rates are low. However, because these procedures do not remove lymph nodes outside of the pelvic plexus, they cannot cure such cases.

Functional results of EAPL were poor, however. The incidences of urinary dysfunction and impotence after EAPL were 42% and 76%, respectively.[15] To deal with these complications, APLANP was created[12,16] on the basis of improved understanding of pelvic neuroanatomy.[12,16,19] Urinary dysfunction is caused not only by neural injury but by preexisting bladder outlet obstruction and deformity of the bladder and urethra. Similarly, sexual dysfunction is caused not only by neural injury but by vascular damage and psychological trauma. Still, the principal cause is neural injury. Therefore, every effort is made to preserve the whole or part of the autonomic nervous system without compromising lymph node dissection.

Urinary and sexual function after complete nerve preservation with mesorectal excision (NP1 + LD1) are excellent. Almost 100% of patients can urinate spontaneously and are potent to a certain degree. Similar operations are also performed by Heald and Karanjia[10] and Enker,[11] who report similar favorable functional results.

If bilateral pelvic plexuses are preserved (NP2 + LD3), urinary function is almost preserved and potency is preserved to some extent, but retrograde ejaculation inevitably occurs. In the case of unilateral pelvic plexus preservation (NP3 + LD3), urination is preserved to a certain extent, but preservation of potency is difficult. Therefore, to preserve urinary function, at least a unilateral pelvic plexus should be preserved. On the other hand, to preserve potency, preservation of bilateral pelvic plexuses is preferred.

In our opinion, complete nerve preservation with mesorectal excision (NP1 + LD1) is best indicated for pretreatment TNM stage I disease, because T1 and T2 tumors without suspect node swelling are rarely accompanied by paraaortic or lateral pelvic lymph node involvement. As this study showed, survival and disease-free survival of pathologic TNM stage I patients with APLANP is excellent.

In cases of T3 and T4 tumors without suspect node swelling (stage II) and suspected stage III disease, the risks of lateral node involvement are about 18%.[14] Therefore, it is safer to perform extended lateral dissection (LD3 to LD4). Combined resection of the IIAV is mandatory if involvement of lateral nodes is obvious. Even in such difficult cases, cure can be expected in almost 50%.[14] Five-year survival rates of pathologic TNM stage II to III patients with APLANP are comparable to those with EAPL (stage II, 80% vs. 88%; stage III, 71% vs. 61%). However, if the number of involved nodes exceeds four, prognosis is poor.[12] Such an advanced tumor is beyond the reach of surgery and necessitates some adjuvant therapy such as chemoradiation therapy.[8,9]

To avoid insufficient and excessive surgery and to gain maximal survival and functional results, accurate preoperative and intraoperative staging is essential. The accuracy of transrectal ultrasonography in T-staging and assessing regional lymph node involvement is about 80%.[20,21] However, as this study showed, the accuracy of our method of staging using physical examination and radiologic diagnosis is still unsatisfactory. Improved diagnostic accuracy in staging is necessary to perform surgery well tailored to the individual patient.

Finally, we well recognize the criticisms against the efficacy of EAPL and APLANP.[22] Studies claiming the efficacy of these operations are retrospective and use historical controls.[12–15] In the retrospective study, there can be many sources of bias, resulting from stage migration due to method of staging and the extent of dissection, patient selection, historical controls, and so forth. We conclude that APLANP seems to be promising, but further investigation evaluating the real benefits of this surgery is still necessary.

REFERENCES

1. Deddish MR. Abdominopelvic lymph-node dissection in cancer of the rectum and distal colon. Cancer 1951;4:1364.
2. Sauer I, Bacon HE. A new approach for excision of carcinoma of the lower portion of the rectum and anal canal. Surg Gynecol Obstet 1952; 95:229.
3. Bacon HE, Dirbas F, Myers TB, Ponce de Leon F. Extensive lymphadenectomy and high ligation of the inferior mesenteric artery for carcinoma of the left colon and rectum. Dis Colon Rectum 1958;1:457.
4. Stearns Jr MW, Deddish MR. Five-year results of abdominopelvic lymph node dissection for carcinoma of the rectum. Dis Colon Rectum 1959;2:169.
5. Glass RE, Ritchie JK, Thompson HR, Mann CV. The results of surgical treatment of cancer of the rectum by radical resection and extended abdominoiliac lymphadenectomy. Br J Surg 1985;72:599.
6. Enker WE, Heilweil ML, Hertz RE, et al. En bloc pelvic lymphadenectomy and sphincter preservation in the surgical management of rectal cancer. Ann Surg 1986;203:426.
7. Michelassi F, Block GE. Morbidity and mortality of wide pelvic lymphadenectomy for rectal adenocarcinoma. Dis Colon Rectum 1992;35: 1143.
8. Gastrointestinal Tumor Study Group. Prolongation of the disease-free interval in surgically treated rectal carcinoma. N Engl J Med 1985; 312:1465.
9. Krook JE, Moertel CG, Gunderson LL, Wieand HS, Collins RT, Beart RW. Effective surgical adjuvant therapy for high-risk rectal carcinoma. N Engl J Med 1991;324:709.
10. Heald RJ, Karanjia ND. Mesenteric considerations for adequate resection. In: Wanebo HJ, ed. Colorectal cancer. St. Louis: Mosby, 1993: 242.
11. Enker WE. Potency, cure, and local control in the operative treatment of rectal cancer. Arch Surg 1992;127:1396.
12. Moriya Y. Pelvic node dissection with autonomic nerve sparing for invasive lower rectal cancer: Japanese experience. In: Wanebo HJ, ed. Colorectal cancer. St. Louis: Mosby, 1993:274.
13. Koyama Y, Moriya Y, Hojo K. Effects of extended systematic lymphadenectomy for adenocarcinoma of the rectum: significant improvement of survival rate and decrease of local recurrence. Jpn J Clin Oncol 1984;14:623.
14. Moriya Y, Hojo K, Sawada T, Koyama Y. Significance of lateral node dissection for advanced rectal carcinoma at or below the peritoneal reflection. Dis Colon Rectum 1989;32:307.
15. Hojo K, Sawada T, Moriya Y. An analysis of survival and voiding, sexual function after wide iliopelvic lymphadenectomy in patients with carcinoma of the rectum, compared with conventional lymphadenectomy. Dis Colon Rectum 1989;32:128.
16. Hojo K, Vernava AM III, Sugihara K, Katsumata K. Preservation of urine voiding and sexual function after rectal cancer surgery. Dis Colon Rectum 1991;34:532.
17. Hermanek P, Sobin LH, editors. TNM classification of malignant tumors. Berlin: Springer-Verlag, 1992.
18. Kaneko S, Bradly WE. Evaluation of erectile dysfunction with continuous monitoring of penile rigidity. J Urol 1986;136:1026.
19. Lee JF, Block GE. Anatomic relations of pelvic autonomic nerves to pelvic operations. Arch Surg 1973;107:324.
20. Akasu T, Sunouchi K, Sawada T, Tsioulias G, Muto T, Morioka Y. Preoperative staging of rectal carcinoma: prospective comparison of transrectal ultrasonography and computed tomography. (Abstract) Gastroenterology 1990;98:268.
21. Rösch T, Classen M. Colorectal carcinoma. In: Elder D, ed. Gastroenterologic endosonography. New York: Thieme Medical Publishers, 1992:170.
22. Scholefield JH, Steup WH. Surgery for rectal cancer in Japan. Lancet 1992;340:1101.

Surgery for Gastrointestinal Cancer: A Multidisciplinary Approach, edited by Harold J. Wanebo.
Lippincott-Raven Publishers, Philadelphia, © 1997.

CHAPTER 62

Preoperative Radiation and Resection With Coloanal Anastomosis for Low-Lying Rectal Cancer

Gerald J. Marks, John H. Marks, and Mohammed Mohiuddin

The threat of locoregional recurrence and the loss of anal sphincter function continue to be the dominant quality-of-life issues in rectal cancer management. Preoperative high-dose external irradiation is gaining acceptance as a valuable surgical adjunct capable of reducing locoregional recurrence, and, in nonrandomized studies, appreciably improving survival in rectal cancer surgery.[1,2] We are capitalizing on the ability of high-dose preoperative external irradiation to downstage and, in theory, sterilize the regional microlymphatics of the low-lying rectal cancer. These effects led us to accept lesser circumferential and distal margins by applying an original method of radical excision and coloanal anastomosis. Sphincter conservation surgery is now being offered to patients with select cancers of the distal rectum including the zone between the 0.5 and 3 cm superior to the anorectal ring. This chapter describes a 10-year experience in the use of coloanal anastomosis by a new technique of radical proctosigmoidectomy and descending coloanal anastomosis after high-dose external radiation for cancers of the distal 3 cm of the rectum that are mobile 5.5 to 8 weeks postradiation. The low rate of locoregional recurrence and the enhanced survival in this subset of patients suggest a real quality-of-life benefit to this multimodality program.

As an outgrowth of the converging experiences with high-dose preoperative irradiation for fixed and inoperable rectal cancer and the surgical reconstruction of the radiation-necrotic rectum dating to the early 1960s, a program of high-dose preoperative irradiation and sphincter preservation surgery for unfavorable and distal rectal cancer was initiated in 1976. With the confidence drawn from having performed an anastomosis in the distal 2 cm of a radiation-injured rectum, it was posited that by following the same surgical principles, an anastomosis could be safely accomplished after irradiating cancers at the greatest risk for local failure (i.e., prospectively staged unfavorable or low-lying rectal cancers).[3,4] As of April 1, 1994, 274 patients have been treated in this program. Data relative to the first consecutive 65 patients with cancers in the distal 3 cm of rectum who underwent transanal abdominal transanal radical proctosigmoidectomy with coloanal anastomosis after high-dose external irradiation are presented.

Initially, the combined abdominotranssacral method was used exclusively to accomplish sphincter preservation.[5] Presuming the need to have a 2- or 3-cm margin distal to the cancer, sphincter preservation was originally limited to those tumors at and above the 4-cm level relative to the anorectal ring. As data accumulated, revealing a local recurrence rate between 10% to 12%, centimeter by centimeter, cancers lower in the rectum were treated with restorative surgery. In 1984, a new method was designed and used that allowed safe resection of tumors below the 2-cm level. We called this procedure the transanal abdominal transanal radical proctosigmoidectomy with direct coloanal anastomosis. It has become the standard technique used for all mobile cancers in the distal 3 cm of the rectum. The benefit of this procedure derives from the initiation of dissection of the distal rectum by the transanal route. This ensures a maximal distal margin to the cancer and avoids the pitfall of not being able, through an abdominal approach, to palpate a postradiated, small, very low-lying rectal cancer. This method also obviates the need to apply a clamp distal to the tumor in what is frequently an uncomfortably narrow and confined space.

All rectal cancer patients seen in the Comprehensive Rectal Cancer Center since 1976 have been examined by both the

Gerald J. Marks: Edgar J. Deissler, Professor of Surgery, Director of Gastrointestinal Surgical Endoscopy, Director of Comprehensive Rectal Cancer Center, Medical College of Pennsylvania Hahnemann University, Broad and Vine Streets, Philadelphia, PA 19104

John H. Marks: Assistant Director, Comprehensive Rectal Cancer Center Department of Surgery, Medical College of Pennsylvania and Hahnemann University, Broad and Vine Streets, Philadelphia, PA 19102

Mohammed Mohiuddin: Professor and Chair, Department of Radiation Oncology, University of Kentucky, 800 Rose Street, Lexington, KY 40536

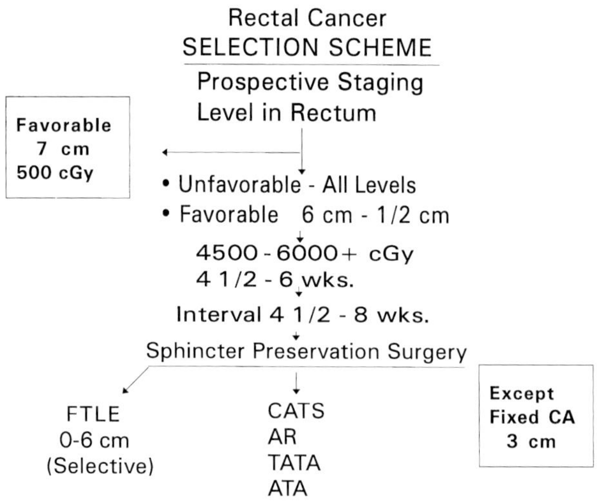

FIG. 62-1. Selection scheme for treatment of rectal cancer. Copyright Gerald Marks.

surgeon and the radiation oncologist. Prospective clinical staging, tumor location in the rectum, and the qualities related to unfavorability (one or more elements including deep ulceration, fixation, obstruction, palpable perirectal lymph nodes, indurated intramural lymphatics, poor histologic differentiation, and full-thickness penetration) were determined and documented. Graphic representations of the tumor configuration and site were recorded in a standard fashion. The site in the rectum was measured in centimeters using the anorectal ring as a reference, except in those instances in which the postradiated tumor was mobile at or below the anorectal ring, in which case the pectinate line was used as the zero point. The selection scheme, which originally limited sphincter preservation to cancers at or above the 4-cm level, as mentioned, evolved to include patients with cancers situated as low as 5 mm above the pectinate line. After prospectively staging the cancer clinically with the aid of endorectal sonography, computed tomography scan, and magnetic resonance imaging with a rectal coil, and determining its level in the rectum, all patients with favorable rectal cancers at or above the 7-cm level were assigned to the selective sandwich program that uses a single treatment of 500 cGy immediately before any suitable sphincter preservation surgery. Those patients with tumors proved histologically to be T3 or N positive were treated with postoperative radiation. All other patients (i.e., those with unfavorable cancers at any level or those with favorable cancers at or below the 6-cm level) were treated before surgery with 4500 to 7000 cGy in fractions of 180 to 250 cGy over a period of 4.5 to 7 weeks (Fig. 62-1). The appreciation of dose-related benefits has led us to select 5580 cGy in 180-cGy fractions as the customary dose.[6]

RADIATION TREATMENT PARAMETERS

Radiation is delivered using high-energy photons, either on the 45-MeV Betatron or the 25-MeV linear accelerator. A minimal tumor dose of 4500 cGy over 5 weeks at 180 cGy per fraction (or an equivalent dose of 4000 cGy at 250 cGy per fraction) is delivered to the whole pelvis. A four-field box technique with shaped anteroposterior/posteroanterior and lateral fields is used. The superior border is at the L5–S1 junction, with the perineum and anal canal included inferiorly. The lateral borders extend 1 cm beyond the bony pelvis. The posterior border encompasses the whole of the sacrum, with adequate margins and lateral fields to include all external and internal iliac lymph nodes. All fields are treated daily, 5 days a week. Patients with tumor fixation are given an additional boost of 1000 to 1500 cGy using a reduced field that encompasses the tumor and presacral tissues.

OPERATIVE TECHNIQUE

The anesthetized patient is placed in a supine lithotomy position with the lower extremities in Allen stirrups, with care taken to protect the common peroneal nerve. Digital rectal examination is performed to confirm the site and characteristics of the tumor, which may be advantageous in planning the dissection strategy. Two povidone–iodine-soaked 4 × 4 gauze sponges are tied together and inserted into the rectum. The skin of the abdomen and perineum is surgically prepared and draped in continuity. The vagina is always prepared. With the buttocks extending over the edge of the table and the patient in an exaggerated lithotomy position, epinephrine solution (1 : 200,000 concentration) is infiltrated into the posterior, lateral, and anterior perirectal tissue, avoiding penetration of the needle into the rectum. Allis-Adair clamps are used to grasp the anal canal stoutly and bring about its gentle eversion. The exposed anal canal is washed with povidone–iodine. Epinephrine solution is injected submucosally and intramurally. The mucosa is incised circumferentially with the electrocautery at a point 3 to 7 mm superior to the pectinate line, allowing for a maximal distal margin (Fig. 62-2). Scissors introduced in the posterior midline are spread to permit penetration through the full thickness of the anorectal wall to reach the interval between the wall and puborectalis muscle (Fig. 62-3). A lighted suction device aids in visualizing the whitish adventitial surface of the puborectalis muscle, which marks the proper plane. This is the key to successful dissection. Blunt fingertip dissection enlarges the plane in both lateral directions (Fig. 62-4). The incision through the full thickness of the wall must be extended circumferentially to avoid a shearing effect when the pressure of finger dissection develops. Completion of the incision through mucosa and muscle anteriorly receives special care because redundant mucosa tends to obscure nonincised segments of mucosa and wall. Failure to recognize an incomplete incision confounds the anterior extrarectal dissection. The transected end of the rectum is grasped with Allis-Adair clamps for proper traction and care is taken to avoid impinging on the very low-lying tumor. Blunt and sharp extrarectal dissection is pursued first in the posterior region, where landmarks are more readily appreciated. It is important not to stray deep or lateral to the puborectalis or the levator ani muscles. The coccyx and the anterior sacrococcygeal ligament are helpful palpable landmarks. The yellow fat that surrounds the rectum is a visual guide. A sweeping motion with the finger frees the perirectal tissue laterally and usually strips the endopelvic fascia, an additional tissue barrier for the rectum, its contained cancer, and the mesorectum. The surgeon must continually be mindful of the need to avoid dissection deep to the levator ani muscle. In the male patient, palpably locating the capsule of the prostate anteriorly and using that as a guide for the development of the proper anterior plane is critical. Avoidance of the urethra is aided by this maneuver. A common

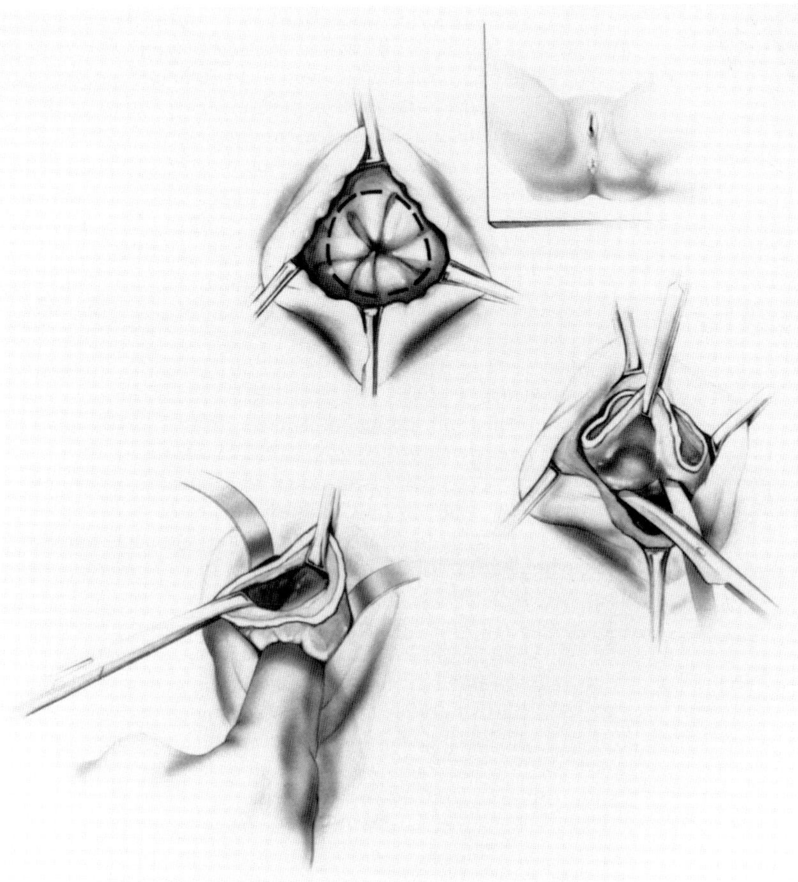

FIG. 62-2. Steps to initiate transanal dissection. Copyright Gerald Marks.

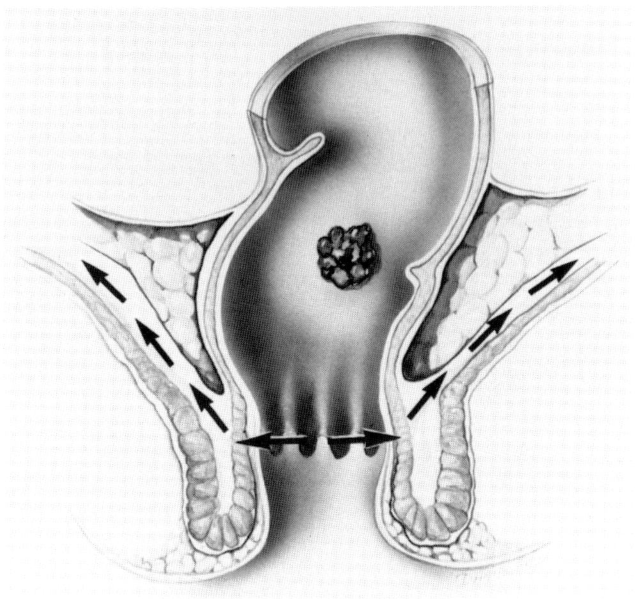

FIG. 62-3. The plane of dissection. Copyright Gerald Marks.

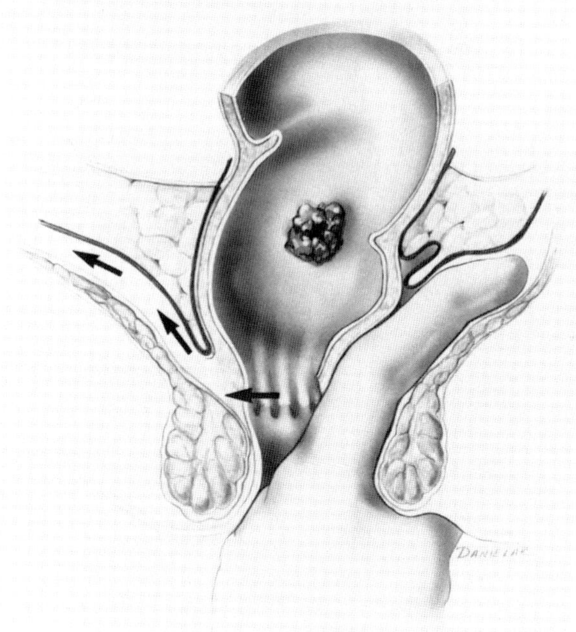

FIG. 62-4. The separation of endopelvic fascia. Copyright Gerald Marks.

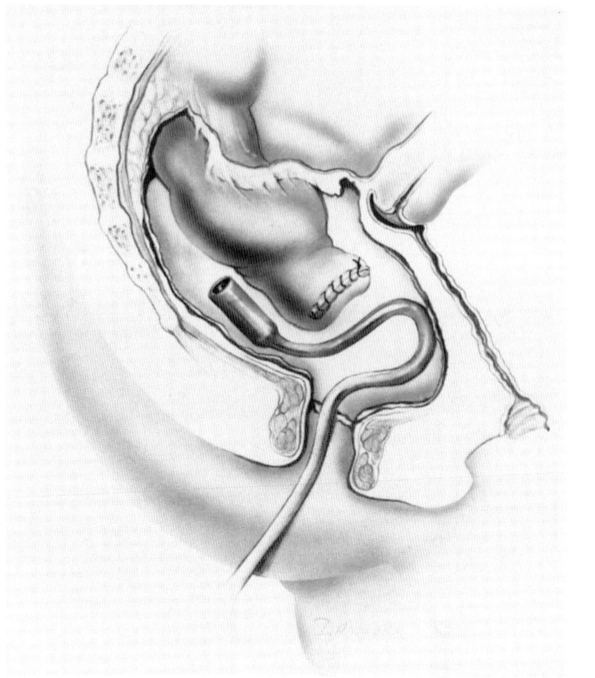

FIG. 62-5. Completion of transanal phase. Copyright Gerald Marks.

pitfall is to dissect in the lateral paraprostatic sulcus. Anterior application of narrow retractors with posterior displacement of the rectum permits appreciation of the arching fibers of the puborectalis muscle, which on transection is one of the few places active bleeding may occur, but this is easily managed with electrocoagulation. Blunt dissection concludes in the region of the seminal vesicles or at the level of the cervix. The transected end of the rectum is then closed with an inverting watertight suture. The pelvis is thoroughly lavaged with topical kanamycin solution, and the pelvis inspected for bleeding. The open end of a #24 red rubber catheter is inserted into the pelvis and fixed externally with a perianal suture (Fig. 62-5). A series of sterile towels covers the perineum and secures the electrocautery probe and suction device for reclaiming during the final perineal phase.

The patient's legs are lowered to 15° of flexion and there is an exchange of instruments, gloves, and gowns, after which the previously prepared and sterile abdomen is addressed by a generous midline or left rectus incision from the symphysis to the xiphoid. Intraperitoneal exploration is carried out with selective intraoperative hepatic sonography. The sigmoidocolic junction is marked with a black silk suture before incising the lateral peritoneal reflection of the sigmoid and left colon. The left colon is mobilized and the splenic flexure released by blunt and sharp retroperitoneal dissection. The omentum is freed to the midpoint of the transverse colon. On total release of the splenic flexure, the colorenal ligament is incised, and the fusion plane between the retroperitoneum and the mesocolon identified. Proceeding along the fusion plane, the retroperitoneum is displaced posteriorly, and the mesocolon is brought medially. The ureter is usually identified without difficulty, but if it is not, it can be found as it crosses the external iliac artery approximately 1 cm lateral to the origin of the hypogastric artery. Once identified, it is gently displaced posteriorly through its course. The lateral peritoneal reflection of the sigmoid colon is incised, and the incision is continued into the pelvis pararectally to the cul-de-sac. The posterior parietal peritoneum to the right of the aorta is incised just inferior to the duodenojejunal junction, and the incision is carried distally over the brim of the pelvis in a pararectal position to the cul-de-sac, where it is brought anteriorly to meet its counterpart. The distal sigmoid colon is encircled with a stout cloth to prevent the sponges that had been introduced into the rectum from migrating proximally. The sigmoid colon is held taut anteriorly, and the hypogastric nerve plexus is visualized and displaced posteriorly. This leads into the plane for the posterior mobilization of the rectum. Once accomplished, the dissection is carried laterally in a usually bloodless plane, and the lateral stalks with the middle hemorrhoidal vessels are identified, transected, and secured. Mobilization of the rectum is remarkably simplified because of the initial transanal stage. The rectum is delivered from the pelvis and covered with an antibiotic-soaked sponge, and the pelvis is filled with antibiotic solution. The inferior mesenteric artery and vein are isolated, and the vein is ligated and interrupted before ligating the artery close to its origin. The inferior mesenteric vein is interrupted again at the level of the duodenojejunal junction as the depth of the mesentery is stepped to provide an adequate length of colon. The ascending branch of the left colic artery and the left branch of the middle colic artery are customarily interrupted. This is performed deep in the mesentery to avoid disturbing the marginal artery.

The site for transection of the descending colon proximal to the previously placed black silk suture is determined, and the mesentery incised to that point. Diverticula noted on the barium enema study should be avoided. The length of bowel necessary to reach the anal canal without tension is determined by a rule of thumb requiring the bowel to lie a comfortable five fingerbreadths distal to the symphysis pubis. A stout cloth tape is tied securely 2 cm proximal to a bowel clamp marking the point of transection (Fig. 62-6). The knot on the tape is usually placed in the left posterior position for subsequent orientation after transection. The end of the bowel is carefully cleansed and covered with a washed glove, and the tape brought through a slit in one of the fingers. The red rubber catheter is retrieved from the pelvis, and the tape is sutured into its open end. After this, the glove finger is brought over the catheter and tied. An assistant moves to the perineal field and places gentle traction on the catheter while the operating surgeon assists by pressing and guiding the bowel into the pelvic floor (Fig. 62-7). The descending colon is passed into, more than pulled into, the pelvis. When the bowel exits the anal canal, it is properly oriented by the knot placement, and the catheter is fixed with a clamp. After an exchange of gowns, gloves, and instruments, the abdomen is redraped and lavaged. A proximal loop transverse colostomy is created and a suction catheter inserted to drain the pelvis. The abdomen is closed and the supported colostomy opened and matured (Fig. 62-8). An effort is made to avoid a diverting loop ileostomy inasmuch as the small bowel may have been exposed to irradiation. On securing the abdominal dressings, the exaggerated lithotomy position is reassumed. The rubber glove covering the colon is carefully teased out of the pelvis, and the anterior wall of the exteriorized bowel is opened transversely from the right to the left lateral positions. The anastomosis is conducted by slight eversion of the anal canal and insertion of a 0-gauge absorbable suture placed first in the anterior mid-

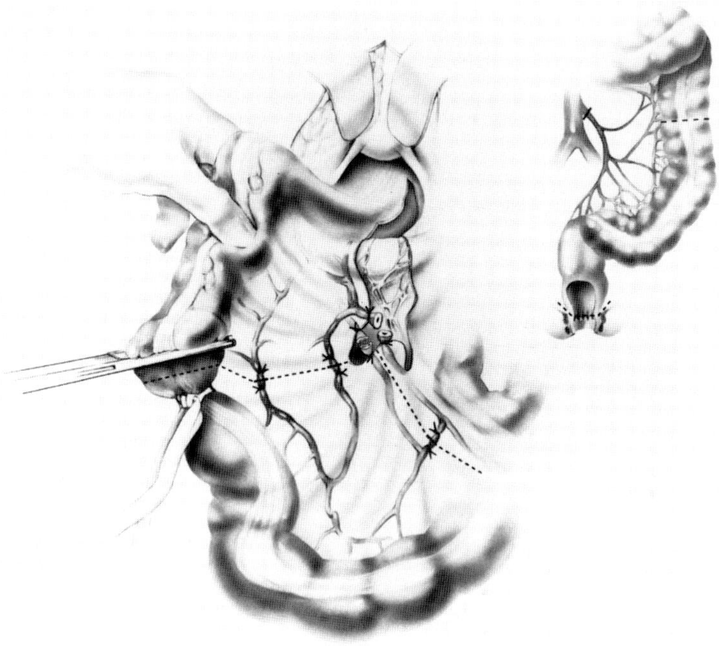

FIG. 62-6. Extent of resection and mesenteric interruption. Copyright Gerald Marks.

line and held (Fig. 62-9). Stout purchases of both the colon and the anal canal wall are considered important. Similar cardinal sutures are placed in the right and left lateral positions and held as well. The transection of the bowel is then completed posteriorly and the last cardinal suture is placed in the posterior midline and held. It is important to avoid inserting a finger or instrument back into the pelvis during this period for fear of contamination. Four intervening sutures are placed in the same manner and tied sequentially. The cardinal sutures are tied to complete the anastomosis. The anastomosis may be checked and additional sutures inserted if required, an uncommon necessity.

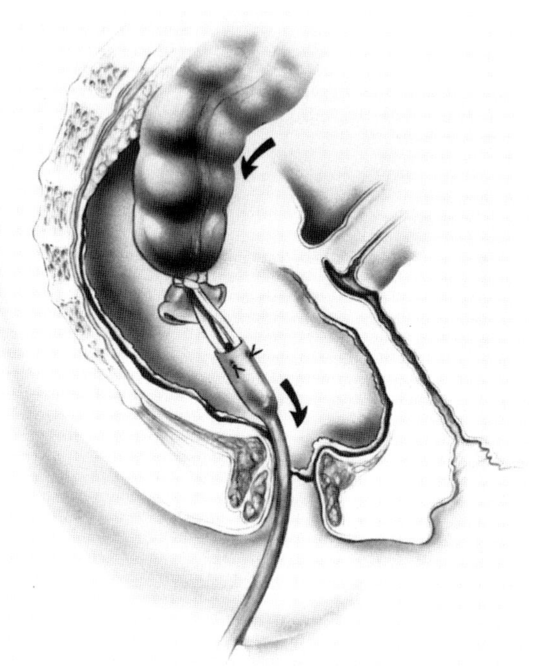

FIG. 62-7. Delivery of proximal bowel. Copyright Gerald Marks.

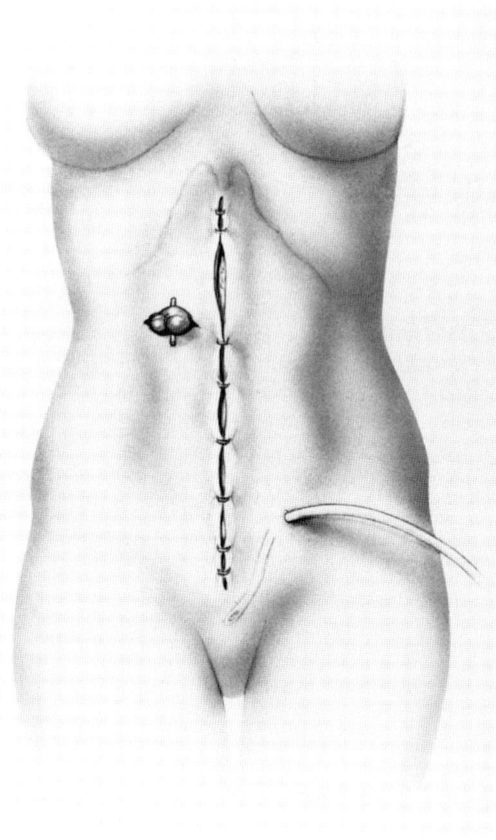

FIG. 62-8. Diverting stoma and pelvic drainage. Copyright Gerald Marks.

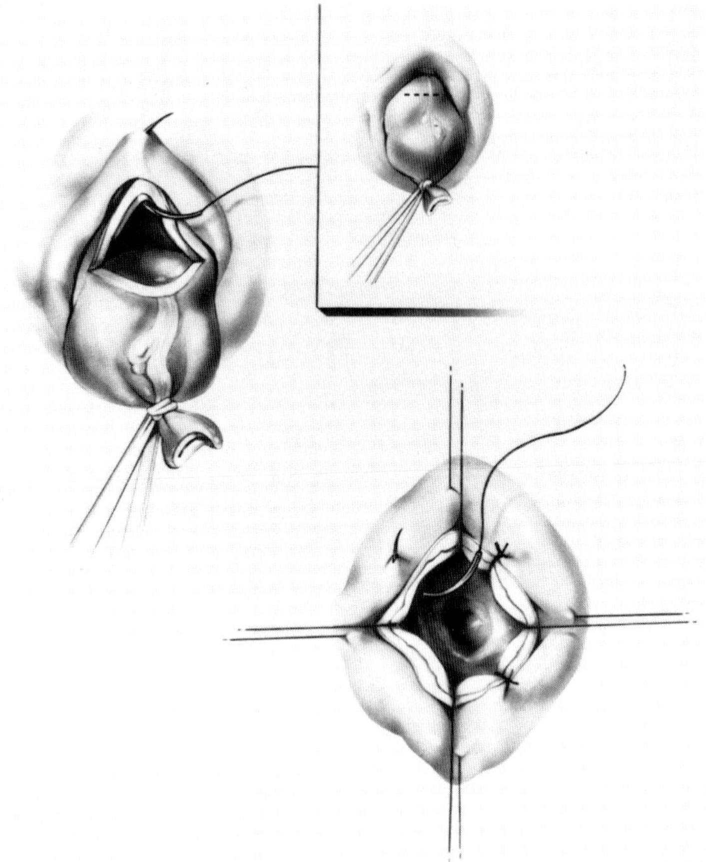

FIG. 62-9. The transanal anastomosis. Copyright Gerald Marks.

PERIOPERATIVE MANAGEMENT

Systemic antibiotics are given for no less than 14 days after surgery because it is our belief that the radiated field is more susceptible to anaerobic infection. The suction catheters are usually removed before the third or fourth day, and it is not uncommon for a small issue of serous fluid to exit through the anal canal between the fourth and seventh day. Irrigation with tap water through the distal stoma begins on the third postoperative week. Digital examination is withheld until the fifth postoperative week, but not delayed beyond the eighth week if stenosis is to be avoided. A water-soluble contrast study performed through the distal stoma is accomplished on the fifth week coincidental to digital rectal examination. Careful narrow-lumen rigid sigmoidoscopy is also performed, allowing inspection for any evidence of purulence, which may be the only hint of a small anastomotic defect. Closure of the stoma is never performed before the eighth postoperative week and only after direct inspection and radiographic studies indicate satisfactory healing. It is mandatory that every digital and rigid sigmoidoscopic examination be conducted with great care. A thoughtlessly rough digital or endoscopic examination may disrupt the anastomosis, an event we have seen as long as 18 months after surgery. Forewarning patients that, immediately after colostomy closure, diarrhea accompanied by temporary incontinence is commonplace, may help avoid emotional trauma. Accommodation to the loss of reservoir rectal function and to the shortened and radiated bowel requires dietary and antidiarrheal measures as well as patience. Maintaining a lactose-free diet is critical. Evaluation of the patient is carried out at 3-month intervals. Digital examination with documentation of extrarectal configuration is desirable to help ensure accurate interpretation of future findings when recurrence is in question. Routine visits are at 3-month intervals for 2 years, then at 4-month intervals until the fifth year, after which 6-month intervals are followed. Carcinoembryonic antigen levels are determined at each visit. Chest roentgenography, computed tomography, and magnetic resonance imaging of the abdomen and pelvis are performed selectively, as is endorectal and endovaginal sonography. Intramural and extrarectal abnormal masses are subjected to endoscopic or computed tomography-guided needle biopsy. Rigid sigmoidoscopy can be accomplished at 6-month intervals and colonoscopy performed at prescribed surveillance intervals. Anal competence is evaluated according to Parks' criteria,[7] which define difficulty in controlling flatus or acute attacks of diarrhea as being in the range of acceptable function.

TABLE 62-1. *Level of cancer in the rectum*

Level (cm)	No. of patients
0.5–1.0	16/65 (25%)
1.1–2.0	25/65 (38%)
2.1–3.0	24 (37%)

TABLE 62-2. *Pattern of local recurrence by postradiation pathologic stage*

Stage	Recurrences/patients
PR STAGE FAVORABLE (N = 35)	
T0 N0	0/10
T1 N0	0/2
T2 N0	0/23
	0/35 (20%)
PR STAGE UNFAVORABLE (N = 30)	
T0 N1	0/1
T2 N1	0/8
T3 N0	2/11
T3 N1	2/6
T2 N2	2/4
	6/30 (20%)
TOTAL	6/65 (9%)

PR, postradiation.

RESULTS

Of the first 82 patients treated by the transanal abdominal transanal radical proctosigmoidectomy with direct coloanal anastomosis procedure, 65 had rectal cancers at or below the 3-cm level. Sixty-six percent were men, and the ages ranged from 29 to 83 years, with a median age of 59 years. Level in the rectum is shown in Table 62-1. Postradiation pathologic stage and local recurrence rates are shown in Table 62-2.

Twenty of the 65 cancers (31%) were fixed at the time of initial examination but became mobile after irradiation. The exclusion of cancers that remain fixed postradiation determines that this select group of patients has a higher percentage of favorable tumors (35/65, 54%) than the series as a whole (78/203, 38%).

Significant perioperative radiation-related morbidity was nonexistent. Radiation therapy was interrupted briefly in less than 5% of patients because of diarrhea. One patient had a small wound infection that responded to antibiotics. Three significant pelvic abscesses occurred; all responded to percutaneous drainage. One major anastomotic disruption occurred and has never been reconstituted. There was one demonstrated radiographic leak that healed spontaneously in which diverticula were presumed to be the source. Mild stricture formations were easily managed by digital dilatation. One patient experienced incontinence attributed to a previously unrecognized obstetrically induced disruption that was repaired with a short-lived benefit. There was one perioperative death from a pulmonary embolism, 55 days from initial surgery. This is the only surgical mortality in the entire series of 274 patients. Age was found to be a factor in the quality of continence. Function is determined by clinical assessment and was satisfactory in all but 5% of patients. There was 100% follow-up in our patients. Six of 65 patients (9%) had local recurrence. The rate of recurrence was less than in the entire series (22/203, 11%). There were no local recurrences among those with postradiation favorable stage (T2 or less) cancers. Kaplan-Meir 5-year actuarial survival for the group is 85%.

The results of the Marks-Mohiuddin program of high-dose preoperative radiation therapy and the transanal abdominal transanal radical proctosigmoidectomy with direct coloanal anastomosis for select cancers of the distal 3 cm of rectum has established the feasibility of radical sphincter preservation surgery with coloanal anastomosis after irradiation for cancers at the very lowest level of the rectum. The enhanced survival and reduced local recurrence rate accomplished with minimal morbidity and mortality attests to the quality-of-life benefits of a selective, multimodality approach to the patient with a postradiated, nonfixed, low-lying rectal cancer.

REFERENCES

1. Marks G, Mohiuddin M, Masoni L, Montori A. High-dose preoperative radiation therapy as the key to extending sphincter-preservation surgery for cancer of the distal rectum. Surgical Oncology Clinics of North America 1992;1:71.
2. Mendenhall WM, Million RR, Bland KI, et al. Preoperative radiation therapy for clinically resectable adenocarcinoma of the rectum. Ann Surg 1985;202:215.
3. Marks G. Combined abdominotranssacral reconstruction of the radiation injured rectum. Am J Surg 1976;131:54.
4. Marks G. Rectal reconstruction by a combined abdominotranssacral approach: report of three cases. Dis Colon Rectum 1973;16:378.
5. Marks G, Mohiuddin M, Borenstein B. Preoperative radiation therapy and sphincter preservation by the combined abdominotranssacral technique for selected rectal cancers. Dis Colon Rectum 1985;28:565.
6. Ahmad N, Marks G, Mohiuddin M. High-dose preoperative radiation for cancer of the rectum: impact of radiation dose on patterns of failure and survival. Int J Radiat Oncol Biol Phys 1993;27:773.
7. Parks AG. Anorectal incontinence. Proc R Soc Med 1975;68:681.

Surgery for Gastrointestinal Cancer: A Multidisciplinary Approach, edited by Harold J. Wanebo.
Lippincott-Raven Publishers, Philadelphia, © 1997.

CHAPTER 63

Management of Rectal Carcinoma

J. Milburn Jessup

Adenocarcinoma of the rectum was diagnosed in approximately 43,000 patients in the United States in 1993, with about 7000 patients dying of their cancer.[1] This common carcinoma constitutes a large part of the oncologic practice of many general surgeons and surgical oncologists. Since the report of Miles[2] in 1908, abdominoperineal resection has been the standard treatment for carcinomas within 12 cm of the anal verge, and involves the resection of anus, rectum, and a portion of the rectosigmoid colon. Abdominoperineal resection has achieved local control of rectal cancer in approximately three quarters of patients. However, it has at least a 10% to 70% incidence of bladder dysfunction, impotence, and infection.[3-12] Older reports suggest that the mortality rate may be as high as 5%,[13,14] although more recent reports indicate that the operative mortality rate is less than 1%.[15] Patients may also find it hard to accept a permanent colostomy.[15] Because conservative surgical procedures combined with chemotherapy and radiation therapy have improved quality of life and yielded survival similar to that for radical resection alone in such other cancers as breast carcinoma and skeletal and soft tissue sarcoma, considerable enthusiasm has been generated for procedures that spare rectal sphincters, avoid a permanent colostomy, and yet achieve both local control and cure at rates similar to that of radical resection. This chapter reviews the conservative management of adenocarcinoma of the rectum: its principles and results. Our focus is on those cancers that are in the low rectum (0 to 6 cm from the anal verge) because lesions that are farther from the anal verge may be treated successfully by anterior resection to achieve sphincter preservation. The chapter first reviews the anatomy that forms the basis for the surgical management of rectal adenocarcinoma. The methods by which the surgeon may objectively select patients for conservative management are reviewed, and the options available for treatment and the current state of results are described. Much of the rationale for a conservative approach to rectal cancer is based on information obtained from radical resection for early stage carcinomas. Therefore, the results of conservative therapy are compared with those of radical resection for similarly staged rectal cancers.

J. Milburn Jessup: Department of Surgery, New England Deaconess Hospital, 110 Francis Street, Boston, MA 02215-6915

SURGICAL ANATOMY OF THE DISTAL RECTUM

The narrow confines of the bony pelvis and the levator ani muscles make a transabdominal approach to the distal rectum difficult. Huber and colleagues[16] have described the surgical anatomy in detail and shown that the rectum lies within a funnel whose neck is formed by the fusion of the levator ani muscles with the muscularis propria of the rectum at the cephalad extent of the internal sphincter muscles, which are approximately 3 cm from the anal verge or 1 cm above the dentate line. This region of the internal sphincter is easily palpable during a digital rectal examination as a muscular band that is termed the anorectal ring (Fig. 63-1). Because the dentate line is approximately 1.5 to 2.0 cm from the anal verge, the anorectal ring is usually 1.5 to 2.0 cm cephalad to the dentate line. Another palpable landmark is the intersphincteric groove, which is 0.5 to 1.0 cm caudad from the dentate line. These landmarks are of practical importance because they represent the boundaries of the anal canal and the rectum. The anal skin is a stratified squamous epithelium that changes to a cuboidal epithelium at the dentate line and extends up the columns of Morgagni.[17] The epithelium then changes to the columnar epithelium that comprises the lining of the rest of the large bowel at the level of the anorectal ring. The extent of this transitional zone of mucosa varies from one person to another, and may extend from the dentate line only to the columns of Morgagni, or further to the level of the anorectal ring. Thus, carcinomas of the anus may be squamous, basaloid, or adenocarcinomas, consistent with the mucosa histologic type. The anatomic landmarks of the anal verge, dentate line, and anorectal ring are confused by many investigators because it is not clear whether proctoscopic or digital landmarks are used. Colorectal surgeons often base their estimates of the location of a rectal carcinoma on the anorectal ring,[18] which is not visible but is palpated, whereas general surgeons often determine location by reference to the anal verge, which is visible but not palpable.[19] It is important to keep this distinction in mind, especially because resection of lesions 1.5 to 3 cm from the anal verge often requires removal of a portion of the anal sphincters with a concomitant increase in complications.[19]

The entrance to the pelvis is 6 cm from the anal verge and extends from the coccyx posteriorly to the bladder or vagina anteriorly and to the levator ani muscles laterally. The funnel

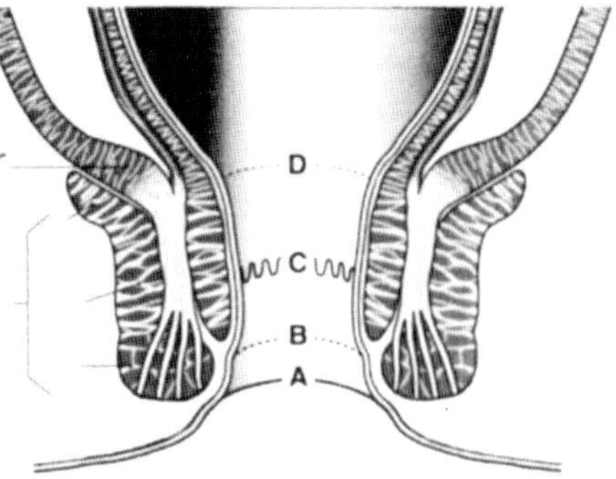

FIG. 63-1. Diagram of anatomy of the rectum and anus. *A*, anal verge; *B*, intersphincteric groove; *C*, dentate line; *D*, anorectal ring. The anal verge and dentate line are identified visually, whereas the intersphincteric groove and the anorectal ring are palpated.

is filled with the adipose tissue of the mesorectum, which is covered by Waldeyer's fascia. Posterior and lateral low rectal cancers that penetrate the rectal wall directly invade the mesorectum and produce micrometastases in the adipose tissue. Low rectal cancers that penetrate the muscularis propria of the anterior rectal wall may invade Denonvillier's fascia and involve either the prostate or bladder in the man or the vagina and uterus in the woman. Thus, most rectal cancer recurrences arise from contiguous spread and occur either at the base of the bladder, prostate, or vagina, or adjacent to the sacrum.[20]

The lymphatic drainage of a carcinoma determines its pattern of nodal metastases and is defined by the distribution of its arterial blood supply. The inferior mesenteric artery terminates in the superior hemorrhoidal artery that supplies the high and middle rectum. In contrast, the low rectum has several sources of arterial supply. The inferior hemorrhoidal and external pudendal arteries supply the distal 2 cm of rectum and anus, whereas the middle hemorrhoidal arteries supply the region 2 to 4 cm from the anal verge, with contributions from the superior hemorrhoidal artery. Because the inferior and middle hemorrhoidal arteries are branches of the internal iliac arteries, lymphatics that course along these arteries drain to lateral pelvic (obturator, iliac) nodes. Lymphatics that follow the external pudendal arteries drain to inguinal nodes associated with the femoral artery, which is the origin of the external pudendal artery. Thus, lymphatic metastases from carcinomas that involve the dentate line may produce metastases in inguinal, iliac, and obturator nodes as well as metastases to the inferior mesenteric and paraaortic nodes.

Invasion of the inferior and the middle hemorrhoidal veins permits rectal carcinoma cells direct access to the systemic circulation and accounts for the higher incidence of lung metastases in rectal cancer compared with colon cancer. Carcinoma cells that invade the superior hemorrhoidal vein from the low rectum enter the portal circulation and traverse the liver first. Thus, the first capillary bed in which a rectal carcinoma metastasis may arrest is either in the lungs or the liver, depending on whether it invades the superior or inferior–middle hemorrhoidal lymphatics or veins.

RECURRENCE PATTERNS IN RECTAL CANCER

Several areas are at high risk for local or regional recurrence of rectal carcinoma based on the anatomy described previously: the obvious regions of contiguous spread in adjacent viscera and sacrum, but also the internal iliac lymph nodes in the pelvic sidewall. Proximal superior hemorrhoidal, inferior mesenteric, or paraaortic nodes may be involved in advanced carcinomas. However, if superior hemorrhoidal or more proximal lymph nodes are involved with metastatic carcinoma, the prognosis is uniformly dismal. The superior hemorrhoidal and inferior mesenteric lymph nodes may be resected as part of the standard abdominoperineal resection by a high ligation of the inferior mesenteric artery, but their resection does not appear significantly to improve survival, and may increase the morbidity of the abdominoperineal resection. The incidence of lateral pelvic lymphatic metastasis in low rectal cancer is as high as 23%.[21–23] This has been used to justify the performance of lateral hypogastric node dissection. However, such a pelvic node dissection has a high morbidity rate, with a 57% incidence of urologic complications (neurogenic bladder, impotence) in patients who have either an abdominoperineal or anterior resection, and incontinence in those patients who have an anterior resection.[24–26] Enker, Block, and their colleagues have suggested that the lateral pelvic node dissection should be part of the standard treatment of rectal cancer.[27,28] However, the benefit in survival may be limited to those stage III patients who have metastases only in pararectal nodes, because none of the patients in their series with lateral pelvic node metastases survived more than 5 years.[28] Similarly, metastasis to lateral pelvic nodes carries a very poor prognosis because only 1 of 48 patients with lateral pelvic node metastasis survived 5 years in the study by Hojo and colleagues.[29] Stearns and Deddish[25] observed that only 1 of 64 patients (2%) with stage I and II lesions subsequently had lateral pelvic nodal metastases, compared with 10 of 58 patients (17%) with stage III lesions. Thus, metastasis to lateral pelvic nodes may occur as a late event after metastasis to pararectal nodes, perhaps because the flow of lymph is altered by the obstruction of lymph flow through pararectal nodal metastases. Surgical clearance of the lateral pelvic nodes would not seem to warrant the morbidity of the extended dissection, because dissemination to systemic sites has probably already occurred if these nodes contain tumor. Even more recent results with parasympathetic node-sparing procedures do not seem significantly to decrease the rate of bladder and sexual dysfunction.[12] Control of lateral pelvic nodal metastases by radiation therapy may be appropriate if the morbidity of such therapy is low.

PROGNOSTIC FACTORS IN RECTAL CARCINOMA

Radical resection of distal rectal cancers may be avoided without compromising cure if objective criteria accurately separate the cancers that are nonmetastatic from those that produce metastases. Those histopathologic characteristics that are directly associated with the production of lymph node and distant metastases are increasing penetration into or through the rectal wall by the primary tumor; progressive loss of differentiation of the neoplastic cells; a high content of mucin in the primary tumor; a border of the tumor that infiltrates rather than pushes into the surrounding margin of tissue; invasion of adjacent blood vessels, lymphatics, or nerves; and ulceration of the tumor. Saclarides and colleagues[30] in a multivariate analysis found that T3 carcinomas, poor differentiation, blood vessel and perineural invasion, and nodes involved with cancer were significant covariates; they did not find that lymphatic involvement was a significant covariate, however, because only a small number of their cancers displayed lymphatic invasion. However, all of the carcinomas that recurred or metastasized had lymphatic invasion! In contrast, Minsky and Cohen[31] found that lymphatic invasion adjacent to the primary cancer was an important indicator of recurrent disease. Cohen and associates[32] demonstrated that the probability of metastasis in regional lymph nodes was only 10% in tumors that were well or moderately differentiated, less than 3 cm in diameter, and exophytic. Similar results were reported by Morson.[33] Further, Jass and colleagues[34] demonstrated that only a 5-mm invasion of the perirectal tissue by the primary carcinoma significantly increased the recurrence of rectal carcinoma. Twenty to 60% of carcinomas that penetrate the serosa (T3) metastasize to regional pararectal lymph nodes, compared with 0% to 20% of carcinomas that invade the submucosa (T1) or the muscularis propria (T2).[32–37] The importance of these prognostic factors in identifying the risk of recurrence is borne out by Pilipshen and coworkers,[38] who reported that 96% of patients who had a pelvic recurrence died of their disease, compared with only 23% of patients who did not have such a local or regional failure. Thus, favorable prognostic markers are defined as T1 or T2 lesions, well or moderately differentiated, without blood vessel, lymphatic or perineural invasion, lacking significant mucin production, without palpable perirectal lymph nodes, and small enough to excise without difficulty (Table 63-1).

Muto and associates[39] and, more recently, molecular biologists[40] suggest that sporadic rectal carcinoma arises from adenomatous polyps that undergo a series of linked genetic mutations and deletions. The precise nature of these genetic alterations is increasingly well understood, and they may serve as prognostic markers to delineate the aggressiveness of colorectal carcinomas. For instance, Jen and colleagues[41] have shown that loss of all or part of an allele of a tumor suppressor gene termed "deleted in colorectal carcinoma" (*DCC*)[42] is associated with a significantly worse outcome in patients with colorectal carcinoma. Thibodeau and coworkers[43] have shown that mutation without loss of *DCC* or *P53*, another tumor suppressor gene, is associated with a significantly better survival than if either gene is deleted. Mutations in other protooncogenes or tumor suppressor genes have not yet been associated convincingly with survival in large prospective series. Thus, in the near future it may be possible to determine the biologic aggressiveness of a rectal cancer by assaying the expression of mutations for selected molecular markers. However, it is not clear at the present time whether such markers should be applied to rectal carcinoma.

TABLE 63-1. *Favorable prognostic factors for local excision of rectal carcinoma*

CURRENTLY ACCEPTED PROGNOSTIC FACTORS
Size <4 cm or 30% circumference of rectum
Lesion above anorectal ring
Lesion is mobile
No palpable perirectal nodes
Well or moderately differentiated
Not mucinous
No invasion of lymphatics, blood vessels, or nerves
PROGNOSTIC FACTORS THAT MAY BE ACCEPTED IN THE FUTURE
Aneuploidy
High proliferation rate
Expression of select phenotypic markers (eg, sucrase-isomaltose)
Genetic alterations (mutation or allelic deletion in *DCC, P53, MSH2, MLH1*)

DNA content, ploidy, and measurement of proliferation by flow cytometry or by static image analysis may be useful prognostic markers. Although several retrospective[44–46] and prospective studies[47–50] suggest that aneuploidy is associated with poor outcome, other studies[51,52] do not show such a significant association. At present, it is not possible to recommend the use of such measures of DNA content of proliferation for determining the metastatic potential of a rectal carcinoma. This may change in the near future, but clinical trials that incorporate these markers of DNA content and proliferation into staging and treatment planning are necessary to determine whether these indices are clinically useful.

THE IMPORTANCE OF THE RADIAL OR LATERAL MARGIN

Performance of a radical resection does not necessarily prevent recurrence of rectal carcinoma. Abdominoperineal resection or anterior resections performed for cure[22,38,53–55] provide 5-year survivals of 72% to 88% for stage I lesions (T1, T2 N0), 57% to 77% for stage II (T3 N0), and 33% to 55% for stage III (T1 to T3 N1 to N2) carcinomas. In addition, local recurrences occur in these patients after radical resections for cure in direct proportion to their stage of disease (0% to 27% for stage I, 12% to 83% for stage II, and 27% to 71% for stage III).[20,22,38,53,56,57] Recurrence does not depend on the proximal and distal margins as much as on the radial or lateral margin in the mesorectum or pararectal tissues closest to adjacent pelvic viscera. Quirke and colleagues[58] observed that 14 of 52 patients who underwent a potentially curative operation for low rectal carcinoma had a positive lateral margin, and that 12 of these patients had a local recurrence. All patients with negative lateral margins remained free of local recurrence for a median of 23 months. An update of this series extended the observations of the lateral margins to 100 rectal carcinomas that had been radically excised.[59] Twenty-six percent had an involved lateral margin, although follow-up was too short to determine whether this translated into local recurrence.[59] Quirke and Scott[59] observed that wide, sharp dissection of the mesorectum did not necessarily clear the lateral margin, because 4 of 20 radically resected rectal cancers had micrometastases within the mesorectum in lymphatic channels and small lymph nodes. Two of these four specimens had tumor involving the lateral margin (10% of the original series). Further, although this is a small series, Quirke and Scott[59] point out that micrometastases more than 3 cm from the primary cancer in the distal mesorectum occurred only in T3 primary cancers that had penetrated more than 4 mm into the perirectal fat. These findings support those of others[34,60–62] that direct extrarectal invasion is associated with greater metastatic potential and poor prognosis. Chan and coworkers[63] report that a lateral margin less than 6 mm for both stage II and III carcinomas was associated with a high recurrence rate in a series of 50 patients who had been resected for cure. In fact, Heald and associates[64] advocate sharp total excision of the mesorectum because they found micrometastases several centimeters beyond the distal edge of the rectal cancer in the mesorectum that would have been left in situ if an extended dissection of the mesorectum was not performed. There were no local recurrences in 50 patients whose mesorectum did not demonstrate any micrometastases. Thus, the amount of tissue removed by an abdominoperineal resection does not guarantee an adequate lateral margin because the narrow confines of the pelvis may not allow the surgeon to achieve a wide resection. As a result, local failure often results from contiguous spread of rectal carcinoma into tissues that are not removed by the surgeon, because removal of such tissues may cause either morbidity or an alteration of lifestyle that is not acceptable to the patient. Further, the presence of micrometastases in the mesorectum is a sign of biologic aggressiveness and poor prognosis. Gunderson and Sosin[20] demonstrated that local recurrence in the perineum or mid-pelvis was a component of 92% of all recurrences in rectal carcinoma, and was the only site of failure in approximately 50% of patients who failed. Because these sites are encompassed within a standard pelvic radiation port, the addition of such other treatment modalities as radiation therapy may sterilize micrometastases in the mesorectum and regional nodes. However, although radiation therapy may decrease local recurrence, the presence of direct tissue invasion and mesorectal metastasis indicates a biologically aggressive carcinoma that may already have metastasized to systemic viscera. Thus, tissue invasion and micrometastases must be considered poor prognostic factors that indicate a need for systemic therapy. Radical surgery alone may not ultimately prevent recurrence or metastasis in these patients.

The role of contiguous spread as the source of recurrence is confirmed by a series of reports on the importance of computed tomography (CT) or magnetic resonance imaging (MRI) in the detection of recurrences after surgery for low rectal carcinoma.[65-69] Most of the lesions in these reports were either at the base of the bladder or the vagina, or in the presacral space at the level of the rectal cancer. Thus, local recurrence is likely to occur if negative lateral margins are not achieved.

PREOPERATIVE IMAGING

Although the evaluation of rectal cancer includes proctoscopy with biopsy to determine whether the cancer is of a favorable size and has good prognostic histologic features, it is important to evaluate the exact location and size of rectal carcinomas as accurately and objectively as possible, especially because even limited penetration into perirectal adipose tissue has significant prognostic consequences. Several studies have attempted to do this with CT or MRI scans. However, it is clear that transrectal ultrasonography (TRUS) appears to be the cheapest and most accurate preoperative imaging modality. Comparison of CT scans to digital examination and TRUS with the final pathologic determination supports the use of both digital examination and TRUS rather than CT scan. Shank and colleagues[70] found that CT imaging of rectal carcinomas could not be used reliably for preoperative staging, whereas Rotte and coworkers[71] reported that TRUS was more reliable than CT scan for preoperative staging. Herzog[72] observed that the accuracy of TRUS was 89% compared with clinical staging and CT imaging, whose accuracies were 71% and 79%, respectively. Although TRUS requires experience and, as a consequence, depends on the skill of the operator, several series[73-77] indicate that use of and familiarity with this technique are increasing. Clearly, TRUS may distinguish those patients whose rectal cancers are limited to the wall (T1 to T2) as opposed to those whose tumors have invaded the wall (T3 to T4). When reports of evaluation of the depth of invasion of the rectal wall by TRUS are combined, the sensitivity for determining T1 to T2 lesions from T3 or T4 lesions is 88%, with a specificity of 96%. This leads to a positive predictive value of 95% and a negative predictive value of 90% (Table 63-2, part A).

TABLE 63-2. *The use of transrectal ultrasonography (TRUS) in evaluating depth of invasion and involvement of perirectal nodes by rectal cancer*

A. Combined analysis of TRUS results in predicting depth of penetration			
	pT1–2	pT3–4	Totals
uT1–2	574	29	603
uT3–4	78	674	752
Totals	652	703	1355
B. TRUS evaluation of perirectal nodal metastases in rectal cancer patients			
	pN0	pN1	Totals
uN0	474	101	575
uN1	103	340	443
Totals	577	441	1018

Results from references 73 through 77 were pooled and arranged as indicated. See text for details of sensitivity, specificity, and predictive values.

However, TRUS is not as precise for the detection of nodal metastases.[73-77] The sensitivity for detecting nodal metastases by TRUS is 77%, with a specificity of 88%, a positive predictive value of 77%, and a negative predictive value of 82% (see Table 63-2, part B). These data are important because TRUS may be used competently to predict which rectal carcinomas may be most amenable to local excision. Although the results of TRUS may be equivalent to the digital examination of an experienced surgeon, it is clear that TRUS aids the surgeon who is less experienced in examining rectal cancers. In addition, as the imaging with TRUS continues to improve, the accuracy of detecting lymph nodes involved with metastasis will also improve. If involved nodes are identified reliably, then patients may receive systemic therapy that is better destined to help them. A conservative approach should not be taken with patients who may have bulky, nonpalpable perirectal nodes. On the other hand, small (<3 mm) perirectal nodes may be sterilized by external beam radiation therapy.[78] Nuclear MRI with an endorectal coil provides excellent and detailed images of the rectal mucosa as well as nodes. However, the added expense of such MRI scans may far outweigh the increased accuracy in preoperative staging. As a result, it is important to compare endorectal MRI scans with images obtained by TRUS. The ability to image nodes accurately would be a major advance in deciding which treatment is best for patients with rectal carcinoma.

PREOPERATIVE RADIATION THERAPY IN RECTAL CANCER

Because neither abdominoperineal nor anterior resection eliminate local recurrence in the pelvis, investigators have attempted to add other treatments to improve local control of rectal cancer. Gunderson and Sosin[20] analyzed patients at the University of Minnesota who underwent second-look surgery and observed that most local recurrences of rectal carcinoma are within the pelvic port of a radiation therapy field and that postoperative radiation therapy should decrease recurrence. Rich and coworkers[79] later demonstrated in a nonrandomized study at the Massachusetts General Hospital that postoperative adjuvant radiation therapy significantly decreased local recurrences for each stage of rectal carcinoma. Romsdahl and Withers[80] observed a similar reduction in local recurrence with postoperative radiation therapy, but did not notice any improvement in patient survival. The administration of 20 to 45 Gy before operation has the theoretic advantage that undisturbed, oxygenated tissues should be more susceptible to ionizing radiation than the relatively avascular planes created by surgery that are treated with postoperative radiation. Further, more than two thirds of nodal metastases are less than 4 mm in diameter,[81] and hence may be controlled by radiation therapy. When preoperative radiation therapy was administered in either a randomized[82] or nonrandomized[83] study, there appeared to be significant downstaging of regional disease because the frequency of lymphatic metastases was decreased in irradiated patients. However, Cedermark and associates[84] did not observe any significant improvement in local control or survival in a randomized trial of preoperative radiation therapy in which patients received 25 Gy to the tumor and pelvis 1 week before surgery; nor did a subsequent trial by the Veterans Administration confirm their first study.[85]

The dose of preoperative radiation therapy may need to be greater than 25 Gy to achieve a measurable biologic effect. Marks and colleagues have aggressively pursued this by irradiating patients with 40 to 55 Gy before surgery and then performing sphincter-saving operations for lower and middle rectal carcinomas that were T3 or T4 lesions, with good results.[86,87] Seven of 43 patients (16%) with carcinoma within 6 cm of the anal verge had a local recurrence, whereas 86% of patients were continent after resection. Fleishman and colleagues[88] reported similar results with anterior resection for rectal carcinomas after 20 to 45 Gy, with a local recurrence rate of less than 2% in a series of 102 patients, 23 of whom had Dukes' C lesions. Fleishman and colleagues[88] stressed that successful healing after preoperative radiation required the advancement of nonirradiated descending colon into the pelvis to provide sufficient blood supply to heal the anastomosis. Papillon and associates[89] reported that 41 patients with more advanced T2 to T4 primary adenocarcinomas in the distal rectum underwent sphincter-saving operations 8 weeks after receiving 30 Gy over 12 days. Anastomotic or rectovaginal fistulas developed in five patients. Thirty of these 41 patients were followed for more than 2 years, and only 1 had a local recurrence, which was salvaged by an abdominoperineal resection. Nine patients did not have any residual cancer in their surgical specimens, whereas 12 patients were T1N0, 5 were T2 to T3N0, and 4 were TN1. None of these patients had local excisions, but underwent either anterior resection or anterior resection with coloanal anastomosis. The results of Papillon and coworkers[89] reinforce those of Fleishman and colleagues[88] in that superior results are obtained in selected patients when the surgeon brings fresh, nonirradiated tissue into the pelvis. In contrast, Marks and associates[87] reported a small series of highly selected patients who received 45 Gy followed 4 to 6 weeks later by a local excision. In the hands of this excellent surgeon, 13 of 14 patients retained good sphincter function. However, three patients had local recurrence. Although these patients may have had unfavorable carcinomas at the beginning of the external beam radiation therapy, it is not clear whether these lesions were downstaged. In addition, these lesions were 0 to 7 cm from the anorectal ring or 3 to 10 cm from the anal verge. Some of these carcinomas may have undergone anterior resection with coloanal anastomosis. It is hard to determine from any of these studies how much reduction in stage actually occurred with preoperative radiation therapy because objective pretreatment and posttreatment staging was not available.

Other trials also indicate that preoperative radiation therapy must be greater than 25 Gy to decrease the incidence of local recurrence, but not improve overall survival. A Japanese study[90] showed that full-course preoperative radiation therapy with 42.6 Gy for low-lying rectal cancers induced a greater than 50% reduction in the volume of the primary cancer in 80% of the patients. Interestingly, preoperative radiation therapy may not significantly change the size and stage of disease when surgery is performed within 2 weeks after 20 Gy delivered in five or fewer fractions, although the radiation effect may make the analysis of the state of differentiation difficult.[91] The ability of preoperative radiation therapy to reduce local recurrence was identified in a prospective, randomized trial performed by the European Organization for the Research and Treatment of Cancer[92] in which local recurrence was significantly decreased in the group of patients who received 34.5 Gy in 19 fractions, from 30% in the surgery alone control subjects to 15% in the preoperative treatment group. The decrease in local recurrence did not translate into a significant improvement in survival at 5 years for the whole group (69% 5-year survival in those who had preoperative radiation therapy and potentially curative surgery, vs. 59% for curative surgery alone, $P = 0.08$). Another randomized, prospective trial[93] was reported from Sweden in which patients with resectable rectal carcinomas were randomized to receive either 25 Gy over 5 to 7 days and radical surgery, or radical surgery alone. A significant reduction in pelvic recurrence was seen for the group of patients who received preoperative radiation therapy as well as for each stage. There was a prolonged time to recurrence in these patients but not a significant improvement in outcome. This is not surprising because the radiation therapy treats only the local disease and does not affect potential micrometastases established outside the surgical field or radiation port. These data also suggest that tissues that have not yet been surgically disturbed may be more susceptible to the lethal effects of external beam radiation than tissues that may be hypoxic after large dissections during radical surgery. As a consequence, these results in stage II and III rectal carcinoma support the concept that external beam radiation therapy applied to undisturbed tissue may improve the control of metastases that exist in regional tissues at the time of treatment of early-stage primary cancer.

COMBINED CHEMOTHERAPY AND RADIATION THERAPY FOR RECTAL CARCINOMA

Although preoperative radiation therapy may decrease local recurrence, it has not been widely accepted, presumably because it may downstage the pathologic specimen and hinder wound healing without altering the potential for metastases outside the pelvis. However, current consensus indicates that radiation therapy should be part of the postoperative adjuvant therapy of rectal cancer that has penetrated the rectal wall or metastasized to regional nodes.[94] The Gastrointestinal Tumor Study Group (GITSG) randomized patients with stage II or III lesions to receive either surgery alone, postoperative radiation therapy (40 to 48 Gy), adjuvant 5-fluorouracil and methyl-CCNU, or combined chemotherapy and radiation therapy. Postoperative radiation therapy combined with 5-fluorouracil and methyl-CCNU significantly decreased local recurrence with an insignificant decrease in distant metastasis.[95] Neither radiation therapy nor chemotherapy alone achieved the same effect on either local or distant recurrence in these patients. The effect of combined chemoradiation therapy has translated into a significant improvement in survival with longer follow-up.[96] A significant effect of adjuvant chemotherapy on survival was observed in the National Surgical Adjuvant Bowel and Breast Project protocol R-01.[97] Patients with stage II or III rectal carcinoma were randomized to either surgery alone, chemotherapy with methyl-CCNU, 5-fluorouracil, and vincristine, or radiation therapy. Both chemotherapy and radiation therapy significantly decreased local recurrence, but only chemotherapy significantly improved the disease-free survival of patients. Unfortunately, this R-01 trial did not contain an arm that combined radiation therapy with chemotherapy. However, a third study from the North Central Cancer Treatment Group supports the GITSG study and demonstrates a decrease in local recurrence and improved disease-free survival in patients with rectal cancer who receive both chemotherapy and radiation therapy.[98] Thus, the standard of practice for adenocarcinomas of the rectum that penetrate the rectal wall (stage II) or involve regional lymph nodes (stage III) is a radical resection followed by chemotherapy and radiation therapy.

RESULTS OF CONSERVATIVE SURGERY ALONE FOR CARCINOMA OF THE DISTAL RECTUM

In the past, patients with carcinoma of the distal rectum were chosen for local excision based on the clinical evaluation of containment of cancer within the rectal wall, the absence of poor prognostic indicators on a pretreatment biopsy, or because patients were medically unfit for radical resection. Patients have undergone a variety of local excision, intraluminal radiation therapy, or repetitive electrocautery desiccation procedures for favorable rectal cancers and have enjoyed 5-year survival rates of 80% to 90%.[99–107] Excision is usually performed by the transanal approach, although several series used a posterior parasacral or transsphincteric technique. Although the transanal approach is easier and may be accomplished with a low complication rate, the posterior sacral approaches have the advantage that the surgeon may evaluate the mesorectum, where small deposits of metastatic carcinoma may be found that would otherwise have escaped detection. The transsphincteric technique was popularized by York Mason,[108,109] although the transsacral method of Kraske[110] provides similar exposure by removing the coccyx. Posterior and lateral rectal cancers within 6 cm of the anal verge are easily excised by either posterior sacral approach, and anterior rectal cancers can be removed through a proctostomy made in the posterior wall of the rectum. One of the earliest series of conservatively managed rectal cancers is from St. Mark's Hospital in England, and was updated by Lock and colleagues in 1993.[111] In this series, 152 patients underwent a local excision of small cancers according to the clinical impression of the "favorability" of the cancer as evaluated by the surgeon. Grade was deemed important because the recurrence rate was highest in poorly differentiated cancers. This observation led to a "policy" that if excision of an otherwise favorable rectal cancer (see Table 63-1) revealed either positive margins or poor grade, the patient was advised to have a radical resection. In an era when patients did not receive chemoradiation, the St. Mark's experience is excellent because locoregional failure occurred in only 12 patients (8%). This British series remains a goal for other conservative trials. Unfortunately, the depth of penetration of the bowel wall is not described, so it is hard to compare this series, which includes pedunculated polypoid cancers along with some colonic lesions, with more recent series in which at least the T stage criterion is objectively measured in distal rectal cancer.

The rates of local control are presented for several series[102,103,112–115] in which local excision without pelvic radiation was performed on rectal carcinomas that were analyzed for depth of bowel wall invasion with a minimum 2.5-year follow-up (Table 63-3). Clearly, local excision alone has an incidence of local failure that is proportional to the depth of wall invasion by the tumor (9% for T1, 20% for T2, and 22% for T3, cumulative results from Table 63-3). Thus, subclinical metastases in pararectal tissues must be treated with another modality to improve local control with conservative surgery.

Does external beam radiation after local excision improve the control of pelvic recurrence in a manner similar to that achieved with preoperative radiation therapy in patients undergoing a radical resection? Can chemotherapy added to radiation therapy improve the local control of rectal cancers that have been locally excised so that the local failure rate matches that achieved by radical resection? Rich and coworkers[99] demonstrated that external beam radiation therapy enhanced local control of rectal cancers removed with microscopically or grossly positive margins. None of the 16 patients failed locally if he or she received more than 45 Gy. These results first suggested that the addition of external beam radiation therapy to local excision of a rectal carcinoma may improve local control. Because multicenter trials had shown that chemotherapy may enhance the effect of radiation therapy to achieve local control, several institutions initiated prospective trials that included systemic chemotherapy with radiation therapy in the conservative management of rectal carcinoma.

The current status of institutional prospective trials of local excision and postoperative radiation therapy suggests that the combination (with or without chemotherapy as a radiosensitizer) improves local control in these patients. When 45 Gy or more is administered to the pelvis, the local and regional failure for T1, T2, and T3 lesions is reduced to 4%, 10%, and 22%, respectively[114–120] (Table 63-4). Radiation therapy has the most impact on T2 lesions because it may decrease locoregional failure by 50%, from 20% to 10% (see Tables 63-3 and 63-4). The impact of radiation therapy on T1 lesions is less dramatic but still represents a 50% reduction. Clearly, the addition of radiation therapy to local excision for T3 lesions does not affect

TABLE 63-3. *Local or regional failure in patients with rectal carcinoma who have only a local excision*

	T stage		
Series	T1	T2	T3
Huber and Koella, 1992[112]	2/9	3/13	2/6
Gall and Hermanek, 1992[113]	4/39	4/19	3/10
Jessup, et al, 1992[114]	2/12	—	—
Coco, et al, 1992[115]	0/20		
Stearns, et al. 1984[102]	1/15	2/14	1/2
Grigg, et al, 1984[103]	1/16		
Totals	10/111 (9%)	9/46 (20%)	4/18 (22%)

Results from individual series in which selected rectal adenocarcinomas were locally excised using a standard transanal or posterior sacral approach. Patients did not receive any other therapy. Mean follow-up is in excess of 3 years. Results are given by depth of invasion (T) as number of failures/total number who underwent excision.

locoregional failure, although the numbers of patients described are small.

Local excision of selected rectal adenocarcinomas, especially when followed by pelvic radiation, appears to have similar locoregional control and overall survival as expected for radically resected stage I rectal cancer. In direct institutional comparisons, both Coco and associates[115] and Willett and colleagues[121] compared the local control and survival of conservatively managed rectal cancers with radically resected cancers. Coco and associates[115] reported that conservatively treated T1 or T2 patients had a 3% locoregional recurrence rate with a 6% cancer-specific death rate, whereas patients with stage I rectal cancer had a 6% locoregional failure rate and a 10% cancer-specific death rate, with both groups followed for a median of at least 5 years. Willett and colleagues[121] presented similar data from the Massachusetts General Hospital, although patients with poor prognostic factors had better local control (89% in 20 patients with abdominoperineal resection vs. 68% in 28 patients with local excision and radiation therapy) and recurrence-free survival (57% at 5 years in the conservative treatment group compared with 79% at 5 years in the abdominoperineal resection group) after radical surgery. Thus, although the outcome of favorable, small rectal cancers treated conservatively was similar to that of radically resected cancers, the outcome of high-risk cancers was improved by radical surgery. The role of chemoradiation added to radical surgery in these high-risk patients is not clear. Nonetheless, the series reported by Willett and colleagues[121] is instrumental in reminding clinicians that the conservative management of rectal cancer depends on the careful, objective selection of favorable lesions. Our current policy at the New England Deaconess Hospital is to attempt local excision of those adenocarcinomas of the distal rectum that clinically are less than 4 cm in diameter or 30% of rectal circumference, mobile, nonulcerated, well or moderately differentiated, and without mucin production. A pelvic CT scan is obtained to exclude patients with detectable pararectal or pelvic lymph node metastases.

ALTERNATIVE APPROACHES TO LOCAL EXCISION OF RECTAL CANCERS

An alternative approach to the local excision of rectal cancers is the use of transanal endoscopic microsurgery. Among the first authors to write about this were Weese and Bruskewitz,[122] who used a urologic resectoscope to remove rectal carcinomas. The cancer was resected in a piecemeal fashion, similar to electrocoagulation, and the procedure suffers from an inability to determine depth of invasion. Because the depth of invasion must be known to estimate the probability of recurrence, this technique is difficult to espouse. However, more recently, several centers in Europe have developed another transanal endo-

TABLE 63-4. *Local failure in patients with rectal cancer treated with local excision with postoperative radiation therapy (± chemotherapy)*

	T stage		
Series	T1	T2	T3
Summers et al, 1992[116]	1/13	1/4	—
Massachusetts General Hospital, 1989[117]	1/10	2/11	1/3
Jessup, et al, 1992[114]	—	0/13	0/2
Ota, et al, 1992[118]	0/16	1/15	3/15
Minsky, 1993[119]	0/4	2/12	2/6
Coco, et al, 1992[115]		1/15	0/1
Rosenthal et al, 1992[120]	0/2	1/9	1/5
Totals	2/45 (4%)	8/79 (10%)	7/32 (22%)

Results from individual prospective series with results presented as described in Table 63-3. Patients in these series received at least 45 Gy to the pelvis, with some patients receiving chemotherapy, usually as a radiation sensitizer.

scopic microsurgery approach. In this, a proctoscope is fitted with three or more channels and a gas casket that allows stereoscopic visualization and the use of instruments while maintaining a gas phase that distends the rectum. The technique was originally developed for the excision of adenomatous polyps in the rectum, but has been applied to the management of rectal carcinomas. The authors are adept at this endoscopic approach and have developed methods of cauterizing blood vessels as well as reapproximating the mucosal defect after a full-thickness excision of a rectal cancer. Buess and coworkers[123] published a series in which 74 carcinomas (51 pT1, 17 pT2, and 6 pT3) were resected using such an endoscopic microsurgery approach. There was one local recurrence in this series. The T3 patients were encouraged to have an abdominoperineal resection. Interestingly, the complication rate was a 9% incidence of rectovaginal fistula or anastomotic fistula; however, only 2 patients required colostomy. Similar results were obtained by Said and colleagues[124] from Cologne, Germany, who performed the transanal endoscopic microsurgery procedure on 233 patients, of whom 22 had T1 rectal carcinomas. The incidence of complications was 6%, but 4.9% of the adenomas recurred. This rate seems high and suggests an incomplete resection even though the authors indicate that they had a 1-cm margin around their tumors on the specimens. Finally, Heintz and associates[125] published another series of 239 endoscopic microsurgical resections that included 66 rectal carcinomas. The complication rate for this series was low at 3%. This series had good pathologic analysis because patients were categorized by T stage as well as other parameters of risk. There was only 1 local recurrence in 21 "Low Risk" T1 lesions, compared with 1 in 5 "High Risk" T1 lesions. Similarly, only 1 of 4 "Low Risk" T2 rectal carcinomas recurred locally, compared with 4 of 6 "High Risk" T2 rectal carcinomas. Adjuvant radiation therapy was not applied, so it was not clear whether the performance of this series is worse than that of other series that include local excision and radiation therapy. Nonetheless, it appears that transanal endoscopic microsurgery is a potentially useful technique that may be applied to the excision of rectal cancers.

MORE RADICAL APPROACHES TO EFFECT SPHINCTER PRESERVATION

Lesions that are above the anorectal ring but penetrate the rectal wall, involve perirectal lymph nodes, or involve more than 30% of the circumference of the rectal wall, usually need more radical surgery than a local excision to achieve negative tissue margins. Although combination chemoradiation therapy may improve local and systemic control, clearly T3NO or T3N1 lesions should have more than a local excision, if only to ensure local control. As a result, surgeons have developed two techniques to perform radical surgery with sphincter preservation. The first was the abdominosacral approach described by Localio and recently updated. Eng and Localio[126] compared their results with 156 patients treated with the abdominosacral approach to their results with anterior resection in 261 patients and 136 abdominoperineal resections. Five-year survival was lowest in the abdominoperineal resection group (51.4%), compared with 67.9% for the abdominosacral group and 67.8% for the anterior resection group. Locoregional recurrences were similar in all three groups. The lower survival in the abdominoperineal resection group may represent patient selection, because only midrectal cancers were considered candidates for the abdominosacral procedure.

The second radical approach involves extending the anterior resection to the level of the internal sphincters and performing coloanal anastomosis. In this procedure, the rectum is excised with sharp dissection of the mesorectum from the levator ani muscles and the descending colon is anastomosed to either the dentate line (after the mucosa and submucosa have been excised by the perineal approach to the level of the anorectal ring) or slightly higher to the level of the anorectal ring. Because the internal sphincter must be left intact, it is important that the anorectal ring not be disturbed. Because rectal carcinomas may spread through the layers of the rectal wall for distances of at least 2 cm,[54] ideally cancers should be 2 cm from the anorectal ring or 4 to 5 cm from the anal verge. The results of surgery, especially if combined with adjuvant chemoradiation therapy, are similar to what can be achieved with abdominoperineal resection. In a pilot study, Cohen and associates[127] found that anterior resection with coloanal anastomosis could be performed safely, and that sphincter function was acceptable even though patients had an increased frequency of stools. Because creating a colonic J-pouch did not alter stool frequency, Cohen and associates[127] suggested that a straight coloanal anastomosis was sufficient. These results are similar to those of Frigell and colleagues,[128] who reported that although patients with conventional anterior resections had increased numbers of stools per day and a several-month period of adaptation to new bowel function, patients overwhelmingly wanted sphincter preservation rather than the colostomy that is produced by the abdominoperineal resection. An update by Paty and coworkers[129] of the Memorial Sloan-Kettering Cancer Center experience indicates that 89% of 134 patients undergoing anterior resection with coloanal anastomosis achieved local control at 5 years. This is an excellent result, especially because 67 (50%) of the patients had T3 lesions! Paty and coworkers[129] also suggest that preoperative radiation therapy may be better tolerated than postoperative radiation therapy, although the data concerning resultant sphincter function were not fully detailed. It is also important to note that a distal margin of less than 2 cm was not associated with local recurrence. One reason for this may be that distal margins may have been closer in T1 or T2 lesions, where the local excision data indicate that a 1-cm margin may be adequate, especially if chemoradiation is added. In addition, local recurrences in this prospective series were associated with T3 invasion, positive nodes, or other poor prognostic factors. The only T2N0 moderately differentiated carcinoma that recurred had a microscopically positive margin (Table 3 in Paty and coworkers[129]). Thus, in selected, bulky T1 to T2 lesions, it may be possible to have closer margins than 2.0 cm. Future studies will be needed before that conclusion is firmly established.

However, there are two situations in which coloanal anastomosis after low anterior resection may not be advantageous. First, involvement of rectal sphincters precludes a coloanal anastomosis if more than 15% to 20% of sphincter is excised, especially if the lateral wall is involved, because patients will be incontinent. Second, patients whose tumors are deeply invasive may not achieve the necessary negative radial margin for good local control. On the other hand, a radical abdominoperineal resection may also not achieve negative margins in patients with these tumors. Thus, although coloanal anastomosis offers an opportunity for rectal sphincter preservation in patients with minimal transmural invasion, it may not be appropriate for more deeply penetrating lesions. The ability to achieve local control with preservation of continence is still preliminary, although the data suggest that coloanal anastomosis preserves continence and has a local failure rate that is similar to that achieved with abdominoperineal resection.

SALVAGE

Despite the most careful selection of patients for conservative management of rectal cancer and advances in multimodality therapy, progressive disease may still develop in some patients. Visceral metastases need to be treated with systemic therapy, but locoregional failure may be salvaged by aggressive surgery if recurrence is detected before it becomes unresectable. The estimate of the incidence of successful salvage of pelvic recurrence is not clear. However, several reports estimate that between 25% and 50% of locoregional failures[111,130–132] may be salvaged by either an abdominoperineal resection or, occasionally, another local excision. In one series with a high locoregional failure rate after electrocoagulation,[130] four of five successfully salvaged patients had an abdominoperineal resection, whereas one had a local excision and remained free of disease for more than 3 years. Bailey and colleagues[131] reported that two of four local recurrences in their series were salvaged by local reexcision. In the St. Mark's series,[111] one third of the local recurrences were salvaged by further surgery, with two of the seven patients undergoing reexcision. Thus, patients must be closely followed by their surgeon, who does a digital rectal examination several times a year. TRUS may also be useful in detecting pararectal recurrences. If recurrences are detected early, then many of these patients may be salvaged by further surgery.

SUMMARY

The data presented in this review suggest that if the surgeon extirpates a primary cancer confined to the rectal wall by a local excision, with negative margins confirmed by the pathologist, then the addition of chemoradiation therapy should provide local control as good if not better than that expected with an abdominoperineal resection. Patients should be objectively selected for this procedure by preoperative histologic characteristics and endorectal ultrasonography. Outcome has not been considered in this review because surgery and radiation therapy are modalities that treat only the local disease and do not have an impact on survival unless there is persistent local failure. Because the incidence of local failure is reasonably low, the outcome should be similar to what is observed with radical resection. However, the various series are still too premature to comment on. The outcome seen to date may reflect selection of patients who have metastases in perirectal nodes limited to 3 mm or less, a tumor volume that may be sterilized by chemoradiation. The validity of the conservative approach to rectal cancer needs to be proven by a large, prospective, multicenter trial such as that currently under investigation as an intergroup trial under the auspices of the Cancer and Acute Leukemia Group B and the Radiation Therapy Oncology Group. In such a setting there are sufficient numbers of patients who are rigorously and objectively selected for study. Local failure, when it occurs, is devastating, especially if it occurs after an abdominoperineal resection. Surgical salvage of patients failing a local excision is feasible and may be easier after local excision than after abdominoperineal resection because tissue planes are not disturbed. The use of coloanal anastomosis with low anterior resection may be appropriate for more advanced lesions, but more experience is required with this procedure before it should be accepted as standard practice.

ACKNOWLEDGMENT

Supported in part by grants CA42587 and CA44704 from the National Institutes of Health, Bethesda, Maryland.

REFERENCES

1. Boring CC, Squires TS, Tong T. Cancer statistics, 1993. CA Cancer J Clin 1993;43:7.
2. Miles WE. A method of performing abdominoperineal excision for carcinoma of the rectum and of the terminal portion of the pelvic colon. Lancet 1988;2:1812.
3. Weinstein M, Roberts M. Sexual potency following surgery for rectal carcinoma. Ann Surg 1977;185:295.
4. Danzi M, Ferulano GP, Abate S, Califano G. Male sexual function after abdominoperineal resection for rectal cancer. Dis Colon Rectum 1983;26:665.
5. Balslev I, Harling H. Sexual dysfunction following operation for carcinoma of the rectum. Dis Colon Rectum 1983;26:785.
6. Williams JT, Slack WW. A prospective study of sexual function after colorectal surgery. Br J Surg 1980;67:772.
7. Yeager ES, van Heerden JA. Sexual dysfunction following proctocolectomy and abdominoperineal resection. Ann Surg 1980;191:169.
8. Kinn A-C, Ohman U. Bladder and sexual function after surgery for rectal cancer. Dis Colon Rectum 1986;29:43.
9. Fowler JW, Bremner DN, Moffat LEF. The incidence and consequences of damage to the parasympathetic nerve supply to the bladder after abdominoperineal resection of the rectum for carcinoma. Br J Urol 1978;50:95.
10. Gerstenberg TC, Nielsen ML, Clausen S, Blaabjerg J, Lindenberg J. Bladder function after abdominoperineal resection of the rectum for anorectal cancer: urodynamic investigation before and after operation in a consecutive series. Ann Surg 1980;191:81.
11. Lea JW, Covington K, McSwain B, Scott HW. Surgical experience with carcinoma of the colon and rectum. Ann Surg 1982;195:600.
12. Hojo K, Vernava AM III, Sugihara K, Katumata K. Preservation of urine voiding and sexual function after rectal cancer surgery. Dis Colon Rectum 1991;34:532.
13. Hughes ESR, McDermott FT, Masterton JP, Cunningham IGE, Polglase AL. Operative mortality following excision of the rectum. Br J Surg 1980;67:49.
14. Payne JE, Chapuis PH, Pheils MT. Surgery for large bowel cancer in people aged 75 years and older. Dis Colon Rectum 1986;29:733.
15. Fick TE, Baeten CG, von Meyenfeldt MF, Obertop H. Recurrence and survival after abdominoperineal and low anterior resection for rectal cancer, without adjunctive therapy. Eur J Surg Oncol 1990;16:105.
16. Huber A, von Hochstetter AHC, Allgower M. Transsphincteric surgery of the rectum: topographical anatomy and operation technique. Berlin: Springer-Verlag, 1984;1.
17. Schrock TR. Examination of the anorectum, rigid sigmoidoscopy, flexible sigmoidoscopy and diseases of the anorectum. In: Sleisenger MH, Fordtran JS, eds. Gastrointestinal disease: pathophysiology, diagnosis, management. 4th ed. Philadelphia: WB Saunders, 1989:1570.
18. Marks G, Mohiuddin M, Goldstein SD. Sphincter preservation for cancer of the distal rectum using high dose preoperative radiation. Int J Radiat Oncol Biol Phys 1988;15:1065.

19. McCready DR, Ota DM, Rich TA, Thielvoldt D, Jessup JM. Prospective phase I trial of conservative management of low rectal lesions. Arch Surg 1989;124:67.
20. Gunderson LL, Sosin H. Areas of failure found at reoperation (second or symptomatic look) following "curative surgery" for adenocarcinoma of the rectum. Cancer 1974;34:1278.
21. Cass AW, Million RR, Pfaff WW. Patterns of recurrence following surgery alone for adenocarcinoma of the colon and rectum. Cancer 1976;37:2861.
22. Brown CE, Warren S. Visceral metastasis from rectal carcinoma. Surg Gynecol Obstet 1938;66:611.
23. Sugarbaker PH, Corlew S. Influence of surgical techniques on survival in patients with colorectal cancer: a review. Dis Colon Rectum 1982; 25:545.
24. Sauer I, Bacon HE. A new approach for excision of carcinoma of the lower portion of the rectum and anal canal. Surg Gynecol Obstet 1952; 95:229.
25. Stearns MW Jr, Deddish MR. Five-year results of abdominopelvic lymph node dissection for carcinoma of the rectum. Dis Colon Rectum 1959;2:169.
26. Glass RE, Ritchie JK, Thompson HR, Mann CV. The results of surgical treatment of cancer of the rectum by radical resection and extended abdominoiliac lymphadenectomy. Br J Surg 1985;72:599.
27. Enker WE, Laffer UT, Block GE. Enhanced survival of patients with colon and rectal cancer is based upon wide anatomic resection. Ann Surg 1979;190:350.
28. Enker WE, Heilweil ML, Hertz RE, et al. En bloc pelvic lymphadenectomy and sphincter preservation in the surgical management of rectal cancer. Ann Surg 1986;203:426.
29. Hojo K, Vernava AM III, Sugihara K, Katumata K. Preservation of urine voiding and sexual function after rectal cancer surgery [see comments]. Comments in: Dis Colon Rectum 1991;34:627.
30. Saclarides TJ, Bhattacharyya AK, Britton-Kuzel C, Szeluga D, Economou SG. Predicting lymph node metastases in rectal cancer. Dis Colon Rectum 1994;37:52.
31. Minsky BD, Cohen AM. Conservative management of invasive rectal cancer: alternative to abdominoperineal resection. Oncology 1989;3: 137.
32. Cohen AM, Wood WC, Gunderson LL, Shinnar M. Pathological studies in rectal cancer. Cancer 1980;45:2965.
33. Morson BC. Factors influencing the prognosis of early cancer of the rectum. Proc R Soc Med 1966;59:607.
34. Jass JR, Atkin WS, Cuzick J, et al. The grading of rectal cancer: historical perspectives and a multivariate analysis of 447 cases. Histopathology 1986;10:437.
35. Schmitz-Mormann P, Himmelmann GW, Baum U, Nilles M. Morphological predictors of survival in colorectal carcinoma: univariate and multivariate analysis. J Cancer Res Clin Oncol 1987;113:586.
36. Spratt JS Jr, Spjut HJ. Prevalence and prognosis of individual clinical and pathologic variables associated with colorectal carcinoma. Cancer 1987;20:1976.
37. Killingback M. Local excision of carcinoma of the rectum: indications. World J Surg 1992;16:437.
38. Pilipshen SJ, Heilweil M, Quan SH, Sternberg SS, Enker WE. Patterns of pelvic recurrence following definitive resections of rectal cancer. Cancer 1984;53:1354.
39. Muto T, Bussey HJR, Morson BC. The evolution of cancer of the colon and rectum. Cancer 1975;36:2251.
40. Vogelstein B, Fearon ER, Hamilton SR, et al. Genetic alterations during colorectal-tumor development. N Engl J Med 1988;319:525.
41. Jen J, Kim H, Piantadosi S, et al. Allelic loss of chromosome 18q and prognosis in colorectal cancer. N Engl J Med 1994;331:213.
42. Fearon ER, Cho KR, Nigro JM, et al. Identification of a chromosome 18q gene that is altered in colorectal cancers. Science 1990;247:49.
43. Thibodeau SN, Bren G, Schaid D. Microsatellite instability in cancer of the proximal colon. Science 1993;260:816.
44. Kokal W, Sheibani K, Terz J, Harada JR. Tumor DNA content in the prognosis of colorectal carcinoma. JAMA 1986;255:3123.
45. Goh HS, Jass JR, Atkin WS, Cuzick J, Northover JMA. Value of flow cytometric determination of ploidy as a guide to prognosis in operable rectal cancer: a multivariate analysis. Int J Colorectal Dis 1987;2:17.
46. Witzig TE, Loprinzi CL, Gonchoroff NJ, et al. DNA ploidy and cell kinetic measurements as predictors of recurrence and survival in stages B2 and C colorectal adenocarcinoma. Cancer 1991;68:879.
47. Schutte B, Reynder MMJ, Wigger T, et al. Retrospective analysis of the prognostic significance of DNA content and proliferative activity in large bowel carcinoma. Cancer Res 1987;47:5494.
48. Jones DJ, Moore M, Schofield PF. Refining the prognostic significance of DNA ploidy status in colorectal cancer: a prospective flow cytometry study. Int J Cancer 1988;41:206.
49. Rognum RO, Lund E, Meling GI, Langmark JF. Aneuploidy and 5-year survival in colorectal cancer. Cancer 1991;68:1077.
50. Armitage NCM, Ballantyne KC, Sheffield JP, Clarke P, Evans DF, Hardcastle JD. Prospective evaluation of the effect of tumor cell DNA content on recurrence in colorectal cancer. Cancer 1991;67:2599.
51. Fisher ERE, Siderits RH, Sass R, Fisher B. Value of assessment of ploidy in rectal cancers. Arch Pathol Lab Med 1989;113:525.
52. Visscher DW, Zarbo RJ, Ma CK, Sakr WA, Crissman JD. Flow cytometric DNA and clinicopathologic analysis of Dukes' A & B colonic adenocarcinomas: a retrospective study. Mod Pathol 1990;3:709.
53. Whittaker M, Goligher JC. The prognosis after surgical treatment for carcinoma of the rectum. Br J Surg 1976;63:384.
54. Williams NS, Dixon MF, Johnston D. Reappraisal of the 5 centimetre rule of distal excision for carcinoma of the rectum: a study of distal intramural spread and of patients' survival. Br J Surg 1983;70:150.
55. Freedman LS, Macaskill P, Smith AN. Multivariate analysis of prognostic factors for operable rectal cancer. Lancet 1984;2:733.
56. Moossa AR, Ree PC, Marks JE, Levin B, Platz CE, Skinner DB. Factors influencing local recurrence after abdominoperineal resection for cancer of the rectum and rectosigmoid. Br J Surg 1975;62:727.
57. McDermott FT, Hughes ES, Pihl E, Johnson WR, Price AB. Local recurrence after potentially curative resection for rectal cancer in a series of 1008 patients. Br J Surg 1985;72:34.
58. Quirke P, Durdey P, Dixon MF, Williams NS. Local recurrence of rectal adenocarcinoma due to inadequate surgical resection. Lancet 1986;2:1.
59. Quirke P, Scott N. The pathologist's role in the assessment of local recurrence in rectal carcinoma. Surgical Oncology Clinics of North America 1992;1:1.
60. Morson BC, Vaughan EG, Bussey HJR. Pelvic recurrences after excision of the rectum for carcinoma. Br Med J 1963;2:13.
61. Cawthorn SJ, Parums DV, Gibbs NM, et al. Extent of mesorectal spread and involvement of lateral resection margin as prognostic factors after surgery for rectal cancer. Lancet 1990;1,335:1055.
62. Wood CB, Gillis CR, Mole D, et al. Local tumor invasion as a prognostic factor in colorectal cancer. Br J Surg 1981;68:326.
63. Chan KW, Bey J, Wong SK. A method of reporting radial invasion and surgical clearance of rectal carcinoma. Histopathology 1985;9: 1319.
64. Heald RJ, Husband EM, Ryall RD. The mesorectum in rectal cancer surgery: the clue to pelvis recurrence? Br J Surg 1982;69:613.
65. Wilking N, Herrera L, Petrelli NJ, Mittelman A. Pelvic and perineal recurrences after abdominoperineal resection for adenocarcinoma of the rectum. Am J Surg 1985;150:561.
66. Thompson WM, Halvorsen RA, Foster WL Jr, Roberts L, Gibbons R. Preoperative and postoperative CT staging of rectosigmoid carcinoma. AJR Am J Roentgenol 1986;146:703.
67. Roman G, de Rosa P, Vallne G, Rotond A, Grassi R, Santangel ML. Intrarectal ultrasound and computed tomography in the pre- and postoperative assessment of patients with rectal cancer. Br J Surg 1985[illegible]17.
68. Freeny PC, Marks WM, Ryan JA, Blen JW. Colorectal carcinoma evaluation with CT: preoperative staging and detection of postoperative recurrence. Radiology 1986;158:347.
69. Schiessel R, Wunderlich M, Herbst F. Local recurrence of colorectal cancer: effect of early detection and aggressive surgery. Br J Surg 1986;73:342.
70. Shank B, Dershaw DD, Caravelli J, Barth J, Enker W. A prospective study of the accuracy of preoperative computed tomographic staging of patients with biopsy-proven rectal carcinoma. Dis Colon Rectum 1990;33:285.
71. Rotte KH, Kluhs L, Kleinau H, Kriedemann E. Computed tomography and endosonography in the preoperative staging of rectal carcinoma. Eur J Radiol 1989;9:187.
72. Herzog U. [Endoluminal sonography as a preoperative staging method in rectal carcinoma]. Die endoluminale Sonographie als preoperative

Staging-Methode beim Rektumkarzinom. Schweiz Med Wochenschr 1990;120:1439.
73. Holdswoth PJ, Johnston D, Chalmers AG, et al. Endoluminal ultrasound and computed tomography in the staging of rectal cancer. Br J Surg 1988;75:1019.
74. Hildebrandt U, Feifel G. Preoperative staging of rectal cancer by intrarectal ultrasound. Dis Colon Rectum 1985;28:42.
75. Mosnier H, Guivarc'h M, Barbagelata M. Endorectal ultrasonography of the rectum: a method of evaluation of locoregional extension of rectal carcinoma. Gastroenterol Clin Biol 1987;11:307.
76. Accarpio G, Scopinaro G, Claudiani F, Davisini D, Mallarini G, Saitta S. Experience with local rectal cancer excision in light of two recent preoperative diagnostic methods. Dis Colon Rectum 1987;30:296.
77. Rifkin MD, McGlynn ET, Marks G. Endorectal sonographic prospective staging of rectal cancer. Scand J Gastroenterol 1986;21(Suppl 123):99.
78. Wong CS, Stern H, Cummings BJ. Local excision and post-operative radiation therapy for rectal carcinoma. Int J Radiat Oncol Biol Phys 1993;25:669.
79. Rich T, Gunderson LL, Lew R, Galdibini JJ, Cohen AM, Donaldson G. Patterns of recurrence of rectal cancer after potentially curative surgery. Cancer 1983;52:1317.
80. Romsdahl MM, Withers HR. Radiotherapy combined with curative surgery. Arch Surg 1978;113:446.
81. Brown MT, Luna-Perez P, Petrelli NJ, Herrera L. Factors associated with nodal involvement of rectal adenocarcinomas. Surgical Oncology Clinics of North America 1992;1:25.
82. Roswit B, Higgins GA Jr, Keehn RJ. Preoperative irradiation for carcinoma of rectum and rectosigmoid colon: report of a National Veterans Administration randomized study. Cancer 1975;35:1597.
83. Mendenhall WM, Bland KI, Rout WR, Pfaff WW, Million RR, Copeland E-M III. Clinically resectable adenocarcinoma of the rectum treated with preoperative irradiation and surgery. Dis Colon Rectum 1988;31:287.
84. Cedermark B, Theve NO, Rieger A, et al. Preoperative short-term radiotherapy in rectal carcinoma: a preliminary report of a prospective randomized study. Cancer 1985;55:1182.
85. Higgins GA, Humphrey EW, Dwight RW, Roswit B, Lee LE, Keehn RJ. Preoperative radiation and surgery for cancer of the rectum: Veterans Administration Surgical Oncology Group Trial II. Cancer 1986; 58:352.
86. Mohiuddin M, Marks GJ. High dose preoperative radiation and sphincter preservation in the treatment of rectal cancer. Int J Radiat Oncol Biol Phys 1987;13:839.
87. Marks G, Mohiuddin MM, Masoni L, Pecchioli L. High-dose preoperative radiation and full-thickness local excision: a new option for patients with select cancers of the rectum. Dis Colon Rectum 1990; 33:735.
88. Fleishman JW, Kodner IJ, Fry RD, Walz B, Gilley MT. Adenocarcinoma of the rectum: results of radiotherapy and resection, endocavitary irradiation, local excision, and preoperative clinical staging. Dis Colon Rectum 1985;28:810.
89. Papillon J, Bobin JY, Papillon M, Berard P. [Role of preoperative radiotherapy in preservation of the anal sphincter in cancer of the lower rectum]. Role de la radiotherapie preoperatoire dans la preservation anale pour les cancers du bas rectum. Bull Cancer (Paris) 1990; 77:15.
90. Sarashina H, Taniyama S, Saitoh N, Nunomura M, Nakayama H, Okui K. Untersuchung zur praoperativen Strahlentherapie beim Rektumkarzinom: I. Einfluss der Bestrahlung auf das Tumorvoluman. Strahlenther Onkol 1990;166:794.
91. James RD, Haboubi N, Schfield PF, Mellor M, Salhab N. Prognostic factors in colorectal carcinoma treated by preoperative radiotherapy and immediate surgery. Dis Colon Rectum 1991;34:546.
92. Gerard A, Buyse M, Nordlinger B, et al. Preoperative radiotherapy as adjuvant treatment in rectal cancer: final results of a randomized study of the European Organization for Research and Treatment of Cancer (EORTC). Ann Surg 1988;208:606.
93. Stockholm Rectal Cancer Study Group. Preoperative short-term radiation therapy in operable rectal carcinoma: a prospective randomized trial. Cancer 1990;66:49.
94. Steele GD Jr, Augenlicht LH, Begg CB, et al. National Institutes of Health Consensus Development Conference Statement: adjuvant therapy for patients with colon and rectal cancer. JAMA 1990;264: 1444.
95. GITSG. Prolongation of the disease-free interval in surgically treated rectal carcinoma: Gastrointestinal Tumor Study Group. N Engl J Med 1985;312:1465.
96. Thomas PR, Lindblad AS. Adjuvant postoperative radiotherapy and chemotherapy in rectal carcinoma: a review of the Gastrointestinal Tumor Study Group experience. Radiother Oncol 1988;13:245.
97. Fisher B, Wolmark N, Rockette H, et al. Postoperative adjuvant chemotherapy or radiation therapy for rectal cancer: results from NSABP protocol R 01. J Natl Cancer Inst 1988;80:21.
98. Moertel CG. Surgical adjuvant treatment of large bowel cancer. J Clin Oncol 1988;6:934.
99. Rich T, Weiss DR, Mies C, Fitzgerald TJ, Chaffey JT. Sphincter preservation in patients with low rectal cancer treated with radiation therapy with local excision or fulguration. Radiology 1985;156:527.
100. Morson BC, Bussey HJR, Samoorian S. Policy of local excision for early cancer of the colorectum. Gut 1977;18:1045.
101. Deddish MR. Local excision. Surg Clin North Am 1974;54:877.
102. Stearns MW Jr, Sternberg SS, DeCosse JJ. Treatment alternatives: localized rectal cancer. Cancer 1984;54:2691.
103. Grigg M, McDermott FT, Pihl EA, Hughes ESR. Curative local excision in the treatment of carcinoma of the rectum. Dis Colon Rectum 1984;27:81.
104. Whiteway J, Nicholls RJ, Morson BC. The role of surgical excision in the treatment of rectal cancer. Br J Surg 1985;72:694.
105. Biggers OR, Beart RW, Ilstrup DM. Local excision of rectal cancer. Dis Colon Rectum 1986;29:374.
106. Killingback MJ. Indications for local excision of rectal cancer. Br J Surg 1985;72:s54.
107. Cuthbertson AM, Simpson RL. Curative local excision of rectal adenocarcinoma. Aust N Z J Surg 1986;56:229.
108. York Mason A. The place of local resection in the treatment of rectal carcinoma. Proc R Soc Med 1970;63:1259.
109. York Mason A. Surgical access to the rectum: a transsphincteric exposure. Proc R Soc Med 1970;63(Suppl):91.
110. Kraske P. Zur extirpation hochsitzenden mastdarmkrebs verhandle deutsch gesellsch. Verh Otsch Gs Chir 1885;14:464.
111. Lock MR, Ritchie JK, Hawley PR. Reappraisal of radical local excision for carcinoma of the rectum. Br J Surg 1993;80:928.
112. Huber AK, Koella C. The Swiss experience with the parasacral-transsphincteric approach to rectal cancer. Surgical Oncology Clinics of North America 1992;1:87.
113. Gall FP, Hermanek P. Update of the German experience with local excision of rectal cancer. Surgical Oncology Clinics of North America 1992;1:99.
114. Jessup JM, Bothe A, Stone MD, et al. Preservation of sphincter function in rectal carcinoma by a multimodality treatment approach. Surgical Oncology Clinics of North America 1992;1:137.
115. Coco C, Magistrelli P, Granone P, Roncolini G, Picciocchi A. Conservative surgery for early cancer of the distal rectum. Dis Colon Rectum 1992;35:131.
116. Summers GE, Mendenhall WM, Copeland EM. Update on the University of Florida experience with local excision and postoperative radiation therapy for the treatment of early rectal carcinoma. Surgical Oncology Clinics of North America 1992;1:125.
117. Wood WD, Willett CG. Update of the Massachusetts General Hospital experience of combined local excision and radiotherapy for rectal cancer. Surgical Oncology Clinics of North America 1992;1:131.
118. Ota DM, Skibber J, Rich T. M. D. Anderson Cancer Center experience with local excision and multimodality therapy for rectal cancer. Surgical Oncology Clinics of North America 1992;1:147.
119. Minsky BD. Clinical experience with local excision and postoperative radiation therapy for rectal cancer. Dis Colon Rectum 1993;36:405.
120. Rosenthal SA, Yeung RS, Weese JL, et al. Conservative management of extensive low-lying rectal carcinomas with transanal local excision and combined preoperative and postoperative radiation therapy: a report of a phase I–II trial. Cancer 1992;69:335.
121. Willett CG, Compton CC, Shellito PC, Efird JT. Selection factors for local excision or abdominoperineal resection of early stage rectal cancer. Cancer 1994;73:2716.
122. Weese JL, Bruskewitz RC. Endoscopic transrectal resection of rectal carcinomas using the urologic resectoscope. Dis Colon Rectum 1984; 27:123.

123. Buess G, Mentges B, Manncke K, Starlinger M, Becker HD. Technique and results of transanal endoscopic microsurgery in early rectal cancer. Am J Surg 1992;163:63, discussion p. 69.
124. Said S, Huber P, Pichlmaier H. Technique and clinical results of endorectal surgery. Surgery 1993;113:65.
125. Heintz A, Braunstein S, Menke-H. [Local excision of rectal tumors. Indications, preoperative diagnosis, surgical technique and results]. Lokale Exzision von Rektumtumoren: Indikationen, praoperative Diagnostik, Operationstechnik und Ergebnisse. Med Klin 1992;87:236.
126. Eng K, Localio SA. Abdominosacral resection for midrectal cancer. Hepatogastroenterology 1992;39:207.
127. Cohen AM, Enker WE, Minsky BD. Proctectomy and coloanal reconstruction for rectal cancer. Dis Colon Rectum 1990;33:40.
128. Frigell A, Ottander M, Stenbeck H, Pahlman L. Quality of life of patients treated with abdominoperineal resection or anterior resection for rectal carcinoma. Ann Chir Gynaecol 1990;79:26.
129. Paty PB, Enker WE, Cohen AM, Lauwers GY. Treatment of rectal cancer by low anterior resection with coloanal anastomosis. Ann Surg 1994;219:365.
130. Stahl TJ, Murray JJ, Coller JA, Schoetz DJ Jr, Roberts PL, Veidenheimer MC. Sphincter-saving alternatives in the management of adenocarcinoma involving the distal rectum: 5-year follow-up results in 40 patients. Arch Surg 1993;128:545, discussion p. 549.
131. Bailey HR, Huval WV, Max E, Smith KW, Butts DR, Zamora LF. Local excision of carcinoma of the rectum for cure. Surgery 1992; 111:555.
132. Graham RA, Garnsey L, Jessup JM. Local excision of rectal carcinoma [see comments]. Am J Surg 1990;160:306. Comment in Am J Surg 1993;165:751.

Surgery for Gastrointestinal Cancer: A Multidisciplinary Approach, edited by Harold J. Wanebo.
Lippincott-Raven Publishers, Philadelphia, © 1997.

CHAPTER 64

Technical Considerations in Local Excision of Rectal Cancers

Theodore John Saclarides

Significant improvements in surgical technique and supportive care over the last century have permitted a variety of radical transabdominal approaches for the treatment of rectal cancer. Nevertheless, there has been a rebirth of interest in conservative local excisions of this malignancy. Initially popularized by Kraske[1] and Lockhart-Mummery,[2] these approaches were soon considered inadequate treatment of cancer because it was recognized that malignant spread in an upward direction along the superior mesenteric lymphatics would be inaccessible to the surgeon.[3] In 1908, Miles therefore postulated that complete rectal excision with removal of the anal sphincter and portions of the levator ani muscle and the rectosigmoid mesentery was mandatory.[4] The subsequent advent of surgical staplers enabled many surgeons to perform a low pelvic anastomosis in patients who would have otherwise undergone a permanent colostomy. Despite becoming what are considered the gold standards for the treatment of rectal cancers, the abdominoperineal and low anterior resection are nevertheless associated with high morbidity, and the former causes significant alterations in body function and image. As such, local excision has remained a viable option for the properly selected patient.

The potential advantages of local excision are obvious. Namely, the morbid complications of a celiotomy are avoided, pain and disability are lessened, hospital stay is shortened, and sphincter function is preserved. The potential disadvantages, however, are equally numerous. Poor exposure through retractors or operating rectoscopes may produce an inadequate resection. Furthermore, possible sites of locoregional disease, namely lymph nodes, are not addressed with these techniques. Therefore, proper patient selection is mandatory if patient survival is not to be compromised for the sake of performing a less morbid operation. In this chapter, patient selection criteria, preoperative evaluation, and currently used techniques for locally excising rectal cancers are reviewed.

Theodore John Saclarides: Associate Professor of Surgery, Head, Section of Colorectal Surgery, Rush-Presbyterian-St. Luke's Medical Center, 1653 West Congress Parkway, Chicago, IL 60612

INDICATIONS

There is little controversy that local excision can be used in certain instances as a palliative means of reducing the local symptoms of a rectal cancer, such as bleeding and tenesmus. Such instances would include the presence of unresectable dissemination to distant sites such as the liver or lungs, and the presence of comorbid medical illnesses that would make a radical operation too hazardous. Similarly, local excision can be used to treat a stoma-phobic patient for whom an abdominoperineal resection would otherwise be indicated. For local excision to be used in a palliative mode, the tumor must be accessible transanally, and not overly large or bulky.

As stated, strict selection criteria must be met if local excision is to be used with curative intent. The tumors should be well differentiated, be no larger than 3 to 4 cm, exhibit minimal penetration of the rectal wall, and lack ominous histologic features such as lymphatic, perineural, or venous invasion.[5–7] If these criteria are not met, the likelihood that there has been spread to regional lymph nodes is unacceptably high, and cure will probably not be achieved by local excision alone.[8–10] A review of prior biopsy specimens and endorectal ultrasonography are essential and extremely helpful in properly selecting patients.

PREOPERATIVE EVALUATION

A digital rectal examination is the initial step and may reveal the degree of tumor mobility or fixation to surrounding structures. Enlarged presacral and pelvic lymph nodes may occasionally be palpable. For anterior lesions in women, simultaneous rectal and vaginal digital palpation is mandatory to assess potential involvement of the rectovaginal septum. Because distal rectal cancers may spread to the inguinal lymphatics, bilateral palpation of the groins must be performed as well.

Rigid proctoscopy is then performed to determine the distalmost aspect of the tumor. This also reveals the extent of circumferential involvement of the rectal wall and the antero-

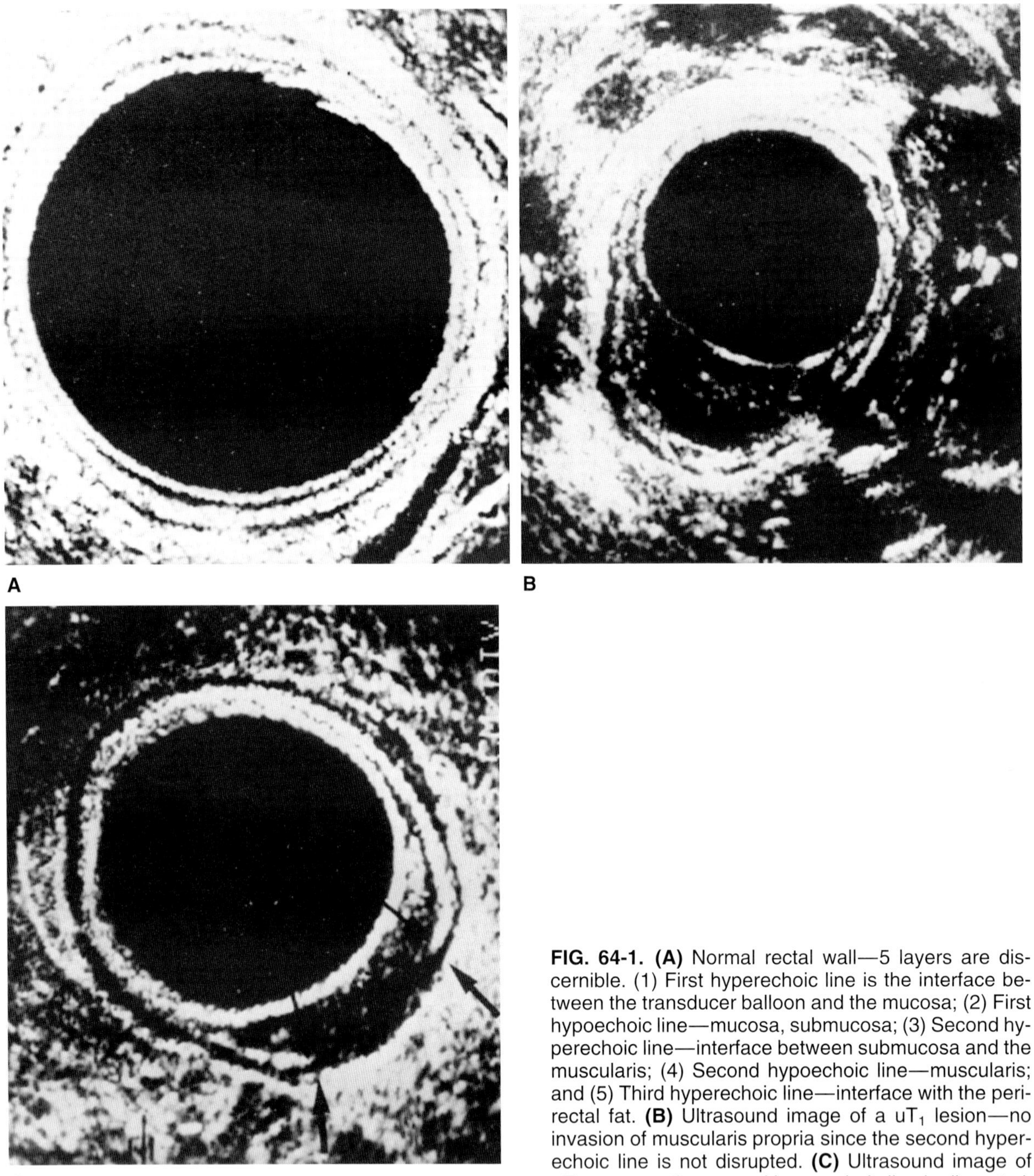

FIG. 64-1. **(A)** Normal rectal wall—5 layers are discernible. (1) First hyperechoic line is the interface between the transducer balloon and the mucosa; (2) First hypoechoic line—mucosa, submucosa; (3) Second hyperechoic line—interface between submucosa and the muscularis; (4) Second hypoechoic line—muscularis; and (5) Third hyperechoic line—interface with the perirectal fat. **(B)** Ultrasound image of a uT_1 lesion—no invasion of muscularis propria since the second hyperechoic line is not disrupted. **(C)** Ultrasound image of uT_2 cancer—the second hyperechoic line is disrupted.

posterior orientation of the tumor. This latter information is important for patient positioning during local excision. If biopsy sampling has not yet been performed, it should now be done and the pathologist asked to comment on the presence of unfavorable histologic features, as outlined earlier. Although tumor size does not correlate with the risk of nodal disease, there is the concern that larger tumors may not be adequately excised locally.[8] As such, the upper limit of acceptable tumor size is 3 to 4 cm. Colonoscopy is advised to rule out the presence of synchronous adenomas or cancers elsewhere in the colon.

Computed tomography or magnetic resonance imaging of the abdomen and pelvis are indicated both to determine involvement of other pelvic viscera and to inspect for metastatic disease within the liver. If unresectable hepatic disease is present, the decision to proceed with a conservative transanal approach is reinforced, provided tumor morphology and accessibility permit. With regard to detecting regional nodal disease, these studies are inferior to endorectal ultrasonography, which has as its main advantage its ability to be placed directly in contact with or in close proximity to the area of interest.

Using a 7- or 10-MHz transducer, the layers of the wall can be examined in detail (Fig. 64-1*A*) and the depth of penetration

TABLE 64-1. *Staging of rectal cancers—depth of invasion*

Reference	Sensitivity	Specificity	Positive Predictive Value	Negative Predictive Value	Overstage	Understage
Herzog et al[11]	98.3%	75%	89.2%	95.4%	10.2%	0.8%
Sentovitch et al[12]	79%	—	uT_2—81% $uT_{3,4}$—90%	uT_2—88% $uT_{3,4}$—100%	17%	4%
Anderson et al[13]	pT_1—70% pT_2—100%	pT_1—100% pT_2—44%	uT_1—100% uT_2—55%	uT_1—85% uT_2—100%	15%	30%
Harnsberger et al[14]	55%	—	—	—	40%	5%
Orrom et al[15]	75%	—	—	—	22%	3%
Glaser et al[16]	96%	—	—	96%	—	—
Hulsmans et al[17]	97%	24%	—	—	"Extensive"	—
Holdsworth et al[18]	96%	50%	—	—	—	—

u, ultrasound staging; p, pathology staging.

by the tumor assessed with high accuracy (see Fig. 64-1*B* and *C*). Lesions penetrating deeply into the muscularis propria or even transmurally into the perirectal fat can therefore be excluded from local excision. Accuracy rates in assessing depth of penetration are shown in Table 64-1. Studies have shown that ultrasound is more likely to overestimate than underestimate tumor penetration, presumably as a result of peritumor inflammation and edema, which can obscure tissue planes. In those instances in which penetration was underestimated, the deeper levels of the rectal wall were usually involved only by microscopic tumor within a small area of the lesion.[17] Our ability to detect metastatic lymph nodes has lagged behind our ability to determine depth of penetration, for several reasons. First, strict reliance on nodal enlargement as the sole criterion produces inaccurate results because, in many instances, metastatic involvement is present only microscopically and may escape ultrasound detection. Diagnostic accuracy is lowest for nodes 5 mm or smaller.[11] Echogenicity and nodal shape also affect accuracy; metastatic nodes are usually hypoechoic and spherical, whereas inflammatory nodes are hyperechoic and oval. If suspect nodes are imaged, ultrasound-guided needle biopsy can be safely performed; however, with currently available instrumentation, nodes above 12 cm from the anal verge are not accessible for needle biopsy.[20] Accuracy rates in detecting metastatic lymph nodes are shown in Table 64-2. Endorectal ultrasonography has the added feature of being able to assess postoperatively for recurrent cancer, which, if it does occur, may be entirely extraluminal and escape endoscopic detection.

SURGICAL PRINCIPLES

Once the selection criteria for local excision have been satisfied, the patient is prepared for surgery. A full mechanical bowel preparation is essential and is accomplished with either a polyethylene glycol oral solution or with enemas and cathartics. Oral and enteral antibiotics are administered as well. Bowel cleansing ensures visibility during the dissection and reduces the potential for infection both within the operative field and the pelvis, should the peritoneal cavity be inadvertently entered during the dissection. Such entry is not likely if the tumor is located in the posterior or lateral quadrants. The anterior peritoneal reflection is variable in its location; however, the surgeon can expect to find it approximately 6 to 8 cm from the anal verge in women and slightly higher in men. The middle valve of Houston is a crude landmark used to identify the approximate location of the anterior peritoneal reflection. If the abdominal cavity is entered, repair can be accomplished transanally; however, if exposure is poor, or if there is concern about the adequacy of repair, laparotomy should be performed. In this regard, preoperative consent should be obtained routinely for conversion to radical resection if unexpected complications are encountered.

Local excision may be performed under a local anesthetic if the tumor is small and located in the distalmost rectum. Otherwise, a regional or general anesthetic should be performed so that patient relaxation is maximized, exposure optimized, and time does not pose any restrictions.

Regardless of which technique is chosen for local excision, patient positioning depends on the exact location of the tumor. If the lesion is anterior, exposure is best if the patient is placed in the prone position. Posterior lesions mandate that the lithotomy position be used; the legs must be well padded to protect them from possible compression injury from the stirrups. If the lesion is located in the lateral quadrants, patients are placed in the necessary lateral position. The exception to these rules is poste-

TABLE 64-2. *Identifying lymph node metastases endorectal ultrasound*

Herzog et al[11]	89.2%	73.4%	71.2%	90.4%	80.2%*
Sentovitch et al[12]	0%	100%	—	73%	—
Fleshman et al[19]	—	—	37.5%	100%	—
Orrom et al[15]	88%	90%	—	—	88%
Glaser et al[16]	—	—	—	—	80%
Holdsworth et al[18]	57%	64%	—	—	61%

* Staging accuracy dependent on node size: if nodes were <5 mm, accuracy was lower ($P <$ .05).

PPV, positive predictive value; NPV, negative predictive value.

rior proctotomy; regardless of which quadrant the tumor is in, the patient must be placed prone. Once excision is undertaken, attention must center on obtaining an adequate lateral and deep margin of resection. If prior biopsy has established that the lesion is malignant, a 1-cm lateral radial margin of normal mucosa is mapped out around the lesion. Adenomas may be excised with a 5-mm margin; however, because large adenomas may harbor an occult cancer, a full-thickness excision with a 1-cm lateral margin is prudent. The depth of excision must be full thickness, incorporating all layers of the bowel wall. Postoperative decisions regarding the need for additional treatment, be it radical surgery or irradiation, can be made only if the depth of penetration is known. This information, along with knowledge of the degree of differentiation and the presence of venous or lymphatic invasion, may help estimate the likelihood of lymph node metastases.[8]

TECHNIQUE

Transanal Excision, Direct Visualization

Visibility of the lesion is obtained with a bivalve retractor, a Park's retractor, or large operating rectoscopes through which are inserted long-shafted instruments (Fig. 64-2). With conventional instruments, the upper limit of resection is approximately 8 cm from the anal verge unless an unusually mobile rectosigmoid can be pulled down into the operative field. Stay sutures placed circumferentially around the lesion can be used to pull the tumor closer into view and for subsequent wound closure after the lesion has been excised. Submucosal injection of 1 : 200,000 epinephrine may aid in hemostasis. Dissection is best done in a distal-to-proximal direction whereby the distal edge of the specimen is grasped and used to provide downward retraction, thus exposing the upper aspect of the tumor (Fig. 64-3). The surgeon should avoid grasping the tumor directly because fragmentation of the specimen may complicate histologic assessment of tumor margins. Care must be exercised that the upper margin does not retract out of reach; therefore, before the upper margin is cut through, stay sutures should be secured. Closure of the wound is performed in a transverse direction to minimize narrowing of the lumen; however, this is not absolutely mandatory (Fig. 64-4). A long-lasting absorbable suture is chosen. After excision, proctoscopy is done to verify a complete excision, lack of bleeding, and maintenance of an adequate lumen. Early discharge can be anticipated in 1 to 2 days; there is no need to confine the bowels or to administer antibiotics for a long period of time.

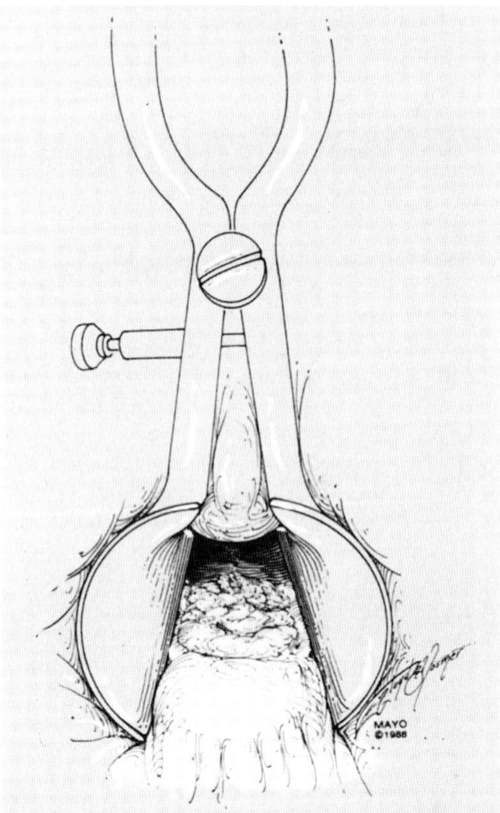

FIG. 64-2. Bivalve retractor inserted into the anus and opened.

The most common complication after local excision is bleeding. Fortunately, most instances stop spontaneously; occasionally, suture ligation or fulguration is needed. Suture line dehiscence probably occurs more frequently than might be thought. Circumstances do not usually dictate that proctoscopic examination of the wound be performed in the early postoperative period, but, when it is done, it is not unusual to find partial or complete separation. No treatment is needed.

Stenosis is uncommon after local excision unless the surgeon has attempted removal of a lesion that encompassed greater than 50% of the rectal circumference or if a large defect was closed longitudinally. If a stenosis does occur, digital or balloon dilatation is usually successful.

Inadvertent injury into the vagina may result in a rectovaginal fistula that, if recognized immediately, may be promptly repaired transanally. Fistulas that become manifest late in the postoperative period may heal spontaneously; however, if healing has not occurred within 6 weeks, either a transanal or transvaginal flap closure will be needed.

Cancer may recur in up to 20% to 25% of patients undergoing local excision without postoperative radiation therapy.[21] Such recurrences may be detected by digital examination, endoscopy, or endorectal ultrasonography. These patients are best treated with salvage abdominoperineal resection; however, if the tumor volume is small, reexcision with radiation therapy or radiation therapy alone may be considered. Approximately 50% of such patients are salvageable, provided the recurrence is not large or disseminated disease has not become manifest in the interim.[21] Occasionally, radiation therapy is administered before or after local excision of tumors thought to be at high risk of harboring nodal metastases. Posttreatment recurrences have been noted in up to 30% of these advanced lesions.[22–25] Such recurrences may be difficult to detect because normal tissue pliability is frequently lost after radiation; as such, the accuracy of digital and sonographic surveillance is diminished.[19]

Transanal Endoscopic Microsurgery

Developed by Professor Gerhard Buess and engineered by the Richard Wolf Company (Germany), transanal endoscopic

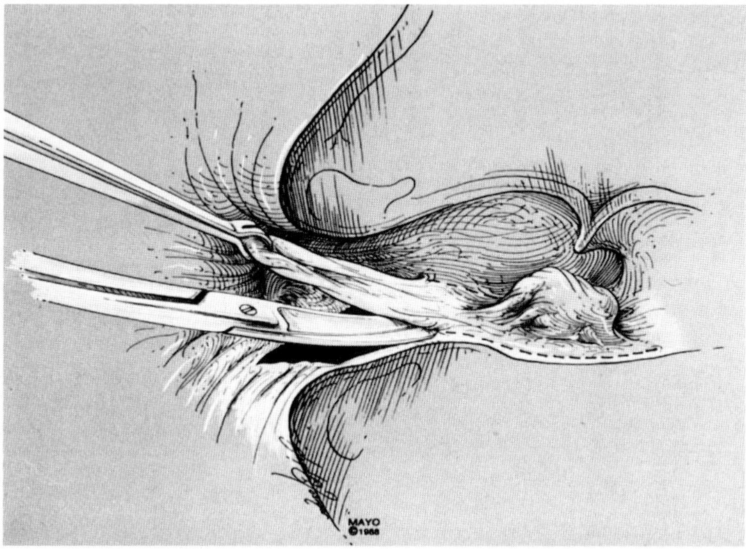

FIG. 64-3. Full thickness dissection in a distal-to-proximal direction.

microsurgery (TEM) has emerged as an alternative means of locally excising selected rectal cancers.[26–28] TEM uses a closed, airtight system, and a 40-mm diameter rectoscope, 20 cm in length, into which CO_2 is constantly insufflated. An intrarectal pressure of 15 cm H_2O is maintained by an endosurgical unit that regulates CO_2 insufflation, suction, and irrigation. The rectoscope is held in place, fixed to the operating room table by a double ball-and-socket support arm. Constant rectal distention and the superior optics provided by stereoscopic magnification are distinct advantages TEM has over conventional instrumentation and retractors. Also, because the rectoscope and instruments necessary to do the dissection are long, access is provided to lesions in the middle and upper rectum, beyond the reach of standard transanal equipment. A variety of instruments are used, including tissue graspers, a high-frequency electrical knife, and needle holders. Because knot tieing is impossible, sutures are anchored into the tissue at the beginning and end of the thread with small silver shots that are placed with a specially designed shot applicator. These instruments are inserted through rubber-sealed ports located in the facepiece at the end of the rectoscope (Fig. 64-5).

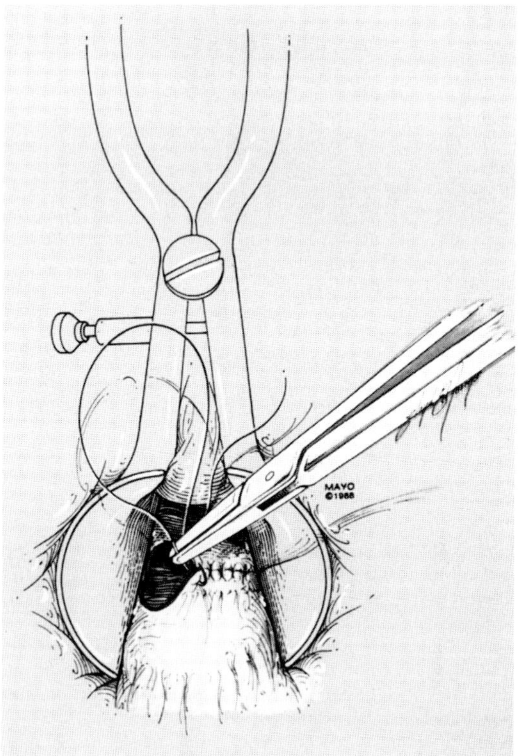

FIG. 64-4. Transanal suture closure of the defect.

Transanal endoscopic microsurgery is technically challenging since the long-shafted instruments are inserted and operated in parallel. As a result, traction and countertraction are difficult to achieve. This is further compounded by the surgeon's natural tendency to cross instruments within the rectoscope which only adds to the difficulty of this technique. These factors, combined with the expense of the equipment and the relatively infrequent nature of the pathology which TEM addresses, will make the technique the domain of but a few surgeons. Widely practiced abroad, TEM has been slow to catch on in the United States. The indications for the procedure as well as patient selection and preparation, the technique of full thickness excision, and post-operative complications are the same as for conventional transanal excision.

POSTERIOR PROCTOTOMY

In an address to the German Surgery Association, Kraske in 1885 presented his results with posterior (transgluteal) proctotomy for locally excising rectal cancers. After resection, either a sacral colostomy was created or bowel continuity was reestablished. Subsequently, Mason and Bevan extended the incision through the sphincter, in effect completely laying open the rectum posteriorly from the anus up to and slightly above the coccyx. After excision, the wound and sphincter muscle were usually reconstructed in layers. These approaches are rarely used today because improvements in anesthetic techniques and sup-

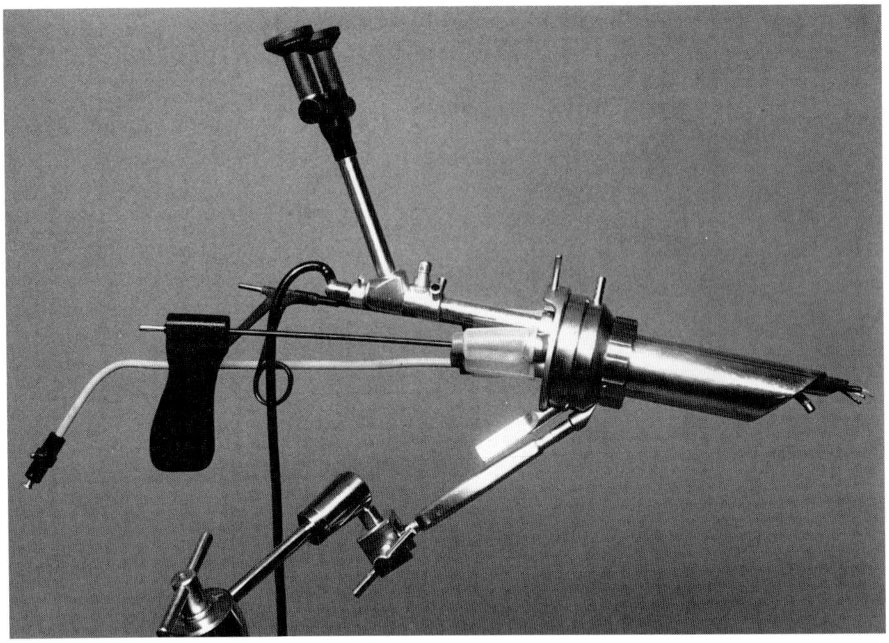

FIG. 64-5. Transanal endoscopic microsurgery (TEM), lateral view.

portive care have rendered a laparotomy and general anesthesia safe and not the highly morbid obstacles they were many years ago. Certainly, the use of surgical staplers and the increasing use of coloanal anastomoses have further reduced the need for a posterior approach to preserve sphincter function. In many cases, therefore, the surgeon does not need to do a posterior proctotomy for distal cancers, in the fear that the lowness of the tumor will mandate a colostomy. It is still possible to reestablish intestinal continuity in these instances. Furthermore, as a result of improved understanding of the pathophysiology of this disease and its modes of spread, as well as improved preoperative staging methods, patients are selected at the onset for either a transabdominal approach for advanced lesions or transanal excision for early lesions. The transanal techniques mentioned in this chapter are the local excision techniques of choice rather than posterior proctotomy, because the sphincter is not disrupted and there is essentially no risk of postoperative incontinence, wound breakdown, or a sacral fistula. The methods of Kraske and Mason have been relegated to the category of esoteric procedures that are rarely seen or used.

SUMMARY

The most important aspect of local excision of rectal cancers is not so much the technique chosen or the instruments used, but rather proper selection of patients so that curability is not compromised. Toward this end, endorectal ultrasonography has emerged as a vital tool in the decision process. Local excision should be viewed as an excisional biopsy sampling procedure that affects whether additional therapy is needed, analogous to lumpectomy for breast cancer. If ominous histologic features are present, such as deep penetration of the rectal wall, tumor present at the margins of resection, poor differentiation, or lymphovascular involvement, further treatment is needed unless comorbid medical illnesses dictate otherwise. Such treatment may include radical surgery or chemoradiation. Ongoing studies may answer whether local excision followed by radiation will yield cure rates for high-risk lesions comparable to those with abdominoperineal or low anterior resection.

REFERENCES

1. Kraske P. Ueber die Entstehung sek undarer Krebsqesch würe durch Impfung. Zentralbl Chir 1884;11:801.
2. Lockhart-Mummery JP. Two hundred cases of cancer of the rectum treated by perineal excision. Br J Surg 1926;14:110.
3. Dukes CE. The spread of cancer of the rectum. Br J Surg 1930;17:643.
4. Miles WE. A method of performing abdominoperineal excision for carcinoma of the rectum and the terminal portion of the pelvic colon. Lancet 1908;2:1812.
5. Morson BC. Histologic criteria for local excision. Br J Surg 1985;72(Suppl P):S53.
6. Killingback MJ. Indications for local excision of rectal cancer. Br J Surg 1985;72(Suppl P):S54.
7. Whiteway J, Nicholls RJ, Morson BC. The role of surgical local excision in the treatment of rectal cancer. Br J Surg 1985;72:694.
8. Saclarides TJ, Bhattacharyya AK, Britton-Kuzel C, Szeluga D, Economou SG. Predicting lymph node metastases in rectal cancer. Dis Colon Rectum 1994;37:52.
9. Gall FP, Hermanek P. Cancer of the rectum: local excision. Surg Clin North Am 1988;68:1353.
10. Minsky BD, Rich T, Recht A, Harvey W, Mies C. Selection criteria for local excision with or without adjuvant radiation therapy for rectal cancer. Cancer 1989;63:1421.
11. Herzog U, von Flüe M, Tondelli P, Schuppisser JP. How accurate is endorectal ultrasound in the preoperative staging of rectal cancer? Dis Colon Rectum 1993;36:127.
12. Sentovitch SM, Blatchford GJ, Falk PM, Thorson AG, Christensen MA. Transrectal ultrasound of rectal tumors. Am J Surg 1993;166:638.
13. Anderson BO, Hann LE, Enker WE, Dershaw DD, Guillem JG, Cohen HM. Transrectal ultrasonography and operative selection for early carcinoma of the rectum. J Am Coll Surg 1994;179:513.
14. Harnsberger JR, Charvat P, Longo WE, et al. The role of intrarectal ultrasound (IRUS) in staging of rectal cancer and detection of extrarectal pathology. Am Surg 1994;60:571.
15. Orrom WJ, Wong WD, Rothenberger DA, Jensen LL, Goldberg SM. Endorectal ultrasound in the preoperative staging of rectal tumors: a learning experience. Dis Colon Rectum 1990;33:654.

16. Glaser F, Friedl P, von Ditfurth B, Schlag P, Herfarth C. Influence of endorectal ultrasound on surgical treatment of rectal cancer. Eur J Surg Oncol 1990;16:304.
17. Hulsmans FJ, Tio TL, Fockens P, Bosma A, Tytgat GN. Assessment of tumor infiltration depth in rectal cancer with transrectal sonography: caution is necessary. Radiology 1994;190:715.
18. Holdsworth PJ, Johnston D, Chalmers AG, et al. Endoluminal ultrasound and computed tomography in the staging of rectal cancer. Br J Surg 1988;75:1019.
19. Fleshman JW, Myerson RJ, Fry RD, Kodner IJ. Accuracy of transrectal ultrasound in predicting pathologic stage of rectal cancer before and after preoperative radiation therapy. Dis Colon Rectum 1992;35:823.
20. Milsom JW, Czyrko C, Hull TL, Strong SA, Fazio VW. Preoperative biopsy of pararectal lymph nodes in rectal cancer using endoluminal ultrasonography. Dis Colon Rectum 1994;37:364.
21. Graham RA, Garnsey L, Jessup JM. Local excision of rectal carcinoma. Am J Surg 1990;160:306.
22. Minsky BD, Cohen Am, Enker WE, Mies C. Sphincter preservation in rectal cancer by local excision and postoperative radiation therapy. Cancer 1991;67:908.
23. Rosenthal SA, Yeung RS, Weese JL, et al. Conservative management of extensive low-lying rectal carcinomas with transanal local excision and combined preoperative and postoperative radiation therapy: a report of a phase I–II trial. Cancer 1992;69:335.
24. Marks G, Mohiuddin MM, Masoni L, Pecchioli L. High dose preoperative radiation and full thickness local excision: a new option for patients with select cancers of the rectum. Dis Colon Rectum 1990;33:735.
25. Jessup JM, Bleday R, Busse P, Steele G Jr. Conservative management of rectal carcinoma: the efficacy of a multimodality approach. Semin Surg Oncol 1993;9:39.
26. Buess G, Kipfmuler K, Ibald R, et al. Clinical results of transanal endoscopic microsurgery. Surg Endosc 1988;2:245.
27. Buess G, Mentges B, Manncke K, Starlinger M, Becker HD. Technique and results of transanal endoscopic microsurgery in early rectal cancer. Am J Surg 1992;163:63.
28. Saclarides TJ, Smith L, Ko ST, Orkin B, Buess G. Transanal endoscopic microsurgery. Dis Colon Rectum 1992;35:1183.

Surgery for Gastrointestinal Cancer: A Multidisciplinary Approach, edited by Harold J. Wanebo.
Lippincott-Raven Publishers, Philadelphia, © 1997.

CHAPTER 65

Adjuvant Chemotherapy of Colorectal Cancer

J. Michael Hamilton and Michael A. Friedman

Adjuvant chemotherapy improves postoperative survival for patients with TNM stage III colon cancer and for those with stage II or III rectal cancer. Compared with treatment with surgery alone, adjuvant therapy reduces the risk of death at 5 years by about 30% (Table 65-1). For the other TNM stages of colorectal cancer, such a clear statement of benefit cannot be made. Patients with stage I colonic or rectal primary tumor are usually curable by surgery alone and have little to be gained by additional chemotherapy. Ambiguity exists in evaluating adjuvant treatment of stage II colon cancer patients. Although these patients have a 15% to 30% death rate 5 years after surgery, clinical trials have not established a significant survival benefit for patients receiving surgery plus chemotherapy, in part because survival of stage II patients is "too good" to show a difference. Stage IV cancers are, in general, incurable. Chemotherapy may have a palliative role in these patients and may extend survival for some, but adjuvant treatment, per se, is not applicable. Even when removal of isolated metastases has rendered a patient free of detectable residual cancer, there are no data from randomized clinical studies that show a benefit for additional chemotherapy.

Although randomized clinical studies of adjuvant treatment for colorectal cancer date from 1957, the statement that adjuvant chemotherapy does have an established role in the management of some colorectal cancers could not have been made as recently as the early 1980s. Only since then have published reports shown that a reduction in cancer recurrence and a lowered risk for death can be achieved by treatment with 5-fluorouracil (5-FU) combined with levamisole or 5-FU combined with leucovorin for therapy of colon cancer, and by 5-FU coupled with radiation therapy for treatment of rectal cancer. Administration of these adjuvant treatments to appropriate candidates may prevent disease recurrence and delay death in up to 10,000 to 15,000 people a year. An appreciation of prognostic factors is emerging within these and other stages of disease that may more precisely distinguish people most at risk for recurrence, thereby identifying the patients with the greatest potential to benefit from perioperative cytotoxic therapy, and increasing the number of people whose lives and cancer-free existence may be extended.

J. Michael Hamilton: NCI-Navy Medical Oncology Branch, DCS, National Cancer Institute, National Naval Medical Center, Bldg 8, Rm 5101, Bethesda, MD 20889-5105

Michael A. Friedman: Office of Operations, Food and Drug Administration, 5600 Fishers Lane, Rockville, MD 20857.

HISTORICAL DEVELOPMENT OF COLORECTAL ADJUVANT THERAPY

The beginning of modern chemotherapy dates from the discovery of the antineoplastic effects of nitrogen mustard in 1943.[1] Within a few years, several other alkylating agents were introduced into the chemotherapy repertoire. The earliest randomized trials of adjuvant chemotherapy for colorectal cancer were multiinstitutional studies by the Veterans Administration Surgical Oncology Group (VASOG)[2] and the Surgical Adjuvant Colorectal Cancer Chemotherapy Study,[3] which tested the alkylator agent thiotepa versus surgery alone in a combined total of more than 1750 patients between 1957 and 1961 (Table 65-2). A detailed review of these and other early studies of adjuvant therapy is available.[4] The importance of these two clinical trials lay not in simply proving that perioperative thiotepa was ineffective for improving survival; their long-term influence came from establishing a multiinstitutional mechanism for testing cancer therapies. These studies developed blueprints for Cooperative Group procedures. They also showed that colon and rectal cancer primaries were distinct clinical entities, deserving independent evaluation, and they identified clear differences in outcome for patients undergoing curative-intent surgeries versus those having palliative or debulking procedures, helping to segregate the groups of patients for whom adjuvant therapy is appropriate to consider. These fundamental points were not self-evident at the time, but came to light through clinical investigation. The progress in identifying effective cancer treatment has involved continued improvements in the process of clinical research as well as the introduction of useful agents.

Antimetabolite chemotherapy development proceeded during the 1950s as the processes of cellular synthesis of nucleic acids and proteins were becoming well defined. The pyrimidine analogues 5-FU and fluorodeoxyuridine were introduced for clinical investigation in 1956.[5] After the completion of the two thiotepa trials in 1960, 5-FU and fluorodeoxyuridine became

TABLE 65-1. *Estimated 5-year survival of colorectal cancer by stage (percent)*

TNM stage	Surgery alone		Surgery plus adjuvant therapy	
	Colon	Rectum	Colon	Rectum
I	90–95	85–90	—	—
II	70–85	55–65	—	75–80
III	45–55	35–45	60–65	55–60
IV	<5	<5	—	—

the focus of adjuvant investigation, and, as single agents, remained the subject of study for 15 years, until the mid-1970s. Three VASOG trials[6,7] and a Central Oncology Group study[8] suggested some degree of benefit for 5-FU, but failed to show statistically convincing results. As the only agents that have shown a consistent, if low level, of activity, fluoropyrimidine-based regimens have continued to be the primary treatment for colorectal cancers. Subsequent clinical investigation has involved modifying routes of drug administration and drug schedules and the addition of other agents to potentiate the effects of 5-FU.

One of these approaches to focus the activity of single-agent

TABLE 65-2. *Early multiinstitutional trials of adjuvant therapy—colon*

Study	Accrual	Regimens	5-Year survival
THIOTEPA STUDIES			
VASOG-1[2] 1957–1960	1064	Thiotepa	55%
		Surgery alone	53%
SACCCS[3] 1957–1960	695	Thiotepa	45%
		Surgery alone	52%
FLUOROPYRIMIDINE STUDIES			
VASOG FUdR[6] 1961–1964	548	FUdR	47%
		Surgery alone	50%
VASOG 5-FU1[7] 1965–1969	308	5-FU	58%
		Surgery alone	48%
VASOG 5-FU2[7] 1969–1973	518	5-FU	49%
		Surgery alone	45%
COG 7041[8] 1971–1976	233	5-FU	55%
		Surgery alone	48%
PORTAL VEIN STUDIES			
NCCTG 784604[10] 1982–1987	224	Portal vein 5-FU	68%
		Surgery alone	68%
NSABP C-02[11] 1984–1988	1158	Portal vein 5-FU	81%*
		Surgery alone	73%*
SAKK 40/81[12] 1981–1987	469	Portal vein 5-FU, mitomyxin-C	70%†
		Surgery alone	57%
MeCCNU/5-FU STUDIES			
VASOG 27A[16] 1973–1979	654	MeCCNU, 5-FU	53%
		Surgery alone	50%
GITSG 6175[17] 1975–1979	572	MeCCNU, 5-FU + BCG-MER	59%
		MeCCNU, 5-FU	61%
		BCG-MER	59%
		Surgery alone	62%
SWOG 7510[18] 1975–1980	559	MeCCNU, 5-FU	55%
		MeCCNU, 5-FU + BCG	60%
		Surgery alone	56%
ECOG 2276[19] 1976–1978	703	MeCCNU, 5-FU	63%
		5-FU	60%
NSABP C-01[20] 1977–1983	1166	MeCCNU, 5-FU, vincristine	67%†
		BCG	67%
		Surgery alone	58%

†$P < 0.05$ compared with control.
* Four-year data.
VASOG, Veterans Administration Surgical Oncology Group; *SACCCS,* Surgical Adjuvant Colorectal Cancer Chemotherapy Study; *FUdR,* fluorodeoxyuridine; *5-FU,* 5-fluorouracil; *COG,* Cooperative Oncology Group; *NCCTG,* North Central Cancer Treatment Group; *NSABP,* National Surgical Adjuvant Breast and Bowel Projects; *SAKK,* Swiss Adjuvant Colorectal Cancer; *MeCCNU,* methyl-CCNU; *GITSG,* Gastrointestinal Tumor Study Group; *BCG-MER,* methanol-extracted residue of bacille Calmette-Guérin; *SWOG,* Southwestern Oncology Group; *ECOG,* Eastern Cooperative Oncology Group.

5-FU has been regional administration, producing higher concentrations of the drug in the liver than could be achieved with systemic administration. A solid rationale exists for perfusing the liver to eliminate micrometastases. About one quarter of patients with resected colon cancer recur with metastatic disease evident only in the liver, and more than half those dying from cancer manifest hepatic metastases. In addition, a large fraction of the dose of 5-FU undergoes first-pass extraction by the liver, thereby reducing systemic toxicity. Taylor and colleagues tested the concept with a randomized trial, comparing surgery alone to surgery plus a 7-day portal vein infusion of 5-FU and heparin.[9] A reduction in the number of recurrences in the liver and an improved survival were noted for the chemotherapy group. Three multiinstitutional clinical trials attempted to validate these observations. The North Central Cancer Treatment Group (NCCTG)[10] and the National Surgical Adjuvant Breast and Bowel Project (NSABP)[11] each evaluated a regimen of 7-day 5-FU portal vein infusion similar to that tested by Taylor and colleagues. The Swiss Adjuvant Colorectal Cancer trial[12] included a dose of mitomycin-C with the 5-FU hepatic perfusate. The Swiss study showed a survival advantage for the treated group compared with the group having surgery alone, and the NSABP observed a disease-free survival advantage. The important finding was that none of these three clinical trials demonstrated a reduction in the frequency of hepatic metastases, even when overall control of disease seemed to be affected by portal vein infusion. That is, the effects of drug infusion in the immediate perioperative period appeared to be on systemic rather than on regional control of disease. This hypothesis is being examined by one of the current, ongoing Intergroup clinical trials, which is described later in this chapter.

Methyl-CCNU (MeCCNU, semustine) is a chloroethyl nitrosourea analogue that was introduced into clinical testing in the early 1970s. Preclinical evaluation showing activity against L1210 leukemia, B16 melanoma, and Lewis lung carcinomas[13] and early phase I and II trials that yielded responses in patients with lymphomas and with solid tumors[14,15] generated enthusiasm for the new compound. Combination with 5-FU for the treatment of gastrointestinal cancers and incorporation into adjuvant studies was rapid. There was hope that this new product of careful preclinical selection plus 5-FU would finally provide the key to successful adjuvant therapy. The decade from the mid-1970s to the mid-1980s saw five large Cooperative Group clinical trials in colon cancer[16–20] and three trials in rectal cancer[21–24] (Table 65-3; see Table 65-2), with nearly 5000 accrued subjects. Various combinations of 5-FU, MeCCNU, BCG (bacille Calmette-Guérin) immunotherapy, and radiation therapy were investigated. Table 65-2 reflects the overall disappointing experience with MeCCNU in colon cancer. Similarly, the initial attempts at adjuvant immunotherapy with BCG or the methanol-extracted residue of BCG showed little promise. For rectal cancer (see Table 65-3), the chemotherapy combinations appeared to be more active. In fact, each of these studies demonstrated a statistically significant advantage for a treatment that contained the drug combination. Yet the essential contribution of MeCCNU to the regimens was not clear. This point was important to clarify because further experience with MeCCNU not only muted the enthusiasm for the drug's antineoplastic activity but revealed serious potential for toxicity and a risk for drug-related, secondary leukemia.[25] More contemporary studies have demonstrated that MeCCNU can be deleted from the treatment of rectal cancer without loss of effectiveness. Gastrointestinal Tumor Study Group (GITSG) 7180[26] and NCCTG 864751[27] compared regimens of 5-FU and radiation therapy with or without MeCCNU. Comparison of outcomes for treatment cohorts in both studies revealed closely apposed survival curves ($P = 0.58$ and $P = 0.61$, respectively) and no suggestion of benefit from the addition of nitrosourea. A third, larger study that addresses the question of MeCCNU in a slightly different manner was NSABP R-02. This study accrued 741 patients between 1987 and 1992. The design included a comparison of a combination of MeCCNU, vincristine, and 5-FU

TABLE 65-3. *Multiinstitutional trials of adjuvant therapy with MeCCNU—rectum*

Study	Accrual	Regimens	5-Year survival
GITSG 7175[21,22] 1975–1980	202	MeCCNU, 5-FU + RT	59%*
		MeCCNU, 5-FU	56%
		RT	52%
		Surgery alone	43%
NCCTG 794651[23] 1980–1986	204	MeCCNU, 5-FU + RT	58%*
		RT	47%
NSABP R-01[24] 1977–1986	555	MeCCNU, 5-FU, vincristine	53%*
		RT	41%
		Surgery alone	43%
GITSG 7180[26] 1981–1985	210	MeCCNU, 5-FU + RT	54%
		5-FU + RT	59%
NCCTG 864751[27] 1986–1990	660	MeCCNU, 5-FU + RT	61%†
		5-FU + RT	60%†
NSABP R-02 (unpub.) 1987–1992	741	MeCCNU, 5-FU, vincristine ± RT	—
		5-FU + leucovorin ± RT	—

*$P < 0.05$ compared with control.

† Four-year data; n.b.: during RT, 5-FU was given as bolus or continuous infusion; see text for survival figures for this portion of the trial.

RT, radiation therapy.

See Table 65-2 for definitions of additional acronyms used.

(MOF) versus 5-FU plus leucovorin chemotherapy. Because of an unexpected apparent detrimental outcome with MOF for female participants in NSABP R-01,[24] only men were randomized to the two chemotherapy regimens, whereas women were assigned to 5-FU plus leucovorin. All patients were further randomized to chemotherapy alone or chemotherapy plus radiation therapy. Results are not yet available. The answers to the questions of the relative activity of MeCCNU-containing treatment to 5-FU plus leucovorin and the contribution of radiation therapy are very relevant to current management decisions in rectal cancer and are discussed further later in this chapter.

Several of these 5-FU studies conducted during the first 25 years of adjuvant research were among the clinical trials subjected to a metaanalysis by Buyse and others.[28] They surveyed 17 randomized clinical trials in colorectal cancer that compared adjuvant chemotherapy to surgery alone in an aggregate of almost 6800 patients. They reported a 2.3% to 5.7% improvement in 5-year survival that could be attributed to 5-FU. The survey concluded that in a common malignancy, such as large bowel cancer, even such a small improvement in survival can be meaningful, because a 5% rise in 5-year survival would translate into a median increase in survival of 10 months. A strong recommendation stated that future clinical trials should be larger than in the past and should have a well characterized subject population. This metaanalysis coincided with efforts in the late 1980s among Cooperative Groups to combined their resources in Intergroup studies and in pooled data to identify incremental improvements in survival that were both statistically and clinically significant. Several groups collaborated in the testing of adjuvant 5-FU plus levamisole and 5-FU plus leucovorin. These investigations have produced not only a more precisely defined effect of adjuvant therapy but increases in survival that are two to three times those reported by Buyse and colleagues for single-agent 5-FU treatment.

5-FLUOROURACIL AND LEVAMISOLE

Levamisole has been used as an effective anthelmintic drug since 1966,[29] and was noted to have apparent immunomodulatory activity in experimental animals in 1971.[30] Since that time, it has been applied extensively to the treatment of nonmalignant and malignant disease. Reviews of the development of levamisole and its combination with 5-FU for adjuvant treatment of colon cancer[31] and a detailed update on more recent clinical experience with the regimen[32] are available. Even after broad laboratory and clinical experience with the agent, the mechanism of levamisole's antitumor activity remains uncertain. Its mode of interaction with 5-FU is unknown. Nevertheless, the clinical data from trials strongly indicate a benefit for the combination that exceeds any activity that might be ascribed to either agent used alone.

One of the earliest studies of levamisole in an adjuvant setting was by Verhaegen and coworkers, who conducted a case–control investigation that assessed the survival of 30 patients with stages I to III colorectal cancer receiving levamisole for 2 years after surgery[33] (Table 65-4). The report of a dramatic difference in 5-year survival compared with a matched control group generated interest in additional studies of this adjuvant therapy.

The European Organization for Research in the Treatment of Cancer attempted to validate the Verhaegen experience with a statistically rigorous protocol design (see Table 65-4).[34] Approximately 300 stage III colon cancer patients were randomized to treatment with levamisole or placebo for 1 year after surgery. Although a survival difference at 5 years was seen in favor of levamisole (51% vs. 39%), this difference was not significant, and, more important, equivalent disease-free survival rates (38% vs. 35%, respectively) indicated that any valid difference in survival was not attributable to a reduction in disease recurrence.

The data from two U.S. Cooperative Group studies served to demonstrate the efficacy of combined levamisole and 5-FU and further confirmed the lack of benefit for single-agent levamisole. The NCCTG and Mayo Clinic compared surgery alone (see Table 65-4), surgery plus levamisole, and surgery plus levamisole and 5-FU in 401 patients with stage II or III colorectal cancer.[35] The drug combination produced a statistically significant improvement in disease-free survival and, for the group of node-positive patients, a survival benefit compared with surgery alone. A follow-up Intergroup study with the participation of the NCCTG, the Eastern Cooperative Oncology Group (ECOG), and the Southwestern Oncology Group (SWOG) accrued 1297 patients with stage II and III cancer.[36,37] More than 900 stage III patients were assigned to surgical control, levamisole, or 5-FU plus levamisole, and 325 stage II patients were randomized to either surgical control or the 5-FU/levamisole combination. This study confirmed the benefit of the two-drug adjuvant regimen for the node-positive patients. After a median follow-up of 5 years, recurrence rates associated with the three treatment options were surgery 53%, levamisole 52%, and 5-FU plus levamisole 37%, and overall survival rates were 51%, 54%, and 64%, respectively.[37] These figures translate into a 39% reduction in risk for recurrence and a 31% reduction in risk of dying. For the patients with stage II disease, there have been too few statistical events (recurrences or deaths) to detect a difference between treatments.

The regimen that was tested in these trials has become an accepted standard adjuvant treatment for patients with node-positive colon cancer. It consists of an intravenous bolus of 5-FU 450 $mg/m^2/d$ for 5 days, and, beginning 4 weeks later, 5-FU 450 mg/m^2 intravenously for one dose each week for 48 weeks, concurrent with levamisole 50 mg (total dose) orally three times a day for 3 days every other week. The adjuvant therapy was to be initiated within about 4 weeks after surgery and after recovery from all surgical complications.

These trials have clearly demonstrated that levamisole alone does not reduce tumor recurrence or enhance survival after surgery, but a persistent point of debate is whether a 5-FU treatment alone would have produced results similar to those achieved with the combination. One study by Windle and colleagues[38] (see Table 65-4) is frequently cited as showing a benefit for adjuvant 5-FU plus levamisole compared with 5-FU alone, but the findings from that trial are controversial because of the small sample size (131 patients randomized to three treatments), the unusual drug dosing (levamisole for only 3 postoperative days and 5-FU orally for 6 months), and the reporting of the survival only as a disease-specific function. There are no trustworthy, prospective data to confirm whether optimally administered, single-agent 5-FU could or could not achieve the results seen with the combination of levamisole and 5-FU. There is, however, the important metaanalysis by Buyse and colleagues that supports the probability that the 31% reduction in risk of death

TABLE 65-4. *Adjuvant trials with levamisole and 5-FU*

Study	Accrual	Regimen	5-Year survival
Verhaegen, et al[33] 1974–1975	30	Surgery + levamisole	70%
	30	Surgery alone (matched control)	43%
EORTC[34] 1978–1985	146	Levamisole	51%
	151	Placebo	39%
NCCTG 784852[35] 1978–1984	136	5-FU + levamisole	62%
	130	Levamisole	59%
	135	Surgery alone	55%
Intergroup 0035[36,37] 1985–1987	304	5-FU + levamisole	64%*
	310	Levamisole	54%*
	315	Surgery alone	51%*
Windle, et al[38]	44	5-FU + levamisole	68%†
	42	5-FU	48%†
	45	Surgery alone	56%†

* Cumulative survival data with 5-year median follow-up of stage III patients; $P < 0.05$ for combination compared with control.

† Disease-specific survival.

EORTC, European Organization for Research in the Treatment of Cancer.

See Table 65-2 for definitions of additional acronyms used.

associated with the combination exceeds that expected with 5-FU by two- to threefold. Of more relevance, the debate has moved from the comparable effects of 5-FU with or without levamisole to a comparison of 5-FU plus levamisole to 5-FU plus leucovorin. Clinical trial data that address the respective activity of these combinations have been reported in abstract form;[38a,38b,38c,38d] full reports of mature data will appear in 1997 and 1998.

5-FLUOROURACIL AND LEUCOVORIN

The basis for the incorporation of 5-FU and leucovorin into an adjuvant treatment plan is more rational than the use of 5-FU plus levamisole, a completely empiric regimen. The primary mechanism of action of 5-FU and leucovorin is understood to be formation of a covalent ternary complex with thymidylate synthase,[39] whereas the basis of the interaction between 5-FU and levamisole is unknown. There are several doses and schedules of 5-FU and leucovorin in common use. The optimal regimen has not been determined, but comparative clinical trials of various doses and schedules have been concluded for both metastatic or adjuvant settings. The regimen of 5-FU and levamisole is based on purely empiric dosing, and theoretic guidelines for further tailoring of the regimen are nonexistent. Finally, one of the principles of adjuvant therapy is to include agents with known activity in the metastatic disease setting. The addition of levamisole to 5-FU in treatment of advanced disease has been shown not to increase response rates or survival.[40,41] In contrast, several clinical trials have demonstrated enhanced response rates with the combination of leucovorin with 5-FU. An overview of randomized trials in stage IV colorectal cancer reported a doubling of the overall response rate from 11% for 5-FU alone to 23% for the combination.[42,43] Although a general increase in survival with 5-FU plus leucovorin was not detected by the overview, an improvement has been seen.[44,45]

A number of published studies have established activity for adjuvant 5-FU and leucovorin in colon cancer. The tabulation of these studies in Table 65-5 reveals a strikingly consistent pattern of benefit, even though different doses, schedules, and durations of chemotherapy were used in individual trials.

The NSABP evaluated postoperative 5-FU and leucovorin versus MOF.[46] The schedule chosen for the 5-FU and leucovorin was modified from the regimen developed by Roswell Park and the GITSG.[47] It consisted of 5-FU 500 mg/m^2 plus leucovorin 500 mg/m^2 administered weekly for 6 weeks followed by a 2-week rest, repeating these 8-week cycles for a total of six cycles or 46 weeks (''GITSG regimen''). The MOF regimen had earlier been noted to be a marginally active adjuvant treatment.[20] Given the suggestion that MeCCNU does not improve the benefit of 5-FU, in assessing the relative activity of 5-FU and leucovorin, MOF might be regarded as a 5-FU-alone control. This study, NSABP C-03, with over 1000 patients followed for a median of 4 years, reported statistically significantly better disease-free and overall survival for patients treated with adjuvant 5-FU and leucovorin. The survival figures shown in Table 65-5 represent a 32% reduction in risk for death within 3 years for the superior chemotherapy group.

The NCCTG led an effort to test postoperative 5-FU and leucovorin compared with surgery alone.[48] Doses of chemotherapy on this study were 5-FU 425 mg/m^2 plus leucovorin 20 mg/m^2 administered for 5 days every 4 to 5 weeks for six monthly cycles (''NCCTG regimen''[45]). This protocol was originally intended to be a follow-up study to the Intergroup INT-0035, 5-FU plus levamisole study. When the information from that previous trial became available showing that treatment was superior to surgery-alone control, it was deemed proper to terminate studies containing an ''observation'' control. Only 309 subjects of the planned total target had been accrued. A significant improvement in recurrence-free survival at 3.5 years ($P = 0.004$) for this small group supports a benefit from adjuvant 5-FU and leucovorin. Survival figures, although slightly higher for the chemotherapy group, do not show a statistically significant difference, but at the time of the preliminary report nearly one third of the anticipated deaths had not yet occurred.

The third summary of results with adjuvant 5-FU plus leuco-

TABLE 65-5. *Adjuvant trials with 5-FU plus leucovorin*

Study	Total accrual	Regimen	3-Year disease-free survival	3-Year survival
NSABP C-03[46] 1987–1989	1041	5-FU + leucovorin	73%*	84%*
		MOF	64%	77%
NCCTG 874651[48]† 1988–1989	309	5-FU + leucovorin	77%*	75%
		Surgery alone	64%	71%
NCIC, GIVIO, FFCD[49] 1987–1992	1493	5-FU + leucovorin	72%*	83%*
		Surgery alone	63%	78%
Siena, Italy[51]‡ 1985–1990	116 (stage III)	5-FU + leucovorin	56%*	69%*
		Surgery alone	41%	43%

*$P < 0.05$ compared with control.
† 3.5-Year data.
‡ Five-year data.
MOF, methyl-CCNU, vincristine, and 5-FU; *GIVIO,* Gruppo Italiano Valutazione Interventi Oncologia; *FFCD,* Foundation Francaise Cancerologie Digestive.
See Table 65-2 for definitions of additional acronyms used.

vorin reflects pooled data from the National Cancer Institute of Canada (NCIC), Gruppo Italiano Valutazione Interventi Oncologia, and Foundation Francaise Cancerologie Digestive.[49] These three groups conducted independent but parallel clinical studies with surgery alone versus a regimen of 5-FU 370 to 400 mg/m^2 plus leucovorin 200 mg/m^2 administered daily for 5 days, monthly for 6 months (''Machover regimen''[50]). In the combined population of almost 1500 patients, both event-free survival and overall survival were significantly improved at 3 years for the group treated with chemotherapy. Treatment reduced relative risk for recurrence by 34% and for death by 22%. Another European study from the University of Siena, Italy, used the Machover regimen given for 12 months compared with surgical control, and has reported its data independently.[51] Among the relatively small total of 236 patients with stage II or III colon cancer, a statistically significant survival advantage for treatment was seen only for the 116 node-positive patients, who experienced roughly a 40% reduced risk for recurrence and for death.

To compare the 5-FU plus leucovorin regimens to a 5-FU plus levamisole control, to rank the degree of benefit from the various drug combinations, and to estimate the contribution of levamisole to a 5-FU-based regimen, three large Cooperative Group colon cancer trials were developed. A fourth study assessed these treatments in resected rectal cancer patients. Accrual of subjects to each of these trials has been completed, but follow-up is not yet mature and the studies have not yet been reported (Tables 65-6 and 65-7).

The NSABP entered more than 2100 patients[38a,38b,38c,38d] between July, 1989 and December, 1990 on a three-arm study (NSABP C-04) to assess treatment with 1 year of 5-FU plus levamisole control versus 46 weeks of the GITSG regimen of 5-FU and leucovorin with or without levamisole. The ECOG, SWOG, and Cancer and Leukemia Group B (CALGB) collaborated on an Intergroup study (INT-0089) that accrued approximately 3700 patients between September, 1989 and August, 1992 and compared 1 year of the 5-FU plus levamisole control, 6 months' therapy with the GITSG regimen, 6 months of the NCCTG regimen, or 6 months of the NCCTG regimen plus levamisole. The NCCTG with the NCIC evaluated two treatments, a 5-FU and levamisole control and an NCCTG 5-FU/leucovorin schedule plus levamisole (NCCTG 894651). In a

TABLE 65-6. *Recently completed multiinstitutional trials with adjuvant chemotherapy*

Study	Total accrual	Regimen
NSABP C-04	2140	5-FU + levamisole
		5-FU + leucovorin weekly
		5-FU + leucovorin weekly + levamisole
Intergroup 0089	3400	5-FU + levamisole
		5-FU + leucovorin weekly
		5-FU + leucovorin monthly
		5-FU + leucovorin monthly + levamisole
NCCTG 894651	915	5-FU + levamisole (6 or 12 mo)
		5-FU + leucovorin monthly + levamisole (6 or 12 mo)
Intergroup 0114	1800	5-FU + pelvic irradiation
		5-FU + levamisole and pelvic irradiation
		5-FU + leucovorin monthly and pelvic irradiation
		5-FU + leucovorin monthly, levamisole and pelvic irradiation
NSABP C-05	2100	5-FU + leucovorin monthly
		5-FU + leucovorin monthly and interferon-α

See Table 65-2 for definitions of acronyms.

TABLE 65-7. *Overlapping design of 5-FU, leucovorin, and levamisole trials (showing approximate duration of therapy)*

Study	5-FU levamisole	5-FU/leucovorin		5-FU–leucovorin–levamisole	
		Weekly	Monthly	Weekly	Monthly
NSABP C-04	12 mo	12 mo		12 mo	
Intergroup 0089	12 mo	6 mo	6 mo		6 mo
NCCTG 894651	6 or 12 mo				6 or 12 mo
Intergroup 0114	6 mo		6 mo		6 mo

See Table 65-2 for definitions of acronyms.

so-called two-by-two factorial design,[52] this trial also addressed a comparison of two durations of treatment by randomizing patients to receive either 6 or 12 months of their assigned therapy. Accrual of 915 subjects was completed within a 3-year time span, similar to that for the other trials. In addition, an Intergroup trial in rectal cancer (INT-0114) in which the ECOG, SWOG, NCCTG, CALGB, and Radiation Therapy Oncology Group (RTOG) participated, tested treatment options generally similar to those of the INT-0089 study, with some exceptions. Each regimen sandwiched pelvic irradiation between two monthly cycles of chemotherapy; the control regimen was considered to be the one that contained single-agent 5-FU, and 5-FU plus levamisole was one of the experimental arms; the design included no GITSG 5-FU plus leucovorin combination; and treatment for all the regimens was completed within 6 months. Accrual began in June, 1990 and was completed in December, 1993 with 1700 patients.

The overlapping design of these four studies (see Table 65-7) should provide concurrent and independent validation of results from each single trial. Average follow-up of patients is now in excess of 3 years. Taken together, the preliminary reports of these 4 studies suggest three conclusions. First, adjuvant 5-FU plus leucovorin is at least equivalent if not marginally superior to 5-FU plus levamisole therapy. Second, while 6 months' treatment with a 5-FU/leucovorin regimen appears to be adequate, a full year's dosing with 5-FU/levamisole is necessary. And, third, the three drug combination of 5-FU, leucovorin, and levamisole is no better and appears to be somewhat more toxic than either doublet.

Moving beyond the generation of studies that compared 5-FU plus leucovorin to 5-FU plus levamisole, the NSABP has more recently focused on trying to improve results with 5-FU and leucovorin, evaluating adjuvant treatment with these two drugs with or without interferon-α (NSABP C-05). The three-drug combination is based on limited in vitro and clinical experience in stage IV disease that seems to show enhanced activity.[53] Accrual of some 2100 patients was completed in the Spring of 1994.

ADJUVANT CHEMOTHERAPY OF RECTAL CANCER

A higher rate of local recurrence after resection accounts for the principal difference in the treatment planning for rectal cancer compared with the management of colon cancers. By definition, the rectum is the portion of the large bowel that extends distally beyond the pelvic peritoneal reflection. The absence of a serosal covering removes one of the anatomic barriers to radial growth of tumor that is present on the rest of the large intestine. The narrow confines of the bony pelvis limit the radial margins that may be obtained at surgery. Therefore, although proximal and distal tumor-free margins may be several centimeters in length, the apparently cancer-free border between the bowel wall and the sacrum, the bladder, or other organs may be only 1 or 2 mm. The structure of the pelvis not only limits successful extirpation of rectal cancers, but the close proximity of the nerves of the sacral plexus, the weight-bearing bones of the pelvic girdle, the vasculature to the legs, and the organs of excretion and reproduction causes the consequences of tumor recurrence to be characterized by extreme morbidity yet, cruelly, by low mortality until months or years of pain and dysfunction have been endured.

Adjuvant radiation therapy is well established as a means for reducing local recurrence after rectal resection. A full discussion of the treatment planning, the toxicities, and the unresolved clinical questions about pelvic irradiation is the subject of Chapter 66 of this text, but neither adjuvant chemotherapy nor radiation therapy of rectal cancer can be discussed without some reference to both modalities. As presented in Table 65-3 and in the discussion earlier in this chapter about historical trials, combinations of 5-FU-based chemotherapy plus radiation treatment have shown benefit in repeated studies when compared to surgery alone or to postoperative radiation without drugs. Consistently, chemotherapy-based adjuvant treatment has yielded 5-year survival rates of 55% to 60%, compared with control rates of 40% to 45%. However, the therapeutic requirement for the inclusion of radiation therapy in an adjuvant plan is not absolutely established. The NSABP R-01 trial demonstrated superior disease-free and overall survival for adjuvant MOF chemotherapy.[24] As described earlier, NSABP R-02 included a comparison of chemotherapy plus radiation to chemotherapy alone (as well as a comparison of MOF versus 5-FU/leucovorin chemotherapy). This as yet unreported study may clarify the extent of the additional contribution that irradiation makes to adjuvant chemotherapy of rectal cancer. Pending the results from that trial, the optimal regimen, drawn from the experience of the Cooperative Groups, seems to be a combination of 5-FU plus radiation. At the time of publication of the NCCTG study 794751, which compared chemotherapy plus radiation to radiation therapy alone,[23] a National Cancer Institute Clinical Announcement[54] recommended the following adjuvant regimen:

> 5-FU 500 mg/m^2/day IV bolus × 5 days in weeks 1 and 5; pelvic radiation 45 Gy plus a 5.4 Gy tumor bed boost (180 cGy per fraction in daily fractions 5 days a week) weeks 9–15, concurrent with 5-FU 500 mg/m^2/day IV bolus × 3 days in the first and fifth week of radiation; beginning 4–8 weeks after completion of radiation, 5-FU 450 mg/m^2/day IV bolus days 1–5 for two cycles 4 weeks apart.

Further attempts to improve chemotherapy for rectal cancer have paralleled avenues of clinical research for colon cancer, as, for example, those questions posed in NSABP R-02, and those in INT-0114 (see Table 65-4). Efforts to enhance the outcome from radiation therapy involve questions of delivery, fraction size, and timing, which are addressed in Chapter 66. Two major areas of overlap addressed here are the use of "radiation-sensitizing" 5-FU and the strategies for integrating adequate and timely doses of both treatments.

Observations that fluoropyrimidines could enhance the cytotoxicity of radiation date from shortly after the introduction of these drugs.[55] Several mechanisms of interaction have been proposed, including depletion by 5-FU of nucleotide substrates used for repair of radiation-induced DNA damage, synchronization of cell cycling by chemotherapy into a phase more susceptible to radiation killing, the incorporation of a fluorinated false nucleotide into DNA, or potentiation of chemotherapy damage by radiation.[56] Without being sure of the precise interaction, the empiric dose, given earlier, of 500 mg/m^2 of 5-FU on the first 3 days of the first and fifth week of a course of irradiation has been shown to be tolerable and has been widely accepted as a standard dose. One study, NCCTG 864751, previously discussed (see Table 65-3) as supporting the lack of benefit for the addition of MeCCNU to adjuvant chemotherapy,[27] compared this bolus schedule of 5-FU to an infusion of 5-FU 225 mg/m^2/24 hours continuously over the 5 to 6 weeks of radiation therapy. In the two-by-two factorial design, 5-FU was also administered (with or without MeCCNU) for two cycles before and two cycles after the course of radiation therapy, but at these times, chemotherapy was given only on a bolus schedule. The results of continuous infusion during the radiation course were dramatic, showing a 27% lower relapse rate and a 31% reduction in death compared with the bolus 5-FU. Interestingly, while recurrences were decreased overall, the change in schedule in radiosensitizing 5-FU did not result in a statistically decreased rate of local recurrence. At 4 years, recurrence-free survival rates for bolus and continuous-infusion 5-FU were 53% and 63%, respectively, and corresponding survival figures were 60% and 70%. (In Table 65-3, note that only the comparisons of survival for 5-FU ± MeCCNU are shown.)

The findings from this study are provocative. The magnitude of benefit from the continuous-infusion treatment is similar to that achieved for chemoradiation compared with control for rectal cancer[23] and for 5-FU plus levamisole for colon cancer.[37] After the positive results from these earlier studies were reported, there was a general consensus that these treatments represented major advances in adjuvant therapy of colorectal cancer.[57] The findings of NCCTG 864751 are further bolstered by evidence from the metastatic disease setting that continuous-infusion 5-FU results in a higher response rate compared with bolus therapy.[58] However, there remains some basis for caution and skepticism in spite of the promise of infusional therapy. First, this is a single study with a subject population of 660 and median follow-up of less than 4 years. The two-by-two factorial design is an accepted statistical tool for exploring multiple issues, but assumes no interaction between the questions being asked (ie, 5-FU vs. 5-FU + MeCCNU and bolus vs. continuous-infusion 5-FU). Consensus about earlier advances rested on validation of preliminary findings by subsequent clinical investigations, providing firm statistical confidence in the results. Administration of a continuous-infusion regimen requires an indwelling intravenous access device and an ambulatory infusion pump. In a cost (risk) : benefit assessment of any treatment, the expense and complications associated with such devices must be considered. Simpler regimens of 5-FU plus leucovorin, for example, may yield the same degree of benefit. Until studies, which are now in progress, can substantiate the superiority of a prolonged infusion schedule of adjuvant 5-FU, this regimen should be implemented in clinical practice only after considering alternative options.

Regarding strategies for scheduling both modalities, integration of drugs and radiation has advantages over sequential delivery of the two treatments. If an entire, 4- to 6-month course of chemotherapy is given before radiation therapy is delivered, the opportunity to eliminate microscopic residual disease from the tumor bed may be jeopardized, especially if the tumor is drug resistant and has, therefore, not received the cytotoxic impact of chemotherapy. On the other hand, general control of disease and extension of survival may be compromised if chemotherapy is delayed for 2 to 3 months to allow time for delivery and recovery from irradiation. It is important to reemphasize that clinical data show that radiation alone contributes to neither systemic tumor control nor survival, but cytotoxic effects of chemotherapy do extend to both systemic and local disease. Not only will the initiation of chemotherapy be delayed, but prior pelvic irradiation may require that, for control of myelosuppression or diarrhea, doses of drugs be attenuated by 10% or more. A schedule of treatment, such as that adopted by the Cooperative Groups, in which initial chemotherapy, followed by radiation plus sensitizing 5-FU, and more chemotherapy are "sandwiched," may allow for optimal benefit from each modality. Evidence in support of this recommendation must be inferred from various past trials. It is exceedingly unlikely and undesirable that a clinical comparison of optimal versus presumed suboptimal treatment would ever be performed to confirm it. In preoperative scheduling of radiation therapy or in a situation in which radiation must be completed before full doses of chemotherapy can begin, an aggressive schedule of radiosensitizing drug might be considered. The direction for clinical research in rectal cancer continues toward determining the best timing of treatments vis-à-vis surgery and refining concurrent delivery of chemotherapy and radiation.

CURRENT DIRECTIONS IN ADJUVANT TRIALS

The current emphasis of Cooperative Group investigation in rectal cancer is to compare preoperative versus postoperative treatment, and is the subject of two new studies, an RTOG-led Intergroup study (INT-0147) and NSABP R-03 (Table 65-8). The major difference in the design of these two trials is in the duration of preoperative therapy, which is about 1 month for INT-0147 and 4 months for NSABP R-03. The rationale for studying preoperative irradiation is laid out in Chapter 66. It seems likely that completion of such studies will require several years because only a small proportion of patients, those accessed before surgery, will be eligible. Patients not available for study in the preoperative setting may be eligible for a trial that addresses chemotherapy issues in postoperative combined-modality treatment (INT-0144). This Intergroup study, to be coordinated by SWOG, compares bolus 5-FU to prolonged infu-

TABLE 65-8. *Current or proposed multiinstitutional adjuvant trials*

Study	Projected accrual	Regimen
RECTAL STUDIES		
Intergroup 0147	800	Postoperative RT and 5-FU + leucovorin Preoperative RT and 5-FU + leucovorin plus postoperative 5-FU + leucovorin
NSABP R-03	900	Postoperative RT and 5-FU + leucovorin Preoperative 5-FU + leucovorin, then concurrent preoperative RT and chemotherapy plus postoperative 5-FU + leucovorin
Intergroup 0144	2400	Bolus 5-FU plus concurrent RT and infusional 5-FU Infusional 5-FU plus concurrent RT and infusional 5-FU Bolus 5-FU + leucovorin plus concurrent RT and 5-FU + leucovorin
COLON STUDIES		
Intergroup 0130 (TNM T4 or N1, 2)	700	5-FU + levamisole 5-FU + levamisole and tumor bed irradiation
Intergroup 0136	2000	5-FU + levamisole Perioperative venous 5-FU infusion followed by 5-FU + levamisole
Intergroup 0153	1800	Bolus 5-FU and leucovorin + levamisole Prolonged infusion 5-FU + levamisole
Intergroup 0135	1400	5-FU + leucovorin and standard-dose levamisole 5-FU + leucovorin and high-dose levamisole

RT, radiation therapy.
See Table 65-2 for definitions of additional acronyms used.

sion 5-FU and to 5-FU plus leucovorin, before, during, and after pelvic irradiation.

The application of radiation therapy to colon cancer is the subject of another Intergroup study, INT-0130. A role for irradiation to improve locoregional control has been postulated for patients with TNM T4 disease (a tumor with direct extension to an adjacent organ), comparable to its role in the management of rectal cancer. INT-0130 is a collaborative study between the NCCTG and RTOG to compare 5-FU and levamisole with or without radiation therapy for completely resected locally advanced colon cancers. This study was activated in mid-1992 and is projected to reach its accrual target of 800 patients over about 7 years.

Another Intergroup study (INT-0136) dealing with a specific clinical subset of colon cancer patients will address patients who are available for immediate perioperative chemotherapy. For these patients, 7-day, perioperative systemic 5-FU infusion will be compared to no perioperative treatment; both groups will subsequently receive 5-FU and levamisole for 1 year. This study is based on the observations of improved systemic disease-free survival seen in trials of perioperative portal vein infusion.[11,12] This study is limited to patients who present to one of the participating Cooperative Group institutions for their primary colon cancer resection. Activated in late 1993, the trial is expected to accrue 800 patients.

A third study, open to patients with resected stage II or III colon cancer, will compare a continuous intravenous infusion schedule versus a bolus schedule of 5-FU in combination with leucovorin and levamisole (INT-0153). The results of this important trial will determine whether the cost and complications of continuous infusion therapy are warranted in the adjuvant setting. This clinical trial, coordinated by SWOG, was activated in late 1994.

Finally, the NCCTG and NCIC have undertaken an investigation of levamisole dose, comparing standard-dose and high-dose levamisole in conjunction with 5-FU plus leucovorin (INT-0135). As noted previously, scarce data exist at present to define the optimal dose of levamisole in the adjuvant setting.

RECOMMENDATIONS FOR THERAPY

Adjuvant treatment of colon or rectal tumors may be initiated as early as 10 to 14 days after surgery, but more commonly begins about 4 weeks after surgery. If therapy has been delayed for more than 8 to 12 weeks, there are no data on which to base an assessment of hypothetical risk or benefit, and discussion with the patient about options for continued follow-up or treatment should reflect this uncertainty.

Candidates for adjuvant therapy should have recovered from surgery to the extent that their wounds are well healing and there is no evidence for infection. Oral intake and bowel function should be normalizing. These patients should not have other medical problems that represent an equal or greater risk to life than does their risk for recurrent cancer. Overall performance status should allow for expected compliance with the therapeutic regimen.

Whenever possible, to contribute to the evolution of better treatment, patients should be considered for clinical trials. Table 65-9 summarizes options for noninvestigational adjuvant therapy.

As noted at the beginning of this chapter, long-term survival for TNM stage I patients with colon or rectal cancer is only slightly lower than that for an age-matched cohort from the general population. Even if a very large clinical trial were to be designed to detect a 3% to 5% improvement in survival for this group, the toxicities and expense of cytotoxic therapy, which would be borne by 100% of the patients, greatly outweigh

TABLE 65-9. *Colorectal cancer: recommendations for adjuvant therapy by stage**

Stage	Options
I—Colon	Observation after curative-intent resection
II—Colon	Postsurgery observation *or* chemotherapy with 5-FU + levamisole or 5-FU + leucovorin
III—Colon	Chemotherapy with 5-FU + levamisole or 5-FU + leucovorin
I—Rectum	Observation after curative-intent resection
II, III—Rectum	Postoperative combined 5-FU (+ leucovorin) chemotherapy plus radiation plus

* See text for doses and duration of regimens.
5-FU, 5-fluorouracil.

the potential benefit to 5%. Only a well tolerated and inexpensive treatment, such as a daily dose of aspirin,[59] would be appropriate even for testing for these patients.

People with stage II or III rectal cancer have a substantial risk for tumor recurrence. Treatment modeled on the 5-FU plus radiation regimen given earlier has been shown to reduce this risk. Incorporation of a schedule of continuous infusion of 5-FU during radiation therapy or inclusion of leucovorin during the cycles of chemotherapy has a rational basis, but still lacks the support of confirmed clinical data. Considerations to use these variations outside of the context of a clinical trial should include a review of treatment options with the patient and awareness that the anticipated toxicity spectrum for treatment may be altered when chemotherapy and irradiation are combined.

Stage II colon cancer presents to the clinician the challenge to determine which patients are most at risk for relapse and which patients have most likely been cured by surgery alone. Current data have failed to prove a benefit from adjuvant chemotherapy in stage II colon cancer, but do not suggest that treatment adversely affects survival for this group.[60] Pooled data from four NSABP studies indicate that benefits observed for stage II patients are comparable to those seen for stage III patients.[61] Some prognostic indicators that may differentiate between high-risk and low-risk patients have been identified. These factors include direct extension of tumor to adjacent structures (TNM T4 or Dukes' B3 disease), tumor associated with bowel perforation or obstruction, and cancer with aneuploid DNA.[62] Several tumor markers, including extent of thymidylate synthase expression,[63] may aid in discriminating candidates for further therapy from those not likely to need adjuvants to surgery. The patient's own enthusiasm for pursuing every means to avoid tumor relapse or total aversion to the idea of chemotherapy are valid factors when discussing the pros and cons of additional treatment. If a decision is made to give adjuvant chemotherapy, the recommendations for stage III colon cancer apply.

For stage III colon cancer, the use of either 5-FU plus levamisole or 5-FU plus leucovorin is supported by clinical data, but the extent of information and the duration of follow-up is greater for 5-FU plus levamisole. Only after the most recently completed studies are reported in detail will there be information about comparative activity of these regimens. To the degree that comparisons can be made across clinical trials, the two combinations appear to have similar effectiveness and tolerance. The doses have been given in the preceding sections. If the clinician chooses to administer adjuvant 5-FU plus leucovorin, there are few data to direct the clinician to the best of these regimens. Familiarity with use of one or the other regimens in the metastatic disease setting may be the best guide. The recommended duration of treatment for 5-FU plus levamisole is 12 months, and for 5-FU plus leucovorin, 6 to 12 months.

REFERENCES

1. Gilman A. The initial trial of nitrogen mustard. Am J Surg 1963;105: 574.
2. Veterans Administration Adjuvant Cancer Chemotherapy Cooperative Group. Status of adjuvant cancer chemotherapy. Arch Surg 1961;82: 466.
3. Holden WD, Dixon WJ. A study of the use of triethylenethiophosphoramide as an adjuvant to surgery in the treatment of colorectal cancer. Cancer Chemotherapy Reports 1962;16:129.
4. Friedman MA, Hamilton JM. Progress in the adjuvant therapy of large bowel cancer. In: DeVita VT, Hellman S, Rosenberg SA, eds. Important advances in oncology 1988. Philadelphia: JB Lippincott, 1988:273.
5. Heidelberger CA, Chaudhari NK, Dannenberg P, et al. Fluorinated pyrimidines: a new class of tumour-inhibitory compounds. Nature 1957;169:663.
6. Dwight RW, Humphrey EW, Higgins GA, et al. FUDR as an adjuvant to surgery in cancer of the large bowel. J Surg Oncol 1973;5:243.
7. Higgins GA, Lee LE, Dwight RW, et al. The case for adjuvant 5-fluorouracil in colorectal cancer. Cancer Clinical Trials 1978;1:35.
8. Grage TB, Moss SE. Adjuvant chemotherapy in cancer of the colon and rectum: demonstration of effectiveness of prolonged 5-FU chemotherapy in a prospectively controlled, randomized trial. Surg Clin North Am 1981;61:1321.
9. Taylor I, Machin D, Mulleet M, et al. A randomized controlled trial of adjuvant portal vein cytotoxic perfusion in colorectal cancer. Br J Surg 1985;72:359.
10. Beart RW Jr, Moertel CG, Wieand HS, et al. Adjuvant therapy for resectable colorectal carcinoma with fluorouracil administration by portal vein infusion: a study of the Mayo Clinic and North Central Cancer Treatment Group. Arch Surg 1990;125:897.
11. Wolmark N, Rockette H, Wickerham DL, et al. Adjuvant therapy of Dukes' A, B, and C adenocarcinoma of the colon with portal-vein fluorouracil hepatic infusion: preliminary results of National Surgical Adjuvant Breast and Bowel Project protocol C-02. J Clin Oncol 1990; 8:1466.
12. Metzger U, Laffer U, Aeberhard P, et al. Randomized multicenter trial of adjuvant intraportal chemotherapy for colorectal cancer SAKK 40/81: an interim report. Acta Chir Scand 1990;156:467.
13. Mayo JG, Lester WR Jr, Andrews CM, et al. Success and failure in the treatment of solid tumors III. Cancer Chemotherapy Reports 1972; 56;183.
14. Young RE, Walker MD, Canellos GP, et al. Initial clinical trials with methyl-CCNU 1-(2-chloroethyl)-3-(4-methyl-cyclohexyl)-1-nitrosourea (MeCCNU). Cancer 1973;31:1164.
15. Moertel CG. Therapy of advanced gastrointestinal cancer with the nitrosoureas. Cancer Chemotherapy Reports 1973;4:27.
16. Higgins GA Jr, Amadeo JH, McElhinney J, et al. Efficacy of prolonged intermittent therapy with combined 5-fluorouracil and methyl-CCNU following resection for carcinoma of the large bowel. Cancer 1984;53: 1.
17. Gastrointestinal Study Group. Adjuvant therapy of colon cancer: results of a prospectively randomized trial. N Engl J Med 1984;310:737.
18. Panettiere FJ, Goodman, PJ Costanzi JJ, et al. Adjuvant therapy in large bowel adenocarcinoma: long term results of a Southwest Oncology Group study. J Clin Oncol 1988;6:947.
19. Mansour E, Ryan L, Lerner H, et al. Lack of effectiveness of 5-FU and methyl CCNU as compared to 5-FU for adjuvant therapy in colon cancer: a randomized trial of the Eastern Cooperative Oncology Group (EST 2276). Proceedings of the American Society of Clinical Oncology 1989;8:115.
20. Wolmark N, Fisher B, Rockette H, et al. Postoperative adjuvant chemotherapy or BCG for colon cancer: results from NSABP C-01. J Natl Cancer Inst 1988;80:14.

21. Gastrointestinal Study Group. Prolongation of the disease-free interval in surgically treated rectal cancer. N Engl J Med 1985;312:1465.
22. Douglass HO, Moertel CG, Mayer RJ, et al. Survival after postoperative combination treatment of rectal cancer. (Letter) N Engl J Med 1986; 315:1294.
23. Krook J, Moertel C, Gunderson LL, et al. Effective surgical adjuvant therapy for high risk rectal carcinoma. N Engl J Med 1991;324:709.
24. Fisher B, Wolmark N, Rockette H, et al. Postoperative adjuvant chemotherapy or radiation therapy for rectal cancer: results from NSABP R-01. J Natl Cancer Inst 1988;80:31.
25. Boice JD, Greene MH, Killen JY, et al. Leukemia and preleukemia after adjuvant treatment of gastrointestinal cancer with semustine (methy-CCNU). N Engl J Med 1983;309:1079.
26. Gastrointestinal Tumor Study Group. Radiation therapy and fluorouracil with or without semustine for the treatment of patients with surgical adjuvant adenocarcinoma of the rectum. J Clin Oncol 1992;10:549.
27. O'Connell MJ, Martenson JA, Wieand HS, et al. Improving adjuvant therapy for rectal cancer by combining protracted-infusion fluorouracil with radiation after curative surgery. N Engl J Med 1994;331:502.
28. Buyse M, Zeleniuch-Jacquotte A, Chalmers TC. Adjuvant therapy of colorectal cancer: why we still don't know. JAMA 1988;259:3571.
29. Raeymaekers AH, Allewjin FTN, Vanderberk J, et al. Novel and broad spectrum anthelmintic tetramisole and related derivatives of 6-arylimidazole[2,1-b]thiazole. J Med Chem 1966;9:545.
30. Renoux G, Renoux M. Stimulation of anti-brucella vaccination in mice by tetramisole, a phenyl-imidothiazole salt. Infect Immunol 1973;8: 544.
31. Hamilton JM, Sznol M, Friedman MA. 5-Fluorouracil plus levamisole: effective adjuvant treatment for colon cancer. In: Devita VT, Hellman S, Rosenberg SA, eds. Important advances in oncology 1990. Philadelphia: JB Lippincott, 1990:115.
32. Hamilton JM, Friedman MA. 5-Fluorouracil plus levamisole update. PPO Updates 1994;11:1.
33. Verhaegen H, DeCree J, DeCock W, et al. Levamisole therapy in patients with colorectal cancer. In: Terry WD, Rosenberg SA, eds. Immunotherapy of human cancer. New York: Excerpta Medica, Elsevier North Holland, Inc., 1982:225.
34. Arnaud J, Buyse M, Nordlinger B, et al. Adjuvant therapy of poor prognosis colon cancer with levamisole: results of an EORTC double-blind randomized clinical trial. Br J Surg 1989;76:284.
35. Laurie JA, Moertel CG, Fleming TR, et al. Surgical adjuvant therapy of large-bowel carcinoma: an evaluation of levamisole and fluorouracil: the North Central Treatment Group and Mayo Clinic. J Clin Oncol 1989;7:1447.
36. Moertel CG, Fleming TR, Macdonald JS, et al. Levamisole and fluorouracil for adjuvant therapy of resected colon carcinoma. N Engl J Med 1990;322:352.
37. Moertel C, Fleming T, Macdonald JS, et al. Fluorouracil plus levamisole after resection of stage III colon carcinoma: a final report. Ann Intern Med 1995;122:321.
38. Windle R, Bell PRF, Shaw D. Five year results of a randomized trial of adjuvant 5-fluorouracil and levamisole in colorectal cancer. Br J Surg 1987;74:569.
38a. Wolmark N, Rockette H, Mamounas EP, et al. The relative efficacy of 5-FU + leucovorin (FU-LV), 5-FU + levamisole (FU-LEV), and 5-FU + leucovorin + levamisole (FU-LV-LEV) in patients with Dukes' B and C carcinoma of the colon: first report of NSABP C-04. Proceedings of the American Society of Clinical Oncology (abstract) 1996;15:205.
38b. Haller DG, Catalano PJ, Macdonald JS, et al. Fluorouracil (FU), leucovorin (LV), and levamisole (LEV) adjuvant therapy for colon cancer: preliminary results of INT-0089. Proceedings of the American Society of Clinical Oncology (abstract) 1996;15:211.
38c. O'Connell MJ, Laurie JA, Shepard, et al. A prospective evaluation of chemotherapy duration and regimen as surgical adjuvant treatment for high-risk colon cancer: a collaborative trial of the North Central Cancer Treatment Group and the National Cancer Institute of Canada Clinical Trials Group. Proceedings of the American Society of Clinical Oncology (abstract) 1996;15:209.
38d. Tepper J, O'Connell M, Petroni G, et al. Toxicity in the adjuvant therapy of rectal cancer: a preliminary report of Intergroup 0114 (CALGB 9081). Proceedings of the American Society of Clinical Oncology (abstract) 1996;15:210.
39. Grem JL, Hoth DF, Hamilton JM, et al. Overview of current status and future directions of clinical trials with 5-fluorouracil in combination with folinic acid. Cancer Treat Rep 1987;71:1249.
40. Bedikian A, Valdivieso M, Mavligit G, et al. Sequential chemoimmunotherapy of colorectal caner: evaluation of methotrexate, Baker's antifol and levamisole. Cancer 1978;42:2169.
41. Buroker T, Moertel C, Fleming T, et al. A controlled evaluation of recent approaches to biochemical modulation or enhancement of 5-fluorouracil therapy in colorectal carcinoma. J Clin Oncol 1985;3:1624.
42. Advanced Colorectal Cancer Meta-analysis Project. Modulation of fluorouracil by leucovorin in patients with advanced colorectal cancer: evidence in terms of response rate. J Clin Oncol 1992;10:896.
43. Piedbois P, Buyse M. What can we learn from a meta-analysis of trials testing the modulation of 5-FU by leucovorin? Ann Oncol 1993; 4(Suppl 2)dʒ5.
44. Poon MA, O'Connell MJ, Moertel CG, et al. Biochemical modulation of fluorouracil: evidence of significant improvement of survival and quality of life in patients with advanced colorectal carcinoma. J Clin Oncol 1989;7:1407.
45. Poon MA, O'Connell MJ, Wieand HS, et al. Biochemical modulation of fluorouracil with leucovorin: confirmatory evidence of improved therapeutic efficacy in advanced colorectal cancer. J Clin Oncol 1991; 9:1967.
46. Wolmark N, Rockette H, Fisher B, et al. The benefit of leucovorin-modulated fluorouracil as postoperative adjuvant therapy for primary colon cancer: results from National Surgical Adjuvant Breast and Bowel Project protocol C-03. J Clin Oncol 1993;11;1879.
47. Petrelli N, Douglass HO Jr, Herrera L, et al for the Gastrointestinal Tumor Study Group. The modulation of fluorouracil with leucovorin in metastatic colorectal carcinoma: a prospective randomized phase III trial. J Clin Oncol 1989;7:1419.
48. O'Connell M, Maillard J, Macdonald J, et al. An intergroup trial of intensive course 5FU and low dose leucovorin as surgical adjuvant therapy for high risk colon cancer. (Abstract) Proceedings of the American Society of Clinical Oncology 1993;12:190.
49. International Multicentre Pooled Analysis of Colon Cancer Trials (IMPACT) Investigators. Efficacy of adjuvant fluorouracil and folinic acid in colon cancer. Lancet 1995;345:939.
50. Machover D, Goldschmidt E, Chollet P, et al. Treatment of advanced colorectal and gastric adenocarcinomas with 5-fluorouracil and high-dose folinic acid. J Clin Oncol 1986;4:685.
51. Francini G, Petroli R, Lorenzini L, et al. Folinic acid and 5-fluorouracil as adjuvant chemotherapy in colon cancer. Gastroenterology 1994;106: 899.
52. Byar DP, Piantadosi S. Factorial designs for randomized clinical trials. Cancer Treat Rep 1985;69:1055.
53. Grem JL, Jordan E, Robson ME, et al. Phase II study of fluorouracil, leucovorin, and interferon alfa-2A in metastatic colorectal cancer. J Clin Oncol 1993;11:1737.
54. National Cancer Institute Clinical Announcement. Adjuvant therapy of rectal cancer. Bethesda, MD: National Cancer Institute, March 14, 1991.
55. Heidelberger C, Grisbach C, Montag BJ. Studies on fluorinated pyrimidines: II. effects on transplanted tumors. Cancer Res 1958;18:305.
56. Lawrence TS, Maybaum J. Fluoropyrimidines as radiation sensitizers. Semin Rad Onc 1993;3:20.
57. NIH Consensus Conference. Adjuvant therapy for patients with colon and rectal cancer. JAMA 1990;264:1444.
58. Lokich JJ, Alhgren JD, Gullo JJ, et al. A prospective randomized comparison of continuous infusion fluorouracil with a conventional bolus schedule in metastatic colorectal carcinoma: a Mid-Atlantic Oncology Program study. J Clin Oncol 1989;7:425.
59. Thun MJ, Namboodiri MM, Calle EE, et al. Aspirin use and risk of fatal cancer. Cancer Res 1993;53:1322.
60. Moertel CG, Fleming TR, Macdonald JS, et al. Intergroup study of fluorouracil plus levamisole as adjuvant therapy for stage II/Dukes' B2 colon cancer. J Clin Oncol 1995;13:2936.
61. Mamounas EP, Rockette H, Jones J, et al. Comparative efficacy of adjuvant chemotherapy in patients with Dukes' B vs Dukes' C colon cancer: results from four NSABP adjuvant studies (C-01, C-02, C-03, C-04). Proceedings of the American Society of Clinical Oncology (abstract) 1996;15:205.
62. Moertel CG, Loprinzi CL, Witzig TE, et al. The dilemma of stage B-2 colon cancer: is adjuvant therapy justified? A Mayo Clinic/North Central Cancer Treatment Group study. Proceedings of the American Society of Clinical Oncology 1990;9:108.
63. Johnston PG, Fisher ER, Rockette H, et al. The role of thymidylate synthase expression in prognosis and outcome of adjuvant chemotherapy in patients with rectal cancer. J Clin Oncol 1994;12 (In press).

Surgery for Gastrointestinal Cancer: A Multidisciplinary Approach, edited by Harold J. Wanebo.
Lippincott-Raven Publishers, Philadelphia, © 1997.

CHAPTER 66

Preoperative and Postoperative Radiation Therapy for Rectal Cancer: Indications and Clinical Trial Results

Tyvin A. Rich

Cancer of the rectum has been managed primarily by surgery since the Miles operation established that en bloc resection of the primary rectal tumor along with the "zone of upward spread" was superior to limited excision through the perineum. This more radical operation, which frequently leaves the patient with a permanent colostomy and disturbed bladder function, does not eliminate the problem of local failure, however. The risk of local failure is related to the stage of disease, and two staging systems are used to classify the degree of tumor extension. One is based on the pathologic extent of disease assessed in the surgical specimen, first proposed by Dukes.[1] The other staging system is the TNM for rectal cancer, and is based on the digital rectal examination or an ultrasonographic assessment of tumor extension through the bowel wall. With careful preoperative clinical staging and abdominopelvic computed tomography scanning, the percentage of patients with occult metastatic disease evident at subsequent intraoperative exploration is very small.[2] In other words, the slight risk of understaging by today's clinical and radiographic standard assessments allows treatment options that do not require immediate surgical resection. The results of primary tumor diagnosis and the accuracy in assigning prognosis are good, but noninvasive means of assessing lymphatic involvement are by comparison still inaccurate for clinical decision making. As more knowledge is gained about the biologic behavior of rectal cancer based on an assessment of tumor "markers," noninvasive staging will become even more widely used.

Although there have been substantial advances in perioperative management, the surgical results alone for cancer of the rectum have changed little over the last several decades.[3] Tumor recurrence in the operative bed is a common problem in nearly all large surgical series, and the frequency of local failure ranges from approximately 15% to 65%, depending on tumor stage.[4] One reason for the high rate of local failure is the inverse correlation between the extent of tumor penetration through the bowel wall and the margin of uninvolved normal tissue between the tumor and the line of surgical resection.[5,6] For rectal cancers lying deep in the pelvic funnel, the ability to obtain an adequate circumferential margin of resection is compromised by the proximity of the pelvic bone. This anatomic reality creates a risk that residual cells remain after a total gross tumor removal and probably is the major cause of pelvic relapse. The time course of pelvic recurrence is also consistent with the notion that some patients have incomplete resections, because local relapse occurs much sooner that does distant metastasis.[7]

Patients with a local recurrence present with pain, bleeding, and alteration of bowel function in the residual rectum and altered bladder function, resulting in difficult management problems.[8] The results of treatment of perineal and pelvic recurrences have historically been very poor compared with the results obtained with immediate adjuvant therapy, leaving most patients with a local recurrence facing death from uncontrolled pelvic disease. After primary resection, pelvic recurrence is a disease that must be and can be prevented. Fortunately, external irradiation has been used more commonly since the early 1980s, and its use in the postoperative adjuvant setting has been recommended by the National Institutes of Health as a standard of care after surgery.[9]

In this chapter, the results of pelvic irradiation sequenced either after or before surgery for operable rectal cancer are reviewed. With both approaches there is evidence that the quality of life and the cure rates of some patients have been improved with adjuvant pelvic irradiation. The pros and cons of each of these methods are currently debated largely because of the paucity of scientific proof that one sequence is superior to the other. Cooperative trials are ongoing in the United States and Europe, and it is hoped that they will shed some light on the question of which is superior, preoperative or postoperative irradiation.

PREOPERATIVE IRRADIATION

Preoperative irradiation is used at many institutions because of the preference of the surgical team. This choice is based on

Tyvin A. Rich: Department of Radiation Oncology, University of Virginia, Circle Drive, P.O. Box 383, Charlottesville, VA 22908 the training and the experience of the surgeon. For example, in one large, retrospective study, patient outcome after preoperative irradiation was associated with specialty training and the experience of the surgeon because there were less grade 3 or higher toxicities and better disease-free survival in patients treated by those with greater surgical experience.[10] This single factor was more important for outcome than were radiation dose or technique, or the timing of surgery. Although surgical experience was an important factor in this one study, its importance in multiinstitutional studies is less clear but must be kept in mind when interpreting the data. Based on these observations, preoperative irradiation should probably be undertaken only in an institution in which cooperation and treatment philosophy are agreed on before embarking on this approach. Although there are some who believe that preoperative irradiation is the best approach to operable rectal cancer, others are unconvinced, and patients are treated with surgical resection first.

Some of the earliest efforts with preoperative radiation for operable rectal cancer patients used either single doses or a short course of low-dose external beam irradiation. Single doses of 5 Gy (100 rads = 1 Gy [gray]) external irradiation were compared with sham irradiation followed by immediate resection in one randomized trial.[11] This single dose of irradiation resulted in a small improvement in survival for stage C patients compared with surgical control subjects. In a follow-up to this approach, the Medical Research Council in England conducted a study of low-dose preoperative radiation giving 5 Gy (single fraction) or 20 Gy in 2 weeks compared with surgery alone.[12] However, this study failed to show any survival advantage for those treated with irradiation over surgical control subjects, although there was a trend for less local failure in those irradiated. One criticism of short-course preoperative irradiation and immediate surgery after the completion of irradiation is that tumor shrinkage or pathologic "downstaging" is minimal. This potential disadvantage may be outweighed by the ability with this approach to assess the pathologic extent of disease in the resected specimen, and thus to gauge prognosis based on the pathologic stage.

In another study of preoperative irradiation reported from Memorial Sloan-Kettering Hospital, patients receiving 20 Gy before surgery in 1 week had a better overall survival than patients treated with surgery alone (43% vs. 27%).[13] However, in a follow-up randomized trial, no benefit was demonstrated in those receiving preoperative radiation compared with surgical control subjects.[14] Similarly, in the Veterans Administration Surgical Adjuvant Group (VASAG) study, 700 patients with histologically proven adenocarcinoma of the rectum and rectosigmoid were randomized to receive either 20 Gy in 2 weeks or surgery alone.[15] The 5-year survival was 48.5% in the group treated before surgery, compared with 38.8% for the control subjects. A survival advantage was found for patients with distal rectal cancers undergoing abdominoperineal resection, where 41% of the treated group survived 5 years compared with 28% treated with surgery alone. In a second trial, the VASAG used a higher preoperative dose of 31.5 Gy given in 18 fractions in patients suitable for abdominoperineal resection; these results showed no improvement in survival with preoperative irradiation because the 5-year survival was 50% in both arms.[16] In contrast, a nonrandomized series from Washington University, St. Louis, reported on the use of 20 Gy preoperative irradiation for 24 patients with mobile rectal cancers that resulted in a 58% 5-year disease-free survival in patients with tumors staged B2 and C.[10]

TABLE 66-1. *The effect of total radiation dose and fractionation pattern on pathologically determined treatment response in operable cancer of the rectum*

Series	Gy/fractions	Pathologic complete response	Dukes' stage (%) A	B	C
MSKCC[13]	20/10	none	23	35	42
Yale[17]	45/25	12%	53	12	22
TJUH[18]	45/25	10%	29	32	29
EORTC[19]	34/15	2%*	11	53	33
Lyon[20]	30/10	17%	25	27	30

* Time interval between the completion of irradiation and surgery was <1 week.

MSKCC, Memorial Sloan-Kettering Cancer Center; *TJUH,* Thomas Jefferson University Hospital; *EORTC,* European Organization for Research and Treatment of Cancer.

Because the doses used in these studies were relatively low compared with those used in tumors of the breast and head and neck, in which preoperative irradiation has been successful in shrinking tumors before complete resection, larger fraction sizes and higher total doses of preoperative irradiation have been investigated. High daily doses, or hypofractionation, is attractive because it results in a treatment schedule that is usually finished in 1 to 3 weeks, thus shortening the overall interval between diagnosis and tumor removal. However, less downstaging occurs with short intervals, even with total doses of 35 Gy; more tumor regression occurs when there is a sufficiently long enough time interval (~4 to 6 weeks) between the end of irradiation and surgical resection (Table 66-1). With the use of daily fractions of 2.4 to 3.5 Gy given to total doses of 34.5 to 45 Gy, there is concern that wound healing problems and late reactions such as excessive scarring will be increased in comparison with the late reactions seen with treatment schedules using daily doses of approximately 2.0 Gy.[21]

Several nonrandomized studies using moderate doses of irradiation (≥45 Gy) have been performed and show roughly a 5% to 10% pathologic complete response and a greater chance of sterilization of the peripheral margins of the tumor (see Table 66-1). This observation is important because low rectal tumors that may be difficult to resect may now be removed with a clean "tangential margin."[22] With these radiation doses there is also the possibility that marginally resectable or initially unresectable tumors may be amenable to curative surgical resection after preoperative irradiation. Moderate-dose preoperative irradiation also allows tumors to be resected with limited longitudinal surgical margins, thereby extending the level at which sphincter-sparing surgical procedures can be performed safely in the distal segment of the rectum.[18] This latter experience is particularly important to the surgeon who would otherwise hesitate to use preoperative irradiation because of reluctance to operate on tissues that have received high doses of radiation. Although a primary anastomosis in an irradiated field can be hazardous, there are abundant data that indicate the feasibility and safety of this approach.[23,24] In summary, preoperative irradiation alone has been shown to decrease the local failure rate after surgical resection, but has only a small positive impact on

TABLE 66-2. *Results of preoperative irradiation alone for operable rectal cancer in selected nonrandomized series*

Series	No. of patients	Total dose (Gy)	Local failure		Survival*	
			Radiation	Surgery	Radiation	Surgery
University of Florida[25]	71	30–45	8%	29%	71%	41%
TJUH[18]	220	45–70	15%		72%	
University of Virginia[24]	56	40–50	16%	40%	52%	48%
Yale[17]	33	45			41%	25%
EORTC[19]	466	34.5	14%	33%	69%	59%

Five-year actuarial survival.

TJUH, Thomas Jefferson University Hospital; *EORTC,* European Organization for Research and Treatment of Cancer.

survival. Several major nonrandomized and randomized trials supporting this position are listed in Table 66-2.

POSTOPERATIVE IRRADIATION ALONE

Adjuvant postoperative irradiation has been used in several nonrandomized studies that have demonstrated a marked improvement in local control in comparison with the results obtained with surgical resection alone. For example, the data from M. D. Anderson Cancer Center[26] and Massachusetts General Hospital[4] demonstrate that for stages B2 and C rectal cancer, local recurrence rates decreased from an expected incidence of 37% to 48% with surgery alone to 6% to 8% in patients receiving postoperative radiation therapy. In the study reported by Hoskins and colleagues, most patients were given postoperative radiation to doses ranging from 45 to 50.4 Gy, with daily fractions of 1.8 to 2.0 Gy.[27] The overall incidence of local failure was 9% in the group treated with postoperative radiation, compared with 39% in similarly staged patients treated with surgery alone; similar results were reported by others[28] (Table 66-3).

Several randomized studies have also been done with adjuvant postoperative irradiation, and the first study to show a benefit for postoperative irradiation was the Gastrointestinal Tumor Study Group (GITSG) protocol GI-7175. Patients with Dukes' stage B and C rectal cancer were randomized to either surgery alone or three arms of adjunctive treatment, consisting of postoperative radiation (40 to 48 Gy), postoperative chemotherapy (5-fluorouracil [5-FU] and methyl-CCNU), or a combination of postoperative radiation and chemotherapy.[29] Although the disease-free survival in all three adjunctive treatment arms was higher than with surgery alone, the only statistically significant improvement in 5-year survival was noted in the combined arm with both chemotherapy and radiation (60%), compared with surgery alone (45%; $P = 0.005$). Although an improvement in survival was observed in the combined modality arm, there was no decrease in the incidence of distant metastases, and only the incidence of local recurrence (9% vs. 25%) was decreased. The incidence of local failure in the radiation-only arm (20%) was almost twice as high as the local recurrence rates (6% to 8%) observed in most institutional studies using similar doses of postoperative radiation. In another study, the National Surgical Adjuvant Breast and Bowel Project (NSABP) protocol R-01 randomized 550 patients with Dukes' B and C rectal cancer to receive either curative resection, postoperative radiation (46 to 51 Gy), or postoperative chemotherapy (5-FU, semustine, and vincristine).[31] There was an overall reduction in locoregional recurrence observed with postoperative radiation (16% vs. 5%; $P = 0.06$), but no significant benefit in overall survival or disease-free survival from postoperative irradiation. A large, randomized study from Denmark also failed to demonstrate a significant improvement in survival with the use of postoperative irradiation alone.[33]

PREOPERATIVE VERSUS POSTOPERATIVE IRRADIATION

Nonrandomized comparisons have been made regarding the relative superiority of preoperative and postoperative irradiation for patients with operable rectal cancer. The hazards in the interpretation of these data regard the selection criteria used and the

TABLE 66-3. *Postoperative irradiation alone or in conjunction with chemotherapy for operable cancer of the rectum*

Series	No. of patients	Total dose (Gy)	Local failure			Survival		
			Surgery	XRT	CXRT	Surgery	XRT	CXRT
GITSG[29]	182	44–48	27%	20%	11%	45%		58%
NCCTG[30]	204	50.4		25%	14%		48%	58%
NSABP[31]	350	47	25%	16%		43%		
Intergroup[32]*	660	50.4–54		8% vs.	12%†		70% vs.	60%

* The Intergroup trial is a multicenter trial under the NCCTG, Eastern Cooperative Oncology Group, Southwestern Oncology Group, and Radiation Therapy Oncology Group.

GITSG, Gastrointestinal Tumor Study Group; *NCCTG,* North Central Cancer Treatment Group; *NSABP,* National Surgical Adjuvant Breast and Bowel Project.

† Surgery; *XRT,* irradiation alone; *CXRT,* chemoradiation.

TABLE 66-4. *Preoperative compared with postoperative irradiation for pathologic stage B2, C1, and C2 patients with operable rectal cancer: nonrandomized and randomized studies*

Series	Local failure		5-Year survival	
	Preop	Postop	Preop	Postop
TJUH[34]	6%	8%	72%	41%
Washington University,[10]	14%	26%	66%	37%
Swedish multicenter trial[35]	12%	21%	42%	38%

Preop, preoperative irradiation; *Postop,* postoperative irradiation; *TJUH,* Thomas Jefferson University Hospital.

potential for noncomparability between the treatment groups. One way of overcoming the differences in the treatment groups is to compare patients on the basis of pathologic stage after local therapy, regardless of the sequence of treatment. The results from two large centers in North America using preoperative and postoperative irradiation have been published, and they provide some useful information. In the report from Washington University, St Louis,[10] better results were obtained in the patients treated with preoperative irradiation compared with those who received postoperative treatment (Table 66-4). In this series, a variety of dose schedules were used, ranging from low doses of 20 Gy in 1 week to doses of 40 to 50 Gy over 5 weeks. Freedom from local relapse and disease-free survival were superior in patients treated with preoperative irradiation, even when pathologic stage A and B1 patients were excluded from the analysis. Local tumor control was better in the patients with N0 tumors treated with preoperative irradiation compared with those treated after surgery (89% vs. 67%, respectively), whereas those with N1 tumors did less well with either treatment (79% vs. 76%, respectively). There was also a benefit in disease-free survival for both N0 and N1 patients who received preoperative irradiation. The patients irradiated before surgery also had fewer treatment-related complications than those treated after surgery (7% vs. 11%; not statistically significant). In general, the late complications associated with preoperative irradiation are associated with wound healing, whereas the complications in those mainly treated with postoperative irradiation are in the small intestine.[36]

In a similar experience reported from the Thomas Jefferson University Hospital,[34] rectal cancer patients were treated with either low-dose preoperative alone or followed by postoperative irradiation if they had transmural tumor invasion or involved lymph nodes; a separate group was treated with postoperative irradiation alone, and were selected for this treatment on the basis of pathologic stage alone (see Table 66-4). There was little difference in the patterns of failure or complications for preoperative compared with postoperative radiation-treated groups of high-risk patients, but there was a large advantage in survival at 5 and 10 years for those treated with a preoperative irradiation component. The authors explain that part of the reason for the relatively poor outcome for the patients treated with postoperative irradiation alone was the high proportion of unfavorable risk factors such as older age and distal tumor location, as well as a higher percentage of patients requiring abdominoperineal resection and who had Dukes' stage C tumors in this group. They concluded that in spite of similar pathologic stages in these groups of patients, selection can significantly affect the outcome of adjuvant therapy.

The lack of a scientifically valid study addressing the question of preoperative versus postoperative radiation prompted a randomized, multicenter trial in Sweden that compared these two approaches directly for patients with operable rectal and rectosigmoid cancers.[35] Included in this trial were patients with rectal and rectosigmoid cancers arising up to 18 to 20 cm from the anal verge who were randomized between preoperative treatment consisting of 25.5 Gy in 5 to 7 days, or 60 Gy in 8 weeks given after surgery with conventional fractionation only to the patients with tumors at high risk for local recurrence (pathologic stages B2, C1, C2). Patients with unresectable tumors, advanced age, poor medical condition, or metastatic disease were excluded from the trial. The surgery was performed within 1 week of the completion of irradiation, and in 89% the surgery was considered curative. The local recurrence rate was 12% in those receiving preoperative irradiation, compared with 21% of those treated with postoperative irradiation ($P = 0.02$; see Table 66-4). Although preoperative irradiation was better tolerated compared with postoperative treatment, the preoperative group had more perineal wound sepsis and had significantly longer hospitalization; these problems resolved in all patients within 3 months. The rates of distant metastasis were identical in these groups, and there was no difference in survival rates at 5 years. These authors concluded that with preoperative doses equivalent to approximately 45 Gy in 5 weeks, although a rapid fractionation schedule was used here, a reduction in the local recurrence rate can be expected.

PREOPERATIVE VERSUS POSTOPERATIVE CHEMORADIATION: RATIONALE AND CURRENT TRIALS

The use of irradiation plus concurrent 5-FU chemotherapy has been studied in gastrointestinal tumors since the early 1960s.[37] There are now data from nonrandomized and randomized trials showing evidence that the addition of chemotherapy to conventionally fractionated external beam irradiation (chemoradiation) improves local control and increases survival in several cancer sites in the gastrointestinal tract.[38,39] In patients with unresectable esophageal cancer, the Radiation Therapy Oncology Group (RTOG) showed that 50 Gy combined with infusional 5-FU (1000 mg/m^2) and bolus cisplatin (75 mg/m^2) was superior to 64 Gy alone.[38] In this trial, chemoradiation treatment resulted in heightened acute toxicity, but this was manageable in the outpatient setting. The late normal tissue toxicity of these treatments was equal in both arms, but because there was a 22% reduction in the total external beam dose in the patients treated with chemoradiation, combination treatment should be done with caution and preferably in prospective studies to evaluate the long-term morbidity before these approaches become standard practice.

More pertinent to the discussion of treatment sequencing of chemoradiation with surgery are the reports on postoperative 5-FU chemoradiation in the adjuvant treatment of operable rectal cancer. The GITSG showed that combination treatment was superior to surgery alone and to either of the single modalities alone, as mentioned earlier.[29] In a follow-up study performed by the North Central Cancer Treatment Group, a benefit in local control and survival for chemoradiation was demonstrated compared with irradiation alone.[30] The improved tumor control was achieved with only minor additional toxicity, thus indicating a real improvement in therapeutic gain with chemoradiation. In a subsequent study, protracted venous infusional (PVI) 5-FU was combined with approximately 55 Gy given after surgery, and was compared with the more standard 5-FU bolus injection schedule during irradiation. These results showed that PVI 5-FU improved both local control ($P = 0.08$) and overall survival ($P = 0.02$) compared with the use of bolus 5-FU given just during the irradiation phase of treatment.[32] In this same study there was no evidence that the use of methyl-CCNU added to survival. These data verify the preclinical studies showing that 5-FU is a time-dependent drug, and that when used as a cytotoxic or as a radioenhancing agent, the prolongation of the exposure time increases its activity. An ongoing postoperative adjuvant rectal cancer trial is assessing the use of PVI 5-FU compared with biomodulated 5-FU (5-FU with leucovorin).

The use of PVI 5-FU chemoradiation has been reported in a preoperative irradiation schedule for cancers of the rectum. In a series of reports from M. D. Anderson Cancer Center, investigators used a dosage of 300 mg/m^2 for 5 days per week for the treatment of T3 rectal cancers[40] and advanced primary rectal cancers.[41] In these two series, pelvic irradiation doses of 45 Gy (25 fractions over 5 weeks) were well tolerated when combined with infusional 5-FU. The local recurrence rate in patients with operable rectal cancers was only 4% (3/77 patients), and two of three patients with local recurrence were surgically salvaged. In comparison, the data on the use of biomodulated 5-FU with leucovorin in the preoperative management of rectal cancer have not been as extensive, nor is there as high a pathologic complete response rate in patients with operable rectal cancer.[42]

Two ongoing national trials in the United States are attempting to assess the use of preoperative biomodulated chemoradiation for patients with operable rectal cancer. In the trial being performed by the RTOG, all patients receive external beam doses of 50 Gy in conjunction with biomodulated 5-FU. The NSABP study is also using preoperative treatment, but differs from the RTOG trial in that all patients on the preoperative therapy arm first receive systemic chemotherapy followed by chemoradiation. These trials have just begun, and results are not yet available.

SUMMARY

The use of adjuvant pelvic irradiation in the management of rectal cancer has been shown significantly to decrease subsequent pelvic relapse in nonrandomized and randomized trials. An improved pelvic relapse rate means that there are fewer pelvic symptoms during the patient's remaining life span, which adds to the quality of life. There are some suggestions that survival is improved marginally in patients given preoperative irradiation alone, but randomized trials were not designed to detect for small differences.

The addition of systemic chemotherapy to external irradiation has been shown to increase the survival rate compared with irradiation or chemotherapy treatment alone in several randomized, postoperative studies. More recent data indicate that preoperative combined therapy for rectal cancer with infusional 5-FU combined with fractionated external beam irradiation are very well tolerated. However, preoperative infusional 5-FU chemoradiation should be used with caution until the standard management of operable rectal cancer is clarified based on the randomized trials.

REFERENCES

1. Dukes CE. The classification of cancer of the rectum. J Pathol 1932; 35:323.
2. Hildebrandt U, Feifel G. Preoperative staging of rectal cancer by intrarectal ultrasound. Dis Colon Rectum 1985;28:24.
3. Sugarbaker P, Gunderson LL, Wittes RE. Surgical treatment of primary colorectal cancer. In: DeVita VT Jr, Hellman S, Rosenberg SA, eds. Cancer: principles and practice of oncology. 2nd ed. Philadelphia: JB Lippincott, 1985:836.
4. Rich T, Gunderson LL, Lew R, Cohen A, Donaldson G, Galdibini J. Patterns of recurrence of rectal cancer after potentially curative surgery. Cancer 1983;52:1317.
5. Chan KW, Boey J, Wong SKC. A method of reporting radial invasion and surgical clearance of rectal carcinoma. Histopathology 1985;9: 1319.
6. Quirke P, Durdey P, Dixon MF, Williams NS. Local recurrence of rectal adenocarcinoma due to inadequate surgical resection: histopathological study of lateral tumor spread and surgical excision Lancet 1986; 1:996.
7. Rich TA, Terry NHA, Meistrich, Cleary K, Ota D. Pathologic, anatomic, and biologic factors correlated with local recurrence of colorectal cancer. Seminars in Radiation Oncology 1993;3:13.
8. Gilbert SG. Symptomatic local tumor failure following abdomino-perineal resection. Int J Radiat Oncol Biol Phys 1978;4:801.
9. National Institutes of Health. Adjuvant therapy for patients with colon and rectum cancer. NIH Consensus Development Conference Statement. Bethesda, MD: National Institutes of Health, 1991:1.
10. Myerson RJ, Michalski JM, King ML, et al. Adjuvant radiation therapy for rectal carcimoma: predictors of outcome. Int J Radiat Oncol Biol Phys 1995;32:41.
11. Rider WD, Palmer JA, Mahoney LJ, et al. Preoperative irradiation in operable cancer of the rectum: report of the Toronto trial. Can J Surg 1977;20:335.
12. Third report of the MRC Trial: clinico-pathological features of prognostic significance in operable rectal cancer in 17 centers on the U.K. Br J Surg 1984;50:435.
13. Quan SHQ, Deddish MR, Stearns MW. The effect of preoperative roentgen therapy upon the 10 and 5 year results of the surgical treatment of cancer of the rectum. Surg Gynecol Obstet 1960;111:507.
14. Stearns MW, Deddish MR, Quan SHQ, et al. Preoperative roentgen therapy for cancer of the rectum and rectosigmoid. Cancer 1974;37: 2866.
15. Roswit B, Higgins GA, Keehn RJ. Preoperative irradiation for carcinoma of the rectum and rectosigmoid colon: report of a National Veterans Administration randomized study. Cancer 1975;35:1597.
16. Higgins GA, Humphrey EQ, Dwight RW, et al. Preoperative radiation and surgery for cancer of the rectum: Veterans Administration Surgical Oncology Group Trial II. Cancer 1986;58:352.
17. Kligerman MM, Urdaneta N, Knowlton A, Vidone R, Hartman PV, Vera R. Preoperative irradiation of rectosigmoid carcinoma including its regional lymph nodes. American Journal of Roentgenology Radium Therapy and Nuclear Medicine 1972;114:498.
18. Mohiuddin M, Marks G. Adjuvant radiation therapy for colon and rectal cancer. Semin Oncol 1991;18:411.
19. Gerard A, Buyse M, Nordlinger B, et al. Preoperative radiotherapy as adjuvant treatment in rectal cancer: final results of a randomized study of the European Organization for Research and Treatment of Cancer (EORTC). Ann Surg 1988;208:606.
20. Papillon J. Present status of radiation therapy in the conservative management of rectal cancer. Radiother Oncol 1990;17:275.
21. Thames HD, Hendry JH, eds. Fractionation in radiotherapy. London: Taylor and Francis, 1987.
22. Kodner IJ, Shemesh EI, Fry RD, et al. Preoperative irradiation for rectal cancer. Ann Surg 1989;209:194.

23. Marks G, Mohiuddin M, Masoni L, Montori A. High-dose preoperative radiation therapy as the key to extending sphincter-preservation surgery for cancer of the rectum. Surgical Oncology Clinics of North America 1992;1:71.
24. Fortier G, Constable WC, Myers H, Wanebo HJ. Preoperative radiation therapy for rectal cancer. Arch Surg 1986;121:1380.
25. Mendenhall WM, Million RR, Bland KI, Pfaff WW, Copeland EM. Preoperative radiation therapy for clinically resectable adenocarcinoma of the rectum. Ann Surg 1985;202:215.
26. Romsdahl M, Withers HR. Radiotherapy combined with curative surgery. Arch Surg 1978;113:446.
27. Hoskins RB, Gunderson LL, Dosoretz DE, et al. Adjuvant postoperative radiotherapy in carcinoma of the rectum and rectosigmoid. Cancer 1985;55:61.
28. Vigliotti A, Rich TA, Romsdahl MM, Withers HR, Oswald MJ. Postoperative adjuvant radiotherapy for adenocarcinoma of the rectum and rectosigmoid. Int J Radiat Oncol Biol Phys 1987;13:999.
29. Gastrointestinal Tumor Study Group. Survival after postoperative combination treatment of rectal cancer. N Engl J Med 1986;315:1294.
30. Krook JE, Moertel CG, Gunderson LL, et al. Effective surgical adjuvant therapy for high-risk rectal carcinoma. N Engl J Med 1991;324:709.
31. Fisher B, Wolmark N, Rockette H, et al. Postoperative adjuvant adjuvant chemotherapy for rectal cancer: results from NSABP protocol R-01. J Natl Cancer Inst 1988;80:21.
32. O'Connell MJ, Martenson JA, Wieand HS, et al. Improved combined modality surgical adjuvant therapy for high risk rectal cancer. N Engl J Med 1994;331:502.
33. Balslev I, Pederen M, Teglbjaerg P, et al. Postoperative radiotherapy in Dukes' B and C carcinoma of the rectum and rectosigmoid: a randomized multicenter study. Cancer 1986;58:22.
34. Lingareddy V, Mohiuddin M, Marks G. The importance of patient selection for adjunctive postoperative radiation therapy for cancer of the rectum. Cancer 1994;73:1805.
35. Pahlman L, Glimelius B. Pre- or postoperative radiotherapy in rectal and rectosigmoid carcinoma. Ann Surg 1990;211:187.
36. Mak AC, Rich TA, Schultheiss TE, Kavanagh B, Ota DM, Romsdahl MM. Late complications of postoperative radiation therapy for cancer of the rectum and rectosigmoid. Int J Radiat Oncol Biol Phys 1994; 28:597.
37. Rich TA. Chemoradiation for gastrointestinal cancer. Front Radiat Ther Oncol 1992;26:115.
38. Herskovic A, Martz K, Al-Sarraf M, et al. Combined chemotherapy and radiotherapy compared with radiotherapy alone in patients with cancer of the esophagus. N Engl J Med 1992;326:1593.
39. Rich TA, Ajani JA, Morrison WH, Ota D, Levin B. Chemoradiation therapy for anal cancer: radiation plus continuous infusion of 5-fluorouracil with or without cisplatin. Radiother Oncol 1993;27:209.
40. Rich TA, Skibber JM, Ajani JA, et al. Preoperative infusional chemoradiation therapy for stage T3 rectal cancer. Int J Radiat Oncol Biol Phys 1995;32:1025.
41. Weinstein GD, Rich TA, Shumate CR, et al. Preoperative infusional chemoradiation and surgery with or without an electron beam intraoperative boost for advanced primary rectal cancer. Int J Radiat Oncol Biol Phys 1995;32:197.
42. Minsky BD. Preoperative combined modality treatment for rectal cancer. Oncology 1994;8:53.

Surgery for Gastrointestinal Cancer: A Multidisciplinary Approach, edited by Harold J. Wanebo.
Lippincott-Raven Publishers, Philadelphia, © 1997.

CHAPTER 67

Anal Canal Cancer: Multimodality Therapy

R. James Koness and Harold J. Wanebo

The treatment of epidermoid cancer of the anal canal has evolved over the last quarter century. Traditionally, patients were treated with abdominoperineal resection (APR) as a logical extension of experience with adenocarcinoma of the rectum. Today, combined modality treatment with chemotherapy and radiation therapy results in anal sphincter preservation in many cases, and an increased possibility of cure. The Wayne State experience originally published in 1974 has served as a paradigm for combined modality approaches to other malignant sites and histologic types.

ANATOMIC CONSIDERATIONS

Disagreements concerning terminology and definition of the anatomy in this complex region lead to frequent confusion. For clinical purposes, the anus can be divided into two regions: the anal canal and the anal margin (Fig. 67-1). The distinction is important because malignant squamous and basal cell tumors of the anal margin are skin cancers from a biologic and therapeutic standpoint. The distal rectum proximal to the anorectal ring is composed of columnar mucosa. Moving distally toward the dentate line, a transitional epithelium is encountered. It contains elements of both columnar and cuboidal epithelium. Extending distally from the pectinate or dentate line to the anal verge is the stratified squamous epithelium of the anal canal. The anal margin is caudal to the anal verge and is covered with keratinized stratified squamous epithelium, which is pigmented and has hair follicles. Anal margin or perianal tumors are defined as those that occur within 5 cm of the anal verge. The intersphincteric groove represents the potential plane between the internal and external sphincter mechanisms, the external sphincter being more superficial and caudal, and is most commonly within the distal anal canal.

Lymphatic drainage from tumors of the anal region is variable and depends to some extent on the anatomic location of the primary tumor. Carcinomas of the anal margin and anal canal proper drain primarily to the superficial inguinal lymph nodes. Tumors in the region of the dentate line can drain through the inferior and middle hemorrhoidal vessels and lymphatics to the iliac (hypogastric) lymph nodes. Cancers that extend superiorly into the distal rectum may drain through the superior hemorrhoidal lymphatics into the inferior mesenteric system, and from there into the portal system. In an analysis of patients undergoing APR with lymph node clearing at Roswell Park, 22% were found to have lymph node metastasis, with almost one half measuring less than 5 mm in diameter.[1] An analysis of maps of lymph nodes showed that lymph nodes are scant in the perianal zone, that the perirectal zone contains an average of nine lymph nodes, and that metastases are most common in this zone. These results supported an unpredictable, rather than orderly, pattern of lymph node involvement.

PATHOLOGY AND PATHOLOGIC STAGING

The histologic differentiation of tumors of the anal canal is related directly to the anatomic site where they develop. Most authors group these neoplasms together as epidermoid carcinomas because they do not demonstrate a difference in prognosis and their response to treatment is similar. *Squamous cell carcinomas* arise most commonly from the nonkeratinizing epithelium of the upper anal canal. The rectal columns (columns of Morgagni) that extend proximal from the dentate line give rise to *transitional cell or cloacogenic cancers.* Each adjacent rectal column is connected at the dentate line by a valve, creating the anal crypts. Small rudimentary glands open into some of the crypts, and the anal glands are thought to give rise to the less common *mucoepidermoid cancers.* When the neoplasm histologically resembles basal cell carcinoma of the skin, it is termed a *basaloid carcinoma.*

In 1987, the International Union Against Cancer staging system was updated and adopted by the American Joint Committee on Cancer (Table 67-1). Unlike carcinomas of other sites in the gastrointestinal tract, the T discriminant for anal cancer is based on tumor size, and accounts for the fact that anal canal cancer often is treated by nonsurgical methods. The N classification

R. J. Koness: Department of Surgical Oncology, Brown University, Roger Williams Medical Center, 825 Chalkstone Avenue, Providence, RI 02908

H. J. Wanebo: Department of Surgical Oncology, Brown University, Roger Williams Medical Center, 825 Chalkstone Avenue, Providence, RI 02908

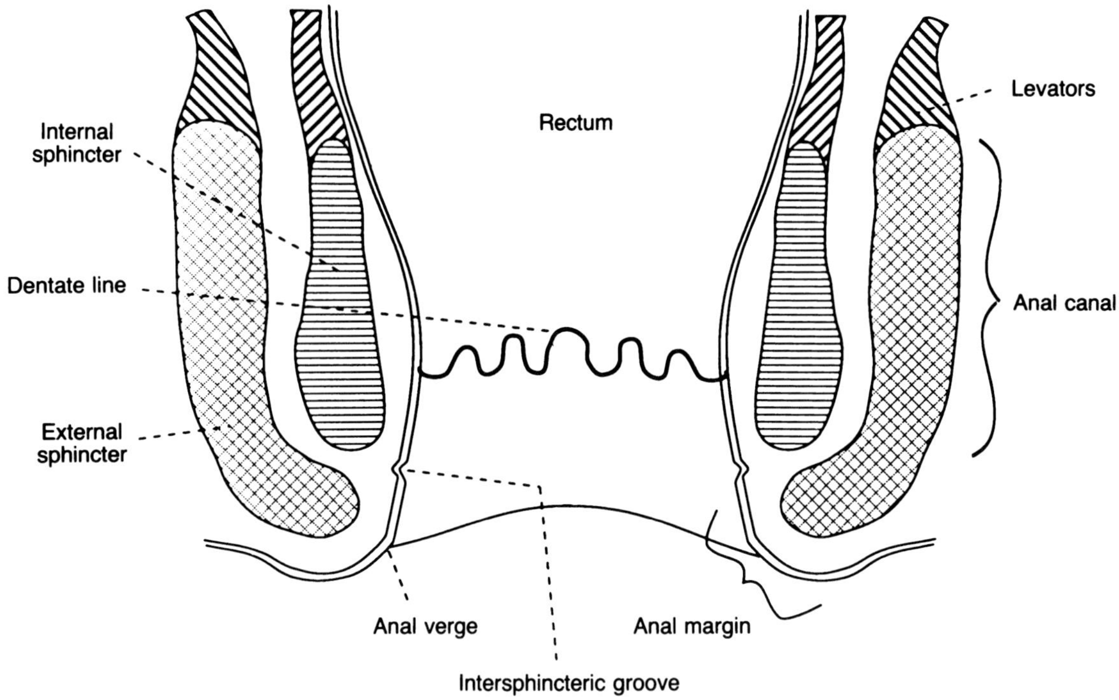

FIG. 67-1. Gross anatomy of the anal region. (With permission from Beck DE, Wexner SD, eds. Anal neoplasms. In: Fundamentals of anorectal surgery, p 223.)

for the anal canal subdivides the regional nodes, taking into account the poor prognosis with involvement of internal iliac or inguinal nodes. Clinical stage correlates strongly with prognosis. Goldman and colleagues found that the 5-year survival rate was 80% for patients with T1 and T2 cancers, but less than 20% for those with T3 and T4 tumors.[2]

ETIOLOGY AND DIAGNOSIS

Epidermoid carcinoma of the anal region usually occurs in the sixth and seventh decades of life, although its incidence is rising among men younger than 45 years. In the United States, anal canal carcinoma is more common in women, whereas anal margin cancer is more common in men. Fewer than 2000 cases occur annually in this country. Human papillomavirus appears to be an important causative agent. The DNA of human papillomavirus type 16 is found most frequently in anal squamous cell carcinomas, and the DNA of types 6 and 18 also is found, whereas the DNA of type 11 has never been detected.[3,4] In men and women without a history of genital warts, other sexually transmitted diseases, cigarette smoking, prior irradiation, immunosuppression, and other benign anorectal disorders may be associated.

TABLE 67-1. *AJCC staging rules for anal canal cancers*

T1	= tumor ≤2 cm
T2	= tumor 2–5 cm
T3	= tumor >5 cm
T4	= tumor of any size invades adjacent organ(s)
N0	= tumor not involved in regional lymph nodes
N1	= perirectal lymph node(s)
N2	= unilateral internal iliac and/or inquinal lymph node(s)
N3	= perirectal and inguinal lymph nodes and/or bilateral internal iliac and/or inguinal lymph nodes
M0	= no distant metastasis
M1	= distant metastasis
STAGE GROUPING	
Stage I	T1 N0 M0
Stage II	T2 N0 M0
	T3 N0 M0
Stage IIIA	T4 N0 M0
	T any N1 M0
Stage IIIB	T4 N1 N0
	T any N2–3 M0
Stage IV	T any N any M1

Bleeding, pain, and a sensation of a mass are the most common symptoms. Because the initial symptoms of anal cancer are similar to those of several benign anorectal conditions, there often is a delay in diagnosis. Associated benign conditions are common. In the Memorial Sloan-Kettering series, almost one third of patients were thought to have benign conditions until a biopsy showed carcinoma.[5] Bleeding occurs in 27% to 74% of patients and usually is more continuous than that associated with hemorrhoids.[6] Twenty-one percent to 39% of patients have pain, but the pain is less severe than that associated with anal fissure.[7] The physical examination should include a digital examination, anoscopy, and palpation of the inguinal lymph nodes. An incisional biopsy is needed to confirm the diagnosis. Excision should not be attempted unless the lesion is small and superficial. Palpable inguinal lymph nodes should be subjected to biopsy, and fine-needle aspiration should be considered as the initial diagnostic maneuver. Computed tomography and transrectal ultrasound may be useful in clinical staging of the tumor.[8,9] To complete the metastatic workup, the patient should have a chest radiograph and liver function studies.

SURGICAL THERAPY

Superficial anal margin skin cancers outside the anal verge can be treated with wide local excision. A 1-cm margin with primary closure usually suffices, a skin graft can be placed if the defect is large, and flaps rarely are necessary. The cure rate for superficial anal margin carcinomas exceeds 80% and local failure is unusual unless the tumor involves the anal canal. Giant condylomata acuminata (Buschke-Löwenstein tumors) with or without histologically confirmed malignancy are treated best with radical wide local excision, rather than conservative approaches.[10] Deeply infiltrating anal margin carcinomas have been treated with wide-field APR, but overall survival is affected most by early control of disease. Regional failure in the inguinal lymph nodes does occur.

Local excision of epidermoid cancers of the anal canal should be limited to tumors that are well differentiated, less than 2 cm in diameter, invade only to the submucosa, and are located in the distal anal canal. In collective series, when this procedure is used in selected patients, the local recurrence rate is about 28% and the 5-year survival rate is about 71%.[6] APR was the standard therapy for anal canal cancers in the United States before 1974. The operation is similar to that used for rectal cancer except that a wide perianal skin margin is removed. In women, the posterior vaginal wall is excised because the incidence of rectovaginal septum invasion is high. In good-risk patients, a radical lymphadenectomy up to and including aortocaval clearance is advocated. This approach is associated with significant morbidity and mortality. Stearns and Quan reported a mortality rate of 1.7% for patients younger than 70 years of age, but a rate of 8.5% for older patients.[5] Although APR offers an aggressive attempt at microscopic control, local recurrence rates after surgery have ranged from 11% to 40%, and such recurrences rarely are treatable. The 5-year survival rate after this form of treatment averages 50%, with a published range of 27% to 71%.[6] The Mayo Clinic reported a 5-year survival rate of 71%.[11] At the Ellis Fischel State Cancer Hospital, 58% of 46 patients survived for 5 years.[12] The M.D. Anderson group reported a 5-year survival rate of 62%, but one in six patients had anal margin cancer.[13] A Memorial Sloan-Kettering update quoted a 55% survival rate for tumors that involved the dentate line.[14] At St. Mark's Hospital, the 5-year survival rate for 83 similar patients was 48%.[15] The wide range in survival rates results in part from the small number of patients in some centers and from case selection in others. With the success of multimodality therapy, APR is indicated only for persistent or locally recurrent disease.

RADIATION THERAPY

Epidermoid carcinomas of the anal canal are radiosensitive tumors, and this method of therapy has been used widely in Europe for many years. The major advantage of radiation therapy over surgery is that 75% of patients retain a functional anus without a long-term colostomy. External-beam radiation, interstitial radiation, and split-course radiation therapy all have been used. The reported 5-year survival rate after external-beam radiation therapy ranges from 46% to 92%, with an average of 68%. The mean local recurrence rate is about 26%.[6] Dubois and associates have stated that survival is related to primary tumor factors such as tumor size and is similar to or better than survival after APR.[16] Complications of radiation therapy include incontinence, anal stricture, and mucosal necrosis, which often is severe enough to require colostomy and rectal excision. Other potential side effects include enterocolitis, lower leg edema, and urethral or vaginal strictures or fistulas. If radiation therapy is the sole treatment modality, high doses (65 to 70 Gy) must be delivered to the primary site to control this disease. The benefit of combined radiation therapy and chemotherapy versus radiation therapy alone has never been reported prospectively, but is being examined in the United Kingdom Co-ordination Committee for Cancer Research anal cancer trial.[17,18]

Interstitial radiation has the potential to cure early lesions that are unlikely to have spread to the inguinal lymph nodes. Most of the early experience involved radium needles; however, implants with ^{192}Ir also have been used. Local control has been achieved in 64% of tumors less than 5 cm in diameter, but in only 23% of larger tumors.[19] Further, of 35 locoregional failures, only 7 could be salvaged by aggressive surgery. Papillon speculated that anal canal carcinomas are ideally suited to split-course therapy, combining external-beam and interstitial irradiation, because these tumors are easily accessible to interstitial therapy and are characterized by a slow rate of shrinkage.[20] Split-course radiation with a dose of 30 to 42 Gy of external-beam irradiation followed 2 months later by a booster dose of 15 to 20 Gy delivered by an ^{192}Ir implant has been used and decreased local recurrence has been achieved. The inability to obtain nodal and distant control with radiation therapy alone and improved local control with large lesions led Papillon to advocate the use of chemotherapy during the initial days of irradiation to reinforce the efficacy of treatment.[21]

COMBINED MODALITY RADIATION THERAPY AND CHEMOTHERAPY

The concept of combined chemotherapy and radiation therapy initially was explored at the Mayo Clinic for unresectable tumors of the gastrointestinal tract after it was recognized that some chemotherapeutic agents have synergy with radiation therapy.[22] In 1974, Nigro and colleagues described three patients treated with a combination of 5-fluorouracil (5-FU), mitomycin C, and radiation therapy (3000 cGy).[23] Two patients subsequently underwent APR, with no viable tumor seen in the pathologic specimen. The third patient refused surgery and was clinically disease-free at 14 months. These investigators believed that most patients have recurrence in the pelvis, and that local failure may be related to a profuse network of blood and lymph vessels in and around the anal canal that are not controlled adequately by surgical therapy, largely because of anatomic constraints. The initial intent was that the chemotherapy and irradiation would be added to surgery to enhance local control; APR was planned 4 to 6 weeks after completion of the protocol (Table 67-2). Over the ensuing 20 years, evidence gathered from single-armed phase II trials has indicated that initial chemotherapy and irradiation yields significant tumor responses, including a high rate of complete response (Table 67-3). Surgery may not be required for most patients, even those

TABLE 67-2. *Nigro's chemoradiation therapy*

EXTERNAL IRRADIATION

3000 rads to the primary carcinoma and pelvic inquinal nodes; start—day 1 (200 rads/day)

SYSTEMIC CHEMOTHERAPY

5-FU 1000 mg/m^2/24 hr as a continuous infusion for 4 days; start—day 1

Mitomycin C, 15 mg/m^2 as an intravenous bolus; start-day 1 only

5-FU, repeat 4-day infusion; start—day 28

With permission from Nigro ND. An evaluation of combined therapy for squamous cell cancer of the anal canal. Dis Colon Rectum 1984; 27:763.

with large tumors at presentation. APR is reserved for patients with residual or recurrent local disease.

Nigro eventually described 104 patients treated at several institutions from 1971 to 1983.[24] Six weeks after chemotherapy and irradiation, gross tumor disappeared in 97 patients. Visible tumor remained in the other 7 patients, all of whom eventually died despite undergoing APR. Twenty-four patients had APR after chemotherapy and irradiation, as specified in the initial protocol. No residual carcinoma was found in 22 patients, and 2 had microscopic disease. The scar was subjected to biopsy in 62 patients, only 1 of whom was found to have microscopic disease, which was treated successfully with local excision. Eleven patients refused to undergo biopsy of the scar after the disappearance of gross disease. Two of these patients died of their disease, but 9 remained free of disease at 2 to 9 years' follow-up. Eight patients had recurrence, which developed 5 to 33 months after chemotherapy and irradiation was completed. Seven of these patients underwent salvage APR resection and 5 remained free of disease a minimum of 4 years after surgery.

Radiation therapy supplemented with chemotherapy is advocated by many as the treatment of choice,[40] although there have been no published randomized trials. Controlled trials comparing radiation therapy with APR are not likely to be conducted, but the benefit of combined radiation therapy and chemotherapy versus radiation therapy alone is being examined in the United Kingdom Co-ordination Committee for Cancer Research anal cancer trial.[18] Although 5-year survival rates for combined treatment are similar to those for radiation therapy alone, the primary control rate may be higher (93% versus 60% for radiation therapy alone) despite increased hematologic and intestinal toxicity.[41] Side effects of combined therapy include dermatitis, mucositis, alopecia, and reversible pancytopenia. Intestinal obstruction, anal incontinence, and chronic pelvic pain may occur, but anal sphincter function is preserved in about 80% of patients.

There has been a trend in clinical trials toward treating patients with higher doses of external-beam radiation than initially specified by Nigro. Influencing this decision are data indicating that higher doses are required to eradicate squamous cell cancers elsewhere in the body, and that some larger anal canal carcinomas are not controlled with 3000 cGy.[42] Of the 85 patients in Nigro's series who had tumors measuring 5 cm or less, only 6% died of their disease, compared with 47% of those with tumors larger than 5 cm. Tumor size as a predictor of survival has been reported by several other investigators.[2,32,34] Nigro recommends additional chemotherapy and radiation therapy for all patients with original tumors larger than 5 cm, regardless of the response after his protocol.[43] Further, he recommends additional therapy for patients with residual tumor after chemotherapy and irradiation because of the poor survival after APR in these patients. Flam and associates also have demonstrated nonsurgical salvage for residual disease at the completion of multimodality therapy.[28] In the Memorial Sloan-Kettering experience, however, a pathologic response to chemotherapy and irradiation did not predict a difference in survival or subsequent salvage with surgery; 55% of patients had residual carcinoma in biopsy samples and clinical evaluation was unable to predict accurately a complete pathologic response.[6] All patients were treated aggressively 4 to 6 weeks after chemotherapy and irra-

TABLE 67-3. *Multimodality therapy for anal canal carcinoma*

Author/Series	Year	No of patients	Radiotherapy dose (GY)	Chemotherapy	Complete regression (%)	Survival (%)	Follow-up (median-mos)
Nigro[24,24a]	1987	104	30	F,M	89	83	24–132*
Cummings[25]	1984	30	50	F,M	93	70	25
Sischy[26]	1985	33	45	F,M	91	78	51
Meeker[27]	1986	19	30	F,M	88	87	30
Flam[28]	1987	30	41–45	F,M	87	90	9–76*
Gilmelius[29]	1987	23	40–65	B	96	79	45
Habr-Gama/Sao Paulo[30]	1989	30	30–45	F,M	73	75	36
Sischy/ROTC[31]	1989	79	41	F,M	90	73	36
Miller/MSK[32]	1991	42	30	F,M	45	82	71
Doci/Milan[33]	1992	51	54–60	F,M	87	81	49
Johnson[34]	1993	24	41–45	F,M	100	87	36
Tanum/Oslo[35]	1993	86	50	F,M	84	72	60
Grabenbauer[37]	1993	44	50	F,M	93	77	38
Beck[36]	1994	35	30–45	F,M	97	87	62
Smith[38]	1994	42	30	F,M	98	90	33
Basser[39]	1994	31	30–60	F,M	77	81	62

F, fluorouracil; M, mitomycin; B, bleomycin; *, range.

diation with wide local excision or APR. The role of biopsy alone versus wide local excision for patients with a complete pathologic response after chemotherapy and irradiation remains controversial.

Deviations from the original combination of 5-FU and mitomycin C have been tried, including the use of bleomycin and cisplatin. Byfield and associates treated 11 patients with a 120-hour infusion of 5-FU and concurrent irradiation (30 to 47.5 Gy), without mitomycin.[44] All patients had complete clinical regression and only 1 had histologically demonstrable disease. In prospective but nonrandomized protocols, Cummings and colleagues found that the addition of mitomycin was associated with improved primary tumor control rates (87% versus 58% at 4 years) and improved actuarial cause-specific survival rates (80% versus 64%).[45] The role of mitomycin in anal cancer is being evaluated in a randomized clinical trial being conducted by the Radiation Therapy Oncology Group. A few trials investigating the use of cisplatin with 5-FU and irradiation have revealed promising results, especially for high-risk patients.[46,47]

INGUINAL LYMPH NODE DISSECTION

At least half of all clinically detectable synchronous inguinal nodes are inflammatory; however, pathologic involvement by tumor is a poor prognostic sign. O'Brien and associates found involved inguinal lymph nodes in 11 of 21 patients.[48] Six cases were apparent at presentation, and none of the patients survived for 3 years. Involvement of the inguinal nodes after APR developed in 5 patients; 2 of these patients lived more than 5 years, but died of disease at 6 and 8 years. In the series by Stearns and Quan, only 2 of 14 patients with synchronous inguinal lymph node metastasis survived 5 years, whereas 15 of 20 patients with metachronous inguinal metastasis survived 5 years after radical groin dissection.[49] Based on these statistics and on the high morbidity and mortality associated with groin dissection, prophylactic lymph node dissection for microscopic involvement is not recommended, despite a positive yield of about 10% to 30%.[50]

In 1982, Cummings and colleagues suggested that elective irradiation (45 to 50 Gy) of clinically normal inguinal nodes carries little morbidity and may reduce the risk of late node failure.[51] It is now a rare circumstance for patients to fail only in their inguinal nodes after receiving radiation therapy or combined chemotherapy and radiation therapy when the lateral fields include the inguinal and internal and external iliac node groups. Further, synchronous inguinal lymph node metastasis is treated best with adjuvant radiation therapy or combined chemotherapy and radiation therapy. In Papillon's series, 19 patients with resectable tumors and synchronous groin metastases were treated with radical groin dissection followed by irradiation, and 11 were alive and well at 3 years.[20] Forty-two percent of these patients died of their cancer, compared with 19% of the patients who had no inguinal node metastasis. Cummings and associates reported that 87% (33 of 38) of the cases of regional lymph node metastasis (predominantly inguinal) were controlled by primary radiation therapy or combined chemotherapy and radiation therapy without groin dissection.[25] Regional lymph node metastases that did not regress completely always were unresectable or associated with failure at another site. The development of unilateral metachronous inguinal nodes after multimodality therapy is not necessarily an ominous sign and should be treated with a formal groin dissection followed by chemotherapy.

RECURRENT CARCINOMA OF THE ANAL CANAL

Relapse after multimodality therapy is most common in the pelvis. In addition, many patients with distant metastasis also have local recurrence. Adjuvant treatment with chemotherapy and a radiation boost offers promise, as demonstrated in a large controlled trial.[52] Thirty-six patients received salvage treatment with radiation therapy plus 5-FU and cisplatin. Twenty-eight patients had additional biopsy information, and 50% had no pathologic evidence of tumor. Mitomycin plus 5-FU also can induce major remissions in previously treated patients who have locally recurrent disease.[53] However, Longo and colleagues found that with long-term follow-up, only 27% of the patients treated with salvage chemotherapy and radiation therapy were long-term survivors, whereas 57% of those who underwent salvage APR were cured.[54] The success rate of surgical salvage averages about 60% in previously reporting centers.[55]

In patients with locally advanced disease, such as those with pelvic sidewall involvement or tumors larger than 10 cm, it may be beneficial to plan extensive resections after the completion of chemotherapy and radiation therapy. Wanebo and associates described seven patients with locally advanced epidermoid carcinoma of the anal canal.[56] Three patients had recurrent or persistent disease and four had advanced primary cancer. All patients received one or two cycles of chemotherapy (5-FU and mitomycin C) before surgery, and four patients (not previously irradiated) received 3000 cGy of radiation. Tumor regression exceeding 50% occurred in five patients, minor regression (25% to 50%) occurred in one patient, and no regression was seen in one patient (on chemotherapy alone). All patients had total resection of all gross tumor with microscopic clear margins, and five had groin dissection. Four of the five patients who underwent inguinal node dissection had residual disease. Three patients were alive and free of disease after 2 years, two patients died of intercurrent disease at 4 and 5 months, and two patients died of disease at 6 and 34 months.

REFERENCES

1. Wade DS, Herrera L, Castillo NB, Petrelli NJ. Metastases to the lymph nodes in epidermoid carcinoma of the anal canal studied by a clearing technique. Surg Gynecol Obstet 1989;169:238.
2. Goldman S, Auer G, Erhardt K, Seiligson U. Prognostic significance of clinical stage, histologic grade, and nuclear DNA content in squamous cell carcinoma of the anus. Dis Colon Rectum 1987;30:444.
3. Beckmann AM, Daling JR, Sherman KJ, et al. Human papillomavirus infection and anal cancer. Int J Cancer 1989;43:1042.
4. Palmer JG, Scholefield JH, Coates PJ, et al. Anal cancer and human papillomaviruses. Dis Colon Rectum 1989;32:1016.
5. Stearns MW, Quan SH. Epidermoid carcinoma of the anorectum. Surg Gynecol Obstet 1970;191:953.
6. Beck DE, Wexner SD. Anal neoplasms. In: Beck DE, Wexner SD, eds. Fundamentals of anorectal surgery. New York: McGraw-Hill, 1992:222.
7. Mitchel EP. Carcinoma of the anal region. Semin Oncol 1988;15:146.
8. Hildebrandt U, Klein T, Feifel G, Schwarz H-P, Koch B, Schmitt RM.

Endosonography of pararectal lymph nodes. In vitro and in vivo evaluation. Dis Colon Rectum 1990;33:863.
9. Roseau G, Palazzo L, Colardelle P, Chaussade S, Couturier D, Paolaggi JA. Endoscopic ultrasonography in the staging and follow-up of epidermoid carcinoma of the anal canal. Gastrointest Endosc 1994;40:447.
10. Chu QD, Vezeridis MP, Libbey NP, Wanebo HJ. Giant condyloma acuminatum (Buschke-Lowenstein tumor) of the anorectal and perianal regions: analysis of 42 cases. Dis Colon Rectum 1994;37:950.
11. Boman BM, Moertel CG, O'Connell MJ, et al. Carcinoma of the anal canal: a clinical and pathologic study of 188 cases. Cancer 1984;54:114.
12. Dillard BM, Spratt JS Jr, Ackerman LV, Butcher HR Jr. Epidermoid cancer of anal margin and canal. Arch Surg 1963;86:772.
13. Frost DB, Richards PC, Montague ED, Giacco GG, Martin RG. Epidermoid cancer of the anorectum. Cancer 1984;53:1285.
14. Greenall MJ, Quan SHQ, Urmacher C, DeCosse JJ. Treatment of epidermod carcinoma of the anal canal. Surg Gynecol Obstet 1985;161:509.
15. Hardcastle JD, Bussey HJR. Results of surgical treatment of squamous cell carcinoma of the anal canal and anal margin seen at St. Mark's Hospital 1928-66. Journal Royal Socirty Medicine 1968;61:629.
16. Dubois JB, Garrigues JM, Pujol H. Cancer of the anal canal: report on the experience of 61 patients. Int J Radiat Oncol Biol Phys 1991;20:575.
17. Northover JMA. Anal cancer: a changing disease. (Editorial) Br J Hosp Med 1990;44:313.
18. United Kingdom Co-ordination Committee for Cancer Research (UKCCR). Anal cancer trial protocol. London: CRC Clinical Trials Centre, 1992.
19. James RD, Pointon RS, Martin S. Local radiotherapy in the management of squamous carcinoma of the anus. Br J Surg 1985;72:282.
20. Papillon J. Radiation therapy in the management of epidermoid carcimoma of the anal region. Dis Colon Rectum 1974;17:181.
21. Papillon J, Montbarbon JF. Epidermoid carcinoma of the anal canal: a series of 276 cases. Dis Colon Rectum 1987;30:324.
22. Moertel CG, Childs DS, Reitemeter RJ, et al. Combined 5-fluorouracil and supervoltage radiation therapy for locally unresectable gastrointestinal cancers. Lancet 1969;2:865.
23. Nigro ND, Vaitkevicius VK, Considine B Jr. Combined therapy for cancer of the anal canal. Dis Colon Rectum 1974;17:354.
24. Nigro ND. Multidisciplinary management of cancer of the anus. World J Surg 1987;1:446.
24a. Nigro ND. An evaluation of combined therapy for squamous cell carcinoma of the oral canal. Dis Colon Rectum 1984:27:763.
25. Cummings B, Keane T, Thomas G, Harwood A, Rider W. Results and toxicity of the treatment of anal canal carcinoma by radiation therapy or radiation therapy and chemotherapy. Cancer 1984;54:2062.
26. Sischy B. The use of radiation therapy combined with chemotherapy in the management of the anus and marginally resectable adenocarcinoma of the rectum. Int J Radiat Oncol Biol Phys 1985;11:1587.
27. Meeker WR, Sickle-Santanello BJ, Philpott G. Combined chemotherapy, radiation, and surgery for epithelial cancer of the anal canal. Cancer 1986;57;525.
28. Flam MS, John MJ, Mowry PA, Lovalvo LJ, Ramalho LD, Wade J. Definitive combined modality therapy of carcinoma of the anus. Dis Colon Rectum 1987;30:495.
29. Glimelius B, Pahlman L. Radiation therapy of anal epidermoid carcinoma. Int J Radiat Oncol Biol Phys 1987;13:305.
30. Habr-Gama A, da Silva e Sousa AH Jr, Nadalin W, Gansl R, da Silva JH, Pinotti HW. Epidermoid carcinoma of the anal canal: results of treatment by combined chemotherapy and radiation therapy. Dis Colon Rectum 1989;32:773.
31. Sischy B, Doggett RSL, Krall JM, et al. Definitive irradiation and chemotherapy for radiosensitization in management of anal carcinoma: interim report on radiation therapy oncology group study No. 8314. J Natl Cancer Inst 1989;81:850.
32. Miller EJ, Quan SHQ, Thaler HT. Treatment of squamous cell carcinoma of the anal canal. Cancer 1991;67:2038.
33. Doci R, Zucali R, Bombelli L, Montalto F, Lamonica G. Combined chemoradiation therapy for anal cancer: a report of 56 cases. Ann Surg 1992;215:150.
34. Johnson D, Lipsett J, Leong L, Wagman LD, Terz JJ. Carcinoma of the anus treated with primary radiation therapy and chemotherapy. Surg Gynecol Obstet 1993;177:329.
35. Tanum G, Tveit KM, Karlsen KO. Chemoradiotherapy of anal carcinoma: tumour response and acute toxicity. Oncology 1993;59:14.
36. Beck DE, Karulf RE. Combination therapy for epidermoid carcinoma of the anal canal. Dis Colon Rectum 1994;37:1118.
37. Grabenbauer GG, Schneider IJF, Gall FP, Sauer R. Epidermoid carcinoma of the anal canal: treatment by combined radiation and chemotherapy. Radiother Oncol 1993;27:59.
38. Smith DE, Shah KH, Rao AR, et al. Cancer of the anal canal: treatment with chemotherapy and low-dose radiation therapy. Radiology 1994;191:569.
39. Basser RL, Smith JG, Worotniuk V, Guiney MJ. Conservative management of squamous cell carcinoma of the anal canal. Aust N Z J Surg 1994;64:754.
40. Deans GT, McAleer JJA, Spence RAJ. Manlignant anal tumours. Br J Surg 1994;81:500.
41. Cummings BJ, Keane TJ, O'Sullivan B, Wong CS, Catton CN. Epidermoid anal cancer: treatment by radiation alone or by radiation and 5-fluorouracil with and without mitomycin C. Int J Radiat Oncol Biol Phys 1991;21:1115.
42. Brown SH, Cohen JL. Chemoradiation therapy for anal cloacogenic cancer. Seminars in Colon and Rectal Surgery 1995;6:156.
43. Nigro ND, Vaitkevicius VK, Herskovic AM. Preservation of function in the treatment of cancer of the anus. In: DeVita VJ, Hellman S, Rosenberg SA, eds. Advances in oncology. Philadelphia: Lippincott, 1989:161.
44. Byfield JE, Barone RM, Sharp TR, Frankel SS. Conservative management without alkylating agents of squamous cell anal cancer using cyclical 5-FU alone and x-ray therapy. Cancer Treat Rep 1983;67:709.
45. Cummings BJ, Keane TJ, O'Sullivan B, Wong CS, Catton CN. Mitomycin in anal canl carcinoma. Oncology 1993;50:63.
46. Roca E, DeSimone G, Barugel M, et al. A phase II study of alternating chemoradiotherapy including cisplatin in anal canal carcinoma. Proc Am Soc Clin Oncol 1990;9:128.
47. Brunet R, Sadek H, Vignoud J, et al. Cisplatine (P) and 5-fluorouracil (5-FU) for the neoadjuvant treatment (Tt) of epidermoid anal canal carcinoma (EACC). Proc Am Soc Clin Oncol 1990;9:104.
48. O'Brien PH, Jenrette JM, Wallace KM, Metcalf JS. Epidermoid carcinoma of the anus. Surg Gynecol Obstet 1982;155:745.
49. Stearns MW Jr, Quan SHQ. Epidermoid carcinoma of the anorectum. Surg Gynecol Obstet 1970;131:953.
50. Nivatvongs S. Perianal and anal canal neoplasms. In: Gordon PH, Nivatvongs S, eds. Principles and practice of surgery for the colon, rectum and anus. St Louis: Quality Medical Publishing, 1992:401.
51. Cummings BJ, Thomas GM, Keane TJ. Primary radiation therapy in the treatment of anal canal carcinoma. Dis Colon Rectum 1982;25:778.
52. Flam MS, John MJ, Peters J, et al. Radiation and 5-fluorouracil (5FU) vs. radiation, 5FU, mitomycin C (MMC), in the treatment of anal canal carcinoma: preliminary results of a phase III randomized RTOG/ECOG intergroup trial. Proc Am Soc Clin Oncol 1993;12:192.
53. Barni S, Frigio F, Lissoni P, Crispino S, Paolorossi F. Anal squamous cell carcinoma arising on radiodermatitis cured with chemotherapy alone: case report. Tumori 1987;73:423.
54. Longo WE, Vernava AM, Wade TP, et al. Recurrent squamous cell carcinoma of the anal canal: predictors of initial treatment failure and results of salvage therapy. Ann Surg 1994;220:40.
55. Shank B, Cohen AM, Kelsen D. Cancer of the anal region. In: DeVita VT Jr, Hellman S, Rosenberg SA, eds. Cancer: principles & practice of oncology. 4th ed. Philadelphia: Lippincott, 1993:1006. 56. Wanebo HJ, Futrell W, Constable W. Multimodality approach to surgical management of locally advanced epidermoid carcinoma of the anorectum. Cancer 1981;47:2817.

Surgery for Gastrointestinal Cancer: A Multidisciplinary Approach, edited by Harold J. Wanebo.
Lippincott-Raven Publishers, Philadelphia, © 1997.

CHAPTER 68

Carcinoembryonic Antigen-Directed Second-Look Operations: Where Do We Stand?

David J. Bertsch and Edward W. Martin, Jr.

HISTORICAL OVERVIEW

Colorectal cancer afflicts 149,000 people in the United States annually.[1] After diagnosis, 70% to 80% of these patients undergo an apparently curative resection. However, only 45% of patients are actually cured. Twenty to 30% of the patients are found to have advanced, incurable disease. The remaining 25% to 45% manifest recurrent disease ranging from locoregional recurrence to widespread metastasis[2,3] (Fig. 68-1). Of those diagnosed with lymph node metastasis, only 50% are alive 5 years later. Traditional systemic treatments have not been able to effect a cure in patients with recurrent colorectal cancer. However, some cures have been obtained with ''second-look'' operations.

This chapter reviews the development of second-look surgery: from the 1950s blind second-look, to traditional carcinoembryonic antigen (CEA)-directed second-look, to radioimmunoguided surgery (RIGS)-augmented, CEA-directed, second-look surgery.

It is now generally believed that recurrent colorectal cancer is a manifestation of the progression of occult, microscopic, residual disease remaining after ''curative'' resection. Because approximately 45% of colorectal cancer patients are cured with primary surgery, the concept of second-look surgery for a repeat attempt at cure for those patients with recurrent disease has waxed and waned in popularity over the last half century. During that time, second-look surgery has undergone developmental refinements.

Credit for the concept and promotion of second-look surgery is given to Dr. Owen Wangensteen.[4,5] Noting a high incidence of recurrent disease in patients with lymph node-positive colorectal cancer or gastric cancer initially treated with ''curative'' resection, he recommended a protocol of repeat laparotomy at approximately 6-month intervals until no tumor was found or inoperable disease was encountered. In analyzing the results of Wangensteen's University of Minnesota second-look program, Griffen and colleagues[6] reported a 6.2% salvage rate for colon cancer and a 4.5% salvage rate for patients with rectal cancer. Ninety-four percent of patients received no benefit from the second-look operations. Because of the many negative laparotomies and their attendant morbidity and mortality, this approach fell out of favor. However, the program gathered valuable information about the location of recurrent tumors. In originally lymph node-positive patients, at second-look operation, ''involvement of the paravena cava and aorta lymph nodes in reentry operation is usual. No surgeons, however, in the initial operation . . . excise regularly this secondary chain of lymph nodes . . ..''[3] Improved selection criteria for second-look surgery were needed to overcome the nontherapeutic laparotomy rate in the Wangensteen approach. The discovery of CEA seemed to provide those criteria.

Carcinoembryonic antigen, a tumor-associated antigen, was detected and described in 1965 by Gold and Freedman.[7,8] By electron microscopy, it is a ''cruller''-shaped glycoprotein with a molecular weight of 200,000 daltons, containing 55% to 65% carbohydrate, with the remainder being protein.[9] CEA is one of a class of oncofetal antigens that can be found in the gastrointestinal tract of fetuses and in increased amounts in the circulation of normal fetuses. During the second trimester, it disappears from fetal circulation and remains measurable in low levels in normal, healthy adults.[9,10]

A higher level of this cell surface glycoprotein is associated with some carcinomas. Elevated serum levels of CEA can be found in patients with malignancies such as medullary thyroid carcinoma and pancreatic, breast, gastric, and esophageal adenocarcinomas. However, measures of CEA levels are clinically most useful in patients with colorectal cancer.[11] Elevated preoperative levels were noted by Thomson and associates[12] to return to normal after curative colon resection. Livingstone and colleagues[13] also noted this tendency, and showed that 65% of 137

David J. Bertsch: Surgical Oncology Fellow, Division of Surgical Oncology, Department of Surgery, Ohio State University and The Arthur G. James Cancer Hospital and Research Institute, 410 West 10th Avenue, Doan N-911, Columbus, OH 43210-1236

Edward W. Martin, Jr.: Professor, Division of Surgical Oncology, Department of Surgery, Ohio State University and The Arthur G. James Cancer Hospital and Research Institute, 410 West 10th Avenue, Doan N-911, Columbus, OH 43210-1236

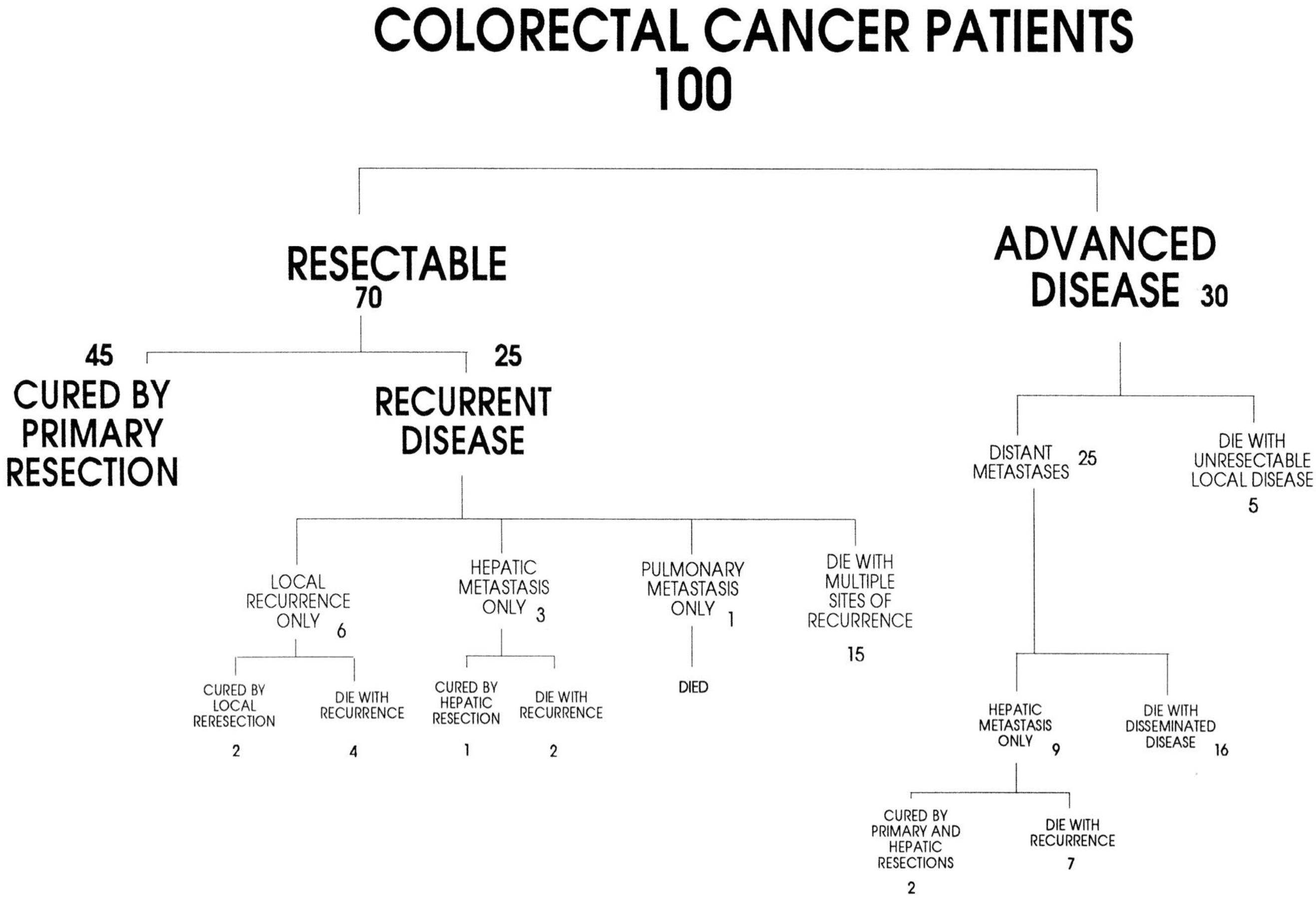

FIG. 68-1. Patterns of failure in 100 patients presenting with large bowel cancer. (August DA, Ottow RT, Sugarbaker PH. Clinical perspectives on human colorectal cancer metastases. Cancer Metastasis Rev 1984;3:303.)

patients had elevated preoperative levels. Other investigators had similar observations. Later, we[14] showed an elevated preoperative CEA level in 81% of patients. After changes in assay methods, allowing more accurate determination of serum level, and taking into account different patient populations, Woolfson reported elevated preoperative CEA levels in 65% of patients with colorectal cancer.[15] Most patients with localized disease have a normal CEA level, yet 30% to 40% in this group show an elevated CEA.[16–18] Wanebo and colleagues[19] and Ladenson and coworkers[20] demonstrated a correlation between advanced stages of colorectal cancer and higher CEA levels (Table 68-1). Wanebo and colleagues also noted that poorly differentiated tumors usually did not produce CEA levels as high as moderately or well differentiated tumors. In addition, higher preoperative levels tended to portend a higher incidence of recurrence.

By 1975, we proposed monitoring the serum level of CEA as a biologic marker of recurrent colorectal carcinoma and using elevated levels to determine the timing of second-look surgery.[21] Ohio State University (OSU) developed a nomogram for interpretation of significant changes in CEA level by 1977[22] (Fig. 68-2). The slope analysis method of Staab and coworkers[23] was another method of evaluating the significance of increasing CEA levels.

Carcinoembryonic antigen became a valuable tool in following patients after their colorectal cancer surgery. Early studies had shown that an elevated preoperative CEA level would return to normal in less than 2 months in patients undergoing a "curative resection."[24,25] A rising CEA level indicates recurrent disease and often does so 2 to 3 months before the patient shows signs, symptoms, or radiologic evidence of recurrence[26–35] (Table 68-2).

TABLE 68-1. *Plasma carcinoembryonic antigen (CEA) concentration according to stage of colorectal carcinoma*

	Dukes' stage			
	A	B	C	D
Patients (n)	58	51	63	31
CEA concentration (%)				
0–2.5 ng/mL	72	55	25	16
2.6–4.0 ng/mL	25	20	30	19
5.1–10.0 ng/mL	3	10	14	3
10.1–20.0 ng/mL	0	15	13	19
>20.0 ng/mL	0	0	18	43

Data from Wanebo HJ, Rao B, Pinsky CM, et al. Preoperative carcinoembryonic antigen level as a prognostic indicator in colorectal cancer. N Engl J Med 1978;229:448; adapted by Ladenson JH, McDonald JM, Landt M, Schwartz MK. Colorectal carcinoma and carcinoembryonic antigen (CEA). Clin Chem 1980;26:1213.

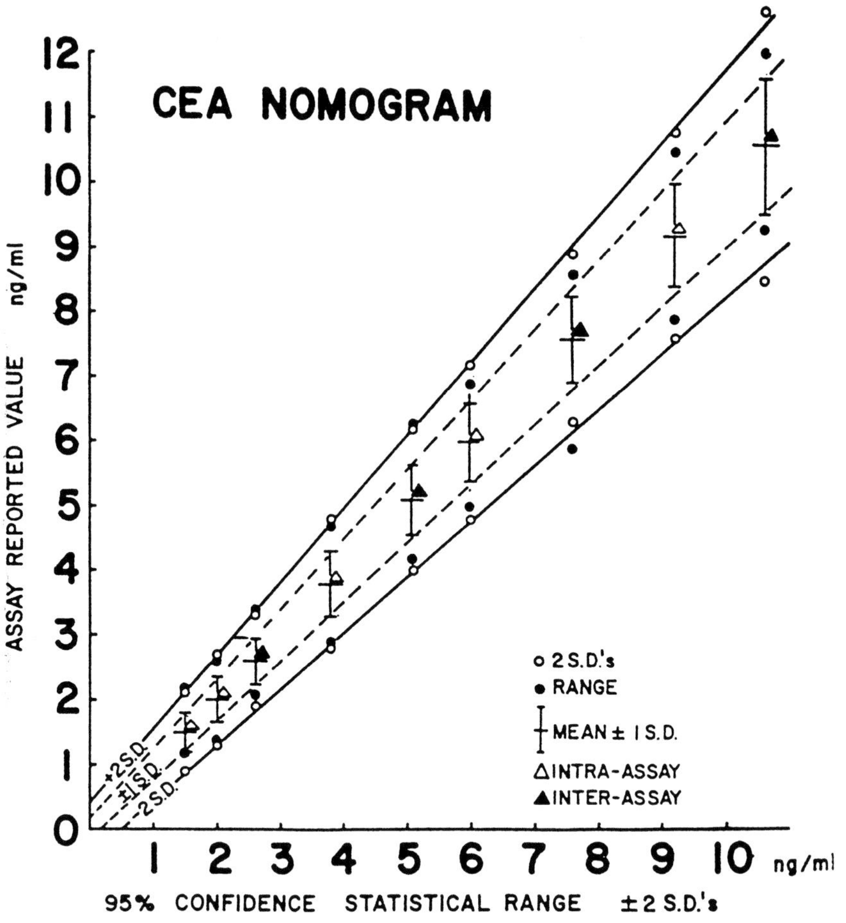

FIG. 68-2. Carcinoembryonic antigen (CEA) nomogram to be used for comparing serial CEA levels to determine if the change is significant (>2 standard deviations) to indicate recurrent gastrointestinal cancer. (Minto JP, James KK, Hurtubise PE, Rinker L, Joyce S, Martin EW Jr. The use of serial carcinoembryonic antigen determinations to predict recurrence of carcinoma of the colon and the time for a second-look operation. Surg Gynecol Obstet 1978;147:208.)

In 1977, we used an elevated CEA greater than two standard deviations by nomogram to confirm suitability for surgery. In this series, 88% (22/25) of the patients had recurrent disease. Seventy-three percent (16/22) of patients had distant metastases, but 27% (6/22) of the patients had localized disease resected for possible cure.[22] Wanebo and colleagues[36] in 1978 reported that 14 of 16 patients explored for elevated CEA levels had recurrent disease. Seven of these 16 patients had disease resected for potential cure.

Multiple second-look studies[22,36–40] from the late 1970s and early 1980s showed that elevated CEA levels predicted tumor recurrence in 85% to 95% of the patients explored. Resectability for possible cure varied from 20% to 50%.

Minton and coworkers[41] reported the results of a 400-patient second-look colorectal cancer study in 1984. This study was carried out by members of the Society of Surgical Oncology. Of 400 patients, 130 had recurrent disease. Seventy-five of these 130 patients underwent a second-look laparotomy. Forty-three of the 75 patients underwent CEA-directed laparotomies, whereas 32 of 75 patients had clinically indicated second-look

TABLE 68-2. *Recurrent colorectal cancer lead time between elevated carcinoembryonic antigen and clinical evidence of disease*

Author	Year	Median time Months	Range	Percentage of positivity preceding detection of recurrence
MacKay, et al[26]	1974	9	3–18	—
Sorokin, et al[27]	1974	—	0–29	—
Mach, et al[28]	1974	—	2–10	89
Holyoke, et al[29]	1975	6.7	6–14	30
Herrera, et al[30]	1976	5.5	—	61
Zamcheck[31]	1975	—	0–29	—
Wood, et al[32]	1980	4	2–28	78
Lunde and Havig[33]	1982	5	—	59
Hine and Dykes[34]	1984	7.5	—	67

From Sardi A. Multiple operations for recurrent colorectal cancer. Semin Surg Oncol 1991;7:146.

laparotomies. Fifty-nine percent (23/43) of the CEA-directed and 50% (16/32) of the clinically indicated operations were judged potentially curative. Martin and associates[42] in 1985 reported on 146 *asymptomatic* patients who, after a curative colorectal cancer operation, underwent a CEA-directed second-look procedure. Ninety-five percent had recurrent cancer and 58% were resected for possible cure. The 5-year survival rate was 31%.

With time, it became apparent that the most beneficial use of CEA was in the postoperative monitoring of colorectal cancer patients. Properly interpreted CEA levels could help assess the completeness of primary surgical therapy and the response to palliative or systemic treatments, and could indicate tumor recurrence before clinical detection.[35,43]

POSTOPERATIVE FOLLOW-UP

Colorectal cancer has the greatest chance for recurrence in the first 2 years after surgery, and nearly all recurrences (≥98%) occur within 4 years.[18] Follow-up should be diligent and maximal during this time. Most surgeons believe the greatest chance for salvage is when the recurrent disease is asymptomatic or minimally evident. Before the primary operation, a baseline CEA level should be obtained. After surgery, the CEA should return to normal within 1 to 2 months for the operation to be considered curative. Failure of the CEA level to fall to normal levels indicates residual cancer.

For postoperative follow-up, the American Cancer Society[44] recommends a history, physical examination including rectal examination and stool guaiac, and CEA level every 4 months. Annually, a chest radiograph and colon examination (ie, air contrast barium enema or total colonoscopy) should be performed. Serum liver function tests and CEA levels also should be obtained at the annual examination. Any abnormalities require further evaluation.

Once the CEA level has returned to a postoperative normal baseline, it is monitored with appropriate frequency. The American Cancer Society recommends checking the CEA level every 3 to 4 months. At OSU, however, we recommend checking it every 6 to 8 weeks. We also perform a computed tomography scan of the liver and a chest radiograph at 6-month intervals for the first 2 years. Rectal ultrasound is performed at 4- to 6-month intervals in rectal cancer patients who have been treated with surgical procedures and modalities other than abdominal perineal resection.

EVALUATION OF AN ELEVATED CARCINOEMBRYONIC ANTIGEN LEVEL

A rising CEA level demands further evaluation. A repeat determination is obtained approximately 2 weeks after the first elevated value is detected. Two or more elevated levels, rising more than two standard deviations on the nomogram, or changes in the level from less than 2.5 ng/mL to greater than 5 to 6 ng/mL, necessitate a full evaluation. It is important to obtain the CEA values from the same laboratory because variations in testing techniques and references between laboratories can affect the significance of an isolated value.

An evaluation is carried out to determine if the patient is a candidate for second-look laparotomy. First, benign conditions that can elevate the CEA level should be ruled out easily with a history and a physical examination. Some benign conditions that can elevate CEA levels are hepatocellular diseases, biliary obstruction, hepatocellular toxicity from 5-fluorouracil and levamisole, pancreatitis, inflammatory bowel disease, heavy smoking, asthmatic conditions, and advanced age.[10,45] Other malignancies such as adenocarcinoma of the breast, pancreas, stomach, esophagus, lung, thyroid, and ovary can increase the CEA.[11] Assuming these causes are ruled out with the history and physical examination, the evaluation focuses on common routes of colorectal cancer metastasis.

The physical examination includes an examination of the lymph nodes—axillary (Irish's), supraclavicular (Virchow's), and umbilical (Sister Mary Joseph's). Biopsy-proven disease found in these areas indicates incurability.

The abdomen is examined for masses. A digital rectal examination is carried out to evaluate for rectal or pelvic recurrence. In female patients, a pelvic examination is performed to assess the ovaries, which comprise 2% to 10% of the incidence of colorectal cancer metastases,[46] and the pelvis.

Laboratory studies should be obtained and include the two or more confirmatory elevated CEA levels, liver function tests, complete blood count, and electrolyte levels.

The colon is examined with a total colonoscopy to look for an anastomotic recurrence or metachronous colorectal cancer. Transrectal ultrasound may be worthwhile in rectal carcinoma patients treated with sphincter preservation (ie, transanal excision and radiation, low anterior or coloanal resection).

A chest radiograph is obtained. If this is negative, a computed tomography scan of the chest is performed. Many times, the chest computed tomography scan reveals mediastinal nodal or pulmonary metastases not evident on chest radiography.

Evaluation of the abdomen and pelvis is carried out with computed tomography scans. Magnetic resonance imaging of the liver is being used with increasing frequency. Hepatic magnetic resonance imaging can often distinguish a benign process, such as a hemangioma, from a metastasis.[47] Three-dimensional reconstruction can be done to demonstrate the relation of one or more lesions to the portal, hepatic, or caval venous systems.

Although uncommon, bone metastases do occur in colorectal cancer.[35] If the history and physical examination suggest bone metastases, a bone scan and traditional radiographs of the symptomatic area should be obtained. Involvement of pelvic bones by recurrent rectal cancer can sometimes be evaluated by magnetic resonance imaging.

The results of all these studies are reviewed to determine if the patient is a candidate for surgery. Obviously, pulmonary or mediastinal disease with intraabdominal disease is incurable. Occasionally, mediastinoscopy or thoracic evaluation of the isolated pulmonary mass in a patient with abdominal disease is warranted to rule out benign disease or a second primary tumor site. An isolated pulmonary mass in a patient with no abdominal disease should be resected. If this is a colorectal cancer metastasis, there is a 20% to 30% chance of 5-year survival after resection.[35,48]

Patients with no evidence of extraabdominal disease are candidates for second-look laparotomies unless they have clearly

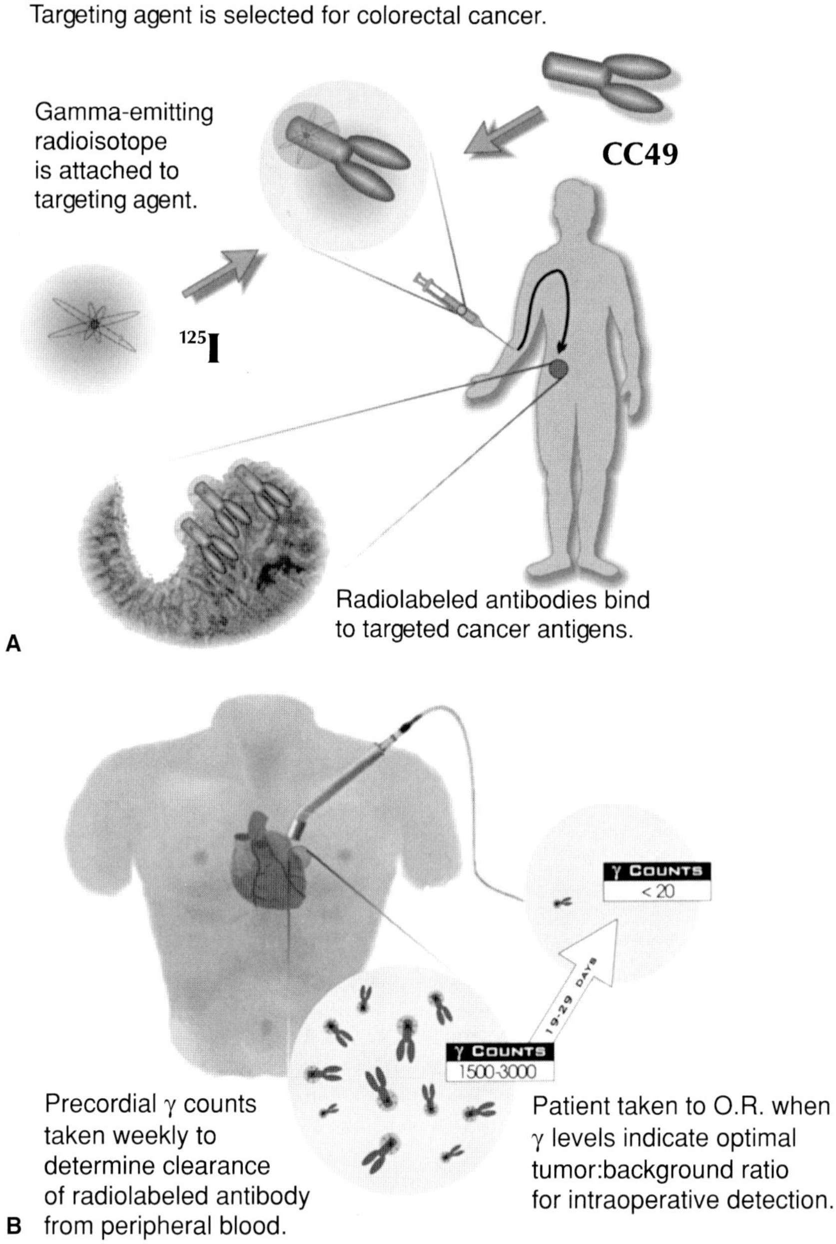

FIG. 68-3. (A) Injection, circulation, and targeting of radiolabeled ^{125}I-CC49 monoclonal antibody. **(B)** Assessment of precordial γ counts of patients undergoing radioimmunoguided surgery.

unresectable liver metastasis or extensive bilobar disease; however, this may not be clearly determined until laparotomy. If the patient's performance status suggests he or she will tolerate the surgery, the operation is undertaken.

At OSU, in an attempt to improve the results of second-look surgery, we have enrolled second-look patients in RIGS-directed second-look laparotomy protocols. The RIGS technique was developed at OSU to provide surgeons with additional intraoperative information, enhanced tumor identification, and the ability to find occult metastatic disease.

The RIGS system uses an intravenously administered iodine 125 (^{125}I)-labeled monoclonal antibody, CC49 (Neoprobe Corporation, Dublin, OH). CC49 is a second-generation anti–tumor-associated glycoprotein (TAG-72) antibody. TAG-72 is a mucin expressed by a large number of human adenocarcinomas, including colorectal, breast, renal, gastric, and pancreatic. The ^{125}I-labeled CC49 is administered after adequate thyroid blockage (Thyro-Block; Wallace Laboratories, Cranbury, NJ) to prevent uptake of ^{125}I in the thyroid. A 2- to 3-week waiting period between injection and surgery allows the antibody to target the cancer cells and bind to the antigen, and the ^{125}I CC49 to clear from the blood. The radioactivity in the blood background is assessed weekly by obtaining precordial (heart blood pool) measurements with a hand-held gamma detector (the Neoprobe 1000 portable radioisotope detector; Neoprobe Corporation). Precordial counts of radioactivity less than 20 counts per 2 seconds represent a low background count that is optimal for the probe to distinguish higher counts of radioactivity in tissue localized by the radiolabeled monoclonal antibody. When the precordial count reaches this level, it is assumed that the tumor-to-background ratio is optimal for RIGS exploration, and the patient goes to surgery (Fig. 68-3).

THE SECOND-LOOK OPERATION

Second-look operations should be performed by those surgeons capable of performing extensive and demanding surgery, including hepatic resection, pelvic exenteration, retroperitoneal node dissection, reconstruction of the urinary tract, and abdominosacral resection. A multimodality approach is often needed; consultation with urologic or orthopedic surgeons and radiation oncologists may be invaluable.

Risks, benefits, and extent of surgery are reviewed with the patient. The patient receives a bowel preparation. The operation is carried out through a midline incision. Even patients suspected of having an isolated hepatic recurrence should be explored through a midline incision to allow complete inspection of the abdomen and pelvis. A xiphoid to symphysis pubis incision, appropriate retractor, and a fully mobilized liver allow all types of lobectomies, partial hepatectomies, and segmentectomies to be performed.

The viscera are prepared for thorough evaluation. All adhesions are lysed, from the ligament of Treitz to the colon. The liver is mobilized, dividing the triangular and falciform ligaments. The lesser sac is opened superior to the stomach.

Traditional examination of the abdomen and pelvis is carried out to look for recurrences on the peritoneal, serosal, and diaphragmatic surfaces. Special attention is directed to nodal areas (ie, celiac, portal, gastrohepatic, and paraaortic; Fig. 68-4). The entire bowel, the anastomosis, previous bed of resection, the uterus, and the ovaries are inspected.

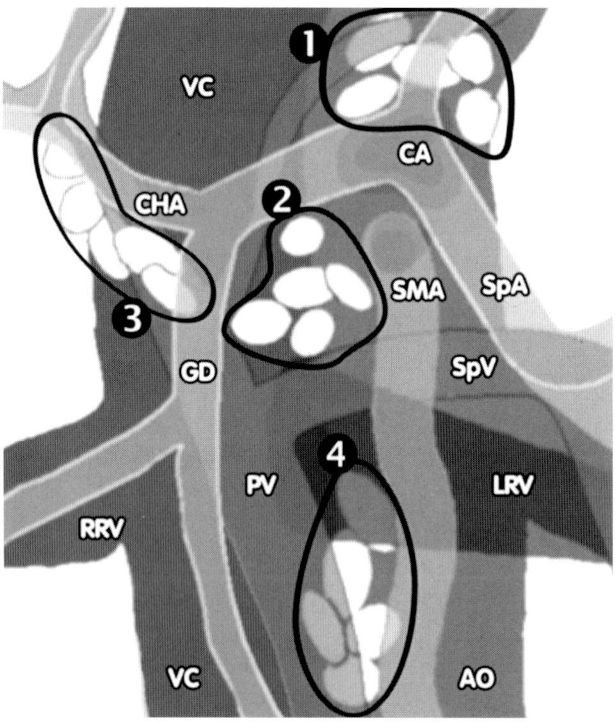

FIG. 68-4. Lymph node areas assessed at second-look surgery: *1*, celiac nodes; *2*, gastrohepatic ligament nodes; *3*, periportal nodes; *4*, paraarotic nodes; *AO*, aorta; *CA*, celiac axis; *CHA*, common hepatic artery; *GD*, gastroduodenal artery; *SMA*, superior mesenteric artery; *SpA*, splenic artery; *LRV*, left renal vein; *PV*, portal vein; *RRV*, right renal vein; *VC*, vena cava.

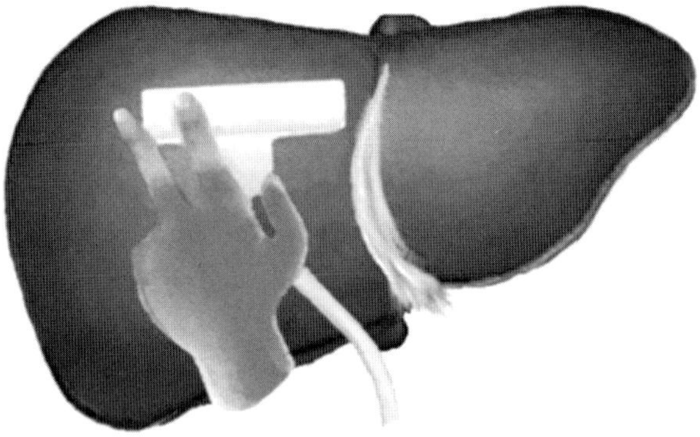

FIG. 68-5. Intraoperative ultrasonography of the liver.

With the liver mobilized, palpation and inspection are performed. Intraoperative ultrasound is used to assess the number of liver metastases and their relation to major vessels (Fig. 68-5). Often, the intraoperative ultrasound reveals more hepatic metastases than evidenced by the preoperative studies or the surgeon's visual and bimanual examination.

After traditional exploration, a RIGS exploration is performed. The areas examined with the probe are shown schematically (Fig. 68-6). RIGS-positive tissue is defined as tissue showing counts greater than three standard deviations above the baseline (background) count. The RIGS survey takes less than 10 to 15 minutes.

After all methods of exploration are completed, an assessment of the extent of disease and possibility of surgical cure is made. The main consideration in this decision is that all disease must be removed for a patient to be cured. Positive margins or residual disease lead to failure.

In traditional second-look surgery, hepatic resection is undertaken for three to four or fewer lesions resectable with anatomic (lobectomy, segmentectomy) or nonanatomic (wedge resection) procedures including negative margins of 1 to 2 cm. Unresectable extrahepatic disease is a contraindication to liver resection. A small volume of resectable extrahepatic disease in the presence of resectable hepatic disease is more controversial. Many surgeons believe this circumstance indicates incurable disease; however, at OSU we would resect these patients. Patients without liver involvement should have their nonhepatic recurrences resected if the procedure can include negative margins.

At OSU, we use the RIGS surveying technique as an adjunct to assess extent of disease, to find occult disease, and to determine margins of resection. Inability to resect RIGS-positive tissue, even if it appears grossly normal, is a contraindication to extensive surgery. Hepatic resection or a curative pelvic exenteration is not undertaken unless all extrahepatic or extrapelvic RIGS-positive tissue can be surgically removed.

If the operative findings demonstrate unresectable disease, palliative procedures may be indicated. Other regional treatments, such as hepatic infusion lines, brachytherapy, or intraop-

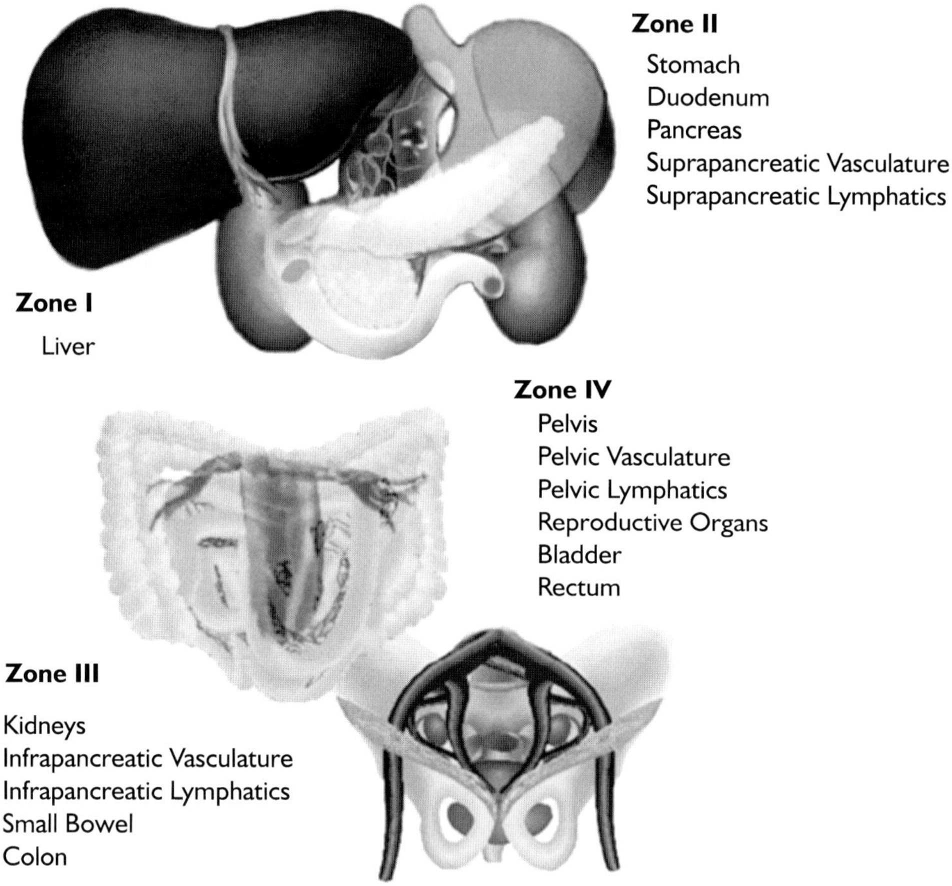

FIG. 68-6. Zones and structures assessed with radioimmunoguided surgery.

erative radiation therapy, may be of benefit or may be indicated as part of a protocol. In cases of carcinomatosis without liver or nodal disease, intraperitoneal hyperthermic perfusion may be considered.

RESULTS

Carcinoembryonic antigen-directed second-look laparotomies reveal recurrent or metastatic disease up to 95% of the time. Common sites of recurrence are usually categorized as local or locoregional, hepatic, nonhepatic intraabdominal, or diffuse[35,40,49–54] (Table 68-3). Rates of resectability for cure vary from 20% to 60%. In the 5% of patients with no evidence of disease, most manifest metastatic colorectal cancer within 12 months.

In general, the 5-year cure rate for second-look surgery is 20% to 40%. This cure rate applies to hepatic and nonhepatic recurrences. What does this 20% to 40% 5-year survival mean? If all patients with colorectal cancer are considered, from 12% to 50% with Dukes' B or Dukes' C (stage II or III) primary disease will have a recurrence.[19,38,55] Twenty-five percent will be evaluated for second-look surgery, and 10% will undergo the procedure. Twenty to 60% of explored patients will be resected for a potential cure, but only 20% to 40% of resected patients will be cured. A salvage rate of 2% to 3% of all colo-

TABLE 68-3. *Colorectal cancer patterns of failure at the time of second-look surgery (%)*

		Locoregional		Liver		
Author	Year	Alone	Combination	Alone	Combination	Location
Gunderson, et al[49]	1971	34	76	30	—	Colon
Gunderson and Sosin[50]	1974	48	92	6	21	Rectum
Wanebo, et al[36]	1978	37	—	37	—	Colon/rectum
Attiyeh and Stearns[40]	1981	40	—	48	—	Colon/rectum
Tong, et al[51]	1983	16	48	5	43	Colon/rectum
Russell, et al[52]	1984	20	47	22	33	Colon
Makela and Kairaluoma[53]	1986	40	—	—	—	Colon/rectum
Sardi, et al[54]	1989	40	59	41	56	Colon/rectum

From Sardi A. Multiple operations for recurrent colorectal cancer. Semin Surg Oncol 1991;7:146.

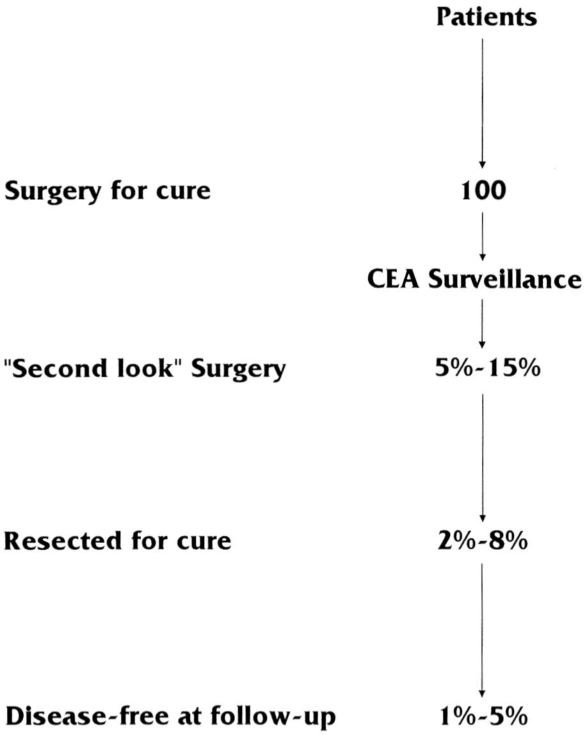

FIG. 68-7. Estimated salvage by second-look surgery of recurrent colorectal cancer patients. The cure rate for colorectal cancer that might be attributed to postoperative monitoring of carcinoembryonic antigen (CEA) levels and second-look surgery. Although often not specified, the median follow-up appears to be a few years in most series. (Fletcher RH. Carcinoembryonic antigen. Ann Intern Med 1986;104:66.)

rectal cancer patients is confirmed in most CEA-directed second-look studies[17,55–57] (Fig. 68-7). Statistical models and estimates yield salvage rates of 1% to 5%.

Is a salvage rate less than 5% worthwhile? Northover[58] stated that cancer cures attributable to CEA monitoring were at best infrequent and questioned the substantial cost of CEA monitoring and associated interventions. The cost in Moertel and colleagues'[59] 1993 study was $1,439,000 for 1017 patients with a median follow-up of 6 years (range, 5 to 8.5 years). Nelson[60] estimates the annual expense of colorectal cancer follow-up to be $650,000,000 per annum for the United States. On top of this, second-look surgery is estimated to cost $50,000 per procedure. If 2% of followed colorectal cancer patients undergo second-look surgery, an additional national cost of $500,000,000 is sustained.

In response to Moertel and colleagues' position, Cohen and Paty[61] eloquently reviewed the benefit of CEA monitoring for colorectal cancer patients in whom isolated hepatic metastases develop. Of the 150,000 patients diagnosed with colorectal cancer each year, 100,000 need close follow-up. Of the 50,000 patients in whom recurrent disease develops, one third, or 17,000, have only hepatic metastases. One third of these, or 5500, can be resected, and one third of resected patients, or 1850, are cured for a salvage rate of 2% in patients undergoing a hepatic metastatectomy. By extension of this principle, if 2% to 4% of the closely monitored 100,000 colorectal cancer patients are cured with second-look surgery, 2000 to 4000 people are saved from an otherwise incurable disease. CEA monitoring should help to salvage these patients.

OHIO STATE UNIVERSITY AND RADIOIMMUNOGUIDED SURGERY RESULTS

Early studies at OSU involved CEA-directed second-look laparotomies in the asymptomatic patient. In a study of 22 patients undergoing second-look surgery between 1971 and 1976, 2 are still alive 20 and 22 years later. The 1976 to 1979 OSU study was a prospective, nonrandomized study of 146 patients who underwent a CEA-directed second-look operation. Tumor was identified in 95% of these patients. Fifty-five percent were resected for cure and the 5-year survival rate was 31%.[42]

The RIGS system has been developed and refined over the last 10 years at OSU. This technique was initially created to improve the results of second-look surgery, but is now also being applied to primary operations for colorectal cancer. The RIGS technology has been developed to detect occult microscopic disease, identify new areas of cancer spread, and improve survival in CEA-directed second-look surgery.

Early RIGS studies at OSU demonstrated the feasibility of using the RIGS system to localize tumor at the time of surgery. An early murine monoclonal antibody, 17-1A, localized tumor in 75% of patients with recurrent colorectal cancer.[62,63] Subsequently, the first-generation anti-TAG antibody B72.3 showed a 78% rate of localization. An initial RIGS study using B72.3 showed that 25% (8/31) of patients with recurrent colorectal cancer had subclinical tumor identified at surgery. This information led to altered surgical plans (ie, more or less surgery in these eight patients).[64]

In 1991, Cohen and associates[65] reported multicenter trial results using RIGS with B72.3. One hundred five patients were enrolled, 78 with recurrent colorectal cancer and 27 with primary colorectal cancer. In the recurrent patients, localization

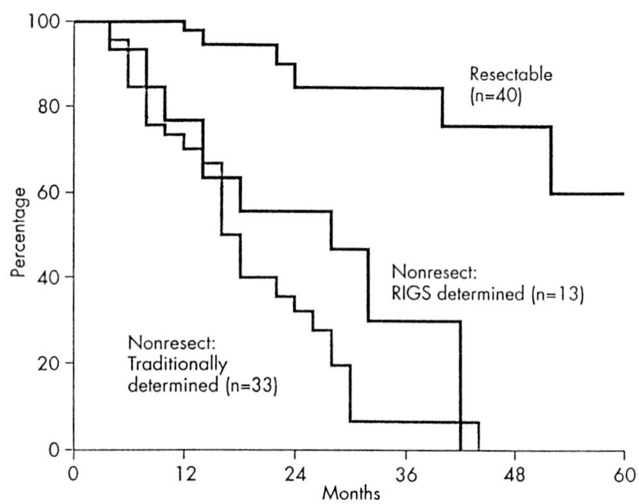

FIG. 68-8. Survival analysis of patients with radioimmunoguided surgery (RIGS)-positive recurrent colon and rectal cancer. (Martin EW Jr, Carey LC. Second-look surgery for colorectal cancer: the second time around. Ann Surg 1991;214: 321.)

TABLE 68-4. *Metastatic sites in 40 resected patients*

Site	Number
Liver	24
Pelvis	4
Anastomosis	2
Right gutter	1
Lymph nodes	17
Periportal	10
Retroperitoneal	5
Peripancreatic	1
Mesenteric	1

with the antibody was 78%. RIGS information at the time of surgery altered the operation in approximately 25% of patients. In 27% of the 36 nonresectable patients, nonresectability was based on RIGS information alone. In the 35 patients undergoing resection, 23% had an extended resection based solely on RIGS information.

A follow-up study with B72.3 carried out in 86 recurrent colorectal cancer patients who underwent RIGS procedures looked at survival rates.[66] Three groups were evaluated as resectable patients (N = 40), nonresectable (N = 33), and RIGS-determined nonresectable (N = 13). Thirty-three of 40 resectable patients (83%) were alive at 2 to 5 years. However, only 21% and 31% in the traditionally nonresectable group and RIGS nonresectable group, respectively, were alive. The actual 5-year survival rate is 60% for the resected group and 0% in the nonresected group[66] (Fig. 68-8). The 5-year survival rate of 60% in the resectable group is significantly higher than the survival rate of 31% in our study of non-RIGS CEA-directed second-look surgery.

Fifty metastatic sites were identified in the 40 resectable patients (Table 68-4). The nodal areas of recurrence were an interesting finding. Periportal, peripancreatic, and retroperitoneal nodes are not often assessed in traditional primary or second-look colorectal surgery, but are often identified with the RIGS system.

A second-generation monoclonal antibody against TAG-72, CC49, has the highest localization of any antibody used with the RIGS system to date, as shown in a phase I CC49 study of 54 evaluable patients started in 1990 at OSU. Eighty-six percent of primary and 97% of recurrent colorectal cancer patients had localization of tumor by ^{125}I-labeled CC49. Nearly 50% of patients in the study had a change in their planned second-look operation based on immediate intraoperative RIGS information.[67]

In these and other clinical trails, the RIGS system has identified occult micrometastatic disease and provided new knowledge about tumor spread. More important, beneficial intraoperative decisions have been made as a result of the information the RIGS system provided to surgeons.

SUMMARY

Since Wangensteen's[4] studies 50 years ago, when 60% of patients had a negative laparotomy, second-look surgery has

TABLE 68-5. *History of second-look surgery for recurrent colorectal cancer*

Type of surgery	Number of patients	Percent resected	Percent negative	Mortality	Survival
PLANNED (BLIND) REOPERATION					
Wangensteen 1964[5]	35	—	57	2.8	2 NED (9–12 mo)
	29	—	52	10	4 NED (18–50 mos) 14% salvage 28% of (+) cases
Griffen et al, 1969[6]	44	—	54	7	4.5% Rectum
	98	—	63	8	17% Salvage (colon)
SYMPTOMATIC SECOND LOOK					
Gunderson and Sosin 1974[50]	74	—	39	5.4	7.7% Rectum
CEA-DIRECTED REOPERATION					
Martin and Minton 1977	22	27	12	NS	1 NED (3 y)
Wanebo 1978[3]	16	44	12	NS	4 NED (12–37 mo) 5 ED (2–12 mo)
Martin et al, 1985[42]	146	58	5	NS	31%
CEA-DIRECTED REOPERATION AND RIGS					
Martin and Carey, 1991[66]*	86	46	0%	NS	60% Resectable group 28% Total group
Martin, Burak, and Bertsch, 1994†‡	168	37	3%	NS	63% (1.5–8 y) Resectable group 35% (20–72 mo) Total group

* B72.3 monoclonal antibody.
† B72.3, CC83, CC49 anti–tumor-associated glycoprotein monoclonal antibodies.
‡ Unpublished data.
NED, no evidence of disease; *ED,* evidence of disease; *NS,* not stated; *CEA,* carcinoembryonic antigen; *RIGS,* radioimmunoguided surgery.
* Martin et al. The use of CEA as an early indicator for gastrointestinal tumor recurrence and second-look procedures. Cancer 1977;39:440–446.

changed significantly (Table 68-5). Today, CEA-directed second-look surgery identifies recurrent tumor 95% of the time. Twenty to 60% of patients undergo a curative resection and 20% to 40% achieve a 5-year cure with traditional surgical methods, for a salvage rate of 2% to 3%. Early RIGS results show promise for increasing the 5-year survival rate toward 60% in selected patients. Results from further studies are forthcoming, such as a multicenter trial in the United Kingdom quantifying the effects on mortality from CEA-directed second-look surgery,[68] and ongoing RIGS studies. These studies will help to clarify which patients benefit from second-look surgery. Postsurgical follow-up of colorectal cancer patients, including CEA monitoring, is expensive, anxiety producing, and time consuming, but it helps to save the lives of 2000 to 4000 people per year (in the United States) who have an otherwise incurable disease.

ACKNOWLEDGMENTS

The authors thank Cheryl Wilson for preparation of the manuscript and Martin Boso for the original illustrations.

REFERENCES

1. American Cancer Society, Inc., Atlanta, GA. Cancer facts and figures 1994.
2. Cohen AM, Minsky BD, Schilsky RL. Colon cancer. In: DeVita VT Jr, Hellman S, Rosenberg SA, eds. Cancer: principles and practice of oncology. 4th ed. Philadelphia: JB Lippincott, 1993:929.
3. August DA, Ottow RT, Sugarbaker PH. Clinical perspectives on human colorectal cancer metastases. Cancer Metastasis Rev 1984;3:303.
4. Wangensteen OH, Lewis FJ, Tongen LA. The "second look" in cancer surgery. Lancet 1951;71:303.
5. Wangensteen OH, Lewis FJ, Arhelger SW, Muller JJ, MacLean LD. An interim report upon the "second look" procedure for cancer of the stomach, colon, and rectum and for "limited intraperitoneal carcinosis." Surg Gynecol Obstet 1954;99:257.
6. Griffen WO Jr, Humphrey L, Sosin H. The prognosis and management of recurrent abdominal malignancies. Curr Probl Surg 1969;6:3.
7. Gold P, Freedman SO. Demonstration of tumor-specific antigens in human colonic carcinoma by immunological tolerance and absorption techniques. J Exp Med 1965;121:439.
8. Gold P, Freedman SO. Specific carcinoembryonic antigens of the human digestive system. J Exp Med 1965;122:467.
9. Slayter HS, Coligan JE. Electron microscopy and physical characterization of the carcinoembryonic antigen. Biochemistry 1975;14:2323.
10. Fletcher RH. Carcinoembryonic antigen. Ann Intern Med 1986;104:66.
11. Chevinsky AH. CEA in tumors of other than colorectal origin. Semin Surg Oncol 1991;7:162.
12. Thomson DM, Krupey J, Freedman SO, Gold P. The radioimmunoassay of circulating carcinoembryonic antigen of the human digestive system. Proc Natl Acad Sci U S A 1969;64:161.
13. Livingstone AS, Hampson LG, Shuster J, Gold P, Hinchey EJ. Carcinoembryonic antigen in the diagnosis and management of colorectal carcinoma: current status. Arch Surg 1974;109:259.
14. Martin EW Jr, Kibbey WE, DiVecchia L, Catalano P, Anderson G, Minton JP. Carcinoembryonic antigen: clinical and historical aspects. Cancer 1976;37:60.
15. Woolfson K. Tumor markers in cancer of the colon and rectum. Dis Colon Rectum 1991;34:506.
16. Go VL. Carcinoembryonic antigen: clinical application. Cancer 1976;37:562.
17. Herberman RB. Immunologic approaches to the diagnosis of cancer. Cancer 1976;37:549.
18. Moertel C. Large bowel. In: Foley J, Vose J, Armitage J, eds. Current therapy in cancer. Philadelphia: WB Saunders, 1994:74.
19. Wanebo HJ, Rao B, Pinsky CM, et al. Preoperative carcinoembryonic antigen level as a prognostic indicator in colorectal cancer. N Engl J Med 1978;299:448.
20. Ladenson JH, McDonald JM, Landt M, Schwartz MK. Colorectal carcinoma and carcinoembryonic antigen (CEA). Clin Chem 1980;26:1213.
21. Nieroda CA, Martin EW Jr. Rising CEA 14 months after colon cancer resection. In: Wanebo HJ, ed. Common problems in cancer surgery. Chicago: Year Book Medical Publishers, 1990;12:75.
22. Martin EW Jr, James KK, Hurtubise PE, Catalano P, Minton JP. The use of CEA as an early indicator for gastrointestinal tumor recurrence and second-look procedures. Cancer 1977;39:440.
23. Staab HJ, Anderer FA, Stumpf E, Fischer R. Slope analysis of postoperative CEA time course and its possible application as an aid in diagnosis of disease progression in gastrointestinal cancer. Am J Surg 1978;136:322.
24. Ewing HP, Newsom BD, Hardy JD. Tumor markers. Curr Probl Surg 1982;19:53.
25. Fortner JG, Silva JS, Cox EB, Golbey RB, Gallowitz H, Maclean BJ. Multivariate analysis of a personal series of 247 patients with liver metastasis from colorectal cancer: II. treatment by intrahepatic chemotherapy. Ann Surg 1984;199:317.
26. MacKay AM, Patel S, Carter S, et al. Role of serial plasma C.E.A. assays in detection of recurrent and metastatic colorectal carcinomas. Br Med J 1974;4:382.
27. Sorokin JJ, Sugarbaker PH, Zamcheck N, Pisick M, Kupchik HZ, Moore FD. Serial carcinoembryonic antigen assays: use in detection of cancer recurrence. JAMA 1974;228:49.
28. Mach JP, Jaeger P, Bertholet MM, Ruegsegger CH, Loosli RM, Pettavel J. Detection of recurrence of large-bowel carcinoma by radioimmunoassay of circulating carcinoembryonic antigen (C.E.A.). Lancet 1974;2:535.
29. Holyoke ED, Chu TM, Murphy GP. CEA as a monitor of gastrointestinal malignancy. Cancer 1975;35:830.
30. Herrera MA, Chu TM, Holyoke ED. Carcinoembryonic antigen (CEA) as a prognostic and monitoring test in clinically complete resection of colorectal carcinoma. Ann Surg 1976;183:5.
31. Zamcheck N. The present status of CEA in diagnosis, prognosis, and evaluation of therapy. Cancer 1975;36:2460.
32. Wood CB, Ratcliffe JG, Burt RW, Malcolm AJ, Blumgart LH. The clinical significance of the pattern of elevated serum carcinoembryonic antigen (CEA) levels in recurrent colorectal cancer. Br J Surg 1980;67:46.
33. Lunde OC, Havig O. Clinical significance of carcinoembryonic antigen (CEA) in patients with adenocarcinoma in colon and rectum. Acta Chir Scand 1982;148:189.
34. Hine KR, Dykes PW. Serum CEA testing in the post-operative surveillance of colorectal carcinoma. Br J Cancer 1984;49:689.
35. Sardi A. Multiple operations for recurrent colorectal cancer. Semin Surg Oncol 1991;7:146.
36. Wanebo HJ, Stearns M, Schwartz MK. Use of CEA as an indicator of early recurrence and as a guide to a selected second-look procedure in patients with colorectal cancer. Ann Surg 1978;188:481.
37. Martin EW Jr, Cooperman M, King G, Rinker L, Carey LC, Minton JP. A retrospective and prospective study of serial CEA determinations in the early detection of recurrent colon cancer. Am J Surg 1979;137:167.
38. Minton JP, James KK, Hurtubise PE, Rinker L, Joyce S, Martin EW Jr. The use of serial carcinoembryonic antigen determinations to predict recurrence of carcinoma of the colon and the time for a second-look operation. Surg Gynecol Obstet 1978;147:208.
39. Steele G Jr, Zamcheck N, Wilson R, et al. Results of CEA-initiated second-look surgery for recurrent colorectal cancer. Am J Surg 1980;139:544.
40. Attiyeh FF, Stearns MW Jr. Second-look laparotomy based on CEA elevations in colorectal cancer. Cancer 1981;47:2119.
41. Minton JP, Hoehn JL, Gerber DM, et al. Results of a 400-patient carcinoembryonic antigen second-look colorectal cancer study. Cancer 1985;55:1284.
42. Martin EW Jr, Minton JP, Carey LC. CEA-directed second-look surgery in the asymptomatic patient after primary resection of colorectal carcinoma. Ann Surg 1985;202:310.
43. Herrera MA, Chu TM, Holyoke ED, Mittelman A. CEA monitoring of palliative treatment for colorectal carcinoma. Ann Surg 1977;185:23.

44. Holleb AI, Fink DJ, Murphy GP. Colorectal cancer. In: Beart RW Jr, ed. American Cancer Society textbook of clinical oncology. Atlanta: The American Cancer Society, 1991:213.
45. Moertel CG, Fleming TR, Macdonald JS, Haller DG, Laurie JA. Hepatic toxicity associated with fluorouracil plus levamisole adjuvant therapy. J Clin Oncol 1993;11:2386.
46. Turk PS, Wanebo HJ. Results of surgical treatment of nonhepatic recurrence in colorectal carcinoma. Cancer 1993;71:4267.
47. Bennett WF, Bova JG. Imaging prior to second-look surgery for carcinoma. Semin Surg Oncol 1991;7:138.
48. Murray KD. Excision of pulmonary metastasis of colorectal cancer. Semin Surg Oncol 1991;7:157.
49. Gunderson LL, Sosin H, Levitt S. Extrapelvic colon—areas of failure in a reoperation series: implications for adjuvant therapy. Int J Radiat Oncol Biol Phys 1985;11:731.
50. Gunderson LL, Sosin H. Areas of failure found at reoperation (second or symptomatic look) following "curative surgery" for adenocarcinoma of the rectum: clinicopathologic correlation and implications for adjuvant therapy. Cancer 1974;34:1278.
51. Tong D, Russell AH, Dawson LE, Wisbeck W. Second laparotomy for proximal colon cancer: sites of recurrence and implications for adjuvant therapy. Am J Surg 1983;145:382-6.
52. Russell AH, Tong D, Dawson LE, Wisbeck W. Adenocarcinoma of the proximal colon: sites of initial dissemination and patterns of recurrence following surgery alone. Cancer 1984;53:360.
53. Makela J, Kairaluoma MI. Reoperation for colorectal cancer. Acta Chir Scand 1986;152:151.
54. Sardi A, Workman M, Mojzisik C, et al. Intra-abdominal recurrence of colorectal cancer detected by radioimmunoguided surgery (RIGS system). Arch Surg 1989;124:55.
55. Bleday R, Steele G Jr. Second-look surgery for recurrent colorectal carcinoma: is it worthwhile? Semin Surg Oncol 1991;7:171.
56. Martin EW Jr, Cooperman M, Carey LC, Minton JP. Sixty second-look procedures indicated primarily by rise in serial carcinoembryonic antigen. J Surg Res 1980;28:389.
57. Steele G, Ellenberg S, Ramming K, et al. CEA monitoring among patients in multi institutional adjuvant GI therapy protocols. Ann Surg 1982:196:162.
58. Northover J. Carcinoembryonic antigen and recurrent colorectal cancer. Gut 1986;27:117.
59. Moertel CG, Fleming TR, Macdonald JS, Haller DG, Laurie JA, Tangen C. An evaluation of the carcinoembryonic antigen (CEA) test for monitoring patients with resected colon cancer. JAMA 1993;270: 943.
60. Nelson RL. The decision to treat patients with recurrent colorectal cancer. Cancer 1993;71:4298.
61. Cohen AM, Paty P. CEA for monitoring colon cancer. JAMA 1994; 271:346.
62. Martin EW, Tuttle SE, Rousseau M, et al. Radioimmunoguided surgery: intraoperative use of monoclonal antibody 17-1A in colorectal cancer. Hybridoma 1986;5:S97.
63. Sardi A, Agnone CM, Nieroda CA, et al. Radioimmunoguided surgery in recurrent colorectal cancer: the role of carcinoembryonic antigen, computerized tomography, and physical examination. South Med J 1989;82:1235.
64. Sickle-Santanello BJ, O'Dwyer PJ, Mojzisik CM, et al. Radioimmunoguided surgery using the monoclonal antibody B72.3 in colorectal tumors. Dis Colon Rectum 1987;30:761.
65. Cohen AM, Martin EW Jr, Lavery I, et al. Radioimmunoguided surgery using iodine ^{125}I B72.3 in patients with colorectal cancer. Arch Surg 1991;126:349.
66. Martin EW Jr, Carey LC. Second-look surgery for colorectal cancer: the second time around. Ann Surg 1991;214:321.
67. Arnold MW, Schneebaum S, Berens A, et al. Intraoperative detection of colorectal cancer with radioimmunoguided surgery (RIGS) and CC49, a second-generation monoclonal antibody (MAb). Ann Surg 1992;216:627.
68. Tornquist A, Ekelund G, Leandoer L. The value of intensive follow up after curative resection for colorectal carcinoma. Br J Surg 1982; 69:725.

Surgery for Gastrointestinal Cancer: A Multidisciplinary Approach, edited by Harold J. Wanebo.
Lippincott-Raven Publishers, Philadelphia, © 1997.

CHAPTER 69

Pelvic Recurrence

Resection and Other Alternatives

Peter S. Turk and Harold J. Wanebo

INCIDENCE OF LOCOREGIONAL RECURRENCE

Locoregional disease is the most common pattern of recurrence from rectal cancer. Surgical series have found isolated local recurrence in 7% to 33% of patients after curative resection of rectal carcinoma, combined local and systemic recurrences in 7% to 30%, and systemic recurrence alone in 6% to 19% of patients.[1–6] The site of recurrence from a rectal cancer depends on the location of the primary lesion. Local recurrence predominates in low- and mid-rectal lesions, whereas systemic recurrence is more prevalent in upper rectal cancers, paralleling the pattern of colon carcinoma.[1] This increased incidence of local disease in the pelvis may be attributable to the more limited margins of clearance possible in the pelvis, as well as to the diffuse lymphatic channels in the mesorectum.

The incidence of local recurrence after an abdominoperineal resection (APR) ranges from 12% to 32%, and after a low anterior resection (LAR), 14% to 43%,[7] and is related to the stage and grade of the initial tumor. The extent and resectability of a local recurrence is determined by the type of initial operation. After APR, only 10% of recurrences present without evidence of pelvic sidewall or combined sidewall with anteroposterior involvement, because most of these are identified at an advanced stage. After LAR, recurrences are more frequently unfixed, with greater potential for surgical resection.[1]

STAGING OF RECURRENCE

Many anastomotic recurrences after LAR are small, apparently isolated lesions that are amenable to local re-resection or APR. The surgeon must be sure, however, that the visible lesion is not the "tip of the iceberg," with a more extensive regional recurrence. Patients with an early stage of recurrence, in whom resection may result in clear margins and a prolonged disease-free interval, are the only appropriate candidates for aggressive surgical resection. This management is analogous to treatment of distantly metastatic disease, in which the benefits of resection of isolated pulmonary and liver metastases are well documented.[8–10] Historically, 7% to 20% of locally recurrent colorectal carcinomas can be reoperated for cure, with most patients having advanced disease at diagnosis, or ultimately recurring again locally or systemically.

Staging of regional recurrences should include computed tomography scans of the chest and abdomen to identify distant metastatic disease and skeletal involvement. Magnetic resonance imaging scanning of the pelvis is complementary to the computed tomography scan in evaluating encasement of pelvic vasculature, as well as local soft tissue extension. Magnetic resonance imaging has been found superior in the differentiation of soft tissue masses,[11] but it has not been consistently found to be superior to computed tomography in differentiating inflammatory tissue from tumor.[12]

Locally unresectable disease includes tumor involving the pelvic sidewalls, growing into the sciatic notch, encasing the bladder or iliac vessels, extending to the sacral promontory, or with significant leg edema secondary to venous obstruction. The presence of deep-seated pelvic pain or sciatica raises the possibility of encasement of sacral nerve roots. This process is considered a contraindication to resection by some authors,[13] but others use this to delineate the extent of resection in isolated recurrences.[14] Extrapelvic disease involving peritoneal implants or liver or lung metastases precludes surgical intervention for cure.

Treatment options depend on the extent of the initial resection (local excision, sphincter-saving resection, or APR), the extent and location of the recurrence, the functional state of the patient, and use of adjuvant chemotherapy or radiation therapy in conjunction with the initial operation.

Peter S. Turk: Randolph Surgical Associates, 2300 Randolph Road, Charlotte, NC 28207.
Harold J. Wanebo: Department of Surgical Oncology, Brown University, Roger Williams Medical Center, 825 Chalkstone Avenue, Providence, RI 02908.

TABLE 69-1. *Resection for recurrent rectal CA*

Author	No. of pts.	1st procedure	2nd procedure	Results
Polk & Spratt[15]	21	APR	Resection of perineal recurrence (8 perineal, 13 combined approach)	21/21 DOD (median 12 mo)
Bacon & Berkley[16]	20	APR/Hartmann	Exenteration/APR	at least 7/20 (35%) alive after 5 yrs
	8	LAR	APR, 5; LAR, 2; Pullthrough, 2	1 postoperative death 4/8 alive, NED at 3 yr
Goligher et al[17]	7	LAR	APR	2 NED (21, 22 mo) 1 AWD (33 mo) 2 DOD (5, 6 mo) 1 unknown
Lofgren et al[18]	35	LAR	Reresection	3/15 (20%) alive at 3 yr
Sanella[19]	11	LAR	APR	2 NED (22 mo, 13 yr) 9 DOD (median 21 mo) 4/9 dead of pelvic recurrence
Segall et al[20]	12	LAR	APR	6/12 NED (median 6 mo) 4 DOD (10, 15, 40, 103 mo)
Hojo[21]	22	LAR	Reresection	1/22 (50%) NED
Schiessel et al[22]	53	LAR/APR	21 APR 9 Sacral excision 8 Abdominal excision 3 Evisceration 10 Reresection	16/53 (30%) alive at 3 yr

APR, abdominoperineal resection; LAR, low anterior resection of the colon; DOD, dead of disease; LWD, living with disease; NED, no evidence of disease

CURATIVE RESECTION OF LOCOREGIONAL RECURRENCE

Localized Re-resection After Low Anterior Resection or Abdominoperineal Resection

Local re-resection after recurrence of a low rectal carcinoma has been shown to produce good palliation, but after an APR for a local recurrence, the cure rate is only 9% to 14%, with the remaining patients eventually experiencing systemic or another pelvic recurrence. Series reporting resection of local recurrence from rectal cancer[15–22] are summarized in Table 69-1. Recurrence after LAR is more commonly unfixed, without involvement of the posterior and lateral pelvic walls.

Willett and colleagues[23] found improved resectability in patients having had an initial LAR (13 of 25 patients) compared with initial APR (3 of 11 patients), as did Bacon and Berkley (47% vs. 40%).[16] The more recent series report a 30% to 50% long-term disease-free survival, most likely related to more accurate preoperative staging as well as more radical resection. Hojo[21] reviewed 30 anastomotic recurrences after 273 sphincter-saving resections for rectal cancer. Re-resection was performed in 22 of the 30 patients, 11 of these without recurrence. Segall and coworkers[20] reported a 50% disease-free survival at early follow-up, and Schiessel and associates[22] found 30% alive 3 years after local re-resection.

Pelvic Exenteration

Exenteration achieves adequate margins if the recurrence involves only the anterior structures, including vagina, prostate, or bladder. Any attempt to remove a more extensive recurrence without obtaining a wide-field resection posteriorly and posterolaterally may result in positive resection margins. Special care must be taken to include mesorectum, iliac, obturator, and perirectal lymph nodes, as well as pelvic adhesions.[24–27] Reoperation after a previous pelvic dissection has little chance of cure: older series quote a 66% incidence of second recurrence, usually in the pelvis.[28,29] Because recurrences in the deep pelvis are often much more extensive than appreciated before surgery, abdominosacral resection (ASR) should always be considered for recurrences in the posterior pelvis.

Despite the wide variety of tumors and resections completed in series reporting pelvic exenteration for recurrent cancer, some conclusions may be drawn from these data.[28–35] Morbidity was highest among patients receiving radiation therapy before exenteration,[32,33] and in those who underwent urinary diversions.[34] The complication rate was higher for those undergoing exenteration for recurrent as opposed to primary disease.[36] Specific complications in all series included wound infections, injuries to ureters or bladder, enteroperineal fistulas, abdominal abscesses, anastomotic leaks from urinary diversions, parastomal hernias, postoperative pancreatitis, and small bowel obstructions.[36,37] The morbidity rate in all series ranged from 26% to 100%, with a median of 58%. The postoperative mortality rate ranged from 0% to 33%, with a median of 9%, and the 5-year survival rate ranged from 23% to 67%, with a median of 39%. Improved survival has been reported in more recent series, attributed to improvements in patient selection and perioperative care.

Abdominosacral Resection

Because resection of the primary rectal cancer by APR or LAR involves dissection in the presacral space posteriorly and to the proximal levator muscles laterally, locoregional recurrence potentially contaminates this area. With recurrence, anatomic planes are distorted, and uninvolved margins are difficult to determine and to maintain during dissection. Therefore, for a patient with a large posterior pelvic recurrence or recurrence after an APR, the composite resection (ASR) is required to encompass the potentially involved sacrum.[38–43] The technique of ASR is briefly illustrated at the end of this chapter, and previously published in detail (see Figs. 69-4 through 69-10, later in this chapter).[14,37]

The most demanding aspect of the resection is the actual sacral transection. The proximal extent of this procedure is limited by the necessity of preserving a stable pelvic ring as well as sacral nerve roots. The S1 roots can be salvaged in almost all patients, and S2 and S3 roots are left intact, at least unilaterally, in most patients. Because the recurrence may encroach on the sacral component of the sciatic nerve, this often must be resected en bloc with a more proximal tumor.

The published series incorporating ASR for recurrent rectal cancer are shown in Table 69-2.[38–43] In a report by Wanebo and colleagues,[38] 47 patients underwent ASR, 41 of these for cure. Twenty-two of these patients required an exenteration or had other organs resected with the sacrum. The surgical margin was clear in 36 patients, whereas 5 patients had microscopic involvement in spite of gross clearance of the tumor. The mean blood loss for these procedures was 10,000 mL. Total mean operative time was 18.5 hours, with most patients undergoing a two-staged procedure, with 2 to 3 days between the abdominal and sacral stages for patient stabilization. A low-lying recurrence, involving only the coccyx and distal sacrum, was approached as a routine pelvic exenteration incorporating the one-stage approach, with lateral positioning of the patient as described by Localio and coworkers,[44] or internal sacrectomy.

The surgical mortality in this series was 8.5%, with one death at 2 days after surgery, and three delayed hospital deaths. Major morbidity included cardiopulmonary insufficiency requiring prolonged endotracheal intubation in 10 patients, postoperative hemorrhage requiring reoperation in 9, intestinal fistulization in 9, and ureteral or bladder fistulization in 5. Wound complications occurred in 25% of patients, with frequent posterior wound infections and flap separations related to the preoperative pelvic radiation and the pelvic devascularization required during the resection.

Results

Long-term survival was obtained in 14 patients (living 46 to 206 months), comprising 33% of the 43 patients who had greater than 48-month follow-up. The overall survival was 33%, and disease-free survival was 27% (Fig. 69-1A,B). Among the survivors, nine patients were alive with no evidence of disease (NED) from 60 to 206 months, of whom one recurred at 61 months and died of disease at 82 months, one recurred and is living with disease at 61 months, and one patient who was NED at 60 months died of disease at 102 months. One patient is NED at the 4.5-year level (55 months), but required a liver resection for metastases at 48 months. There were four patients who died between the fourth and fifth year (46, 51, 53, and 57 months).

The following prognostic factors were examined. Disease-free interval after the initial surgery, Dukes' stage of the primary cancer, type of initial operative procedures for the primary cancer, and the carcinoembryonic antigen (CEA) level before resection of the recurrence. The disease-free interval using either the 12-month break point or the 24-month break point showed no significant relation to outcome. There were 22 patients who previously had an APR, versus 16 with an LAR, all of whom were followed for more than 4 years. The median survival in the patients having previous APR was 22 months (5-year = 15%) versus 57 months (5-year = 46%) in the LAR group ($P < 0.001$; see Fig. 69-1C). Comparison of the Dukes' stage of the primary cancer with outcome after ASR showed an approximate equivalent failure rate overall. The median survival was 51 months in patients who were initially Dukes' B, versus 31 months in the patients who were initially Dukes' C (P = NS). The preoperative CEA level as measured before ASR was related to outcome. A significantly more favorable survival rate was seen in patients with low CEA levels. Patients with CEA levels less than 10 ng/mL had a median survival of 57 months (5-year = 44%) compared with those with CEA greater than 10 ng/mL, in whom the median survival was 31 months (5-year = 17.8%; $P = 0.04$ by log rank, and 0.07 by Wilcoxon). A very high-risk group consisted of 10 patients who had combination marrow invasion (4 patients), positive margins (4 patients), or who had peripelvic nodal metastases, (2 patients), in whom median survival was 10 months. Re-recurrence after ASR was documented in 27 patients. One third were local failure, and 15% each had liver, intraabdominal, or lung metastases

TABLE 69-2. *Results of abdominal sacral resection for cure for locally recurrent rectal cancer*

Author	No. of patients	Results
Wanebo, et al[38]	41	Median disease-free survival—24 months Median overall survival—36 months 5-yr estimated survival—24%
Takagi, et al[39]	7	4 patients NED; 1 patient LWD at 3–32 months
Pearlman, et al[40]	8	3 patients NED; 1 patient dead of other causes at 46 months
Temple and Ketcham[41]	9	local control—45% 5-yr disease-free survival—18%
Touran, et al[42]	12	12 month survival—62% 24 month survival—14%
Maetani, et al[43]	23	5-year survival—23%

Revised with permission from Turk PS, and Wanebo HJ Treatment of locoregional recurrence of rectal carcinoma. In Wanebo HJ (ed), Colorectal Cancer. Mosby-Yearbook: St. Louis, 1993;443

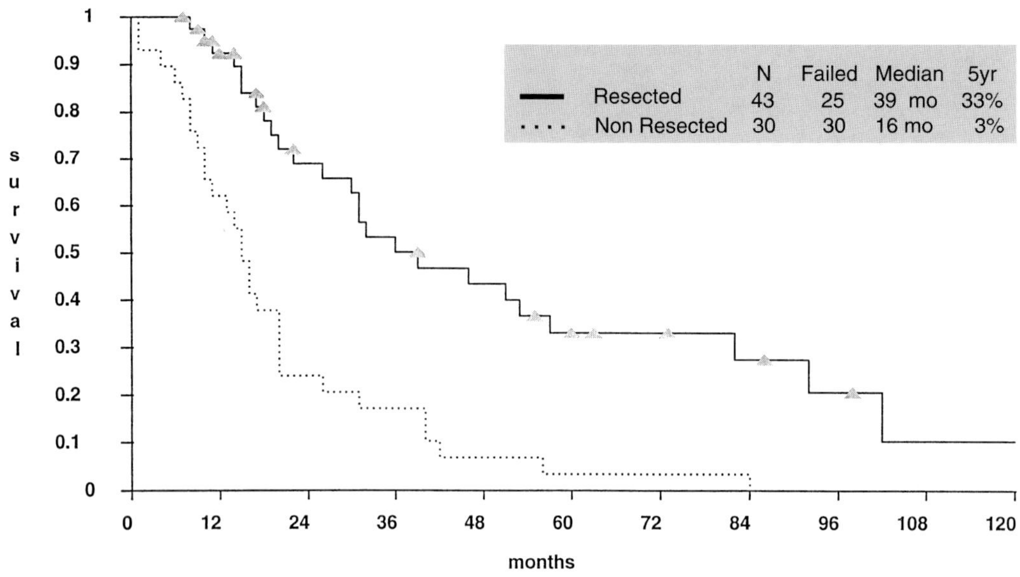

A

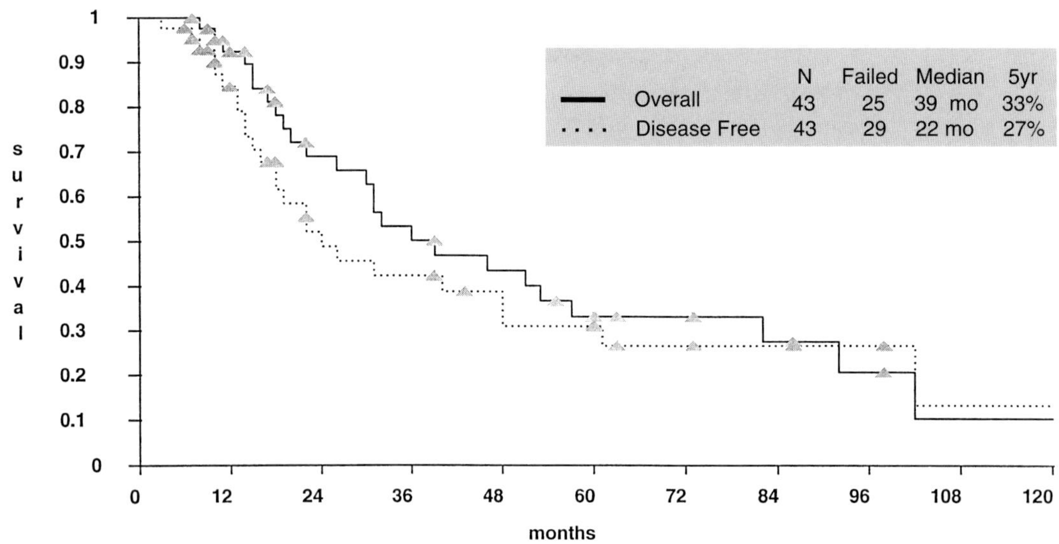

B

FIG. 69-1. Survival after abdominosacral resection for recurrent rectal cancer with curative intent (41 patients). Median disease-free survival was 24 months, median overall survival was 36 months. **(A)** Overall survival. **(B)** Overall survival and disease-free survival. *(continued)*

(± other organ involvement). Four patients (15%) had bone metastases.

Of the six patients with palliative resections, the survival ranged from 2 to 12 months (mean, 7 months). In the 41 patients with curative resections, the median disease-free survival was 24 months, and median overall survival was 36 months. The 5-year estimated survival for the patients undergoing resection for cure was 24% (see Fig. 69-1). Five patients achieved long-term survival (67 to 168 months).

The functional result after ASR for recurrent rectal cancer depended on the extent of resection. Sacral transection at the S3 level, appropriate for low-lying tumors, was an uncomplicated procedure allowing normal urinary continence if the bladder was retained. Proximal transection to the level of the mid-S1 body, a more formidable procedure required for more extensive lesions, still maintained pelvic stability. At this level, S1 and S2 nerve roots unilaterally or bilaterally were spared, producing only mild urinary dysfunction. If both S2 roots were incised, bladder function was compromised, with increased bladder residuals and decreased detrusor tone. Division of the S1 nerve root bilaterally resulted in complete bladder denervation (necessitating cystectomy), as well as peroneal nerve injury with loss of plantar flexion. A neurogenic bladder, resulting from division of proximal sacral roots, was treated by Crede's method of voiding, α agonists, or by self-catheterization (in severe cases).

Although long-term neurologic sequelae were unusual, many

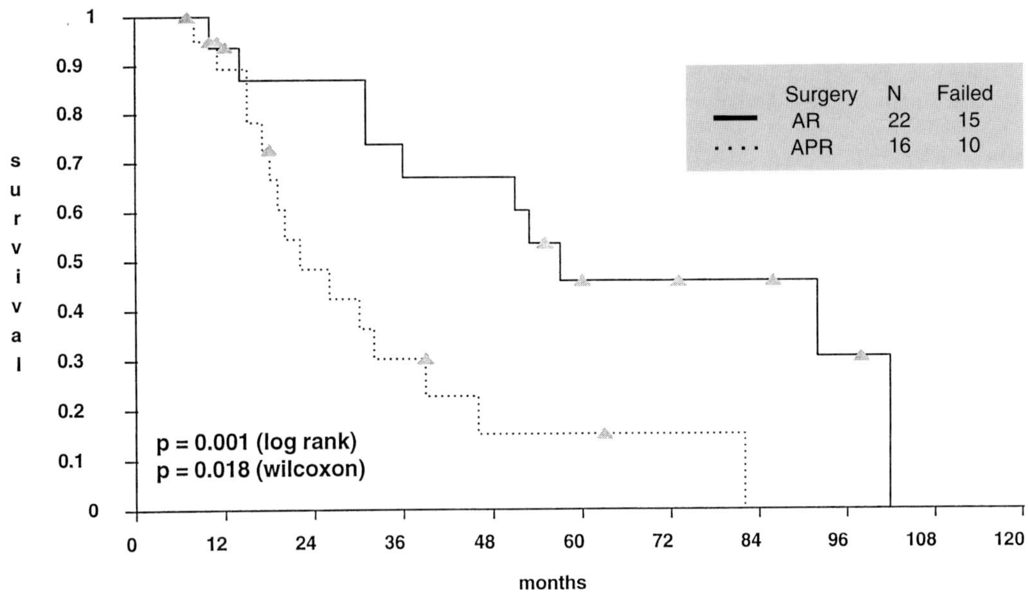

C

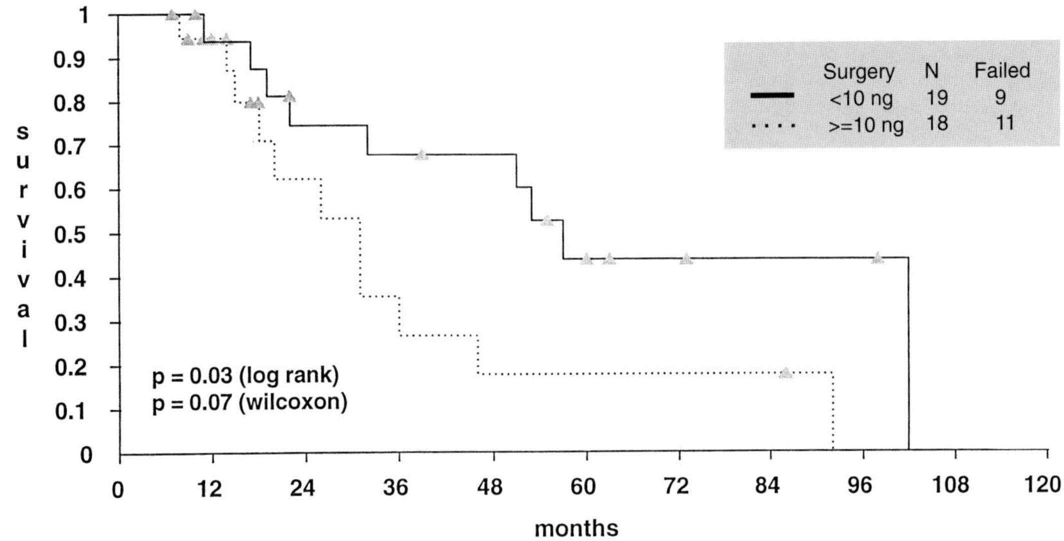

D

FIG. 69-1. *(Continued).* **(C)** Relation of initial primary surgery to survival after pelvic resection. *AR,* anterior resection; *APR,* abdominoperineal resection. **(D)** Relation of preoperative carcinoembryonic antigen level to survival. (From Wanebo HJ, Koness RJ, Turk PS, Cohen SI. Composite resection of posterior pelvic malignancy. Ann Surg 1992; 215:685, with permission.)

patients did incur short-term lower extremity weakness. Patients complained of unsteadiness, diminished lower leg strength (particularly diminished plantar flexion), and sensory deficits in the foot. Overall, serious locomotive dysfunction was evident only in patients having resections involving the S1 and S2 roots bilaterally.

Overall, 66% of the patients returned to their previous lifestyles, and 43% returned to work. In general, the extent of impaired function was 3 months. Of patients with long-term follow-up (>6 months), 30 of 31 (97%) had relief of initial symptoms during the initial 3 to 6 months after resection. Twelve of 34 (35%) had persistent postoperative pain, typically new phantom-like or causalgic pain, or local symptoms related to the delayed wound healing.

Takagi and colleagues[39] treated seven patients with localized recurrence of rectal cancer by ASR. Mean blood loss was 6200 mL, and the resections averaged 8.8 hours. There were no operative deaths, and complications included one perineal abscess and one intestinal fistula. All patients realized pain relief. Three patients have died of recurrent disease (pulmonary and hepatic, pulmonary, and pelvic wall recurrences), two patients are alive with recurrent disease (pulmonary and pelvic wall), and two are alive without evidence of disease. Pearlman and associates[40] reported on 12 patients undergoing ''sacropelvic resections,''

8 for cure and 4 in the presence of known extrapelvic disease. Four patients were cured of their disease, with three patients alive without disease at 46 months, whereas four patients had a second local recurrence. Appreciable pain relief was noted in seven patients.

Temple and Ketcham[41] reported on nine patients with local recurrence undergoing curative resection by a combined approach. All resections were between the S1 and S3 levels, mean blood loss was 4 to 6 units, and there was one perioperative death. Three patients had recurrences in the perineal wound, with an overall 45% local control rate and 18% 5-year disease-free survival. All patients reported excellent palliation of pelvic pain.

Finally, Touran and coworkers[42] treated 12 patients by single-stage ASR, with a median operative time of 5 hours and mean blood loss of 1400 mL. All patients reported good palliation. Nevertheless, only one patient (living with local and metastatic disease) was alive longer than 2 years after surgery. Five of the seven patients with follow-up eventually experienced local recurrence, reflecting the questionable resection margins inherent in a less aggressive operation. This recurrence rate underscores the necessity of clear pathologic margins for any potential of extended disease-free survival.

Resection of Recurrence After Initial Local Excision

Conservative surgery for low rectal carcinoma has become increasingly popular. This limited type of resection balances the benefit of decreased short- and long-term operative morbidity against the increased risk of local recurrence. The question of optimal selection criteria for local excision is as yet unanswered. In the published series, the incidence of locoregional recurrence after local excision is 3% to 25%; it is directly related to the stage and grade of the initial tumor, and probably influenced by the addition of adjuvant chemotherapy or radiation. Recurrences after local excision of rectal carcinoma are far more resectable than those after APR or LAR. Cuthbertson and Simpson,[45] Willett and coworkers,[46] Otmezguine and associates,[47] and Hoffman and colleagues[48] all found 100% resectability in this setting, and the overall resectability rate appears to be over 70%.[45–52] Selected series of treatment of local recurrence after local excision of rectal cancer are given in Table 69-3. The treatment for the recurrence was usually APR, and the overall salvageability for the combined groups was 70% (24 of 34 patients) with 17 to 50 months of follow-up.

TREATMENT OF UNRESECTABLE LOCOREGIONAL RECURRENCE

Most retrospective series underscore the difficulty of identifying a locoregional recurrence at a resectable stage, particularly when symptomatic. These recurrences, therefore, often require other modalities for optimal palliation.

Primary Irradiation

Historically, external beam radiation has been the primary modality used in this setting, with subjective improvement (initial pain control and improvement of quality of life) in 80% to 90% of patients.[53,54] Nevertheless, few patients experience long-term relief of pain (>6 to 8 months); many of these patients outlive the palliative attempts, and die of local progression of disease.[55]

TABLE 69-3. *Results of treatment for isolated local recurrence after primary local excision (LE)*

Source	No. of recurrences (treatment of primary cancer)	No. of patients undergoing resection of recurrence	Type of resection of recurrence	Results
Cuthbertson and Simpson[45]	6 (LE alone)	6	APR, 5 repeat LE, 1	all NED after 50 mos
Willett et al[46]	5 (LE alone)	5	APR	all DOD at 50 mos
	2 (LE + RT 45 Gy)	2	APR	1 NED, 1 DOD
Otmezguine et al[47]	3 (preop RT 35GY + LE + postop Interstitial RT 20 Gy)	3	APR	3 NED (mean 40 mos)
Killingback et al[49]	17	7	APR, 2; LAR, 3 perineal excision, 1 repeat LE, 1	4 alive >5 yr (2 NED) 1 dead NED 36 mos
Minsky[50]	3 (LE + RT 46–55 Gy)	2	APR	2 NED (2, 28 mos)
Bennett[51]	3 (LE + RT 45 Gy)	2	APR	2 NED
Hoffman[48]	4 (LE alone)	4	LAR, 1	3 NED (20, 22, 30 mos); 1 AWD (21 mos)
Bailey et al[52]	4 (LE alone)	3	LE + RT, 1 APR, 2	2 NED (17, 62 mos) 1 DOD of CNS mets at 42 mos

APR, abdominoperineal resection; LAR, low anterior resection of the colon; DOD, dead of disease; LWD, living with disease; NED, no evidence of disease

Combined Chemoradiation

Despite the lack of objective benefit of combined chemoradiation for recurrent rectal cancer, this has become the standard treatment for patients who have never been radiated. This is based mostly on the proven benefit of combined treatment in the adjuvant setting for primary rectal cancer.[56–58] Prospective trials have been undertaken to examine the role of chemoradiation therapy for residual, recurrent, or inoperable rectal cancer, using 5-fluorouracil (5-FU)-based chemotherapy. A Radiation Therapy Oncology Group trial randomized patients to receive external beam radiation alone or radiation therapy with concurrent 5-FU, followed by maintenance 5-FU and methyl-CCNU.[59] Sixty-four percent of the entire group ultimately experienced local failure, with no significant difference in disease control seen between the two arms. A second prospective trial, by the Eastern Cooperative Oncology Group,[60] also evaluated the efficacy of combined chemoradiation in the face of recurrent or unresectable disease. Patients received either continuous radiation plus 5-FU or split-course radiation plus 5-FU, and some also received postradiation maintenance 5-FU plus methyl-CCNU. Again, there was no appreciable difference in the results of the two treatment groups, with an overall objective response rate of 10%; median survival in each group was 17 months. In both of these prospective trials, toxicity was substantial, especially in patients treated with combined modality therapy. Intestinal complications including severe diarrhea and small intestinal obstruction and perforation were the most important causes of treatment-related morbidity.

Intraoperative Radiation

Because current protocols commit most advanced-stage primary tumors to perioperative chemoradiation, other therapies have been adopted to treat local recurrence in the face of previous external beam irradiation. The use of adjuvant intraoperative radiation has been shown to enhance survival in selected series. Beart and colleagues[61] reported on 24 patients treated for locally recurrent rectal cancer. All patients underwent resection of the pelvic disease, but had gross or microscopic residual disease. They then underwent intraoperative radiation therapy during a separate surgical procedure. At mean follow-up of 20 months, 13 patients were alive without evidence of disease. Among the 8 patients (alive or deceased) who recurred, three had isolated local recurrence and five had disseminated disease. With further follow-up,[62] the 4-year actuarial disease-free survival was 28%, and was related to the extent of resection. In a second series, by Willett and associates,[23] 30 patients with locally recurrent rectal or rectosigmoid carcinoma underwent a multimodality approach of preoperative external beam radiation, surgical resection, and intraoperative electron beam radiation therapy. The 5-year actuarial local control and disease-free survival of all 30 patients were 26% and 19%, respectively, and correlated directly with completeness of tumor resection. The toxicities included soft tissue or sacral injury (three patients) and pelvic neuropathy (three patients).

Palliative Resection and Debulking

Although radical pelvic resection is not indicated for incurable tumors,[38] palliative resection may benefit patients with uncontrollable disease ulcerating through the perineum. Temple and Ketcham[63] reported on seven patients with uncontrolled local recurrence treated with resection of tumor, including a portion of the sacrum, to obtain all but deep margins clear of tumor. All patients experienced significant pain relief. Three patients returned to work for 6 to 12 months after surgery. Mean postoperative survival was 13 months.

Intraluminal tumor debulking is an alternative to diverting colostomy in patients with an obstructing, unresectable local recurrence after an LAR. Techniques including cryotherapy,[64] laser,[65] electrocoagulation,[66] and urologic resectoscope[67] have been used, with good palliation in most cases.

Regional Chemotherapy

Regional chemotherapy has produced effective palliation as well as tumor shrinkage, in some cases to the point of resectability in some series.[68] Intraarterial infusion of chemotherapy has been used for palliation of pelvic tumors, attaining one to two times the local drug exposure possible with intravenous dosing, and resulting in a 20% to 75% palliation rate and 20% to 31% objective response rate.[69–71]

To maximize the therapeutic potential of high-dose local chemotherapy, a protocol for isolated pelvic perfusion chemotherapy was undertaken at Brown University/Roger Williams Cancer Center.[72] The 10 patients initially evaluated and treated were symptomatic with recurrent pelvic malignancy, either as isolated disease or as the major symptomatic component of recurrence. They presented either with progressive disease on aggressive systemic chemotherapy regimens or after multimodality treatment of their recurrent tumors. The primary diseases included six recurrent rectal cancers, three recurrent anal carcinomas, and one recurrent anorectal melanoma.

The procedure, completed in the operating room, required bilateral common femoral artery and saphenous vein cannulation of double-lumen, high-flow dialysis catheters, as well as placement of aortic and vena caval Fogarty occlusion balloon catheters (Fig. 69-2). The balloons were inflated at the level of the L3–L4 vertebral interspace, bilateral thigh tourniquets were inflated to 250 mm Hg, and the extracorporeal circuit flow was maintained at 250 mL/minute. The chemotherapy was infused over 25 minutes, and the isolated perfusion was continued for a total of 45 minutes after start of drug infusion.

A total of 17 treatments was administered, 12 with multiple chemotherapeutic agents. One to three courses were completed per patient. The resultant mean ratios of pelvic : systemic drug exposure during the procedures were 9.8 : 1 for 5-FU, 4.8 : 1 for cisplatinum, and 4.4 : 1 for mitomycin (Fig. 69-3).

Six patients had externally visible pelvic disease, and all six had early objective response, including hyperemia, necrosis, and tumor shrinkage, with three patients (all having received multiple-agent perfusions) obtaining a partial response, and three patients a minor response. Two patients presenting with marginally resectable recurrent pelvic disease obtained a partial response, and subsequently underwent surgical resection of the remaining disease. Nine patients presented with pelvic pain. Improvement or resolution of pain was immediate after the perfusion in seven patients (78%), and ranged in duration from 1 week to greater than 6 months (median duration, 4 months) after the final treatment. Extended pain relief was more durable

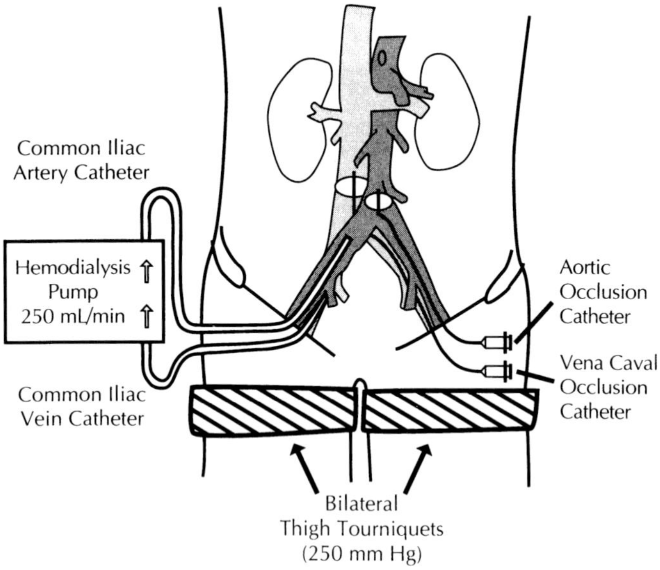

FIG. 69-2. Isolated pelvic perfusion incorporating transfemoral access and vascular isolation, and the extracorporeal circuit using standard hemodialysis technology. (From Turk PS, Belliveau JF, Darnowski JW, Weinberg MC, Wanebo HJ. Isolated pelvic perfusion for unresectable malignancy using the balloon occlusion technique. Arch Surg 1993;128: 533, with permission.)

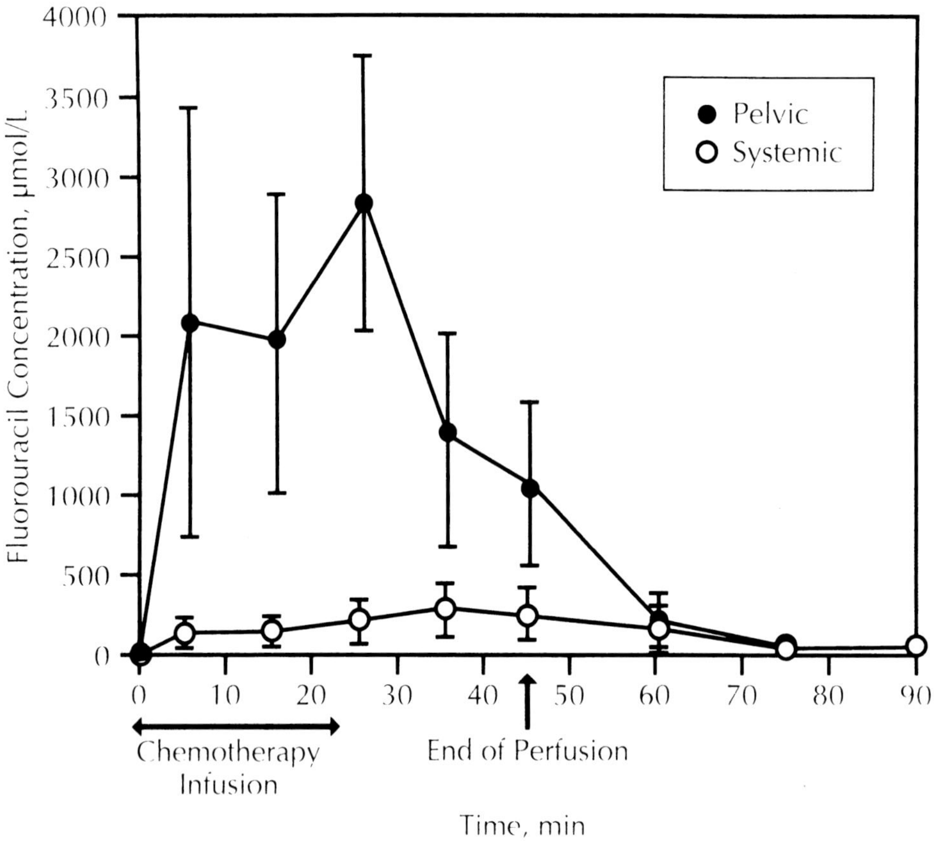

FIG. 69-3. 5-Fluorouracil concentration over time, during isolated pelvic perfusion (12 courses included, 1100–2000 mg/m^2). (From Turk PS, Belliveau JF, Darnowski JW, Weinberg MC, Wanebo HJ. Isolated pelvic perfusion for unresectable malignancy using the balloon occlusion technique. Arch Surg 1993128:533, with permission.)

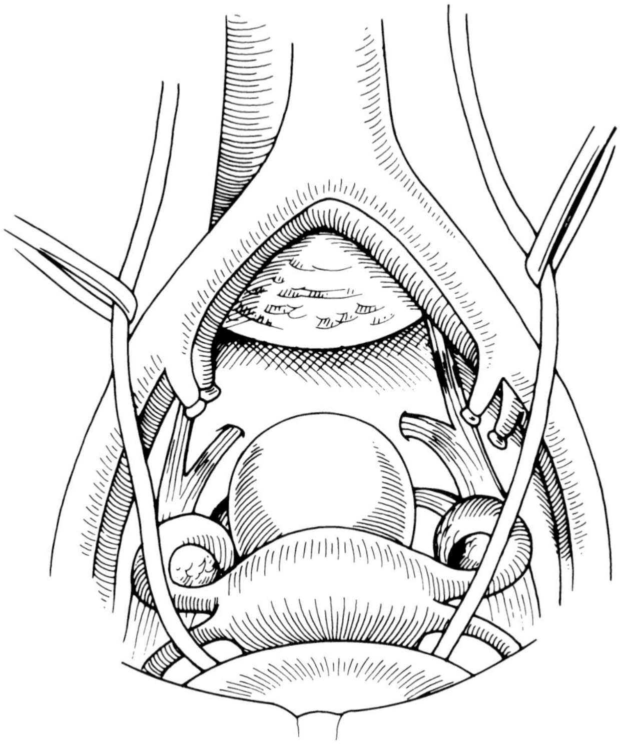

FIG. 69-4. The internal iliac artery and vein are divided and ligated with sutures bilaterally to accomplish devascularization of the pelvis. (From Wanebo HJ, Turk PS. Abdominosacral resection for recurrent rectal cancer. In: Bauer JJ, Gorfine SR, Kreel I, Gelernt IM, Rubin P, eds. Colorectal surgery illustrated: a focused approach. St. Louis: Mosby Year Book, 1993:243, with permission.)

after multiple-agent perfusion, and was again attained in three patients undergoing repeated perfusions. Of the three patients having isolated pelvic disease (unresected) and elevated CEA levels, all realized a reduction to a mean 20% of the original CEA value 2 to 8 months after the perfusion regimen.

Using limited access, isolated pelvic perfusion produces high pelvic : systemic concentration gradients, and results in increased resectability in selected patients. Because few palliative modalities are effective in these previously irradiated patients with severe local symptoms, this procedure produces unequaled palliation for symptomatic recurrent pelvic cancers.

CONCLUSION

Locally recurrent rectal cancer is typically unresectable at the time of presentation, either because of the extent of local extension or the presence of distantly metastatic disease. Close follow-up regimens after the primary resection incorporating

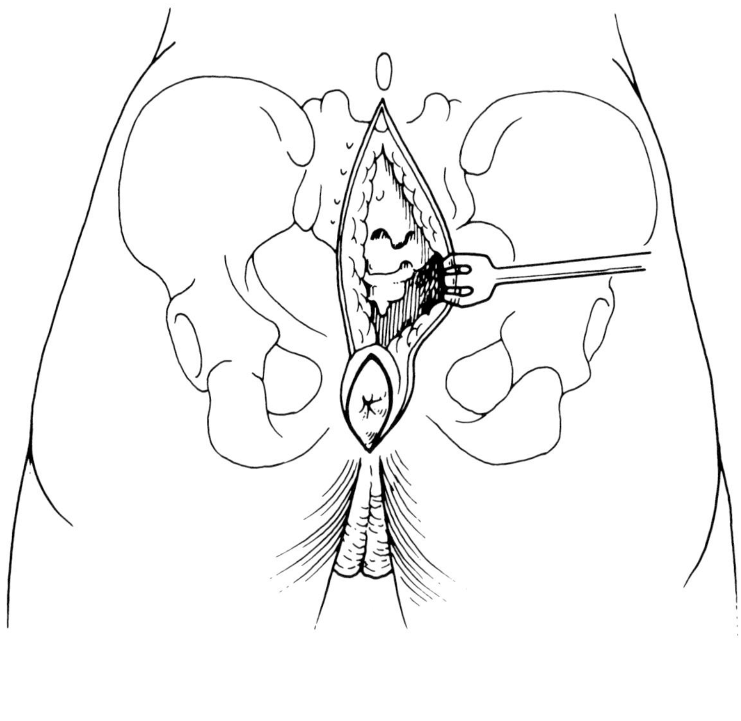

FIG. 69-5. A posterior sacral incision is made from the spinous process of L5 to the perineum and the flaps are raised to the level of the sacral periosteum. (From Wanebo HJ, Turk PS. Abdominosacral resection for recurrent rectal cancer. In: Bauer JJ, Gorfine SR, Kreel I, Gelernt IM, Rubin P, eds. Colorectal surgery illustrated: a focused approach. St. Louis: Mosby Year Book, 1993:244, with permission.)

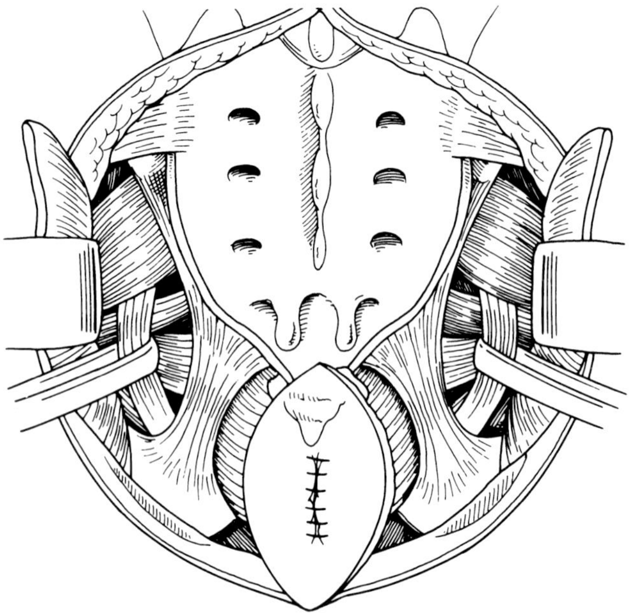

FIG. 69-6. After the gluteus maximus and medius muscles are dissected from their sacral origins, the sciatic nerve is identified bilaterally and encircles with a vessel loop. (From Wanebo HJ, Turk PS. Abdominosacral resection for recurrent rectal cancer. In: Bauer JJ, Gorfine SR, Kreel I, Gelernt IM, Rubin P, eds. Colorectal surgery illustrated: a focused approach. St. Louis: Mosby Year Book, 1993:245, with permission.)

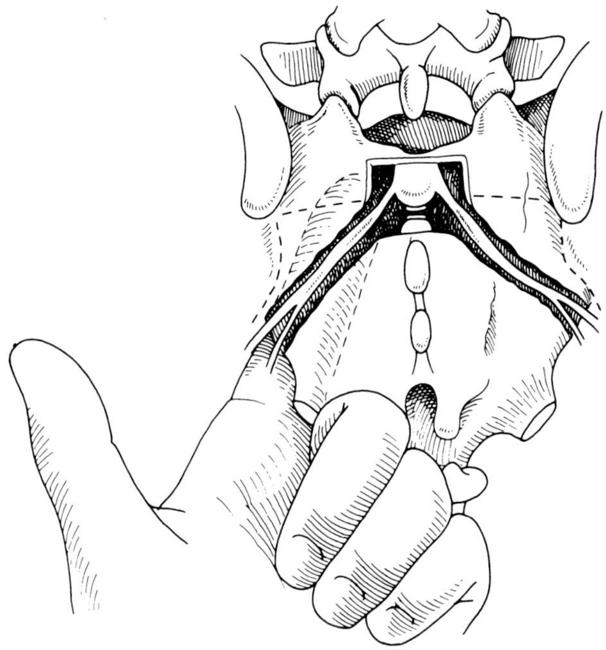

FIG. 69-8. The sacrum is divided with an osteotome or an oscillating saw; the surgeon's finger is positioned anteriorly to protect the underlying intraabdominal contents. (From Wanebo HJ, Turk PS. Abdominosacral resection for recurrent rectal cancer. In: Bauer JJ, Gorfine SR, Kreel I, Gelernt IM, Rubin P, eds. Colorectal surgery illustrated: a focused approach. St. Louis: Mosby Year Book, 1993:247, with permission.)

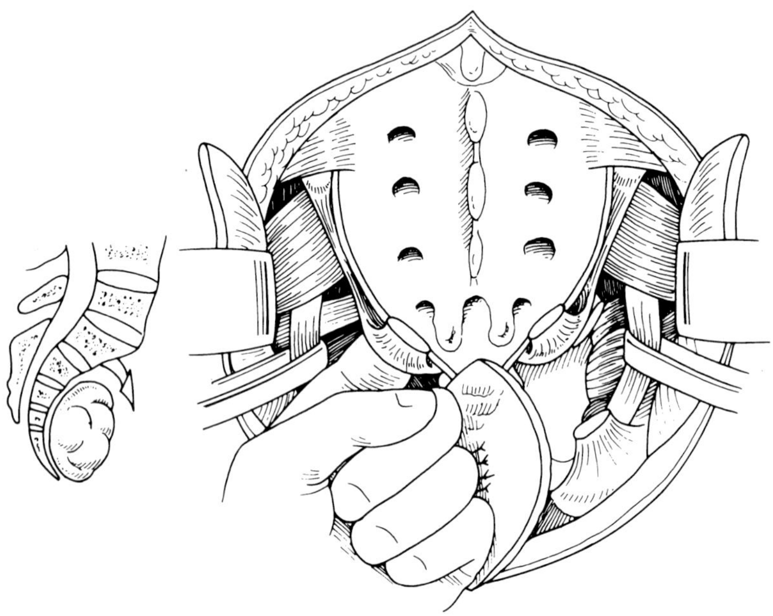

FIG. 69-7. The surgeon's finger is inserted anteriorly from the medial aspect of the sciatic nerve and advanced deeply beneath the piriformis muscle and through the underlying endopelvic fascia to reach the anterior surface of the rectum. (From Wanebo HJ, Turk PS. Abdominosacral resection for recurrent rectal cancer. In: Bauer JJ, Gorfine SR, Kreel I, Gelernt IM, Rubin P, eds. Colorectal surgery illustrated: a focused approach. St. Louis: Mosby Year Book, 1993:245, with permission.)

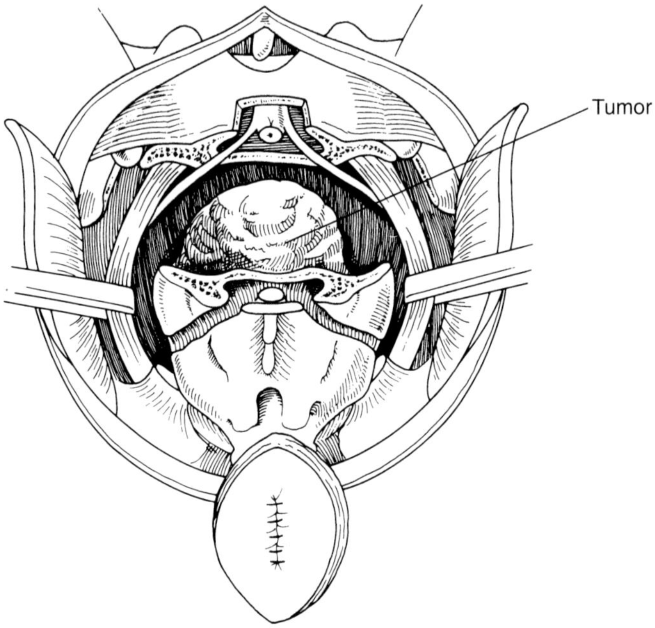

FIG. 69-9. The sacrum, pelvic sidewalls, tumor, and attached pelvic structures are removed en bloc. (From Wanebo HJ, Turk PS. Abdominosacral resection for recurrent rectal cancer. In: Bauer JJ, Gorfine SR, Kreel I, Gelernt IM, Rubin P, eds. Colorectal surgery illustrated: a focused approach. St. Louis: Mosby Year Book, 1993:248, with permission.)

careful clinical examinations and more sensitive radiologic studies may improve survival rates, especially after sphincter-preserving operations. Initial local excision allows for identification of locally recurrent disease at a much earlier stage, resulting in greater resectability and overall survival after resection of recurrence in this setting.

If the recurrent tumor is operable, the extent of operation depends on the type of initial resection and the structures now involved. Thorough preoperative and intraoperative evaluations should be completed before an aggressive resection of a locoregional recurrence, because resection leaving gross residual disease is of no survival benefit.

The recurrence may be eradicated with local re-resection, but wide-field resection results in improved local control and greater long-term survival (Figs. 69-4 through 69-10). The only opportunity for long-term survival occurs if the disease is truly isolated, diagnosed at an early stage, and treated in an aggressive manner with clear surgical margins. With these criteria fulfilled, long-term survival can be expected for resection of local recurrence in 50% to 80% of patients after local resection, 30% to 50% after LAR, and 20% to 35% after APR.

In cases of unresectable recurrence, palliation may be achieved by a combination of radiation and systemic chemotherapy, local surgical maneuvers, regional chemotherapy, or a variety of analgesic regimens. Unfortunately, most of these patients die with symptoms from the locally advanced disease.

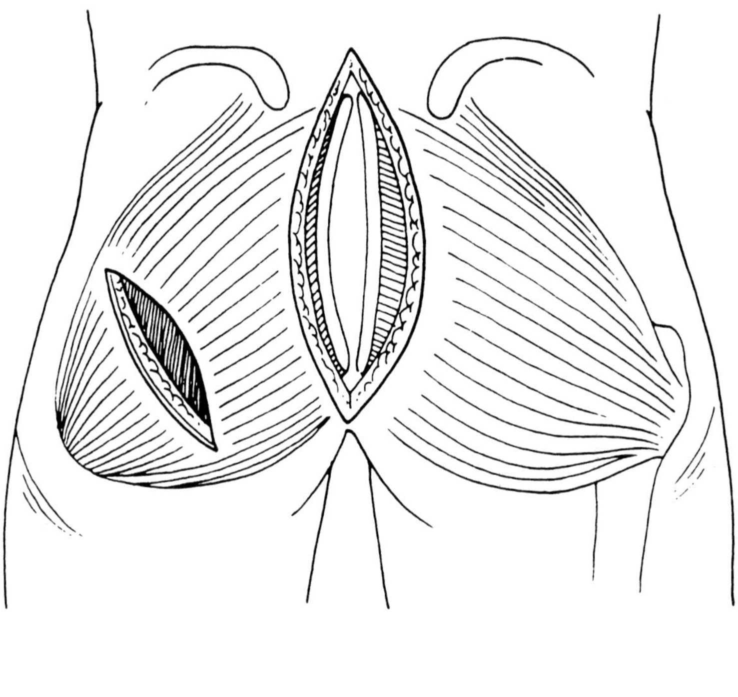

FIG. 69-10. The muscles are approximated in the midline. The lateral insertion of the gluteus maximus may have to be incised to allow medial advancement of the muscle. (From Wanebo HJ, Turk PS. Abdominosacral resection for recurrent rectal cancer. In: Bauer JJ, Gorfine SR, Kreel I, Gelernt IM, Rubin P, eds. Colorectal surgery illustrated: a focused approach. St. Louis: Mosby Year Book, 1993:249, with permission.)

REFERENCES

1. Pilipshen SJ, Heilweil M, Quan SH Sternberg SS, Enker WE. Patterns of pelvic recurrence following definitive resections of rectal cancer. Cancer 1984:53:1354.
2. Berge T, Ekelund G, Mellner C, Pihl B, Wenckert A. Carcinoma of the colon and rectum in a defined population. Acta Chir Scand 1973; Suppl 438):1.
3. Gunderson LL, Sosin H. Areas of failure found at reoperation following curative surgery for adenocarcinoma of the rectum. Cancer 1974;34: 1278.
4. Rao AR, Kagan AR, Chan PM, Gilbert HA, Nussbaum H, Hintz BL. Patterns of recurrence following curative resection alone for adenocarcinoma of the rectum and sigmoid colon. Cancer 1981;48:1492.
5. McDermott FT, Hughes ESR, Pihl E, Johnson WR, Price AB. Local recurrence after potentially curative resection for rectal cancer in a series of 1,008 patients. Br J Surg 1985;72:34.
6. Carlsson U, Lasson A, Ekelund G. Recurrence rates after curative surgery for rectal carcinoma with special reference to their accuracy. Dis Colon Rectum 1987;30:431.
7. Pilipshen S. Cancer of the rectum: local recurrence. In: Fazio VW, ed. Current therapy in colon and rectal surgery. Toronto: Brian C. Decker, 1990:137.
8. McCormick PM, Bains MS, Beattie EJ, Martini N. Pulmonary resection in metastatic carcinoma. Chest 1978;73:163.
9. Hughes KS, Simon R, Songhorabodi MS, et al. Resection of the liver for colorectal carcinoma metastasis: a multiinstitutional study of indications for resection. Surgery 1986;100:278.
10. Wanebo HJ, Semoglou C, Attiyeh F, Stearns MJ. Surgical management of patients with primary operable colorectal cancer and synchronous liver metastases, Am J Surg 1978;135:81.
11. Johnson RJ, Jenkins JPR, Isherwood I, James RD, Schofield PF. Quantitative magnetic resonance imaging in rectal carcinoma. Br J Radiol 1987;60:76.
12. deLange EE, Fechner RE, Wanebo HJ. Suspected recurrent rectosigmoid carcinoma and abdominoperineal resection: MR imaging and histopathologic findings. Radiology 1989;170:323.
13. Ketcham AS. The management of recurrent rectal cancer. Can J Surg 1985;28:422.
14. Wanebo HJ, Gaker DL, Whitehill E, Morgan RF, Constable WC. Pelvic recurrence of rectal cancer: options for curative resection. Ann Surg 1987;205:482.
15. Polk HC, Spratt JJ. Results of treatment of perineal recurrence of cancer of the rectum. Cancer 1979;43:952.
16. Bacon HE, Berkley JL. The rationale of re-resection for recurrent cancer of the colon and rectum. Dis Colon Rectum 1959;2:549.
17. Goligher JC, Dukes CE, Bussey HJR. Local recurrences after sphincter-saving excisions for carcinoma of the rectum and rectosigmoid. Br J Surg 1951;39:199.
18. Lofgren EP, Waugh JM, Dockery MB. Local recurrence of carcinoma after anterior resection of the rectum and sigmoid. Arch Surg 1957; 74:825.
19. Sanella NA. Abdominoperineal resection following anterior resections. Cancer 1976;38:378.
20. Segall MM, Goldberg SM, Nivatvongs S, et al. Abdominoperineal resection for recurrent cancer following anterior resection. Dis Colon Rectum 1981;24:80.
21. Hojo K. Anastomotic recurrence after sphincter saving resection for rectal cancer: length of distal clearance of the bowel. Dis Colon Rectum 1986;29:11.
22. Schiessel R, Wunderlich M, Herbst F. Local recurrence of colorectal cancer: effect of early detection and aggressive surgery. Br J Surg 1986; 73:342.
23. Willett CG, Shellito PC, Tepper JE, Eliseo R, Convery K, Wood WC. Intraoperative electron beam radiation therapy for recurrent locally advanced rectal or rectosigmoid carcinoma. Cancer 1991;67:1504.
24. Heald RJ, Husband EM, Ryall RDH. The mesorectum in rectal cancer surgery: the clue to pelvic recurrence? Br J Surg 1982;69:613.
25. Enker WE, Pilipshen SJ, Heilweil ML, et al. En bloc pelvic lymphadenectomy and sphincter preservation in the surgical management of rectal cancer. Ann Surg 1986;203:426.
26. Wolmark N, Fisher B, Wieand HS. The prognostic value of the modifications of the Dukes' C class of colorectal cancer: an analysis of the NSABP clinical trials. Ann Surg 1986;203:115.
27. Hatch KD, Gelder MS, Soong SJ, et al. Pelvic exenteration with low rectal anastomosis: survival, complications, and prognostic factors. Gynecol Oncol 1990;38:462.
28. Olsson CA, Deckers PH, Williams LF, et al. New look at pelvic exenteration. Urology 1976;7:355.
29. Cole WH. Recurrence in carcinoma of the colon and proximal rectum following resection for carcinoma. Arch Surg 1952;65:264.
30. Hafner GH, Herrera L, Petrelli NJ. Patterns of recurrence after pelvic exenteration for colorectal adenocarcinoma. Arch Surg 1991;126:1510.
31. Hafner GH, Herrera L, Petrelli NJ. Morbidity and mortality after pelvic exenteration for colorectal adenocarcinoma. Ann Surg 1992;215:63.
32. Petros JG, Lopez MJ. Pelvic exenteration for carcinoma of the colon and rectum. Surgical Oncology Clinics of North America 1994;3:257.
33. Vezeridis MP, Wanebo HJ. Extended radical pelvic surgery including sacral resection. Surgical Oncology Clinics of North America 1994;3: 291.
34. Lopez MJ, Kraybill WG, Downey RS, et al. Exenterative surgery for locally advanced rectosigmoid cancer: is it worthwhile? Surgery 1987; 102:644.
35. Jakowatz JG, Porudominsky D, Riihimaki DU, et al. Complications of pelvic exenteration, Arch Surg 1985;120:1261.
36. Pearlman NW, Donohue RE, Wettlauter JN, et al. Continent ileocolonic urinary reservoirs for filling and lining the postexenterative pelvis. Am J Surg 1990;160:634.
37. Wanebo HJ, Koness RJ, Vezeridis MP, et al. Pelvic resection of recurrent rectal cancer. Ann Surg 1994;220:586.
38. Wanebo HJ, Koness RJ, Turk PS, Cohen SI. Composite resection of posterior pelvic malignancy. Ann Surg 1992;215:685.
39. Takagi H, Morimoto T, Hara S, Suzuki R, Horio S. Seven cases of pelvic exenteration combined with sacral resection for locally recurrent rectal cancer. J Surg Oncol 1986;32:184.
40. Pearlman NW, Donahue RE, Stiegmann GV, Ahnen DJ, Sedlacek SM, Braun TJ. Pelvic and sacropelvic exenteration for locally advanced or recurrent anorectal cancer. Arch Surg 1987;122:537.
41. Temple WJ, Ketcham AS. Sacral resection for control of pelvic tumors. Am J Surg 1992;163:370.
42. Touran T, Frost DB, O'Connell TR. Sacral resection: operative technique and outcome. Arch Surg 1990;125:911.
43. Maetani S, Nishikawa T, Yasnynki I, et al. Extensive en bloc resection to regionally recurrent carcinoma of the rectum. Cancer 1992;69:2876.
44. Localio AS, Eng K, Ransom NHC. Abdominosacral approach for retrorectal tumors. Am Surg 1980;179:555.
45. Cuthbertson A, Simpson R. Curative local excision of rectal adenocarcinoma. Aust N Z Surg 1986;56:229.
46. Willett CG, Tepper JE, Donnelly S, et al. Patterns of failure following local excision and local excision and postoperative radiation therapy for invasive rectal adenocarcinoma. J Clin Oncol 1989;7:1003.
47. Otmezguine Y, Grimard L, Calitchi E. A new combined approach in the conservative management of rectal cancer. Int J Radiat Oncol Biol Phys 1989;17:539.
48. Hoffman JP, Riley L, Carp NZ, Litwin S. Isolated locally recurrent rectal cancer: a review of incidence, presentation, and management. Semin Oncol 1993;20:5a6.
49. Killingback M. Local excision of carcinoma of the rectum: indications. World J Surg 1992;16:437.
50. Minsky BD, Cohen AM, Enker WE, Mies C. Sphincter preservation in rectal cancer by local excision and postoperative radiation therapy. cancer 1991;67:908.
51. Bennett CJ, Sombeck MD, Mendenhall WM, Million RR, Bland KI, Copeland EM. Conservative alternatives in the management of early adenocarcinoma of the rectum. South Med J 1993;86:4 9.
52. Bailey HR, Huval WV, Max E, et al. Local excision of carcinoma of the rectum for cure. Surgery 1992;111:555.
53. Dobrowski W, Schmid AP. Radiotherapy of presacral recurrences following radical surgery of rectal cancer. Dis Colon Rectum 1985;28: 917.
54. Pacini P, Cionini L, Pirtoll L, et al. Symptomatic recurrence of carcinoma of the rectum and sigmoid: the influence of radiotherapy on the quality of life. Dis Colon Rectum 1986;29:865.
55. Rostock RA, Zajac AJ, Gallagher MJ, et al. Radiation therapy in the treatment of colorectal cancer. In: Ahlgren J, MacDonald J, eds. Gastrointestinal oncology. Philadelphia: JB Lippincott, 1992:366.
56. Gastrointestinal Tumor Study Group. Prolongation of disease-free interval in surgically treated rectal cancer. N Engl J Med 1985;312:1465.

57. Gastrointestinal Tumor Study Group, Douglass HO, Moertel CG, Mayer RJ, et al. Survival after post-operative combination treatment of rectal cancer. N Engl J Med 1986;315:1294.
58. Krook JE, Moertel CG, Gunderson LL, et al. Effective surgical adjuvant therapy for high risk rectal cancer. N Engl J Med 1991;324:709.
59. Rominger CJ, Gelber RD, Gunderson LL, Conner N. Radiation therapy alone or in combination with chemotherapy in the treatment of residual or inoperable carcinoma of the rectum and rectosigmoid or pelvic recurrence following colorectal surgery: Radiation Therapy Oncology Group Study (76-16). Am J Clin Oncol 1985;8:118.
60. Danjoux CE, Gelber RD, Catton GE, Klassen DJ. Combination chemotherapy for residual, recurrent, or inoperable carcinoma of the rectum: ECOG Study (EST 3276). Int Radiat Oncol Biol Phys 1985;11:765.
61. Beart RW, Martin JK, Gunderson LL. Management of recurrent rectal cancer. Mayo Clin Proc 1986;61:448.
62. Gunderson LL, Martin KJ, Beart RW, et al. Intraoperative and external beam irradiation for locally advanced colorectal cancer. Ann Surg 1988; 207:52.
63. Temple WJ, Ketcham AS. Surgical palliation for recurrent rectal cancers ulcerating in the perineum. Cancer 1990;65:1111.
64. Fritsch A, Seidl W, Walzel C, Moser K, Schiessel R. Palliative and adjunctive measures in rectal cancer. World J Surg 1982;6:569.
65. Wodnicki H, Goldenberg R, Kaplan S, Yahr WZ, Kreiger B, Russin D. The laser: an alternative for palliative treatment of obstructing intraluminal lesions. Am Surg 1988;54:227.
66. Christiansen J, Kirkegaard P. Treatment of recurrent rectal cancer by electroresection/coagulation after low anterior resection. Dis Colon Rectum 1983;26:656.
67. Kurz KR, Pitts WR, Speer D, Vaughan ED. Palliation of carcinoma of the rectum and pararectum using the urologic resectoscope. Surg Gynecol Obstet 1988;166:60.
68. Wile A, Smolin M. Hyperthermic pelvic isolation-perfusion in the treatment of refractory pelvic cancer. Arch Surg 1987;122:1321.
69. Carlsson C, Hafstrom L, Jonsson P-E, Ask A, Kallum B, Lunderquist A. Unresectable and locally recurrent rectal cancer treated with radiotherapy or bilateral internal iliac artery infusion of 5-FU. Cancer 1986; 58:336.
70. Oberfield RA. Intra-arterial infusion in tumors of the pelvis. Recent Results Cancer Res 1983;10:15.
71. Heim ME, Eberwein S, Georgi M. Palliative therapy of pelvic tumors by intra-arterial infusion of cytotoxic drugs. Recent Results Cancer Res 1983;10:37.
72. Turk PS, Belliveau JF, Darnowski JW, Weinberg MC, Wanebo HJ. Isolated pelvic perfusion for unresectable malignancy using the balloon occlusion technique. Arch Surg 1993;128:533.

Surgery for Gastrointestinal Cancer: A Multidisciplinary Approach, edited by Harold J. Wanebo.
Lippincott-Raven Publishers, Philadelphia, © 1997.

CHAPTER 70

Pain Control for Pelvic and Abdominal Cancers

Nathan I. Cherny and Kathleen M. Foley

Patients with gastrointestinal malignancies are heterogeneous in their experience of pain and symptom distress, and clinicians who care for these patients must be prepared to manage a diverse spectrum of problems, ranging from the treatment of acute procedure-related pain to the management of chronic unremitting pain in patients with advanced disease.[1]

In general, about one third of patients with cancer who are undergoing active therapy and as many as 70% to 90% of those who have advanced disease experience pain.[2] A survey of 106 patients receiving outpatient treatment found that 96 (91%) of those with cancer of the gastrointestinal tract had tumor-related pain. The pain was inadequately relieved in 58% of cases.[3] Among patients with advanced cancer, pain is more prevalent with gastric and pancreatic tumors than with colorectal tumors.[4] In a survey of 181 ambulatory patients with colon cancer, "persistent or frequent" pain during the previous 2 weeks was reported by 52 patients (28.7%), the median duration of pain was 4 weeks (range, less than 1 to 468 weeks), about 90% of the patients experienced pain more than 25% of the time, and the average pain severity was "moderate." More than half the patients interviewed reported that pain interfered at least moderately with their enjoyment of life, general activity, sleep, and mood.[5] In a study of patients admitted for hospice care, 49% of those with colorectal cancer had severe pain.[6]

The prevalence of acute and chronic cancer pain, and the burden of distress and suffering engendered by this symptom oblige the treating clinician to be skilled in its assessment and treatment. Relief of pain is an ethical imperative. It is incumbent on clinicians to maximize the knowledge, skill, and diligence needed to attend to this task.[7–9] Although established analgesic strategies can benefit most patients,[10] undertreatment is common.[3,11,12] The success of cancer pain therapy depends on the ability of the clinician to assess the presenting problems, identify and evaluate pain syndromes, and formulate a comprehensive care plan with provision for reevaluation and follow-up. Cancer pain is a dynamic problem, and successful management requires a continuity of care that provides an appropriate level of vigilance and responds quickly, flexibly, and expertly to the changing needs of the patient.[13–15] This approach recognizes the need to incorporate pain treatment within a broader therapeutic agenda, in which needs for tumor control, symptom palliation (physical and psychological), and functional rehabilitation are addressed concurrently.[13,16]

PAIN: GENERAL PRINCIPLES

Pain and Nociception

Nociception

Nociception is the activity produced in the nervous system by potentially tissue-damaging stimuli. This process cannot be observed directly, but is assumed to occur when a tissue-damaging stimulus impinges on a pain-sensitive structure.

Pain

The International Association for the Study of Pain has defined pain as "an unpleasant sensory and emotional experience associated with actual or potential tissue damage or described in terms of such damage."[17] As such, pain is the perception of nociception, and like other perceptions, it is determined by an interaction between activity in sensorineural pathways and a variety of behavioral and psychological factors.

Three broad categories of pain mechanisms usually are recognized: ongoing nociception, neuropathic processes, and psychological influences. From information acquired through the assessment process, these mechanisms can be used to label pains according to the predominant pathophysiology that is inferred to exist.

Nathan I. Cherny: Pain and Palliative Medicine Physician, Department of Cancer Medicine, Shaare Zedek Medical Center, Jerusalem, ISRAEL

Kathleen M. Foley: Chief, Pain Service, Department of Neurology, Memorial Sloan-Kettering Cancer Center, 1275 York Avenue, New York, NY 10021-6094

Nociceptive Pain

The term *nociceptive pain* is applied to pain that is perceived to be commensurate with tissue damage associated with an identifiable somatic or visceral lesion. The persistence of pain is related to ongoing activation of nociceptors. Nociceptive pain that originates from somatic structures (also known as somatic pain) tends to be well localized and described as sharp, aching, burning, or throbbing. Pain originating from visceral structures (visceral pain) often is more diffuse, and usually is described as gnawing or cramping when caused by obstruction of a hollow viscus, and as aching, sharp, or throbbing when caused by involvement of organ capsules or other mesentery. From the clinical perspective, nociceptive pains (particularly somatic pains) usually respond to opioid drugs[18,19] or to interventions that ameliorate or denervate the peripheral lesion.[20]

Neuropathic Pain

Neuropathic pain refers to pain that is caused by injury to, or diseases of, the peripheral or central neural structures, or that is perceived to be sustained by aberrant somatosensory processing at these sites.[21,22] Clinically, it is suggested most strongly when an abnormal sensation (dysesthesia) occurs in a region of motor, sensory, or autonomic dysfunction that is attributable to a discrete neurologic lesion.[22] This diagnosis often is inferred from the characteristics and distribution of the pain or the identification of a lesion in neural structures that innervate this region.

Neuropathic pain syndromes are categorized according to the presumed site of the aberrant neural activity (''generator'') that sustains the pain.[22] So-called peripheral neuropathic pain is caused by injury to a peripheral nerve or nerve root and is sustained by aberrant processes originating in the nerve root, plexus, or nerve. Neuropathic pains believed to be sustained by a central generator include sympathetically maintained pain and a group of syndromes traditionally known as the deafferentation pains. Sympathetically maintained pain (also known as reflex sympathetic dystrophy or causalgia) may occur after injury to soft tissue, peripheral nerve, viscera, or central nervous system, and is characterized by focal autonomic dysregulation in a painful region (eg, vasomotor or pilomotor changes, swelling, sweating abnormalities) or trophic changes.[23] For example, a patient with locally advanced rectal tumor involving the lumbosacral plexus can have foot pain associated with anhidrosis and thermal dysregulation.[24,25]

The diagnosis of neuropathic pain has important clinical implications. The response of neuropathic pain to opioid drugs is less predictable and, in general, less than that observed for nociceptive pain.[18,19,26,27] Optimal treatment may depend on the use of so-called adjuvant analgesics[22,28] or other specific approaches, such as sympathetic nerve block.

Idiopathic Pain

Idiopathic pain is a term used to describe pain that is perceived to be excessive for the extent of identifiable organic pathology. Some patients with idiopathic pain have affective and behavioral disturbances that are severe enough to infer a predominating psychological pathogenesis, in which case a specific psychiatric diagnosis of somatoform disorder can be applied.[29] When this inference cannot be made, an occult organic process may be responsible and assessments should be repeated at appropriate intervals. Although psychological processes can strongly influence the expression and effect of pain,[30–32] nociceptive and neuropathic factors predominate in the cancer population.[33]

Pain Pathways

Primary Afferent Neurons

The primary afferent neurons transmit nociceptive stimuli from peripheral nociceptors to the first central synapse in the dorsal horn. They have their cell bodies in the dorsal root ganglion; their axons enter the spinal cord through the dorsal root and, usually, ascend for one or two segments in Lissauer's tracts before synapsing in the laminae of the dorsal horn.

Somatic Nociceptors

Somatic nociceptors are distributed widely in skin, muscle, and connective tissues.[34–38] In skin, a variety of subtypes have been identified, the best characterized of which are the thinly myelinated A-delta mechanoreceptors and mechanothermal receptors, and the unmyelinated C-polymodal receptors that respond to mechanical, thermal, and chemical stimuli in the skin.[38] The nociceptor nomenclature for joint and muscle afferent nerves is different: small myelinated axons are designated group III and unmyelinated axons are designated group IV.[38] Visceral nociceptors are similar morphologically and likewise respond to discrete sets of noxious stimuli.[35,39]

Nociceptors may become sensitized by noxious stimuli, and thereafter demonstrate spontaneous activity, a lower threshold, and a more intense response.[36] This process of peripheral sensitization can be triggered by the release of inflammatory mediators into the environment of the nociceptor terminals, and some nociceptors are relatively unresponsive until they are sensitized.[38]

Visceral Pathways

Contrary to conventional teaching, it is now known that pain impulses arising from most viscera are transmitted to the dorsal horn by unmyelinated afferent fibers in the sympathetic and parasympathetic nerves.[39] At the dorsal horn, visceral afferent nerves account for about 2% to 10% of afferent fibers (the others arise from somatic structures). The visceral afferent fibers terminate in the dorsal horn, where they synapse with ascending viscerosomatic neurons in the spinothalamic tracts.

The First Central Synapse

The Dorsal Horn

The neuroanatomy and neurochemistry of the dorsal horn are extraordinarily complex.[37,40,41] Many putative neurotransmitters or neuromodulators, including peptides, amino acids, monoamines, and other compounds, have been implicated in the processing of nociceptive input at the first central synapse.[42]

Central Sensitization

The responsiveness of spinothalamic cells can increase after mechanical, thermal, or chemical nociceptive stimulation, and a state of hyperresponsiveness to otherwise innocuous stimuli can develop. Sensitization of the central nociceptive neurons is mediated by activation of the *N*-methyl-D-aspartate receptor by excitatory amino acids and nitric oxide released by the synaptic terminals of nociceptors or excitatory interneurons.[38,43]

Segmental and Supraspinal Pain Modulation

Nociception is modulated by both segmental and suprasegmental systems, a concept originally modeled in the gate control theory.[44] Segmental processes at the level of the dorsal horn may involve the activation of inhibitory interneurons by myelinated non-nociceptive afferent fibers. The most important of the descending inhibitory pathways arises in the periaqueductal gray nuclei of the midbrain, synapses in the raphae magnus nucleus of the medulla, and projects to the dorsal horn through the dorsal longitudinal fasciculus.[41,45] Neurotransmitters, such as dopamine, serotonin, norepinephrine, and the endogenous opioid peptides (ie, enkephalin, β-endorphin, and dynorphin), play a significant role in this modulatory system. Endogenous opioids are involved in this modulatory system at multiple sites through many distinct compounds and receptor subtypes.[46,47]

Subpopulations of opioid receptors are localized in the ascending and descending pain pathways. These receptors mediate the multiple pharmacologic effects of the opioid analgesics. The periaqueductal gray region in the midbrain and the dorsal horn in the spinal cord are rich in opioid receptors and represent the supraspinal and spinal sites that mediate opioid analgesia. Direct administration of opioids into the periaqueductal gray region or spinal cord[48] inhibits pain transmission.

Ascending Pathways

Several ascending pathways arise from second-order neurons and decussate in the central gray spinal cord to become the neospinothalamic and paleospinothalamic tracts.[37,40] The neospinothalamic tract, which projects monosynaptically to the ventrobasal complex of the thalamus, subserves pain intensity and localization. Multiple polysynaptic pathways (together termed the paleospinothalamic tracts), which connect with various brain stem and subcortical sites, contribute to autonomic and affective responses and to the activation of pain-modulating systems.

Pain, Psychological Distress, and Suffering

Pain and Psychological Distress

The presence of cancer pain can disturb normal processes of coping and adjustment, which are fundamental reactions to the stresses imposed by the cancer and its treatment.[49–51] Pain may augment a sense of vulnerability, contributing to a preoccupation with the potential for catastrophic outcomes.[49] In some cases, unrealistic or distorted attitudes toward the pain problem (eg, assumptions, beliefs, expectations) can undermine the ability to cope so that the patient becomes utterly helpless and desperate.[49] This situation can be reflected in the development of pain behaviors characterized by increasing passivity and dependency, or the uncontrolled expression of negative attitudes and feelings. These behaviors, in turn, can exacerbate social isolation.[49]

The relation between pain and psychological well-being is complex. Mood disturbance and beliefs about the meaning of pain in relation to illness have been shown to be significant predictors of perceived pain intensity,[52,53] and the perceived meaning of the pain is a major determinant of function and mood.[54] In a prospective study of the prevalence of psychiatric disorders among patients with cancer,[30] Derogatis and colleagues found that the prevalence of cancer-related pain was 39% in those who had a psychiatric diagnosis and only 19% in those without such a diagnosis. In the group with pain, the most important psychiatric diagnoses included adjustment disorders with depressed mood, mixed depression and anxiety, and major depression.[30] The relation between pain and psychological distress is demonstrated further by the observation that uncontrolled pain is a major factor in cancer-related suicide[55–58] and that psychiatric symptoms commonly have been observed to disappear with adequate pain relief.[59]

Suffering

Suffering can be described as an aversive emotional experience characterized by the perception of personal distress that is generated by adverse factors that undermine quality of life.[60] Pain may contribute profoundly to suffering, but numerous other factors, such as the experience of other symptoms, progressive physical impairment, or psychosocial disturbances, may be equally or more important.[60–62] Suffering and pain, therefore, are regarded best as related but discrete experiences that have distinct clinical implications. Pain therapy must be a critical component of a more comprehensive therapeutic plan designed to address the diverse factors that impair quality of life.[16,60]

PAIN FEATURES AND SYNDROME IDENTIFICATION

Pain Syndrome Classification

In the context of cancer pain, syndromes are defined by the association of particular pain characteristics and physical signs with specific complications of the underlying disease or its treatment. These specific syndromes are associated with distinct causes, pathophysiologies, and prognostic and therapeutic implications.

Acute Pain Syndromes

Acute pain syndromes are characterized by a well-defined onset and a readily identifiable cause. Among patients with cancer, acute pains usually are related to diagnostic and therapeutic interventions, such as chemotherapy-induced stomatitis or headache after lumbar puncture (Table 70-1). Although some tumor-related pains have an acute onset (eg, pain from a bowel perforation), most are chronic or recurrent unless effective therapy for the underlying lesion is provided. Acute cancer-related pain often is associated with overt pain behaviors (eg, moaning, grimacing, and splinting), anxiety, or signs of generalized sympathetic hyperactivity, including diaphoresis, hypertension, and tachycardia.

Chronic Pain Syndromes

Chronic pain has been defined by persistence for 3 months or more beyond the usual course of an acute illness or injury, a pattern of recurrence at intervals over months or years, or association with a chronic pathologic process.[63] Chronic tumor-related pain usually is insidious in onset and has a course that is characterized by fluctuations in intensity. About two thirds of cases are caused by direct tumor infiltration of pain-sensitive structures (Table 70-2). Pain often increases progressively with tumor growth, and may regress with tumor shrinkage (in response to anticancer therapy). Adverse consequences of cancer therapy, including surgery, chemotherapy, and radiation therapy, account for 15% to 25% of chronic cancer pain problems, and a small proportion of the chronic pains experienced by patients with cancer are caused by pathology unrelated to the cancer or its therapy.[64–68] Chronic pain caused by cancer may be associated with affective disturbances (anxiety or depression) or vegetative symptoms (eg, asthenia, anorexia, sleep disturbance); overt pain behaviors and sympathetic hyperactivity often are absent.[69]

TABLE 70-1. *Acute pain syndromes in patients with gastrointestinal cancer*

ACUTE PAIN ASSOCIATED WITH DIAGNOSTIC AND THERAPEUTIC INTERVENTIONS

- Acute pain associated with diagnostic interventions
  - Arterial or venous blood sampling
  - Lumbar puncture
  - Colonoscopy
  - Myelography
  - Percutaneous biopsy
- Acute postoperative pain
- Acute pain caused by other therapeutic interventions
  - Pleurodesis
  - Tumor embolization
  - Suprapubic catheterization
  - Intercostal catheterization
  - Nephrostomy insertion
- Acute pain associated with analgesic techniques
  - Injection pain
  - Opioid headache
  - Spinal opioid hyperalgesia syndrome
  - Epidural injection pain

ACUTE PAIN ASSOCIATED WITH ANTICANCER THERAPIES

- Acute pain associated with chemotherapy infusion techniques
  - Intravenous infusion pain
  - Hepatic artery infusion pain
  - Intraperitoneal chemotherapy abdominal pain
- Acute pain associated with chemotherapy toxicity
  - Mucositis
  - Corticosteroid-induced perineal discomfort
  - Steroid pseudorheumatism
  - Colony-stimulating factor–induced bone pain
  - 5-Fluorouracil–induced anginal chest pain
  - Palmar-plantar erythrodysesthesia
- Acute pain associated with immunotherapy
  - Interferon-induced acute pain
- Acute pain associated with radiation therapy
  - Incidence pains
  - Acute radiation enteritis and proctocolitis
  - Subacute radiation myelopathy

ACUTE PAIN ASSOCIATED WITH INFECTION

- Acute herpetic neuralgia
- Abdominal or pelvic abscess

Adapted from Cherny NI, Portenoy RK. Cancer pain: principles of assessment and syndromes. In: Wall PD, Melzack R, eds. Textbook of pain. 3rd ed. Edinburgh: Churchill Livingstone, 1994:787.

TABLE 70-2. *Chronic pain syndromes in patients with gastrointestinal cancer*

TUMOR-RELATED PAIN SYNDROMES

- Visceral pain syndromes
  - Hepatic distention syndrome
  - Midline retroperitoneal syndrome
  - Chronic intestinal obstruction
  - Peritoneal carcinomatosis
  - Malignant perineal pain
  - Malignant pelvic floor myalgia
  - Ureteric obstruction
- Pain syndromes caused by tumor involvement of the peripheral nervous system
  - Malignant lumbosacral plexopathy and radiculopathy
- Bone pain syndromes
  - Vertebral syndromes
  - Back pain and epidural (spinal cord and cauda equina) compression
  - Pain syndromes of the bony pelvis and hip
- Headache and facial pain syndromes
  - Intracerebral tumor
  - Leptomeningeal metastases
  - Base of skull metastases
  - Painful cranial neuralgias

CHRONIC PAIN SYNDROMES ASSOCIATED WITH CANCER THERAPY

- Postchemotherapy pan syndromes
  - Avascular necrosis of femoral or humeral head
  - Plexopathy associated with intraarterial infusion
- Chronic postsurgical pain syndromes
  - Phantom anus pain
  - Postsurgical pelvic floor myalgia
- Chronic postradiation pain syndromes
  - Radiation-induced lumbosacral plexopathy
  - Chronic radiation enteritis and procititis
  - Burning perineum syndrome
  - Chronic radiation myelopathy
  - Osteoradionecrosis

Adapted from Cherny NI, Portenoy RK. Cancer pain: principles of assessment and syndromes. In: Wall PD, Melzack R, eds. Textbook of pain. 3rd ed. Edinburgh: Churchill Livingstone, 1994:787.

Breakthrough Pain

Transitory exacerbations of severe pain over a baseline of moderate pain or less may be described as breakthrough pain.[70]

Breakthrough pain can occur in acute or chronic pain states. In a survey of patients with chronic cancer pain, almost two thirds experienced severe or excruciating breakthrough pain.[70] These exacerbations may be precipitated by volitional actions of the patient, such as movement, micturition, cough, or defecation (incident pains), or by nonvolitional events, such as bowel distention. Spontaneous fluctuations in pain intensity also can occur without an identifiable precipitant. Clinicians should be aware of this phenomenon when formulating therapeutic plans for pain control.

Pain Characteristics

Evaluation of pain characteristics provides some of the raw data essential for syndrome identification. The most important of these characteristics are outlined below.

Pain Intensity

In the cancer population, evaluation of pain intensity is pivotal to therapeutic decision-making. The selection of an analgesic drug, route of administration, and rate of dose titration all may be influenced by reported pain intensity.[71,72] Furthermore, intensity may help characterize the pain mechanism and underlying syndrome. For example, clinical observation strongly suggests that the pain associated with radiation-induced nerve injury rarely is severe; therefore, the occurrence of severe pain in a previously irradiated region suggests the existence of recurrent neoplasm or a radiation-induced second primary tumor.[73]

Pain Quality

The quality of the pain often suggests its pathophysiology. Somatic nociceptive pains usually are well localized and described as sharp, aching, throbbing, or pressure-like. Visceral nociceptive pains usually are diffuse and may be gnawing or cramping when caused by obstruction of a hollow viscus, or aching, sharp, or throbbing when caused by involvement of organ capsules or mesentery. Neuropathic pains may be described as burning, tingling, or shock-like.[74]

Pain Distribution

Patients with cancer pain commonly experience pain at more than one site.[5,64,68,75] The number of pain sites has been identified as a salient determinant of the effect of pain on mood and function.[5] The distinction between focal, multifocal, and generalized pain may be important in the selection of therapy, such as nerve blocks, radiation therapy, or surgical approaches.

The distribution of the pain often clarifies its relation to the underlying organic lesion. In contrast to *focal pain,* which describes pain that is experienced in the region of the underlying lesion, the term *referred pain* is applied when pain is experienced in a distribution remote to the lesion. Pain referral patterns, which have been characterized for both nociceptive (somatic and visceral) pain and neuropathic pain,[35,76,77] must be recognized to evaluate the underlying organic cause. For example, neuropathic pain is associated with several characteristic patterns, including pain referred anywhere in the distribution of peripheral nerves from a lesion involving the nerve itself or the plexus from which it arises, pain referred to the dermatome innervated by a damaged nerve root (radicular pain), pain referred anywhere in the region of the body innervated by a damaged central pathway, and symmetric extremity pain from a peripheral neuropathy. Somatic and visceral nociceptive stimuli similarly may be associated with characteristic pain referral patterns. For example, a patient with a past history of gastric cancer who has progressive shoulder pain and no evidence of focal pathology needs to undergo evaluation of the region above and below the diaphragm to exclude the possibility of referred pain from diaphragmatic irritation. Familiarity with pain referral patterns is essential to target appropriate diagnostic and therapeutic maneuvers (Table 70-3).)

ASSESSMENT OF CANCER PAIN PROBLEMS

General Considerations

The objectives of cancer pain assessment are accurate characterization of the pain, including the pain syndrome and inferred pathophysiology, and evaluation of the effect of the pain and the role it plays in the overall suffering of the patient. This process requires the establishment of a trusting relationship with the patient in which the clinician projects the attitude that relief of pain and suffering are central to the goals of therapy. This approach encourages open and effective communication about symptoms. Even with such a relationship, however, the clinician should not be cavalier about the potential for symptom underreporting. Symptoms frequently are described as complaints, and there is a common perception that the ‘‘good patient’’ refrains from complaining.[78] If the patient is unable or unwilling to describe the pain, a family member may need to be questioned to assess the distress or disability of the patient. The prevalence of pain is so great that an open-ended question about the presence of pain should be included at each patient visit in routine oncologic practice.

A practical approach to cancer pain assessment incorporates a stepwise approach that begins with data collection and ends with a clinically relevant formulation (Fig. 70-1).

Data Collection

The Patient History

A review of the past medical history and the chronology of the cancer is important to place the pain problem in context. The pain-related history must include the relevant pain characteristics and the responses of the patient to previous disease-modifying and analgesic therapies. Patients often have multiple pain problems, and each must be assessed independently. Patient self-report is the gold standard for the assessment of pain intensity.[3,79–81] The use of a validated pain assessment tool such as 10-point verbal scale or a 100-mm visual analogue scale for pain intensity,[82] or an instrument such as the Memorial Pain Assessment Card[83] or the Brief Pain Inventory[84] can provide a format

TABLE 70-3. *Common patterns of pain referral*

Pain mechanism	Site of lesion	Referral site
Visceral	Esophageal	Epigastric, chest, arm, interscapular
	Diaphragmatic irritation	Shoulder
	Urothelial tract	Inguinal region and genitalia
Somatic	C-7–T-1 vertebrae	Interscapular
	L1-2	Sacroiliac joint and hip
	Hip joint	Knee
	Pharynx	Ipsilateral ear
Neuropathic	Nerve or plexus	Anywhere in the distribution of a peripheral nerve
	Nerve root	Anywhere in the corresponding dermatome
	Central nervous system	Anywhere in the region of the body innervated by the damaged structure

for communication between the patient and health care professionals, and also can be used to monitor the adequacy of therapy. A pain history at each visit and routine recording of pain intensity along with other vital signs is recommended[85,86] (Fig. 70-2).

The consequences of the pain also must be assessed. These may include impairment in activities of daily living; psychological, familial, and professional dysfunction; disturbed sleep, appetite, and vitality; and financial concerns. The psychiatric history, current level of anxiety or depression, suicidal ideation, and perceived meaning of the pain all are relevant to therapy. It is important to assess the patient-family interaction, and to observe both the kind and frequency of pain behaviors and the nature of the family response.

Most patients with cancer pain have multiple other symptoms.[75,87,88] It is incumbent on the clinician to evaluate the severity and distress caused by symptoms other than pain. Symptom checklists and quality of life measures may contribute to this comprehensive evaluation.[89–91]

The Physical Examination

The physical examination should attempt to identify the underlying cause of the pain problem, clarify the extent of the underlying disease, and discern the relation of the pain complaint to the disease. A physical examination, including a neurologic evaluation, is a necessary part of the initial pain assessment. The high prevalence of painful neurologic conditions in patients with cancer pain[33,92] justifies the need for a thorough neurologic assessment.

Review of Previous Investigations

Careful review of previous laboratory and imaging studies can provide important information about the cause of the pain and the extent of the underlying disease.

Provisional Assessment

The information derived from the initial data collection provides the basis for a provisional pain diagnosis, assessment of global disease status, and identification of other concurrent concerns. The provisional pain diagnosis includes an assessment of the probable pathophysiology and pain syndrome. An understanding of disease status requires an evaluation of the extent of the disease, the prognosis, and the anticipated goals of therapy.[93] Evaluation of concurrent concerns includes other symptoms and related psychosocial problems.

Diagnostic Investigations and Additional Assessment

Additional investigations often are required to clarify areas of uncertainty in the provisional assessment.[33] The extent of the diagnostic investigation must be appropriate to the patient's general status and the overall goals of care.

The lack of a definitive finding on an investigation should not be used to override a compelling clinical diagnosis. In the evaluation of hip pain, for example, plain radiographs provide only a crude assessment of bony lesions, and further investigation with bone scintigrams or computed tomography (CT), including soft tissue and bone windows, may be indicated. To minimize the risk of error, the physician ordering the diagnostic procedures should review the results personally with the radiologist to correlate pathologic changes with the clinical findings.

Pain must be managed during the diagnostic evaluation. Comfort improves compliance and reduces the distress associated with procedures. No patient should be evaluated inadequately because of poorly controlled pain.

Additional Assessments

The comprehensive assessment also may require additional evaluation of other physical or psychosocial problems identified during the initial assessment. Expert assistance from other physicians, nurses, social workers, or others may be essential.

Formulation and Therapeutic Planning

The evaluation should enable the clinician to appreciate the nature of the pain, its effect, and concurrent concerns that further undermine quality of life. The findings of this evaluation should be reviewed with the patient. Through candid discussion, current problems can be prioritized to reflect their importance to the patient.

This evaluation also may identify potential outcomes that would benefit from contingency planning. Examples include advanced medical directives, evaluation of resources for home care, pre-bereavement interventions with the family, and provision of assistive devices in anticipation of compromised ambulation.

STEP 1: DATA COLLECTION

Pain related history
- Other relevant history
- Disease related
- Other symptoms
- Psychiatric history
- Social resources

Other relevant history
- Disease related
- Other symptoms
- Psychiatric history
- Social resources

Physical examination

Available laboratory and imaging data
- Radiographs and scans
- Tumor markers
- Hematologic parameters
- Biochemical parameters

STEP 2: PROVISIONAL ASSESSMENT

Provisional pain diagnosis
1) syndrome identification
2) inferred pathophysiology

Global assessment
1) extent of disease
2) goals of care:
   prolonging survival
   optimizing function
   optimizing comfort

Concurrent concerns
1) other symptoms
2) untreated concurrent diseases
3) psychosocial needs
4) rehabilitative needs
5) financial needs

STEP 3: DIAGNOSTIC INVESTIGATIONS AND OTHER ASSESSMENTS

Diagnostic investigations
1) symptom specific
2) extent of disease

Other assessments
1) psychological
2) social
3) financial
4)functional

STEP 4: INITIAL FORMULATION AND PROBLEM LIST

1) pain syndromes and pathophysiology
2) extent of disease
3) concurrent concerns
4) anticipated contingencies

STEP 5: PATIENT REVIEW AND FORMULATION OF PRIORITIZED PROBLEM LISTS

1) current problems
2) anticipated contingencies

STEP 6: MULTIMODALITY THERAPEUTIC PLAN

1) primary anti-cancer treatment:
- Chemotherapy
- Radiotherapy
- Surgery
- Immunotherapy
- Other

2) treatment of concurrent disease processes
3) symptom directed pharmacotherapy
4) rehabilitative approaches
5) psychological approaches
6) anesthetic approaches
7) neurostimulatory approaches

FIG. 70-1. Stepwise assessment of the patient with cancer pain. (Adapted from Cherny NI, Portenoy PRK. Cancer pain: principles of assessment and syndromes. In: Wall PD, Melzack R, eds. Textbook of pain. 3rd ed. Edinburgh: Churchill Livingstone. 1994: 787.)

ACUTE PAIN SYNDROMES

Acute Pain Associated With Diagnostic and Therapeutic Interventions

Acute Postoperative Pain

Acute postoperative pain is universal unless adequately treated. Undertreatment remains a problem despite the availability of adequate analgesic and anesthetic techniques.[94–96] Although the duration and severity of postoperative pain is variable, it usually is transient. Postoperative pain that exceeds the normal duration or severity should prompt a careful evaluation for the possibility of infection (eg, wound infection, abscess in the pelvis or subphrenic space) or other complications. The management of postoperative pain has been reviewed and guidelines have been published.[95,97]

Acute Procedure-Related Pain

For some patients, procedures can be associated with incident pain that is precipitated by manipulation of the patient during transport or positioning. Many invasive investigations are asso-

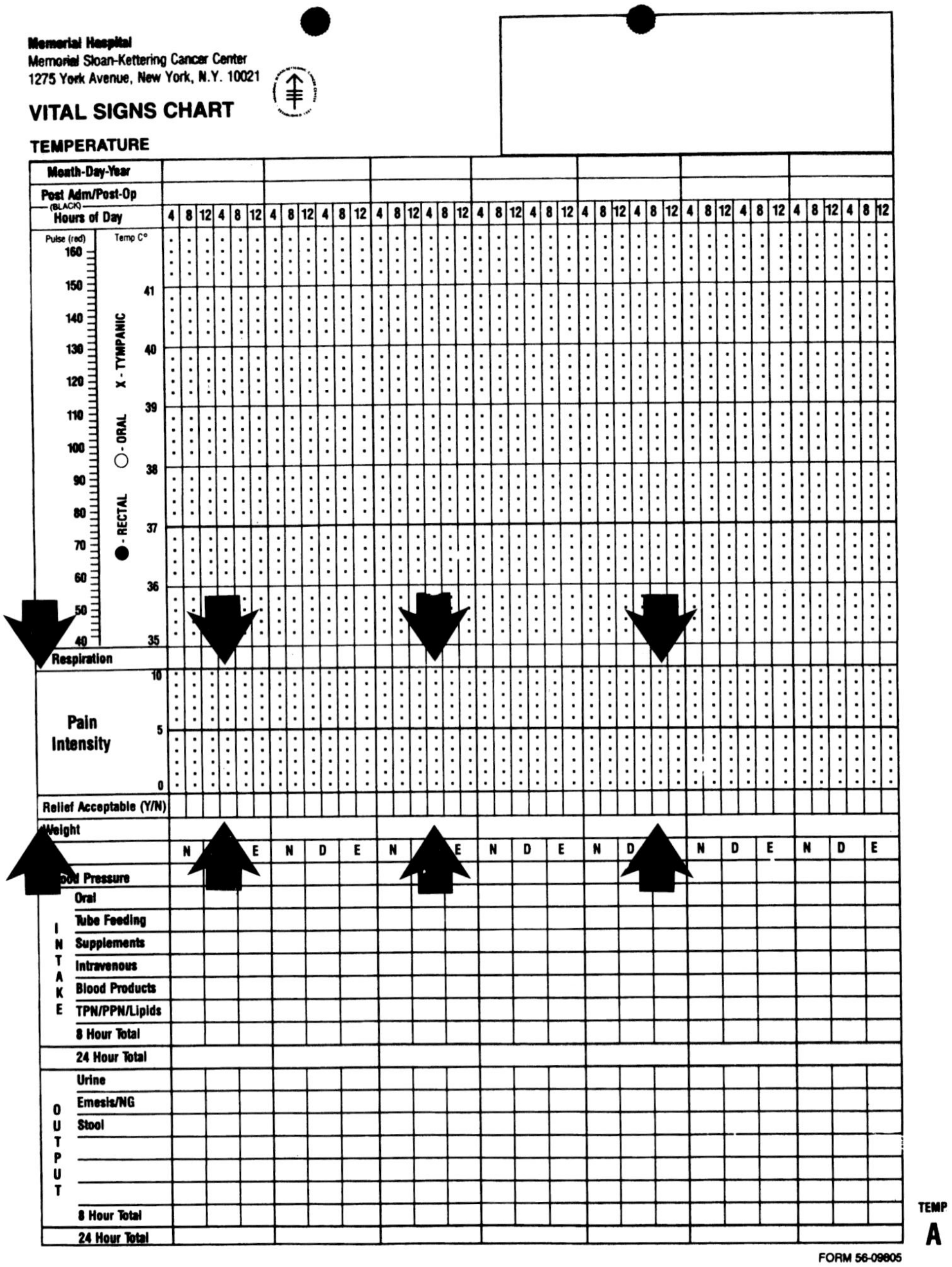

FIG. 70-2. The modified vital sign chart used at Memorial Sloan Kettering Cancer Center, illustrating the incorporation of a 10-point pain scale (*arrows*).

ciated with predictable, transient, traumatic pain. The pain caused by colonoscopy is produced by mesenteric tension (caused by progression of the colonoscope) and excessive air insufflation.[98,99] Further examples of acute procedure-related pain include that associated with fine-needle aspiration cytology of abdominal masses,[100] tumor embolization techniques,[101,102] percutaneous alcohol injection of hepatic metastases,[103] and chemical pleurodesis.

Acute Pain Associated With Analgesic Techniques

Injection Pain

Intramuscular (IM) and subcutaneous (SC) injections are painful. When repetitive dosing is required, the IM route of administration is not recommended.[95] If the volume of analgesic is small, repetitive SC boluses can be administered through a 27-gauge "butterfly" that is maintained in situ,[104,105] or continual infusion techniques can be considered.

Opioid Headache

The development of a reproducible generalized headache after opioid administration has been observed. It can be speculated that this may be caused by opioid-induced histamine release.

Spinal Opioid Hyperalgesia Syndrome

Intrathecal and epidural injection of high opioid doses occasionally is complicated by a paradoxical response characterized by pain (typically perineum, buttock, or leg), hyperalgesia, and associated manifestations, including segmental myoclonus, piloerection, and priapism. This is an uncommon phenomenon that remits after discontinuation of the drug.[106–108]

Epidural Injection Pain

Back, pelvic, and leg pain precipitated by epidural injection or infusion is a well-recognized complication of this technique. In an overview of epidural-associated side effects, the overall incidence of this problem was estimated at about 20%.[108] It is speculated that it may be caused by the injected fluid compressing an adjacent nerve root.[108]

Acute Pain Associated With Anticancer Therapies

Acute Pain Associated With Cancer Chemotherapy

Infusion Pain

Infusion site pain is a common problem in patients receiving cancer chemotherapy. Four intravenous (IV) infusion-related pain syndromes are recognized: venous spasm, chemical phlebitis, vesicant extravasation, and anthracycline-associated flare.[109,110] Pain caused by venous spasm is not associated with inflammation or phlebitis and may be modified by the application of a warm compress or a reduction in the rate of infusion.[109] Chemical phlebitis can be caused by cytotoxic medications, including amasarcine, dacarbazine, and carmustine,[111,112] and by the infusion of potassium chloride and hyperosmolar solutions. The pain and linear erythema associated with chemical phlebitis must be distinguished from the more serious complication of a vesicant cytotoxic extravasation.[113] Vesicant extravasation may produce intense pain followed by desquamation and ulceration. Finally, a brief venous flare reaction often is associated with IV administration of the anthracycline, doxorubicin. The flare typically is associated with local urticaria and occasional patients report pain or stinging.[110]

Chemotherapy infusion into the hepatic artery often is associated with the development of a diffuse abdominal pain.[114,115] In patients receiving continual infusions, the pain can be persistent. In some patients, the pain is caused by the development of gastric ulceration or erosions, or of cholangitis.[116] In patients with no evidence of gastric pathology, the pain has been observed to resolve with discontinuation of the infusion. A dose relation is suggested by the observation that some patients can tolerate recommencement of the infusion at a lower dose without pain.[114]

Abdominal pain is a common complication of intraperitoneal chemotherapy. A transient mild abdominal pain, associated with sensations of fullness or bloating, is reported by about 25% of patients receiving intraperitoneal chemotherapy.[117] A further 25% of patients report moderate or severe pain necessitating opioid analgesia or discontinuation of therapy.[117] Moderate or severe pain in intraperitoneal chemotherapy usually is caused by chemical serositis or infection.[118] Drug selection may be a factor in the incidence of chemical serositis; it is a common complication of intraperitoneal anthracycline agents such as mitoxantrone[119,120] and doxorubicin,[121,122] but is relatively infrequent with 5-fluorouracil.[123] Abdominal pain, associated with fever and rising peripheral and peritoneal fluid leukocyte counts, is suggestive of infectious peritonitis.[124]

Mucositis

Mucositis is a complication of chemotherapy that frequently is observed with 5-fluorouracil and other cytotoxic drugs. Although the clinical syndrome usually involves the oral cavity and pharynx, the underlying pathology may extend to other gastrointestinal mucosal surfaces, and symptoms may occur as a result of involvement of the esophagus and stomach (eg, odynophagia, dyspepsia). Damaged mucosal surfaces may become superinfected with microorganisms such as *Candida albicans* and herpes simplex. Numerous prophylactic programs have been described, including the use of cryotherapy,[125] surface-coating agents,[126,127] antibiotics,[128] antiviral agents,[129] and disinfectant mouthwashes.[130,131] Severe mucositis in this setting is uncommon, and usually requires local and systemic analgesic therapy.[132,133]

Palmar-Plantar Erythrodysesthesia Syndrome

Protracted infusion of 5-fluorouracil can be complicated by the development of a tingling or burning sensation in the palms and soles, followed by the appearance of an erythematous rash. The rash is characterized by a painful, sharply demarcated, intense erythema of the palms, soles, or both, followed by bulla formation, desquamation, and healing. Continuous low-dose 5-fluorouracil infusion (200 to 300 $mg/m^2/d$) produces this palmar-plantar erythrodysesthesia syndrome in 40% to 90% of patients.[134–136] It occurs rarely in patients undergoing 96- to 120-hour infusions.[137] The pathogenesis is unknown. The eruption is self-limiting in nature and usually does not require discontinuation of therapy. Symptomatic measures often are necessary,[137] and treatment with pyridoxine has been reported to induce resolution of the lesions.[135]

5-Fluorouracil–Induced Anginal Chest Pain

Patients receiving continual infusions of 5-fluorouracil may experience ischemic chest pain.[138–140] Continuous ambulatory electrocardiographic monitoring of patients undergoing 5-fluorouracil infusion demonstrated a nearly threefold increase in ischemic episodes over pretreatment recordings.[141] Electrocardiographic changes are more common among patients with known coronary artery disease.[141] It is widely speculated that coronary vasospasm may be the underlying mechanism.[139–141]

Corticosteroid Pain Syndromes

A transient burning sensation in the perineum is described by some patients after the rapid infusion of large doses of dexamethasone (20 to 100 mg) administered as an antiemetic or in the setting of spinal cord compression. Patients need to be warned that such symptoms may occur. This syndrome is attenuated with slow infusion. The complaint is self-limiting and rarely requires treatment.[142]

Corticosteroid withdrawal pseudorheumatism presents with diffuse myalgias, arthralgias, and tenderness of muscles and joints after dosage reduction. Treatment consists of reinstituting the corticosteroids at a higher dosage, then withdrawing them more slowly.[143]

Interferon-Induced Acute Pain

Virtually all patients treated with interferon experience an acute syndrome consisting of fever, chills, myalgias, arthralgias, and headache. The acute syndrome usually begins shortly after initial dosing and frequently improves with continued administration of the drug.[144,145] The severity of the symptoms is related to the type of interferon, route of administration, schedule, and dose.[144] Doses of 1 to 9 million units of interferon-α usually are well tolerated, but doses of 18 million units or more yield moderate to severe toxicity.[144] Acetaminophen pretreatment often is useful in ameliorating these symptoms.[145]

Acute Pain Associated With Radiation Therapy

Acute pain syndromes associated with radiation therapy can be incidental or toxic. Incident pains can be precipitated by transport and positioning of the patient for radiation therapy. Pain caused by acute radiation toxicity is associated most commonly with inflammation and ulceration of mucous membranes, and rarely skin, within the radiation port. The syndrome produced depends on the involved field; pelvic therapy can cause a proctitis, cystitis-urethritis, or vaginal ulceration.

Acute Radiation Enteritis and Proctocolitis

Acute radiation enteritis is observed in as many as 50% of patients receiving abdominal or pelvic radiation therapy. Involvement of the small intestine can present with cramping abdominal pain associated with nausea and diarrhea.[146,147] Pelvic radiation therapy can cause a painful proctocolitis with tenesmic pain in association with diarrhea, mucous discharge, and bleeding.[146] These complications usually resolve shortly after completion of therapy, but may have a slow resolution over 2 to 6 months.[146,147] Acute enteritis is associated with an increased risk of late-onset radiation enteritis (see later).[146]

Acute Pain Syndromes Associated With Infection

Acute Herpetic Neuralgia

The incidence of acute herpetic neuralgia is five times higher in patients with cancer than in the general population.[148] Pain or itch usually precedes the development of the rash by several days and occasionally occurs without the development of skin eruption.[149] The pain, which may be continuous or lancinating, may persist for several weeks after the resolution of the rash and usually resolves within 2 months.[149] Pain persisting beyond this interval is referred to as postherpetic neuralgia. Postherpetic neuralgia is two or three times more frequent in the cancer population than in the general population.[148] Patients with postherpetic neuralgia and cancer who describe changes in the pattern of pain, or the development of new neurologic deficits, may have tumor-related pain that exacerbates the existing neuropathic pain. The dermatomal location of the varicella zoster infection shows a significant correlation with the site of the malignancy, and exacerbations occur twice as frequently in previously irradiated dermatomes as in nonirradiated areas.[148] Dissemination of the infection is twice as frequent in patients with active tumor compared with patients in remission.[150] In patients receiving chemotherapy, the infection usually develops at a median time of less than 1 month after the completion of treatment.

CHRONIC PAIN SYNDROMES

Pain Syndromes Caused by Tumor Involvement of Viscera and Adjacent Structures

Pain may be caused by pathology involving the luminal organs of the gastrointestinal or genitourinary tracts, the parenchymal organs, the peritoneum, or the retroperitoneal soft tissues. Obstruction of a hollow viscus, such as the intestine, biliary tract, or ureter, produces visceral nociceptive syndromes that are well described in the surgical literature.[151] Pain arising from retroperitoneal and pelvic lesions may involve mixed nociceptive and neuropathic mechanisms if both somatic structures and nerve plexuses are involved.

Hepatic Distention Syndrome

The liver is the most common visceral site of metastases arising from gastrointestinal cancers. Pain-sensitive hepatic structures include the liver capsule, vascular structures, and biliary tract.[152,153] Nociceptive afferent nerves that innervate these structures travel through the celiac plexus, the phrenic nerve, and the lower right intercostal nerves. Extensive intrahepatic metastases, or gross hepatomegaly associated with cholestasis, may produce discomfort in the right subcostal region of the abdomen, and less commonly in the right midback or flank.[152,153] Referred pain may be experienced in the right neck or shoulder, or in the region of the right scapula.[152] The pain, which usually is described as a dull aching, may be exacerbated by movement, pressure in the abdomen, and deep inspiration. It commonly is accompanied by symptoms of anorexia and nausea. Physical examination may reveal a hard, irregular subcostal mass that descends with respiration and is dull to percussion. Other features of hepatic failure may be present. Imaging of the hepatic parenchyma by ultrasound or CT usually identifies the presence of space-occupying lesions and cholestasis.

Occasional patients have an acute subcostal pain exacerbated by respiration. Physical examination may demonstrate a palpable or audible rub. These findings suggest the development of an overlying peritonitis, which may occur in response to some acute event, such as a hemorrhage into a metastasis.

Midline Retroperitoneal Syndrome

Cancers of the pancreas and biliary tree or retroperitoneal lymphadenopathy involving the upper abdomen may produce pain by invasion into deep somatic structures of the posterior abdominal wall, distortion of pain-sensitive connective tissue and vascular structures, local inflammation, and direct infiltration of the celiac plexus. The pain is experienced in the epigastrium, the low thoracic region of the back, or both. It usually is dull and boring in character, exacerbated with recumbency, and improved by sitting. The retroperitoneum is well imaged using CT techniques. Because tumors in the paravertebral space can extend through the intervertebral canal into the epidural space, when paravertebral tumors are identified, consideration should be given to imaging the epidural space.

Chronic Intestinal Obstruction

Abdominal pain is an almost invariable manifestation of chronic intestinal obstruction.[154–156] The factors that contribute to this pain include smooth muscle contractions, mesenteric tension, and mural ischemia. Obstructive symptoms can be caused primarily by the tumor, or more commonly, by a combination of mechanical obstruction and other processes, such as autonomic neuropathy and ileus from metabolic derangements and drugs. Both continuous and colicky pain occur.[154,155] The pain is referred to the dermatomes corresponding to the spinal segments supplying the affected viscera. Vomiting, anorexia, and constipation are important associated symptoms. Abdominal radiographs taken in supine and erect positions may demonstrate the presence of air–fluid levels and intestinal distention. CT or magnetic resonance imaging (MRI) of the abdomen can assess the extent and distribution of intraabdominal neoplasm, which has implications for subsequent treatment options.

Peritoneal Carcinomatosis

Gastrointestinal malignancies are among the most common causes of peritoneal carcinomatosis.[157] Peritoneal carcinomatosis occurs most often by transcoelomic spread of abdominal or pelvic tumors.[157,158] It can cause peritoneal inflammation, mesenteric tethering, malignant adhesions, and ascites,[158] all of which can cause pain. Mesenteric tethering and tension can cause a diffuse abdominal or low back pain. Tense malignant ascites may produce a diffuse abdominal discomfort and a distinct stretching pain in the anterior abdominal wall. Adhesions also can cause obstruction of a hollow viscus, with intermittent colicky pain.[159] CT may demonstrate evidence of ascites, omental infiltration, and peritoneal nodules.

Perineal Pain

Colorectal and anal cancers are the neoplastic diseases most commonly responsible for perineal pain.[160–163] The pain, which typically is described as constant and aching, often is aggravated by sitting or standing, and may be associated with tenesmus or bladder spasms.[160] Perineal pain most commonly is caused by local extension or local recurrence of tumor,[160,163] and postoperative recurrence of perineal pain is highly suggestive of local recurrence.[160,163] In one pain clinic, perineal pain was the reason for referral for 50 of 85 patients with a diagnosis of carcinoma of the rectum.[163] Local tumor recurrence or other types of tumor dissemination in the pelvis were diagnosed in 47 of these patients. A non-neoplastic cause of perineal pain could be confirmed in only 1 patient.[163] The pathologic finding of perineural invasion in resected tumor is highly predictive of the probability of local recurrence (80%), and most such recurrences (90%) are associated with pain as the predominant symptom.[161,162,164]

Tumor invasion of the musculature of the deep pelvis also can result in a syndrome that resembles tension myalgia of the pelvic floor.[165] Patients with this syndrome typically describe a constant ache or heaviness in the perineum that is exacerbated with upright posture. When caused by tumor, the pain may be concurrent with other types of perineal pain. Digital examination of the pelvic floor may reveal local tenderness or palpable tumor.

Ureteric Obstruction

Ureteric obstruction most frequently is caused by tumor compression or infiltration within the true pelvis.[166] Less commonly, it is caused by more proximal obstruction associated with retroperitoneal lymphadenopathy, isolated retroperitoneal metastasis, or intramural or mucosal metastases.[166] Carcinoma of the rectum is one of the most common tumors associated with this complication.[166,167]

Pain may or may not accompany ureteric obstruction. When present, it typically is a dull, chronic discomfort in the flank. Colicky pain and pain radiation into the groin or genitalia also can occur. More frequently, unilateral obstruction is discovered after an incidental finding of unilateral hydronephrosis. Bilateral obstruction typically presents with symptoms of nausea, anorexia, lethargy, delirium, or anuria. Ureteric obstruction can be complicated by pyelonephritis or pyonephrosis, which often present with features of sepsis, loin pain, and dysuria. The diagnosis of ureteric obstruction can be confirmed by the demonstration of hydronephrosis on renal sonography.[168,169] The level of obstruction can be demonstrated by pyelography, and CT techniques usually demonstrate the cause[167,169] (Fig. 70-3).

Pain Syndromes Involving the Peripheral Nervous System

Lumbosacral Plexopathy

The lumbar plexus, which lies in the paravertebral psoas muscle, is formed primarily by the ventral rami of L1-4. The sacral plexus forms in the sacroiliac notch from the ventral rami of S1-3 and the lumbosacral trunk (L4-5), which courses caudally over the sacral ala to join the plexus.[170] Among patients with gastrointestinal malignancies, lumbosacral plexopathy usually is caused by neoplastic infiltration or compression. Polyradiculopathy from leptomeningeal metastases or epidural metastases can mimic lumbosacral plexopathy, and these lesions also must be considered in the evaluation (see later).

Malignant Lumbosacral Plexopathy

Cancers of the distal gastrointestinal tract are among the most common causes of malignant lumbosacral plexopathy.[73,171] In

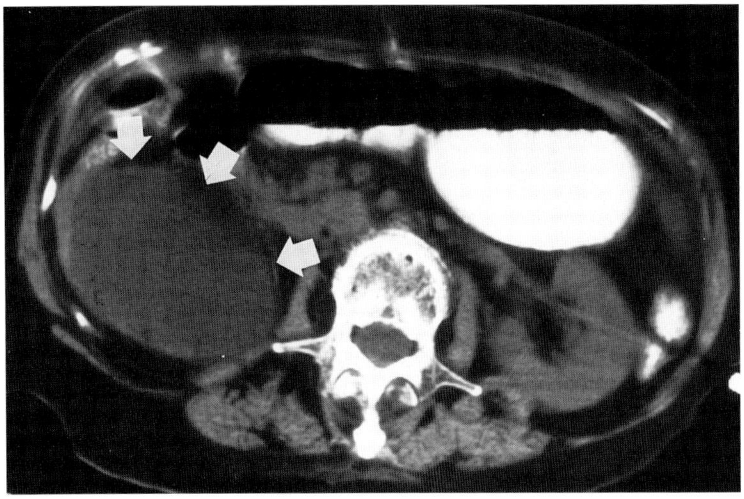

FIG. 70-3. Abdominal computed tomographic scan demonstrating massive right-sided hydronephrosis with marked cortical thinning (*arrows*) from a patient with a pelvic recurrence of rectal carcinoma who had right-sided loin pain. (Cherny NI, Portenoy RK. Cancer pain: principles of assessment and syndromes. In: Wall PD, Melzack R, eds. Textbook of pain. 3rd ed. Edinburgh: Churchill Livingstone, 1994:787.)

general, tumors involve the plexus by direct extension from intrapelvic neoplasms; metastases account for only one fourth of cases.[171] In one study, two thirds of patients had plexopathy within 3 years of their primary diagnosis and one third had plexopathy within 1 year.[171]

Pain in the lower abdomen, inguinal region, buttock, or leg is the first symptom reported by most patients with malignant lumbosacral plexopathy, and is experienced by almost all patients during the course of the disease.[171] The quality usually is aching, pressure-like, or stabbing. Most patients also experience numbness, paresthesias, and weakness weeks to months after the pain begins. Common signs include leg weakness that involves multiple myotomes, sensory loss that crosses dermatomes, reflex asymmetry, focal tenderness, leg edema, and positive direct or reverse straight leg-raising signs.

Upper plexus involvement occurs in almost one third of patients,[171] and most commonly is caused by direct extension from a colorectal tumor. Pain may be experienced in the lower abdomen, flank, or iliac crest, or in the anterolateral thigh. Physical examination findings include sensory, motor, and reflex changes in an L1-4 distribution. A subgroup of these patients have a syndrome characterized by pain and paresthesias limited to the lower abdomen or inguinal region, with occasional sensory loss and no motor findings. CT in these patients may show tumor adjacent to the L-1 vertebra (the L-1 syndrome),[171] or along the pelvic sidewall, where it presumably damages the ilioinguinal, iliohypogastric, or genitofemoral nerve. The so-called malignant psoas syndrome occurs in patients who have neoplastic involvement of the psoas muscle and experience a syndrome characterized by upper lumbosacral plexopathy and painful flexion of the ipsilateral hip with a positive psoas muscle stretch test.[172]

A lower plexopathy occurs in a little more than 50% of patients,[171] and in this population usually is caused by direct extension from a rectal cancer. Pain may be localized in the buttocks and perineum, or referred to the posterolateral thigh and leg. Associated symptoms and signs conform to an L4-S1 segmental distribution. Physical examination may reveal weakness or sensory changes in the L-5 and S-1 dermatomes and depressed ankle jerks. Other findings include leg edema, bladder or bowel dysfunction, sacral or sciatic notch tenderness, and a positive straight leg-raising test. A pelvic mass may be palpable.

Sacral plexopathy may occur from direct extension of a sacral lesion or a presacral mass. This may present with predominant involvement of the lumbosacral trunk, characterized by pain over the dorsal medial foot and sole, and weakness of knee flexion, ankle dorsiflexion, and inversion. Other patients demonstrate particular involvement of the coccygeal plexus, with prominent sphincter dysfunction and perineal pain.

A panplexopathy with involvement in an L1-S3 distribution occurs in almost one fifth of patients with lumbosacral plexopathy.[171] Local pain may occur in the lower abdomen, buttocks, or perineum. Referred pain can be experienced anywhere in the distribution of the plexus. Leg edema is extremely common. Neurologic deficits may be confluent or patchy over the L1-S3 distribution, and a positive straight leg-raising test usually is present.

Cross-sectional imaging, with CT or MRI, is the usual diagnostic procedure to evaluate lumbosacral plexopathy (Figs. 70-4 and 70-5). Scanning should be done from the level of the L-1 vertebral body, through the sciatic notch.[173] When using CT techniques, images should include bone and soft-tissue windows. Definitive imaging of the epidural space adjacent to the plexus should be considered in the patient who has features indicative of a relatively high risk of epidural extension, such as bilateral symptoms or signs, unexplained incontinence, or a prominent paraspinal mass.[171,173,174]

Uncommon Causes of Lumbosacral Plexopathy

In occasional patients, lumbosacral plexopathy develops as a result of surgical trauma, radiation therapy, infarction, cytotoxic damage, infection in the pelvis or psoas muscle, abdominal aneurysm, or idiopathic lumbosacral neuritis.[170,175–178]

Bone Pain

In an autopsy study, 20% of bony metastases observed had derived from tumors of the gastrointestinal tract.[179] Bone metastases potentially cause pain by endosteal or periosteal nociceptor activation that is sustained by mechanical distortion or release of chemical mediators such as prostaglandins, bradykinin,

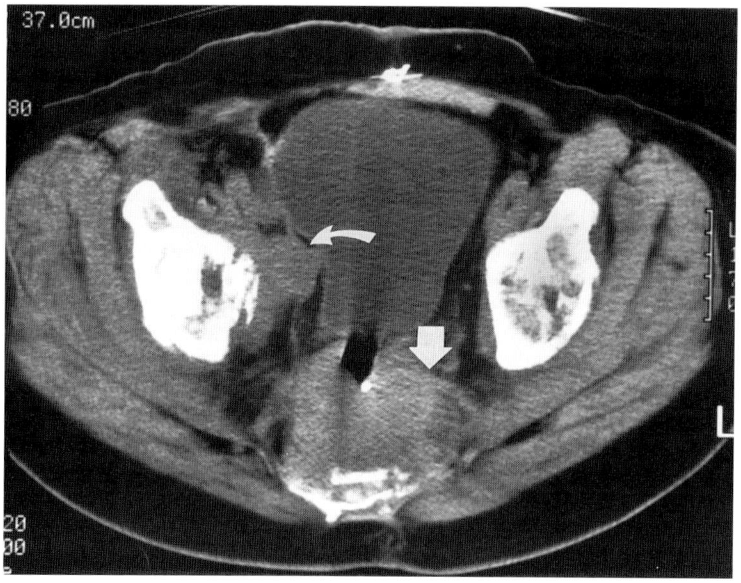

FIG. 70-4. Pelvic computed tomographic scan demonstrating a presacral mass that erodes the sacrum (*large arrow*) and involves the plexus in the right pelvic sidewall (*small arrow*).

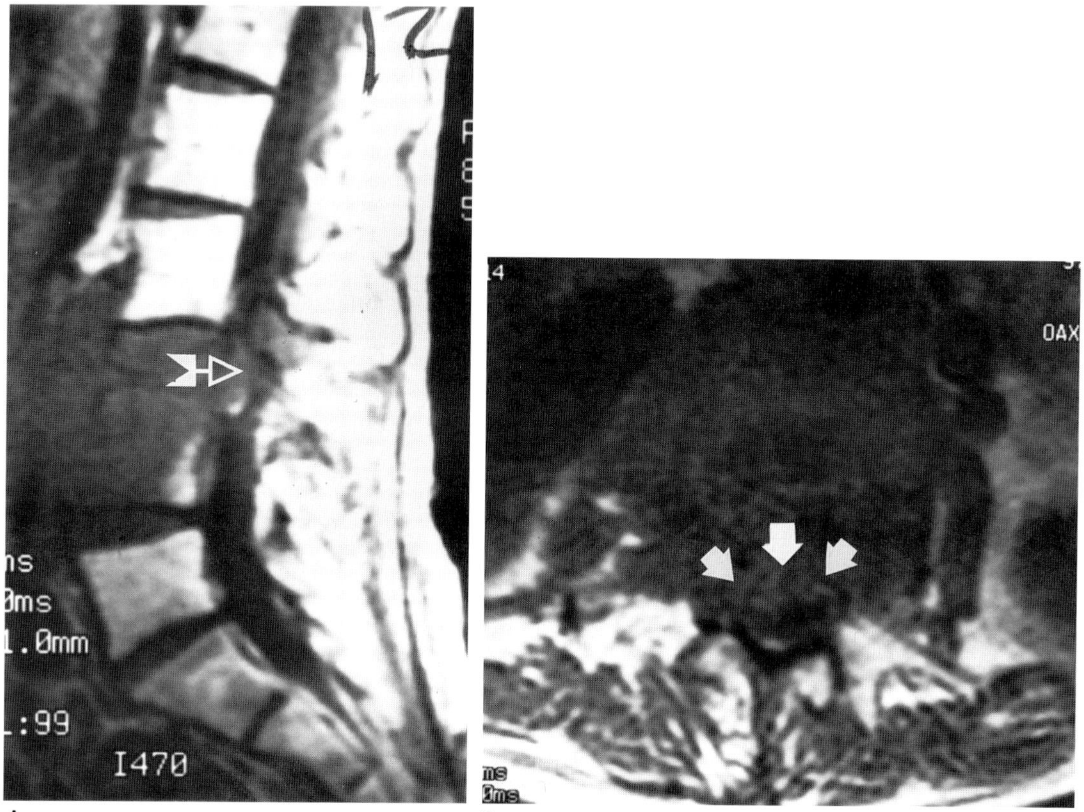

A B

FIG. 70-5. Sagittal and axial magnetic resonance imaging scans of the lumbar spine in a 56-year-old woman with carcinoma of the colon who had back pain and L3 radicular pain in the right leg. **(A)** The sagittal scan demonstrates extensive destruction of both L3 and L4 vertebral bodies. There is posterior extension of the tumor into the epidural space, which compresses the spinal cord (*horizontal arrow*). **(B)** The axial scan performed through L3 demonstrates complete obliteration of the epidural space (*arrows*) and severe compression of the thecal sac. (Cherny NI, Portenoy RK. Cancer pain: pathophysiology, assessment and syndromes. In: Wall PD, Melzack R, eds. Textbook of pain. 3rd ed. Edinburgh: Churchill Livingstone, 1994.)

TABLE 70-4. *Vertebral pain syndromes*

Syndrome	Pain	Significance
Atlantoaxial destruction, odontoid fractures	Nuchal or occipital pain that radiates over the posterior aspect of the skull to the vertex and is exacerbated by flexion of the neck	Pathologic fracture may result in secondary subluxation with ensuing compression of the spinal cord at the cervicomedullary junction
C-7–T-1 syndrome	Pain referred to the interscapular region	May be missed if radiographic evaluation is mistakenly targeted to the painful area caudal to the site of damage; may be obscured by overlying bone and mediastinal shadows; bone scintigraphy may assist in targeting additional diagnostic imaging procedures, particularly computed tomography or magnetic resonance imaging
T-2–L-1 syndrome	T-12 or L-1 vertebral lesions can refer pain to the ipsilateral iliac crest or the sacroiliac joint	Imaging procedures directed at pelvic bones miss the source of the pain
Sacral syndrome	Severe focal pain radiating to the buttocks, perineum, or posterior thighs may accompany destruction of the sacrum; often exacerbated by sitting or lying and relieved by standing or walking	Local extension of the tumor mass also may involve the sacral plexus, resulting in neurologic deficits, most importantly sphincter dysfunction (see later); lateral spread to involve muscles that rotate the hip (eg, the piriformis muscle) may produce a malignant piriformis syndrome, characterized by buttock or posterior leg pain that is exacerbated by internal rotation of the hip

substance P, and histamine, and or by tumor growth into adjacent soft tissues and nerves.[180]

Bone pain caused by metastatic tumor needs to be differentiated from less common causes of chronic bone pain in patients with cancer. Non-neoplastic causes in this population include osteoporotic pathologic fractures and focal osteonecrosis, which may be idiopathic or related to corticosteroids or radiation therapy.

In general, the vertebrae are the most common sites of bony metastases.[181,182] Vertebral metastases of colorectal tumors occur most commonly in the lumbosacral spine.[181,183] Vertebral metastases can be associated with specific clinical syndromes (Table 70-4).

The early recognition of pain syndromes caused by neoplastic invasion of vertebral bodies is essential, because pain usually precedes compression of adjacent neural structures and prompt primary therapy directed at the lesion may prevent the subsequent development of neurologic deficits. This recognition often requires substantial clinical acumen; referral of pain is common, and the associated symptoms and signs can mimic a variety of other disorders, both malignant (eg, paraspinal masses) and nonmalignant.

Back Pain and Epidural Spinal Cord Compression

In general, epidural compression of the spinal cord or cauda equina is a common neurologic complication of cancer, occurring in up to 10% of patients[184]; gastrointestinal tumors account for less than 10% of these episodes.[181,183,185] Most epidural compression is caused by posterior extension of vertebral body metastasis to the epidural space; some is caused by tumor extension from the posterior arch of the vertebra or infiltration of a paravertebral tumor through the intervertebral foramen.

Because the most salient determinant of treatment efficacy is the degree of neurologic impairment at the time therapy is initiated, early identification is essential.[174] Although 75% of patients who are ambulatory when they begin treatment remain so, this proportion declines to 30% to 50% for those who begin treatment while markedly paretic, and is less than 10% for those who are paralyzed.[174,181,184,186,187]

Back pain, however, is a nonspecific symptom that can result from bony or paraspinal metastases without epidural encroachment, from retroperitoneal or leptomeningeal tumors, or from a large variety of other benign conditions, including musculoskeletal disorders.[184] Because it is impracticable to pursue an extensive evaluation in every patient who has back pain, the assessment of this symptom must include a systematic evaluation that determines the probability of epidural compression and selects patients appropriate for further investigation of the epidural space. The selection process is based on symptoms and signs and on the results of simple and inexpensive imaging techniques. The clinical features suggestive of epidural extension are listed in Table 70-5.

The evaluation (and, if appropriate, treatment) of patients with emerging symptoms and signs indicative of spinal cord or cauda equina dysfunction should proceed on an emergency basis. Unless contraindicated, these patients should receive an IV dose of corticosteroid before epidural imaging is performed. High-dose dexamethasone is used customarily. One regimen advocates an initial IV bolus of 100 mg followed by 96 mg/d in divided doses, which is tapered over 3 to 4 weeks. Patients with symptoms and signs of radiculopathy or stable or mild signs of spinal cord or cauda equina dysfunction also usually are treated presumptively with a corticosteroid (typically with a more moderate dose) and are scheduled for definitive imaging of the epidural space as soon as possible.

Among patients who have back pain without symptoms or

signs suggesting epidural compression, radiographic abnormalities consistent with neoplasm at the appropriate level indicate a high probability (60%) of epidural compression.[188] Definitive imaging of the epidural space is indicated strongly for patients with greater than 50% vertebral body collapse, and usually is recommended for patients with pedicle erosion. In patients with back pain and normal bone radiographs, a positive scintigram at the site of pain is associated with a 12% to 17% probability of epidural disease.[174,189] If both radiographs and scintigraphy are normal but the patient has severe or progressive pain, evaluation with CT, or preferably MRI, still may be warranted.

Definitive imaging of the epidural space confirms the existence of epidural compression (indicating the necessity and urgency of treatment), determines the extent of epidural encroachment (influencing the prognosis and perhaps altering the therapeutic approach), and defines the appropriate radiation portals.[190] The options for definitive imaging include MRI, myelography, and CT-myelography (Fig. 70-6). MRI, which is noninvasive and offers accurate soft-tissue imaging and multiplanar views, usually is preferred. Myelography remains the investigation of choice for patients who lack access to MRI and those who are unable to undergo the procedure. MRI is relatively contraindicated in patients with severe claustrophobia and absolutely contraindicated in patients with some forms of metallic implants.

TABLE 70-5. *Clinical features suggestive of epidural spinal cord and cauda equina compression*

Clinical features	Notes
Rapid progression of back pain	Ominous occurrence
Radicular pain	Can be intermittent, constant, or lancinating
	Usually unilateral in cervical and lumbosacral regions
	Usually bilateral in the thorax
	Exacerbated by recumbency, coughing, sneezing, or Valsalva maneuver
Weakness	Segmental: suggestive of radiculopathy
	Lumbosacral multisegmental: suggesting of cauda equina compression
	Pyramidal distribution: suggestive of spinal cord compression
	Variable rate of progression
	After development of weakness, 30% have paraplegia within 7 days
Sensory abnormalities	Also may begin segmentally
	Ultimately may evolve to a sensory level
	Upper level of sensory findings may correspond to the location of the epidural tumor
Bladder and bowel dysfunction	Usually occurs late
	Early symptom of conus medullaris or cauda equina lesion
Musculoskeletal features	Scoliosis
	Asymmetric wasting of paravertebral musculature
	Gibbus (palpable step) in the dorsal spines
	Spinal tenderness to percussion

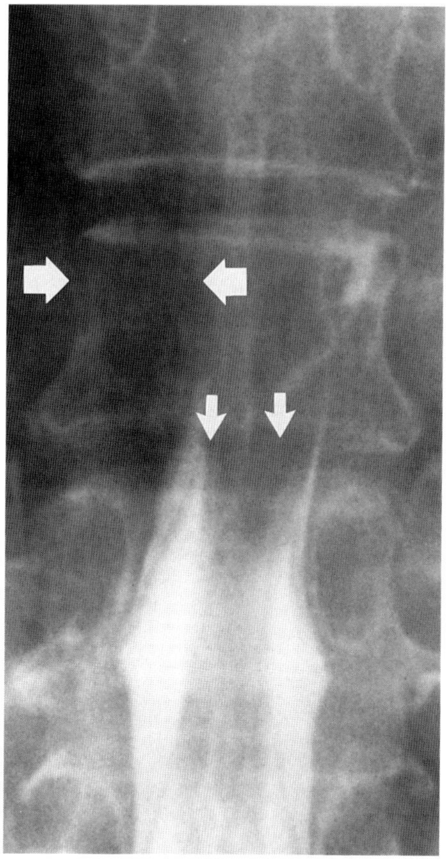

FIG. 70-6. Segment of a thoracic myelogram (T-8 through T-11) performed on a 54-year-old woman with severe mid-back pain. There is a complete block to the flow of contrast medium at the T9 level (*vertical arrows*). The left pedicle of the T9 vertebra is absent as a result of metastatic erosion (*horizontal arrows*). (Cherny NI, Portenoy RK. Cancer pain: pathophysiology, assessment and syndromes. In: Wall PD, Melzack R, eds. Textbook of pain. 3rd ed. Edinburgh: Churchill Livingstone, 1994.)

Treatment usually involves the administration of corticosteroids and radiation therapy.[191,192] Surgical decompression is considered for some patients with radiation-resistant tumors, those who previously have received maximal radiation therapy to the involved field, those with spinal instability, and those for whom no other tissue is available for histologic diagnosis.[184,185] Decompressive laminectomy for posteriorly located lesions and anterior vertebrectomy with spinal stabilization for lesions arising from the vertebral body are the recommended procedures.[193–195] Decompressive laminectomy in the setting of vertebral body collapse is not recommended because of the risk of neurologic deterioration or spinal instability (22% to 25%) induced by the procedure.[196,197]

Pain Syndromes of the Bony Pelvis and Hip

The pelvis and hip are common sites of metastatic involvement. The weight-bearing function of these structures, essential for normal ambulation, contributes to the propensity of disease at these sites to cause incident pain with ambulation.

Hip Joint Syndrome

Tumor involvement of the acetabulum or head of the femur typically produces localized hip pain that is aggravated by weight bearing and movement of the hip. The pain may radiate to the knee or medial thigh, and occasionally this is the only site of pain.[198] Medial extension of an acetabular tumor can involve the lumbosacral plexus as it traverses the pelvic sidewall. Plain radiographs and bone scintigraphy usually demonstrate bony involvement. CT and MRI techniques are more sensitive, and they also demonstrate the extent of adjacent soft-tissue involvement.[199]

Headache and Facial Pain

Tumor-related headache is a relatively uncommon cancer pain problem in patients with gastrointestinal cancers. Cancer-related headache results from traction, inflammation, or infiltration of pain-sensitive structures in the head and neck.[200]

Brain Metastases

The incidence of cerebral metastases in patients with gastrointestinal cancer is about 5%.[201] Headache is a common presenting symptom in patients with brain metastases, occurring in 60% to 90%; patients with multiple metastases and those with posterior fossa metastases are most likely to report this symptom.[200,202,203] The quality of the headache may be throbbing or steady, and the intensity usually is mild to moderate. The location may be local or generalized; when lateralized, it usually overlies the site of the lesion, but posterior fossa lesions often cause a bifrontal headache.[204] The headache often is worse in the morning and is exacerbated by stooping, sudden head movements, or Valsalva maneuvers (coughing, sneezing, or straining).

Base of Skull Metastases

Bony metastases to the base of the skull are associated with well-described clinical syndromes,[205] named according to the site of metastatic involvement: orbital, parasellar, middle fossa, jugular foramen, occipital condyle, clivus, and sphenoid sinus (Table 70-6). When base of the skull metastases are suspected, CT with bone window settings is the diagnostic procedure of choice to evaluate bony disease.[205] MRI is most sensitive for assessing soft-tissue extension. Cerebrospinal fluid analysis may be needed to exclude leptomeningeal metastases.[142]

Painful Cranial Neuralgias

Glossopharyngeal and trigeminal neuralgias can occur from metastases in the base of the skull or leptomeninges. Each of these syndromes has a characteristic presentation.[142] Early diagnosis is critical to prevent progressive neurologic injury.

Leptomeningeal Metastases

Leptomeningeal metastases, characterized by diffuse or multifocal involvement of the subarachnoid space by metastatic tumor, are an uncommon complication of gastrointestinal cancers. Generalized headache and radicular pain in the low back and buttocks are the most common painful manifestations of this syndrome.[206,207] The headache may be associated with changes in mental status, nausea, vomiting, tinnitus, and nuchal rigidity. Focal or multifocal neurologic symptoms or signs may involve any level of the neuraxis.[208,209] The diagnosis is confirmed through analysis of the cerebrospinal fluid, which may reveal elevated pressure, elevated protein level, depressed glucose concentration, lymphocytic pleocytosis, and positive cytology. Ninety percent of patients ultimately show positive cytology, but multiple analyses may be required.[206,207,210] MRI of the cranium and spinal cord with gadolinium enhancement is the most sensitive imaging modality.[211,212] CT or MRI of the head may demonstrate enhancement of the dural membranes or ventricular enlargement,[213,214] and myelography is abnormal in up to 30% of patients.

Chronic Pain Syndromes Associated With Cancer Therapy

Most treatment-related pains caused by tissue-damaging procedures are acute, and are remarkable for their predictability and self-limited natural history. Chronic treatment-related pain syndromes are associated with a persistent nociceptive complication of an invasive treatment, such as a postsurgical abscess, or more commonly, a neural injury.[142] In some cases, these

TABLE 70-6. *Base of skull pain syndromes*

Syndrome	Clinical features
Orbital	Progressive ipsilateral, retroorbital, and supraorbital pain
Parasellar	Unilateral supraorbital and frontal headache ± diplopia, ophthalmoparesis, papilledema, hemianopsia, or quadrantinopsia
Middle cranial fossa	Facial numbness or paresthesias in the distribution of the second or third divisions of the trigeminal nerve referred to the cheek or jaw
Jugular foramen	Hoarseness or dysphagia, pain referred to the ipsilateral ear or mastoid, occasionally glossopharyngeal neuralgia, with or without syncope
Occipital condyle	Unilateral occipital pain worsened with neck flexion ± stiffness of the neck
Clivus	Vertex headache, which often is exacerbated by neck flexion; lower cranial nerve (VI–XII) dysfunction (may become bilateral)
Sphenoid sinus	Bifrontal headache radiating to the temporal region, and intermittent retroorbital pain

syndromes occur long after the therapy is completed, resulting in a difficult differential diagnosis between recurrent disease and a complication of therapy.

Chronic Postsurgical Pain Syndromes

Phantom Anus Syndrome

Phantom pain is perceived to arise from a resected body structure, as if the structure were still contiguous with the body. A phantom anus pain syndrome occurs in about 15% of patients who undergo abdominoperineal resection of the rectum.[215,216] Phantom anus pain may develop in the early postoperative period or after a latency of months to years.[161,215] Late-onset pain almost always is associated with tumor recurrence.[161,163] In a series of 29 patients with perineal pain caused by recurrent rectal cancer, the pain began a median of 5.5 months before the tumor recurrence was diagnosed.[163]

Postsurgical Pelvic Floor Myalgia

Surgical trauma to the pelvic floor can cause a residual pelvic floor myalgia that, like the neoplastic syndrome described previously, mimics so-called tension myalgia.[165] The risk of disease recurrence associated with this condition is not known, and its natural history has not been defined. In patients who have undergone anorectal resection, this condition must be differentiated from the phantom anus syndrome (see earlier).

Postsurgical Lumbosacral Plexopathy

Surgical trauma to the lumbosacral plexus during deep pelvic resection can result in persistent neurologic dysfunction and pain.

Postesophagectomy Pain

A Japanese study evaluating the quality of life of patients after esophagectomy for esophageal cancer reported that 40% of patients complained of dysphagia, abdominal pain, or diarrhea after meals.[217]

Chronic Postradiation Pain Syndromes

Chronic pain occurring as a complication of radiation therapy tends to occur late in the course of a patient's illness. These syndromes always be must differentiated from recurrent tumor.

Radiation-Induced Lumbosacral Plexopathy

Radiation fibrosis of the lumbosacral plexus is rare and may occur from 1 to more than 30 years after radiation therapy. Radiation-induced plexopathy typically presents with progressive weakness and leg swelling; pain usually is not a prominent feature.[218] Weakness begins distally in the L5-S1 segments and is slowly progressive. The symptoms and signs often are bilateral.[218] If CT demonstrates a lesion, it usually is a nonspecific diffuse infiltration of the tissues. Electromyography may show myokymic discharges.[218]

Chronic Radiation Enteritis and Proctitis

Chronic enteritis and proctocolitis occur as a delayed complication in 2% to 10% of patients who undergo abdominal or pelvic radiation therapy.[146,147] The rectum and rectosigmoid are involved more commonly than the small bowel,[146] a pattern that may relate to the retroperitoneal fixation of those structures. The latency is variable (3 months to 30 years).[146,147] Chronic radiation injury to the rectum can present as proctitis (with bloody diarrhea, tenesmus, and cramping pain), obstruction resulting from stricture formation, or fistulas to the bladder or vagina.[146,147] Small-bowel radiation damage typically causes colicky abdominal pain, which can be associated with chronic nausea or malabsorption.[146,147] Barium studies may demonstrate a narrow tubular bowel segment resembling Crohn's disease or ischemic colitis. Endoscopic imaging and biopsy may be necessary to distinguish suspicious lesions from recurrent cancer.[146]

Burning Perineum Syndrome

Persistent perineal discomfort is an uncommon delayed complication of pelvic radiation therapy. After a latency period of 6 to 18 months, persistent burning pain develops in the perianal region; the pain may extend anteriorly to involve the vagina or scrotum.[219] In patients who have had abdominoperineal resection, phantom anus pain and recurrent tumor are major elements in the differential diagnosis. Appropriate studies must be done to exclude recurrent neoplasm.

Chronic Radiation Myelopathy

Chronic radiation myelopathy is a late complication of spinal cord irradiation that rarely is seen in this population. The latency interval is highly variable, but is most commonly 12 to 14 months. Common presentations include a progressive Brown-Séquard syndrome[220] and partial transverse myelopathy.

Osteoradionecrosis

Osteoradionecrosis is a late complication of radiation therapy that, although usually painless, may be characterized by the development of a painful focus of necrotic bone. Overlying tissue breakdown can occur spontaneously or as a result of trauma.[221,222] Delayed development of a painful ulcer must be differentiated from tumor recurrence.

Postchemotherapy Pain Syndromes

Avascular Necrosis of the Femoral or Humeral Head

Avascular necrosis of the femoral or humeral head may occur spontaneously or as a complication of intermittent or continuous corticosteroid therapy. Involvement of the femoral head is most common and typically causes pain in the hip, thigh, or knee that is exacerbated by movement and relieved by rest.[223] Bone scintigraphy and MRI are sensitive and complementary diagnostic procedures.

MANAGEMENT OF CHRONIC CANCER PAIN

General Considerations

Optimal management of pain problems in patients with cancer requires familiarity with a range of therapeutic options, including antineoplastic therapies, analgesic pharmacotherapy, and anesthetic, neurosurgical, psychological, and physiatric techniques (Fig. 70-7). Successful pain management is characterized by the implementation of the techniques with the most favorable therapeutic indices for the prevailing circumstances, along with provision for repeated evaluations so that a favorable balance between pain relief and adverse effects is maintained.[224,225] Currently available techniques can provide adequate relief to most patients.

Primary Therapy

The assessment process may reveal a cause for the pain that is amenable to etiologically directed primary therapy. For pain produced by tumor infiltration or compression, antineoplastic

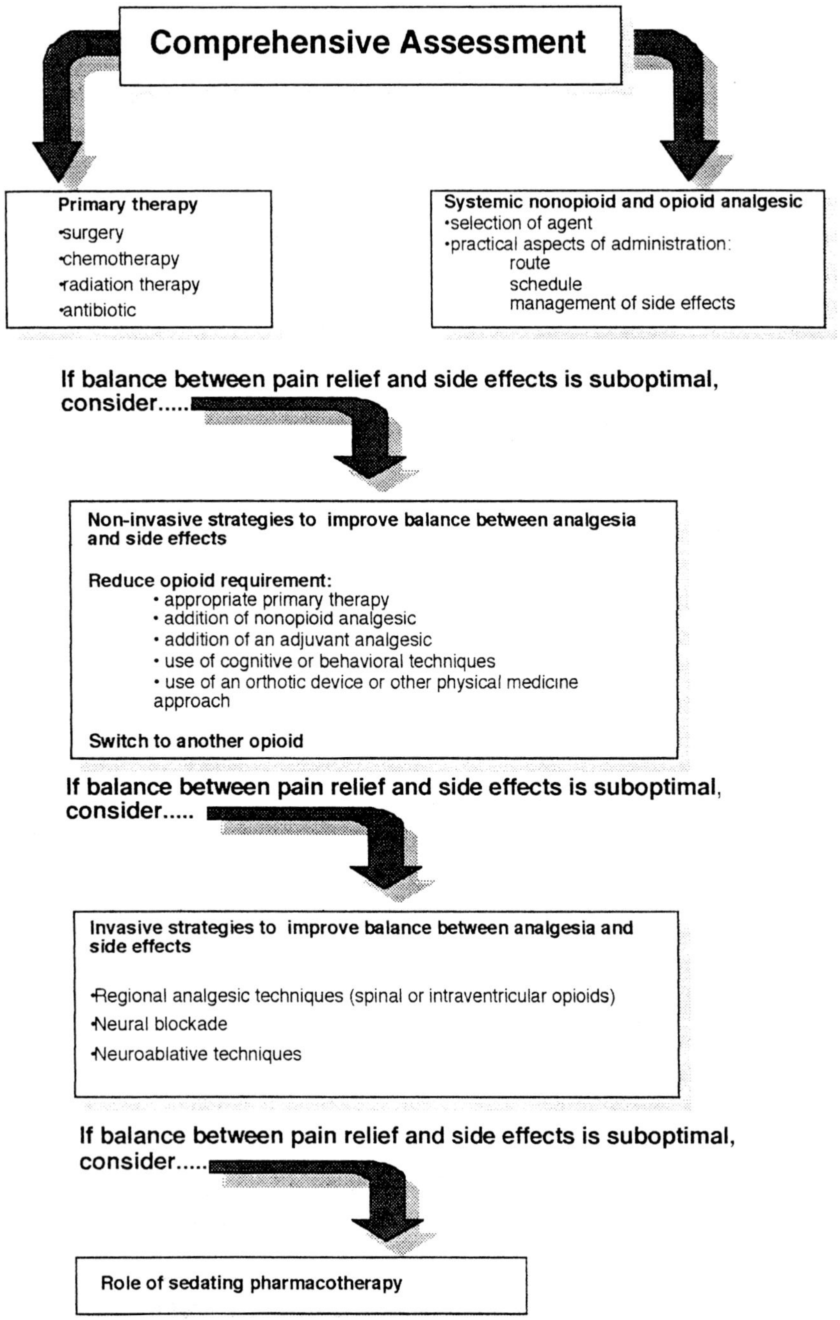

FIG. 70-7. Overview of an integrated approach to the management of cancer pain. (Adapted from Cherny NI, Portenoy RK. Cancer pain management: current strategy. Cancer 1993;72(Suppl):3393.)

treatment with surgery, radiation therapy, chemotherapy, or other novel approaches may be considered. Pain caused by infections may be amenable to antibiotic therapy or drainage procedures. If successful, such primary therapy can have profound analgesic consequences.

Radiation Therapy

Although in general it is true that radiation therapy has a pivotal role in the palliative treatment of bony metastases,[226,227] epidural spinal cord compression,[226] and cerebral metastases,[228] data specific to metastases arising from tumors of the gastrointestinal tract are not available. Guidelines for the evaluation of the role of palliative radiation therapy have been described: a high probability of efficacy should be anticipated, the treatment should not entail significant risk of adverse effects, the duration of treatment should be short, and the treatment should offer a greater palliative index than other available therapeutic modalities.[229] There is a paucity of data regarding the efficacy of radiation therapy in the management of pelvic plexopathy pain. There an impression that palliative radiation therapy for malignant lumbosacral plexopathy often yields partial relief of short duration.[229] The results with perineal pain caused by low sacral plexopathy and the phantom anus syndrome are more encouraging.[229–231] Hepatic radiation therapy, with 20 to 30 Gy, usually is well tolerated and can relieve the pain of hepatic capsular distention in 50% to 90% of patients,[232–236] and limited experience has been reported with simultaneous radiation and chemotherapy.[236] Radiation therapy may be of palliative value for some patients with unresectable pancreatic cancer.[237]

Chemotherapy

The therapeutic index of chemotherapy in the management of cancer pain is related to the balance between its antineoplastic efficacy and cost factors of toxicity and out-of-hospital opportunity cost.[238] In general, patients with advanced esophageal,[239] gastric,[240] colorectal,[241,242] pancreatic,[243] or hepatocellular[244,245] cancers have a relatively low probability of major tumor response to chemotherapy. Despite this, even among tumors that usually are considered relatively refractory, tumor response can be associated with a significant degree of pain relief.[246–249] If palliative chemotherapy is considered appropriate, it should be administered as a trial of therapy, additional to specific analgesic treatment. Squamous cell cancer of the anus, in contrast, can be highly responsive to combined modality treatment, and an impressive cure rate is reported even with advanced disease.[250,251] The response to salvage chemotherapy for recurrent anal cancer is variable, and long duration of the initial response is predictive of a higher probability of a second response.

Surgery

Surgery may have a role in relieving symptoms caused by specific mechanical problems, such as an obstructed hollow viscus, unstable bony structures, and compressed neural structures.[252–256] Against the potential benefits must be weighed the probability and duration of benefit, the direct risks of surgery, and the anticipated length of hospitalization and convalescence.[252] Clinical experience suggests that the surgical interventions of high palliative index include stabilization of pathologic fractures, relief of remediable bowel obstructions, and drainage of symptomatic ascites. Paracentesis may provide prompt relief from the pain and discomfort of tense ascites. The duration of relief usually is short unless large volumes are drained. Large-volume paracentesis, up to 5 to 10 L, can provide more durable palliation[252,257] and can be performed with small risk of hypotension[257,258] or diminution of serum protein levels.[259] Peritoneovenous shunts palliate malignant ascites in as many as 75% of patients with tolerable and acceptable morbidity.[260–262] The outlook for patients with ascites caused by gastric cancer is substantially better than that for patients with ascites caused by pancreatic or colorectal neoplasms.[263] Radical surgery to excise locally advanced disease in patients with no evidence of metastatic spread may be of both palliative and survival value in some patients.[264–266] Successful management of pain associated with uncontrollable recurrent pelvic tumors ulcerating through the perineum after radical surgical debridement with perineal reconstruction has been reported.[267]

Antibiotic Therapy

Antibiotics may be analgesic when the source of the pain involves infection. Illustrative examples include chronic sinus infections, pelvic abscesses, pyonephrosis, and osteitis pubis.[268,269] In some cases, infection is occult and confirmed only by the symptomatic relief provided by empiric treatment with these drugs.[270,271]

Analgesic Therapy: An Overview

For most patients, pain management involves the use of specific analgesic approaches. Systemic pharmacologic therapy is the mainstay and should be integrated with psychological and physiatric techniques.[16,65,272] Anesthetic and neurosurgical techniques should be considered for patients who have not obtained satisfactory pain relief. These analgesic treatments always must be integrated skillfully with the management of other symptoms.

The "Analgesic Ladder" Approach to Systemic Pharmacotherapy

An expert committee convened by the Cancer Unit of the World Health Organization has proposed a useful approach to drug selection for cancer pain, which has become known as the *analgesic ladder*.[272] When combined with appropriate dosing guidelines, this approach is capable of providing adequate relief to 70% to 90% of patients.[273–277] Emphasizing that pain intensity should be the prime consideration in analgesic selection, the approach advocates three basic steps (Fig. 70-8):

Step 1: Patients with mild to moderate cancer-related pain should be treated with a nonopioid analgesic, which should be combined with an adjuvant analgesic if a specific indica-

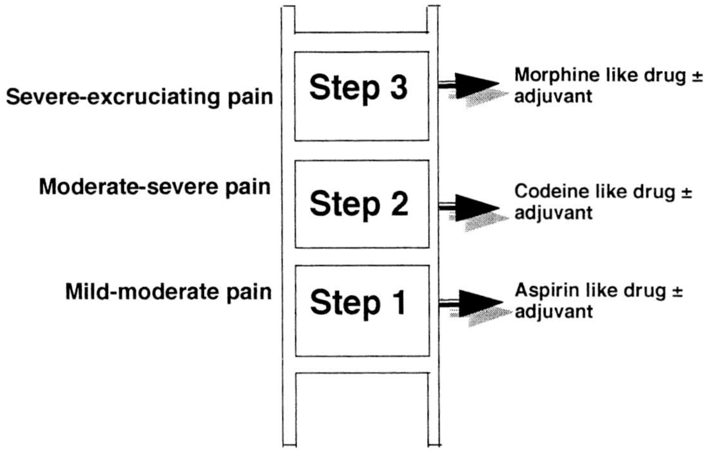

FIG. 70-8. World Health Organization three-step analgesic ladder. (Adapted from World Health Organization. Cancer pain relief. Geneva: World Health Organization, 1986.)

tion for one exists. For example, a patient with continual leg pains of mild to moderate intensity caused by postradiation lumbosacral plexopathy may benefit from a tricyclic antidepressant agent in addition to acetaminophen.

Step 2: Patients who are relatively nontolerant and have moderate to severe pain, or who fail to achieve adequate relief after a trial of a nonopioid analgesic, should be treated with a so-called weak opioid (eg, codeine, oxycodone, propoxyphene); this drug typically is combined with a nonopioid and may be coadministered with an adjuvant analgesic.

Step 3: Patients who have severe pain, or fail to achieve adequate relief after appropriate administration of drugs on the second rung of the analgesic ladder, should receive a so-called strong opioid, which also may be combined with a nonopioid analgesic or an adjuvant drug.

Systemic Analgesic Pharmacotherapy

Nonopioid Analgesics

General Considerations

The nonopioid analgesics are useful alone for mild to moderate pain (step 1 of the analgesic ladder) and provide additive analgesia when combined with opioid drugs in the treatment of more severe pain. Unlike opioid analgesics, these drugs have a ''ceiling'' effect for analgesia and produce neither tolerance nor physical dependence. The nonopioid analgesics comprise numerous subclasses (Table 70-7). Some of these agents, such as aspirin and the nonsteroidal antiinflammatory drugs (NSAIDs), inhibit the enzyme cyclooxygenase and consequently block the biosynthesis of prostaglandins, inflammatory mediators known to sensitize peripheral nociceptors.[278] A central mechanism also is probable,[279] and appears to predominate in acetaminophen analgesia.[280]

Dosing

The optimal administration of nonopioid analgesics requires an understanding of their clinical pharmacology,[281] including potential adverse effects. To reduce the risk of therapy, it is reasonable to begin treatment with a relatively low dosage and then explore the dose-response relation through gradual dosage escalation.

Drug Selection

The great variability in the response to different NSAIDs suggests that the patient's prior experience with one or more agents should be considered when a drug is selected. If cost is a factor in selection, aspirin and acetaminophen are far less expensive than the NSAIDs. In a patient who has a bleeding diathesis and a strong indication for an antiinflammatory drug, the nonacetylated salicylates, such as choline magnesium trisalicylate and salsalate, are preferred. These drugs have less effect on platelet aggregation and no effect on bleeding time at usual clinical dosages.[282] Fixed dosing regimens are not required by all patients, and the availability of drugs with short half-lives, including aspirin, acetaminophen, and ibuprofen, allows ''as-needed'' administration for those who would benefit from this approach.

Adverse Effects

Safe administration of these agents requires familiarity with their potential adverse effects.[281] Aspirin and the other NSAIDs have a broad spectrum of potential toxicities; bleeding diathesis caused by inhibition of platelet aggregation, peptic ulcer disease, and renal impairment are the most common. Uncommon adverse effects include confusion, precipitation of cardiac failure, and exacerbation of hypertension. Patients at increased risk for adverse effects, including those with blood-clotting disorders, predilection to peptic ulceration, impaired renal function, concurrent corticosteroid therapy, and advanced age, require particular caution when these agents are administered. Acetaminophen has fewer adverse effects than the acidic nonopioid analgesics; gastrointestinal toxicity is rare and there are no adverse effects on platelet function. Hepatic toxicity is possible, however, and patients with chronic alcoholism and liver disease can experience severe hepatotoxicity even when the drug is given in the usual therapeutic dosages.[283]

TABLE 70-7. *Commonly used nonopioid analgesics*

Chemical class	Generic name	Half-life (h)	Starting dosage (mg)	Maximum recommended dose (mg/d)	Comments
Nonacidic	Acetaminophen	3–4	750 q4h	6000	Available over the counter
Salicylates	Aspirin	3–12*	650 q4–6h	6000	Available over the counter
	Diflunisal	8–12	500 q12h	1500	Less GI toxicity than aspirin
	Choline magnesium trisalicylate	8–12	1000 q12h	4000	Minimal GI toxicity; no effect on platelet function at usual dosages
	Salsalate	8–12	1000 q12h	4000	Minimal GI toxicity; no effect on platelet function at usual dosages; available over the counter
Propionic acids	Ibuprofen	3–4	400 q6h	4200	
	Naproxen	1–3	250 q12h	1000	
	Fenoprofen	2–3	200 q6h	3200	
Acetic acids	Indomethacin	4–5	25 q12h	200	Sustained-release and rectal preparations
	Sulindac	14	150 q12h	400	
	Diclofenac	2	25 q8h	200	
	Ketorolac	4–7	30 q6h	240	Oral or parenteral preparation
Oxicams	Piroxicam	45	20 q24h	40	

GI, gastrointestinal.

Adapted from Cherny NI, Portenoy RK. Pharmacotherapy of cancer pain. In: Arbit E, ed. Management of cancer-related pain. Mount Kisko, NY: Futura, 1993:65.

Opioid Analgesics: Introductory Remarks

A trial of opioid therapy should be administered to all patients with pain of moderate or greater severity, irrespective of the pathophysiologic mechanism underlying the pain.[26,284–286]

Opioid Classification

The pure agonist opioid drugs have no ceiling effect to analgesia. As the dosage is increased, analgesic effects increase, until analgesia is achieved or intolerable adverse effects (eg, confusion, sedation, myoclonus, respiratory depression) supervene. Furthermore, the increase in analgesic effect occurs as a log-linear function: dosage increments on a semi-logarithmic scale yield linear increases in analgesia.[26] The efficacy of any particular drug in a specific patient is determined by the degree of analgesia produced after dosage escalation before the development of unmanageable side effects.

The mixed agonist-antagonist opioids (pentazocine, nalbuphine, and butorphanol) and the partial agonist opioids (buprenorphine and probably dezocine) play a minor role in the management of cancer pain.[65,287] The factors limiting their utility in this setting include the existence of a ceiling effect for analgesia, the precipitation of withdrawal in patients physically dependent on opioid agonists, and the problem of dose-dependent psychotomimetic side effects.[287]

Relative Potency and Equianalgesic Doses

Relative analgesic potency is the ratio of the dose of two analgesics required to produce the same analgesic effect. By convention, the relative potency of each of the commonly used opioids is based on a comparison with 10 mg of parenteral morphine.[288] Knowledge of equianalgesic doses (see Chap. 95, Table 70-8) is essential for dose selection when the drug or route of administration is changed.

Commonly Used Opioid Agonist Drugs (Table 70-8)

Codeine

Codeine is the most commonly used opioid analgesic for the management of mild to moderate pain. It is the standard drug against which all drugs for mild or moderate pain are compared. It is used most commonly in combination with aspirin or acetaminophen.[289] Thirty milligrams of oral codeine is equivalent to 650 mg of aspirin, and the combination of 30 mg of codeine and 650 mg of aspirin yields an analgesic effect that equals or exceeds that produced by 60 mg of codeine.[290] The plasma half-life of codeine is 2 to 4 hours and its duration of action is 3 to 6 hours. The predominant metabolite of codeine is codeine-6-glucuronide. Minor metabolites include norcodeine, morphine, morphine-3-glucuronide, morphine-6-glucuronide, and normorphine.[291]

TABLE 70-8. *Opioid agonist drugs*

Drug	Dosage equianalgesic to 10 mg of intramuscular morphine			Duration of action
	IM (Mg)	PO (mg)	Half-life (h)	
Codeine	130	200	2–3	2–4
Oxycodone	15	30	2–3	2–4
Propoxyphene	100	50	2–3	2–4
Morphine	10	30 (repeated dose) 60 (single dose)	2–3	3–4
Hydromorphone	1.5	7.5	2–3	2–4
Methadone	10	20	15–190	4–8
Meperidine	75	300	2–3	2–4
Oxymorphone	1	10 (PR)	2–3	3–4
Levorphanol	2	4	12–15	4–8
Fentanyl transdermal system		*		48–72

IM, intramuscularly; *PO,* orally. *PR,* Rectally.
* Transdermal fentanyl 100 μg/h; morphine 4 mg/h.

Oxycodone

Oral oxycodone has an analgesic potency that is comparable to morphine.[292,293] Oral oxycodone, in combination with aspirin or acetaminophen in products that provide 5 mg of oxycodone per tablet, is a useful drug for moderate pain in step 2 of the analgesic ladder. It also is available as a single tablet or syrup, however, and doses can be escalated to effectively manage severe pain.[294] In some countries, oxycodone pectinate is available as a rectal suppository. Using available oral formulations, this drug usually requires 3- to 4-hour dosing, although a sustained-release formulation of oral oxycodone is under development and should be available soon.

Propoxyphene (Dextropropoxyphene)

Propoxyphene is a congener of methadone. It is metabolized to norpropoxyphene, which has a long half-life and is associated with excitatory effects, including tremulousness and seizures.[295] These effects are dose-related and do not appear to pose a clinical problem at the doses of propoxyphene typically administered for moderate pain in the nontolerant patient.[289]

Morphine

Based on its availability and clinician familiarity with its use, morphine has been designated the prototypical agent for step III of the analgesic ladder.[272] The World Health Organization has placed oral morphine on the Essential Drug List, and preparations are available for oral, rectal, parenteral, and intraspinal administration.

Morphine undergoes glucuronidation at the 3 and 6 positions. Morphine-3-glucuronide is the major metabolite.[296] Morphine-3-glucuronide is not an analgesic and may be an opioid antagonist.[297] There is increasing evidence that morphine-3-glucuronide levels may be associated with adverse effects.[298] Morphine-6-glucuronide binds to opioid receptors[299] and produces potent opioid effects in animals[299–301] and man.[299,302–305] Morphine-6-glucuronide excretion by the kidney is related directly to calculated creatinine clearance.[304] In patients with impaired renal function, high concentrations of morphine-6-glucuronide have been associated with toxicity.[302,306,307] Although further studies are needed to clarify the clinical importance of this and other metabolites, the data available are adequate to recommend caution when administering morphine to patients with renal impairment.

Single-dose studies of morphine in postoperative patients with cancer demonstrated an IM-to-oral potency ratio of 1 : 6.[308] However, both bioavailability data[293,309–311] and surveys of patients receiving the drug long-term suggest that a ratio of 1 : 3 or 1 : 2 is more appropriate.[312,313]

The development of slow-release morphine preparations, which can be administered on an 8- or 12-hour schedule, has had a major effect on clinical practice. These preparations provide improved convenience of dosing and can be particularly useful in eliminating the need for frequent dosing during the nighttime hours.[314] Controlled-release morphine should not be used to titrate the dose rapidly in patients with severe pain. At least 24 hours is required to approach steady-state plasma concentrations after dosing is initiated or changed, and these kinetics may complicate efforts to identify the appropriate dose rapidly. Dose finding in these situations is performed more efficiently with an immediate-release morphine preparation.[315] When the effective dose is identified, the patient can be changed over to a controlled-release preparation using a milligram-to-milligram conversion.[315]

Hydromorphone

Hydromorphone is another morphine congener with a short half-life that is a useful alternative to morphine. Hydromorphone is a versatile drug that can be administered by the oral, rectal, parenteral, and intraspinal routes. Because of its significant solubility and the availability of a high-concentration preparation (10 mg/mL), it has been used widely by SC infusion. A study has demonstrated that its bioavailability by continuous SC infusion is about 78% of its bioavailability by the IV route.[316] A sustained-release formulation of hydromorphone is under development and should be available soon.[317,318]

Meperidine (Pethidine)

Meperidine is a synthetic opioid agonist with a short half-life and a profile of potential adverse effects that limits its utility as an analgesic for chronic cancer pain. Meperidine is *N*-demethylated to normeperidine, which is an active metabolite that is twice as potent as a convulsant and half as potent as an analgesic compared with its parent compound. The accumulation of normeperidine after repetitive dosing of meperidine can result in central nervous system excitability characterized by subtle mood effects, tremors, multifocal myoclonus, and, occasionally, seizures.[319–321] Although the accumulation of normeperidine is most likely to affect patients with overt renal disease, toxicity sometimes is observed in patients with normal renal function.[319,322] These potential adverse effects are a relative contraindication to the use of meperidine in the management of chronic cancer pain.[82] Given the availability of alternative drugs that lack these toxicities, its use in the management of acute pain also can be questioned.[95]

Fentanyl

Fentanyl is a semi-synthetic opioid characterized by high potency and lipophilia. Fentanyl has been used parenterally and intraspinally to manage postoperative and obstetric pain. The development of a transdermal system (see later) has broadened its clinical utility to the treatment of patients with chronic cancer pain.[323–325] A transmucosal preparation is under development and may be useful in the management of acute pain, including "breakthrough" pain in the cancer population.[326]

Oxymorphone

Oxymorphone is another congener of morphine with a short half-life. Injectable and rectal formulations are available in the United States. Oxymorphone is less likely to produce histamine release than is morphine,[327,328] and may have particular utility for patients who experience itching in response to other opioids.[329]

Levorphanol

Levorphanol is a morphine congener with a long half-life (12 to 16 hours). Similar to methadone, drug accumulation may follow the initiation of therapy or dosage escalation. Levorphanol is used commonly as a second-line agent in patients with chronic pain who cannot tolerate morphine. The possibility that this drug may be particularly useful in morphine-tolerant patients has been proposed on the basis of its affinity for receptors (kappa-3 and delta) that presumably are not involved in morphine analgesia.[330]

Methadone

Methadone is a synthetic opioid with a long plasma half-life, which averages about 24 hours (range, 13 hours to more than 100 hours).[331] This long half-life notwithstanding, most patients require dosing at 4- to 8-hour intervals to maintain analgesic effects.[332] After treatment is initiated or the dosage is increased, the plasma concentration rises for a prolonged period, and this may be associated with delayed onset of side effects.[333,334] Serious adverse effects can be avoided if the initial period of dosing is accomplished with as-needed administration and patients are monitored carefully. When a steady state has been achieved, the scheduled dose frequency should be determined by the duration of analgesia after each dose. Oral and parenteral preparations of methadone are available. However, the SC route usually is not recommended because the infusion of methadone often is associated with the development of local skin toxicity.[335]

Practical Guidelines in Opioid Therapy

Optimal use of opioid analgesics requires a sound understanding of the pharmacologic characteristics of each of the commonly used drugs and principles of administration, including drug selection, routes of administration, dosing and dose titration, and adverse effects and their management.

Opioid Selection

Moderate Pain

Patients with moderate pain commonly are treated with a combination product containing acetaminophen or aspirin plus a conventional step 2 opioid (codeine, oxycodone, or propoxyphene).[16,272] The doses of these combination products can be increased until the maximum dose of the nonopioid coanalgesic is attained (e.g. 4000 mg of acetaminophen); beyond this dose, the opioid contained in the combination product could be increased as a single agent, or the patient could be switched to an opioid conventionally used in step 3.

Severe or Excruciating Pain

Patients who have severe pain usually are treated with an opioid customarily used in step 3 of the analgesic ladder. For patients without major organ failure who are opioid-naive, any of the available agonist opioids can be selected. Opioid agonists with short half-lives (morphine, hydromorphone, fentanyl, oxycodone, and oxymorphone) usually are favored because they are easier to titrate than drugs with long half-lives, which require a longer period to approach steady-state plasma concentrations. Among the opioids with short half-lives, the range of available formulations often influences specific drug selection. For example, although oxycodone is a versatile opioid agonist, when patients require high doses, the oral formulations available in the United States cannot be administered conveniently and no parenteral formulation is available. For ambulatory patients who are able to tolerate oral opioids, morphine sulfate often is preferred because it has a short half-life and is easy to titrate in its immediate-release form, and it also is available as a controlled-release preparation that allows an 8- to 12-hour dosing interval. The drugs with long half-lives (methadone and levorphanol) usually are not considered first-line therapy because they can be difficult to titrate and present challenging management problems if delayed toxicity develops as plasma concentrations rise gradually after dose increments.

It always is important to review the response to previous trials of opioid therapy. If the current opioid is well tolerated, it usually is continued unless difficulties in dose titration occur or the required dose cannot be administered conveniently. If dose-limiting side effects develop, a trial of an alternative opioid should be considered. In a prospective survey of 100 consecutive inpatients treated by pain service physicians at Memorial Sloan-Kettering Cancer Center, 44 required trials of two or more systemically administered opioid drugs, and 20 required sequential trials of three or more opioids to optimize the balance between analgesia and side effects. Switches were made when dose-limiting toxicity developed in the setting of uncontrolled (43%) or controlled pain (27%), or when a more convenient opioid regimen was desirable (25%). The existence of different degrees of incomplete cross-tolerance to various receptor-mediated opioid effects (analgesia and side effects) may explain the utility of these sequential trials.[336–339] To implement the technique of sequential opioid trials, clinicians should be familiar with at least three opioid drugs used in the management of severe pain and have the ability to calculate appropriate starting doses using equianalgesic dosing data.

Patients with renal impairment may accumulate the active metabolites of propoxyphene (norpropoxyphene), meperidine (normeperidine), and morphine (morphine-6-glucuronide). Particular caution is required in the administration of these drugs to such patients.[302,306,340–343]

Routes of Systemic Opioid Administration

Opioids should be administered by the least invasive and safest route capable of providing adequate analgesia. In a survey of patients with advanced cancer, more than half required two or more routes of administration before death, and almost one fourth required three or more routes.[75] Changes in the route of administration, particularly between the oral and parenteral routes, require careful attention to relative potency (see Table 70-8). Whenever possible, it is prudent to perform the switch in a gradual, stepwise manner over a 2- to 3-day period.

Oral

The oral route of opioid administration remains the most important and appropriate in routine practice. Most patients can use the oral route throughout most of their illness. Orally administered drugs have a slower onset of action, delayed peak time, and longer duration of effect than parenterally administered drugs. Although the time to peak effect depends on the drug and the nature of the formulation, for most immediate-release oral formulations, peak effect typically is achieved after 60 minutes.[344,345] The oral route of drug administration is not appropriate in patients who have impaired swallowing or gastrointestinal obstruction, and some patients who require the rapid onset of analgesia after each dose may not benefit significantly from this route.

Rectal

The rectal route is a noninvasive alternative to the parenteral route for patients who are unable to take oral opioids.[346,347] Rectal suppositories containing hydromorphone, oxymorphone, and morphine are available in the United States (oxycodone suppositories are available in Australia), and controlled-release morphine tablets also can be administered rectally.[348] The potency of opioids administered rectally approximates that achieved with oral dosing.[349]

Transdermal

The transdermal route of administration is another noninvasive alternative for patients who are unable to tolerate oral medication.[325] The first opioid available by the transdermal route is fentanyl. The transdermal system consists of a drug reservoir that is separated from the skin by a copolymer membrane that controls the rate of drug delivery to the skin surface. Drug is released into the skin at a nearly constant amount per unit time. The dosing interval for each system usually is 72 hours, but interindividual pharmacokinetic variability is large,[324,350,351] and some patients require a dosing interval of 48 hours. Empirically, the indications for the transdermal route include intolerance of oral medication, poor compliance with oral medication, and, occasionally, the desire to provide a trial of fentanyl to patients who have reacted unfavorably to other opioids.[325] The 12-hour delay until peak effect limits the utility of this route for patients with unstable pain problems.

Sublingual

The sublingual approach has limited utility because of the lack of true sublingual formulations in the United States, poor absorption of most drugs, and the inability to deliver high doses or prevent swallowing of the dose.[346,352] Sublingual administration of an injectable formulation occasionally is used in relatively nontolerant patients who transiently lose the option of oral dosing. On the basis of bioavailability data, sublingual absorption appears to be best with lipophilic opioids such as fentanyl or methadone.[352]

Parenteral

Parenteral routes of administration should be considered for patients who have impaired swallowing or gastrointestinal obstruction, patients who require the rapid onset of analgesia, and highly tolerant patients who require doses that cannot be administered conveniently otherwise. Repeated bolus injections can be administered by the IV, IM, or SC routes. However, they may be associated with prominent "bolus" effects (toxicity at peak concentration or pain breakthrough at the trough). Although repetitive IM injections are a common practice, they are painful and offer no pharmacokinetic advantage, and are not recommended.[82,95] Repeated bolus doses, if required, can be accomplished without frequent skin punctures through the use of an indwelling IV or SC infusion device. To deliver repeated

SC injections, a 27-gauge infusion device (a butterfly) can be left under the skin for up to a week.[105,353,354]

Continuous infusions avoid the problems associated with the bolus effect and may be administered by the IV or SC route.[105,353–357] Ambulatory infusion devices vary in complexity, cost, and ability to provide patient-controlled "rescue doses" as an adjunct to a continuous basal infusion (see later). Opioids suitable for continuous SC infusion must be soluble, well absorbed, and nonirritating. Extensive experience has been reported with heroin, hydromorphone, oxymorphone, and morphine.[316,354,356–360] Methadone often produces a local inflammatory reaction and is not recommended for SC infusion.[335] Studies suggest that dosing with SC administration can proceed in a manner identical to continuous IV infusion: a postoperative study that compared patients who received an identical dose of morphine by IV or SC infusion found no difference in blood levels,[361] and a controlled study of hydromorphone calculated a bioavailability of 78% for the SC route and observed that analgesic outcome was identical during IV or SC infusion.[316] To maintain the comfort of an infusion site, the SC infusion rate should not exceed 5 mL/h. Patients who require high doses may benefit from the use of concentrated solutions, which, in selected cases, can be compounded specifically for continuous SC infusion.

Continuous IV infusion may be the most appropriate way of delivering an opioid when a large volume of solution is needed or when methadone is used. If continuous IV infusion must be continued on a long-term basis, a permanent central venous port is recommended.

Continuous infusions of drug combinations may be indicated when pain is accompanied by nausea, anxiety, or agitation. In such cases, an antiemetic, neuroleptic, or anxiolytic can be combined with an opioid provided it is nonirritant, miscible, and stable in combined solution. Experience has been reported with infusions of an opioid combined with metoclopramide, haloperidol, scopolamine, cyclizine, methotrimeprazine, chlorpromazine, and midazolam.[354,362–364]

Opioid Scheduling and Dosing

Schedule of Administration

Patients with continuous or frequently recurring pain usually benefit from scheduled "around-the-clock" dosing. Clinical vigilance is required, however, in patients with no previous opioid exposure and in those who are given drugs with long half-lives. With drugs that have long half-lives, such as methadone, delayed toxicity may develop as the plasma concentration rises slowly toward steady-state levels.[331]

All patients who receive an around-the-clock opioid regimen also should be offered a rescue dose, a supplemental dose given on an as-needed basis to treat pain that breaks through the regular schedule. The integration of scheduled dosing with rescue doses provides a method for safe and rational stepwise dosage escalation and is applicable to all routes of opioid administration (Table 70-9). The rescue drug typically is identical to that administered on a continuous basis, with the exception of transdermal fentanyl and methadone; the use of an alternative opioid with a short half-life is recommended for the rescue dose when these drugs are used. The frequency with which the rescue dose can be offered depends on the time to peak effect for the drug and on the route of administration. Oral rescue doses can be offered as often as every 1 to 2 hours and parenteral rescue doses can be offered as often as every 15 to 30 minutes. Clinical experience suggests that the size of the rescue dose should be equivalent to about 5% to 15% of the 24-hour baseline dose.

Controlled-release formulations can lessen the inconvenience associated with around-the-clock drug administration.[314] These formulations should not be used to titrate the dose rapidly in patients with severe pain. Controlled-release oral morphine sulfate and transdermal fentanyl are used widely, and new controlled-release formulations of oxycodone and hydromorphone are under development.[317,318] Although controlled-release preparations of morphine sulfate typically achieve peak plasma levels 3 to 5 hours after a dose and have a duration of effect of 8 to 12 hours,[365] newer formulations achieve lower peak levels and have a longer duration of effect.[366] An immediate-release formulation of an opioid with a short half-life (usually the same drug) usually is used as the rescue medication (see Table 70-9). Controlled-release and immediate-release formulations of oral morphine are dose-equivalent; a switch from one to the other is done on a milligram-to-milligram basis when the effective around-the-clock dose is identified.

In some limited situations, an as-needed dosing regimen alone can be recommended. This type of dosing provides additional safety during the initiation of opioid therapy in the opioid-naive patient, particularly when rapid dosage escalation is needed or a drug with a long half-life is administered. This technique is strongly recommended when initiating methadone therapy.

Patient-controlled analgesia is a technique of parenteral drug administration in which the patient controls a pump that delivers bolus doses of an analgesic according to parameters set by the physician. Use of a patient-controlled analgesia device allows the patient to titrate the opioid dose carefully to his or her individual analgesic needs. The technique is used most commonly to manage acute postoperative pain. Long-term patient-controlled analgesia in patients with cancer is accomplished by the SC or IV route using an ambulatory infusion device. The more technologically advanced of these devices have programmable variables, including infusion rate, rescue dose, and lockout interval.[105] The option for bolus dosing typically is administered in conjunction with a continuous opioid infusion.[357,367]

Starting Dose

A patient who is relatively nontolerant, having had only some exposure to a weak opioid, usually should begin taking one of the strong opioids at a dose equivalent to 5 to 10 mg of IM morphine every 3 to 4 hours. If morphine is used, an IM-to-oral relative potency ratio for morphine of 1 : 3 is conventional. If a switch from one opioid drug to another is required, the equianalgesic dose table (see Table 70-8) is used as a guide. For patients with good pain control but unacceptable side effects, the starting dose of the new drug should be reduced to 50% to 75% of the equianalgesic dose to account for incomplete cross-tolerance. For patients with poor pain control and unacceptable side effects, the starting dose of the new drug usually can be 75% to 100% of the equianalgesic dose. Clinical experi-

TABLE 70-9. *Examples of stepwise close escalation of morphine sulfate administered as oral immediate-release preparation, oral controlled-release preparation, and continuous infusion*

	Oral immediate release		Oral controlled-release (with immediate-release rescue closing)		Subcutaneous infusion (with subcutaneous rescue doses)	
Step*	"Around the clock" dose (mg q4h)	Rescue dose (mg q1h prn)	"Around the clock" dose (mg)	Rescue dose (mg q1h prn)	Around the clock" infusion (mg/h)	Rescue dose (mg q20 min prn)
1	10	5	30 q12h	7.5	3	2.0
2	15	7.5	30 q8h	15.0	5	2.5
3	30	15.0	60 q12h	15.0	7	3.5
4	45	22.5	100 q12h	30.0	10	5.0
5	60	30.0	100 q8h	30.0	15	7.5
6	90	45.0	200 q12h	45.0	20	10.0
7	120	60.0	200 q8h	60.0	30	15.0

* Indications for progression from one step to the next: requirement of >2 rescue doses in any 4-h interval; and requirement of >6 rescue doses in 24 h.

Adapted from Cherny NI, Portenoy RK. Cancer pain management: current strategy. Cancer 1993;72 (Suppl): 3393.

ence suggests that additional caution is needed when the change is to methadone; a reduction to 25% to 50% of the equianalgesic dose is prudent. After any change from one opioid to another, the patient must be monitored to assess the adequacy of analgesia and to detect the development of side effects. Subsequent dose adjustments usually are necessary.

Dose Titration

The persistence of inadequate pain relief should be addressed through a stepwise escalation of the opioid dosage until adequate analgesia is reported or unmanageable side effects supervene. Because opioid response increases linearly with the log of the dose, dosage escalations of less than 30% to 50% are not likely to improve analgesia significantly. In most cases, gradual dosage escalation identifies a favorable balance between analgesia and side effects that remains stable for a prolonged period.[6,368] Although doses can become extremely large during this process, the absolute dose is immaterial as long as the balance between analgesia and side effects remains favorable. In one retrospective study of patients with advanced cancer, the average daily opioid requirement was equivalent to 400 to 600 mg of IM morphine, but about 10% of patients required more than 2000 mg and one patient required more than 35,000 mg per 24 hours.[75] Patients who experience dose-limiting side effects during dose titration require the use of another analgesic approach or a technique to reduce opioid toxicity (see later).

The severity of the pain should determine the rate of dose titration. Patients with severe pain can be treated by repeated parenteral dosing every 15 to 30 minutes until the pain is partially relieved. Guidelines have been proposed for the calculation of hourly maintenance dosing after parenteral loading with an opioid with a short half-life.[369] These guidelines recommend that the starting hourly maintenance dosage be approximated by dividing the total loading dose by twice the elimination half-life of the drug. For example, the starting maintenance dosage for a patient who has required an IV loading dose of morphine sulfate of 30 mg (half-life, about 3 hours) would be 5 mg/h. Patients with moderate pain, who are treated with opioids with short half-lives, can undergo dosage increases as often as twice daily. The dosage of controlled-release preparations of oral morphine or transdermal fentanyl can be increased every 24 to 48 hours.

The Development of Tolerance

Physicians and patients frequently are concerned that tolerance will develop to the analgesic effect of the drug and that this will necessitate rapid dosage escalation, which may continue until the drug is no longer useful. However, most patients who require an escalation in dosage to manage increasing pain have demonstrable progression of disease.[368,370,371] True pharmacologic tolerance to the analgesic effect of an opioid, in which exposure to the opioid is inferred to be the "driving force" for dosage escalation, can be said to occur only if a patient manifests the need for increasing opioid doses in the absence of other factors that would be capable of explaining the increase in opioid requirement (eg, progressive disease, psychological factors, pharmacokinetic factors). Analgesic tolerance does occur, but it seldom is the dominant factor in the need for opioid dosage escalation. There are two important implications of this observation: concern about tolerance should not impede the use of opioids early in the course of the disease, and worsening pain in a patient receiving a stable dosage of opioids usually should be assessed as presumptive evidence of disease progression or, less commonly, increasing psychological distress or delirium.[372]

Adverse Effects and Their Management

Successful opioid therapy requires that the benefits of analgesia and other desirable effects clearly outweigh treatment-related adverse effects. This implies that a detailed understanding of adverse opioid effects, and strategies to prevent and manage them, are essential skills for all involved in cancer pain management.

Respiratory Depression

Respiratory depression is potentially the most serious adverse effect of opioid therapy. Respiratory depression occurs as a consequence of the activation of specific receptors (mu-2) in the lower brain stem,[373] and may result in the impairment of all phases of respiratory activity (rate, minute volume, and tidal exchange). With repeated administration, tolerance to this effect develops, and it is a rare event in the patient with cancer whose opioid dosage is titrated carefully against pain.

Clinically significant respiratory depression always is accompanied by other signs of central nervous system depression, including sedation and mental clouding. Respiratory compromise accompanied by tachypnea and anxiety never is a primary opioid event. When respiratory depression occurs in such patients, alternative explanations (eg, pneumonia, pulmonary embolism) should be sought. Opioid-induced respiratory depression also can occur if the stimulus of the pain is removed suddenly (eg, after neurolytic procedures) and the opioid dosage is not reduced.

If clinically significant respiratory depression occurs, naloxone should be used to improve ventilation. The goal of this therapy is to improve respiration without causing systemic withdrawal. A small bolus injection of dilute naloxone (0.4 mg in 10 mL of saline solution) should be titrated against the respiratory rate. In the comatose patient, an endotracheal tube should be placed to assist ventilation and prevent aspiration. Specific caution is required for the patient who has received long-term meperidine therapy, because naloxone may precipitate seizures by blocking the depressant action of meperidine and allowing the convulsant activity of normeperidine to be manifest.[374] If the patient can be aroused, and the peak plasma levels of the opioid already have been reached, the opioid dose should be withheld and the patient monitored until improvement is observed.

Sedation, Cognitive Impairment, and Delirium

The initiation of opioid therapy or significant dosage escalation often is associated with somnolence or cognitive impairment that usually persists for days to weeks.[375] Although tolerance usually develops, some patients continue to have intolerable effects, particularly if other contributing factors exist. These factors include the use of other sedating drugs, and coexistent diseases such as dementia, metabolic encephalopathy, or brain metastases.

A stepwise management strategy is useful:

1. Eliminate nonessential central nervous system depressant medications and evaluate the patient for concurrent causes, including sepsis, metabolic derangement, and intracerebral or leptomeningeal metastases.
2. If analgesia is satisfactory, reduce the opioid dosage by 25%.
3. If analgesia is unsatisfactory, switch to a different opioid drug.
4. If analgesia is satisfactory and lethargy persists, consider the addition of a psychostimulant, such as methylphenidate (starting dose, 5 to 10 mg twice daily),[376,377] dextroamphetamine (starting dose, 5 to 10 mg twice daily),[378] or pemoline (starting dose, 18.75 to 35.5 mg twice daily).[379]
5. If the patient is hallucinating or delirious, switch to a different opioid drug and consider a trial of haloperidol (starting dose, 0.5 mg three times daily).
6. If these problems persist, consider the addition of a nonopioid or adjuvant analgesic (which may allow a reduction in the opioid dosage), a switch to a different opioid drug, or an anesthetic or neurolytic technique.[71]

Constipation

Constipation is the most common adverse effect encountered during long-term opioid therapy.[65,68,224,380,381] Opioids bind to peripheral receptors in the gut, prolonging colonic transit time by increasing segmental contractions and decreasing propulsive peristalsis, and reducing intraluminal fluid content by increasing salt and water absorption across the intestinal mucosa. Central opioid receptors also presumably are involved in colonic transit and the urge to defecate.[382,383] The probability of opioid-induced constipation is so great that laxative medications should be prescribed prophylactically to most patients.[65,68,224,343,380,381,384,385] The differential diagnosis of constipation includes ileus and mechanical obstruction (caused by tumor or adhesions). Rectal impaction by fecal matter and the finding of extensive fecal shadowing on abdominal radiographs suggest a diagnosis of constipation.

Recommendations for laxative therapy are empiric.[386] A combination of a softening agent (docusate) and a cathartic (eg, senna, bisocodyl, phenolphthalein) frequently is used. The dosages of these drugs should be increased as necessary, and an osmotic laxative (eg, lactulose, a magnesium-containing product) can be added if needed. Occasional patients are managed with intermittent colonic lavage using an oral bowel preparation such as Golytely. Rare patients who are refractory to laxative therapy can undergo a trial of oral naloxone, which has a bioavailability of less than 3% and presumably acts selectively on opioid receptors in the gut.[380,387] Because there is a small risk of systemic withdrawal from oral naloxone,[387] the initial dosage should be conservative (0.8 to 1.2 mg once or twice daily); this dosage can be escalated slowly until favorable effects occur or abdominal cramps, diarrhea, or any other adverse effect develops. Naloxone should not be used in any patient with bowel obstruction.

Nausea and Vomiting

In ambulatory patients, the incidence of nausea and vomiting has been estimated to be 10% to 40% and 15% to 40%, respectively.[388] Three putative mechanisms may produce nausea and vomiting: a direct effect on the chemoreceptor trigger zone, enhanced vestibular sensitivity, and delayed gastric emptying. If nausea is associated with early satiety, bloating, or postprandial vomiting, all of which are features of delayed gastric emptying, metoclopramide is the most reasonable initial treatment. Patients with vertigo, or prominent movement-induced nausea, may benefit from the use of an antivertiginous drug, such as scopolamine or meclizine. If there are no prominent signs of gastroparesis or vestibular dysfunction, treatment usually is begun with a neuroleptic, such as prochlorperazine or metoclopramide. If these drugs are ineffective at relatively high dosages, other options include a trial of an alternative opioid or treatment with an antihistamine (eg, diphenhydramine, hydroxyzine); a neuroleptic (eg, haloperidol, chlorpromazine, droperidol); a benzodiazepine (eg, lorazepam); a corticosteroid (eg, dexamethasone); or a serotonin antagonist (eg, ondansetron, tropisetron).

Myoclonus

Myoclonus is a dose-related adverse effect of all opioids. Mild and infrequent myoclonus is common, and may resolve spontaneously with the development of tolerance to this effect. Myoclonus can be symptomatic and distressing. In this situation, benzodiazepines, particularly clonazepam,[389] may be of value in the management of this symptom. If symptomatic myoclonus is refractory to treatment, the opioid should be changed and consideration should be given to alternative strategies for pain management.

Urinary Retention

Opioid analgesics increase smooth muscle tone and occasionally cause bladder spasm or an increase in sphincter tone. The latter effect can lead to urinary retention.[390] This is an infrequent problem that usually is observed in elderly men. Tolerance can develop rapidly, but catheterization may be necessary to manage transient problems.

Physical Dependence and Psychological Dependence (Addiction)

Concern about physical dependence, psychological dependence, and abusive drug-related behaviors augments the fear of opioid drugs and contributes substantially to the undertreatment of pain.[78,385,391–394]

Physical dependence is a pharmacologic property of opioid drugs that is defined by the development of an abstinence (withdrawal) syndrome after abrupt dosage reduction or the administration of an antagonist. Physical dependence is not a clinical problem if patients are warned to avoid abrupt discontinuation of the drug, a tapering schedule is used if treatment cessation is indicated, and opioid antagonist drugs (including agonist-antagonist analgesics) are avoided.

Psychological dependence (addiction) refers to a psychological and behavioral syndrome characterized by loss of control over drug use, compulsive use, and continued use despite harm to self or others. Addicts crave the opioid to achieve a psychic effect and manifest aberrant drug-related behaviors, such as unsanctioned dosage escalation, acquisition of drug from multiple providers, or use of illicit drugs. The medical use of opioids rarely is associated with the development of addiction.[391,395,396] In the largest prospective study, only four cases of iatrogenic addiction could be identified among 11,882 patients with no prior history of addiction who received at least one opioid dose in the hospital setting.[396] Extensive clinical experience in the use of opioids for patients with chronic cancer pain affirms that the risk of addiction in this population is extremely low.[16,272,395,397,398]

The distress engendered in patients who have a therapeutic requirement for analgesic drugs but who continue to experience unrelieved pain occasionally is expressed in behaviors that are reminiscent of patients with psychological dependence, such as intense concern about opioid availability. The absence of use despite harm and the elimination of these behaviors by sustained pain relief, usually produced by dosage escalation, distinguishes these patients from true addicts. Misunderstanding of these phenomena may lead clinicians to stigmatize patients inappropriately with the label ''addiction,'' which may compromise care and erode the doctor-patient relationship.[399] In the setting of unrelieved pain, abnormal drug-related behaviors require careful assessment, renewed efforts to manage the pain, and the avoidance of stigmatizing labels.

Adjunctive Techniques: Noninvasive Interventions

Even with optimal management of adverse effects, some patients do not attain an acceptable balance between pain relief and side effects. Several types of noninvasive interventions should be considered for their potential to improve this balance by reducing the opioid requirement. These include the concurrent use of an appropriate primary therapy; alternative pharmacologic approaches (nonopioid analgesics, adjuvant analgesics, or a switch to another opioid); and the use of psychological, physiatric, or noninvasive neurostimulatory techniques.

Adjuvant Analgesics

Adjuvant analgesics are drugs that have a primary indication other than pain, but have analgesic effects in some painful conditions. Combined with primary analgesics in any of the three steps of the analgesic ladder, these drugs play an important role for some patients who otherwise cannot attain an acceptable balance between relief and opioid side effects. Adjuvant analgesics can be divided broadly into general-purpose analgesics and those with specific utility for neuropathic, bone, or visceral pain.

General Purpose

Corticosteroids

Corticosteroids are the most widely used general-purpose adjuvant analgesics.[400] These drugs may ameliorate pain and produce beneficial effects on appetite, nausea, mood, and malaise.[401–406] The painful conditions that commonly respond to corticosteroids include raised intracranial pressure, acute spinal cord compression, superior vena cava syndrome, metastatic bone pain, neuropathic pain caused by infiltration or compression by tumor, and hepatic capsular distention. Patients with advanced cancer who experience pain and other symptoms that may respond to corticosteroids usually are given relatively small dosages (eg, dexamethasone 1 to 2 mg twice daily). A short course of relatively high dosages (eg, dexamethasone 100 mg IV followed initially by 96 mg/d in divided doses) can be used to manage an acute episode of severe pain that is related to a neuropathic lesion (eg, plexopathy, epidural spinal cord compression) or bony metastasis and cannot be reduced promptly with opioids. The dosage always should be decreased gradually after pain reduction to the minimum needed to sustain relief.

Topical Local Anesthetics

Topical local anesthetics can be used in the management of painful cutaneous and mucosal lesions, and as a premedication before skin puncture. Controlled studies have demonstrated the effectiveness of a eutectic mixture of 2.5% lidocaine and 2.5% prilocaine (EMLA) in reducing pain associated with venipuncture,[407–411] lumbar puncture,[408,412] and arterial puncture.[413] For optimal effect, the cream should be applied thickly 1 hour before the procedure and covered with an occlusive dressing (plastic wrap can be used). EMLA also can be applied to painful cutaneous lesions such as postherpetic neuralgia and painful ulcers. Lidocaine viscous frequently is used in the management of oropharyngeal ulceration.[414–417] Although the risk of aspiration appears to be small, caution with eating is required after oropharyngeal anesthesia.

Neuroleptic Drugs

Neuroleptic drugs have a limited role in the management of cancer pain. Methotrimeprazine has been useful in bedridden patients with advanced cancer, who experience pain associated with anxiety, restlessness, nausea, or a propensity to bowel obstruction.[418,419] In the United States, methotrimeprazine is approved only for repetitive IM administration, but extensive experience has affirmed that it also can be given by continuous SC administration,[354,419] SC bolus injection, or brief IV infusion (administration over 20 to 30 minutes).

Adjuvants for Neuropathic Pain

Neuropathic pain, such as painful lumbosacral plexopathy, can present a major therapeutic challenge. The use of adjuvant analgesics can contribute substantially to the successful management of these problems. Numerous drugs are used empirically for this indication, including selected antidepressants, oral local anesthetics, anticonvulsants, and others. For the purpose of drug selection, it is useful to distinguish between continuous, lancinating, and sympathetically maintained neuropathic pain[28] (Table 70-10). Given the great interpatient and intrapatient variability in the response to adjuvants in this setting (including those within the same class), sequential trials frequently are required.

Antidepressants

The tricyclic antidepressants typically are used to manage continuous dysesthesias that have not responded adequately to an opioid, and lancinating neuropathic pains that are refractory to other specific adjuvant drugs.[28,420] These compounds also are useful in patients with pain complicated by depression and insomnia.[28,420] Although the evidence for analgesic efficacy is greatest for the tertiary amine tricyclic drugs, such as amitriptyline, doxepin, and imipramine,[421–425] the secondary amine drugs, such as desipramine and nortriptyline, may be preferred when concern about sedation, anticholinergic effects, or cardiovascular toxicity is high. There also is some evidence that selective serotonin uptake inhibitor antidepressants, such as trazodone, maprotiline, and paroxetine, are analgesic.[28] The starting dosage of a tricyclic antidepressant should be low (eg, amitriptyline 10 mg in the elderly and 25 mg in younger patients). Dosages can be increased every few days by increments equal to the starting dosage. The usual effective dosage for the most widely used of these drugs, amitriptyline, is 50 to 150 mg/d. It is reasonable to continue upward dosage titration beyond this range, however, when patients fail to achieve benefit and have no limiting side effects. Plasma drug concentrations, if available, may provide useful information and should be followed up during the course of therapy. Extremely low levels in nonresponders suggest poor compliance or an unusually rapid metabolism. In the latter case, dosages can be increased while repeatedly monitoring the plasma drug level. Likewise, nonresponders whose plasma concentrations are not extremely low, but are lower than the antidepressant range, should be considered for a trial of higher dosages if side effects are not a problem.

TABLE 70-10. *A guide to the selection of adjuvant analgesics for neuropathic pain based on clinical characteristics*

Continuous pain	Lancinating pain	Sympathetically maintained pain
Tricyclic antidepressants	Anticonvulsant drugs	Phenoxybenzamine
Amitriptyline	Carbamazepine	Prazosin
Doxepin	Phenytoin	Corticosteroids
Imipramine	Clonazepam	Nifedipine
Desipramine	Valproate	
Nortriptyline	Baclofen	
	Oral local anesthetics	
Oral local anestheics		
Mexiletine		
Clonidine		
Capsaicin		

Adapted from Cherny NI, Portenoy RK. Cancer pain management: current strategy. Cancer 1993;72 (Suppl): 3393.

Anticonvulsants

Anticonvulsant drugs appear to be analgesic for diverse types of lancinating (shooting) neuropathic pain.[28,426] Although carbamazepine often is preferred because of the high response rate observed in trigeminal neuralgia,[427–430] caution is required in patients with cancer who have thrombocytopenia, those at risk for marrow failure (eg, after chemotherapy), and those whose blood counts must be monitored to determine disease status. If carbamazepine is used, a complete blood count should be obtained before the initiation of therapy, after 2 and 4 weeks, and then every 3 to 4 months thereafter. A leukocyte count below 4000 usually is considered to be a contraindication to treatment, and a decline to less than 3000, or an absolute neutrophil count of less than 1500 during therapy, should prompt discontinuation of the drug. Published reports and clinical experience also support trials with other anticonvulsant drugs, including phenytoin,[431–434] clonazepam,[433,435] and valproate.[433,436,437] Dosing guidelines for the use of these drugs as adjuvant analgesics customarily are identical to those used in the treatment of seizures. Low initial dosages are appropriate for carbamazepine, valproate, and clonazepam, and the administration of phenytoin often begins with the presumed therapeutic dosage (eg, 300 mg/d) or a prudent oral loading regimen (eg, 500 mg twice, separated by hours). When low initial dosages are used, dosage escalation should ensue until a favorable effect occurs, intolerable side effects supervene, or the plasma drug concentration reaches a predetermined level, which customarily is at the upper end of the therapeutic range for seizure management.

Baclofen

Baclofen, a gamma-aminobutyric acid agonist effective for trigeminal neuralgia,[438–440] often is used in the management of lancinating pains resulting from neural injury of any type. A starting dosage of 5 mg two or three times per day is escalated gradually until analgesia is achieved or adverse effects of sedation or confusion emerge.

Systemic Local Anesthetics

Notwithstanding anecdotal support[441–445] and controlled studies[446,447] that demonstrated analgesic effects from brief IV infusions of local anesthetics, this technique has not been applied widely in the cancer population.

Oral local anesthetic drugs can be considered in the management of neuropathic pains characterized by continuous or lancinating dysesthesias.[448–451] The evidence in support of this therapy is less abundant than that available for other drug classes; therefore, it is reasonable to undertake a trial with an oral local anesthetic in patients with continuous dysesthesias who fail to respond to tricyclic antidepressants, and in patients with lancinating pains refractory to trials of anticonvulsant drugs and baclofen. Mexiletine is the safest of these drugs and is preferred over flecainide and tocainide.[452,453] Dosing with mexiletine usually should start at 100 to 150 mg/d. If intolerable side effects do not occur, the dosage can be increased by a similar amount every few days, until the usual maximum dosage of 300 mg three times per day is reached.

Other Agents

Experience with other drugs in the treatment of cancer-related neuropathic pain is limited. Clonidine, an α_2-adrenergic agonist available in oral or transdermal formulations, has antinociceptive effects in the management of diverse pains, but like the tricyclic antidepressants, is used conventionally for continuous neuropathic pain in the cancer population.[454,455] Calcitonin (200 IU/d) has been shown to be an active analgesic in the management of some neuropathic pains,[456] and pimozide, a phenothiazine neuroleptic, has activity against lancinating neuropathic pain.[457] The latter drug is not preferred because of a high incidence of adverse effects, including physical and mental slowing, tremor, and parkinsonian symptoms.

Adjuvant Drugs for Sympathetically Maintained Pain

Anecdotal reports suggest that trials of phenoxybenzamine,[458] prazosin,[459] propranolol,[460] and nifedipine[461] can be considered in the setting of sympathetically maintained pain.

Adjuvants for Bone Pain

The management of bone pain frequently requires the integration of opioid therapy with multiple ancillary approaches. Although a metanalysis of NSAID therapy in cancer pain that reviewed data from 1615 patients in 21 trials found no specific efficacy in bone pain and analgesic effects equivalent only to weak opioids,[462] some patients appear to benefit greatly from the addition of such a drug.

Radiopharmaceuticals

The radiopharmaceutical strontium-89 has been approved for the treatment of bone pain caused by metastatic disease.[463–468] Although data specific to bone pain caused by metastases from gastrointestinal malignancies is lacking, analgesic response can be anticipated in a substantial proportion of patients who have radionuclide avid metastatic disease. Because treatment with this agent can compromise marrow reserve and irreversibly lower platelet count, its use is not recommended if future myelosuppressive chemotherapy is under consideration or if significant thrombocytopenia is present. Among responding patients, pain relief usually develops within 6 weeks and is sustained for a median duration of 6 months.[469] Relapsing patients can be retreated unless clinically significant thrombocytopenia occurs.[470] Other radiopharmaceuticals with similar activity that are under investigation include samarium-153-ethylenediaminetetramethylene phosphonic acid[471–475] and rhenium-186-hydroxyethylidene diphosphonate.[476,477]

Bisphosphonates and Other Agents

The bisphosphonate drugs, pamidronate and clodronate, inhibit osteoclast activity and also have been demonstrated to relieve malignant bone pain.[478–484] Parenteral administration of pamidronate every 2 weeks usually is well tolerated and the risk of symptomatic hypocalcemia is low. Other agents worthy of consideration include corticosteroids, calcitonin,[485] and gallium nitrate.[486]

Adjuvants for Visceral Pain

Bladder Spasm

Limited data support the potential efficacy of a range of adjuvant agents for the management of bladder spasm, tenesmic pain, and colicky intestinal pain. Based on limited clinical experience and in vitro evidence that prostaglandins play a role in bladder smooth-muscle contraction, a trial of NSAIDs may be justified for patients with painful bladder spasms.[487–489]

Rectal Spasm

Rectal spasm can be a difficult symptom to treat. Diltiazem[490,491] and clonidine[492] have been effective in the management of proctalgia fugax and are worthy of consideration. Chlorpromazine[493] and benzodiazepines[494] have been used anecdotally.

Bowel Obstruction

Pain caused by inoperable bowel obstruction has been treated empirically with IV scopolamine (hyoscine) butylbromide,[154,155,495] sublingual scopolamine (hyoscine) hydrobromide,[496] and the somatostatin analogue, octreotide.[497] Despite the theoretic advantages of antimuscarinic drugs in these conditions, and some limited support for the use of emepronium bromide,[498] dicyclomine, and flavoxate,[499] anticholinergic adverse effects are frequent and benefit rarely is observed.[489]

Pancreatic Cancer

In the management of pain caused by pancreatic cancer, there is limited evidence supporting the effectiveness of the octreotide[500] and the oral administration of trypsin.[501] It is speculated that these effects are mediated by a reduction in pancreatic exocrine secretion.

Adjuvant Agents in the Management of Lymphedema

Benzopyrone drugs stimulate proteolysis and can remove excess protein and its consequent edema.[502] This effect results in a slow reduction of lymphedema and an associated reduction in its clinical sequelae, such as pain and discomfort, chronic inflammation, and secondary infections. In a randomized, double-blind, placebo-controlled, crossover trial of 5,6-benzo-α-pyrone involving 21 patients with lymphedema of the leg, patients received 400 mg of the active drug or placebo, each for 6 months.[503] During the placebo period, lymphedema often worsened. Treatment with benzo-α-pyrone reduced the mean amount of edema fluid in the legs from 25% to 17% above normal, the circumference of the legs from 11% to 7% above normal, and the frequency of secondary acute inflammation. Bursting pains and feelings of hardness were decreased, as were feelings of tightness, tension, swelling, and heaviness; limb mobility also improved. The active drug was preferred to the placebo by 93% of the patients. Active treatment was well tolerated; side effects of mild nausea or diarrhea were infrequent.

Other Noninvasive Analgesic Techniques

Psychological Therapies

All patients with cancer benefit from psychological assessment and support. Some also benefit from specific psychological interventions used in the management of pain. Cognitive-behavioral interventions can help reduce pain-related distress through the development of coping skills and the modification of thoughts, feelings, and behaviors.[49] Some patients may be able to use relaxation techniques to reduce muscular tension and emotional arousal or to enhance pain tolerance.[504] Other approaches reduce anticipatory anxiety that may lead to avoidance behaviors. Successful application of these therapies requires a cognitively intact patient and a dedicated, well-trained clinician. In a controlled study, a structured nondrug program in which elderly patients were educated in the use of various strategies, including heat, cold, massage or vibration, distraction, and relaxation, was shown to diminish pain and enhance patient satisfaction.[505]

Physiatric Techniques

Physiatric techniques can be used to enhance analgesia and optimize the function of patients with chronic cancer pain. Therapeutic modalities such as electrical stimulation (including transcutaneous electrical neurostimulation), heat, or cryotherapy can be useful adjuncts to standard analgesic therapy. The treatment of lymphedema by the use of wraps, pressure stockings, or pneumatic pump devices may improve function and relieve pain and heaviness.[506] Orthotic devices can immobilize and support painful or weakened structures, and assistive devices can enhance comfort for patients with pain precipitated by weight bearing or ambulation.

Invasive Interventions in Pain Therapy

Patients who are unable to achieve a satisfactory balance between analgesia and side effects from systemic analgesic therapies may be candidates for the use of invasive anesthetic and neurosurgical techniques. These approaches (Table 70-11) may reduce the requirement for systemically administered opioids. Techniques such as intraspinal opioid and local anesthetic administration can achieve this end without compromising neurologic integrity. The use of neurodestructive procedures should be based on an evaluation of the probability and duration of analgesic benefit, the immediate and long-term risks, the probable duration of survival, and the anticipated length of hospitalization. In the Italian validation study of the World Health Organization analgesic ladder, anesthetic and neurosurgical techniques were required in less than 30% of patients. Even

TABLE 70-11. *Anesthetic and neurosurgical analgesic techniques*

Class	Technique	Clinical situation
Regional analgesia	Spinal opioids and/or local anesthetics	Systemic opioid analgesia complicated by unmanageable supraspinally mediated adverse effects
	Intrapleural local anesthetic	Persistent chest wall or upper abdominal pain
Sympathetic blockade and neurolysis	Celiac plexus block	Refractory malignant pain involving the upper abdominal viscera, including the upper retroperitoneum, liver, small bowel, and proximal colon
	Superior hypogastric plexus block	Persistent pelvic visceral pain
	Lumbar sympathetic blockade	Sympathetically maintained pain involving the legs
Somatic neurolysis or pathway ablation	Chemical rhizotomy	Intercostal nerve pain, chest wall pain Refractory bilateral pelvic or lumbosacral plexus pain in a patient with urinary diversion who is confined to bed
	Transacral neurolysis	Refractory pain limited to the perineum
	Cordotomy	Refractory unilateral pain arising in the torso or lower extremity
High center ablation	Pituitary ablation	Refractory multifocal pain
	Cingulotomy	Refractory multifocal pain

when these methods are implemented, concurrent systemic pharmacotherapy is required.[274] The major indications for these techniques are presented in Table 70-12.

Regional Analgesia

Intraspinal (Epidural and Intrathecal) Opioids

The delivery of low opioid doses near the sites of action in the spinal cord may decrease supraspinally mediated adverse effects. In the absence of randomized trials that compare the various intraspinal techniques with other analgesic approaches, the indications for the spinal route remain empiric.[507] Persistent dose-limiting toxicity from systemic opioid therapy is the usual indication for the selection of these routes.[508] Hogan and colleagues, who described similar guidelines for patient selection, reported that only 16 of 1205 patients with cancer pain required the use of these routes.[509] Particularly in the management of pelvic and perineal pain, spinal opioids have the advantage of preserving sensation, strength, and sympathetic function compared with neuroablative therapies.[510] Contraindications include bleeding diathesis, profound leukopenia, and sepsis. A temporary trial of spinal opioid therapy should be performed to assess the potential benefits of this approach before the implantation of a permanent catheter.[508]

TABLE 70-12. *A guide to the selection of invasive analgesic techniques according to the site of pain*

Site	Procedure
Chest wall	Spinal opioid ± local anesthetic Intercostal neurolysis Paravertebral neurolysis Intrapleural local anesthetic ± phenol Chemical thizotomy Surgical rhizotomy
Abdominal somatic	Spinal opioid ± local anesthetic Chemical rhizotomy Surgical rhizotomy Cordotomy (unilateral pain)
Upper abdomen: visceral	Celiac plexus neurolysis Intrapleural local anesthetic ± phenol
Lower abdomen: visceral	Superior hypogastric neurolysis
Perineum	Spinal opioid ± local anesthetic Chemical rhizotomy Surgical rhizotomy Transsacral S4 neurolysis
Pelvis and lower limb	Spinal opioid ± local anesthetic Chemical rhizotomy Surgical rhizotomy
Unilateral lower quadrant	Cordotomy
Multifocal or generalized pain	Pituitary ablation Cingulotomy

Opioid selection for intraspinal delivery is influenced by several factors. Hydrophilic drugs, such as morphine and hydromorphone, have a prolonged half-life in cerebrospinal fluid and significant rostral redistribution.[511–514] Lipophilic opioids, such as fentanyl and sufentanil, have less rostral redistribution[515] and may be preferable for segmental analgesia at the level of spinal infusion. The addition of a low concentration of a local anesthetic, such as 0.125% to 0.25% bupivacaine, to an epidural opioid has been demonstrated to increase analgesic effect without increasing toxicity.[509,516–518] The potential morbidity for these procedures indicates the need for a well-trained clinician and long-term monitoring.

Intrapleural Analgesia

Several authors have described the use of intrapleural local anesthetics in the management of cancer-related pains involving the head, neck, chest, arms, and upper abdominal viscera.[519–521] Although a single bolus may provide a prolonged analgesia, continuous infusion of a local anesthetic has been recommended for patients with chronic pain caused by advanced cancer.[519] Intrapleural phenol and bupivacaine were used successfully to relieve pain caused by metastatic esophageal cancer. Postmortem studies revealed no macroscopic or microscopic changes to the viscera, spinal cord, or sympathetic chain.[520]

Anesthetic Techniques for Sympathetically Maintained Pain and Visceral Pain

Celiac Plexus Block

Neurolytic celiac plexus blockade can be considered in the management of pain caused by neoplastic infiltration of the upper abdominal viscera, including the pancreas, upper retroperitoneum, liver, gallbladder, and proximal small bowel.[522–524] In addition to an extensive anecdotal experience, this technique is supported by a small controlled study of the percutaneous approach[525] and a controlled trial of intraoperative neurolysis.[526] Reported analgesic response rates in patients with pancreatic cancer are 50% to 90%, and the reported duration of effect is about 1 to 12 months.[522–525] Given the overall favorable response to this approach, most clinicians recommend it as the next intervention for patients with an appropriate pain syndrome who fail to obtain an adequate balance between analgesia and side effects from an oral opioid. Common transient complications include postural hypotension and diarrhea.[522–524] Posterior spread of the neurolytic solution occasionally can lead to the involvement of lower thoracic and lumbar somatic nerves, which potentially can result in a neuropathic pain syndrome. Other uncommon complications include pneumothorax, retroperitoneal hematoma, and paraparesis.

Superior Hypogastric Nerve Plexus Block

The superior hypogastric nerve plexus, which lies anterior to the sacral promontory, transmits sensation from pelvic visceral structures. Bilateral percutaneous neurolytic superior hypogastric plexus blocks with 10% phenol can relieve chronic cancer-related pelvic pain in 40% to 80% of patients.[527,528]

Lumbar Sympathetic Blockade

Lumbar sympathetic blockade should be considered for sympathetically maintained pain involving the legs. The risk of sphincter dysfunction with this technique is small.[523]

Neuroablative Techniques for Somatic and Neuropathic Pain

Chemical Rhizotomy

Chemical rhizotomy is an effective method of pain control for patients with advanced malignancy and otherwise refractory pelvic, perineal, or plexopathy pain.[529,530] The aim of subarachnoid and epidural neurolysis is to produce a chemical rhizotomy, interrupting the afferent pathways from the affected area. Because of the significant risk of increasing the patient's disability through motor weakness, sphincter incompetence, and loss of positional sense, chemical rhizotomy is reserved best for patients who already are confined to bed and have urinary and fecal diversion.

Subarachnoid techniques involving the use of absolute alcohol and phenol are well described.[523] Alcohol is hypobaric and is administered with the patient placed in the lateral oblique position with the painful side uppermost. Phenol solutions are hyperbaric and viscous, and the technique requires that the patient lie on the painful side in a semi-lateral or supine position so that the posterior nerve roots are dependent. In addition to its neurolytic effect, phenol has an initial local anesthetic action, producing warmth, tingling, or a prickling sensation over the distribution of the affected nerve. The hyperbaric nature of phenol is of particular advantage in the production of saddle block anesthesia in patients with midline pain caused by pelvic cancer.

Epidural rhizotomy is an alternative technique that involves epidural catheter placement with the tip close to the center of the segmental area to be blocked. After a local anesthetic test dose is injected to confirm placement, small doses of phenol or alcohol are injected at 1-day intervals, until the desired analgesic result is obtained. About 1 to 3 mL is injected on each occasion. With phenol-in-saline solutions, the onset of pain relief is rapid (1 to 2 minutes).

Satisfactory analgesia is achieved in about 30% to 50% of patients.[523,531] Adverse effects can be related to the injection technique (spinal headache, mechanical neural damage, infection, and arachnoiditis) or to the neurolysis of nerve fibers not concerned in the mediation of pain. Complications include motor paresis (5% to 20%), sphincter dysfunction (5% to 60%), impairment of touch and proprioception, and dysesthesias.[523] Fortunately, neurologic deficits usually are transient, although fatal meningitis, paraplegia, and permanent impairment of sphincteric function have been recorded.[523] Patient counseling regarding the risks involved in these techniques is essential.

Transsacral Neurolysis

Refractory pain limited to the perineum may be amenable to neurolysis of the S-4 nerve root through the ipsilateral posterior sacral foramen.[532] This technique is associated with minimal risk of motor impairment.

Cordotomy

Cordotomy involves the ablation of the anterolateral spinothalamic tract to produce contralateral hypesthesia to pain and temperature.[533,534] The patient with severe unilateral pain arising in the torso or lower extremity, such as that caused by tumor involving the pelvic sidewall, is most likely to benefit from this procedure.[530] The percutaneous cervical cordotomy is performed under local anesthesia, with biplane fluoroscopic monitoring. A miniature electrode is inserted into the anterolateral quadrant of the cervical spine through a C1-2 puncture. With the patient awake, it is possible to test the placement of the electrode to ensure adequate somatotopic localization before an ablative thermal lesion is made with a radiofrequency generator.[533] The open cordotomy is performed through a posterior laminectomy or by an anterior low cervical approach. Open cordotomy usually is reserved for patients who are unable to lie in the supine position or who are not cooperative enough to undergo a percutaneous procedure.[533]

Significant pain relief is achieved in more than 90% of patients during the period immediately after the procedure.[530,533–535] Fifty percent of surviving patients have recurrent pain after 1 year and repeated cordotomy may be necessary. The neurologic complications of cordotomy include paresis, ataxia, and bladder dysfunction.[535] The complications usually are transient, but are protracted and disabling in about 5% of cases. Rarely, patients with a long duration of survival (more than 12 months) experience a delayed-onset dysesthesia pain. The most serious potential complication is respiratory dysfunction, which may occur in the form of phrenic nerve paralysis or as sleep-induced apnea.[536] The latter is a result of the interruption of ascending reticular pathways. Because of these concerns, bilateral high cervical cordotomies or a unilateral cervical cordotomy ipsilateral to the site of a solely functioning lung are not recommended.

Other Techniques

Pituitary ablation by chemical or surgical hypophysectomy has been reported to relieve diffuse and multifocal pain syndromes that have been refractory to opioid therapy and are unsuitable for any regional neuroablative procedure.[524,537] Pain relief has been observed in patients with hormone-dependent and hormone-independent tumors.[524,537]

Anecdotal reports also support the efficacy of cingulotomy[538] or cervical midline myelotomy in the management of diffuse pain syndromes that have been refractory to opioid therapy. The mechanisms of action of these procedures are unknown and they rarely are considered.

Therapy for Patients With Refractory Pain: The Role of Sedation

For some patients with advanced disease, adequate relief of physical pain may be achieved only at the cost of profound sedation.[87] The incidence of this situation is controversial, and has been estimated variably at 5% to 52% of patients with far-advanced cancer.[539] Increasing attention has been focused on the use of sedation to manage intractable pain and suffering in the population who fail to benefit from optimal therapy.[539] The patient with advanced cancer and uncontrolled symptoms may choose the transitory use of sedating therapy while continuing trials of analgesic approaches. Alternatively, a strategy can be designed to provide adequate sedation until death.

The literature describing the use of sedation in the management of refractory pain is anecdotal and guidelines for drug selection are empiric. When sedation is desired by a patient who already is receiving an opioid for pain, an attempt usually is made first to escalate the opioid dosage. Although some patients benefit from this intervention, inadequate sedation or the development of neuroexcitatory side effects, such as myoclonus or agitated delirium, often necessitates the addition of a second agent.[540,541] The addition of a benzodiazepine usually is effective in this situation. Drugs with short half-lives, such as lorazepam,[542] midazolam,[363,543–547] or flunitrazepam,[548] are easy to titrate and tend to be preferred. When a rapid effect is required, the selected drug should be administered by a parenteral route, preferably IV or SC. In patients who lack IV access, the water-soluble benzodiazepines, midazolam and flunitrazepam, can be administered by the SC route, or alternatively, diazepam can be administered as a suppository.[549–551] Patients suffering from an agitated delirium who are sedated inadequately by a neuroleptic agent such as haloperidol, methotrimeprazine, or chlorpromazine also can benefit from the addition of a benzodiazepine.[542]

Rarely, benzodiazepine drugs cause a paradoxical agitation, and an alternative strategy is required. Experience in the management of refractory physical symptoms using barbiturates alone has been described. Greene and Davis[552] treated 17 imminently dying terminally ill patients with amobarbital (9 cases) or thiopental (8 cases), reporting adequate symptom relief in all cases. This approach has been endorsed by Truog and associates,[553] who also described the potential utility of barbiturates for terminal agitation or terminal anguish.

The ethical basis of this approach is predicated on informed consent and an acknowledgment of the ''principle of double effect,'' which distinguishes between the compelling primary therapeutic intent (to relieve suffering) and unavoidable untoward consequences (the potential for accelerating death).[554] This approach recognizes the right of dying patients to adequate relief of pain, and the right of all patients to choose between appropriate therapeutic options.[539] No patient should have to ask to be killed because of persistently unrelieved pain, and contrariwise, no patient should be sedated without appropriate informed consent of the patient or proxy. The process of informed decision-making requires candid discussion that clarifies the prevailing clinical predicament and presents the alternative analgesic options (including sedation).

CONCLUSION

Among patients with tumors of the gastrointestinal tract, the experience of acute pain is virtually universal, and a large proportion have chronic pain in the setting of incurable disease. The individual practitioner can treat most pain problems effectively by attending to careful pain assessment and implementing analgesic therapy. Currently available analgesic techniques can provide adequate relief to most patients, most of whom respond to systemic pharmacotherapy alone. Comprehensive continuing care requires the integration of this expertise with management of other symptoms and the psychosocial needs of the patient. The successful ongoing treatment of patients with chronic cancer pain requires a continuity of care that provides an appropriate level of monitoring and responds quickly, flexibly, and expertly to the changing needs of the patient. Patients with refractory pain or unremitting suffering related to other losses or distressing symptoms should have access to specialists in pain management or palliative medicine who can provide an approach capable of addressing these complex problems.

REFERENCES

1. Balch CM. The surgeon's expanded role in cancer care. Cancer 1990; 3:604.
2. Foley KM. Scope of the cancer-pain problem. In: Arbit E, ed. Management of cancer-related pain. Mount Kisko, NY: Futura, 1993:3.
3. Cleeland CS, Gonin R, Hatfield A, et al. Pain and its treatment in outpatients with metastatic cancer. N Engl J Med 1994;330:592.
4. Portenoy RK. Cancer pain: epidemiology and syndromes. Cancer 1989;63:2298.

5. Portenoy RK, Miransky J, Thaler HT, et al. Pain in ambulatory patients with lung or colon cancer: prevalence, characteristics and impact. Cancer 1992;70:1616.
6. Brescia FJ, Portenoy RK, Ryan M, Krasnoff L, Gray G. Pain, opioid use, and survival in hospitalized patients with advanced cancer. J Clin Oncol 1992;10:149.
7. Edwards RB. Pain management and the values of health care providers. In: Hill CS, Fields WS, eds. Drug treatment of cancer pain in a drug oriented society. Advances in pain research and therapy. 11th vol. New York: Raven Press, 1989:101.
8. Wanzer SH, Federman DD, Adelstein SJ, et al. The physicians responsibility toward hopelessly ill patients—a second look. N Engl J Med 1989;120:844.
9. Martin RS. Mortal values: healing, pain and suffering. In: Hill CS, Fields WS, eds. Drug treatment of cancer pain in a drug oriented society. Advances in pain research and therapy. 11th vol. New York: Raven Press, 1989:19.
10. Jorgensen L, Mortensen MB, Jensen NH, Eriksen J. Treatment of cancer pain patients in a multidisciplinary pain clinic. Pain Clinic 1990;3:83.
11. Stjernsward J, Teoh N. The scope of the cancer pain problem. In: Foley KM, Bonica JJ, Ventafridda V, eds. Second international congress on cancer pain. Advances in pain research and therapy. 16th vol. New York: Raven Press, 1990:7.
12. Solomon MZ, O'Donnell L, Jennings B, et al. Decisions near the end of life: professional views on life-sustaining treatments. Am J Public Health 1993;83:14.
13. Ventafridda V. Continuing care: a major issue in cancer pain management. Pain 1989;36:137.
14. Shegda LM, McCorkle R. Continuing care in the community. J Pain Symptom Manage 1990;5:279.
15. Coyle N. A model of continuity of care for cancer patients with chronic pain. Med Clin North Am 1987;71:259.
16. World Health Organization. Cancer pain relief and palliative care. Geneva: World Health Organization, 1990.
17. International Association for the Study of Pain, Subcommittee on Taxonomy. Pain terms: A list with definitions and notes on usage. Pain 1980;8:249.
18. Arner S, Meyerson BA. Lack of analgesic effect of opioids on neuropathic and idiopathic forms of pain. Pain 1988;33:11.
19. Cherny NI, Thaler HT, Friedlander-Klar H, et al. Opioid responsiveness of cancer pain syndromes caused by neuropathic or nociceptive mechanisms: a combined analysis of controlled single dose studies. Neurology 1994;44:857.
20. Tasker R. Management of nociceptive, deafferentation, and central pain by surgical intervention. In: Fields HL, ed. Pain syndromes in neurology. Butterworths international medical reviews: neurology. 10th vol. London: Butterworths, 1990:143.
21. Devor M, Basbaum AI, Bennett GJ, et al. Group report: mechanisms of neuropathic pain following peripheral injury. In: Basbaum A, Besson J-M, eds. Towards a new pharmacotherapy of pain. New York: John Wiley & Sons, 1991:417.
22. Portenoy RK. Issues in the management of neuropathic pain. In: Basbaum A, Besson J-M, eds. Towards a new pharmacotherapy of pain. New York: John Wiley & Sons, 1991:393.
23. Janig W, Blumberg H, Boas RA, Campbell JN. The reflex sympathetic dystrophy syndrome: consensus statement and general recommendations for diagnosis and clinical research. In: Bond MR, Charlton JE, Woolf CJ, eds. Proceedings of the VIth World Congress on Pain. Pain research and clinical management. 4th vol. Amsterdam: Elsevier, 1991:373.
24. Dalmau J, Graus F, Marco M. "Hot and dry foot" as initial manifestation of neoplastic lumbosacral plexopathy. Neurology 1989;39:871.
25. Aguilera NJ, Lopez DJ, Gil NE, Gil PA. [Neoplastic lumbosacral plexopathy and "hot foot"]. Neurologia 1993;8:271.
26. Portenoy RK, Foley KM, Inturrisi CE. The nature of opioid responsiveness and its implications for neuropathic pain: new hypotheses derived from studies of opioid infusions. Pain 1990;43:273.
27. Dubner R. A call for more science, not more rhetoric, regarding opioids and neuropathic pain. Pain 1991;47:1.
28. Portenoy RK. Adjuvant analgesics in pain management. In: Doyle D, Hanks GW, MacDonald N, eds. Oxford textbook of palliative medicine. Oxford: Oxford University Press, 1993:187.
29. American Psychiatric Association. Somatoform disorders. In: Diagnostic and statistical manual of mental disorders. 3rd ed. Washington, DC: American Psychiatric Association, 1987:255.
30. Derogatis LR, Morrow GR, Fetting J, Penman D, Piasetsky S, Schmale AM. The prevalence of psychiatric disorders among cancer patients. JAMA 1983;249:751.
31. Breitbart W. Psychiatric management of cancer pain. Cancer 1989; 63:2336.
32. Chapman CR, Gavrin J. Suffering and its relationship to pain. J Palliat Care 1993;9:5.
33. Gonzales GR, Elliot KJ, Portenoy RK, Foley KM. The impact of a comprehensive evaluation in the management of cancer pain. Pain 1991;47:141.
34. Mense S, Stahnke M. Responses in muscle afferent fibers of slow conduction velocity to contractions and ischaemia in the cat. J Physiol (Lond) 1983;342:343.
35. Ness TJ, Gebhart GE. Visceral pain: a review of experimental studies. Pain 1990;41:167.
36. Perl ER. Characterization of nociceptors and their activation of neurons in the superficial dorsal horn: first step for the sensation of pain. In: Kruger L, Liebeskind JC, eds. Advances in pain research and therapy. 6th vol. New York: Raven Press, 1984:23.
37. Besson JM, Chaouch A. Peripheral and spinal mechanisms of nociception. Physiol Rev 1987;67:67.
38. Willis WD. Mechanisms of somatic pain. In: Chapman CR, Foley KM, eds. Current and emerging issues in cancer pain: research and practice. New York: Raven Press, 1993:67.
39. Gebhart GF. Visceral pain mechanisms. In: Chapman CR, Foley KM, eds. Current and emerging issues in cancer pain: research and practice. New York: Raven Press, 1993:99.
40. Willis WD. The pain system: the neural basis of nociceptive transmission in the mammalian nervous system. Basel: Karger, 1985.
41. Duggan AW, Weihe E. Central transmission of impulses in the nociceptor events in the superficial dorsal horn. In: Basbaum AL, Besson J-M, eds. Towards a new pharmacotherapy of pain. New York: John Wiley & Sons, 1991:35.
42. Kocher L, Anton F, Reeh PW, Handwerker HO. The effect of carrageenan-induced inflammation on the excitability of unmyelinated skin nociceptors in the rat. Pain 1987;29:363.
43. Dickenson AH, Sullivan AF. Evidence for the role of the NMDA receptor in the frequency of rodent potentiation of deep dorsal horn neurones following C-fiber stimulation. Neuropharmacology 1987; 26:1235.
44. Melzack R, Wall PD. Pain mechanism: a new theory. Science 1965; 150:971.
45. Basbaum AI, Fields HL. Endogenous pain control systems: brainstem spinal pathways and endorphin circuitry. Annu Rev Neurosci 1984; 7:309.
46. Evans CJ, Hammond DL, Fredrickson RCA. The opioid peptides. In: Pasternak GW, ed. The opiate receptors. Clifton, NJ: Humana Press, 1988:23.
47. Dickenson AH. Mechanisms of the analgesic actions of opiates and opioids. BMJ 1991;47:690.
48. Yaksh TL. Direct evidence that spinal serotonin and noradrenaline terminals mediate the spinal antinociceptive effects of morphine in the periaqueductal gray. Brain Res 1979;160:180.
49. Fishman B. The treatment of suffering in patients with cancer pain: cognitive behavioral approaches. In: Foley KM, Bonica JJ, Ventafridda V, eds. Second international congress on cancer pain. Advances in pain research and therapy. 16th vol. New York: Raven Press, 1990: 301.
50. Lazarus RS, Folkman C. Stress, appraisal and coping. New York: Springer, 1984.
51. Syrjala KL. Integrating medical and psychological treatments for cancer pain. In: Chapman CR, Foley KM, eds. Current and emerging issues in cancer pain: research and practice. New York: Raven Press, 1993:393.
52. Bond MR, Pearson IB. Psychosocial aspects of pain in women with advanced cancer of the cervix. J Psychosom Res 1969;13:13.
53. Barkwell DP. Ascribed meaning: a critical factor in coping and pain attenuation in patients with cancer-related pain. J Palliat Care 1991; 7:5.
54. Daut RL, Cleeland CS. The prevalence and severity of pain in cancer. Cancer 1982;50:1913.

55. Bolund C. Medical and care factors in suicides by cancer patients in Sweden. Journal of Psychosocial Oncology 1985;3:31.
56. Breitbart W. Suicide in the cancer patient. Oncology 1987;1:49.
57. Cleeland CS. The impact of pain on the patient with cancer. Cancer 1984;54:2635.
58. Baile WF, Di Maggio JR, Schapira DV, Janofsky JS. The request for assistance in dying. The need for psychiatric consultation. Cancer 1993;72:2786.
59. Breitbart W. Cancer pain and suicide. In: Foley KM, Bonica JJ, Ventafridda V, eds. Second international congress on cancer pain. Advances in pain research and therapy. 16th vol. New York: Raven Press, 1990: 399.
60. Cherny NI, Coyle N, Foley KM. Suffering in the advanced cancer patient: a definition and taxonomy. J Palliat Care 1994;10:57.
61. Cassell EJ. The nature of suffering and the goals of medicine. N Engl J Med 1982;306:639.
62. Ventafridda V, DeConno F, Ripamonti C, Gamba A, Tamburini M. Quality of life assessment during a palliative care program. Ann Oncol 1990;1:415.
63. Bonica JJ, Ventafridda V, Twycross RG. Cancer pain. In: Bonica JJ, ed. The management of pain. 2nd ed. Philadelphia: Lea & Febiger, 1990:400.
64. Banning A, Sjogren P, Henriksen H. Pain causes in 200 patients referred to a multidisciplinary cancer pain clinic. Pain 1991;45:45.
65. Foley KM. The treatment of cancer pain. N Engl J Med 1985;313: 84.
66. Foley KM. Clinical assessment of pain. Acta Anaesthica Scandinavia 1982;74(Suppl):91.
67. Twycross RG, Fairfield S. Pain in far-advanced cancer. Pain 1982; 14:303.
68. Twycross RG, Lack SA. Symptom control in far-advanced cancer: pain relief. London: Pitman, 1984.
69. McCaffery M, Thorpe DM. Differences in perception of pain and the development of adversarial relationships among health care providers. In: Hill CS, Fields WS, eds. Drug treatment of cancer pain in a drug oriented society. Advances in pain research and therapy. 11th vol. New York: Raven Press, 1989:19.
70. Portenoy RK, Hagen NA. Breakthrough pain: definition, prevalence and characteristics. Pain 1990;41:273.
71. Cherny NI, Portenoy RK. Practical issues in the management of cancer pain. In: Wall PD, Melzack R, eds. Textbook of pain. 3rd ed. Edinburgh: Churchill Livingstone, 1994:1437.
72. Cherny NI, Portenoy RK. Cancer pain management: current strategy. Cancer 1993;72(Suppl):3393.
73. Jaeckle KA. Nerve plexus metastases. Neurol Clin 1991;9:857.
74. Boureau F, Doubrere JF, Luu M. Study of verbal description in neuropathic pain. Pain 1990;42:145.
75. Coyle N, Adelhardt J, Foley KM, Portenoy RK. Character of terminal illness in the advanced cancer patient: pain and other symptoms during the last four weeks of life. J Pain Symptom Manage 1990;5:83.
76. Kellgren JG. On distribution of pain arising from deep somatic structures with charts of segmental pain areas. Clin Sci (Colch) 1939;4: 35.
77. Torebjork HE, Ochoa JL, Schady W. Referred pain from intraneural stimulation of muscle fascicles in the median nerve. Pain 1984;18: 145.
78. Cleeland CS. Pain control: public and physician's attitudes. In: Hill CS, Fields WS, eds. Drug treatment of cancer pain in a drug-oriented society. Advances in pain research and therapy. 11th vol. New York: Raven Press, 1989:81.
79. Grossman SA, Sheidler VR, Swedeen K, Mucenski J, Piantadosi S. Correlation of patient and caregiver ratings of cancer pain. J Pain Symptom Manage 1991;6:53.
80. Baillie L. A review of pain assessment tools. Nursing Standards 1993; 7:25.
81. Jensen MP, Karoly R. Measurement of cancer pain by self report. In: Chapman CR, Foley KM, eds. Current and emerging issues in cancer pain: research and practice. New York: Raven Press, 1993:193.
82. Agency for Health Care Policy and Research, Acute Pain Management Panel. Management of cancer pain. Clinical practice guideline number 9. Washington, DC: US Department of Health and Human Services, 1994.
83. Fishman B, Pasternak S, Wallenstein SL, Houde RW, Holland JC, Foley KM. The Memorial Pain Assessment Card: a valid instrument for the evaluation of cancer pain. Cancer 1987;60:1151.
84. Daut RL, Cleeland CS, Flanery RC. Development of the Wisconsin Brief Pain Questionnaire to assess pain in cancer and other diseases. Pain 1983;17:197.
85. McCaffery M, Ferrell BR. How vital are vital signs? Nursing 1992; 22:42.
86. American Pain Society Committee of Quality Assurance Standards. American Pain Society quality assurance standards for the relief of acute pain and cancer pain. In: Bond MR, Charlton JE, Woolf CJ, eds. Proceedings of the VIth World Congress on Pain. Pain research and clinical management. 4th vol. Amsterdam: Elsevier, 1991:185.
87. Ventafridda V, Ripamonti C, De Conno F, Tamburini M, Cassileth BR. Symptom prevalence and control during cancer patients' last days of life. J Palliat Care 1990;6:7.
88. Reuben DB, Mor V, Hiris J. Clinical symptoms and length of survival in patients with terminal cancer. Arch Intern Med 1988;148:1586.
89. Moinpour CM, Feigl P, Metch B, Hayden KA, Meyskens FJ, Crowley J. Quality of life endpoints in cancer clinical trials: review and recommendations. J Natl Cancer Inst 1989;81:485.
90. Moinpour CM, Hayden KA, Thomson IM, Feigl P, Metch B. Quality of life assessment in Southwest Oncology Group trials. In: Tchekmedyian NS, Cella D, eds. Quality of life in oncology practice and research. Williston Park, Dominus Publishing, 1991:43.
91. Portenoy R, Thaler HT, Kornblith AB, et al. The Memorial Symptom Assessment Scale: an instrument for the evaluation of symptom prevalence, characteristics and distress. European Journal of Clinical Oncology 1994;30:1326.
92. Clouston P, De Angelis L, Posner JB. The spectrum of neurologic disease in patients with systemic cancer. Ann Neurol 1992;31:268.
93. Haines IE, Zalcberg J, Buchanan JD. Not-for-resuscitation orders in cancer patients: principles of decision making. Med J Aust 1990;153: 225.
94. Marks RM, Sachar EJ. Undertreatment of medical inpatients with narcotic analgesics. Ann Intern Med 1973;78:173.
95. Agency for Health Care Policy and Research, Acute Pain Management Panel. Acute pain management: operative or medical procedures and trauma. Clinical practice guideline. Washington: US Department of Health and Human Services, 1992.
96. Edwards WT. Optimizing opioid treatment of postoperative pain. J Pain Symptom Manage 1990;5(Suppl 1):24.
97. Ready LB. The treatment of post operative pain. In: Bond MR, Charlton JE, Woolf CJ, eds. Proceedings of the VIth World Congress on Pain. Pain research and clinical management. 4th vol. Amsterdam: Elsevier, 1991:53.
98. Nivatvongs S. Diagnosis. In: Gordon PH, Nivatvongs S, eds. Principles and practice of surgery for the colon, rectum and anus. St Louis: Quality Medical Publishing, 1992:81.
99. McCarthy BD, Moskowitz MA. Screening flexible sigmoidoscopy: patient attitudes and compliance. J Gen Intern Med 1993;8:120.
100. Khanna AK, Misra MK, Khanna A, Misra VK, Khanna S. Fine-needle aspiration cytology of abdominal masses. J Surg Oncol 1990;44:15.
101. Borner M, Castiglione M, Triller J, et al. Considerable side effects of chemoembolization for colorectal carcinoma metastatic to the liver. Ann Oncol 1992;3:113.
102. Kolmannskog F, Kolbenstvedt AN, Schrumpf E, Hanssen LE. Side effects and complications after hepatic artery embolization in the carcinoid syndrome. Scand J Gastroenterol 1991;26:557.
103. Amin Z, Bown SG, Lees WR. Local treatment of colorectal liver metastases: a comparison of interstitial laser photocoagulation (ILP) and percutaneous alcohol injection (PAI). Clin Radiol 1993;48:166.
104. Mather LE. Novel methods of analgesic drug delivery. In: Bond MR, Charlton JE, Woolf CJ, eds. Proceedings of the VIth World Congress on Pain. Pain research and clinical management. 4th vol. Amsterdam: Elsevier, 1991:159.
105. Coyle N, Cherny NI, Portenoy RK. Subcutaneous opioid infusions in the home. Oncology 1994;8:21.
106. De Conno F, Caracenti A, Martini C, Spoldi E, Salvetti M, Ventafridda V. Hyperalgesia and myoclonus with intrathecal infusion of high-dose morphine. Pain 1991;47:337.
107. Stillman MJ, Moulin DE, Foley KM. Paradoxical pain following high-dose spinal morphine. Pain 1987;(Suppl 4):389.
108. De Castro MD, Meynadier MD, Zenz MD. Regional opioid analgesia.

Developments in critical care medicine and anesthesiology. 20th vol. Dordrecht (Germany) Kluwer Academic Publishers, 1991.
109. Molloy HS, Seipp CA, Duffey P. Administration of cancer treatments: practical guide for physicians and oncology nurses. In: De Vita VT, Hellman S, Rosenberg SA, eds. Cancer: principles & practice of oncology. 3rd ed. Philadelphia: JB Lippincott, 1989:2369.
110. Curran CF, Luce JK, Page JA. Doxorubicin-associated flare reactions. Oncol Nurs Forum 1990;17:387.
111. Mrozek-Orlowski M, Christie J, Flamme C, Novak J. Pain associated with peripheral infusion of carmustine. Oncol Nurs Forum 1991;18: 942.
112. Hundrieser J. A non-invasive approach to minimizing vessel pain with DTIC or BCNU. Oncol Nurs Forum 1988;15:199.
113. Schneider SM, Distelhorst CW. Chemotherapy-induced emergencies. Semin Oncol 1989;16:572.
114. Kemeny N, Cohen A, Bertino J, Sigurson ER, Botet J, Oderman P. Continuous intrahepatic infusion of floxuridine and leucovorin through an implantable pump for the treatment of hepatic metastases from colorectal carcinoma. Cancer 1990;65:2446.
115. Metzger U, Weder W, Rothlin M, Largiader F. Phase II study of intra-arterial fluorouracil and mitomycin-C for liver metastases of colorectal cancer. Recent Results Cancer Res 1991;121:198.
116. Botet JF, Watson RC, Kemeny N, Daly JM, Yeh S. Cholangitis complicating intraarterial chemotherapy in liver metastasis. Radiology 1985;156:335.
117. Almadrones L, Yerys C. Problems associated with the administration of intraperitoneal therapy using the Port-A-Cath system. Oncol Nurs Forum 1990;17:75.
118. Markman M. Cytotoxic intracavitary chemotherapy. Am J Med Sci 1986;291:175.
119. Dufour P, Maloisel F, Bergerat JP, et al. Intraperitoneal mitoxantrone as consolidation treatment for stage III ovarian carcinoma: a pilot study. Bull Cancer (Paris) 1991;78:273.
120. Gitsch E, Sevelda P, Schmidl S, Salzer H. First experiences with intraperitoneal chemotherapy in ovarian cancer. Eur J Gynaecol Oncol 1990;11:19.
121. Deppe G, Malviya VK, Boike G, Young J. Intraperitoneal doxorubicin in combination with systemic cisplatinum and cyclophosphamide in the treatment of stage III ovarian cancer. Eur J Gynaecol Oncol 1991; 12:93.
122. Markman M, Howell SB, Lucas WE, Pfeifle CE, Green MR. Combination intraperitoneal chemotherapy with cisplatin, cytarabine, and doxorubicin for refractory ovarian carcinoma and other malignancies principally confined to the peritoneal cavity. J Clin Oncol 1984;2: 1321.
123. Schilsky RL, Choi KE, Grayhack J, Grimmer D, Guarnieri C, Fullem L. Phase I clinical and pharmacologic study of intraperitoneal cisplatin and fluorouracil in patients with advanced intraabdominal cancer. J Clin Oncol 1990;8:2054.
124. Kaplan RA, Markman M, Lucas WE, Pfeifle C, Howell SB. Infectious peritonitis in patients receiving intraperitoneal chemotherapy. Am J Med 1985;78:49.
125. Mahood DJ, Dose AM, Loprinzi CL, et al. Inhibition of fluorouracil-induced stomatitis by oral cryotherapy. J Clin Oncol 1991;9:449.
126. Barker G, Loftus L, Cuddy P, Barker B. The effects of sucralfate suspension and diphenhydramine syrup plus kaolin-pectin on radiotherapy-induced mucositis. Oral Surg Oral Med Oral Pathol 1991;71: 288.
127. Pfeiffer P, Madsen EL, Hansen O, May O. Effect of prophylactic sucralfate suspension on stomatitis induced by cancer chemotherapy. A randomized, double-blind cross-over study. Acta Oncol 1990;29: 171.
128. Spijkervet FK, Van Saene HK, Van Saene JJ, et al. Effect of selective elimination of the oral flora on mucositis in irradiated head and neck cancer patients. J Surg Oncol 1991;46:167.
129. Redding SW. Role of herpes simplex virus reactivation in chemotherapy-induced oral mucositis. National Cancer Institute Monograph 1990;1990:103.
130. Ferretti GA, Raybould TP, Brown AT, et al. Chlorhexidine prophylaxis for chemotherapy- and radiotherapy-induced stomatitis: a randomized double-blind trial. Oral Surg Oral Med Oral Pathol 1990; 69:331.
131. Spijkervet FK, van Saene HK, van Saene JJ, Panders AK, Vermey A, Mehta DM. Mucositis prevention by selective elimination of oral flora in irradiated head and neck cancer patients. J Oral Pathol Med 1990;19:486.
132. Hill HF, Chapman CR, Kornell J, Sullivan K, Saeger L, Benedetti C. Self-administration of morphine in bone marrow transplant patients reduces drug requirement. Pain 1990;40:121.
133. Hill HF, Mackie AM, Coda BA, Iverson K, Chapman CR. Patient-controlled analgesic administration. A comparison of steady-state morphine infusions with bolus doses. Cancer 1991;67:873.
134. Lokich JJ, Moore C. Chemotherapy-associated palmar-plantar erythrodysesthesia syndrome. Ann Intern Med 1984;101:798.
135. Fabian CJ, Molina R, Slavik M, Dahlberg S, Giri S, Stephens R. Pyridoxine therapy for palmar-plantar erythrodysesthesia associated with continuous 5-fluorouracil infusion. Invest New Drugs 1990;8: 57.
136. Grem JL, McAtee N, Balis F, et al. A phase II study of continuous infusion 5-fluorouracil and leucovorin with weekly cisplatin in metastatic colorectal carcinoma. Cancer 1993;72:663.
137. Bellmunt J, Navarro M, Hidalgo R, Sole LA. Palmar-plantar erythrodysesthesia syndrome associated with short-term continuous infusion (5 days) of 5-fluorouracil. Tumori 1988;74:329.
138. Collins C, Weiden PL. Cardiotoxicity of 5-fluorouracil. Cancer Treatment Reports 1987;71:733.
139. Freeman NJ, Costanza ME. 5-Fluorouracil-associated cardiotoxicity. Cancer 1988;61:36.
140. Eskilsson J, Albertsson M. Failure of preventing 5-fluorouracil cardiotoxicity by prophylactic treatment with verapamil. Acta Oncol 1990; 29:1001.
141. Rezkalla S, Kloner RA, Ensley J, et al. Continuous ambulatory ECG monitoring during fluorouracil therapy: a prospective study. J Clin Oncol 1989;7:509.
142. Elliott K, Foley KM. Neurologic pain syndromes in patients with cancer. Neurol Clin 1989;7:333.
143. Rotstein J, Good RA. Steroid pseudorheumatism. Arch Intern Med 1957;99:545.
144. Quesada JR, Talpaz M, Rios A, Kurzrock R, Gutterman JU. Clinical toxicity of interferons in cancer patients: a review. J Clin Oncol 1986; 4:234.
145. Jones GJ, Itri LM. Safety and tolerance of recombinant interferon alfa-2a (Roferon-A) in cancer patients. Cancer 1986;8:1709.
146. Earnest DL, Trier JS. Radiation enteritis and colitis. In: Sleisenger MH, Fordtran JS, eds. Gastrointestinal disease: pathophysiology diagnosis management. 2nd vol. Philadelphia: WB Saunders, 1989:1369.
147. Buchi K. Radiation proctitis: therapy and prognosis. JAMA 1991; 265:1180.
148. Rusthoven JJ, Ahlgren P, Elhakim T, et al. Risk factors for varicella zoster disseminated infection among adult cancer patients with localized zoster. Cancer 1988;62:1641.
149. Portenoy RK, Duma C, Foley KM. Acute herpetic and postherpetic neuralgia: clinical review and current management. Ann Neurol 1986; 20:651.
150. Rusthoven JJ, Ahlgren P, Elhakim T, et al. Varicella-zoster infection in adult cancer patients: a population study. Arch Intern Med 1988; 148:1561.
151. Silen W. Cope's early diagnosis of the acute abdomen. 16th ed. New York: Oxford, 1983.
152. Mulholland MW, Debas H, Bonica JJ. Diseases of the liver, biliary system and pancreas. In: Bonica JJ, ed. The management of pain. 2nd vol. Philadelphia: Lea & Febiger, 1990:1214.
153. Coombs DW. Pain due to liver capsular distention. In: Ferrer-Brechner T, ed. Common problems in pain management. Common problems in anesthesia. Chicago: Year Book Medical Publishers, 1990:247.
154. Ventafridda V, Ripamonti C, Caraceni A, Spoldi E, Messina L, De Conno F. The management of inoperable gastrointestinal obstruction in terminal cancer patients. Tumori 1990;76:389.
155. Baines M. The pathophysiology and management of malignant intestinal obstruction. In: Doyle D, Hanks GW, MacDonald N, eds. Oxford textbook of palliative medicine. Oxford: Oxford University Press, 1993:311.
156. Ripamonti C, De CF, Ventafridda V, Rossi B, Baines MJ. Management of bowel obstruction in advanced and terminal cancer patients. Ann Oncol 1993;4:15.
157. Walsch D, Williams G. Surgical biopsy studies of omental and peritoneal nodules. Br J Surg 1971;58:428.
158. Bender MD. Diseases of the peritoneum, mesentery and diaphragm.

In: Sleisenger MH, Fordtran JS, eds. Gastrointestinal disease: pathophysiology diagnosis management. 4th ed. Philadelphia: WB Saunders, 1989:1932.
159. Lynch MA, Cho KC, Jeffrey RJ, Alterman DD, Federle MP. CT of peritoneal lymphomatosis. AJR Am J Roentgenol 1988;151:713.
160. Stillman M. Perineal pain: diagnosis and management, with particular attention to perineal pain of cancer. In: Foley KM, Bonica JJ, Ventafrida V, eds. Second international congress on cancer pain. Advances in pain research and therapy. 16th vol. New York: Raven Press, 1990: 359.
161. Boas RA, Schug SA, Acland RH. Perineal pain after rectal amputation: a 5-year follow-up. Pain 1993;52:67.
162. Boas RA. Post-surgical perineal pain in cancer: a 5 year follow-up. Pain 1990;(Suppl 5):376.
163. Radbruch L, Zech D, Grond S, Meuser T, Lehmann KA. [Perineal pain and rectal cancer—prevalence in local recurrence]. Med Klin 1991;86:180.
164. Seefeld PH, Bargen JA. The spread of carcinoma of the rectum: invasion of lymphatics, veins and nerves. Ann Surg 1943;118:76.
165. Sinaki M, Merritt JL, Stilwell GK. Tension myalgia of the pelvic floor. Mayo Clin Proc 1977;52:717.
166. Talner LB. Specific causes of obstruction. In: Pollack HM, ed. Clinical urography. 2nd vol. Philadelphia: WB Saunders, 1990:1629.
167. Greenfield A, Resnick MI. Genitourinary emergencies. Semin Oncol 1989;16:516.
168. Frohlich EP, Bex P, Nissenbaum MM, Epstein BM, Sonnendecker EW. Comparison between renal ultrasonography and excretory urography in cervical cancer. Int J Gynaecol Obstet 1991;34:49.
169. Fair WR. Urologic emergencies. In: DeVita VT, Hellman S, Rosengerg SA, eds. Cancer: principles and practice of oncology. 3rd ed. Philadelphia: JB Lippincott, 1989:2016.
170. Chad DA, Bradley WG. Lumbosacral plexopathy. Semin Neurol 1987;7:97.
171. Jaeckle KA, Young DF, Foley KM. The natural history of lumbosacral plexopathy in cancer. Neurology 1985;35:8.
172. Stevens MJ, Gonet YM. Malignant psoas syndrome: recognition of an oncologic entity. Australas Radiol 1990;34:150.
173. Krol G. Evaluation of neoplastic involvement of brachial and lumbar plexus: imaging aspects. J Back and Musculoskel Rehab 1993;3:35.
174. Portenoy RK, Galer BS, Salamon O, et al. Identification of epidural neoplasm. Radiography and bone scintigraphy in the symptomatic and asymptomatic spine. Cancer 1989;64:2207.
175. Garcia-Diaz J, Balseiro J, Calandre L, Bermejo F. Aortic dissection presenting with neurologic signs. N Engl J Med 1988;318:1070.
176. Brown MJ, Asbury AK. Diabetic neuropathy. Ann Neurol 1984;15: 2.
177. Evans BA. Lumbosacral plexus neuropathy. Neurology 1981;31: 1327.
178. Bradley WG, Chad D, Verghese JP, et al. Painful lumbosacral plexopathy with elevated erythrocyte sedimentation rate: a treatable inflammatory syndrome. Ann Neurol 1984;15:457.
179. Abrams HL, Spiro R, Goldstein N. Metastases in carcinoma. Analysis of 1000 autopsied cases. Cancer 1950;23:74.
180. Nielsen OS, Munro AJ, Tannock IF. Bone metastases: pathophysiology and management policy. J Clin Oncol 1991;9:509.
181. Gilbert RW, Kim JH, Posner JB. Epidural spinal cord compression from metastatic tumor: diagnosis and treatment. Ann Neurol 1978;3: 40.
182. Sorensen S, Borgesen SE, Rohde K, et al. Metastatic epidural spinal cord compression. Results of treatment and survival. Cancer 1990; 65:1502.
183. Stark RJ, Henson RA, Evans SJW. Spinal metastases: a retrospective survey from a general hospital. Brain 1982;105:189.
184. Posner JB. Back pain and epidural spinal cord compression. Med Clin North Am 1987;71:185.
185. Grant R, Papadopoulos SM, Greenberg HS. Metastatic epidural spinal cord compression. Neurol Clin 1991;9:825.
186. Ruff RL, Lanska DJ. Epidural metastases prospectively evaluated in veterans with cancer and back pain. Cancer 1989;63:2234.
187. Barcena A, Lobato RD, Rivas JJ, et al. Spinal metastatic disease: analysis of factors determining functional prognosis and choice of treatment. Neurosurgery 1984;15:820.
188. Rodichok LD, Harper GR, Ruckdeschel JC, et al. Early diagnosis of spinal epidural metastases. Am J Med 1981;70:1181.
189. O'Rourke T, George CB, Redmond J. Spinal computed tomography and computer tomographic metrimazide myelography in the early diagnosis of spinal metastatic disease. J Clin Oncol 1986;4:576.
190. Portenoy RK, Lipton RB, Foley KM. Back pain in the cancer patient: an algorithm for evaluation and management. Neurology 1987;37: 134.
191. Zelefsky MJ, Scher HI, Krol G, Portenoy RK, Leibel SA, Fuks ZY. Spinal epidural tumor in patients with prostate cancer. Clinical and radiographic predictors of response to radiation therapy. Cancer 1992; 70:2319.
192. Flynn DF, Shipley WU. Management of spinal cord compression secondary to metastatic prostatic carcinoma. Urol Clin North Am 1991; 18:145.
193. Sundaresan N, Galicich JH, Lane JM, Bains MS, McCormack P. Treatment of neoplastic epidural cord compression by vertebral resection and stabilization. J Neurosurg 1985;63:676.
194. Sundaresan N, Galicich JH, Bains MS, Martini N, Beattie E. Vertebral body resection in the treatment of cancer involving the spine. Cancer 1984;53:1393.
195. Harrington KD. Anterior cord decompression and spinal stabilization for patients with metastatic lesions of the spine. J Neurosurg 1984; 61:107.
196. Brice J, McKissock W. Surgical treatment of malignant extradural tumors. BMJ 1965;1:1341.
197. Findlay GF. The role of vertebral body collapse in the management of malignant spinal cord compression. J Neurol Neurosurg Psychiatry 1987;50:151.
198. Sim FH. Metastatic bone disease: lesions of the pelvis and hip. In: Sim FH, ed. Diagnosis and management of metastatic bone disease. A multidisciplinary approach. New York: Raven Press, 1988:183.
199. Beatrous TE, Choyke PL, Frank JA. Diagnostic evaluation of cancer patients with pelvic pain: comparison of scintigraphy, CT, and MR imaging. AJR Am J Roentgenol 1990;155:85.
200. Forsyth PA, Posner JB. Headache associated with intracranial neoplasms. In: Olesen J, Tfelt-Hansen P, Welch KMA, eds. The headaches. New York: Raven Press 1993:705
201. Wright DC, Delaney TF. Treatment of metastatic cancer to the brain. In: DeVita VT, Hellman S, Rosenberg SA, eds. Cancer: principles and practice of oncology. 3rd ed. Philadelphia: JB Lippincott, 1989: 2245.
202. Fadul C, Misulis KE, Wiley RG. Cerebellar metastases: diagnostic and management considerations. J Clin Oncol 1987;5:1110.
203. Posner JB, Chernik NL. Intracranial metastases from systemic cancer. Adv Neurol 1978;19:575.
204. Posner JB. Headache and other head pain. In: Wyngaaden JB, Smith LH, Claude Bennett J, eds. Cecil's textbook of medicine. 19th ed. Philadelphia: WB Saunders, 1992:2117.
205. Greenberg HS, Deck MDF, Vikram B, et al. Metastasis to the base of the skull: clinical findings in 43 patients. Neurology 1981;31:530.
206. Wasserstrom WR, Glass JP, Posner JB. Diagnosis and treatment of leptomeningeal metastasis from solid tumors: experience with 90 patients. Cancer 1982;49:759.
207. Kaplan JG, DeSouza TG, Farkash A, et al. Leptomeningeal metastases: comparison of clinical features and laboratory data of solid tumors, lymphomas and leukemias. J Neurooncol 1990;9:225.
208. Glass PJ, Foley KM. Carcinomatous meningitis. In: Harris JR, Hellman S, Henderson IC, Kinne D, eds. Breast diseases. Philadelphia: Lippincott, 1991:700.
209. Henson RA, Urich H. Cancer and the nervous system. Boston: Blackwell Scientific Publications, 1982:100.
210. Olsen ME, Chernik NL, Posner JB. Infiltration of the leptomeninges by systemic cancer. Arch Neurol 1974;30:122.
211. Dillon WP. Imaging of central nervous system tumors. Current Opinion in Radiology 1991;3:46.
212. Manelfe C. Imaging of the spine and spinal cord. Current Opinion in Radiology 1991;3:5.
213. Lee YY, Glass JP, Geoffray A, et al. Cranial computed tomographic abnormalities in leptomeningeal metastasis. American Journal of Neuroradiology 1984;5:559.
214. Krol G, Sze G, Malkin M, Walker R. MR of cranial and spinal meningeal carcinomatosis. American Journal of Neuroradiology 1988;9: 709.
215. Boas RA. Phantom anus syndrome. In: Bonica JJ, Lindblom U, Iggo A, eds. Proceedings of the third world congress on pain. Advances

in pain research and therapy. 5th vol. New York: Raven Press, 1983: 947.
216. Ovesen P, Kroner K, Ornsholt J, Bach K. Phantom-related phenomena after rectal amputation: prevalence and characteristics. Pain 1991;44: 289.
217. Noguchi Y, Baba M, Nakano S, et al. Quality of life of patients after esophagectomy for esophageal cancer. Nippon Geka Gakkai Zasshi 1991;92:281.
218. Thomas JE, Cascino TL, Earl JD. Differential diagnosis between radiation and tumor plexopathy of the pelvis. Neurology 1985;35:1.
219. Minsky B, Cohen A. Minimizing the toxicity of radiation therapy in rectal cancer. Oncology 1988;2:21.
220. Jellinger K, Strum KW. Delayed radiation in myelopathy in man. J Neurol Sci 1971;14:389.
221. Epstein JB, Wong FLW, Stephenson-Moore P. Osteoradionecrosis: clinical experience and a proposal for classification. J Oral Maxillofac Surg 1987;45:104.
222. Epstein JB, Schubert MM, Scully C. Evaluation and treatment of pain in patients with orofacial cancer. The Pain Clinic 1991;4:3.
223. Foley KM. Pain syndromes in patients with cancer. Med Clin North Am 1987;71:169.
224. Foley KM, Inturrisi CE. Analgesic drug therapy in cancer pain: principles and practice. Med Clin North Am 1987;71:207.
225. Ferrell BR, Wisdom C, Wenzl C. Quality of life as an outcome variable in the management of cancer pain. Cancer 1989;11:2321.
226. Bates T. A review of local radiotherapy in the treatment of bone metastases and cord compression. Int J Radiat Oncol Biol Phys 1992; 23:217.
227. Bates T, Yarnold JR, Blitzer P, Nelson OS, Rubin P, Maher J. Bone metastasis consensus statement. Int J Radiat Oncol Biol Phys 1992; 23:215.
228. Coia LR. The role of radiotherapy in the treatment of brain metastases. Int J Radiat Oncol Biol Phys 1992;23:239.
229. Bosch A. Radiotherapy. Clin Oncol (R Coll Radiol) 1984;3:47.
230. Dobrowsky W, Schmidt AP. Radiotherapy for presacral recurrence following radical surgery for rectal carcinoma. Dis Colon Rectum 1985;28:917.
231. Allum WH, Mack P, Priestman TJ, Fielding JW. Radiotherapy for pain relief in locally recurrent colorectal cancer. Ann R Coll Surg Engl 1987;69:220.
232. Borgelt BB, Gelber R, Brady LW, Griffin T, Hendrickson FR. The palliation of hepatic metastases. Results of a Radiation Therapy Oncology Group pilot study. Int J Radiat Oncol Biol Phys 1981;7:587.
233. Prassad B, Lee M, Hendrickson FR. Irradiation of hepatic metastases. Int J Radiat Oncol Biol Phys 1977;2:129.
234. Sherman DM, Weichselbaum R, Order SE, Cloud L, Trey C, Piro AJ. Palliation of hepatic metastases. Cancer 1978;41:2013.
235. Minsky BD, Leibel S. The treatment of hepatic metastases from colorectal cancer with radiation therapy alone or combined with chemotherapy or misonidazole. Cancer Treat Rev 1989;16:213.
236. Eble MJ, Gademann G, Wannenmacher M. [The value of radiotherapy for liver metastases]. Strahlenther Onkol 1993;169:459.
237. Dobelbower RR, Bronn DG. Radiotherapy in the treatment of pancreatic cancer. Baillieres Clin Gastroenterol 1990;4:969.
238. MacDonald N. Principles governing the use of cancer chemotherapy in palliative medicine. In: Doyle D, Hanks GW, MacDonald N, eds. Oxford textbook of palliative medicine. Oxford: Oxford University Press, 1993:105.
239. Ilson DH, Kelson DP. Chemotherapy in esophageal cancer. Anticancer Drugs 1993;4:287.
240. Findlay M, Cunningham D. Chemotherapy of carcinoma of the stomach. Cancer Treat Rev 1993;19:29.
241. Herrmann R. Systemic treatment of colorectal cancer. Eur J Cancer 1993;30A:404.
242. Findlay M, Cunningham D. Current advances in the treatment of gastrointestinal malignancy. Crit Rev Oncol Hematol 1993;14:127.
243. Douglass HO. Current approaches to multimodality management of advanced pancreatic cancer. Hepatogastroenterology 1993;40:433.
244. Luporini G, Labianca R, Pancera G. Medical treatment of hepatocellular carcinoma. J Surg Oncol Suppl 1993;3:115.
245. Moore DJ, Pazdur R. Systemic therapies for unresectable primary hepatic tumors. J Surg Oncol Suppl 1993;3:112.
246. Saltzburg D, Foley KM. Management of pain in pancreatic cancer. Surg Clin North Am 1989;69:629.
247. Carlsson G, Hafstrom L, Jonsson PE, Ask A, Kallum B, Lunderquist A. Unresectable and locally recurrent rectal cancer treated with radiotherapy or bilateral internal iliac artery infusion of 5-fluorouracil. Cancer 1986;58:336.
248. Turk PS, Belliveau JF, Darnowski JW, Weinberg MC, Leenen L, Wanebo HJ. Isolated pelvic perfusion for unresectable cancer using a balloon occlusion technique. Arch Surg 1993;128:533.
249. Young N, Hollands M, Wong KP. Symptom relief and survival after chemo-embolization with adriamycin, lipiodol and gelfoam for hepatocellular carcinoma. Australas Radiol 1993;37:173.
250. Cummings BJ. Anal cancer. Int J Radiat Oncol Biol Phys 1990;19: 1309.
251. Tanum G, Tveit K, Karlsen KO, Hauer JM. Chemotherapy and radiation therapy for anal carcinoma. Survival and late morbidity. Cancer 1991;67:2462.
252. Boraas M. Palliative surgery. Semin Oncol 1985;12:368.
253. MacDonald N. The role of medical and surgical oncology in the management of cancer pain. In: Foley KM, Bonica JJ, Ventafrida V, eds. Second international congress on cancer pain. Advances in pain research and therapy. 16th vol. New York: Raven Press, 1990:27.
254. Sundaresan N, DiGiacinto GV. Antitumor and antinociceptive approaches to control of cancer pain. Med Clin North Am 1987;71:329.
255. Williams MR. The place of surgery in terminal care. In: Saunders C, ed. The management of terminal disease. London: Edward Arnold, 1984:148.
256. Petrelli NJ, Velez A, Herrera L, Walsh D, Mittelman A. Ileal conduits for recurrent unresectable colorectal adenocarcinoma. Am J Surg 1985;150:239.
257. Ross GJ, Kessler HB, Clair MR, Gatenby RA, Hartz WH, Ross LV. Sonographically guided paracentesis for palliation of symptomatic malignant ascites. AJR Am J Roentgenol 1989;153:1309.
258. Cruikshank DP, Buchsbaum HJ. Effects of rapid paracentesis. Cardiovascular dynamics and body fluid composition. JAMA 1973;225: 1361.
259. Lifshitz S, Buchsbaum HJ. The effect of paracentesis on serum proteins. Gynecol Oncol 1976;4:347.
260. Edney JA, Hill A, Armstrong D. Peritoneovenous shunts palliate malignant ascites. Am J Surg 1989;158:598.
261. Gough IR, Balderson GA. Malignant ascites. A comparison of peritoneovenous shunting and nonoperative management. Cancer 1993;71: 2377.
262. Holm A, Halpern NB, Aldrete JS. Peritoneovenous shunt for intractable ascites of hepatic, nephrogenic, and malignant causes. Am J Surg 1989;158:162.
263. Smith DA, Weaver DW, Bouwman DL. Peritoneovenous shunt (PVS) for malignant ascites. An analysis of outcome. Am Surg 1989;55:445.
264. Montesani C, Ribotta G, De MR, et al. Extended resection in the treatment of colorectal cancer. Int J Colorectal Dis 1991;6:161.
265. Williams LJ, Huddleston CB, Sawyers JL, Potts J, Sharp KW, McDougal SW. Is total pelvic exenteration reasonable primary treatment for rectal carcinoma? Ann Surg 1988;207:670.
266. Takagi H, Morimoto T, Yasue M, Kato K, Yamada E, Suzuki R. Total pelvic exenteration for advanced carcinoma of the lower colon. J Surg Oncol 1985;28:59.
267. Temple WJ, Ketcham AS. Surgical palliation for recurrent rectal cancers ulcerating in the perineum. Cancer 1990;65:1111.
268. Burney RE, Faulkner DJ. Recurrent abdominal abscess caused by retained colorectum after proctocolectomy. Surgery 1988;104:580.
269. Butch RJ, Wittenberg J, Mueller PR, Simeone JF, Meyer JE, Ferrucci JJ. Presacral masses after abdominoperineal resection for colorectal carcinoma: the need for needle biopsy. AJR Am J Roentgenol 1985; 144:309.
270. Bruera E, McDonald N. Intractable pain in patients with advanced head and neck tumors: a possible role of local infection. Cancer Treatment Report 1986;70:691.
271. Coyle N, Portenoy RK. Infection as a cause of rapidly increasing pain in cancer patients. J Pain Symptom Manage 1991;6:266.
272. World Health Organization. Cancer pain relief. Geneva: World Health Organization, 1986.
273. Walker VA, Hoskin PJ, Hanks GW, White ID. Evaluation of WHO analgesic guidelines for cancer pain in a hospital-based palliative care unit. J Pain Symptom Manage 1988;3:145.
274. Ventafridda V, Tamburini M, Caraceni A, DeConno F, Naldi F. A

validation study of the WHO method for cancer pain relief. Cancer 1987;59:851.
275. Takeda F. Results of field-testing in Japan of WHO draft interim guidelines on relief of cancer pain. The Pain Clinic. 1986;1:83.
276. Schug SA, Zech D, Dorr U. Cancer pain management according to WHO analgesic guidelines. J Pain Symptom Manage 1990;5:27.
277. Grond S, Zech D, Schug SA, Lynch J, Lehman KA. Validation of World Health Organization guidelines for cancer pain relief during the last days and hours of life. J Pain Symptom Manage 1991;6:411.
278. Vane JR. Inhibition of prostaglandin synthesis as a mechanism of action for aspirin-like drugs. Nature 1971;234:231.
279. Willer J, DeBroucker T, Bussel B, Robi-Brami A, Harrewyn J. Central analgesic effect of ketoprofen in humans: electrophysiologic evidence for a supraspinal mechanism in a double-blind and cross-over study. Pain 1989;38:1.
280. Piletta P, Porchet HC, Dayer P. Central analgesic effect of acetaminophen but not of aspirin. Clin Pharmacol Ther 1991;49:350.
281. Brooks PM, Wood AJJ. Nonsteroidal antiinflammatory drugs—differences and similarities. N Engl J Med 1991;324:1716.
282. Insel PA. Analgesic-antipyretics and antiinflammatory agents: drugs employed in the treatment of rheumatoid arthritis and gout. In: Gilman AG, Rall TW, Nies AS, Teylor P, eds. The pharmacological basis of therapeutics. 8th ed. New York: Pergamon Press, 1990:638.
283. Seeff LB, Cuccherini BA, Zimmerman HI, Adler E, Benjamin S. Acetaminophen hepatotoxicity in alcoholics. Ann Intern Med 1986; 104:399.
284. McQuay HJ, Jadad AR, Carroll D, et al. Opioid sensitivity of chronic pain: a patient controlled analgesia method. Anaesthesia 1992;47:757.
285. Jadad AR, Carroll D, Glynn CJ, Moore RA, McQuay HJ. Morphine responsiveness of chronic pain: double blind randomised crossover study with patient controlled analgesia. Lancet 1992;339:1367.
286. Cherny NI, Thaler HT, Friedlander-Klar H, Lapin J, Portenoy RK. Opioid responsiveness of neuropathic cancer pain: combined analysis of single-dose analgesic trials. (Abstract) In: Proceedings of the American Society of Clinical Oncology. 1992:11.
287. Hanks GW. The clinical usefulness of agonist-antagonistic opioid analgesics in chronic pain. Drug Alcohol Depend 1987;20:339.
288. Houde RW, Wallenstein SL, Beaver WT. Evaluation of analgesics in patients with cancer pain. In: Lasagna L, ed. International encyclopedia of pharmacology and therapeutics. 1st vol. New York: Pergamon Press, 1966:59.
289. De Conno F, Ripamonti C, Sbannotto A, et al. A clinical study on the use of codeine, oxycodone, dextropropoxyphene, buprenorphine and pentazocine in cancer pain. J Pain Symptom Manage 1991;6:423.
290. Beaver W. Combination analgesics. Am J Med 1984;77:38.
291. Vree TB, Verwey vWC. Pharmacokinetics and metabolism of codeine in humans. Biopharm Drug Dispos 1992;13:445.
292. Poyhia R, Vainio A, Kalso E. A review of oxycodone's clinical pharmacokinetics and pharmacodynamics. J Pain Symptom Manage 1993; 8:63.
293. Kalso E, Vainio A. Morphine and oxycodone hydrochloride in the management of cancer pain. Clin Pharmacol Ther 1990;47:639.
294. Glare PA, Walsh TD. Dose-ranging study of oxycodone for chronic pain in advanced cancer. J Clin Oncol 1993;11:973.
295. Inturrisi CE, Colburn WN, Verebey K, Dayton HE, Woody GE, O'Brien CP. Propoxyphene and norpropoxyphene kinetics after single and repeated doses of propoxyphene. Clin Pharmacol Ther 1982;31: 157.
296. Sawe J, Svensson JO, Rane A. Morphine metabolism in cancer patients on increasing oral doses—no evidence for autoinduction or dose dependence. J Clin Pharmacol 1983;16:85.
297. Smith MT, Watt JA, Cramond T. Morphine-3-glucuronide—a potent antagonist of morphine analgesia. Life Sci 1990;47:579.
298. Ashby MA, Flemming BG, van Crugten J, Somogyi A. Plasma morphine, morphine-3-glucuronide (M3G) and morphine-6-glucuronide (M6G) concentrations in hospice patients receiving morphine for cancer pain: absence of relationship to opioid side effects. (Abstract) In: Seventh world congress on pain: abstracts. Seattle: IASP Publications, 1993;1002.
299. Paul D, Standifer KM, Inturrisi CE, Pasternak GW. Pharmacological characterization of morphine-6 beta-glucuronide, a very potent morphine metabolite. J Pharmacol Exp Ther 1989;251:477.
300. Pasternak GW, Bodnar RJ, Clarke JA, Intorrisi CE. Morphine-6-glucuronide, a potent mu agonist. Life Sci 1987;41:2845.
301. Shimomura K, Kamata O, Ueki S, et al. Analgesic effects of morphine glucuronides. Tohoku J Exp Med 1971;105:45.
302. Osborne RJ, Joel SP, Slevin ML. Morphine intoxication in renal failure: the role of morphine-6-glucuronide. BMJ 1986;292:1548.
303. Hanna MH, Peat SJ, Woodham M, Knibb A, Fung C. Analgesic efficacy and CSF pharmacokinetics of intrathecal morphine-6-glucuronide: comparison with morphine. Br J Anaesth 1990;64:547.
304. Osborne R, Thompson P, Joel S, Trew D, Patel N, Slevin M. The analgesic activity of morphine-6-glucuronide. Br J Clin Pharmacol 1992;34:130.
305. Portenoy RK, Thaler HT, Inturrisi CE, Friedlander-Klar H, Foley KM. The metabolite, morphine-6-glucuronide, contributes to the analgesia produced by morphine infusion in pain patients with normal renal function. Clin Pharmacol Ther 1992;51:422.
306. Hagen N, Foley KM, Cerbones DJ, Portenoy RK, Inturrisi CE. Chronic nausea and morphine-6-glucuronide. J Pain Symptom Manage 1991;6:125.
307. Lehmann KA, Zech D. Morphine-6-glucuronide, a pharmacologically active morphine metabolite: a review of the literature. European Journal of Pain 1993;12:28.
308. Houde RW, Wallenstein SL, Beaver WT. Clinical measurement of pain. In: de Stevens G, ed. Analgesics. New York: Academic Press, 1965:75.
309. Hasselstrom J, Eriksson LS, Persson A, Rane A, Svensson J, Sawe J. The metabolism and bioavailability of morphine in patients with severe liver cirrhosis. Br J Clin Pharmacol 1990;29:289.
310. Sawe J, Dahlstrom B, Paazlow L, Rane A. Morphine kinetics in cancer patients. Clin Pharmacol Ther 1981;30:629.
311. Gourlay GK, Plummer JL, Cherry DA, Purser T. The reproducibility of bioavailability of oral morphine from solution under fed and fasted conditions. J Pain Symptom Manage 1991;6:431.
312. Kaiko RF. Commentary: equianalgesic dose ratio of intramuscular/oral morphine, 1:6 versus 1:3. In: Foley KM, Inturrisi CE, eds. Opioid analgesics in the management of clinical pain. Advances in pain research and therapy. 8th vol. New York: Raven Press, 1986:87.
313. Twycross RG. Opioid analgesics in cancer pain: current practice and controversies. Cancer Surv 1988;7:29.
314. Arkinstall WW, Goughnour BR, White JA, Stewart JH. Control of severe pain with sustained-release morphine tablets v. oral morphine solution. Can Med Assoc J 1989;140:653.
315. Warfield CA. Guidelines for the use of MS Contin tablets in the management of cancer pain. Postgrad Med J 1991;67:12.
316. Moulin DE, Kreeft JH, Murray PN, Bouquillon AI. Comparison of continuous subcutaneous and intravenous hydromorphone infusions for management of cancer pain. Lancet 1991;337:465.
317. Hagen N, Dhaliwal H, Hays H, et al. Crossover evaluation of the clinical efficacy and safety of controlled (cr) and immediate release (ir) hydromorphone in cancer pain. (Abstract) In: Seventh world congress on pain: congress abstracts. Seattle: IASP Publications, 1993; 898.
318. Bruera E, Sloan P, Scott J, Mount B. Slow release (SR) versus intermediate release (IR) hydromorphone (HM) in patients with cancer pain: a controlled, crossover trial. (Abstract) In: Seventh world congress on pain: congress abstracts. Seattle: IASP Publications, 1993;899.
319. Szeto HH, Inturrisi CE, Houde R, Saal R, Cheigh J, Reidengerg MM. Accumulation of normeperidine, an active metabolite of meperidine, in patients with renal failure or cancer. Ann Intern Med 1977;86:738.
320. Eisendrath SJ, Goldman B, Douglas J, Dimatteo L, Van DC. Meperidine-induced delirium. Am J Psychiatry 1987;144:1062.
321. Hagmeyer KO, Mauro LS, Mauro VF. Meperidine-related seizures associated with patient-controlled analgesia pumps. Ann Pharmacother 1993;27:29.
322. Kaiko RF, Foley KM, Grabinski PV, et al. Central nervous system excitatory effects of meperidine in cancer patients. Ann Neurol 1983; 13:180.
323. Varvel JR, Shafer SL, Hwang SS, Coen PA, Stanski DR. Absorption characteristics of transdermally administered fentanyl. Anesthesiology 1989;70:928.
324. Gourlay GK, Kowalski SR, Plummer JL, et al. The efficacy of transdermal fentanyl in the treatment of postoperative pain; a double blind comparison of fentanyl and placebo systems. Pain 1990;40:21.
325. Calis KA, Kohler DR, Corso DM. Transdermally administered fentanyl for pain management. Clinical Pharmacology 1992;11:22.
326. Fine PG, Marcus M, DeBoer AJ, Van der Oord B. An open label

study of oral transmucosal fentanyl citrate (OTFC) for the treatment of breakthrough cancer pain. Pain 1991;45:149.
327. Sinatra RS, Hyde NH, Harrison DM. Oxymorphone revisited. Seminars in Anesthesia 1988;8:208.
328. Hermens JM, Hanifin JM, Hirshman CA. Comparison of histamine release in human skin mast cells by morphine, fentanyl and oxymorphone. Anesthesiology 1985;62:124.
329. Rogers A. Considering histamine release in prescribing opioid analgesics. J Pain Symptom Manage 1991;6:44.
330. Moulin DE, Ling GS, Pasternak GW. Unidirectional cross tolerance between morphine and levorphanol in the rat. Pain 1988;33:233.
331. Fainsinger R, Schoeller T, Bruera E. Methadone in the management of cancer pain: a review. Pain 1993;52:137.
332. Grochow L, Sheidler V, Grossman S, Green L, Enterline J. Does intravenous methadone provide longer lasting analgesia than intravenous morphine? A randomized double-blind study. Pain 1989;38:151.
333. Inturrisi CE, Portenoy RK, Max MB, Colburn WA, Foley KM. Pharmacokinetic-pharmacodynamic (PK-PD) relationships of methadone infusions in patients with cancer pain. Clin Pharmacol Ther 1990;47: 565.
334. Inturrisi CE, Colburn WA, Kaiko RF, Houde RW, Foley KM. Pharmacokinetics and pharmacodynamics of methadone in patients with chronic pain. Clin Pharmacol Ther 1987;41:392.
335. Bruera E, Fainsinger R, Moore M, Thibault R, Spoldi E, Ventafridda V. Local toxicity with subcutaneous methadone. Experience of two centers. Pain 1991;45:141.
336. Galer BS, Coyle N, Pasternak GW, Portenoy RK. Individual variability in the response to different opioids: report of five cases. Pain 1992; 49:87.
337. de Stoutz ND, Bruera E, Suarez-Almazor M. Opiate rotation (OR) for toxicity reduction in terminal cancer patients. In: Seventh world congress on pain: congress abstracts. Seattle: IASP Publications, 1993.
338. Crews JC, Sweeney NJ, Denson DD. Clinical efficacy of methadone in patients refractory to other mu-opioid receptor agonist analgesics for management of terminal cancer pain. Case presentations and discussion of incomplete cross-tolerance among opioid agonist analgesics. Cancer 1993;72:2266.
339. MacDonald N, Der L, Allan S, Champion P. Opioid hyperexcitability: the application of alternate opioid therapy. Pain 1993;53:353.
340. Chan GL, Matzke GR. Effects of renal insufficiency on the pharmacokinetics and pharmacodynamics of opioid analgesics. Drug Intelligence and Clinical Pharmacology 1987;21:773.
341. Sawe J, Svensson JO, Odar-Cederlof I. Kinetics of morphine in patients with renal failure. (Letter) Lancet 1985;2:211.
342. Portenoy RK, Foley KM, Stulman J, et al. Plasma morphine and morphine-6-glucuronide during chronic morphine therapy for cancer pain: plasma profiles, steady state concentrations and the consequences of renal failure. Pain 1991;47:13.
343. McQuay HJ, Carroll D, Faura CC, Gavaghan DJ, Hand CW, Moore RA. Oral morphine in cancer pain: influences on morphine and metabolite concentration. Clin Pharmacol Ther 1990;48:236.
344. Hoskin PJ, Hanks GW, Aherne GW, Chapman D, Littleton P, Filshie J. The bioavailability and pharmacokinetics of morphine after intravenous, oral and buccal administration in healthy volunteers. Br J Clin Pharmacol 1989;27:499.
345. Hanks GW. Morphine pharmacokinetics and analgesia after oral administration. Postgrad Med J 1991;67 suppl 2:60.
346. Ripamonti C, Bruera E. Rectal, buccal, and sublingual narcotics for the management of cancer pain. J Palliat Care 1991;7:30.
347. Cole L, Hanning CD. Review of the rectal use of opioids. J Pain Symptom Manage 1990;5:118.
348. Wilkinson TJ, Robinson BA, Begg EJ, Duffull SB, Ravenscroft PJ, Schneider JJ. Pharmacokinetics and efficacy of rectal versus oral sustained-release morphine in cancer patients. Cancer Chemother Pharmacol 1992;31:251.
349. Hanning CD. The rectal absorption of opioids. In: Benedetti C, Chapman CR, Giron G, eds. Opioid analgesia. Advances in pain research and therapy. 14th vol. New York: Raven Press, 1990:259.
350. Portenoy PK, Southam M, Gupta SK, et al. Transdermal fentanyl for cancer pain: repeated dose pharmacokinetics. Anesthesiology 1993; 78:36.
351. Holley FO, Van-Steennis C. Postoperative analgesia with fentanyl: pharmacokinetics and pharmacodynamics of constant-rate I.V. and transdermal delivery. Br J Anaesth 1988;60:608.
352. Weinberg DS, Inturrisi CE, Reidenberg B, et al. Sublingual absorption of selected opioid analgesics. Clin Pharmacol Ther 1988;44:335.
353. Bruera E, Brenneis C, Michaud M, et al. Use of the subcutaneous route for the administration of narcotics in patients with cancer pain. Cancer 1988;62:407.
354. Storey P, Hill HH, St Louis R, Tarver EE. Subcutaneous infusions for control of cancer symptoms. J Pain Symptom Manage 1990;5:33.
355. Portenoy RK. Continuous intravenous infusions of opioid drugs. Med Clin North Am 1987;71:233.
356. Coyle N, Mauskop A, Maggard J. Continuous subcutaneous infusions of opiates in cancer patients with pain. Oncol Nurs Forum 1986;13: 53.
357. Swanson G, Smith J, Bulich R, New P, Shiffman R. Patient-controlled analgesia for chronic cancer pain in the ambulatory setting: a report of 117 patients. J Clin Oncol 1989;7:1903.
358. Bruera E, Brenneis C, Michaud M, MacMillan K, Hanson J, MacDonald RN. Patient-controlled subcutaneous hydromorphone versus continuous subcutaneous infusion for the treatment of cancer pain. J Natl Cancer Inst 1988;80:1152.
359. Bruera E, Macmillan K, Selmser P, MacDonald RN. Decreased local toxicity with subcutaneous diamorphine (heroin): a preliminary report. Pain 1990;43:91.
360. Moulin DE, Johnson NG, Murray PN, Geoghegan MF, Goodwin VA, Chester MA. Subcutaneous narcotic infusions for cancer pain: treatment outcome and guidelines for use. Can Med Assoc J 1992;146: 891.
361. Waldmann CS, Eason JR, Rambohu LE, Hanson GC. Serum morphine levels. A comparison between continuous subcutaneous infusions and intravenous infusions in postoperative patients. Anaesthesia 1984;39: 768.
362. Dover SB. Syringe driver in terminal care. BMJ 1987;294:553.
363. Amesbury BDW. Use of SC midazolam in the home care setting. Palliat Med 1989;3:299.
364. Oliver DJ. Syringe drivers in palliative care: a review. Palliat Med 1988;2:21.
365. Shepherd K. Review of a controlled-release morphine preparation. In: Foley KM, Bonica JJ, Ventafridda V, eds. Second international congress on cancer pain. Advances in pain research and therapy. 16th vol. New York: Raven Press, 1990:191.
366. West RJ, Maccarrone FH. Single dose pharmacokinetics of a new oral sustained-release morphine formlation, Kapanol capsules. (Abstract) In: Seventh world congress on pain: congress abstracts. Seattle: IASP Publications, 1993:997.
367. Citron ML, Kalra JM, Seltzer VL, Chen S, Hoffman M, Walczak MB. Patient-controlled analgesia for cancer pain: a long-term study of inpatient and outpatient use. Cancer Invest 1992;10:335.
368. Kanner RM, Foley KM. Patterns of narcotic drug use in a cancer pain clinic. Ann NY Acad Sci 1981;362:161.
369. Edwards WT, Breed RJ. Treatment of postoperative pain in the post anesthesia care unit. Anesthesiology Clinics of North America 1990; 8:235.
370. Collin E, Poulain P, Gauvain-Piquard A, Petit G, Pichard-Leandri E. Is disease progression the major factor in morphine "tolerance" in cancer pain treatment? Pain 1993;55:319.
371. Coyle N, Adelhardt J, Foley KM. Disease progression and tolerance in the cancer pain patient. Second international congress on cancer pain. J Pain Symptom Manage 1988;3:S25.
372. Coyle N, Breitbart W, Weaver S, Portenoy RK. Delirium as a contributing factor to "crescendo" pain: three case reports. J Pain Symptom Manage 1994;9:44.
373. Ling GSFF, Spiegel K, Lockhart SH, Pasternak GW. Separation of opioid analgesia from respiratory depression: evidence for different receptor mechanisms. J Pharmacol Exp Ther 1985;232:149.
374. Umans JG, Inturrisi CE. Antinociceptive activity and toxicity of meperidine and normeperidine in mice. J Pharmacol Exp Ther 1982;223: 203.
375. Bruera E, Macmillan K, Hanson J, MacDonald RN. The cognitive effects of the administration of narcotic analgesics in patients with cancer pain. Pain 1989;39:13.
376. Bruera E, Brenneis C, Paterson AH, MacDonald RN. Use of methylphenedate as an adjuvant to narcotic analgesics in patients with advanced cancer. J Pain Symptom Manage 1989;4:3.

377. Bruera E, Chadwich S, Brenneis C, Hanson J, MacDonald RN. Methylphenidate associated with narcotics for the treatment of cancer pain. Cancer Treatment Report 1987;71:67.
378. Forrest WH, Brown BW, Brown CR, et al. Dextroamphetamine with morphine for the treatment of postoperative pain. N Engl J Med 1977; 296:712.
379. Breitbart W, Mermelstein H. Pemoline: an alternative psychostimulant for the management of depressive disorders in cancer patients. Psychosomatics 1992;33:352.
380. Sykes NP. Oral naloxone in opioid associated constipation. Lancet 1991;337:1475.
381. Walsh TD. Prevention of opioid side effects. J Pain Symptom Manage 1990;5:363.
382. Kaufman PN, Krevsky B, Malmud LS, et al. Role of opiate receptors in the regulation of colonic transit. Gastroenterology 1988;94:1351.
383. Rogers M, Cerda JJ. The narcotic bowel syndrome. J Clin Gastroenterol 1989;11:132.
384. Inturrisi CE. Management of cancer pain. Cancer 1989;63:2308.
385. Hill CS, Fields WS, eds. Drug treatment of cancer pain in a drug-oriented society. Advances in pain research and therapy. 11th vol. New York: Raven Press, 1989.
386. Sykes NP. Constipation and diarrhoea. In: Doyle D, Hanks GW, MacDonald N, eds. Oxford textbook of palliative medicine. Oxford: Oxford University Press, 1993:299.
387. Culpepper-Morgan JA, Inturrisi CE, Portenoy RK, et al. Treatment of opioid induced constipation with oral naloxone: a pilot study. Clin Pharmacol Ther 1992;52:90.
388. Campora E, Merlini L, Pace M, et al. The incidence of narcotic induced emesis. J Pain Symptom Manage 1991;6:428.
389. Eisele JH, Grigsby EJ, Dea G. Clonazepam treatment of myoclonic contractions associated with high dose opioids: a case report. Pain 1992;49:231.
390. Jaffe JH, Martin WR. Opioid analgesics and antagonists. In: Gilman AG, Rall TW, Nies AS, Teylor P, eds. The pharmacological basis of therapeutics. 8th ed. New York: Pergamon Press, 1990:485.
391. Schuster CR. Does treatment of cancer pain with narcotics produce junkies? In: Hill CS, Fields WS, eds. Drug treatment of cancer pain in a drug-oriented society. Advances in pain research and therapy. 11th vol. New York: Raven Press, 1989:1.
392. Foley KM. The decriminalization of cancer pain. In: Hill CS, Field H, eds. Drug treatment of cancer pain in a drug-oriented society. Advances in pain research and therapy. 11th vol. New York: Raven Press, 1989:5.
393. Jaffe JH. Misinformation: euphoria and addiction. In: Hill CS, Fields WS, eds. Drug treatment of cancer pain in a drug-oriented society. Advances in pain research and therapy. 11th vol. New York: Raven Press, 1989:163.
394. Morgan JP. American opiophobia: customary underutilization of opioid analgesics. In: Hill CS, Fields WS, eds. Drug treatment of cancer pain in a drug-oriented society. 11th vol. New York: Raven Press, 1989:181.
395. Chapman CR, Hill HF. Prolonged morphine self-administration and addiction liability. Cancer 1989;63:1636.
396. Porter J, Jick H. Addiction rare in patients treated with narcotics. (Letter) N Engl J Med 1980;302:123.
397. American College of Physicians Health and Public Policy Committee. Drug therapy for severe chronic pain in terminal illness. Ann Intern Med 1983;99:870.
398. American Pain Society. Principles of analgesic use in the treatment of acute pain and chronic cancer pain. A concise guide to medical practice. 3rd ed. Skokie, IL: American Pain Society, 1992.
399. Weissman DE, Haddox JD. Opioid pseudoaddiction—an iatrogenic syndrome. Pain 1989;36:363.
400. Ettinger AB, Portenoy RK. The use of corticosteroids in the treatment of symptoms associated with cancer. J Pain Symptom Manage 1988; 3:99.
401. Della Cuna GR, Pellegrini A, Piazzi M. Effect of methylprednisolone sodium succinate on quality of life in preterminal cancer patients. A placebo-control multicenter study. European Journal of Cancer and Clinical Oncology 1989;29:1817.
402. Tannock I, Gospodarowicz M, Meakin W, Panzarella T, Stewart L, Rider W. Treatment of metastatic prostatic cancer with low-dose prednisone: evaluation of pain and quality of life as pragmatic indices of response. J Clin Oncol 1989;7:590.
403. Popiela T, Lucchi R, Giongo F. Methylprednisolone as palliative therapy for female terminal cancer patients. The Methylprednisolone Female Preterminal Cancer Study Group. European Journal of Cancer and Clinical Oncology 1989;25:1823.
404. Moertel CG, Shutte A, Reitemeier R, et al. Corticosteroid therapy of preterminal gastrointestinal cancer. Cancer 1974;33:1607.
405. Wilcox JC, Corr J, Shaw J, Richardson M, Calman KC. Prednisolone as appetite stimulant in patients with cancer. BMJ 1984;288:27.
406. Bruera E, Roca E, Cedaro L, Carraro S, Chacon R. Action of oral methylprednisolone in terminal cancer patients: a prospective randomized double-blind study. Cancer Treatment Report 1985;69:751.
407. Wig J, Johl KS. Our experience with EMLA Cream (for painless venous cannulation in children). Indian J Physiol Pharmacol 1990; 34:130.
408. Halperin DL, Koren G, Attias D, Pellegrini E, Greenberg ML, Wyss M. Topical skin anesthesia for venous, subcutaneous drug reservoir and lumbar punctures in children. Pediatrics 1989;84:281.
409. Soliman IE, Broadman LM, Hannallah RS, McGill WA. Comparison of the analgesic effects of EMLA (eutectic mixture of local anesthetics) to intradermal lidocaine infiltration prior to venous cannulation in unpremedicated children. Anesthesiology 1988;68:804.
410. Cooper CM, Gerrish SP, Hardwick M, Kay R. EMLA cream reduces the pain of venipuncture in children. Eur J Anaesthesiol 1987;4:441.
411. Maunuksela EL, Korpela R. Double-blind evaluation of a lignocaine-prilocaine cream (EMLA) in children. Effect on the pain associated with venous cannulation. Br J Anaesth 1986;58:1242.
412. Kapelushnik J, Koren G, Solh H, Greenberg M, De Veber L. Evaluating the efficacy of EMLA in alleviating pain associated with lumbar puncture; comparison of open and double-blinded protocols in children. Pain 1990;42:31.
413. Nilsson A, Danielson K, Engberg G, Henneberg S. EMLA for pain relief during arterial cannulation. A double-blind, placebo-controlled study of a lidocaine-prilocaine cream. Ups J Med Sci 1990;95:87.
414. Shortsleeve MJ, Levine MS. Herpes esophagitis in otherwise healthy patients: clinical and radiographic findings. Radiology 1992;182:859.
415. Carnel SB, Blakeslee DB, Oswald SG, Barnes M. Treatment of radiation- and chemotherapy-induced stomatitis. Otolaryngol Head Neck Surg 1990;102:326.
416. Watts SJ, Alexander LC, Fawcett K, Check FJ, Abnrashed A. Herpes simplex esophagitis in a renal transplant patient treated with cyclosporine A: a case report. Am J Gastroenterol 1986;81:185.
417. Welling LR, Watson WA. The emergency department treatment of dyspepsia with antacids and oral lidocaine. Ann Emerg Med 1990; 19:785.
418. Beaver WT, Wallenstein S, Houde RW, Rogers A. A comparison of the analgesic effects of methotrimeprazine and morphine in patients with cancer. Clin Pharmacol Ther 1966;7:436.
419. Oliver OJ. The use of methotrimeprazine in terminal care. Br J Clin Pract 1985;39:339.
420. Walsh TD. Antidepressants in chronic pain. Clin Neuropharmacol 1983;6:271.
421. Breivik H, Rennemo F. Clinical evaluation of combined treatment with methadone and psychotropic drugs in cancer patients. Acta Anaesthetica Scandanavica 1982;74:135.
422. Magni G, Arsie D, DeLeo D. Antidepressants in the treatment of cancer pain. A survey in Italy. Pain 1987;29:347.
423. Hugues A, Chauvergne J, Lissilour T, Lagarde C. L'imipramine utilisee comme antalgique majeur en carcinologie: etude de 118 cas. Presse Med 1963;71:1073.
424. Walsh TD. Controlled study of imipramine and morphine in chronic pain due to cancer. Proceedings of the American Society of Clinical Oncology 1986;5:237.
425. Panerai AE, Bianchi M, Sacerdote P, Ripamonti C, Ventafridda V, De Conno F. Antidepressants in cancer pain. J Palliat Care 1991;7: 42.
426. Swerdlow M. Anticonvulsant drugs and chronic pain. Clin Neuropharmacol 1984;7:51.
427. Lloyd-Smith DL, Sachdev KK. A long-term, low dosage study of carbamazepine in trigeminal neuralgia. Headache 1969;9:64.
428. Rockliff BW, Davis EH. Controlled sequential trials of carbamazepine in trigeminal neuralgia. Arch Neurol 1966;15:129.
429. Taylor JC, Brauer S, Espir MLE. Long-term treatment of trigeminal neuralgia with carbamazepine. Postgrad Med J 1980;57:16.

430. Tomson T, Bertilsson L. Potent therapeutic effects of carbamazepine 10,11-epoxide in trigeminal neuralgia. Arch Neurol 1984;41:598.
431. Braham J, Saia A. Phenytoin in the treatment of trigeminal and other neuralgias. Lancet 1960;2:892.
432. Ramsey RE, Wilder BJ, Berger JR, Bruni J. A double-blind study comparing carbamazepine and phenytoin as initial seizure therapy in adults. Neurology 1983;33:904.
433. Swerdlow M, Cundill JG. Anticonvulsant drugs used in the treatment of lancinating pain. A comparison. Anaesthesia 1981;36:1129.
434. Yajnik S, Singh GP, Singh G, Kumar M. Phenytoin as a coanalgesic in cancer pain. J Pain Symptom Manage 1992;7:209.
435. Caccia MR. Clonazepam in facial neuralgia and cluster headache: clinical and electrophysiological study. Eur Neurol 1975;13:560.
436. Raftery H. The management of postherpetic pain using sodium valproate and amitriptyline. Journal of the Irish Medical Association 1979;72:399.
437. Peiris JB, Perera GLS, Davendra SV, Lionel NDW. Sodium valproate in trigeminal neuralgia. Med J Aust 1980;2:278.
438. Fromm GH, Terrence CF, Chattha AS. Baclofen in the treatment of trigeminal neuralgia: double-blind study and long-term follow-up. Ann Neurol 1984;15:240.
439. Fromm GH. Trigeminal neuralgia and related disorders. In: Portenoy RK, ed. Pain: mechanisms and syndromes. Neurologic clinics. 7th vol. Philadelphia: WB Saunders, 1989:305.
440. Parmar BS, Shah KH, Gandhi IC. Baclofen in trigeminal neuralgia—a clinical trial. Indian J Dental Research 1989;1:109.
441. Barbour CM, Tovell RM. Experiences with procaine administered intravenously. Ann Intern Med 1948;10:514.
442. Edwards WT, Habib F, Burney RG, Begin G. Intravenous lidocaine in the management of various chronic pain states. Reg Anesth 1985; 10:1.
443. Graubaud DJ, Peterson MC. The therapeutic uses of intravenous procaine. Ann Intern Med 1949;10:175.
444. Glazer S, Portenoy RK. Systemic local anesthetics in pain control. J Pain Symptom Manage 1991;6:30.
445. Devulder JE, Ghys L, Dhondt W, Rolly G. Neuropathic pain in a cancer patient responding to subcutaneously administered lignocaine. Clin J Pain 1993;9:220.
446. Birch K, Jorgensen B, Chraemer-Jorgensen B, Kehlet H. Effect of i.v. lignocaine on pain and the endocrine metabolic responses after surgery. Br J Anaesth 1987;59:721.
447. Ellemann K, Sjogren P, Banning AM, Jensen TS, Smith T, Geertsen P. Trial of intravenous lidocaine on painful neuropathy in cancer patients. Clin J Pain 1989;5:291.
448. Pascual J, Berciano J. Failure of mexiletine to control trigeminal neuralgia. Headache 1989;29:517.
449. Kubota K, Joshita Y, Tamura J, et al. Relief of severe diabetic truncal pain with mexiletine. J Med 1991;22:307.
450. Chabal C, Russell LC, Burchiel KJ. The effect of intravenous lidocaine, tocainide and mexiletine on spontaneously active fibers originating in rat sciatic neuromas. Pain 1989;38:333.
451. Dejgard A, Petersen P, Kastrup J. Mexiletine for treatment of chronic painful diabetic neuropathy. Lancet 1988;1:9.
452. CAST (Cardiac Arrhythmia Suppression Trial) Investigators. Preliminary report: effect of encainide and flecainide on mortality in a randomized trial of arrhythmia suppression after acute myocardial infarction. N Engl J Med 1989;321:406.
453. Horn HR, Hadidian Z, Johnson JL, Vasallo HG, Williams JH, Young MD. Safety evaluation of tocainide in an American emergency use program. Am Heart J 1980;100:1037.
454. Quan DB, Wandres DL, Schroeder DJ. Clonidine in pain management. Ann Pharmacother 1993;27:313.
455. Tan Y-M, Croese J. Clonidine and diabetic patients with leg pains. Ann Intern Med 1986;105:633.
456. Jaeger H, Maier C. Calcitonin in phantom limb pain: a double-blind study. Pain 1992;48:21.
457. Lechin F, van der Dijs B, Lechin ME, et al. Pimozide therapy for trigeminal neuralgia. Arch Neurol 1989;9:960.
458. Ghostine SY, Comair YG, Turner DM, Kassell NF, Azar CG. Phenoxybenzamine in the treatment of causalgia. J Neurosurg 1984;60:1263.
459. Abram SE, Lightfoot RW. Treatment of longstanding causalgia with prazosin. Reg Anesth 1981;6:79.
460. Simson G. Propranolol for causalgia and Sudek's atrophy. JAMA 1974;227:327.
461. Prough DS, McLeskey CH, Poehling GG, et al. Efficacy of oral nifedipine in the treatment of reflex sympathetic dystrophy. Anesthesiology 1985;62:796.
462. Berkey CS, Eisenberg E, Carr DB, Chalmers TC, Mosteller F. Nonsteroidal anti-inflammatory drugs (NSAIDS) for cancer pain: meta-analysis. (Abstract) In: Seventh world congress on pain: congress abstracts. Seattle: IASP Publications, 1993:5.
463. Robinson RG, Preston DF, Spicer JA, Baxter KG. Radionuclide therapy of intractable bone pain: emphasis on strontium-89. Semin Nucl Med 1992;22:28.
464. Porter AT, McEwan AJ, Powe JE, et al. Results of a randomized phase-III trial to evaluate the efficacy of strontium-89 adjuvant to local field external beam irradiation in the management of endocrine resistant metastatic prostate cancer. Int J Radiat Oncol Biol Phys 1993; 25:805.
465. Lewington VJ, McEwan AJ, Ackery DM, et al. A prospective, randomised double-blind crossover study to examine the efficacy of strontium-89 in pain palliation in patients with advanced prostate cancer metastatic to bone. Eur J Cancer 1991;27:954.
466. Laing AH, Ackery DM, Bayly RJ, et al. Strontium-89 chloride for pain palliation in prostatic skeletal malignancy. Br J Radiol 1991;64: 816.
467. Fossa SD, Paus E, Lochoff M, Backe SM, Aas M. Strontium-89 in bone metastases from hormone resistant prostate cancer: palliation effect and biochemical changes. Br J Cancer 1992;66:177.
468. Dearnaley DP, Bayly RJ, A'Hern RP, Gadd J, Zivanovic MM, Lewington VJ. Palliation of bone metastases in prostate cancer. Hemibody irradiation or strontium-89? Clin Oncol (R Coll Radiol) 1992;4:101.
469. Laing AH, Ackery DM, Bayly RJ, et al. Strontium-89 chloride for pain palliation in prostatic skeletal malignancy. Br J Radiol 1991;64: 816.
470. Robinson RG. Strontium 89: precursor targeted therapy for relief of blastic metastatic disease. Cancer 1993;72(Suppl):3433.
471. Holmes RA. [153Sm]EDTMP: a potential therapy for bone cancer pain. Semin Nucl Med 1992;22:41.
472. Sandeman TF, Budd RS, Martin JJ. Samarium-153-labelled EDTMP for bone metastases from cancer of the prostate. Clin Oncol (R Coll Radiol) 1992;4:160.
473. Turner JH, Claringbold BG, Heatherington EL, Sorby P, Martindal AA. A phase I study of samarium-153 ethylenedi-amenetetramethylene phosphonate therapy for disseminated skeletal metastases. J Clin Oncol 1989;7:1926.
474. Turner JH, Claringbold PG. A phase II study of treatment of painful multifocal skeletal metastases with single and repeated dose samarium-153 ethylenediaminetetramethylene phosphonate. Eur J Cancer 1991;27:1084.
475. Collins C, Eary JF, Donaldson G, et al. Samarium-153-EDTMP in bone metastases of hormone refractory prostate carcinoma: a phase I/II trial. J Nucl Med 1993;34:1839.
476. Maxon H, Thomas SR, Hertzberg VS, et al. Rhenium-186 hydroxyethylidene diphosphonate for the treatment of painful osseous metastases. Semin Nucl Med 1992;22:33.
477. Maxon H3, Schroder LE, Hertzberg VS, et al. Rhenium-186(Sn)HEDP for treatment of painful osseous metastases: results of a double-blind crossover comparison with placebo. J Nucl Med 1991; 32:1877.
478. Coleman RE, Woll PJ, Miles M, Scrivener W, Rubens RD. Treatment of bone metastases with (3 amino-1-hydroxyprpylidene)-1, 1-bisphosphonate (APD). Br J Cancer 1988;58:621.
479. Thiebaud D, Leyvraz S, von Fliedner V, et al. Treatment of bone metastases from breast cancer and myeloma with pamidronate. Eur J Cancer 1991;27:37.
480. Morton AR, Cantrill JA, Pillai GV, McMahon A, Anderson DC, Howell A. Sclerosis of lytic bony metastases after aminohydroxyprpylidene bisphosphonate (APD) in patients with breast cancer. BMJ 1988; 297:772.
481. van Holten Verzantvoort ATM, Zwinderman AH, Aaronson NK, et al. The effect of supportive pamidronate treatment on aspects of quality of life of patients with advanced breast cancer. Eur J Cancer 1991;27: 544.
482. Ernst DS, MacDonald RN, Paterson AHG, Jensen J, Brasher P, Bruera E. A double blind, crossover trial of I.V. clodronate in metastatic bone pain. J Pain Symptom Manage 1992;7:4.
483. Clemens MR, Fessele K, Heim ME. Multiple myeloma: effect of daily

dichloromethylene bisphosphonate on skeletal complications. Ann Hematol 1993;66:141.
484. van Holten-Verzantvoort AT, Kroon HM, Bijvoet OL, et al. Palliative pamidronate treatment in patients with bone metastases from breast cancer. J Clin Oncol 1993;11:491.
485. Roth A, Kolaric K. Analgesic activity of calcitonin in patients with painful osteolytic metastases of breast cancer. Oncology 1986;43:283.
486. Warrell RP, Lovett D, Dilmanian FA, Schnieder R, Heelan RT. Low-dose gallium nitrate for prevention of osteolysis in myeloma: results of a pilot randomized study. J Clin Oncol 1993;11:2443.
487. Abrams P, Fenely R. The action of prostaglandins on smooth muscle of the human urinary tract in vitro. Br J Urol 1976;47:909.
488. Cardozo LD, Stanton SL. A comparison between bromocriptine and indomethacin in the treatment of detrusor instability. J Urol 1981;73: 236.
489. Hanks GWC, Portenoy RK, MacDonald N, O'Niel WM. Difficult pain problems. In: Doyle D, Hanks GW, MacDonald N, eds. Oxford textbook of palliative medicine. Oxford: Oxford University Press, 1993:257.
490. Boquet J, Moore N, Lhuintre JP, Boismare F. Diltiazem for proctalgia fugax. (Letter) Lancet 1986;1:1493
491. Castell DO. Calcium blocking agents for gastrointestinal disorders. Am J Cardiol 1986;55:210.
492. Swain R. Oral clonidine for proctalgia fugax. Gut 1987;28:1039.
493. Twycross RG, Lack SA. Therapeutics in terminal cancer. 2nd ed. Edinburgh: Churchill Livingstone, 1990.
494. Hanks GW. Psychotropic drugs. Clin Oncol (R Coll Radiol) 1984;3: 135.
495. De Conno F, Carraceni A, Zecca E, Spoldi E, Ventafridda V. The continuous subcutaneous infusion of hyoscine butyl bromide reduces secretions in patients with gastrointestinal obstruction. J Pain Symptom Manage 1991;6:484.
496. Baines MJ. Management of malignant intestinal obstruction in patients with advanced cancer. In: Foley KM, Bonica JJ, Ventafridda V, eds. Second international congress on cancer pain. Advances in pain research and therapy. 16th vol. New York: Raven Press, 1990: 327.
497. Mercadante S, Spoldi E, Caraceni A, Maddaloni S, Simonetti MT. Octreotide in relieving gastrointestinal symptoms due to bowel obstruction. Palliat Med 1993;7:295.
498. Syversen JH, Mollestad E, Semb LS. Emepronium bromide (Cetiprin) as a postoperative spasmolytic agent in transvesical prostatectomy. Scand J Urol Nephrol 1976;10:201.
499. Bradley DV, Cazort RJ. Relief of bladder spasm by flavoxate. A comparative study. J Clin Pharmacol 1970;10:65.
500. Canobbio L, Boccardo F, Cannata D, Gallotti P, Epis R. Treatment of advanced pancreatic carcinoma with the somatostatin analogue BIM 23014. Preliminary results of a pilot study. Cancer 1992;69:648.
501. Ihse I, Permerth J. Enzyme therapy and pancreatic pain. Acta Chirurgica Scandinavica 1990;156:281.
502. Casley-Smith JR, Casley-Smith JR. Modern treatment of lymphoedema. II. The benzopyrones. Australas J Dermatol 1992;33:69.
503. Casley-Smith J, Morgan RG, Piller NB. Treatment of lymphedema of the arms and legs with 5,6-benzo-[alpha]-pyrone. N Engl J Med 1993;329:1158.
504. Linton SL, Melin L. Applied relaxation in the management of cancer pain. Behavioral Psychotherapy 1983;11:337.
505. Rhiner M, Ferrell BR, Ferrell BA, Grant MM. A structured nondrug intervention program for cancer pain. Cancer Practice 1993;1:137.
506. Brennan MJ. Management of lymphedema: review of pathophysiology and treatment. J Pain Symptom Manage 1992;7:110.
507. Plummer JL, Cherry DA, Cousins MJ, Gourlay GK, Onley M, Evans KHA. Long term spinal administration of morphine in cancer and non-cancer pain: a retrospective study. Pain 1991;44:212.
508. Krames ES. Intrathecal infusional therapies for intractable pain: patient management guidelines. J Pain Symptom Manage 1993;8:36.
509. Hogan Q, Haddox JD, Abram S, Weissman D, Taylor ML, Janjan N. Epidural opiates and local anesthetics for the management of cancer pain. Pain 1991;46:271.
510. Patt R, Jain S. Long-term management of a patient with perineal pain secondary to rectal cancer. J Pain Symptom Manage 1990;5:127.
511. Moulin DE, Inturrisi CE, Foley KM. Epidural and intrathecal opioids: cerebrospinal fluid and plasma pharmacokinetics in cancer pain patients. In: Foley KM, Inturrisi CE, eds. Opioid analgesics in the management of clinical pain. Advances in pain research and therapy. 8th vol. New York: Raven Press, 1986:369.
512. Max MB, Inturrisi CE, Kaiko RF, Grabinski PY, Li CH, Foley KM. Epidural and intrathecal opiates: cerebrospinal fluid and plasma profiles in patients with chronic cancer pain. Clin Pharmacol Ther 1985; 38:631.
513. Brose WG, Tanalian DL, Brodsky JB, Mark JBD, Cousins MJ. CSF and blood pharmacokinetics of hydromorphone and morphine following lumbar epidural administration. Pain 1991;45:11.
514. Kroin JS, Ali A, York M, Penn RD. The distribution of medication along the spinal canal after chronic intrathecal administration. Neurosurgery 1993;33:266.
515. Chrubasik J, Wust H, Schulte MJ, Thon K, Zindler M. Relative analgesic potency of epidural fentanyl, alfentanil, and morphine in treatment of postoperative pain. Anesthesiology 1988;68:929.
516. Du Pen SL, Ramsey DH. Compounding local anaesthetics and narcotics for epidural analgesia in cancer outpatients. Anesthesiology 1988; 69:A404.
517. Nitescu P, Appelgren L, Linder LE, Sjoberg M, Hultman E, Curelaru I. Epidural versus intrathecal morphine-bupivicaine: assessment of consecutive treatment in advanced cancer pain. J Pain Symptom Manage 1990;5:18.
518. Van Dongen RT, Crul BJ, De BM. Long-term intrathecal infusion of morphine and morphine/bupivacaine mixtures in the treatment of cancer pain: a retrospective analysis of 51 cases. Pain 1993;55:119.
519. Myers DP, Lema MJ, de Leon-Casasola OA, Bacon DR. Intrapleural analgesia for the treatment of severe cancer pain in terminally ill patients. J Pain Symptom Manage 1993;8:505.
520. Lema MJ, Myers DP, De LCO, Penetrante R. Pleural phenol therapy for the treatment of chronic esophageal cancer pain. Reg Anesth 1992; 17:166.
521. Waldman SD, Allen ML, Cronen MC. Subcutaneous tunneled intrapleural catheters in the long-term relief of right upper quadrant pain of malignant origin. J Pain Symptom Manage 1989;4:86.
522. Brown DL, Bulley CK, Quiel EC. Neurolytic celiac plexus blockade for pancreatic cancer pain. Anesth Analg 1987;66:869.
523. Cousins MJ, Dwyer B, Gibb D. Chronic pain and neurolytic blockade. In: Cousins MJ, Bridenbaugh PO, eds. Neural blockade in clinical anesthesia and management of pain. 2nd ed. Philadelphia: JB Lippincott, 1988:1053.
524. Bonica JJ, Buckley FP, Moricca G, Murphey TM. Neurolytic blockade and hypophysectomy. In: Bonica JJ, ed. The management of pain. 2nd vol, 2nd ed. Philadelphia: Lea & Febiger, 1990:1980.
525. Mercadante S. Celiac plexus block versus analgesics in pancreatic cancer pain. Pain 1993;52:187.
526. Lillemoe KD, Cameron JL, Kaufman HS, Yeo CJ, Pitt HA, Sauter PK. Chemical splanchnicectomy in patients with unresectable pancreatic cancer. A prospective randomized trial. Ann Surg 1993;217:447.
527. Plancarte R, Amescua C, Patt RB, Aldrete JA. Superior hypogastric plexus block for pelvic cancer pain. Anesthesiology 1990;73:236.
528. de Leon Casasola OA, Kent E, Lema MJ. Neurolytic superior hypogastric plexus block for chronic pelvic pain associated with cancer. Pain 1993;54:145.
529. Hellendoorn SM, Overweg van Kints J. Perineal pain: a case report. Eur J Surg Oncol 1988;14:197.
530. Ischia S, Luzzani A, Ischia A, Magon F, Toscano D. Subarachnoid neurolytic block (L5-S1) and unilateral percutaneous cervical cordotomy in the treatment of pain secondary to pelvic malignant disease. Pain 1984;20:139.
531. Rodriguez-Bigas M, Petrelli NJ, Herrera L, West C. Intrathecal phenol rhizotomy for management of pain in recurrent unresectable carcinoma of the rectum. Surg Gynecol Obstet 1991;173:41.
532. Robertson DH. Transsacral neurolytic nerve block. An alternative approach to intractable perineal pain. Br J Anaesth 1983;55:873.
533. Arbit E. Neurosurgical management of cancer pain. In: Foley KM, Bonica JJ, Ventafrida V, eds. Second international congress on cancer pain. Advances in pain research and therapy. 16th vol. New York: Raven Press, 1990:289.
534. Rosomoff HL, Carroll F, Brown J. Percutaneous radiofrequency cervical cordotomy: technique. J Neurosurg 1965;23:639.
535. Tasker RR, Tsuda T, Howrylyshn P. Percutaneous cordotomy—the lateral high cervical technique. In: Schmidek HH, Sweet WH, eds. Operative neurosurgical technique: indications, methods and results. New York: Grune & Stratton, 1988:1191.

536. Polatty RC, Cooper KR. Respiratory failure after percutaneous cordotomy. South Med J 1986;79:367.
537. Levin AB, Ramirez LL. Treatment of cancer pain with hypophysectomy: surgical and chemical. In: Benedetti C, Chapman CR, Moricca G, eds. Recent advances in the management of pain. Advances in pain research and therapy. 7th vol. New York: Raven Press, 1984:631.
538. Hassenbusch SJ, Pillay PK, Barnett GM. Radiofrequency cingulotomy for intractable cancer pain using stereotaxis guided by magnetic resonance imaging. Neurosurgery 1990;27:220.
539. Cherny NI, Portenoy RK. Sedation in the treatment of refractory symptoms: guidelines for evaluation and treatment. J Palliat Care 1994;10:31.
540. Portenoy RK, Moulin DE, Rogers A, Inturrisi CE, Foley KM. IV infusion of opioids for cancer pain: clinical review and guidelines for use. Cancer Treatment Reports 1986;70:575.
541. Dunlop RJ. Excitatory phenomena associated with high dose opioids. Curr Ther Endocrinol Metab 1989;30:121.
542. Breitbart W, Passik SD. Psychiatric aspects of palliative care. In: Doyle D, Hanks GW, MacDonald N, eds. Oxford textbook of palliative medicine. Oxford: Oxford University Press, 1993:609.
543. Burke AL, Diamond PL, Hulbert J, Yeatman J, Farr EA. Terminal restlessness—its management and the role of midazolam. Med J Aust 1991;155:485.
544. Johanson GA. Midazolam in terminal care. Am J Hospice and Palliative Care 1993;10:13.
545. Enck RE. The last few days. Am J Hospice Palliative Care 1992;9:11.
546. McNamara P, Minton P, Twycross RG. The use of midazolam in palliative care. Palliat Med 1991;5:244.
547. Bottomly DM, Hanks G. Subcutaneous midazolam infusion in palliative care. J Pain Symptom Manage 1990;5:259.
548. Smales OR, Smales EA, Sanders HG. Flunitrazepam in terminal care. J Paediatr Child Health 1993;29:68.
549. Twycross RG, Lichter I. The terminal phase. In: Doyle D, Hanks GW, MacDonald N, eds. Oxford textbook of palliative medicine. Oxford: Oxford University Press, 1993:651.
550. Gusterson FR, Kay J, Kingsbury AW. Analgesia in terminal malignant disease. (Letter) BMJ 1979;2:6181.
551. Lichter I, Hunt E. The last 48 hours of life. J Palliat Care 1990;6:7.
552. Greene WR, Davis WH. Titrated intravenous barbiturates in the control of symptoms in patients with terminal cancer. South Med J 1991;84:332.
553. Truog RD, Berde CB, Mitchell C, Greir HE. Barbiturates in the care of the terminally ill. N Engl J Med 1992;327:1678.
554. Latimer EJ. Ethical decision-making in the care of the dying and its applications to clinical practice. J Pain Symptom Manage 1991;6:329.

Surgery for Gastrointestinal Cancer: A Multidisciplinary Approach, edited by Harold J. Wanebo.
Lippincott-Raven Publishers, Philadelphia, © 1997.

CHAPTER 71

Peritoneal Carcinomatosis: Rational Therapeutic Interventions Using Intraperitoneal Chemotherapy

Paul H. Sugarbaker

ETIOLOGY OF PERITONEAL CARCINOMATOSIS

Gastrointestinal cancer is a disease of malignancies that arises in the epithelial lining of the gut. Tumors progress by invading the surrounding normal tissues and finally reaching the serosal surface or mesenteric fat. During the course of this invasion, gastrointestinal cancer may disseminate by three routes.[1] If the primary cancer invades into venules, it may travel through the portal vein to the liver sinusoids. Within the liver, cancer cells that implant develop into liver metastases.[2] Similarly, lymphatic channels may be invaded and lymph nodes become involved by the malignant process. This usually occurs as an orderly progression of cancerous nodes along the nodal chain.[3] Full-thickness invasion of the bowel wall may result in tumor penetration through this structure. This causes seeding of cancer on peritoneal surfaces adjacent to the primary malignancy, or direct extension to tissues surrounding the cancer. The distribution of these tumor implants is proximal to the primary tumor but randomly distributed on the nearby surfaces.[4]

In two of these three routes of cancer dissemination, metastases from metastases can occur. Hematogenous and lymphatic metastases progress as a cascade phenomenon, so that tumor at other "systemic" sites (especially the lungs) develops.[2] As peritoneal implants grow into larger nodules, these nodules exfoliate malignant cells into the peritoneal space to increase exponentially the number of cancerous nodules on peritoneal surfaces. For high-grade cancer, a matting together of structures within the abdomen and pelvis occurs.

The progression of gastrointestinal cancer is slow during the early phases of primary tumor growth. With the development of secondary tumor deposits, the pace of the disease increases markedly as metastases from metastases develop and implants exfoliate within the peritoneal cavity. A preponderance of metastases develop in the tissue whose capillary bed receives venous blood directly from the primary cancer. For gastrointestinal cancer, this is the liver. Exponential progression rapidly brings about the patient's demise. The secondary liver tumors disseminate to the lung and then to other systemic sites. The secondary lymph node tumors disseminate through the thoracic duct to the lung and then to other systemic sites. If intraarterial malignant emboli occur, they bring about metastases to virtually all capillary beds.[5] At systemic sites, there may be a preferential appearance of metastases in organs with less rapid blood flow (puddling) and little extrinsic motion (eg, bone marrow, adrenal gland, brain).[2] Metastases to organs in vigorous motion (eg, skeletal muscle, heart muscle) are rare. Metastases to nodes in the small bowel mesentery and pelvic sidewall may result from cancerous nodules on peritoneal surfaces.

The requirements for intraperitoneal spread of cancer are considerably different than for vascular or lymphatic dissemination. For peritoneal carcinomatosis to occur, the integrity of the bowel wall must be violated. This can result from tumor pushing through bowel wall, especially thin-walled structures such as the appendix, or from invasion. Mucinous cancers seem to dissect through the layers of a visceral structure, such as the stomach wall, and more frequently gain access to the peritoneal space. Even the lowest-grade mucinous tumors, if they seed the peritoneal cavity, develop into peritoneal carcinomatosis. In contrast, for hematogenous or lymphatic metastases to occur, the cancer must be a high-grade invasive tumor. Venular and lymphatic invasion requires a high-grade tumor, and implantation on endothelium-lined and basement membrane intact surfaces requires an invasive capability. Peritoneal carcinomatosis does not require this high-grade tumor biology. Even grade I mucinous tumors that never metastasize by hematogenous or lymphatic routes disseminate within the peritoneal cavity. In addition, these low-grade tumors do not move from the peritoneal cavity to systemic sites in the cascade phenomenon. Therefore, if local control of low-grade cancer can be achieved on peritoneal surfaces, these malignancies can be cured. Peritoneal

Paul H. Sugarbaker: Director—Surgical Oncology, The Washington Cancer Institute, Washington Hospital Center, 110 Irving Street, NW, Washington, DC 20010-2975 carcinomatosis should not be considered evidence of systemic disease.

CAUSES OF PERITONEAL SEEDING

The original seeding from a primary cancer may occur at two different times in the course of the disease. First, dissemination may occur before operation through full-thickness penetration of the bowel wall by cancer. The early seeding is proximal to the primary cancer and limited in its extent. If there is an inflammatory component to the perforation, the exfoliated cells may be walled off and not cause more widespread peritoneal seeding. An exception is the spread of mucinous tumors, which disseminate widely within the peritoneum.[4] Alternatively, intraoperative trauma may result in cancer dissemination within the peritoneal cavity. Peritoneal seeding occurs by both natural and iatrogenic mechanisms.

As a result of tumor contamination of the abdominal and pelvic surfaces, two distinct patterns of recurrent disease after surgical removal of the primary cancer are evident. Low-density seeding of tumor away from the resection site of the primary tumor causes peritoneal carcinomatosis. At the resection site, especially if there were narrow margins of resection of a lymph node–positive cancer, a higher density of tumor emboli accumulation can be expected. This results in the plaque of tumor that frequently is observed in the resection site of a recurrent rectal cancer. Often, patients with rectal cancer have a confluence of cancer in the hollow of the pelvis. Other examples of resection site recurrence include recurrent local cancer in the resection bed of a pancreatic malignancy and a layering of recurrent gastric cancer on the undersurface of the left hemidiaphragm.

Perhaps one of the most unambiguous demonstrations of both peritoneal implantation (low-density seeding) and resection site recurrence (high-density seeding) occurs with retroperitoneal sarcoma (Fig. 71-1). When this disease recurs, sarcomatosis nearly always is a part of the surgical treatment failure. Sarcomatous nodules of uniform size are found scattered throughout the abdomen and pelvis, sometimes with a slightly increased density close to the site of the tumor. Frequently, tumor nodules also are found within abdominal adhesions (sites of previous surgical trauma) or within the abdominal incision. Along the aorta and vena cava, the site for narrow margins of excision, a layering of recurrent sarcoma occurs.[6] This author's hypothesis suggests that this results from high-density seeding from tumor spillage that occurred at the time of resection of the primary tumor mass. The mechanisms for peritoneal sarcomatosis and local recurrence of retroperitoneal sarcoma are the same, and both types of recurrence often are seen in the same patient. In summary, individual tumor emboli disseminated around the peritoneal cavity result in tumor nodules that are diagnosed as peritoneal carcinomatosis or sarcomatosis. Higher-density seeding of tumor that accumulates in a traumatized cancer bed develops into a confluence of disease that conforms to the anatomy of the operative site from which the primary tumor was removed.

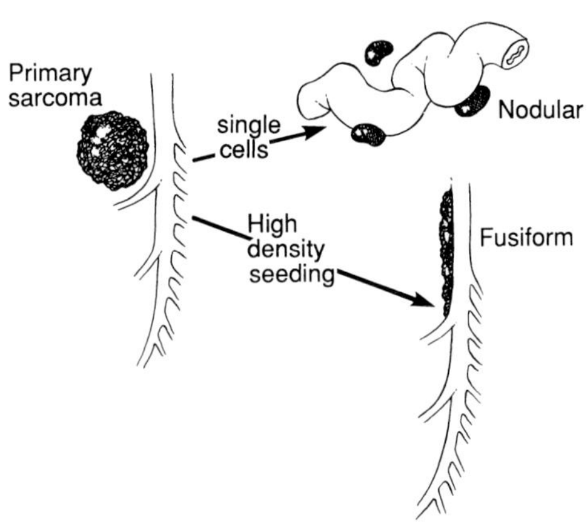

FIG. 71-1. Intraperitoneal dissemination of retroperitoneal sarcoma. Tumor cells traumatically dislodged from the primary tumor disseminate into the abdominal cavity and result in two types of recurrent cancer. Low-density seeding at a distance from the primary tumor results in nodular recurrences. High-density seeding along major vascular and other vital structures results in recurrences in and around the resection site of the primary sarcoma.

An unsolved problem in the surgical management of abdominal and pelvic malignancy is the unacceptably high incidence of local recurrence. This is especially true for pancreatic cancer, gastric cancer, rectal cancer, and retroperitoneal sarcoma. In the past, most oncologists related resection site recurrence to disease persistence in lymph nodes or within unresected lymphatic channels. However, there is no evidence for these mechanisms of local recurrence,[7] and no alternative theories have been proposed. The pattern of disease recurrence in retroperitoneal sarcoma is virtually identical to that in the adenocarcinomas. The progression of adult-onset sarcoma through lymph nodes or lymphatic channels is extremely unusual. The pattern of retroperitoneal sarcoma recurrence cannot be explained rationally as a problem of lymphatic disease persistence. Instead, an integrated mechanism for resection site recurrence of sarcoma and sarcomatosis is intraoperative sarcoma seeding to the narrow margins of excision and to peritoneal surfaces. By analogy, this also may explain the resection site disease seen with pancreatic, gastric, and rectal cancer.

MECHANISMS FOR INTRAPERITONEAL TUMOR EMBOLI

The most obvious way that tumor emboli seed the peritoneal cavity is by full-thickness invasion of the bowel wall and penetration of the cancer through the serosa. However, other mechanisms of seeding may occur at the time of cancer resection. Perhaps the most prominent is leakage of tumor cells from lymphatic channels that have been traumatically divided during the operation (Fig. 71-2). Undoubtedly, cancer cells are present in the lymph nodes and malignant tumor emboli are present in the lymphatic channels. As the specimen is handled and removed, the lymphatic channels on the specimen side of the dissection can seed the resection site and other portions of the abdominopelvic cavity with tumor cells.

It is well known that cancer cells are present in the venous blood draining a malignancy. In every cancer operation, blood is lost into the free abdominal cavity from the specimen. Most of the blood lost during a cancer resection is from the incompletely resected specimen. As the blood is infused peripherally by the

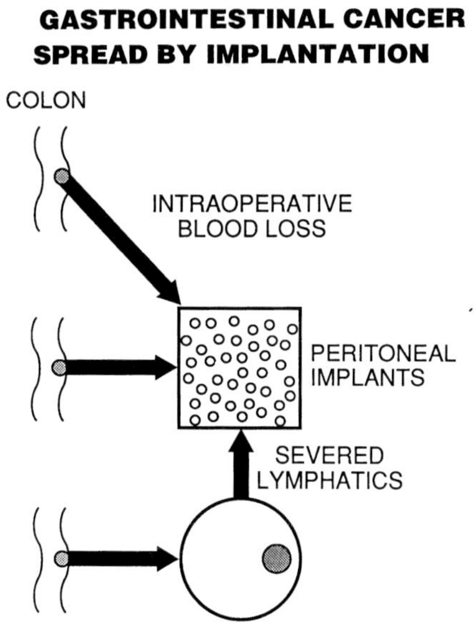

FIG. 71-2. Spread of gastrointestinal cancer by implantation. Three mechanisms of intraperitoneal cancer dissemination are suggested: cancer cells in the blood lost into the peritoneal cavity; cancer cells leaking from lymphatic channels that have been transected; and cancer cells traumatically disrupted from the primary tumor as a result of narrow margins of resection and rough handling of the cancer specimen.

anesthesiologist, it enters the specimen, floods the cancerous tissue, and is lost from venous channels not secured on the cancer specimen. Intraoperative blood loss may cause the intraperitoneal dissemination of viable tumor cells.

Trauma to the specimen, combined with a narrow margin of excision, can force cancer cells through tissue planes and result in free intraabdominal tumor emboli.

Evidence suggests that free intraperitoneal tumor emboli readily implant within raw surfaces. They cannot be washed away easily with saline or water irrigation solutions. Tumor cells are most likely to be entrapped at sites of trauma. At these sites, blood clot and fibrin accumulations may surround large numbers of free intraperitoneal tumor emboli. These entrapped tumor cells grow. In some instances, their growth is enhanced by soluble factors responsible for wound healing.[8] Growth factors may be responsible for the high incidence and rapid progression of recurrent tumors seen at special sites within the abdomen and pelvis. The abdominal incision, the suture lines, the ligatures around blood vessels, and the vaginal cuff in patients who undergo hysterectomy result in compression of tumor cells between tissue planes at these sites; along with intense wound healing, cancer recurrence at these sites occurs repeatedly and progresses rapidly.

PREVENTION OF PERITONEAL CARCINOMATOSIS AND LOCAL RECURRENCE USING INTRAOPERATIVE AND EARLY POSTOPERATIVE INTRAPERITONEAL CHEMOTHERAPY

If the hypothesis regarding peritoneal carcinomatosis and resection site recurrence presented earlier is correct, the most profitable time to intervene in the natural history of these processes is during the perioperative period. Protocols to deliver chemotherapy into the abdomen and pelvis after the complete resection of a gastrointestinal cancer have been initiated.

Pancreatic Cancer

Pancreatic cancer has a high incidence of locoregional recurrence. It may recur as an isolated surgical treatment failure or in combination with disease at other sites.[9,10]

Ettinghausen has used heated intraoperative intraperitoneal cisplatin and mitomycin C.[11] The abdomen is lavaged for 2 hours with these drugs in 3 L of fluid. The lavage is carried out after the pancreatic malignancy has been resected, but before the reconstruction is performed. This ensures that no cancer cells are trapped in tissues compressed by sutures during the performance of an anastomosis or with closure of the abdominal cavity. The same tubes and drains that are used to deliver intraoperative chemotherapy with cisplatin and mitomycin are used for early postoperative intraperitoneal administration of 5-fluorouracil. This protocol does not help control the disease in residual contaminated lymph nodes and perineural lymphatics. It also does not prevent the progression of hematogenous metastases in the liver or other systemic sites. However, it may have a significant effect on the high incidence of resection site recurrence with pancreatic cancer.

Gastric Cancer

Gastric cancer is another abdominopelvic malignancy that often presents in an advanced state. About 70% of patients have lymph node involvement. Consequently, resection often results in tumor cell dissemination through the transected lymphatic channels. In addition, gastric cancer frequently penetrates through the serosal surface of the stomach, and free intraperitoneal tumor emboli often are present even before resection of the primary tumor.[12] Several controlled trials have suggested that perioperative treatment can diminish the incidence of peritoneal seeding and improve the results of surgical therapy for gastric cancer. Takahashi and colleagues used mitomycin C in activated charcoal. They distributed the drug around the upper portion of the abdomen after gastrectomy. This approach resulted in improved survival in a randomized, controlled study.[13] Similarly, in a prospective, randomized study, Koga and colleagues used heated intraoperative perfusion to treat patients with mitomycin C.[14,15] This technique was designed to eliminate stray tumor cells from the abdominal cavity after definitive resection of the primary gastric cancer. These investigators demonstrated a statistically significant improvement in survival. Yu and colleagues used early postoperative intraperitoneal mitomycin C and 5-fluorouracil in patients with stage II and III gastric cancer.[16] A survival advantage of 11% was seen in the treated patients. A greater incidence of peritonitis was seen in the patients who received early postoperative intraperitoneal chemotherapy. These authors postulated that small leaks in the esophagojejunal anastomosis resulted in generalized peritonitis in some patients who underwent lavage. The leaks remained more localized in patients who did not receive intraperitoneal chemotherapy and resulted in less morbidity.

Several trials with gastric cancer have demonstrated no benefit to delayed intraperitoneal chemotherapy. Schiessel and colleagues administered intraperitoneal mitomycin C and cisplatin 1 month after surgery.[17] Three other trials of delayed intraperitoneal chemotherapy for gastric cancer were unsuccessful.[18–20]

Colon and Rectal Cancer

Nordlinger and associates have instituted a controlled trial in patients with colon cancer using intraperitoneal 5-fluorouracil as an adjuvant therapy. Treatment is begun on the fourth postoperative day and continued through the ninth postoperative day. The morbidity and mortality of this technique have been acceptable.[21] Survival results are not available. Fujimoto and colleagues have introduced a heated pelvic perfusion technique for the prevention of local recurrence and peritoneal seeding with rectal cancer. The pelvis is filled with a small volume of drug-containing fluid. The solution contains mitomycin C and is heated to 45°C. Treatment of the pelvic surfaces is continued for 1 hour. An absence of pelvic recurrence has been reported in these patients.[22]

MANAGEMENT OF ESTABLISHED PERITONEAL CARCINOMATOSIS

Appendiceal Cancer

Spratt and colleagues were the first to use intraperitoneal chemotherapy to treat peritoneal carcinomatosis.[23] They performed lavage with a solution of thiotepa and methotrexate in a patient with pseudomyxoma peritonei. Appendiceal cancer may be the ideal malignancy in which to test these techniques. Figure 71-3 compares the natural history of colorectal malignancy with that of grade I mucinous appendiceal cancer. Even when surgery and intraperitoneal chemotherapy eradicate cancer on peritoneal surfaces in patients with colon cancer, disease within the liver or at other distant sites often results in death. In patients with appendiceal cancer, lymphatic and hematogenous metastases rarely occur. Consequently, successful eradication of peritoneal surface disease results in long-term disease-free survival. Sugarbaker and colleagues introduced a therapeutic strategy for peritoneal carcinomatosis from appendiceal cancer that included cytoreductive surgery and early postoperative intraperitoneal administration of mitomycin C and 5-fluorouracil. These regional chemotherapeutic treatments were used after maximal surgical efforts to remove gross disease from the abdominal cavity.[24] In patients with biopsy-proven appendiceal cancer, survival depended greatly on the presence or absence of lymph node metastases (Fig. 71-4). However, long-term survival did occur in some patients with both peritoneal seeding and lymph node metastases.

Colon and Rectal Cancer

A cytoreductive approach to the treatment of peritoneal carcinomatosis from adenocarcinoma of the colon was reported by Schellinx and associates.[25] Fifty-six patients were treated and

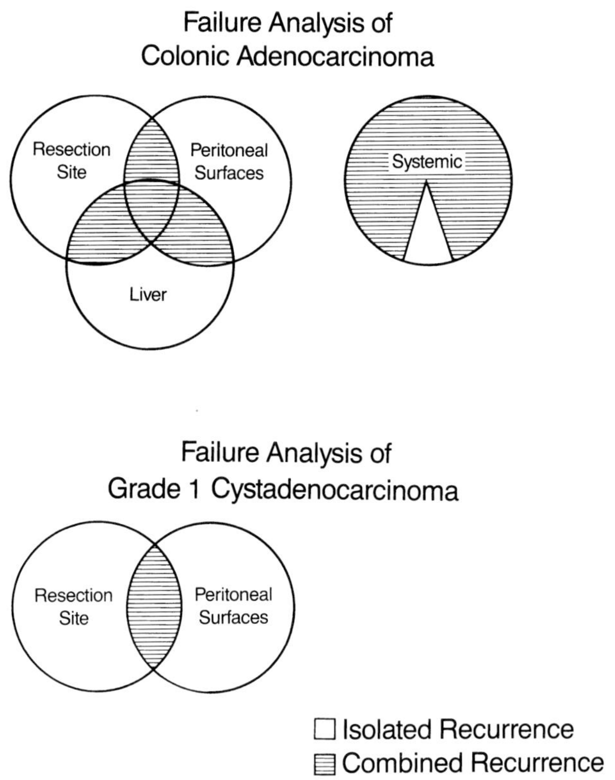

FIG. 71-3. Failure analysis of high-grade and low-grade adenocarcinoma. High-grade tumors disseminate by cancer spread on peritoneal surfaces and resection sites, and through hematogenous and lymphatic metastases to liver and systemic sites. Low-grade mucinous tumors do not metastasize; however, they readily implant on peritoneal surfaces if allowed to find access to the free peritoneal cavity.

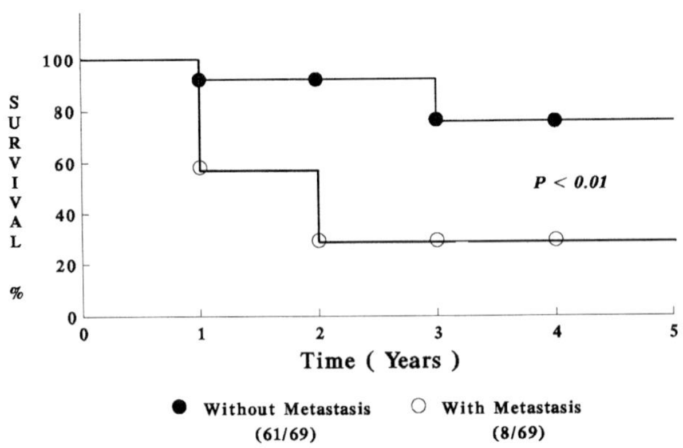

FIG. 71-4. Survival of patients with appendiceal cancer who have peritoneal seeding after cytoreductive surgery and intraperitoneal chemotherapy with mitomycin C and 5-fluorouracil. Survival is improved in those patients who do not have lymph node metastases. (Surgarbaker PH, Bowei Z, Banez Sase G, Shmookler B. Peritoneal carcinomatosis from appendiceal cancer: results in 69 patients treated by cytoreductive surgery and intraperitoneal chemotherapy. Dis Colon Rectum 1993; 36:323.)

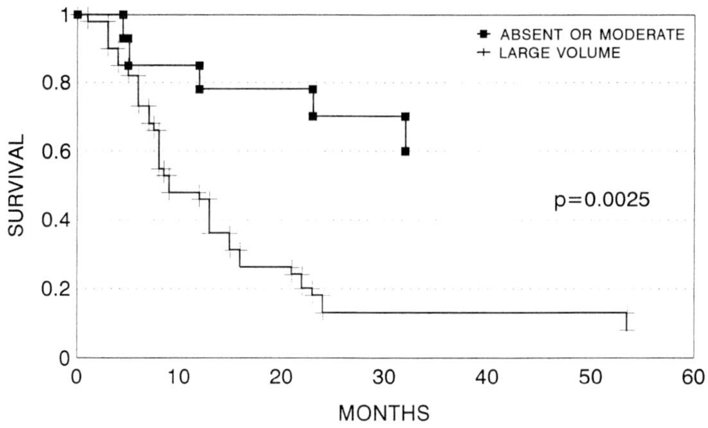

FIG. 71-5. Survival of patients with colon cancer by preresection tumor volume. Patients with a small or moderate tumor volume showed a statistically significant improved survival when compared with patients with a large tumor volume. All patients were treated by cytoreductive surgery and intraperitoneal chemotherapy.

the results were subjected to statistical analysis. A small volume of tumor present in the abdomen and pelvis at the time of exploration correlated with a good prognosis. Other positive prognostic features included complete cytoreduction of tumor nodules to a size of 2.5 mm or less and limited involvement of the abdominal region. A mucinous histologic type of high-grade adenocarcinoma correlated adversely with prognosis when compared with adenocarcinoma. This was a result of the widespread involvement of abdominal and pelvic surfaces by mucinous cancers. Figure 71-5 outlines the results of this study. Long-term survival depended greatly on a low volume of cancer at the time of cytoreduction. These data strongly suggest that early definitive intervention should be pursued in patients with peritoneal carcinomatosis from colon or rectal cancer. With a "watch and wait" approach using only systemic chemotherapy, treatment is impossible by the time the patient becomes symptomatic.

Gastric Cancer

Treatment protocols for patients with gastric cancer who have biopsy-proven peritoneal implants have been instituted by several Japanese and European investigators. In a case-controlled study, Fujimoto and colleagues evaluated the survival of patients treated with intraoperative heated mitomycin C combined with palliative resection.[26] In their most recent report, they reviewed the results of this approach in 20 patients and 10 control subjects.[27,28] The overall 3-year survival rate was 40% after intraperitoneal hyperthermic chemotherapy and 0% after surgery alone. In patients with low-volume peritoneal carcinomatosis (P1 according to the General Rules for Gastric Cancer Study in Surgery and Pathology), 10% of the patients who received combined treatment survived 3 years, whereas all those who underwent surgery alone died within a year. Patients with more advanced peritoneal spread (P2 to P3) survived a median of 440 days after combined treatment, compared with only 125 days for patients in the control group.

Fujimura and associates and Yonemura and colleagues modified the technique of intraperitoneal hyperthermic perfusion with cisplatin and mitomycin C. They administered intraoperative chemotherapy through a device that allowed access to the peritoneal cavity to ensure even and controlled drug distribution within the peritoneal cavity.[29,30] Among 41 patients with established peritoneal carcinomatosis but no liver metastasis, cytoreductive surgery was assessed as complete in 83% of cases. Heated peritoneal perfusion was conducted for 2 hours. As a result of treatment, malignant ascites disappeared in 78% of patients. In 16 cases, a second-look surgery was performed to evaluate treatment response and deliver a second cycle of heated intraperitoneal chemotherapy. The overall response rate was 41% in evaluated cases, and 50% of responders survived 2 years.

In 1993, Panteix and associates reported the results of a pilot study of hyperthermic peritoneal perfusion with mitomycin C. This is the only gastric cancer study that has been conducted outside Japan. Palliative resection was performed in 9 of 20 patients. Forty-seven percent of the patients survived 1 year.[31]

In all reported trials, no excessive postoperative morbidity or mortality was observed and the treatment was well tolerated by the patients with advanced neoplastic disease.

INDICATIONS FOR INTRAPERITONEAL CHEMOTHERAPY

Table 71-1 presents the current indications for the use of intraperitoneal chemotherapy in patients with gastrointestinal cancer. Adenocarcinoma or sarcoma of low malignant potential may arise from many different intraabdominal sites and seed the abdominal or pelvic cavity extensively. Most of these noninvasive malignancies can be eradicated from the abdomen. Cytoreductive surgery followed by intraperitoneal chemotherapy should be considered the standard therapy for patients with malignant pseudomyxoma peritonei, recurrent grade I sarcoma,

TABLE 71-1. *Current indications for intraperitoneal chemotherapy for gastrointestinal cancer*

1. Large-volume, low-grade peritoneal carcinomatosis, or sarcomatosis, or nonaggressive mesothelioma after definitive cytoreductive surgery.
2. Limited volume and limited distribution of peritoneal seeding of high-grade cancer.
3. Perforated gastrointestinal cancers.
4. Cancers adherent to adjacent structures.
5. Tumor spill during surgery.
6. Positive intraperitoneal cytology.

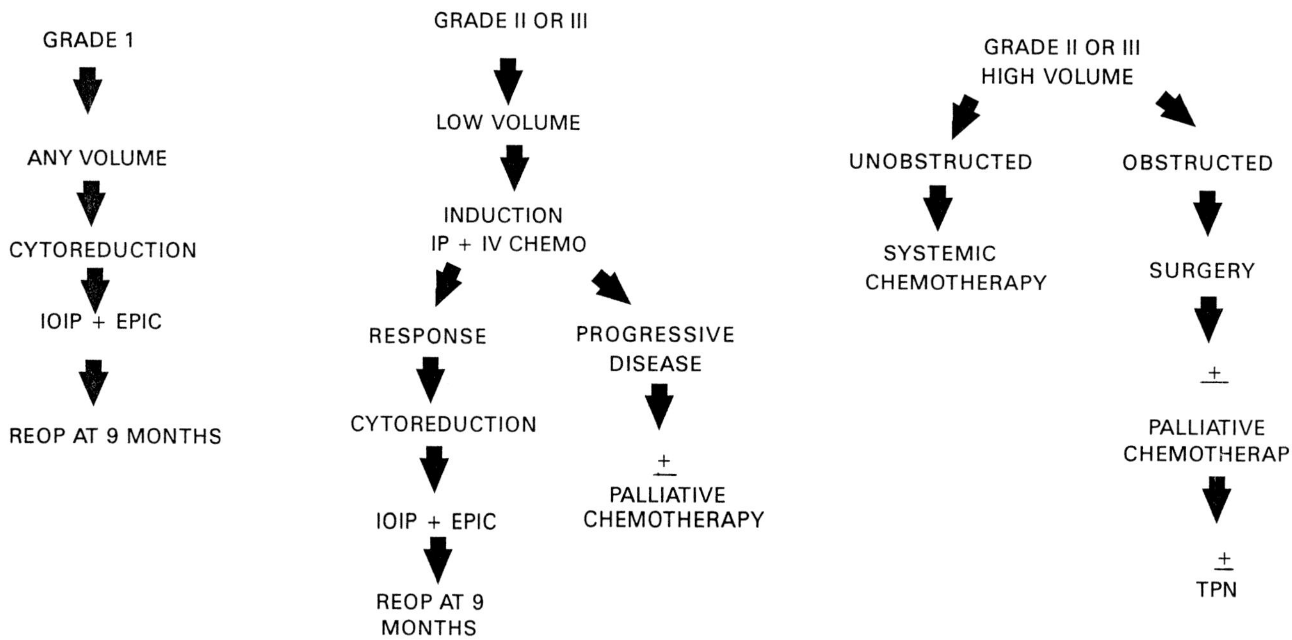

FIG. 71-6. Four treatment plans for patients with peritoneal carcinomatosis. Patients are separated into groups by the grade of the malignancy and by its preresection tumor volume. *EPIC*, early postoperative intraperitoneal chemotherapy; *IOIP*, intraoperative intraperitoneal chemotherapy; *REOP*, reoperation, *TPN*, total parenteral nutrition, *IP*, intraperitoneal; *IV*, intravenous.

and nonaggressive mesothelioma. This approach also has proven beneficial in patients with peritoneal carcinomatosis from grade I cystadenocarcinoma.

Higher-grade adenocarcinomas of gastric, colonic, or appendiceal origin are treated selectively. Management begins with induction intraperitoneal chemotherapy, followed by cytoreductive surgery. In patients with large-volume, high-grade cancer, only palliative therapy for peritoneal carcinomatosis should be considered. In patients with low-volume, high-grade peritoneal seeding, three cycles of intraperitoneal chemotherapy are used routinely before definitive cytoreductive surgery. About 10% of all patients with colon and rectal cancer have peritoneal seeding at the time of resection of the primary cancer. This warrants the use of induction intraperitoneal chemotherapy and cytoreductive surgery. The treatment plans shown in Figure 71-6 outline the current therapeutic options for peritoneal carcinomatosis from colonic, rectal, and appendiceal cancer.

In the standard approach, tumor volume is a fundamental selection criterion for the sequencing of therapy for intraabdominal cancer. The treatment of large-volume disease in the abdominal cavity by intraperitoneal chemotherapy should be avoided. Only patients with low-volume peritoneal surface cancer and minimal abdominopelvic adhesions should receive intraperitoneal chemotherapy. Low-volume disease limited to one or two abdominal regions should be expected to respond and constitutes an indication for induction chemotherapy. If large-volume, low-grade disease is present, a complete surgical cytoreduction must precede the administration of intraperitoneal chemotherapy.[32]

This treatment strategy represents a major departure from standard practice for patients with gastrointestinal cancer in whom peritoneal seeding is documented at the time of primary tumor resection. The standard approach in patients with peritoneal carcinomatosis includes resection of the primary cancer and administration of systemic chemotherapy after full recovery is achieved. Some surgeons do not recommend chemotherapy, in the belief that it diminishes the quality of life in patients who have limited life expectancy. This author performs an extended resection of the primary cancer plus cytoreduction of all peritoneal surface nodules using laser mode electrosurgery.[33] Peritonectomy procedures of visceral or parietal peritoneum are indicated.[34] For example, a rectosigmoid cancer with pelvic seeding and omental nodules requires a complete pelvic peritonectomy and a greater omentectomy. A gastric cancer with seeding on the surface of the stomach and on the underpart of the peritoneal surface of the left hemidiaphragm requires a formal lesser omentectomy with stripping of the omental bursa and a left subdiaphragmatic peritonectomy.

Intraperitoneal chemotherapy plays a major role in the prevention of subsequent peritoneal carcinomatosis or sarcomatosis. Peritoneal carcinomatosis develops in virtually every patient who has a free intraabdominal perforation of gastrointestinal cancer through the malignancy itself. This author recommends intraperitoneal chemotherapy in the early postoperative period for all patients with perforated gastrointestinal cancers.

Frequently, patients who are undergoing resection of large intraabdominal tumors have tumor spills. Tumor spills are extremely common with advanced primary or recurrent rectal malignancies. With resection of advanced primary or recurrent colon cancers, traumatic dispersal of tumor emboli occurs almost routinely. The same is true for large retroperitoneal sarcomas. If a tumor spill occurs, this author recommends the use of intraperitoneal chemotherapy to prevent the subsequent development of peritoneal carcinomatosis or sarcomatosis. Limited peritoneal seeding, perforation, and tumor spill are absolute indications for the use of intraperitoneal chemotherapy.

Peritoneal fluid that is cytologically positive for cancer is an indication for intraperitoneal chemotherapy. Traditionally, this is accomplished using a large volume of fluid, which is recovered by suction aspiration of all dependent parts of the abdomen and subjected to centrifugation. Another technique is more likely to reveal cancer cells on the surface of the primary cancer. A surgical knife blade is used to scrape gently the serosal surface of the primary cancer after it has been passed off the operative field. The cells that accumulate on the blade are plated out onto a glass side and immediately sent to be stained and read by a pathologist. Limited peritoneal seeding can be detected in this manner that cannot be documented using the lavage technique.

TECHNICAL CONSIDERATIONS IN THE USE OF INTRAPERITONEAL CHEMOTHERAPY

To interrupt the implantation of tumor cells on intraabdominal and pelvic surfaces, the abdominal cavity is flooded with chemotherapeutic agents in a large volume of fluid during surgery and in the early postoperative period. This strategy for the prevention and treatment of peritoneal carcinomatosis and sarcomatosis involves a change in both the route and the timing of chemotherapy.

INTRAOPERATIVE MITOMYCIN C OR CISPLATIN

This new approach to the surgical treatment of intraabdominal malignancies begins in the operating room with proper placement of tubes and drains for intraoperative delivery of intraperitoneal chemotherapy (Fig. 71-7).

Closed-suction drains are placed in the dependent portions of the abdomen. This includes the right subhepatic space, the left subdiaphragmatic space, and the pelvis. A Tenckhoff catheter (Quinton spiral peritoneal catheter, Quinton Incorporated, Seattle, WA) with the end sealed off is placed through the abdominal wall and secured with stitches at the site the surgeon judges to be at highest risk for recurrent cancer. This provides the treatment with a regional intensity. The hottest and most turbulent lavage fluid is at the site where the catheter infuses into the peritoneal cavity. All transabdominal drains and tubes are secured with a pursestring suture at the peritoneal level and at the skin. If stripping of the hemidiaphragm has occurred, right-angle thoracostomy tubes (Deknatel, Floral Park, NY) are inserted into the right and left chest after the intraoperative chemotherapy is completed. This prevents postoperative fluid accumulation in the chest.

The skin, but not the fascia, of the abdomen is closed with a running monofilament suture. Lavage of the abdomen is instituted with 3 L of 1.5% dextrose peritoneal dialysis solution to which chemotherapeutic drugs have been added. Mitomycin (10 mg/m^2) is used routinely if colorectal, pancreatic, or gastric cancer is being treated. If ovarian cancer or sarcoma is being treated, cisplatin (50 to 75 mg/m^2) is used.

IMMEDIATE POSTOPERATIVE ABDOMINAL LAVAGE

To keep the catheters used for drug instillation and abdominal drainage clear of blood clots and tissue debris, abdominal lavage is begun in the operating room as soon as the abdominal incision is closed. In this way, the tubes and drains positioned for the intraoperative chemotherapy can be used. This author has used large volumes of fluid infused rapidly and then drained from the abdomen after a short dwell time. During the 12 to 24 hours of abdominal lavage, the patient's hemodynamic and respiratory status is allowed to stabilize. The standardized orders for postoperative lavage are given in Table 71-2.

EARLY POSTOPERATIVE INTRAPERITONEAL 5-FLUOROURACIL CHEMOTHERAPY FOR ADENOCARCINOMA

Intraperitoneal chemotherapy is given in the first 5 days after complete cytoreduction. In patients with colon cancer, rectal

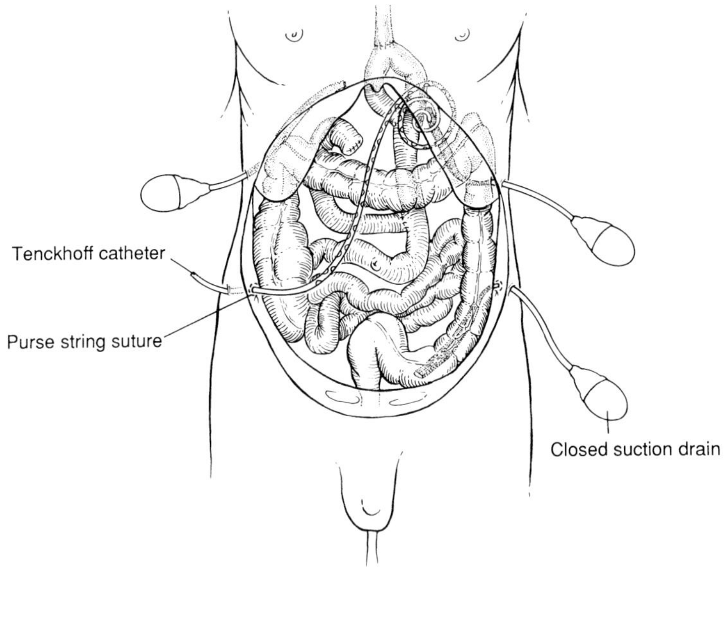

FIG. 71-7. Tubes and drains positioned within the abdominal cavity for the delivery of intraoperative or early postoperative intraperitoneal chemotherapy. A Tenckhoff catheter is used to infuse the drugs. Drains beneath the right hemidiaphragm, beneath the left hemidiaphragm, and within the pelvis drain the drugs. Pursestring sutures at the peritoneal level are used to prevent leakage of fluid from the peritoneal cavity.

TABLE 71-2. *Immediate postoperative abdominal lavage*

Day of operation
1. Run in 1000 mL of 1.5% dextrose peritoneal dialysis solution as rapidly as possible. Warm to body temperature before instillation. Clamp all abdominal drains during infusion.
2. No dwell time.
3. Drain as rapidly as possible through Tenckhoff catheter and abdominal drains.
4. Repeat irrigations every hour for 4 hours, then every 4 hours until returns are clear, then every shift until chemotherapy begins.
5. Change dressing at Tenckhoff catheter and abdominal drain skin exit sites using sterile technique once daily and as needed.
6. Record intake and output of dialysis fluid by weight.

cancer, appendiceal cancer, or other gastrointestinal adenocarcinomas, 5-fluorouracil has been used. The standardized orders for early postoperative administration of intraperitoneal 5-fluorouracil are outlined in Table 71-3.

EARLY POSTOPERATIVE INTRAPERITONEAL DOXORUBICIN (ADRIAMYCIN) CHEMOTHERAPY FOR SARCOMA AND MESOTHELIOMA

In many patients, the abdominal surfaces and resection sites are at high risk for recurrent cancer, but 5-fluorouracil and mitomycin C do not produce the necessary responses. In these patients, the drugs that show the highest response rates often are cisplatin and doxorubicin (Adriamycin). Patients with sarcomatosis and mesothelioma are treated with heated intraoperative intraperitoneal cisplatin and early postoperative intraperitoneal doxorubicin if complete cytoreduction can be accomplished. Both primary and recurrent sarcomas involving the abdomen or pelvis are treated. Patients with a low biologically aggressive mesothelioma are treated by this regimen even if complete cytoreduction cannot be accomplished, because long-term survival has been reported with debulking plus intraperitoneal chemotherapy.[35] In addition, intraperitoneal chemotherapy palliates ascites even when gross mesothelioma is left behind after surgery. Table 71-4 outlines the standardized orders for early postoperative intraperitoneal doxorubicin chemotherapy.

TABLE 71-3. *Early postoperative intraperitoneal chemotherapy with 5-fluorouracil*

Postoperative days 1 to 5:
1. Add to ____ mL of 1.5% dextrose peritoneal dialysis solution: (a) ____ mg of 5-fluorouracil (15 mg/kg × ____ kg) (maximal dose 1500 mg) and (b) 50 mEq of sodium bicarbonate. Use 1000 mL of 1.5% Dianeal for patients $<$1.5 m^2; use 1500 mL for patients $>$1.5 but $<$20 m^2; use 2000 mL for patients $>$2 m^2.
2. Drain all fluid from the abdominal cavity before instillation, then clamp abdominal drains.
3. Run into abdominal cavity as rapidly as possible the 1 L of chemotherapy solution. Dwell for 23 hours and repeat chemotherapy instillation.
4. Continue to drain abdominal cavity after final 23-hour dwell until Tenckhoff catheter is removed.
5. Use 25% dose reduction for age greater than 65 years or prior radiation therapy.

TABLE 71-4. *Early postoperative intraperitoneal chemotherapy with Doxorubicin (Adriamycin)*

Postoperative days 1 to 5:
1. Doxorubicin (Adriamycin) ____ mg (0.1 mg/kg) maximal dose 10 mg/d) in ____ mL of 1.5% Dianeal through Tenckhoff catheter on ________ to ________. Last dose ________. Dwell for 23 hours and drain for 1 hour before next instillation. Use 1000 mL of 1.5% Dianeal for patients $<$1.5 m^2; use 1500 mL for patients $>$1.5 but $<$20 m^2; use 2000 mL for patients $>$2 m^2.
2. Continue to drain abdominal cavity after last dose until Tenckhoff catheter is removed.
3. Use 1000.

RATIONALE FOR EARLY POSTOPERATIVE INTRAPERITONEAL CHEMOTHERAPY

Cancer cells that remain in the abdominal cavity can be destroyed by pharmacologic concentrations of intraperitoneal chemotherapeutic agents instilled on postoperative days 1 through 5. Drugs such as 5-fluorouracil are used over a prolonged period because they are cell-cycle specific. Drugs such as doxorubicin are used in a large volume of fluid over a long period to decrease their sclerotic effects. The timely use of intraperitoneal chemotherapy during surgery and in the early postoperative period eliminates tumor cells from the abdomen before they become fixed within the scar tissue (adhesions) that results from wound healing.

The chemotherapy directly destroys tumor cells and also eliminates viable platelets, leukocytes, and monocytes from the peritoneal cavity. This diminishes or at least delays the accumulation of growth factors associated with the wound healing process. The use of intraperitoneal chemotherapy reduces resection site recurrence and peritoneal surface recurrence in patients with intraabdominal cancer. However, the removal of leukocytes and monocytes decreases the ability of the abdomen to resist infectious processes. For this reason, strict aseptic technique must be used when administering chemotherapy or handling abdominal tubes and drains.

INDUCTION INTRAPERITONEAL AND SYSTEMIC CHEMOTHERAPY

The standardized orders for induction intraperitoneal and systemic chemotherapy in patients with adenocarcinomas are shown in Table 71-5. The standardized orders for induction chemotherapy in patients with sarcomatosis or mesothelioma are outlined in Table 71-6.

Intraperitoneal chemotherapy is given only to patients who have low-volume disease that is not confluent at any site within the abdomen or pelvis.[33] After the three cycles of combined intraperitoneal and systemic chemotherapy have been delivered, all treatments are discontinued for at least 2 months. The complication rate is increased when surgery is performed too soon

TABLE 71-5. *Induction intraperitoneal 5-fluorouracil and intravenous mitomycin C chemotherapy, standardized orders*

Cycle # ________

1. Complete blood count, platelets, profile A, and appropriate tumor marker before treatment, and complete blood count and platelets 10 days after initiation of treatment.
2. 5-Fluorouracil _____ mg (20 mg/kg) (maximum dose 1600 mg) and 50 mEq of sodium bicarbonate in 1000 mL of 1.5% dextrose peritoneal dialysis solution through intraperitoneal catheter every day for 5 days. Last dose ________. Dwell for 23 hours; drain for 1 hour. Continue with next administration even if no drainage is obtained.
3. On day 3 (date ________): 500 mL of lactated ringer's solution intravenously over 2 hours before mitomycin C infusion. Mitomycin C _____ mg (10 mg/m^2 × _____ m^2) (maximum dose 20 mg) in 200 mL of 5% dextrose and water intravenously over 2 hours.
4. Follow routine procedure for peripheral extravasation of a vesicant if extravasation should occur.
5. Prochlorperazine (Compazine) 25 mg per rectum every 4 hours as needed for nausea.
   OUTPATIENT ONLY: May dose times 4 for use at home.
6. Oxycodone and acetaminophen (Percocet) 1 tablet orally every 3 hours as needed for pain.
   OUTPATIENT ONLY: May dose times 4 for use at home.
7. Routine vital signs.
8. Out of bed at liberty.
9. Diet: Regular as tolerated.
10. Daily dressing change to intraperitoneal catheter skin exit site.
11. Use 25% dose reduction for age greater than 65 years or prior radiation therapy.

after intraperitoneal chemotherapy. When patients have returned to full activity, a complete exploratory laparotomy is performed, with meticulous cytoreduction of all residual cancer.[36–38] A final cycle of intraoperative and early postoperative intraperitoneal chemotherapy is administered.

Morbidity and mortality are high in patients with intestinal obstruction who are candidates for cytoreductive surgery.[36,37] In these cases, any small bowel that remains after surgery must be free of seromuscular tears. In addition, only small bowel anastomosis should be performed. A jejunostomy or ileostomy often is required in patients with preoperative intestinal obstruction. The bowel used to construct the ostomy must be sutured circumferentially to the peritoneal surface to prevent postoperative leakage of the chemotherapeutic solution.

Patients who have received prior intraabdominal radiation therapy or intraperitoneal chemotherapy are at increased risk for postoperative bowel perforation and anastomotic leakage.[38] A high temporary ostomy may be indicated if there is extensive trauma to the small bowel as a result of lysis of adhesions or dissection of cancer from small bowel surfaces.

CLINICAL RESEARCH METHODS USED IN THE TREATMENT OF PERITONEAL CARCINOMATOSIS AND SARCOMATOSIS

The progress of research in patients with peritoneal carcinomatosis has been limited, largely because of the lack of standardized statistical techniques for reliable evaluation of treatment response. Clinical research has shown that the prognosis of these patients depends on preoperative and intraoperative variables that can be measured reliably. These include the histologic grade of the malignancy, the preoperative volume of the tumor as assessed at surgery, the distribution of the tumor at surgery, and the completeness of cytoreductive surgery. In addition, preoperative abdominal and pelvic computed tomography (CT) have demonstrated predictive value in assessing the completeness of cytoreduction in patients with mucinous carcinomatosis.

The assessment of the abdominopelvic region is designed to produce a conscientious, clinically relevant, and statistically measurable recording of involvement by peritoneal carcinomatosis (Fig. 71-8). The anatomic boundaries of these regions are defined by anatomic landmarks that surround the abdominal and pelvic cavities. Two transverse planes and two sagittal planes are used to divide the abdomen into nine abdominopelvic regions (AR-0 through AR-8). The upper transverse plane is the lowest aspect of the costal margin. The lower transverse plane is the anterosuperior iliac spine. The sagittal planes divide the abdomen into three equal sectors. The regions are numbered 0 through 8, starting at the umbilical region and proceeding in a clockwise manner. Different anatomic structures are found in the nine abdominopelvic regions:

Abdominopelvic region 0 (AR-0 or central region) includes the midline abdominal incision, the entire greater omentum, and the transverse colon.

TABLE 71-6. *Induction intraperitoneal cisplatin and intravenous doxorubicin (Adriamycin) chemotherapy, standardized orders*

Cycle # ________

1. Complete blood count, platelets, profile A, and appropriate tumor marker before treatment, and complete blood count and platelets 10 days after initiation of treatment.
2. Cisplatin _____ mg (15 mg/m^2, maximum dose 30 mg) in 1000 mL of 1.5% dextrose peritoneal dialysis solution through intraperitoneal catheter every day for 5 days. Last dose ________. Dwell for 23 hours; drain for 1 hour. Continue with next administration even if no drainage is obtained.
3. On day 3 (date ________): 500 mL of lactated Ringer's solution intravenously over 2 hours before doxorubicin (Adriamycin) infusion. Doxorubicin (Adriamycin) _____ mg (50 mg/m^2, maximum dose 100 mg) in 200 mL of 5% dextrose and water intravenously over 2 hours.
4. Follow routine procedure for peripheral extravasation of a vesicant if extravasation should occur.
5. Prochlorperazine (Compazine) 25 mg every 4 hours as needed for nausea.
   OUTPATIENT ONLY: May dose times 4 for use at home.
6. Oxycodone and acetaminophen (Percocet) 1 tablet orally every 3 hours as needed for pain.
   OUTPATIENT ONLY: May dose times 4 for use at home.
7. Routine vital signs.
8. Out of bed at liberty.
9. Diet: Regular as tolerated.
10. Daily dressing change to intraperitoneal catheter skin exit site.
11. Use 25% dose reduction for age greater than 65 years or prior radiation therapy.

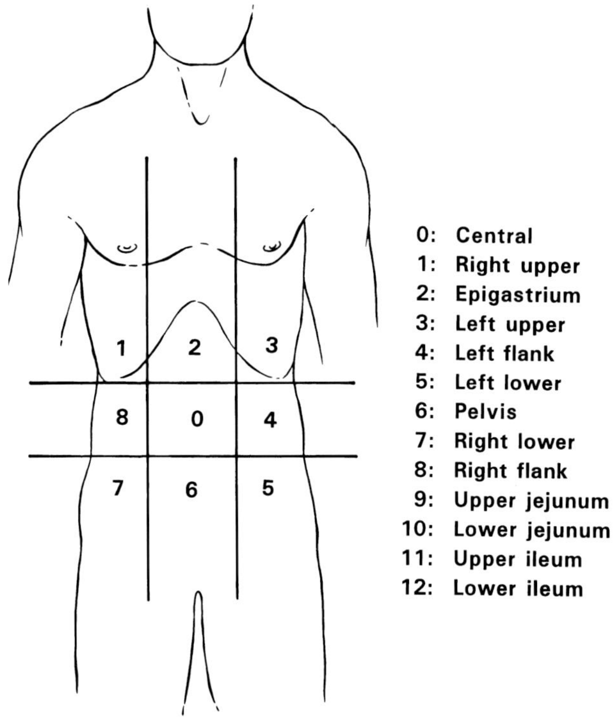

FIG. 71-8. Abdominopelvic regions (AR = 0 to AR = 9). Each region was scored for cancer volume from V-0 to V-3.)

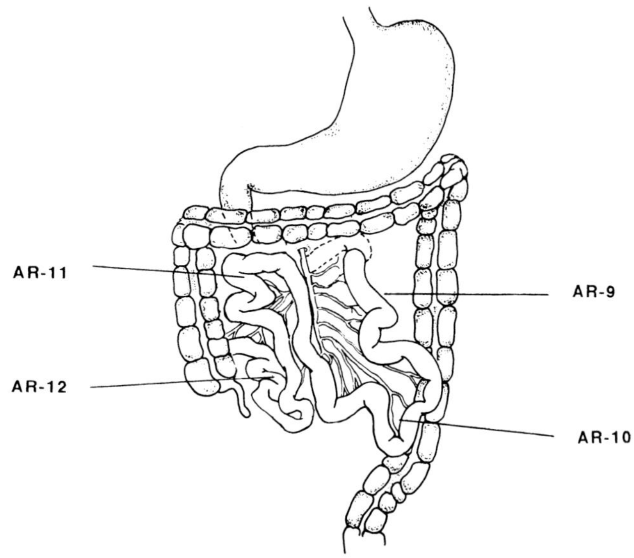

FIG. 71-9. Abdominopelvic regions related to the small bowel (AR = 9 to AR = 11). Each region can be scored for cancer volume from V-0 to V-3.

Abdominopelvic region 1 (AR-1 or right upper region) includes the superior surface of the right lobe of the liver and the undersurface of the right hemidiaphragm. It also includes the right retrohepatic space.

Abdominopelvic region 2 (AR-2 or epigastric region) includes the epigastric fat pad, the left lobe of the liver, the lesser omentum, and the falciform ligament.

Abdominopelvic region 3 (AR-3 or left upper region) includes the undersurface of the left hemidiaphragm, the spleen, the tail of the pancreas, and the anterior and posterior surfaces of the stomach.

Abdominopelvic region 4 (AR-4 or left flank region) includes the descending colon and the left abdominal gutter.

Abdominopelvic region 5 (AR-5 or left lower region) includes the pelvic sidewall lateral to the sigmoid colon and the sigmoid colon itself.

Abdominopelvic region 6 (AR-6 or pelvic region) includes the female internal genitalia (ovaries, tubes and uterus, bladder, cul-de-sac of Douglas) and the rectosigmoid colon.

Abdominopelvic region 7 (AR-7 or right lower region) includes the right pelvic sidewall and the base of the cecum, including the appendix.

Abdominopelvic region 8 (AR-8 or right flank region) includes the right abdominal gutter and the ascending colon.

The small bowel is assessed as a separate entity and designated AR-9 through AR-12 (Fig. 71-9). AR-9 includes the upper jejunum and is located in the left upper abdomen, AR-10 includes the lower jejunum and is located in the left lower abdomen, AR-11 includes the upper ileum and is located in the right upper abdomen just below the liver, and AR-12 includes the lower ileum, encompassing the terminal ileum located in the right lower abdomen. The large bowel is scored along with the abdominal region, but the small bowel is scored separately. In each of these regions, a volume score (V-0 through V-3) may be obtained. Often, the region simply is scored for the presence or absence of cancer.

Simplified Assessment of Cancer Distribution

A more simplified system of assessing cancer distribution in the abdomen and pelvis also has been used (Fig. 71-10). This system divides the abdomen into four quadrants and a pelvic region. The designations are as follows: 1 is the right upper

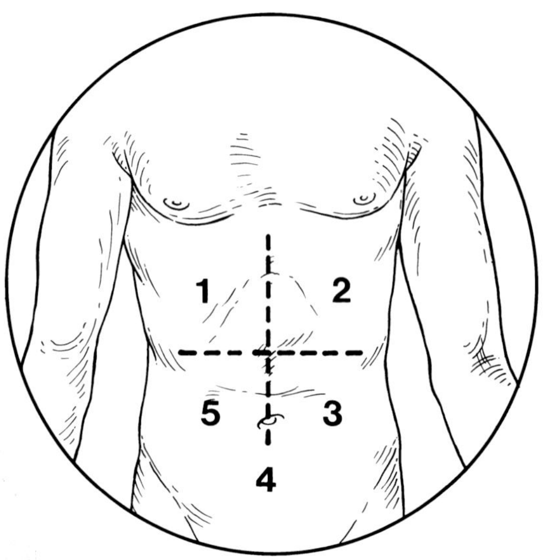

FIG. 71-10. Simplified scoring of cancer distribution in the abdomen and pelvis. Each region can be scored for cancer volume from V-0 to V-3.

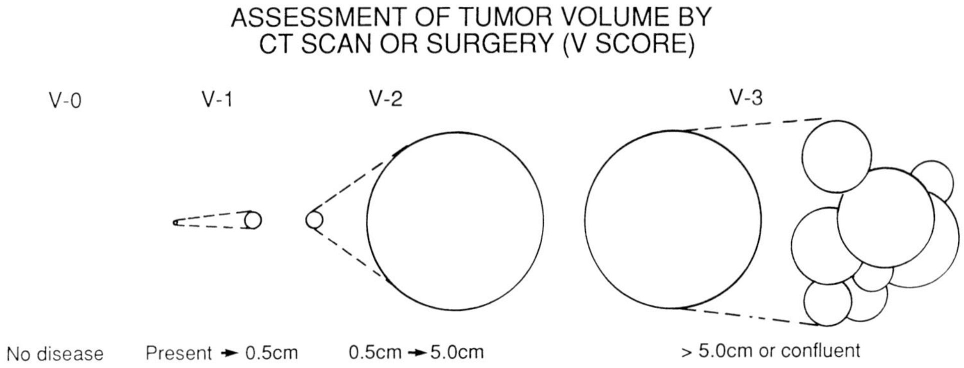

FIG. 71-11. Volume of disease from V-0 to V-3. *CT*, computed tomography.

quadrant, 2 is the left upper quadrant, 3 is the left lower quadrant, 4 is the pelvis, and 5 is the right lower quadrant.[5] In each of these regions, a volume score (V-0 through V-3) may be assigned.

Assessment of Tumor Volume Using Preoperative Computed Tomography or Intraoperative Evaluation

For each region, tumor volume is estimated using four categories: V-0 indicates an absence of cancer at a particular abdominopelvic region or anatomic site; V-1 indicates tumor nodules less than 0.5 cm in diameter (minimal volume); V-2 indicates tumor nodules 0.5 to 5 cm in diameter (moderate volume); and V-3 indicates tumor nodules greater than 5 cm in diameter (gross volume). If an organ is coated by a mat of tumor (confluent disease), this region or site is scored as V-3 (Fig. 71-11). The same volume estimates are used after surgery by the radiologist for CT and at laparotomy by the surgical team. Using this quantitative system for distribution and volume assessment, peritoneal carcinomatosis can be scored on numerous occasions. Responses to treatment in all parts of the abdomen and pelvis can be assessed after each therapeutic intervention.

Preoperative Computed Tomographic Assessment of Tumor Extent (Distribution and Volume)

For preoperative assessment of peritoneal carcinomatosis and sarcomatosis, CT is the only radiologic study that provides useful quantitative information.[39] Its limitations have been documented in several studies.[40–42] Even though the size threshold for the detection of liver lesions and retroperitoneal lesions by CT is about 1 cm, Jacquet and associates demonstrated an accuracy rate of only 50% for lesions measuring 0.5 to 5 cm. For lesions larger than 5 cm, the accuracy rate was 90%.[40]

Preoperative Computed Tomographic Assessment of Resectability in Patients With Mucinous Peritoneal Carcinomatosis

The selection criteria for cytoreductive surgery in patients with mucinous peritoneal carcinomatosis have been defined. CT may play an important role in the selection of patients with mucinous peritoneal carcinomatosis for definitive treatment. One study showed that six CT findings are common in patients with incomplete resection[39]: bowel segments obstructed by tumor, mesentery drawn together by tumor, tumor located in small bowel mesentery, tumor located in AR-9, tumor located in AR-10, and tumor located in AR-11. A statistical analysis of these parameters showed that the probability of incomplete resection was 94% in patients with bowel segments obstructed by tumor on preoperative CT and with tumor located in AR-11. In patients without these two CT findings, the probability of complete resection was 92%. Extension of this preoperative CT assessment to the selection of patients with adenocarcinoma for reoperation is needed.

Grading of Mucinous Peritoneal Carcinomatosis

Tumors that produce mucin are identified by a variety of descriptive terms, all of which have about the same meaning: mucinous tumors, mucoid tumors, colloid adenocarcinomas, and cystadenocarcinomas. Although there is a fairly uniform histologic description of mucin, there is no consensus regarding the location or percentage of the colloid pattern in an adenocarcinoma that must be present to define a mucinous carcinoma. Umpleby and colleagues defined a moderate mucinous adenocarcinoma of the colon as a tumor containing 60% to 80% of the colloid pattern, and a high mucinous adenocarcinoma as a tumor containing more than 80% of the colloid pattern.[43] Symonds and Vickery defined a mucinous carcinoma as a tumor containing more than 60% colloid.[44] Minsky and associates defined mucinous cancer as an adenocarcinoma of which more than two thirds was growing in a colloid pattern.[45]

Mucin exists in two states: an extracellular form that is secreted by epithelial cells and an intracellular form. Intracellular mucin is detected most commonly in signet cell or signet-ring cell carcinoma. This tumor has a poor prognosis in most series.[46–48] Frequently, patients have both extracellular and intracellular mucoid components to the malignancy. The changes in intracellular metabolism that result in signet-ring cell carcinoma have not been defined.

Grading of Mucinous Adenocarcinomas

Mucinous adenocarcinomas from the appendix and colon are graded according to a histopathologic classification.[49] The survival of patients treated by cytoreductive surgery and intraperi-

TABLE 71-7. *Criteria for histologic grading of colonic and appendiceal carcinomas*

	Grade 0	Grade 1	Grade 2	Grade 3
Malignant differentiation of cell	−	+	+ +	+ + +
Histologic glandular morphology	−	Pools of mucin lined by a single layer of cells	Several layers of cells surrounding the mucin	Solid area of cells with necrosis
Stromal pattern	−	Minimal	Present	Cribriform
Intracellular mucin	−	−	−	+ + +
Evidence of tissue invasion	−	−	±	+

toneal chemotherapy is influenced strongly by the histologic grade of their tumors.[50] Mucinous tumors are graded from 0 to 3 (MTG-0 to MTG-3). This classification depends on the histologic appearance of the malignant cells (differentiation), the glandular morphology, the stroma on which the epithelial cells are based, the presence or absence of signet-ring cells, and evidence of tissue invasion (Table 71-7). With some tumors, mixed patterns of MTG-1 through MTG-3 are present in the same patient. However, the tumors are scored by the highest grade of malignancy visualized.

The histology of MTG-0 tumors is similar to that of benign pseudomyxoma peritonei. Pools of mucin are seen without identifiable malignant cells. Careful searching through the mucus by light microscopy away from the primary tumor does not reveal epithelial cells. With extensive sampling, regression of these tumors can be predicted. The origin of this condition usually is a ruptured mucocele of the appendix.

MTG-1 cancers show abundant mucin with free-floating malignant cells arranged individually or in small clusters. These cells are columnar or goblet in nature, but do not show the signet-ring configuration. Pools of mucin may be lined by a predominantly single layer of cells. The cells are bland-appearing and there are no mitotic figures and no atypia. This is the characteristic histology of pseudomyxoma peritonei.

MTG-2 cancers show increased numbers of cell layers surrounding the mucin follicles. There is mitotic activity, nuclear atypia, and a complex stromal pattern. Tumors of similar cytology (moderate differentiation) with less than 80% mucin in a field of view are referred to as grade 2 adenocarcinomas rather than mucinous adenocarcinomas. These cancers may invade the seromuscular layers of the bowel, but rarely cause intestinal obstruction.

MTG-3 cancers are of two general types. Both mucinous (MTG-3) and nonmucinous cancers (grade 3 adenocarcinomas) show solid areas of cells with marked atypia. There is necrosis and mitotic figures. Solid areas of tumor invade into the soft tissues of the omentum, mesentery, or bowel wall. MTG-3 cells usually show a signet-ring configuration in multiple fields.

SURGERY

Scoring of Prior Surgical Interventions

In assessing the prognosis of a patient with mucinous peritoneal carcinomatosis, the histologic grade of the malignancy may be the dominant independent variable. Patient survival varies as tumor grade progresses. However, within each tumor grade, there is a proportion of patients who do not respond to treatment and a proportion who are long-term survivors. The volume of mucinous cancer present is an important prognostic factor, especially in high-grade tumors. With minimally invasive MTG-1 tumors, even with a large volume, complete cytoreduction is possible. However, with high-grade tumors, complete cytoreduction is possible only with a low volume of malignancy. When a high-grade tumor has a high volume in the peritoneal cavity, complete resection is not possible and the results of surgery are poor.

However, even with MTG-1 cancers, complete cytoreduction occasionally is not possible. Studies indicate that cytoreduction fails in patients who have undergone extensive prior surgical interventions. Therefore, the number and extent of prior surgical procedures should be determined in each case and a surgery score assigned. A prior surgery score of 3 (PSS-3) indicates that at least five of the nine abdominopelvic regions have been dissected without the use of intraoperative or early postoperative intraperitoneal chemotherapy. PSS-2 indicates that between two and five abdominopelvic regions have been dissected. PSS-1 means that only one region (usually a biopsy) has been dissected. The number of abdominopelvic regions is, by convention, additive for all prior surgical procedures. In this regard, the prior surgery score is a composite of all prior surgeries.

Scoring of Cancer Extent (Distribution and Volume) by Surgical Exploration

The extent of peritoneal carcinomatosis is based on the location of disease (AR-0 through AR-12) found at surgical exploration and on the volume of disease observed at each location (V-0 through V-3). The initial exploration must be thorough and methodical, with lysis of all adhesions. The location and volume of any tumor implant within the peritoneal cavity must be scored at the time of dissection in a prospective manner.

Two tumor assessments that have prognostic importance must be recorded prospectively by the surgeon in the management of peritoneal carcinomatosis:

1. Tumor matting of organs. The scoring system previously described uses the size of tumor nodules to describe the extent of peritoneal carcinomatosis. If a confluence of cancer matting together organs or structures is found, tumors are scored as V-3, even though the thickness of the cancer is minimal. Confluent disease implies high-grade cancer that has coated an organ or a resection site. It frequently is seen in patients with PSS-3 as a result of high-density seeding of cancer within a resection site.
2. Tumor redistribution and small bowel sparing. Distinct patterns of cancer dissemination to peritoneal surfaces have been observed.[4,50] The degree of biologic invasiveness and the extent of extracellular mucus production influence the

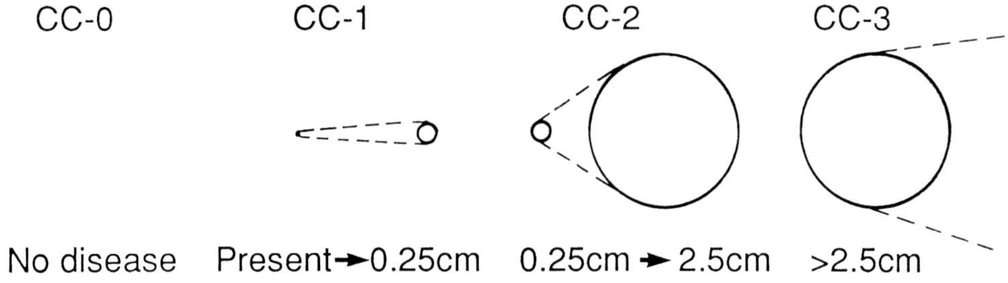

FIG. 71-12. Completeness of cytoreduction from CC-0 through CC-3.

type of tumor distribution. Low-grade cancers with a high content of extracellular mucin show a redistributed spread of malignancy. Redistribution means that large volumes of tumor are found at some predetermined anatomic sites within the peritoneal cavity, but are absent or greatly reduced in volume at other sites. Low-grade mucinous tumor cells do not necessarily adhere to the surfaces they initially contact. Tumor cells are mobile and left to accumulate at other sites within the abdomen. Peritoneal fluid resorption and gravity account for tumor accumulation within the greater omentum, on the undersurface of the right hemidiaphragm, in the right retrohepatic space, and in the pelvic and abdominal gutters. The bowel surfaces and mesentery may remain completely free of tumor because these structures are moved continuously by peristaltic activity. They are not involved extensively unless there have been numerous prior surgical dissections and tumor cells have become entrapped on traumatized surfaces.

Residual Disease After Surgery Assessed by Completeness of Cytoreduction

All sites of residual disease after cytoreductive surgery must be recorded. A scoring system is used to indicate the volume of disease that remains after surgery. The completeness of cytoreduction is designated by a score ranging from CC-0 to CC-3 (Fig. 71-12). A score of CC-0 indicates that no tumor was visualized during the course of the complete resection. These patients have walled-off tumor nodules, tumors encased within scar tissue, or a complete response to induction chemotherapy. A score of CC-1 means that no tumor nodules greater than 2.5 mm in both diameters were left behind. A score of CC-2 indicates the presence of residual tumor measuring 2.5 mm to 2.5 cm in diameter. A score of CC-3 is used when tumor larger than 2.5 cm in diameter is left behind. Patients with tumor nodules less than 2.5 mm (CC-0 and CC-1) in both directions are considered to have undergone complete resection. Theoretically, optimal intraperitoneal chemotherapy can penetrate through a 2.5-mm tumor nodule and prevent its recurrence.[31] Patients who have tumors measuring 2.5 mm or greater left behind within the abdomen or pelvis at the completion of surgery are considered to have undergone incomplete resection.

The size of residual tumor nodules after cytoreduction profoundly influences the efficiency of intraperitoneal chemotherapy. A major factor determining the benefits of intraperitoneal therapy is the depth of penetration of cytostatic drugs by diffusion directly into the tumor. Incomplete drug penetration into solid tumors is an important explanation for failure to achieve total eradication of residual disease after surgery. The penetration of cytostatic drugs has been examined in vitro and in vivo in several experimental systems using multiple agents.[51–53] The conclusion of such studies was that direct penetration of the drugs into tissue is extremely limited, ranging from several cell layers to perhaps 1 to 3 mm from the surface. Because of this limited penetration, the residual disease to be treated should have a diameter of less than 2 to 3 mm. The experience of this author confirms these data, in that the 3-year survival rate was 75% after complete resection (R-0 to R-1) compared with 20% after incomplete resection in a series of patients treated by cytoreductive surgery and early postoperative chemotherapy for peritoneal carcinomatosis from colonic and appendiceal cancers.[50]

TABLE 71-8. *Assessment of response after cytoreductive surgery*

Complete response (CR):	Maintenance of a disease-free status for 6 months after completion of the treatment.
Partial response (PR):	Greater than 50% reduction in the sum of the parts of the largest perpendicular diameters of indicator lesion(s) for 6 months after completion of the treatment, with no progression in any lesion or appearance of a new lesion.
Stable disease (SD):	Failure to qualify for CR, PR, or PD.
Progressive disease (PD):	Greater than 25% increase in the sum of the parts of the largest perpendicular diameters of indicator lesion(s).

Assessment of Response

In performing clinical research on peritoneal carcinomatosis, the criteria for measuring treatment response must be modified. Reliable quantitative end points are difficult to achieve by radiologic criteria. This is not surprising when the inaccuracy of CT in patients with peritoneal carcinomatosis is considered. The most reliable monitoring technique often is serial measurement of levels of tumor markers. Unfortunately, a progressive increase in the levels of tumor markers does not occur in all patients. A continuous rise is evidence of progressive disease, but the volume of disease that tumor markers reflect varies from patient to patient. Some patients, even with large-volume recurrences, do not have elevated levels of tumor markers. The truism for the clinical use of tumor markers, ''negative means nothing,'' must be applied.

A complete response after a complete cytoreduction with

TABLE 71-9. *Evolution of strategies for the prevention and treatment of peritoneal carcinomatosis*

1. Spratt et al. (1980): Suggested a hyperthermic peritoneal perfusion system with the administration of intraperitoneal chemotherapy. University of Louisville, Kentucky.[22]
2. Koga et al. (1984): Experimental study with prophylactic continuous hyperthermic peritoneal perfusion with mitomycin C. A significant prolongation of survival was observed when 41.5°C hyperthermia was combined with mitomycin C. Tottori University, Japan.[39]
3. Flessner et al. (1984): Pharmacokinetic studies established the peritoneal-plasma barrier. National Institutes of Health, Bethesda, Maryland.[38]
4. Sugarbaker et al. (1985): Randomized controlled study of intravenous versus intraperitoneal 5-fluorouracil. First trial to document a diminished incidence of peritoneal carcinomatosis in patients receiving intraperitoneal 5-fluorouracil chemotherapy. National Institutes of Health, Bethesda, Maryland.[40]
5. Koga et al. (1988): First study on adjuvant intraoperative hyperthermic peritoneal perfusion with mitomycin C in gastric cancer. Totori University, Japan.[13]
6. Fujimoto et al. (1989): Used intraoperative hyperthermic peritoneal perfusion with mitomycin C combined with extended surgery in patients with gastric cancer and established peritoneal carcinomatosis. After the treatment, 12.8% survived 1 year as compared with 0% after surgery alone. Chiba University, Japan.[25]
7. Sugarbaker et al. (1990): Trial of early postoperative intraperitoneal mitomycin C and 5-fluorouracil. First trial to integrate cytoreductive surgery and chemotherapy as a single event. Washington Hospital Center, Washington, DC.[41]
8. Fujimura et al. and Yonemura et al. (1990): Suggested peritoneal cavity expander for optimization of intraoperative intraperitoneal hypethermochemotherapy delivery in patients with gastric cancer. Kanazawa University, Japan.
9. Sugarbaker (1991): First large phase II trial that combined complete cytoreduction with early postoperative intraperitoneal mitomycin C and 5-fluorouracil. Washington Hospital Center, Washington, DC.[42]
10. Wansik Yu et al. (1994): Positive results of randomized study on adjuvant early postoperative intraperitoneal chemotherapy for gastric cancer. Taegeu, Korea.[15]
11. Sugarbaker (1994): Medical illustrations of peritonectomy procedures. Washington Hospital Center, Washington, DC.[33]
12. Sugarbaker et al. (1994): Protocol for induction chemotherapy for low-volume peritoneal carcinomatosis from colorectal cancer. Washington Hospital Center, Washington, DC.[31]

intraperitoneal chemotherapy is defined more accurately as maintenance of a complete cytoreduction by chemotherapy. No matter how meticulous the dissection, viable tumor cells are left behind. A complete response to treatment of peritoneal carcinomatosis means maintenance of a clinically disease-free state (Table 71-8).

SUMMARY

The theoretical basis for treatment strategies for peritoneal carcinomatosis have continued to gain prominence over the last decade. A definitive role for intraperitoneal chemotherapy in the management of gastrointestinal cancer has not been established, but early studies are promising. The significant contributions are summarized in Table 71-9. Continued quantitative studies are necessary to refine further the selection and treatment of patients with peritoneal carcinomatosis or sarcomatosis.

REFERENCES

1. Sugarbaker PH, MacDonald JS, Gunderson LL. Colorectal cancer. In: DeVita VT, Hellman S, Rosenberg SA, eds. Cancer: principles and practice of oncology. Philadelphia: JB Lippincott, 1982.
2. Weiss L. Principles of metastasis. Orlando: Academic Press, 1985.
3. Dukes CE, Bussey HJR. The spread of rectal cancer and its effect on prognosis. Br J Cancer 1958;12:309.
4. Sugarbaker PH, ed. Observations concerning cancer spread within the peritoneal cavity and concepts supporting an ordered pathophysiology. In: Peritoneal carcinomatosis. Principles of management. Norwell, MA: Kluwer Academic Publishers, 1996.
5. Murphy P, Alexander P, Kerkhamn N, Fleming J, Taylor I. Pattern of spread of bloodborne tumour. Br J Surg 1986;73:829.
6. Sugarbaker TA, Chaney D, Koslowe P, Sugarbaker PH. Patterns of spread of recurrent intraabdominal sarcoma. In: Surgarbaker PH, ed. Peritoneal carcinomatosis. Diagnosis and treatment. Norwell, MA: Kluwer Academic Publishers, 1995:65.
7. Lofgren EP, Waugh JM, Dockerty MB. Local recurrence of carcinoma after anterior resection of the rectum and the sigmoid. Arch Surg 1957; 74:825.
8. Zoetmulder FAN. Model studies over the colorectale carcinoma. Amsterdam: Rodopi, 1982.
9. Tepper J, Nardi G, Suit H. Carcinoma of the pancreas. Review of MGH experience from 1963 to 1973. Cancer 1976;37:1519.
10. Griffin JF, Smalley SR, Jewell W, et al. Patterns of failure after curative resection of pancreatic carcinoma. Cancer 1990;66:56.
11. Ettinghausen SE. Rationale for intraperitoneal chemotherapy in the treatment of adenocarcinoma of the pancreas. In: Sugarbaker PH, ed. Peritoneal carcinomatosis: drugs and diseases. Norwell, MA: Kluwer Academic Publishers, 1996:227.
12. Douglass HO. Gastric cancer. Overview of current therapies. Semin Oncol 1985;12:57.
13. Takahashi T, Sawai K, Hagiwara A, Takahashi S, Seiki K, Tokuda H. Type-oriented therapy for gastric cancer effective for lymph node metastasis. Management of lymph node metastasis using activated carbon particles adsorbing an anticancer agent. Semin Oncol 1991;7:378.
14. Koga S, Hamazoe R, Maeta M, et al. Prophylactic therapy for peritoneal recurrence of gastric cancer by continuous hyperthermic peritoneal perfusion with mitomycin C. Cancer 1988;61:232.
15. Hamazoe R. Experimental studies of continuous hyperthermic peritoneal perfusion in the treatment of peritoneal metastases of cancer (in Japanese with English abstract). Journal Japanese Surgical Society 1983;84:1117.
16. Yu W, Sugarbaker PH, Whang I. Randomized controlled trial of early postoperative intraperitoneal chemotherapy in gastric cancer. A preliminary report. J Regional Cancer Treat 1994;7.2:90.
17. Schiessel R, Funovics J, Schick B, et al. Adjuvant intraperitoneal cisplatin therapy in patients with operated gastric carcinoma. Results of a randomized trial. Acta Med Austriaca 1989;16:68.
18. Sautner T, Hoflbauer F, Depisch D, Schiessel R, Jakesz R. Adjuvant intraperitoneal cisplatin chemotherapy does not improve long-term survival after surgery for advanced gastric cancer. J Clin Oncol 1994;12: 970.
19. Jones AL, Trott P, Cunningham D, et al. A pilot study of intraperitoneal cisplatin in the management of gastric cancer. Ann Oncol 1994;5:126.
20. Atiq OT, Kelsen DP, Shiu MH, et al. Phase Ii trial of postoperative adjuvant intraperitoneal cisplatin and fluorouracil and systemic fluorouracil chemotherapy in patients with resected gastric cancer. J Clin Oncol 1993;11:425.
21. Nordlinger B, Bouteloup PY, Favre JP, et al. Early postoperative intraperitoneal chemotherapy is feasible and well tolerated in colon cancer. A prospective randomized study. J Cancer Res Clin Oncol 1990;116: 686.

22. Fujimoto S, Takahashi M, Endoh F, et al. A clinical pilot study combining surgery with intraoperative pelvic hyperthermochemotherapy to prevent the local recurrence of rectal cancer. Ann Surg 1991;213:43.
23. Spratt JS, Adcock RA, Muskovin M, Sherrill W, McKeown J. Clinical delivery system for intraperitoneal hyperthermic chemotherapy. Cancer Res 1980;40:256.
24. Sugarbaker PH, Bowei Z, Banez Sese G, Shmookler B. Peritoneal carcinomatosis from appendiceal cancer. Results in 69 patients treated by cytoreductive surgery and intraperitoneal chemotherapy. Dis Colon Rectum 1993;36:323.
25. Schellinx MET, von Meyenfeldt MF, Sugarbaker PH. Peritoneal carcinomatosis from adenocarcinoma of the colon. In: Sugarbaker PH, ed. Peritoneal carcinomatosis: drugs and diseases. Norwell, MA: Kluwer Academic Publishers, 1996:247.
26. Fujimoto S, Shrestha RD, Kokubun M, et al. Clinical trial with surgery and intraperitoneal hyperthermic perfusion for peritoneal recurrence of gastrointestinal cancer. Cancer 1989;64:154.
27. Fujimoto S, Shrestha RD, Kokubun M, et al. Intraperitoneal hyperthermic perfusion combined with surgery effective for gastric cancer patients with peritoneal seeding. Ann Surg 1988;208:36.
28. Fujimoto S, Shrestha RD, Kokuban M, et al. Positive results of combined therapy of surgery and intraperitoneal hyperthermic perfusion for far-advanced gastric cancer. Ann Surg 1990;212:592.
29. Fujimura T, Tonemura Y, Fushida S, et al. Continuous peritoneal perfusion for the treatment of peritoneal dissemination in gastric cancer and subsequent second-look operation. Cancer 1990;65:65.
30. Yonemura Y, Fujimura T, Fushida S, et al. Hyperthermochemotherapy combined with cytoreductive surgery for the treatment of gastric cancer with peritoneal dissemination. World J Surg 1991;15:530.
31. Panteix G, Guillanumont M, Cherpin L, et al. Study of the pharmacokinetics of mitomycin C in humans during intraperitoneal chemohyperthermia with special mention of the concentration in local tissues. Oncology 1993;50:366.
32. Sugarbaker PH, Steves MA, Hafner GH. Treatment of peritoneal carcinomatosis from colon or appendiceal cancer with induction intraperitoneal chemotherapy. Regional Cancer Treatment 1993;4:183.
33. Sugarbaker PH. Dissection by electrocautery with a ball tip. J Surg Oncol 1994;56:246.
34. Sugarbaker PH. Peritonectomy procedures. Ann Surg 1995;221:29.
35. Averbach AM, Sugarbaker PH. Peritoneal mesothelioma: treatment approach based on natural history. In: Sugarbaker PH, ed. Peritoneal carcinomatosis: drugs and diseases. Norwell, MA: Kluwer Academic Publishers, 1996:193.
36. Moreno E, Sugarbaker PH. Gastrointestinal fistula following cytoreductive procedures for peritoneal carcinomatosis. Incidence and outcome. Journal of Experimental and Clinical Cancer Research 1993;12:153.
37. Fernandez-Trigo V, Sugarbaker PH. Diagnosis and management of postoperative gastrointestinal fistula. A kinetic analysis. Journal of Experimental and Clinical Cancer Research 1994;13.3:233.
38. Esquivel J, Vidal-Jove J, Steves MA, Sugarbaker PH. Morbidity and mortality of cytoreductive surgery and intraperitoneal chemotherapy. Surgery 1994;113:631.
39. Archer A, Sugarbaker PH, Jelinek J. Radiology of peritoneal carcinomatosis. In: Sugarbaker, ed. Peritoneal carcinomatosis. Principles of management. Norwell, MA: Kluwer Academic Publishers, 1995.
40. Jacquet P, Jelinek JS, Steves MA, Sugarbaker PH. Evaluation of computed tomography in patients with peritoneal carcinomatosis. Cancer 1993;72:1631.
41. Walkey MM, Friedman AC, Sohotra P, Radecki PD. CT manifestations of peritoneal carcinomatis. AJR Am J Roentgenol 1988;150:1035.
42. Nelson RC, Chezmar JL, Hoel MJ, Buck DR, Sugarbaker PH. Peritoneal carcinomatosis. Preoperative CT with intraperitoneal contrast material. Radiology 1992;182:133.
43. Umpleby HC, Ranson DL, Williamson RC. Peculiarities of mucinous colorectal carcinoma. Br J Surg 1985;72:715.
44. Symonds DA, Vickery AL. Mucinous carcinoma of the colon and rectum. Cancer 1976;37:1891.
45. Minsky BD, Mies C, Rich TA, Recht A, Chaffey JT. Colloid carcinoma of the colon and rectum. Cancer 1987;60:3103.
46. Almagro US. Primary signet ring carcinoma of the colon. Cancer 1983;52:1453.
47. Giacchero A, Aste H, Barrachini P, et al. Primary signet ring carcinoma of the large bowel. Report of nine cases. Cancer 1985;56:2723.
48. Sugarbaker PH. Cancer of the appendix and pseudomyxoma. In: Fazio VW, ed. Current therapy in colon and rectal surgery. Philadelphia: BC Decker, 1989:295.
49. Sugarbaker PH, Jablonski KA. Prognostic features of 51 colorectal and 130 appendiceal cancer patients with peritoneal carcinomatosis treated by cytoreductive surgery and intraperitoneal chemotherapy. Ann Surg 1995;221:124.
50. Sugarbaker PH. Pseudomyxoma peritonei. A cancer whose biology is characterized by a redistribution phenomenon. Ann Surg 1994;219:109.
51. Kerr DJ, Kaye SB. Aspects of cytotoxic drug penetration with particular reference to anthracyclines. Cancer Chemother Pharmacol 1987;9:1.
52. Los G, Smals OA, Van Vight MJ. A rationale for carboplatin treatment and abdominal hyperthermia in cancers restricted to the peritoneal cavity. Cancer Res 1992;52:1252.
53. Ozols RF, Locker GY, Doroshow JH, et al. Pharmacokinetics of adriamycin and tissue penetration in murine ovarian cancer. Cancer Res 1979;39:3209.

Surgery for Gastrointestinal Cancer: A Multidisciplinary Approach, edited by Harold J. Wanebo.
Lippincott-Raven Publishers, Philadelphia, © 1997.

CHAPTER 72

Chemotherapy for Advanced Gastrointestinal Cancer: Current Best and Future Hopes

Miguel A. Rodriguez-Bigas, Neal J. Meropol, and Nicholas J. Petrelli

This year in the United States, about 143,500 new cases and 56,000 cancer-related deaths will occur from colorectal carcinoma.[1] Metastases will develop in about 50% of the patients who undergo primary resection for cure, of whom only a few will benefit from resection.[2] 5-Fluorouracil (5-FU) and leucovorin (LV) is the treatment of choice for patients with unresectable stage IV colorectal cancer. With this modulation, objective response rates of up 48% have been reported, with some evidence of improved survival and quality of life.[3,4] However, in spite of clear increases in response rate with 5-FU and LV modulation, the finding of improved survival has not been universal.[5] Therefore, in an attempt to improve on these results, efforts are focusing on optimizing the biochemical and biologic modulation of 5-FU and developing new drugs and novel therapeutic approaches to this disease. In this chapter, chemotherapy for advanced colorectal cancer is discussed, with an emphasis on biochemical and biologic modulation of 5-FU. Hepatic regional chemotherapy was discussed in Chapter 49.

5-FLUOROURACIL

5-Fluorouracil, a fluorinated pyrimidine, has been the treatment of choice in advanced colorectal carcinoma for many years.[6] However, alone, 5-FU has a response rate of 10% to 20%, with no clear survival benefit. 5-FU can inhibit the synthesis of RNA and DNA. To exert its antitumor activity, 5-FU must be activated within the cell to fluorodeoxyuridine monophosphate (FdUMP), an analogue of deoxyuridine, and to fluoridine triphosphate, a nucleotide derivative.[6] In the presence of 5,10-methylenetetrahydrofolate, FdUMP binds to thymidylate synthase, forming a stable ternary complex that results in the inhibition of de novo synthesis of thymidylates.[6–10] Although inhibition of thymidylate synthase is thought to be the primary mechanism of cytotoxicity, FdUMP can impair RNA processing, providing an alternate tumoricidal pathway.

It still is not clear whether intravenous (IV) bolus or continuous infusion (CI) is the preferred method of administering 5-FU. However, response rates of 25% to 52% have been reported for CI 5-FU.[11] Because its half-life is 11 minutes and its cytotoxic activity is S-phase specific, IV bolus administration of 5-FU targets only a small fraction of the tumor cells.[12] With CI, the number of cells exposed to the drug is higher, and a dose-response curve has been suggested.[13] A dose intensity of about 2.5 g/m^2/wk can be achieved with CI 5-FU, compared with 750 mg/m^2/wk with IV bolus dosing.[12]

Several randomized trials have compared CI 5-FU with IV bolus 5-FU. In 70 patients, Seifert and associates compared 5 days of CI 5-FU at 30 mg/kg/d every 29 days to 5 days of IV bolus 5-FU at 12 mg/kg/d every 29 days and found response rates of 44% and 22%, respectively.[14] Lokich and colleagues, in a Mid-Atlantic Oncology Program Study Group, reported a 30% response rate for CI 5-FU at 300 mg/m^2/d for 10 weeks versus a 7% response rate for IV bolus 5-FU at 500 mg/m^2/d for 5 days every 29 days.[15] Survival was 13 months with the former approach and 12 months with the latter. Weinerman and associates described 170 patients, 88 of whom received CI 5-FU at 350 mg/m^2/d for 14 days every 28 days and 82 of whom received IV bolus 5-FU at 450 mg/m^2/d for 5 days every 28 days.[16] The response rate was 12% in the former group and 7% in the latter, with no difference in survival. Rougier and colleagues reported a statistically significant improvement in response rate (19% versus 8%) but not in overall survival (10 months versus 9 months) in 155 patients with measurable metastatic disease who were randomly assigned to treatment with CI 5-FU or IV bolus 5-FU.[17] CI 5-FU was administered at 750 mg/m^2/d for 7 days every 3 weeks. IV bolus 5-FU was given at 500 mg/m^2/d for 5 days every 4 weeks. Dose escalation of 50 mg was allowed in both groups of patients, depending on

M. A. Rodriguez-Bigas: Assistant Professor of Surgery, State University of New York at Buffalo; Associate Chief, Colorectal Surgery, Roswell Park Cancer Institute, Buffalo, NY 14263.

N. J. Meropol: Assistant Professor of Medicine, State University of New York at Buffalo; Department of Medicine, Roswell Park Cancer Institute, Buffalo, NY 14263.

N. J. Petrelli: Associate Professor of Surgery, State University of New York at Buffalo; Chief, Department of Surgical Oncology, Roswell Park Cancer Institute, Buffalo, NY 14263.

toxicity. The median total dose intensity was 1369 mg/m^2/wk for the CI group versus 558 mg/m^2/wk for the IV bolus group. The incidence of stomatitis and the hand-foot syndrome was significantly higher in the CI group. Diarrhea occurred in 25% and 20% of the patients in the CI and IV bolus groups, respectively.

Randomized studies of CI 5-FU have yielded increased response rates and higher total dose intensity, but no improvement in survival. Toxicity usually consists of mucositis and the hand-foot syndrome, which are reversible when the drug is stopped. Myelosuppression and diarrhea are rare.

Evidence suggests that CI 5-FU results in improved survival when compared with IV bolus 5-FU in the adjuvant treatment of rectal cancer.[18]

BIOCHEMICAL AND BIOLOGIC MODULATION

Studies of 5-FU alone or in combination with alkylating agents, *Vinca* alkaloids, and biochemical and biologic modulators have reported objective tumor response rates ranging from 9.5% to 63%.[19–40] The concept of biochemical modulation has been applied to 5-FU. When administered, a modulator manipulates the metabolic activity of an antitumor agent so as to selectively increase the agent's antineoplastic effect.[41] By itself, a biochemical modulator may or may not have an antitumor effect. 5-FU has served as the prototype for successful application of biochemical modulation to the treatment of patients with cancer.

5-FLUOROURACIL AND INTERFERONS

Interferons (IFNs) by themselves have not shown a significant antitumor effect in adenocarcinomas of the gastrointestinal tract.[42] However, IFNs can produce concentration-dependent modulation of the cytotoxic effects of 5-FU.[43] Although the mechanism of action of this synergism is unknown, possibilities include enhancement of the conversion of 5-FU to FdUMP, inhibition of thymidine salvage pathways, and inhibition of the intracellular rise in thymidylate synthase after exposure to 5-FU.[6] IFNs also can produce changes in the pharmacokinetics of 5-FU, such as elevation in the serum 5-FU concentration, decrease in 5-FU clearance, increase in the elimination half-life of 5-FU, and increase in the area under the curve (plasma concentration time curve).[42]

A report by Wadler and Wiernik in which 63% of 32 previously untreated patients with advanced colorectal cancer experienced a partial response to treatment with 5-FU and IFNα encouraged other groups to pursue investigations using these agents.[39] Using similar regimens, Kemeny and associates[34] and Pazdur and colleagues[36] reported response rates of 26% and 35% in groups of 34 and 52 patients, respectively. In the study by Kemeny and associates, significant neurotoxicity was observed.[34] Wek and colleagues reported a partial response rate of 31% in 55 analyzable patients using CI 5-FU at 750 mg/m^2/d for 5 days followed by IV bolus 5-FU at 750 mg/m^2/wk starting at day 15 and IFN-α2b at 9 million U subcutaneously three times per week.[44] In this study, the number of metastatic sites had a significant influence on the response; 14 of 32 patients with one metastatic site had a partial response. There also were no differences between the total amount of 5-Fluorouracil administered and the response rates.[44] About one third of the patients experienced drug toxicity, which consisted mainly of leukopenia, fever, diarrhea, and mucositis.[44]

In summary, response rates using the combination of 5-FU and IFN-α in previously untreated patients have varied from 26% to 42%.[34,36,44–46] Newer approaches combining 5-FU and IFN-α with other modulators have been reported and are discussed later in this chapter.

5-FLUOROURACIL AND LEUCOVORIN

5-Fluorouracil can interfere with the synthesis of RNA and DNA. The therapeutic activity of 5-FU is enhanced by increasing the reduced folate pools through the administration of calcium LV (folinic acid).[8,9] The strength and duration of the ternary complex formed by thymidylate synthase, 5,10-methylene tetrahydrofolate (CH_2FH_4), and FdUMP occurs at extracellular folate concentrations of 10 μmol/L.[8] The cytotoxicity of 5-FU is potentiated by polyglutamate forms of CH_2FH_4, whose formation is a function of the duration of exposure to LV.[47] Because the ternary complex dissociates slowly, the cytotoxic activity of 5-FU is potentiated by expanding the folate pool with LV, which increases the formation of the ternary complex.

Several randomized phase III clinical trials in advanced colorectal cancer have been performed (Table 72-1), and a metanalysis of nine trials has been done in which 5-FU alone was compared with 5-FU modulated with LV.[3–5,48–56] Response rates (partial and complete) ranged from 16% to 48% for the combined 5-FU and LV regimens and from 5% to 16% for 5-FU alone. Two of the studies demonstrated a modest but significant improvement in survival for the 5-FU and LV group. In the first study, reported by Erlichman and colleagues,[49] a 13-week survival advantage was observed for the 5-FU and LV group. However, on longer follow-up, the survival advantage was not maintained.[57] In the North Central Cancer Treatment Group study, a 19-week survival advantage was observed in the 5-FU and LV group.[3] Although the North Central Cancer Treatment Group trial was not included, the metanalysis revealed that the response rate of patients receiving 5-FU and LV in weekly or monthly regimens (23%) was statistically better than that of patients receiving 5-FU alone (11%).[5] This improved response rate did not result in improved survival. Median survival was 11 months for the 5-FU group and 11.5 months for the 5-FU and LV group.[5] Three combined 5-FU and LV regimens have shown activity in prospectively randomized trials in advanced colorectal cancer: the Roswell Park regimen (500 mg/m^2 of LV in a 2-hour infusion with a 600-mg/m^2 IV push of 5-FU 1 hour into the LV infusion weekly for 6 weeks with a 2-week rest period); the Mayo Clinic high-dose LV regimen (a 200-mg/m^2 IV bolus of LV followed by a 370- to 400-mg/m^2 IV infusion of 5-FU over 15 minutes daily for 5 days every 28 to 35 days); and the Mayo Clinic low-dose LV regimen (a 20-mg/m^2 IV bolus of LV followed by a 425-mg/m^2 IV bolus of 5-FU daily for 5 days every 28 to 35 days).

The toxicity profile of 5-FU combined with LV varies depending on the regimen used. With the Roswell Park regimen, the dose-limiting toxicity is diarrhea, which occurs most commonly in weeks 5 to 6 of the first 6-week course.[48,52] The diarrhea must be treated aggressively because deaths related to this

TABLE 72-1. *Prospective randomized phase III clinical trials of 5-fluorouracil (5-FU) and leucovorin (LV)*

Schedule	Response* (%)	Reference
5-FU 450 mg/m² IV bolus days 1–5, then 200 mg/m² every other day for 6 doses every 28 days	11	48
LV 500 mg/m² (2-h infusion), 5-FU 600 mg/m² at mid infusion weekly × 6 every 8 wk	48 (P = .0009)	
5-FU 370 mg/m² IV bolus days 1–5 every 28 days	7	49
LV 200 mg/m² IV, 5-FU 370 mg/m² IV days 1–5 every 28 days	33 (P < .0005)	
5-FU 600 mg/m² IV every week	5	50
LV 500 mg/m² (2-h infusion), 5-FU 600 mg/m² at mid infusion weekly	16 (P = .05)	
5-FU 13.5 mg/kg bolus days 1–5 every 28 days	15	51
LV 200 mg/m² IV, 5-FU 400 mg/m² IV in 15 minutes days 1–5 every 28 days	16 (P = NS)	
5-FU 500 mg/m² IV bolus days 1–5 every 28 days	12	52
LV 500 mg/m² (2-h infusion), 5-FU 600 mg/m² at mid infusion weekly × 6 every 8 wk	30	
LV 25 mg/m² IV bolus, 5-FU 600 mg/m² 1 h after LV infusion weekly × 6 every 8 weeks	19	
5-FU 12 mg/kg IV bolus days 1–5, then 15 mg/m² IV bolus weekly	16	53
LV 200 mg/m² IV, 5-FU 400 mg/m² days 1–5 every 28 days	18 (P > .4)	
5-FU 12 mg/kg IV bolus days 1–5 every 35 days	10	3
LV 200 mg/m², 5-FU 370 mg/m² days 1–5 every 28 days × 2, then every 35 days	26	
LV 20 mg/m² IV, 5-FU 425 mg/m² days 1–5 every 28 days × 2, then every 35 days	43 (P = .001)	
5-FU 370 mg/m² days 1–5 every 28 days	13	54
LV 500 mg/m² (24-h infusion), 5-FU 370 mg/m² days 1–5 every 28 days	44 (P = .0002)	
5-FU 400 mg/m² IV bolus days 1–5 every 28 days	13	55
LV 200 mg/m² IV, 5-FU 400 mg/m² days 1–5 every 28 days	21 (P = .046)	
LV 200 mg/m², 5-FU 370 mg/m² days 1–5 every 28 days × 2, then every 35 days	31	4
LV 20 mg/m², 5-FU 425 mg/m² days 1–5 every 28 days × 2, then every 35 days	42	
LV 20 mg/m², 5-FU 425 mg/m² days 1–5 every 28–35 days	33	56
LV 500 mg/m² (2-h infusion), 5-FU at mid infusion weekly × 6 every 8 wk	28 (P = .47)	

* Complete and partial responses.

toxicity have been reported.[52] Many investigators have used octreotide acetate to treat this chemotherapy-induced diarrhea, with encouraging results.[58,59] The dose-limiting toxicity is stomatitis when the LV regimen is given daily for 5 days,[3,4,56] and diarrhea when it is given weekly. Although uncommon, morbidity and mortality related to neutropenic sepsis can occur with 5-day schedules.[3,4]

The optimal dosage and schedule of 5-FU and LV have not been established. A prospective randomized trial comparing the Roswell Park high-dose and Mayo Clinic low-dose regimens in advanced colorectal carcinoma attempted to address this question.[60] Both regimens were equally effective in producing tumor responses (35% versus 31%, respectively), and median survival was similar (9.3 months versus 10.7 months, respectively). However, when financial costs were tallied to include drugs, administration charges, and hospitalization expenses to manage toxicity, the balance favored the low-dose LV daily regimen ($4216 versus $8144, respectively).

Another approach to the modulation of 5-FU with LV is the use of CI 5-FU with weekly IV boluses of LV.[61,62] This schedule attempts to take advantage of continuous exposure of the cells to 5-FU with the proven ability of LV to stabilize the ternary complex, increasing the duration and degree of thymidylate synthase inhibition with resultant cell destruction. Sinnige and colleagues reported a phase I to II study using this schedule.[62] In the phase I study, 10 patients were given CI 5-FU at 300 mg/m²/d for 14 days with IV bolus LV at 200 mg/m²/d on days 2 and 8 every 28 days. This LV dosage produced significant toxicity and had to be decreased by half. The most common toxicity was the hand-foot syndrome, which occurred in 40 of 54 courses. Grade 3 to 4 mucositis occurred in 24 of 54 courses, and diarrhea occurred in 7 of 54 courses.[62] Three of 8 evaluable patients after two courses had a response, and the other patients had stable disease. No decrease in the incidence and grade of toxicity was observed after reduction of the LV dosage. Therefore, in the phase II study, the LV dosage remained at 200 mg/m² on days 2 and 8, whereas the 5-FU dosage was reduced to 200 mg/m². Twenty-one previously untreated patients were studied. The response rate was 23.8%. Toxicity consisted of the hand-foot syndrome, which occurred in 19 of 113 courses, and conjunctivitis, which occurred in 9 of 113 courses; no grade 3 to 4 mucositis or diarrhea was observed.[62]

5-FU and oral LV regimens also have been shown to have activity in metastatic colorectal cancer.[63,64] Laufman and associates reported a randomized double-blind trial of 5-FU and placebo versus 5-FU and oral LV.[63] In 198 analyzable patients,

TABLE 72-2. *Southwest Oncology Group Screening Trial*[65]

Regimen/schedule	Response rate* (%)
5-FU 500 mg/m^2 IV bolus days 1–5 every 5 wk	23
LV 20 mg/m^2 + 5-FU 425 mg/m^2 IV bolus days 1–5 every 4 wk	15
LV 500 mg/m^2 as a 3-h infusion + 5-FU 600 mg/m^2 IV bolus weekly for 6 wk every 8 wk	9
5-FU 300 mg/m^2 d CI days 1–28 every 5 wk	24
LV 20 mg/m^2 IV bolus weekly + 5-FU 200 mg/m^2 CI days 1–28 every 35 days	26
5-FU 2600 mg/m^2 24-h CI every week	14
PALA 250 mg/m^2 IV bolus day 1 + 5-FU 2600 mg/m^2 24-h CI × 2 every week	10

* In patients with measurable disease.
5-FU, 5-fluorouracil; *LV,* leucovorin; *CI,* continuous infusion; *PALA, N-* (phosphonacetyl)-L-aspartate.

the response rate was better, but not statistically significant, using the 5-FU and LV regimen (32% versus 23%, respectively). Median survival was 44 weeks versus 54 weeks, favoring the 5-FU and placebo group. The mean 5-FU weekly dose intensity was significantly better in the 5-FU and placebo group (472 mg/m^2/wk) compared with the 5-FU and LV group (400 mg/m^2/wk). Toxicity was the same in both groups, with a 37% incidence of grade 3 and 4 mucositis in the 5-FU and placebo group (mainly asthenia [21%], neutropenia [11%], and diarrhea [10%]) versus a 45% incidence in the 5-FU and LV group (mainly diarrhea [24%], asthenia [18%], and nausea and vomiting [14%]).[63]

In an attempt to determine the optimal dosage and schedule of 5-FU with and without LV, the Southwest Oncology Group randomly assigned 560 patients (75% with measurable and 25% with nonmeasurable disease) to one of seven regimens in a phase II trial.[65] As illustrated in Table 72-2, all regimens were active in patients with measurable disease, with preliminary response rates varying from 9% to 26%. Survival rates were reported to be nearly identical in the IV bolus schedule groups. However, in terms of survival, when compared with IV bolus 5-FU alone, the regimens of CI 5-FU alone and CI 5-FU and LV revealed the hazard ratios favoring the CI regimens.[65]

LV commonly is prepared as a racemic mixture. The 6S-isomer is transported more readily within the cell, binds to thymidylate synthase with greater affinity than the 6R-isomer, and is viewed as the active component of LV.[66,67] At Roswell Park, the combination of 6S-isomer LV and 5-FU has been investigated in a phase II study (Meropol and associates, unpublished data, April 1994). IV bolus 5-FU at 600 to 750 mg/m^2 was administered midway through a 2-hour infusion of 6S-isomer LV at 250 mg/m^2 weekly for 4 of every 5 weeks. Thirty previously untreated patients (except for adjuvant therapy in 6 patients) were studied. The overall response rate was 40%. Diarrhea, leukopenia, and stomatitis were the most common toxicities.

5-FLUOROURACIL AND *N*-(PHOSPHONACETYL)-L-ASPARTATE

N-(phosphonacetyl)-L-aspartate (PALA) is a synthetic inhibitor of aspartate transcarbamylase, which is an enzyme involved in the de novo synthesis of pyrimidines.[68] By inhibiting de novo pyrimidine synthesis, PALA can increase the incorporation of 5-FU into RNA.[69] Since 1978, clinical studies involving PALA have been performed. PALA has no antitumor activity as a single agent.[70–72] When used as a single agent, PALA's dose-limiting toxicities are dermatitis, diarrhea, and stomatitis occurring 5 to 10 days after its administration.[73] Other toxicities include nausea, vomiting, mild myelosuppression, paresthesias, facial tingling, seizures, and minor elevations in aspartate aminotransferase and uric acid levels.[73–77]

PALA produces maximal inhibition of pyrimidine synthesis at a dose of 250 mg/m^2, which is one-tenth its maximal tolerated dose.[78] The combination of PALA and 5-FU has been reported to produce response rates of 35% to 43%.[79–81] Ardalan and colleagues conducted a phase I to II study evaluating the combination of 5-FU and PALA in previously untreated patients.[79] IV PALA (250 mg/m^2) was administered over 15 minutes, 24 hours before CI 5-FU (750 to 3400 mg/m^2/wk). The maximal tolerated dose of 5-FU was 2600 mg/m^2. The response rate was 40% in patients with advanced colorectal carcinoma. In this study, the dose-limiting toxicity was ataxia, which was reversible on discontinuation of therapy.[79] Diarrhea occurred in 25% of the patients, but the exact grades of the toxicities were not stated by the authors. The addition of PALA to 5-FU did not increase toxicity. O'Dwyer and associates reported a response rate of 43% in 37 previously untreated patients who were given PALA and 5-FU.[80] PALA was administered weekly by IV bolus 24 hours before a 24-hour CI of 5-FU at 2600 mg/m^2. Grade 3 and 4 diarrhea and neurotoxicity occurred in 15% and 5% of the patients, respectively. Kemeny and colleagues reported a response rate of 35% in 43 analyzable patients with advanced colorectal cancer who were treated with PALA and 5-FU.[81] However, these investigators administered 5-FU as an IV bolus (600 to 800 mg/m^2) 24 hours after IV PALA (250 mg/m^2/wk for 6 weeks with a 2-week rest period). Grade 4 neutropenia occurred in 4 patients at an 5-FU dosage of 800 mg/m^2; however, no patients had grade 3 to 4 cytopenia at lower 5-FU dosages. Grade 3 to 4 diarrhea occurred in 36% and 24% of the patients treated at 5-FU dosages of 800 mg/m^2 and 700 mg/m^2, respectively. Grade 4 neurotoxicity and skin toxicity occurred in 1 patient each at the highest 5-FU dosage. Ascites occurred in 13% of the patients and aminoaspartate transaminase levels were twice as high as baseline or bilirubin levels were greater than 1.3 mg/dL in 36% of the patients. The overall response rate was 35% and was not dependent on the 5-FU dosage.[81] The combination of PALA and 5-FU has been demonstrated to be active in colorectal cancer when 5-FU is given by CI or IV bolus.

Modulation of PALA and 5-FU with other drugs, such as 6-mercaptopurine riboside,[82] thymidine,[83] and LV, has been reported.[84] The rationale is to exploit the use of biochemical modulators that act on different pathways of 5-FU anabolism and catabolism. Response rates have been 7%, 33%, and 29% with PALA, 5-FU, and 6-mercaptopurine riboside; PALA, 5-FU, and thymidine; and PALA, 5-FU, and LV, respectively.

5-FLUOROURACIL AND METHOTREXATE

By inhibiting the enzyme dihydrofolate reductase, methotrexate (MTX) precludes the replenishment of tetrahydrofolate cofactors that are essential in de novo purine synthesis.[85] At the intracellular level, levels of phosphoribosylpyrophosphate, a cofactor in the conversion of 5-FU to FdUMP, are increased, which results in the formation of 5-FU metabolites.[86]

The timing of MTX administration can affect its antineoplastic effects. Because 5-FU impedes the generation of dihydrofolate, which is necessary for MTX toxicity, it is speculated that less than additive antineoplastic activity occurs when 5-FU is administered before MTX.[87] 5-FU also decreases the polyglutamation of MTX, preventing the formation of antifolate.[87,88] However, when MTX is administered before 5-FU, enhanced activity occurs, probably secondary to the increased formation of 5-FU metabolites.[89] In spite of the fact that MTX inhibits the formation of reduced folates, this inhibition causes less than 100% depletion of 5,10-methylene tetrahydrofolate (CH_2CH_4) and causes a rise in dihydrofolate that can replace CH_2CH_4 in the ternary complex with FdUMP and thymidylate synthase.[90]

Table 72-3 illustrates phase III trials using combinations of sequential MTX and 5-FU with or without LV. Two of these studies revealed a significant improvement in survival.[91,92] In 249 evaluable patients, the Nordic group demonstrated a statistically significant advantage in both response (17% versus 2%) and survival (8.5 months versus 6 months) associated with MTX, 5-FU, and LV compared with 5-FU alone.[91] There was no difference in the incidence of grade 3 and 4 toxicities, except for stomatitis, which was more common with the combination of MTX, 5-FU, and LV. Other toxicities that occurred more commonly with the sequential MTX regimen were diarrhea, conjunctivitis, and renal failure. Marsh and colleagues reported a study in which both treatment regimens included MTX, 5-FU, and LV.[92] The only difference was in the timing of administration of 5-FU and LV. In one regimen, 5-FU and LV were administered 24 hours after MTX; in the other regimen, they were administered 1 hour after MTX. A statistically significant improvement in response rate (29% versus 14.5%) and survival (15.3 months versus 11.4 months) was observed when MTX was administered 24 hours before 5-FU and LV. In this trial, the improved response rate and survival were observed only in patients with colonic primary tumors.[92] Stomatitis was more common and severe when MTX was administered 24 hours before 5-FU and LV. Of four deaths associated with neutropenia, three occurred when 5-FU and LV were administered 1 hour after MTX. Three other drug-related deaths occurred.[92]

COMBINATION OF 5-FLUOROURACIL AND ITS MODULATORS

The activity of 5-FU can be modulated by several drugs. Some investigators have attempted to take advantage of the different mechanisms of action of these modulators by using them in combination. Grem and associates[93] reported an overall response rate of 54% in 44 analyzable patients in a phase II study using IFN-α (5 million U/m^2 subcutaneously on days 1

TABLE 72-3. *Selected prospective randomized phase III studies of methotrexate and 5-fluorouracil with or without leucovorin*

Schedule	Response* (%)	Reference
5-FU 450 mg/m^2 IV bolus days 1–5, then every other day × 6 every 28 d	11	48
MTX 50 mg/m^2 IV over 4 h, then 5-FU 600 mg/m^2 weekly × 4, then every 2 wk	5 (*P* = NS)	
5-FU 12 mg/kg IV bolus days 1–5 (800 mg maximum), then 15-mg/kg bolus every week	17	49
MTX 50 mg/m^2 po every 6 h × 5; 5-FU 500 mg/m^2 IV bolus at 24 h; LV 10 mg/m^2 po every 6 h × 5 doses every 2 wk	20 (*P* = NS)	
5-FU 500 mg/m^2 days 1–5 every 5 wk	10	3
MTX 40 mg/m^2 IV bolus; 5-FU 700 mg/m^2 IV bolus at 24 h; repeat day 8, then every 4 wk	26 (*P* = .04)	
MTX 200 mg/m^2 IV (over 4 h); 5-FU 900 mg/m^2 at 7 h; LV 14 mg/m^2 po every 6 h × 8 (24 h after MTX); repeat at 3 and 6 wk, then every 4 wk	(*P* = NS from 5-FU)	
MTX 200 mg/m^2 IV (over 4 h); 5-FU 1100 mg/m^2 at 7 h; LV 14 mg/m^2 po every 6 h × 8 (24 h after MTX); repeat at 3 and 6 wk, then every 4 wk	14	4
LV 200 mg/m^2; 5-FU 370 mg/m^2 days 1–5 every 28 d × 2, then every 35 d	31 (*P* < .01)	
LV 20 mg/m^2; 5-FU 425 mg/m^2 days 1–5 every 28 d × 2, then every 35 d	42 (*P* < .01)	
5-FU 600 mg/m^2 IV bolus days 1 and 2 every 2 wk × 8 every 3–4 wk	2	91
MTX 250 mg/m^2 IV (over 2 h); 5-FU 500 mg/m^2 IV bolus at hours 3 and 23; LV 15 mg IM followed by 15 mg po every 6 h × 7 (at hour 24) evey 2 wk × 8, then every 3–4 wk	17 (*P* = .001)	
MTX 200 mg/m^2 IV (30-minute infusion); 5-FU 600 mg/m^2 IV bolus at hour 24; LV 10 mg/m^2 po 6 h after MTX every 2 wk	29	92
Same as above, except 1-h interval between MTX and 5-FU	14 (*P* = .026)	

* Complete and partial responses.
MTX, methotrexate; *LV,* leucovorin; *5-FU,* 5-fluorouracil.

to 7), 5-FU (370 mg/m^2/day IV on days 2 to 6), and LV (500 mg/m^2 IV on days 2 to 6). These patients had no prior chemotherapy except adjuvant 5-FU alone or with levamisole at least 1 year before inclusion in the study. Response rates were associated with the Eastern Cooperative Oncology Group performance status. Overall response rates were 65%, 54%, and 0% in patients with Eastern Cooperative Oncology Group performance status 0, 1, and 2, respectively.[93] Grade 3 to 4 mucositis and diarrhea occurred in 37% and 40% of patients, respectively. In another phase II study involving 30 analyzable previously untreated patients with colorectal cancer who were given IFN-α2a, LV, and 5-FU, the overall response rate was 57%.[94] Mucositis and leukopenia occurred in 57% and 27% of patients, respectively, but the grade of toxicity was not mentioned.[94] In a study of 95 previously untreated patients with colorectal cancer who were randomly assigned to receive either 5-FU and LV or 5-FU, LV, and IFN-α2b, response rates were 19% and 6%, respectively.[95] Sobrero and colleagues reported an overall response rate of 13.6% in 44 analyzable patients in a phase II trial with IFN-α2b, 5-FU, and LV.[96] In this study, the response rate was 20% in previously untreated patients and 10% in previously treated patients. Five patients discontinued treatment because of adverse reactions. Four of these patients had severe influenza-like symptoms and the others had diarrhea.[96] Further studies are needed to evaluate the potential benefit and toxicity of combining the different 5-FU modulators in a single regimen.

OTHER MODULATION APPROACHES

The use of other drugs, such as uridine, dipyridamole, hydroxyurea, and uracil/ftorafur, has been reported in clinical studies.[97–108]

Dipyridamole is a nucleoside transport inhibitor that curbs the cellular uptake of uridine and thymidine, and the efflux of active 5-FU metabolites.[109–112] In a phase I trial, the use of dipyridamole and 5-FU produced a 10% response rate, with stomatitis being the dose-limiting toxicity.[97] In two phase I studies, the combination of dipyridamole, 5-FU, and LV was not shown to have activity against colorectal cancer.[98,99] In these trials, toxicities included stomatitis, headaches, neutropenia, nausea, and vomiting.

Hydroxyurea inhibits ribonucleotide reductase, with the subsequent production of deoxyuridine monophosphate, which competes with FdUMP for binding with thymidylate synthase.[113] In metastatic colorectal cancer, response rates of 0% and 21% with no improvement in survival have been reported with the use of bolus 5-FU and hydroxyurea.[31,100,113–115] In 28 analyzable previously untreated patients, the combination of hydroxyurea, 5-FU, and LV produced a response rate of 36%.[116] Toxicities were nausea, diarrhea, and the hand-foot syndrome. Grade 3 toxicities occurred in 3 patients. This combination requires further study before incorporation into standard practice.

Ftorafur is a 5-FU prodrug that is converted gradually in vivo into 5-FU after oral administration.[117–119] Uracil is a pyrimidine base that inhibits competitively the degradation of 5-FU by dihydrouracil dehydrogenase.[120,121] Alone, uracil has no antitumor activity.[122,123] Uracil/ftorafur is a combination with a molar ratio of 1:4 that is attractive because it is administered orally and shows a spectrum of activity similar to that of 5-FU. These authors have evaluated the combination of oral uracil/ftorafur plus oral LV in patients with advanced colorectal cancer in a phase II trial. The dose-limiting toxicity with this regimen is diarrhea. Given encouraging results, a phase III comparison of oral uracil/ftorafur and LV with 5-FU and LV is underway.

Another approach has been to use uridine rescue to attempt to ameliorate toxicity. One hypothesis is that the incorporation of 5-FU into RNA contributes substantially to the toxicity of 5-FU.[105,106] When uridine is administered, the binding of FdUMP to thymidylate synthase is not affected, but uridine triphosphate replaces fluorouridine triphosphate in RNA.[107,108]

PLATINUMS

Cisplatin has been investigated extensively in combination with 5-FU. In phase II trials, response rates of up to 64% have been reported with cisplatin and CI 5-FU.[11,124,125] However, these results were not confirmed in randomized trials using either IV push 5-FU or CI 5-FU.[11] A new platinum analogue, oxaliplatin, has been reported to have activity in patients with colorectal cancer, both as a single agent and in combination with 5-FU and LV.[126,127] There is preclinical and clinical evidence that oxaliplatin is not cross-resistant with cisplatin or 5-FU. In 57 previously treated patients, a 38% response rate was obtained using 5-FU, LV, and oxaliplatin.[127] Grade 3 to 4 toxicities included reversible peripheral neuropathy (18%), vomiting (8%), and diarrhea (6%).

NEW DRUGS

Camptothecin (CPT) is a plant alkaloid that has antineoplastic activity against several experimental tumors.[128] Irinotecan hydrochloride (CPT-11), a water-soluble semisynthetic derivative of CPT, is converted in the liver to SN-38, an active metabolite that inhibits DNA topoisomerase I.[129,130] In phase I and II studies, the overall response rates in patients with advanced colorectal cancer who were treated with CPT-11 have ranged from 19% to 27%.[131–133] In a study by Shimada and associates, an overall response rate of 27% was obtained in 63 analyzable patients.[132] In this study, CPT-11 was administered in two schedules: as a weekly IV infusion of 100 mg/m^2 over more than 90 minutes, or every 2 weeks at a dosage of 150 mg/m^2. The response rates were 22.6% and 31.3%, respectively. Ten of 46 patients (22%) who previously had been treated with 5-FU responded. Pulmonary metastases responded better than did hepatic metastases. Leukopenia (16%) was the most common grade 3 to 4 toxicity encountered; other grade 3 to 4 toxicities were anemia (14.5%), diarrhea (12.9%), nausea and vomiting (12.7%), and alopecia (11.1%). Leukopenia was encountered more frequently with the weekly CPT-11 schedule, but there were no significant differences between the two schedules with regard to other toxicities.[132] The combination of CPT-11 and 5-FU has been shown to have synergistic activity in four cell lines[134] and is under active investigation.

Although the dominant target of 5-FU activity is thymidylate synthase, 5-FU catabolites interact with multiple metabolic pathways, which may contribute to toxicity and antitumor activity. Several highly potent specific inhibitors of thymidylate synthase have become available for clinical use. The furthest along in clinical development is tomudex (ZD 1694), a quinazoline folate analogue. Cunningham and associates reported a phase II study in which 124 previously untreated patients (except for adjuvant therapy) with advanced measurable colorectal cancer received tomudex (ZD 1694) at a dosage of 3 mg/m^2 IV every 3 weeks.[135] The objective response rate was 25% (31 of 124 patients). Grade 3 and 4 toxicities included neutropenia (13%), diarrhea (11%), nausea and vomiting (10%), fatigue (7%), and reversible elevation of liver transaminase levels (7%).

SUMMARY

Application of the concepts of biochemical and biologic modulation offers hope for patients with advanced colorectal carcinoma. A modest improvement in survival has been demonstrated with the combination of 5-FU and LV, although the optimal dosages and schedule remain undefined. An Intergroup trial that randomly assigns patients to 5-FU as a 24-hour infusion alone, 5-FU as a 24-hour infusion plus PALA, 5-FU plus oral LV, 5-FU plus high-dose IV LV, and 5-FU plus IFN-α is accruing patients. This study and others exploring new agents will enhance further the treatment of patients with advanced colorectal carcinoma. Elevated levels of thymidylate synthase protein and gene ratios have been correlated with a decreased response to combined 5-FU and LV chemotherapy in patients with colorectal and gastric cancer.[136] These assays may help select those patients who may benefit from 5-FU and LV modulation.

Another question that has been answered only partially is whether asymptomatic patients with advanced metastatic disease should be treated. The Nordic Gastrointestinal Tumor Adjuvant Therapy Group randomly assigned 183 previously untreated patients to expectant treatment or treatment with MTX, 5-FU, and LV.[137] This study demonstrated that early treatment of patients with advanced asymptomatic metastatic colorectal cancer prolonged the time to the appearance of symptoms, and suggested a median survival difference of 5 months in treated patients.

The use of chemoprotectant agents also holds promise for patients with colorectal cancer. The ability to reduce toxicity could allow for dose intensification of current regimens. There is some evidence of a clinically significant dose-response relation in patients with colorectal cancer,[13] and therefore, safe delivery of higher doses could improve outcome. Many investigators have been exploring the use of the so-called hematopoietic growth factors as mucosal protectants in patients being treated with combined 5-FU and LV, based on early observations of decreased stomatitis in phase I trials with these agents.[138–141]

Other investigational approaches to the treatment of patients with advanced colorectal cancer include early trials of immunotherapies directed at tumor antigens or molecular targets. These and other avenues derived from our understanding of colorectal tumor biology must continue to be translated into the clinical arena.

REFERENCES

1. Parker SL, Tong T, Bolden S, Wingo PA. Cancer statistics 1996. CA Cancer J Clin 1996;46:5.
2. Cohen AM, Shank B, Friedman MA. Colorectal cancer. In: De Vita VT Jr, Hellman S, Rosenberg SA, eds. Cancer: principles and practice of oncology. 3rd ed. Philadelphia: JB Lippincott, 1989:895.
3. Poon MA, O'Connell MJ, Moertel CG, et al. Biochemical modulation of fluorouracil. Evidence of significant improvement of survival and quality of life in patients with advanced colorectal carcinoma. J Clin Oncol 1989;7:1407.
4. Poon MA, O'Connell MJ, Wieand HS, et al. Biochemical modulation of fluorouracil with leucovorin: confirmatory evidence of improved therapeutic efficacy in advanced colorectal cancer. J Clin Oncol 1991; 9:1967.
5. Advanced Colorectal Meta-analysis Project. Modulation of fluorouracil by leucovorin in patients with advanced colorectal cancer: evidence in terms of response rate. J Clin Oncol 1992;10:896.
6. Kobayashi K, Schilsky RL. Update on biochemical modulation of chemotherapeutic agents. Oncology 1993;7:99.
7. Heidelberger C. Fluorinated pyrimidines and their nucleosides. In: Santorelli AC, Johns DG, eds. Antineoplastic and immunosuppressive agents, part 2. Handbook of experimental pharmacology. 38th vol. New York: Springer Verlag, 1974.
8. Evans RM, Laskin JD, Hakala MT. Effect of excess folates and deoxyinosine on the activity and site of action of 5-fluorouracil. Cancer Res 1981;41:3288.
9. Houghton JA, Houghton PJ. On the mechanism of cytotoxicity of fluorinated pyrimidines in four colon adenocarcinoma xenografts maintained in immune-deprived mice. Cancer 1980;45:1159.
10. Hakala MT. Basis for the effect of leucovorin on the activity and site of action of 5-fluorouracil in human cells. In: Bruckner HW, Rustum YW, eds. Advances in cancer chemotherapy: the current status of 5-fluorouracil-leucovorin calcium combinations. New York: J Wiley, 1984.
11. Kohne-Wompner C-H, Schmoll H-J, Hrstrick A, Rustum YM. Chemotherapeutic strategies in metastatic colorectal cancer: an overview of current clinical trials. Semin Oncol 1992;2(Suppl 3):105.
12. Wils JA. High-dose fluorouracil: a new perspective in the treatment of colorectal cancer? Semin Oncol 1992;(Suppl 3):126.
13. Hryniuk WM, Figueredo A, Goodyear M. Applications of dose intensity to problems in chemotherapy of breast and colorectal cancer. Semin Oncol 1987;14(Suppl 4):3.
14. Seifert P, Baker LH, Reed ML, Vaitkevicius VK. Comparison of continuously infused 5 fluorouracil with bolus injection in the treatment of patients with colorectal adenocarcinoma. Cancer 1975;36: 123.
15. Lokich JJ, Ahlgren JD, Gullo JJ, Phillips JA, Fryer JG. Prospective randomized comparison of continuous infusion fluorouracil with a conventional bolus schedule in metastatic colorectal carcinoma. A Mid-Atlantic Oncology Program Study. J Clin Oncol 1989;7:425.
16. Weinerman B, Shah A, Fields A, et al. A randomized trial of continuous systemic infusion fluorouracil (SI) vs bolus (B) with 5-fluorouracil (5-FU) in metastatic measurable colorectal cancer. (Abstract) Proceedings of the American Society of Clinical Oncology 1990;9:103.
17. Rougier PH, Paillot B, Laplanche A, et al. End results of a multicenter randomized trial comparing 5-FU in continuous systemic infusion (CI) to bolus administration (B) in measurable metastatic colorectal cancer. (Abstract) Proceedings of the American Society of Clinical Oncology 1992;11:163.
18. O'Connell M, Martenson J, Rich T, et al. Protracted venous infusion (PVI) 5-fluorouracil (5-FU) as a component of effective combined modality postoperative surgical adjuvant therapy for high-risk rectal cancer. (Abstract) Proceedings of the American Society of Clinical Oncology 1993;12:193.
19. Ansfield FJ, Curreri AR. Further clinical studies with 5-fluorouracil. J Natl Cancer Inst 1959;22:497.
20. Ansfield FJ, Curreri AR. Further clinical comparison between 5-fluorouracil (5FU) and 5-fluoro-2'deoxyuridine (FUDR). Cancer Chemotherapy Reports 1963;32:101.
21. Ansfield F, Klotz J, Nealon T. A phase III study comparing the clinical utility of four regimens of 5-fluorouracil: a preliminary report. Cancer 1977;39:34.
22. Baker LH, Talley RW, Matter R, et al. Phase III comparison of the treatment of advanced gastrointestinal cancer with bolus weekly 5-FU vs methyl-CCNU plus bolus weekly 5-FU. Cancer 1976;38:1.
23. Baker LH, Vaitkevicius VK, Gehan E, the Gastrointestinal Committee of the Southwest Oncology Group. Randomized prospective trial com-

paring 5-fluorouracil (NSC 19893) to 5-fluorouracil and methyl-CCNU (NSC 95441) in advanced gastrointestinal cancer. Cancer Treatment Reports 1976;60:737.

24. Bellet RE, Engstrom PF, Catalano RB, Creech RH, Mastrangelo MJ. Phase II study of ICRF-159 in patients with metastatic colorectal carcinoma previously exposed to systemic chemotherapy. Cancer Treatment Reports 1976;50:1395.
25. Douglass HO, Lavin PT, Moertel CG. Nitrosoureas. Useful agents for the treatment of advanced gastrointestinal cancer. Cancer Treatment Reports 1976;50:769.
26. Falkson G, Falkson HC. Fluorouracil, methyl-CCNU + vincristine in cancer of the colon. Cancer 1976;38:1468.
27. Moertel CG, Reitemeier RJ, Hahn RG. Therapy with the fluorinated pyrimidines. In: Moertel CG, Reitemeier RJ, eds. Advanced gastrointestinal cancer: clinical management & chemotherapy. New York: Harper & Row, 1969.
28. Moertel CG, Schutt AJ, Hahn RG, Reitemier RJ. Therapy of advanced colorectal cancer with a combination of 5-fluorouracil, methyl-1,3-cis(2 chloroethyl)-1-nitrosourea + vincristine. J Natl Cancer Inst 1975;54:69.
29. Moertel CG. Chemotherapy of gastrointestinal cancer. N Engl J Med 1978;299:1049.
30. Moertel CG. Therapy of advanced gastrointestinal cancer with the nitrosoureas. Cancer Chemotherapy Reports 1973;4:27.
31. Lavin P, Mittelman A, Douglass H Jr, Engstrom P, Klaassen D. Survival & response to chemotherapy for advanced colorectal adenocarcinoma. An Eastern Cooperative Oncology Group report. Cancer 1980; 46:1536.
32. Kemeny N, Yagoda A, Golbey R. A prospective randomized study of methyl CCNU, 5-fluorouracil and vincristine (MOF) vs MOF plus streptozotocin (MOF-strep) in patients with metastatic colorectal carcinoma. (Abstract) Proceedings of American Association for Cancer Research and American Society of Clinical Oncology 1980;21:417.
33. Posner MR, Belliveau JF, Weitberg AB, Sabbath K. Continuous-infusion cisplatin and bolus 5-fluorouracil in colorectal carcinoma. Cancer Treatment Reports 1987;71:1975.
34. Kemeny NE, Schneider A, Martin DS. Phase I trial of PALA, methotrexate, fluorouracil, leucovorin, and uridine rescue in patients with advanced cancer. The use of uridine to decrease fluorouracil toxicity. Cancer Invest 1990;8:263.
35. Padilla F, Correa J, Buroker T, Vaitkevicius VK. Phase II of Baker's Antifol in advanced colorectal cancer. Cancer Treatment Reports 1978;62:553.
36. Pazdur R, Ajani JA, Patt YZ, et al. Phase II study of fluorouracil and recombinant interferon alfa-2a in previously untreated advanced colorectal carcinoma. J Clin Oncol 1990;8:2027.
37. Petrelli NJ, Mittelman A. An analysis of chemotherapy for colorectal carcinoma. J Surg Oncol 1984;25:201.
38. Schutt AJ, Hahn RG, Reitemeier RJ, Moertel CG. A phase 2 study of intermittent high dose cyclophosphamide therapy of advanced gastrointestinal cancer. Cancer Res 1973;33:2218.
39. Wadler S, Wiernik PH. Clinical update on the role of fluorouracil and recombinant interferon alfa-2a in the treatment of colorectal carcinoma. Semin Oncol 1990;17:16.
40. Wasserman TH, Comis RL, Goldsmith M, et al. Tabular analysis of the clinical chemotherapy of solid tumors. Cancer Chemotherapy Reports 1975;5:399.
41. Martin DS, Stolfi RL, Sawyer RC, Young CW. Application of biochemical modulation with a therapeutically inactive modulating agent in clinical trials of cancer chemotherapy. Cancer Treatment Reports 1985;69:421.
42. Grem JL, McAtee N, Murphy RF, et al. A pilot study of interferon alfa-2a in combination with fluorouracil plus high-dose leucovorin in metastatic gastrointestinal carcinoma. J Clin Oncol 1991;9:1811.
43. Elias L, Crissman HA. Interferon effects upon the adenocarcinoma 38 and HL-60 cell lines. Antiproliferative responses and synergistic interactions with halogenated pyrimidine antimetabolites. Cancer Res 1988;48:4868.
44. Wek HJ, Platz D, Braumann D, et al. Phase II trial of 5-fluorouracil and recombinant interferon alfa-2B in metastatic colorectal carcinoma. Eur J Cancer 1992;28A:1820.
45. Wadler S, Lembersky B, Kirkwood J, Atkins M, Petrelli N. Phase II trial of fluorouracil (5FU) and recombinant alpha-2 interferon (IFN) in patients (pts) with advanced colorectal cancer: an Eastern Cooperative Oncology Group study. (Abstract) Proceedings of the American Society Clinical Oncology 1991;10:136.
46. Fornasiero A, Daniele O, Ghiotto C, Aversa SML, Morandi P, Florentino MV. Alfa-2 interferon and 5-fluorouracil in advanced colorectal cancer. Tumori 1990;76:385.
47. Rustum YM. Modulation of fluoropyrimidines by leucovorin: rationale and status. In: Taguchi T, ed. Cancer update II: latest developments in oncology. Tokyo, Japan: PMSI, 1993:13.
48. Petrelli N, Herrera L, Rustum Y, et al. A prospective randomized trial of 5-fluorouracil versus 5-fluorouracil and high dose leucovorin versus 5-fluorouracil and methotrexate in previously untreated patients with advanced colorectal carcinoma. J Clin Oncol 1987;5:1559.
49. Erlichman C, Fine S, Wong A, Elhakim T. A randomized trial of fluorouracil and folinic acid in patients with metastatic colorectal carcinoma. J Clin Oncol 1988;6:469.
50. Nobile MT, Vidili MG, Sobrero MG, et al. 5-Fluorouracil (FU) alone or combined with high dose folinic acid (FA) in advanced colorectal cancer patients. A randomized trial. (Abstract) Proceedings of the American Society of Clinical Oncology 1988;7:97.
51. Di Costanzo F, Bartolucci R, Sofra M, et al. 5-Fluorouracil (5-FU) alone vs high dose folinic acid (FA) and 5-FU in advanced colorectal cancer (CA). A randomized trial of the Italian Oncology Group for Clinical Research (GOIRC). (Abstract) Proceedings of the American Society Clinical Oncology 1989;8:106.
52. Petrelli N, Douglass HO, Herrera L, et al. The modulation of fluorouracil with leucovorin in metastatic colorectal carcinoma. A prospective randomized phase III trial. J Clin Oncol 1989;7:1419.
53. Valone FH, Friedman MA, Wittlinger PS, et al. Treatment of patients with advanced colorectal carcinomas with fluorouracil alone, high-dose leucovorin plus fluorouracil, or sequential methotrexate, fluorouracil, and leucovorin. A randomized trial of the Northern California Oncology Group. J Clin Oncol 1989;7:1427.
54. Doroshow JH, Multhauf P, Leong L, et al. Prospective randomized comparison of fluorouracil versus fluorouracil and high-dose continuous infusion leucovorin calcium for the treatment of advanced measurable colorectal cancer in patients previously unexposed to chemotherapy. J Clin Oncol 1990;8:491.
55. Labianca R, Pancera G, Aitini E, et al. Folinic acid + 5-fluorouracil (5-FU) versus equidose 5-FU in advanced colorectal cancer. Phase III study of 'GISCAD' (Italian Group for the Study of Digestive Tract Cancer). Ann Oncol 1991;2:673.
56. Gerstner J, O'Connell MJ, Wieand HS, Buroker TR, Krook J. A prospectively randomized clinical trial comparing 5-FU combined with either high or low dose leucovorin for the treatment of advanced colorectal cancer. (Abstract) Proceedings of the American Society Clinical Oncology 1991;10:134.
57. Erlichman C. Fluorouracil/leucovorin study update. J Clin Oncol 1991;9:2076.
58. Cascinu S, Fedeli A, Fedeli SL, Catalano G. Octreotide versus loperamide in the treatment of fluorouracil-induced diarrhea. A randomized trial. J Clin Oncol 1993;10:148.
59. Petrelli NJ, Rodriguez-Bigas M, Rustum Y, Herrera L, Creaven P. Continuous infusion somatostatin analogue (Sandostatin) for the treatment of chemotherapy induced diarrhea in patients with colorectal carcinoma. Cancer 1993;72:1543.
60. Buroker TR, O'Connell MJ, Wieand HS, et al. Randomized comparison of two schedules of fluorouracil and leucovorin in the treatment of advanced colorectal cancer. J Clin Oncol 1994;12:14.
61. Ardalan B, Chua L, Tian E, et al. A phase II study of weekly 24-hour infusion with high-dose fluorouracil with leucovorin in colorectal cancer. J Clin Oncol 1991;9:625.
62. Sinnige HAM, Nanninga AG, Verscheren RCJ, et al. A phase I-II study of 14-days continuous infusion of 5-fluorouracil with weekly bolus leucovorin in metastatic colorectal carcinoma. Eur J Cancer 1992;28A:885.
63. Laufman LR, Bukowski RM, Collier MA, et al. A randomized, double blind trial of fluorouracil plus placebo versus fluorouracil plus oral leucovorin in patients with metastatic colorectal cancer. J Clin Oncol 1993;11:1888.
64. Hines JD, Adelstein DJ, Spiess JL, Carter SG, Troy JE. High-dose weekly oral leucovorin and 5-fluorouracil in previously untreated patients with advanced colorectal carcinoma. A phase I study. In: Rustum YW, McGuire JJ, eds. Advances in experimental medicine and biology. 244th vol. New York: Plenum Press, 1988:167.

65. Leichman CG, Fleming TR, Muggia FM, et al. Fluorouracil (5-FU) schedules and modulation in advanced colorectal cancer (CRC): a Southwest Oncology Group (SWOG) screening trial. (Abstract) Proceedings American Society Clinical Oncology 1993;12:198.
66. Lee PP, Schilsky RL. Inhibition of thymidylate synthase by the diastereoisomers of leucovorin. Cancer Chemother Pharmacol 1990;26: 273.
67. White JC, Bailey BD, Goldman ID. Lack of stereospecificity at carbon 6 of methyltetrahydrofolate. Transport in Ehrlich ascites tumor cells. J Biol Chem 1978;253:242.
68. Collins KD, Staik GR. Aspartate transcarbamylase. Interaction with the transition state analogue N-(phosphonacetyl)-L-aspartate. J Biol Chem 1971;246:6599.
69. Speigelman S, Sawyer R, Nayak R, Ritzi E, Stolfi R, Martin D. Improving the anti-tumor activity of 5-fluorouracil by increasing its incorporation into RNA via metabolic modulation. Proc Natl Acad Sci USA 1980;77:4966.
70. Rubin J, Purvis J, Britell JC, Hahn RG, Moertel CG, Schuti AG. Phase II study of PALA in advanced large bowel carcinoma. Cancer Treatment Reports 1981;65:335.
71. Van Echo DA, Diggs CH, Scoltock M, Wiernik PH. Phase II evaluation of N-(phosphonacetyl)-L-aspartic acid (PALA) in metastatic adenocarcinoma of the colon or rectum. Cancer Treatment Reports 1980; 64:339.
72. Carroll DS, Gralla RJ, Kemeny NE. Phase II evaluation of N-(phosphonacetyl)-L-aspartic acid (PALA) in patients with advanced colorectal carcinoma. Cancer Treatment Reports 1980;64:349.
73. Grem JL, King SA, O'Dwyer PJ, et al. Biochemistry and clinical activity of N-(phosphonacetyl)-L-aspartate. A review. Cancer Res 1988;48:4441.
74. Gralla RJ, Casper ES, Natale RB, et al. Phase I trial of PALA. Cancer Treatment Reports 1980;64:1301.
75. Valdivieso M, Moore EL, Burgess AM, et al. Phase I clinical study of N-(phosphonacetyl)-L-aspartate (PALA). Cancer Treatment Reports 1980;64:285.
76. Erlichman C, Strong JM, Wiernik PH, et al. Phase I trial of N-(phosphonacetyl)-L-aspartate. Cancer Res 11979;39:3992.
77. Kovach JS, Schutt AJ, Moertel CG, O'Connell MJ. Phase I study of N-(phosphonacetyl)-L-aspartic acid (PALA). Cancer Treatment Reports 1979;63:1909.
78. Casper ES, Vale K, Williams LJ, Martin DS, Young CW. Phase I and clinical pharmacological evaluation of biochemical modulation of 5-fluorouracil with N-(phosphonacetyl)-L-aspartic acid. Cancer Res 1983;43:2324.
79. Ardalan B, Singh G, Silberman H. A randomized phase I and II study of short-term infusion of high-dose fluorouracil with or without N-(phosphonacetyl)-L-aspartic acid in patients with advanced pancreatic and colorectal cancers. J Clin Oncol 1988;6:1053.
80. O'Dwyer PJ, Paul AR, Walczak J, Weiner LM, Litwin S, Comis RL. Phase II study of biochemical modulation of fluorouracil by low-dose PALA in patients with colorectal cancer. J Clin Oncol 1990;8:1497.
81. Kemeny N, Conti JA, Seiter K, et al. Biochemical modulation of bolus fluorouracil by PALA in patients with advanced colorectal cancer. J Clin Oncol 1992;10:747.
82. O'Dwyer PJ, Hudes GR, Colofiore J, et al. Phase I trial of fluorouracil modulation by N-phosphonacetyl-L-aspartate and 6-methylmercaptopurine riboside dose and schedule through biochemical analysis of sequential tumor biopsy specimens. J Natl Cancer Inst 1991;83:1235.
83. Windschitl HE, O'Connell MJ, Wieand HS, et al. A clinical trial of biochemical modulation of 5-fluorouracil with N-phosphonacetyl-L-aspartate and thymidine in advanced gastric and anaplastic colorectal cancer. Cancer 1990;66:853.
84. Ardalan B, Sridhar KS, Benedetto P. A phase I,II study of high-dose 5-fluorouracil and high-dose leucovorin with low-dose phosphonacetyl-L-aspartic acid in patients with advanced malignancies. Cancer 1991;68:1242.
85. Bertino JR, Mini E, Fernandez DJ. Sequential methotrexate and 5-fluorouracil: mechanisms of synergy. Semin Oncol 1983;10(Suppl 2): 2.
86. Doroshow JH, Newman EM. Fluoropyrimidines biochemical modulation in colon cancer: pharmacology relevant in both the laboratory and the clinic. J Clin Oncol 1991;9:365.
87. Chabner BA. Biochemical modulation of 5-fluorouracil with methotrexate and leucovorin in colon cancer trials. In: Satellite Symposium of Biochemical Modulation, Walsh Japan Co., Tokyo, Japan 1990: 33.
88. Cown KH, Jolivet J. A methotrexate-resistant human breast cancer cell line with multiple defects, including diminished formation of methotrexate polyglutamates. J Biol Chem 1984;259:10793.
89. Leyland-Jones B, O'Dwyer PJ. Biochemical modulation: application of laboratory model to the clinic. Cancer Treatment Reports 1986;70: 219.
90. Allegra CJ, Fine RL, Drake JC. The effect of methotrexate on intracellular folate pools in human MCF-7 breast cancer cells: evidence for direct inhibition of purine synthesis. J Biol Chem 1986;261:6478.
91. Nordic Gastrointestinal Tumor Adjuvant Study Group. Superiority of sequential methotrexate, fluorouracil, and leucovorin to fluorouracil alone in advanced symptomatic colorectal carcinoma: a randomized trial. J Clin Oncol 1989;7:1437.
92. Marsh JC, Bertino J, Katz KH, et al. The influence of drug interval on the effect of methotrexate and fluorouracil in the treatment of advanced colorectal cancer. J Clin Oncol 1991;9:371.
93. Grem JL, Jordan J, Robson ME, et al. Phase II study of fluorouracil, leucovorin and interferon alfa-2a in metastatic colorectal carcinoma. J Clin Oncol 1993;11:1737.
94. Sinnige HAM, Buter J, Sleijter D Th, et al. Update of a phase II study of 5-fluorouracil (5-FU), leucovorin and alfa-2a interferon (IF) in advanced colorectal cancer. (Abstract) Proceedings of the American Society Clinical Oncology 1993;12:206.
95. Kosmidis P, Tsavaris T, Skarlos D, et al. Fluorouracil (5-FU) and folinic acid (FA) with or without a-2b-interferon (IFN) in advanced colorectal cancer. A prospective randomized trial. (Abstract) Proceedings of the American Society Clinical Oncology 1993;12:211.
96. Sobrero A, Nobile MT, Guglielmi A, et al. Phase II study of 5-fluorouracil plus leucovorin and interferon alpha 2B in advanced colorectal cancer. Eur J Cancer 1992;28A:850.
97. Remick SC, Grem JL, Fischer PH, et al. Phase I trial of 5-fluorouracil and dipyridamole administered by seventy-two-hour concurrent continuous infusion. Cancer Res 1990;50:2667.
98. Budd GT, Jayaraj A, Grabowski D, et al. Phase I trial of dipyridamole with 5-fluorouracil and folinic acid. Cancer Res 1990;50:7206.
99. Bailey H, Wilding G, Tutsch KD, et al. A phase I trial of 5-fluorouracil, leucovorin, and dipyridamole given by concurrent 120-h continuous infusion. Cancer Chemother Pharmacol 1992;30:297.
100. Lokich J, Anderson N, Bern M, et al. Dual modulation of 5-fluorouracil using leucovorin and hydroxyurea: a phase I trial. Cancer 1991; 68:744.
101. Nakajima O, Ihara K, Isoda T, et al. Phase I and II studies on a mixture of 1-(2-tetrahydrofuryl)-5-fluorouracil and uracil (UFT). Cancer Chemother 1980;7:1558.
102. Nakano Y, Taguchi T, Sakai K, et al. Clinical phase II study on UFT by cooperative study group. Cancer Chemother 1980;7:1569.
103. Murakami M, Ota K. Clinical results of UFT therapy for malignant tumors under cooperative study (phase II study). Cancer Chemother 1980;7:1579.
104. Watanabe H, Yamamoto S, Naito T. Clinical results of oral UFT therapy under cooperative study. Cancer Chemother 1980;7:1588.
105. Houghton JA, Houghton PJ, Wooten RS. Mechanism of induction of the gastrointestinal toxicity in the mouse by 5-fluorouracil, 5-fluorouridine and 5-fluoro-2'deoxyuridine. Cancer Res 1979;39:2406.
106. Sawyer RC, Stolfi RL, Spiegelman S, et al. Effect of uridine on the metabolism of 5-fluorouracil in the CD8F1 murine mammary carcinoma system. Pharm Res 1984;2:69.
107. Martin DS, Stolfi RL, Sawyer RC, Spiegelman S, Young CW. High-dose 5-fluorouracil with delayed uridine "rescue" in mice. Cancer Res 1982;42:3964.
108. Klubes P, Cerna I, Meldon MA. Uridine rescue from the lethal toxicity of 5-fluorouracil in mice. Cancer Chemother Pharmacol 1982;8:17.
109. O'Connell MJ, Poon MA, Moertel CG. What is the value of methotrexate in the treatment of advanced colorectal cancer? J Clin Oncol 1991;9:1322.
110. Grem JL, Fisher PH. Augmentation of 5-fluorouracil cytotoxicity in human colon cancer cells by dipyridamole. Cancer Res 1985;45:2967.
111. Grem JL, Fisher PH. Alteration of fluorouracil metabolism in human colon cancer cells by dipyridamole with a selective increase in fluorodeoxyuridine monophosphate levels. Cancer Res 1986;46:6191.
112. Alberts DS, Einsphahr J, Peng YM, Spears P. Dipyridamole (D) poten-

tiation of FUDR antitumor activity. Clin Pharmacol Ther 1987;41: 247.
113. Kao AK, Muggia FM, Dubin N, et al. Evaluation of a sequential 5-FU and hydroxyurea combination in advanced bowel cancer. Cancer Treatment Reports 1984;68:1383.
114. Lokich JJ, Pitman SW, Skarin AT. Combined 5-fluorouracil and hydroxyurea therapy for gastrointestinal cancer. Oncology 1975;32:34.
115. Engstrom PF, MacIntyre JM, Mittelman A, Klaassen DJ. Chemotherapy of advanced colorectal carcinoma. Fluorouracil alone vs drug combinations using fluorouracil, hydroxyurea, semustine, dacarbazine, razoxane, and mitomycin. A phase III trial by the Eastern Cooperative Oncology Group. Am J Clin Oncol 1984;7:313.
116. de Gramont A, Louvet C, Bennamoun M, et al. Dual modulation of 5-fluorouracil (5-FU) with folinic acid (LV) and hydroxyurea (HU) in metastatic colorectal cancer. (Abstract) Proceeding of the American Society of Clinical Oncology 1993;12:228.
117. Hiller SA, Zhuk RA, Lidak M. Analogues of pyrimidine nucleosides: I. N1-(-furanidyl) derivatives of natural pyrimidine basis and their antimetabolites. Dokl Akad Nauk 1975;176:332.
118. Toide H, Akiyoshi H, Minato Y, Okuda H, Fujii S. Comparative studies on the metabolism of 2-(tetrahydrofuryl)-5-fluorouracil and 5-fluorouracil. Gann 1977;68:553.
119. Benvenuto JA, Lu K, Hall SW, Benjamin RS, Loo T. Disposition and metabolism of 1-(tetrahydro-2-furanyl)-5-fluorouracil (Ftorafur) in humans. Cancer Res 1978;38:3867.
120. Fujii S, Ikenaka K, Fukushima M, Shirasaka T. Effect of uracil and its derivatives on antitumor activity of 5-fluorouracil and 1-(2-tetrahydrofuryl)-5-fluorouracil. Gann 1978;69:763.
121. Kimura K, Suga S, Shimaji T. Clinical basis of chemotherapy for gastric cancer with uracil and 1-(2-tetrahydro-furyl)-5-fluorouracil. Gastroenterologia Japonica 1980;15:324.
122. Kasai Y, Inokuchi K, Hattori T, et al. Randomized study on the long term adjuvant chemotherapy with ftorafur and mitomycin C for gastric cancer. The secondary study. Cancer Chemother 1982;9:1449.
123. Wenzel DG, Keplinger ML. Central depressant properties of uracil and related oxypyrimidines. Journal Pharmacological Association 1955;44:56.
124. Cantrell JEJ, Hart RD, Taylor RF, et al. Pilot trial of prolonged continuous infusion 5-fluorouracil and weekly cisplatin in advanced colorectal cancer. Cancer Treatment Reports 1987;71:615.
125. Krizan Z, Dimitrov D, Suhrland G, et al. Six week cycles of continuous infusion (CI) 5-FU and weekly low dose cisplatin (DDP) in metastatic colorectal carcinoma. (Abstract) Proceedings of the American Society of Clinical Oncology 1990;9:103.
126. Brienza S, Levi F, Valori VM, et al. Intensified (every two week) chronotherapy with 5-fluorouracil (5-FU), folinic acid (FA) and oxaliplatin (L-OHP) in previously treated patients (pts) with metastatic colorectal cancer. (Abstract) Proceedings of the American Society of Clinical Oncology 1993;12:197.
127. Moreau S, Machover D, de Gramont A, et al. Phase II trial of oxaliplatin. L-OHP in patients with colorectal carcinoma (CRC) previously resistant to 5 fluorouracil (5-FU) and folinic acid (FA). (Abstract) Proceedings of the American Society of Clinical Oncology 1993;12:214.
128. Gallo RC, Whang-Peng J, Adamson RH. Studies on the antitumor activity, mechanism of action, and cell cycle effects of camptothecin. J Natl Cancer Inst 1971;46:789.
129. Kunimoto T, Nitta K, Tanaka T. Antitumor activity of 7-ethyl-10-[4-(1-piperidino)-1-piperidino] carbonyloxy-camptothecin, a novel water-soluble derivative of camptothecin, against murine tumors. Cancer Res 1987;47:5944.
130. Kawato Y, Aonuma M, Hirota Y, Kuga H, Sato K. Intracellular roles of SN-38, a metabolite of the camptothecin derivative CPT-11, in the antitumor effect of CPT-11. Cancer Res 1991;51:4187.
131. Sakata Y, Nakao I, Futatsuki K, et al. An early phase II trial of CPT-11, in patients with advanced gastrointestinal cancer. Journal of Japan Society for Cancer Therapy 1992;27:2028.
132. Shimada Y, Yoshino M, Wakui A, et al. Phase II study of CPT-11, a new camptothecin derivative in colorectal cancer. J Clin Oncol 1993; 11:909.
133. Shimada Y, Sasaki Y, Sugano K, et al. Combination phase I study of CPT 11 (Irinotecan) combined with continuous infusion 5-fluorouracil (5FU) in metastatic colorectal cancer. (Abstract) Proceedings of the American Society of Clinical Oncology 1993;12:196.
134. Funakoski S, Aiba K, Shibata H, et al. Enhanced antitumor activity of SN-38, an active metabolite of CPT 11 and 5'fluorouracil combination for human colorectal cancer cell lines. (Abstract) Proceedings of the American Society of Clinical Oncology 1993;12:193.
135. Cunningham D, Zalcberg J, Francois E, et al. Tomudex (ZD1694): a new thymidylate synthase inhibitor with good antitumor activity in advanced colorectal cancer (ACC). (Abstract) Proceedings of the American Society of Clinical Oncology 1994;13:199.
136. Johnston PG, Lenz HJ, Danenberg KD, et al. Thymidylate synthase protein and gene expression predicts for response to 5-fluorouracil, leucovorin chemotherapy in patients with colorectal and gastric cancer. (Abstract) Procedings of the American Society of Clinical Oncology 1994;13:196.
137. Nordic Gastrointestinal Tumor Adjuvant Therapy Group. Expectancy or primary chemotherapy in patients with advanced asymptomatic colorectal cancer: a randomized study. J Clin Oncol 1992;10:904.
138. Gabrilove JL, Jakubowski A, Scher H, et al. Effect of granulocyte colony-stimulating factor on neutropenia and associated morbidity due to chemotherapy for transitional-cell carcinoma of the urothelium. N Engl J Med 1988;318:1414.
139. Meropol NJ, Miller LL, Korn EL, Braitmain LE, MacDermott ML, Schchter LM. The coadministration of granulocyte colony-stimulating factor and cytotoxic chemotherapy results in severe myelosuppression. J Natl Cancer Inst 1992;84:1201.
140. Schuchter LM, Luginbuhl WE, Meropol NJ. The current status of toxicity protectants in cancer therapy. Semin Oncol 1992;19:742.
141. Grem JL, McAtee N, Murphy RF, et al. Phase I and pharmacokinetic study of recombinant human granulocyte-macrophage colony-stimulating factor given in combination with fluorouracil plus calcium leucovorin in metastatic gastrointestinal carcinoma. J Clin Oncol 1994; 12:560.

Surgery for Gastrointestinal Cancer: A Multidisciplinary Approach, edited by Harold J. Wanebo.
Lippincott-Raven Publishers, Philadelphia, © 1997.

CHAPTER 73

Biological Therapy: Current and Future Considerations

Michael T. Lotze and James S. Goydos

Over the past 30 years, our understanding of the cause, pathophysiology, and genetics of cancer has progressed rapidly. We have refined our surgical techniques and markedly improved our ability to deliver radiation therapy. We have developed new cytotoxic chemotherapies and become more skilled at their use. However, our ability to extend the survival of patients with advanced solid tumors has been disappointing. Study is ongoing in the three traditional fields of cancer treatment, cancer prevention, and early detection.

As our understanding of the role the immune system plays in tumor surveillance and tumor eradication has grown, we have embarked on a fourth field of cancer treatment, namely, immunotherapy. The exploitation of the immune system's ability to distinguish minor alterations in expressed gene products gives us a powerful weapon with which to combat cancer. The major problem with conventional cancer therapies is that they exploit differences in location or gross cell growth alterations between tumors and normal cells. The side effects of treatment often limit the ability to deliver sufficient doses of cytolytic or cytostatic agents to control tumor growth. The immune system can target tumors specifically because it can be exquisitely sensitive to the minor differences between tumors and normal cells. The modern history of immunotherapy dates back to the early part of the 20th century, when W.B. Coley observed that a patient with a sarcoma had a better prognosis if a wound infection developed. He tested this theory by developing a treatment using bacterial products consisting of mixed toxins of *Streptococcus erysipelas* and *Bacillus prodigiosus* (now known as *Serratia marcescens*) in patients with metastatic sarcoma.[1] Coley's toxins had anecdotal success and were the direct antecedents of many bacterial and synthetic products used as immunostimulants in later trials. From this modest beginning, the field of immunotherapy has expanded concomitant with a far more profound understanding of immunoreactivity. The types of immunotherapy are categorized in Table 73-1. For ease of understanding, we classify immunotherapies as active or passive and as specific or nonspecific. This simple classification system is not perfect, and many types of immunotherapy could be cross-classified into more than one category. As the chapter proceeds, we discuss the areas of crossover and how they are applied.

CANCER AS A GENETIC DISORDER

Cancer is the result of genetic alterations leading to mutations or overexpression of functional proteins important in regulating growth, such as p53, p16, and ras. The changes in these molecules could be identified by cells within the patient's immune system, and evidence to support this notion has accumulated for ras and p53. A relative state of immunosuppression has been documented in many studies. Takao and colleagues demonstrated the immunosuppressive effects of serum factors from patients with gastric cancer.[2] They attributed some of the effects to molecules such as ferritin, α-fetoprotein, and other poorly characterized factors. The cytotoxicity of peripheral blood lymphocytes was decreased when they were cultured with these serum-derived factors. Another study conducted by Reynolds and associates showed that recombinant interleukin-2 (IL-2)–activated lymphocytes from normal donors had decreased cytotoxicity (lymphokine-activated killer [LAK] cell reactivity) against Daudi cells in a standard 4-hour chromium release assay when the lymphocytes first were cultured in the sera from patients with advanced cancers. When the sera used to incubate the lymphocytes was from patients with localized "early" cancers, decreased cytotoxicity was not observed.[3] These authors postulated that the sera of patients with advanced cancers contained factors not present in normal individuals or patients with early cancers. They suggested that biologic therapy could be more useful in patients with less advanced malignancies. Others have suggested a role for immunosuppressor cells, potentially pro-

Michael T. Lotze, Professor of Surgery and Molecular Genetics and Biochemistry, Chief, Section of Surgical Oncology, Department of Surgery, University of Pittsburgh School of Medicine, Biomedical Science Tower, W1543, Pittsburgh, PA 15261-2004

James S. Goydos, Section of Surgical Oncology, Cancer Institute of New Jersey, 303 George Street, Suite 501, New Brunswick, NJ 08901

TABLE 73-1. *A nosology of immunotherapy*

	Active	Passive
Specific	Tumor vaccines Synthetic vaccines Monoclonal antiidiotypic Ab Gene therapies	Monoclonal Ab Unconjugated Immunoconjugates T lymphocytes (TIL, TDL)
Nonspecific	Cytokines (IL1–15; IFNα,β,γ; TNFα,β; GM-CSF, G-CSF, M-CSF) Immunostimulants Biologic (BCG, OK432 Chemical (levamisole, cimetidine)	LAK cells ANK cells

Ab, antibody; *IL,* interleukin; *IFN,* interferon; *TNf,* tumor necrosis factor; *GM-CSF,* granulocyte-macrophage colony-stimulating factor; *G-CSF,* granulocyte colony-stimulating factor; *M-CSF,* macrophage colony-stimulating factor; *BCG,* bacillus Calmette-Guérin; *TIL,* tumor-infiltrating lymphocyte; *TDL,* tumor derived lymphocyte; *LAK,* lymphokine-activated killer; *ANK,* activated natural killer.

ducing nominal immunosuppressive factors such as prostaglandin E_2, transforming growth factor-β, or IL-10, in patients with advanced cancers. Malnutrition also has been suggested as a possible contributing factor to the immunosuppression observed in patients with cancer. Global T-cell defects observed primarily at the site of tumor, but also in the periphery, associated with defects in T-cell signaling and of the ζ chain, have been observed in mice[4] and in patients with renal cell cancer[5] and colorectal cancer.[6] Further studies are needed to identify the cause, and find a means to reverse, the immunosuppression found in patients with advanced malignancies.

A PRIMER ON THE NATURAL AND ADAPTIVE IMMUNE RESPONSE

Innate or natural immunoreactivity is mediated by host natural killer cells, macrophages, and mast cells. These cells are distributed through normal tissues and are sensitive to tissue injury or destruction. This damage causes cells to elaborate chemokines (eg, RANTES, MCP-1α, MIP-1α, IL-8) that promote traffic of inflammatory cells and lymphocytes into the tissues and cause the release of other inflammatory cytokines (eg, IL-1, IL-6, tumor necrosis factor-α [TNFα]). These inflammatory cytokines alter the hepatic acute-phase reactants, induce fever (which presumably enhances immunoreactivity), and promote local vascular congestion and procoagulant activity (which compartmentalizes the immune response). These cytokines also promote the production of later-acting cytokines, such as interferon-α (IFNα) and interferon-γ (IFNγ), IL-4, and IL-12. These later cytokines, coupled with specific antigenic stimulation, promote the local or regional development of so-called adaptive immune responses largely mediated by B cells and T cells. These are the cells imbued with "memory," allowing a heightened immune response at disparate locations and times of antigenic challenge. B-cell diversity, allowing greater than 10^{21} possible targets, is generated by recombination of multiple genetic elements and by somatic mutations. Further, so-called affinity maturation allows enhanced selectivity of B cells for carbohydrate or protein antigens based on tertiary structure, widely regarded as a "lock-and-key" mechanism by which immunoglobulins bind to their target. The humoral immune response, tightly regulated by T helper cells, is particularly sensitive and keyed to external microbial pathogens. Cellular immunoreactivity, mediated largely by TH1 cells and CD8 cells, allows responses to endogenous cellular pathogens such as viruses or other facultative organisms and to the subtle genetic alterations found in tumor cells. T-cell diversity, similar to B-cell diversity, is keyed to changes in the structure of two chains expressed on the cell surface known as the heterodimeric T-cell receptor. T-cell receptors interact with small (8 to 25 amino acids) linear peptides presented by the molecular scavengers, the major histocompatibility complex (MHC) class I and class II molecules. $CD4^+$ cells usually recognize peptide in conjunction with class II molecules and $CD8^+$ cells with class I molecules. Many tumors, including colorectal cancers, evade immune recognition by altering class I molecules.

MECHANISMS OF ESCAPE FROM IMMUNOREACTIVITY

The regulation of T-cell reactivity is extremely complex. Confirmation of the role of immunoreactivity in tumor cells comes from the identification of tumor-specific T cells capable of specifically killing or releasing effector cytokines after encounter with tumor, and from studies of the escape mechanisms used by tumor cells. These mechanisms include altering MHC molecules or their diversity to decrease the expression of nominal tumor antigens and releasing substances locally to prevent immunoreactivity. An example of the former mechanism is the selective loss of expression of human leukocyte antigen (HLA)-A, -B, or -C alleles (class I molecules) that has been observed in gastric and colon carcinomas. This represents some of the best evidence we have that tumors coevolve with the host immune response and have found ways to evade it. Means to promote or restore immunoreactivity now represent the major goals of effective immunotherapies.

ACTIVE, NONSPECIFIC IMMUNOTHERAPY

Active, nonspecific immunotherapy probably induces cytokines that enhance immunoreactivity. This can be accomplished by administering biologic or chemical immunostimulants to the patient, or directly with systemic or local cytokines themselves. Coley's toxins, described earlier, were a form of biologic immunostimulation. The most commonly used form of biologic immunostimulant is bacillus Calmette-Guérin (BCG), a mycobacterium attenuated by more than 230 passages in culture. A large amount of data has accrued in the use of BCG, in both animal and human studies. The BCG bacteria are viable when used in vaccines and have been shown to enhance resistance to experimental tumors and infections. They also can accelerate graft rejection and improve the survival of animals with various

TABLE 73-2. *Trials using levamisole in patients with colorectal cancer*

Author (year)	Arms of trial	Number of patients	Conclusions
Verhagen et al.[17] (1982)	Levamisole No levamisole	60	Increased survival in levamisole group
Borden et al.[18] (1982)	Chemotherapy Chemotherapy + levamisole	72	Increased survival in levamisole group
Laurie et al.[19] (1989)	No treatment 5-FU + levamisole Levamisole	401	Increased disease-free survival in levamisole + 5-FU group versus no treatment
Moertel et al.[20] (1990)	No treatment 5-FU + levamisole Levamisole	1296	Increased survival and disease-free survival in 5-FU + levamisole group versus no treatment
Chlebowski et al.[21] (1994)	Levamisole Placebo	78	No difference in relapse-free survival and overall survival in the first 5 years; increased late mortality in levamisole group

5-FU, 5-fluorouracil.

transplanted tumors.[7–10] The methanol-extracted residue of BCG has been shown to mimic BCG's immunostimulation, but can be prepared in a stable, standardized dosage form.[11,12] Mathe and colleagues showed that BCG was able to prolong survival in uncontrolled studies of patients with acute lymphocytic leukemia, and this led to trials in many other tumor types.[13] These studies in general failed to show a significant benefit in patients with advanced cancers. A single trial of BCG used as an adjuvant in resected colorectal cancer revealed improvement, primarily by a reduction in cardiac mortality,[14] but this trial remains unconfirmed. BCG has not been shown to affect survival in patients with advanced cancers of the gastrointestinal tract, although this is still controversial. It is approved only for use in the treatment of superficial bladder tumors.

Another immunomodulator, widely used in Japan and Korea, is OK432. It is a lyophilized preparation of an attenuated strain of *Streptococcus pyogenes* used as an immunostimulant. It has been administered intramuscularly, intradermally, subcutaneously, orally, intralesionally, and instilled directly into the peritoneal and pleural cavities. Many studies have been done in the Pacific Rim nations that have shown increased overall and disease-free survival in patients with a variety of tumors. Studies in North America and Europe have not substantiated these claims, and some of these approaches have been associated with a poorer outcome in treated populations as compared with control subjects.[15] Other microbial products used as immunostimulants include PSK, a protein-bound polysaccharide derived from a fungus, and *Corynebacterium parvum.*

Levamisole has been used as an anthelminthic drug for more than 20 years. It was found to have immunostimulant effects in the 1970s and showed antitumor effects in animal studies.[16] Levamisole's method of action is unknown and it has few side effects when given systemically. Studies were performed using levamisole as a single agent and in combination with cytotoxic chemotherapeutic agents, mainly 5-fluorouracil (5-FU; Table 73-2). Levamisole in combination with 5-FU now represents a first line of adjuvant therapy for the treatment of resected, regional colorectal cancer.

Cytokines also are used as nonspecific immunomodulators. Cytokines are soluble proteins largely produced by monocytes and lymphocytes that regulate cells involved in immunity. The five main groups of cytokines are the ILs, IFNs, colony-stimulating factors, chemokines, and TNFs (see Table 73-1). Cytokines also could be classified as passive, nonspecific immunotherapies because some (eg, TNFα, IFN) can directly cause tumor destruction or involution.

PASSIVE, NONSPECIFIC IMMUNOTHERAPY

Passive, nonspecific immunotherapy entails the transfer of immunocompetent natural killer cells to a patient after they have been stimulated by lymphokines outside the body. The conventional source of such cells has been the patient's own peripheral blood, and the activating agents are cytokines with or without other stimulating substances. LAK cell activity conventionally is mediated by lymphocytes incubated in IL-2, IL-4, IL-7, IL-10, IL-12, or IL-15 for 3 to 5 days.[22–27] Cells with LAK activity are capable of lysing fresh tumor cells in a nonspecific (non-MHC–restricted) fashion.[27] Murine studies have shown that the adoptive transfer of LAK cells coupled with the systemic administration of IL-2 can cause regression of established tumor metastases of the lung, liver, and subdermal tissues early after tumor inoculation. It is probable that their natural role is to delay or impede tumor implantation at distant sites.[27] Antigen-presenting cells also can be primed and adoptively transferred. These cells include the macrophages and dendritic cells that present antigens to the MHC-restricted effector cells of the immune system. When pulsed with specific antigen, these presenting cells would act as activated specific immunotherapies.

PASSIVE, SPECIFIC IMMUNOTHERAPY

Passive, specific immunotherapy is the transfer of humoral or cellular immune components that are specific for a patient's tumor. T cells found in the resected tumor and those found in the draining lymph nodes of the tumor presumably have been activated by the tumor and often are specific for it. The selective activation and clonal expansion of these tumor-infiltrating lymphocytes (TILs) or tumor-draining lymphocytes (TDLs) in vitro followed by their adoptive transfer back to the patient is a form of passive, specific immunotherapy.[28]

TABLE 73-3. *Representative Monoclonal Antibodies to Human Gastrointestinal Tumor Antigens*

Monoclonal antibody	Antigen	Tumor types	Source	References
17-1A	37–41–kD gp	Colon, pancreatic	Murine	30–35
B72.3	TAG-72, HMW gp	Colon	Murine	35–37
19-9	Sialyated Le^a	Colon	Murine	38
ST-4-39	HMW mucin-like gp	Adenocarcinoma	Murine	39
DuPan-2	HMW mucin-like gp	Adenocarcinoma	Murine	40
Col 1-15	CEA	Colon	Murine	41
VII 23	CEA, 180-kD gp	Colon	Murine	42
T84.66	CEA, 180-kD gp	Colon	Murine	43
NCC-ST-421	Dimeric Le^a	Colon, gastric	Murine	44
KM10	180–200–kD protein	Colon, gastric, pancreatic	Murine	45
KM231	Sialyl Le^a	Colon, gastric	Murine	46
e21	ErbB-2	Gastric, other	Murine	47
e23	ErbB-2	Gastric, other	Murine	47
Hepama-1	43-kD gp	Hepatoma	Murine	48
BW494	200-kD gp	Pancreatic	Murine	49–51
L6	Ganglioside	Carcinomas	Murine	52, 53
YJ-37	Sialylated lacto-carbohydrate	Colon, gastric	Human	54
28A32	Membrane/cytoplasmic Ag	Colon	Human	35
16.88	Cytoplasmic Ag	Colon	Human	55

kD, kilodalton; *gp*, glycoprotein; *HMW*, high molecular weight; *CEA*, carcinoembryonic antigen; *Ag*, antigen.

Another form of passive, specific immunotherapy is the production and transfer of monoclonal antibodies (MoAbs). A MoAb is a homogeneous antibody preparation of a single specificity produced by the fusion of an antigen-specific B cell and a myeloma cell.[29] The result is an immortal cell that produces large quantities of antibodies with the same idiotype (the antigen-binding portion of the molecule). The antibodies used most often are specific for tumor-specific antigen. MoAbs can be used to coat cells and set in motion antibody-dependent cellular cytotoxicity and complement-mediated cell lysis. These cytolytic mechanisms can be augmented by the addition of various cytokines, including IL-2. Table 73-3 lists some of the MoAbs that have been developed to gastrointestinal targets. Early development of human antimouse antibody reactions causing rapid elimination is one of the major obstacles to this form of treatment. The mouse antibodies are foreign proteins, and the patient's development of neutralizing antibodies is not unexpected. There is some controversy regarding the significance of the human antimouse antibody reaction, but research is continuing on ways to circumvent it and other problems associated with this type of therapy. Human MoAbs, in theory, would be tolerated better, but are more complex and difficult to produce. Another way around the human antimouse antibody reaction is "humanization" of mouse antibodies. This is done by fusing the genes that produce the mouse variable region of the antibody with a human constant region.[56] Clinical trials of such reagents are in progress at many centers.

Another way to use MoAbs in cancer treatment is by attaching various moieties to the constant end of the antibodies so they can be delivered preferentially to the tumor. This has been done with some success in the imaging of occult tumors using radioisotopes.[57] Radionuclides, toxins, and cytotoxic chemotherapeutic agents all have been conjugated to MoAbs. Table 73-4 lists some of the immunoconjugates undergoing evaluation.

ACTIVE, SPECIFIC IMMUNOTHERAPY

Active, specific immunotherapy involves strategies designed to "immunize" a patient to his or her own tumor. The patient's immune system should be capable of recognizing alterations in

TABLE 73-4. *Representative immunoconjugates*

Immunoconjugate	Type	Use	Conjugate molecule	References
XMMCO-791-RTA	Immunotoxin	Tx	Ricin A chain	58, 59
A7-NCS	Immunochemotherapeutic	Tx	Neocarzinostatin	60
A7-MMC	Immunochemotherapeutic	Tx	Mitomycin C	60
KS1/4-DAVLB	Immunochemotherapeutic	Tx	*Vinca* alkaloid	61
e23-LysPE40	Immunotoxin	Tx	*Pseudomonas* exotoxin	62
MGb2-Da	Immunochemotherapeutic	Tx	Daunomycin	63
90Y.B72.3	Radioimmunoconjugate	Tx	Yttrium-90	64
QC1054	Radioimmunoconjugate	Tx	Yttrium-90 or I-131	65
COU-1-131I	Radioimmunoconjugate	Dx	I-131	66
17-1A-1251	Radioimmunoconjugate	Dx	I-125	67

Tx, treatment; *Dx,* diagnosis.

the tumor and responding appropriately, but it presumably has failed to do so for a variety of potential reasons. The immunization process is designed to present nominal tumor antigens to the host's immune system in an effective immunogenic milieu that stimulates an immune response. Several different strategies have been developed to accomplish this presentation of antigen. One of the first tested was a tumor vaccine that contained the patient's own tumor cells with an adjuvant such as BCG, which then was injected back into the patient.[68] This whole-cell vaccine approach stimulates both a humoral and a cellular immune response, but results have been mixed, with only transient responses in most series (see later). Another strategy is to manufacture the specific antigenic determinants and inject them along with an adjuvant. The advantage of this type of vaccination is that it elicits a largely cellular immune response. A mucin vaccine developed at the University of Pittsburgh is an example of a synthetic antigen vaccine that is undergoing trial.[69] Another form of "immunization" involves the transfer of modified tumor cells admixed with autologous cells into which cytokine genes have been introduced. Cytokine gene therapy is based on the premise that the cytokine-producing cells will locally activate the immune system in the vicinity of the injected tumor cells and elicit a systemic immune response to the tumor. The genes for IL-4 and IL-12 have been introduced into fibroblasts, and IL-4 and IL-12 gene therapy is being assessed.[70] Trials using similar strategies involving IL-2, IFNγ, TNFα, granulocyte-macrophage colony-stimulating factor, and IL-7 have begun or will begin soon.

An alternate strategy of active, specific immunotherapy is the transfer of antiidiotypic (AB2) antibodies. The antiidiotypic antibody recognizes the antigen-binding portion of antitumor antibodies (AB1), mimicking the tumor antigens themselves. The hope is that the patient's immune response (AB3) to these tumor-mimicking antibodies will attack and destroy the original tumor.

The remainder this chapter is devoted to published studies of immunotherapy for gastrointestinal tract cancers, organized by organ and tumor type. Many trials overlap, and the same trial can include patients with different gastrointestinal tumors. When this occurs, the overlap is remarked, but discussion of the therapy is confined to the type of tumor under consideration. Many of the trials available for assessment were based on previous incomplete understanding of immunoreactivity, but hopefully presage more effective regimens.

IMMUNOTHERAPY FOR ESOPHAGEAL CANCER

Cancer of the esophagus is less common than other cancers of the gastrointestinal tract, particularly lethal, and less accessible to trials using experimental immune-based therapies. Patients with esophageal cancer often show profound depression of immunity and would seem to be one of the best groups in which to study immunotherapy.[71] However, few trials have been done and most of the data on the immunotherapy for esophageal cancer come from trials in which cancers arising in other sites in the gastrointestinal tract are included. As improved methods of preparing immunotherapeutic agents are developed and multicenter trials are conducted, a better understanding of the role of immunotherapy in the treatment of esophageal cancer will evolve.

Specific immunotherapies, active or passive, for the treatment of esophageal cancer have not been reported. Most gene therapies and vaccines being tested in other forms of gastrointestinal malignancies could include patients with esophageal cancer.[70] The development of MoAbs also is progressing rapidly.[72] The development of TIL therapy has been hampered by the difficulty in obtaining uncontaminated specimens that have not been irradiated, and by the poor physical condition of the patients. Review of the literature suggests that TIL and TDL transfer protocols have not been pursued actively.

Several trials have been done to test nonspecific immunotherapies in patients with esophageal cancer. The biologic response modifiers BCG and PSK were studied by Koga and associates.[73] They found increased survival in patients with esophageal cancer who were treated with standard radiation therapy and chemotherapy when BCG and PSK were added to the regimen. Similar results were obtained by Ogoshi when he treated 140 patients with esophageal cancer using a combination of radiation therapy and PSK.[74] This author went on to show that the pretreatment levels of certain glycoproteins and HLA antigens could help in the selection of patients to undergo this radioimmunotherapy.

The results of two phase II trials of chemotherapy and IFNα-2a have been reported.[75,76] A 27% response rate was obtained and has led to more widespread testing of this combination. The University of Pittsburgh is among the institutions involved in testing IFNα in the combined treatment of esophageal cancer. An ongoing trial uses 5-FU, cisplatin, IFN, and radiation therapy followed by surgical resection in patients with locally advanced esophageal cancer.[77] Preliminary results have shown eradication or substantial regression of treated tumors in a large percentage of cases.

Patients with esophageal cancer have been included in trials using IL-2 and LAK cell transfer.[78] No responses were observed, but a reversal of the immunodepression often observed in patients with advanced cancer was found. The use of adoptive immunotherapy in combination with cytotoxic chemotherapy and radiation therapy needs to be tested, and advances in LAK cell production may make this approach more effective.

IMMUNOTHERAPY FOR GASTRIC CANCER

The incidence of gastric cancer is declining in Europe and North America. It remains common in Asia, although even there, the incidence has plateaued and may be dropping. Early detection programs and more extensive surgical procedures have been applied with considerable enthusiasm and suggested benefit. Immunotherapy also has been studied extensively. Many trials using both passive and active strategies have been tried. An association of gastric cancer with Epstein-Barr virus infection has been observed in about one third of patients tested, again suggesting a reason for considering immune reagents.

Active, Nonspecific Immunotherapy

Many trials have been done using nonspecific immunostimulants in the treatment of gastric cancer, a list of which can be found in Table 73-5. A trial using BCG cell wall skeleton was performed in Japan between January 1976 and December

TABLE 73-5. *Trials involving cytotoxic chemotherapy and active, nonspecific immunotherapeutic agents in patients with gastric cancer*

Author (year)	Treatment arms	Number of patients	Author's conclusions
Ochiai et al.[79] (1983)	Surgery alone BCG-CWS + mitomycin + 5-FU + Ara C MFC alone	98	BCG-CWS is an effective immunotherapeutic agent
Yamamura et al.[80] (1986)	Surgery alone Mitomycin + 5-FU OK432 + mitomycin + 5-FU	122	Chemotherapy plus immunotherapy may be effective, but further data needed
Popiela et al.[81] (1988)	BCG + 5-FU 5-FU Surgery alone	322	Immunotherapy plus chemotherapy may be a safe and effective adjuvant
Italian Gastrointestinal Tumor Study Group[82] (1988)	Surgery alone MeCCNU + 5-FU + levamisole MeCCNU + 5-FU	213	No survival advantage with either immunotherapy or chemotherapy
Kyoto Research Group for Digestive Organ Study[83] (1991)	CS + oral FP CS + FP + oral OK432 CS + FP + IT OK432 PS + FP PS + FP + oral OK432 PS + FP + IT OK432	970	No survival difference in PS groups; significantly increased survival in CS group given oral immunotherapy
	PS + FP PS + FP + oral OK432 PS + FP + IT OK432		Significantly increased survival in immunotherapy groups if spleen left in place
Merrouche et al.[84] (1991)	BCNU + autologous bone marrow transplant + IL-2	15	20% response rate warrants further study
Kim et al.[85] (1992; Two trials reported)	Surgery alone MF MFC MF + OK432 MFC + OK432	468	Significantly increased survival in the immunotherapy groups (all curative resections)
Tsujitani et al.[86] (1992)	Curative resection + MMC + Tegafur Curative resection + MMC + Tegafur + PSK	53	Significantly increased survival in immunotherapy group when tumors had only slight infiltration with dendritic cells
Nakazato et al.[87] (1993)	Curative resection + MMC + 5-FU Curative resection + MMC + 5-FU + PSK	253	Addition of PSK increases both overall and disease-free survival

BCG-CWS, bacillus Calmette-Guérin cell wall skeleton; *5-FU,* 5-fluorouracin; *Ara C,* cytarabine; *MFC,* X; *BCG,* bacillus Calmette-Guérin; *MeCCNU,* semustine; *CS,* curative surgery; *FP,* fluoropyrimidine; *IT,* intratumoral; *PS,* palliative surgery; *BCNU,* carmustine; *IL-2,* interleukin-2; *MF,* methyl CCNU, 5-fluorouracil; *MFC,* MF + cyclophosphamide; *MMC,* mitomycin C.

1978.[79] The investigators randomly assigned patients with both curatively and noncuratively resected gastric cancer to surgery alone, surgery plus cytotoxic chemotherapy, or surgery plus intradermal injections of BCG cell wall skeleton plus cytotoxic chemotherapy. They found a significant difference in the BCG cell wall skeleton–treated group as compared with the control groups in terms of survival rates. These results led to widespread testing of BCG and other immunostimulants. A trial by Popiela and associates used BCG plus 5-FU versus 5-FU alone versus no chemotherapy in postoperative patients with advanced gastric cancer.[81] They found a slight improvement in survival among patients receiving BCG plus 5-FU. Bonfanti and colleagues reported on the trials of the Italian Gastrointestinal Tumor Study Group.[82] They tested a combination of cytotoxic chemotherapy plus levamisole administered after surgery compared with surgical resection alone in patients with gastric cancer and found no survival difference between the two groups.

OK432 also has been used in gastric cancer trials in Asia.[80,83,85] It has been given intravenously, intradermally, intratumorally, and orally. A slight survival advantage often has been found in the treated groups compared with historical or randomized control groups, especially in patients with stage III disease. Extensive testing of the patient's immunoreactivity to determine which alterations occur with the addition of immunostimulants has been performed.[85,86] Modest response rates have been reported (see Table 73-5).

Cytokines also have been studied in the treatment of gastric cancer. Failures with single cytokine treatments of other gastrointestinal malignancies led to combination trials for gastric cancer. Merrouche and associates treated 15 patients with metastatic or unresectable gastric cancer with high-dose BCNU (carmustine) with autologous bone marrow transplant followed by IL-2 infusion at 18 × 10^6 IU/m^2/d in a phase II trial.[84] They found an overall response rate of 20%, with one complete

TABLE 73-6. *Trials involving intrahepatic infusion of cytotoxic chemotherapeutic agents and active, nonspecific immunotherapeutic agents in patients with gastric cancer*

Author (year)	Agents used	Number of patients	Author's conclusions
Miya et al.[89] (1991)	Doxorubicin (Adriamycin); MMC, or 5-FU + IL-2 or OK432	9	44% response rate warrants further study
Okuno et al.[90] (1992)	MMC, 5-FU, and IL-2	20 (both colorectal and gastric cancer patients)	70% response rate and little toxicity; further studies are needed
Sugiyama et al.[91] (1993)	Doxorubicin or MMC alone	30	Improved survival in the immunotherapy group
	Doxorubicin or MMC + OK432 + IL-2	12	

MMC, mitomycin C; *5-FU,* 5-fluorouracil; *IL-2,* interleukin-2.

response. The duration of the complete response was 21 months and the partial responses lasted an average of 6 months. The treatment had significant toxicity, with no patients receiving more than 8 days of therapy. Trials combining cytokines with cytotoxic agents are ongoing, and newer cytokines, such as IL-12, are being tested here and elsewhere.

The treatment of hepatic and peritoneal metastases from gastric cancer with local cytokine therapy also has been attempted. As with colorectal cancer, the intraperitoneal infusion of cytokines to treat carcinomatosis is an attractive alternative, but results have been disappointing. Work by Uchiyama and colleagues suggests that the intraperitoneal administration of OK432 followed by incubation of peritoneal-derived lymphocytes in IL-2 and IFNγ increases the tumoricidal activity of the lymphocytes against autologous tumor cells and a natural killer cell–resistant gastric cancer cell line (KAT03).[88] Trials using the intrahepatic infusion of IL-2, other immunostimulants, and cytotoxic chemotherapeutic agents in patients with hepatic metastases from gastric cancer are shown in Table 73-6. Trials using IL-2 and newer cytokines in Ethiodol emulsions (based on similar trials of cytotoxic chemotherapeutic emulsions[92]) infused into the liver in patients with hepatic metastases from gastrointestinal malignancies have begun at the University of Pittsburgh Medical Center.

Passive, Nonspecific Immunotherapy

The adoptive transfer of nonspecific, immunocompetent cells has been studied extensively in patients with gastric cancer. Fujimoto and associates outlined the basic procedures for adoptive immunotherapy for gastric cancer.[93] Results in general have been poor, and some of the more recent trials using adaptive transfer of cells with LAK activity have stressed the immunosuppressive effects of this tumor type and its significance for adoptive immunotherapy.[2,3,94] Many of the trials with LAK cells in gastric cancer are aimed at correcting this immunosuppression. In one of these studies, Okuno and colleagues cultured spleen cells in both IL-3 and IL-2, and obtained more potent cytotoxic cells than when IL-2 was used alone.[95] Monson and associates attempted to correct the immunosuppression by giving total parenteral nutrition for 7 days before the initiation of treatment. They hoped to counteract any nutritionally based immunosuppression, but found that the treated patients surprisingly had apparent "worsening" of their measured cellular immune responses when compared with the control subjects.[96,97] Many studies have been done using immunostimulants such as OK432 and PSK in combination with adoptive immunotherapy to correct the immunosuppression.[98–100]

Passive, Specific Immunotherapy

One of the largest areas of study in the treatment of gastric cancer has been the production of MoAbs and immunoconjugates. Table 73-3 lists some of the antigens and MoAbs being studied for the treatment of gastric cancer. Immunoconjugates are shown in Table 73-4. New tumor antigens are being characterized and MoAbs produced in may laboratories around the world. None of the available MoAbs or immunoconjugates have proven useful in the treatment of gastric cancer. The problems of toxicity and delivery are being addressed and novel dosing methods are being developed.[47] TILs have been produced and adoptively transferred in patients with gastric cancer. Yamaue and colleagues treated seven patients with advanced gastrointestinal malignancies and obtained a partial response in one patient with gastric cancer.[101]

Active, Specific Immunotherapy

No vaccine protocols appear in the literature involving patients with gastric cancer. However, synthetic vaccines such as mucin could include these patients in future phase II trials.[69] Gene therapy protocols also easily could enroll patients with gastric cancer. Shou and associates have developed an animal model of an antiidiotypic antibody to gastric cancer,[102] but have not applied it clinically.

IMMUNOTHERAPY FOR HEPATIC CANCER

Worldwide, hepatocellular carcinoma (HCC) probably is the most common lethal tumor, predominantly affecting individuals in areas where hepatitis B is endemic, including sub-Saharan Africa and Asia. Surgical resection still offers the only hope for cure, but often is not possible because of the extent of the tumor or the presence of advanced cirrhosis. Much work has been done to develop nonsurgical therapies for HCC, and immunotherapy appears to represent a promising approach. Little work has been done testing immunotherapies in patients with the other major form of hepatic cancer, namely cholangiocarcinoma. Goydos and colleagues have shown extremely high serum levels of IL-6 in patients with cholangiocarcinoma, suggesting its possible role, as in myeloma and renal cell carcinoma, as an autocrine growth factor.[103]

Active, Nonspecific Immunotherapy

Immunostimulants have been used in the treatment of patients with HCC.[104–106] No benefit in the form of improved overall or disease-free survival has been found when BCG, OK432, or other immunostimulants have been used in patients with HCC. Most of the trials have grouped HCC with metastatic liver tumors, and results consequently are difficult to interpret. Controlled trials using immunostimulants in this patient population have not been performed.

Cytokines also have been used in the treatment of patients with HCC. IL-2 has been used systemically and locally in patients with HCC, but no lasting effect was found and no change in survival obtained.[107–109] Yamamoto and associates used a continuous infusion pump to deliver IL-2.[110] The patients underwent cytoreductive therapy before the administration of IL-2. These investigators obtained four complete and two partial responses among 11 patients, but all patients eventually relapsed and 1- and 2-year cumulative survival rates were 41% and 16%, respectively.

IFNα has been applied widely in the treatment of hepatitis B, hepatitis C, and HCC. Objective tumor regression has been observed in 10% of patients treated with IFNα.[111] The Gastrointestinal Study Group tested IFNα-2a in patients with HCC and obtained two short-lived responses among 28 patients treated.[112] These studies showed that IFNα has only weak antitumor effects and, consequently, combination therapy studies were suggested. Carr has added intramuscular injections of IFNα to the intrahepatic chemotherapeutic regimen with possibly improved antitumor effects.[113]

Passive, Nonspecific Immunotherapy

Adoptive immunotherapy has undergone extensive testing in patients with HCC. Ishikawa and associates treated 3 patients with advanced HCC using hepatic artery infusion of LAK cells and systemic administration of IL-2.[114] They obtained a partial response in 1 patient and reported little toxicity. Intrahepatic LAK cell infusion and systemic IL-2 treatment also was used with minimal toxicity by Onishi and colleagues in 10 patients with HCC.[115] They obtained a partial response in 2 patients with small tumor burdens and stable disease in 7 patients with more advanced tumors. Komatsu and associates described 9 patients with HCC treated with LAK cells and IL-2.[116] They obtained one partial response that lasted 6 months. They also found stable disease in 5 patients, and the patients with stable disease or a partial response had significant reductions in their α-fetoprotein levels. These studies suggest that there may be some value in the intrahepatic infusion of LAK cells in this patient population, and that further studies using combination therapies are warranted. Cytoreduction with surgery, embolization, or alcohol injection also could be combined with adoptive immunotherapy.

Passive, Specific Immunotherapy

The use of TILs in patients with HCC has been tried, but has met with little success. Takayama and colleagues described three patients treated with a regimen of chemotherapy and TILs, one of whom had HCC.[117] They showed that the TILs localized to the tumors and were able to obtain a greater than 55% reduction in the tumor burden in a single patient with HCC.

MoAbs also have been tested in patients with HCC. Fuhrer and associates reported on a MoAb specific for a 43-kilodalton antigen expressed uniquely on human HCC cell surfaces.[48] It could be useful for localization and possible treatment of this disease. Chen and colleagues developed a bispecific MoAb formed by coupling a MoAb for hepatoma cells with one for IL-2–activated T cells.[118] They have observed lysis of hepatoma cells when the bispecific antibody and cytotoxic T cells are added to the medium. The cross-linking of the T-cell receptor to a cell-surface antigen of the hepatoma cells is thought to be the method of action of this and other bispecific MoAbs, ultimately leading to enhanced cytotoxicity or the release of effector cytokines such as IL-2 and IFNγ.

Immunoconjugates also have undergone testing in animal models of HCC. Klein and associates used a human hepatoblastoma animal model to test polyclonal and monoclonal immunoconjugates.[119] They found increased survival with iodine-131–labeled and yttrium-90–labeled MoAb and polyclonal antibody treatments, with acceptable toxicity. Complete responses were obtained only with the MoAb immunoconjugates.

Active, Specific Immunotherapy

The literature contains no trials of vaccines, antiidiotypic antibodies, or gene therapies in the treatment of HCC. Trials of these immunotherapies are being pursued actively in other gastrointestinal malignancies, and these immunotherapeutic techniques could be adopted easily for use in patients with HCC.

IMMUNOTHERAPY FOR PANCREATIC CANCER

Pancreatic cancer is perhaps the most aggressive and lethal cancer of the gastrointestinal tract. Only surgical resection offers hope for cure or long-term survival, and most patients have unresectable disease at presentation. Standard cytotoxic chemotherapy and radiation therapy offer little hope of significant palliation or cure. Because of the dismal prognosis in most cases of pancreatic cancer, alternate therapies have been sought. Many trials using different forms of immunotherapy have been performed.

Active, Nonspecific Immunotherapy

Because of the relatively short survival of patients with advanced pancreatic cancer, trials using nonspecific therapies are difficult to perform. A few studies using biologic and chemical immunostimulants in patients with pancreatic cancer have been done.[120–122] These studies grouped the patients with pancreatic cancer together with patients with other types of malignancies, and the results are difficult to interpret. Studies testing immunostimulants in animal models of human pancreatic cancer are now possible because of advances in the development of these models.[123–125] It is hoped that this will lead to new trials using agents proven effective in preclinical trials.

Croghan and colleagues performed a phase I trial of IL-2 with or without cyclophosphamide (Cytoxan) in patients with disseminated carcinoma.[126] They obtained a partial response in one patient with advanced pancreatic cancer and were reported to be investigating means to modify their protocol to obtain a higher response rate. Another study by Schwartzberg and associates in 1990 used IL-2 and TNF in patients with advanced malignancies.[127] This was a phase II trial and the investigators obtained a partial response in one of the two patients with pancreatic cancer. In an interesting application of a cytokine therapy, Moriai and colleagues used an animal model of human pancreatic cancer to demonstrate a synergistic effect of IL-2 and irradiation.[128] They found that irradiation followed by the intratumoral injection of IL-2 after the restoration of immunologic competence (18 days later) led to enhanced tumor inhibition. The most impressive results in the cytokine treatment of pancreatic cancer involve the use of TNFα and IFNγ. Raitano and associates found TNF and IFN receptors in pancreatic cell lines and showed how these receptors correlated with the inhibitory effects of the cytokines.[129] This laid the groundwork for further trials using this cytokine combination. Abbruzzese and colleagues performed a trial using TNF and IFN in patients with advanced gastrointestinal malignancies, but found the combination too toxic.[130] Watanabe and colleagues were able to show a marked antiproliferative effect of the TNF/IFN combination in pancreatic cell lines,[131] and have demonstrated a similar antiproliferative effect in an animal model.[132] They and others are analyzing the actions of TNF and IFN on pancreatic cancer cell lines in hopes of finding a therapeutic regimen that lacks the toxic side effects of this combination.[133]

Passive, Nonspecific Immunotherapy

The use of LAK cells in the treatment of pancreatic cancer has been studied. LAK cells have been given to patients with pancreatic cancer, but no responses have been observed.[134] Work has continued on adoptive immunotherapy, mostly in animal models. Sugiura showed tumor inhibition in pancreatic cell lines exposed to LAK cells.[135] A series of experiments was performed by Marincola and colleagues showing that LAK cells injected into a mouse model of pancreatic cancer localized to tumors, and that animals treated with LAK cells and IL-2 had prolonged survival.[136,137] More potent lymphocytes and perhaps direct infusion are needed if adoptive immunotherapy is to be feasible in patients with pancreatic cancer.

Passive, Specific Immunotherapy

One promising approach for patients with pancreatic cancer is the use of MoAbs. Table 73-3 lists some currently used MoAbs and their target antigens. Early success in the characterization of pancreatic tumor antigens, the production of MoAbs to these antigens, and the promising preclinical trials led to many human trials. The phase I trials showed that antibodies could be given to patients with pancreatic cancer, and that the side effects were tolerable in most cases.[31,49] Stabilization of disease for short periods was obtained in these phase I trials, but partial responses were rare and no complete responses have been reported.[31,49] Based on these data, phase II trials have been initiated. Buchler and associates reported on a trial using the murine MoAb 494/32 in patients with resectable pancreatic cancer.[51] All patients underwent a Whipple procedure and then received the antibody treatments. They found no survival advantage in the treatment group as compared with a control group, and concluded that this therapy was not helpful in patients with resectable pancreatic cancer. Weiner and colleagues reported the results of a multicenter trial of the MoAb 17-1A in patients with unresectable pancreatic cancer.[33] They found that repetitive dosing of this murine MoAb was feasible and had acceptable toxicity, but that it lacked efficacy. These results seem to indicate that unconjugated murine MoAb is not effective against advanced or resectable pancreatic cancer, and that other approaches are needed. Tempero and associates used the MoAb 17-1A mixed with autologous mononuclear leukocytes in combination with IFNγ.[32] One complete response lasted 4 months and 6 patients with stable disease lasting 4 to 48 months were observed among 26 analyzable patients. Newer trials are continuing using different combinations, different murine MoAbs, and human and "humanized" murine MoAbs.

The failure of MoAbs alone to improve survival in patients with pancreatic cancer has led to several trials of immunoconjugates. Radiolabeling of MoAbs specific for pancreatic cancer antigens is being developed to help in early diagnosis and planning of surgical treatment.[67,138] Immunoconjugates also are being developed for use in treatment. Mehta and colleagues used a nude mouse model of human pancreatic cancer to study a yttrium-90–labeled MoAb.[64] They studied the distribution of the radioisotope and showed a 26-fold increase in the delivery of the isotope to the tumor targets when it was conjugated to the MoAb B72.3. Bosslet and associates performed a study using a bispecific MoAb.[139] They could demonstrate binding to the tumor target and a radiolabeled chelate, delivering a radioactive dose to the tumor in a specific manner. Further studies of this unique delivery system are ongoing. Another group has conjugated MoAb A7 to neocarzinostatin, an anticancer drug.[60] They hope to use this combination in future human trials.

The other forms of passive, specific immunotherapy, TILs and TDLs, also have been studied in the treatment of pancreatic cancer. Problems that arise when preparing TILs in patients with pancreatic cancer include the rapid course of the disease and the frequent difficulty of obtaining tumor samples. Yamaue and colleagues tried to avoid these problems by using lymphocytes found in ascitic fluid in patients with pancreatic and gastric cancers.[140] They could obtain regression of the ascites using direct infiltration of expanded TILs and IL-2. Further studies are continuing, and it is hoped that newer culture techniques and harvesting strategies will make the delivery of TILs to these patients feasible.

Active, Specific Immunotherapy

Little has been done with antiidiotypic MoAbs and gene therapies in pancreatic cancer, but vaccines are being studied. Our group at the University of Pittsburgh is testing a synthetic mucin vaccine in patients with pancreatic cancer and other gastrointestinal malignancies.[69] Preliminary results reveal no responses, but stabilization of disease in 2 of 20 patients and little toxicity. The final results of this and other trials are necessary before the usefulness of specific vaccines in this disease can be evaluated.

IMMUNOTHERAPY FOR COLORECTAL CANCER

The use of adjuvant and neoadjuvant chemotherapy and radiation therapy has improved survival. In advanced cancer of the colon and rectum, the application of such agents has not led to cure or long-term regression. Most immunotherapeutic regimens have been tried with limited success and newer trials are ongoing.

Active, Nonspecific Immunotherapy

The ability to upregulate a relatively immunodeficient immune response has been explored extensively in the treatment of colon and rectal cancers. The first agents tried were attenuated bacteria and purified bacterial wall products in an adjuvant. Trials using BCG or the methanol-extracted residue of BCG have been reported. No survival advantage, a modest survival advantage, or an inferior disease-free survival has been found in these trials (Table 73-7).

Levamisole is an anthelminthic drug used in veterinary medicine. It has no direct antitumor effect, but seems to augment host cellular defense by restoring T-cell proliferation, lymphokine production, and macrophage and neutrophil functions in immunocompromised patients. Clinical trials have been done, and the results are mixed (see Table 73-2). There may be a benefit in patients with Duke's B2 and C lesions when levamisole is given with 5-FU. Confusion regarding its mechanism of activity has precluded widespread enthusiasm for the use of levamisole.

OK432 is a lyophilized preparation of an attenuated strain of *S pyogenes* used as an immunostimulant. It has found wide use in many different types of cancer, mostly in the Pacific Rim nations. The literature contains many articles dealing with the use of OK432 in gastric cancer (see earlier), but its use in colorectal cancer also has been reported.[152,153] Intramuscular injection, oral dosing, intratumoral injection, and intraperitoneal instillation all have been tried with varying results. Some studies have shown tumor shrinkage and superior local control,[153] but no conclusive evidence of increased survival has been demonstrated.

Other immunostimulants, such as PSK and *Propionibacterium granulosum,* also have been studied. Results have shown the study groups having an increased disease-free and overall survival.[154,155] Combination therapy involving standard cytotoxic chemotherapy and immunostimulants may prove effective.

Cytokines have been tested in patients with colorectal cancer in multiple trials. IL-2 by itself has been tested in more than 50 patients with colorectal cancer in six trials, with no responses reported.[156–161] IFN can cause morphologic differentiation and increased carcinoembryonic antigen production in colorectal tumor cell lines. Brown and colleagues conducted a phase II

TABLE 73-7. *Clinical trials using bacillus Calmette-Guérin (BCG) or the methanol-extracted residue of BCG (MER) in patients with colorectal cancer*

Author (year)	Arms of trial	Agent	Number of patients	Conclusions
Mavligit et al.[141] (1978)	BCG versus historical controls	BCG	88	Improved disease-free survival
Engstrom et al.[142] (1978)	Chemotherapy Chemotherapy + BCG	BCG	47	No difference in response rates
Moertel et al.[143] (1978)	Chemotherapy Chemotherapy + BCG-MER	BCG MER		No difference
Lokich[144] (1979)	Chemotherapy Chemotherapy + BCG-MER	BCG MER	394	No difference
Richards et al.[145] (1979)	Chemotherapy Chemotherapy + BCG-MER	BCG MER		No difference
Panettiere & Chen[146] (1982)	Chemotherapy Chemotherapy + BCG	BCG	317	Improved disease-free interval
Robinson et al.[147] (1982)	Chemotherapy + radiation Chemotherapy + radiation + BCG-MER	BCG MER	53	Increased survival in BCG-MER group
Higgins et al.[148] (1984)	No treatment BCG-MER Chemotherapy Chemotherapy + BCG-MER	BCG MER	204	No difference; possible negative effect of BCG-MER
Gastrointestinal Tumor Study Group[149] (1984)	No treatment BCG-MER Chemotherapy Chemotherapy + BCG-MER	BCG MER	621	No difference
Wolmark et al.[150] (1988)	No treatment BCG-MER Chemotherapy	BCG MER	1161	No difference
Abdi et al.[151] (1989)	No treatment Chemotherapy Chemotherapy + BCG	BCG	253	No difference; possible negative effect of BCG

trial using IFNγ in patients with advanced colorectal cancer.[162] They observed no antitumor responses and significant toxicity. Other trials support a poor response when IFNs are used as single agents, with response rates of less than 2%. TNF can cause the in vivo necrosis of tumors in murine models, but the maximal tolerated dose in human trials is lower and would seem to preclude efficacy. A trial by Kemeny and associates showed no responses in 14 patients with colorectal cancer, and major toxicities were observed.[163] Single-cytokine therapy has little effect on colorectal cancers. Trials have been done using combination therapies.

The rationale behind the use of combination cytokine therapies is the same as for combination cytotoxic chemotherapies. Using multiple agents with different actions and toxicities theoretically could increase the efficacy and decrease the side effects of the treatment.

IL-2 and IFNα was one of the first combinations tried because it displayed synergistic effects both in vitro and in animal models.[164–167] We reported the use of IL-2 and IFNα in patients with advanced cancers.[168] Of 9 patients with colorectal cancer, 1 had a partial response. Mittleman and colleagues reported a study using low-dose IL-2 and IFNα-2a in patients with melanoma, renal cell cancer, or colorectal cancer. They observed a 22% response rate in the patients with renal cell cancer, but no responses in the 10 patients with colorectal cancer.[169]

Combinations of IL-2 and TNF or IFN and TNF also have been applied. Combinations of two or all three cytokines showed synergy, with increased antitumor effects in preclinical tests.[170–177] Abbruzzese and associates began a trial of IFNγ and TNF in patients with advanced gastrointestinal tract malignancies, but had to terminate the study because of excessive toxicity.[178] They observed no objective responses in those patients who received the therapy. Fiedler and colleagues used TNF and IFNγ in a phase II trial of 14 patients with colorectal cancer.[179] They had 1 patient with a mixed response, 4 patients with stable disease, and 9 patients with progressive disease. We used a combination of TNF and IL-2 in a phase I trial and had one complete and three partial responses in patients with colorectal cancer. These results were somewhat better than those expected using IL-2 alone.[180,181] Further trials using combination cytokine therapy are ongoing, and newer cytokines such as IL-12 are being developed based on successful animal models.[182] We have treated 2 patients with lower gastrointestinal tract malignancies with up to 15 doses of IL-12 at 30 to 100 ng/kg/d. These patients are being observed for a response.

Combination therapies using cytokines and cytotoxic chemotherapies also are being tested. The combination of cyclophosphamide and IL-2 was one of the first to be tried. It was thought that the cyclophosphamide would decrease the number of suppressor cells and potentiate the effects of IL-2.[183] Preclinical trials were promising,[184] but human trials have failed to show a benefit beyond that observed with IL-2 alone.[185–187] The combination of 5-FU and cytokines also has been studied. West and colleagues treated patients with IL-2 and LAK cells (see later). Two patients who previously had not responded to 5-FU therapy responded after the cytokine treatment.[188] This finding, in part, led to trials using 5-FU and IL-2 as combination therapy. Hamblin and associates treated 7 patients with metastatic colorectal cancer using IL-2 and 5-FU.[189] Two patients had a greater than 50% tumor regression and 3 patients had stabilization of their disease. Yang and colleagues treated 25 patients with metastatic colorectal cancer with a combination of 5-FU, leucovorin, and high-dose IL-2 in a phase II trial.[190] Of 23 analyzable patients, the overall response rate was 46%, with two complete responses. They concluded that most responses were attributable to the cytotoxic chemotherapy, but that the few complete and durable responses were the result of the IL-2 therapy. Hiddemann and colleagues treated patients with colorectal cancer with IL-2, 5-FU, and folinic acid.[191] Of 22 analyzable patients, 8 showed partial responses or stabilization of disease. Further studies using 5-FU and IL-2 in combination are ongoing.

The use of 5-FU and IFN also has been studied. Preclinical trials showed synergy, with increased tumor regression.[192,193] Wadler and associates treated patients with colorectal cancer with continuous-infusion 5-FU and IFNα-2a.[194] Seventeen patients were analyzable and 13 showed a response, including one complete response. Four other trials using 5-FU and IFNα have been reported and summarized.[195] An objective response rate of 41% was found when the results of these trials were combined, and the toxicities reported were not worse than with cytotoxic therapy alone. Pazdur and colleagues reported a different dosing schedule using 5-FU and IFNα-2a.[196] They entered 39 patients in a phase II trial using continuous-infusion 5-FU over 5 days at a dosage of 750 mg/m^2/d, and IFNα at a dosage of 9×10^6 IU subcutaneously on days 1, 3, and 5. They gave four courses of this therapy to each patient and found a 31% response rate with toxicity similar to that reported in other trials. This response was similar, but not superior, to other published schedules. These results show the efficacy of modulating 5-FU with cytokines. Further trials are ongoing to better define the role of this therapy. Other cytotoxic chemotherapy regimens combined with cytokines also are under study. A combination of etoposide and IFNα has been studied by Ajani and associates at the M.D. Anderson Cancer Center.[197] They treated 14 consecutive patients with previously untreated metastatic colorectal cancer, none of whom had responses to this therapy.

Newer cytokines also are being tested. IL-4 has been studied in patients with gastrointestinal malignancies, but has been associated with no antitumor effects. IL-12 has entered clinical trials. Preclinical trials suggest promise for this cytokine in the treatment of patients with a wide variety of cancers.[198,199] It is being tested as an parenteral agent, but a depot preparation and a gene therapy should enter trials soon. Depot preparations of IL-2 also are being studied. A mixture of poppy seed oil (Ethiodol) and IL-2 is being studied at the University of Pittsburgh as a way to introduce the cytokine into the peritoneal and pleural cavities in a depot form. Introduction of this combination into the hepatic artery in patients with liver metastases also is being studied.

Passive, Nonspecific Immunotherapy

The adoptive transfer of cytokine-activated, nonspecific, immunocompetent LAK cells to treat colorectal cancer first was attempted by Rosenberg and colleagues at the National Cancer Institute.[200] They treated 14 patients with advanced colorectal cancer with LAK cells and high-dose IL-2, and obtained a 17% response rate. The IL-2/LAK Working Group treated 19 patients with advanced colorectal cancer and had a 16% response rate, with one complete response.[201] Attempts to increase the response rate led to identification of the more cytolytic activated natural killer cells[202] (also known as adherent LAK), which have been used in multiple trials. Our trials are focusing on administering the activated natural killer/LAK cells locally by infusing them into the hepatic artery in patients with hepatic metastases or into the peritoneal cavity in patients with carcinomatosis. Steis and associates introduced LAK cells and IL-2 into the peritoneal cavity in patients with malignancies limited to the peritoneal cavity.[203] Five of 12 patients with colorectal cancer had a laparoscopically proven partial response (42%). The treatment was limited by intraperitoneal fibrosis.

Passive, Specific Immunotherapy

In an attempt to increase the response rate of adoptive immunotherapy, Rosenberg and colleagues took lymphocytes directly from the resected tumor specimen and activated them with IL-2. These TILs are MHC-restricted and nominally a tumor-specific therapy. Two patients with colorectal cancer have been treated with TILs and IL-2, with one of the patients obtaining a minor response (25% tumor shrinkage). This patient with disseminated carcinomatosis has undergone a resection of residual disease and has been without evidence of disease for 4 years. TILs that have been cultured with both IL-2 and TNFα were studied by Stolfi and associates.[204] They found increased expansion and cytotoxicity of such cultured TILs. Administration of these cells could lead to greater efficacy in vivo. Trials using genetically engineered TILs are under way.[205]

Another way to obtain tumor-reactive cells is to culture cells from the draining lymph nodes of a tumor. Satho and colleagues treated patients who had liver metastases from gastric or colorectal cancers with activated TDLs and OK432.[100] Of 19 analyzable patients, 2 had a complete response and 4 had a partial response. Five patients had their liver metastases resected and remained without recurrence from 7 to 40 months. TDLs are obtained more easily and are less likely to be contaminated by bacteria. Further studies are needed to better define the role of TDLs in the clinical setting.

The transfer of MoAbs to patients with colorectal cancer has been explored. Several MoAbs specific for colorectal cancers have been developed (see Table 73-3). The MoAb 17-1A is perhaps the most widely studied antibody. This MoAb is of mouse origin and recognizes the tumor-associated antigen CO17-1A found on the surface of adenocarcinoma cells.[30–34] Mellstedt and colleagues used 17-1A to treat 52 patients with metastatic colorectal carcinomas.[206] They obtained a 19% response rate and believed that the major obstacle to more effective therapy was delivery of antibody to tumor. They found that the amount of antibody in the tumor and the degree of mononuclear infiltrate was directly proportional to the amount of antibody given. They concluded that the cellular response was an important treatment-related factor and that it could be enhanced by the addition of cytokines. A surprising study by Riethmuller and associates used 17-1A as adjuvant treatment in 189 patients with curatively resected Dukes' C colorectal carcinoma.[34] Patients were assigned randomly to an observation regimen or a postoperative treatment regimen consisting of the 17-1A antibody. They obtained a 30% decrease in the overall

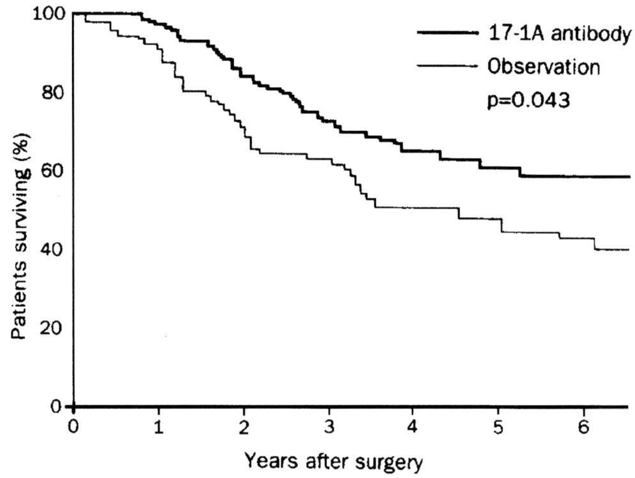

FIG. 73-1. Overall survival. (Riethmuller G, Schneider-Gadicke E, Schlimok G, et al. Randomized trial of monoclonal antibody for adjuvant therapy of resected Dukes' C colorectal carcinoma. Lancet 1994;343:1177.)

death rate (Fig. 73-1) and a 27% decrease in the recurrence rate in the treatment group (Fig. 73-2). The patients treated with the MoAb experienced little toxicity. The authors state that the problem of delivery of the MoAb to the tumor site was circumvented by removing all gross disease, leaving only microscopic disease for the antibody to deal with. Further studies are needed to confirm these findings and to determine the role of this and other MoAbs in the adjuvant setting.

A trial by Douillard and associates used 17-1A and transfer of autologous mononuclear cells to 20 patients.[207] These investigators obtained one complete response, four partial responses, and stabilization of disease in five cases. A study by Markoe and colleagues used radiation therapy to the liver to potentiate the effects of MoAbs in patients with hepatic metastases.[208] They had three responses among 8 patients treated, and theorized that increased delivery through capillary leak caused by

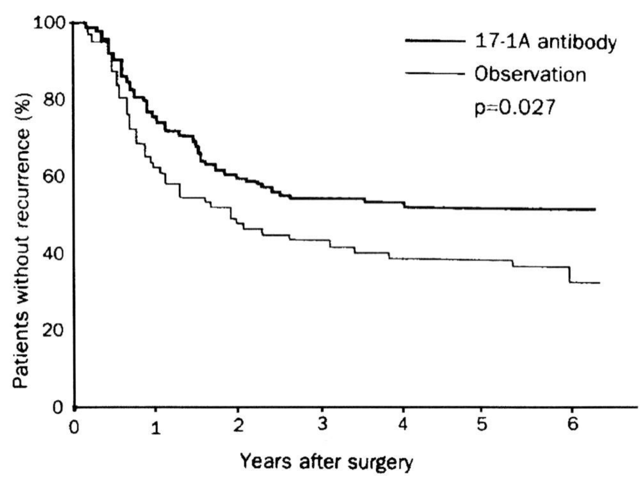

FIG. 73-2. Recurrence-free survival. (Riethmuller G, Scheider-Gadicke E, Schlimok G, et al. Randomized trial of monoclonal antibody for adjuvant therapy of resected Dukes' C colorectal carcinoma. Lancet 1994;343:1177.)

the radiation or decreased suppressor cell activity may explain the high response rate in their study. Studies using combinations of MoAbs and cytokines have been done, but the results have been poor.[209] Response rates of 5% or less have been obtained, and these responses have been short-lived. Ziegler and associates used a different MoAb, L6, which they administered along with IL-2.[53] In a phase I trial, they treated a group of patients who had advanced adenocarcinomas. They obtained one response among 5 patients and reported little toxicity.

In an attempt to increase the efficacy of MoAb treatment, numerous immunoconjugates have been developed. Toxins, cytotoxic drugs, and radioisotopes all have been conjugated to MoAbs and the results of several trials have been reported (see Table 73-4). One of the first uses of conjugated MoAbs was to detect microscopic metastatic disease or recurrences in patients with colorectal cancer, and most studies obtained 50% to 80% response rates.[43,57,210] The preoperative and intraoperative use of these radiolabeled MoAbs has been used to determine which patients should undergo conventional therapies and to guide more extensive resections. Preclinical trials of immunotoxins have shown antitumor efficacy in human colorectal tumor grafts in vitro and in nude mice.[211,212] A conjugate of the mouse MoAb and ricin toxin was used in a phase I trial by Byers and colleagues.[58] They had 17 analyzable patients with metastatic colorectal cancer, of whom 5 had a partial response. Zaleberg and associates reported the results of a phase I to II trial involving 17 patients with analyzable colon cancer.[213] They also used a mouse MoAb-ricin immunoconjugate, but injected the conjugate directly into hepatic metastases under computed tomographic guidance. They obtained two minor responses among 10 analyzable patients. The level of toxicity was minor in this study. Newer MoAb-toxin conjugates are being developed to try and combat the toxicity problems found with the systemic use of immunotoxins and the human antimouse antibody effect they elicit.

Conjugating MoAbs and cytotoxic drugs also has been tried. Takahashi and associates conjugated the mouse MoAb A7 with neocarzinostatin and obtained three minor responses among eight patients with liver metastases from colorectal cancer.[60] The low response rate was attributed to inability to deliver enough of the drug per molecule of antibody. A similar problem was found by Schneck and colleagues when they used a *Vinca* alkaloid immunoconjugate (KS1/4-DAVLB).[61] Senter tried to get around this drawback by conjugating a MoAb with an enzyme that activated a prodrug given systemically.[214] He has been successful in animal models, and clinical studies are planned.

The use of radioimmunoconjugates for the treatment of colorectal cancer also has been tested. Preclinical studies have shown inhibition of tumor growth and increased survival in experimental animals with human colon cancer xenografts with the use of yttrium-90–labeled MoAbs.[215,216] The major drawback to the use of these conjugates has been bone marrow suppression. Experiments are under way with bone marrow transplants to help alleviate this toxicity.[217]

Active, Specific Immunotherapy

Vaccinating patients to their own colorectal tumors was championed by Hoover, Hanna, and associates. They developed tumor cell/BCG vaccines that were shown to eliminate small tumor burdens in experimental animal models.[218,219] Clinical trials in patients with colorectal cancer first were reported by this group in 1989.[220] An update of a subsequent trial was published in 1992 with 80 patients enrolled.[221] These investigators found a modest increase in overall and disease-free survival in 24 patients with Dukes' stage B_2 to C_3 colon cancer, but no overall or disease-free survival advantage in 17 patients with rectal cancer. They explained the difference in the two groups by pointing out that the patients with rectal cancer all underwent radiation therapy that could suppress the immune response to the vaccine.

Attempts have been made to increase the response to autologous tumor vaccines by modifying the tumor cells to make them more immunogenic. Gray and colleagues modified colorectal tumor cells by treating them with the enzyme *Vibrio cholera* neuraminidase, and then used these modified cells in a BCG vaccine.[222] They treated 148 patients with stage B or C colorectal cancer with this vaccine, but were unable to show a benefit in overall or disease-free survival over the control group. They concluded that this modification of tumor cells did not affect the natural history of advanced colorectal cancer. Other types of tumor cell modification have been done, including infecting the tumors with various viruses, such as Newcastle disease virus.[223]

In an attempt to elicit a cell-mediated immune response, Steele and associates used a butanol-extraction technique to extract tumor-associated antigens and then incorporate them into liposomes.[224] They used liposomes because it previously has been shown that liposomes stimulate a T-cell–dependent immune response.[225] Preclinical trials were promising, and this may lead to an effective allogeneic vaccine. In another attempt to elicit a T-cell–dependent immune response, Kotera and colleagues have developed a mucin/BCG vaccine.[69] Mucin is a glycosylated protein made by most epithelial tissues. Most tumors make a hypoglycosylated form of mucin, and this abnormal mucin has been shown to elicit a non-MHC–restricted cell-mediated immune response. A phase I trial is ongoing at the University of Pittsburgh Medical Center in patients with breast, pancreatic, and colorectal cancers.

Another type of active, specific immunotherapy is gene therapy. Our group is involved in a trial using radiated autologous tumor cells and autologous fibroblasts engineered to produce IL-4 in a vaccination protocol.[70] This is a phase I trial and results are not available. Future gene therapies are planned using fibroblasts engineered to produce IL-12 and possibly other cytokines.

SUMMARY

Many novel therapies are being tested, and many more are being developed, for the treatment of gastrointestinal cancers. As our knowledge of the workings of the immune system and its role in tumor surveillance increases, ever more precise tuning of biologic therapies will be possible. Our modest success to date should not deter us from continued research in this exciting field.

REFERENCES

1. Coley WB. The treatment of inoperable sarcoma with the mixed toxins of erysipelas and bacillus prodigiosus. JAMA 1898;31:389.

2. Takao H, Saji S, Sugiyama Y, et al. Effects of serum immunosuppressive factors on the cytotoxicity of lymphokine-activated killer (LAK) cells induced by recombinant interleukin-2 (R-IL-2). Jpn Surg Society 1988;89:992.
3. Reynolds JV, Somers S, Guillou PJ. Serum from patients with advanced but not localized visceral cancer suppresses LAK cell generation. Br J Cancer 1990;62:17.
4. Mizoguchi H, O'Shea JJ, Longo DL, et al. Alterations in signal transduction molecules in T lymphocytes from tumor-bearing mice. Science 1992;258:1795.
5. Finke JH, Zea AH, Stanley J, et al. Loss of T-cell receptor zeta chain and p561ck in T-cells infiltrating human renal cell carcinoma. Cancer Res 1993;53:5613.
6. Nakagomi H, Petersson M, Magnusson I, et al. Decreased expression of the signal-transducing zeta chains in tumor-infiltrating T-cells and NK cells of patients with colorectal carcinoma. Cancer Res 1993;53:5610.
7. Mitchell MS, Murhata RI. Modulation of immunity by bacillus Calmette-Guerin. Pharmacol Ther 1979;4:329.
8. Vitale B, Allegreth N. Influence of BCG infection on the intensity of homograft reaction in rats. Nature 1963;199:507.
9. Weiss DW, Bonhag R, Leslie P. Studies on the heterologous immunogenicity of a methanol-insoluble fraction of attenuated against tumor isografts. J Exp Med 1966;124:1039.
10. Hersh EM, Taylor CW. Immunotherapy by active immunization: use of nonspecific stimulants and modulators. In: Devita VT, Hellman S, Rosenberg SA, eds. Biologic therapy of cancer. Philadelphia: JB Lippincott, 1991.
11. Enker WE, Jacobitz JL, Craft K, Wissler RW. Surgical adjuvant immunotherapy for colorectal cancer. J Surg Oncol 1978;10:389.
12. Weiss DW. MER and other mycobacterial fractions in the immunotherapy of cancer. Med Clin North Am 1976;60:473.
13. Mathe G, Amiel JL, Schwarenberg L, et al. Active immunotherapy for acute lymphoblastic leukemia. Lancet 1969;2:697.
14. Wolmark N, Fisher B, Rockette H, et al. Postoperative adjuvant chemotherapy or BCG for colon cancer: results from NSABP Protocol C-01. J Natl Cancer Inst 1988;80:30.
15. Kirkwood JM. Adjuvant therapy for high-risk melanoma: current strategies for biological therapy. Melanoma Res 1993;3(Suppl 1):27.
16. Goldin A, Chirigos MA, MacDonald JS, et al. Biologic-response modifiers and adjuvant chemotherapy. Recent Results Cancer Res 1982; 80:351.
17. Verhagen H, DeCree J, DeCock W, et al. Levamisole therapy in patients with colorectal cancer. In: Terry WD, Rosenberg SA, eds. Immunotherapy of human cancer. New York: Elsevier/North Holland, 1982.
18. Borden EC, Davis TE, Crowley JJ, et al. Interim analysis of a trial of levamisole and 5-fluorouracil in metastatic colorectal carcinoma. In: Terry WD, Rosenberg SA, eds. Immunotherapy of human cancer. New York: Elsevier/North Holland, 1982.
19. Laurie JA, Moertel CG, Fleming TR, et al. Surgical adjuvant therapy of bowel carcinoma: an evaluation of levamisole and the combination of levamisole and fluorouracil: The North Central Cancer Treatment Group and the Mayo Clinic. J Clin Oncol 1989;7:1447.
20. Moertel CG, Fleming TR, McDonald JS, et al. Levamisole and fluorouracil for adjuvant therapy of resected colon carcinoma. N Engl J Med 1990;322:352.
21. Chlebowski RT, Lillington L, Nystrom JS, Sayre J. Late mortality and levamisole adjuvant therapy in colorectal cancer. Br J Surg 1994; 69:1094.
22. Stotter H, Lotze MT. Human lymphokine-activated killer cell activity. Role of IL-2, IL-4, and IL-7. Arch Surg 1991;126:1525.
23. Stotter H, Custer MC, Bolton ES, et al. IL-7 induces human lymphokine-activated killer cell activity and is regulated by IL-4. J Immunol 1991;146:150.
24. Berman RM, Zeh HJ, Storkus WJ, Lotze MT. Interleukin-10 induces lymphokine activated killer (LAK) cell activity. J Immunotherapy 1993;13:56.
25. Naume B, Gately MK, Desai BB, et al. Synergistic effects of interleukin 4 and interleukin 12 on NK cell proliferation. Cytokine 1993;5: 38.
26. Lotze MT, Zeh HJ, Elder EM, et al. Use of T-cell growth factors (IL-2 to IL-12) in the investigation and treatment of melanoma. J Immunotherapy 1992;12:212.
27. Rosenberg SA, Lotze MT, Muul LM, et al. A new approach to the therapy of cancer based on the systemic administration of autologous lymphokine-activated killer cells and recombinant interleukin-2. Surgery 1986;100:71.
28. Spiess PJ, Yang JC, Rosenberg SA. In vivo antitumor activity of tumor infiltrating lymphocytes expanded in recombinant interleukin-2. J Natl Cancer Inst 1987;79:1067.
29. Schlom J. Basic principles and applications of monoclonal antibodies in the management of carcinomas: the Richard and Linda Rosenthal Foundation Award Lecture. Cancer Res 1986;46:3225.
30. Verrill H, Goldberg M, Rosenbaum R, et al. Clinical trial of Wistar Institute 17-1A monoclonal antibody in patients with advanced gastrointestinal adenocarcinoma: a preliminary report. Hybridoma 1986;1: S175.
31. Tempero MA, Pour PM, Uchida E, et al. Monoclonal antibody CO17-1A and leukapheresis in immunotherapy of pancreatic cancer. Hybridoma 1986;1:S133.
32. Tempero MA, Haga Y, Sivinski C, et al. Immunotherapy with monoclonal antibody (Mab) in pancreatic adenocarcinoma. Int J Pancreatol 1991;9:125.
33. Weiner LM, Harvey E, Padavic-Shaller K, et al. Phase II multicenter evaluation of prolonged murine monoclonal antibody 17-1A therapy in pancreatic carcinoma. J Immunother 1993;13:110.
34. Riethmuller G, Schneider-Gadicke E, Schlimok G, et al. Randomized trial of monoclonal antibody for adjuvant therapy of resected Dukes' C colorectal carcinoma. Lancet 1994;343:1177.
35. Kaplan EH. The diagnostic and therapeutic use of monoclonal antibodies in colorectal cancer. Med Clin North Am 1989;3:125.
36. Colcher D, Mineeli MF, Roselli M, Muraro R, Simpson-Milenic D, Schlom J. Radioimmunolocalization of human carcinoma xenografts with B72.3 second generation MABs. Cancer Res 1988;48:4597.
37. Filella X, Molina R, Jo J, et al. Tumor associated glycoprotein-72 (TAG-72) levels in patients with non-malignant and malignant disease. Bull Cancer (Paris) 1992;79:271.
38. Koprowski H, Steplewski Z, Mitchell K, et al. Colorectal carcinoma antigens detected by hybridoma antibodies. Somat Cell Genet 1979; 5:957.
39. Watanabe M, Hirohasi S, Shimosato Y, et al. Carbohydrate antigen defined by a monoclonal antibody raised against a gastric cancer xenograft. Jpn J Cancer Res 1985;76:43.
40. Hollingsworth MA, Metzgar RS. Antigens of normal and malignant human exocrine pancreatic cells. In: Sells S, Reisfeld RA, eds. Monoclonal antibodies in cancer. Clifton, NJ: Humana Press, 1985:279.
41. Muraro R, Wunderlich D, Thor A, et al. Definition by monoclonal antibodies of a repertoire on carcinoembryonic antigen differentially expressed in human colon carcinomas versus normal adult tissues. Cancer Res 1985;45:5769.
42. Mach JP, Buchegger F, Forni M, et al. Use of radiolabeled monoclonal anti-CEA antibodies for the detection of human carcinomas by external photoscanning and tomoscintigraphy. Immunol Today 1981;2: 239.
43. Beatty JD, Duda RB, Williams LE, et al. Preoperative imaging of colorectal carcinoma with indium-III labeled anti-CEA monoclonal antibody. Cancer Res 1986;46:6494.
44. Watanabe M, Kubota T, Kitajima M, et al. Synergetic effect of interleukin-2 and cellular cytotoxicity against a novel tumor-associated carbohydrate antigen Le^a/Le^a (dimeric Le^a) mediated by monoclonal antibody NCC-ST-421 in adoptive immunization using SCID mice. Cancer Immunol Immunother 1993;37:245.
45. Ohyanagi H, Ishida H, Ishida T, et al. A monoclonal antibody, KM10 reactive with human gastrointestinal cancer and its application for immunotherapy. Jpn J Cancer Res 1988;79:1349.
46. Shitara K, Hanai N, Kusano A, et al. Application of Anti-Sialyl Le^a monoclonal antibody, KM231, for immunotherapy of cancer. Anticancer Res 1991;11:2003.
47. Kasprzyk PG, Song SU, Di Fiore PP, et al. Therapy of an animal model of human gastric cancer using a combination of anti-erbB-2 monoclonal antibodies. Cancer Res 1992;52:2771.
48. Fuhrer JP, Xie H, Murphy MJ Jr, et al. Characterization of a membrane-associated glycoprotein (gp 43) on human hepatocellular carcinoma by a monoclonal antibody. Cancer Res 1991;51:2158.

49. Schulz G, Buchler M, Muhrer KH, et al. Immunotherapy of pancreatic cancer with monoclonal antibody BW 494. Int J Cancer 1988;2:89.
50. Buchler M, Friess H, Malfertheiner P, et al. Studies of pancreatic cancer utilizing monoclonal antibodies. Int J Pancreatol 1990;7:151.
51. Buchler M, Friess H, Schultheiss KH, et al. A randomized controlled trial of adjuvant immunotherapy (murine monoclonal antibody 494/32) in resectable pancreatic cancer. Cancer 1991;68:1507.
52. Hellstrom I, Beaumier P, Hellstrom K, et al. Antitumor effects of L6, an IgG2a antibody that reacts with most human carcinomas. Proc Natl Acad Sci USA 1986;83:7059.
53. Ziegler LD, Palazzolo P, Cunningham J, et al. Phase I trial of murine monoclonal antibody L6 in combination with subcutaneous interleukin-2 in patients with advanced carcinoma of the breast, colorectum and lung. J Clin Oncol 1992;10:1470.
54. Yagyu T, Monden T, Baba M, et al. A cancer-reactive human monoclonal antibody derived from a colonic cancer patient treated with local immunotherapy. Jpn J Cancer Res 1993;84:75.
55. Taddei-Peters WC, Haspel MV, Vente P, et al. Quantitation of human tumor-reactive monoclonal antibody 16.88 in the circulation and localization of 16.88 in colorectal metastatic tumor tissue using murine antiidiotypic antibodies. Cancer Res 1992;52:2603.
56. Hand PH, Kashmiri SV, Schlom J. Potential for recombinant immunoglobulin constructs in the management of cancer. Cancer 1994; 73(Suppl 3):1105.
57. Duda RB, Beatty JD, Sheibani K, et al. Imaging of human colorectal adenocarcinoma with indium-labeled anticarcinoembryonic antigen monoclonal antibody. Arch Surg 1986;121:1315.
58. Byers VS, Rodvien R, Grant K, et al. Phase I study of monoclonal antibody-ricin A chain immunotoxin xomazyme-791 in patients with metastatic colon cancer. Cancer Res 1989;49:6153.
59. Durrant LG, Byers VS, Scannon PJ, et al. Humoral immune responses to XMMCO-791-RTA immunotoxin in colorectal cancer patients. Clin Exp Immunol 1989;75:258.
60. Takahashi T, Yamaguchi T, Kitamura K, et al. Clinical application of monoclonal antibody-drug conjugates for immunotargeting chemotherapy of colorectal carcinoma. Cancer 1988;61:881.
61. Schneck D, Butler F, Dugan W, et al. Disposition of a murine monoclonal antibody vinca conjugate (KS1/4-DAVLB) in patients with adenocarcinomas. Clin Pharmacol Ther 1990;47:36.
62. Batra JK, Kasprzyk PG, Bird RE, et al. Recombinant anti-ERBB2 immunotoxins containing pseudomonas exotoxin. Proc Natl Acad Sci USA 1992;89:5867.
63. Li S, Zhang XY, Qiao TD, et al. Enhanced antitumor activity of daunomycin conjugated with antigastric cancer monoclonal antibody MGb2. Oncol Res 1992;4:447.
64. Mehta MP, Kubsad SS, Fowler JF, et al. 90Y.B72.3 against pancreatic cancer: dosimetric and biological analysis. Int J Radiat Oncol Biol Phys 1990;19:627.
65. Klein JL, Nguyen TH, Laroque P, et al. Yttrium-90 and iodine-131 radioimmunoglobulin therapy of an experimental human hepatoma. Cancer Res 1989;49:6383.
66. Ditzel H, Rasmussen JW, Borup-Christensen P, et al. Immunoscintigraphy of colon cancers with the human monoclonal antibody COU-1. Cancer 1994;73:858.
67. Maeda M, Shoji M, Kawagoshi T, et al. Distribution of 111In- and 125I-labeled monoclonal antibody 17-1A in mice bearing xenografts of human pancreatic carcinoma HuP-T4. Cancer 1994;73:800.
68. Hanna MG Jr, Peters LC. Immunotherapy of established micrometastases with a bacillus Calmette-Guerin tumor cell vaccine. Cancer Res 1978;38:204.
69. Kotera Y, Fontenot D, Pecher G, Finn O. Humoral immunity against a tandem repeat epitope of human mucin MUC-1 in sera from breast, pancreatic and colon cancer patients. Cancer Res 1994;54:2856.
70. Lotze MT, Rubin JT, Carty S, et al. Gene therapy of cancer: a pilot study of IL-4-gene modified fibroblasts admixed with autologous tumor to elicit an immune response. Hum Gen Ther 1994;5:41.
71. Saito T, Shimoda K, Kinoshita T, et al. Prediction of operative mortality based on impairment of host defense systems in patients with esophageal cancer. J Surg Oncol 1993;52:1.
72. Jamasbi RJ, Kennel SJ, Stoner GD. Production of monoclonal antibodies with selective immuno-reactivity for human esophageal carcinomas. (Abstract) Proc Annu Meet Am Assoc Cancer Res 1991;32: A1425.
73. Koga Y, Ishigami K, Inokuchi K. Effectiveness of multidisciplinary treatment combined with immunotherapy in esophageal cancer—analysis of 287 cases of carcinoma of the thoracic part of the esophagus in Kyushu and Yamaguchi districts. Jpn J Cancer Clin 1987;33:777.
74. Ogoshi K. Evaluation of immunotherapy with PSK in esophageal cancer. Gan To Kagaku Ryoho 1988;15:3143.
75. Strack M, Wadler S, Lyver A, et al. Phase II trial of fluorouracil (5FU) and recombinant alpha-2a-interferon (rIFN-alpha-2a) in patients (pts) with advanced carcinoma of the esophagus. (Abstract) Proc Annu Meet Am Soc Clin Oncol 1990;9:A462.
76. Lovett D, Kelsen D, Heelan R, et al. 5-Fluorouracil and alpha-interferon (IFN) in the treatment of esophageal carcinoma (EC). (Abstract) Proc Am Soc Clin Oncol 1990;9:121.
77. Posner MC, Lembersky B, Landreneau RJ, Mullen E, Oppenheim M, Lotze MT. Combined modality therapy for operable carcinoma of the esophagus and gastroesophageal (GE) junction. Proc Annu Meet Am Soc Clin Oncol 1993;12:A686.
78. Toge T, Yamaguchi Y. Lymphokine-activated killer cell adoptive immunotherapy for cancer treatment and its significance. Hum Cell 1992;5:218.
79. Ochiai T, Sato H, Okuyama K, et al. Immunotherapy of gastric cancer with special reference to Japanese randomized trials. Int J Immunotherapy 1986;2:87.
80. Yamamura Y, Nishimura M, Sakamoto J, et al. A randomized controlled trial of surgical adjuvant therapy with mitomycin C, 5-fluorouracil, and OK-432 in patients with gastric cancer. Gan To Tagaku Ryoho 1986;13:2134.
81. Popiela T, Zembala M, Kulig J, et al. Postoperative immunochemotherapy (BCG + 5-FU) in advanced gastric cancer. Anticancer Res 1988;8:1423.
82. The Italian Gastrointestinal Tumor Study Group. Adjuvant treatments following curative resection for gastric cancer. Br J Surg 1988;75: 1100.
83. Kyoto Research Group for Digestive Organ Surgery. A comprehensive multi-institutional study on postoperative adjuvant immunotherapy with oral streptococcal preparation OK-432 for patients after gastric cancer surgery. Ann Surg 1992;216:44.
84. Merrouche Y, Negrier S, Rebattu P, et al. A phase II study of interleukin-2 (IL-2) following high-dose BCNU and autologous bone marrow transplantation (ABMT) in the treatment of metastatic gastric cancer. Proc Annu Meet Am Soc Oncol 1991;10:A510.
85. Kim J-P, Kwon OJ, Oh ST, et al. Results of surgery on 6589 gastric cancer patients and immunochemosurgery as the best treatment of advanced gastric cancer. Ann Surg 1992;216:269.
86. Tsujitani S, Kakeji Y, Orita H, et al. Postoperative adjuvant immunochemotherapy and infiltration of dendritic cells for patients with advanced gastric cancer. Anticancer Res 1992;12:645.
87. Nakazato H, Koike A, Saji S, et al. A randomized clinical trial on adjuvant immunochemotherapy with protein bound polysaccharide (PSK) in gastric cancer with curative resection. Proc Annu Meet Am Soc Clin Oncol 1993;12:A550.
88. Uchiyama A, Yoshida T, Torisu M. Enhancement of tumoricidal activity in peritoneal exudate lymphocytes (PELS) from patients with malignant ascites by the combined use of IL-2 and IFN gamma. FASEB J 1990;4:A1946.
89. Miya K, Saji S, Furata T, et al. Significance of antitumor effects and immunological response on endogenously induced LAK therapy for primary or metastatic liver tumor. Gan To Kagaku Ryoho 1992;19: 1453.
90. Okuno K, Ohnishi H, Nakajimi I, et al. Intrahepatic infusion of interleukin-2 (IL-2) with mitomycin C (MMC)/5-fluorouracil (5-fu) through an implantable pump for the treatment of liver metastases. Proc Annu Meet Am Assoc Cancer Res 1992;33:A1475.
91. Sugiyama Y, Kato M, Takao H, et al. Immunological effects of locoregional immunochemotherapy for liver metastases of gastric cancer. Gan To Kagaku Ryoho 1993;20:1461.
92. Stuart K, Stokes K, Jenkins R, et al. Treatment of hepatocellular carcinoma using doxorubicin/ethiodized oil/gelatin powder chemoembolization. Cancer 1993;72:3202.
93. Fujimoto T, Omote K, Mai M, et al. Evaluation of basic procedures for adoptive immunotherapy for gastric cancer. Biotherapy 1992;5: 153.
94. Ebihara T, Koyama S, Fukao K, et al. Lymphokine-activated suppres-

sor (LAS) cells in patients with gastric carcinoma. Cancer Immunol Immunother 1989;28:218.
95. Okuno K, Ohnishi H, Shilayama YL, et al. Augmentation of human lymphokine-activated killer cell activity in splenic lymphocytes by the combination of low-dose interleukin-2 plus interleukin-3. Molecular Biotherapy 1992;4:83.
96. Monson JRT, Ramsden CW, Macfie J, et al. Immunorestorative effect of lipid emulsions during total parenteral nutrition. Br J Surg 1986; 73:843.
97. Monson JRT, Sedman PC, Ramsden CW, et al. Total parenteral nutrition adversely influences tumor-directed cellular cytotoxic responses in patients with gastrointestinal cancer. Eur J Surg Oncol 1988;14: 435.
98. Kan N, Okino T, Nakanishi M, et al. Clinical therapeutic effect of adoptive immunotherapy using IL-2 cultured autologous lymphocytes. Hum Cell 1988;1:289.
99. Kan N, Ohgaki K, Okino T, et al. Immunotherapy of gastric cancer. Gan To Kagaku Ryoho 1988;15:755.
100. Satho K, Kan N, Okino T, et al. The therapeutic effect of OK-423-combined adoptive immunotherapy against liver metastases from gastric or colorectal cancers. Biotherapy 1993;6:41.
101. Yamaue H, Tanimura H, Tsunoda T, et al. Clinical application of adoptive immunotherapy by cytotoxic T lymphocytes induced from tumor-infiltrating lymphocytes. J Jpn Soc for Cancer Therapy 1990; 25:978.
102. Shou CC, Dong ZW, Liu PN. Anti-FD4 idiotypic antibody mimicking human gastric cancer-associated antigen. Chin Med J (Engl) 1991; 104:711.
103. Goydos JS, Carty SE, Brumfield A, Frezza E, Lotze MT. IL-6 as a serum marker in hepatic malignancies. (Submitted for publication).
104. Imaoka S, Sasaki Y, Ishikawa O, et al. Immunochemotherapy in human hepatocellular carcinoma using the streptococcal agent OK-432. J Clin Oncol 1986;4:1645.
105. Hazama S, Oka M, Shimizu R, et al. Intra-arterial combination immunotherapy in hepatocellular carcinoma. Gan To Kagaku Ryoho 1990; 17:1638.
106. Park BC, Lee SK, Suh SY. Chemoimmunotherapy for advanced primary hepatocellular carcinoma. Second International Conference on Gastrointestinal Cancer. Jerusalem: 1989:32.
107. Ito T, Ikeda N, Sue K, et al. Immunotherapy using Freund's adjuvant and recombinant interleukin-2 combined with transarterial chemoembolization for hepatocellular carcinoma. Gastroenterologia Japonica 1989;24:386.
108. Yamamoto M, Iizuka H, Kono T, et al. Significance of reduction surgery for stage IV hepatocellular carcinoma (HCC) and postoperative immunochemotherapy for extension of survival period. J Jpn Surg Soc 1991;92:1334.
109. Chien CH, Hsieh KH, Yang PM. Immunochemotherapy with recombinant interleukin-2 and adriamycin in primary hepatocellular carcinoma. Asian Pac J Allergy Immunol 1991;9:75.
110. Yamamoto M, Iizuka H, Fuhi H, et al. Hepatic arterial infusion of interleukin-2 in advanced hepatocellular carcinoma. Acta Oncol 1993; 32:43.
111. Lai CL, Wu PC, Lok ASF, et al. Recombinant alpha 2 interferon is superior to doxorubicin for inoperable hepatocellular carcinoma: a prospective randomized trial. Br J Cancer 1987;60:928.
112. Gastrointestinal Tumor Study Group. A prospective trial of recombinant human interferon alpha 2b in previously untreated patients with hepatocellular carcinoma. Cancer 1990;66:135.
113. Carr BI. High-objective response rates of advanced hepatocellular carcinoma (HCC) to IA chemotherapy. (Abstract) Proc Annu Meet Am Soc Clin Oncol 1992;11:A470.
114. Ishikawa T, Imawari M, Moriyama T, et al. Immunotherapy of hepatocellular carcinoma with autologous lymphokine-activated killer cells and/or interleukin-2. Cancer Res Clin Oncol 1988;114:283.
115. Onishi S, Saibara T, Fujikawa M, et al. Adoptive immunotherapy with lymphokine-activated killer cells plus recombinant interleukin-2 in patients with unresectable hepatocellular carcinoma. Hepatology 1989;10:349.
116. Komatsu T, Yamauchi K, Furukawa T, et al. Transcatheter arterial injection of autologous lymphokine-activated killer (LAK) cells into patients with liver cancers. J Clin Immunol 1990;10:167.
117. Takayama T, Makuuchi M, Sekine T, et al. Distribution and therapeutic effect of intraarterially transferred tumor-infiltrating lymphocytes in hepatic malignancies. Cancer 1991;68:2391.
118. Chen Q, Sun P, Prigione I, et al. Targeting of T lymphocytes against human hepatoma cells by a bispecific monoclonal antibody: role of different lymphocyte subsets. Tumori 1992;78:79.
119. Klein JL, Nguyen TH, Laroque P, et al. Yttrium-90 and iodine-131 radioimmunoglobulin therapy of an experimental human hepatoma. Cancer Res 1989;49:6383.
120. Axelrod RS, Havas HF, Murasko DM, et al. Effect of the mixed bacterial vaccine on the immune response of patients with non-small cell lung cancer and refractory malignancies. Cancer 1988;61:2219.
121. Yagita A, Hosaka N, Itoh H, et al. Clinical effects of multidrug immunotherapy (OK-432, PSK and SPG) and its cytotoxic factor differing from TNF. First Shanghai International Symposium on Gastrointestinal Cancers. Shanghai, China: 1988:179.
122. Kuninobu H, Toge T, Takayama T, et al. Clinical efficacy of intratumoral administration of BRM in advanced cancer and its mechanism of action. Gan To Kagaku Ryoho 1989;16:2769.
123. Goldrosen MH, Loftus R, Lloyd F Jr, et al. Localization of monoclonal antibody in a novel nude mouse model of pancreatic cancer. Proc Annu Meet Am Assoc Cancer Res 1988;29:A1668.
124. Marincola FM, Drucker BJ, Siao DY, et al. The nude mouse as a model for the study of human pancreatic cancer. J Surg Res 1989; 47:520.
125. Kay HD, Haga Y, Uhl B, et al. The Syrian hamster as a preclinical model for pancreatic cancer: in vitro antitumor IL-2-boosted cell-mediated cytotoxicity. Proc Annu Meet Am Assoc Cancer Res 1990; 31:A1466.
126. Croghan M, Hersh EM, Meyskens F, et al. A phase I study of interleukin-2 (IL-2) with or without cytotoxan for the treatment of disseminated carcinoma. Proc Annu Meet Am Soc Clin Oncol 1988;7:A272.
127. Schwartzberg L, West W, Birch R, et al. A phase II study of recombinant tumor necrosis factor (RTNF) and recombinant interleukin-2 (RIL-2) in advanced malignancy. Proc Annu Meet Am Soc Clin Oncol 1990;9:A767.
128. Moriai T, Makino I, Kikuchi Y. Synergistic antitumor effect of interleukin-2 and irradiation on pancreatic cancer in syrian golden hamsters. In Vivo 1990;4:127.
129. Raitano AB, Scuderi P, Korc M. Binding and biological effects of tumor necrosis factor and gamma interferon in human pancreatic carcinoma cells. Pancreas 1990;5:267.
130. Abbruzzese JL, Levin B, Ajani JA, et al. A phase II trial of recombinant human interferon-gamma and recombinant tumor necrosis factor in patients with advanced gastrointestinal malignancies: results of a trial terminated by excessive toxicity. J Biol Response Modifiers 1990;9:522.
131. Watanabe T, Fuchimoto S, Matsubara N, et al. Anti-proliferative effect on human pancreatic cancer cells of natural human tumour necrosis factor-β combined with natural human interferon-α or interferon-γ. J Int Med Res 1992;20:112.
132. Watanabe T, Fuchimoto S, Iwagaki H, et al. Anti-proliferative effect of combined tumour necrosis factor-α and interferon-α on human pancreatic cancer in vitro and in vivo. Anticancer Res 1993;13:1501.
133. Schmiegel W, Roeder C, Schmielau J, et al. Tumor necrosis factor α induces the expression of transforming growth factor α and the epidermal growth factor receptor in human pancreatic cancer cells. Proc Natl Acad Sci USA 1993;90:863.
134. Oldham RK, Bartal AH, Yannelli JR, et al. Intra-arterial and intracavitary administration of lymphokine activated killer cells in patients with advanced cancer: feasibility and laboratory results. Proc Annu Meet Am Assoc Cancer Res 1988;29:A1578.
135. Sugiura H. LAK sensitivity of human pancreas carcinoma cell lines. Hokkaido Igaku Zasshi 1993;68:921.
136. Marincola FM, DaPozzo LF, Howick JC, et al. Prolonged survival of nude mice bearing human pancreatic cancer and treated with lymphokine-activated killer cells and interleukin-2. Current Surgery 1989; 22:304.
137. Marincola FM, DaPozzo LF, Drucker BJ, et al. Adoptive immunotherapy of human pancreatic cancer with lymphokine-activated killer cells and interleukin-2 in a nude mouse model. Surgery 1990;108:919.
138. Jakowatz JG, Gan K, Ulich TR, et al. Murine monoclonal antibodies to human pancreatic cancer: specificity and sensitivity. Oncology 1990;47:149.
139. Bosslet K, Steinstraesser A, Hermentin P, et al. Generation of bispec-

ific monoclonal antibodies for two phase radioimmunotherapy. Br J Cancer 1991;63:681.
140. Yamaue H, Tanimura H, Tsunoda T, et al. Clinical application of adoptive immunotherapy by cytotoxic T lymphocytes induced from tumor-infiltrating lymphocytes. J Japanese Society for Cancer Therapy 1990;25:978.
141. Mavligit G, Malahy M, Hersh E. Systemic adjuvant therapy with BCG vs. BCG plus 5-FU in colorectal cancer Dukes' class C: updated analysis. (Abstract) Proc Am Assoc Cancer Res 1978;19:312.
142. Engstrom PF, Paul RA, Catalano RB, et al. Fluorouracil versus fluorouracil plus BCG in colorectal adenocarcinoma. In: Terry WD, Windhorst D, eds. Immunotherapy of cancer: present status of trials in man. New York: Raven Press, 1978.
143. Moertel CG, O'Connell MJ, Ritts RE, et al. A controlled evaluation of combined immunotherapy (MER-BCG) and chemotherapy for advanced colorectal cancer. In: Terry WD, Windhorst D, eds. Immunotherapy of cancer: present status of trials in man. New York: Raven, 1978.
144. Lokich JJ. Adjuvant therapy for surgically curable colon cancer: a controlled study of chemo and immune therapy. (Abstract) Proc Am Assoc Cancer Res 1979;20:423.
145. Richards F, Muss HB, Cooper MR, et al. Chemotherapy versus chemoimmunotherapy in advanced adenocarcinoma of the colon and rectum: a prospective randomized study. Cancer 1979;43:91.
146. Panettiere FJ, Chen TT. SWOG study of adjuvant chemotherapy with and without oral BCG in the postoperative treatment of cancer of the colon: an update. In: Terry WD, Rosenberg SA, eds. Immunotherapy of human cancer. New York: Elsevier/North Holland, 1982.
147. Robinson E, Bartal A, Cohen Y, et al. Treatment of radically operated colorectal cancer patients with combined adjuvant therapy: radiotherapy, chemotherapy and methanol extraction residue of BCG. In: Terry WD, Rosenberg SA, eds. Immunotherapy of human cancer. New York: Elsevier/North Holland, 1982.
148. Higgins GA, Donaldson RC, Rogers LS. Efficacy of MER immunotherapy when added to a regimen of 5-fluorouracil and methyl-CCAV following resection for carcinoma of the large bowel: a Veterans Administration Surgical Oncology Group report. Cancer 1984;54:193.
149. GITSG. Adjuvant therapy of colon cancer: results of a prospectively randomized trial. N Engl J Med 1984;310:737.
150. Wolmark N, Fisher B, Rockette H, et al. Postoperative adjuvant chemotherapy or BCGT for colon cancer: results from NSABP Protocol C-01. J Natl Cancer Inst 1988;80:30.
151. Abdi EA, Hanson J, Harbora DE. Adjuvant chemoimmuno and immunotherapy in Dukes' stage B2 and C colorectal carcinoma: a 7-year follow-up analysis. J Surg Oncol 1989;40:205.
152. Nio Y, Ohgaki K, Tsuchitani T, et al. Orally administered streptococcal preparation OK-432 augments the antitumor immunity of patients with gastric or colorectal cancer. Biotherapy 1990;2:213.
153. Monden T, Morimoto H, Murotani M, et al. Intratumoral injection of OK-432 in conjunction with fibrinogen greatly enhances antitumor effect on colorectal carcinomas. Nippon Geka Gakkai Zasshi 1991; 92:31.
154. Grundmann R, Weber F, Kluger J, et al. Preoperative nonspecific immunostimulation with propionibacterium granulosum KP-45 in patients with colorectal cancer. A prospective randomized study. Chirurg 1988;59:272.
155. Mitomi T, Tsuchiya S, Iijima N, et al. Randomized, controlled study on adjuvant immunochemotherapy with PSK in curatively resected colorectal cancer. The cooperative study group of surgical adjuvant immunochemotherapy for cancer of colon and rectum. Dis Colon Rectum 1992;35:123.
156. Creekmore SP, Harris JE, Ellis TM, et al. A phase I clinical trial of recombinant interleukin-2 by periodic 24-hour intravenous infusions. J Clin Oncol 1989;7:276.
157. Sarna GP, Figlin RA, Pertcheck M, et al. Systemic administration of recombinant methionyl human interleukin-2 (Ala 125) to cancer patients: clinical results. J Biol Response Mod 1989;8:16.
158. Rosenberg SA, Lotze MT, Mule J. New approaches to the immunotherapy of cancer using interleukin-2. Ann Intern Med 1988;108:853.
159. Lotze MT, Frana LW, Sharrow SO, et al. Systemic administration of interleukin-2 in humans. J Biol Response Mod 1984;3:475.
160. Allison MAK, Jones SE, McGuffey P. Phase II trial of outpatient interleukin-2 in malignant lymphoma, chronic lymphocytic leukemia and selected solid tumors. J Clin Oncol 1989;7:75.
161. Mitchell MS, Oettgen HF, eds. Progress in cancer research and therapy. 21st vol. Hybridomas in cancer diagnosis and treatment. New York: Raven Press, 1982.
162. Brown TD, Goddman PJ, Fleming T, et al. Phase II trial of recombinant DNA gamma-interferon in advanced colorectal cancer: a Southwest Oncology Group study. J Immunother 1981;10:379.
163. Kemeny N, Childs B, Larchian W, et al. A phase II trial of recombinant tumor necrosis factor in patients with advanced colorectal carcinoma. Cancer 1990;66:659.
164. Rosenberg SA, Schwarz SL, Spiess PJ. Combination immunotherapy for cancer: synergistic antitumor interaction of interleukin-2, alpha interferon and tumor infiltrating lymphocytes. J Natl Cancer Inst 1988; 80:1393.
165. Cameron RB, McIntosh JY, Rosenberg SA. Synergistic antitumor effects of combination immunotherapy with recombinant interleukin-2 and a recombinant hybrid interferon alpha in the treatment of established murine hepatic metastases. Cancer Res 1988;48:5810.
166. Brunda MY, Tarrowski D, Davatelis V. Interaction of recombinant interferon with recombinant interleukin-2: differential effects on natural killer cell activity and interleukin-2-activated killer cells. Int J Cancer 1986;37:787.
167. Igo M, Sakurai M, Tamura T, et al. In vivo activity of multiple injections of recombinant interleukin-2: alone and in combination with three different types of recombinant interferons on various syngeneic murine tumors. Cancer Res 1988;48:260.
168. Rosenberg SA, Lotze MT, Yang JC, et al. Combination therapy with interleukin-2 and alpha-interferon for the treatment of patients with advanced cancer. J Clin Oncol 1989;7:1863.
169. Mittleman A, Huberman M, Puccio C, et al. A phase I study of recombinant human interleukin-2 and alpha-interferon-2a in patients with renal cell cancer, colorectal cancer and malignant melanoma. Cancer 1990;66:664.
170. McIntosh JK, Mule JJ, Marino MJ, et al. Synergistic antitumor effects of immunotherapy with recombinant interleukin-2 and recombinant tumor necrosis factor-alpha. Cancer Res 1988;48:4011.
171. Agah R, Malloy B, Sherrod A, et al. Therapy of disseminated NK-resistant tumor by the synergistic effects of recombinant tumor necrosis factor and recombinant interleukin-2 in mice. Int J Cancer 1987; 40:255.
172. Winkelhate JL, Sramph LS, Zimmerman RJ. Synergistic effects of combination therapy with human recombinant interleukin-2 and tumor necrosis factor in murine tumor models. Cancer Res 1987;47:3948.
173. Talmadge JE, Tribble HR, Pennington RW, et al. Immunomodulatory and immunotherapeutic properties of gamma-interferon and recombinant tumor necrosis factor in mice. Cancer Res 1987;47:2563.
174. Heidenrich S, Weyers M, Crong JH, et al. Potentiation of lymphokine-induced macrophage activation by tumor necrosis factor alpha. J Immunol 1988;140:1511.
175. Balkwill FR, Ward BG, Moodie E, et al. Therapeutic potential of tumor necrosis factor-alpha and gamma-interferon in experimental human ovarian cancer. Cancer Res 1987;47:4755.
176. Shalaby MR, Aggarwal BB, Rinderknecht E. Activation of human polymorphonuclear functions by interferon-gamma and tumor necrosis factors. J Immunol 1985;135:2069.
177. McIntosh JK, Mule JJ, Krosnick JA, et al. Combination cytokine immunotherapy with tumor necrosis factor-alpha, interleukin-2 and alpha-interferon and its synergistic antitumor effects in mice. Cancer Res 1989;49:1408.
178. Abbruzzese JL, Levin B, Ajani JA, et al. A phase II trial of recombinant human interferon-gamma and recombinant tumor necrosis factor in patients with advanced gastrointestinal malignancies: results of a trial terminated by excessive toxicity. J Biological Response Modifiers 1990;9:522.
179. Fiedler W, Zeller W, Peimann CJ, et al. A phase II combination trial with recombinant human tumor necrosis factor and gamma-interferon in patients with colorectal cancer. Klin Wochenschr 1991;69:261.
180. Rosenberg SA, Lotze MT, Yang JC, et al. Experience with the use of high-dose interleukin-2 in the treatment of 652 cancer patients. Ann Surg 1989;210:474.
181. Mule JJ, Rosenberg SA. Combination cytokine therapy: experimental and clinical trials. In: DeVita VT, Hellman S, Rosenberg SA, eds. Biologic therapy of cancer. Philadelphia: JB Lippincott, 1991.
182. Pappo I, Tahara H, Nishihara K, et al. Administration of systemic or

local interleukin 2 enhances the antitumor effects of interleukin 12 gene therapy. J Surg Res 1994;57.
183. North RJ. Cyclophosphamide-facilitated adoptive immunotherapy of established tumor-induced suppressor cells. J Exp Med 1982;155: 1063.
184. Papa MZ, Yang JC, Velto JT, et al. Combined effects of chemotherapy and interleukin-2 in the therapy of mice with advanced pulmonary tumors. Cancer Res 1988;48:122.
185. Rosenberg SA. Cancer therapy with interleukin-2: immunologic manipulation can mediate the regression of cancer in human. J Clin Oncol 1988;6:403.
186. Koliz JE, Wong GY, Welte K, et al. Phase I trial of recombinant interleukin-2 and cyclophosphamide: augmentation of cellular immunity and T cell mitogenic response with long-term administration of IL-2. J Biol Response Mod 1988;7:457.
187. Mitchell MS, Kempf RA, Harel W, et al. Effectiveness and tolerability of low-dose cyclophosphamide and low-dose intravenous interleukin-2 in disseminated melanoma. J Clin Oncol 1988;6:409.
188. West WH, Taner KW, Yanelli JR, et al. Constant infusion recombinant interleukin-2 in adoptive immunotherapy of advanced cancer. N Engl J Med 1987;316:898.
189. Hamblin TJ, Sadullah S, Williamson P, et al. A phase III study of recombinant interleukin-2 and 5-fluorouracil chemotherapy in patients with metastatic colorectal cancer. Br J Cancer 1993;68:1186.
190. Yang JC, Shlasko E, Ritchey JL, et al. Combination chemoimmunotherapy for metastatic colorectal cancer using 5-fluorouracil, leucovorin and interleukin-2. Eur J Cancer 1993;29A:355.
191. Hiddemann W, Ruelfs C, Ottensmeier C, et al. Interleukin-2 followed by fluorouracil and folinic acid in refractory colorectal cancer—results of a clinical phase II study. Semin Oncol 1992;19:225.
192. Wadler S, Schwartz EL, Goldman M, et al. Preclinical and clinical studies of 5-fluorouracil (FUra) and recombinant alpha-2-a-interferon (IFN) against gastrointestinal (GI) malignancies. (Abstract) Clin Res 1988;36:803A.
193. Stolfi RL, Martin DS, Sawyer RC, et al. Modulation of 5-fluorouracil-induced toxicity in mice with interferon or with the interferon inducer, polyinsinicpolycytidylic acid. Cancer Res 1983;43:561.
194. Wadler S, Schwartz EL, Goldman M, et al. Fluorouracil and recombinant alpha-2a-interferon, an active regimen against advanced colorectal carcinoma. J Clin Oncol 1989;7:1769.
195. Walder S. The role of immunotherapy in colorectal cancer. Semin Oncol 1991;18:27.
196. Pazdur R, Ajani JA, Yehuda Z, et al. Phase II evaluation of recombinant alpha-2a-interferon and continuous infusion fluorouracil in previously untreated metastatic colorectal adenocarcinoma. Cancer 1993; 71:1214.
197. Ajani JA, Abbruzzese JL, Markowitz AB, et al. Phase II study of etoposide and alpha-interferon in patients with advanced measurable colorectal carcinoma. Invest New Drugs 1993;11:67.
198. Zeh HJ, Hurd S, Storkus WJ, Lotze MT. Interleukin-12 promotes the proliferation and cytolytic maturation of immune effectors: implications for the immunotherapy of cancer. J Immunother 1993;14:155.
199. Tahara H, Zeh HJ 3rd, Storkus WJ, et al. Fibroblasts genetically engineered to secrete interleukin 12 can suppress tumor growth and induce antitumor immunity to a murine melanoma in vivo. Cancer Res 1994; 54:182.
200. Rosenberg SA, Lotze MT, Muul LM, et al. A new approach to the therapy of cancer based on the systemic administration of autologous lymphokine-activated killer cells and recombinant interleukin-2. Surgery 1986;100:262.
201. Hawkin MJ. IL-2/LAK. PPO updates 1989;3:1.
202. Melder RJ, Whiteside TL, Vujanovic NL, et al. A new approach to generating antitumor effectors for adoptive immunotherapy using human adherent lymphokine-activated killer cells. Cancer Res 1988; 48:3461.
203. Steis RG, Urba WJ, VanderMolen LA, et al. Intraperitoneal lymphokine-activated killer-cell and interleukin-2 therapy for malignancies limited to the peritoneal cavity. J Clin Oncol 1990;8:1618.
204. Stolfi VM, Milsom JW, Finke JH, et al. Resident research award: tumor necrosis factor alpha selectively enhances growth and cytotoxic activity of tumor infiltrating lymphocytes from human colorectal cancer. J Surg Res 1992;52:39.
205. Rosenberg SA, Aebersold P, Cornetta K, et al. Gene transfer into humans: immunotherapy of patients with advanced melanoma, using tumor-infiltrating lymphocytes modified by retroviral gene transduction. N Engl J Med 1990;323:570.
206. Mellstedt H, Frodin JE, Ragnhammar P, et al. The clinical use of monoclonal antibodies, Mab 17-1A, in the treatment of patients with metastatic colorectal carcinomas. Med Oncol Tumor Pharmacother 1989;6:99.
207. Douillard JY, Lehur PA, Vighoud J, et al. Monoclonal antibodies: specific immunotherapy of gastrointestinal tumors. Hybridoma 1986; 5:139.
208. Markoe AM, Brady LW, Amendola BE, et al. Treatment of gastrointestinal cancer using monoclonal antibodies. In: Vaeth JM, Meyer JL, eds. Frontiers of radiation therapy and oncology: the present and future roles of monoclonal antibodies in management of cancer. Basel, Switzerland: Karger, 1990.
209. Wadler S. The role of immunotherapy in colorectal cancer. Semin Oncol 1991;18:27.
210. Beatty JD, Williams LE, Yamauchi D, et al. Presurgical imaging with indium-labeled anti-CEA for colon cancer staging. Cancer Res 1990; 50:922.
211. Byers VS, Pimm MV, Scannon PJ, et al. Inhibition of growth of human tumor xenografts in athymic mice treated with ricin toxic A chain-monoclonal antibody 791T/36 conjugates. Cancer Res 1987; 47:5042.
212. Byers VS, Pawluczyk IZ, Hooi DS, et al. Endocytosis of immunotoxin-791T/36-RTA by tumor cells in relation to its cytotoxic action. Cancer Res 1991;51:1990.
213. Zaleberg JR, Pielersz G, Toohey B, et al. Phase I–II study of a ricin monoclonal antibody conjugate in colon cancer. (Abstract) In: Fourth International Conference on Monoclonal Antibody Immunoconjugates for Cancer. March 30-April 1, 1989. San Diego, USCD Cancer Center. :47.
214. Senter P. Activation of prodrugs by antibody-enzyme conjugates: a new approach to cancer therapy. FASEB J 1990;4:188.
215. Hyams DM, Esteban JM, Beatty BG, et al. Therapy of peritoneal carcinomatosis of human colon cancer xenografts with 90Y-labeled anti-CEA antibody ZCE025. Arch Surg 1987;122:1333.
216. Hyams DM, Esteban JM, Beatty BG, et al. Prolongation of survival of nude mice bearing human colon cancer by treatment with 90yttrium-labeled anti-CEA antibody. Arch Surg 1989;124:175.
217. Beatty JD. Immunotherapy of colorectal cancer. Cancer 1992;70: 1425.
218. Hanna MG, Brandhorst JS, Peters LC. Active specific immunotherapy of residual micrometastasis: an evaluation of sources, closes and ratios of BCG with tumor cells. Cancer Immunol Immunother 1979;7:165.
219. Peters LC, Hanna MG Jr. Active-specific immunotherapy of established micrometastasis: effect of cryopreservation procedures on tumor cell immunogenicity in guinea pigs. J Natl Cancer Inst 1980; 64:1521.
220. Hoover HC Jr, Hanna MG. Active immunotherapy in colorectal cancer. Semin Surg Oncol 1989;5:436.
221. Hoover HC Jr, Brandhorst JS, Peters LC, et al. Adjuvant active specific immunotherapy for human colorectal cancer: 6.5-year median follow-up of a phase III prospectively randomized trial. J Clin Oncol 1993;11:390.
222. Gray BN, Walker C, Andrewartha L, et al. Controlled clinical trial of adjuvant immunotherapy with BCG and neuraminidase-treated autologous tumour cells in large bowel cancer. J Surg Oncol 1989;40: 34.
223. Lehner B, Schlag P, Liebrich W, et al. Postoperative active specific immunization in curatively resected colorectal cancer patients with a virus-modified autologous tumor cell vaccine. Cancer Immunol Immunother 1990;32:173.
224. Steele G Jr, Ravikumar T, Ross D, et al. Specific active immunotherapy with butanol-extracted, tumor-associated antigens incorporated into liposomes. Surgery 1984;96:352.
225. Beatty JD, Beatty BG, Paraskevas F. Liposomes: T-cell dependent immune adjuvant property. Surg Forum 1982;33:346.

Index

Entries followed by *f* indicate figures; entries followed by *t* indicate tabular material.

R